UNIT 1 Medical Terminology, Anatomy, and Physiology

1. **Medical Terminology Basics**, 1
2. **Anatomy and Physiology Basics**, 13
3. **Musculoskeletal System**, 35
4. **Integumentary System**, 69
5. **Digestive System**, 94
6. **Urinary System**, 122
7. **Reproductive System**, 145
8. **Blood**, 166
9. **Lymphatic and Immune Systems**, 187
10. **Cardiovascular System**, 207
11. **Respiratory System**, 238
12. **Nervous System and Mental Health**, 260
13. **Sensory System**, 295
14. **Endocrine System**, 324

UNIT 2 Professional Medical Assistant

15. **Professionalism in Healthcare**, 342
16. **Legal Basics**, 361
    PROCEDURE 16.1 Apply the Patient's Bill of Rights, 373
    PROCEDURE 16.2 Locate the Medical Assistant's Legal Scope of Practice, 378
17. **Healthcare Laws**, 380
    PROCEDURE 17.1 Protecting a Patient's Privacy, 385
    PROCEDURE 17.2 Completing a Release of Record Form for a Release of Information, 387
    PROCEDURE 17.3 Perform Disease Reporting, 392
    PROCEDURE 17.4 Report Illegal Activity, 395
    PROCEDURE 17.5 Complete Incident Report, 398
18. **Healthcare Ethics**, 400
    PROCEDURE 18.1 Developing an Ethics Separation Plan, 403
    PROCEDURE 18.2 Demonstrate Appropriate Response to Ethical Issues, 407

UNIT 3 Administrative Ambulatory Care

19. **The Health Record**, 412
    PROCEDURE 19.1 Register a New Patient Using the Practice Management Software, 417
    PROCEDURE 19.2 Upload Documents to the Electronic Health Record, 423
    PROCEDURE 19.3 Protect the Integrity of the Medical Record, 423
    PROCEDURE 19.4 Create and Organize a Patient's Paper Health Record, 433
    PROCEDURE 19.5 File Patient Health Records, 434
20. **Telephone Techniques and Scheduling**, 438
    PROCEDURE 20.1 Demonstrate Professional Telephone Techniques, 443
    PROCEDURE 20.2 Document Telephone Messages and Report Relevant Information Concisely and Accurately, 446
    PROCEDURE 20.3 Establish the Appointment Matrix, 454
    PROCEDURE 20.4 Schedule a New Patient, 458
    PROCEDURE 20.5 Schedule an Established Patient, 460
    PROCEDURE 20.6 Schedule a Patient Procedure, 462
21. **Technology and Written Communication**, 468
    PROCEDURE 21.1 Compose a Professional Business Letter, 485
    PROCEDURE 21.2 Compose a Professional Email, 491
22. **Reception and Daily Operations**, 493
    PROCEDURE 22.1 Coach Patients Regarding Office Policies, 501
    PROCEDURE 22.2 Perform an Equipment Inventory With Documentation, 504
    PROCEDURE 22.3 Perform Routine Maintenance of Equipment, 505
    PROCEDURE 22.4 Perform a Supply Inventory With Documentation While Using Proper Body Mechanics, 508
    PROCEDURE 22.5 Prepare a Purchase Order, 509
    PROCEDURE 22.6 Evaluate the Work Environment, 515
    PROCEDURE 22.7 Participate in a Mock Exposure Event, 517
    PROCEDURE 22.8 Use a Fire Extinguisher, 519
23. **Health Insurance Basics**, 521
24. **Diagnostic Coding Basics**, 532
    PROCEDURE 24.1 Perform Coding Using the Current ICD-10-CM Manual or Encoder, 540
25. **Procedural Coding Basics**, 548
    PROCEDURE 25.1 Perform Procedural Coding: Surgery, 556
    PROCEDURE 25.2 Perform Procedural Coding: Office Visit and Immunizations, 558
    PROCEDURE 25.3 Working With Providers to Ensure Accurate Code Selection, 564
26. **Billing and Reimbursement**, 565
    PROCEDURE 26.1 Interpret Information on an Insurance Card, 567
    PROCEDURE 26.2 Show Sensitivity When Communicating With Patients Regarding Third-Party Requirements, 569
    PROCEDURE 26.3 Perform Precertification With Documentation, 570
    PROCEDURE 26.4 Complete an Insurance Claim Form, 578
    PROCEDURE 26.5 Use Medical Necessity Guidelines: Respond to a "Medical Necessity Denied" Claim, 582
    PROCEDURE 26.6 Inform a Patient of Financial Obligations for Services Rendered, 584
27. **Accounts, Collections, and Banking**, 587
    PROCEDURE 27.1 Post Charges and Payments to a Patient's Account, 592
    PROCEDURE 27.2 Post Payments and Adjustments to a Patient's Account, 603
    PROCEDURE 27.3 Prepare a Bank Deposit, 610

UNIT 4 Basic Clinical Procedures

28. **Infection Control**, 616
    PROCEDURE 28.1 Perform Hand Hygiene, 623
    PROCEDURE 28.2 Remove Contaminated Gloves and Discard Biohazardous Material, 626
    PROCEDURE 28.3 Sanitizing Soiled Instruments, 633
29. **Vital Signs**, 636
    PROCEDURE 29.1 Obtain an Oral Temperature Using a Digital Thermometer, 641
    PROCEDURE 29.2 Obtain an Axillary Temperature Using a Digital Thermometer, 642
    PROCEDURE 29.3 Obtain a Rectal Temperature of an Infant Using a Digital Thermometer, 642
    PROCEDURE 29.4 Obtain a Temperature Using a Tympanic Thermometer, 643
    PROCEDURE 29.5 Obtain a Temperature Using a Temporal Artery Thermometer, 644
    PROCEDURE 29.6 Obtain an Apical Pulse, 647
    PROCEDURE 29.7 Assess the Patient's Radial Pulse and Respiratory Rate, 648
    PROCEDURE 29.8 Determine a Patient's Blood Pressure, 655
    PROCEDURE 29.9 Perform Pulse Oximetry, 658
    PROCEDURE 29.10 Measuring a Patient's Weight and Height, 659
30. **Physical Examination**, 662
    PROCEDURE 30.1 Obtain and Document Patient Information, 667
    PROCEDURE 30.2 Respond to Nonverbal Communication, 670
    PROCEDURE 30.3 Use Proper Body Mechanics, 681
    PROCEDURE 30.4 Fowler and Semi-Fowler Positions, 682
    PROCEDURE 30.5 Supine (Horizontal Recumbent) and Dorsal Recumbent Positions, 683
    PROCEDURE 30.6 Lithotomy Position, 684
    PROCEDURE 30.7 Sims Position, 685
    PROCEDURE 30.8 Prone Position, 686
    PROCEDURE 30.9 Knee-Chest Position, 687
    PROCEDURE 30.10 Assist Provider With a Patient Exam, 692
    PROCEDURE 30.11 Measuring Distance Visual Acuity, 694
    PROCEDURE 30.12 Assess Color Acuity Using the Ishihara Test, 697
    PROCEDURE 30.13 Measuring Hearing Acuity With an Audiometer, 700
    PROCEDURE 30.14 Demonstrate Appropriate Self-Boundaries, 701
31. **Assisting With Obstetrics and Gynecology**, 703
    PROCEDURE 31.1 Set Up for and Assist the Provider With a Gynecology Examination, 705

PROCEDURES

32 **Assisting in Pediatrics,** 722
    PROCEDURE 32.1 Document Immunizations, 731
    PROCEDURE 32.2 Measure the Head Circumference of an Infant, 737
    PROCEDURE 32.3 Measure an Infant's Length and Weight, 737

33 **Assisting in Geriatrics,** 742
    PROCEDURE 33.1 Understand the Sensorimotor Changes of Aging, 743

34 **Assisting With Minor Surgery,** 757
    PROCEDURE 34.1 Wrap Instruments and Supplies for Sterilization in an Autoclave, 772
    PROCEDURE 34.2 Operate the Autoclave, 775
    PROCEDURE 34.3 Perform Skin Prep for Surgery, 779
    PROCEDURE 34.4 Perform a Surgical Hand Scrub, 780
    PROCEDURE 34.5 Prepare a Sterile Field, Use Transfer Forceps, and Pour a Sterile Solution Into a Sterile Field, 782
    PROCEDURE 34.6 Two-Person Sterile Tray Setup, 784
    PROCEDURE 34.7 Put on Sterile Gloves, 785
    PROCEDURE 34.8 Assist With Minor Surgery, 787
    PROCEDURE 34.9 Apply a Sterile Dressing, 791
    PROCEDURE 34.10 Remove Sutures and/or Surgical Staples, 794

UNIT 5 Advanced Clinical Procedures

35 **Patient Coaching With Health Promotion,** 799
    PROCEDURE 35.1 Coach a Patient on Disease Prevention, 808
    PROCEDURE 35.2 Coach a Patient on Breast Self-Exam, 809
    PROCEDURE 35.3 Coach a Patient on Testicular Self-Exam, 811
    PROCEDURE 35.4 Perform a Monofilament Foot Exam, 816
    PROCEDURE 35.5 Apply a Cold Pack, 822
    PROCEDURE 35.6 Coach a Patient to Use Axillary Crutches, 826
    PROCEDURE 35.7 Coach a Patient to Use a Walker, 828
    PROCEDURE 35.8 Coach a Patient to Use a Cane, 830
    PROCEDURE 35.9 Develop a List of Community Resources and Facilitate Referrals, 831

36 **Patient Coaching With Nutrition,** 833
    PROCEDURE 36.1 Instruct a Patient on a Dietary Change, 850

37 **Pharmacology Basics,** 853
    PROCEDURE 37.1 Prepare a Prescription, 869
    PROCEDURE 37.2 Calculate Medication Dosages, 881

38 **Administering Medication,** 884
    PROCEDURE 38.1 Administer Oral Medications, 891
    PROCEDURE 38.2 Instill an Eye Medication, 894
    PROCEDURE 38.3 Instill Ear Drops, 895
    PROCEDURE 38.4 Irrigate a Patient's Eye, 897
    PROCEDURE 38.5 Irrigate a Patient's Ear, 898
    PROCEDURE 38.6 Prepare Medication From an Ampule, 905
    PROCEDURE 38.7 Prepare Medication Using a Prefilled Sterile Cartridge, 907
    PROCEDURE 38.8 Prepare Medication From a Vial, 909
    PROCEDURE 38.9 Reconstitute Powdered Medication, 911
    PROCEDURE 38.10 Mixing Two Insulins, 913
    PROCEDURE 38.11 Administer an Intradermal Injection, 918
    PROCEDURE 38.12 Administer a Subcutaneous Injection, 924
    PROCEDURE 38.13 Administer an Intramuscular Injection, 929
    PROCEDURE 38.14 Administer an Intramuscular Injection Using the Z-Track Technique, 931

39 **Cardiopulmonary Procedures,** 933
    PROCEDURE 39.1 Perform Electrocardiography, 944
    PROCEDURE 39.2 Apply a Holter Monitor, 952
    PROCEDURE 39.3 Measure the Peak Flow Rate, 955
    PROCEDURE 39.4 Perform Spirometry Testing, 957
    PROCEDURE 39.5 Administer a Nebulizer Treatment, 959
    PROCEDURE 39.6 Administer Oxygen Per Nasal Cannula or Mask, 961

40 **Medical Emergencies,** 963
    PROCEDURE 40.1 Provide First Aid for a Patient With Insulin Shock, 976
    PROCEDURE 40.2 Incorporate Critical Thinking Skills When Performing Patient Assessment, 979
    PROCEDURE 40.3 Provide First Aid for a Patient With Seizure Activity, 979
    PROCEDURE 40.4 Provide First Aid for a Choking Patient, 982
    PROCEDURE 40.5 Provide First Aid for a Patient With a Bleeding Wound, Fracture, and Syncope, 984
    PROCEDURE 40.6 Provide First Aid for a Patient With Shock, 985
    PROCEDURE 40.7 Provide Rescue Breathing, Cardiopulmonary Resuscitation (CPR), and Automated External Defibrillator (AED), 986

UNIT 6 Medical Laboratory

41 **Assisting in the Clinical Laboratory,** 990
    PROCEDURE 41.1 Perform a Quality Control Measure on a Glucometer and Record the Results on a Flow Sheet, 998
    PROCEDURE 41.2 Use of the Eyewash Equipment: Perform an Emergency Eyewash, 1002
    PROCEDURE 41.3 Evaluate the Laboratory Environment, 1004
    PROCEDURE 41.4 Perform Routine Maintenance on Clinical Equipment (Microscope), 1011

42 **Assisting in the Analysis of Urine,** 1014
    PROCEDURE 42.1 Instruct a Patient in the Collection of a 24-Hour Urine Specimen, 1018
    PROCEDURE 42.2 Collect a Clean-Catch Midstream Urine Specimen, 1020
    PROCEDURE 42.3 Assess Urine for Color and Turbidity: Physical Test, 1022
    PROCEDURE 42.4 Perform Quality Control Measures: Differentiate Between Normal and Abnormal Test Results While Determining the Reliability of Chemical Reagent Strips, 1026
    PROCEDURE 42.5 Test Urine With Chemical Reagent Strips, 1026
    PROCEDURE 42.6 Prepare a Urine Specimen for Microscopic Examination, 1031
    PROCEDURE 42.7 Test Urine for Glucose Using the Clinitest Method, 1039
    PROCEDURE 42.8 Perform a CLIA-Waived Urinalysis: Perform a Pregnancy Test, 1040

43 **Assisting in Blood Collection,** 1046
    PROCEDURE 43.1 Perform a Venipuncture: Collect a Venous Blood Sample Using the Vacuum Tube Method, 1058
    PROCEDURE 43.2 Perform a Venipuncture: Collect a Venous Blood Sample Using the Syringe Method, 1061
    PROCEDURE 43.3 Perform Venipuncture: Obtain a Venous Sample With a Safety Winged Butterfly Needle Assembly, 1064
    PROCEDURE 43.4 Perform a Capillary Puncture: Obtain a Blood Sample by Capillary Puncture, 1071

44 **Assisting in the Analysis of Blood,** 1076
    PROCEDURE 44.1 Perform Preventive Maintenance for the Microhematocrit Centrifuge, 1078
    PROCEDURE 44.2 CLIA-Waived Hematology Testing: Perform a Microhematocrit Test, 1079
    PROCEDURE 44.3 Perform CLIA-Waived Hematology Testing: Perform a Hemoglobin Test, 1082
    PROCEDURE 44.4 Perform CLIA-Waived Hematology Testing: Determine the Erythrocyte Sedimentation Rate Using a Modified Westergren Method, 1084
    PROCEDURE 44.5 Perform a CLIA-Waived PT/INR Test, 1087
    PROCEDURE 44.6 Assist the Provider with Patient Care: Perform a Blood Glucose TRUEresult Test, 1095
    PROCEDURE 44.7 Perform a CLIA-Waived Chemistry Test: Determine the Cholesterol Level or Lipid Profile Using a Cholestech Analyzer, 1098

45 **Assisting in Microbiology and Immunology,** 1104
    PROCEDURE 45.1 Instruct Patients in the Collection of Fecal Specimens to Be Tested for Ova and Parasites, 1112
    PROCEDURE 45.2 Collect a Specimen for a Throat Culture, 1117
    PROCEDURE 45.3 Perform a CLIA-Waived Microbiology Test: Perform a Rapid Strep Test, 1118
    PROCEDURE 45.4 Perform a CLIA-waived Immunology Test: Perform a QuickVue+ Infectious Mononucleosis Test, 1119

UNIT 7 Employment Seeking

46 **Career Development,** 1126
    PROCEDURE 46.1 Prepare a Chronologic Resume, 1133
    PROCEDURE 46.2 Create a Cover Letter, 1137
    PROCEDURE 46.3 Complete a Job Application, 1139
    PROCEDURE 46.4 Create a Career Portfolio, 1141
    PROCEDURE 46.5 Practice Interview Skills During a Mock Interview, 1143
    PROCEDURE 46.6 Create a Thank-You Note for an Interview, 1144

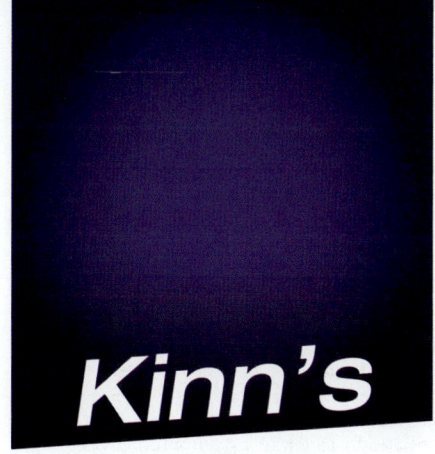

Kinn's
MEDICAL ASSISTING
FUNDAMENTALS

Administrative and Clinical Competencies
with Anatomy & Physiology

Brigitte Niedzwiecki, RN, MSN, RMA
Medical Assistant Program Director & Instructor
Chippewa Valley Technical College
Eau Claire, Wisconsin

Julie Pepper, BS, CMA (AAMA)
Medical Assistant Instructor
Chippewa Valley Technical College
Eau Claire, Wisconsin

P. Ann Weaver, MSEd, MT (ASCP)
Medical Assistant Instructor
Chippewa Valley Technical College
Eau Claire, Wisconsin

ELSEVIER

ELSEVIER

3251 Riverport Lane
St. Louis, Missouri 63043

KINN'S MEDICAL ASSISTING FUNDAMENTALS: ADMINISTRATIVE
AND CLINICAL COMPETENCIES WITH ANATOMY & PHYSIOLOGY,
FIRST EDITION
ISBN: 978-0-323-55119-9
Copyright © 2019, Elsevier Inc. All Rights Reserved.

No part of this publication may be reproduced or transmitted in any form or by any means, electronic or mechanical, including photocopying, recording, or any information storage and retrieval system, without permission in writing from the publisher. Details on how to seek permission, further information about the Publisher's permissions policies and our arrangements with organizations such as the Copyright Clearance Center and the Copyright Licensing Agency, can be found at our website: www.elsevier.com/permissions.

Notices

Practitioners and researchers must always rely on their own experience and knowledge in evaluating and using any information, methods, compounds or experiments described herein. Because of rapid advances in the medical sciences, in particular, independent verification of diagnoses and drug dosages should be made. To the fullest extent of the law, no responsibility is assumed by Elsevier, authors, editors or contributors for any injury and/or damage to persons or property as a matter of products liability, negligence or otherwise, or from any use or operation of any methods, products, instructions, or ideas contained in the material herein.

International Standard Book Number: 978-0-323-55119-9

Publishing Director, Education Content: Kristin Wilhelm
Content Development Manager: Ellen Wurm-Cutter
Senior Content Development Specialist: Becky Leenhouts
Publishing Services Manager: Julie Eddy
Senior Project Manager: Richard Barber
Design Direction: Paula Catalano

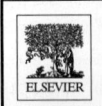

Working together
to grow libraries in
developing countries

www.elsevier.com • www.bookaid.org

Printed in Canada

Last digit is the print number: 9 8 7 6 5 4 3 2 1

PREFACE

Medical assisting as a profession has dramatically changed over the last 60 years. You are entering the profession at an exciting time. With the advances in technology, the medical assistant role has expanded. With those changes, medical assistants need a strong foundation in anatomy, disease, medical terminology, math, and soft skills as they apply to administrative and clinical responsibilities.

This textbook was a team effort, and was created utilizing significant content from Shiland: *Mastering Healthcare Terminology,* ed. 5 and Proctor: *Kinn's The Medical Assistant,* ed. 13. The borrowed content includes but is not limited to text, boxes, and illustrations.

FEATURES OF THIS TEXTBOOK FOR STUDENTS

Following in the tradition of *Kinn's* product suite, *Kinn's Medical Assisting Fundamentals: Administrative and Clinical Competencies with Anatomy & Physiology* offers a comprehensive, up-to-date, and innovated approach to learning the medical assistant role. The easy-to-understand writing style and the tables with concise information will help you build a strong foundation of knowledge. The extensive figures provide examples, illustrate skills, and showcase ambulatory equipment and supplies. Features we have incorporated into the textbook include:
- *Emphasis on anatomy, physiology, and pathology*, including signs/symptoms, diagnostic procedures, and treatments.
- *Strong focus on medical terminology* including a chapter focused on the basics of medical terminology and feature boxes highlighting chapter-related medical terminology throughout the textbook.
- *Embedded math exercises* to help you build your math skills.
- *Customer service boxes* that will help you develop the soft skills that employers seek when hiring medical assistants.
- *Applied learning approach* introduces a case scenario at the beginning of each chapter and then revisits it throughout the chapter to help you understand new concepts as they are presented.
- *Chapter learning tools* include vocabulary with definitions, critical thinking applications, and content that ties directly to the order of learning objectives.
- *Pharmacology glossary* of the top 100-150 most common over-the-counter and prescription medications gives you quick access to pronunciation guides, generic and trade names, and drug classification.
- **Trusted *Kinn's* content** supports the following exam plans: CMA from the American Association of Medical Assistants; RMA and CMAS from American Medical Technologist; CCMA and CMAA from the National Healthcareer Association; NCMA from the National Center for Competency Testing; and CMAC from the American Medical Certification Association.

ORGANIZATION OF THIS TEXTBOOK

To provide you with a solid understanding of the basics, Unit 1 addresses medical terminology, anatomy, physiology, and pathology. Unit 2 focuses on the professional medical assistant. This content is critical to you as you begin your career. Being professional starts in the classroom and extends into practicum and beyond. Besides professional attributes, communication skills and legal and ethical concepts will be discussed.

Unit 3 covers administrative medical assistant topics. Reception duties including working with the health record, answering telephones, and scheduling appointments are addressed. Insurance, coding, billing, collections, and banking principles are also discussed. Often in larger ambulatory care facilities, these activities are done in the business department.

Units 4 through 6 address the clinical medical assistant duties. Unit 4 covers skills related to infection control procedures, obtaining vital signs, assisting with physical exams, and assisting with minor surgery. Unit 5 includes advanced clinical procedures. The medical assistant's role with advanced clinical procedures depends on the state's law and the agency where the medical assistant is employed. Advanced clinical procedures include coaching patients, administering medications, performing cardiopulmonary procedures, and assisting with medical emergencies. Unit 6 address procedures performed in the medical laboratory setting. These skills include collecting specimens, performing CLIA-waived laboratory tests on urine, blood, and other body fluids.

Unit 7 focuses on employment. As you complete your program, learning how to market yourself to potential employers is important. This unit addresses the skills to secure employment.

STUDY GUIDE FEATURES FOR STUDENTS AND INSTRUCTORS

The Study Guide provides students with the opportunity to review and build on information they have learned in the text through medical terminology and vocabulary reviews, review of concepts, chapter review multiple choice questions, case scenarios, and online activities. Students also have the opportunity to review and practice procedures for psychomotor and affective competencies, with clear steps and behaviors indicated.

For instructors, the Study Guide offers unique, time-saving tools, including specific mapping of assessments to both CAAHEP and ABHES competencies.
- Specific assessment questions and procedure steps are mapped to competencies, helping to eliminate hours of program management for national accreditation.
- Procedures are designed to be conveniently performed in the classroom.
- Procedure Checklists for psychomotor competencies are easy to use and address multiple competencies in many cases.
- Uniquely designed Procedure Checklists for affective competencies allow instructors to quickly identify a student's professional and nonprofessional behaviors while assessing the range of performance with ease.
- Clearly written Procedure Checklists for psychomotor and affective competencies help students identify what steps and behaviors are required for success.

EVOLVE

The Evolve site features a variety of student resources, including Chapter Review Quizzes, Procedure Videos, practice CMA and RMA exams, and much more! The Instructor Resources consists of TEACH Instructor Resources, including Lesson Plans, PowerPoint Presentations, Answer Keys for Chapter Review Quizzes, and a Test Bank.

PREFACE

FEATURES

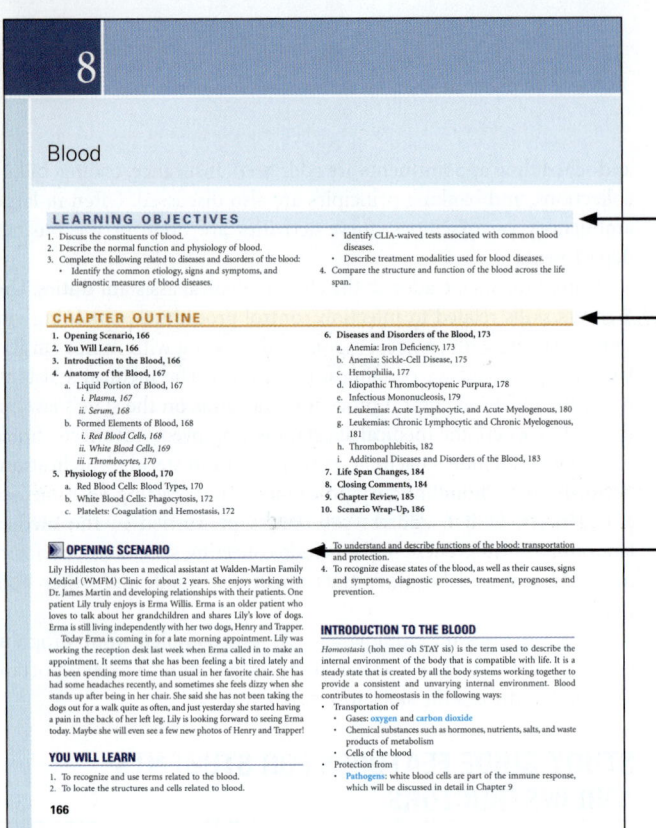

Learning Objectives emphasize the cognitive and performance objectives presented in the chapter.

Chapter Outlines present a guide for the chapter content and a quick reference for the topics covered.

Opening Scenarios present a real-world situation for students to envision while reading the chapter content.

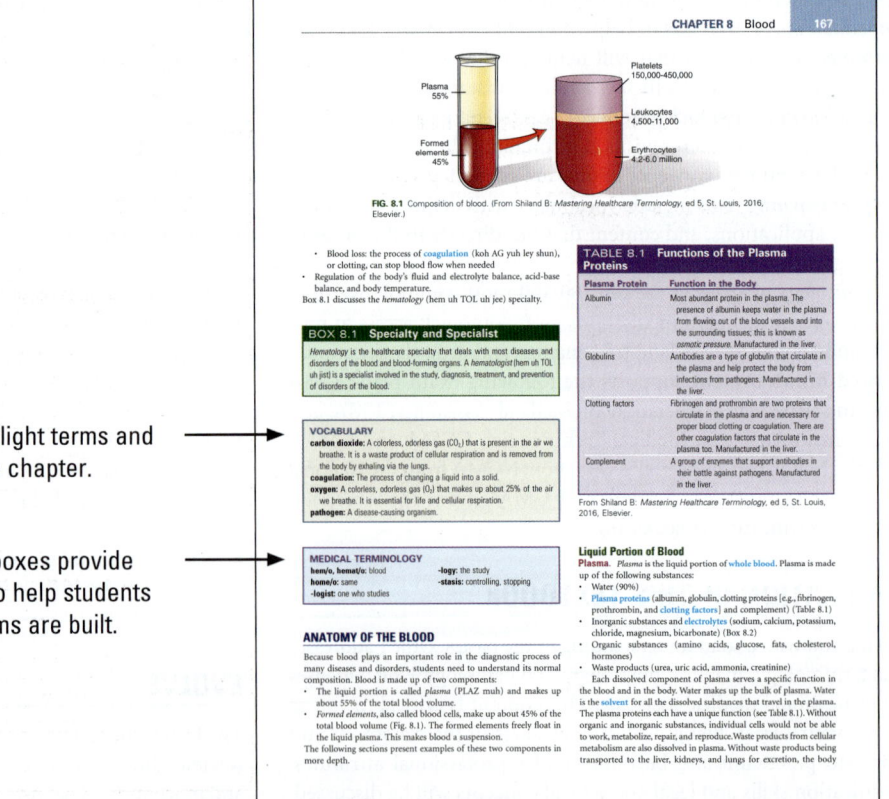

Vocabulary boxes highlight terms and definitions found in the chapter.

Medical Terminology boxes provide review of word parts to help students learn how medical terms are built.

PREFACE

Safety Alert boxes alert students to vital safety information and reinforce the importance of safety in the profession.

Critical Thinking boxes prompt students to apply what they have learned as they read and study the chapter.

Study Tip boxes provide pointers and tips on remembering and distinguishing topics that are easily confused in practice.

PREFACE

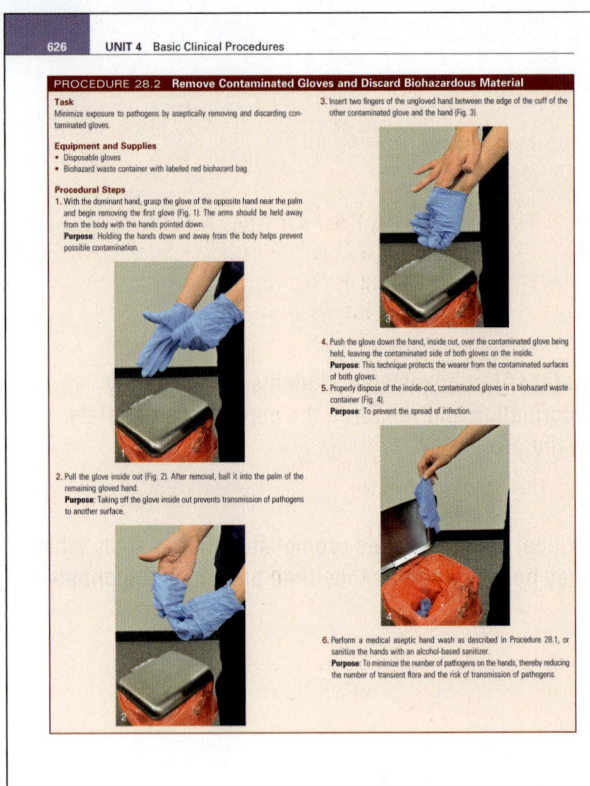

Step-by-step Procedure boxes demonstrate how to perform and document procedures encountered in the healthcare setting.

The Scenario Wrap-Up brings together the content of the chapter and the opening scenario in a real-world context.

The Chapter Review at the end of each chapter reviews and reinforces the important points of the chapter's focus to help students with content mastery.

Exceptional Customer Service boxes provide tips on customer service that are specific to each chapter's content.

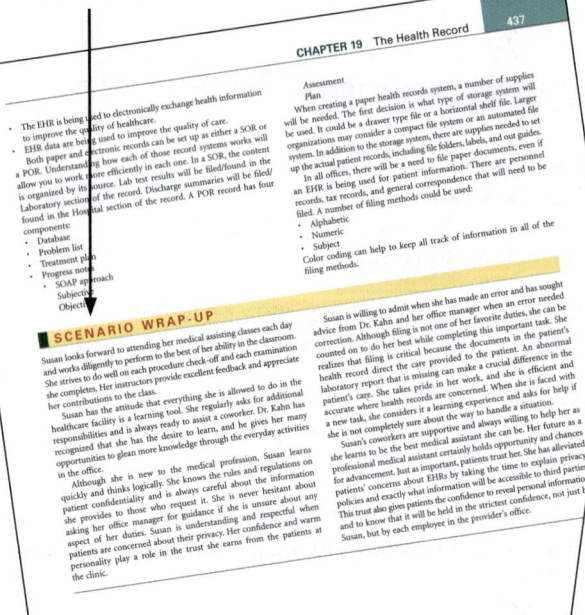

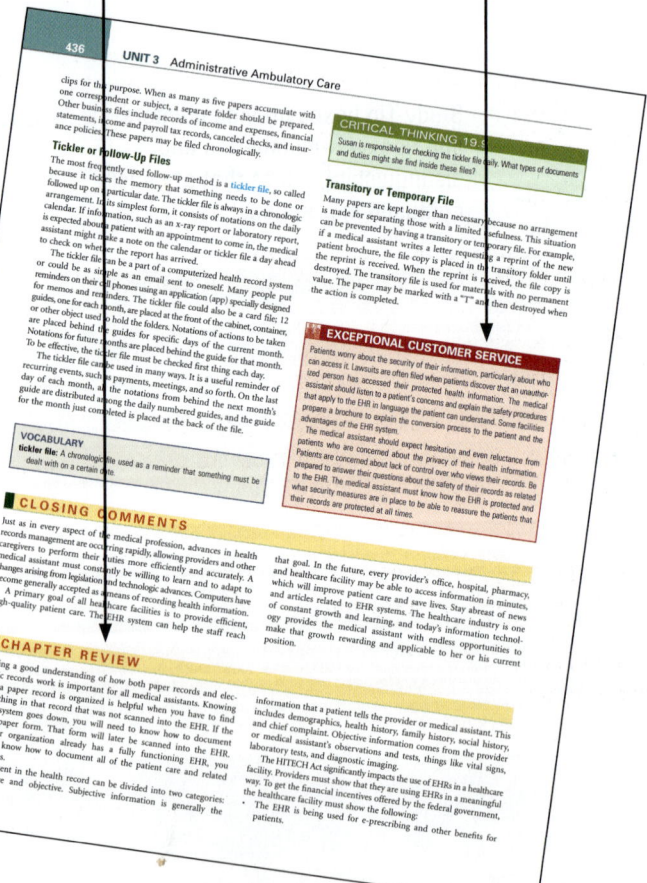

REVIEWERS

Angela Belnap, MS, CMA(AAMA)
Masters of Science in Integrated Healthcare Management
Bachelor of Science in Applied Management
Associate of Applied Science in Medical Assistant
Doctoral student in Health Professional Education
Certified Medical Assistant through the AAMA since 2005
Assistant Professor of Health Science
Medical Assisting Department
Salt Lake Community College
School of Health Sciences
Division of Allied Health
Department of Medical Assisting
Salt Lake Community College
Salt Lake City, Utah

Amber Dunn, LPN, RMA, AHI
BS Health Science, Community Development,
Director of the Medical Assistant Program
Allied Health
East Central College
Union, Missouri

Bryan Quincy Edmonds, Sr., MBA-H, RMA (AMT), EMT
Medical Assisting Program Coordinator/Instructor
Medical Assisting
Milwaukee Area Technical College
Milwaukee, Wisconsin

Lyndsay Evans, CMAA, CBCS, CEHRS
CTT Instructor
Medical Administrative Assisting
Sierra Nevada Job Corps Center
Reno, Nevada

Deborah S. Gilbert, RHIA, MBA, CMA
Program Director Health Information Management
Health Professions
Dalton State College
Dalton, Georgia

Pamela Harvey, RN, ASN, BSN, MSN, BLS
Instructor in the Medical Assistant Program
Bradford Union Career Technical Center
Starke, Florida

Kimberly Head, BA, BS, DC
Director of Healthcare Programs
Continuing Education
Collin College
Plano, Texas

Starra R. Herring, BSAH, BSHA, CMA (AAMA)-MA, AHI
Medical Assisting Program Director & Practicum Coordinator
 of the Medical Assisting Program &
Billing and Coding Program Director
Medical Assisting/ Allied Health and Public Service
Stanly Community College
Locust, North Carolina

Judith Kimelman Kline, NCRMA
Medical Assistant Instructor
Health Science
Miami Lakes Educational Center And Technical
 College- Miami Dade Public School
Miami Lakes, Florida

LaToya Nicole Mason, CMA(AAMA), MBA, MHA
Director, Healthcare Education Institute
Health Sciences
Lake Michigan College
Benton Harbor, Michigan

Jillian J. McDonald BS, RMA (NHA), EMT, CPT(NPA)
Medical Assisting Program Director
Health and Natural Sciences (Medical Assisting)
Goodwin College
East Hartford, Connecticut

Melody A. Miller, LPN
Medical Assistant Instructor
Lancaster County Career and Technology Center
Willow Street, Pennsylvania

Kristen Schoville, RN/BSN
Medical Assistant Instructor
Southwest Wisconsin Technical College
Fennimore, Wisconsin

Kathy Elisa Smith-Stillson, PhD, MSN, RN
Doctor of Philosophy in Human Resource Development and
 Educational Leadership
Nursing
Colorado Christian University
Northglenn, Colorado

Bobbi Jane Steelman, BSEd, MAEd, CPhT
Director of Education, Pharmacy Technician Program
 Director
Academics
Daymar College
Bowling Green, Kentucky

REVIEWERS

Audrey Jean Theisen, BS, RHIA, MSCIS, PhD
Adjunct Professor
Medical Assistant Program
Community College of Denver
Denver, Colorado

Debra Van Den Bussche
Instructor
Medical Office Assisting/Unit Clerk
Bredin College of Business and Health Care
Spruce Grove, Alberta, Canada

Shaili N. Vora, MD
Manager of Training & Development
Staff Training
Baylor Scott & White Health
Temple, Texas

Jessica Weinoldt, RT(R)(M)(CMA)
Radiographer, Medical Assistant Instructor
Medical Assistant Class
Lancaster County Career and Technology Center
Willow Street, Pennsylvania

Petra M. York, BS, CMA (AAMA), CET, CPT, AHI, CMAA, CPhT
Program Director
Medical Assistant
Western Technical College
El Paso, Texas

CONTENTS

UNIT 1 Medical Terminology, Anatomy, and Physiology

1. **Medical Terminology Basics**, 1
   - Opening Scenario, 1
   - You Will Learn, 1
   - Where Does Medical Terminology Come From?, 1
   - Types of Medical Terms, 2
   - Decoding Terms, 3
   - Building Terms, 4
   - Singular/Plural Rules, 9
2. **Anatomy and Physiology Basics**, 13
   - Opening Scenario, 13
   - You Will Learn, 13
   - Anatomy Basics, 14
   - Acid-Base Balance, 24
   - Pathology Basics, 25
3. **Musculoskeletal System**, 35
   - Opening Scenario, 35
   - You Will Learn, 35
   - Anatomy of the Musculoskeletal System, 36
   - Physiology of the Musculoskeletal System, 46
   - Diseases and Disorders of the Musculoskeletal System, 52
   - Life Span Changes, 63
4. **Integumentary System**, 69
   - Opening Scenario, 69
   - You Will Learn, 69
   - Anatomy of the Integumentary System, 70
   - Physiology of the Integumentary System, 73
   - Diseases and Disorders of the Integumentary System, 73
   - Life Span Changes, 92
5. **Digestive System**, 94
   - Opening Scenario, 95
   - You Will Learn, 95
   - Anatomy of the Digestive System, 96
   - Physiology of the Digestive System, 99
   - Diseases and Disorders of the Digestive System, 102
   - Lifespan Changes, 119
6. **Urinary System**, 122
   - Opening Scenario, 122
   - You Will Learn, 122
   - Anatomy of the Urinary System, 123
   - Physiology of the Urinary System, 126
   - Diseases and Disorders of the Urinary System, 128
   - Life Span Changes, 141
7. **Reproductive System**, 145
   - Opening Scenario, 145
   - You Will Learn, 146
   - Anatomy of the Reproductive System, 146
   - Physiology of the Reproductive System, 148
   - Diseases and Disorders of the Reproductive System, 151
   - Life Span Changes, 162
8. **Blood**, 166
   - Opening Scenario, 166
   - You Will Learn, 166
   - Anatomy of the Blood, 167
   - Physiology of the Blood, 170
   - Diseases and Disorders of the Blood, 173
   - Life Span Changes, 184
9. **Lymphatic and Immune Systems**, 187
   - Opening Scenario, 187
   - You Will Learn, 187
   - Anatomy of the Lymphatic and Immune Systems, 188
   - Physiology of the Lymphatic and Immune Systems, 190
   - Diseases and Disorders of the Lymphatic and Immune Systems, 195
   - Life Span Changes, 204
10. **Cardiovascular System**, 207
    - Opening Scenario, 207
    - You Will Learn, 207
    - Anatomy of the Cardiovascular System, 208
    - Physiology of the Cardiovascular System, 215
    - Diseases and Disorders of the Cardiovascular System, 217
    - Life Span Changes, 235
11. **Respiratory System**, 238
    - Opening Scenario, 238
    - You Will Learn, 238
    - Anatomy of the Respiratory System, 238
    - Physiology of the Respiratory System, 242
    - Diseases of the Respiratory System, 242
    - Life Span Changes, 258
12. **Nervous System and Mental Health**, 260
    - Opening Scenario, 261
    - You Will Learn, 261
    - Anatomy of the Nervous System, 261
    - Physiology of Mental and Behavioral Health, 270
    - Diseases and Disorders of the Nervous System, 271
    - Diseases and Disorders of Mental and Behavioral Health, 279
    - Life Span Changes, 288
13. **Sensory System**, 295
    - Opening Scenario, 295
    - You Will Learn, 295
    - Anatomy of the Eye, 296
    - Anatomy of the Ear, 299
    - Physiology of the Eye, 301
    - Physiology of the Ear, 301
    - Diseases and Disorders of the Eye, 309
    - Diseases and Disorders of the Ear, 313
    - Life Span Changes, 315
14. **Endocrine System**, 324
    - Opening Scenario, 324
    - You Will Learn, 324
    - Anatomy of the Endocrine System, 325
    - Physiology of the Endocrine System, 329
    - Diseases and Disorders of the Endocrine System, 330
    - Life Span Changes, 339

ix

UNIT 2 Professional Medical Assistant

15 Professionalism in Healthcare, 342
- Opening Scenario, 343
- You Will Learn, 343
- Introduction, 343
- Professionalism, 343
- Nonverbal Communication, 350
- Verbal Communication, 353
- Understanding Behavior, 357

16 Legal Basics, 361
- Opening Scenario, 361
- You Will Learn, 362
- Introduction to the Law, 362
- Sources of Law, 362
- Criminal and Civil Law, 362
- Tort Law, 363
- Contracts, 369
- Consent, 371
- Patient's Bill of Rights, 372
- Practice Requirements, 372
- PROCEDURE 16.1 Apply the Patient's Bill of Rights, 373
- PROCEDURE 16.2 Locate the Medical Assistant's Legal Scope of Practice, 378

17 Healthcare Laws, 380
- Opening Scenario, 380
- You Will Learn, 381
- Introduction to Law, 381
- Privacy and Confidentiality, 381
- PROCEDURE 17.1 Protecting a Patient's Privacy, 385
- PROCEDURE 17.2 Completing a Release of Record Form for a Release of Information, 387
- Additional Healthcare Laws and Regulations, 387
- Compliance Reporting, 391
- PROCEDURE 17.3 Perform Disease Reporting, 392
- PROCEDURE 17.4 Report Illegal Activity, 395
- PROCEDURE 17.5 Complete Incident Report, 398

18 Healthcare Ethics, 400
- Opening Scenario, 400
- You Will Learn, 401
- Introduction to Ethics, 401
- Personal and Professional Ethics, 401
- PROCEDURE 18.1 Developing an Ethics Separation Plan, 403
- Principles of Healthcare Ethics, 403
- Ethical Issues, 404
- PROCEDURE 18.2 Demonstrate Appropriate Response to Ethical Issues, 407

UNIT 3 Administrative Ambulatory Care

19 The Health Record, 412
- Opening Scenario, 413
- You Will Learn, 413
- Introduction, 413
- Types of Records, 413
- Importance of Accurate Health Records, 414
- Contents of the Health Record, 414
- PROCEDURE 19.1 Register a New Patient Using the Practice Management Software, 417
- Ownership of the Health Record, 419
- Technologic Terms in Health Information, 419
- Health Information Technology for the Economic and Clinical Health Act (HITECH Act) and Meaningful Use, 420
- Capabilities of Electronic Health Record Systems, 420
- Maintaining A Connection With the Patient When Using the Electronic Health Record, 422
- PROCEDURE 19.2 Upload Documents to the Electronic Health Record, 423
- PROCEDURE 19.3 Protect the Integrity of the Medical Record, 423
- Backup Systems for the Electronic Health Record, 424
- Retention and Destruction of Health Records, 424
- Releasing Health Record Information, 425
- Organization of the Health Record, 425
- Documenting in an Electronic Health Record, 428
- Documenting in A Paper Health Record, 428
- Making Corrections and Alterations to Health Records, 428
- Dictation and Transcription, 429
- Creating an Efficient Paper Health Records Management System, 430
- Indexing Rules, 432
- Filing Methods, 432
- PROCEDURE 19.4 Create and Organize a Patient's Paper Health Record, 433
- PROCEDURE 19.5 File Patient Health Records, 434
- Organization of Files, 435

20 Telephone Techniques and Scheduling, 438
- Opening Scenario, 439
- You Will Learn, 439
- Introduction, 439
- Telephone Techniques, 440
- PROCEDURE 20.1 Demonstrate Professional Telephone Techniques, 443
- PROCEDURE 20.2 Document Telephone Messages and Report Relevant Information Concisely and Accurately, 446
- Scheduling Appointments, 452
- PROCEDURE 20.3 Establish the Appointment Matrix, 454
- PROCEDURE 20.4 Schedule a New Patient, 458
- PROCEDURE 20.5 Schedule an Established Patient, 460
- PROCEDURE 20.6 Schedule a Patient Procedure, 462

21 Technology and Written Communication, 468
- Opening Scenario, 468
- You Will Learn, 469
- Introduction, 469
- Electronic Technology in the Ambulatory Care Center, 469
- Fundamentals of Written Communication, 480
- Written Correspondence, 482
- PROCEDURE 21.1 Compose a Professional Business Letter, 485
- PROCEDURE 21.2 Compose a Professional Email, 491

22 Reception and Daily Operations, 493
- Opening Scenario, 494
- You Will Learn, 494
- Introduction, 494

Opening the Healthcare Facility, 494
Patient Processing Tasks, 497
PROCEDURE 22.1 Coach Patients Regarding Office Policies, 501
Closing the Healthcare Facility, 502
Equipment and Supplies, 503
PROCEDURE 22.2 Perform an Equipment Inventory With Documentation, 504
PROCEDURE 22.3 Perform Routine Maintenance of Equipment, 505
PROCEDURE 22.4 Perform a Supply Inventory With Documentation While Using Proper Body Mechanics, 508
PROCEDURE 22.5 Prepare a Purchase Order, 509
Handling Mail, 511
Safety and Security, 512
PROCEDURE 22.6 Evaluate the Work Environment, 515
PROCEDURE 22.7 Participate in a Mock Exposure Event, 517
PROCEDURE 22.8 Use a Fire Extinguisher, 519

23 Health Insurance Basics, 521
Opening Scenario, 521
You Will Learn, 522
Introduction, 522
Benefits, 522
Health Insurance Plans, 522
Health Insurance Models, 526
Participating Provider Contracts, 527
The Medical Assistant's Role, 528
Other Types of Insurance, 529
The Affordable Care Act, 530

24 Diagnostic Coding Basics, 532
Opening Scenario, 532
You Will Learn, 533
Introduction, 533
What Is Diagnostic Coding?, 533
Getting to Know the ICD-10-CM, 533
Preparing for Diagnostic Coding, 538
Steps in ICD-10-CM Coding, 539
PROCEDURE 24.1 Perform Coding Using the Current ICD-10-CM Manual or Encoder, 540
Understanding Coding Guidelines, 543
Maximizing Third-Party Reimbursement, 546
Providers and Accurate Coding, 546

25 Procedural Coding Basics, 548
Opening Scenario, 549
You Will Learn, 549
Introduction to Procedural Coding, 549
Introduction to the CPT Manual, 549
Code Categories in the CPT Manual, 549
Organization of the CPT Manual, 550
Unlisted Procedure or Service Code, 550
CPT Coding Guidelines, 551
CPT Conventions, 552
Documentation for CPT Coding, 552
Using the Alphabetic Index, 552
Using the Tabular List, 554
Common CPT Coding Guidelines: Evaluation and Management Section, 555
PROCEDURE 25.1 Perform Procedural Coding: Surgery, 556
PROCEDURE 25.2 Perform Procedural Coding: Office Visit and Immunizations, 558
Common CPT Coding Guidelines: Surgical Section, 561
Common CPT Coding Guidelines: Pathology and Laboratory Section, 562
HCPCS Code Set and Manual, 562
Common HCPCS Coding Guidelines, 563
PROCEDURE 25.3 Working With Providers to Ensure Accurate Code Selection, 564

26 Billing and Reimbursement, 565
Opening Scenario, 566
You Will Learn, 566
Introduction, 566
Medical Billing Process, 566
PROCEDURE 26.1 Interpret Information on an Insurance Card, 567
Types of Information Found in the Patient's Billing Record, 567
PROCEDURE 26.2 Show Sensitivity When Communicating With Patients Regarding Third-Party Requirements, 569
Managed Care Policies and Procedures, 569
PROCEDURE 26.3 Perform Precertification With Documentation, 570
Submitting Claims to Third-Party Payers, 571
Generating Electronic Claims, 571
Completing the CMS-1500 Health Insurance Claim Form, 572
Accurate Coding to Prevent Fraud and Abuse, 577
PROCEDURE 26.4 Complete an Insurance Claim Form, 578
Preventing Rejection of a Claim, 580
Checking the Status of a Claim, 581
Explanation of Benefits, 581
Denied Claims, 581
The Patient's Financial Responsibility, 582
PROCEDURE 26.5 Use Medical Necessity Guidelines: Respond to a "Medical Necessity Denied" Claim, 582
PROCEDURE 26.6 Inform a Patient of Financial Obligations for Services Rendered, 584

27 Accounts, Collections, and Banking, 587
Opening Scenario, 588
You Will Learn, 588
Introduction, 588
Managing Funds in the Healthcare Facility, 588
Bookkeeping in the Healthcare Facility, 589
Accounts Receivable (A/R), 589
PROCEDURE 27.1 Post Charges and Payments to a Patient's Account, 592
PROCEDURE 27.2 Post Payments and Adjustments to a Patient's Account, 603
Accounts Payable (A/P), 604
PROCEDURE 27.3 Prepare a Bank Deposit, 610
Employee Payroll, 614

UNIT 4 Basic Clinical Procedures

28 Infection Control, 616
Opening Scenario, 616

You Will Learn, 616
Introduction, 617
Disease, 617
Chain of Infection, 617
Inflammatory Response, 620
Types of Infection, 621
Occupational Safety and Health Administration Standards for the Healthcare Setting, 622
PROCEDURE 28.1 Perform Hand Hygiene, 623
PROCEDURE 28.2 Remove Contaminated Gloves and Discard Biohazardous Material, 626
Aseptic Techniques: Preventing Disease Transmission, 630
PROCEDURE 28.3 Sanitizing Soiled Instruments, 633
Role of the Medical Assistant in Asepsis, 634

29 Vital Signs, 636
Opening Scenario, 637
You Will Learn, 637
Introduction, 637
Factors That May Influence Vital Signs, 637
Temperature, 637
Sites, 638
PROCEDURE 29.1 Obtain an Oral Temperature Using a Digital Thermometer, 641
Pulse, 641
PROCEDURE 29.2 Obtain an Axillary Temperature Using a Digital Thermometer, 642
PROCEDURE 29.3 Obtain a Rectal Temperature of an Infant Using a Digital Thermometer, 642
PROCEDURE 29.4 Obtain a Temperature Using a Tympanic Thermometer, 643
PROCEDURE 29.5 Obtain a Temperature Using a Temporal Artery Thermometer, 644
PROCEDURE 29.6 Obtain an Apical Pulse, 647
PROCEDURE 29.7 Assess the Patient's Radial Pulse and Respiratory Rate, 648
Respiration, 649
Blood Pressure, 651
PROCEDURE 29.8 Determine a Patient's Blood Pressure, 655
Pulse Oximetry, 658
Anthropometric Measurements, 658
PROCEDURE 29.9 Perform Pulse Oximetry, 658
PROCEDURE 29.10 Measuring a Patient's Weight and Height, 659

30 Physical Examination, 662
Opening Scenario, 663
You Will Learn, 663
Introduction, 663
Medical History, 664
Understanding and Communicating With Patients, 665
PROCEDURE 30.1 Obtain and Document Patient Information, 667
PROCEDURE 30.2 Respond to Nonverbal Communication, 670
Interviewing the Patient, 670
Assessing the Patient, 674
Documentation, 675
Physical Examination, 675
Principles of Body Mechanics, 679
Assisting With the Physical Examination, 680

PROCEDURE 30.3 Use Proper Body Mechanics, 681
PROCEDURE 30.4 Fowler and Semi-Fowler Positions, 682
PROCEDURE 30.5 Supine (Horizontal Recumbent) and Dorsal Recumbent Positions, 683
PROCEDURE 30.6 Lithotomy Position, 684
PROCEDURE 30.7 Sims Position, 685
PROCEDURE 30.8 Prone Position, 686
PROCEDURE 30.9 Knee-Chest Position, 687
Vision and Hearing Screenings, 691
PROCEDURE 30.10 Assist Provider With a Patient Exam, 692
PROCEDURE 30.11 Measuring Distance Visual Acuity, 694
PROCEDURE 30.12 Assess Color Acuity Using the Ishihara Test, 697
PROCEDURE 30.13 Measuring Hearing Acuity With an Audiometer, 700
PROCEDURE 30.14 Demonstrate Appropriate Self-Boundaries, 701

31 Assisting With Obstetrics and Gynecology, 703
Opening Scenario, 704
You Will Learn, 704
Introduction, 704
Gynecology, 704
PROCEDURE 31.1 Set Up for and Assist the Provider With a Gynecology Examination, 705
Obstetrics, 713
Recognizing Domestic Abuse, 719

32 Assisting in Pediatrics, 722
Opening Scenario, 722
You Will Learn, 722
Introduction, 722
Normal Growth and Development, 723
Pediatric Diseases and Disorders, 725
Immunizations, 727
The Pediatric Patient, 729
PROCEDURE 32.1 Document Immunizations, 731
The Medical Assistant's Role in Pediatric Procedures, 733
PROCEDURE 32.2 Measure the Head Circumference of an Infant, 737
PROCEDURE 32.3 Measure an Infant's Length and Weight, 737
The Adolescent Patient, 739
Injury Prevention, 739
Child Abuse, 740

33 Assisting in Geriatrics, 742
Opening Scenario, 742
You Will Learn, 742
Introduction, 742
PROCEDURE 33.1 Understand the Sensorimotor Changes of Aging, 743
Changes in Anatomy and Physiology, 744
The Medical Assistant's Role in Caring for the Older Patient, 755

34 Assisting With Minor Surgery, 757
Opening Scenario, 758
You Will Learn, 758
Introduction, 758
Minor Surgery Room, 758
Surgical Solutions and Medications, 758

Surgical Instruments, 759
Classifications of Surgical Instruments, 761
Miscellaneous Instruments, 766
Drapes, Sutures, and Needles, 767
Surgical Asepsis and Assisting With Surgical Procedures, 769
Care and Handling of Instruments, 769
PROCEDURE 34.1 Wrap Instruments and Supplies for Sterilization in an Autoclave, 772
PROCEDURE 34.2 Operate the Autoclave, 775
PROCEDURE 34.3 Perform Skin Prep for Surgery, 779
PROCEDURE 34.4 Perform a Surgical Hand Scrub, 780
PROCEDURE 34.5 Prepare a Sterile Field, Use Transfer Forceps, and Pour a Sterile Solution Into a Sterile Field, 782
PROCEDURE 34.6 Two-Person Sterile Tray Setup, 784
PROCEDURE 34.7 Put on Sterile Gloves, 785
PROCEDURE 34.8 Assist With Minor Surgery, 787
PROCEDURE 34.9 Apply a Sterile Dressing, 791
PROCEDURE 34.10 Remove Sutures and/or Surgical Staples, 794

UNIT 5 Advanced Clinical Procedures

35 Patient Coaching With Health Promotion, 799
Opening Scenario, 800
You Will Learn, 800
Introduction, 800
Coaching, 800
Making Changes for Health, 801
Basics of Teaching and Learning, 802
Coaching on Disease Prevention, 806
PROCEDURE 35.1 Coach a Patient on Disease Prevention, 808
Coaching on Health Maintenance and Wellness, 809
PROCEDURE 35.2 Coach a Patient on Breast Self-Exam, 809
PROCEDURE 35.3 Coach a Patient on Testicular Self-Exam, 811
PROCEDURE 35.4 Perform a Monofilament Foot Exam, 816
Coaching on Diagnostic Tests, 817
Coaching on Treatment Plans, 817
PROCEDURE 35.5 Apply a Cold Pack, 822
PROCEDURE 35.6 Coach a Patient to Use Axillary Crutches, 826
Care Coordination, 828
PROCEDURE 35.7 Coach a Patient to Use a Walker, 828
PROCEDURE 35.8 Coach a Patient to Use a Cane, 830
PROCEDURE 35.9 Develop a List of Community Resources and Facilitate Referrals, 831

36 Patient Coaching With Nutrition, 833
Opening Scenario, 834
You Will Learn, 834
Introduction, 834
Metabolism, 834
Dietary Nutrients, 834
Dietary Guidelines, 840
Reading Food Labels, 840
Medically Ordered Diets, 842
Nutritional Needs for Various Populations, 847
Eating Disorders, 848
Instructing Patients on Dietary Changes, 849
PROCEDURE 36.1 Instruct a Patient on a Dietary Change, 850

37 Pharmacology Basics, 853
Opening Scenario, 854
You Will Learn, 854
Introduction, 854
Pharmacology Basics, 854
Drug Legislation and the Ambulatory Care Setting, 857
Drug Names, 859
Drug Reference Information, 860
Types of Medication Orders, 862
PROCEDURE 37.1 Prepare a Prescription, 869
Over-the-Counter Medications and Herbal Products, 871
Math for Medications, 871
PROCEDURE 37.2 Calculate Medication Dosages, 881

38 Administering Medication, 884
Opening Scenario, 885
You Will Learn, 885
Introduction, 885
Nine Rules of Medication Administration, 885
Forms of Medications, 887
Routes of Medications, 889
PROCEDURE 38.1 Administer Oral Medications, 891
PROCEDURE 38.2 Instill an Eye Medication, 894
PROCEDURE 38.3 Instill Ear Drops, 895
PROCEDURE 38.4 Irrigate a Patient's Eye, 897
PROCEDURE 38.5 Irrigate a Patient's Ear, 898
Needles and Syringes, 899
Preparing Parenteral Medication, 904
PROCEDURE 38.6 Prepare Medication From an Ampule, 905
PROCEDURE 38.7 Prepare Medication Using a Prefilled Sterile Cartridge, 907
PROCEDURE 38.8 Prepare Medication From a Vial, 909
PROCEDURE 38.9 Reconstitute Powdered Medication, 911
PROCEDURE 38.10 Mixing Two Insulins, 913
Giving Parenteral Medications, 914
Intradermal Injections, 915
PROCEDURE 38.11 Administer an Intradermal Injection, 918
Subcutaneous Injections, 922
PROCEDURE 38.12 Administer a Subcutaneous Injection, 924
Intramuscular Injections, 926
PROCEDURE 38.13 Administer an Intramuscular Injection, 929
Monitoring Intravenous Therapy, 931
PROCEDURE 38.14 Administer an Intramuscular Injection Using the Z-Track Technique, 931

39 Cardiopulmonary Procedures, 933
Opening Scenario, 934

You Will Learn, 934
Introduction, 934
Cardiovascular System Review, 934
ECG Tracing, 937
12-Lead ECG, 939
ECG Supplies and Equipment, 939
ECG Procedure, 942
PROCEDURE 39.1 Perform Electrocardiography, 944
Additional ECG Testing, 951
PROCEDURE 39.2 Apply a Holter Monitor, 952
Respiratory System, 954
PROCEDURE 39.3 Measure the Peak Flow Rate, 955
PROCEDURE 39.4 Perform Spirometry Testing, 957
PROCEDURE 39.5 Administer a Nebulizer Treatment, 959
PROCEDURE 39.6 Administer Oxygen Per Nasal Cannula or Mask, 961

40 Medical Emergencies, 963
Opening Scenario, 963
You Will Learn, 963
Introduction, 964
Emergencies in Healthcare Settings, 964
Emergency Equipment and Supplies, 964
Handling Emergencies, 968
PROCEDURE 40.1 Provide First Aid for a Patient With Insulin Shock, 976
PROCEDURE 40.2 Incorporate Critical Thinking Skills When Performing Patient Assessment, 979
PROCEDURE 40.3 Provide First Aid for a Patient With Seizure Activity, 979
PROCEDURE 40.4 Provide First Aid for a Choking Patient, 982
PROCEDURE 40.5 Provide First Aid for a Patient With a Bleeding Wound, Fracture, and Syncope, 984
PROCEDURE 40.6 Provide First Aid for a Patient With Shock, 985
PROCEDURE 40.7 Provide Rescue Breathing, Cardiopulmonary Resuscitation (CPR), and Automated External Defibrillator (AED), 986

UNIT 6 Medical Laboratory

41 Assisting in the Clinical Laboratory, 990
Opening Scenario, 991
You Will Learn, 991
Introduction: The Clinical Laboratory and Patient Care, 991
Government Legislation Affecting Clinical Laboratory Testing, 994
Quality Assurance Guidelines, 996
Quality Control Guidelines, 997
PROCEDURE 41.1 Perform a Quality Control Measure on a Glucometer and Record the Results on a Flow Sheet, 998
Laboratory Safety, 999
PROCEDURE 41.2 Use of the Eyewash Equipment: Perform an Emergency Eyewash, 1002
Specimen Collection, Processing, and Storage, 1004
PROCEDURE 41.3 Evaluate the Laboratory Environment, 1004
Laboratory Mathematics and Measurement, 1007
Laboratory Equipment, 1008
PROCEDURE 41.4 Perform Routine Maintenance on Clinical Equipment (Microscope), 1011

42 Assisting in the Analysis of Urine, 1014
Opening Scenario, 1015
You Will Learn, 1015
Introduction, 1015
Urine Formation, 1015
Collecting A Urine Specimen: Patient Sensitivity, 1017
PROCEDURE 42.1 Instruct a Patient in the Collection of a 24-Hour Urine Specimen, 1018
PROCEDURE 42.2 Collect a Clean-Catch Midstream Urine Specimen, 1020
Routine Urinalysis, 1021
PROCEDURE 42.3 Assess Urine for Color and Turbidity: Physical Test, 1022
PROCEDURE 42.4 Perform Quality Control Measures: Differentiate Between Normal and Abnormal Test Results While Determining the Reliability of Chemical Reagent Strips, 1026
PROCEDURE 42.5 Test Urine With Chemical Reagent Strips, 1026
Microscopic Preparation and Examination of Urine Sediment, 1030
PROCEDURE 42.6 Prepare a Urine Specimen for Microscopic Examination, 1031
Additional CLIA-Waived Tests Performed on Urine, 1038
PROCEDURE 42.7 Test Urine for Glucose Using the Clinitest Method, 1039
PROCEDURE 42.8 Perform a CLIA-Waived Urinalysis: Perform a Pregnancy Test, 1040

43 Assisting in Blood Collection, 1046
Opening Scenario, 1046
You Will Learn, 1047
Introduction, 1047
Venipuncture Equipment, 1047
Order of the Draw, 1052
Needles and Supplies Used in Phlebotomy, 1052
Needle Safety, 1054
Routine Venipuncture, 1056
PROCEDURE 43.1 Perform a Venipuncture: Collect a Venous Blood Sample Using the Vacuum Tube Method, 1058
PROCEDURE 43.2 Perform a Venipuncture: Collect a Venous Blood Sample Using the Syringe Method, 1061
PROCEDURE 43.3 Perform Venipuncture: Obtain a Venous Sample With a Safety Winged Butterfly Needle Assembly, 1064
Problems Associated With Venipuncture, 1066
Capillary Puncture, 1067
Routine Capillary Puncture, 1069
Pediatric Phlebotomy, 1071
PROCEDURE 43.4 Perform a Capillary Puncture: Obtain a Blood Sample by Capillary Puncture, 1071
Handling the Specimen After Collection, 1074

44 Assisting in the Analysis of Blood, 1076
Opening Scenario, 1077
You Will Learn, 1077
Introduction, 1077
Hematology, 1077
Hematology in the Physician Office Laboratory (POL), 1078
PROCEDURE 44.1 Perform Preventive Maintenance for the Microhematocrit Centrifuge, 1079
PROCEDURE 44.2 CLIA-Waived Hematology Testing: Perform a Microhematocrit Test, 1080
PROCEDURE 44.3 Perform CLIA-Waived Hematology Testing: Perform a Hemoglobin Test, 1082
PROCEDURE 44.4 Perform CLIA-Waived Hematology Testing: Determine the Erythrocyte Sedimentation Rate Using a Modified Westergren Method, 1084
Hematology in the Reference Laboratory, 1086
PROCEDURE 44.5 Perform a CLIA-Waived PT/INR Test, 1087
Immunohematology, 1093
Blood Chemistry in the Physician Office Laboratory, 1094
PROCEDURE 44.6 Assist the Provider with Patient Care: Perform a Blood Glucose TRUEresult Test, 1095
PROCEDURE 44.7 Perform a CLIA-Waived Chemistry Test: Determine the Cholesterol Level or Lipid Profile Using a Cholestech Analyzer, 1098
Reference Laboratory Chemistry Panels and Single Analyte Testing and Monitoring, 1099

45 Assisting in Microbiology and Immunology, 1104
Opening Scenario, 1105
You Will Learn, 1105
Introduction, 1105
Classification of Microorganisms, 1106
Characteristics of Bacteria, 1107
Unusual Pathogenic Bacteria: Chlamydia, Mycoplasma, and Rickettsia, 1108
Pathogenic Fungi, 1109
Pathogenic Protozoa, 1110
Pathogenic Parasites, 1110
Pathogenic Helminths (Worms), 1111
Pathogenic Viruses, 1111
Specimen Collection and Transport in the Physician Office Laboratory, 1111
PROCEDURE 45.1 Instruct Patients in the Collection of Fecal Specimens to Be Tested for Ova and Parasites, 1112
CLIA-Waived Microbiology Testing, 1116
PROCEDURE 45.2 Collect a Specimen for a Throat Culture, 1117
PROCEDURE 45.3 Perform a CLIA-Waived Microbiology Test: Perform a Rapid Strep Test, 1118
CLIA-Waived Immunology Testing, 1119
PROCEDURE 45.4 Perform a CLIA-waived Immunology Test: Perform a QuickVue+ Infectious Mononucleosis Test, 1119
Microbiology Reference Laboratory: Identification of Pathogens, 1122

UNIT 7 Employment Seeking

46 Career Development, 1126
Opening Scenario, 1127
You Will Learn, 1127
Introduction to Career Development, 1127
Understanding Personality Traits Important to Employers, 1127
Assessing Your Strengths and Skills, 1128
Developing Career Objectives, 1129
Identifying Personal Needs, 1130
Finding a Job, 1130
Developing a Resume, 1131
PROCEDURE 46.1 Prepare a Chronologic Resume, 1133
Developing a Cover Letter, 1136
PROCEDURE 46.2 Create a Cover Letter, 1137
Completing Online Profiles and Job Applications, 1138
PROCEDURE 46.3 Complete a Job Application, 1139
Creating a Career Portfolio, 1140
Job Interview, 1140
PROCEDURE 46.4 Create a Career Portfolio, 1141
PROCEDURE 46.5 Practice Interview Skills During a Mock Interview, 1143
PROCEDURE 46.6 Create a Thank-You Note for an Interview, 1144
Improving Your Opportunities, 1145
You Got the Job!, 1146

Appendix A: Word Parts and Definitions, 1149
Appendix B: Definitions and Word Parts, 1157
Appendix C: Abbreviations, 1164
Appendix D: Medication Classifications, 1169
Glossary, 1180
Index, 1192

1

Medical Terminology Basics

LEARNING OBJECTIVES

1. Describe where medical terminology comes from, and discuss the difference between decodable and nondecodable terms.
2. Describe how to decode terms using the check, assign, reverse, and define (CARD) method.
3. Use the rules given to build, spell, and pronounce healthcare terms.

CHAPTER OUTLINE

1. Opening Scenario, 1
2. You Will Learn, 1
3. Where Does Medical Terminology Come From? 1
4. Types of Medical Terms, 2
   a. Decodable Terms, 2
   b. Nondecodable Terms, 2
   c. Abbreviations and Symbols, 3
5. Decoding Terms, 3
   a. Check, Assign, Reverse, and Define (CARD) Method, 3
6. Building Terms, 4
   a. Spelling Rules, 4
   b. Suffixes, 5
      i. Noun-Ending Suffixes, 5
      ii. Adjective Suffixes, 5
      iii. Pathology Suffixes, 8
      iv. Diagnostic Procedures Suffixes, 8
      v. Therapeutic Intervention Suffixes, 8
      vi. Instrument Suffixes, 8
      vii. Specialty and Specialist Suffixes, 9
   c. Prefixes, 9
7. Singular/Plural Rules, 9
8. Closing Comments, 11
9. Chapter Review, 12
10. Scenario Wrap-Up, 12

▶▶ OPENING SCENARIO

As a new medical assistant student, Emma Davis is just starting to learn about medical terminology. Her instructors have told her that medical terminology is an important part of communication in a healthcare setting, and Emma is excited to get started. She understands that learning medical terminology is very much like learning a foreign language. She also understands that by learning the meanings of different word parts, she can easily figure out the meaning of a new medical term.

YOU WILL LEARN

1. To decode medical terms using the CARD method.
2. To identify combining forms, suffixes, and prefixes used in medical terminology.
3. To apply spelling rules to medical terminology.

WHERE DOES MEDICAL TERMINOLOGY COME FROM?

Medical terminology is a specialized vocabulary that has its root in Greek and Latin word components. Professionals in healthcare use this terminology to communicate with each other. By applying the process of "decoding," or recognizing the word components and their meanings, anyone will be able to interpret literally thousands of medical terms.

The English language and medical terminology share many common origins. This proves to be an additional bonus for those who put in the time and effort to learn hundreds of new word parts. Two examples are the **combining forms** gloss/o (Greek) and lingu/o (Latin), which mean "tongue." Because the word tongue is instrumental in creating spoken language, Greek and Latin equivalents appear, not surprisingly, in familiar English vocabulary. Table 1.1 shows the intersection of our everyday English language with the ancient languages of Greek and Latin, which can help us to clearly see the connections. **Suffixes** and **prefixes** also are presented in this table. Make note of the pronunciation key provided directly under the examples: You will have to use your tongue to say them! *Please remember that terminology is spoken as well as written and read.* Taking advantage of the many resources provided throughout this text will help you to fully communicate as a healthcare professional.

VOCABULARY
combining forms: The "subjects" of most terms. They consist of the word root with its respective combining vowel.
suffixes: Word parts that appear at the end of some terms.
prefixes: Word parts that appear at the beginning of some terms.

Did you notice that medical terms use the word origins literally, whereas English words are related to word origins but are not exactly

UNIT 1 Medical Terminology, Anatomy, and Physiology

TABLE 1.1 Ancient Word Origins in Current English and Medical Terminology Usage

Term	Word Origins	Definition
glossary (GLAH sur ee)	*gloss/o* tongue (Greek) *-ary* pertaining to	An English term meaning "an alphabetical list of terms with definitions"
glossitis (glah SYE tiss)	*gloss/o* tongue (Greek) *-itis* inflammation	A medical term meaning "inflammation of the tongue"
bi**lingu**al (by LIN gwal)	*bi-* two *lingu/o* tongue (Latin) *-al* pertaining to	An English term meaning "pertaining to two languages"
sub**lingu**al (sub LIN gwal)	*sub-* under *lingu/o* tongue (Latin) *-al* pertaining to	A medical term meaning "pertaining to under the tongue"

From Shiland B: *Mastering Healthcare Terminology*, ed 5, St. Louis, 2016, Elsevier.

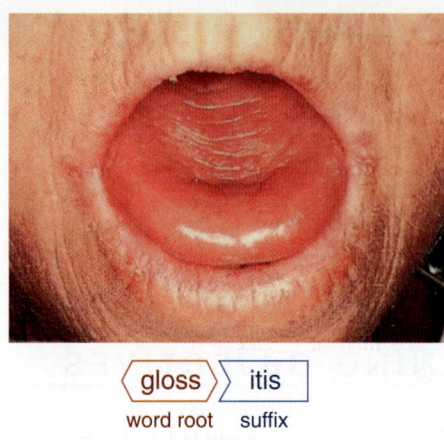

FIG. 1.1 Decoding of the term *glossitis*. (From Feldman M, Friedman LS, Brandt LJ: *Sleisenger and Fordtran's Gastrointestinal and Liver Disease*, ed 8, Philadelphia, 2006, Saunders/Elsevier.)

the same? Fortunately, most medical terms may be assigned a simple definition through the use of their word parts.

TYPES OF MEDICAL TERMS
Decodable Terms
Decodable terms are those that can be broken into their Greek and Latin word parts and given a working definition based on the meanings of those word parts. Most medical terms are decodable, so learning word parts is important. The word parts are as follows:
- **Combining form:** Word root with its respective combining vowel.
  - **Word root:** Foundation of the medical term.
  - **Combining vowel:** A letter sometimes used to join word parts. Usually an "o" but occasionally an "a," "e," "i," or "u."
- **Suffix:** Word part that appears at the end of a term. Suffixes are used to modify the meaning of the combining form.
- **Prefix:** Word part that sometimes appears at the beginning of a term. Prefixes also modify the meaning of the combining form. They usually are used to further define the absence, location, number, quantity, or state of the term.

In our first examples, gloss/ and lingu/ are word roots with an "o" as their combining vowel. Therefore gloss/o and lingu/o are combining forms; -ary, -al, and -itis are suffixes, and bi- and sub- are prefixes. Figs. 1.1 and 1.2 demonstrate the decoding of the terms *glossitis* and *sublingual*. Throughout the text, we will be using combining forms so that you will learn the appropriate combining vowel for that particular term.

Nondecodable Terms
Not all terms are composed of word parts that can be used to determine the definition. These terms are known as **nondecodable terms**. For these types of terms the meaning must be memorized. A medical dictionary is an excellent tool to help with finding the definition of nondecodable terms. Examples of nondecodable terms include the following:

> **VOCABULARY**
> **nondecodable terms:** Words used in healthcare whose definitions must be memorized without the benefit of word parts.

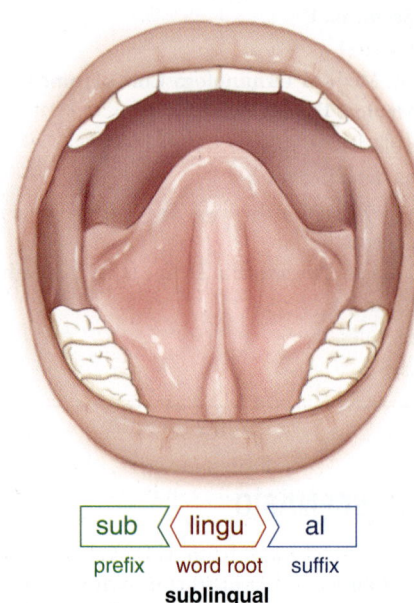

FIG. 1.2 Decoding of the term sublingual. (From Shiland B: *Mastering Healthcare Terminology*, ed 5, St. Louis, 2016, Elsevier.)

- **Cataract** (KAT ah rakt): From the Greek term meaning "waterfall." In healthcare language, this means the condition in which the lens becomes progressively opaque (loss of transparency). (This is explained in more detail in Chapter 13.)
- **Asthma** (AZ mah): From the Greek term meaning "panting." Although this word origin is understandable, the definition is a respiratory disorder characterized by recurring episodes of paroxysmal dyspnea (difficulty breathing). (This is explained in more detail in Chapter 11.)
- **Diagnosis** (dy ag NOH sis): The disease or condition that is determined after a healthcare provider evaluates a patient's signs, symptoms, and history. Although the term is built from word parts (dia-, meaning "through," "complete," and -gnosis, meaning "state of knowledge"), using these word parts to form the definition of diagnosis, which is "a state of complete knowledge," is not very helpful.

- **Prognosis** (prawg NOH sis): Similar to *diagnosis*, the term *prognosis* can be broken down into its word parts (pro-, meaning "before" or "in front of," and -gnosis, meaning "state of knowledge"), but this does not give the true definition of the term, which is "a prediction of the probable outcome of a disease or disorder."
- **Sequela** (suh KWELL ah): A condition that follows and is the result of an injury or disease.
- **Acute** (ah KYOOT): A term that describes a sudden, severe onset (acu- means "sharp") to a disease.
- **Chronic** (KRAW nik): Developing slowly and lasting for 6 months or longer (chron/o means "time"). Diagnoses may be additionally described as being either acute or chronic.
- **Sign:** An objective finding of a disease state (e.g., fever, high blood pressure, rash).
- **Symptom** (SIMP tom): A subjective report of a disease (pain, itching).

Other types of terms that are not built from word parts include the following:
- **Eponym** (EP uh nim): Terms that are named after a person or place associated with the term. Examples include the following:
  - **Alzheimer disease** (AWLZ hy mer), which is named after Alois Alzheimer, a German neurologist (nyoor AW loh jist). The disease is a progressive mental deterioration.
  - **Achilles tendon** (uh KIL eez), which is a body part named after a figure in Greek mythology whose one weak spot was this area of his anatomy. Tendons are bands of tissue that attach muscles to bone. The Achilles tendon is the particular tendon that attaches the calf muscle to the heel bone (calcaneus, kal KAY nee us). Unlike some eponyms, this one does have a medical equivalent, the calcaneal tendon.

This text presents eponyms without the possessive. This practice is in accordance with the American Medical Association (AMA) and the American Association of Transcriptionists (AAMT).

Abbreviations and Symbols

Abbreviations are terms that have been shortened to letters or numbers for the sake of convenience, such as AAMA for the American Association of Medical Assistants. Symbols are graphic representations of a term, such as @ for *at*. Abbreviations and symbols are common in written and spoken medical terminology but can pose problems for healthcare workers. The Joint Commission has published a "DO NOT USE" list of dangerously confusing abbreviations, symbols, and acronyms that should be avoided (see Appendix C). The Institute of Safe Medical Practice, Inc., has provided a more extensive list. Each healthcare organization should have an official list, which includes the single meaning allowed for each abbreviation or symbol. Examples of acceptable abbreviations and symbols include the following:
- **Simple abbreviations:** A combination of letters (often, but not always the first of significant word parts) and sometimes numbers
  - IM: Abbreviation for *intramuscular* (pertaining to within the muscles)
  - C2: Second cervical vertebra (second bone in neck)
- **Acronyms:** Abbreviations that are also pronounceable
  - CABG (KAB ij): Coronary artery bypass graft (a detour around a blockage in an artery of the heart)
  - TURP: Transurethral (trans yoor EE thral) resection of the prostate (a surgical procedure that removes the prostate through the urethra)
- **Symbols:** Graphic representations of terms
  - ♂ stands for male
  - ♀ stands for female
  - ↑ stands for increased
  - ↓ stands for decreased
  - + stands for present
  - − stands for absent

DECODING TERMS

Check, Assign, Reverse, and Define (CARD) Method

Using Greek and Latin word components to break down the meanings of medical terms requires a simple four-step process—the check, assign, reverse, and define (CARD) method. You need to do the following:
- *Check* for the word parts in a term.
- *Assign* meanings to the word parts.
- *Reverse* the meaning of the suffix to the front of your definition.
- *Define* the term.

Using Fig. 1.3, see how this process is applied to your first patient, Alex.

In the tables that follow, the term and its pronunciation appear in the first column, the word origin in the second, and a definition in the third. Table 1.2 introduces six common combining forms and six common suffixes. (The use of prefixes will be introduced later.) Table 1.3 introduces six medical terms that use six different combining forms and suffixes. Success in decoding these terms depends on how well you remember the word parts presented in Table 1.2. Once you have mastered these 12 word parts, you will be able to recognize and define many other medical terms that use these same word parts.

Table 1.3 demonstrates how terms are presented in this book. Notice that the first column includes the term and its pronunciation. The

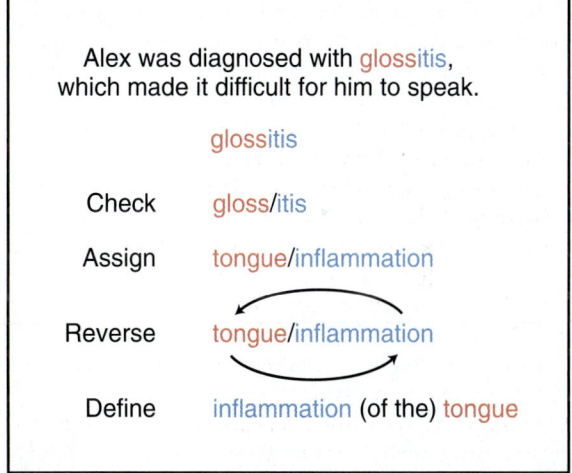

FIG. 1.3 How to decode a medical term using the check, assign, reverse, and define (CARD) method. (From Shiland B: *Mastering Healthcare Terminology*, ed 5, St. Louis, 2016, Elsevier.)

TABLE 1.2 Common Combining Forms and Suffixes

Combining Forms	Suffixes
arthr/o = joint	**-algia** = pain
gastr/o = stomach	**-tomy** = incision
ophthalm/o = eye	**-scope** = instrument to view
ot/o = ear	**-logy** = study of
rhin/o = nose	**-plasty** = surgical repair
hepat/o = liver	**-itis** = inflammation

From Shiland B: *Mastering Healthcare Terminology*, ed 5, St. Louis, 2016, Elsevier.

UNIT 1 Medical Terminology, Anatomy, and Physiology

TABLE 1.3	Samples of Decodable Terms	
Term	**Word Origins**	**Definition**
arthralgia (ar THRAL jah)	**arthr/o** joint **-algia** pain of	Pain of a joint; also called **arthrodynia** (-dynia means pain)
gastrotomy (gass TROT uh mee)	**gastr/o** stomach **-tomy** incision	Incision of the stomach
ophthalmoscope (off THAL muh skohp)	**ophthalm/o** eye **-scope** instrument to view	Instrument used to view the eye
otology (oh TALL uh jee)	**ot/o** ear **-logy** study of	Study of the ear
rhinoplasty (RYE noh plass tee)	**rhin/o** nose **-plasty** surgical repair	Surgical repair of the nose
hepatitis (heh peh TYE tiss)	**hepat/o** liver **-itis** inflammation	Inflammation of the liver

From Shiland B: *Mastering Healthcare Terminology*, ed 5, St. Louis, 2016, Elsevier.

second column breaks the term down into word parts and their meanings. The third column includes the definition of the term and any synonyms.

The "wheel of terminology" included in Fig. 1.4 demonstrates how the different suffixes in Table 1.2 can be added to a combining form to make a variety of terms.

BUILDING TERMS

Now that you've seen how terms are decoded, we will talk about how they are built. First, here are a few rules on how to spell medical terms correctly.

Spelling Rules

With a few exceptions, decodable medical terms follow five simple rules.

1. If the suffix starts with a vowel, a combining vowel is *not* needed to join the parts. For example, it is simple to combine the combining form **arthr/o** and suffix **-itis** to build the term **arthritis**, which means "an inflammation of the joints." The combining vowel "**o**" is not needed because the suffix starts with the vowel "**i**."
2. If the suffix starts with a consonant, a combining vowel *is* needed to join the two word parts. For example, when building a term using **arthr/o** and **-plasty**, the combining vowel is used and the resulting

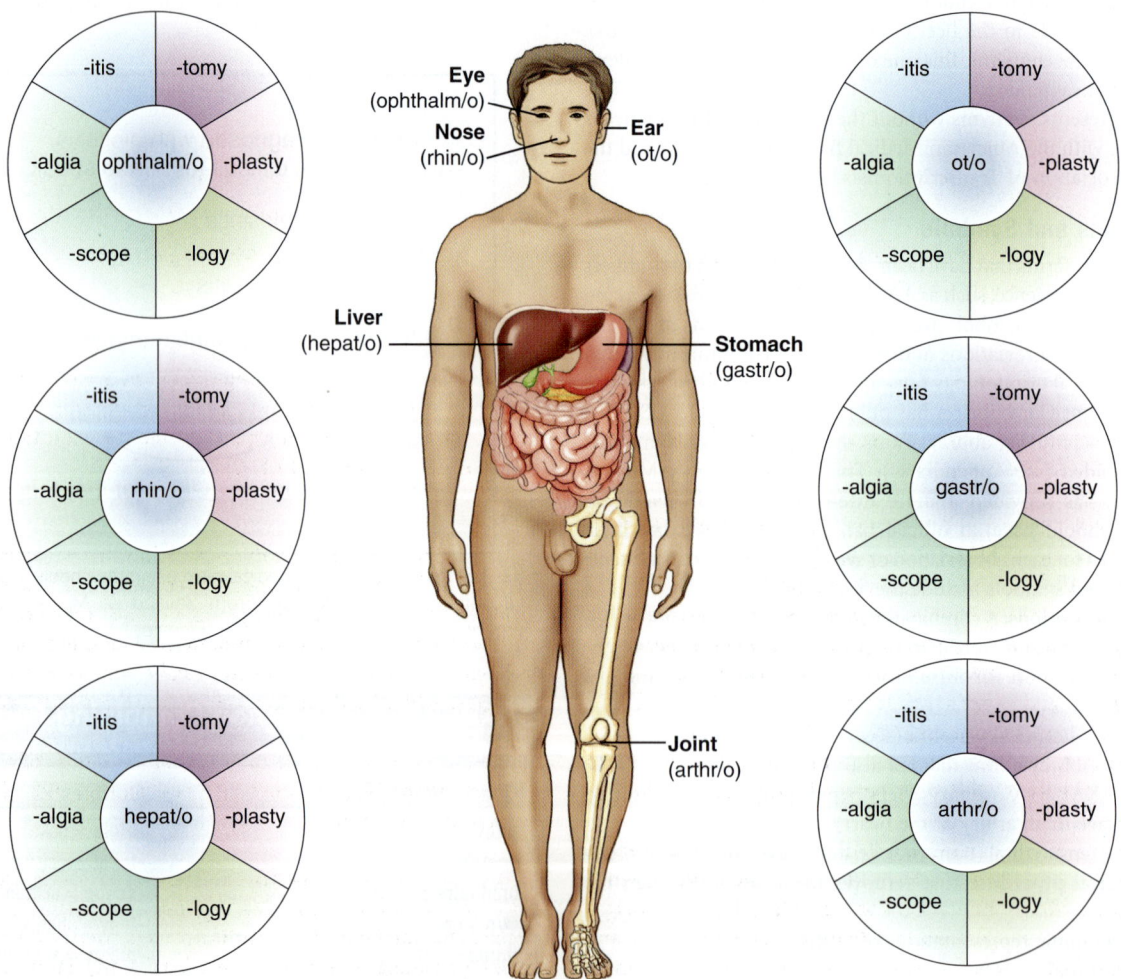

FIG. 1.4 Body parts and their combining forms. Surrounding the figure are "terminology wheels" that show how different suffixes can be added to a combining form to make a variety of terms. (From Shiland B: *Mastering Healthcare Terminology*, ed 5, St. Louis, 2016, Elsevier.)

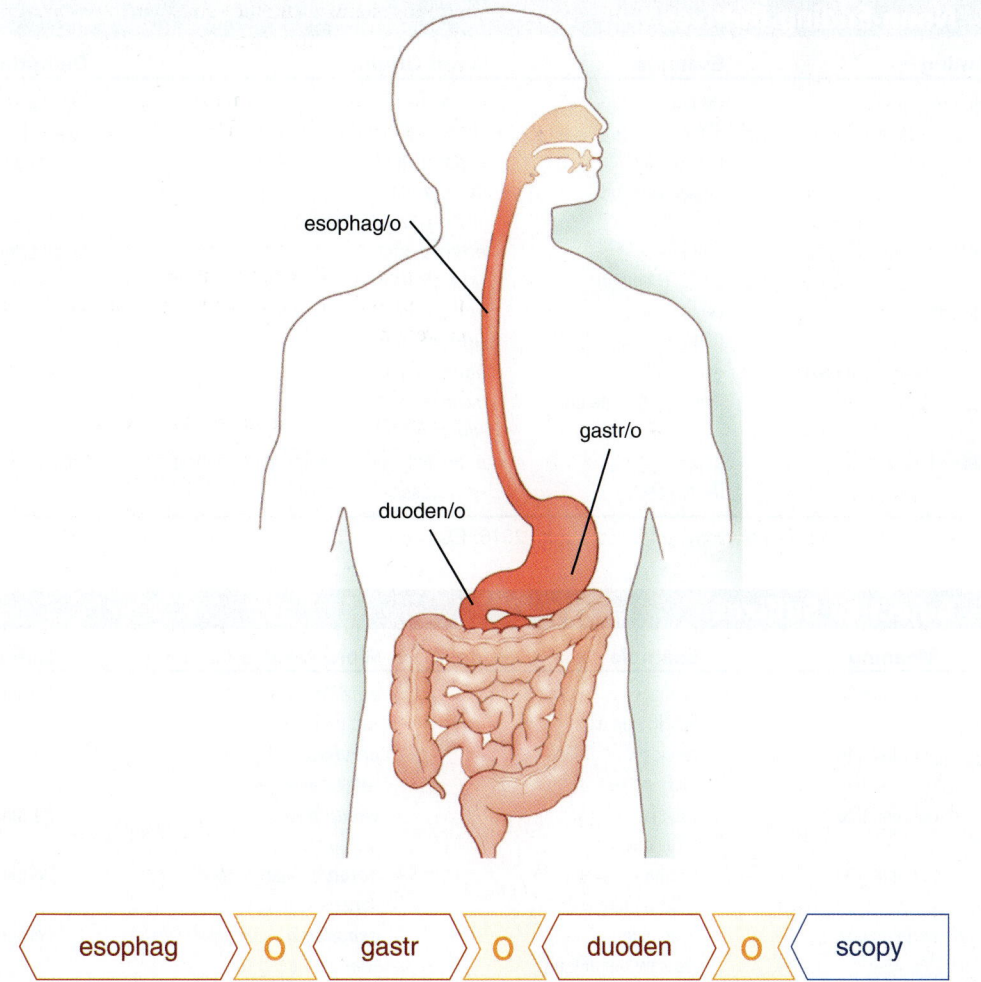

FIG. 1.5 The decoding of the term esophagogastroduodenoscopy (EGD). (From Shiland B: *Mastering Healthcare Terminology*, ed 5, St. Louis, 2016, Elsevier.)

term is spelled **arthroplasty**, which refers to a surgical repair of a joint.
3. If a combining form ends with the same vowel that begins a suffix, one of the vowels is dropped. The term that means "inflammation of the inside of the heart" is built from the suffix **-itis** (inflammation), the prefix **endo-** (inside), and the combining form **cardi/o**. Endo- + cardi/o + -itis would result in *endocardiitis*. Instead, one of the "i"s is dropped, and the term is spelled **endocarditis**.
4. If two or more combining forms are used in a term, the combining vowel is retained between the two, regardless of whether the second combining form begins with a vowel or a consonant. For example, joining **gastr/o** and **enter/o** (small intestine) with the suffix **-itis**, results in the term **gastroenteritis**. Notice that the combining vowel is *kept* between the two combining forms (even though **enter/o** begins with the vowel "e"), and the combining vowel is *dropped* before the suffix **-itis**.
5. Sometimes when two or more combining forms are used to make a medical term, special notice must be paid to the order in which the combining forms are joined. For example, joining **esophag/o** (which means esophagus), **gastr/o** (which means stomach), and **duoden/o** (which means duodenum, the first part of the small intestines) with the suffix **-scopy** (process of viewing), produces the term *esophagogastroduodenoscopy*. An esophagogastroduodenoscopy (EGD) is a visual examination of the esophagus, stomach, and duodenum. In this procedure, the examination takes place in a specific sequence (that is, esophagus first, stomach second, and then the duodenum). Thus the term reflects the direction from which the scope travels through the body (Fig. 1.5).

Suffixes

The body system chapters in this text include many combining forms that are used to build terms specific to each system. These combining forms will not be seen in other places, except as a sign or symptom of a particular disorder. **Suffixes**, however, are used over and over again throughout the text. Suffixes usually can be grouped according to their purposes. Tables 1.3 through 1.9 cover the major suffix categories.

Noun-Ending Suffixes. Noun endings are used most often to describe anatomic terms. Noun endings such as -icle, -ole, and -ule describe a small or tiny structure.

Adjective Suffixes. Adjective suffixes such as those listed in Table 1.4 usually mean "pertaining to." For example, when the suffix **-ac** is added to the combining form **cardi/o**, the term *cardiac* is formed, which means "pertaining to the heart." Remember that when you see an adjective term, you need to see what it is describing. For example, cardiac pain is pain of the heart, and cardiac surgery is surgery done on the heart. An adjective tells only half of the story.

TABLE 1.4 Noun-Ending Suffixes

Suffix	Meaning	Example	Word Origins	Definition
-icle	small, tiny	cuticle (KYOO tih kl)	cut/o skin -icle small	Small skin (surrounding the nail)
-is	structure, thing	Hypodermis (hi poh DER mis)	hypo- under derm/o skin -is structure	Structure under the skin
-ole	small, tiny	arteriole (ar TEER ee ohl)	arteri/o artery -ole small	Small artery
-ule	small, tiny	venule (VEN ule)	ven/o vein -ule small	Small vein
-um	structure, thing, membrane	endocardium (end oh KAR dee um)	endo- within cardi/o heart -um structure	Structure within the heart
-y	process of, condition	atrophy (A truh fee)	a- no, not, without troph/o development -y process of	Process of no development

From Shiland B: *Mastering Healthcare Terminology*, ed 5, St. Louis, 2016, Elsevier.

TABLE 1.5 Adjective Suffixes

Suffix	Meaning	Example	Word Origins	Definition
-ac	pertaining to	cardiac (KAHR dee ak)	cardi/o heart -ac pertaining to	Pertaining to the heart
-al	pertaining to	cervical (SER vih kal)	cervic/o neck -al pertaining to	Pertaining to the neck
-ar	pertaining to	valvular (VAL vyuh ler)	valvul/o valve -ar pertaining to	Pertaining to a valve
-ary	pertaining to	coronary (KOR oh nair ee)	coron/o[a] heart, crown -ary pertaining to	Pertaining to the heart
-eal	pertaining to	esophageal (ee saw fah JEE al)	esophag/o esophagus -eal pertaining to	Pertaining to the esophagus
-ic	pertaining to	hypodermic (hi puh DUR mik)	hypo- below derm/o skin -ic pertaining to	Pertaining to below the skin
-ous	pertaining to	subcutaneous (sub kyoo TAY nee us)	sub- under cutane/o skin -ous pertaining to	Pertaining to under the skin

[a]Coron/o literally means "crown," but it is used most frequently to describe the arteries that supply blood to the heart, so the meaning "heart" has been added.
From Shiland B: *Mastering Healthcare Terminology*, ed 5, St. Louis, 2016, Elsevier.

TABLE 1.6 Pathology Suffixes

Suffix	Meaning	Example	Word Origins	Definition
-algia	pain	cephalalgia (sef al AL jah)	cephal/o head -algia pain	Pain in the head
-cele	herniation	cystocele (SIS toh seel)	cyst/o bladder, sac -cele herniation, protrusion	Herniation of the bladder
-dynia	pain	cardiodynia (kar dee o DIN ee uh)	cardi/o heart -dynia pain	Pain in the heart
-emia	blood condition	hyperlipidemia (hy per lip ih DEE mee ah)	hyper- excessive lipid/o fats -emia blood condition	Condition of excessive fats in the blood
-ia	condition	agastria (aa GAS tree uh)	a- without gastr/o stomach -ia condition	Condition of having no stomach

TABLE 1.6 Pathology Suffixes—cont'd

Suffix	Meaning	Example	Word Origins	Definition
-itis	inflammation	gastroenteritis (gas troh en ter EYE tis)	**gastr/o** stomach **enter/o** small intestine **-itis** inflammation	Inflammation of the stomach and small intestine
-malacia	softening	chondromalacia (con droh mah LAY sha)	**chondr/o** cartilage **-malacia** softening	Softening of the cartilage
-megaly	enlargement	splenomegaly (spleh noh MEG ah lee) (Fig. 1.6)	**splen/o** spleen **-megaly** enlargement	Enlargement of the spleen
-oma	tumor, mass	osteoma (aw stee OH mah)	**oste/o** bone **-oma** tumor, mass	Tumor of a bone
-osis	abnormal condition	psychosis (sy KOH sis)	**psych/o** mind **-osis** abnormal condition	Abnormal condition of the mind
-pathy	disease process	gastropathy (gas TROP a thee)	**gastr/o** stomach **-pathy** disease process	Disease process of the stomach
-ptosis	prolapse, drooping, sagging	hysteroptosis (HIS ter oh pa toh sis)	**hyster/o** uterus **-ptosis** prolapse	Prolapse of the uterus
-rrhage, -rrhagia	bursting forth	hemorrhage (HEM oh rij)	**hem/o** blood **-rrhage** bursting forth	Bursting forth of blood
-rrhea	discharge, flow	otorrhea (oh toh REE ah)	**ot/o** ear **-rrhea** discharge, flow	Discharge from the ear
-rrhexis	rupture	cystorrhexis (SIS toh rek sis)	**cyst/o** bladder, sac **-rrhexis** rupture	Rupture of the bladder
-sclerosis	abnormal condition of hardening	arteriosclerosis (ar teer ee oh skleh ROH sis)	**arteri/o** artery **-sclerosis** abnormal condition of hardening	Abnormal condition of hardening of an artery
-stenosis	abnormal condition of narrowing	tracheostenosis (tray kee oh steh NOH sis)	**trache/o** trachea, windpipe **-stenosis** abnormal condition of narrowing	Abnormal condition of narrowing of the trachea or windpipe

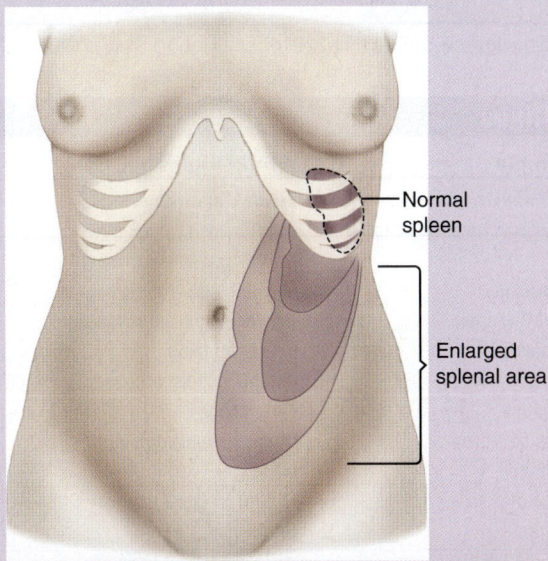

FIG. 1.6 Splenomegaly. (From Shiland B: *Mastering Healthcare Terminology*, ed 5, St. Louis, 2016, Elsevier.)

From Shiland B: *Mastering Healthcare Terminology*, ed 5, St. Louis, 2016, Elsevier.

UNIT 1 Medical Terminology, Anatomy, and Physiology

TABLE 1.7 Diagnostic Procedure Suffixes

Suffix	Meaning	Example	Word Origins	Definition
-graphy	process of recording	mammography (mah MAW grah fee)	mamm/o breast -graphy process of recording	Process of recording the breast
-metry	process of measuring	spirometry (spih RAW meh tree)	spir/o breathing -metry process of measuring	Process of measuring breathing
-opsy	process of viewing	biopsy (BY awp see)	bi/o living, life -opsy process of viewing	Process of viewing living tissue
-scopy	process of viewing	esophagogastroduodenoscopy (eh saw fah goh gas troh doo oh den AW skoh pee)	esophag/o esophagus gastr/o stomach duoden/o duodenum -scopy process of viewing	Process of viewing the esophagus, stomach, and duodenum

From Shiland B: *Mastering Healthcare Terminology,* ed 5, St. Louis, 2016, Elsevier.

TABLE 1.8 Therapeutic Intervention Suffixes

Suffix	Meaning	Example	Word Origins	Definition
-ectomy	removal, resection, excision	tonsillectomy (tawn sil EK toh mee)	tonsill/o tonsil -ectomy removal, excision	Removal of the tonsils
-plasty	surgical repair	rhinoplasty (RY noh plas tee)	rhin/o nose -plasty surgical repair	Surgical repair of the nose
-rrhaphy	suture, repair	splenorrhaphy (spleh nor rha FEE)	splen/o spleen -rrhaphy suture, repair	Suture of the spleen
-stomy	new opening	colostomy (koh LAW stoh mee)	col/o colon, large intestine -stomy new opening	New opening of the colon or large intestine
-tomy	incision, cutting	osteotomy (AW stee aw toh mee)	oste/o bone -tomy incision	Incision into the bone
-tripsy	crushing	lithotripsy (LITH oh trip see)	lith/o stone -tripsy crushing	Crushing of stones

From Shiland B: *Mastering Healthcare Terminology,* ed 5, St. Louis, 2016, Elsevier.

TABLE 1.9 Instrument Suffixes

Suffix	Meaning	Example	Word Origins	Definition
-graph	instrument to record	electrocardiograph (ee lek troh kar dee AW graf)	electr/o electricity cardi/o heart -graph instrument to record	Instrument to record the electricity of the heart
-meter	instrument to measure	thermometer (ther MOM i ter)	therm/o temperature, heat -meter instrument to measure	Instrument to measure temperature
-scope	instrument to view	ophthalmoscope (of thal MO skohp)	ophthalm/o eye -scope instrument to view	Instrument to view the eye
-tome	instrument to cut	osteotome (AW stee oh tohm)	oste/o bone -tome instrument to cut	Instrument to cut bone
-tripter	machine to crush	lithotripter (lith oh TRIP tor)	lith/o stone -tripter machine to crush	Machine to crush stone
-trite	instrument to crush	lithotrite (LITH oh trahyt)	lith/o stone -trite instrument to crush	Instrument to crush stone

From Shiland B: *Mastering Healthcare Terminology,* ed 5, St. Louis, 2016, Elsevier.

Pathology Suffixes. Pathology suffixes describe a disease process or a sign or symptom. The meanings vary according to the conditions that they describe.

Diagnostic Procedure Suffixes. Diagnostic procedure suffixes point to a procedure that helps to determine the diagnosis. Although a few diagnostic procedures also can help to treat a disease, most are used to establish which particular disease or disorder is occurring.

Therapeutic Intervention Suffixes. Therapeutic intervention suffixes indicate types of treatment. Treatments may be medical or surgical in nature.

Instrument Suffixes. Instruments are indicated by yet another set of suffixes. Note the obvious similarities to their diagnostic and therapeutic cousins. For example, electrocardiography is a diagnostic procedure that is done to measure the electrical activity in the heart; an electrocardiograph is the instrument used to perform electrocardiography.

Specialty and Specialist Suffixes. Specialties and specialists require yet another category of suffixes (Table 1.10). Someone who specializes in the study of the heart would be called a *cardiologist*. **Cardi/o** means "heart," and **-logist** means "one who specializes in the study of."

> ### CRITICAL THINKING 1.1
> Emma understands that by breaking a medical term into word parts (combining forms, suffixes, and prefixes) it will be easier to figure out the meaning of the term. She decides to spend some time reviewing suffixes. She quickly learns that -ia means condition and -itis means inflammation, because they are parts of terms she has heard before. However, she has never heard terms that use the following suffixes: -sclerosis, -malacia, -ptosis, -rraphy, and -trite. Can you figure out the meaning of each of those suffixes?

Prefixes

Prefixes modify a medical term by indicating a structure's or a condition's
- Absence
- Location
- Number or quantity
- State

Sometimes, as with other word parts, a prefix can have more than one meaning. For example, the prefix **hypo-** can mean "below" or "deficient." To spell a term with the use of a prefix, simply add the prefix directly to the beginning of the term. No combining vowels are needed (Table 1.11).

> ### CRITICAL THINKING 1.2
> Emma has mastered suffixes and is ready to move on to prefixes. She concentrates most on prefixes that are similar to one another in spelling or meaning. Can you explain the difference between inter- and intra-? Para- and peri-? Ante- and anti-?

SINGULAR/PLURAL RULES

Because most medical terms end with Greek or Latin suffixes, making a medical term singular or plural is not always done the same way as it is in English. Table 1.12 gives the most common singular/plural endings and the rules for using them.

TABLE 1.10 Specialty and Specialist Suffixes

Suffix	Meaning	Example	Word Origins	Definition
-er	one who	polysomnographer (paw lee sawm NAW grah fer)	*poly-* many, much, excessive, frequent *somn/o* sleep *graph/o* record *-er* one who	One who records many (aspects of) sleep
-iatrician	one who specializes in treatment	geriatrician (jair ee ah TRIH shun)	*ger/o* old age *-iatrician* one who specializes in treatment	One who specializes in treatment of old age (patients)
-iatrics	treatment	pediatrics (pee dee ah TRICKS)	*ped/o* children *-iatrics* treatment	The treatment of children
-iatrist	one who specializes in treatment	psychiatrist[a] (sy KY ah trist)	*psych/o* mind *-iatrist* one who specializes in treatment	One who specializes in treatment of the mind
-iatry	process of treatment	psychiatry (sy KY ah tree)	*psych/o* mind *-iatry* process of treatment	Process of treatment of the mind
-ist	one who specializes	dentist	*dent/i* teeth *-ist* one who specializes	One who specializes in the teeth
-logist	one who specializes in the study of	psychologist[b] (sy KAW loh jist)	*psych/o* mind *-logist* one who specializes in the study of	One who specializes in the study of the mind
-logy	study of	neonatology (nee oh nay TAW loh jee)	*neo-* new *nat/o* born, birth *-logy* study of	The study of the newborn

[a] A psychiatrist holds a medical degree.
[b] A psychologist usually has a master's or a doctoral degree.
From Shiland B: *Mastering Healthcare Terminology*, ed 5, St. Louis, 2016, Elsevier.

TABLE 1.11 Prefixes

Prefix	Meaning	Example	Word Origins	Definition
a-	no, not, without	apneic (AP nee ik)	a- without pne/o breathing -ic pertaining to	Pertaining to without breathing
an-	no, not, without	anophthalmia (an OF thal me a)	an- without ophthalm/o eye -ia condition	Condition of without an eye
ante-	forward, in front of, before	anteversion (an tee VUR zhuh n)	ante- forward vers/o turning -ion process of	Process of turning forward
anti-	against	antibacterial (an tee bak TEER ee uh l)	anti- against bacteri/o bacteria -al pertaining to	Pertaining to against bacteria
dys-	abnormal, difficult, bad, painful	dystrophy (DIS truh fee)	dys- abnormal -trophy process of nourishment	Process of abnormal nourishment
endo-, end-	within	endoscopy (en DAW skoh pee)	endo- within -scopy process of viewing	Process of viewing within
epi-	above, upon	epigastric (ep ih GAS trik)	epi- above gastr/o stomach -ic pertaining to	Pertaining to above the stomach
hyper-	excessive, above	hyperglycemia (hy per gly SEE mee ah)	hyper- excessive glyc/o sugar, glucose -emia blood condition	Blood condition of excessive sugar
hypo-	below, deficient	hypoglossal (hy poh GLAW sal)	hypo- below gloss/o tongue -al pertaining to	Pertaining to below the tongue
inter-	between	intervertebral (in ter VER teh bral)	inter- between vertebr/o vertebra, backbone -al pertaining to	Pertaining to between the backbones
intra-	within	intramuscular (in trah MUS kyoo lar)	intra- within muscul/o muscle -ar pertaining to	Pertaining to within the muscle
neo-	new	neonatal (nee oh NAY tal)	neo- new nat/o birth, born -al pertaining to	Pertaining to a newborn
par-	near, beside	parotid (pah RAW tid)	par- near ot/o ear -id pertaining to	Pertaining to near the ear
para-	near, beside, abnormal	paraphilia (par uh FIL ee uh)	para- abnormal phil/o attraction -ia condition	Condition of abnormal attraction
per-	through	percutaneous (per kyoo TAY nee us)	per- through cutane/o skin -ous pertaining to	Pertaining to through the skin, as in a nephrolithotomy
peri-	surrounding, around	pericardium (pair ih KAR dee um)	peri- surrounding cardi/o heart -um structure	Structure surrounding the heart
poly-	many, much, excessive, frequent	polyneuritis (paw lee nyoor EYE tis)	poly- many neur/o nerve -itis inflammation	Inflammation of many nerves
post-	after, behind	postnatal (post NAY tal)	post- after nat/o birth, born -al pertaining to	Pertaining to after birth

TABLE 1.11 Prefixes—cont'd

Prefix	Meaning	Example	Word Origins	Definition
pre-	before, in front of	prenatal (pre NAY tal)	**pre-** before **nat/o** birth, born **-al** pertaining to	Pertaining to before birth
sub-	under, below	subhepatic (sub HEE pat ik)	**sub-** under **hepat/o** liver **-ic** pertaining to	Pertaining to under the liver
trans-	through, across	transurethral (trans yoor EE thral)	**trans-** through **urethr/o** urethra **-al** pertaining to	Pertaining to through the urethra

From Shiland B: *Mastering Healthcare Terminology*, ed 5, St. Louis, 2016, Elsevier.

TABLE 1.12 Rules for Using Singular and Plural Endings

If a Term Ends in:	Form the Plural by:	Singular Example	Plural Example
-a	dropping the -a and adding -ae	vertebr**a** (a bone in the spine) (VUR tuh brah)	vertebr**ae** (VUR tuh bray)
-is	dropping the -is and adding -es	arthros**is** (an abnormal condition of a joint) (ar THROH sis)	arthros**es** (ar THROH seez)
-ix or -ex	dropping the -ix or -ex and adding -ices	append**ix** (ap PEN dicks)	append**ices** (ap PEN dih seez)
-itis	dropping the -itis and adding -itides	arthr**itis** (inflammation of a joint) (ar THRY tiss)	arthr**itides** (ar THRIH tih deez)
-nx	dropping the -nx and adding -nges	phala**nx** (a bone in the fingers or toes) (FAY lanks)	phala**nges** (fuh LAN jeez)
-um	dropping the -um and adding an -a	endocardi**um** (the structure inside the heart) (en doh KAR dee um)	endocardi**a** (en doh KAR dee ah)
-us	dropping the -us and adding an -i	digit**us** (a finger or toe) (DIJ ih tus)	digit**i** (DIJ ih tye)
-y	dropping the -y and adding -ies	therap**y** (a treatment) (THAIR ah pee)	therap**ies** (THAIR ah peez)

From Shiland B: *Mastering Healthcare Terminology*, ed 5, St. Louis, 2016, Elsevier.

CLOSING COMMENTS

Communication is key to providing the best possible patient care. Learning how medical terms are put together (and as well as how to decode them) will help with that communication process. Tables 1.13 and 1.14 are resources to help you learn how to use medical terminology both verbally and in a written format. Using medical terminology correctly is key to communicating in an ambulatory care setting.

TABLE 1.13 Pronunciation of Unusual Letter Combinations

Spelling	Pronunciation	Term	Meaning
eu	you	**eu**thyroid (yoo THIGH royd)	Good, healthy thyroid function
ph	f (fill)	**ph**alanx (FAY lanks)	One of the bones of the fingers or toes
pn	n (no)	**pn**eumonitis (noo moh NYE tis)	Inflammation of the lungs
ps	s (sort)	**ps**ychology (sye KALL uh jee)	Study of the mind
pt	t (top)	**pt**osis (TOH sis)	Prolapse, drooping
rh, rrh	r (row)	**rh**initis (rye NYE tis)	Inflammation of the nose
x	z (zoo)	**x**eroderma (zeer oh DUR mah)	Condition of dry skin

From Shiland B: *Mastering Healthcare Terminology*, ed 5, St. Louis, 2016, Elsevier.

TABLE 1.14 Common Combining Forms

Combining Form	Meaning	Combining Form	Meaning
arteri/o	artery (AR ter ee)	lingu/o	tongue
arthr/o	joint	lipid/o	lipid, fat
bacteri/o	bacteria (bak TEER eah)	lith/o	stone
		mamm/o	breast
bi/o	living, life	muscul/o	muscle
cardi/o	heart	my/o	muscle
cephal/o	head	nat/o	birth, born
cervic/o	neck, cervix (SER viks)	neur/o	nerve
chondr/o	cartilage (KAR tih lij)	ophthalm/o	eye
		oste/o	bone
col/o	large intestine, colon	ot/o	ear
coron/o	crown, heart	path/o	disease
cut/o	skin	ped/o	child
cutane/o	skin	phil/o	attraction
cyst/o	bladder, sac	pne/o	breathing
dent/i	tooth	psych/o	mind
derm/o	skin	rhin/o	nose
duoden/o	duodenum (doo oh DEE num)	somn/o	sleep
		spir/o	breathing
electr/o	electricity	splen/o	spleen
enter/o	small intestine	therm/o	heat, temperature
esophag/o	esophagus (eh SAW fah gus)	tonsill/o	tonsil (TAWN sil)
gastr/o	stomach	trache/o	trachea (TRAY kee ah), windpipe
gloss/o	tongue	troph/o	nourishment
glyc/o	glucose, sugar	urethr/o	urethra (yoor EE thrah)
hem/o	blood		
hepat/o	liver	valvul/o	valve
hyster/o	uterus (YOO ter us)	ven/o	vein
		vers/o	turning
		vertebr/o	backbone, vertebra (VER the brah)

From Shiland B: *Mastering Healthcare Terminology,* ed 5, St. Louis, 2016, Elsevier.

CHAPTER REVIEW

Medical terminology has its roots in Greek and Latin, like much of the English language. As you learn more medical terms, you will begin to recognize English terms that contain those same word parts. This should be helpful in memorizing the meaning of those Latin and Greek word parts.

Many medical terms can be decoded or broken down into word parts: combining forms, suffixes, and prefixes. Decoding terms can help with determining the meaning of that term. Appendixes A and B can help with the decoding process. There are also some medical terms that cannot be decoded, as they are not built using word parts. For these nondecodable terms you must memorize the meaning. A medical dictionary is a valuable tool for clarifying those nondecodable terms.

When learning medical terminology, it is important to understand how terms are built, using combining forms, suffixes, and prefixes. By learning the meanings of the most common suffixes and prefixes, you will be able to determine the meaning of many medical terms.

It is also important to be able to use and spell the medical terms correctly. Being familiar with the spelling rules and the correct way to create a plural medical term from a singular medical term will increase the effectiveness of your communication in the ambulatory care setting.

SCENARIO WRAP-UP

Emma is excited to be able understand so many medical terms. When she comes across a new term, she is now able to decode it by breaking it down into word parts. With her knowledge of the most common prefixes and suffixes, she can get a general idea of what the term means even if she does not know the meaning of all of the word parts. She can already see how she will be able to use her knowledge of medical terminology in other classes in her medical assistant program.

Anatomy and Physiology Basics

LEARNING OBJECTIVES

1. Describe the structural organization of the human body.
2. Use surface anatomy, positional, and directional terminology.
3. Describe body cavities, abdominopelvic quadrants, and body planes.
4. Discuss the acid-base balance in the human body.
5. Discuss pathology basics, including pathology terminology, protection mechanisms, predisposing factors, and the causes of disease.

CHAPTER OUTLINE

1. Opening Scenario, 13
2. You Will Learn, 13
3. Anatomy Basics, 14
    a. Structural Organization of the Body, 14
        i. *Cells*, 14
        ii. *Tissues*, 15
        iii. *Organs*, 16
        iv. *Body Systems*, 16
        v. *Organism*, 16
    b. Surface Anatomy Terminology, 18
    c. Positional and Directional Terminology, 18
    d. Body Cavities, 22
        i. *Abdominopelvic Quadrants and Regions*, 22
    e. Body Planes, 23
4. Acid-Base Balance, 24
5. Pathology Basics, 25
    a. Pathology Terminology, 25
    b. Protection Mechanisms, 25
    c. Predisposing Factors, 25
    d. Causes of Disease, 28
        i. *Genetics*, 28
        ii. *Infectious Pathogens*, 28
        iii. *Inflammatory Response*, 28
        iv. *Immunity*, 29
        v. *Nutritional Imbalances*, 29
        vi. *Trauma and Environmental Agents*, 30
        vii. *Neoplasms*, 30
6. Closing Comments, 32
7. Chapter Review, 33
8. Scenario Wrap-Up, 34

OPENING SCENARIO

Daniela Garcia was just hired as a part-time float receptionist at Walden-Martin Family Medical (WMFM) Clinic. As a float receptionist, she will be working in many different departments. She will also be assisting in the specialty clinic, where providers from other agencies hold outreach clinics. During outreach, these providers see patients and provide specialty services not offered by WMFM providers.

Daniela was excited to accept this position. She has just started the medical assistant program at the local community college. She is currently taking a human body and disease course and a medical terminology course. She felt this job would give her a foot in the door for a possible medical assistant position in the future. She also felt the experience would be helpful on her résumé. It will also allow her to learn more about healthcare. Having just graduated from high school in May, she did not have a lot of previous work experience.

During her first week on the job, Daniela realized there was a lot to learn. Not only did she have to learn new computer software, she also had to learn the medical terminology used. From patients to providers, everyone seemed to use medical terminology. She was happy to know a bit from her course, but she realized she had a lot more learning to do.

During her training, she will be shadowing receptionists, insurance coders, and medical assistants. She looks forward to learning the clinic's routines and learning more about healthcare.

YOU WILL LEARN

1. To recognize and use terms related to the basic anatomy and pathology concepts.
2. To describe the organization of the body.
3. To describe body systems.
4. To recognize and use surface anatomy, directional, and positional terms.
5. To describe body cavities and abdominopelvic quadrants.
6. To describe predisposing factors and causes of disease.

It is important for medical assistants to understand the anatomy and physiology of the body. *Anatomy* (ah NAT uh mee) is the study of how the body is shaped and structured. It includes the structures, levels of organization, and the relationships between different body parts.

Physiology (fi zee ALL uh jee) is the study of body functions. Anatomy and physiology information is used in many ways in clinical and administrative settings. From coding and billing to entering diagnostic orders, having a strong understanding will help medical assistants perform their roles more efficiently.

This chapter discusses the organization of the body, along with body cavities and directional terms. In the coming body system chapters, you will learn the anatomy and physiology of each body system. You will also be introduced to diseases that impact each system. To help you understand this content, this chapter also provides the basics for understanding **pathology** (pah THOL uh jee), **diagnostic procedures**, and treatments.

ANATOMY BASICS

Structural Organization of the Body

If we were to break apart the body, we would have many body systems. Examples include the digestive, cardiovascular, musculoskeletal, and respiratory systems. Each system is composed of different organs. For instance, the stomach and intestines are digestive system organs. Each organ is made up of combinations of tissues, and these tissues are composed of cells. So when studying the organization of the body, it is easier to start at the level of cells and work up to the organism (human body) level.

Cells. The basic unit of life is the *cell*. Cells determine the functional and structural characteristics of the entire body. Cells are microscopic in size. They have a variety of shapes and perform a vast array of functions. A cell is covered by a plasma membrane. The cell contains cytoplasm and **organelles** (ORE ga nels). See Table 2.1 and Fig. 2.1 for the parts of the cells.

Most human cells reproduce by **mitosis** (my TOE sis). Mitosis is a process where one cell splits into two identical daughter cells. The two cells are genetically identical to the parent cell. Prior to the mitosis process, the cell enters the interphase stage. During this stage, the genetic

---

MEDICAL TERMINOLOGY
- **ana-**: apart, away, up
- **-logy**: study of
- **path/o**: disease
- **physi/o**: growth
- **-tomy**: cutting, incision

VOCABULARY
- **diagnostic procedures**: Tests and procedures used to help diagnose or monitor a condition.
- **organelles**: Structures inside of the cell.
- **pathology**: Study of disease.

TABLE 2.1 Cell Parts

Cell Parts	Word Parts	Description
Plasma membrane (PLAZ ma mem BRAIN)		Outer covering surrounding the cell that allows certain substances to enter the cell and blocks other substances. Can also be called cell membrane.
Cytoplasm (SYE toh plaz um)	**cyt/o** cell **-plasm** formation	Jelly-like substance the surrounds the nucleus and fills the cells. *Organelles* (structures in the cell) are suspended in the cytoplasm.
Ribosome (RYE boh sohm)	**rib/o** ribose **-some** body	Free-floating organelle that makes enzymes and proteins. Contains ribonucleic acid (RNA). Considered the cell's "protein factories."
Rough endoplasmic reticulum (ER) (en doe PLAZ mik ri TIK ue lum)	**endo-** within, inner	Organelle that is a network of membranes; connects to the nucleus. Ribosomes are attached to the ER, causing the rough appearance. Involved with making protein.
Smooth endoplasmic reticulum (ER) (en doe PLAZ mik ri TIK ue lum)		Tube-like organelle; role differs based on the type of cell. Roles may include storage of calcium and making steroids and lipids.
Golgi apparatus (GOLE jee)		Organelle that processes and packages the proteins and lipids made by the cell. Considered to be the cell's "processing plant."
Lysosomes (LYE soh sohm)	**lys/o** dissolving **-some** body	Organelles that contain enzymes and are involved with digesting nutrients and other substances in the cell. Considered to be the cell's "waste collectors."
Mitochondrion (pl. mitochondria) (mye toh KAHN dree un)	**mitochondri/o** mitochondria **-on** structure	Organelle that produces the energy for the cell. Called the cell's "power plant."
Nucleus (pl. nuclei) (NOO klee us)	**nucle/o** nucleus **-us** structure	Control center of cell; contains chromosomes that are made up of deoxyribonucleic acid (DNA), which carries genetic information. Called the "control center."
Nucleolus (NOO klee o lus)		Inside of the nucleus; produces ribosomes.
Centrioles (SEN tree ol)		Tube-like structures that help with cell division and with the formation of the *spindle fibers* (a type of microtubules).
Cilia (SIL ee ah)		Fine, hair-like extensions on the surface of the cell. Used to detect surroundings or chemicals.
Microvilli	**micro-** small	Small projections on the surface of the cell. This increases the surface area, which allows for additional absorption.
Flagellum (fla JEL uhm)		Single long hairlike extension on the surface of the cell. Used to propel or move cell.

From Shiland B: *Mastering Healthcare Terminology,* ed 5, St. Louis, 2016, Elsevier.

CHAPTER 2 Anatomy and Physiology Basics

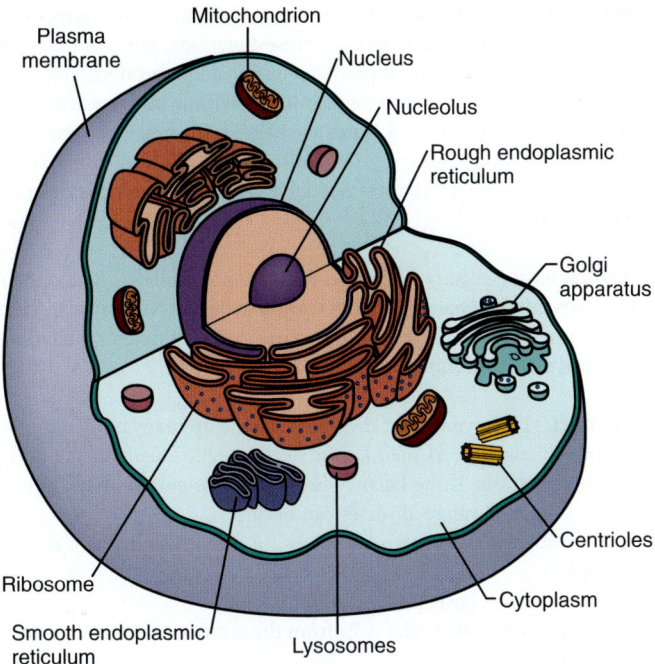

FIG. 2.1 Cell structure.

CRITICAL THINKING 2.1

Daniela was learning about the cell structures in school. While on break one night, she talked to Bella. Bella is a new CMA (AAMA) who just graduated. Daniela mentioned she was learning about cell parts. Bella encouraged Daniela to associate the cell parts to the things she might see in a city. For instance, she stated, "The plasma membrane could be the walls around the city." What other associations could be made between the cell structures and a city?

- *Epithelial* (eh puh THEE lee ul) *tissue*: Acts as an internal or external covering for organs. Examples of epithelial tissue include the outer layer of the skin, glands, and linings of body cavities and organs. Epithelial tissue has the cells packed so closely together that there is little to no intercellular material. *Simple epithelium* is a single layer of the same shaped cells. *Stratified epithelium* contains multiple layers of cells. Epithelial tissue is classified according to shape. See Table 2.2 for epithelial classification and appearance.
- *Connective tissue*: Supports and binds other body tissues. Examples of connective tissue include bone, blood, fat, fibrous, areolar, and cartilage. Connective tissue is the most frequently occurring tissue in the body.
- *Muscle tissue*: Produces movement. Table 2.3 shows the classification, characteristics, and role of the types of muscle tissue.
- *Nervous tissue*: Includes cells that provide transmission of information to control a variety of functions. Nervous tissue controls the body's functions to maintain homeostasis (hoh mee oh STAY sis). Nervous tissue is made up of neurons and supportive structures called *neuroglial cells*.

information (i.e., chromosomes [KROE mah somes]) replicate. Each sister pair of chromosomes (called *chromatids*) are joined together until they are pulled apart later in the mitosis process. The point where the two chromatids are joined is called the *centromere*. The centromere is also the attachment point for spindle fibers, which will be involved in the mitosis process. The mitosis process consists of the following four phrases:

- *Prophase*: The membrane around the nucleus starts to break down. Centrioles produce spindle fibers and start to move toward opposite sides of the cell.
- *Metaphase*: Each pair of chromatids lines up, and each chromatid is attached to a spindle fiber.
- *Anaphase*: Spindle fibers pull the sister chromatids apart.
- *Telophase*: Nucleus reforms around each set of chromosomes. The cell continues to separate into two daughter cells.

Tissues. *Tissue* is a group of similar cells from the same source that together carry out a specific function. The study of body tissues is known as histology (hi STOL uh jee). All of the body tissues are grouped into four types. The four types of tissue include the following:

TABLE 2.2 Epithelial Tissue Shapes

Classification	Appearance
Squamous	Flat
Cuboidal	Square
Columnar	Long and narrow
Transitional	Varying shapes that can stretch

VOCABULARY

chromosomes: Rod-shaped structures found in the cell's nucleus; they contain genetic information.
mitosis: A cell division process by which two daughter cells are formed from one parent cell; each daughter has a complete copy of parent's chromosomes.
histology: The microscopic study of body tissues.
homeostasis: The internal environment of the body that is compatible with life. A steady state that is created by all the body systems working together to provide a consistent and unvarying internal environment.
intercellular: Located between cells.
neurons: Nerve cells.
peristalsis: Rhythmic contraction of involuntary muscles lining the gastrointestinal tract.
striated: Striped in appearance.
vasoconstriction: Contraction of the muscles causing the narrowing of the inside tube of the vessel.

❋ STUDY TIP

Remember the phases of mitosis as PMAT:
Prophase—**PREPARES**
Metaphase—chromosomes **MEET** in the **MIDDLE**
Anaphase—chromosome pull **APART**
Telophase—the cell **TEARS** in **TWO**

MEDICAL TERMINOLOGY
hist/o: tissue neur/o: nervous
home/o: same -stasis: controlling
my/o: muscle

TABLE 2.3 Classification of Muscle Tissue

Classification	Characteristics	Role
Skeletal	Striated, voluntary	Attached to bones and produces voluntary body movements when contracted
Cardiac	Striated, involuntary	Forms the heart muscle wall
Smooth	Nonstriated, involuntary	Lines the blood vessel walls and hollow organs; causes peristalsis (per uh STAHL suhs) and vasoconstriction (va zo kuhn STRIK shun)

Organs. An *organ* is a structure composed of two or more types of tissue. An organ may have one or more functions. For instance, the pancreas has two functions. It produces insulin and it produces digestive enzymes (EN zimes). Organs are grouped within body systems. An organ may be part of one or more systems. For instance, the pancreas is part of the endocrine system and also part of the digestive system. Organs can be divided into parts. See Table 2.4 for the terms that describe parts of organs.

Body Systems. A *body system* is composed of several organs and their related structures. These structures work together to perform a specific function in the body. Table 2.5 summarizes the body systems, including their structures and functions.

Organism. The *organism* of the body is made up many body systems. These work together to maintain a steady environment in the body called homeostasis. If the balance is off or if the environment moves out of the normal range, diseases can occur.

To summarize the structural organization of the body from simple to complex:
- Cells: the most basic unit.
- Tissues: groups of similar cells from the same source that carry out a specific function

TABLE 2.4 Parts of Organs

	Term	Combining Form	Definition
	apex (pl. apices) (A pecks)	apic/o	The pointed extremity of a cone-shaped structure
	corporis or body (KOR por iss)	corpor/o som/o somat/o	The largest or most important part of an organ
	fornix (pl. fornices) (FOR nicks)	fornic/o	Any vaultlike or arched structure
	fundus (pl. fundi) (FUN dis)	fund/o	The base or deepest part of a hollow organ that is farthest from the mouth of the organ
	hilum (pl. hila) (HYE lum)	hil/o	Exit or entrance of a duct into a gland, or of a nerve and vessels into an organ
	lumen (pl. lumina) (LOO min)	lumin/o	The space within an artery, vein, intestine, or tube

TABLE 2.4 Parts of Organs—cont'd

	Term	Combining Form	Definition
	sinus (pl. sinuses) (SYE nus)	sin/o, sinus/o	A cavity or channel in bone, a dilated channel for blood, or a cavity that permits the escape of purulent (pus-filled) material
	vestibule (VES tih byool)	vestibul/o	A small space or cavity at the beginning of a canal

From Shiland B: *Mastering Healthcare Terminology,* ed 5, St. Louis, 2016, Elsevier.

TABLE 2.5 Summary of Body Systems

Body System	Cells, Structures, and Organs	Functions
Blood	Arteries, arterioles, veins, venules, white blood cells, red blood cells, platelets, plasma	Transports materials (e.g., oxygen, nutrients) and collects waste throughout the body; involved with fighting infection and forming clots
Cardiovascular (kar dee oh VASS kyoo lur)	Heart, valves, arteries, arterioles, veins, venules	Transports materials in the blood throughout the body
Endocrine (EN doh krin)	Pituitary, pineal gland, hypothalamus, thyroid, pancreas, adrenal cortex and medulla, parathyroid, thymus, ovaries, testes	Produces hormones that circulate in the blood to target tissue that stimulates a particular action
Gastrointestinal (gass troh in TESS tih nul)	Mouth, tongue, teeth, pharynx, esophagus, stomach, small intestine, large intestine, liver, gallbladder, pancreas, appendix	Breakdown, digestion, and absorption of nutrients
Integumentary (in teg yoo MEN tuh ree)	Skin, subcutaneous tissue, sweat and sebaceous glands, hair, nails, sense receptors	Protection, temperature regulation; senses organ activity
Lymphatic and immune (lim FAT tick)	Lymph, lymph vessels, lymph nodes, thymus, tonsils, spleen, lymphocytes, antibodies	Maintains fluid balance; protects internal environment; provides immunity to some diseases
Musculoskeletal (muss kyoo loh SKELL uh tul)	Bones, joints, muscles, tendons, ligaments, cartilage	Movement, heat production, support, protection
Nervous (NER vus)	Brain, spinal cord, neurons, neuroglial cells, peripheral nerves, autonomic nerves	Controls body structures to maintain homeostasis; receives and processes information
Reproductive	Female: estrogen and progesterone, ovum, ovaries, fallopian tubes, uterus, vagina, vulva, mammary glands Male: testosterone, sperm, epididymis, vas deferens, prostate gland, testes, scrotum, penis, urethra	Produces hormones; reproduction
Respiratory (RESS pur ah tore ee)	Nose, sinuses, pharynx, larynx, trachea, bronchi, lungs, bronchioles, alveoli	Delivers oxygen to cells and removes carbon dioxide
Sensory	Eyes, ears, taste buds, olfactory receptors, sensory receptors	Gathers information through vision, hearing, balance, taste, and smell
Urinary (YUUR ih nair ee)	Nephron unit, kidneys, ureters, bladder, urethra	Eliminates nitrogenous waste; maintains electrolyte, water, and acid-base balances

- Organ: a structure made up of two or more types of tissues
- Body system: made up of several organs and their related structures
- Organism: made up of many body systems that work together for homeostasis in the body

CRITICAL THINKING 2.2

Bella's tip really helped Daniela with the cell structures. Now Daniela needs to remember the organization of the body in order from the simplest to the most complex. Bella encouraged Daniela to create a phrase or word that would help her remember cells, tissues, organs, body system, and organism. What might be a way to remember these five items in order?

Surface Anatomy Terminology

In healthcare we use surface anatomy terminology to describe locations on the body. For instance, when you take a blood pressure reading, you need to place the stethoscope over the brachial artery in the antecubital space. The radial artery is used when taking a radial pulse. Knowing the surface anatomy terminology will help you understand what is being asked of you and allow you to communicate professionally to others.

The *anatomical position* is a standard frame of reference. This means the body stands erect with the face forward, arms at the sides, palms forward, and toes pointed forward. Fig. 2.2 shows the body in this position. Tables 2.6 through 2.9 provide additional information on front (ventral) and back (dorsal) surface anatomy terminology.

CRITICAL THINKING 2.3

As Daniela was learning about surface anatomy terminology, she tried to relate it to things she knew or learned about at her receptionist position. For instance, *palmar* sounds like *palm* and refers to the palm. For Tables 2.6 through 2.9, which words have you heard before? How might you remember these surface anatomy terms?

Positional and Directional Terminology

Positional and directional terms are used to describe up/down, middle/side, and front/back. Many times patients will be in different positions depending on the situation. Having a standard method to communicate directions and positions allows for clear communication between healthcare professionals. These terms are used commonly in healthcare. For example, x-rays may be taken from the front of the body to the back—an anteroposterior (AP) view—or from the back to the front—a posteroanterior (PA) view.

The *midline* of the body is an imaginary line drawn from the crown of the head down between the eyes, through the chest, and separating the legs. Several of the directional terms use the midline as a reference. Table 2.10 lists directional and positional terms as opposite pairs with their respective combining forms or prefixes and illustrations.

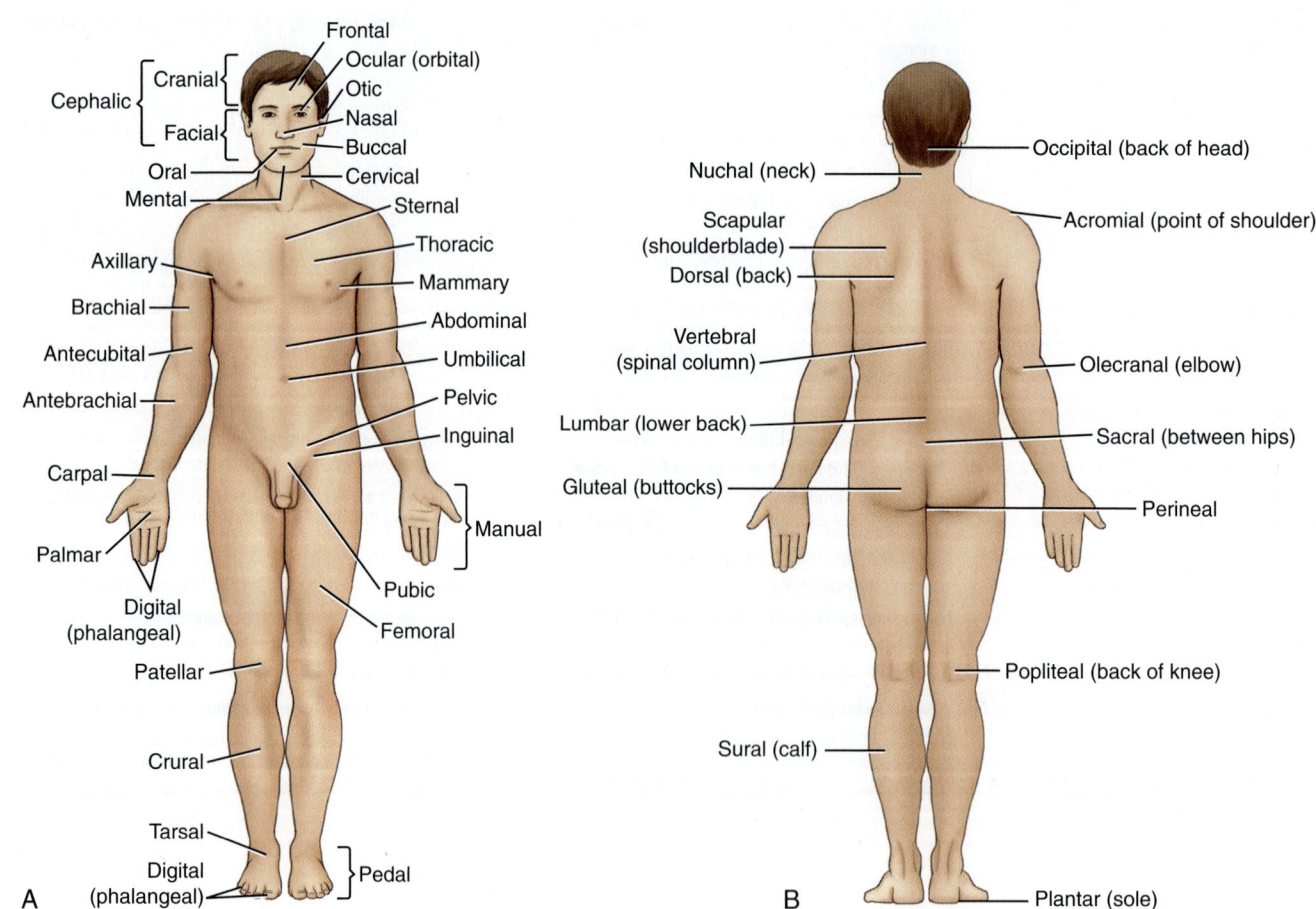

FIG. 2.2 (A) Ventral surface anatomy. (B) Dorsal surface anatomy. (From Shiland B: *Mastering Healthcare Terminology*, ed 5, St. Louis, 2016, Elsevier.)

TABLE 2.6 Ventral Surface Anatomy Terms for the Head

Term	Word Origin	Definition
buccal (BUCK uhl)	bucc/o cheek -al pertaining to	Pertaining to the cheek
cephalic (seh FAL ik)	cephal/o head -ic pertaining to	Pertaining to the head
cervical (SUR vik uhl)	cervic/o neck -al pertaining to	Pertaining to the neck. **Collum** is a term that refers to the entire neck
cranial (KRAY nee uhl)	crani/o skull -al pertaining to	Pertaining to the skull.
facial (FAY shuhl)	faci/o face -al pertaining to	Pertaining to the face
frontal (FRUN tuhl)	front/o front -al pertaining to	Pertaining to the front, the forehead
mental (MEN tuhl)	ment/o chin -al pertaining to	Pertaining to the chin (and can also pertain to the mind)
nasal (NAY zuhl)	nas/o nose -al pertaining to	Pertaining to the nose
ocular (AHK you lar)	ocul/o eye -ar pertaining to	Pertaining to the eye
oral (OR uhl)	or/o mouth -al pertaining to	Pertaining to the mouth
otic (OH tik)	ot/o ear -ic pertaining to	Pertaining to the ear; also called **auricular**

From Shiland B: *Mastering Healthcare Terminology*, ed 5, St. Louis, 2016, Elsevier.

TABLE 2.7 Ventral Surface Anatomy Terms for the Trunk

Term	Word Origin	Definition
abdominal (ab DOM ih nuhl)	abdomin/o abdomen -al pertaining to	Pertaining to the abdomen
axillary (AKS ih lay ree)	axill/o axilla (armpit) -ary pertaining to	Pertaining to the armpit
coxal (KOKS uhl)	cox/o hip -al pertaining to	Pertaining to the hip
deltoid (DELL toyd)	delt/o triangular -oid resembling	The triangular muscle covering the shoulder joint; the combining form **om/o** is often used for the shoulder
inguinal (IN gwin uhl)	inguin/o groin -al pertaining to	Pertaining to the groin
mammary (MAM ah ree)	mamm/o breast -ary pertaining to	Pertaining to the breast
pelvic (PELL vik)	pelv/o, pelv/i pelvis -ic pertaining to	Pertaining to the pelvis
pubic (PEW bik)	pub/o pubis -ic pertaining to	Pertaining to the pubis
sternal (STIR nuhl)	stern/o sternum (breastbone) -al pertaining to	Pertaining to the breastbone
thoracic (thor AS ik)	thorac/o chest -ic pertaining to	Pertaining to the chest; also called **pectoral**
umbilical (um BILL ih kuhl)	umbilic/o umbilicus (navel) -al pertaining to	Pertaining to the umbilicus

From Shiland B: *Mastering Healthcare Terminology*, ed 5, St. Louis, 2016, Elsevier.

TABLE 2.8 Ventral Surface Anatomy Terms for the Arms and Legs

Term	Word Origin	Definition	Term	Word Origin	Definition
antecubital (an tee KYOO bit uhl)	ante- forward, in front of, before cubit/o elbow -al pertaining to	Pertaining to the front of the elbow	femoral (FEM or uhl)	femor/o thigh -al pertaining to	Pertaining to the thigh
brachial (BRAY kee uhl)	brachi/o arm -al pertaining to	Pertaining to the arm; **antebrachial** means pertaining to the forearm	manual (MAN you uhl)	man/u hand -al pertaining to	Pertaining to the hand
			palmar (PALL mar)	palm/o palm -ar pertaining to	Pertaining to the palm; also termed **volar**
carpal (KAR puhl)	carp/o wrist -al pertaining to	Pertaining to the wrist	patellar (pah TELL ar)	patell/o, patell/a kneecap -ar pertaining to	Pertaining to the kneecap
crural (KRUR uhl)	crur/o leg -al pertaining to	Pertaining to the leg	pedal (PED uhl)	ped/o foot -al pertaining to	Pertaining to the foot
digital (DIJ ih tuhl)	digit/o finger/toe -al pertaining to	Pertaining to the finger/toe; **phalangeal** means pertaining to the bones in the fingers/toes	tarsal (TAR suhl)	tars/o ankle -al pertaining to	Pertaining to the ankle

From Shiland B: *Mastering Healthcare Terminology*, ed 5, St. Louis, 2016, Elsevier.

TABLE 2.9 Dorsal Surface Anatomy Terms

Term	Word Origin	Definition	Term	Word Origin	Definition
acromial (ak ROH mee uhl)	**acromi/o** acromion **-al** pertaining to	Pertaining to the acromion (highest point of shoulder)	plantar (PLAN tur)	**plant/o** sole **-ar** pertaining to	Pertaining to the sole of the foot
dorsal (DOR suhl)	**dors/o** back **-al** pertaining to	Pertaining to the back	popliteal (pop lih TEE uhl)	**poplit/o** back of knee **-eal** pertaining to	Pertaining to the back of the knee
gluteal (GLOO tee uhl)	**glute/o** buttocks **-al** pertaining to	Pertaining to the buttocks	sacral (SAY kruhl)	**sacr/o** sacrum **-al** pertaining to	Pertaining to the sacrum
lumbar (LUM bar)	**lumb/o** lower back, loin **-ar** pertaining to	Pertaining to the lower back	scapular (SKAP yoo luhr)	**scapul/o** scapula, shoulderblade **-ar** pertaining to	Pertaining to the scapula
nuchal (NOO kull)	**nuch/o** neck **-al** pertaining to	Pertaining to the neck, especially the back of the neck	sural (SOO ruhl)	**sur/o** calf **-al** pertaining to	Pertaining to the calf
olecranal (oh LEK rah nuhl)	**olecran/o** elbow **-al** pertaining to	Pertaining to the elbow	ventral (VEN truhl)	**ventr/o** belly **-al** pertaining to	Pertaining to the belly side
perineal (pair ih NEE uhl)	**perine/o** perineum **-al** pertaining to	Pertaining to the perineum; the perineum is the space between the external genitalia and the anus	vertebral (ver TEE bruhl)	**vertebr/o** vertebra, spine **-al** pertaining to	Pertaining to the spine

From Shiland B: *Mastering Healthcare Terminology*, ed 5, St. Louis, 2016, Elsevier.

TABLE 2.10 Positional and Directional Terms

Term	Word Origin	Definition
anterior (ant) (an TEER ee or) ventral (VEN truhl)	**anter/o** front **-ior** pertaining to **ventr/o** belly **-al** pertaining to	Pertaining to the front Pertaining to the belly side
posterior (pos) (poss TEER ee or) dorsal (DOOR sul)	**poster/o** back **-ior** pertaining to **dors/o** back **-al** pertaining to	Pertaining to the back Pertaining to the back of the body
superior (sup) (soo PEER ee or) cephalad (SEFF uhl add)	**super/o** upward **-ior** pertaining to **cephal/o** head **-ad** toward	Pertaining to upward Toward the head
inferior (inf) (in FEER ee or) caudad (CAW dad)	**infer/o** downward **-ior** pertaining to **caud/o** tail **-ad** toward	Pertaining to downward Toward the tail

CHAPTER 2 Anatomy and Physiology Basics

TABLE 2.10 Positional and Directional Terms—cont'd

Term	Word Origin	Definition
medial (MEE dee uhl)	**medi/o** middle **-al** pertaining to	Pertaining to the middle (midline)
lateral (lat) (LAT ur uhl)	**later/o** side **-al** pertaining to	Pertaining to the side
ipsilateral (ip see LAT er uhl)	**ipsi-** same **later/o** side **-al** pertaining to	Pertaining to the same side
contralateral (kon trah LAT er uhl)	**contra-** opposite **later/o** side **-al** pertaining to	Pertaining to the opposite side
unilateral (you nee LAT er uhl)	**uni-** one **later/o** side **-al** pertaining to	Pertaining to one side
bilateral (bye LAT er uhl)	**bi-** two **later/o** side **-al** pertaining to	Pertaining to two sides
superficial (external) (soo per FISH uhl)		On the surface of the body
deep (internal)		Away from the surface of the body

Continued

TABLE 2.10 Positional and Directional Terms—cont'd

	Term	Word Origin	Definition
	proximal (PROCK sih muhl)	**proxim/o** near **-al** pertaining to	Pertaining to near the origin
	distal (DISS tuhl)	**dist/o** far **-al** pertaining to	Pertaining to far from the origin
	dextrad (DEKS trad)	**dextr/o** right **-ad** toward	Toward the right
	sinistrad (SIN is trad)	**sinistr/o** left **-ad** toward	Toward the left
	afferent (AF fur ent)	**af-** toward **fer/o** to carry **-ent** pertaining to	Pertaining to carrying toward a structure
	efferent (EF fur ent)	**ef-** away from **fer/o** to carry **-ent** pertaining to	Pertaining to carrying away from a structure
	supine (SOO pine)		Lying on one's back
	prone (PROHN)		Lying on one's belly

Modified from Shiland B: *Mastering Healthcare Terminology*, ed 5, St. Louis, 2016, Elsevier.

CRITICAL THINKING 2.4

Bella continued to help Daniela on breaks during work. Today, Daniela was learning directional terms. Bella encouraged Daniela to repeat the term and definition as she pointed to that part of her body. How else might Daniela learn the directional terms and the opposite pairs?

Body Cavities

The body contains *cavities* or hollowed areas that are filled with organs. The body is separated into the dorsal (posterior) and ventral (anterior) body cavities. The *dorsal body cavity* protects nervous system organs. It contains the cranial cavity and the spinal cavity. The *ventral body cavity* is divided into the thoracic and abdominopelvic cavities. The diaphragm (DYE uh fram) creates a physical separation between the thoracic and the abdominopelvic cavities. Table 2.11 summarizes the structures found in each body cavity.

> **VOCABULARY**
> **diaphragm**: A broad dome-shaped muscle used for breathing that separates the thoracic and abdominopelvic cavities.

Abdominopelvic Quadrants and Regions. The abdominopelvic cavity is extensive. To help describe a location in the abdominopelvic area, either the four quadrants or the nine regions can be used. Descriptions that focus on the quadrants are simpler to understand and may be used with patients. The regions are more specific and are typically used by healthcare providers.

TABLE 2.11 Body Cavities

Main Body Cavities	Subcategories	Description
Dorsal body cavity	Cranial cavity	Contains the brain; surrounded and protected by the cranium (skull)
	Spinal cavity	Contains the spinal cord; surrounded and protected by the vertebrae (bones of the spine)
Ventral body cavity	Thoracic cavity	Contains the heart, lungs, esophagus and trachea (windpipe). Protected by the ribs, the sternum (breastbone), and the vertebrae (backbones)
	Abdominopelvic cavity	Can be divided as follows: • Abdominal cavity—contains the abdominal organs (e.g., stomach, liver, gallbladder, intestines). • Pelvic cavity—contains the urinary bladder and the reproductive organs Nothing separates the abdominal and pelvic cavities.

With the abdominopelvic quadrants, an imaginary line is drawn down the midline of the body. A horizontal line is drawn across the abdominopelvic cavity, intersecting at the naval (Fig. 2.3). These quadrants are referred to as either right or left and upper or lower. Typically, abbreviations are used when documenting information about the patient. The four quadrants are as follows:
- *Right upper quadrant* (RUQ): includes the right lobe of liver, gallbladder, right kidney, small intestine (duodenum), large intestine (ascending and transverse colon), head of pancreas
- *Left upper quadrant* (LUQ): includes the stomach, spleen, left lobe of liver, pancreas, left kidney, and large intestine (transverse and descending colon)
- *Right lower quadrant* (RLQ): includes the appendix, cecum, right ovary, right ureter, right spermatic cord, large intestine (ascending colon), right kidney
- *Left lower quadrant* (LLQ): includes the small intestine, large intestine (descending and sigmoid colon), left ovary, left ureter, left spermatic cord, and left kidney

The nine abdominopelvic regions lie over the abdominopelvic cavity. They provide a more specific location than the quadrants. Refer to Fig. 2.4 and Table 2.12 for the nine regions and the related organs.

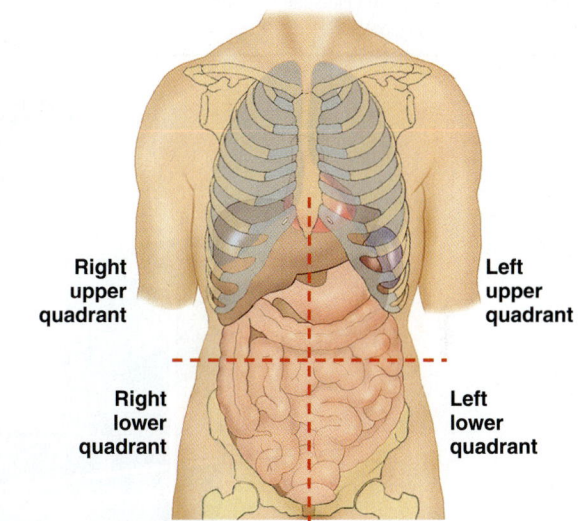

FIG. 2.3 Abdominopelvic quadrants. (From Shiland B: *Mastering Healthcare Terminology*, ed 5, St. Louis, 2016, Elsevier.)

CRITICAL THINKING 2.5

Tonight, Bella was helping Daniela practice positional and directional terms with the regions. Bella asked Daniela the following questions:
- What regions are lateral to the umbilical region?
- What regions are superior to the lumbar regions?
- What region is medial to the hypochondriac regions and superior to the umbilical region?
- What region is inferior to the umbilical region?
- What regions are lateral to the sides of the hypogastric region?

What should Daniela's answers be to the above questions?

MEDICAL TERMINOLOGY

abdomin/o: abdomen
chondr/o: cartilage
epi-: above, upon
gastr/o: stomach
hypo-: under
-ic, -iac: pertaining to
pelv/o: pelvis

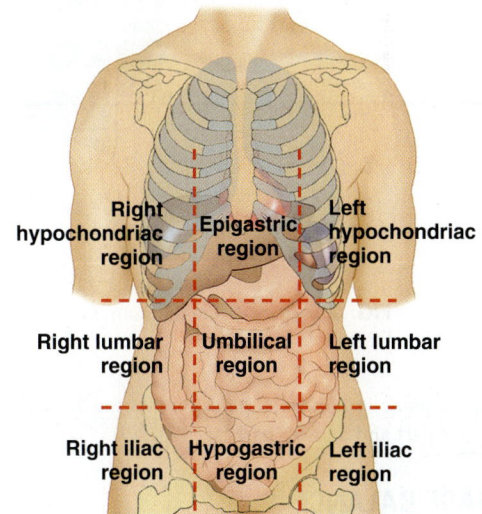

FIG. 2.4 Abdominopelvic regions. (From Shiland B: *Mastering Healthcare Terminology*, ed 5, St. Louis, 2016, Elsevier.)

Body Planes

Another way of describing the body is by dividing it into planes. *Planes* are imaginary cuts or sections through the body. The use of plane terminology is common when discussing diagnostic imaging (e.g., computed tomography [CT] or computerized axial tomography [CAT] scan) of the body. Diagnostic imaging will be discussed in more detail later in the chapter.

A *midsagittal* (mid SAJ ih tul) *plane* or *median plane* separates the body into equal right and left halves. The *coronal* (koh ROH nul) *plane* or *frontal plane* divides the body into front and back portions.

TABLE 2.12 Abdominopelvic Regions With the Underlying Organs

Right Hypochondriac Region (hye poh KON dree ack) Liver, gallbladder, right kidney	Epigastric Region (eh pee GASS trick) Kidneys, pancreas, liver, stomach	Left Hypochondriac Region (hye poh KON dree ack) Stomach, liver, left kidney, spleen
Right Lumbar Region (LUM bar) Small intestine, large intestine (ascending colon), liver, right kidney	Umbilical Region (um BILL ih kul) Small intestine, large intestine (transverse colon), pancreas, stomach	Left Lumbar Region (LUM bar) Small intestine, large intestine (descending colon), left kidney
Right Iliac Region (ILL ee ack) Appendix, small intestine, large intestine (cecum and ascending colon)	Hypogastric Region (hye poh GASS trick) Small intestine, large intestine (sigmoid colon), bladder	Left Iliac Region (ILL ee ack) Small intestine, large intestine (descending and sigmoid colon)

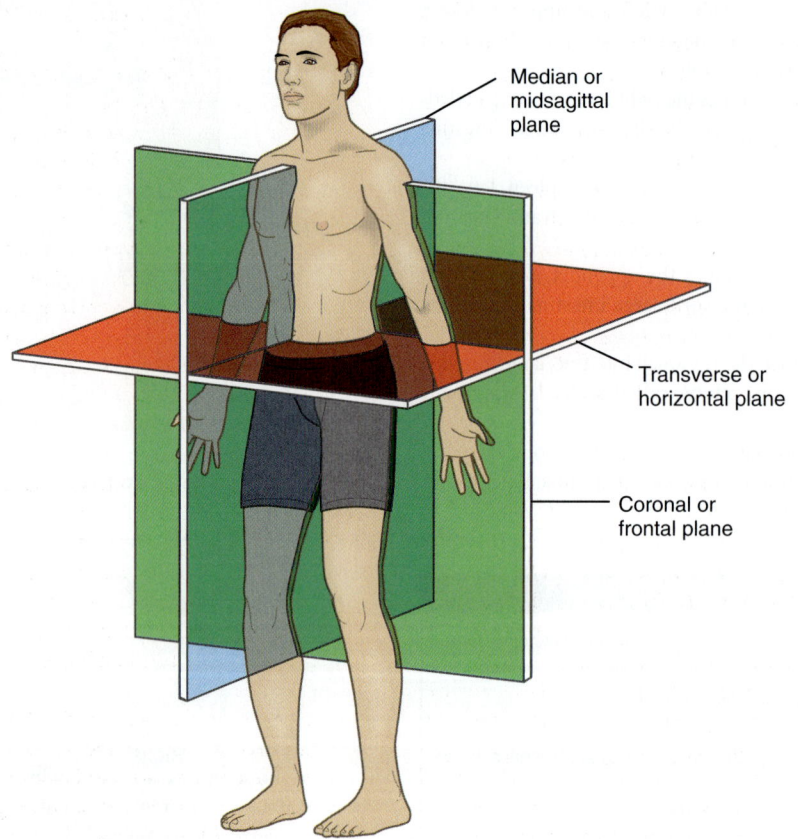

FIG. 2.5 Body planes. (From Proctor D, et al: *Kinn's The Medical Assistant*, ed 13, St. Louis, 2017, Elsevier.)

The *transverse plane* or *horizontal plane* divides the body horizontally into an upper part and a lower part (see Fig. 2.5).

ACID-BASE BALANCE

The *pH* refers to the acid-base level of a solution on a scale of 1 to 14. A neutral pH is 7. An acidic solution has a pH under 7 and contains more hydrogen ions. A base or alkaline solution has a pH over 7 and contain fewer hydrogen ions. To maintain homeostasis, the body attempts to keep the pH between 7.35 and 7.45. To maintain the acid-base range in the body, the concentration of hydrogen ions must remain constant. If the pH moves outside of this range, serious illness or even death can occur.

The pH of our bodies can change based on the food we eat, the air we breathe, and the urine we excrete. To help maintain the pH range, the urinary system, the respiratory system, and chemical buffers must all work together. *Buffers* (like bicarbonate) work to prevent changes in the pH. If there are more hydrogen ions, lowering the pH, buffers will absorb some of the hydrogen ions. This will raise the pH. If the pH is too high, the buffers will "donate" hydrogen ions, bringing the pH down to the normal range.

The respiratory system regulates the carbon dioxide (CO_2) in our blood. CO_2 in the blood can combine with water to form the buffer bicarbonate. If a person *hyperventilates* (breathes rapidly), the CO_2 levels in the blood decrease, which also causes a decrease in the bicarbonate levels in the blood. This causes the pH of the body to rise.

The urinary system also has a role in the acid-base levels. The kidneys can absorb more base or more acid depending on what the body needs for homeostasis. The kidneys can also produce bicarbonate if needed.

PATHOLOGY BASICS

Pathology is the study of diseases. In the ambulatory care setting, many of the patients' visits relate to the diagnosis or treatment of one or more disease processes. As a person ages, it is common to have more than one chronic illness. Having an understanding of common diseases is important for medical assistants. The body system chapters that follow will cover the most common diseases impacting the system discussed. This chapter provides you with the basics to help you understand the concepts discussed in the future chapters. Common pathology terminology, protective mechanisms in the body, predisposing factors for disease, and causes of disease will be discussed.

Pathology Terminology

As you learn more about diseases, you will notice different terms used. Here is a list of terms commonly used when discussing pathology:

- *Disease*: a specific illness with a recognizable group of signs and symptoms and a clear cause (e.g., infection, environment).
- *Syndrome*: a group of signs and symptoms that occur together and are associated with it.
- *Disorder*: a disruption of the function or structure of the body. Many times the words *disorder* and *disease* are used interchangeably in healthcare.
- *Prevalence*: how often the disease occurs.
- *Incidence*: reflects the number of newly diagnosed people with the disease.
- *Morbidity*: illness.
- *Mortality*: death.
- *Acute*: a severe, sudden onset of a disease.
- *Chronic*: a disease, disorder, or syndrome that lasts longer than 6 months.

The coming chapters regarding the body systems will discuss common diseases. For most of the diseases, the following sections will be discussed. It is important for the medical assistant to be familiar with the terminology used:

- *Etiology*: the cause of the disorder or disease.
- *Sign*: something that is measured or observed by others; also called *objective data*. Examples of signs include redness, swelling or edema, blood pressure, and pulse.
- *Symptom*: something that is only perceived by the patient; also called *subjective data*. Examples include pain, headache, dizziness, and nausea. Many times *signs* and *symptoms* are used interchangeably, but there is a difference in their definitions.
- *Diagnostic procedures*: tests and procedures that are used to help diagnose or monitor a condition. See Table 2.13 for common diagnostic procedures.
- *Treatments*: management of a disease or disorder; can include follow-up care and home treatments (e.g., medications, special diets, testing).
- *Prognosis*: medical prediction of the outcome of the disease or disorder process.
- *Prevention*: methods to avoid getting the disease.

> **CRITICAL THINKING 2.6**
>
> Daniela was struggling to remember the difference between signs and symptoms. What might be ways to remember these two terms? What are some examples of signs and symptoms?

> **MEDICAL TERMINOLOGY**
> **-gram**: record, recording
> **-graphy**: process of recording
> **-scope**: instrument to view
> **-scopy**: process of viewing
> **tom/o**: section

Protection Mechanisms

The body has built-in mechanisms that protect against infection. The body's first line of defense includes chemical and physical barriers such as the following:

- Skin: forms a waterproof barrier.
- Tears and saliva: contain an enzyme that breaks the **pathogen's** (PATH oe jens) cell wall.
- Mucus: a slick secretion produced in the respiratory, reproductive, and gastrointestinal systems. It protects the tissues and traps substances (e.g., bacteria, dust).
- Cilia: fine hairs that work closely with the mucus in the respiratory tract, trapping substances.
- Stomach acid: a very strong acid that kills bacteria, parasites, and other invaders that are swallowed.
- "Good" bacteria: found on the skin and in the gastrointestinal system and prevents bad bacteria from taking over.
- Urine: flushes pathogens from the bladder and urethra.

If the structures are altered (e.g., a cut in the skin), then pathogens can get into the body. When this happens, the second line of defense, the immune system, kicks in. White blood cells and the lymphatic system work together to protect the body. The immune system will be covered in Chapter 9.

Predisposing Factors

Predisposing factors are risk factors for disease. These factors make it more likely or increase the risk that the person may develop the disease or condition. Some predisposing factors can be changed to decrease the risk of developing a disease, whereas others cannot be changed. Predisposing factors include the following:

- Hereditary or genetic factors: certain diseases can be inherited, or members of a family have a higher-than-normal risk for getting that specific disease.
- Age: certain diseases occur in childhood, whereas others occur more often in older adults. Some diseases occur due to changes in the body structures with age. For instance, the ear structures are different in an infant compared with an older person. Degenerative diseases occur in the older generations due to the wear and tear on the structures.
- Gender: certain diseases occur more in one gender than the other. For instance, testicular cancer impacts males whereas uterine cancer affects females. Sometimes both genders may get a disease, but one gender has a higher risk factor. Women are at higher risk for breast cancer than men.

> **VOCABULARY**
> **endoscope**: A scope with a camera attached to a long, thin tube that can be inserted into the body.
> **endoscopy**: A nonsurgical procedure that uses an endoscope to view inside of the body.
> **pathogen**: A disease-causing organism.

TABLE 2.13 Common Diagnostic Procedures and Tests in Ambulatory Healthcare

Done by/Type of Test	Procedure	Description
Medical laboratory blood tests	Blood glucose	Used to detect high or low blood sugar (glucose)
	C-reactive protein (CRP)	Detects inflammation
	Complete blood count (CBC)	Measures red blood cells (RBCs) and white blood cells (WBCs), hemoglobin (Hgb), hematocrit (HCT), and platelets; CBC with differential test provides a breakdown of the number of each type of white blood cell
	Comprehensive metabolic panel (CMP)	Includes different tests that evaluate, for instance, liver function, kidney function, glucose, and electrolytes
	Electrolyte panel (Lytes)	Used to check for electrolyte (e.g., sodium, potassium, chloride) imbalances
	Erythrocyte sedimentation rate (ESR)	Used to measure the degree of inflammation in the body
	Follicle-stimulating hormone (FSH)	Measures the follicle-stimulating hormone, a reproductive hormone
	Glycated hemoglobin test or hemoglobin glycosylated test (HbA$_{1C}$ or A$_{1C}$)	Measures the average blood glucose (sugar) over 2 to 3 months
	Lipid profile	Used to check cholesterol and triglycerides
	Liver function panel	Measures specific proteins and enzymes to provide information on the liver's functioning; also called the hepatic function test
	Partial thromboplastin time (PTT), prothrombin time (PT), and international normalized ratio (INR)	Measures blood clotting time
	Thyroid-stimulating hormone (TSH) test	Measures the amount of thyroid stimulating hormone in the blood; also part of the thyroid panel, which includes additional tests
Medical laboratory tests	Culture and sensitivity (C and S)	Culture detects organism in body fluid (e.g., blood, sputum, urine) and sensitivity testing to determine antibiotics that would inhibit organism
	Fecal immunochemical test (FIT)	Uses antibodies to detect human hemoglobin protein
	Guaiac fecal occult blood test (gFOBT)	Used to detect blood in stool
	Stool parasitic examination (O & P)	Used to detect ova and parasites in the stool
	Urinalysis (UA)	Detects abnormalities in the urine that can be used to diagnose many conditions
Endoscopy	Arthroscopy	An arthroscope is inserted in a small incision to view a joint
	Bronchoscopy	A bronchoscope is inserted through the mouth to visualize the trachea and bronchi
	Capsule endoscopy	A camera in a capsule is swallowed and provides pictures of the gastrointestinal tract
	Colonoscopy and sigmoidoscopy	An endoscopye is inserted through the anus and used to visualize the large intestine and colon
	Colposcopy	A colposcope is inserted into the vagina to visualize the cervix and vagina
	Cystoscopy and ureteroscopy	An **endoscope** is inserted into the urethra and used to look at the urinary system
	Endoscopic retrograde cholangiopancreatography (ERCP)	An endoscope is inserted into the mouth and passed to the duodenum; a thin tube, called a catheter, is passed through the endoscope and is used to inject dye into the ducts that lead to the pancreas and gallbladder, then x-rays are used to detect narrowing of structures
	Esophagogastroduodenoscopy (EGD)	An endoscope is inserted through the mouth to visualize the lining of the esophagus, stomach, and duodenum (small intestine)
Imaging procedures	Computed tomography (CT, CAT) scan	A computerized x-ray imaging modality that provides axial and three-dimensional scans; the patient lies on a table that slides into the circular device that takes the x-rays
	Fluoroscopy (floor OS ko pee)	Direct observation of an x-ray image in motion

TABLE 2.13 Common Diagnostic Procedures and Tests in Ambulatory Healthcare—cont'd

Done by/Type of Test	Procedure	Description
	Magnetic resonance imaging (MRI)	An imaging modality that uses a magnetic field and radiofrequency pulses to create computer images of both bones and soft tissues in multiple planes.
	Nuclear scans	A radioactive substance is injected or ingested and then is detected by a special camera as it to moves through a body structure
	Positron emission tomography (PET) scan	Imaging test that uses a radioactive drug (tracer) to show the activity of tissues and organs
	Ultrasound (US) (also called sonography)	A transducer is moved over the body and sends out high-frequency sound waves; waves bounce off of tissues and the transducer captures the waves • 2D US: creates a flat two-dimensional picture (Fig. 2.6) • 3D US: creates a three dimensional (3D) picture (Fig. 2.7) • 4D US: creates a 3D picture with sound and motion • Doppler US: assesses blood flow through blood vessels

	X-ray (also called radiograph)	Uses electromagnetic waves to take pictures of the inside structures of the body; creates black-and-white images based on the amount of radiation that is absorbed
		• White areas: absorb more radiation (e.g., bones)
		• Gray areas: absorb less (e.g., soft tissue and fat)
		• Black: absorbs none (e.g., air)
		• Different views can be ordered
		  • PA (posteroanterior) films: x-ray passes from the back to the front of the person
		  • AP (anteroposterior) films: x-ray passes from the front to the back of the person

	Contrast media	Can be used with x-rays, CT, MRI, and US to improve the clarity of the soft tissue picture; ingested, administered by enema, or by injection (via blood vessels) and eliminated via the urine or stool; common contrast media include the following: • X-rays and CT scans: barium and iodine • MRIs: gadolinium • US: saline (salt water) and air

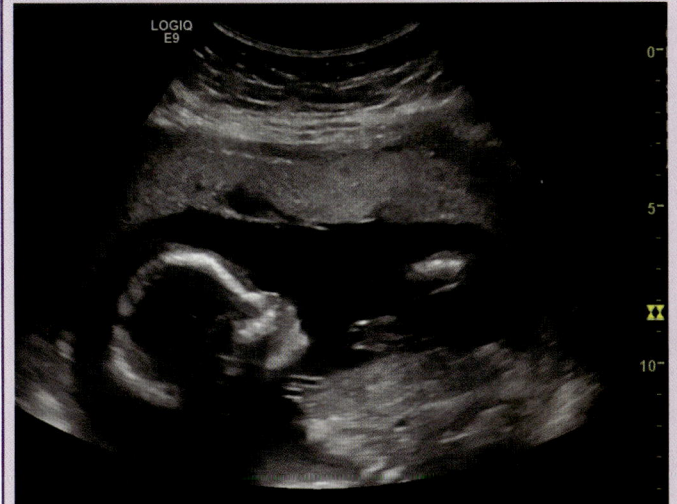

FIG. 2.6 Two-dimensional fetal ultrasound.

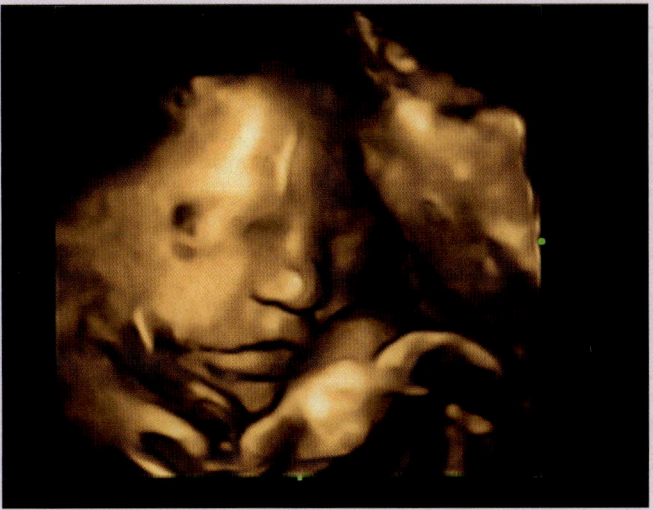

FIG. 2.7 Three-dimensional fetal ultrasound.

- Environmental factors: certain diseases are more common when a person has been exposed to pollutants in the air, land, or water. Though pesticides can reduce the risk of disease (e.g., West Nile and rabies), exposure to certain pesticides has been found to increase the risk of cancer.
- Lifestyle: stress, poor diet, infrequent exercise, or abusing nicotine, alcohol, or drugs can increase the risk for disease.

> **CRITICAL THINKING 2.7**
>
> While on break at work, Daniela worked on an assignment. She needed to determine which predisposing factors could be changed and how they could be changed. What could be her answers?

Causes of Disease

Disease can result from a change in homeostasis or be the result of the body's response to a perceived threat. There are several common causes of diseases, including genetics, infectious pathogens, inflammatory processes, immunity, nutritional imbalance, trauma and environmental agents, and neoplasms. The following sections describe these causes.

Genetics. Each person is made up of 46 chromosomes, which carry genetic information (genes). We get 23 chromosomes from each of our parents. *Genes* are the basic units of heredity or the instructions on how our bodies should develop and function. Genes provide the differences among us and the similarities in families. From genes, we get our physical appearance as well as our susceptibility to disease.

If you recall, chromosomes are found in the cell's nucleus. During the process of conception and the cell division that follows, an extra chromosome or a change in the chromosome structure may occur. A genetic disease may result from a chromosomal error or from the patient inheriting a defective gene from either parent. Types of genetic disease include the following:
- *Monogenic disorders*: a defective gene is inherited from one or both parents. See Table 2.14 for genetic diseases and how a child could get the disease.
- *Chromosomal disorders*: an abnormal number of chromosomes or a change in the chromosomal structure causes a disease like Klinefelter syndrome or Turner syndrome.

Infectious Pathogens. Many microorganisms are *nonpathogenic*, which means they do not cause disease. They can be found in our body maintaining the homeostasis. Other microorganisms are *pathogenic*, which means disease causing (Table 2.15). These pathogens enter our bodies through direct contact, indirect contact, or by vectors (Table 2.16).

When a pathogen enters our body and starts to multiply, we have an infection. Changes occur in our body, yet we do not feel any different. This is the *incubation period*. It starts at the time of exposure and ends when the signs and symptoms appear. The incubation period is different for each disease. For instance, strep throat has an incubation period of 2 to 5 days, whereas varicella (chicken pox) has an incubation period of 14 to 16 days. As our body tissues become damaged from the infection, we start to see the signs and symptoms. This is when disease occurs.

Some diseases are *noncommunicable*. They cannot be transmitted from one person to another. For instance, a person with tetanus cannot spread the disease to another person. Other diseases are *communicable*. These diseases are transmitted from one person to another. If a communicable disease is known to be easily transmitted, it is called a *contagious disease*. Strep throat and influenza are examples of contagious diseases. For instance, people with strep throat are contagious from the start of the fever until they are on the appropriate antibiotics for 24 hours. The period during which a disease can spread to another is called the *contagious period*. It is important for people in healthcare to understand the ways diseases are spread. Taking required precautions will minimize the risk of you "catching something" from your patients.

> **VOCABULARY**
>
> **toxins**: Substances created by microorganisms, plants, or animals and poisonous to humans.

> **CRITICAL THINKING 2.8**
>
> At school, Daniela learned about the transmission of pathogens. As a receptionist, she sees a lot of sick people stopping at her desk. She encourages those who cough to wear a mask. Hand sanitizer and tissue are also available. Thinking about disease transmission, why are these three items important in the prevention of disease?

Inflammatory Response. The inflammatory response is the body's efficient way of protecting itself. Inflammation occurs when the tissues are injured. The injury could be the result of bacteria, trauma, heat, toxins, or other causes. The cells damaged release chemicals called

TABLE 2.14 Inherited Genetic Diseases

Requirements for the Child to Get the Disease or Trait	Examples of Genetic Diseases
One copy of the defective dominant gene	Huntington disease
Two copies (one from each parent) of the defective recessive gene	Cystic fibrosis Tay-Sachs disease Sickle cell anemia Phenylketonuria (PKU)

TABLE 2.15 Common Pathogens

Pathogen	Description	Related Diseases
Fungi	Yeast and molds; only a few cause fungal disease or mycoses	Tinea corporis (ringworm) Tinea pedis (athlete's foot) Thrush
Protozoa	One-celled organism	Trichomoniasis Malaria Amebic dysentery
Viruses	Smallest microorganism; requires a host cell to multiply.	Common cold Measles, mumps Chicken pox, influenza
Bacteria	Single-celled organisms; classified by shape: bacilli (rod shaped), spirilla (spiral shaped), cocci (dot shaped) Many disease-causing bacteria produce **toxins** (TOK sins) that create the illness	Bacilli: tuberculosis, whooping cough Spirilla: cholera, syphilis Cocci: gonorrhea, meningitis
Helminths	A group of larger parasites that enter the body and live off the food you eat	External: lice, mites Internal: pinworms, tapeworms, flukes

TABLE 2.16 Modes of Transmission for Pathogens

Modes of Transmission	Definition	Examples of Diseases
Direct contact	Susceptible person comes in contact with an infected person; spread via contact with blood, body fluids, and excretions (e.g., stool, urine, and saliva) Methods of direct contact include the following: • Person to person (sneezing, touching, coughs) • Animal to person (being bitten or scratched or handling animal waste) • Mother to unborn child	Influenza Pertussis Chicken pox Rabies Gonorrhea Tuberculosis
Indirect Contact	Through contact with a contaminated object (e.g., water, food, drinking glass, airborne transmission)	E. coli Botulism
Vectors (insects)	Most blood-sucking insects consume the disease-causing microorganism from one host and transmit it during a "meal" to another host	Mosquitoes: yellow fever, malaria, West Nile fever, Zika Ticks: Lyme disease, tick-borne encephalitis, rickettsial diseases Fleas: plague, rickettsiosis

BOX 2.1 Five Key Signs of Inflammation
- Erythema (redness)
- Edema (swelling)
- Pain
- Warmth
- Loss of function

histamine, prostaglandins, and bradykinin. These chemicals cause the following responses:
- Blood vessels at the site dilate. This causes more local blood flow. With the increase in blood flow, *erythema* (ER i thee mah), or redness and warmth, occur in that area.
- Blood vessel walls allow more white blood cells and plasma to move out of the vessel into the surrounding tissues. The white blood cells work to protect the cells and clean up the dead tissue. The extra fluid from the blood causes *edema* (eh DEE mah), or swelling, pain, and loss of movement. For instance, if the injury occurred in the finger joint area, the edema may be so great that it prevents you from moving your finger.

Even though the inflammatory process can be efficient, it can also be the cause of disease. *Autoinflammatory diseases* (like familial Mediterranean fever) differ from autoimmunity diseases, which will be described later in the chapter. Autoinflammatory diseases result from a genetic mutation that causes the inflammatory process to activate without a reason. The person may experience recurring brief attacks of pain and fevers, and blood work indicates systemic inflammation (Box 2.1).

Immunity. Our immune system protects our bodies against potentially harmful substances. Our immune system "remembers" the **antigens** (an TIE jens) from diseases and responds with specific **antibodies** (AN tih bod ees). The antibodies destroy or attempt to destroy the harmful substances. Like with the autoinflammatory conditions, at times the immune response can work against us. These malfunctions are classified as follows:
- *Allergies* (AL ur jee): reactions occur if a person is exposed to a food (e.g., milk, tree nuts, peanuts, eggs, soy, and wheat), pollen, dust mites, mold, pet dander, inhalants, or other substances.
- *Autoimmunity*: the immune system does not recognize the body's own antigens and starts attacking itself. Rheumatoid arthritis, lupus, and psoriasis are examples of autoimmune disorders.
- *Immunodeficiency* (ih myoo noh deh FIH shun see): caused by a deficiency in one or more of the immune system key players (e.g., white blood cells like the B cells and T cells). A person with immunodeficiency has impaired resistance to infections.

VOCABULARY
antibodies: Protein substances produced in the blood or tissues in response to a specific antigen, that destroy or weaken the antigen. Part of the immune system.
antigens: Substances that stimulate the production of an antibody when introduced into the body. Antigens include toxins, bacteria, viruses, and other foreign substances.

MEDICAL TERMINOLOGY
allo-: different, other
anti-: against
auto-: self
erg/o: work
-gen: producing
immun/o: safety, protection
-y: condition

Nutritional Imbalances. Nutritional imbalances include too little or too much of a nutrient. Nutritional imbalances can impact growth, disease, and death. The following are causes of nutritional imbalances:
- Vitamin and mineral deficiencies: Some of these deficiencies can be caused by alcoholism, disease, dietary deficiencies (and poverty), weight loss surgery, and metabolic disorders.
- Vitamin and mineral excesses: Vitamin excesses can occur when a person takes too much of a vitamin. The water-soluble vitamins (vitamins B and C) pass through the body fairly quickly. The fat-soluble vitamins (vitamins A, D, E, and K) can accumulate in the body. This can lead to toxic conditions. Mineral excess can be caused by diet, medication, or a metabolic error.
- Obesity: Causes include the following:
  - Eating too many calories
  - Getting too little exercise
  - Having an endocrine or metabolic condition

Obesity can increase a person's risk for other diseases, including heart disease, diabetes, hypertension (high blood pressure), and stroke.
- Starvation: Eating too little food can result from a disease or poverty.

TABLE 2.17 Differences Between Benign and Malignant Tumors

Characteristic	Benign Tumor	Malignant Tumor
Cellular structure	Same as surrounding tissue	Anaplastic (a NAH plas tik) changes and poorly differentiated (dif EH ren shee ated)
Type of growth	Grows within a "shell" (encapsulated)	Infiltrates and metastasizes (MEH tas tuh sizes); spreads to distant site(s) in the body via the bloodstream or lymph system
Rate of growth	Usually slow; rarely fatal	May be slow, rapid, or very rapid; almost always fatal if left untreated
Destruction of localized tissue	None	Common; invades and takes over the surrounding tissue

Trauma and Environmental Agents. Trauma from auto accidents, violence, falls, and other events can cause disease. Common traumatic injuries include fractures, lacerated and ruptured organs, bleeding, neck and spinal injuries, and head injuries. Psychological trauma can also cause disorders.

Environmental changes like severe heat or cold temperatures and extremes of atmospheric pressures can impact health. Poisonings, insect and animal bites, burns, electric shock, and near drownings can also cause diseases.

Neoplasms. When cells grow quicker than normal or do not die as fast as they should, an abnormal mass is created. This mass is called a *neoplasm* (NEE oh plaz uhm) or *tumor* (too mohr). Tumors can be *benign* (bi NINE) (noncancerous) or *malignant* (mah LIG nahnt) (cancerous). Table 2.17 shows the difference between benign and malignant tumors.

There are more than 100 different types of cancer. Cancers are classified based on the type of tissue from which they originate (Fig. 2.8). See Table 2.18 for the classifications of cancer. (See also Figs. 2.9 and 2.10.)

As the malignant cells grow, they can break through the *basement membrane*. This delicate membrane separates the epithelial cells from connective tissues. Once this occurs, the cancerous cells can invade blood and lymph vessels. The circulating fluid (blood, lymph fluid) can then carry the cancerous cells to another location in the body. Thus cancerous cells from the primary or original tumor can metastasize to another location in the body, creating a secondary tumor.

If a provider suspects a patient may have cancer, a number of blood tests and imaging tests will be ordered. A biopsy (bye OP see) may be performed. The surgeon may also take a biopsy of nearby lymph nodes so the tissue can be checked for malignant cells. Based on the diagnostic results, the oncologist (on KOL uh jest) or pathologist (pa THOL uh jest) will grade and stage the cancer.

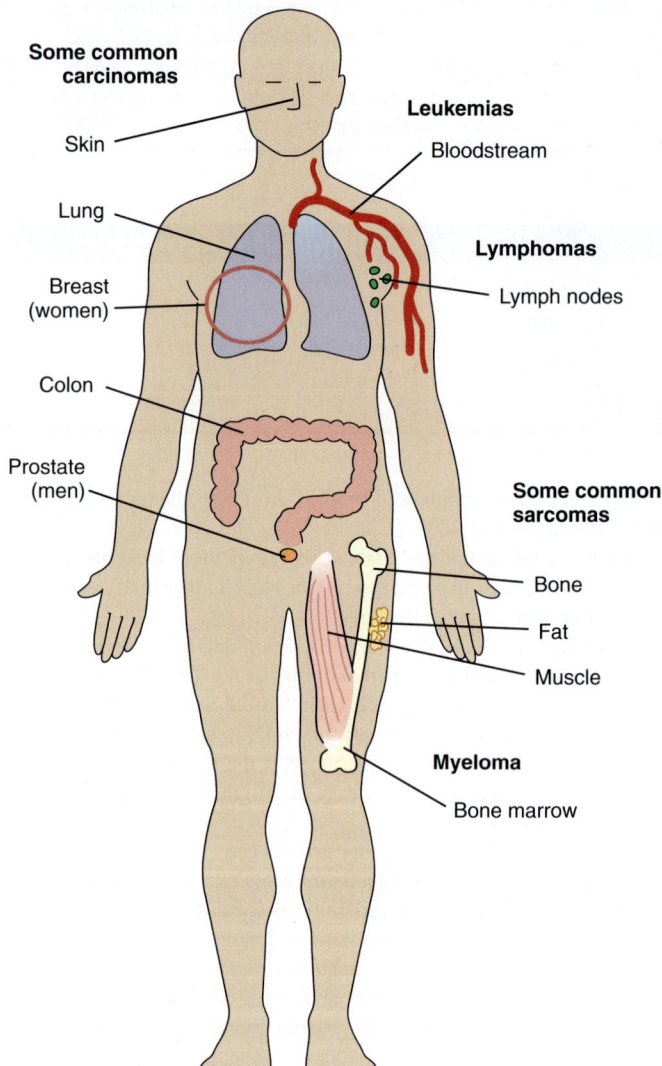

FIG. 2.8 Common cancers and where they occur. (From Shiland B: *Mastering Healthcare Terminology*, ed 5, St. Louis, 2016, Elsevier.)

VOCABULARY
- **anaplastic**: A rapidly dividing cancer cell that has little to no similarity to normal cells.
- **biopsy**: Process of viewing living tissue that has been removed for the purpose of diagnosis or treatment.
- **differentiated**: Describes how malignant tissue looks like the normal tissue it came from; poorly differentiated means it does not look like the normal tissue, and well differentiated means it looks like the normal tissue.
- **metastasizes**: To spread from one part of the body (the primary tumor) to another part of the body, forming a secondary tumor.
- **oncologist**: A specially trained doctor who diagnoses and treats cancer.
- **pathologist**: A physician specially trained in the nature and cause of disease.

MEDICAL TERMINOLOGY
- **ana-**: apart, up
- **bi/o**: living, life
- **neo-**: new
- **onc/o, -oma**: tumor
- **-opsy**: process of viewing
- **-plasia**: condition of formation
- **-plasm**: formation:

TABLE 2.18 Classification of Cancer

Classification	Medical Terminology	Description	Disease Examples
Carcinoma (kar sih NOH mah) Types:	**carcin/o** cancer **-oma** tumor, mass	Impact skin, lungs, breast, colon, prostate	
Squamous cell carcinoma (SKWAY muss) (see Fig. 2.9)	**-carcinoma** cancer of epithelial origin **squamo/o** scaly	Derived from squamous epithelium	Squamous cell carcinoma of the lung
Adenocarcinoma (ad en noh kar seh NOH mah)	**aden/o** gland	Derived from an organ or gland	Gastric adenocarcinoma
Sarcomas (sar KOH mah)	**-sarcoma** **sarc/o** connective tissue cancer	Impact connective tissue (bones, muscle, cartilage, blood vessels, and fat)	Osteosarcoma, chondrosarcoma, hemangiosarcoma, mesothelioma, and glioma
Lymphomas (limf OH mah) Types:	**lymph/o** lymph **-oma** tumor, mass	Impact lymphatic tissue (vessels, nodes, and organs, including the spleen, tonsils, and thymus gland)	
Hodgkin lymphoma		Diagnosed by the detection of Reed-Sternberg cell, a cell specific only to this disease	
Non-Hodgkin lymphoma		All other lymphomas with the exception of Hodgkin lymphoma.	
Leukemia (loo KEE me ah)	**leuk/o** white **-emia** blood condition	Impacts the bone marrow causing lots of abnormal blood cells to be created	Acute myelocytic leukemia
Myeloma (mye eh LOH mah) (see Fig. 2.10)	**myel/o** bone marrow, spinal cord **-oma** tumor, mass	Impacts the plasma cells (a type of white blood cells) in the bone marrow	Multiple myeloma
Mixed tumors		Combination of cells from within one classification or between two cancer classifications	Teratocarcinoma carcinosarcoma

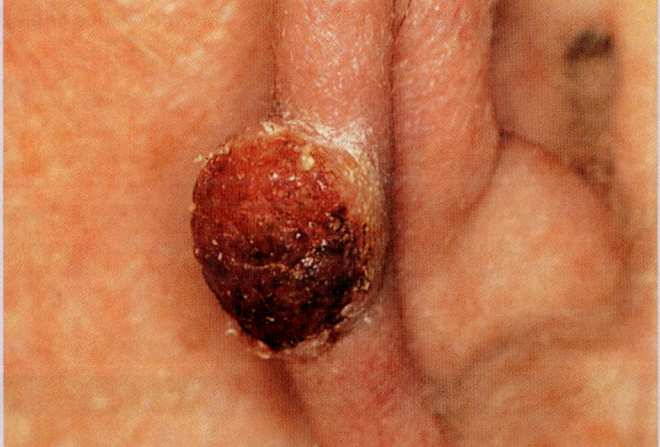

FIG. 2.9 Squamous cell carcinoma on the ear. (From McCance KL, Huether SE: *Pathophysiology: The Biologic Basis for Disease in Adults and Children,* ed 6, St. Louis, 2010, Mosby.)

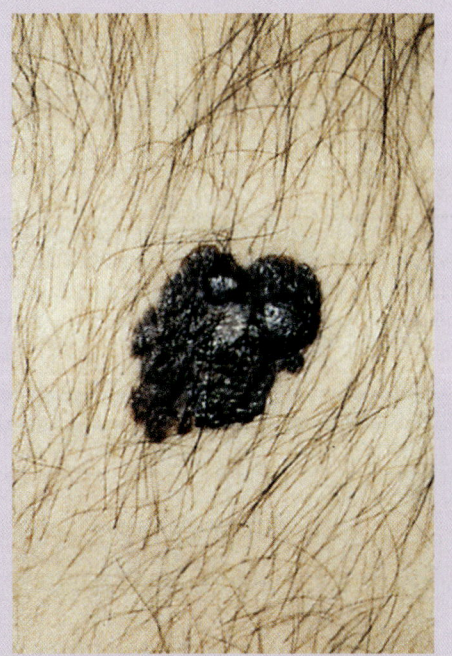

FIG. 2.10 Malignant melanoma on the arm. (From Damjanov I: *Anderson's Pathology,* ed 10, St. Louis, 2000, Mosby.)

Grade refers to how abnormal the malignant cells look. If the malignant cells and tissues closely resemble normal cells and tissue, the tumor is called "well differentiated." These are more slow-growing tumors. If the malignant cells and tissues do not look like normal cells and tissue, they are called "undifferentiated" or "poorly differentiated." The microscopic look of the cell is graded using 1, 2, 3, or 4 to indicate the appearance. Grade 1 means well-differentiated or the cells and organization of the malignant tissue looks close to normal tissue. Grade 2 means moderately differentiated, or the tissue does not look like normal tissue. The cells are growing at a faster rate than normal. Grades 3 and 4 do not look like normal tissue and tend to spread quicker.

Stage refers to the extent of the cancer, including the size and if it has spread. A cancer is referred to by this stage. Several staging systems are used, and various factors must be taken into consideration with staging systems:
- Location of the tumor
- Type of cell
- Size of the tumor
- If it has spread to nearby lymph nodes
- If it has spread to other locations in the body
- Tumor grade or how abnormal the cells look compared with normal sizes and how quickly it grows and spreads

The TNM staging system is widely used. The letters T, N, and M will be followed by a number or letter. For instance, a patient may have T1N0M0. It is important to have an understanding of what this means:
- T: refers to the size and extent of the primary tumor
  - TX: primary tumor cannot be measured
  - T0: primary tumor cannot be found
  - T1, T2, T3, and T4: refers to the size and extent of the primary tumor; the higher the number the larger or more extensive the tumor
- N: refers to the number of nearby lymph nodes impacted by the malignant cells

TABLE 2.19 Stages of Cancer

Stage	Definition
Stage 0	Abnormal cells are present; no spreading has occurred.
Stages I, II and III	Malignancy is present. The number is greater for larger tumors and tumors that have spread to nearby tissues.
Stage IV	Cancer has metastasized.

TABLE 2.20 Stages of Cancer

Stage	Definition
In situ	Abnormal cells are present; no spreading has occurred.
Localized	Cancer cells are present; no spreading has occurred.
Regional	Cancer has spread to nearby lymph nodes, organs, or tissues.
Distant	Cancer has metastasized.
Unknown	Not enough information is available.

- NX: nearby lymph node cancer cannot be measured
- N0: no cancer in the nearby lymph nodes
- N1, N2, and N4: refers to the location and quantity of nearby lymph nodes that have cancer; the higher the number, the more nodes are impacted
- M: refers to if the tumor has metastasized
  - MX: metastasis cannot be measured
  - M0: no metastasis has occurred
  - M1: metastasis has occurred

Other systems can be used in healthcare to stage cancer. Tables 2.19 and 2.20 provide two additional methods. This information will help you understand references to cancer.

CLOSING COMMENTS

Having an understanding of the structural organization of the body will help as you learn about each system. Tables 2.21 and 2.22 contain medical terminology that relate to body organization, cavities, quadrants, regions, and planes. As a medical assistant, you will be communicating with providers and peers. Using correct medical terminology and having a strong understanding of the body systems will help you communicate clearly and accurately in the ambulatory care setting.

TABLE 2.21 Medical Terminology Related to Body Organization

Word Part	Meaning	Word Part	Meaning
adip/o	fat	epitheli/o	epithelium
-al	pertaining to	hem/o	blood
ana-	up, apart, away	hemat/o	blood
ara-	near, beside, abnormal	hist/o	tissue
bol/o	to throw, throwing	home/o	same
cardi/o	heart	-ia	condition, state of
cata-	down	-ism	condition, state of
cellul/o	cell	kary/o	nucleus
chym/o	juice	lys/o	breakdown, dissolve
cyt/o	cell	meta-	beyond, change
en-	in	muscul/o	muscle
endo-	within	my/o	muscle
epi-	above, upon	myocardi/o	heart muscle

TABLE 2.21 Medical Terminology Related to Body Organization—cont'd

Word Part	Meaning	Word Part	Meaning
neur/o	nerve	-stasis	controlling, stopping
nucle/o	nucleus	strom/o	stroma
-on	structure	supra-	upward, above
organ/o	organ	system/o	system
osse/o	bone	thel/e	nipple
oste/o	bone	-um	structure, thing, membrane
-ous	pertaining to	-us	structure
-plasm	formation	viscer/o	viscera
-some	body		

From Shiland B: *Mastering Healthcare Terminology*, ed 5, St. Louis, 2016, Elsevier.

TABLE 2.22 Medical Terminology Related to Body Cavities, Abdominopelvic Quadrants and Regions, and Planes

Word Part	Meaning	Word Part	Meaning
abdomin/o	abdomen	lumb/o	lower back, loin
-ant	pertaining to	mediastin/o	mediastinum
celi/o	abdomen	mid-	middle
chondr/o	cartilage	omphal/o	umbilicus (navel)
crani/o	cranium (skull)	pariet/o	wall
diaphragm/o	diaphragm	pelv/i	pelvis
diaphragmat/o	diaphragm	pelv/o	pelvis
dors/o	back	peritone/o	peritoneum
epi-	above, upon	phren/o	diaphragm
front/o	front, belly side	pleur/o	pleura
gastr/o	stomach	sagitt/o	separating the sides
hyper-	excessive, above	spin/o	spine
hypo-	deficient, below, under	stern/o	sternum
-iac	pertaining to	thorac/o	thorax (chest)
-ic	pertaining to	trans-	through, across
ile/o	ileum	umbilic/o	umbilicus (navel)
ili/o	ilium	ventr/o	front, belly side
inguin/o	groin	-verse	to turn
lapar/o	abdomen	vertebr/o	vertebra

From Shiland B: *Mastering Healthcare Terminology*, ed 5, St. Louis, 2016, Elsevier.

CHAPTER REVIEW

Cells are the basic units of life. Groups of similar cells from the same source that carry out a specific function are called tissues. A structure composed of two or more types of tissues is an organ. Several organs and their related structures make up a body system. The most complex level, the organism (body), is made up of many body systems that work together to maintain homeostasis in the body.

The anatomical position provides a reference when using directional and positional terms. The anatomical position is when the body stands erect with the face forward, arms at the sides, palms forward, and toes pointed forward.

Body cavities are hollowed areas filled with organs. The body has dorsal (posterior) and ventral (anterior) body cavities. The dorsal body cavity protects nervous system organs and contains the cranial cavity and spinal cavity. The ventral body cavity is divided into the thoracic cavity and the abdominopelvic cavity.

With the abdominopelvic quadrants, an imaginary line is drawn down the midline of the body. A horizontal line is drawn across the abdominopelvic cavity, intersecting at the naval. These quadrants are referred to as either right or left and upper or lower. The abdominopelvic regions are nine regions that lie over the abdominopelvic cavity. They provide a more specific location than the quadrants.

The body's first line of defense includes chemical and physical barriers. These include skin, tears, saliva, mucus, cilia, stomach acid, good bacteria, and urine. If the structures are altered, then pathogens can get into the body. When this happens, the second line of defense, the immune system, kicks in. White blood cells and the lymphatic system work together to protect the body.

Predisposing factors include genetic factors, age, gender, environmental factors, and lifestyle. Diseases can be caused by genetics, pathogens, nutritional imbalances, trauma, environmental agents, and neoplasms. Normal body processes including the inflammatory processes and immunity can function improperly and cause disease.

SCENARIO WRAP-UP

Daniela continues her position as a float receptionist. She is gaining a lot of experience in the Walden-Martin Family Medical Clinic. Bella continues to help Daniela with her medical terminology and human body courses. Daniela really appreciates the study tips and reviewing assistance that Bella gives her. Some of her favorite ways to study these courses include the following:

- Making flashcards with the term or word part on one side and the definition on the other. Bella warned her to keep the definition short and simple. For nonmedical terminology, Daniela figured out that she learned more when she wrote her own definition. She realized the tests did not always use the exact words used in the textbook.
- Daniela realized that she learned better when she listened to the content. So she recorded herself going through her flashcards and review sheets. She found that if she stated the term or question and then paused, when she listened she could fill in the blank before hearing the answer.
- Lastly, Daniela learned that she sometimes felt she knew the content but was not always sure until it came to the test. So she decided to test herself on the content during her study times to see what she really knew.

Daniela is very excited to complete her human body and disease course and medical terminology course. She is also excited to apply the study practices she is learning to her future medical assistant courses.

3

Musculoskeletal System

LEARNING OBJECTIVES

1. Discuss the anatomy of the musculoskeletal system, list the major structures for the musculoskeletal system, and identify the anatomic location of the major muscles and bones of the musculoskeletal system.
2. Describe the normal function and physiology of the musculoskeletal system.
3. Complete the following for diseases and disorders related to the musculoskeletal system:
   - Identify the common signs and symptoms, etiology, and diagnostic measures of the musculoskeletal system.
   - Identify CLIA-waived tests associated with common musculoskeletal system diseases.
   - Describe treatment modalities used for musculoskeletal diseases.
4. Compare the structure and function of the musculoskeletal system across the life span.

CHAPTER OUTLINE

1. Opening Scenario, 35
2. You Will Learn, 35
3. **Anatomy of the Musculoskeletal System, 36**
   a. Skeleton, 36
      i. *Bone: Formation and Structure*, 36
      ii. *Types of Bones*, 37
      iii. *Axial Skeleton*, 37
      iv. *Appendicular Skeleton*, 39
   b. Joints, 40
   c. Muscles, 45
      i. *Structure of a Skeletal Muscle*, 46
      ii. *Muscle Naming Conventions*, 46
      iii. *Skeletal Muscles of the Human Body*, 46
4. **Physiology of the Musculoskeletal System, 46**
   a. Muscle Cell in Action, 46
   b. Types of Muscle Contractions, 51
   c. Impact of Exercise on Skeletal Muscles, 51
   d. Types of Muscle Action, 51
5. **Diseases and Disorders of the Musculoskeletal System, 52**
   a. Fractures, 54
   b. Additional Musculoskeletal Traumas, 58
      i. *Definition of Additional Traumas*, 58
      ii. *Etiology*, 58
   c. Arthritis, 59
   d. Bursitis, 59
   e. Carpal Tunnel Syndrome, 61
   f. Degenerative Joint Disorder: Osteoarthritis, 62
   g. Muscular Dystrophy, 62
   h. Osteoporosis, 63
   i. Skeletal Deformities: Lordosis, Kyphosis, Scoliosis, 63
   j. Additional Musculoskeletal Diseases and Disorders, 63
6. **Life Span Changes, 63**
7. **Closing Comments, 66**
8. **Chapter Review, 68**
9. **Scenario Wrap-Up, 68**

OPENING SCENARIO

Patsy Mulhern, CMA (AAMA), works with Dr. James Martin at the Walden-Martin Family Medical Clinic (WMFM). Today is Patsy's 20th anniversary at WMFM! Dr. Martin hired Patsy right out of school as a new graduate. She has seen a lot in her years as a medical assistant (MA). Many aspects of her day have changed from when she first started as an MA, but one thing that has not changed is her love for helping patients.

Another busy day is scheduled, and Patsy's first patient is Walter Biller. Walter is in his late 40s, is in good general health, is near his ideal weight, and has no chronic conditions. He saw Dr. Martin a few weeks ago when he experienced worsening pain in his hands and knees. He had been planting in his garden and noticed that the next day that he had more pain and stiffness in his hands than usual. He also experienced pain in the muscle on the front of his forearm, just below the elbow. Bending down on his hands and knees in the garden was not as easy as it used to be. Dr. Martin performed a physical exam and ordered lab tests. He asked Walter to make a follow-up appointment to go over the results. Today Walter is back at the clinic, and Patsy is ready to room him for his appointment.

YOU WILL LEARN

1. To recognize and use terms related to the skeleton, muscles, and joints.
2. To locate the bones of the skeleton and muscles of the body.
3. To understand and describe the movement of joints in the body.

4. To recognize disease states of the skeleton including their causes, signs and symptoms, diagnostic processes, treatment, prognosis, and prevention.
5. To recognize disease states of the muscles including their causes, signs and symptoms, diagnostic processes, treatment, prognoses, and prevention.
6. To recognize disease states of the joints including their causes, signs and symptoms, diagnostic processes, treatment, prognoses, and prevention.

ANATOMY OF THE MUSCULOSKELETAL SYSTEM

The musculoskeletal (muss skyoo loh SKELL uh tul) system (MS) consists of three interrelated parts: bones, joints, and muscles. Imagine a body without bones, muscles, and joints. How could we move, bend, twist, or stretch? The musculoskeletal system is responsible for the following functions:
- Body movement
- Support and framework for the organ systems of the body
- Protection for the core internal organs, brain, and spinal cord
- Storage for important minerals such as calcium and phosphorous
- Continually forming new blood cells by the process of *hematopoiesis* (hee mah toh poh EE sis), which occurs in the red bone marrow inside some bones; red blood cells, white blood cells, and platelets are all made in the bone marrow

Let's learn more about the musculoskeletal system (Box 3.1).

BOX 3.1 Specialties/Specialists

Orthopedics (or thoh PEE diks) is the healthcare specialty that deals with most musculoskeletal disorders. An *orthopedist* (or thoh PEE dist) is a specialist involved in the diagnosis, treatment, and prevention of disorders of the musculoskeletal system.

Rheumatology (roo muh TOL uh jee) is a specialty that deals with disorders of connective tissue, including bone and cartilage. Rheumatology also deals with many diseases that are classified as **autoimmune**. The specialist is called a *rheumatologist* (roo muh TOL uh jist).

VOCABULARY
autoimmune: A disease that causes the body to produce antibodies that attack its own tissues, leading to the deterioration of tissue.
ossification: The natural process of bone formation and hardening.

MEDICAL TERMINOLOGY
arthr/o, articul/o: joint	**orth/o:** straight
-cyte: cell	**oste/o, oss/i, osse/o:** bone
hemat/o: blood	**ped/o:** child
-ist: one who specializes	**-poiesis:** formation
-logy: study of	**rheumat/o:** watery flow
muscul/o, my/o, myos/o: muscle	**skelet/o:** skeleton

Skeleton
When babies are born, their bones are not mature. The bones go through a process called ossification (ah sih fih KAY shun) to eventually mature and harden. Ossification is gradual. It will take place from infancy through adolescence. The adult skeleton contains 206 bones.

Bones are composed of mature bone cells called *osteocytes* (OS tee oh sytes). The material between the bone cells is called the matrix (MAY tricks). The matrix stores calcium (Ca) and phosphorus (P) for the body to use as needed. Mineral storage is a very important function of the bones, especially the storage of calcium. Once a bone is mature it may not grow in size, but it will continue to change. Bone is a living tissue that is continuously remodeled throughout a person's lifetime.

Bone: Formation and Structure. About 10% of a mature skeleton is broken down and then remodeled each year. There are specific cells that are responsible for this activity, *osteoclasts* (os tee oh KLAST) and *osteoblasts* (os tee oh BLAST). Calcium is an important mineral in the body and is necessary for proper muscle and nerve function. In order for the body to use calcium stored in the bones, osteoclasts break down old or damaged bone tissue. This releases needed calcium into the blood. Once blood calcium is high enough, osteoblasts are then responsible for using extra blood calcium to build new bone tissue. This continuous process of breaking down and building up bone tissue is called *remodeling*. It is an important process that maintains proper blood calcium levels and promotes skeletal strength and healing.

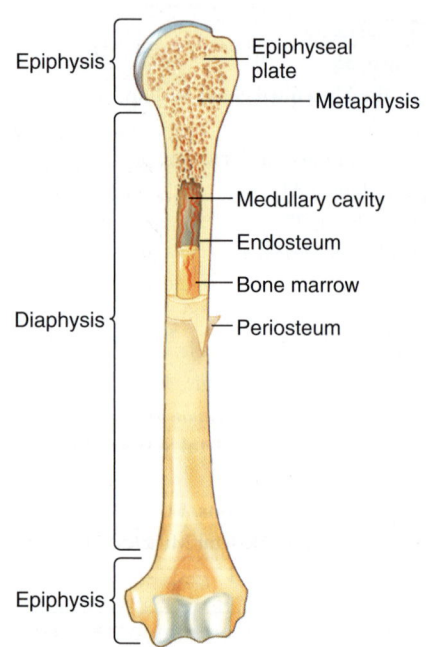

FIG. 3.1 Long bone. (From Shiland B: *Mastering Healthcare Terminology*, ed 5, St. Louis, 2016, Elsevier.)

Each long bone (Fig. 3.1) is composed of a long shaft called the *diaphysis* (dye AFF ih sis). The diaphysis is a long hollow tube of hard **compact bone**. The hollow space inside the diaphysis is called the *medullary* (MEH dyoo lair ee) *cavity* and contains **yellow bone marrow**. Yellow marrow is an inactive, fatty form of bone marrow. Each end of a long bone is called an *epiphysis* (eh PIFF ih sis) and is made up of **spongy** or **cancellous** (KAN seh lus) **bone**. Spongy bone is less dense than compact bone and has a network of open spaces that contain **red bone marrow**. Blood cells are produced in the red bone marrow. Below

CHAPTER 3 Musculoskeletal System

VOCABULARY

compact bone: Bone tissue that is the rigid, dense outer layer of bone that consists mostly of calcium and minerals.
ossicles: The three small bones of the middle ear that transmit sound vibrations from the eardrum to the inner ear: the malleus, incus, and stapes.
red bone marrow: An active form of bone marrow that produces red and white blood cells and platelets.
spongy bone: Light and porous bone tissue that contains bone marrow; also called **cancellous bone**.
yellow bone marrow: An inactive, fatty form of bone marrow, it does not produce blood cells.

CRITICAL THINKING 3.1

Patsy was thinking about Walter as she prepared the exam room for his appointment. Walter's hands and knees were bothering him. The hands and knees are both part of the appendicular skeleton. She thought for a moment and quickly named the major structures in the appendicular and axial skeleton. Can you name them too?

MEDICAL TERMINOLOGY

-al: pertaining to
appendic/o-: appendages, limbs, or appendix
axi/o-: at the center
-blast: embryonic
chondr/o, cartilag/o: cartilage
-clast: breaking down
crani/o: skull, cranium
dia-: through
endo-: within
epi-: above
epiphyseal (singular), **epiphyses** (plural)
ethmoid/o: ethmoid
faci/o: face
fasci/o: fascia
front/o: frontal
ligament/o, syndesm/o: ligament:
mastoid/o: mastoid
meta-: change
myel/o: bone marrow
nas/o: nose
occipit/o: occipital
para-: near
pariet/o: parietal
peri-: surrounding
-physis: growth, nature
sphenoid/o: sphenoid
tempor/o: temporal
tendin/o, tend/o, ten/o: tendon
-um: structure

Types of Bones. Bones are divided into two categories:
- *Axial* (ACK see ul) *skeleton:* made up of the skull, rib cage, and spine
- *Appendicular* (ap pen DICK yoo lur) *skeleton:* made up of the shoulder girdle, collar bones, arms, pelvic girdle, and legs (Fig. 3.2)

Human bones appear in a variety of shapes and sizes that suit their function in the body. See Fig. 3.2 and Table 3.1 for the locations and descriptions of these bones.

The shape of a bone enables practitioners to speak specifically about an area on that bone. For instance, any groove, opening, or hollow space is called a *depression*. Depressions provide an entrance and exit for vessels and protection for the organs they hold. Raised or projected areas are called *processes*. These are often areas of attachment for ligaments or tendons.

Using Table 3.2 and Fig. 3.2, locate the bones of the body described on the following pages. Note the blue color of the axial skeleton and the tan color of the appendicular skeleton.

Axial Skeleton.
The skull is made up of two parts:
- *Cranium* (KRAY nee um), which encloses and protects the brain
- *Facial bones* (Fig. 3.3)

See Table 3.3 for a list of the bones of the skull.

The last three bones of the skull, the **ossicles**, are tiny bones within the middle ear cavity of the temporal bone. The ossicles are small and vital structures, which will be discussed in more detail in Chapter 13. Use Table 3.4 to become familiar with the names of the facial bones. Then, look at Fig. 3.3 to locate the most common facial bones and the **sinuses**.

There are 12 pairs of *ribs*. Ribs are thin, flat bones. They attach in the back to the *thoracic* (thor AS ik) vertebrae in the back and curve around and attach to **costochondral** (kost toh KON drul) tissue in the front (Fig. 3.4C). The ribs can be categorized as follows:
- *True ribs:* seven pairs attached directly to the sternum (STUR num) in the front of the body
- *False ribs:* five pairs attached to the *sternum* by cartilage; the last two pairs of false ribs are called *floating ribs* because they are not attached in the front of the body at all

the epiphyses are the *epiphyseal* (eh pee FIZZ ee ul) *plates or growth plates*, which is where bone growth normally occurs. Between the ages of 16 and 25, the epiphyseal plates close and bone growth stops. The epiphysis and epiphyseal plates together form the *metaphysis* (meh TAFF ih sis).

Compact bone, unlike spongy bone, does not contain a network of open spaces. Instead, compact bone is made up of structural units called *osteons* (OS tee ohns). These circular structural units are composed of osteocytes and calcified matrix. Osteons are arranged in many layers, like the layers of an onion. There are small passageways in compact bone where blood vessels supply osteocytes with nutrients. Because bones have a good blood supply, they easily heal after trauma or a fracture.

The outer covering of the bone is called the *periosteum* (pair ee OS tee um), and the inner lining of the bone is known as the *endosteum* (en DOS tee um). Between the two coverings, osteoblasts and osteoclasts continuously remodel bones, making them strong, durable, and able to heal.

Box 3.2 describes the terms for the different types of musculoskeletal connections.

BOX 3.2 Musculoskeletal Connections

Summary of the connections in the musculoskeletal system:
- *Ligaments* (LIH gah ments) connect bones to bones.
- *Tendons* (TEN duns) connect muscles to bone.
- *Fascia* (FASH ee ah) is a tough fibrous covering of the muscles.
- *Cartilage* (KAR tih lij) is a flexible connective tissue that covers the ends of many bones at the joint.

UNIT 1 Medical Terminology, Anatomy, and Physiology

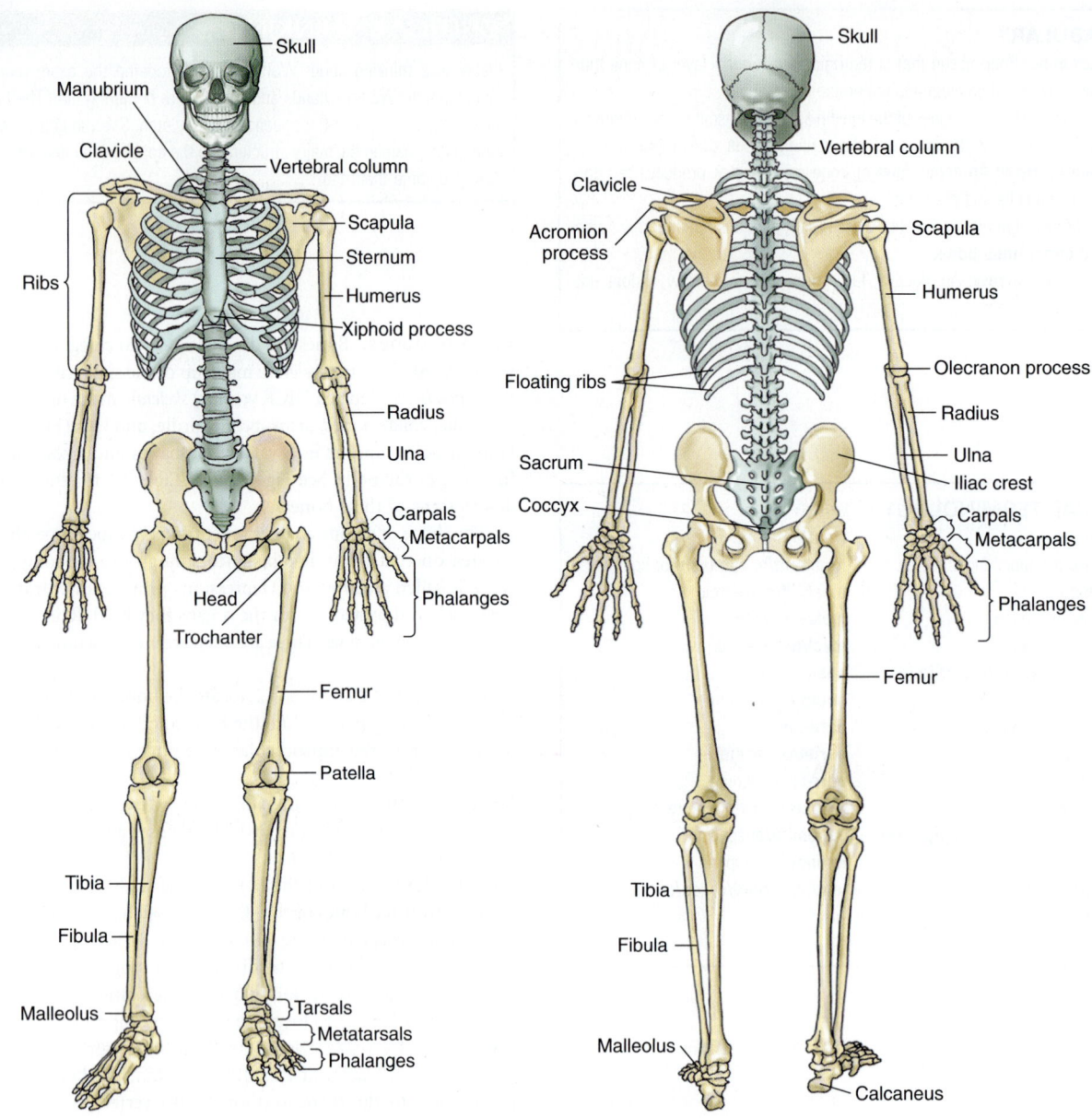

FIG. 3.2 Axial and appendicular skeleton. The structures that constitute the axial skeleton are in blue. (From Shiland B: *Mastering Healthcare Terminology*, ed 5, St. Louis, 2016, Elsevier.)

TABLE 3.1	Shapes of Human Bones
Types	**Examples**
Long bones	Humerus (upper arm bone), femur (thigh bone)
Short bones	Carpal (wrist bone), tarsal (ankle bone)
Flat bones	Sternum (breastbone), scapula (shoulder blade)
Irregular bones	Vertebra (backbone), stapes (a bone of the ear)
Sesamoid (SEH sah moyd) bones	Patella (kneecap)

From Shiland B: *Mastering Healthcare Terminology*, ed 5, St. Louis, 2016, Elsevier.

TABLE 3.2	Two Divisions of the Skeleton
Axial Skeleton (80 Bones Total)	**Appendicular Skeleton (126 Bones Total)**
Skull • Face • Ear bones • Cranium	**Upper Appendicular** • Shoulder girdle–collar bone and shoulder blade • Arms • Wrist
Spine • Vertebrae	**Lower Appendicular** • Pelvic girdle–hip bones • Legs • Ankles • Feet
Rib Cage • Ribs • Sternum	
Hyoid Bone • At the base of the tongue	

From Shiland B: *Mastering Healthcare Terminology*, ed 5, St. Louis, 2016, Elsevier.

CHAPTER 3 Musculoskeletal System

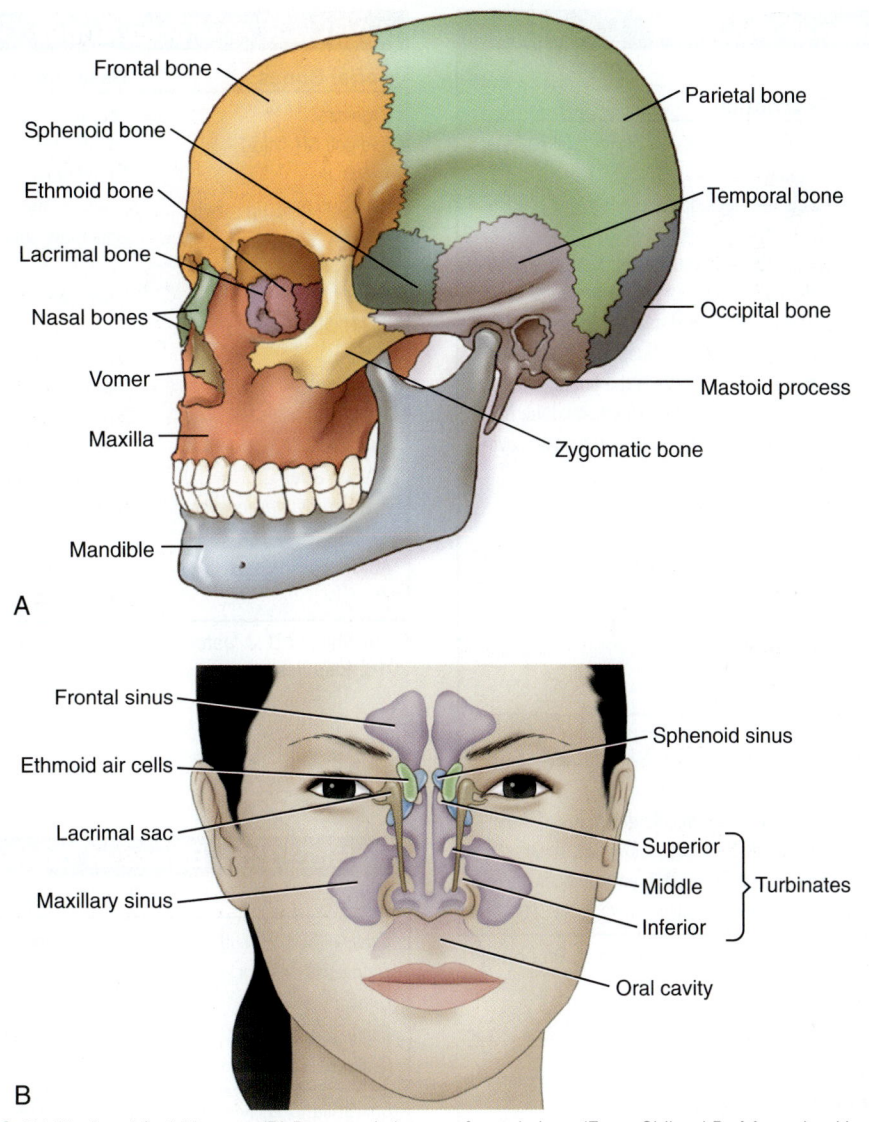

FIG. 3.3 (A) Skull and facial bones. (B) Paranasal sinuses, frontal view. (From Shiland B: *Mastering Healthcare Terminology*, ed 5, St. Louis, 2016, Elsevier.)

In addition to ribs, the rib cage includes the sternum, also known as the breastbone. There are three portions of bone that make up the sternum. The top portion is called the *manubrium* (mah NOO bree um). The middle portion is called the *sternum* or may be referred to as the *body of the sternum*. The sharp point at the bottom of the sternum is called the *xiphoid* (ZIH foyd) *process*. The combining form *xiph/o* means "sword" in Greek, and the xiphoid process resembles the tip of a sword. When performing cardiopulmonary resuscitation (CPR), the sternum is compressed.

The *spinal*, or *vertebral*, column is divided into five regions from the neck to the tailbone. It is composed of 26 bones called the **vertebrae** (VUR teh bray) (Fig. 3.4A). Table 3.5 lists the bones in the spine. Fig. 3.4B illustrates a vertebra with the *laminae* (LAM uh nee), *spinous* and *transverse processes*, and *facets* (FAS its). Laminae are thin, platelike arches in the vertebrae. Facets are processes that articulate between vertebrae.

Appendicular Skeleton. The appendicular skeleton is composed of the upper appendicular and lower appendicular skeletons. Tables 3.6

MEDICAL TERMINOLOGY
cost/o: rib
lacrim/o: lacrimal
mandible/o: mandible
maxill/o: maxilla
palat/o: palatine

sinus (singular), **sinuses** (plural)
stern/o: sternum
vomer/o: vomer
zygom/o, zygomat/o: zygoma

VOCABULARY
costochondral: The cartilage that joins the ribs and the sternum on the front of the rib cage.
sinus: An air-filled cavity in a dense portion of a skull bone, lined with mucous-secreting cells.

TABLE 3.3 Bones of the Skull

Bones of the Cranium	Description
Frontal	Forms the anterior part of the skull and the forehead
Parietal (puh RYE uh tul)	Forms the sides of the cranium
Occipital (ock SIP ih tul)	Forms the back of the skull; a large hole at the ventral surface, the *foramen magnum*, allows spinal cord to enter the cranium
Temporal (TEM poor ul)	Forms the lower two sides of the cranium; the *mastoid process* is the bump at the posterior part of the bone behind the ear
Ethmoid (EHTH moyd)	Forms the roof and walls of the nasal cavity
Sphenoid (SFEE noyd)	Anterior to the temporal bones
Paranasal sinuses	Air-filled cavities that are named for the bones in which they are located; each is lined with a mucous membrane (see Fig. 3.3B)

Bones of the Ear	Description
Malleus (MAL ee us)	Tiny bone of the middle ear cavity of the temporal bone; also known as the *hammer*
Incus (ING kus)	Tiny bone of the middle ear cavity of the temporal bone; also known as the *anvil*
Stapes (STAY peez)	Tiny bone of the middle ear cavity of the temporal bone; also known as the *stirrup*

From Shiland B: *Mastering Healthcare Terminology,* ed 5, St. Louis, 2016, Elsevier.

TABLE 3.4 Facial Bones

Facial Bones	Description
Zygomatic (zye goh MAT tick)	Cheekbone; also called the *zygoma* (zye GOH mah)
Lacrimal (LACK rih mul)	Paired bones at the corner of each eye that cradle the tear ducts
Maxilla (MACK sill ah)	Upper jaw bone—unable to move
Mandible (MAN dih bul)	Lower jaw bone—movable
Vomer (VOH mur)	Bone that forms the posterior/inferior part of the nasal septal wall between the nostrils
Palatine (PAL eh tyne)	Shell-shaped structures that make up part of the roof of the mouth
Nasal turbinates (conchae) (KON kee)	Make up part of the interior of the nose
Nasal bones	Pair of small bones that make up the bridge of the nose

From Shiland B: *Mastering Healthcare Terminology,* ed 5, St. Louis, 2016, Elsevier.

TABLE 3.5 Bones of the Spine

Region	Type and Abbreviation
Cervical (SUR vih kul)	Neck bones (C1–C7)
Thoracic (thor AS ick)	Upper back (T1–T12)
Lumbar (LUM bar)	Lower back (L1–L5)
Sacral (SAC rul)	Sacrum (S1–S5) (five bones, fused)
Coccygeal (kock sih JEE ul)	Coccyx (KOCK sicks) or tailbone

From Shiland B: *Mastering Healthcare Terminology,* ed 5, St. Louis, 2016, Elsevier.

MEDICAL TERMINOLOGY

cervic/o: neck
coccyg/o: coccyx
lamina (singular), laminae (plural)
lamin/o: lamina
lumb/o: lumbar (lower back)
sacr/o: sacrum
spin/o: spine
thorac/o: thorax (chest)
vertebr/o, spondyl/o: vertebra
xiph/o: xiphoid

VOCABULARY

vertebrae: A series of small, irregular-shaped bones that form the backbone or spine. Each vertebra has several projections, joint surfaces, areas for muscle attachment, and a hole where the spinal cord passes.

CRITICAL THINKING 3.2

Patsy rooms Walter, and they have a few moments to talk. She goes about collecting vital signs. After she finishes the respiratory rate she asks, "Walter, did you know that there are three parts to the breastbone, or sternum?" He replies, "Yes, I do. I can even name them!" Can you name the three parts of the sternum? Share any memory tips with your instructor and classmates.

and 3.7 list and explain the bones of the upper and lower appendicular skeleton. Figs. 3.5 and Fig. 3.6 correlate each bone's description with its location. Box 3.3 compares the male and female pelvis.

Joints

Joints, or articulations as they are sometimes called, are the parts of the body where two or more bones of the skeleton join. Examples of joints include the following:
- The knee, which joins the tibia and the femur
- The elbow, which joins the humerus with the radius and ulna

Joints provide *range of motion* (ROM), the range through which a joint can be extended and flexed. Different joints have different ROM, from no movement at all to full range of movement. Categorized by ROM, they are as follows:

No Range of Motion
- *Synarthroses* (sin ar THROH sees) are immovable joints held together by fibrous cartilaginous tissue—for example, the suture lines of the skull.

CHAPTER 3 Musculoskeletal System

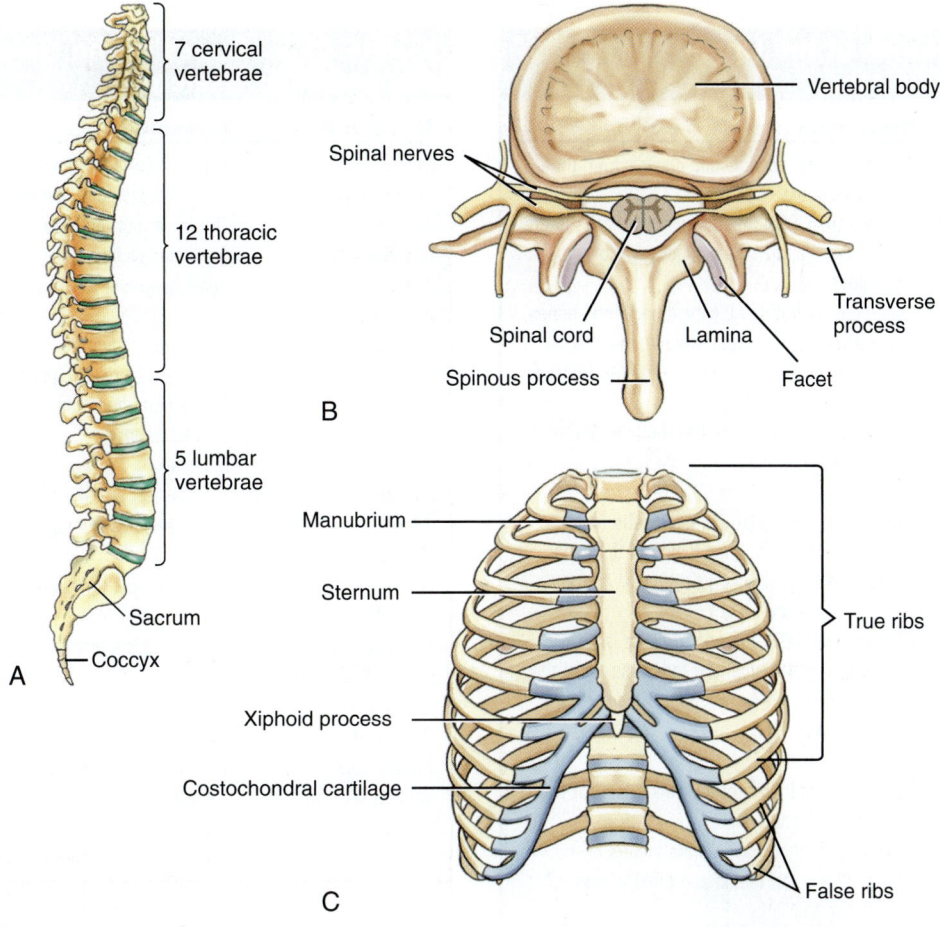

FIG. 3.4 (A) Spine. (B) Vertebrae. (C) Ribs. (From Shiland B: *Mastering Healthcare Terminology*, ed 5, St. Louis, 2016, Elsevier.)

STUDY TIP

Remember the "T" of Tarsals is by the Toes! This is a quick way to remember tarsals and metatarsals are in the feet. Carpals are in the wrist and hand.

VOCABULARY

pelvic girdle: A bowl-shaped complex of bones that connects the trunk and the legs. The pelvic girdle consists of the ilium, ischium, and pubis.

shoulder girdle: The set of bones that connects the arm to the axial skeleton on each side. Also called the pectoral girdle, it consists of the clavicle and the scapula.

MEDICAL TERMINOLOGY

acromial/o: acromion
calcane/o: calcaneus
carp/o: carpal (wrist)
carpus (singular), **carpals** (plural)
clavicul/o, clad/o: clavicle
femor/o: femur
fibul/o, perone/o: fibula
humer/o: humerus
ili/o: ilium
ischi/o: ischium
malleol/o: malleolus
metacarp/o: metacarpal
metacarpus (singular), **metacarpals** (plural)
metatarsus (singular), **metatarsals** (plural)
metatars/o: metatarsal
olecran/o: olecranon
patell/o, patell/a: patella
pelv/i, pelv/o: pelvis
phalang/o: phalanx
phalanx (singular), **phalanges** (plural)
pub/o: pubis
radi/o: radius
scapul/o: scapula
tarsus (singular), **tarsals** (plural)
tars/o: tarsal
tibi/o: tibia
uln/o: ulna

UNIT 1 Medical Terminology, Anatomy, and Physiology

TABLE 3.6 Bones of the Upper Appendicular Skeleton

Name of Bone	Description
Scapula (SKAP yoo lah)	Shoulder blade; *scapula* and *clavicle* form the shoulder girdle. *Acromion* (ack ROH mee un) *process* is the lateral tip of the scapula, the highest point of the shoulder
Clavicle (KLA vih kul)	Collarbone; pair of long, curved horizontal bones that attach to the upper sternum and the acromion process; add stability to the front of the shoulder. Scapula and clavicle form the shoulder girdle
Humerus (HYOO mur us)	Upper arm bone
Radius (RAY dee us)	Lower lateral arm bone parallel to the ulna; articulates with the thumb side of the hand
Ulna (UL nuh)	Lower medial arm bone; articulates with the little finger side of the hand. *Olecranon* (oh LECK ruh non) *process* is a projection of the ulna that forms the tip of the elbow; commonly known as the *funny bone*
Carpals (KAR pals)	The eight wrist bones
Metacarpals (meh tuh KAR pals)	The five bones that form the middle part of the hand; palm of the hand
Phalanges (fah-LAN-jeez)	The 14 bones that make up the fingers of the hand, two in the thumb and three in each of the other four fingers

From Shiland B: *Mastering Healthcare Terminology*, ed 5, St. Louis, 2016, Elsevier.

TABLE 3.7 Bones of the Lower Appendicular Skeleton

Name of Bone	Description
Ilium (ILL ee um)	The superior and widest bone of the pelvis. The ilium, ischium, and pubis form the pelvic girdle
Ischium (ISS kee um)	The lower portion of the pelvic bone. The ilium, ischium, and pubis form the pelvic girdle
Pubis (PYOO bis)	*Pubic bone*: the lower anterior part of the pelvic bone. The ilium, ischium, and pubis form the pelvic girdle
Femur (FEE mur)	Thigh bone, upper leg bone. The femoral head fits into a socket called the *acetabulum*
Patella (puh TELL uh)	Kneecap
Tibia (TIB ee uh)	Shin bone, lower medial leg bone
Fibula (FIB yuh luh)	Smaller, lower lateral leg bone
Malleolus (mah LEE oh lus)	Process on the distal ends of tibia and fibula
Tarsals (TAR sals)	The seven bones of the ankle, hindfoot, and midfoot; the *calcaneus* is the heel bone
Metatarsals (met uh TAR sals)	The five foot bones between the tarsals and the phalanges
Phalanges	The 14 toe bones, two in the great toe and three in each of the other four toes

From Shiland B: *Mastering Healthcare Terminology*, ed 5, St. Louis, 2016, Elsevier.

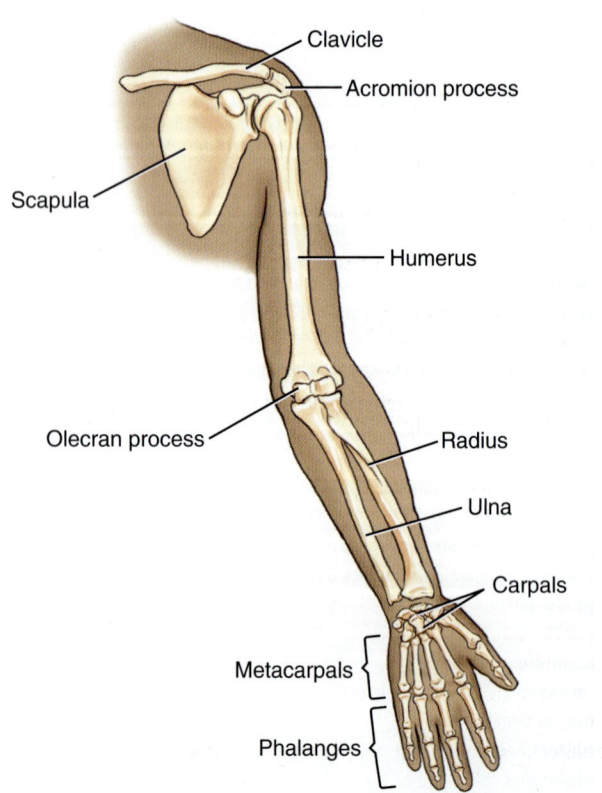

FIG. 3.5 Shoulder girdle and upper extremity. (From Shiland B: *Mastering Healthcare Terminology*, ed 5, St. Louis, 2016, Elsevier.)

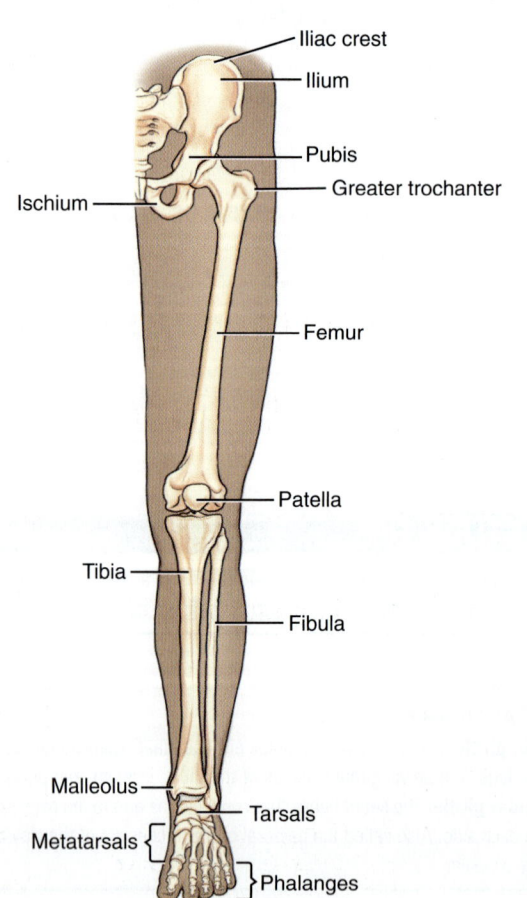

FIG. 3.6 Pelvic girdle and lower extremity. (From Shiland B: *Mastering Healthcare Terminology*, ed 5, St. Louis, 2016, Elsevier.)

BOX 3.3 Comparison of Male and Female Pelvis

The male and female pelvises are different in the human skeleton. The male pelvis is generally deep and narrow. The female pelvis is generally broad and shallow, and the pelvic inlet is wider to accommodate the birth of a baby. Also, note in Fig. 3.7 that the angle between the pubic bones in the female skeleton is wider.

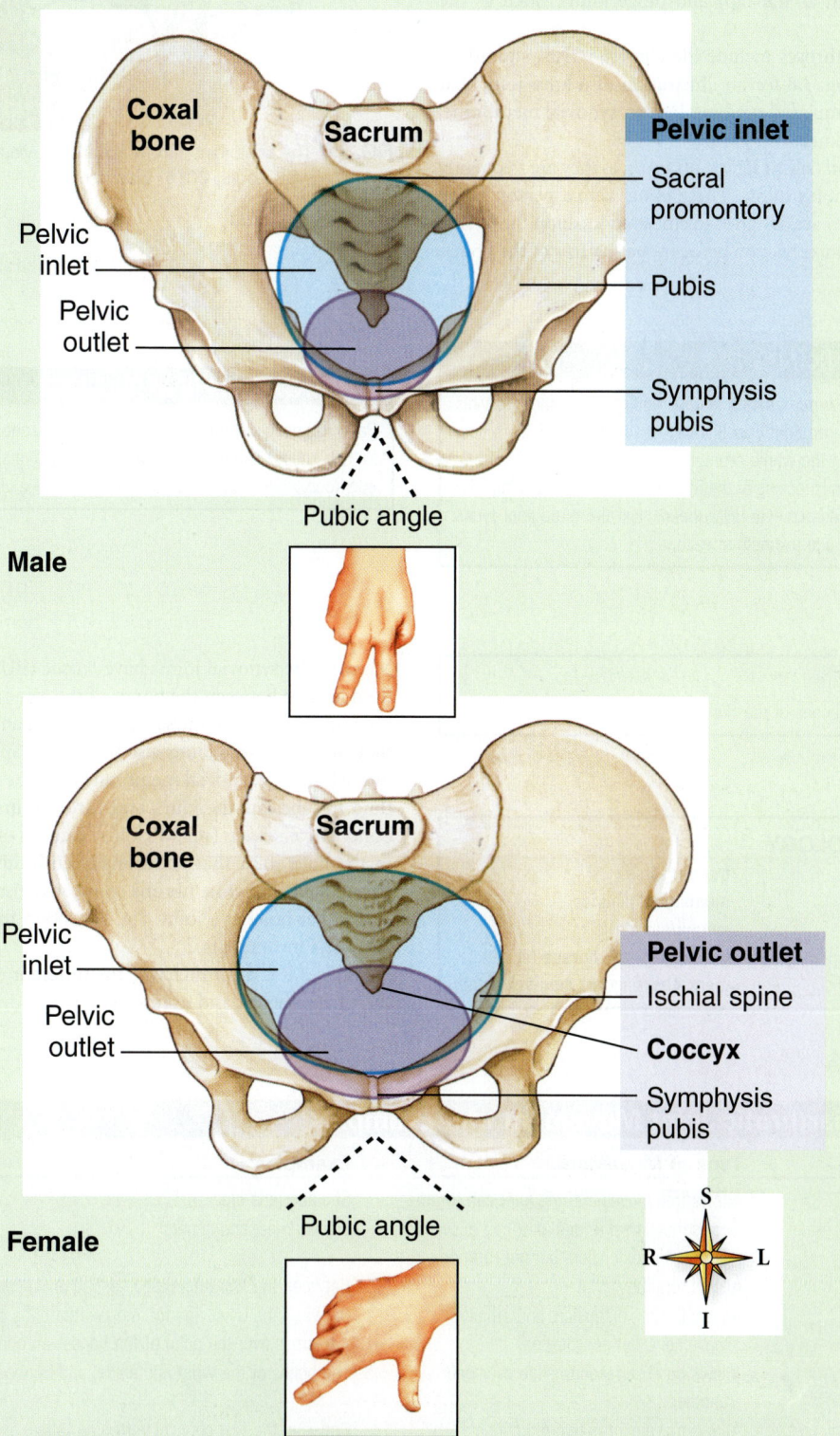

FIG. 3.7 Comparison of the male and female pelvis. (From Patton K: *Structure and Function of the Body*, ed 15, St. Louis, 2016, Elsevier.)

Limited Range of Motion
- *Amphiarthroses* (am fee ar THROH sees) are joints joined together by cartilage that are slightly movable—for example, the vertebrae of the spine or the pubic bones of the pelvic girdle.

Full Range of Motion
- *Diarthroses* (dye ar THROH sees) are joints that have free movement. Types of joints that have free movement include ball-and-socket joints (such as the hip) and hinge joints (such as the knees).
- Examples of diarthroses include the elbows, wrists, shoulders, and ankles. See Fig. 3.8 for an illustration of a knee joint that shows the bones, muscles, tendons, bursae, synovial membrane, and cavity in the knee.

Diarthroses, or *synovial* (sih NOH vee ul) *joints*, as they are frequently called, are the most complex joints. These joints help a person move around for a lifetime. They are designed to efficiently cushion the jarring of the bones and to minimize friction between the surfaces of the bones.

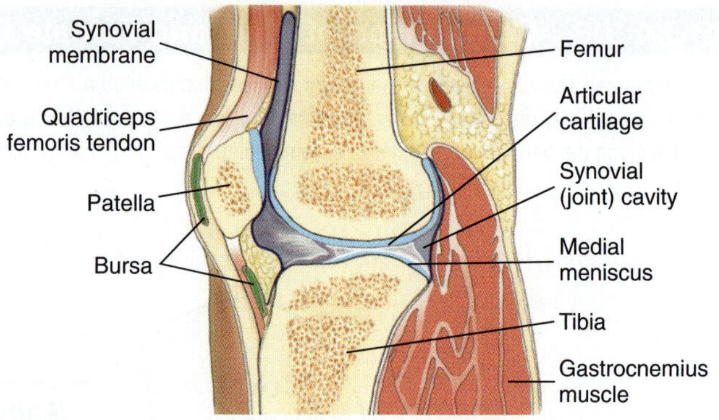

FIG. 3.8 The knee joint. (From Shiland B: *Mastering Healthcare Terminology*, ed 5, St. Louis, 2016, Elsevier.)

CRITICAL THINKING 3.3

As Dr. Martin examines Walter's hands, he has Walter open and close his hands, wiggle his fingers, grip tightly around two of Dr. Martin's fingers, and move his wrist. Throughout the whole exam, Dr. Martin is watching Walter's hands and wrist. Dr. Martin is looking at the ROM in Walter's hands. Describe in your own words what the acronym ROM means. List the three joint types (based on ROM), and give one example of each.

CRITICAL THINKING 3.4

Patsy has been a runner for years, but recently she was diagnosed with bursitis in her knees. Explain how Patsy's running may have contributed to this condition.

VOCABULARY
suture lines: Where the bones of the skull meet.

MEDICAL TERMINOLOGY
amphi-: both
articul/o, arthr/o: joint
dia-: through
-sis: condition
syn-: together
burs/o: bursa
menisc/o: meniscus
synovi/o: synovial
bursa (singular), **bursae** (plural)
meniscus (singular), **menisci** (plural)

Many of the synovial joints have *bursae* (BURR see). These are sacs of fluid located between the bones of the joint and the tendons that hold the muscles in place. Bursae help cushion and support the joints when they move. Synovial joints also have joint capsules that enclose the ends of the bones. A synovial membrane lines the joint capsules and secretes fluid to lubricate the joint, and cartilage that covers and protects the bone. The *meniscus* (mi NIS kuhs) consists of crescent-shaped cartilage in the knee joint that additionally cushions the joint. *Ligaments* are strong bands of white fibrous connective tissue that connect one bone to another bone at a joint. Fig. 3.9 shows the different types of joints and their movements.

Table 3.8 is a summary of the different types of diarthrotic joints, their movements, and examples in the body.

TABLE 3.8 Diarthrotic Joint Movement and Examples

Joint Name	Type of Movement	Examples
Ball-and-socket	Allows free movement, the joint can rotate	Shoulder and hip
Hinge	Allows movement in one axis, can allow for flexion and extension, but not rotation	Elbow, knee, and fingers
Pivot	Allows rotation	Between the first (atlas) and second (axis) cervical vertebrae of the spine
Saddle	Allows flexion, extension, and other movement, but not rotation	Between the wrist and the metacarpal bone of the thumb; allows thumb to cross over the palm of the hand—an opposable thumb
Gliding	Allows bone surfaces to slide over one another	The bones of the wrist and ankle, and between vertebrae
Condyloid (or ellipsoidal joints)	Allows movement is two directions: flexion-extension and circular motion	Between the first cervical vertebrae (atlas) and the base of the occipital bone of the skull

From Shiland B: *Mastering Healthcare Terminology*, ed 5, St. Louis, 2016, Elsevier.

CHAPTER 3 Musculoskeletal System   45

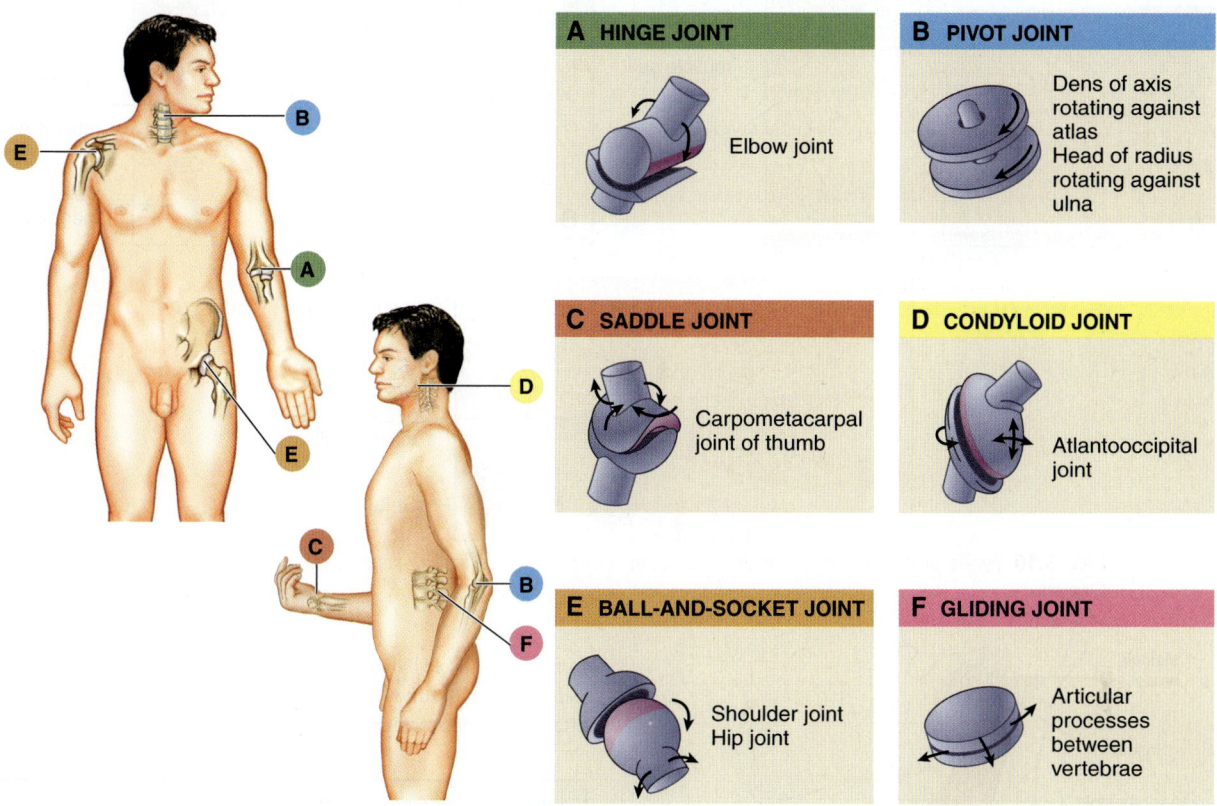

FIG. 3.9 Types of diarthrotic joints. (From Patton K: *Structure and Function of the Body*, ed 15, St. Louis, 2016, Elsevier.)

Muscles

A muscle is a tissue composed of cells that are able to contract and relax. Because of these two specialized actions, muscles along with joints and bones help move the body. The muscles in the human body are specialized into three different functions:

1. *Skeletal muscle* makes up about 40% of a person's body weight. It is *striated* (STRY aa ted), or striped in appearance and is attached to the bones of the skeleton by tendons. Most skeletal muscle allows the body to move voluntarily at the joints. There are more than 600 individual skeletal muscles on the body, but many of our muscles work in groups to bring about voluntary movement. Skeletal muscles have three primary functions:
   - Movement of the skeleton—primarily at the joints
   - Maintenance of posture—to maintain good muscle tone so muscles are ready to be active when needed
   - Generation of body heat—through the use of muscle groups, or shivering
2. *Cardiac muscle* is designed to allow the heart to contract and relax consistently. Cardiac muscle is also striated and has prominent dark bands called *intercalated* (inter CAH lait ed) *disks*. The intercalated disks are areas where plasma membranes from several cardiac muscle fibers meet. This allows electrical impulses to travel through the cardiac muscle in an efficient manner. Cardiac muscle also branches and then recombines to create long interconnected fibers. Because cardiac muscle contains intercalated disks and interconnected fibers, it is able to consistently create an efficient and coordinated contraction of the heart.
3. *Smooth muscle* makes up the walls of hollow internal organs, blood vessels, respiratory system passageways, and other structures in the body. Smooth muscle does not have striations like skeletal and cardiac muscle. Smooth muscle moves in a wavelike motion called *peristalsis* (pair ih STAL sis). This unique movement helps substances move through the body's internal organs easily and effectively.

Fig. 3.10 shows examples of each type of muscle in the human body.

Muscles are attached to bones by strong fibrous bands of connective tissue called *tendons*. The *origin* of a muscle is attached to a bone that does not move. The *insertion* of a muscle is attached to a bone that does move when the muscle contracts or relaxes. A muscle often crosses a joint between the origin and insertion. This joint is where movement will occur (Fig. 3.11). Some muscles work as opposites: when one muscle contracts, the other muscle relaxes. These are called *antagonistic muscles*. As an example of this process, a *flexor* (FLEK sor) muscle bends a joint, and an *extensor* (eks TEN sor) muscle stretches out a joint. *Synergistic muscles* work together to refine a movement. An example is the Hamstring muscle group. All three muscles that make up the Hamstring work together to properly flex the knee.

MEDICAL TERMINOLOGY

ex-: out	**muscul/o, my/o, myos/o:** muscle
flex/o: bending	**myocardi/o:** heart muscle
insert/o: introduce, put in	**peri-:** around
inter-: between	**-sis:** condition, process
-ion: action, condition, process of	**stal/o:** contraction
leiomy/o: smooth muscle	**tens/o:** stretching

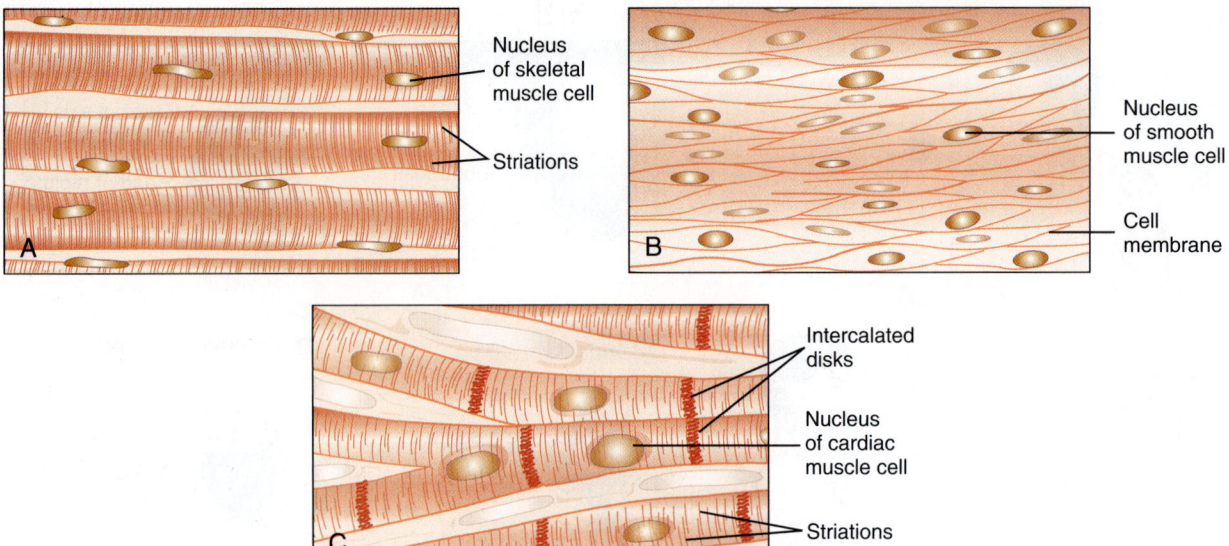

FIG. 3.10 Types of muscle. (From Proctor D, et al: *Kinn's The Medical Assistant*, ed 13, St. Louis, 2017, Elsevier.)

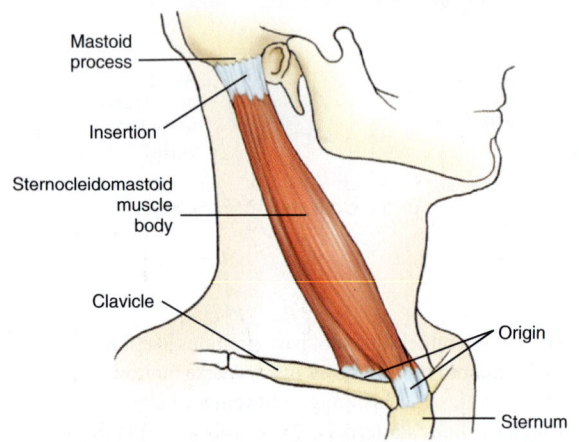

FIG. 3.11 Attachments of a skeletal muscle. (From Shiland B: *Mastering Healthcare Terminology*, ed 5, St. Louis, 2016, Elsevier.)

Structure of a Skeletal Muscle. In a skeletal muscle, individual muscle fibers are bundled together to form *fascicles* (FAS ih kuls). The individual muscles in the bundle lay parallel to each other so that when they contract, they all move in the same direction. Every muscle fiber is made up of **myofibrils** that contain thick strands of protein called *myosin* and thin strands of a protein called *actin*. Fascicles are held together with layers of tough connective tissue. All the layers of connective tissue join to form a tendon, which then secures a muscle to a bone.

> **VOCABULARY**
> **myofibrils:** A contractile fiber of skeletal muscle made up of mostly actin and myosin.

Muscle Naming Conventions. Although the principles used to name all the muscles in the body are too numerous to cover in this text, there are a few helpful conventions that can be followed. Refer to the Table 3.9 for examples of how muscles are named by their location, number of insertions, size, shape, and muscle action. Some muscles get their names from their general location. For instance, the pectoralis muscle is a large muscle in the chest (pector/o: chest). Another convention is to name a muscle by its origins and insertion. For example, the *sternocleidomastoid* (stur noh kly doh MASS toyd) muscle (see Fig. 3.11) attaches to the sternum, the clavicle, and the mastoid process.

> **MEDICAL TERMINOLOGY**
> **cleid/o-:** clavicle **rhabdomy/o:** skeletal muscle
> **mastoid/o:** mastoid **stern/o:** sternum
> **pector/o:** chest

Skeletal Muscles of the Human Body. The illustrations in Fig. 3.12 show anterior and posterior views of the major skeletal muscles of the body. Fig. 3.13 shows the muscles of the head and neck. Fig. 3.14 shows the muscles of the trunk. In addition, Table 3.10 lists the major muscles of the body grouped by their location and function.

> **CRITICAL THINKING 3.5**
> Which large leg muscles would Patsy use when she runs? Name some of the arm, back, and leg muscles Walter would use when he gardens.

PHYSIOLOGY OF THE MUSCULOSKELETAL SYSTEM

Muscle Cell in Action

Before a skeletal muscle can contract, it must be stimulated by an impulse that comes from the brain or spinal cord. The impulse moves away from the brain toward the muscle via a nerve cell. This type of nerve cell is called a *motor neuron*. The point of contact between the nerve ending and the muscle fiber is called a *neuromuscular junction (NMJ)*. An NMJ is an example of a *synapse*. A synapse is a point of communication between two cells. In this case, the two cells are the motor neuron and the muscle fiber. At the synapse, there is a very small gap called a *synaptic cleft*. Chemical messengers called *neurotransmitters* are released by the motor neuron in response to a nerve impulse. Neurotransmitters must travel across the synaptic cleft to continue the stimulus and generate a muscle contraction.

TABLE 3.9 Muscle Naming Conventions

Naming Device	Name of Muscle	Word Origin	Definition
Location	Zygomaticus	zygomatic/o zygoma -us noun ending	Cheek muscle that covers the zygomatic bone of the face
Number of insertions	Biceps brachii	bi- two ceps heads[a] brachi/o arm -i plural noun ending	Muscle that flexes upper arm
Size	Gluteus maximus	glute/o buttock -us noun ending maxim/o large -us noun ending	Large buttock muscle
Shape	Deltoid	delt/o triangle -oid like	Triangular muscle in upper back
Muscle action	Adductor longus	ad- toward duct/o carrying -or one who long/o long -us noun ending	Long upper leg muscle that carries one leg back to the midline
Origin/insertion	Sternocleidomastoid (see Fig. 3.11)	stern/o breastbone cleid/o collarbone mastoid/o mastoid process	Muscle that originates in the sternum and collarbone and inserts on the mastoid process

[a]ceps is a variation of cephal/o, the combining form for head. These word parts are used for "the head" or the beginning of a structure and also are used for bones (bone heads), as well as muscle heads.
From Shiland B: *Mastering Healthcare Terminology*, ed 5, St. Louis, 2016, Elsevier.

TABLE 3.10 Muscles of the Human Body

MUSCLES OF THE HEAD AND NECK

Muscle Name	Muscle Action
Frontal	Raises eyebrows
Orbicularis oculi (or bih kyoo LAIR is AW kyoo lie)	Closes eye
Orbicularis oris (or bih kyoo LAIR is OR is)	Draws lips together
Zygomaticus	Elevates corners of the lips and mouth
Masseter (MAS eh ter)	Closes jaws
Buccinator (buk sih NAY tor)	Flattens cheek, aids in chewing, allows a person to whistle or blow
Temporal	Closes jaws
Sternocleidomastoid (ster noh kly doh MAS toyd)	Rotates and flexes head and neck
Trapezius (trah PEE zee us)	Extends head and neck

MUSCLES OF THE UPPER EXTREMITIES

Muscle Name	Muscle Action
Pectoralis major (pek toh RAH lis)	Flexes and helps adduct the upper arm
Latissimus dorsi (lah TIH sih mus DOR sigh)	Extends and helps adduct upper arm
Deltoid (DEL toyd)	Abducts upper arm
Biceps brachii (BY seps BRAY kee eye)	Flexes elbow
Triceps brachii (TRY seps BRAY kee eye)	Extends elbow

MUSCLES OF THE TRUNK

Muscle Name	Muscle Action
External oblique (eks TER nal oh BLEEK)	Compresses abdomen
Internal oblique (in TER nal oh BLEEK)	Compresses abdomen
Transversus abdominis (trans ver sus ab DAW mih nis)	Compresses abdomen
Rectus abdominis	Flexes trunk
Diaphragm (DIE ah fram)	Expands thoracic (chest) cavity during inspiration

MUSCLES OF THE LOWER EXTREMITIES

Muscle Name	Muscle Action
Iliopsas (ill ee AWP sus)	Flexes thigh or trunk
Sartorius (sar TOR ee us)	Flexes thigh and rotates leg (allows a person to cross their legs)
Gluteus maximus (gloo TEE us MAK sih mus)	Extends thigh
Adductor group (ahd DUK tor)	Adducts thigh
Hamstring group (HAM string)	Flexes knee
Quadriceps group (KWAD rih seps)	Extends knee
Tibialis anterior (tib ee AL is)	Dorsiflexes ankle
Gastrocnemius (gas trawk NEE mee us)	Plantar flexes ankle
Soleus (SEW lee us)	Plantar flexes ankle
Peroneus group (also known as fibularis group) (pair oh NEE us)	Everts and plantar flexes ankle

From Shiland B: *Mastering Healthcare Terminology*, ed 5, St. Louis, 2016, Elsevier.

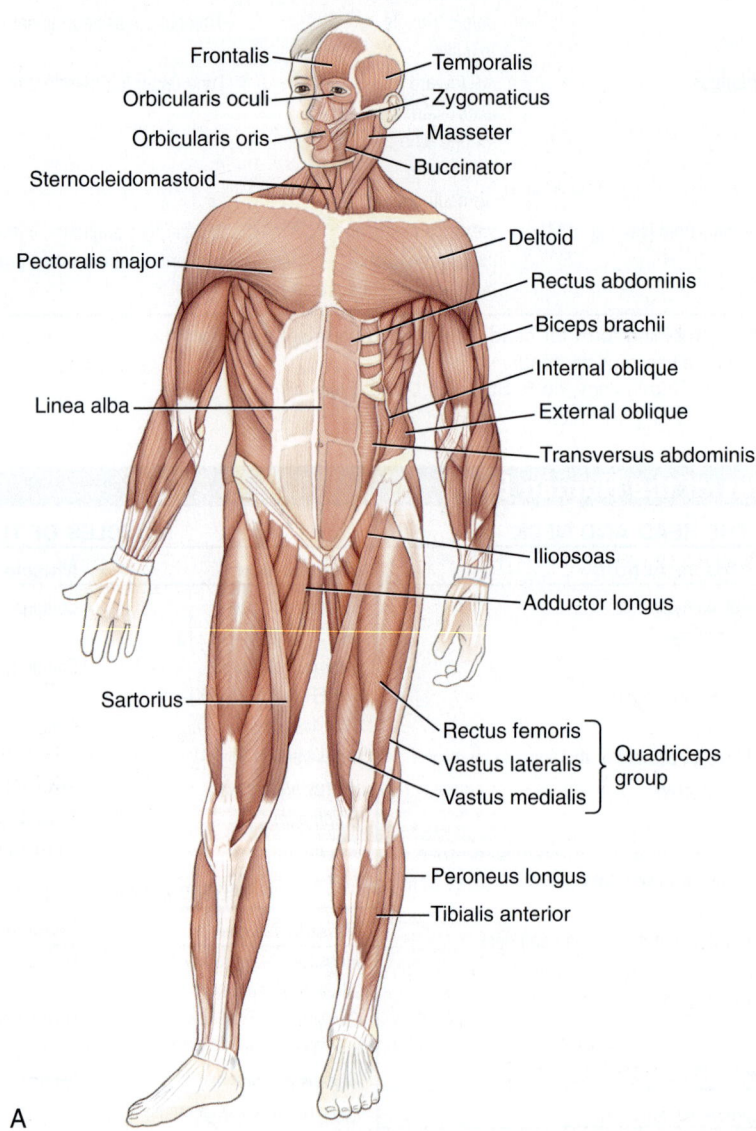

FIG. 3.12 Major muscles of the body, anterior (A) and posterior (B) views. (From Shiland B: *Mastering Healthcare Terminology*, ed 5, St. Louis, 2016, Elsevier.)

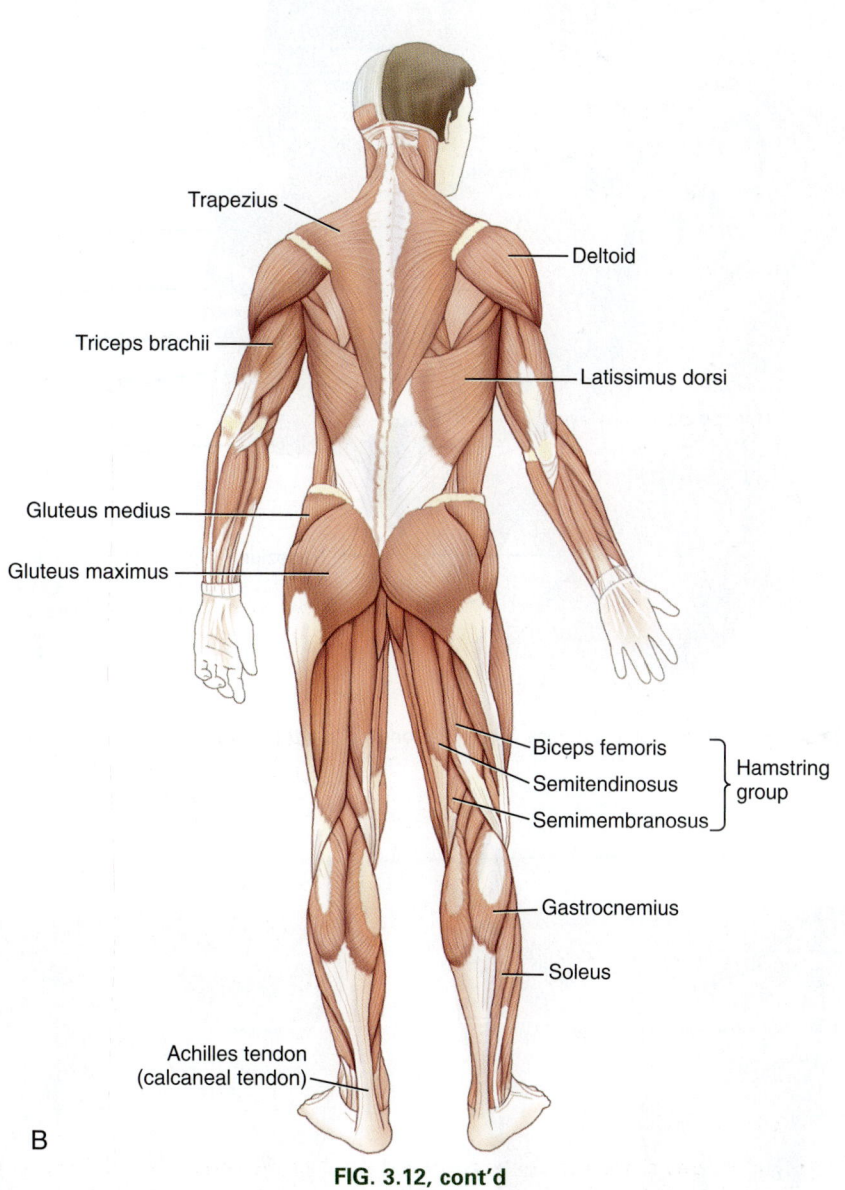

FIG. 3.12, cont'd

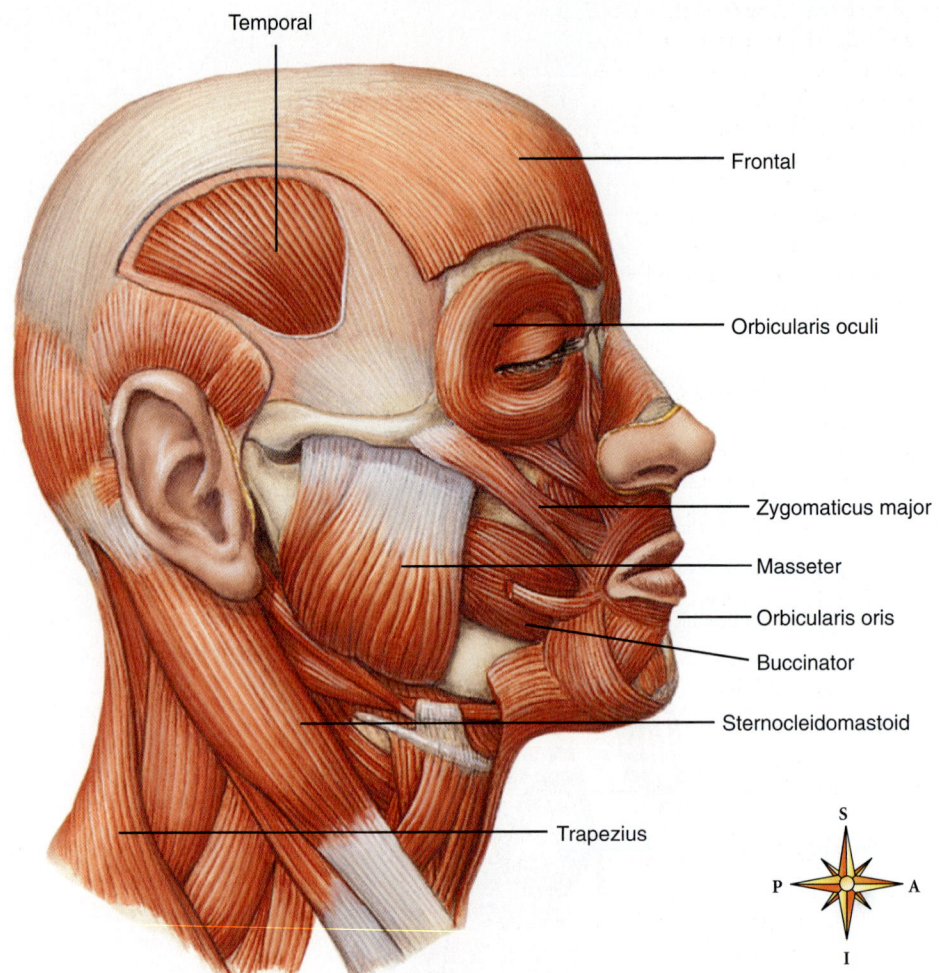

FIG. 3.13 Muscles of the head and neck. (From Patton K: *Structure and Function of the Body*, ed 15, St. Louis, 2016, Elsevier.)

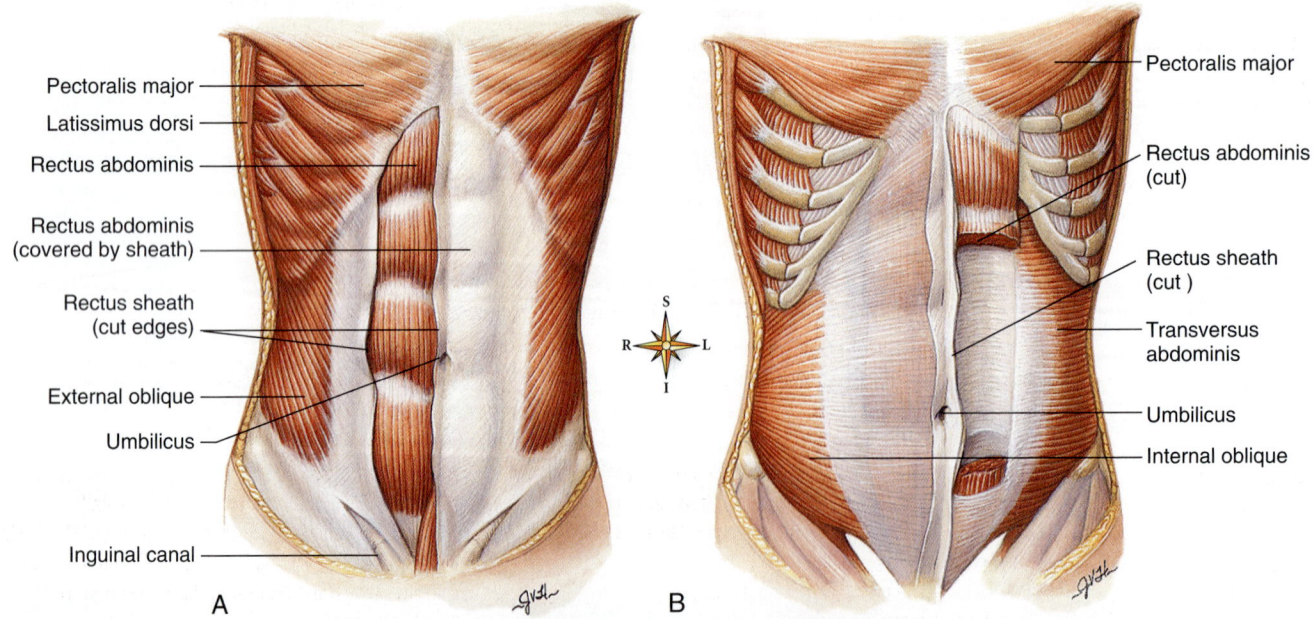

FIG. 3.14 Muscles of the trunk. (From Patton K: *Structure and Function of the Body*, ed 15, St. Louis, 2016, Elsevier.)

The neurotransmitter most often acting on skeletal muscle is acetylcholine (ACh). The released ACh triggers a change in the permeability of the individual muscle fiber. Then sodium ions flow into the fibers. This causes calcium to be released from their storage area in the muscle fiber. When calcium is released, the thin actin fibers slide between the thick myosin fibers, causing the muscle to shorten or *contract*. Without appropriate calcium levels, actin and myosin are unable to interact properly. Not only is calcium needed for muscle contraction, but the muscles also use energy in the form of ATP (adenosine triphosphate). The muscle will relax once the ACh is inactivated and the calcium ions are back in their storage areas of the muscle.

Types of Muscle Contractions

Think of how many times each day we use our muscles and how many chemical changes take place for just one muscle to contract. Even when we are not actively moving, our muscles are in a state of partial contraction called *muscle tone*. Nerve impulses help maintain muscle tone so that muscles are ready to act when needed. Muscle tone is an important factor in proper posture too.

The two types of muscle contractions that the body most frequently uses are *isotonic* (i so TON ick) and *isometric* (i so MEH trick) contractions:
- Isotonic: muscle contraction that usually produces movement at a joint. The muscle usually shortens and thickens (bulges), and a task is done. Examples include walking, running, lifting weight, and twisting.
- Isometric: muscle contraction usually does not produce movement. There is no change in muscle length, but there is an increase in muscle tension. Examples include pushing against an immovable object, pushing against a wall, and pushing palms together—there is no movement, but there is an increase in muscle tension.

Using muscles with regular exercise provides many benefits to our bodies as a whole. Box 3.4 describes some of them.

Impact of Exercise on Skeletal Muscles

Exercise affects the muscles in different ways depending on the type of exercise. There are three main constituents of exercise:
- Stretching
- Aerobic conditioning
- Resistance training

All three types of exercise are beneficial and affect muscles in unique ways. See Table 3.11 for an explanation of the benefits of each type of exercise. Box 3.5 describes the impact of aging on muscles.

CRITICAL THINKING 3.6

Walter tells Dr. Martin about his love of gardening. He loves being outdoors and feeling the dirt on his hands. Dr. Martin palpates the sore muscle on Walter's forearm and asks about the gardening activities that make the pain worse. Walter replies, "The activities that hurt the most are digging, pulling weeds, and pushing dirt in around the small plants." Which of these three actions are an isotonic contraction of the muscle, and which are isometric?

MEDICAL TERMINOLOGY
a-: without, away from,
hyper-: above, more than normal
neur/o: nerve
troph/o: development

VOCABULARY
acetylcholine (ACh): A substance that is released at the junction between neurons and muscle fibers; a chemical messenger.
ATP (adenosine triphosphate): A high-energy molecule, found in every cell, that supplies large amounts of energy for various biochemical processes.
metabolism: The chemical processes that occur within a living organism in order to maintain life.
permeability: A quality or characteristic of a material that allows another substance to pass through it.

Types of Muscle Action

Table 3.12 summarizes the types of muscle action. Stand up and go through the muscle action as a class or with a friend.

BOX 3.4 Benefits of Regular Exercise

Benefits of regular exercise include the following:
- Improved muscle tone and size (*hypertrophy*)
- Better posture
- More efficient heart and lung function
- Less fatigue
- Looking and feeling better

Prolonged inactivity causes disuse *atrophy*.

TABLE 3.11 Benefits of Exercise

Type of Exercise	Example	Benefits to Muscles
Stretching	Yoga, active stretching, static stretching	Muscles can interact over a greater length Improves flexibility at the joints Improves overall balance
Aerobic conditioning	Running, biking, swimming, or any continuous, rhythmic movement of large muscle groups to strengthen the heart and lungs (cardiovascular system)	Improved endurance Increased number of capillaries, brings more blood to cells Increased number of mitochondria, increase in energy (ATP) to cells Oxygen and glucose delivery can become more efficient to muscles
Resistance training	Free weights, weight machines, body weight workout, resistance bands	Muscle cells increase in size, hypertrophy (hahy-PUR-truh-fee) Increased muscle strength

From Shiland B: *Mastering Healthcare Terminology*, ed 5, St. Louis, 2016, Elsevier.

BOX 3.5 Impact of Aging on the Muscles

As people age and their activity levels decrease, the skeletal muscles of the body can be affected in the following ways:
- Gradual loss of muscle cells resulting in decreased muscle size
- Decreased muscle tone
- Disuse atrophy
- Decreased overall metabolism
- Poor posture that may contribute to kyphosis, also known as a humpback posture; affects the skeleton and muscles of the upper back; may be caused by osteoporosis

DISEASES AND DISORDERS OF THE MUSCULOSKELETAL SYSTEM

The skeleton, muscles, and joints together work as a unit to move the body. Diseases of the musculoskeletal system often affect the ability to move with ease. Some conditions may be temporary and inconvenient. Other disease states are chronic conditions that affect a person's quality of life. Box 3.6 describes some of the common symptoms of diseases and disorders of the musculoskeletal system. As with each system we will explore, there are some disease states that can be fatal. Tables 3.13 and 3.14 describe imaging technologies and diagnostic testing related to the musculoskeletal system.

TABLE 3.12 Muscle Actions

Action	Word Origin	Description
Extension (ecks TEN shun)	**ex-** out **tens/o** stretching **-ion** process of	Process of stretching out; increasing the angle of a joint
Flexion (FLEK shun)	**flex/o** bending **-ion** process of	Process of decreasing the angle of a joint
Abduction (ab DUK shun)	**ab-** away from **duct/o** carrying **-ion** process of	Process of carrying away from the midline
Adduction (ad DUK shun)	**ad-** toward **duct/o** carrying **-ion** process of	Process of carrying toward the midline
Supination (soo pin NAY shun)		Turning the palm upward
Pronation (proh NAY shun)		Turning the palm downward
Dorsiflexion (DOOR sih flek shun)	**dors/i** back **flex/o** bending **-ion** process of	Process of bending back

TABLE 3.12 Muscle Actions—cont'd

	Action	Word Origin	Description
	Plantar flexion (PLAN tar FLEK shun)	**plant/o** sole **-ar** pertaining to **flex/o** bending **-ion** process of	Lowering the foot; pointing the toes away from the shin
	Eversion (ee VER shun)	**e-** out **vers/o** turning **-ion** process of	Process of turning out
	Inversion (in VER shun)	**in-** in **vers/o** turning **-ion** process of	Process of turning in
	Protraction (proh TRAK shun)	**pro-** forward **tract/o** pulling **-ion** process of	Process of pulling forward; the forward movement of a muscle
	Retraction (ree TRAK shun)	**re-** backward **tract/o** pulling **-ion** process of	Process of backward pulling; the backward movement of a muscle
	Rotation (roh TAY shun)	**rot/o** wheel **-ation** process of	Process of a bone turning on its axis (like a wheel)
	Circumduction (ser KUM duk shun)	**circum-** around **duct/o** carrying **-ion** process of	Process of carrying around; the circular movement of the distal end of a limb around its point of attachment

From Shiland B: *Mastering Healthcare Terminology*, ed 5, St. Louis, 2016, Elsevier.

TABLE 3.13 Imaging Technologies Related to Musculoskeletal Diagnosis

Term	Definition
Arthrography (ar THRAH gruh fee)	X-ray recording of a joint
Arthroscopy (ar THRAHS kuh pee)	Visual examination of a joint, accomplished by use of an arthroscope
Bone scan	A small amount of radioactive material is injected into a vein; the radioactive material is attracted to damaged area of bone; fractures show up as bright spots on the image
Computerized tomography (CT) scan	Imaging technology that records transverse planes of the body for diagnostic purposes
Dual energy x-ray absorptiometry (DEXA) scan (DECK suh)	A procedure that measures the density of bone at the hip and spine. Also called *bone mineral density studies*
Electromyography (EMG) (ee leck troh mye AH gruh fee)	Procedure that records the electrical activity of muscles
Magnetic resonance imaging (MRI)	Procedure that uses magnetic properties to record detailed information about internal structures
Myelogram (MYE eh loh gram)	X-ray of spinal canal done after injection of contrast medium
X-ray (radiograph)	Imaging technique using electromagnetic radiation for recording internal structures; images from several different angles may be taken so that abnormalities can be detected

From Shiland B: *Mastering Healthcare Terminology*, ed 5, St. Louis, 2016, Elsevier.

BOX 3.6 Common Symptoms of Musculoskeletal Diseases and Disorders

Common symptoms of musculoskeletal disease and disorders include the following:
- Pain or swelling in the joints, muscles, or bones
- Fatigue, malaise
- Myalgia, myositis, muscle tenderness
- Inflammation
- Temporary loss of function or loss of normal mobility

CRITICAL THINKING 3.7

As Dr. Martin finishes his exam with Walter, he asks Patsy to join them as they discuss Walter's test results. Dr. Martin ordered an RF test, Lyme disease antibody test, ESR, and C-reactive protein (CRP) through the clinical laboratory. He also ordered a series of hand x-rays and knee x-rays. What information will each of the lab tests tell Dr. Martin? What will the x-rays of the hands and knees show him?

VOCABULARY

density: Describes how compact or concentrated something is.
inflammation: A localized reaction that produces redness, warmth, swelling, and pain because of infection, irritation, or injury. Inflammation can be external or internal. It can become chronic and affect the body as a whole.
malaise: A condition of general bodily weakness or discomfort, often marking the onset of a disease.
myalgia: Pain in a muscle or group of muscles.
myositis: Inflammation of a muscle or group of muscles.

MEDICAL TERMINOLOGY

goni/o: angle
-gram: record, recording
-graphy: process of recording
-metry: process of measuring
myel/o: spinal cord
-oid: resembling
rheumat/o: watery flow
-scopy: process of viewing
tom/o: section
trauma: A physical injury or wound caused by an external force or violence.

Fractures

Trauma to the body can cause a variety of injuries. The following pages will identify and describe some musculoskeletal conditions that can be caused by trauma or an accident.

A *fracture* is a broken bone. However, there are a few different types of breaks. Broken bones need to be realigned and repaired so that proper movement can be recovered. All fractures are first classified as *simple* or *compound*:

- A simple fracture does not break through the skin.
- A compound fracture does break through the skin. Bone can be seen protruding at the site of the break.
- Compound fractures generally are considered more complicated. There is a greater opportunity for infection, and repairing the break is often more difficult.
- See Table 3.15 for a summary of the different types of fractures.

Etiology. Most fractures occur because of physical trauma or an accident. Some fractures result from an underlying disease, such as osteoporosis or cancer. A fracture that results from an existing disease is called a *pathologic fracture* or a *spontaneous fracture*.

Signs and Symptoms. Symptoms of a simple bone fracture include the following:
- Pain, often immediately after an injury that increases with activity
- Swelling, tenderness, and bruising at or near the break site
- Throbbing pain that increases with activity and decreases with rest

TABLE 3.14 Diagnostic Testing Related to Musculoskeletal Diagnosis

Term	Definition
Cyclic citrullinated peptide antibody (anti-CCP)	Anti-CCP is an autoantibody produced by the immune system. This test is used to help diagnose rheumatoid arthritis and evaluate the severity and likely prognosis of an individual patient.
C-reactive protein (CRP)	CRP is a nonspecific marker for inflammation in the body. CRP is produced in the liver and measured by testing the blood. CRP levels rise in response to inflammation.
Erythrocyte sedimentation rate (ESR)	Sometimes called a sed rate, an ESR measures the rate that red blood cells (RBCs) settle to the bottom of a calibrated tube. Inflammation causes abnormal proteins to appear in the blood. When this happens, RBCs clump and settle faster than normal. A higher than normal sed rate is a nonspecific indicator of inflammation in the body. This is a CLIA-waived test.
Goniometry (goh nee AH meh tree)	The process of measuring a joint's ROM. The instrument used is called a *goniometer* (Fig. 3.15).
Lyme disease blood antibodies	Lab test that looks for antibodies to *Borrelia burgdorferi* in the blood. Used in combination with physical signs and symptoms to diagnose Lyme disease. Some CLIA-waived tests.
Phalen test (FAY lin)	A diagnostic test in which the back (dorsal surfaces) of the patient's hands are pressed together to elicit the symptoms of carpal tunnel syndrome (Fig. 3.16).
Range of motion (ROM) testing	An assessment of the degree to which a joint can be extended and flexed.
Rheumatoid factor (RF) test (ROO mah toyd)	Lab test that looks for RF present in the blood of those who may have rheumatoid arthritis.
Serum calcium (Ca)	Test to measure the amount of calcium in the blood.

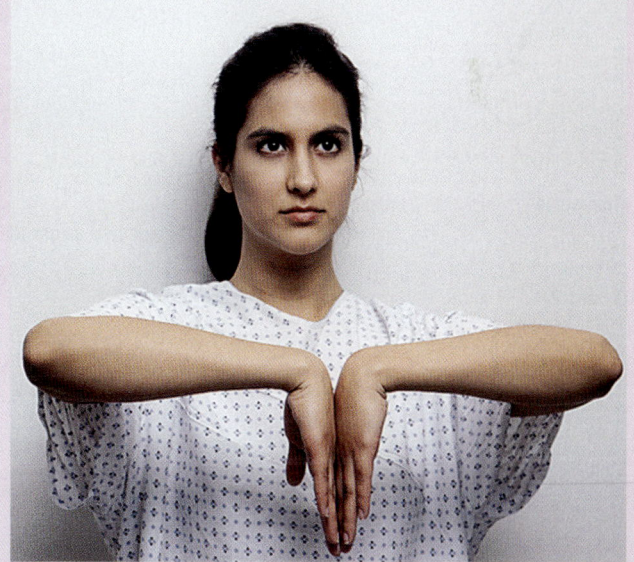

FIG. 3.15 Goniometry using a goniometer. (From Wilson SF, Giddens JF: *Health Assessment for Nursing Practice,* ed 4, St. Louis, 2012, Mosby.)

FIG. 3.16 Phalen test. (From Shiland B: *Mastering Healthcare Terminology,* ed 5, St. Louis, 2016, Elsevier.)

From Shiland B: *Mastering Healthcare Terminology,* ed 5, St. Louis, 2016, Elsevier.

- Deformity or distortion of a limb
- Difficulty using the affected area; difficulty walking or lifting an object

Symptoms of a compound bone fracture include the following:
- Severe pain
- Deformity or distortion of a limb
- Difficulty or inability to use the affected area; difficulty walking or lifting an object
- Bleeding at the site of bone breaking through the skin

Diagnostic Procedures. Most fractures require imaging. The provider may order one or more of the following imaging tests: x-rays, bone scan, computed tomography (CT) scan, or magnetic resonance imaging (MRI) (see Table 3.13). Many fractures can be seen on x-rays; however, some, like stress fractures, may not show up on x-rays until the bones have started to heal. Images from several different angles may be taken so that the fracture can be detected. See Chapter 2 or Table 3.13 for more detail on CT scans.

Treatment. Treatments for fracture can range from rest and over-the-counter (OTC) medication to surgery. Broken bones must be "set"—that is, aligned and immobilized; the most common method is with a plaster or fiberglass cast. If a bone does not mend and realign correctly, it is said to be a *malunion*. If no healing takes place, it is a *nonunion*. A piece of bone that does not have a renewed blood supply will die; this tissue then is called a sequestrum (seh KWES trum). Removal of dirt, damaged tissue, or foreign objects from a wound is one of the first steps in repairing a compound fracture. The removal of debris is called

TABLE 3.15 Types of Fractures

Fracture	Definition	Fracture	Definition
Closed, or simple	Broken bone is contained within intact skin.	Comminuted	Break is caused by a severe, direct force, which creates a fracture with multiple fragments.
Open, or compound	Skin is broken above the fracture; open to the external environment creating the potential for infection.	Impacted	Break is caused by strong forces that drive bone fragments firmly together.
Longitudinal	Fracture extends along the length of the bone.	Pathologic	Break results from weakening of the bones by disease, as in osteoporosis or sarcoma.
Transverse	Break is caused by direct force applied perpendicular to a bone; fracture runs across the bone.	Nondisplaced	Bone ends remain in alignment.
Oblique	Break is caused by a twisting force with an upward thrust; fracture ends are short and run at an oblique angle across the bone.	Displaced	Bone ends are moved out of alignment.
Greenstick	Break is caused by compression or angulation forces in the long bones of children under age 10; because of its softness, the bone is cracked on one side and intact on the other side.		

TABLE 3.15 Types of Fractures—cont'd

Fracture	Definition	Fracture	Definition
Spiral	Break is caused by a twisting or rotary force, which results in long, sharp, pointed bone ends; suspicious as a child abuse injury.	Avulsion	Break is caused by forceful contraction of a muscle against resistance, and a bone fragment tears at the site of muscle insertion.
		Depression	Bone fragments of the skull are driven inward.
Compression	Break is caused by forces that drive bones together; typically seen in the vertebrae.		

From Chester GA: *Modern Medical Assisting,* Philadelphia, 1999, Saunders.

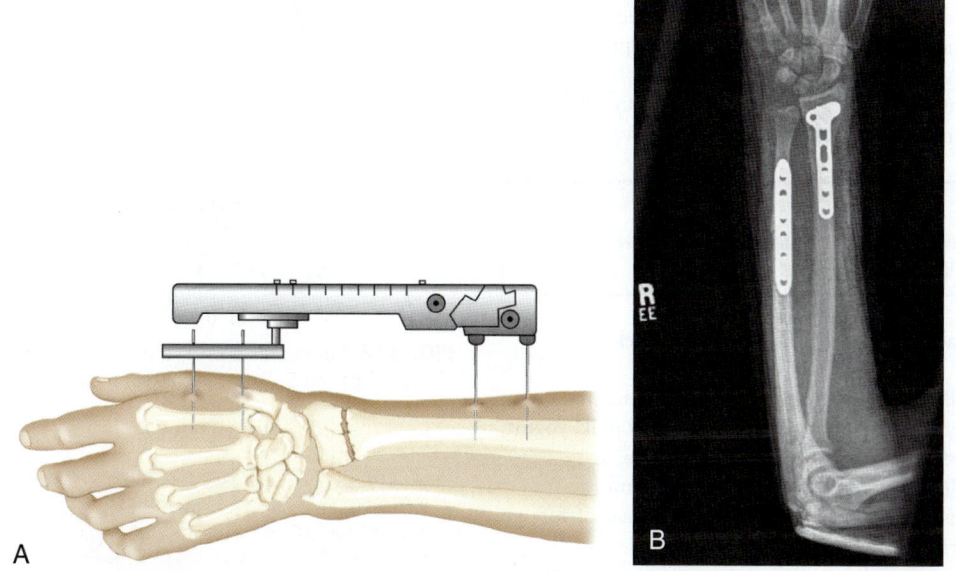

FIG. 3.17 Fixation. (A) External. (B) Internal. (From Kowalczyk N: *Radiographic Pathology for Technologists,* ed 5, St. Louis, 2009, Mosby.)

débridement (de breed MONT). Methods of *fixation* and alignment are described as follows:
- *Reduction.* A displaced fracture may require the manipulation of bones to correctly align their position. Depending on the fracture, this may be done with or without surgery. Muscle relaxants, sedatives, or even general anesthetic may be used to perform this procedure. A closed reduction (CR) does not require an incision. A *CREF* is a closed reduction using external fixation (Fig. 3.17A).
- *Surgical procedures.* If a fracture is compound, comminuted, impacted, or displaced, surgery may be performed to accurately align the bones (called open reduction). Without correct bone alignment, the fracture will not heal properly. An orthopedic surgeon may need to use internal fixation hardware (e.g., screw, pins, or plates) to properly position bones during healing. This type of surgery is called open reduction and internal fixation (*ORIF*). The hardware may be removed after the fracture has healed if it is causing problems (Fig. 3.17B).
- *Immobilization.* To heal, a fractured bone, once in place, must be immobilized so that its ends can heal. A fracture may require the use of the following:
  - An elastic wrap bandage with or without a splint
  - Taping and padding the affected area
  - A removable brace, boot, or shoe with a stiff sole
  - A splint to stabilize the break until the initial swelling goes down; then a hard plaster or fiberglass cast is applied
- *Medications.* Depending on the severity of the fracture, the provider may recommend medications such as the following:
  - Analgesics: morphine, hydrocodone, acetaminophen
  - Antiinflammatory drugs: nonsteroidal antiinflammatory drugs (NSAIDs) and steroids
  - Muscle relaxants

TABLE 3.16 Additional Musculoskeletal Traumas

Feature/Trauma	Sprain Strain Dislocation Subluxation
Signs and symptoms	Swelling, pain, and possible discoloration or bruising at the site of injury
Diagnostic procedures	Physical exam, x-rays, or MRI
Treatment: nondrug treatment	A range of treatments may be used starting with: elevation, rest, ice to affected area Crutches, braces, boots, and other aids may be required to stabilize the affected joint Physical therapy Torn ligaments, tendons, severe or repeated dislocations, and subluxations may require surgical repair
Treatment: medications	Depending on the severity of the trauma, one of the following medications may be recommended: Analgesics: morphine, hydrocodone, acetaminophen Antiinflammatory drugs: NSAIDs and steroids Muscle relaxants
Prognosis	Good with treatment and follow-up Grade III sprains, dislocations, and subluxations with surgery may take a year or longer to heal completely
Prevention	Try to avoid traumas that may cause injuries Try to avoid traumas and activities that cause the injury Avoid overuse and repetitive movements of ligaments and tendons if possible

From Shiland B: *Mastering Healthcare Terminology*, ed 5, St. Louis, 2016, Elsevier.

- *Physical therapy*. After a fracture has healed, muscles, ligaments, and tendons may need to be strengthened and stretched. Structured physical therapy and home exercises may be used to improve strength and flexibility.

Follow-up is usually required during the healing process and then again after the completion of any required physical therapy treatment.

> **VOCABULARY**
> **sequestrum**: A fragment of bone that has died as a result of disease or injury and has separated from the normal bone structure.

Prognosis. Most fractures heal well within 6 to 12 weeks.

Prevention. The following helpful tips may prevent fractures:
- Build bone strength. Eat calcium-rich foods, such as milk, yogurt, and cheese.
- Talk to the provider about vitamin D supplementation.
- Keep walkways inside and outside of a residence clear of foreign objects to avoid tripping and falling.
- Use safety equipment and precautions for exercise and athletic activities.
- Alternate exercise activities to prevent stress fractures.

Additional Musculoskeletal Traumas

Musculoskeletal trauma is not always a fracture. Damage to tendons, ligaments, and joints are defined here. See Table 3.16 for more information regarding additional traumas.

Definition of Additional Traumas

- *Sprain*: traumatic injury to a ligament, further categorized as the following (Fig. 3.18B):
  - Grade I: stretching of a ligament
  - Grade II: partial tearing of a ligament
  - Grade III: complete tear of a ligament
- Strain (Fig. 3.18A): tear, partial tear, overuse, or overstretching of a muscle or tendon
- Dislocation (Fig. 3.19): bone that is completely displaced out of its joint socket
- Subluxation: a partial dislocation

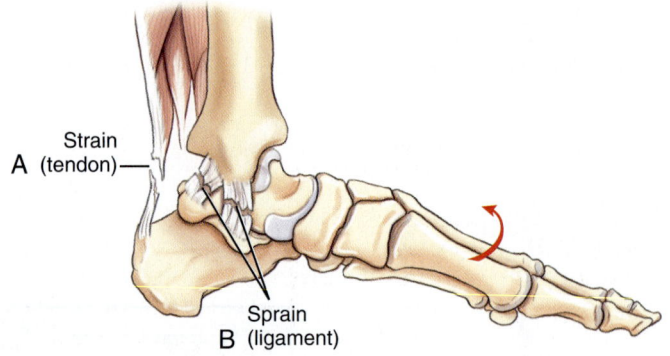

FIG. 3.18 Strain and sprain. (From Shiland B: *Mastering Healthcare Terminology*, ed 5, St. Louis, 2016, Elsevier.)

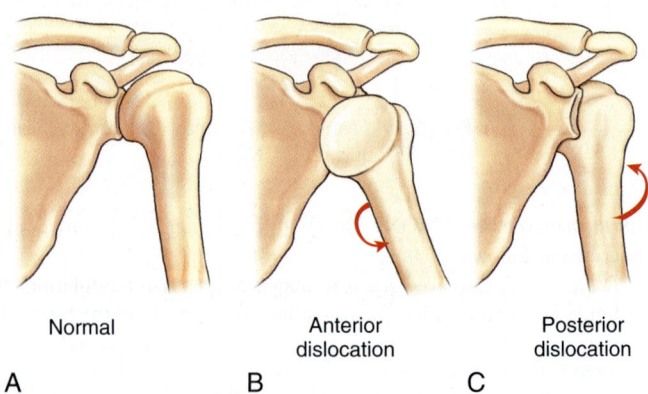

FIG. 3.19 Joint dislocation. (From Shiland B: *Mastering Healthcare Terminology*, ed 5, St. Louis, 2016, Elsevier.)

Etiology. The cause of most nonfracture trauma to the musculoskeletal system is accidental. Traumas can be associated with repetitive use, overstretching, a blow to a specific area of the body, or a fall. Many activities can cause trauma; see Table 3.16 for additional information. Box 3.7 describes an option for treatment using complementary medical practices.

BOX 3.7 Chiropractic Care

Some people find chiropractic care to be a very useful complementary treatment method for musculoskeletal conditions. Chiropractic adjustments involve gentle and precise manipulations of the skeleton. Make sure to ask about chiropractic care when taking the patient's history.

CRITICAL THINKING 3.8

Dr. Martin did not order x-rays on Walter's arm because Walter is feeling muscle pain. What type of muscle trauma could Walter be experiencing? What would the recommendations for treatment be?

Arthritis

Arthritis is a term that refers to any inflammatory joint condition. There are about 100 types of arthritis, and proper diagnosis is needed to develop an effective treatment plan. Arthritis can have a variety of causes:
- Autoimmunity
- Infection
- Injury
- Genetic conditions

Table 3.17 presents three of the most common types of arthritis.

CRITICAL THINKING 3.9

Dr. Martin has asked Patsy to come into the exam room as he and Walter discuss his test results. Patsy brings up Walter's electronic health record (EHR) and takes notes during the discussion. The RF test is negative, and the CRP and ESR are only slightly elevated. What do these test results indicate?

Bursitis

Bursitis (bur-SY-tis) is a painful inflammation of small, fluid-filled sacs called bursae. The sacs help cushion bones, tendons, and muscles near the joints. Bursitis occurs when bursae become irritated and inflamed. The most common locations for bursitis are in the shoulder, elbow, and hip. The knee, heel, and base of the big toe can also be affected. Bursitis often occurs near joints that perform frequent repetitive motion.

Etiology. Repetitive motions or positions that irritate the bursae around a joint are the most common causes of bursitis. Examples include repetitive lifting and throwing, or leaning or kneeling for long periods of time. Other causes include injury or trauma to an affected joint. Inflammatory arthritis, such as rheumatoid arthritis or gout, can also cause bursitis.

TABLE 3.17 Arthritis: Rheumatoid, Gout, and Infection

Feature/Arthritis	Rheumatoid Arthritis	Gout	Infection
Etiology	Autoimmune disease Antibodies attack the synovial lining of joints causing chronic inflammation Inflammation spreads to affect cartilage, connective tissue Eventually can affect blood vessels, eyes, lungs, and heart	Metabolic condition where uric acid increases in the blood Sodium urate crystals (needle-like in shape) are deposited in the joints, which causes inflammation Can be chronic and cause continued inflammation and tissue damage	Lyme disease is caused by the bite of a tick infected with the bacteria *Borrelia burgdorferi*
Signs and symptoms	Joint pain, especially in the morning Fatigue Fever Weight loss Anemia As the disease progresses, additional signs and symptoms can be seen in the eyes, skin, lungs, heart, kidneys, nerve tissue, blood vessels Joint deformity including ulnar deviation or shift (see Fig. 3.20)	Joint pain—intense Red, tender, inflamed Pain often starts in the joint of the big toe, but can occur in any joint Pain is most intense in the first 4–12 hours of occurrence Pain may last a few days or weeks Recurrent pain tends to last longer and involve more joints Limited range of motion (ROM)	Joint pain—possible early in the infection, possible throughout the course of the disease if initial infection is not diagnosed/treated Early symptoms include bull's eye red rash at the area of tick bite and flulike symptoms If undiagnosed and untreated, symptoms can progress to arthritis, numbness or tingling in hands and feet, malaise, trouble concentrating or focusing, numbness or paralysis in facial muscles (Bell palsy); skin, heart, and nervous system complications
Diagnostic procedures	**Laboratory Tests** ESR, CRP, RF, and anticyclic citrullinated peptide (see Table 3.14) Imaging X-ray and MRI	**Laboratory Tests** Microscopic joint fluid examination may reveal urate crystals Blood test-uric acid and creatinine RF, CRP, and blood test for Lyme's disease antibodies Imaging X-ray, ultrasound, and CT scan	**Laboratory Tests** Blood test for Lyme disease antibodies Imaging X-ray or MRI in undiagnosed and untreated cases to see the extent of joint damage RF and CRP

TABLE 3.17 Arthritis: Rheumatoid, Gout, and Infection—cont'd

Feature/Arthritis	Rheumatoid Arthritis	Gout	Infection
Treatment: nondrug therapy	Physical and occupational therapy Assistive aids for daily living Exercise that is gentle on joints: tai chi, swimming, yoga Surgery to repair or replace joints and tendons, joint fusion	Limit alcoholic and fructose-sweetened drinks Drink plenty of water daily Limit intake of red meat, poultry, and seafood Exercise regularly and maintain desired weight Home remedy: sour cherry juice during flare-ups Check with healthcare provider first	See prevention
Treatment: medications	Antiinflammatory drugs (NSAIDs and steroids) Disease-modifying antirheumatic drugs (DMARDs) Biologic response modifiers, this newer class of DMARDs	Antigout Antiinflammatory drugs (NSAIDs and steroids)	Antibiotics Analgesics Antiinflammatory drugs (NSAIDs and steroids)
Prognosis	Prognosis for all three conditions is good with early intervention and patient compliance with medication and lifestyle changes Prognosis for all three can be poor if early intervention does not take place and with patient noncompliance for medication and lifestyle changes; chronic inflammation brings many serious complications over time		
Prevention	Rheumatoid arthritis is an autoimmune disease. It cannot be prevented but can be managed through medication and lifestyle adjustments	Once gout has been diagnosed, do the following to limit or eliminate recurrences: high fluid intake, especially water; avoid alcohol; limit intake of meat, fish, and poultry; maintain a desirable body weight; avoid fasting or rapid weight loss.	Prevent tick bites when in wooded or grassy areas: cover skin with light-colored clothing; wear a hat, long-sleeved shirt, long pants with the legs tucked into socks; use a bug repellent that contains DEET, IR3535, or Picaridin; treat and check pets for ticks

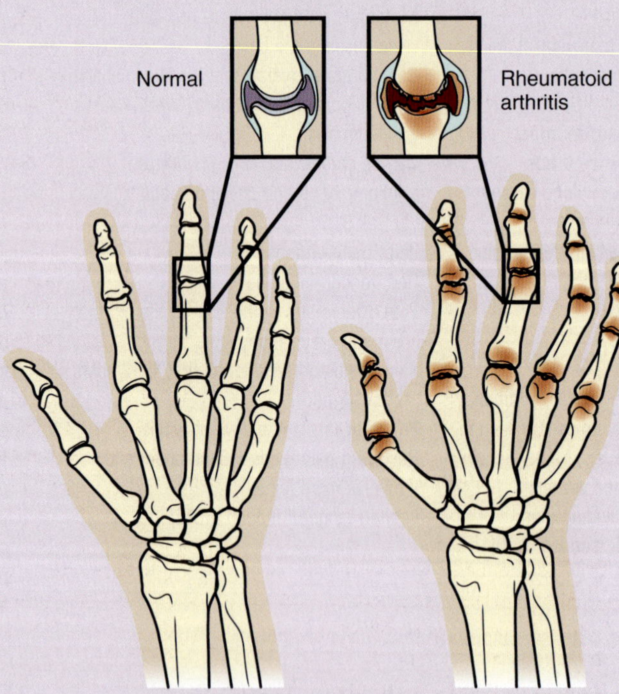

FIG. 3.20 Rheumatoid arthritis.

From Shiland B: *Mastering Healthcare Terminology,* ed 5, St. Louis, 2016, Elsevier.

Signs and Symptoms. Someone with bursitis may experience the following signs and symptoms:
- Affected joint may be stiff or achy
- Joint may look swollen or red
- Pain with movement, feels better with rest
- Joint may hurt more if the patient/provider presses on the area

Diagnostic Procedures
- History and physical exam
- X-rays may be used to exclude other possible conditions
- Ultrasound or MRI may be recommended

Treatment
- Resting the joint and ice at the site of inflammation
- Medications include acetaminophen, NSAIDs; ibuprofen and naproxen sodium
- Provider may recommend physical therapy to strengthen the joint and prevent a recurrence
- Injection of corticosteroids into the bursa can help relieve inflammation, especially in the shoulder or hip
- Assistive devices such as a cane or walker to take pressure off the affected joint
- Surgical drainage or removal of the affected bursa is rare but may be necessary for a severely damaged bursa

Prognosis. The prognosis is generally good. Usually bursae heal within 1 to 6 months. Repeated damage may lengthen the healing process.

Prevention. Not all types of bursitis can be prevented. To reduce the risk of bursitis and its recurrence, patients are educated about the following activities:
- Lifting properly
- Taking frequent breaks when doing repetitive tasks, such as lifting, kneeling, or carrying heavy loads
- Using kneeling pads, wheeled carts, wheelbarrows, and other assistive devices for repetitive tasks
- Avoiding sitting for too long; getting up and moving to relieve pressure on the bursae of the hips and buttocks
- Exercising to strengthen muscles and stay flexible
- Maintaining a healthy weight

Carpal Tunnel Syndrome

Carpal tunnel syndrome is caused by a pinched nerve in the wrist (Fig. 3.21). The carpal tunnel is a narrow passageway located on the palm side of the wrist and is surrounded by bones and ligaments. This tunnel protects the median nerve to the hand and the nine tendons that bend the fingers.

Etiology. Anything that compresses or irritates the median nerve in the carpal tunnel space can lead to carpal tunnel syndrome. For example, rheumatoid arthritis can cause inflammation or a fracture of the wrist can irritate the median nerve. Repetitive motion can also irritate the nerve or cause inflammation in the carpal space. Sometimes one specific cause cannot be found, and a combination of factors contribute to the condition.

Signs and Symptoms
- Starts as a gradual tingling or numbness of the thumb, index, and middle fingers; no tingling or numbness in the little finger
- Symptoms can come and go initially but can worsen and become more persistent with time

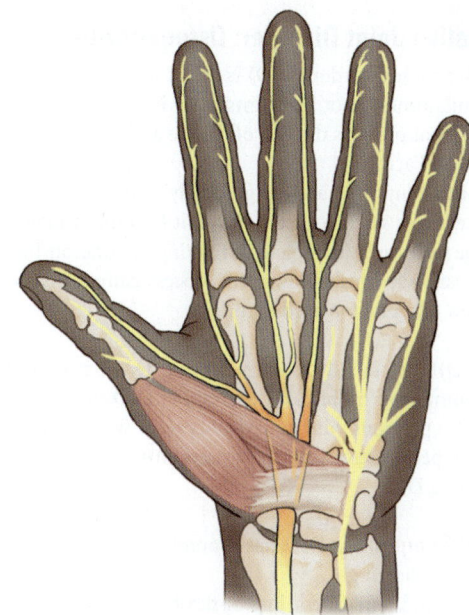

FIG. 3.21 Carpal tunnel syndrome. (From Lewis SM: *Medical-Surgical Nursing: Assessment and Management of Clinical Problems*, ed 8, St. Louis, 2011, Mosby.)

- Weakness in the hands; may drop items more frequently and be unable to pinch or grasp due to weakness of the thumb and index finger

Diagnostic Procedures
- History of symptoms and the timing of symptoms (to determine during what type of activity the symptoms occur)
- Physical exam that may include bending the wrist, tapping or pressing on the nerve
- X-rays may be recommended to rule out other causes of wrist pain
- Electromyogram (see Table 3.13)

Treatment
- Taking a break during repetitive tasks
- Cold packs to reduce swelling
- Wrist splinting, daytime or nighttime
- Medication include NSAIDs; ibuprofen and naproxen sodium
- Injection of corticosteroids into the carpal tunnel can help relieve inflammation and pain
- Surgery may be performed to relieve pressure on the median nerve
- Follow-up with the provider will continue until the condition is resolved

Prognosis. The prognosis is good if patient compliance is consistent. A timetable of 2 to 12 months for resolution is achievable.

Prevention. There are some lifestyle and preventive actions patients can take:
- Take quick breaks for repetitive tasks that involve the hands.
- Rotate the wrists and stretch out hands and palms.
- Keep hands and wrists warm.
- When gripping an item, relax the grip. Hold items gently.
- Take OTC pain relievers such as NSAIDs: ibuprofen or aspirin.
- Wear a wrist splint at night.
- Sleep with the hands in a position that does not cause pain, stiffness, numbness, or tingling in the morning.

Degenerative Joint Disorder: Osteoarthritis

Degenerative joint disorder (DJD) is called osteoarthritis, but it really is not an inflammation of the joints. DJD is a gradual destruction of the cartilage that protects the end of a bone at the joint. It is also called "wear and tear" arthritis.

Signs and symptoms appear gradually and get worse over time. Once the cartilage starts to break down, it becomes rough. Over time the cartilage wears away completely, resulting in bone-on-bone contact. When the cartilage breaks down the process cannot be reversed, but the joint can often be replaced surgically.

Etiology. DJD is caused by the wear and tear on joints through a lifetime. Women are more likely to develop DJD than men. Someone who has had a previous joint injury, is obese, or works in an occupation that places repeated stress on particular joints may have a greater risk for developing DJD.

Signs and Symptoms. DJD has a number of signs and symptoms including the following:
- Joint pain and tenderness, loss of flexibility
- Joint stiffness, especially after a time of inactivity
- A grinding or grating feeling when the joint moves
- The development of Heberden and Bouchard nodes in the joints of the fingers
- Development of bone spurs

Diagnostic Procedures
- X-ray and MRI imaging tests
- Rheumatoid factor testing on blood may be done to rule out rheumatoid arthritis (see Table 3.14)
- Joint fluid analysis will help rule out gout and infectious arthritis

Treatment. The following treatments are used for DJD:
- Maintaining a healthy weight and moderate exercise
- Medications such as acetaminophen, NSAIDs, and duloxetine
- Injection therapy
  - Cortisone injections—directly into the joint
  - Lubrication injections—*hyaluronic acid* may provide relief with additional cushioning in the joint
- Physical therapy to strengthen muscles around the joint
- Occupational therapy to teach the patient how to do everyday tasks while putting less stress on the affected joint
- Realigning bones with an osteotomy (a surgical procedure in which the damaged area of a joint is removed; a bone wedge is added to shift the weight away from the damaged part of the joint.)
- Joint replacement (*arthroplasty*) during which the surgeon removes the damaged surface of the joint and then replaces the surface with plastic or metal parts
- Alternative therapies include acupuncture and glucosamine and chondroitin supplements

DJD is a chronic condition that has to be treated over time. Treatment may change as the condition progresses. Follow-up care with a healthcare provider will probably be ongoing.

Prognosis. DJD is an ongoing complaint, but with proper treatment and patient compliance, it can be a well-managed condition.

Prevention
- Maintaining a proper weight and including moderate exercise in one's daily routine
- Avoiding joint injuries and seeking proper treatment if injured
- Eating omega-3 fatty acid-rich foods
- Adequate vitamin D intake from the sun, foods, and supplements

> **CRITICAL THINKING 3.10**
>
> Dr. Martin has ruled out rheumatoid arthritis and Lyme disease, but Walter's x-rays show damage to his knee joints and joints of the fingers. Dr. Martin also observed the beginning of Heberden and Bouchard nodes on his right hand. What joint condition would this information indicate?

Muscular Dystrophy

Muscular dystrophy is a collection of muscle diseases that cause progressive muscle weakness and loss of muscle mass (atrophy). This group of diseases interferes with a person's ability to make the proteins necessary to form healthy muscles.

There are many different types of muscular dystrophy. Some are diagnosed when a child is an infant or toddler, and some forms of the disease are not apparent until adolescence or even adulthood. The most common form is Duchenne muscular dystrophy, which is usually diagnosed by the age of 3. About half of the people with muscular dystrophy have Duchenne type. Boys are affected much more frequently than girls.

Etiology. For muscles to grow and be strong, the body needs to produce specific proteins that will protect muscle fibers from damage. Muscular dystrophy may be congenital or caused by a genetic mutation that disrupts the body's ability to make muscle-protecting proteins.

Each particular type of muscular dystrophy is caused by a specific genetic mutation. Many of these mutations are inherited, but some occur spontaneously.

Signs and Symptoms. Typically signs and symptoms for Duchenne muscular dystrophy start to appear around age 2 or 3. Depending on the type of muscular dystrophy, the age of onset and specific symptoms may be slightly different:
- Frequent tripping and falling
- Trouble running, jumping, and getting up from a lying or sitting position
- Waddling gait when walking and walking on tip toes
- Large calf muscles
- Muscle pain and stiffness
- Learning disabilities

Diagnostic Procedures. Diagnostic procedures include the following:
- *Enzyme tests.* Damaged muscles release enzymes into the blood, the most common with muscular dystrophy is creatine kinase (CK). Without trauma, high levels of CK suggest muscle disease, such as muscular dystrophy.
- *Electromyography.* See Table 3.13.
- *Genetic testing.* Blood samples are examined for genetic mutations that cause the different types of muscular dystrophy.
- *Muscle biopsy.* A small muscle tissue sample is removed through a needle. Biopsy can distinguish muscular dystrophy from other muscle diseases.

Treatment. There is no cure for muscular dystrophy. Treatments can help improve quality of life, help people to remain mobile for as long as possible, and reduce or prevent bone and spinal complications. Treatments include the following:
- Corticosteroid medications, such as prednisone. Helps to maintain muscle strength and may help delay disease progression.

- Heart medications, such as angiotensin-converting enzyme (ACE) inhibitors or beta-blockers. These are used if heart damage has occurred.
- Range-of-motion and stretching exercises. These types of exercise can keep the joints and muscle as flexible as possible.
- Low-impact aerobic exercises like swimming and walking. These exercises help maintain overall health, mobility, and muscle strength.
- Braces help to maintain muscle and tendon flexibility. They can also give needed support to weakened muscles.
- Mobility aids. Canes, walkers, and wheelchairs all help the person maintain mobility and independence as long as possible.
- Breathing assistance. As muscular dystrophy progresses, breathing issues will occur. As respiratory muscles weaken, people may benefit from oxygen delivery during the night. Some people with severe muscular dystrophy need a ventilator to force air in and out of the lungs.
- Surgery may be required to correct spinal deformities that would make breathing more difficult.
- Some dietary changes can be beneficial to slow the progression of muscular dystrophy. The most commonly recommended diet for a person with muscular dystrophy is high-fiber, high-protein, low-calorie diet.
- Muscular dystrophy is a lifelong condition, so lifelong medical care and follow-up is required.

Prognosis. Depending on the type of muscular dystrophy, people can live until their 20s or even as long as their 40s or 50s. With good medical care and patient compliance, people with Duchenne muscular dystrophy can survive into their 30s or even 40s. Advances in treatment have extended the life span.

Prevention. Muscular dystrophy is a genetic condition that cannot be prevented.

Osteoporosis

Osteoporosis is a condition that causes bones to become brittle and weak. Healthy bone is constantly being broken down and remodeled. When a person has osteoporosis, bones are being broken down quicker than new bone can be created. This leads to weak bones that are easily fractured. Fractures are most common in the wrist, hip, and spine. In advanced osteoporosis, even a cough can cause fractures to brittle bones.

Etiology. Peak bone mass is reached during a person's 20s. As people age, their bone mass is lost faster than it can be produced. The loss in bone mass leads to osteoporosis. Increased risks for osteoporosis include the following:
- Being a woman past menopause
- Family history, small body frame
- Race: white or of Asian descent
- Medical conditions: hormonal imbalance, dietary deficiencies (low calcium intake), long-term corticosteroid use, celiac disease, kidney or liver disease, cancer, and some autoimmune conditions
- Sedentary lifestyle, tobacco use, and excessive alcohol consumption

Signs and Symptoms. In early osteoporosis, there are no overt signs and symptoms, but as the bones become weak the following may occur:
- Back pain that may be caused by collapsed or fractured vertebrae
- Loss of height
- A stooped posture with an exaggerated thoracic curve; kyphosis
- A bone fracture that happens easily or without trauma

Diagnostic Procedures. A bone density test is the only diagnostic test for osteoporosis. A low-level x-ray machine is used to measure bone density. The x-ray determines the mineral content of the bone. This is a painless test that checks the proportion of mineral in the bone of the hip, wrist, and spine.

Treatment. Treatment for osteoporosis may include the following:
- Weight-bearing exercise to maintain bone density
- Modifying risk factors to prevent falls
- Appropriate calcium and vitamin D intake from food or supplements
- Medications: bisphosphonates, hormone replacement therapy (estrogen)

Prognosis. Osteoporosis is a chronic condition that can be managed, but it does progress with age. If a person does not have a fracture from a fall, the prognosis is much better. A person's prognosis becomes much worse with a fall and fracture, especially a hip fracture.

Prevention
- Build up as much bone density as possible by a person's mid-20s.
- Maintain an active lifestyle that includes weight-bearing exercise.
- Do not smoke or consume alcohol in excess.
- Maintain a diet rich in calcium, vitamin D, and protein.
- Maintain a proper body weight.
- Prevent falls.

Building and maintaining strong bones throughout the life span is the best prevention for osteoporosis as you age.

Skeletal Deformities: Lordosis, Kyphosis, Scoliosis

Abnormal curvatures of the spine deprive the body of important features related to spinal strength, balance, and posture. The three most common curvatures are as follows:
- *Lordosis*: an exaggerated curve in the lumbar region of the spine sometimes called swayback
- *Kyphosis*: an exaggerated curve in the thoracic region of the spine sometime called hunchback; most common in older adults and in female patients with osteoporosis
- *Scoliosis*: an abnormal side-to-side curvature that could be in both the thoracic and lumbar regions of the spine; most common in adolescents; girls tend to develop a progressive or worsening curve as they go through adolescence

Table 3.18 describes the etiology, signs and symptoms, diagnosis, and treatment of abnormal curvatures of the spine. See Fig. 3.22.

Additional Musculoskeletal Diseases and Disorders

Tables 3.19 through 3.25 list a number of musculoskeletal diseases and disorders that are grouped by similar characteristics. Each condition listed is accompanied by a brief description.

> **MEDICAL TERMINOLOGY**
> **-algia:** pain
> **gnath/o:** jaw

LIFE SPAN CHANGES

As the table of congenital disorders demonstrates, there are several musculoskeletal conditions that a child may be born with: achondroplasia, muscular dystrophy, two disorders of the phalanges (syndactyly and

TABLE 3.18 Abnormal Curvatures of the Spine

Feature/Spinal Curvature	Lordosis	Kyphosis	Scoliosis
Etiology	Poor posture Congenital Secondary to osteoporosis	Secondary to osteoporosis and spinal disk degeneration Birth defects, cancer and cancer treatments	Congenital (muscular dystrophy, cerebral palsy) Spinal injury, infection, or idiopathic in adolescent girls
Signs and symptoms	Significant inward curve in the lower back (sway back) Back pain, stiffness in the lower back Pain and fatigue in the lower back, hips, and legs	Abnormally rounded curve of the upper back (hunchback) Pain and fatigue in the lower back, hips, and legs Severe cases: breathing problems and digestive issues	Sideways curve of the back, sometimes S or C shaped One shoulder or hip higher than the other, uneven waistline, rotation of trunk in some severe cases Pain and fatigue in the lower back, hips, and legs
Diagnostic procedures	Physical exam of the spine and neurologic exam Imaging: x-ray, MRI, CT scan		
Treatment: nondrug treatment	Depends on the severity of the curve and the patient age; may include physical therapy, exercise, weight loss, medication, and spinal fusion surgery Scoliosis may require additional treatment including back brace and surgical placement of metal stabilizing rods		
Treatment: medications	Depending on the severity of the spinal curvature, the provider may recommend medications such as analgesics, antiinflammatory drugs (NSAIDs, steroids) and muscle relaxants		
Prognosis	*Mild and moderate curves*—good prognosis *Severe curves with greater abnormalities*—prognosis varies		
Prevention	Use good posture for noncongenital Weight loss for obese patients	Prevention of osteoporosis Maintain good blood calcium levels Weight-bearing exercise	None

From Shiland B: *Mastering Healthcare Terminology,* ed 5, St. Louis, 2016, Elsevier.

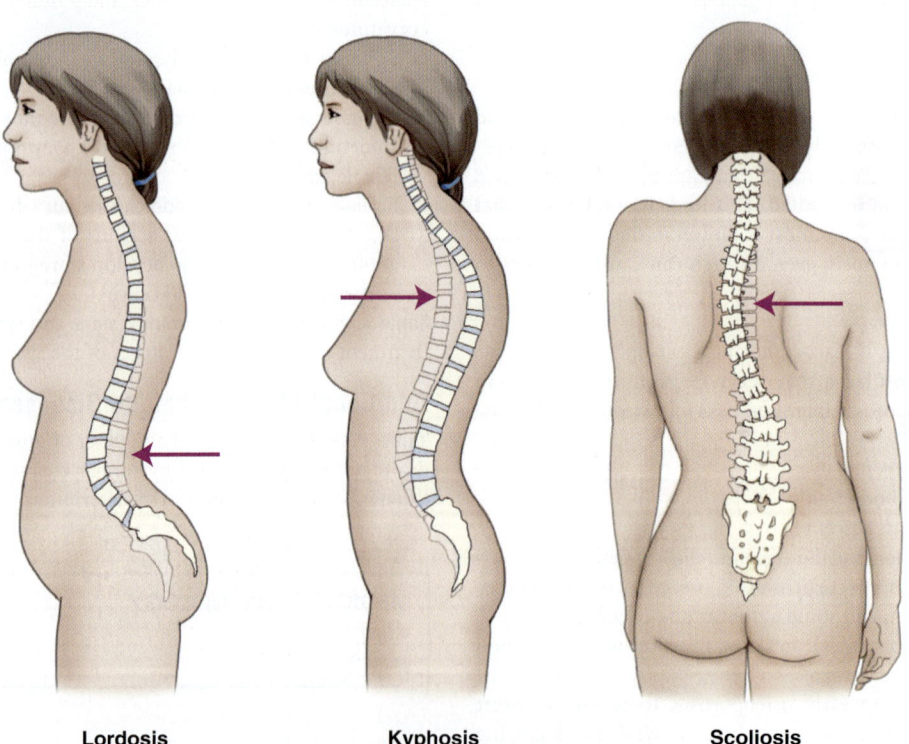

Lordosis **Kyphosis** **Scoliosis**

FIG. 3.22 Abnormal curvatures of the spine. (From Shiland B: *Mastering Healthcare Terminology,* ed 5, St. Louis, 2016, Elsevier.)

TABLE 3.19 Congenital Diseases and Disorders

Term	Definition
Achondroplasia (a kon droh PLAY zha)	Disorder of the development of cartilage at the epiphyses of the long bones and skull, resulting in dwarfism
Congenital hip dysplasia	The hip socket that does not fully cover the ball portion of the upper femur; this allows the hip joint to become partially or completely dislocated
Osteogenesis imperfecta	Caused by a defect in the gene that produces type 1 collagen, which is necessary to build strong bones
Polydactyly (pall ee DACK tih lee)	Condition of more than five fingers or toes on each hand or foot
Spina bifida occulta (SPY nah BIFF ih dah ah KULL tah)	Congenital malformation of the bony spinal canal without involvement of the spinal cord
Syndactyly (sin DACK tih lee)	Condition of the joining of the fingers or toes, giving them a webbed appearance
Talipes (TALL ih peez)	Deformity resulting in an abnormal twisting of the foot; also called *clubfoot*; may also be acquired
Torticollis (TOR tih kah lis)	Prolonged congenital or acquired condition that manifests itself as a contraction of the muscles of the neck; also called *wryneck*

From Shiland B: *Mastering Healthcare Terminology*, ed 5, St. Louis, 2016, Elsevier.

TABLE 3.20 Additional Bone Diseases and Disorders

Term	Definition
Osteitis deformans (ahs tee EYE tis dee FOR menz)	Misshaped bone resulting from excessive breakdown and formation of bone tissue; also known as *Paget disease*
Osteomalacia (ahs tee oh mah LAY sha)	Softening of bone caused by loss of minerals from the bony matrix as a result of vitamin D deficiency; when osteomalacia occurs in childhood, it is called *rickets*
Osteomyelitis (ahs tee oh mye eh LYE tis)	Inflammation or infection of the bone and bone marrow

From Shiland B: *Mastering Healthcare Terminology*, ed 5, St. Louis, 2016, Elsevier.

TABLE 3.21 Terms Related to Arthropathies and Related Disorders

Term	Definition
Baker cyst (BAY kur sist)	Cyst of synovial fluid in the popliteal area of leg; often associated with rheumatoid arthritis (RA)
Bunion (BUN yun)	Fairly common, painful enlargement and inflammation of the first metatarsophalangeal joint (the base of the great toe)
Scleroderma (SKLAIR oh dur mah)	Autoimmune connective tissue disorder that causes hardening and thickening of the skin
Systemic lupus erythematosus (SLE) (siss TEM ick LOO pus eh rith mah TOH sis)	Autoimmune disorder characterized by systemic inflammation, arthritis, and a distinctive red butterfly-like rash on the nose, forehead, and cheeks; also called *disseminated lupus erythematosus (DLE)*
Temporomandibular joint disorder (TMJ) (tem pore oh man DIB byoo lur)	Dysfunctional temporomandibular joint, accompanied by gnathalgia, or jaw pain
Tendinitis	Inflammation of a tendon; also called *tendonitis*

From Shiland B: *Mastering Healthcare Terminology*, ed 5, St. Louis, 2016, Elsevier.

TABLE 3.22 Terms Related to Deforming Dorsopathies and Spondylopathies

Term	Definition
Ankylosing spondylitis (ang kih LOH sing spon dill LYE tis)	Chronic inflammatory disease of idiopathic origin, which causes a fusion of the spine
Herniated intervertebral disk	Protrusion of the central part of the disk that lies between the vertebrae, resulting in compression of the nerve root and pain
Spinal stenosis (SPY nul steh NOH sis)	Abnormal condition where the spinal canal narrows; chronic pain, sometimes caused by DJD or spondylolisthesis
Spondylolisthesis (spon dih loh liss THEE sis)	Condition resulting from the partial forward dislocation of one vertebra over the one below it

From Shiland B: *Mastering Healthcare Terminology*, ed 5, St. Louis, 2016, Elsevier.

TABLE 3.23 Terms Related to Muscle Disorders

Term	Definition
Contracture (kun TRACK chur)	Chronic fixation of a joint in flexion (such as a finger) caused by atrophy and shortening of muscle fibers after a long period of disuse
Fibromyalgia (fye broh mye AL jah)	Disorder characterized by musculoskeletal pain, fatigue, muscle stiffness and spasms, and sleep disturbances
Myasthenia gravis (mye ah STHEE nee ah GRAV us)	Autoimmune condition characterized by fatigue and progressive muscle weakness, especially of the face and throat
Plantar fasciitis (plan tur fass ee EYE tis)	Inflammation of the fascia on the sole of the foot; the chronic form is called *plantar fasciosis* (plan tur fass ee OH sis)
Polymyalgia rheumatica (pol e my AL juh rue MAT ih kuh)	An inflammatory disorder that causes muscle pain and stiffness, especially in the shoulders
Polymyositis (pahl ee mye oh SYE tis)	Chronic, idiopathic inflammation of skeletal muscles

From Shiland B: *Mastering Healthcare Terminology*, ed 5, St. Louis, 2016, Elsevier.

TABLE 3.24 Terms Related to Benign Neoplasms

Term	Definition
Chondroma (kon DROH mah)	Benign tumor of the cartilage, usually occurring in children and adolescents
Leiomyoma (lye oh mye OH mah)	Benign tumor of smooth muscle; the most common leiomyoma is in the uterus and is termed a *fibroid*
Osteoma (ahs tee OH mah)	Benign bone tumor, usually of compact bone
Rhabdomyoma (rab doh mye OH mah)	Benign tumor of striated/voluntary/skeletal muscle

From Shiland B: *Mastering Healthcare Terminology*, ed 5, St. Louis, 2016, Elsevier.

TABLE 3.25 Terms Related to Malignant Neoplasms

Term	Definition
Chondrosarcoma (kon droh sar KOH mah)	Malignant tumor of the cartilage; occurs most frequently in adults
Leiomyosarcoma (lye oh mye oh sar KOH mah)	Malignant tumor of smooth muscle, most commonly appearing in the uterus
Osteosarcoma (ahs tee oh sar KOH mah)	Malignant tumor of bone; also called *Ewing sarcoma*; most common bone cancer in children
Rhabdomyosarcoma (rab doh mye OH sar koh mah)	Highly malignant tumor of skeletal muscle; also called *rhabdosarcoma* or *rhabdomyoblastoma*

From Shiland B: *Mastering Healthcare Terminology*, ed 5, St. Louis, 2016, Elsevier.

polydactyly), spina bifida occulta, talipes, and congenital torticollis. Although not exclusive to childhood, pediatric statistics reveal high numbers of children treated each year for the effects of physical trauma. Fractures are common, beginning with clavicular fractures (the result of birth trauma) to fractures of the arms (humerus, radius, and ulna) and the legs (femur, tibia, and fibula). Sprains, strains, dislocations, and subluxations are other pediatric diagnoses that appear with regularity for this system.

Statistics collected on the geriatric population of patients also report a high number of fractures. These, however, are mainly fractures of the hip and femur and are often preceded by bone loss caused by osteoporosis or cancer. DJD, often referred to as "wear and tear disease," is another disorder that afflicts many patients as they age. The high numbers of total knee replacement (TKR) surgeries today are often the result of this disease.

CLOSING COMMENTS

When working in an ambulatory care setting, assisting patients with musculoskeletal trauma and disease is common. It is important for the medical assistant to understand the anatomic structures of all three components of this system: the skeleton, joints, and muscles. The physiology of bone repair and growth, and how muscles contract is important for understanding many disease states and traumas. Medical terminology related to the musculoskeletal system will be invaluable in your career. Knowing word parts, definitions, and common abbreviations is vital when working with patients and providers (Tables 3.26 through 3.29). The medical assistant should also know about the etiology, signs and symptoms, diagnostic procedures, treatments, prognoses, and prevention of common musculoskeletal diseases and traumas.

TABLE 3.26 Combining and Adjective Forms for the Anatomy of the Musculoskeletal System

Meaning	Combining Form	Adjective Form	Meaning	Combining Form	Adjective Form
bone	oste/o, osse/o, oss/i	osseous, osteal	metatarsus (foot bone)	metatars/o	metatarsal
bone marrow	myel/o		muscle	my/o, myos/o, muscul/o	muscular
bursa	burs/o	bursal	muscle (heart)	myocardi/o, cardiomy/o	myocardial
calcaneus (heel bone)	calcane/o	calcaneal	muscle (skeletal)	rhabdomy/o	
carpal bone	carp/o	carpal	muscle (smooth)	leiomy/o	
cartilage	chondr/o, cartilag/o	cartilaginous, chondral	neck	cervic/o	cervical
clavicle (collarbone)	clavicul/o, cleid/o	clavicular, cleidal	occiput	occipit/o	occipital
coccyx (tailbone)	coccyg/o	coccygeal	palatine bone	palat/o	palatine
condyle	condyl/o	condylar	parietal bone	pariet/o	parietal
elbow (olecranon)	olecran/o	olecranal	patella (kneecap)	patell/o, patell/a	patellar
epicondyle	epicondyl/o	epicondylar	pelvis	pelv/i, pelv/o	pelvic
ethmoid	ethmoid/o	ethmoidal	phalanx (one of the bones of the fingers or toes)	phalang/o	phalangeal
fascia	fasci/o	fascial			
femur (thigh bone)	femor/o	femoral			
fibula (lower lateral leg bone)	fibul/o, perone/o	fibular, peroneal	pubis (pubic bone)	pub/o	pubic
			radius (lower lateral arm bone)	radi/o	radial
finger, toe, (whole), digitus	dactyl/o, digit/o	digital			
			rib (costa)	cost/o	costal
foramen	foramin/o	foraminal	sacrum	sacr/o	sacral
frontal bone	front/o	frontal	scapula (shoulderblade)	scapul/o	scapular
humerus (upper arm bone)	humer/o	humeral	skeleton	skelet/o	skeletal
			skull (cranium)	crani/o	cranial
ilium	ili/o	iliac	sole	plant/o	plantar
ischium	ischi/o	ischial	sphenoid	sphenoid/o	sphenoidal
jaw	gnath/o		spinal column, spine	spin/o, rachi/o, vertebr/o	spinal, vertebral, rachial
joint (articulation)	arthr/o, articul/o	articular			
lacrima	lacrim/o	lacrimal	sternum, breastbone	stern/o	sternal
lamina	lamin/o	laminar	tarsus (anklebone)	tars/o	tarsal
ligament	ligament/o, syndesm/o	ligamentous, syndesmal	temporal bone	tempor/o	temporal
lower back	lumb/o	lumbar	tendon	tendin/o, tend/o, ten/o	tendinous
malleolus	malleol/o	malleolar	thorax (chest)	thorac/o	thoracic
mandible (lower jaw bone)	mandibul/o	mandibular	tibia (shinbone)	tibi/o	tibial
			ulna	uln/o	ulnar
mastoid process	mastoid/o	mastoid	vertebra (backbone)	vertebr/o, spondyl/o	vertebral
maxilla (upper jaw bone)	maxill/o	maxillary	vomer	vomer/o	
			xiphoid process	xiph/o	xiphoid
meniscus	menisc/o	meniscal	zygoma (cheekbone)	zygomat/o	zygomatic
metacarpus (hand bone)	metacarp/o	metacarpal			

From Shiland B: *Mastering Healthcare Terminology*, ed 5, St. Louis, 2016, Elsevier.

TABLE 3.27 Prefixes for the Anatomy of the Musculoskeletal System

Prefix	Meaning	Prefix	Meaning
ab-	away from	ex-, e-	out
ad-	toward	in-	in
amphi-	both	inter-	between
bi-	two	intra-	within
circum-	around	peri-	surrounding, around
dia-	through, complete	pro-	forward
endo-, end-	within	re-	back
epi-	above, upon	syn-	together, joined

From Shiland B: *Mastering Healthcare Terminology*, ed 5, St. Louis, 2016, Elsevier.

TABLE 3.28 Suffixes for the Anatomy of the Musculoskeletal System

Suffix	Meaning	Suffix	Meaning
-ar, -al, -ic, -ous, -eal	pertaining to	-physis	growth
-blast	embryonic	-poiesis	formation
-clast	breaking down	-sis	condition
-cyte	cell	-um	structure
-oid	full of, like		

From Shiland B: *Mastering Healthcare Terminology*, ed 5, St. Louis, 2016, Elsevier.

TABLE 3.29 Abbreviations

Abbreviation	Meaning	Abbreviation	Meaning
A	action	MRI	magnetic resonance imaging
C1–C7	first cervical through seventh cervical vertebrae	NSAID	nonsteroidal antiinflammatory drug
CR	closed reduction	O	origin
CREF	closed reduction external fixation	OA	osteoarthritis
CT	computed tomography	OR	open reduction
CTS	carpal tunnel syndrome	ORIF	open reduction internal fixation
DEXA	dual energy x-ray absorptiometry	PIP	proximal interphalangeal joint
DIP	distal interphalangeal joint	RA	rheumatoid arthritis
DJD	degenerative joint disease	RF	rheumatoid factor
EF	external fixation	ROM	range of motion
EMG	electromyography	S1–S5	first sacral through fifth sacral segments
Fx, #	fracture	SLE	systemic lupus erythematosus
I	insertion	T1–T12	first thoracic through twelfth thoracic vertebrae
L1–L5	first lumbar through fifth lumbar vertebrae	THR	total hip replacement
MD	muscular dystrophy	TKR	total knee replacement

From Shiland B: *Mastering Healthcare Terminology*, ed 5, St. Louis, 2016, Elsevier.

CHAPTER REVIEW

The musculoskeletal system is divided into three components: the skeleton, the joints, and the muscles. The main functions of the musculoskeletal system are movement, protection, support, mineral storage, and hematopoiesis.

In a healthy individual, the bones are immature at birth. Then, through the process of ossification, bones mature to become strong and stable. When we are in our early 20s, bone growth stops and the growth plates close. Bone remodeling continues throughout a person's lifetime as a constant building up and breaking down of bone. This remodeling process is vital to maintain proper blood calcium levels and keep bones strong and healthy.

The joints of the body are also a part of the musculoskeletal system. Joints are an important factor in body movement. Many joints in the body are diarthrotic joints, which are freely movable. Joints allow us to bend, twist, walk, chew, and perform other movements that affect the body as a whole.

The muscles of the body are the last component of the musculoskeletal system. There are three types of muscles: skeletal, cardiac, and smooth. Skeletal muscles help the body move. Cardiac muscle aids in the maintenance of an efficient and coordinated heartbeat. Smooth muscle makes up part of our internal organs and vessels. Smooth muscle helps us breath, dilate and constrict blood vessels, and move food through the digestive system, to name just a few of its functions. All muscles are stimulated by the nervous system, which initiates muscle contraction. Through the processes of contraction and relaxation, all three types of muscles perform their specific functions within the human body.

Many musculoskeletal diseases were presented in the chapter. Common signs and symptoms include pain, tenderness, fatigue, and possible loss of mobility. Common etiology includes trauma, infection, autoimmune conditions, congenital abnormalities, and structural changes in the skeleton, muscles, and joints. Typical diagnostic tests include a variety of imaging technologies and laboratory testing. CLIA-waived tests include rheumatoid factor (RF) testing, Lyme disease antibody testing, and erythrocyte sedimentation rate (ESR) tests. The musculoskeletal system changes with age. Infants and children are at risk for congenital conditions, degenerative disorders, and traumas. Older adults are also at risk for degenerative disorders, inflammatory joint disorders, and wear-and-tear (or overuse) conditions and traumas.

SCENARIO WRAP-UP

Dr. Martin, Patsy, and Walter wrap up the appointment. Dr. Martin has recommended that Walter garden for shorter stretches of time, use a knee cushion when weeding, and take acetaminophen when he needs pain relief. Degenerative joint disease is manageable, and with a few changes in Walter's gardening routine, the prognosis is good. As for the muscle strain that Walter is feeling in his forearm, that too can be managed with muscle rest, ice, and acetaminophen.

Patsy walks Walter out to the lobby. As she returns to the exam room, she reflects back on 20 years as a medical assistant and is so happy with the choice she made so many years ago.

4

Integumentary System

LEARNING OBJECTIVES

1. Discuss the anatomy of the integumentary system, list the major structures of the integumentary system, and identify the anatomic location of the major structures of the integumentary system.
2. Describe the normal function and physiology of the integumentary system.
3. Complete the following for diseases and disorders related to the integumentary system:
   - Identify the common signs and symptoms, etiology, and diagnostic measures of the integumentary diseases.
   - Identify CLIA-waived tests associated with common integumentary diseases.
   - Describe treatment modalities used for integumentary diseases.
4. Compare the structure and function of the integumentary system across the life span.

CHAPTER OUTLINE

1. Opening Scenario, 69
2. You Will Learn, 69
3. Anatomy of the Integumentary System, 70
   a. Membranes of the Body, 70
   b. Skin, 70
      i. *Epidermis, 70*
      ii. *Dermal-Epidermal Junction, 71*
      iii. *Dermis, 72*
      iv. *Subcutaneous Tissue, 72*
   c. Accessory Structures, 72
      i. *Glands, 72*
      ii. *Hair, 72*
      iii. *Nails, 72*
4. Physiology of the Integumentary System, 73
   a. Protection, 73
   b. Sensory Organ Activity, 73
   c. Temperature Regulation, 73
   d. Excretion, 73
   e. Synthesis of Vitamin D, 73
5. Diseases and Disorders of the Integumentary System, 73
   a. Acne Vulgaris, 77
   b. Burns, 78
   c. Carcinomas of the Skin, 80
   d. Decubitus Ulcers, 83
   e. Dermatophytosis (Tenia Fungal Infections), 84
   f. Eczema (Atopic Dermatitis), 85
   g. Psoriasis, 86
   h. Shingles (Herpes Zoster), 87
   i. Skin Infestations (Scabies and Pediculosis), 88
   j. Additional Diseases and Disorders of the Integumentary System, 89
6. Life Span Changes, 92
7. Closing Comments, 92
8. Chapter Review, 93
9. Scenario Wrap-Up, 93

OPENING SCENARIO

Mai Vang is a medical assistant who has been working at the Walden Martin Family Medical Clinic (WMFM) for 2 years. She really wanted to work in a family practice clinic so that she could see patients of varying ages and medical conditions. Mai has noticed that skin conditions are a frequent reason for patient visits. When she was in high school, she visited her physician to get help for an acne breakout that would not go away. She remembers feeling self-conscious about the condition, so she tries to be especially sensitive to patients with skin diseases and disorders.

Today Mai's first patient after lunch is Casey Hernandez. She is coming in to see Jean Burke, the WMFC nurse practitioner.

YOU WILL LEARN

- To recognize and use terms related to the membranes of the body.
- To understand and describe the functions of epithelial and connective tissue membranes.
- To recognize and use terms related to the integumentary system.
- To locate the integumentary system structures.
- To understand and describe the functions of the integumentary system: protection, heat regulation, sensory organ activity, excretion, and vitamin D synthesis.
- To recognize disease states of the integumentary system: their causes, signs and symptoms, diagnostic processes, treatment, prognoses, and prevention.

TABLE 4.1 Membranes of the Body

Name	Composition	Location	Function	Secretion
Epithelial-cutaneous (kyoo TAY nee us)	Two-layered membrane (epidermis and dermis) made up of epithelial tissue and an underlying layer of fibrous connective tissue	Skin that covers the outside of the body	Protection, heat regulation, excretions, vitamin D synthesis, sensory organ activity	Sebum (oil), perspiration (sweat)
Epithelial-serous (Seer us)	Epithelial and connective tissue	Line the surfaces of closed cavities of the body	Line the surfaces of closed body cavities and cover internal organs Produce serous fluid	Serous fluid-thin, watery fluid that provides lubrication for internal organs and internal body cavities
Epithelial-mucous (MYOO cus)	Epithelial and connective tissue	Line many of the internal hollow organs and openings to the external environment Examples include respiratory and digestive systems	Protect the tissue, keep it moist and soft Aid passage of materials within the hollow organs of the body or external body openings Produce mucus Part of the first line of defense of the immune system	Mucus: thick and slimy fluid that provides protection, aids movement, and is part of immune system's first line of defense
Connective	Connective tissue only	Covers the ends of bones and lines the joint capsule for articulating bones	To help reduce friction between the articulating bones in a movable joint	*Synovial* (sih NOH vee al) fluid, thick and clear Helps reduce friction in movable joints

From Shiland B: *Mastering Healthcare Terminology*, ed 5, St. Louis, 2016, Elsevier.

> **BOX 4.1 Specialty and Specialist**
>
> *Dermatology* (der mah TAW loh jee) is the healthcare specialty that deals with most skin diseases and disorders. A *dermatologist* (der mah TAW loh jist) is a specialist involved in the diagnosis, treatment, and prevention of disorders of the *integumentary* (in te gyoo MEN tair ee) system.

ANATOMY OF THE INTEGUMENTARY SYSTEM

The most important function of the skin (or integument [in TE gyoo ment]) is protecting the body from disease. The skin provides a physical barrier that is our first line of defense against **pathogens**. It is the largest organ of the body, and, in addition to physically protecting the body, is also helps to do the following:
- Regulate the body temperature
- Provide information about the environment through sensory activity
- Assist in the **synthesis** of vitamin D
- Eliminate some waste products through the skin

The skin functions together with accessory structures that include hair, nails, *sebaceous* (seh BAY shus) glands, or *oil glands*, and *sudoriferous* (soo doh RIF er us) glands, or *sweat glands*. Any damage or injury to the skin has the potential to lessen its ability to carry out these functions, which can lead to disease (Box 4.1).

Membranes of the Body

The membranes of the body are very thin layers of tissue that have many functions throughout the body. There are two classifications of body membranes: *epithelial* (ep i THEE lee al) and connective. Each type of membrane functions to protect the covered structures. See Table 4.1 for more information on membranes of the body.

Skin

The *skin* is considered a *cutaneous membrane* made up of **epithelial cells**, which covers the entire body. The skin is composed of two layers: the *epidermis* (eh pih DUR mis), which forms the outermost layer, and the *dermis*, which forms the inner layer (Fig. 4.1). The dermis is attached to a layer of connective tissue called the *subcutaneous* (sub kyoo TAY nee us) layer, or hypodermis, which is mainly composed of fat or *adipose* (AD ih pohs) tissue.

> **VOCABULARY**
> **epithelial cells:** Form cellular sheets that cover surfaces, both inside and outside the body. Epithelial cells are closely packed, take on different shapes, and strongly stick to each other.
> **pathogen:** A disease-causing organism.
> **synthesis:** Formation of a chemical compound from simpler compounds or elements.

> **MEDICAL TERMINOLOGY**
> **adip/o:** fat
> **cutane/o:** skin
> **derm/o:** skin
> **epi-:** above, upon
> **hypo-:** under, below
> **-is:** structure
> **-ous:** pertaining to
> **sub-:** under, below

Epidermis. The epidermis is the top layer of the skin and is composed of several different **strata** of epithelial tissue. This type of tissue covers many of the external and internal surfaces of the body and has a

CHAPTER 4 Integumentary System

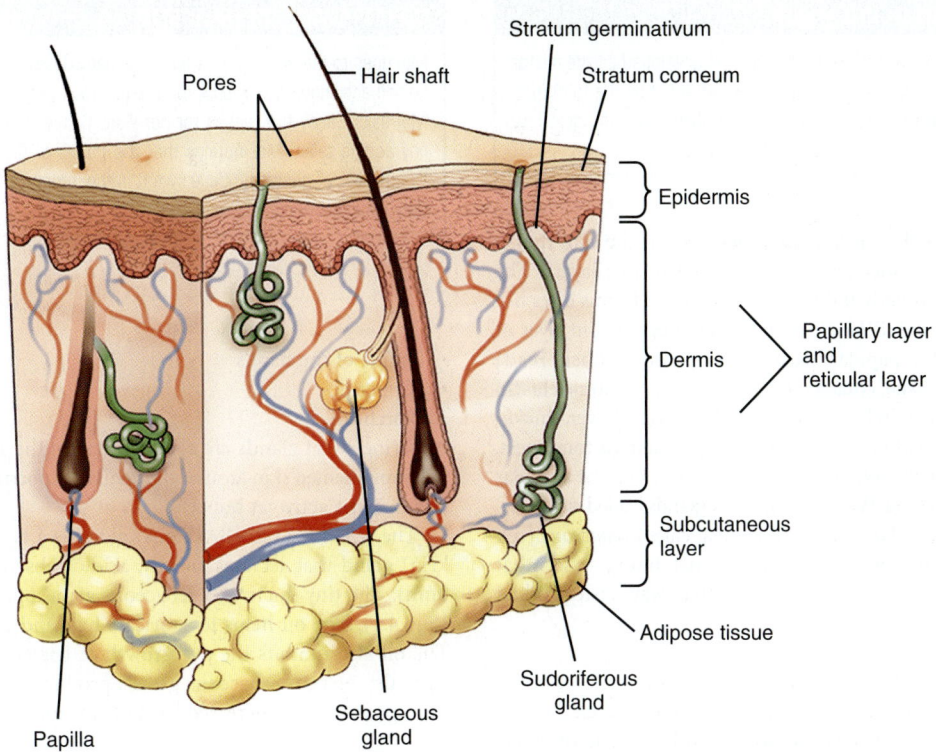

FIG. 4.1 Diagram of the skin. (From Shiland B: *Mastering Healthcare Terminology*, ed 5, St. Louis, 2016, Elsevier.)

microscopic scaly appearance. The cellular arrangement is referred to as *stratified* because the cells are organized in layers. The oldest cells make up the external layer of the skin. The proper description of epidermal cells is stratified *squamous epithelium* (SKWAY muss eh pih THEE lee um).

The epidermis is *avascular* (a VAS kyoo lur), which means it contains no blood vessels. New skin cells are formed in the **basal** (BAY sul) layer of the epidermis, called the *stratum germinativum* (STRAH tum jur mih nuh TIH vum). This layer is also where *melanin* (MEL ah nin), which is a pigment, is produced by **melanocytes** (meh LAN oh sites). When the skin is exposed to ultraviolet (UV) light, the melanocytes secrete more melanin. Birthmarks, age spots, and freckles result from clumps of melanin. Individuals have different skin colors because of varying numbers of melanocytes in the stratum germinativum of the skin.

New cells produced in the stratum germinativum move upward toward the top layer, or *stratum corneum* (kor NEE um). During the transition from the basal layer to the upper layer, the cell's cytoplasm is replaced with *keratin* (KAIR ah tin). Once this process is complete, the cells are called *keratinocytes* (KAIR ah tin oh sites). Keratin is a hard protein material that enhances the skin by making it waterproof, abrasion resistant, and able to retain moisture in the body. These properties add to the protective nature of the skin.

Dermal-Epidermal Junction. The *dermal-epidermal junction* is where the two layers of the skin meet. The top layer of the dermis contains *dermal papillae* (pah PILL ee), which are peglike projections that help fasten the dermis and epidermis together. This unique junction not only uses dermal papillae to create a bond, but it also uses a specialized gel that acts as a glue to keep the two layers of the skin connected.

If the dermal-epidermal junction is damaged by a burn, irritation, abrasion, or friction, a blister may occur. If the dermal-epidermal junction is destroyed, the skin will fall apart. If this happens in a small area, the body can heal the damage. If a large area of the junction is destroyed, it would result in an overwhelming infection that would be serious, possibly fatal.

VOCABULARY
basal: Bottom layer.
melanocytes: Cells of the stratum germinativum that produce a brownish pigment called melanin. Melanin gives us our skin color.
strata: Naturally or artificially formed layers of material, usually multiple layers.

MEDICAL TERMINOLOGY
a-: without
-ar: pertaining to
bas/o: basal
-cyte: cell
-in: substance

kerat/o: hard, horny
melan/o: black
vascul/o: vessel
squam/o: scaly
strata (singular), **stratum** (plural)

> **CRITICAL THINKING 4.1**
>
> Yesterday Mai wore a new pair of shoes to work and developed a little blister on the heel of her right foot. What skin layers are affected by the formation of a blister? How should Mai properly care for her blister over the next few days?

Dermis. The *dermis* is the thick, underlying layer of the skin that is composed of vascular connective tissue arranged in two layers. The dermis gives the skin strength and stretch that the epidermis does not possess. The *papillary (pah PILL air ee) layer* is the upper thin layer of the dermis. Much of the papillary layer is composed of fibers made from loose connective tissue, collagen (KAW lah jen), and some elastin (ee LAS tin). The *reticular (reh TIC koo lahr) layer* is the lower, thicker layer, which is composed of dense collagen that gives skin its toughness. There are also elastin fibers that help give the layer stretch. The reticular layer holds the *hair follicles* (FAW lih kuls), sweat glands, called *sudoriferous* (soo doh RIF er us) *glands*, and oil glands, called *sebaceous* (seh BAY shus) *glands*. The dermis contains many small blood vessels that supply the skin with nutrients and oxygen and take away waste product and carbon dioxide.

Subcutaneous Tissue. The subcutaneous tissue is not a layer of the skin. It lies below the dermis and creates a connection between the skin and the structures that are below the skin, such as muscle or bone. Subcutaneous tissue is made up of loose connective tissue and adipose (fat) tissue. This tissue is not rigid but rather movable and pliable. The subcutaneous tissue can slip over underlying structures. Without subcutaneous tissue, our skin would tear with movement.

Accessory Structures

Glands. The *sudoriferous* glands are also called sweat glands. They are in the dermis and provide a means of temperature regulation for the body (see Fig. 4.1). They secrete sweat through tiny openings in the surface of the skin called pores. The secretion of sweat is called *perspiration*. There are two types of sweat glands: *eccrine* (EK rin) and *apocrine* (AP uh krin). Eccrine sweat glands are dispersed throughout the body but are seen in greater numbers in the following locations:
- Soles of the feet

> **VOCABULARY**
>
> **collagen:** The most abundant structural protein found in skin and other connective tissues. It provides strength and cushioning to many parts of the body.
> **elastin:** A highly elastic protein in connective tissue that allows tissues to resume their shape after stretching or contracting. It is found abundantly in the dermis of the skin.
> **pores:** Tiny openings in the surface of the skin that allow gases, liquids, or microscopic particles to pass.

> **MEDICAL TERMINOLOGY**
>
> **axillae** (singular), **axilla** (plural)　**seb/o:** sebum
> **-ferous:** pertaining to carrying　**sebac/o:** oil
> **follicul/o:** follicle　**sudor/i:** sweat
> **papill/o:** papilla　**trich/o, pil/o:** hair

> **CRITICAL THINKING 4.2**
>
> Mai goes to the waiting area and calls back Casey Hernandez. She introduces herself and shows Casey back to the exam room. After vital signs are completed, Mai asks Casey the reason for her visit. Casey is looking down and is a bit shy as she talks. Mai notices that the palms of Casey's hands are sweaty. What types of glands produce sweat in the integumentary system? Where are they concentrated in the body?

- Palms of the hands
- Upper lip
- Forehead

Apocrine sweat glands are concentrated in the axillae, or armpits, and in the pigmented skin around the genitals. Apocrine sweat glands enlarge and become active at puberty.

The *sebaceous* (seh BAY shus) gland is a type of *exocrine* (EK suh krin) gland that secretes an oily, acidic substance called *sebum* (SEE bum). The tiny ducts of a sebaceous gland open into the hair follicle (Fig. 4.1). The oil helps to lubricate hair and the surface of the skin. The oil also inhibits the overgrowth of bacteria and keeps structures from drying out. Sebaceous glands produce more oil during puberty in response to the increased level of sex hormones.

> **CRITICAL THINKING 4.3**
>
> Casey tells Mai that today she is going to talk to Jean Burke, the nurse practitioner, about her persistent acne. She does not really want to look up, and Mai senses Casey is not at ease. Mai comments, "I really struggled with acne in high school, and I finally went to the doctor. I was so glad that I did." Casey looks at Mai and comments on her beautiful skin.
> If a person has acne, what skin glands are affected by the condition? Use the pronunciation guide in the text if needed and say the names of the skin glands aloud. How can you remember the names of the skin glands? Share any tips you have with your classmates.

Hair. Hair has its roots in the dermis (Fig. 4.1). The hair roots, together with their coverings, are called *hair follicles* (FALL ih kuls). The visible part of hair is called the *hair shaft*. Underneath the follicle is a nipple-shaped structure called the *papilla* (puh PIL uh). Dermal blood vessels nourish the papilla. Epithelial cells on top of the papilla are responsible for the formation of the hair shaft. When these cells die, the hair can no longer regenerate, and hair loss occurs. The term for any type of hair loss is *alopecia* (al oh PEE sha).

The main function of hair is to assist in temperature regulation by holding heat near the body. When it is cold, hair stands on end, holding a layer of air as insulation near the body. This process is called *piloerection* (py loh ee REK shun). There is a small smooth muscle at the base of every dermal papilla that also attaches to the side of a hair follicle. This little muscle is called the *arrector pili* (ah REK tor pil ee). When the muscle contracts, piloerection occurs. This usually only happens when a person is cold or scared.

Nails. Nails cover and protect the dorsal surfaces of the distal bones of the fingers and toes (Fig. 4.2). The visible part of the nail is the *nail body*. The *nail root* is in a groove under a small fold of skin at the base of the nail called the *cuticle* (KYOO tih kul). The *nail bed* is the highly

CHAPTER 4 Integumentary System

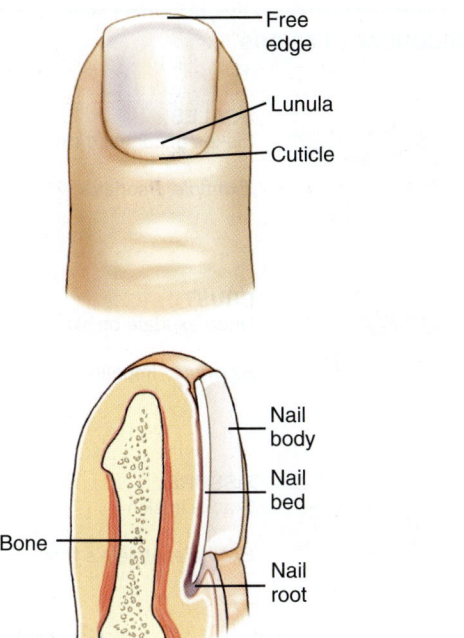

FIG. 4.2 The nail. (From Shiland B: *Mastering Healthcare Terminology*, ed 5, St. Louis, 2016, Elsevier.)

vascular tissue under the nail that normally appears pink. If the nail bed appears blue or purple, it indicates that the person is oxygen deficient. The moonlike white area at the base of the nail is called the *lunula* (LOON yoo lah). The fold of skin near the sides of the nail is called the *paronychium* (pair ih NICK ee um).

> **MEDICAL TERMINOLOGY**
> **epi-**: above
> **-ium**: structure
> **onych/o**: nail
> **par-**: near

PHYSIOLOGY OF THE INTEGUMENTARY SYSTEM

The five functions of the integumentary system are listed and discussed next:
- Protection
- Sensory organ activity
- Temperature regulation
- Excretion
- Synthesis of vitamin D

Protection
The skin protects the internal organs by providing a flexible, waterproof barrier to the outside environment. It is part of the first line of defense from microbial pathogens, toxic chemicals, and physical tears, cuts, and abrasions. The keratin in our skin cells protects us from excessive fluid loss and dehydration. Finally, the melanin in the epidermis of the skin protects the body from damaging UV light. Skin is so amazing!

Sensory Organ Activity
The skin has many sensory receptors scattered throughout the tissue. Sensory receptors can feel pain, pressure, heat, and cold. This allows us to respond to the environment and make appropriate changes to keep ourselves from harm.

Temperature Regulation
The skin is a very good thermoregulator. When we are cold, it constricts blood vessels close to the skin's surface. This preserves body heat and lessens the heat loss to the surrounding environment. When we are hot, it can produce sweat that evaporates and cools us off. Because of the extensive blood supply to the skin, the body can help regulate and maintain a consistent body temperature. This is all part of homeostasis (hoh mee uh STEY sis).

Excretion
The body can regulate the amount of sweat produced and the chemical content of the sweat. When we sweat, we lose water, electrolytes, and small amounts of other waste products. The integumentary system can excrete substances through the skin to help maintain the necessary chemical balance in the body as a whole.

Synthesis of Vitamin D
The *synthesis* (SIN thuh sis) of vitamin D is a vital function of the body, and it all starts in the skin. When skin is exposed to the sun's ultraviolet rays, it manufactures a vitamin D precursor molecule (MOL uh kyool). The molecule is carried to the liver and kidneys by way of the blood. The precursor molecule is then converted to the active form of vitamin D that the body can use. Research has uncovered many body functions affected by vitamin D, a few of which are as follows:
- Proper absorption of calcium
- Maintaining normal calcium and phosphorus levels in the blood; calcium helps maintain strong bones, proper blood clotting, muscle function, and immunity
- Protection against osteoporosis (os tee oh puh ROH sis), high blood pressure, and some forms of cancer
- Consistently low vitamin D levels put a person at a higher risk for developing multiple sclerosis (skli ROH sis), heart disease, osteoporosis, and depression

> **CRITICAL THINKING 4.4**
>
> As Casey is waiting for Jean Burke to come into the exam room, she takes a mirror out of her purse and looks at the acne on her face. She is hopeful that coming to see the nurse practitioner is a good idea. As a medical assistant, how could you show sensitivity to Casey on her visit today?

DISEASES AND DISORDERS OF THE INTEGUMENTARY SYSTEM

Diseases of the integumentary system are varied in appearance and cause. Fig. 4.3 shows examples of many common lesions of the skin. Many factors can cause skin diseases, disorders, and infections. Bacterial, fungal, viral, and parasitic infections can cause skin infections. Box 4.2

> **BOX 4.2 Common Signs and Symptoms of Integumentary Diseases and Disorders**
>
> Common signs and symptoms seen in patients with skin diseases and disorders include the following:
> - Skin discoloration or redness
> - Itching, weeping, or bleeding lesions
> - Blisters, macules, papules (see Fig. 4.3 for examples)
> - Scaly or flaky skin surface
> - New or changing lesions

PRIMARY LESIONS

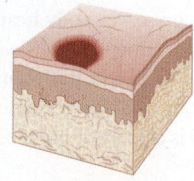

MACULE
Flat area of color change (no elevation or depression)

Example: Freckles

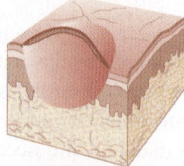

PAPULE
Solid elevation less than 0.5 cm in diameter

Example: Allergic eczema

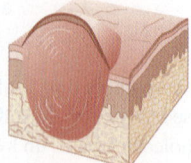

NODULE
Solid elevation 0.5 to 1 cm in diameter. Extends deeper into dermis than papule

Example: Mole

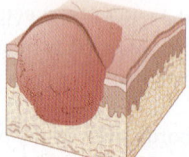

TUMOR
Solid mass—larger than 1 cm

Example: Squamous cell carcinoma

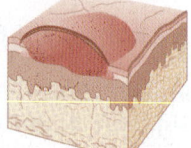

PLAQUE
Flat elevated surface found on skin or mucous membrane

Example: Thrush

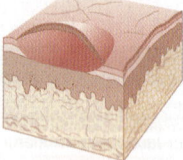

WHEAL
Type of plaque. Result is transient edema in dermis

Example: Intradermal skin test

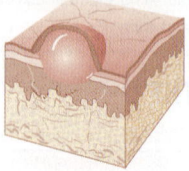

VESICLE
Small blister—fluid within or under epidermis

Example: Herpesvirus infection

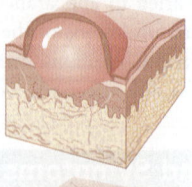

BULLA
Large blister (greater than 0.5 cm)

Example: Burn

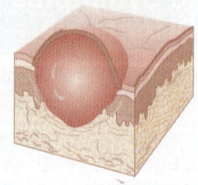

PUSTULE
Vesicle filled with pus

Example: Acne

SECONDARY LESIONS

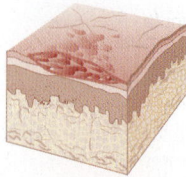

SCALES
Flakes of cornified skin layer

Example: Psoriasis

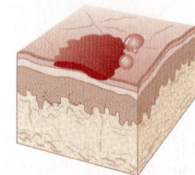

CRUST
Dried exudate on skin

Example: Impetigo

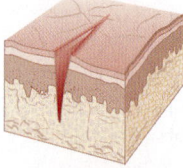

FISSURE
Cracks in skin

Example: Athlete's foot

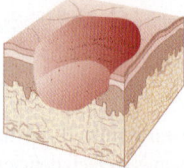

ULCER
Area of destruction of entire epidermis

Example: Decubitus (pressure sore)

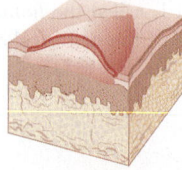

SCAR
Excess collagen production after injury

Example: Surgical healing

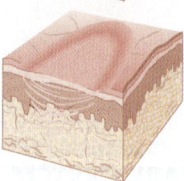

ATROPHY
Loss of some portion of the skin

Example: Paralysis

FIG. 4.3 Lesions of the skin. (From Proctor D, et al: *Kinn's The Medical Assistant*, ed 13, St. Louis, 2017, Elsevier.)

describes the common signs and symptoms of integumentary diseases and disorders. Determining the cause will vary and likely dictate the type of treatment needed.

A skin *lesion* (LEE zhun) is any visible, localized abnormality of skin tissue. It can be described as either primary or secondary. Primary lesions are early skin changes that have not yet undergone natural evolution or change caused by manipulation. Secondary lesions are the result of natural evolution or the manipulation of a primary lesion (Fig. 4.3). Other terms related to skin lesions, diagnostic testing, and therapies are found in Tables 4.2 to 4.5.

TABLE 4.2 Terms Related to Primary Skin Lesions

Term	Definition
Cyst (sist)	Nodule filled with a semisolid material, such as a keratinous or sebaceous cyst
Ecchymosis (eck ih MOH sis)	Hemorrhage or extravasation (leaking) of blood into the subcutaneous tissue; the resultant darkening is commonly described as a bruise
Hematoma (hee mah TOH mah)	Collection of blood trapped in the tissues and palpable to the examiner
Macule (MACK yool)	Flat blemish or discoloration less than 1 cm, such as a freckle, port-wine stain, or tattoo
Nodule (NOD yool)	Palpable, solid lesion less than 2 cm, such as a very small lipoma
Papule (PAP yool)	Solid skin lesion raised less than 1 cm, such as a pimple
Patch	Large, flat, nonpalpable macule, larger than 1 cm
Petechia (peh TEEK ee ah)	Tiny ecchymosis within the dermal layer
Plaque (plack)	Raised plateau-like papule greater than 1 cm, such as a psoriatic lesion or seborrheic keratosis
Purpura (PUR pur ah)	Massive hemorrhage into the tissues under the skin
Pustule (PUS tyool)	Superficial, elevated lesion containing pus that may be the result of an infection, such as acne
Telangiectasia (tell an jee eck TAY zsa)	Permanent dilation of groups of superficial capillaries and venules; also known as spider veins
Tumor (TOO mur)	Nodule more than 2 cm; any mass or swelling, including neoplasms
Vesicle (VESS ih kul)	Circumscribed, elevated lesion containing fluid and smaller than one-half cm, such as an insect bite; if larger than one-half cm, it is termed a bulla; commonly called a blister
Wheal (hweel)	Circumscribed, elevated papule caused by localized edema, which can result from a bug bite; *urticaria*, or *hives*, results from an allergic reaction

From Shiland B: *Mastering Healthcare Terminology,* ed 5, St. Louis, 2016, Elsevier.

TABLE 4.3 Terms Related to Secondary Skin Lesions

Term	Definition
Eschar (ES kar)	Dried serum, blood, or pus; may occur in inflammatory and infectious diseases, such as impetigo, or as the result of a burn; also called a *scab*
Fissure (FISH ur)	Cracklike lesion of the skin, such as an anal fissure
Keloid (KEE loyd)	Type of scar that is an overgrowth of tissue at the site of injury in excess of the amount of tissue necessary to repair the wound; the extra tissue is partially due to an accumulation of collagen at the site
Ulcer	Circumscribed craterlike lesion of the skin or mucous membrane resulting from *necrosis* (neck KROH sis), or tissue death, that can accompany an inflammatory, infectious, or malignant process; an example is a *decubitus ulcer* (deh KYOO bih tus) seen sometimes in bedridden patients

From Shiland B: *Mastering Healthcare Terminology,* ed 5, St. Louis, 2016, Elsevier.

TABLE 4.4 Terms Related to Laboratory Tests

Term	Definition
Fungal tests	Cultures of scrapings of lesions used to identify fungal infections
Wood light examination	Method used to identify a variety of skin infections using a Wood light, which produces UV light; tinea capitis and pseudomonas infections in burns are two of the disorders that it can reveal (Fig. 4.4)
Wound and abscess cultures	Lab samplings that can identify pathogens in wounds, such as diabetic or decubitus ulcers, postoperative wounds, or abscesses

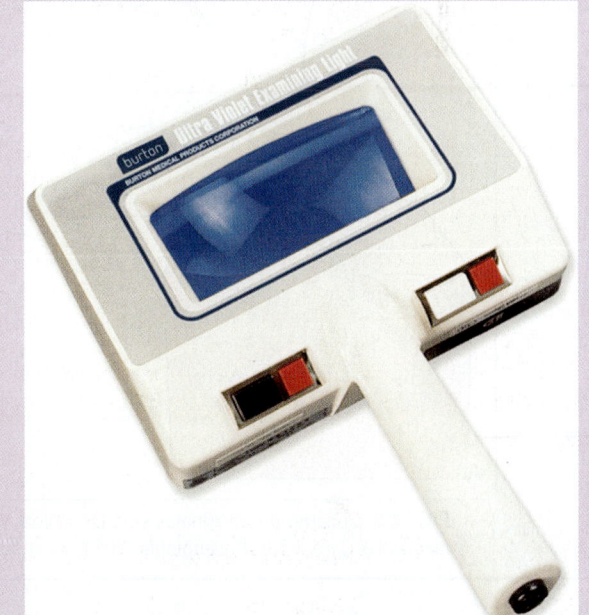

FIG. 4.4 Wood light. (From Seidel HM, Ball JW, Dains JE, et al: *Mosby's Guide to Physical Examination,* ed 7, St. Louis, 2011, Mosby.)

From Shiland B: *Mastering healthcare terminology,* ed 5, St. Louis, 2016, Elsevier.

TABLE 4.5 Terms Related to Tissue Removal and Other Therapies

Term	Definition
Cauterization (kah tur ih ZAY shun)	Destruction of tissue by burning with heat
Cryosurgery (KRY oh sur juh ree)	Destruction of tissue through the use of extreme cold, usually liquid nitrogen
Curettage (kyoo ruh TAJZ)	Scraping of material from the wall of a cavity or other surface to obtain tissue for microscopic examination; this is done with an instrument called a *curette* (Fig. 4.5)
Débridement (dah breed MON)	First step in wound treatment, involving removal of dirt, foreign bodies (FBs), damaged tissue, and cellular debris from the wound or burn to prevent infection and to promote healing
Escharotomy (ess kar AH tuh mee)	Surgical incision into necrotic tissue resulting from a severe burn; this may be necessary to prevent edema leading to ischemia (loss of blood flow) in underlying tissue
Incision and drainage (I&D)	Cutting open and removing the contents of a wound, cyst, or other lesion
Laser therapy	Procedure to repair or destroy tissue, particularly in the removal of tattoos, warts, port wine stains, and psoriatic lesions
Mohs surgery (MOHZ)	Repeated removal and microscopic examination of layers of a tumor until no cancerous cells are present (Fig. 4.6)
Occlusive therapy	Use of a nonporous occlusive dressing to cover a treated area to enhance the absorption and effectiveness of a medication; used to treat psoriasis, lupus erythematosus, and chronic hand dermatitis
Onychectomy (ah nick ECK tuh mee)	Removal of a fingernail or toenail because of trauma or disease
Photodynamic therapy (PDT)	Photodynamic therapy is a cancer treatment that uses medications to make cancer cells vulnerable to special lights; PDT involves applying a drug that makes the cells light sensitive, then the cancer cells are exposed to a certain wavelength of light; the light kills the cells that have absorbed the light-sensitive medication
Phototherapy	The use of light in the treatment of disease, especially of the skin; can be sunlight, ultraviolet light, or infrared light; can be in combination with a topical treatment
Psoralen plus ultraviolet A (PUVA) therapy (SORE ah lin)	Directing a type of UV light onto psoriatic lesions
Shaving (paring)	Slicing of thin sheets of tissue to remove lesions

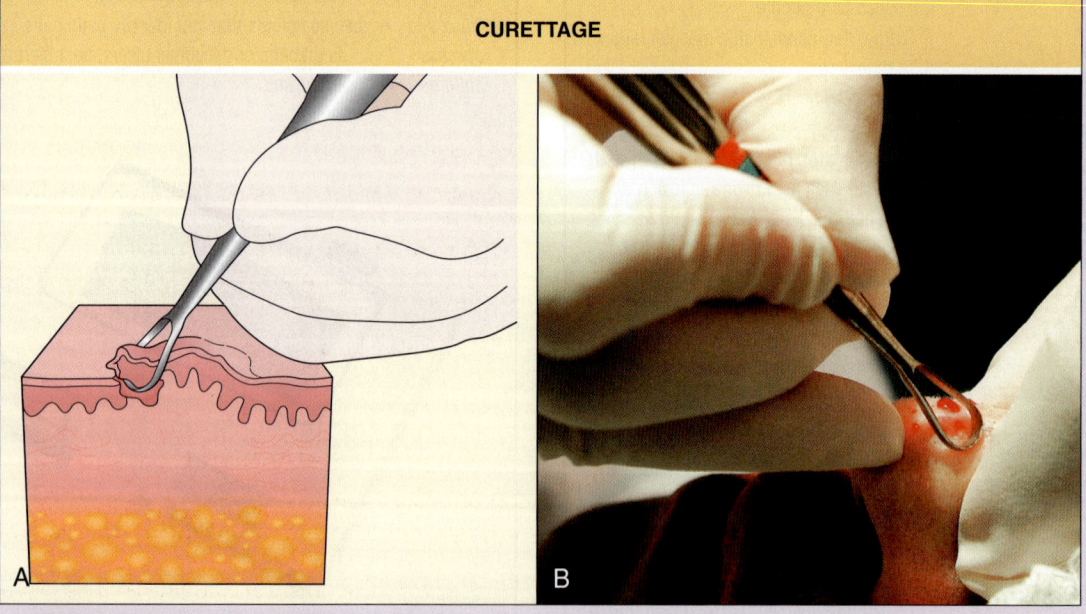

FIG. 4.5 Curette. (From Ignatavicius DD, Workman ML: *Medical-Surgical Nursing: Critical Thinking for Collaborative Care,* ed 6, Philadelphia, 2011, Saunders.)

CHAPTER 4 Integumentary System

TABLE 4.5 Terms Related to Tissue Removal and Other Therapies—cont'd

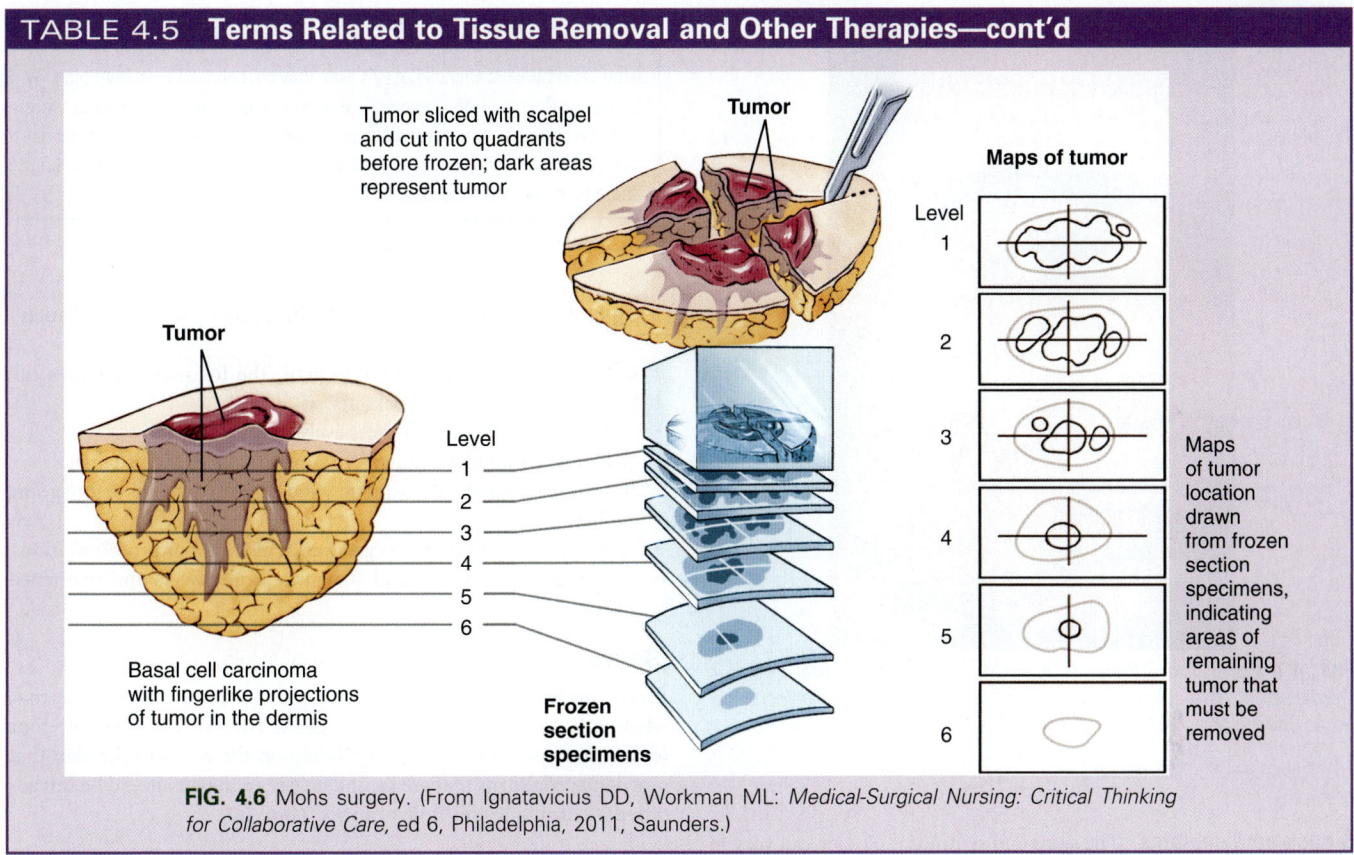

FIG. 4.6 Mohs surgery. (From Ignatavicius DD, Workman ML: *Medical-Surgical Nursing: Critical Thinking for Collaborative Care*, ed 6, Philadelphia, 2011, Saunders.)

From Shiland B: *Mastering Healthcare Terminology*, ed 5, St. Louis, 2016, Elsevier.

MEDICAL TERMINOLOGY

angi/o: vessel	**-oma:** mass
cauter/i: burn	**onych/o:** nail
chym/o: juice	**-osis:** abnormal condition
cry/o: extreme cold	**papul/o:** pimple
cyst/o: sac, bladder	**purpur/o:** purple
ec-: out	**pustul/o:** pustule
-ectasia: dilation	**teal/e:** far
-ectomy: removal, excision	**-tomy:** incision
hemat/o: blood	**troph/o:** development
-ive: pertaining to	**-ule:** small
macul/o: spot	**vesicul/o:** blister or small sac
nod/o: knot	**-y:** process
occlus/o: to close	**-zation:** process of

CRITICAL THINKING 4.5

Jean Burke comes into the exam room and greets Casey. Jean sits down, and she and Casey talk about the reason for the visit and what improvements Casey would like to see in her skin. Jean mentions that she had issues with acne as a teenager and assures Casey that they will develop a plan together. What type of lesions could Casey have with acne? Review Fig. 4.3 and share your thoughts with the class.

Acne Vulgaris

Acne is a skin condition that occurs when a hair follicle becomes plugged with oil and dead skin cells (Fig. 4.7). Acne is most common on the face, but it can occur on other sites of the body such as neck, chest, shoulders, and back. Acne is most common during adolescence, but it can occur at any age. Because acne can cause scarring, it is best treated as early as possible to minimize scars and emotional distress.

Etiology. The main causes of acne include excess oil production, pores clogged with dead skin cells and oil, and bacterial infections. Once a pore is clogged, bacteria that are trapped in the pore multiply and cause inflammation. Risk factors for acne include the following:
- Age: adolescents are most prone due to hormonal changes
- Medications: corticosteroids, androgens, oral contraceptives, and lithium
- Stress and diet: a diet that is high in dairy products and simple carbohydrates such as refined sugars, processed foods, and sweets can make acne worse

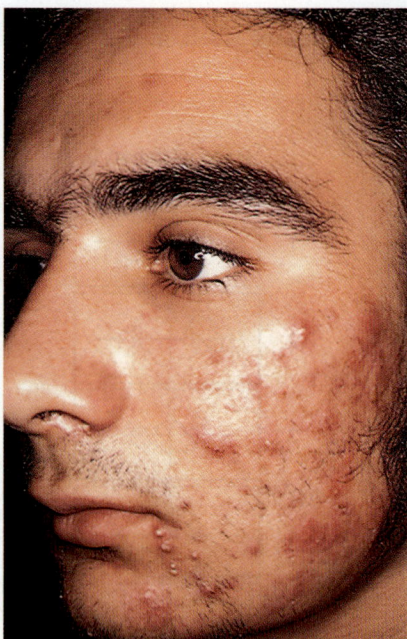

FIG. 4.7 Acne. (From Paller A, Mancini A: *Hurwitz Clinical Pediatric Dermatology: A Textbook of skin Disorders in Childhood and Adolescence*, ed 4, Philadelphia, 2011, Saunders.)

Signs and Symptoms. The signs and symptoms of acne can vary in severity. Common signs include the following:
- Whiteheads and blackheads
- Papules and pustules (Fig. 4.3)
- Large solid painful nodules
- Painful, pus-filled lumps beneath the skin's surface, known as *cystic acne*

Diagnostic Procedures. Acne that does not respond to over-the-counter (OTC) medications should be looked at by a physician. A physician will look at the lesions and will also ask questions related to the following:
- Diet, duration of acne, OTC remedies used
- Medications, including oral contraceptives
- Pregnancy status
- Use of lotions, sunscreen, soaps, and cosmetics

Treatment. There are many treatments used for acne, from simple OTC lotions to more extensive use of medications, antibiotics, and dermatologic procedures:
- Common medications include topical prescription-strength benzoyl peroxide, antibiotics, retinoids, and oral contraceptives.
- Common dermatologic procedures include light therapy, chemical peels, extraction of whiteheads and blackheads by a provider, and steroid injections.
- Common dietary changes recommended include reducing or eliminating dairy products, refined sugar, and simple carbohydrate foods. Examples include juice, soda, sweets, pasta, and bread.
- More extensive treatments include dermabrasion, laser resurfacing, and minor skin surgery to repair area of damage or excessive scarring.

Acne often requires extended treatment and follow-up, depending on the severity of the condition.

> **CRITICAL THINKING 4.6**
>
> After Jean Burke examines Casey's skin, they chat about a treatment plan. By reviewing the materials presented on acne in this chapter, write down what could be included in the treatment plan for Casey. Include dietary recommendations, OTC medications, and any other treatments you think may be helpful. Share your plan with the class.

Prognosis. The prognosis is good with proper patient compliance.

Prevention. For people prone to acne, the following activities can help reduce or eliminate breakouts:
- Keep skin clean and not excessively dry.
- Use medications or products recommended by the provider.
- Use noncomedogenic cosmetics, and remove makeup before going to bed.
- Eat a healthy diet rich in vegetables, fruit, and nonprocessed foods.
- Drink plenty of water, and stay away from sweets and sweetened drinks.

Burns

Burns are injuries to tissues that result from exposure to thermal, chemical, electrical, or radioactive agents. They are classified into four different degrees of severity, depending on the layers of the skin that are damaged. Burns that are second degree or higher should be categorized according to the "rule of nines" (Box 4.3).

Etiology. Because burns are injuries, the cause is trauma of some kind. Many risk factors could be included in this discussion, but caution should be taken when participating in activities that involve fire, chemicals, or electrical hazards. Proper safety equipment should always be available and ready to use when burns are a possibility.

Signs and Symptoms. The bulleted information that follows describes each category of burn:
- First-degree burn (superficial burn): A burn in which only the first layer of the skin, the epidermis, is damaged. It is characterized by redness (*erythema*), tenderness, and physical sensitivity (*hyperesthesia*), with no scar development.
- Second-degree burn (partial-thickness burn): A burn in which only the first and second layers of the skin (the epidermis and part of the dermis) are affected. If the burn extends to the papillary level, it is classified as a *superficial partial-thickness burn*. If it extends farther, to the reticular layer, it is classified as a *deep partial-thickness burn*. This type of burn is characterized by redness, blisters, and pain, with possible scar development.
- Third-degree burn (full-thickness burn): A burn that damages the epidermis, dermis, and subcutaneous tissue. Pain is not present because the nerve endings in the skin have been destroyed. The skin may appear deep red, pale gray, brown, or black. Scar formation is likely.
- Fourth-degree burn (deep full-thickness burn): Although not a universally accepted category, some burn specialists use this category to describe a rare burn that extends beyond the subcutaneous tissue into the muscle and bone.

Diagnostic Procedures. Burns may not uniformly affect an injured area, so determining the depth of a burn and the extent of tissue damage is important. Burns are treated differently depending on the depth of damage. Treatment is based on the category of burn (Fig. 4.6).

CHAPTER 4 Integumentary System

BOX 4.3 Burns: The Rule of Nines

The rule of nines regarding burns divides the body into percentages that are, for the most part, multiples of nine: the head and neck equal 9%, each upper limb 9%, each lower limb 18%, the front and back of the torso 36%, and the genital area 1% (Fig. 4.8). Fig. 4.9 illustrates the different degrees of burns.

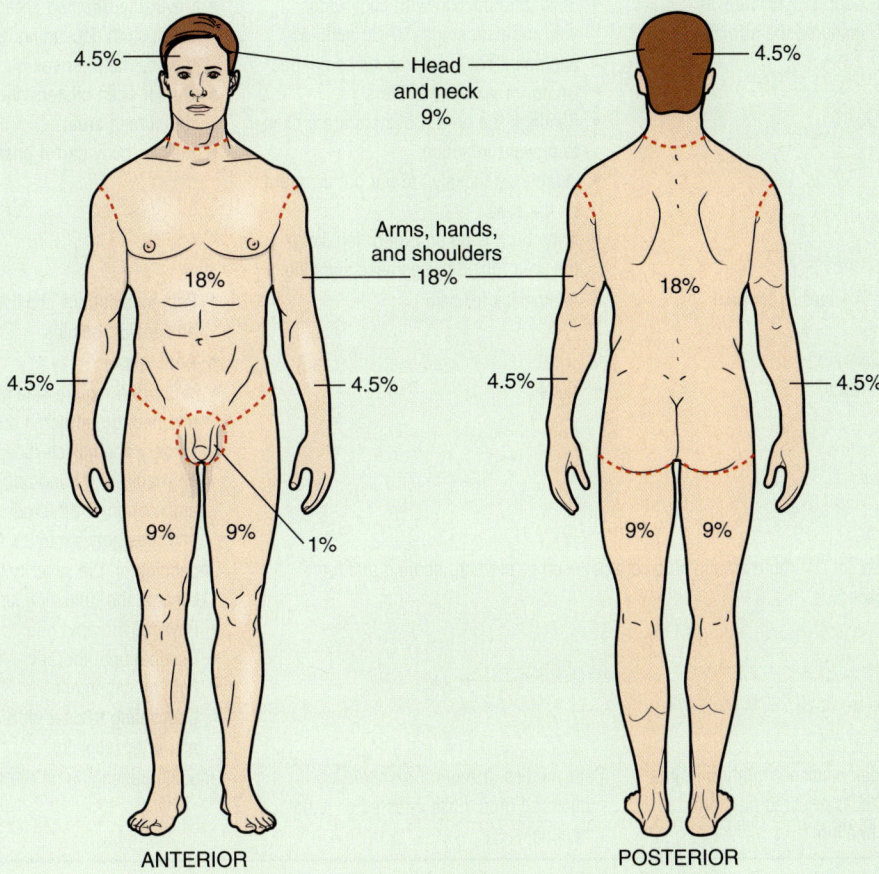

FIG. 4.8 Rule of nines for estimating the extent of burns.

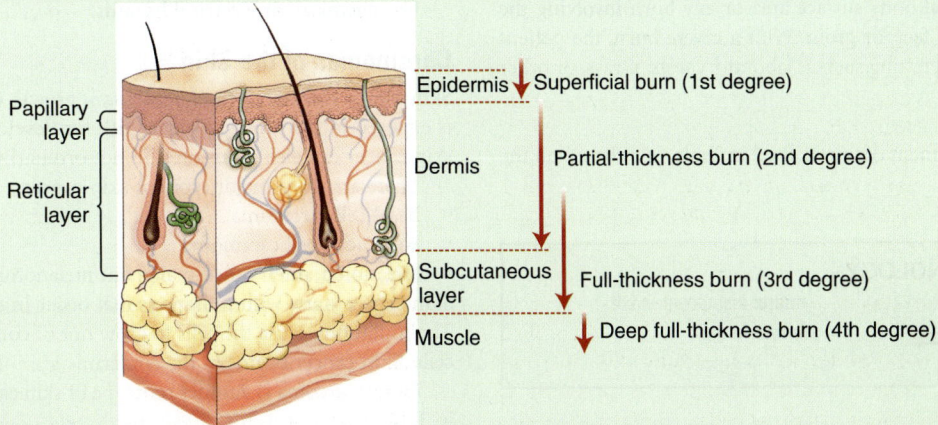

FIG. 4.9 Burn category tissue involvement. (From Shiland B: *Mastering Healthcare Terminology*, ed 5, St. Louis, 2016, Elsevier.)

TABLE 4.6 Treatment of Burns

	First-Degree Burn	Second-Degree Burn	Third- and Fourth-Degree Burns (this category of burn will need immediate and ongoing medical attention)
Treatment, nondrug	• Cool to cold water to immerse the affected area	• Rinse burned skin with cool water until the pain stops, 10–30 minutes; additional cool compresses as needed • Do not break open blisters • Bandage the area if blisters are broken to prevent infection • Wrap area loosely; do not put pressure on the area • If the burn is on an arm or leg, keep the area raised to decrease swelling	• Cover the affected area with sterile gauze or a clean cloth depending on the size of the burn until medical help arrives • Do not open blisters or remove clothing stuck to the burned area • Elevate body part if possible
Treatment, medications	• Analgesics for pain	• Analgesics for pain	• Pain medications consistent with pain needs; analgesics, opioids • Antibiotics
Surgical intervention	• None	• None	• Will often require skin grafts to close the wound and heal the affected area (Table 4.7); plastic surgery and muscle/bone surgical restoration may be required; if bone and muscle are destroyed, amputation of affected areas may be necessary and prosthetics may be required
Other treatments	Topical OTC burn cream, aloe vera gel used to promote healing and limit scarring		Depending on the severity of the burn and tissue damage, the following services may be needed: • Physical therapy • Occupational therapy • Pain management • Counseling to deal with emotional issues during and after recovery
Follow-up treatments	Seek medical attention if area looks infected or is not healing	Seek medical attention *immediately* if blistered area looks infected or is not healing	Ongoing depending on the extent of tissue damage

From Shiland B: *Mastering Healthcare Terminology*, ed 5, St. Louis, 2016, Elsevier.

The American Burn Association defines a severe burn as a burn that affects 25% of the total body surface area or any burn involving the eyes, ears, face, hands, feet, or groin. With a severe burn, the patient may require additional testing such as laboratory tests, x-rays, or other diagnostics.

Treatment. The treatment of burns listed in Table 4.6 is based on the category of burn.

> **MEDICAL TERMINOLOGY**
> **all/o:** other
> **auto-:** self
> **dermat/o:** skin
> **-tome:** instrument to cut
> **xen/o:** foreign

Prognosis. The prognosis for first- and second-degree burns is very good. The prognosis for third- and fourth-degree burns depends on the percentage of the body affected and the cause and location of the tissue damage.

Prevention
- Proper safety equipment should always be available and ready to use when burns are a possibility.
- Caution should be used when participating in activities that involve fire, chemical, or electrical hazards.

Carcinomas of the Skin

Skin cancer is the abnormal, **malignant** growth of skin cells. Skin that is exposed to the sun is at higher risk for developing skin cancer, but skin cancer can also occur on skin not ordinarily exposed to sunlight.

There are three major types of skin cancer:
- Basal cell carcinoma
- Squamous cell carcinoma
- Melanoma, often called malignant melanoma

Skin cancer starts with mutations that occur in the DNA of skin cells. The mutations cause the cells to grow out of control and form cancer cells. Skin cancer begins in the epidermis.

Kaposi sarcoma is another rare type of skin cancer that is addressed in Table 4.10.

> **VOCABULARY**
> **malignant:** A descriptive term for things or conditions that threaten life or well-being. Malignant is the opposite of benign.

TABLE 4.7 Terms Related to Grafting Techniques

Term	Definition
Allograft (AL oh graft)	Harvest of skin from another human donor for temporary transplant until an autograft is available; also called a *homograft*
Autograft (AH toh graft)	Harvest of the patient's own skin for transplant (Fig. 4.10)
Dermatome (DUR mah tohm)	Instrument used to remove split-thickness skin grafts (Fig. 4.11)
Flap	Section of skin transferred from one location to an immediately adjacent one; also called a skin graft (SG)
Full-thickness graft	Skin graft in which full portions of both the epidermis and the dermis are used
Skin graft (SG)	Skin transplant performed when normal skin cover has been lost as a result of burns, ulcers, or operations to remove cancerous tissue
Split-thickness skin graft (STSG)	Skin graft in which the epidermis and parts of the dermis are used
Xenograft (ZEE noh graft)	Temporary skin graft from another species, often a pig, used until an autograft is available; also called a *heterograft*

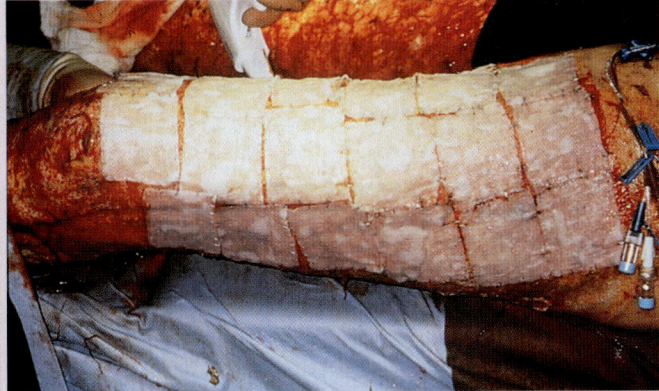

FIG. 4.10 Autograft. (From McCance KL, Huether SE: *Pathophysiology: The Biologic Basis for Disease in Adults and Children,* ed 6, St. Louis, 2010, Mosby.)

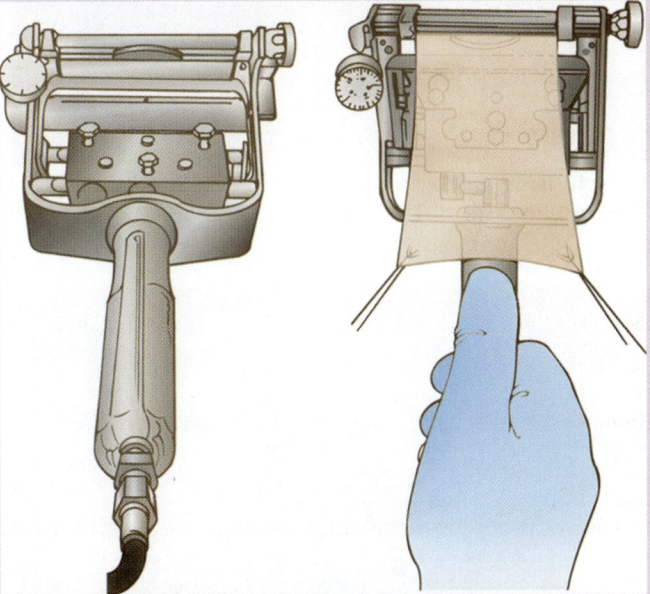

FIG. 4.11 Dermatome. (From Shiland B: *Mastering Healthcare Terminology,* ed 5, St. Louis, 2016, Elsevier.)

From Shiland B: *Mastering Healthcare Terminology,* ed 5, St. Louis, 2016, Elsevier.

Etiology. Skin cancer can happen in three different types of cells in the epidermis:
- *Squamous cells* lie just below the outer surface of the skin.
- *Basal cells* produce new skin cells and are located beneath the squamous cells.
- *Melanocytes* produce melanin, the pigment that gives skin its normal color. They are located in the lower part of the epidermis.

These cancers are thought to be caused by exposure to UV rays of the sun. UV rays can damage DNA in the skins cells, which starts a mutation. Although not all cancers develop in areas of the body exposed to the sun. It is still unknown what other specific factors influence the start of a malignant mutation.

Additional risk factors for skin cancer include the following:
- Fair skin with blond or red hair and light-colored eyes, and skin that freckles or sunburns easily
- History of sunburns that have blistered
- Moles that look irregular and are generally larger than normal moles
- A family history of skin cancer; if one parent or a sibling has had skin cancer, there may be an increased risk of the disease

Signs and Symptoms. Basal cell carcinoma most frequently appears on sun-exposed areas (Fig. 4.12) and may appear as follows:
- A pearly or waxy bump
- A flat, flesh-colored or brown scarlike lesion

Squamous cell carcinoma most frequently appears on sun-exposed areas (Fig. 4.13) and may appear as follows:
- A firm, red nodule
- A flat lesion with a scaly, crusted surface

Melanoma can develop anywhere on the body (Fig. 4.14). It can start in normal-looking skin or in an existing mole. Skin that has not been exposed to sunlight can still develop melanoma. Melanoma can affect people of any skin color. People with darker skin can develop melanoma on the palms of hand or soles of their feet, or even under fingernails or toenails. Melanoma may appear as follows:
- A large brownish spot with darker speckles
- A mole that changes in color, size, feel, or that bleeds

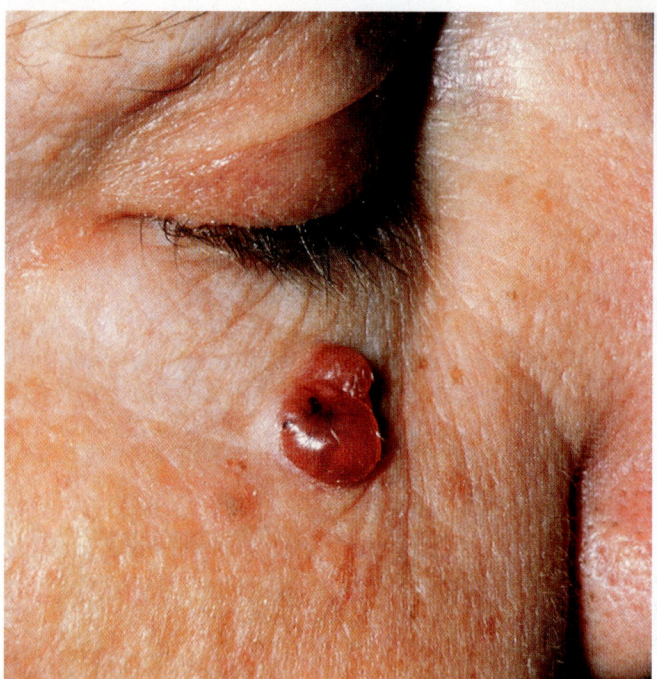

FIG. 4.12 Basal cell carcinoma. (From James WD, et al: *Andrews' Diseases of the Skin,* ed 11, Philadelphia, 2011, Saunders.)

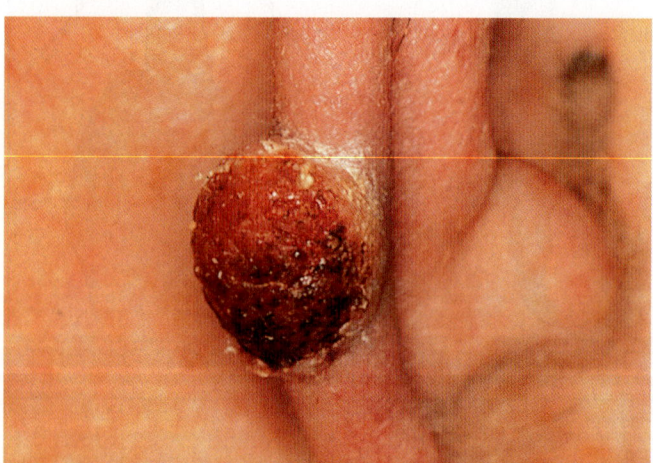

FIG. 4.13 Squamous cell carcinoma. (From McCance KL, Huether SE: *Pathophysiology: The Biologic Basis for Disease in Adults and Children,* ed 6, St. Louis, 2010, Mosby.)

- A small lesion with an irregular border and portions that appear red, white, blue, or blue-black
- Dark lesions on the palms of the hands, soles of the feet, fingertips, or toes

Box 4.4 describes the melanoma self-examination process.

Diagnostic Procedures. To diagnose any type of skin cancer, the provider will do the following:
- The provider will examine the skin and look for changes that are likely to be skin cancer.
- If abnormal areas of the skin are found, a skin biopsy will be performed (Table 4.8). A biopsy will determine whether skin cancer is present. If cancer is found, a pathologist will determine what type of skin cancer is present.

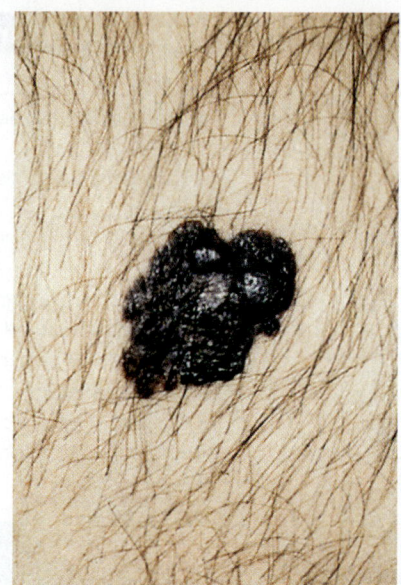

FIG. 4.14 Malignant melanoma. (From Damjanov I: *Anderson's Pathology,* ed 10, St. Louis, 2000, Mosby.)

BOX 4.4   Melanoma Self-Examination

A nevus, also called a mole, is a pigmented lesion often present at birth. Various abnormal changes of a mole raise concern that there is development of a malignancy. The American Academy of Dermatology advises that everyone watch skin spots for these features:
  Asymmetry: one area of the mole is changing
  Borders: moles are becoming irregular
  Colors: changes or uneven pigmentation
  Diameter: increasing size, more than 6 mm or one-fourth of an inch
  Evolving: changing
Follow this **ABCDE** guide to determine if a spot on the skin may be melanoma.

- If there is skin cancer, additional tests may be done to determine the extent or stage of the skin cancer.
- Additional tests might include the following:
  - Imaging tests to examine nearby lymph nodes for signs of cancer
  - Removal of a nearby lymph node that will be tested for signs of cancer and staged; skin cancer's stage helps determine which treatment options will be most effective

CRITICAL THINKING 4.7

After Jean Burke and Casey go over the proposed treatment plan, Jean takes out a brochure on skin cancer. She shows the brochure to Casey and reminds her of how important her skin is. Even though Casey is young, precautions taken now could help prevent skin cancer in her future. List five preventive measures that she can take now in order to protect her skin from cancer. Share with the class.

Treatment. Treatment for skin cancer varies greatly depending on the type of skin cancer and stage. Early detection and treatment is always the best option for any type of skin cancer, but that is not always possible.

TABLE 4.8   Terms Related to Biopsies

Term	Definition
Excisional biopsy	Biopsy (Bx) in which the entire tumor may be removed with borders as a means of diagnosis and treatment (Fig. 4.15)
Exfoliation (ECKS foh lee A shun)	Scraping or shaving off samples of friable (easily crushed) lesions for a laboratory examination called *exfoliative cytology*
Incisional biopsy	Biopsy in which larger tissue samples may be obtained by excising a wedge of tissue and suturing the incision (see Fig. 4.15)
Needle aspiration	Aspiration of fluid from lesions to obtain samples for culture and examination
Punch biopsy	Biopsy in which a tubular punch is inserted through to the subcutaneous tissue and the tissue is cut off at the base (Fig. 4.16)

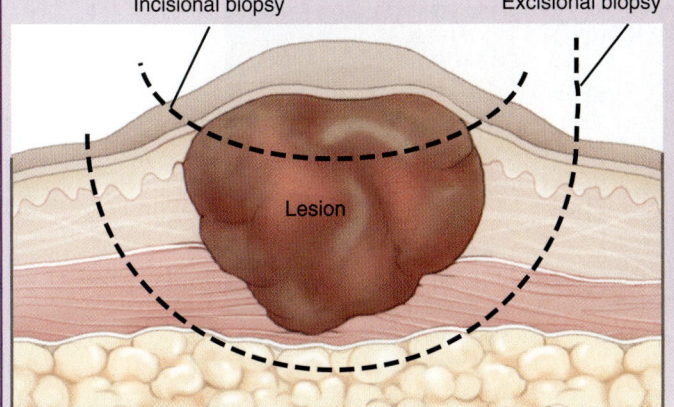

FIG. 4.15 Incisional and excisional biopsies. (From Shiland B: *Mastering Healthcare Terminology,* ed 5, St. Louis, 2016, Elsevier.)

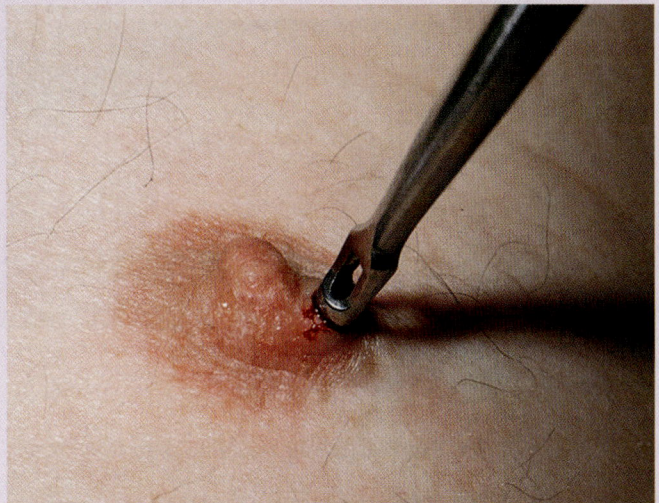

FIG. 4.16 Punch biopsy. (From Shiland B: *Mastering Healthcare Terminology,* ed 5, St. Louis, 2016, Elsevier.)

Common treatments for basal cell and squamous cell carcinomas include the following:
- Mohs micrographic surgery (see Table 4.5)
- Excisional surgery (Table 4.5)
- Topical medications and photodynamic therapy (PDT) (see Table 4.5)
- Electrosurgery, cryosurgery, or laser surgery (see Table 4.5)

Treatment for melanoma varies greatly depending on the location and stage of the cancer. Treatment ranges from minor localized surgery to major surgery, radiation, and chemotherapy.

Prognosis. Prognosis for any type of malignancy is dependent on the type of cancer, location, and stage. Basal cell and squamous cell cancers rarely, if ever, spread beyond the skin. The prognosis for these two cancers is usually very good.

Melanoma, if detected and treated early, also has a good prognosis. But if melanoma is detected once the cancer has spread to the lymph nodes or other tissue, the prognosis is much more cautious.

Prevention. Most skin cancers are preventable. The prevention tips that follow will help protect a patient against possible skin cancer:
- Avoid the sun during the middle of the day from 10 a.m. and 4 p.m.
- Wear sunscreen, at least SPF 15, even in the winter months or on cloudy days.
- Wear protective clothing. Clothing should cover the arms and legs. Wear a broad-brimmed hat to protect the face, neck, nose, and ears. Photoprotective clothing is available; ask a dermatologist to recommend an appropriate brand. Wear sunglasses. Look for protection against UVA and UVB rays.
- Examine your own skin regularly; report changes to your provider. Examine skin for changes to moles, freckles, bumps, and birthmarks.
- Avoid tanning beds.

Decubitus Ulcers

The terms *bedsores* and *pressure ulcers* are also names for decubitus ulcers (Fig. 4.17). These sores are injuries to the skin and underlying tissue from prolonged pressure to the skin. This type of injury is most common on the skin that covers bony areas of the body, such as heels, ankles, hips, tailbone, elbows, and shoulders.

Patients who are confined to beds or wheelchairs or who have limited ability to change position are at greatest risk for bedsores. They can develop quickly and are often difficult to treat. This type of wound may not look like much superficially, but underneath there may be significant damage down to the bone.

Etiology. Decubitus ulcers are caused by prolonged pressure against the skin that limits blood flow. The affected area is deprived of nutrients and oxygen, causing damage to the skin. Various risk factors contribute to bedsores:
- Prolonged pressure to one area of the body because of an inability to move independently and infrequent repositioning
- Paralysis, general poor health and weakness, friction against fragile skin
- Injury, illness, or surgery that causes immobility
- Limited awareness of one's surroundings

Signs and Symptoms. Decubitus ulcers are categorized by the National Pressure Ulcer Advisory Panel into one of four stages based

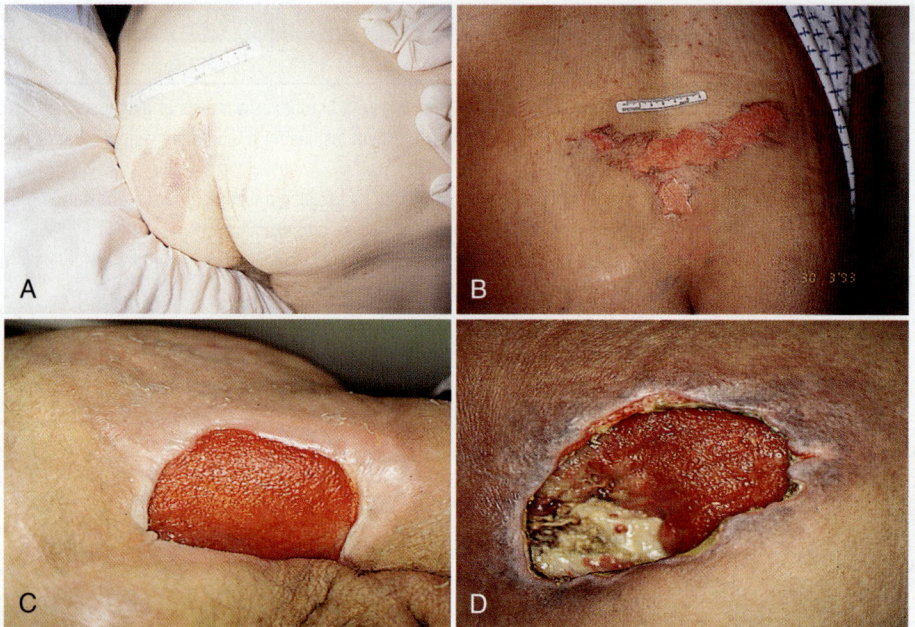

FIG. 4.17 Decubitus ulcers. (From Elkin MK, Perry AG, Potter PA: *Nursing Intervention and Clinical Skills*, ed 4, St. Louis, 2008, Mosby.)

on the severity of tissue damage. See the following abbreviated stage definitions:
- *Stage I*: The skin is unbroken but appears red with lighter skin and may show discoloration with darker skin. The site may be tender or painful.
- *Stage II*: The epidermis and part of the dermis is damaged or missing. The wound may be shallow pinkish or red. It may appear like a fluid-filled blister or ruptured blister.
- *Stage III*: The ulcer is a deep wound with skin loss and some underlying fat is exposed. The bottom of the wound may have some yellowish dead tissue and extend beyond the primary wound.
- *Stage IV*: The ulcer shows large-scale tissue loss. The wound may expose muscles, bone, or tendons. The bottom of the wound is likely dead yellowish, dark, or crusty in appearance.

An unstageable decubitus ulcer surface is covered in yellow, brown, black, or dead tissue. It is not possible to see how deep the wound is.

Diagnostic Procedures. To evaluate a bedsore, the provider examines the patient to do the following:
- Determine the size and depth of the ulcer
- Check for bleeding and debris in the wound
- Look for signs of infection, dead tissue, and odors that indicate infection
- Check the area for signs of spreading tissue damage or infection
- Check for other pressure sores on the body

Laboratory tests may include the following:
- Blood tests to check overall health
- Wound cultures to diagnose bacterial or fungal infection in a wound that does not heal with treatment or is already at stage IV
- Tissue cultures to check for cancerous tissue in a chronic, nonhealing wound

Treatment
- Reducing pressure by doing the following:
  - Repositioning the patient more frequently and in different positions
  - Using support surfaces such as special cushions to support fragile skin
- Cleaning and dressing wounds
  - Removing damaged tissue may require surgical débridement that involves cutting away dead tissue for stage III and IV ulcers
- Managing pain, which includes the use of nonsteroidal antiinflammatory drugs (NSAIDs) and topical pain medications
- Using antibiotics, topical or oral, if the ulcer is infected
- Administering negative pressure therapy (vacuum-assisted closure [VAC]), which uses a device that applies suction to a clean wound and may help healing in some types of pressure sores
- Performing surgery if a pressure sore fails to heal

Prognosis. If a decubitus ulcer is detected in stage I or II, the prognosis is good. If the ulcer is at stage III or IV, the prognosis is varied.

Prevention. The best prevention for a decubitus ulcer is frequent position change, if a person can move independently. If a person has limited mobility, frequent repositioning is critical. Good skin care, daily skin inspection, and a proper diet and hydration will also help to discourage the formation of decubitus ulcers or bedsores.

Dermatophytosis (Tenia Fungal Infections)

Dermatophytosis, when it affects the body, is more commonly known as ringworm. These infections are called ringworm because of the appearance of the infected area. Ringworm infections start as a flat, scaly area that may be red and itchy. This small area then develops into a round, red rash with a clear center and slightly raised red border. There is no worm involved in this infection, just fungus.

Etiology. Tenia is the general term for a fungal infection, or *mycoses*, on the body. There are several tenia infections that can occur on the body (Box 4.5). Fungal infections are spread by skin contact with another infected person, animal, or surface that is harboring a fungus.

BOX 4.5 Common Tenia Infections and Locations

Here is a list of the different types of common fungal infections and their location:
- Ringworm: tenia corporis, located on the trunk and limbs
- Jock itch: tenia cruris, located in the groin
- Ringworm on the scalp (Fig. 4.18): tenia capitis
- Athlete's foot (Fig. 4.19): tenia pedis
- Fingernail and toenail infections: tenia unguium

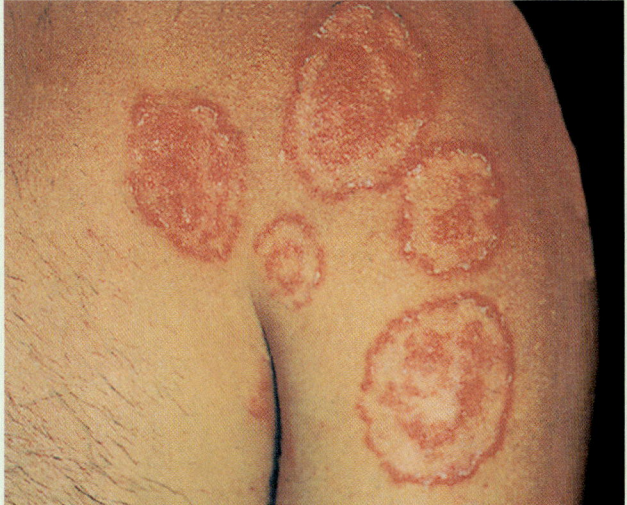

FIG. 4.18 Tinea corporis (ringworm). (From Habif TP: *Clinical Dermatology*, ed 4, St. Louis, 2004, Mosby.)

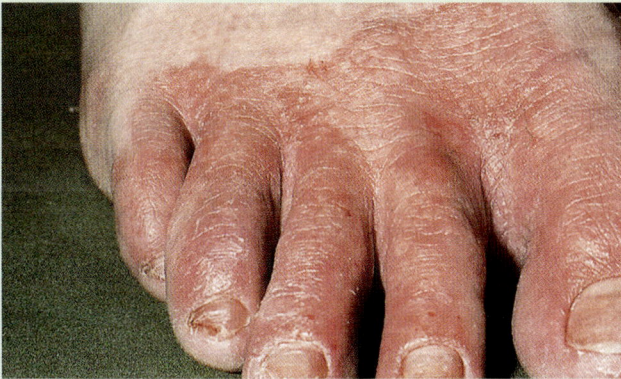

FIG. 4.19 Tinea pedis (athlete's foot). (From Gawkrodger D: *Dermatology*, ed 5, New York, 2012, Churchill Livingstone.)

Signs and Symptoms. Ringworm and other fungal infections may appear as follows:
- Red, flat, scaly patches emerge, which are itchy at first.
- As the infection spreads, the patch continues to grow and has a clear center that may have red, scaly patches with a red, raised circular border.
- Red, scaly patches with itching, burning, or cracking skin also characterize other fungal infection sites.
- Fungal infections rarely spread to areas below the skin surface, but individuals who are immune compromised or who have a weakened immune system may find it hard to successfully treat fungal infections.

BOX 4.6 Common Fungal Over-the-Counter Treatments

OTC medicated creams include antifungal ingredients such as miconazole, clotrimazole, ketoconazole, and terbinafine.

Diagnostic Procedures. Most healthcare providers can diagnose ringworm and other fungal skin infections by sight. If there is any doubt about the cause of the infection, a skin scraping from the affected area can be collected and viewed under a microscope for diagnosis. Fungal cultures are rarely done.

Treatment. Antifungal creams and lotions are the most common treatment for fungal infections and are very effective (Box 4.6). Most OTC topical fungal treatments should be used for 2 to 3 weeks until the infected area is completely healed. If OTC strength applications are not effective, a prescription-strength antifungal cream, lotion, or oral medication may be recommended. Treatment should be continued until the entire affected area is completely healed; this may take 2 to 3 weeks.

Prognosis. The prognosis is good if treatment directions are followed.

Prevention. To prevent dermatophytosis:
- Do not have skin contact with infected individuals or animals or with objects that have touched an infected person or animal.

Eczema (Atopic Dermatitis)

Eczema, also known as *atopic dermatitis*, is a group of conditions that will make skin irritated, inflamed, red, and itchy. It is more common in children but can occur at any age. Eczema is a chronic condition that may become worse occasionally and then subside.

Eczema is a group of conditions with an inherited tendency. It is often seen in combination with asthma or hay fever. Most infants who develop eczema outgrow it by their 10th birthday. Some adults continue to have symptoms throughout their lifetime. The disease often can be controlled with proper treatment.

Etiology. The cause of eczema in unknown, but it is more common in families with a history of allergies and asthma. Flare-ups can occur in response to specific substances, conditions, or triggers. Temperature, exposure to certain chemicals, fabric texture, and pet dander are all examples of possible irritants. Stress can also be a trigger.

Signs and Symptoms. Some of the common signs and symptoms of eczema are listed here:
- Itchy skin is a common symptom for anyone with eczema.
- Rash often appears on the face, back of knees, hands, wrists, or feet.
- Skin may have a dry, thickened, or scaly appearance that starts out pink or red but can turn brownish with time.

Diagnostic Procedures. A pediatrician, dermatologist, or primary care provider will observe the rash and ask specific questions about the signs and symptoms. Sometimes the provider will perform allergy tests to try to pinpoint a specific trigger or irritant. Most frequently, observation and patient history are sufficient to diagnose eczema.

Treatment. The treatment of eczema is focused on relieving itching and preventing scratching of the skin, which can lead to infection. Using a provider-recommended lotion or cream to keep the skin moist is the most common treatment. Applying topical treatments when the skin is damp (i.e., after a bath or shower) may help the skin to retain moisture. Cold compresses and 1% hydrocortisone cream are also common treatments.

If OTC remedies are not providing relief, creams and ointments that contain corticosteroids can be prescribed to lessen inflammation of the skin. Antibiotics may also be prescribed if an area becomes infected after vigorous itching.

Other treatments include the following:
- Antihistamines are prescribed to lessen severe itching.
- Phototherapy is administered, during which a UV light is applied to affected areas of the skin.
- For patients with moderate to unresponsive eczema, cyclosporine or topical immunomodulators (TIM) may be prescribed. Both drugs are immunosuppressants, which means they work by altering the immune system response to help prevent flare-ups. Cyclosporine is an oral medication; TIM is a skin cream. There are concerns about side effects, so caution should be used with either of these medications.

Prognosis. The prognosis for eczema is good, especially with irritant avoidance and proper ongoing skin care.

Prevention. Eczema flare-ups can be diminished or prevented with good ongoing skin care, which includes the following:
- Keep skin clean and frequently moisturize to avoid dry skin.
- Avoid sudden changes in temperature or humidity, and avoid sweating or overheating
- Reduce stress as much as possible.
- Avoid scratchy fabrics, harsh soaps or detergents, and solvents.
- Avoid any foods that may cause a flare-up.

Psoriasis

Psoriasis is an autoimmune disease that affects the life cycle of skin cells. Psoriasis causes skin cells to build up rapidly on the surface of the skin. The extra skin cells form thick, silvery scales and itchy, dry, red patches that are sometimes painful. There may be times when symptoms improve, alternating with times when they worsen.

Etiology. Psoriasis is caused by a malfunction in the immune cells called T lymphocytes (T cells). T lymphocytes normally travel through the body looking for pathogens (bacteria and viruses) to destroy. That is their job. But for people who have psoriasis, their T lymphocytes attack healthy skin cells. This T cell overactivity causes the skin to produce too many new skin cells and the immune system to produce too many T cells.

It is unclear why the immune system of people with psoriasis acts this way. It can become a vicious cycle of rapid skin cell production, which leads to the characteristic psoriasis plaques. Anyone can develop psoriasis, but risk factors include the following:
- A family history of psoriasis
- Stress
- A history of recurring streptococcal infections
- Obesity
- Smoking

Box 4.7 describes some of the conditions that can cause psoriasis to worsen.

Signs and Symptoms. Psoriasis signs and symptoms can vary, but plaques have a characteristic appearance and tend to be as follows:
- Red patches of skin covered in silvery scales
- Dry, cracked skin that may bleed and small patches of scaly spots

---

> **BOX 4.7 Conditions That Cause Psoriasis to Worsen**
>
> Here is a list of some conditions that can cause psoriasis to get worse:
> - Injury to the skin, such as a scrape, cut, bug bite, abrasion, or severe sunburn
> - Stress, physical or emotional
> - Cold weather
> - Smoking tobacco products or heavy alcohol consumption
> - Streptococcal infections of the throat and skin

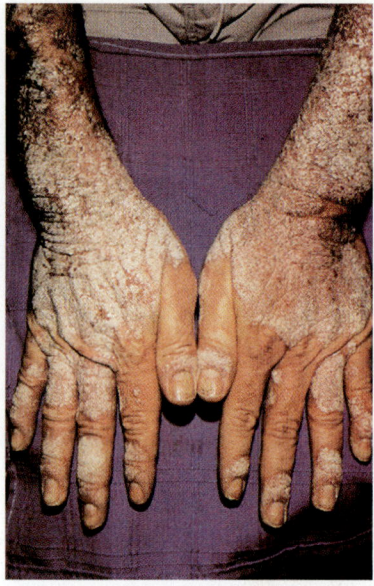

FIG. 4.20 Psoriasis. (From Bork K, Brauninger W: *Skin Disease in Clinical Practice*, ed 2, Philadelphia, 1999, Saunders.)

- Itching, burning, and pain in and around plaques
- Thick, pitted, or ridged finger- and toenails
- Swollen and stiff joints

Some people may only have a few spots of psoriasis; others may have large skin eruptions that may cover large areas of the body. Psoriasis may erupt, then get better, and continue this cycle for years.

Some of the most common forms of psoriasis are plaque, nail, scalp, and psoriatic arthritis, which also affects the joints (Figs. 4.20 and 4.21).

> **CRITICAL THINKING 4.8**
>
> As Casey and Jean Burke finish their appointment, Jean calls Mai back into the exam room to go over Casey's treatment plan and asks Mai to put together a treatment plan packet for Casey. As all three women talk, Casey comments about how she was nervous coming in to talk about her acne because she was embarrassed, but she feels so much better after knowing that Mai and Jean had acne issues in the past. How can you help put your patients at ease when they have sensitive or embarrassing issues to discuss with the provider? Why can skin issues be difficult for people to talk about? Share your thoughts with the class.

Diagnostic Procedures. Common diagnostic procedures include, but are not limited to, the following:
- History and physical examination, which should include skin, nails, and scalp
- Skin biopsy

CHAPTER 4 Integumentary System 87

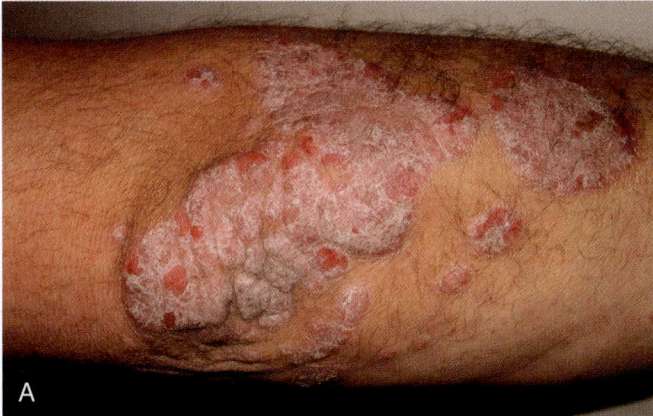
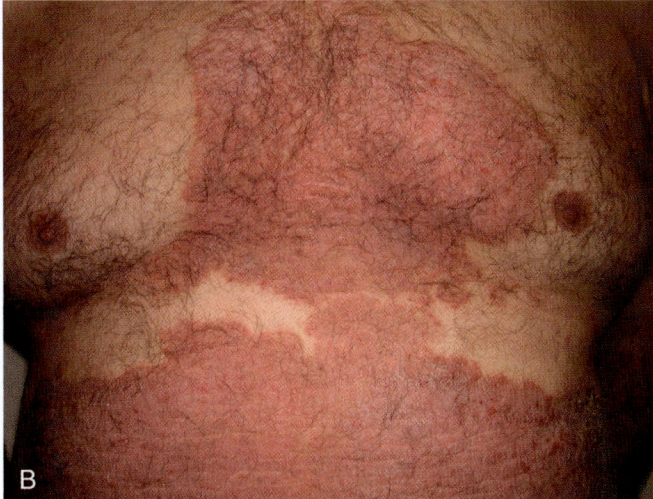

FIG. 4.21 Psoriasis. (From Marks J, Miller J: *Lookingbill and Marks' Principles of Dermatology*, ed 5, Philadelphia, 2014, Saunders.)

TABLE 4.9	Laboratory Testing Related to Psoriasis (Autoimmune Diseases)
Term	**Definition**
C-reactive protein (CRP)	CRP is a nonspecific marker for inflammation in the body; it is produced in the liver and measured by testing the blood; CRP levels rise in response to inflammation
Erythrocyte sedimentation rate (ESR)	Sometimes called a sed rate, an ESR measures the rate that red blood cells (RBCs) settle to the bottom of a calibrated tube; inflammation causes abnormal proteins to be appear in the blood; when this happens, RBCs clump and settle faster than normal; a higher than normal sed rate is a nonspecific indicator of inflammation in the body; CLIA-waived test
Rheumatoid factor (RF) test (ROO mah toyd)	Lab test that looks for RF present in the blood of those who may have rheumatoid arthritis

From Shiland B: *Mastering Healthcare Terminology*, ed 5, St. Louis, 2016, Elsevier.

- Laboratory tests that may include erythrocyte sedimentation rate (ESR) and C-reactive protein (CRP) testing, and, if joints are involved, a rheumatoid factor (RF) test to rule out rheumatoid arthritis. (Table 4.9)

Treatment. The goals of psoriasis treatment are as follows:
- To stop the skin from overproducing skin cells
- To reduce inflammation
- To improve the scaly patches of skin and returning it to a normal appearance

There are three main areas of treatment for psoriasis: topical treatments, light therapy, and systemic medications. Using a combination of all three types of treatment will help to return effected skin to its normal function and appearance:
- Topical treatments: examples include topical corticosteroids, synthetic vitamin D creams, topical retinoids, salicylic acid, coal tar, and moisturizers
- Light therapy treatments: examples include natural sunlight, ultraviolet B therapy, and Goeckerman therapy (a combination of coal tar therapy and UVB phototherapy)
- Systemic medications: examples include retinoids, methotrexate, cyclosporine, and biologics or immunomodulators to alter the immune system

Prognosis. The prognosis for psoriasis is as varied as the disease. It is a chronic autoimmune condition that requires ongoing treatment and patient compliance.

Prevention. Because psoriasis is an autoimmune condition that seems to have family history links, it may not be entirely possible to prevent it. Staying away from known triggers that can cause psoriasis flare-ups is recommended. Proper and ongoing skin care will help to lessen flare-ups. Keeping stress levels low and not consuming alcohol to excess will also help.

Shingles (Herpes Zoster)

Shingles is a viral infection that causes a painful, burning rash. Shingles can occur anywhere on the body, but it most often appears as a stripe of blisters that wraps around either side of the torso at the lower part of the ribs. This is a painful condition that can disrupt a person's quality of life.

Etiology. Shingles is caused by a herpes virus known as varicella-zoster. This same virus is the causative agent for chickenpox. After a person has had chickenpox, the virus stays in the body in an inactive form. It lays dormant on nerve tissue near the spinal cord and brain. Years later, the virus may reactivate as shingles. Some people can have more than one reactivation in their life. Vaccines can help reduce the risk of shingles, whereas early treatment can help shorten the active infection and lessen the chance of complications.

Some people have a greater risk for developing shingles:
- People who have had chickenpox and are 50 years old or older
- People who are immunocompromised or have conditions such as HIV/AIDS and cancer
- People who are undergoing chemotherapy or radiation for cancer treatment
- People who are taking certain types of medications such as antirejection medication for organ transplant patients and long-term use of steroids such as prednisone

Signs and Symptoms. Common signs and symptoms for shingles usually occur in a localized area (around the ribs, at the hairline on the forehead, behind the ear) (Figs. 4.22 and 4.23) and include the following:
- Pain, burning, numbness, or tingling; pain can be intense
- Skin that is sensitive to the touch

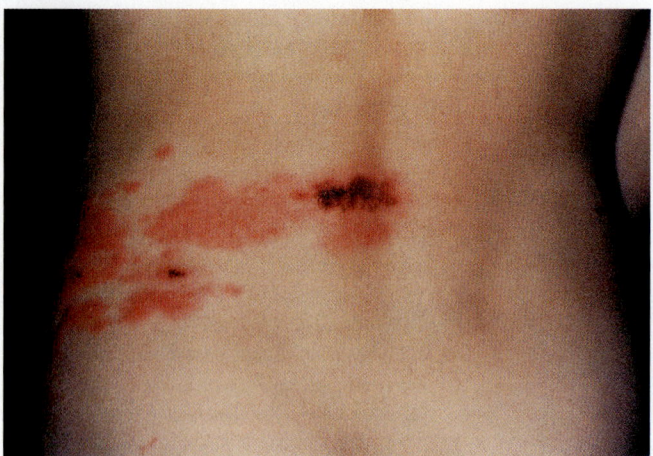

FIG. 4.22 Shingles. (From Callen JP, Greer KE, Saller AS, et al: *Color Atlas of Dermatology*, ed 2, Philadelphia, 2000, Saunders.)

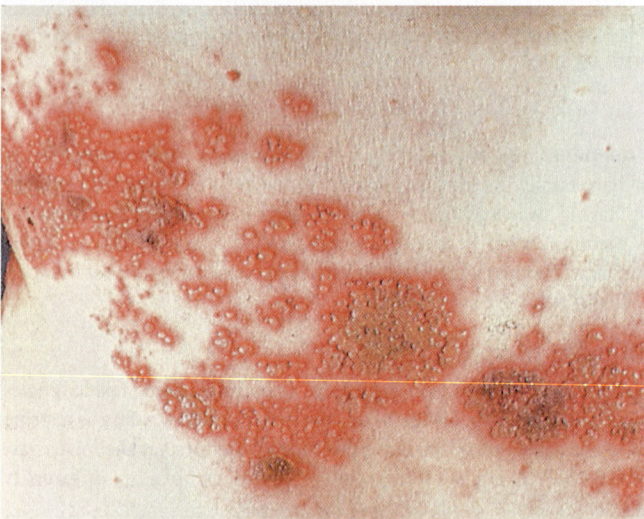

FIG. 4.23 Shingles. (From Swartz MH: *Textbook of Physical Diagnosis*, ed 7, Philadelphia, 2014, Saunders.)

- A red rash that develops a few days after the pain starts
- Fluid-filled blisters that break open and become crusty (look like chickenpox)
- Itching skin in the area of the rash
- Fever, headache, or fatigue may accompany any of these symptoms

Diagnostic Procedures. Diagnosis is usually based on a physical exam and history. The lesions and location of shingles is characteristic of the disease. Also, pain that precedes the appearance of the rash is important to note in the diagnosis.

Treatment. Treating shingles quickly helps to lessen the duration of the disease. Prescription antiviral medications can be administered and can be effective in speeding up the healing process, as well as reducing the risks of complications from shingles.

Shingles can also cause severe pain, so the provider may prescribe one or more of the following types of medication:
- Capsaicin cream
- Anticonvulsants
- Tricyclic antidepressants

> **BOX 4.8 Home Remedies for Shingles**
>
> Home remedies that may lessen the pain or duration of shingles include the following:
> - Eliminating sugar, chocolate, nuts, and processed foods made with white flours; not eating these foods may help
> - Taking cool baths or applying cool compresses to painful areas of the skin
> - Reducing stress

- Numbing agents
- Corticosteroid injections or local anesthetics

Box 4.8 lists some home remedies that may help with the signs and symptoms of shingles.

Prognosis. Shingles usually last from 2 to 6 weeks. Most people only get shingles once, but it can occur multiple times. Some people experience lingering shingles pain, but most people do not. Overall, the prognosis is very good.

Prevention. Preventing shingles can be accomplished by receiving the chickenpox vaccine as a child. If the patient never had chickenpox as a child, receiving the vaccine as an adult is also effective. Two shingles vaccines are available for adults. After the age of 60, people can receive the varicella-zoster vaccine (Zostavax) to help prevent shingles. A second shingles vaccine is also available after the age of 50 (Shingrix). No vaccine is 100% effective, but the vaccines mentioned decrease the chances of developing shingles or shorten the duration of symptoms and reduce related complications.

Skin Infestations (Scabies and Pediculosis)

Parasitic infestations of the skin can occur at any age. They are spread in group settings such as among families or in childcare groups, school classes, nursing homes, prisons, and dormitories. The two most common types of skin parasites seen are scabies (itch mites) and pediculosis (lice). Both parasites infect the skin and cause itching. Both parasites can be treated and the infection resolved.

Etiology. Scabies is caused by the itch mite *Sarcoptes scabiei* (Fig. 4.24). This little mite burrows under the skin, causing intense itching.

Pediculosis is caused by lice that populate three specific areas of the body (Fig. 4.25). A person can have head lice (*Pediculus capitis*), body

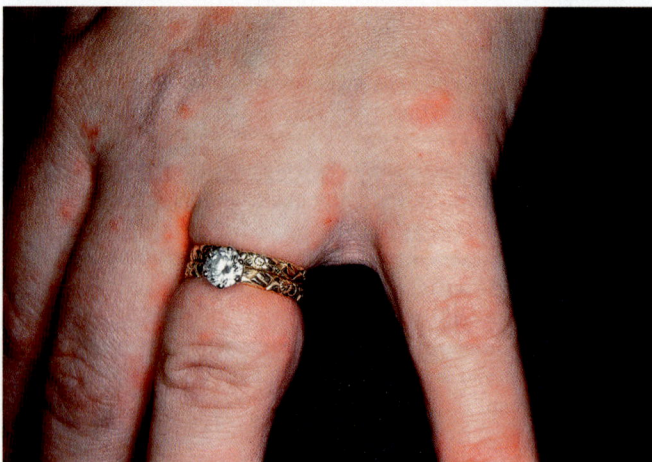

FIG. 4.24 Scabies on the hand. (From James WD, et al: *Andrews' Diseases of the Skin*, ed 11, Philadelphia, 2011, Saunders.)

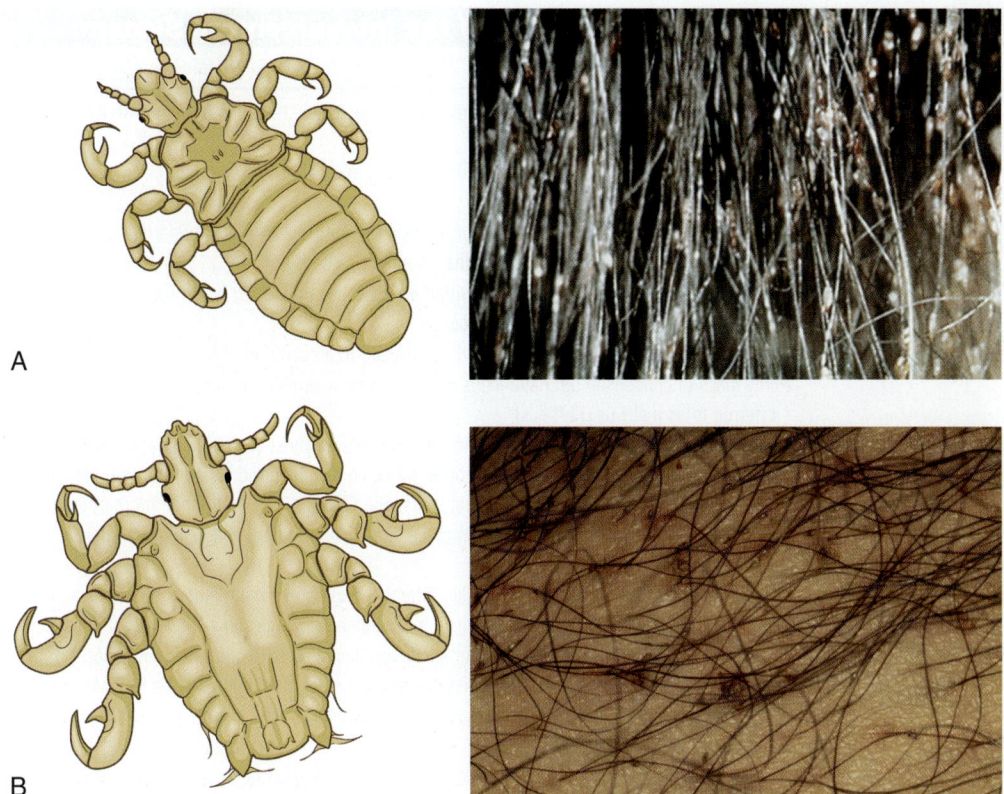

FIG. 4.25 Types of lice. (A from Lissauer T, et al: *Illustrated Textbook of Paediatrics,* ed 4, London, 2012, Mosby. B from Long SS, et al: *Principles and Practice of Pediatric Infectious Diseases,* ed 4, Philadelphia, 2012, Saunders.)

lice *(Pediculus corporis),* or pubic lice or crabs *(Pthirus pubis).* Lice crawl but cannot fly or hop. Both parasites can move from person to person through close physical contact as well as by sharing inanimate objects or *fomites* such as combs, brushes, clothes, and bedding.

> **MEDICAL TERMINOLOGY**
> **pedicul/i:** lice
> **scab/i:** mites

Signs and Symptoms. Signs and symptoms of scabies or pediculosis are similar and are listed here:
- Intense itching
- Tickling feeling as parasites move hair on the skin
- Lice: small red bumps on the skin and nits (eggs) on body, facial, or pubic hair
- Scabies: little burrows or tunnels can be seen under the skin, frequently in areas of the skin that fold such as between fingers and toes, around the waist, in the armpits, and on knees and elbows

Diagnostic Procedures. For lice, physical examination often involves the use of a magnifying lens to see the lice and nits on hair. A Wood light (Table 4.4 and Fig. 4.4) can also be used to detect the nits—they look pale blue.

For scabies, physical examination involves looking for characteristic burrows under the skin. The provider may scrape the skin and exam it under the microscope to look for eggs.

Treatment. Prescription shampoo, body wash, and lotion can be used to kill the parasites on the head, hair, and body. The lice and mites are generally killed quickly, but the patient must follow all instructions to make sure eggs are also killed. There may be some itching after the parasites are killed, but that does not necessarily indicate a continued infection. Women who are pregnant and the parents of infants should consult their provider before applying antiparasitic products. They are strong chemicals that may cause complications for the very young and for pregnant women.

In addition to properly washing the hair and body, all clothing, bedding, personal items, furniture should also be cleaned with hot, soapy water. If all the eggs are not removed, reinfections can occur.

Prognosis. The prognosis is good if treatment is properly done and the living environment is decontaminated.

Prevention. Parasitic infections can be prevented by taking certain precautions:
- Not sharing personal items such as combs, hats, scarves, clothing, blankets, or bedding
- Avoiding the placement of personal items in shared spaces such as baskets, bins, lockers, or backpacks

Additional Diseases and Disorders of the Integumentary System

There are many other diseases and disorders of the integumentary system, too many to cover in depth. Tables 4.10 through 4.12 briefly describe a variety of additional conditions that may be of interest.

TABLE 4.10 Additional Diseases and Disorders of the Integumentary System

Term	Definition
Albinism (AL bih niz um)	Complete lack of melanin production by existing melanocytes, resulting in pale skin, white hair, and pink iris of the eye
Callus (KAL us)	Common painless thickening of the stratum corneum at locations of external pressure or friction
Candidiasis (kan dih DYE ah sis)	Yeast infection in moist, creased areas of the skin (armpits, inner thighs, underneath pendulous breasts) and mucous membranes; also called moniliasis (mah nih LYE ah sis)
Cellulitis (sell yoo LYE tis)	Diffuse, spreading, acute inflammation within solid tissues (lower leg is the most common site); the most common cause is a *Streptococcus pyogenes* infection
Contact dermatitis (DUR muh tahy tis)	Irritated or allergic response of the skin that can lead to an acute or chronic inflammation
Corn	Horny mass of condensed epithelial cells overlying a bony prominence as the result of pressure or friction; also referred to as a clavus (KLA vus)
Discoid lupus erythematosus (DLE) (DIS koid LOO puhs er uh THEE muh toe sus)	A chronic autoimmune disease of the skin that presents as sores with inflammation and scarring favoring the face, ears, and scalp, and at times on other body areas; coin-shaped red lesions that are inflamed patches with scaly or crusty appearance; can cause disfiguring scars; see Chapter 9 for additional information on autoimmune diseases
Folliculitis (foh lick yoo LYE tis)	Inflammation of the hair follicles, which may be superficial or deep, and acute or chronic
Furuncle (FYOOR ung kul)	Localized, **suppurative** staphylococcal skin infection originating in a gland or hair follicle and characterized by pain, redness, and swelling; if a subcutaneous pocket connects two or more furuncles, it is called a carbuncle
Herpes simplex virus (HSV) (HUR peez sim PLEKS)	Viral infection characterized by clusters of small vesicles filled with clear fluid on raised inflammatory bases on the skin or mucosa; HSV-1 causes fever blisters (herpetic stomatitis) and keratitis, an inflammation of the cornea. HSV-2 is more commonly known as genital herpes, which causes blisters in the genital area
Hidradenitis (hye drah din EYE tis)	Inflammation of the sweat glands
Hyperhidrosis (hye pur hye DROH sis)	Excessive perspiration caused by heat, strong emotion, menopause, hyperthyroidism, or infection
Hypertrichosis (hye pur trih KOH sis)	Abnormal excess of hair; also known as *hirsutism* (HER soo tih zum)
Impetigo (im peh TYE goh)	Superficial vesiculopustular bacterial skin infection, normally seen in children, but possible in adults (Fig. 4.26). Causative agents are *Streptococcus* spp. and *Staphylococcus* spp. Also called *Streptococcal pyoderma,* if caused by Streptococcus spp.

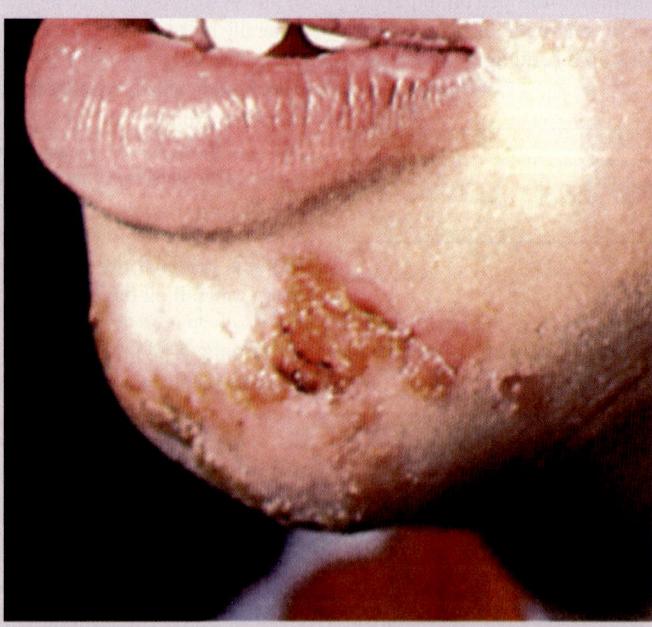

FIG. 4.26 Impetigo. (From Marks JG Jr, Miller JJ: *Lookingbill & Marks' Principles of Dermatology,* ed 4, London, 2006, Saunders.)

TABLE 4.10 Additional Diseases and Disorders of the Integumentary System—cont'd

Term	Definition
Kaposi sarcoma (KS) (KAP uh see sar KOH mah)	A rare skin cancer that takes the form of red/purple nodules, usually on the extremities; one form appears most often in patients with deficient immune systems, such as those with acquired immunodeficiency syndrome (AIDS); causative agent is human herpes virus-8 (HHV8)
Keratinous cyst (kur AT tin us)	**Benign** cavity lined by keratinizing epithelium and filled with sebum and epithelial debris; also called a sebaceous cyst
Pilonidal cyst (pye loh NYE duhl)	Growth of hair in a cyst in the sacral region
Pruritus (proo RYE tuss)	Itching; the marks that result from intense scratching are called excoriations
Rosacea (roh ZAY shuh)	Redness on the nose, cheeks, chin, and forehead; can also cause burning and soreness in the eyes; most common in people over 30; not an infection
Scleroderma (SKLER uh dur muh)	An autoimmune disease characterized by chronic hardening and contraction of the skin and connective tissue; can either affect skin locally or systemic throughout the body, affecting internal organs; see Chapter 9 for additional information on autoimmune diseases
Seborrheic dermatitis (seb uh REE ick DUR muh tahy tis)	Inflammatory scaling disease of the scalp and face; in newborns, this is known as cradle cap
Systemic lupus erythematosus (SLE)	An autoimmune disease that can affect the skin, joints, kidneys, brain, and other organs; see Chapter 9 for additional information on autoimmune diseases
Urticaria (ur ti KAIR ee uh)	Rash of round, red welts on the skin that itch intensely; sometimes caused by an allergic reaction, typically to specific foods or topical irritants; also called hives
Vitiligo (vit I AHY goh)	Benign autoimmune disease of unknown origin, consisting of irregular patches of skin that vary in size and lack pigment (Fig. 4.27)
Warts	Common, contagious epithelial growths usually appearing on the skin of the hands, feet, legs, and face; can be caused by any of 60 types of the human papillomavirus (HPV)

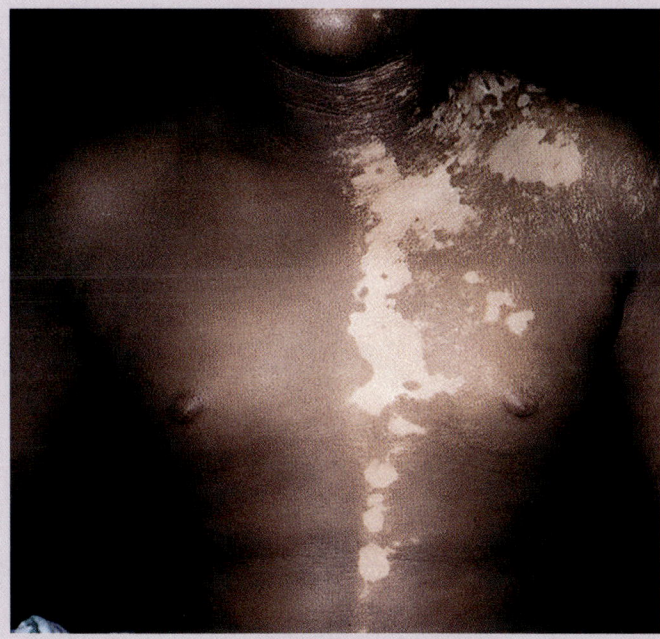

FIG. 4.27 Vitiligo. (From Shiland B: *Mastering Healthcare Terminology*, ed 5, St. Louis, 2016, Elsevier.)

From Shiland B: *Mastering Healthcare Terminology*, ed 5, St. Louis, 2016, Elsevier.

TABLE 4.11 Additional Diseases and Disorders of the Integumentary System: Benign Skin Growths

Term	Definition
Angioma (an jee OH mah)	Localized vascular lesion that includes hemangiomas, vascular nevi, and lymphangiomas
Dermatofibroma (dur mat toh fye BROH mah)	Fibrous tumor of the skin that is painless, round, firm, and usually found on the extremities
Lipoma (lih POH mah)	Fatty tumor that is a soft, movable, subcutaneous nodule
Seborrheic keratosis (seh boh REE ick kair ah TOH sis)	Benign, circumscribed, pigmented, superficial warty skin lesion; an *actinic keratosis* is a lesion caused by sun exposure
Skin tags	Small, soft, pedunculated (with a stalk) lesions that are harmless outgrowths of epidermal and dermal tissue, usually occurring on the neck, eyelids, armpits, and groin; usually occur in multiples; also known as *acrochordons* (ack roh KORE dons)

From Shiland B: *Mastering Healthcare Terminology,* ed 5, St. Louis, 2016, Elsevier.

TABLE 4.12 Cosmetic Procedures of the Integumentary System

Term	Definition
Blepharoplasty (BLEF ar oh plas tee)	Surgical repair of the eyelid
Chemical peel	Use of a mild acid to produce a superficial burn; normally done to remove wrinkles
Dermabrasion (dur mah BRAY zhun)	Surgical procedure to resurface the skin; used to remove acne scars, nevi, wrinkles, and tattoos
Dermatoplasty (DUR mat tuh plas tee)	Transplant of living skin to correct the effects of injury, operation, or disease
Lipectomy (lih PECK tuh mee)	Removal of fatty tissue
Liposuction (LYE poh suck shun)	Technique for removing adipose tissue with a suction pump device
Rhytidectomy	Surgical operation to remove wrinkles; commonly known as a "face-lift"

From Shiland B: *Mastering Healthcare Terminology,* ed 5, St. Louis, 2016, Elsevier.

> **VOCABULARY**
> **benign:** A noncancerous condition; not malignant, harmless.
> **suppurative:** Characterized by the formation or discharge of pus.

> **MEDICAL TERMINOLOGY**
> **nevus** (singular), **nevi** (plural)
> **verruca** (singular), **verrucae** (plural)

LIFE SPAN CHANGES

Children routinely appear at physician offices with skin disorders. Some of the most common are impetigo, acne, seborrheic dermatitis, cellulitis, and pediculosis. Although none of these are serious disorders, impetigo and pediculosis are highly contagious. Also seen are the different degrees of burns, usually accidental, but potentially life threatening.

Older patients have a completely different set of diagnoses. The disorders categorized as those related to cornification, especially corns and calluses, are seen routinely in medical offices. These masses or thickenings of the skin are formed as a defensive response to constant friction, usually within shoes. Pressure sores (also called *bedsores* or *decubitus ulcers*) are seen most often in bedridden patients whose skin may already be atrophied and thin. Eczema, cellulitis, and fungal infections are also common complaints. The last category of skin disorders often seen in older adults is skin cancers. Although younger patients with skin cancers are often seen, older patients have had a longer time to be exposed to the sun and develop malignancies.

> **CRITICAL THINKING 4.9**
> Mai goes over the treatment packet with Casey to wrap up her appointment. Casey is comfortable with some of dietary recommendations and the OTC medications she will be using for her acne. On Casey's way out of the clinic, she makes a follow-up appointment for 2 months later. Why is a follow-up appointment a good idea for Casey and her condition? Share your thoughts with the class.

CLOSING COMMENTS

When working in an ambulatory care setting, assisting patients with skin diseases and disorders is common. It is important for the medical assistant to understand the anatomy of the skin and the functions of the integumentary system as a whole. The skin has amazing qualities that allow it to repair and recover from injury and disease. Dermatology is the specialty that focuses on the skin, but medical assistants working in urgent care and primary care (e.g., pediatrics, internal medicine, and family practice) will see many skin-related diseases and disorders too. Medical terminology related to the integumentary system will be invaluable in your career. Knowing word parts, definitions, and common abbreviations is vital when working with patients and providers (Tables 4.13 through 4.16). The medical assistant should also know about the etiology, signs and symptoms, diagnostic procedures, treatments, prognoses, and prevention of common integumentary diseases, disorders, and traumas.

TABLE 4.13 Combining and Adjective Forms for the Anatomy of the Integumentary System

Meaning	Combining Form	Adjective Form
base, bottom	bas/o	basal
black, dark	melan/o	melanotic
fat	adip/o	adipose
follicle	follicul/o	follicular
gland	aden/o	adenal
hair	trich/o, pil/o	pilar
hard, horny	kerat/o	keratic
nail	ungu/o, onych/o	ungual, onychia
papilla	papill/o	papillary
scaly	squam/o	squamous
sebum, oil	seb/o, sebac/o	sebaceous
skin	derm/o, dermat/o, cut/o, cutane/o	cutaneous, dermic, dermatic
sudoriferous gland	hidraden/o	
sweat	hidr/o, sudor/i	hidrotic, sudorous
vessel	vascul/o	vascular

From Shiland B: *Mastering Healthcare Terminology*, ed 5, St. Louis, 2016, Elsevier.

TABLE 4.14 Prefixes for the Anatomy of the Integumentary System

Prefix	Meaning
a-	no, not, without
epi-	above
hypo-, sub-	under, below

From Shiland B: *Mastering Healthcare Terminology*, ed 5, St. Louis, 2016, Elsevier.

TABLE 4.15 Suffixes for the Anatomy of the Integumentary System

Suffix	Meaning
-al, -ar, -ous, -ic	pertaining to
-cyte	cell
-ferous	pertaining to carrying
-is	structure

From Shiland B: *Mastering Healthcare Terminology*, ed 5, St. Louis, 2016, Elsevier.

TABLE 4.16 Abbreviations

Abbreviation	Meaning
BCC	basal cell carcinoma
Bx	biopsy
FB	foreign body
H	hypodermic
HPV	human papillomavirus
HSV-1	herpes simplex virus 1
HSV-2	herpes simplex virus 2
I&D	incision and drainage
ID	intradermal
KS	Kaposi sarcoma
PPD	purified protein derivative
PUVA	psoralen plus ultraviolet A
SCC	squamous cell carcinoma
SG	skin graft
STSG	split-thickness skin graft
TB	tuberculosis
TTS	transdermal therapeutic system

From Shiland B: *Mastering Healthcare Terminology*, ed 5, St. Louis, 2016, Elsevier.

CHAPTER REVIEW

The integumentary system is divided into four components: the epidermis, the dermis, the subcutaneous layer, and the appendages. The main functions of the integumentary system are protection, temperature regulation, sensory organ activity, vitamin D synthesis, and excretion.

In a healthy individual, the skin and its appendages are present and fully functional at birth. The skin is rejuvenated with a constant supply of new cells that are formed and moved to the outer layer of the skin as they become less effective. This constant renewal and change of skin cells allows the integumentary system to heal quickly and keep the body protected from the outside environment.

The appendages of the integumentary system are the glands, hair, and nails. They are an accessory structure of the integumentary system and help to maintain body temperature, keep the skin moisturized and soft, and protect the ends of the fingers and toes.

Many integumentary diseases and disorders were presented in this chapter. Common signs and symptoms include discoloration, itching, weeping, flaky or scaly patches of the skin, and the appearance of or change in skin lesions. Common etiology includes injury, infection, autoimmune conditions, and allergic reactions. Typical diagnostic tests include physical observation of the condition, medical history, biopsy, and laboratory testing. CLIA-waived tests include rheumatoid factor (RF) testing and erythrocyte sedimentation rate (ESR) tests.

The integumentary system changes with age. Infants and children are at risk for infections, allergic reactions, and injuries. Older adults are also at risk for fungal infections, skin cancers, and lesions or conditions due to older, thinning skin.

SCENARIO WRAP-UP

Casey is back at WMFM for her follow-up visit. In the past 2 months, she has followed the treatment plan and is happy to show Mai and Jean Burke the improvements that have taken place. Her acne has improved greatly. She is pleased with the results and glad that she decided to visit WMFM about her skin issues. Casey also thanks Mai and Jean for being understanding on her first visit. How did Mai and Jean help Casey on her first visit? List three things that they did to help make Casey's experience positive.

5

Digestive System

LEARNING OBJECTIVES

1. Discuss the anatomy of the digestive system, list the major organs for the digestive system, and identify the anatomic location of major digestive system organs.
2. Describe the normal function and physiology of the digestive system.
3. Complete the following for diseases and disorders to the digestive system:
   - Identify the common signs and symptoms, etiology, and diagnostic measures for the digestive system.
   - Identify CLIA-waived tests associated with common digestive diseases.
   - Describe treatment modalities used for digestive diseases.
4. Compare the structure and function of the digestive system across the life span.

CHAPTER OUTLINE

1. Opening Scenario, 95
2. You Will Learn, 95
3. Introduction to the Digestive System, 95
4. Anatomy of the Digestive System, 96
   a. Oral Cavity, 96
   b. Throat, 97
   c. Esophagus, 97
   d. Stomach, 97
   e. Small Intestine, 98
   f. Large Intestine, 98
5. Physiology of the Digestive System, 99
   a. Chemical Digestion, 99
   b. Absorption and Excretion, 101
6. Diseases and Disorders of the Digestive System, 102
   a. Acute Appendicitis, 102
   b. Cancers of the Digestive System, 106
      i. *Etiology*, 106
   c. Cholelithiasis (Gallstones), 107
   d. Crohn Disease, 108
   e. Diverticulitis, 109
   f. Gastroesophageal Reflux Disease, 110
   g. Hemorrhoids, 111
   h. Hepatitis, Viral, 112
   i. Hiatal Hernia, 113
   j. Pancreatitis, 114
   k. Ulcers: Peptic Ulcers, 115
7. Additional Diseases and Disorders of the Digestive System, 116
8. Lifespan Changes, 119
9. Closing Comments, 119
10. Chapter Review, 120
11. Scenario Wrap-Up, 120

CHAPTER 5 Digestive System

OPENING SCENARIO

This is the first day on the job at Walden-Martin Family Medical (WMFM) Clinic for Samuel Lyman, CMA (AAMA). He has completed his orientation and today he starts his career as a medical assistant. He will be working with Dr. Martin today, and the morning looks busy. The first patient this morning is Al Neviaser, who has had gastrointestinal symptoms over the past few months.

Al had an appointment with Dr. Martin about a month ago. At that time, Dr. Martin performed a physical exam, went over Al's history, and ordered some preliminary lab work. Al came back to see Dr. Martin a week later, they discussed the lab results, and Dr. Martin recommended a colonoscopy for Al. Today Al will find out the results of the colonoscopy.

YOU WILL LEARN

- To recognize and use terms related to the digestive system.
- To locate the digestive system structures.
- To understand and describe the functions of the digestive system.
- To recognize disease states of the digestive system: their causes, signs and symptoms, diagnostic processes, treatment, prognoses, and prevention.

INTRODUCTION TO THE DIGESTIVE SYSTEM

The digestive system provides the nutrients needed for cells to replicate themselves continually and build new tissue (Fig. 5.1). This is done through several distinct processes:

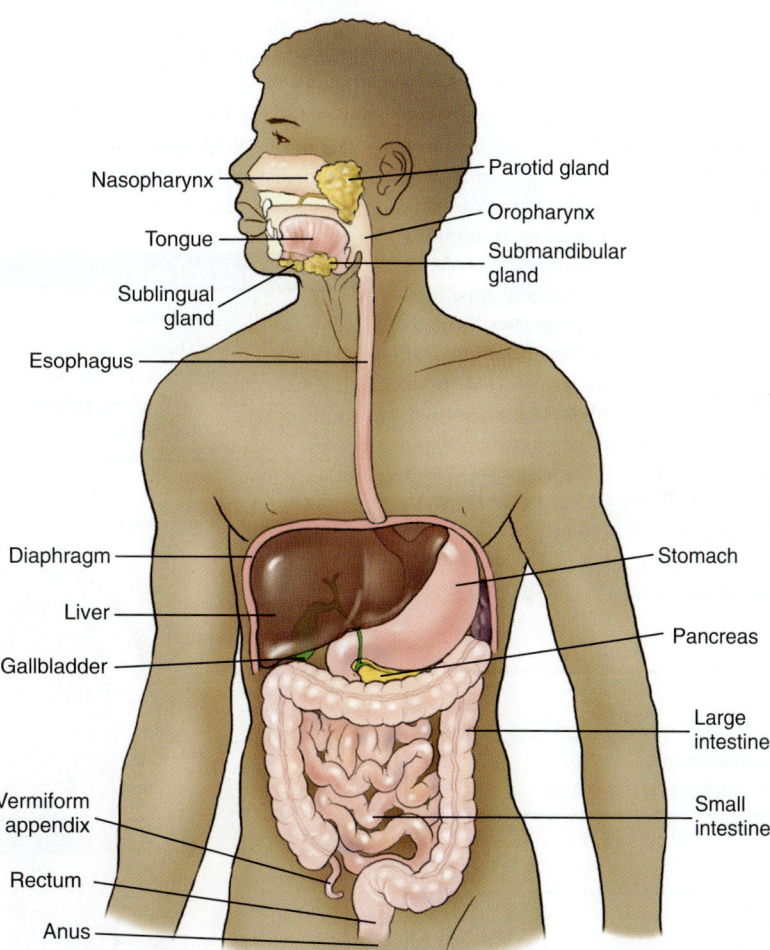

FIG. 5.1 The digestive system. (From Shiland B: *Mastering Healthcare Terminology*, ed 5, St. Louis, 2016, Elsevier.)

- *Ingestion:* the intake of food
- *Digestion:* the breakdown of food
- *Absorption:* the process of extracting nutrients
- *Elimination:* the excretion of any waste products

Other names for this system are the *gastrointestinal* (gas troh in TES tuh nl) *system,* or *gastrointestinal (GI) tract,* and the *alimentary* (al uh MEN tair ee) *canal.* Box 5.1 contains definitions of the digestive system specialty and the specialists.

The GI tract refers to the two main structures of the system: the stomach and the intestines. The alimentary canal refers to the tubelike nature of the digestive system, starting at the mouth and continuing in varying diameters to the anus.

BOX 5.1 Specialty and Specialist

Gastroenterology (gas-troh-en-tuh-ROL-uh-jee) is the healthcare specialty that deals with most digestive diseases and disorders. A *gastroenterologist* (gas-troh-en-tuh-ROL-uh-jist) is a specialist involved in the diagnosis, treatment, and prevention of disorders of the digestive system. A *proctologist* (prok-TOL-uh-jist) is a subspecialist that treats disorders of the rectum and anus.

ANATOMY OF THE DIGESTIVE SYSTEM

The digestive system is made up of structures that direct food in a continuous flow from organ to organ. These are the *primary organs* of the digestive system: mouth, pharynx, esophagus, stomach, small and large intestines, rectum, and anal canal. There are also structures that play a vital role in the digestive system but are not part of the continuous arrangement. These are the *accessory organs* of the digestive system: teeth, tongue, salivary glands, liver, gallbladder, pancreas, and appendix.

The digestive system begins in the oral cavity, progresses through the **mediastinum** (mee-dee-a-STAHY-nuh m) and the *abdominal* and *pelvic* cavities, and finally exits at the anus. The stomach and intestines lie within the abdominal cavity. They are attached to the body wall by a rich vascular membrane called the *mesentery* (MEZ-uh n-ter-ee).

Internally, the alimentary canal is made of three layers, or **tunics** (TOO-niks). The inner layer is the *tunica mucosa* (myoo-KOH-suh), which secretes gastric juices, absorbs nutrients, and protects the tissue through the production of mucus. The next tunic is the *submucosa,* which contains the blood vessels, lymphatic vessels, and nervous tissue.

VOCABULARY
mediastinum: The space in the thoracic cavity that lies between the lungs, containing the heart, trachea, and esophagus.
tunics: A coat or layer covering an organ or part of an organ.

MEDICAL TERMINOLOGY
abdomin/o, lapar/o, celi/o: abdomen
enter/o: small intestine
gastr/o: stomach
-logist: one who specializes
mucos/o, myx/o: mucus, mucosa
peri-: surrounding
proct/o: rectum and anus
-stalsis: contraction

The deepest layer is the *tunica muscularis,* which contracts and relaxes around the tube, in a wavelike movement called *peristalsis,* to move food through the tract.

The following sections explain the digestive system organs in more detail. Both primary and accessory organs are discussed.

CRITICAL THINKING 5.1

As Samuel prepares the exam room for Dr. Martin's patient, he tries to remember the anatomy of the digestive system. Can you name the primary organs of the digestive system? Now what about the accessory organs?

Oral Cavity

Food normally enters the body through the mouth, or *oral cavity* (Fig. 5.2). In the mouth, *mechanical digestion* starts as food is broken down by chewing, or *mastication.* The addition of saliva also lubricates food to make swallowing, or *deglutition* (dee gloo TIH shun), easier.

The oral cavity begins at the *lips,* the two fleshy structures surrounding the opening of the mouth. The inside of the mouth is bounded by the *cheeks,* the *tongue* at the floor, and an anterior *hard palate* (PAL it) and posterior *soft palate,* which form the roof of the mouth. The upper and lower jaws of an adult hold 32 permanent *teeth* (Box 5.2). The teeth are set in the flesh of the *gums,* also called the *gingivae* (jin JAHY vee). The *uvula* (YOO vyoo lah) is the tag of flesh that hangs down from the medial surface of the soft palate.

BOX 5.2 Teeth

The 20 baby (deciduous or primary) teeth are temporary. Most children lose all their baby teeth by the time they are about 12 years old. As the baby teeth are lost, permanent teeth replace them. Permanent teeth are larger than baby teeth, and there are 32 permanent teeth. Fig. 5.2 shows the location and type of permanent teeth in the adult mouth.

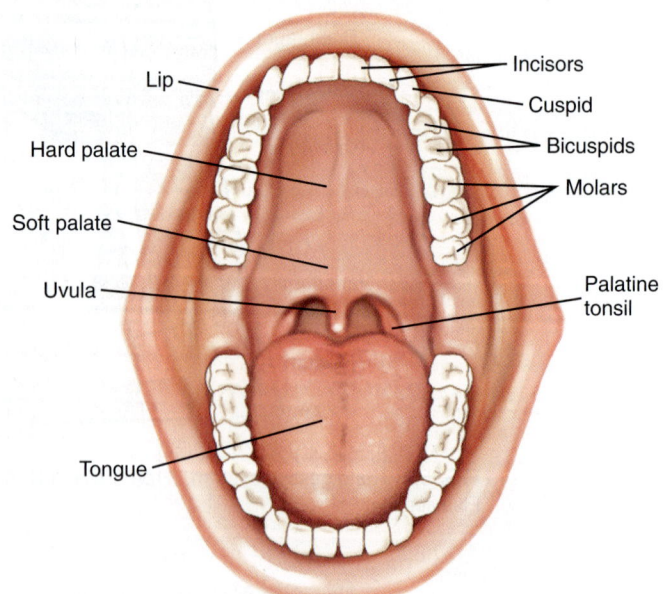

FIG. 5.2 The oral cavity. (From Shiland B: *Mastering Healthcare Terminology,* ed 5, St. Louis, 2016, Elsevier.)

CHAPTER 5 Digestive System

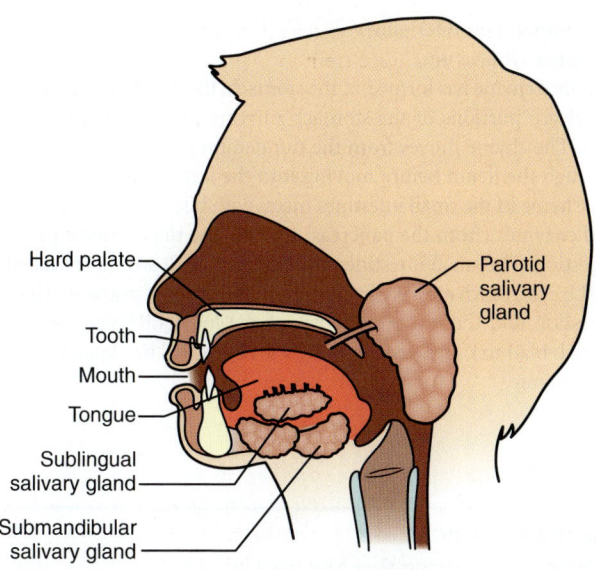

FIG. 5.3 The salivary glands.

> **BOX 5.3 Two Systems**
>
> The pharynx or throat is part of two body systems. Food and drink pass through the throat on the way to the esophagus of the digestive system. Air passes through the throat on the way to the trachea of the respiratory system. The *epiglottis* is a flap of tissue that keeps air from entering the digestive system and food and drink from entering the respiratory system.

Throat

The throat, or *pharynx* (FAIR inks), is a tube that connects the oral cavity with the *esophagus* (Box 5.3). The pharynx is divided into three main parts:
- *Nasopharynx* (nay soh FAIR inks): the most superior part, located behind the nasal cavity
- *Oropharynx* (oh roh FAIR inks): located directly adjacent to the oral cavity
- *Laryngopharynx* (luh-ring-goh-FAR-inks): located below the oropharynx (Fig. 5.4); also called the *hypopharynx* (hye poh FAIR inks)

Esophagus

The esophagus (eh SAH fah gus) is a muscular, mucus-lined tube that extends from the throat to the *stomach*. It carries a masticated lump of food, called a *bolus* (BOH lus), from the oral cavity to the stomach by peristalsis. The glands in the lining of the esophagus produce mucus, which eases the passage of food to the stomach. The muscle that relaxes to let food enter the stomach is called the *lower esophageal* (eh sah fah JEE ul) *sphincter* (SFINK tur) *(LES)*. The LES is also known as the gastroesophageal sphincter and the cardiac sphincter. *Sphincters* are ringlike muscles that appear throughout the digestive system and throughout the body.

Three pairs of *salivary* (SAL ih vair ee) *glands* are in the oral cavity (Fig. 5.3). They are named for their location and include the following:
- *Parotid* (pair AH tid): near the ear
- *Submandibular* (sub man DIB yoo lur): under the *mandible* (lower jaw)
- *Sublingual* (sub LEENG gwul): under the tongue

The salivary glands produce and secrete *saliva* into the mouth. Saliva moistens the mouth and aids in chewing and swallowing food. It contains an enzyme called *salivary amylase*, which is discussed later in the chapter.

Stomach

The stomach is divided into three sections:
- *Fundus* (FUN dus): sits just below the diaphragm (Fig. 5.5)
- *Body* (or *corporis*): central part of the stomach
- *Pylorus* (pye LORE us) (or *gastric antrum*): at the distal end of the stomach, where the small intestine begins

The body and pylorus of the stomach contain acid-producing cells. A small muscle, the *pyloric sphincter*, regulates the gentle release of food from the stomach into the small intestine.

> **CRITICAL THINKING 5.2**
>
> Can you name the three pairs of salivary glands? Do you have a fun way to remember the names and locations of the salivary glands? If you do, please share it with the class.

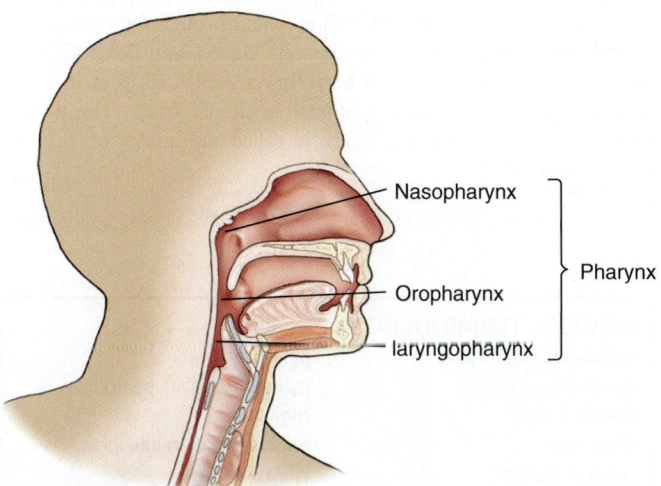

FIG. 5.4 The pharynx. (From Shiland B: *Mastering Healthcare Terminology*, ed 5, St. Louis, 2016, Elsevier.)

MEDICAL TERMINOLOGY	
-al: pertaining to	mandibul/o: lower jaw, mandible
-ar: pertaining to	maxill/o: upper jaw or/o, stomat/o,
bol/o: bolus	stom/o: mouth, oral cavity
bucc/o: cheek	nas/o: nose
cheil/o, labi/o: lips	ot/o: ear
dent/i, odont/o: teeth	palat/o: palate
esophag/o: esophagus	par-: near
gingiv/o: gums	pharyng/o: throat, pharynx
gloss/o, lingu/o: tongue	sial/o: saliva
hypo-: below	sialaden/o: salivary gland
-id: pertaining to	sub-: under
laryng/o: larynx, voice box	

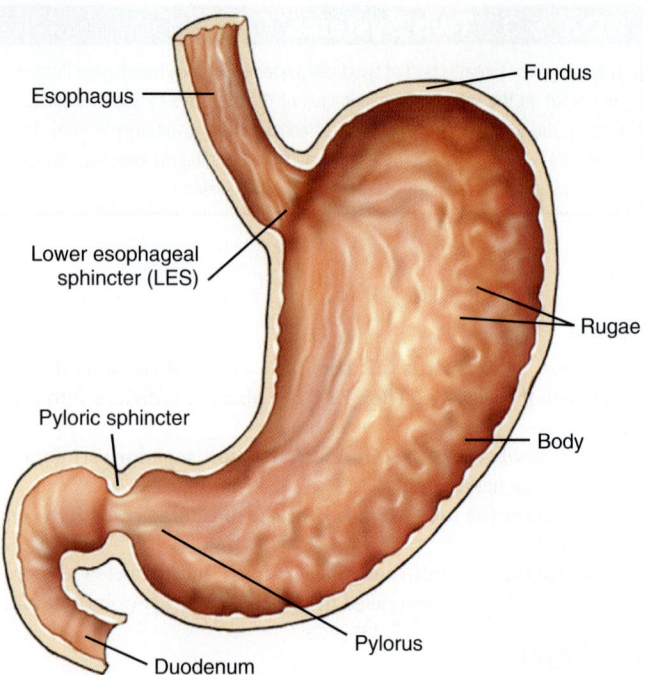

FIG. 5.5 The esophagus and stomach. (From Shiland B: *Mastering Healthcare Terminology*, ed 5, St. Louis, 2016, Elsevier.)

When the stomach is empty, it has an appearance of being lined with many ridges. These ridges, or wrinkles, are called *rugae* (ROO jee). The stomach contains rugae that allow the stomach to expand in size. The stomach enlarges to about 1 liter after a normal meal. If pushed to the limit, the stomach can expand to almost 4 liters in size.

The function of the stomach is to temporarily store chewed food from the esophagus. This food is mixed with gastric juices and hydrochloric acid to start the process of digestion. This mixture is called *chyme* (kyme). The smooth muscles of the stomach contract to aid in the mechanical digestion of the food. A continuous coating of mucus protects the stomach and the rest of the digestive system from the acidic nature of chyme and the gastric juices.

Small Intestine

The small intestine is about 20 feet long. The diameter of its **lumen** (LOO mun) is small compared with the large intestine. The small intestine is divided into three sections:
- *Duodenum* (doo AH deh num)
- *Jejunum* (jeh JOO num)
- *Ileum* (ILL ee um)

Once chyme has formed in the stomach, the pyloric sphincter relaxes to release portions of the stomach mixture into the duodenum (Fig. 5.6). The chyme moves from the duodenum to the jejunum and then through the ileum before moving into the large intestine.

Chyme in the small intestines mixes with bile (from the gallbladder) and enzymes (from the pancreas) to continue the chemical process of digestion. The small intestines also contain small structures called *villi* (VILL eye), which are a vital part of the absorption of nutrients. Chemical digestion and the important roles of the *liver* (LIH vur), *gallbladder* (GALL blad ur), and *pancreas* (PAN kree us) will be explained later in the chapter.

> **VOCABULARY**
> **lumen:** The cavity, channel, or open space within a tube or tubular organ.

Large Intestine

The *large intestine* or *colon* is about 5 feet long. It has a much larger diameter than the small intestine (see Fig. 5.6). The primary function of the large intestine is to eliminate waste products from the body. Unlike the small intestine, the large intestine has no villi and is not well suited to absorb nutrients, but it does reabsorb water.

The *ileocecal* (ILL ee oh SEE kul) valve is the exit from the small intestine and the entrance to the colon. The first part of the large intestine is the *cecum* (SEE kum). A small wormlike appendage, called the *vermiform appendix* (VUR mih form ah PEN dicks), is located near the beginning of the cecum. Although the function of the appendix is not fully known, scientific research suggests that it harbors "good bacteria," which will repopulate the intestines after an illness. The appendix is also believed to have a role in the immune system throughout a person's lifetime.

Waste products, fiber, and water move from the small intestine into the large intestines. The substance that continues through the large intestine changes from chyme to *feces* (FEE sees). Feces pass from the cecum to the *ascending colon* (KOH lin), through the *transverse colon,* down the *descending colon,* through the curve of the *sigmoid colon,* and on to the *rectum* (see Fig. 5.6 and Box 5.4). Once in the rectum, feces are stored until they are released from the body through the *anus* (the final sphincter in the GI tract.) The process of releasing feces from the body is called *defecation,* or a bowel movement (BM).

> **CRITICAL THINKING 5.3**
> Mucous! Not a very pleasant word, but such a useful substance in the body. What is the function of mucous in the stomach? Share your thoughts with the class.

> **CRITICAL THINKING 5.4**
> Can you name the three parts of the small intestine and pronounce them correctly? Using medical terminology correctly gives a patient confidence in your abilities. Practice pronouncing terms perfectly.

> **MEDICAL TERMINOLOGY**
> **corpor/o:** body, corporis
> **duoden/o:** duodenum
> **fund/o:** fundus
> **ile/o:** ileum
> **jejun/o:** jejunum
> **lumin/o:** lumen
> **plic/o:** fold, plica
> **pylor/o:** pylorus
> **pylorus** (singular), **pylori** (plural)
> **rug/o:** rugae
> **ruga** (singular), **rugae** (plural)
> **vill/o:** villus
> **villus** (singular), **villi** (plural)

CHAPTER 5 Digestive System

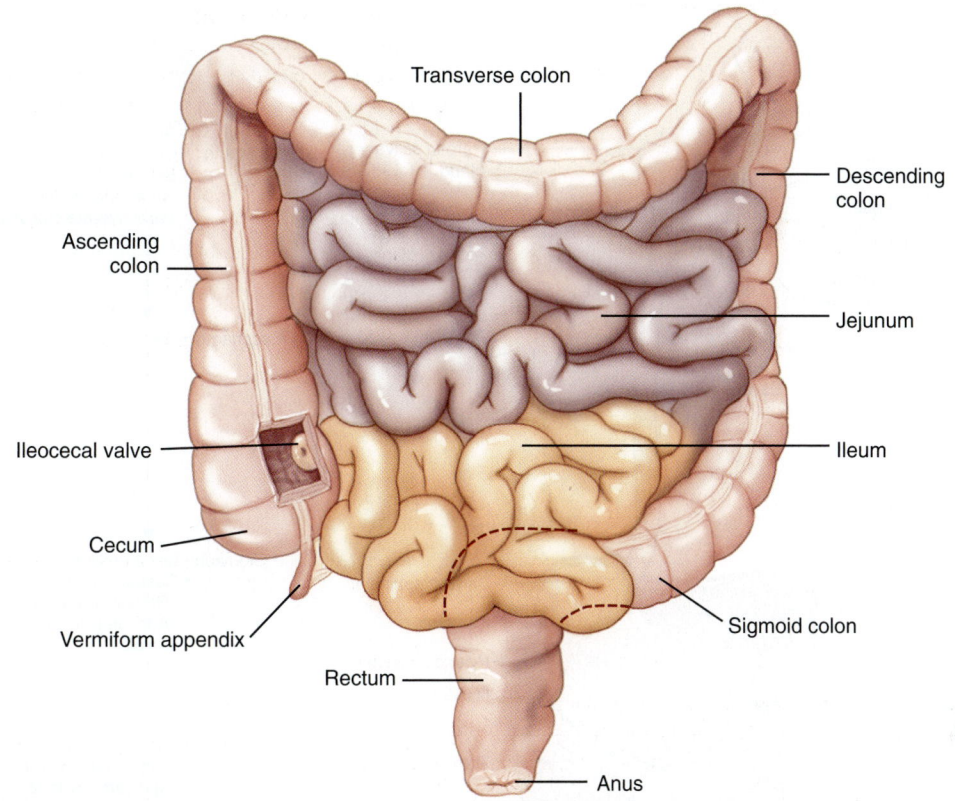

FIG. 5.6 The small and large intestines. (From Shiland B: *Mastering Healthcare Terminology*, ed 5, St. Louis, 2016, Elsevier.)

BOX 5.4 Sigmoid Colon
The sigmoid colon has a curve that resembles an "S" shape. In the Greek alphabet, the letter "S" is called sigma. Because the curve looks like the Greek letter sigma, it is called the sigmoid colon.

BOX 5.5 Intrinsic Factor
Intrinsic factor (IF) is produced in the lining of the stomach. Intrinsic factor is necessary to properly absorb vitamin B_{12} from food. People who do not produce intrinsic factor must receive monthly B_{12} injections.

MEDICAL TERMINOLOGY
an/o: anus
appendic/o, append/o: appendix
appendix (singular), **appendices** (plural)
cec/o: cecum
col/o, colon/o: large intestine, colon
fec/a: feces
-oid: like, similar to
rect/o: rectum, straight
sigm/o: S-shaped
sigmoid/o: sigmoid colon

PHYSIOLOGY OF THE DIGESTIVE SYSTEM

The prior sections discussed the physical changes that our food undergoes. This is *mechanical digestion*. The physical change that takes place is very important, but digestion is not finished yet. The smaller physical particles of food must be further chemically broken down to usable molecules. Without *chemical digestion*, the food eaten would not be available to individual cells and the cells would starve.

Chemical Digestion
Chemical digestion starts in the mouth. Food is chewed and moistened with saliva. Saliva contains an enzyme called salivary amylase. Salivary amylase starts to break down complex carbohydrate molecules into smaller usable molecules (Fig. 5.7).

Once food reaches the stomach, it mixes and churns with the acidic *gastric juice*. The acidic pH of the gastric juice helps in the chemical breakdown of food. *Hydrochloric acid*, *pepsin*, and *intrinsic factor* are found in the gastric juice (Box 5.5). Hydrochloric acid softens and dissolves tough connective tissue and fibrous cell walls. It starts to break down complex molecules into smaller, simpler molecules. Pepsin in the stomach starts to break down large protein molecules into smaller, absorbable molecules (Fig. 5.7). A thick liquid, called chyme, develops as the food particles break down. Chyme leaves the stomach by way of the pyloric sphincter muscle and moves into the small intestine.

Most chemical digestion takes place in the small intestine. Chyme entering the small intestine triggers the release of several chemical substances that help in the process of chemical digestion. The gallbladder, liver, and pancreas secrete substances into the small intestine, which makes chemical digestion possible. They are known as accessory organs, digestive adnexa (ad NECK sah), or GI adnexa (Fig. 5.8).

VOCABULARY
adnexa: Structures that are attached, adjacent, or adjoining to another structure.

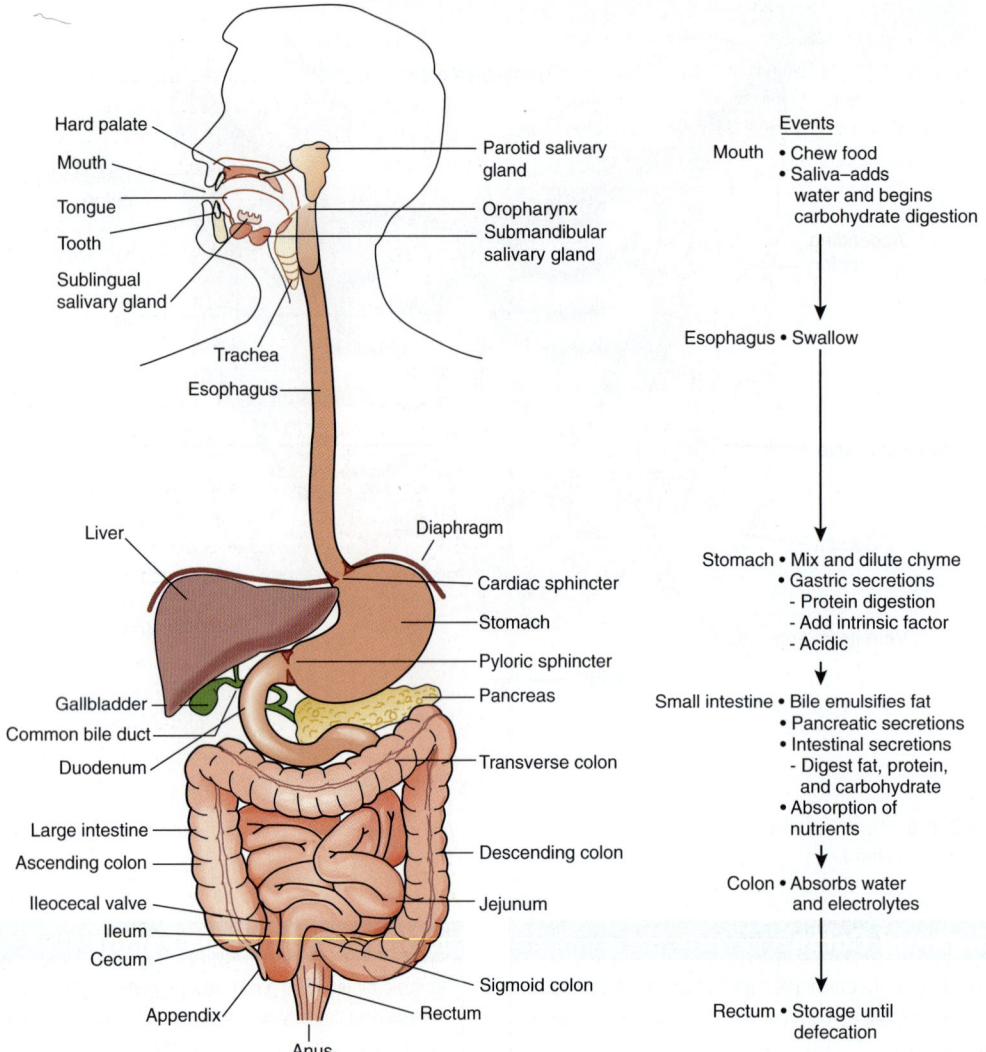

FIG. 5.7 The anatomy of the digestive system and associated events. (From VanMeter KC, Hubert RJ: *Gould's Pathophysiology for the Health Professions,* ed 5, Philadelphia, 2015, Saunders.)

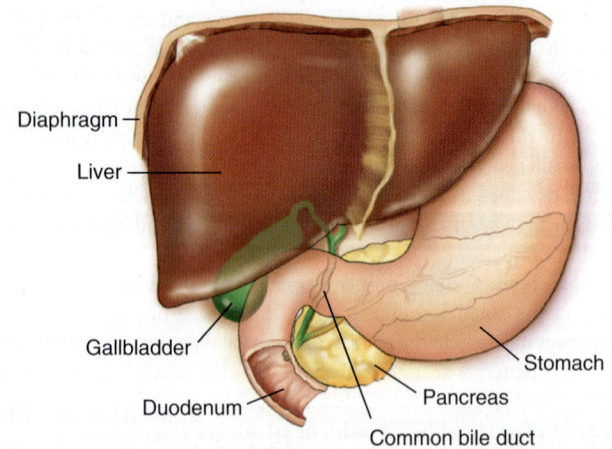

FIG. 5.8 Digestive adnexa. (From Shiland B: *Mastering Healthcare Terminology,* ed 5, St. Louis, 2016, Elsevier.)

> **BOX 5.6 Bile**
>
> Bile is composed of the following:
> - *Bilirubin* (BILL ee roo bin), a breakdown product of red blood cells
> - Bile acid (also called bile salts)
> - *Cholesterol* (koh LESS tur all) substance eaten in food and made by the liver
> - Water
> - Body salts (e.g., sodium, potassium) and metals (e.g., copper)

The liver and gallbladder work together to help the process of chemical digestion. The liver filters and stores blood. The liver also forms *bile*, which **emulsifies** (ee MUL sih fyez) fats into smaller particles (Boxes 5.6 and 5.7). Bile is released from the liver and stored in the gallbladder. When fatty food contained in chyme enters the duodenum, a hormone called *cholecystokinin (CCK)* (koh lee sis to KYE nin) is secreted by the small intestine. CCK causes the gallbladder to contract and release bile into the duodenum through the common bile duct. CCK also increases secretion of pancreatic juices.

BOX 5.7 Liver

The liver is the largest internal organ in the body. It has an important role in maintaining homeostasis, but it does not belong to any one body system. In addition to making bile for the digestive system, the liver has many other functions, including the following:
- Produces blood proteins, including albumin and blood clotting factors
- Manufactures triglycerides and cholesterol
- Converts glucose to glycogen to be stored in the muscles and liver
- Helps detoxify the body and metabolizes medications, drugs, and alcohol
- Stores vitamins B_{12}, B_9 (folic acid), A, D, K, and iron for future use

BOX 5.8 Pancreas

The pancreas is a busy and complex organ. It is involved in the digestive system as an **exocrine** (ECK soh krin) gland. Pancreatic enzymes enter the duodenum through a duct. The pancreas is also involved in the endocrine system as an **endocrine** (EN doh krin) gland. Pancreatic hormones are carried directly in the bloodstream, so no ducts are involved. The pancreas is one organ, but it is busy working in two different body systems and as two distinct glands. The pancreas will also be discussed in Chapter 14.

BOX 5.9 Interesting Suffixes

The suffix *-ase* is used to form the name of an enzyme. It is frequently added to the name of the substance upon which the enzyme acts—for example, lipase, which acts on lipids. The chemical suffix *-ose* indicates that a substance is a carbohydrate, such as *glucose* or *fructose*.

The pancreas produces pancreatic juice that contains enzymes and sodium bicarbonate. This juice passes through the pancreatic duct and common bile duct and empties into the duodenum (Box 5.8). Pancreatic juice is **alkaline**, which helps to neutralize the acidity of the chyme. The pancreatic enzymes chemically break down molecules until they can be absorbed into the bloodstream. The pancreatic enzymes include the following:
- *Lipase*: breaks down fats into fatty acids and glycerol (Box 5.9)
- *Amylase*: breaks down carbohydrates (starches) into sugars (mostly glucose) and food fibers
- *Proteases*: break down proteins into amino acids

With the help of pancreatic enzymes chemical digestion continues to break down large complex molecules into small absorbable molecules that the cells can use.

CRITICAL THINKING 5.5

Name the enzymes released from the pancreas into the small intestines. Which nutrient is digested by each of the enzymes?

Absorption and Excretion

Once chemical digestion is complete, small nutrient molecules need to move from the small intestines into the bloodstream through the process of *absorption*. As chyme continues through the small intestines, multiple circular folds, called *plicae* (PLY see), contain thousands of tiny villi. The villi are then covered by epithelial cells called microvilli that have a brushlike shape. The villi and microvilli increase the surface area of the small intestine and make absorption of nutrients more efficient.

The villi contain lymphatic vessels, known as *lacteals* (LACK tee uls) that absorb *lipids* (LIH pid), or fats. Villi contain blood capillaries that can absorb glucose and amino acids. Some carbohydrates may not completely break down to glucose in the small intestine. If that is the case, the villi produce an enzyme (lactase) that will break down carbohydrates to glucose so that they can be absorbed.

Chemical digestion and nutrient absorption is completed by the time chyme leaves the small intestine. As chyme moves through the large intestine, water and electrolytes are reabsorbed to prevent dehydration. The consistency of chyme changes to a soft-formed solid, called feces. The composition of feces is water, bacteria, undigested carbohydrates, fiber, and some protein and fat.

Besides the reabsorption of water and electrolytes, the large intestine also has an important role with vitamin K. The bacteria that live in the large intestines **synthesize** vitamin K, which is needed for blood clotting, strong bones, and overall heart health.

CRITICAL THINKING 5.6

Why do you think absorption is such a critical role of the digestive system? What is absorbed in the small intestines? What is absorbed in the large intestines? Share your thoughts with the class.

VOCABULARY

alkaline: A substance that has a pH greater than 7.0 on the pH scale (0–14).
emulsifies: When a substance suspends tiny droplets of one liquid into a second liquid. By creating an emulsion, you can mix two liquids that usually do not mix well, such as oil and water.
endocrine: A glandular secretion that is released into the blood or lymph directly (does not go through a duct).
exocrine: A glandular secretion released through a duct.
synthesize: To make whole by combining parts or constituents.

MEDICAL TERMINOLOGY

adnex/o: accessory
chol/e, bil/i: bile
cholecyst/o: gallbladder
choledoch/o: common bile duct
cholesterol/o: cholesterol
chulengo/o: bile vessel
-crine: to secrete
diaphragmat/o, phren/o: diaphragm
endo-: within
exo-: outside
hepat/o: liver
-kinin: movement substance
lipid/o, lip/o: lipid, fat
pancreat/o: pancreas

DISEASES AND DISORDERS OF THE DIGESTIVE SYSTEM

Diseases of the digestive system are diverse and have many causes. Numerous factors can be associated with digestive system conditions. Causes of digestive system diseases and disorders can be related to infections, structural abnormalities, trauma, malignant and benign growths, and congenital conditions.

Table 5.1 describes digestive system signs and symptoms. Common signs and symptoms of digestive system diseases and disorders include the following:
- Pain, nausea, vomiting, and lack of appetite
- Diarrhea with or without blood or mucous, constipation
- Abdominal tenderness and bloating
- Fever, fatigue
- Chest pain, heartburn, difficulty swallowing

Tables 5.2 and 5.3 provide common diagnostic imaging and laboratory testing used for digestive system conditions. Table 5.4 contains therapeutic interventions for the digestive system.

MEDICAL TERMINOLOGY

aliment/o: nutrition
-ation: process of
bi/o: life, living
-centesis: surgical puncture
cutane/o: skin
-ectomy: removal
hem/o: blood
hemorrhoid/o: hemorrhoid
herni/o: hernia
hyper-: excessive
lapar/o: abdomen
ligat/o: tying
lys/o: breakdown
my/o: muscle
nas/o: nose
para-: near, beside
per-: through
polyp/o: polyp
-plasty: surgical repair
-rrhaphy: suture
-scopic: pertaining to viewing
stomat/o: mouth
-stomy: new opening
-tion: the process of
-tomy: incision

CRITICAL THINKING 5.7

Samuel has completed Al's vital signs and has charted the information in the electronic health record (EHR). Samuel comments that Al has lost 5 pounds since his last appointment and asks if he has been trying to lose weight, but Al says "No, just haven't been hungry lately." Al has had some digestive system complaints. What signs and symptoms might he be having? Think of three or four possible symptoms, and share them with the class.

Acute Appendicitis

Appendicitis is an inflamed and infected appendix (Fig. 5.12). The appendix is located at the beginning of the large intestine (*cecum*). The

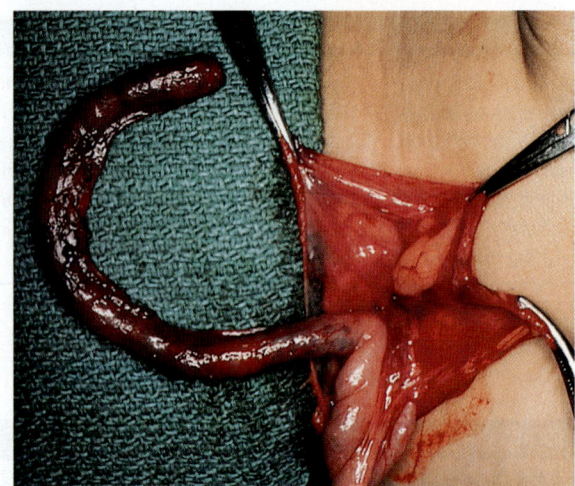

FIG. 5.12 Appendicitis. Note the darker pink color of the appendix, indicating inflammation. (From Zitelli BJ, Davis HW: *Atlas of Pediatric Physical Diagnosis*, ed 5, St. Louis, 2007, Mosby.)

TABLE 5.1 Digestive System Signs and Symptoms

Term	Definition
Constipation (kon stih PAY shun)	Infrequent, incomplete, or delayed BMs; obstipation is intractable (difficult to manage) constipation or intestinal obstruction
Diarrhea (dye ah REE ah)	Abnormal discharge of watery, semisolid stools
Dyspepsia (dis PEP see ah)	Feeling of epigastric discomfort that occurs shortly after eating; the discomfort may include feelings of nausea, fullness, heartburn, or bloating; also called *indigestion*
Flatus (FLAY tus)	Gas expelled through the anus
Halitosis (hal ih TOH sis)	Bad-smelling breath
Hematemesis (hee mah TEM ah sis)	Vomiting of blood
Hematochezia	Bright red, lower GI bleeding from the rectum that may originate in the distal colon; passage of bloody stools
Melena (mah LEE nah)	Black, tarry stools caused by the presence of partially digested blood
Nausea (NAH see ah)	Sensation that accompanies the urge to vomit but does not always lead to vomiting; the abbreviation N&V refers to nausea and vomiting; the term is derived from a Greek word meaning "seasickness"
Pyrosis (pye ROH sis)	Painful burning sensation in esophagus, usually caused by reflux of stomach contents, hyperactivity, or peptic ulcer; also known as *heartburn*
Vomiting (VAH mih ting)	Forcible or involuntary emptying of the stomach through the mouth; the material expelled is called vomitus or emesis

From Shiland B: *Mastering Healthcare Terminology*, ed 5, St. Louis, 2016, Elsevier.

TABLE 5.2 Terms Related to Imaging the Digestive System

Term	Definition
Barium enema (BE) (BAIR ee um EN nuh mah)	Introduction of a barium sulfate suspension through the rectum for imaging of the lower digestive tract to detect obstructions, tumors, and other abnormalities
Barium swallow (BaS)	Radiographic imaging done after oral ingestion of a barium sulfate suspension; used to detect abnormalities of the esophagus and stomach
Cholecystography (koh lee sis TAH gruh fee)	Contrast study in which iodine is ingested orally; the gallbladder is then imaged at different time intervals to assess its functioning; this procedure is used to diagnose cholecystitis, cholelithiasis, tumors, and other abnormalities of the gallbladder
Computed tomography (CT) scan	Radiographic technique that produces detailed images of "slices," or cross sections of the body, used in the digestive system to diagnose tumors or abnormal accumulations of fluid
Endoscopic retrograde cholangiopancreatography (ERCP) (en doh SKAH pik REH troh grade koh LAN jee oh pan kree ah TAH grah fee)	Radiographic imaging of the bile and pancreatic ducts through the placement of a duodenoscope in the common bile duct and injection of a contrast medium into the common bile duct; a series of x-rays are then taken to show the backward flow (retrograde) of dye into the bile vessels
Endoscopy (en DAH skuh pee)	General term for any internal visualization of the body with an instrument called an *endoscope*, which has its own fiber optic light source; the endoscope enters the GI tract through the oral cavity (esophagoscopy, gastroscopy, and esophagogastroduodenoscopy [EGD]), through the anus (proctoscopy, colonoscopy, or sigmoidoscopy), or through an incision in the abdominal wall (laparoscopy or lap)
Hepatobiliary (HIDA) scan (HEP ah toe bill e airy)	Known as a cholescintigraphy and hepatobiliary scintigraphy; a radioactive tracer is injected into a vein in the arm and travels to the bile-producing cells of the liver; the tracer is incorporated into bile and can be followed through the bile ducts into the small intestines; a nuclear medical scanner tracks the flow of bile and creates computer images
Magnetic resonance imaging (MRI)	Procedure that uses magnetic properties to record detailed information about internal structures
Manometry (mah NAH met tree)	Test that measures the motor function (muscle pressure) of the esophagus; a *manometer* is used to measure pressure
Percutaneous transhepatic cholangiography (PTC) (pur kyoo TAY nee us trans heh PAT ick koh lan jee AH gruh fee)	Radiographic procedure to image the bile vessels using a contrast medium introduced into the hepatic duct by an approach through the skin
Ultrasound, abdominal sonography (soh NAH gruh fee)	Use of high-frequency sound waves to image deep structures of the body; used in the digestive system to detect gallstones and tumors

From Shiland B: *Mastering Healthcare Terminology*, ed 5, St. Louis, 2016, Elsevier.

TABLE 5.3 Terms Related to Laboratory Tests for the Digestive System

Term	Definition
Biopsy (BYE op see)	Removal and examination of living tissue from the body for diagnostic purposes
Complete blood count (CBC)	A CBC is used as a screening test to determine an individual's general health status; it can be used to monitor specific blood cells and evaluate ongoing therapies; used to help diagnose conditions such as anemia, infection, inflammation, bleeding disorders, and cancer
Comprehensive chemistry panel	Used as a screening test to determine an individual's general health status; can be used to monitor specific blood constituents and ongoing therapies; used to help diagnose conditions related to the digestive system; measures protein levels, liver enzymes, and bilirubin levels; some CLIA-waived tests are available
C-reactive protein (CRP)	A nonspecific marker for inflammation in the body; produced in the liver and measured by testing the blood; CRP levels rise in response to inflammation; some CLIA-waived tests are available
Helicobacter pylori testing; antibody, stool antigen, breath, or rapid urease test (HE lih coh back ter pie loh ree)	Testing for *Helicobacter pylori* is done to diagnose a bacterial infection that can cause peptic ulcers; samples for testing include serum, stool, tissue biopsy, or breath; CLIA-waived tests are available
Hepatic function panel or liver function panel	Used to help detect, diagnose, evaluate, and monitor conditions related to the liver: acute and chronic liver inflammation, liver infections, disease or damage; tests liver enzymes, bilirubin, albumin, total protein, and possibly additional enzymes and blood clotting function; some CLIA-waived tests available
Human chorionic gonadotropin (hCG)—urine or serum (KOHR ee oh ick goh nad uh TROH pin)	hCG testing is routinely used to screen for a pregnancy; this test may be used to rule out pregnancy, as it relates to abdominal pain and the digestive system; CLIA-waived test (urine only)
Ova and parasite examination (O&P)	A stool examination that uses a microscope to look for parasites that may infect the lower digestive tract
Stool culture	Fecal exam to test for pathogenic bacteria in the feces

Continued

TABLE 5.3 Terms Related to Laboratory Tests for the Digestive System—cont'd

Term	Definition
Stool guaiac, fecal occult blood test, hemoccult test (GWEYE ack HEEM oh kult)	Fecal specimen exam to detect occult or hidden blood, which may indicate GI bleeding; CLIA-waived test
Total bilirubin (BILL lee roo bin)	Blood test to detect possible jaundice (yellowing of the skin), cirrhosis, or hepatitis; some CLIA-waived tests available
Urinalysis (UA) (yoo ruh NAL uh sis)	Tests different components of urine; can help to rule out conditions that may cause abdominal pain such a urinary tract infection (UTI), kidney stones, and some kidney and liver diseases; CLIA-waived test
Viral hepatiti–serum antibody and antigen testing	Testing for specific viral hepatitis antibodies and antigens is done to accurately diagnose viral hepatitis; this type of testing is also used to determine if hepatitis B or C infections are acute or chronic conditions

From Shiland B: *Mastering Healthcare Terminology*, ed 5, St. Louis, 2016, Elsevier.

TABLE 5.4 Terms Related to Therapeutic Interventions for the Digestive System

Term	Definition
Anastomosis (ah nas tih MOH sis)	New connection created between two (usually hollow) structures (Fig. 5.9)
Bariatric surgery (bair ee AT rick)	A variety of surgical procedures done to control morbid obesity by reducing the size of the stomach or by rerouting the small intestine to reduce the absorption of nutrients; these procedures include gastric stapling (gastroplasty), gastric banding (Lap-Band), and gastric bypass (Roux-en-Y)
Cholecystectomy (koh lee sis TECK tuh mee)	Surgical removal of the gallbladder
Colostomy (koh LOSS tuh mee)	Surgical redirection of the bowel to a *stoma* (STOH mah), an artificial opening on the abdominal wall (Fig. 5.10)

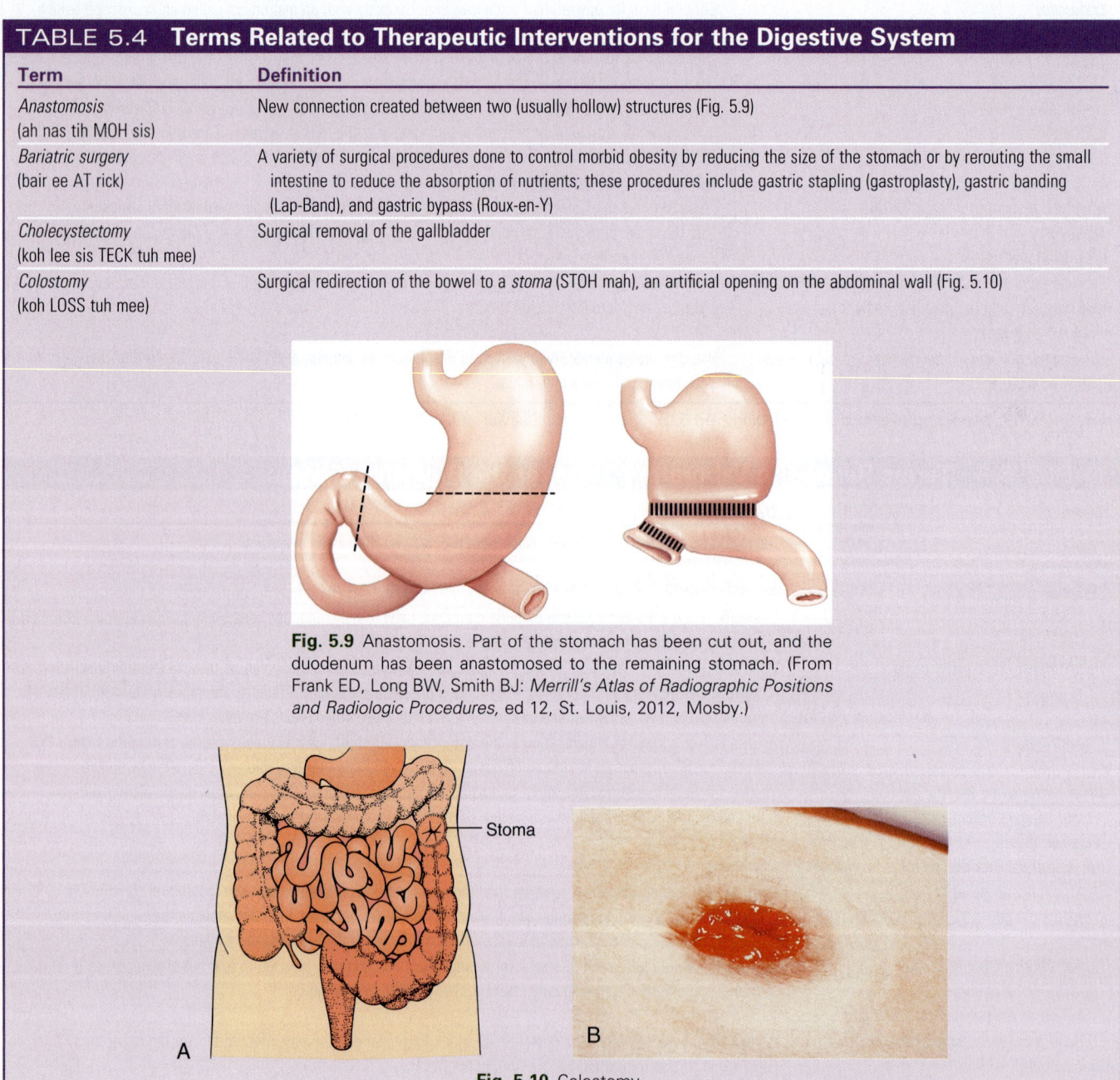

Fig. 5.9 Anastomosis. Part of the stomach has been cut out, and the duodenum has been anastomosed to the remaining stomach. (From Frank ED, Long BW, Smith BJ: *Merrill's Atlas of Radiographic Positions and Radiologic Procedures,* ed 12, St. Louis, 2012, Mosby.)

Fig. 5.10 Colostomy.

TABLE 5.4 Terms Related to Therapeutic Interventions for the Digestive System—cont'd

Term	Definition
Enema (EH nih mah)	Method of introducing a solution into the rectum for therapeutic (relief of constipation) or hygienic (preparation for surgery) reasons
Feeding tubes	*Enteral nutrition*—introduced through a digestive structure *Parenteral nutrition*—introduced through a structure outside of the alimentary canal, usually intravenously
Gastrectomy (gass TRECK tuh mee)	Surgical removal of all or part of the stomach
Gastric gavage (gah VAHZH)	Feeding through a tube in the stomach
Hemorrhoidectomy (heh moh roy DECK tuh mee)	Surgical excision of hemorrhoids
Herniorrhaphy (hur nee OR rah fee)	Hernia repair; suture of a hernia
Hyperalimentation (hye pur al ih men TAY shun)	The therapeutic use of nutritional supplements that exceed recommended daily requirements
Laparoscopic surgery (lap uh roh SCAH pick)	Surgery done through several small incisions in the abdominal wall with the aid of an instrument called a laparoscope; a laparoscopic cholecystectomy is the removal of the gallbladder
Laparotomy (lap uh RAH tuh mee)	Any surgical incision in the abdominal wall for an operative approach or for exploratory purposes
Ligation (lye GAY shun)	Tying off a blood vessel or duct (e.g., the cystic duct is ligated when the gallbladder is removed during a cholecystectomy)
Lysis of adhesions (LYE sis)	Surgical destruction of adhesions (scar tissue that binds two anatomic surfaces) (e.g., in the peritoneal cavity)
Nasogastric intubation (nay soh GASS trick in too BAY shun)	Placement of a tube from the nose, down the back of the throat, then into the stomach, for enteral feeding or removing gastric contents; the tube is sometimes called an *NG tube*
Odontectomy (oh don TECK tuh mee)	Surgical excision of a tooth
Paracentesis (pair ah sen TEE sis)	Procedure for withdrawing fluid from a body cavity, most commonly to remove fluid accumulated in the abdominal cavity
Percutaneous endoscopic gastrostomy (PEG) (pur kew TAY nee us en doh SKOP ick gass TROSS tuh mee)	A new opening of the stomach through the skin that allows the surgeon to place a tube for enteral feeding
Polypectomy (poll ih PECK tuh mee)	Surgical removal of a sessile or pedunculated polyp
Pyloromyotomy (pye lor oh mye AH tuh mee)	An incision of the pyloric sphincter to correct an obstruction, such as pyloric stenosis
Stomatoplasty (STOH mat toh plass tee)	Surgical repair of the mouth
Trocar (TROH kar)	A surgical instrument that is a sharp rod inside of a tube used to puncture a body cavity (Fig. 5.11); each access point formed is called a "port"

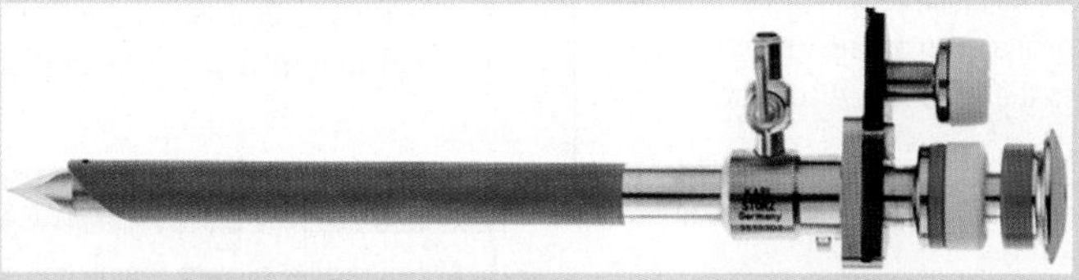

Fig. 5.11 Trocar. (From Fuller JK: *Surgical Technology*, ed 4, Philadelphia, 2000, Saunders.)

From Shiland B: *Mastering healthcare terminology*, ed 5, St. Louis, 2016, Elsevier.

pain associated with appendicitis initially starts near the navel (belly button or *umbilicus*) then moves to the lower right abdomen.

Etiology. If there is a blockage in the lining of the appendix, an infection can occur. As the infection gets worse, the appendix becomes swollen, painful, and filled with pus. If left untreated, an appendix can burst, which can lead to serious complications. Risk factors for acute appendicitis include the following:

- The common age for appendicitis is 10 to 30 years old, but it can occur at any age.
- It is more common in individuals who have chronic constipation, intestinal parasites, obstructive bowel disease, or hard, infrequent bowel movements.

It is thought that chronic constipation obstructs the opening of the appendix, and infection and inflammation are more likely to occur.

Signs and Symptoms. Common signs and symptoms of appendicitis include the following:

- Sudden abdominal pain starting near the navel and then moving to the right lower quadrant of the abdomen
- Nausea, vomiting, and loss of appetite after pain has begun
- Low-grade fever
- Constipation, diarrhea, or abdominal bloating before or after the onset of pain
- If appendicitis is even suspected, medical attention should be sought immediately; a burst appendix can be a serious condition if not treated quickly; without prompt care, it can be fatal

Diagnostic Procedures. Diagnostic procedures for appendicitis start with a history and physical exam. The provider will look for abdominal tenderness, rebound pain, and possibly a low-grade fever upon exam.

- Certain laboratory tests commonly accompany a physical exam:
  - Complete blood count (CBC): specifically looking for elevated white blood cell count and neutrophilia
  - C-reactive protein (CRP) testing
  - Urinalysis: to rule out urinary tract infections or kidney stones
  - Urine hCG: to rule out pregnancy or ectopic pregnancy
- The provider may recommend certain imaging tests:
  - Abdominal x-ray, ultrasound, or computed tomography (CT) scan to confirm appendicitis or rule out other abdominal causes for the pain

> **VOCABULARY**
> **ectopic pregnancy:** The development of a fertilized ovum outside the uterus, as in a fallopian tube.
> **neutrophilia:** An increase of neutrophilic white blood cells in blood or tissues.
> **rebound pain:** When a person feels abdominal pain as pressure is removed, rather than when pressure is applied to the abdomen. Also known as the *Blumberg sign*.

Treatment. Once the appendix has developed an infection, the usual treatment is surgical removal of the appendix. Frequently, antibiotics will be given before surgery to prevent further infection. The most common type of appendectomy performed is a laparoscopic procedure. A small incision is made in the abdomen, and then specialized tools and a small flexible camera are used to remove the appendix. Recovery time and scarring is reduced with laparoscopic procedures. Not all cases of appendicitis can be done laparoscopically, and the surgeon will make the final decision on surgical methods.

If the appendix has burst and an abscess has formed around it, surgery may be delayed while the abscess is drained. A tube is placed through the skin and into the abscess, which drains fluids and infection from the abscess. At the same time, the patient will be taking antibiotics to control the infection. Usually surgery is performed a few weeks after the abscess has been drained. Postoperative treatments include the following:

- Limited activity for about 10 to 14 days, no strenuous activities
- Antibiotic therapy and pain medication
- Extra rest, movement as the patient is able, abdominal support when coughing or sneezing
- Return to work or school after a postsurgery follow-up with the provider

Prognosis. The prognosis for appendicitis is very good for a simple appendectomy without abscess. The prognosis for appendicitis that has burst, or that has formed an abscess, is more complicated. It depends on the severity of the condition and infection. The prognosis also depends on the promptness of diagnosis and treatment.

Prevention. Measures that can be taken to lessen a person's chances of developing appendicitis and any complications include the following:

- A diet high in fiber and adequate water intake to avoid constipation
- Avoiding a sedentary lifestyle, again to avoid constipation
- Prompt medical attention if experiencing any abdominal pain near the navel or lower right quadrant of the abdomen

Cancers of the Digestive System

Cancer or malignancies all begin with a normal cell whose DNA mutates for some reason. The *mutation* creates a cell that acts differently than its parent cell. Cancer cells generally reproduce at a rapid rate, and if the immune system cannot destroy the malignant cells, cancer will develop. These rapidly growing cells can invade nearby tissue, and they can also spread to other parts of the body, which is called metastasis.

There are primary organ and accessory organ cancers that affect the digestive system. Table 5.5 describes five of these cancers. Much more information can be found at www.cdc.gov/cancer, www.cancer.gov, and www.cancer.org/cancer on any type of cancer including digestive system cancers.

Etiology. The causes of cancers can be difficult to determine, but there are factors that seem to affect the development of cancer in the digestive system in general. Risk factors include the following:

- Using tobacco products, but especially smoking tobacco products
- Chronic inflammation in the digestive system
- Family history of digestive system cancer
- Obesity
- Heavy alcohol consumption over time
- Diet low in fruits, vegetables, and fiber

> **CRITICAL THINKING 5.8**
>
> Al's digestive system complaints are abdominal pain, frequent constipation, loss of appetite, and abdominal bloating. He also has had a job change from a field sales representative to an in-house position for the same company. He misses being on the road and seeing customers each day, but the promotion was too good to pass up.
>
> With this information about Al, Samuel is starting to think about why Dr. Martin ordered a colonoscopy. Al is about 50 years old, so it was about time to have his first one done. With Al's symptoms and age, why do you think Dr. Martin wanted him to have a colonoscopy? Share your thoughts with the class.

TABLE 5.5 Cancers of the Digestive System

	Oral Cancer	Stomach Cancer	Pancreatic Cancer	Liver Cancer	Colon Cancer
Unique risk factors	Exposure to certain strains of HPV (human papillomavirus) Excessive sun exposure to lips	Diet high in salty, smoked foods Infection with *Helicobacter pylori*	Diabetes Family history of genetic syndromes including BRCA2 mutation	Cirrhosis Diabetes Nonalcoholic fatty liver disease	Age, older than 50 typically African American race History of colon polyps Radiation therapy for a past cancer
Signs and symptoms	Sore that does not heal, bleeds, or is painful anywhere in the oral cavity Difficulty chewing, swallowing, or a persistent sore throat	Fatigue Feeling full after eating small amounts of food Pain, heartburn, indigestion Persistent vomiting Weight loss	Pain in the upper abdomen and back Weight loss, and loss of appetite Jaundice Fatigue New-onset diabetes	Weight loss and loss of appetite Upper abdominal pain Fatigue Abdominal swelling Jaundice Nausea Chalky, whitish stools	Change in bowel habits Rectal bleeding or blood in stool Fatigue Weight loss Persistent abdominal discomfort; cramps, gas, pain
Diagnostic testing	Physical exam Biopsy of sore/lesion	Endoscopy Biopsy CT scan X-ray with barium swallow	Ultrasound CT scan MRI Biopsy	Blood test; chemistry or liver function panel Ultrasound CT scan MRI Biopsy	Colonoscopy Biopsy CT scan
Treatment	Depending on the stage of cancer at the time of diagnosis, some or all of the following treatments may be used: • Surgical removal of the cancerous growth • Radiation therapy • Chemotherapy • Palliative care				
Prognosis	For any cancer diagnosis, prognosis depends on the following factors: • Stage of cancer at the time of diagnosis • Cancer's response to treatment • Patient's desire and ability to tolerate or continue treatment				
Prevention	The following changes may reduce the risk of developing digestive system cancers: • Not smoking or using tobacco products in any form • Maintaining a healthy weight • Following a diet high in fruits, vegetables, lean protein, and fiber • Not consuming alcohol to excess • Exercising regularly Additional preventive measures unique to each cancer are listed next				
	Avoid excessive sun exposure on the lips See the dentist regularly	Reduce the amount of salty or smoked foods eaten	No additional preventive measures	Use caution when working with chemicals Vaccinate against hepatitis B Take measures to prevent hepatitis C	Be screened for colon cancer beginning at age 50 if there is no family history of colon cancer, younger if there are additional risk factors

From Shiland B: *Mastering Healthcare Terminology*, ed 5, St. Louis, 2016, Elsevier.

Cholelithiasis (Gallstones)

Cholelithiasis (gallstones) refers to deposits of digestive fluid that have hardened in the gallbladder. Gallstones can be as tiny as a grain of sand or as large as a walnut (Fig. 5.13). Some people only develop one gallstone, whereas other people may develop many smaller stones.

Etiology. Specific reasons for why gallstones form are not certain, but the following risk factors seem to increase a person's chances for cholelithiasis:

- Being female, especially if pregnant
- Losing weight quickly
- Being overweight or obese, having a sedentary lifestyle, and eating a high-fat, high-cholesterol, low-fiber diet
- Being over 40 years old, having diabetes or liver disease, or a family history of gallstones
- Being Native American or Mexican American

Signs and Symptoms. Gallstones may be asymptomatic. Gallstone pain may last several minutes to a few hours. If a gallstone lodges in a duct and causes a blockage, the resulting signs and symptoms may include the following:

- Rapidly intensifying pain in the upper right portion or center of the abdomen
- Back pain between the shoulder blades or pain in the right shoulder
- Nausea or vomiting

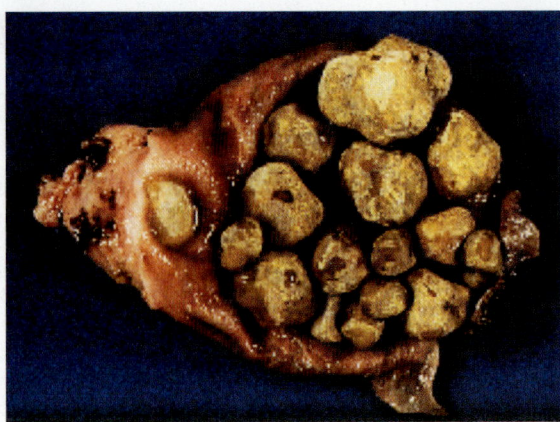

FIG. 5.13 Cholelithiasis (gallstones). (From Damjanov I: *Pathology: A Color Atlas*, St. Louis, 2000, Mosby.)

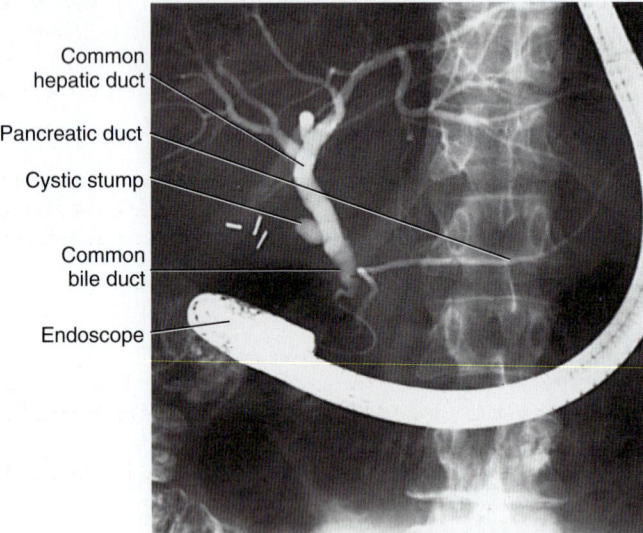

FIG. 5.14 Endoscopic retrograde cholangiopancreatography (ERCP). (From Frank ED, Long BW, Smith BJ: *Merrill's Atlas of Radiographic Positions and Radiologic Procedures*, ed 12, St. Louis, 2012, Mosby.)

- Inflammation of the gallbladder (cholecystitis), which can cause severe pain and fever
- Jaundice and bile duct infection
- Pancreatitis, which can cause constant and intense abdominal pain, usually requiring hospitalization

Diagnostic Procedures. The following tests and procedures may be used to diagnose gallstones:
- Imaging procedures such as the following:
  - Abdominal ultrasound, CT scan, and cholecystography to visualize the gallbladder and look for signs of gallstones
  - Hepatobiliary iminodiacetic acid (HIDA) scan, magnetic resonance imaging (MRI), or endoscopic retrograde cholangiopancreatography (ERCP); gallstones discovered using ERCP can be removed during the procedure (Fig. 5.14)
- Blood tests may be done to look for complications. Testing may include the following:
  - CBC, blood chemistry panel, or hepatic function panel

Treatment. Many patients with gallstones are asymptomatic, so no treatment is needed. If symptoms occur and intensify, one or more of the following treatments may be recommended:
- *Medications to help dissolve gallstones.* These medications are often reserved for people who cannot undergo surgery.
- *Surgery to remove the gallbladder (cholecystectomy).* When the gallbladder is removed, bile flows from the liver into the small intestine directly.

Prognosis. The prognosis for gallstones is good, but if complications occur, the prognosis can deteriorate. With any surgery, there is always a risk of complications.

Prevention. To help reduce the risk of gallstones:
- Do not skip meals or fast frequently, as this can increase the risk of gallstones.
- Lose weight slowly. Weight loss of about 1 or 2 pounds per week is safest.
- Maintain a healthy weight.

Crohn Disease

Crohn disease is an inflammation of the lining of the digestive tract, most commonly the small and large intestine. Crohn disease is classified as an inflammatory bowel disease (IBD). The inflammation caused by Crohn disease can seriously affect the layers of digestive system tissue, causing pain, malnutrition, and sometimes serious complications.

Etiology. The exact cause of Crohn disease remains unknown. Some scientists suspect a bacterial or viral trigger starts an abnormal immune response, which causes the chronic inflammation seen in Crohn disease. Heredity may also play a role; about 20% of people with Crohn have a close relative with the disease or ulcerative colitis.

Risk factors may include the following:
- Although a person can be diagnosed at any age, a diagnosis of Crohn disease is most common in those younger than 30 years old.
- People of Eastern European (Ashkenazi) Jewish descent have a higher risk.
- Living in an urban area, an industrialized country, or in northern climates increases the risk of developing Crohn disease.

Crohn disease can affect just the last segment of the small intestine (ileum), the colon, or both areas of the digestive system.

Signs and Symptoms. Signs and symptoms of Crohn disease can range from mild to severe. They may develop gradually or happen suddenly without warning. Symptoms frequently come and go and do not usually remain constant. When the disease is asymptomatic, it is referred to as being *in remission*.

When the disease is symptomatic, signs and symptoms may include the following:
- Diarrhea, possibly with loose stools, blood (visible or occult), or mucous
- Abdominal pain (may be severe), cramping, nausea, vomiting
- Low-grade fever, fatigue, mouth sores, reduced appetite, and weight loss
- Inability to properly digest food and absorb nutrients; possible malnutrition
- Perianal pain, drainage, infection, or fistula
- Signs and symptoms secondary to Crohn disease include inflammation of skin, eyes, joints, liver, and bile ducts, and delayed development in children

> **VOCABULARY**
> **fistula:** An abnormal connection or passage, caused by disease or injury, between different body parts.
> **occult:** Hidden or unseen.

Diagnostic Procedures. There is no one diagnostic test for Crohn disease, so the provider will likely use a combination of tests to rule out conditions and narrow the diagnosis to Crohn disease. Diagnostic testing may include a combination of the following:
- Imaging tests including CT scan, CT enterography, barium x-rays, MRI
- Laboratory tests including CBC, comprehensive chemistry panel, and fecal occult blood testing (Fig. 5.15)
- Procedural tests including colonoscopy, flexible sigmoidoscopy, and endoscopy

Treatment. The treatment of Crohn disease can be complicated and ever-changing depending on the person's symptoms at any given time. Treatment usually involves a combination of medications and diet to quiet symptoms. For some patients, surgery is necessary, especially if complications occur. There is no cure for Crohn disease, and there is no therapy that relieves symptoms for everyone. Each patient responds differently. The overall goal of treatment is to reduce inflammation, improve symptom severity, limit or eliminate complications, and hopefully achieve long-term remission.

Treatment for Crohn disease may include a combination of any or all of the following:
- Antiinflammatory drugs are prescribed, which frequently include corticosteroids, immune system suppressor medications, antibiotics, antidiarrheal medications, pain relievers, iron supplements, vitamin B_{12} shots, and calcium and vitamin D supplements.
- Nutrition therapy: eating small meals, drinking plenty of water, supplementing with a multivitamin, and consulting with a dietician. It may also include limiting or eliminating dairy products, high-fat foods, trigger foods, or foods that have caused flare-ups in the past. Common trigger foods include high-fiber foods, raw fruits and vegetables, nuts, seeds, popcorn, alcohol, spicy foods, and caffeine-containing food or drink. Refraining from alcohol and carbonated beverages is also recommended.
- Patients are encouraged to stop smoking, try to reduce stress, and incorporate exercise into one's daily routine.

Prognosis. Well-controlled Crohn disease has a good prognosis. Predicting the prognosis can be difficult with Crohn disease, as it can lead to many complications, including the following:
- Chronic bowel inflammation that may increase the risk of colon cancer
- Bowel obstructions, ulcers, fistulas, anal fissure (see Table 5.10, presented later in the chapter)
- Malnutrition, anemia, and osteoporosis
- Gallbladder or liver disease
- Surgery increases risk of complications beyond Crohn disease

Prevention. The cause of Crohn disease is not known, so prevention is difficult to describe. Avoiding chronic inflammation in any part of the body will help maintain a healthy immune system. This can decrease the possibility of any inflammatory immune condition.

Diverticulitis

Diverticula are small, bulging sacs that can form in the wall of the large intestine. This condition is not uncommon, especially after age 40, and it often does not cause problems. However, if one or more of the diverticula become inflamed or infected, then a condition develops called *diverticulitis* (die-vur-tik-yoo-LIE-tis) (Fig. 5.16). Diverticulitis can be a mild condition that is relatively easy to treat, or it can become a severe recurring condition that may require surgery.

Etiology. Diverticulitis develops when weak spots in the colon bulge through the intestinal wall and tear. The damage to the intestinal wall results in inflammation, infection, or both. Risk factors for diverticulitis are as follows:
- As a person ages, diverticulitis is more common
- Obesity, smoking, and a sedentary lifestyle
- A diet that is low in fiber, high in animal fat
- Some medications, such as steroids, opiates, and nonsteroidal antiinflammatory drugs (NSAIDs), increase the risk of diverticulitis

Signs and Symptoms. Signs and symptoms of diverticulitis include the following:

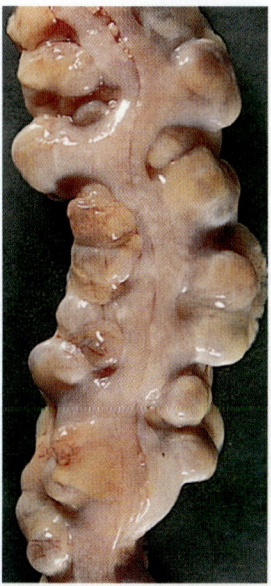

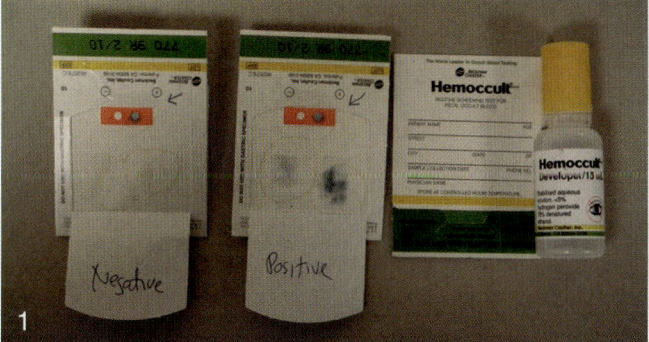

FIG. 5.15 Fecal occult blood testing. (From Roberts J, Hedges J: *Clinical Procedures in Emergency Medicine,* ed 5, Philadelphia, 2010, Saunders.)

FIG. 5.16 Diverticulitis. (From Damjanov I: *Pathology: A Color Atlas,* St. Louis, 2000, Mosby.)

- Pain in the lower left side of the abdomen that is constant for 2 to 3 days
- Fever, abdominal tenderness, nausea, and vomiting
- Constipation (most common) or diarrhea

Diagnostic Procedures. Diverticulitis is frequently diagnosed during an acute, painful attack. Because abdominal pain can be caused by a variety of conditions, diagnostic testing is needed to determine the cause of the signs and symptoms.

A provider will perform a physical exam that should include checking the abdomen for tenderness, bloating, and increased pain upon pressure. If the patient is in a woman, a pelvic exam should be included. Once the physical exam is completed, the following tests may be recommended:
- Laboratory tests, which may include CBC, urinalysis, hCG serum or urine pregnancy test, liver function panel, and stool culture (for patients with diarrhea)
- Imaging tests, which may include a CT scan

Treatment. Depending on findings, the provider may recommend the following treatments. This treatment regimen is effective for most patients with simple diverticulitis. If signs and symptoms are mild, the following is recommended:
- Oral antibiotic treatment for infection and over-the-counter pain medication
- A bland, liquid diet until the infection and inflammation have healed in the bowel, 2 to 4 days; a move to low-fiber solid food only as symptoms improve and the diet can be tolerated
- As solid food is reintroduced, meals should be very small for 2 to 4 weeks; gradually increase fiber content and meal size

For diverticulitis that is severe, or in patients with preexisting or chronic conditions, the following is recommended:
- Complicated cases of diverticulitis will require hospitalization
- Intravenous antibiotics
- Surgery if there is a perforation, abscess, fistula, or bowel obstruction, or if this is a recurrent condition with complications
- Surgery can include the removal of damaged portions of the intestine (anastomosis) or, in severe cases, a colostomy

Follow-up care with the provider after nonsurgical treatment takes place in about 3 to 4 weeks. Follow-up postsurgical care depends on the type of surgery and any postoperative complications.

Prognosis. The prognosis is good for most cases of diverticulitis, but in about 25% of cases, some complications do occur. As with any condition, complications worsen the prognosis. Possible complications include the following:
- Formation of an abscess or fistula
- Blockage in the colon or small intestine caused by scar tissue
- Peritonitis, which is an inflammation of the membranes in the abdominal cavity usually caused by infection; peritonitis is a medical emergency and requires immediate care

Prevention. To help prevent diverticulitis; exercise regularly, eat a diet rich in high-fiber foods, and drink plenty of fluids, especially water.

> **CRITICAL THINKING 5.9**
>
> Samuel is happy to know that Al's colonoscopy was normal; no polyps or abnormalities were found. But Al still has digestive issues. What possible conditions could cause his digestive symptoms? Discuss your thoughts with the class.

Gastroesophageal Reflux Disease

Gastroesophageal reflux disease (GERD) happens when stomach acid or stomach content flows back up (reflux) into the esophagus (Fig. 5.17). Reflux irritates the lining of the esophagus and causes GERD. Acid reflux is a common digestive condition that can happen from time to time. When acid reflux occurs at least twice each week, interferes with daily life, or has damaged the esophagus, the expected diagnosis is GERD.

Etiology. GERD results when frequent acid reflux causes the backup of stomach acid or stomach content into the esophagus. Normally a ring-shaped muscle, the lower esophageal sphincter, closes after food passes from the esophagus to the stomach. If a person has GERD, the lower esophageal sphincter may not close properly or it may be weak. This allows acid reflux to happen.

Constant acid reflux can irritate the lining of the esophagus, causing inflammation or esophagitis. If this continues over time, it can wear away the lining of the esophagus, which may cause bleeding, narrowing of the esophagus, or a precancerous condition called Barrett esophagus.

Risk factors for developing GERD include the following:
- An existing hiatal hernia
- Obesity, smoking, or dry mouth
- Pregnancy, asthma, or diabetes
- Delayed stomach emptying
- Infants can also develop GERD (see Chapter 32).

Signs and Symptoms. Signs and symptoms of GERD may include the following:
- A burning sensation in the chest (heartburn) or throat and a sour taste in the mouth
- Difficulty swallowing (*dysphagia*), chest pain, and dry cough
- A hoarse voice and sore throat
- Regurgitation of food or acid reflux (sour taste)
- Sensation of a lump in the throat

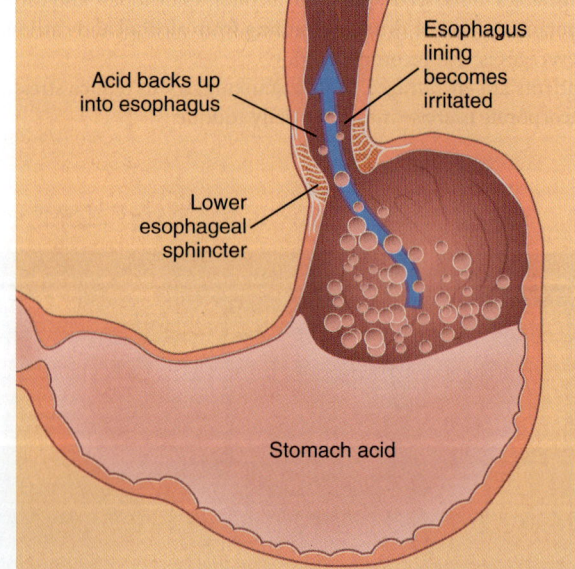

FIG. 5.17 Gastroesophageal reflux disease (GERD). (From Black JM, Hawks JH, Keene A: *Medical Surgical Nursing: Clinical Management for Positive Outcomes*, ed 8, Philadelphia, 2009, Saunders.)

> **VOCABULARY**
> **regurgitation:** Return of partly digested food or stomach contents from the stomach to the mouth.

Diagnostic Procedures. A provider may diagnose GERD based on signs, symptoms, and physical exam. This is the most common first step in GERD diagnosis and treatment. Additional tests may include the following:
- Acid levels in the esophagus are monitored. This can be done using several different varieties of ambulatory acid (pH) probes. Data are collected and examined for 24 hours.
- If GERD is diagnosed and is not well controlled over time, additional testing may be done if surgical repair seems necessary. The following tests may be recommended before deciding on surgery:
  - Barium swallow with or without an upper gastrointestinal (UGI) series (Fig. 5.18)
  - Endoscopy: useful when looking for complications of reflux, such as Barrett esophagus
  - Esophageal motility testing (manometry)

Treatment. Treatment for GERD usually begins with over-the-counter medications that control stomach acid production. If there is no relief, the provider may recommend other treatments, including prescription medications and surgery. Treatments that may help control GERD include the following:
- Medications to neutralize stomach acid (antacids) or reduce acid production (proton pump inhibitors)
- Surgery if medications are not successful; surgeries to reinforce or strengthen the lower esophageal sphincter are most common

Chronic inflammation in the esophagus can lead to complications, including the following:
- Narrowing of the esophagus (esophageal stricture)
- An open sore in the esophagus (esophageal ulcer)

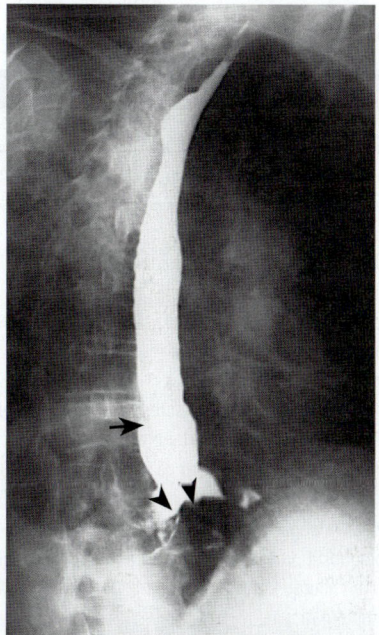

FIG. 5.18 X-ray after barium swallow. (From Shiland B: *Mastering Healthcare Terminology*, ed 5, St. Louis, 2016, Elsevier.)

- Precancerous changes to the esophagus (Barrett esophagus); this condition shows tissue damage in the lower esophagus, and these changes are associated with an increased risk of esophageal cancer

Treatment is ongoing until relief of GERD has been successful.

Prognosis. The prognosis for GERD is generally good without complications. Anytime surgery is necessary, the prognosis is more difficult.

Prevention. Lifestyle changes that may help reduce GERD include the following:
- Maintaining a healthy weight and not smoking
- Avoiding foods and beverages that trigger heartburn or GERD, such as fatty or fried foods, tomato sauce, alcohol, chocolate, mint, garlic, onion, and caffeine
- Eating smaller meals and trying not to overeat; not eating close to bedtime; trying to sit or stand for 3 hours after the last meal of the day
- Elevating the head of the bed at night when lying down

Hemorrhoids

Hemorrhoids (HEM-uh-roids) are swollen veins in the anus and lower rectum, almost like varicose veins, just at a different location in the body. Hemorrhoids are very common. About 75% of adults will have hemorrhoids at some point in their lifetime. Hemorrhoids can be asymptomatic and resolve quickly without treatment. Frequently they do cause symptoms that may be uncomfortable. Hemorrhoids that are located inside the rectum are referred to as internal hemorrhoids. Those that are located under the skin around the anus are referred to as external hemorrhoids.

Etiology. The veins around the anus can stretch under pressure and can become swollen and painful. Hemorrhoids develop from increased pressure in the lower rectum due to the following:
- Straining during bowel movements or sitting on the toilet for extended periods of time
- Pregnancy or obesity
- A low-fiber diet that may lead to infrequent, hard-to-move stools
- Chronic diarrhea or constipation

Hemorrhoids are more frequent in older adults because the muscles and tissues that support the veins in the rectum and anus can weaken and stretch with age and inactivity.

Signs and Symptoms. Signs and symptoms of hemorrhoids may include the following:
- Itching or irritation near the anus
- Pain, discomfort, or swelling around the anus
- Bleeding during bowel movements, which may be painless; patients may see small amounts of bright red blood on toilet tissue or in the toilet
- Swelling near the anus, which may be sensitive, tender, or painful

Symptoms may be different for internal, external, or thrombosed hemorrhoids:
- Internal hemorrhoids cannot be seen or felt and they do not often cause discomfort or pain. But straining when passing a stool can irritate an internal hemorrhoid's surface and cause it to bleed. Straining can also push an internal hemorrhoid through the anal opening, causing a prolapsed or protruding hemorrhoid. This can be painful.
- External hemorrhoids can become irritated more easily with a bowel movement. Common symptoms of external hemorrhoids are pain, itching, and bleeding.

- A thrombosed hemorrhoid occurs when blood pools in an external hemorrhoid and a clot (thrombus) forms. The formation of a clot can cause severe pain, swelling, and a hard bump near the anus.

It is rare to have complications associated with hemorrhoids, but they can occur. Anemia due to chronic blood loss is a possible complication. Also, a strangulated hemorrhoid is possible. This is caused when the blood supply to an internal hemorrhoid is inadequate, and it may result in severe pain.

Diagnostic Procedures. A provider should be able to see external hemorrhoids during a physical exam. Internal hemorrhoids require a physical examination of the anal canal and rectum:

- A digital examination is performed by inserting a gloved, lubricated finger into the patient's rectum. The provider feels for anything unusual, such as growths, lumps, bumps, or swelling in the area.
- Because internal hemorrhoids may be difficult to feel during a rectal exam if they are small or too soft, a provider may recommend an examination of the lower portion of the colon and rectum with an anoscope, proctoscope, or sigmoidoscope. This will allow internal hemorrhoids to be visualized.

Treatment. Patients can relieve mild hemorrhoid pain and swelling with over-the-counter (OTC) or home treatments. Often this is the only action needed to resolve hemorrhoids. Treatments include the following:

- Using OTC topical treatments: hemorrhoid creams and suppositories containing hydrocortisone, or pads containing a numbing agent
- Eating a diet high in fiber: high-fiber foods include fruits, vegetables, and whole grains; also, drinking plenty of water helps soften the stool, making it easier to pass
- Using a warm bath or sitz bath to soothe and heal the anal area to relieve pain and swelling of hemorrhoids: a sitz bath is a basin that fits over a toilet seat and can be filled with clean, warm water; sitting in a sitz bath for 10 to 15 minutes two to three times a day will ease the discomfort of hemorrhoids
- Applying cool or cold compresses to the anal area to bring down swelling
- Taking OTC pain relievers to lessen pain
- Keeping the area clean after a bowel movement by using moist towelettes or wet toilet paper that does not contain perfume or alcohol; dry toilet paper may irritate the area

If symptoms continue, recur, or worsen, the provider may recommend additional treatment such as the following:

- Incision and draining an external hemorrhoid
- Rubber band ligation, injections, or coagulation techniques; all to shrink hemorrhoids and relieve discomfort
- Surgical hemorrhoid removal (hemorrhoidectomy) or stapled hemorrhoidectomy

Prognosis. The prognosis is good in most cases of hemorrhoids. Complications may require additional treatment.

Prevention. The best way to prevent hemorrhoids is to eat a diet adequate in fiber and water. This will keep stools soft and easy to pass. Additional tips to prevent hemorrhoids include the following:

- Eat a diet rich in high-fiber foods. Recommended fiber intake is at least 25 grams per day for women and 38 grams per day for men. Eat fruits, vegetables, and whole grains. A fiber supplement may be recommended.
- Drink plenty of fluids, especially water, six to eight glasses per day.
- Exercise and be active to prevent constipation. Avoid extended periods of sitting or standing in one place.
- Do not strain when passing a bowel movement.

Hepatitis, Viral

Hepatitis is an inflammation of the liver. Inflammation can damage the liver and cause impaired liver function. There are many causes for hepatitis in general, but this material will specifically cover hepatitis that has a viral cause. Viral hepatitis is an infectious disease that in most cases can be prevented. Viral hepatitis can be caused by five main viral strains; A, B, C, D, and E. Hepatitis A and E are both transmitted primarily through fecal-oral contact. Hepatitis B, C, and D are transmitted as blood-borne pathogens. Table 5.6 provides detailed information on viral hepatitis.

TABLE 5.6 Viral Hepatitis

	Hepatitis A and E	Hepatitis B, C, and D
Etiology and risk factors	Person-to-person transmission through fecal-oral contamination. Ingesting something that has been contaminated with the feces of an infected person. Ingesting contaminated food or water Food handler who is infected and did not follow proper hand hygiene Undercooked foods that are contaminated: examples include raw shellfish, vegetables, and fruits Close contact with someone who is infected Sexual/intimate contact with an infected person Use of injection and noninjection illegal drugs	Person-to-person transmission through activities that involve **percutaneous** or mucosal contact with infected blood or body fluids (semen, saliva) Contact with blood or body fluids Sex with an infected partner Injection drug use that involves sharing needles, syringes, or drug-preparation equipment Birth to an infected mother Contact with blood or open sores of an infected person Needle sticks or sharp instrument exposure Sharing personal items such as razors or toothbrushes with an infected person
Signs and symptoms	Some people, especially young children are asymptomatic; children younger than 6 years are frequently asymptomatic; older children and adults are frequently symptomatic If symptoms occur, they can include the following: fever, fatigue, loss of appetite, nausea, vomiting, abdominal pain, dark urine, jaundice, joint pain, clay-colored feces	Children younger than 5 years and newly infected immunosuppressed adults are frequently symptomatic Among children older than 5 years, only about 30%–50% are symptomatic

TABLE 5.6 Viral Hepatitis—cont'd

	Hepatitis A and E	Hepatitis B, C, and D
Diagnostic procedures	A provider will perform a history and physical exam; if there is any indication of hepatitis, blood testing will most likely be done; for hepatitis A, B, C, and D, specific antibody testing is done to confirm the presence and type of hepatitis (see Table 5.2) There is no reliable antibody testing for hepatitis E; history, physical, recent travel, and signs and symptoms are used to diagnose hepatitis E	
Treatment	Lots of rest Eat and drink tiny amounts at one time to cope with nausea Be kind to the liver, do not drink alcohol, and consult the provider about any existing medications that may affect the liver; this includes OTC medications With any type of viral hepatitis, serious complications can occur, including liver failure or death; liver failure requires a liver transplant For hepatitis A and E, treatment is generally supportive	*Hepatitis B—acute infection:* treatment is supportive *Hepatitis B—chronic infection:* antiviral medications to prevent liver damage or liver cancer *Hepatitis C—acute infection:* treated aggressively with antiviral medications to minimize the possibility of developing chronic hepatitis C *Hepatitis C—chronic infection:* treated with antiviral medications to minimize the possibility of liver damage, cirrhosis, liver cancer, or organ failure; chronic hepatitis infections may require a liver transplant in the course of the disease *Hepatitis D—acute infection:* treatment is supportive *Hepatitis D—chronic infection:* antiviral medications to prevent liver damage and liver failure Liver transplant may be required if liver failure occurs
Prognosis	Hepatitis A: good for most healthy individuals; for hepatitis A, middle-aged and older adults run a greater risk of complications, liver failure, or death Hepatitis E: good for most healthy, nonpregnant persons; see prevention below	*Hepatitis B, C, and D* as acute or chronic diseases can range from mild to fulminant during an individual's illness; many factors are involved in the management of hepatitis; patients who develop chronic hepatitis infections face lifelong disease management and the possible development of complications over time; many people manage these conditions well and live normal lives; patient compliance and provider involvement improve the long-term outlook
Prevention	Hepatitis A vaccine is available; consult the provider for vaccination guidelines Hepatitis E does not have a vaccine; pregnant women should restrict travel to hepatitis E–infected areas; hepatitis E can be **fulminant** in pregnant women, causing liver failure and death to the mother and fetus	Hepatitis B vaccine is available; consult the provider for vaccination guidelines Hepatitis C does not have a vaccine; avoid unprotected contact with infected individuals, their blood, body fluids, or personal items (razors and toothbrushes) Hepatitis D vaccine is not available, but anyone vaccinated to hepatitis B cannot acquire hepatitis D; consult the provider regarding hepatitis B vaccination guidelines
Can it become a chronic condition?	Both hepatitis A and E do not become chronic conditions	Hepatitis B, C, and D can become chronic conditions
Comments	Hepatitis E is **endemic** in areas of Africa, the Middle East, Asia, and Mexico; if pregnant, consult the provider for travel recommendations	Hepatitis D is only possible as a co-infection with hepatitis B; if a co-infection occurs, it can develop into a superinfection; a superinfection can cause liver failure and death; to prevent hepatitis D, vaccinate against hepatitis B

Information summarized from the Centers for Disease Control and Prevention; https://www.cdc.gov/hepatitis/index.htm.

VOCABULARY
endemic: Part of the normal pathogen makeup of a specific geographic area.
fulminant: A rapid and aggressive disease state. Can cause complications, organ failure, rapid health decline, and death in a short period of time.
percutaneous: Puncture through the skin.

Hiatal Hernia

A hiatal hernia is when the upper part of the stomach pushes up through the diaphragm. The diaphragm normally has a small opening (*hiatus*) where the esophagus passes through on its way to connect to the stomach. Sometimes the stomach will push up through the hiatus and cause a hiatal hernia. A small hiatal hernia does not usually cause issues, but

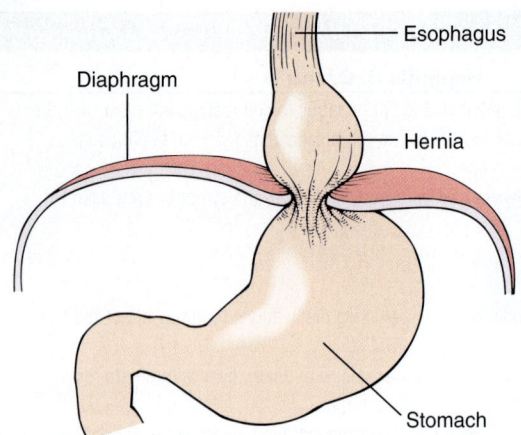

FIG. 5.19 Hiatal hernia. (From Frazier MS, Drzymkowski JW: *Essentials of Human Diseases and Conditions*, ed 4, Philadelphia, 2008, Saunders.)

larger ones can cause problems. With a larger hiatal hernia, food or stomach contents can move back into the esophagus, leading to heartburn, pain, and discomfort.

Etiology. A hiatal hernia happens when weakened muscle tissue lets the stomach move up through the opening in the diaphragm (Fig. 5.19). Causes of hiatal hernia are listed here:
- Repeated and intense pressure on the muscles surrounding the hiatus—for example, coughing, vomiting, straining during a bowel movement, or while lifting heavy objects
- More common in individuals who are over the age of 50 and/or obese
- Injury to the area diaphragm or abdomen
- Being born with an unusually large hiatus

Signs and Symptoms. Most small hiatal hernias go unnoticed and cause no signs or symptoms. Larger hiatal hernias can cause signs and symptoms that include the following:
- Heartburn, belching, and difficulty swallowing
- Chest or abdominal pain
- Feeling especially full after meals
- Vomiting blood or passing black stools, which may indicate gastrointestinal bleeding

Diagnostic Procedures. A hiatal hernia is often diagnosed during a procedure to determine the cause of heartburn, chest pain, or upper abdominal pain. Tests or procedures may include the following:
- Blood tests, possibly including CBC to check for anemia if blood loss was suspected
- Endoscopy, manometry, and x-rays (e.g., barium swallow)

Treatment. Most patients with a hiatal hernia are asymptomatic and will not need treatment. If symptoms are recurrent and include heartburn and acid reflux, treatment may include the following:
- Medications to neutralize stomach acid (antacids) or reduce acid production (proton pump inhibitors)
- Surgical repair in a small percentage of cases; usually only done in emergency cases or for people who are not helped by medications at all

Making the following lifestyle changes can also help to control signs and symptoms of hiatal hernia:
- Avoid eating large meals; instead eat smaller meals more frequently.
- Overweight or obese patients should try to lose weight. It is useful to stop smoking and to avoid alcoholic beverages.
- Avoid foods that may trigger heartburn. Examples include chocolate, onions, spicy foods, citrus fruits, and tomato-based foods.
- Eat the last meal of the day at least 2 to 3 hours before lying down or going to bed.
- Elevate the head of the bed 6 inches, if possible.

Prognosis. The prognosis is good for a hiatal hernia. Although, if surgery is involved, the prognosis is more difficult to predict.

Prevention. Prevention for hiatal hernia includes maintaining a good weight, not smoking, not drinking alcoholic beverages, avoiding trigger foods, and eating smaller, more frequent meals.

Pancreatitis

Pancreatitis is inflammation of the pancreas. The pancreas sits behind the stomach in the left upper quadrant of the abdomen. It is a flat, oblong gland that produces enzymes that aid digestion and hormones that control the way sugar (glucose) is processed in the body.

Pancreatitis can present as an acute condition, meaning it appears suddenly and only lasts for days. Or pancreatitis can present as a chronic condition, which means that it may occur for months or years. Mild cases of pancreatitis generally resolve without treatment, but severe cases can cause life-threatening complications.

Etiology. Pancreatitis occurs when digestive enzymes become activated while they are still in the pancreas. The activated enzymes irritate the cells of the pancreas and cause inflammation. If a person has repeated attacks of acute pancreatitis, the pancreas can become damaged, which may lead to chronic pancreatitis. Inflammation can cause the formation of scar tissue, which may lead to a loss of pancreatic function. An inefficient pancreas can cause digestion problems and diabetes.

Risk factors for developing pancreatitis include the following:
- Alcoholism, cigarette smoking, and certain medications
- Gallstones, injury to the abdomen, abdominal surgery, and infection
- Cystic fibrosis or pancreatic cancer
- High triglyceride or calcium levels in the blood
- Endoscopic retrograde cholangiopancreatography (ERCP), a procedure used to treat gallstones
- Family history of pancreatitis

Signs and Symptoms. Signs and symptoms of acute pancreatitis may include some or all of the following:
- Upper abdominal pain that may radiate to the back and feel worse after eating
- Fever, rapid pulse, nausea, or vomiting
- Abdomen that feels tender when palpated

Signs and symptoms of chronic pancreatitis may include the following:
- Upper abdominal pain
- Losing weight without trying
- Oily, smelly stools (*steatorrhea*)

Complications of pancreatitis may include the following:
- Formation of a *pseudocyst*, infection, internal bleeding
- Malnutrition, diabetes, and kidney failure
- Chemical changes in the body that affect lung function, causing oxygen levels to fall very low
- Chronic inflammation in the pancreas increases the risk of developing pancreatic cancer

> **VOCABULARY**
> **pseudocyst:** The formation of cystlike pockets in the pancreas that are filled with fluid and debris. Acute pancreatitis can lead to the formation of pseudocysts that can rupture, causing complications such as internal bleeding and infection.

Diagnostic Procedures. Tests and procedures used to diagnose pancreatitis include the following:
- Laboratory tests: blood tests to look for elevated levels of pancreatic enzymes, chemistry profile
- Imaging procedures:
  - CT scan and abdominal ultrasound to visualize gallstones
  - Ultrasound and MRI to look for inflammation and blockages in the pancreatic duct or bile duct and abnormalities in the gallbladder or pancreas

Treatment. Initial treatments (hospital) for acute pancreatitis may include the following:
- Fasting and intravenous (IV) fluids or nutrition to help the pancreas rest and heal
- Pain management with medication
- ERCP can be used as a diagnostic procedure and to make repairs to the bile and pancreatic ducts; may cause acute pancreatitis in some cases
- Surgery to remove the gallbladder (*cholecystectomy*)
- Surgery to drain fluid from the pancreas or remove diseased tissue
- Treatment for alcoholism

Additional treatments for chronic pancreatitis may include pain management, supplemental pancreatic enzymes to improve digestion, and a low-fat, high-nutrient eating plan.

Alternative therapies may be recommended to help patients cope with the pain of chronic pancreatitis. Alternative therapies may include the following:
- Meditation, yoga, and relaxation exercises
- Acupuncture therapy and deep-breathing exercises

Prognosis. The prognosis for pancreatitis can be good with proper patient compliance and a willingness to change one's diet and lifestyle if needed. Chronic pancreatitis that is not well controlled, and when the patient is not compliant, will have a varied outcome.

Prevention. If there is a history of pancreatitis or if a patient wants to avoid chronic pancreatitis, the following lifestyle changes can help:
- Stop drinking alcohol and stop smoking.
- Drink more fluids, especially water, throughout the day.
- Choose a low-fat diet, high-nutrient diet. Choose vegetables, fruits, whole grains, and lean proteins for meals. Limit processed foods, fats, and sweets to an occasional treat.

Ulcers: Peptic Ulcers

Peptic ulcers can develop in the stomach or upper portion of the small intestines. Peptic ulcers are open sores in the stomach or small intestines (Fig. 5.20). They appear when acid from the digestive tract eats away at the mucous lining of the stomach or small intestines. These sores can be very painful and may even bleed.

Peptic ulcers include gastric ulcers, which occur in the stomach, and duodenal ulcers, which occur in the first part of the small intestine (duodenum), closest to the stomach.

Etiology. The mucous layer of the digestive tract normally protects the tissues from the strong acids that are produced in the stomach.

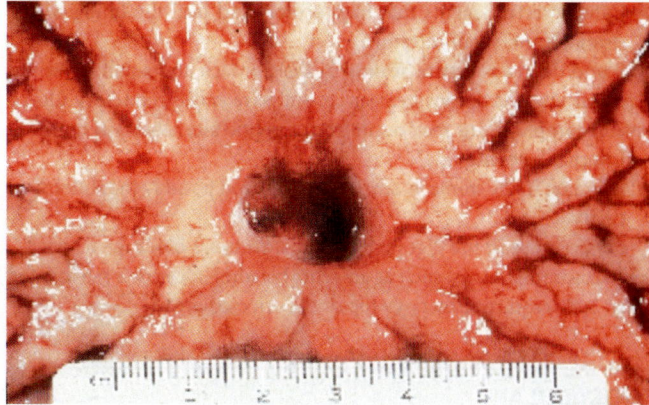

FIG. 5.20 Chronic peptic ulcer. (From Damjanov I: *Pathology: A Color Atlas*, St. Louis, 2000, Mosby.)

Mucous also protects the small intestines from acidic chyme that moves from the stomach to the small intestines. If the quantity of acid in the stomach increases, or the quantity of mucous decreases in the stomach and small intestines, an ulcer can develop. Common causes include the following:
- *Helicobacter pylori* (*H. pylori*) is a bacterium that lives in the mucous layer of the stomach and small intestine. Most of the time *H. pylori* does not cause problems, but sometimes it can cause inflammation that leads to an ulcer.
- Long-term use of NSAID pain relievers such as aspirin, ibuprofen, and naproxen sodium can lead to the formation of ulcers.
- Taking NSAIDs along with other medications such as steroids, anticoagulants, low-dose aspirin, and osteoporosis medications can significantly increase the chance of developing ulcers.
- Additional risk factors that prolong healing time of a peptic ulcer include smoking, drinking alcohol, eating spicy foods, and experiencing untreated emotional stress.

Signs and Symptoms. Signs and symptoms of peptic ulcers include the following:
- Burning stomach pain or heartburn
- Feeling of fullness, bloating, belching, or nausea
- Stomach pain that is most noticeable when the stomach is empty, in between meals, or at night
- Unexplained weight loss, change or loss of appetite, difficulty eating fatty foods

More severe signs and symptoms may include the following:
- Vomiting or vomiting blood, which may appear red or black
- Dark blood in stools, or stools that are black or tarry
- Trouble breathing, feeling faint

Diagnostic Procedures. Diagnostic procedures may include the following tests:
- Provider should conduct a history, physical, and vital signs
- Laboratory tests for *Helicobacter pylori*
- Biopsy of the stomach
- Imaging tests may include endoscopy, x-rays after a barium swallow

Treatment. Treatment for peptic ulcers depends on the cause of the ulcers. The following treatments may be used:
- Antibiotics, if *H. pylori* is found to be the causative agent
- Medications to neutralize stomach acid (antacids) or reduce acid production (proton pump inhibitors, histamine [H-2] blockers)

- Cytoprotective agents that help protect and heal the lining of the stomach and small intestine
- Bland diet to promote healing of the stomach and small intestines

Peptic ulcers that do not heal successfully are called refractory ulcers. Several complications may result from a peptic ulcer that will not heal:
- Internal bleeding
- Infection in the stomach, small intestines, and possibly the abdominal cavity
- Obstruction in the digestive tract that causes a blockage

Serious complications, such as an acute bleeding ulcer or a **perforated ulcer**, may require surgery to repair the affected area.

> **VOCABULARY**
>
> **perforated ulcer:** A condition in which an untreated ulcer can damage the wall of the stomach or small intestine, creating a hole that allows digestive juices and food to leak into the abdominal cavity. Treatment generally requires immediate surgery.

Prognosis. If the treatments are followed, the prognosis for a peptic ulcer is generally good. Patients with refractory ulcers will have a varied prognosis.

Prevention. To help prevent a peptic ulcer or to prevent a reoccurrence, the following recommendations are helpful:
- Choose a diet rich in vegetables, fruits, lean protein, and fiber. Avoid processed foods.
- Avoid or limit dairy products, which can cause excess acid in the stomach.
- Eat probiotic-containing foods such as yogurt, aged cheeses, and miso.
- Control stress. Stress can increase the production of stomach acids. Learn to manage stress through positive activities such as exercise, getting enough sleep, hobbies, spending time with friends, being outdoors, or writing/journaling.
- Do not smoke, and avoid or at least limit alcoholic beverages.
- Use pain-relieving medications with caution and only when necessary.

ADDITIONAL DISEASES AND DISORDERS OF THE DIGESTIVE SYSTEM

There are many diseases and disorders of the digestive system that cannot be presented in detail within this chapter. Tables 5.7 through 5.13 briefly describe additional diseases and disorders of the digestive system.

TABLE 5.7 Terms Related to Congenital Disorders of the Digestive System

Term	Definition
Cleft palate (kleft PAL it)	Failure of the palate to close during embryonic development, creating an opening in the roof of the mouth; cleft palate often is accompanied by a cleft lip (Fig. 5.21)
Esophageal atresia (eh soff uh JEE ul ah TREE zsa)	Esophagus that ends in a blind pouch and therefore lacks an opening into the stomach (Fig. 5.22)
Hirschsprung disease (HERSH sprung)	Congenital absence of normal nervous function in part of the colon, which results in an absence of peristaltic movement, accumulation of feces, and an enlarged colon; also called *congenital megacolon*
Pyloric stenosis (pye LORE ick sten OH sis)	Condition in which the muscle between the stomach and the small intestine narrows or fails to open adequately to allow partially digested food into the duodenum

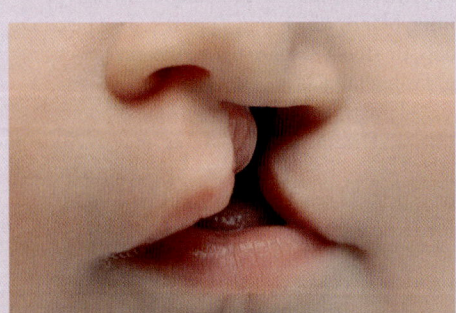

Fig. 5.21 Cleft palate. (Courtesy Maos/iStock/Thinkstock.)

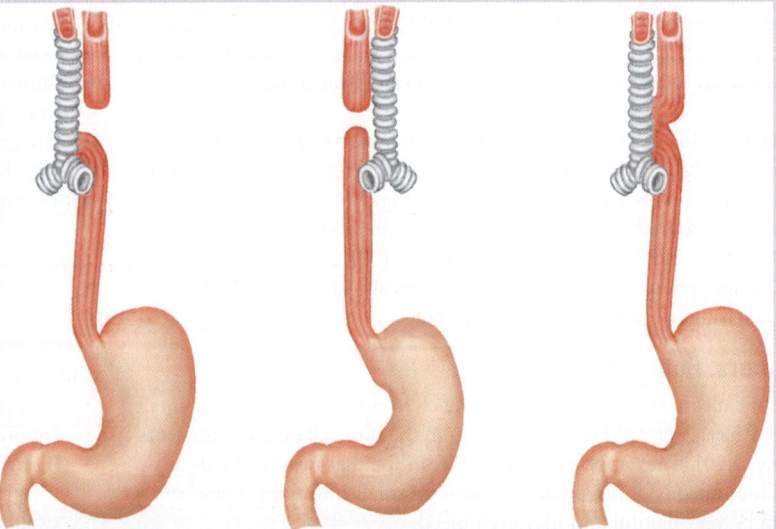

Fig. 5.22 Esophageal atresia. (From Shiland B: *Mastering Healthcare Terminology*, ed 5, St. Louis, 2016, Elsevier.)

From Shiland B: *Mastering Healthcare Terminology*, ed 5, St. Louis, 2016, Elsevier.

TABLE 5.8 Terms Related to Oral Cavity Disorders

Term	Definition
Dental caries (KARE ees)	Plaque disease caused by an interaction between food and bacteria in the mouth, leading to tooth decay; also called cavities
Gingivitis (jin jih VYE tis)	Inflammatory disease of the gums characterized by redness, swelling, and bleeding
Herpetic stomatitis (hur PET ick stoh mah TYE tis)	Inflammation of the mouth caused by the herpes simplex virus (HSV); also known as a *cold sore* or *fever blister*
Leukoplakia (loo koh PLAY kee ah)	Condition of white patches that may appear on the lips, tongue, and buccal mucosa (Fig. 5.23); usually associated with tobacco use and may be precancerous
Periodontal disease (pair ee oh DON tul)	Pathologic condition of the tissues surrounding the teeth
Pyorrhea (pye or REE yah)	Purulent discharge from the tissue surrounding the teeth; often seen with gingivitis

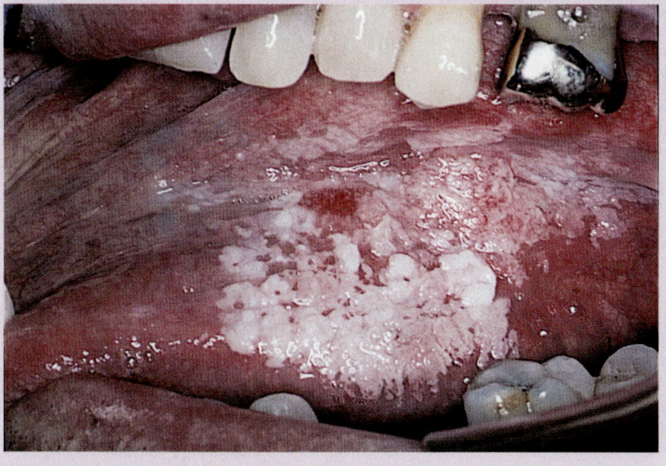

Fig. 5.23 Leukoplakia. (From Eisen D, Lynch DP: *The Mouth: Diagnosis and Treatment*, St. Louis, 1998, Mosby.)

From Shiland B: *Mastering Healthcare Terminology*, ed 5, St. Louis, 2016, Elsevier.

TABLE 5.9 Terms Related to Disorders of the Esophagus, Stomach, and Intestines

Term	Definition
Achalasia ack uh LAY zsa	Impairment of esophageal peristalsis along with the lower esophageal sphincter's inability to relax; also called cardiospasm, esophageal *aperistalsis* (a per rih STALL sis), and megaesophagus
Anal fissure (A null FISH ur)	Cracklike lesion of the skin around the anus
Anorectal abscess (an oh RECK tul AB sess)	Circumscribed area of inflammation in the anus or rectum, containing pus
Colitis (koh LYE tis)	Inflammation of the large intestine
Gastritis (gass TRY tis)	Acute or chronic inflammation of the stomach that may be accompanied by anorexia, nausea and vomiting, or indigestion
Ileus (ILL ee us)	Obstruction; paralytic ileus is lack of peristaltic movement in the intestinal tract; also called adynamic ileus
Inflammatory bowel disease (IBD)	Chronic inflammation of the lining of the intestine characterized by bleeding and diarrhea
Intussusception (in tuh suh SEP shun)	Inward telescoping of the intestines
Irritable bowel syndrome (IBS)	Diarrhea, gas, or constipation resulting from stress with no underlying disease
Mucositis (myoo koh SYE tis)	Inflammation of the mucous membranes; GI mucositis may be an adverse effect of chemotherapy and can occur throughout the GI tract
Peritonitis (pair ih tuh NYE tis)	Inflammation of the peritoneum that most commonly occurs when an inflamed appendix ruptures
Proctitis (prock TYE tis)	Inflammation of the rectum and anus; also called rectitis
Ulcerative colitis (UL sur uh tiv koh LYE tis)	Chronic inflammation of the colon and rectum manifesting with bouts of profuse watery diarrhea; a form of IBD
Volvulus (VAWL vyoo lus)	Twisting of the intestine

From Shiland B: *Mastering Healthcare Terminology*, ed 5, St. Louis, 2016, Elsevier.

TABLE 5.10 Terms Related to Digestive System Accessory Organ Disorders

Term	Definition
Cholangitis (koh lan JYE tis)	Inflammation of the bile vessels
Cholecystitis (koh lee sis TYE tis)	Inflammation of the gallbladder, either acute or chronic; may be caused by cholelithiasis
Cirrhosis (sur OH sis)	Chronic degenerative disease of the liver, commonly associated with alcohol abuse, chronic liver disease, and biliary tract disorders (Fig. 5.24)
Jaundice (JAHN diss)	Yellowing of the skin and sclerae (whites of the eyes) caused by elevated levels of bilirubin; also called icterus

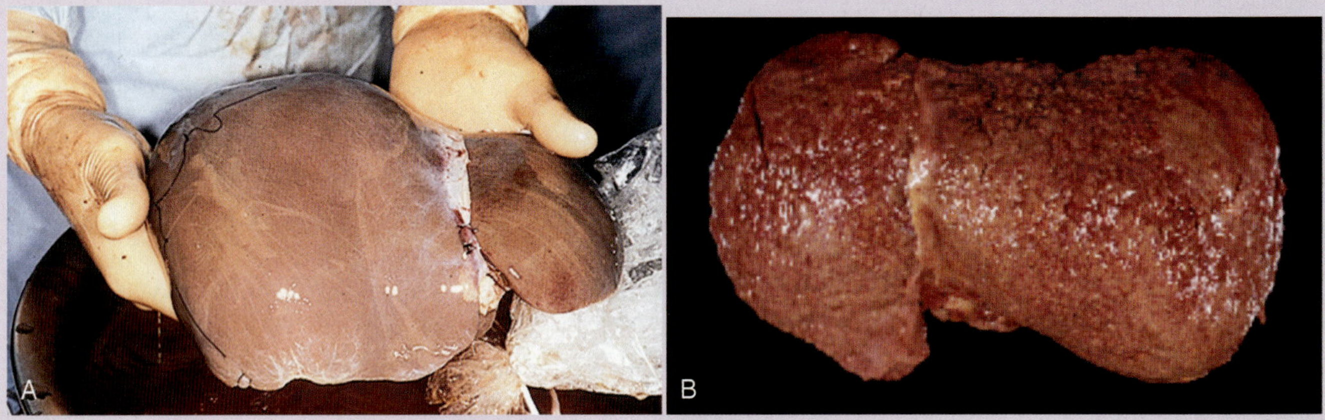

Fig. 5.24 (A) Normal liver. (B) Cirrhosis of the liver. (A, from Mahan LK, Escott-Stump S: *Krause's Food and Nutrition Therapy*, ed 12, Philadelphia, 2008, Saunders/Elsevier. B, from Damjanov I: *Pathology: A Color Atlas*, St. Louis, 2000, Mosby.)

From Shiland B: *Mastering Healthcare Terminology*, ed 5, St. Louis, 2016, Elsevier.

TABLE 5.11 Terms Related to Hernias

Term	Definition
Femoral hernia (FEM uh rull HER nee ah)	Protrusion of a loop of intestine through the femoral canal into the groin; also called a crural hernia
Incarcerated hernia (in KAR sih ray tid HER nee ah)	Loop of bowel with ends occluded (blocked) so that solids cannot pass, and the herniated bowel can become strangulated; also called an irreducible hernia
Inguinal hernia (IN gwin null HER nee ah)	Protrusion of a loop of intestine into the inguinal canal; may be indirect (through a normal internal passage) or direct (through a muscle wall)
Strangulation	Constriction of a tubular structure, including intestines, leading to lack of circulation and resulting very poor blood supply (ischemia) and possible tissue death
Umbilical hernia (um BILL ih kull HER nee ah)	Protrusion of the intestine and omentum through a weakness in the abdominal wall; also known as an *omphalocele* (AHM fah loh seel)

From Shiland B: *Mastering Healthcare Terminology*, ed 5, St. Louis, 2016, Elsevier.

TABLE 5.12 Terms Related to Benign Neoplasms of the Digestive System

Term	Definition
Cystadenoma (sist ad en OH mah)	Glandular tumors that are filled with cysts; these are the most common benign tumors in the pancreas
Leiomyoma (lye oh mye OH mah)	Smooth muscle tumor that may occur in the digestive tract
Odontogenic tumor (oh don toh JEN ick)	Benign tumors that arise around the teeth and jaw
Polyps, adenomatous or hyperplastic (POLL ups ad eh noh MAH tuss hye per PLASS tick)	Adenomatous (growths that arise from glandular tissue and have potential to become malignant) or hyperplastic tumors (generally, small growths that have no tendency to become malignant) occurring throughout the digestive tract

From Shiland B: *Mastering Healthcare Terminology*, ed 5, St. Louis, 2016, Elsevier.

TABLE 5.13 Terms Related to Malignant Neoplasms of the Digestive System

Term	Definition
Adenocarcinoma (ad en noh kar seh NOH mah)	A malignant tumor of epithelial origin that either originates from glandular tissue or has a glandular appearance; adenocarcinomas occur throughout the GI tract, but especially in the esophagus, stomach, pancreas, and colon
Hepatocellular carcinoma/ hepatoma (heh pat oh SELL you lur kar seh NOH mah heh puh TOH mah)	Malignant tumors of epithelial origin that originate in the liver cells; hepatocellular carcinoma (also called hepatoma) is the most common type of primary liver cancer worldwide

From Shiland B: *Mastering Healthcare Terminology*, ed 5, St. Louis, 2016, Elsevier.

LIFESPAN CHANGES

In children, digestive system congenital disorders are cleft palate, esophageal atresia, Hirschsprung disease, and pyloric stenosis. Although none of these are common, they do require medical intervention. Infants can develop GERD, which can lead to weight loss and nutritional issues. Gastroenteritis and appendicitis—with their possible complications, respectively, of dehydration and peritonitis—are the most common reasons for hospital admissions of children.

An aging digestive system is more likely to develop new dysfunctional cell growths (both benign and malignant), so statistics for polyps and colorectal cancer are high for the senior age group. Other diagnoses that appear more often are GERD and dysphagia, hemorrhoids, gallstones, and diverticulitis.

CLOSING COMMENTS

When working in an ambulatory care setting, assisting patients with digestive system diseases and disorders is common. It is important for the medical assistant to understand the anatomy and function of the digestive system. The digestive system has functions that allow the body to break down food so that nutrients, vitamins, and minerals can be absorbed and used throughout the body. Gastroenterology is the specialty that focuses on the digestive system, but medical assistants working in urgent care and primary care (e.g., pediatrics, internal medicine, and family practice) will see many digestive system–related diseases and disorders too. Medical terminology related to the digestive system will be invaluable in your career. Knowing word parts, definitions, and common abbreviations is vital when working with patients and providers (Tables 5.14 through 5.17). The medical assistant should also know about the etiology, signs and symptoms, diagnostic procedures, treatments, prognoses, and prevention of common digestive system diseases, disorders, and traumas.

TABLE 5.14 Combining and Adjective Forms for the Digestive System

Meaning	Combining Form	Adjective Form	Meaning	Combining Form	Adjective Form
abdomen	abdomin/o, celi/o, lapar/o	abdominal, celiac	lips	cheil/o, labi/o	labial
accessory	adnex/o	adnexal	liver	hepat/o	hepatic
anus	an/o	anal	lobe	lob/o	lobular
appendix	appendic/o, append/o	appendicular	lower jaw	mandibul/o	mandibular
bile	chol/e, bil/i	biliary	lumen	lumin/o	luminal
bile vessel	cholangi/o		mouth, oral cavity	or/o, stom/o, stomat/o	oral, stomal, stomatic
bolus	bol/o		nose	nas/o, rhin/o	nasal
cecum	cec/o	cecal	nutrition	aliment/o	alimentary
cheek	bucc/o	buccal	palate	palat/o	palatine
cholesterol	cholesterol/o		pancreas	pancreat/o	pancreatic
common bile duct	choledoch/o	choledochal	pharynx, throat	pharyng/o	pharyngeal
corporis, body	corpor/o	corporeal	pylorus	pylor/o	pyloric
duodenum	duoden/o	duodenal	rectum	rect/o	rectal
epiglottis	epiglott/o	epiglottal	rectum and anus	proct/o	
esophagus	esophag/o	esophageal	rugae	rug/o	rugous
fat, lipid	lip/o, lipid/o	lipid	saliva	sial/o	salivary
feces	fec/a	fecal	salivary gland	sialaden/o	
fold, plica	plic/o	plical	sigmoid colon	sigmoid/o	sigmoidal
fundus	fund/o	fundal	small intestine	enter/o	enteral
gallbladder	cholecyst/o	cholecystic	starch	amyl/o	
glucose, sugar	gluc/o		stomach	gastr/o	gastric
gums	gingiv/o	gingival	teeth	dent/i, odont/o	dental
ileum	ile/o	ileal	tongue	gloss/o, lingu/o	glossal, lingual
intestines	intestin/o	intestinal	upper jaw	maxill/o	maxillary
jejunum	jejun/o	jejunal	uvula	uvul/o	uvular
large intestine, colon	col/o, colon/o	colonic	villus	vill/o	villous

From Shiland B: *Mastering Healthcare Terminology*, ed 5, St. Louis, 2016, Elsevier.

TABLE 5.15 Prefixes for the Digestive System

Prefix	Meaning
endo-	within
exo-	outside
hypo-	below
par-	near
peri-	surrounding
sub-	under

From Shiland B: *Mastering Healthcare Terminology*, ed 5, St. Louis, 2016, Elsevier.

TABLE 5.16 Suffixes for the Digestive System

Suffix	Meaning
-al, -ar, -eal, -ic, -id, -ine, -ous	pertaining to
-crine	to secrete
-kinin	movement substance
-stalsis	contraction

From Shiland B: *Mastering Healthcare Terminology*, ed 5, St. Louis, 2016, Elsevier.

TABLE 5.17 Abbreviations for the Digestive System

Abbreviation	Definition
BaS	barium swallow
BE	barium enema
BM	bowel movement
CT scan	computed tomography scan
EGD	esophagogastroduodenoscopy
ERCP	endoscopic retrograde cholangiopancreatography
GB	gallbladder
GERD	gastroesophageal reflux disease
GGT	gamma-glutamyl transferase
GI	gastrointestinal
HAV	hepatitis A virus
HBV	hepatitis B virus
IBD	inflammatory bowel disease
IBS	irritable bowel syndrome
Lap	laparoscopy, laparotomy
LES	lower esophageal sphincter
N&V	nausea and vomiting
PEG	percutaneous endoscopic gastrostomy
PTC	percutaneous transhepatic cholangiography
PUD	peptic ulcer disease

From Shiland B: *Mastering Healthcare Terminology*, ed 5, St. Louis, 2016, Elsevier.

CHAPTER REVIEW

The digestive system is divided into two types of organs: the primary organs and the accessory organs. The functions of the digestive system are mechanical digestion, chemical digestion, nutrient absorption, and excretion.

The digestive system starts the process of mechanical digestion in the mouth. This process breaks down food into smaller pieces as it passes from the mouth, into the throat, and down the esophagus into the stomach. In the stomach, mechanical digestion continues to happen, turning food into smaller and smaller particles until a slurry called chyme is formed. Chyme is a mixture of food and gastric juices that has the consistency of a smoothie. Once acidic chyme is well mixed, it moves into the small intestines, where most of the chemical digestion takes place. In the small intestine, bile and pancreatic enzymes are added to chyme to continue the process of chemical digestion until food is broken down into small, absorbable molecules. In the small intestines, nutrients are absorbed through villi and then pass into the blood capillaries and are distributed throughout the body. By the time chyme has reached the end of the small intestine, all the nutrients have been absorbed. All that remains is indigestible material and water. The remains of digestion move onto the large intestine where water and electrolytes are reabsorbed. The remaining indigestible waste is called feces. Feces pass from the large intestine to the rectum and then out of the body through the anus.

CRITICAL THINKING 5.10

Describe the difference between mechanical digestion and chemical digestion. Why is each process important?

Many digestive system diseases and disorders were presented in the chapter. Common signs and symptoms of digestive issues include abdominal pain, nausea, vomiting, diarrhea, constipation, bloating, fatigue, heartburn, and difficulty swallowing. Common etiology includes infection, autoimmune conditions, anatomic changes, and malignancies. Typical diagnostics include physical exam and history, biopsy, imaging procedures, and laboratory testing. CLIA-waived tests include urinalysis, urine hCG pregnancy testing, fecal occult blood testing, and some *Helicobacter pylori* testing kits.

The digestive system changes with age. Infants and children are most at risk for infections and anatomic abnormalities. Older adults are at risk for infections, reflux diseases and disorders, and malignancies throughout the digestive system.

SCENARIO WRAP-UP

After Al finishes his appointment with Dr. Martin, Samuel comes back into the exam room. Dr. Martin has given Samuel some literature for Al and asks him to go over the changes in diet that Dr. Martin and Al had discussed. It seems that Al's change in activity level with his new job, long hours sitting at work, and low-fiber sweets at the office (Tuesday and Thursday are donut days) have caused some problems for his digestive system.

Al's colonoscopy was normal, and his blood work was normal, but his digestive issues needed to be addressed. Dr. Martin has recommended a diet high in fruits, vegetables, lean protein, and plenty of water throughout the day. He has also suggested that Al take a short walk during lunch and after work if possible. Samuel goes over the literature that Dr. Martin provided and reminds Al to keep a journal of what he eats and how many minutes he walks each day for the next month. Dr. Martin will see Al in a month, and hopefully he will be able to report better digestive health.

Samuel is glad to see that Al can make positive lifestyle changes to improve his health. He feels good about being part of the WMFM healthcare team. So far, his first day as a medical assistant is going well.

6

Urinary System

LEARNING OBJECTIVES

1. Discuss the anatomy of the urinary system, which will include listing the major organs of the urinary system and identifying the anatomic location of major urinary system organs.
2. Describe the physiology and normal functions of the urinary system.
3. List common diseases and disorders of the urinary system, and discuss the following:
   - Identify the common etiology of each urinary disease.
   - Identify the common signs and symptoms of each urinary disease.
   - Describe diagnostic measures used for each urinary disease.
   - Identify CLIA-waived tests associated with urinary diseases.
   - Describe treatment modalities used for each urinary disease.
   - Discuss the prognosis and prevention of each urinary disease.
4. Compare the structure and function of the urinary system across the life span.

CHAPTER OUTLINE

1. Opening Scenario, 122
2. You Will Learn, 122
3. Anatomy of the Urinary System, 123
   a. Kidneys, 123
   b. Ureters, 125
   c. Bladder, 125
   d. Urethra, 125
4. Physiology of the Urinary System, 126
   a. Filtration, 126
   b. Reabsorption, 126
   c. Secretion, 128
   d. Renin and Blood Pressure, 128
   e. Erythropoietin, 128
   f. Vitamin D, 128
5. Diseases and Disorders of the Urinary System, 128
   a. Bladder Cancer, 128
   b. Cystitis, Acute, 130
   c. End-Stage Renal Disease, 131
   d. Glomerulonephritis, 133
   e. Kidney Cancer, 133
   f. Nephrotic Syndrome, 135
   g. Neurogenic Bladder, 135
   h. Polycystic Kidney Disease, 136
   i. Prostate Cancer, 137
   j. Pyelonephritis, 138
   k. Renal Calculi, 139
   l. Urinary Incontinence, 140
   m. Additional Urinary System Diseases, 141
6. Life Span Changes, 141
7. Closing Comments, 143
8. Chapter Review, 144
9. Scenario Wrap-Up, 144

OPENING SCENARIO

Hannah Yang, CMA (AAMA), was hired 4 months ago as a certified medical assistant. She assists the specialists who hold outreach clinics at Walden-Martin Family Medical (WMFM) Clinic. She has been training with the urology staff that comes for the outreach clinics four times a month.

Hannah's role with the urology staff is to help room patients and assist the staff. To prepare for working with the specialist, Hannah spent some time reviewing her medical assistant textbook. She had forgotten the process of urine formation. She had to brush up on the way the urinary system impacts the homeostasis of the body. Hannah knows that the urinary system is important and that if a person's kidneys are not functioning, he or she will need to go on dialysis. As part of her orientation to this specialty, she was able to spend 4 hours at the local dialysis clinic. There, the "regular" patients enjoyed telling her their experiences. Their experiences and the information from the dialysis technicians helped Hannah understand what patients go through with kidney disease.

When she assists the urologist, Dr. Ubert Riney, and his team, Hannah learns a great deal. She knows she has more to learn with this specialty.

YOU WILL LEARN

1. To recognize and use terms related to the urinary system.
2. To locate the urinary system structures.

CHAPTER 6 Urinary System

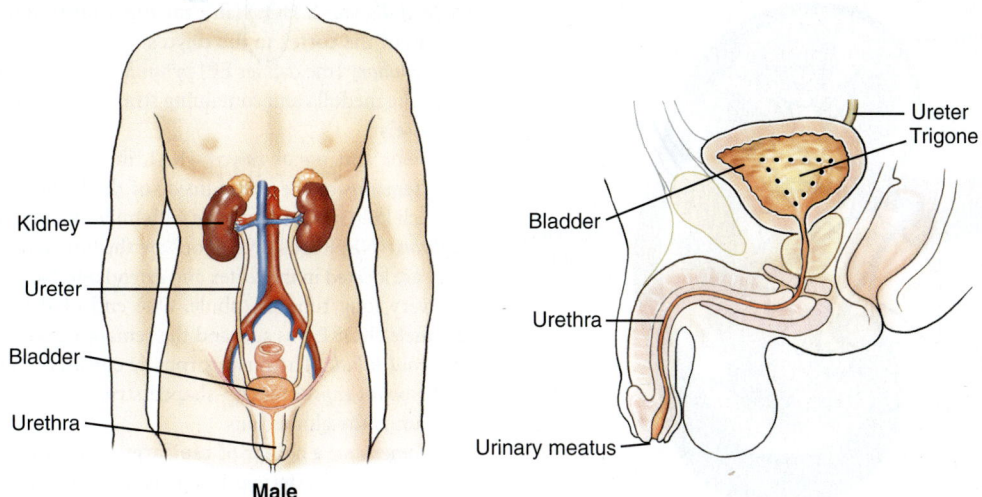

FIG. 6.1 Male urinary system. (From Shiland B: *Mastering Healthcare Terminology*, ed 5, St. Louis, 2016, Elsevier.)

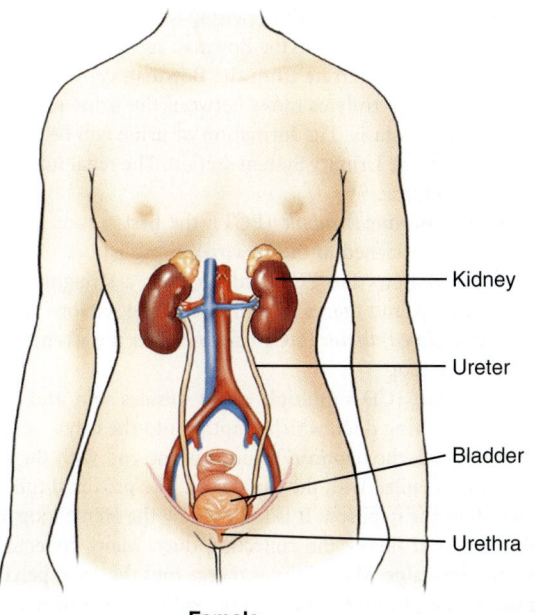

FIG. 6.2 Female urinary system. (From Shiland B: *Mastering Healthcare Terminology*, ed 5, St. Louis, 2016, Elsevier.)

3. To understand and describe the process required to make urine.
4. To recognize disease states of the urinary system, including their etiology, signs and symptoms, diagnostic procedures, treatment, prognosis, and prevention.

ANATOMY OF THE URINARY SYSTEM

The urinary system is composed of two kidneys, two ureters, a urinary bladder, and a urethra (Figs. 6.1 and 6.2). The kidneys filter the blood and eliminate waste through the passage of urine. The ureters (YOOR eh turs) move urine from the kidneys to the bladder. The urinary bladder stores the urine until it is excreted. The urethra (yoo REE thrah) is the tube that conducts the urine out of the bladder (Box 6.1).

> **BOX 6.1   Specialty and Specialist**
>
> Urology (yoo ROL ah jee) is the healthcare specialty that deals with most urinary disorders. A urologist (yoo ROL ah jist) is a specialist involved in the diagnosis, treatment, and prevention of disorders of the urinary system.

Kidneys

The kidneys are bean-shaped organs with an indentation, called the *hilum* (HYE lum). The hilum is the location on the kidney where the ureter and renal vein leave the kidney and the renal artery (AR tur ree) enters. The kidneys are about the size of a fist and are located posterior to the **peritoneum** (PER i tn ee hum) and against the muscles of the back. They are roughly between the T12 and L3 vertebrae. The left kidney is situated about 1 inch (2 cm) higher than the right because of the location of the liver.

> **VOCABULARY**
> **peritoneum**: A serous membrane lining of the abdominal cavity, which folds inward to enclose the viscera (internal organs).

The kidneys remove unwanted substances from the blood and form urine for excretion. Blood is delivered to the two kidneys by the renal arteries, which branch off of the abdominal aorta (Fig. 6.3). Blood flows from the renal arteries into **afferent** (AF fur ent) **arterioles** (ar TEER ee olez) (smaller arteries) and then through a network of capillaries (CAP ih lair eez) called the *glomeruli* (gloh MER yoo lie). Filtration of the blood occurs in the glomerulus (gloh MER yoo lus). Blood from the glomerulus moves into the **efferent** (EF fur ent) arterioles and then into the **peritubular** (PER i too bu lar) **capillaries**. As the blood leaves the kidneys, it moved from the peritubular capillaries to **venules** (VEN yuhls) and then empties into the renal veins. The renal veins take the blood out of the kidneys. Blood from the renal veins flows into the inferior vena cava as it heads to the heart to become oxygenated again (Fig. 6.4).

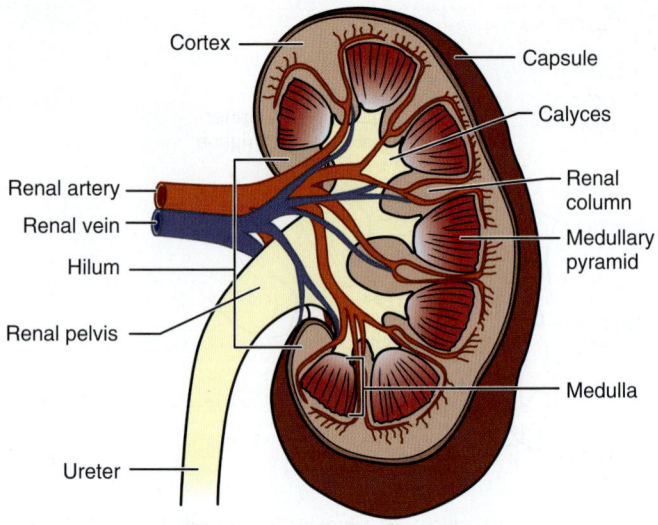

FIG. 6.3 Cross section of a kidney.

- *Medulla* (muh DOO lah): the inner portion that extends from the end of the cortex to the calyces
- *Medullary* (me dah ler EE) *pyramid*: a cone-shaped structure located in the medulla and containing straight tubular structures and blood vessels
- *Minor* and *major calyces* (KAL ih seez) and the renal pelvis are extensions of the ureter inside of the kidney

Each kidney contains tissue with millions of microscopic units called *nephrons* (NEFF rons). Nephrons are the functional units of the kidneys. They are located in the cortex and extend into the medulla. Each nephron is a very long tube or tubule. One end of the nephron is the *renal corpuscle* (KORE pus sul) and the remaining section of the nephron is the *renal tubule*. The renal corpuscle consists of the following:

- *Bowman capsule*: a cup-shaped structure of the nephron that surrounds the glomerulus
- *Glomerulus*: a cluster of capillaries inside of the Bowman capsule

The afferent arteriole brings blood into the glomerulus, and the efferent arteriole takes blood away from the glomerulus. The diameter of the afferent arteriole is much larger than the diameter of the efferent arteriole. The importance of the narrowed diameter will be discussed in the Physiology of the Urinary System section of this chapter.

The renal tubule is a long, thin, twisted tube that brings the **filtrate** (which will become urine) from the Bowman capsule to the renal pelvis. During the passage of filtrate from the Bowman capsule to the renal pelvis, water and electrolytes move between the urine and the blood to maintain homeostasis. The formation of urine will be discussed in the Physiology of the Urinary System section. The renal tubule is made up of the following:

- *Proximal* (*convoluted*) *tubule* (PCT): the first section of the renal tubule that is attached to the Bowman capsule
- *Henle loop*: follows the PCT and includes a straight descending section, a loop, and then a straight ascending section
- *Distal* (*convoluted*) *tubule* (DCT): follows after the ascending section of the Henle loop
- *Collecting duct* (CD): multiple distal tubules join and form this straight collecting duct, which empties into the calyx

To summarize, the nephron begins on one end with the Bowman capsule, which is filled with the capillaries. The proximal tubule is the next section of the nephron. It is followed by the Henle loop, then the distal tubule, and finally the collecting duct. Many collecting ducts empty into one calyx. Many calyces merge into the renal pelvis, which is an extension of the ureter inside of the kidney. The Bowman capsule, proximal tubules, and distal tubes are in the cortex. The Henle loop and the collecting ducts are in the medulla of the kidney.

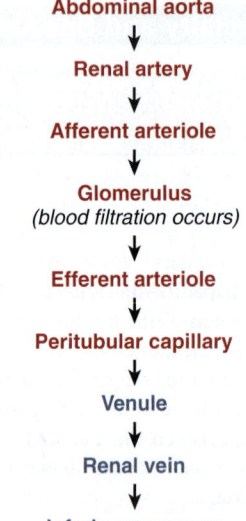

FIG. 6.4 Blood flow to and from the kidney.

If a kidney were sliced open, you would see the following:
- *Capsule*: the fibrous outer covering of the kidney
- *Cortex* (KORE tecks): the outer portion of the kidney
- *Renal column*: extensions of the cortex that dip down between the medullary pyramids

VOCABULARY
afferent: Pertaining to carrying toward a structure.
arterioles: Small arteries.
efferent: Pertaining to carrying away from a structure.
filtrate: Fluid and substances that are filtered out of the blood in the Bowman capsule.
peritubular capillaries: Blood capillaries surrounding the proximal and distal convoluted tubules in the kidneys.
venules: Very small veins.

MEDICAL TERMINOLOGY
af-: toward
calic/o, cali/o, calyc/o: calyx
calyx (singular), **calyces** (plural)
cortex (singular), **cortices** (plural)
cortic/o: cortex
ef-: away from
-ent: pertaining to
fer/o: to carry
glomerul/o: glomerulus
glomerulus (singular), **glomeruli** (plural)
hil/o: hilum
medull/o: medulla
medulla (singular), **medullae** (plural)
peri-: surrounding
pyel/o: pelvis
-ule: small
ven/o: vein

> **CRITICAL THINKING 6.1**
> Hannah is working with Mrs. Green, a urology patient. Mrs. Green has kidney disease and asks Hannah what the kidneys do. How should Hannah explain the role of the kidneys to Mrs. Green?

> **MEDICAL TERMINOLOGY**
> **cysto/o, vesic/o**: bladder
> **trigon/o**: trigone
> **ureter/o**: ureter

Ureters

The bilateral ureters are thin, muscular tubes approximately 10 inches long. The tube's muscular layer creates peristaltic waves that help move the urine to the bladder. The ureters' walls are made of **transitional epithelium**, which allows the ureters to stretch to accommodate urine flow. Many nerve endings are also in the walls. A stone in the ureter can cause severe pain.

The point where the ureter enters the bladder is called the *ureterovesical* (you REE ter oh ves i kal) *junction*. The ureters enter the bladder at an angle. This creates a flap over the end of the ureter. The flap serves as a valve. Urine can empty into the bladder, but it cannot back up from the bladder and reenter the ureter. This mechanism also prevents bacteria from moving from the bladder up to the kidneys.

> **VOCABULARY**
> **residual urine**: Urine that remains in the bladder after micturition or urination.
> **rugae**: Folds in the wall of the organ; when the organ (e.g., stomach, bladder, uterus) fills or needs to expand, the rugae unfold.
> **stretch receptor**: A sensory nerve ending that responds to a stretch stimulus.
> **transitional epithelium**: A type of cell found in the lining of hollow organs; it has the ability to stretch with the contraction and distention of the organ.

> **STUDY TIP**
> The body has two ureters, and there are two "e"s in the word "ureter." The body has one urethra, and only one "e" is in "urethra."

Urethra

The urethra (yoo REE thrah) is a mucous membrane–lined tube that drains urine out of the bladder. In males, the internal urethral sphincter (SFINK tur) is located at the bladder end (or proximal end) of the urethra. The sphincter is made of smooth involuntary muscles. The external sphincter is located in different places in males and in females (Table 6.1). The external sphincter is made of skeletal muscles and is a voluntary muscle. A voluntary muscle provides you the ability to control when you urinate. The distal end of the urethra is called the *urinary meatus* (mee ATE us). The urinary meatus is the final point before the urine leaves the body.

The *prostate* is a walnut-sized gland found below the bladder in males. It surrounds part of the urethra. This gland produces fluid for semen. The prostate is considered a reproductive organ, but it also impacts the urinary system. As men get older, the prostate grows. This condition is known as benign prostatic hyperplasia (BPH). When the prostate increases in size, it can obstruct the urethra, blocking the urine flow.

Bladder

The urinary bladder is a hollow organ in the pelvic cavity. It serves as a holding tank for urine. Urine enters the bladder through the ureters and leaves the bladder through the urethra. The triangular area in the bladder between the ureters' entrance and the urethral outlet is called the *trigone* (TRY gohn).

Transitional epithelium creates the inner lining of the bladder. When the bladder is empty, it flattens and the walls overlap in folds, also known as **rugae** (ROO gee). This creates a wrinkled appearance. As the bladder starts to fill with urine, the rugae and transitional epithelium allow for greater bladder volume. Think of a balloon that was blown up and then emptied of air. The balloon is smaller and wrinkly in appearance. When inflated, the wrinkles are gone and it can accommodate a large volume of air. The same thing happens with the bladder and urine.

The bladder is also composed of smooth muscle fibers that make up the *detrusor* (de TROO ser) muscle. The detrusor muscle relaxes when the bladder fills. It contracts to push urine out of the bladder and into the urethra. Normally, the bladder holds about 1.5 to 2 cups (360–480 mL) of urine during the day and doubles that amount at night. As the bladder fills to about 150 mL, **stretch receptors** in the detrusor send a message to the central nervous system. As more urine enters the bladder, the urge to urinate increases. After urination or *micturition*, **residual urine** remains (usually less than 50 mL) in the bladder.

TABLE 6.1 Difference in the Urethra Between the Genders

	Female	Male
Length	1–1.5 inches	8 inches
Function	Urination	Urination and ejaculation
Location of Internal Sphincter	None	At the proximal end (bladder end) of the urethra, may prevent semen from moving into the bladder
Location of External Sphincter	Extends up to the bladder, encircles the vagina and urethra	Under the prostate gland

> **CRITICAL THINKING 6.2**
>
> Hannah is working with Mr. Endl, who has prostate cancer. He asks Hannah why the prostate cancer impacts his urine flow. How should Hannah respond to Mr. Endl?

> **MEDICAL TERMINOLOGY**
> **meat/o**: meatus
> **urethr/o**: urethra

> **CRITICAL THINKING 6.3**
>
> Hannah is working with Katrina, the urology medical assistant. Hannah asks Katrina what the major differences were between male and female urinary systems. How would Katrina respond to Hannah's question?

PHYSIOLOGY OF THE URINARY SYSTEM

The urinary system has several important roles that help regulate homeostasis in the body:

- Maintains fluid volume. The urinary system increases fluid loss in urine when fluid volume is high. It decreases the fluid loss when the fluid volume is low (e.g., with dehydration).
- Maintains the normal composition of body fluids. The urinary system can increase or decrease the loss of certain electrolytes in the urine as it regulates the normal makeup of the body fluids. This helps to keep the pH of the blood within normal limits.
- Maintains an adequate blood pressure. Renin, an enzyme, is secreted in the urinary system and is involved with increasing the blood pressure.
- Controls the red blood cell production. **Erythropoietin** (eh rith roh POY ee tin) is secreted by the urinary system, which is involved with red blood cell production.
- Activates vitamin D. The kidneys are involved with the final step of vitamin D activation. Vitamin D is important in the absorption of calcium and phosphorus.

Many of these roles are performed during the formation of urine. The body rids itself of unneeded substances produced during the metabolic process. The process of urine formation includes three steps: filtration, reabsorption, and secretion. Each step will be described in more detail in the coming sections.

> **VOCABULARY**
> **erythropoietin**: A hormone that is produced by the kidney cells and travels to the bone marrow to stimulate red blood cell formation.
> **interstitial**: Between the cells.
> **metabolites**: By-products of drug metabolism.
> **permeability**: A quality or characteristic of a material that allows another substance to pass through it.

Filtration

Filtration is the first step in urine formation. It is a continual process that involves the renal corpuscle. If you recall, the renal corpuscle consists of a cup-shaped structure (Bowman capsule) that surrounds the network of capillaries (glomerulus).

The blood is brought to the kidneys by the renal arteries. The arteries branch into smaller vessels that transport the blood throughout the kidney. As the blood gets to the nephron, an afferent arteriole brings the blood into the glomerulus, and an efferent arteriole takes the blood away. Eventually the blood moves into the renal vein and out of the kidney.

Let us focus on what occurs in the glomerulus. The diameter of the afferent arteriole is larger than the efferent arteriole's diameter. This means the blood moves into the glomerulus faster than it leaves. The pressure inside the glomerulus is high, with the increase of blood moving into the glomerulus. This forces water and dissolved substances through the one-celled wall of the capillary and into the Bowman capsule. The substance in the Bowman capsule is known as filtrate. (Think of a garden hose that is wide at one part and then narrowed at another. The pressure builds up behind the narrowed section. Water can leak from any weakened areas in the wall. This is similar to what occurs in the glomerulus.)

Several dissolved substances can move through the capillary wall:
- Electrolytes (i.e., sodium, chloride, and potassium)
- Waste products (i.e., urea, **metabolites** [muh TAB uh lites])
- Other substances (i.e., amino acids and glucose)

White blood cells, red blood cells, and plasma proteins are too large to pass through the capillary wall. With normal kidney function, they remain in the capillary.

If the blood pressure falls (i.e., with hemorrhaging), the pressure in the glomerulus is not high enough to cause movement of the fluids, so little to no filtrate is created and the person will have little to no urine output.

Reabsorption

Reabsorption means substances move from the filtrate back into the blood in the peritubular capillaries. As the filtrate moves out of the Bowman capsule and into the proximal tubule, the reabsorption process starts. Water (H_2O) and solutes (e.g., sodium [Na^+] ions and glucose) move back into the blood (Fig. 6.5). See Table 6.2 for the list of solutes that move back into the blood.

In the Henle loop, the reabsorption process is a bit different. The Henle loop dips down into the medulla and then moves back up. The countercurrent flow occurs as the filtrate flows down and then moves back up. During this time, the chloride (Cl^-) and sodium ions move out of the filtrate and into the **interstitial** (in ter STISH uh l) fluid and blood. This creates a salty interstitial fluid, which then helps pull water from the distal tubule filtrate. Water, chloride, and sodium are reabsorbed back into the blood as the filtrate passes through the distal tubule.

> **STUDY TIP**
> Remember, "water follows sodium."

In the distal tubules, some sodium and chloride ions are reabsorbed from the filtrate. The walls of the distal tubules do not allow water to move out of the filtrate without special help. This help is *antidiuretic hormone* (ADH). ADH is a hormone produced by the posterior pituitary gland. This hormone increases the water **permeability** of the walls of the distal tubule and collecting duct. With the help of ADH, water moves out of the filtrate into the bloodstream. Without ADH a person would pass vast quantities of urine. This condition is called diabetes insipidus.

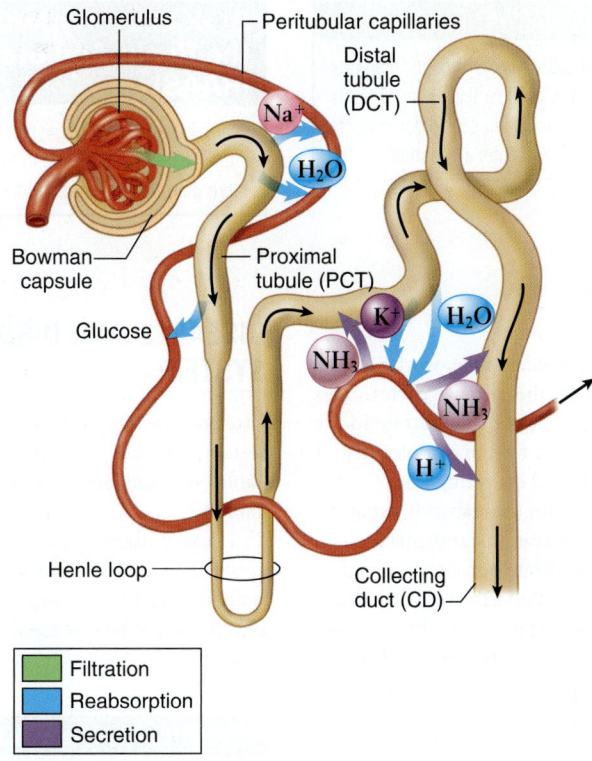

FIG. 6.5 Formation of urine. Diagram shows examples of steps in urine formation in successive parts of a nephron: filtration, reabsorption, and secretion. (From Patton KT, Thibodeau G: *The Human Body in Health and Disease*, ed 6, St. Louis, 2014, Mosby.)

TABLE 6.2	Movement of Substances Between the Blood and Filtrate in the Nephron				
Nephron Sections Processes	Renal Corpuscle (Bowman Capsule and Glomerulus)	Proximal Tubule (PCT)	Henle Loop	Distal Tubule (DCT)	Collecting Duct (CD)
Filtration (moves from blood to create filtrate)	Water, electrolyte ions (sodium, chloride, potassium), urea, glucose, and amino acids				
Reabsorption (moves from filtrate to blood)		Water, glucose, amino acids, urea, and electrolyte ions (sodium, chloride, phosphate)	Water and electrolytes ions (chloride, sodium)	Electrolytes ions (chloride, sodium) and water (only in the presence of ADH)	Electrolytes ions (sodium), urea, water (only in the presence of ADH)
Secretion (moves from blood to filtrate)			Urea	Ammonium, potassium, hydrogen, como drugs	Ammonium, potassium, hydrogen, some drugs

> **CRITICAL THINKING 6.4**
>
> Hannah is confused about diabetes insipidus. She always thought diabetes related to insulin and blood glucose. She does not recall learning about diabetes insipidus in school. She asks Katrina to explain how diabetes insipidus impacts the urinary system. How might Katrina respond to Hannah's question?

> **BOX 6.2 Hypertensive Medications and the Renin-Angiotensin Aldosterone System (RAAS)**
>
> Many hypertensive (high blood pressure) medications impact the RAAS at various points in the hope of lowering the blood pressure. Sometimes it takes more than one medication to lower a person's blood pressure to a safe level.

Besides ADH, another hormone, called *aldosterone*, works on the urinary system. Aldosterone is secreted by the adrenal cortex. This hormone increases the movement of sodium out of the filtrate in the distal tubule and collecting duct. See Table 6.2 for the complete list of substances reabsorbed in the distal tubule and collecting duct.

To maintain homeostasis, the kidneys retain (or reabsorb) what the body needs. Substances in excessive concentrations and metabolism waste products remain in the filtrate. The filtrate becomes more concentrated as water is reabsorbed back into the bloodstream. The kidneys create about 48 gallons (about 182 L) of filtrate a day. By the time reabsorption occurs, they produce only 1 to 2 quarts (about 0.9–1.9 L) of urine a day.

Secretion

Secretion means that substances move from the blood to the filtrate. This allows the body to maintain homeostasis and move unneeded substances back into the filtrate. Urea moves back to the filtrate in the Henle loop. As the filtrate moves through the distal tubule and collecting duct, more adjustments are made. Ammonia (NH_3), certain drugs, hydrogen (H^+), and potassium (K^+) move from the blood into the filtrate. The movement of potassium into the filtrate can be caused by aldosterone. After the filtrate or urine leaves the collecting ducts, no more adjustments are made. The urine then flows to the calyces and to the ureter before going through the rest of the urinary system structures.

Renin and Blood Pressure

As mentioned before, the kidneys have an important role in maintaining blood pressure. The *juxtaglomerular* (JUKS tah glo MER you lar) *cells* are smooth muscle cells in the afferent arterioles. These cells make and secrete the enzyme *renin*. When the arterial blood pressure decreases or when there is a decrease in sodium, renin is released. Secreting renin is one of the first steps in the complex renin-angiotensin aldosterone system (RAAS). Ultimately when renin is secreted, a series of events occur. The outcome impacts the blood plasma volume and the constriction of blood vessels. An increase in the blood plasma volume or the constriction of blood vessels can increase blood pressure (Box 6.2).

Erythropoietin

As the blood is moving through the kidneys, specialized kidney cells can detect low oxygen levels in the blood. When this occurs, a hormone called *erythropoietin* is released from the kidney cells. Erythropoietin travels to the bone marrow and stimulates the marrow to make more red blood cells.

Vitamin D

Vitamin D assists with calcium absorption and helps maintain calcium and phosphorus levels. These minerals are important for strong bones. We get vitamin D from exposure to sunlight, as well as from the consumption of supplements and food. The kidneys must convert vitamin D to an active form so that the body can use it.

DISEASES AND DISORDERS OF THE URINARY SYSTEM

Urologic diseases are conditions that impact one or more of the urinary system structures. Common urinary signs and symptoms are listed in Tables 6.3 and 6.4. Common urinary diagnostic tests are listed in Table 6.5.

Urinary diseases can include infections, stones, kidney problems, cancer, and bladder control problems. A urinary tract infection (UTI) is an infection in one or more of the urinary tract structures. Specific infections will be discussed in the following section, along with other diseases.

> **CRITICAL THINKING 6.5**
>
> Hannah is confused about the terms *azotemia* and *azoturia*. How might she remember which term relates to blood and which relates to urine?

> **CRITICAL THINKING 6.6**
>
> Hannah is working with Dr. Riney. He ordered an antibiotic for Mrs. Williams, who has a UTI. When the urine culture and sensitivity (C&S) report came back to the department, he asked Hannah to call Mrs. Williams regarding a change in the antibiotic. Why might the provider change the antibiotic once the urine C&S report became available?

> **VOCABULARY**
> **intravenously (IV)**: Through a vein; fluids and medications can be given through a vein.

Bladder Cancer

Bladder cancer is the sixth most common cancer in the United States. Bladder cancer tends to recur, so follow-up testing is critical. There are several types of bladder cancer:
- Transitional cell carcinoma or urothelial carcinoma: the most common cause; involves the transitional (epithelium) cells that change and stretch as the bladder fills with urine
- Squamous cell carcinoma: occurs with frequent infections, especially parasitic infections; rare in the United States
- Adenocarcinoma: involves the cells that make and release fluids like mucus in the bladder wall; rare in the United States

Etiology. Risk factors for developing bladder cancer include the following:
- Smoking: due to the harmful chemicals excreted in the urine
- Chemical exposure: arsenic and chemicals used in the manufacturing process of different products (e.g., paint, rubber, dyes)

TABLE 6.3 Terms Related to Urinary Signs

Term	Word Origin	Definition
abscess (AB ses), urinary		Cavity containing pus and surrounded by inflamed tissue in the urinary system
albuminuria (al byoo mih NOOR ee ah)	albumin/o protein -uria urinary condition	Albumin (a protein) in the urine; also called proteinuria (pro teen NOOR ee ah)
azotemia (a zoh TEE mee ah)	azot/o nitrogen -emia blood condition	Condition of excessive urea in the blood indicating nonfunctioning kidneys; also called uremia
azoturia (a zoh TOOR ee ah)	azot/o nitrogen -uria urinary condition	Excessive nitrogenous compounds, including urea, in the urine
bacteriuria (back tur ee YOOR ee ah)	bacteri/o bacteria -uria urinary condition	Bacteria in the urine
edema (eh DEE mah)		Accumulation of fluid in the tissues; can result from kidney failure
glycosuria (gly kohs YOOR ee ah)	glycos/o sugar, glucose -uria urinary condition	Sugar in the urine
hematuria (hee mah TOOR ee ah)	hemat/o blood -uria urinary condition	Blood in the urine
hypertension (hye pur TEN shun)	hyper- excessive tens/o stretching -ion process of	Condition of high blood pressure
pyuria (pye YOOR ee ah)	py/o pus -uria urinary condition	Pus in the urine

From Shiland B: *Mastering Healthcare Terminology*, ed 5, St. Louis, 2016, Elsevier.

- Family history of the disease
- Chronic bladder infections and inflammation
- Increasing age: rarely seen in people younger than 40
- Caucasian: greatest risk compared with other races
- Males: greater risk than females
- Medications: certain chemotherapy products and diabetes mellitus drugs

Signs and Symptoms. Common symptoms of bladder cancer include the following:
- Hematuria
- Frequency (urinating often) and urgency to urinate
- Dysuria, pelvic pain, and low back pain

Diagnostic Procedures. Several procedures can be used to diagnose bladder cancer:
- Urine testing
- Cystoscopy (Fig. 6.6)
- Biopsy

TABLE 6.4 Terms Related to Urinary Symptoms

Term	Word Origin	Definition
anuria (a NOOR ee ah)	an- without -uria urinary condition	Condition of no urine
diuresis (dye yoor EE sis)	di- through, complete ur/o urine -esis state of	Condition of increased formation and excretion of urine, of large volumes of urine; caffeine and alcohol are diuretics (dye yoor RET icks)—that is, they increase the amount of urine produced
dysuria (dis YOOR ee ah)	dys- painful, abnormal -uria urinary condition	Condition of painful urination
enuresis (en yoor EE sis)	en- in ur/o urine -esis state of	Also commonly known as "bed wetting," enuresis can be nocturnal (at night) or diurnal (during the day)
nocturia (nock TOOR ee ah)	noct/i night -uria urinary condition	Condition of excessive urination at night
oliguria (ah lig GYOOR ee ah)	olig/o scanty, few -uria urinary condition	Condition of scanty urination
polydipsia (pah lee DIP see ah)	poly- excessive, frequent -dipsia condition of thirst	Condition of excessive thirst (usually accompanied by polyuria)
polyuria (pah lee YOOR ee ah)	poly- excessive, frequent -uria urinary condition	Condition of excessive urination
urgency		Intense sensation of the need to urinate immediately
urinary incontinence (in KON tih nense)		Inability to hold urine
urinary retention		Inability to release urine

From Shiland B: *Mastering Healthcare Terminology*, ed 5, St. Louis, 2016, Elsevier.

To identify if the cancer spread to other parts of the body, the provider may order any of the following tests:
- Computed tomography (CT) scan
- Magnetic resonance imaging (MRI)
- Positron emission tomography (PET) scan

Treatment. Treatments used for bladder cancer include surgery, radiation therapy, and chemotherapy. *Biologic therapy* or *immunotherapy* is also a treatment option. Biologic therapy can be useful, as it increases the body's ability to help fight the cancer.

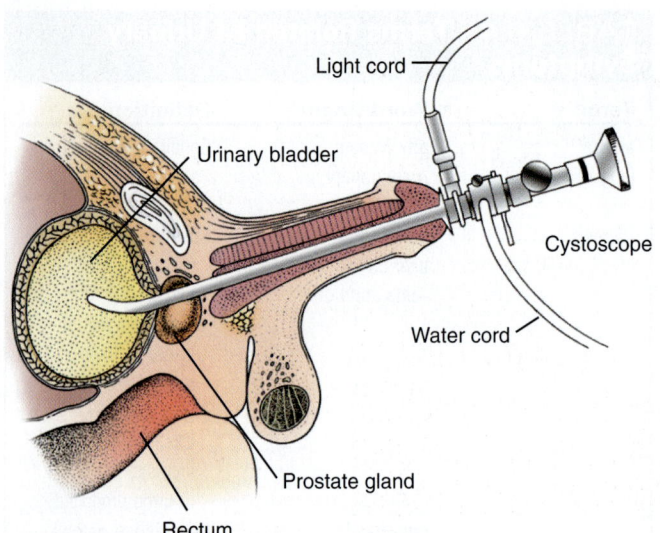

FIG. 6.6 Cystoscopy. (From Shiland B: *Mastering Healthcare Terminology*, ed 5, St. Louis, 2016, Elsevier.)

Prognosis. The prognosis of bladder cancer depends on the stage of the cancer. Stage 0 has a 5-year survival rate of about 98% according to the American Cancer Society. Stage IV has a 15% 5-year survival rate.

Prevention. To lower the bladder cancer risk, it is important to decrease the risk factors. To help lower the risk, patients should stop smoking, decrease exposure to industrial chemicals, and maintain a healthy diet.

Cystitis, Acute

Acute cystitis (si STIE tis) is an inflammation of the bladder.

Etiology. In many cases, inflammation is related to a bacterial infection. One of the most common causes is *Escherichia coli (E. coli)*. Due to the shorter urethra, women are more at risk than men to get infections. Box 6.3 lists the risk factors for getting cystitis. Besides bacteria, inflammation can be caused by medications, radiation therapy, spermicidal jellies, and long-term catheterization.

TABLE 6.5 Common Diagnostic Procedures Used for Urinary Diseases

Done by/Type of Test:	Procedure	Description
Provider during the exam	Digital rectal examination (DRE)	Done during the physical examination. The provider inserts a gloved, lubricated finger into the rectum to feel for abnormalities in the prostate, bladder, ovaries, or uterus. For urinary tract issues, the DRE may be done to check if the prostate gland is swollen and obstructing the urinary tract structures.
Endoscopy	Cystoscopy and ureteroscopy	An endoscope is inserted into the urethra and used to look at the urinary system.
Imagining procedures	Computerized tomography (CT) scan	Images can show urinary tract obstructions. (See Chapter 2 for more information.)
	DMSA scan	A renal scan that uses the radioisotope, Technetium-99m dimercaptosuccinic acid (DSMA), to evaluate the kidneys. The function, shape, position, size, and scarring can be observed. The radioisotope is injected, and a gamma camera is used to take pictures of the kidney.
	Intravenous pyelogram (IVP)	Iodine contrast is given **intravenously (IV)**. Then x-ray images will be taken to see how the kidneys filter the contrast from the blood. The test can provide information on the functioning of the kidneys, bladder, and ureters.
	Postvoid residual (PVR) urine test	Measures the amount of urine in the bladder after urination. A straight catheter can be inserted to drain the remaining urine so the volume can be measured, but this procedure can increase the risk of UTIs. A portable ultrasound unit can also be used as a noninvasive test. The scan identifies the urine left, and the unit automatically calculates the volume of residual urine.
	Ultrasound (US)	Images can show urinary tract obstructions. (See Chapter 2 for more information.)
	Voiding cystourethrogram (VCUG)	A minimally invasive test that involves fluoroscopy to visualize the urinary tract and bladder. Images are taken while the bladder is full and during urination. Contrast medium is used to help visualize the urinary structures on the x-ray image (Fig. 6.7).
Medical laboratory	Blood urea nitrogen (BUN test)	Urea is a waste product in the blood that is filtered out by the kidneys. If the kidney function is abnormal, the blood level of urea will be increased.
	Creatinine and creatinine clearance tests	Creatinine is a waste product from normal muscle breakdown. Creatinine is filtered out of the blood by the kidneys. The blood creatinine level indicates kidney function. The creatinine clearance rate shows how the kidneys filter creatinine from the blood.
	Urinalysis (UA)	A urine sample is collected in a special container. The urine is analyzed in the lab for abnormal levels of substances. Some of the substances that may be found in urine include blood, ketones, bilirubin, glucose, protein, and nitrites. The urinalysis is a CLIA-waived test.
	Urine culture	A urine sample is collected in a special container. The urine is analyzed in the lab for bacterial growth over a period of days (usually 1–3 days). Specific bacteria grown in the sample will be listed on the urine culture report.
	Urine culture and sensitivity (C&S)	A urine culture is done as discussed above. The sensitivity results indicate if the pathogen is susceptible or resistant to specific antibiotics.

TABLE 6.5 Common Diagnostic Procedures Used for Urinary Diseases—cont'd

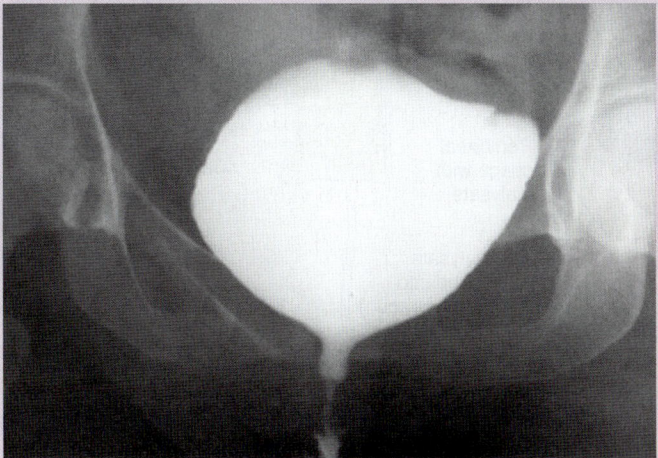

FIG. 6.7 Female voiding cystourethrogram (VCUG). (From Bontrager KL: *Textbook of Radiographic Positioning and Related Anatomy*, ed 7, St. Louis, 2009, Mosby.)

BOX 6.3 Risk Factors for Cystitis

- **Catheter** (KATH uh tur): indwelling (remains in) or straight (removed after urine has drained out of the bladder)
- Urinary tract procedure
- Pregnancy, menopause
- Obstructions (bladder, urethra, or due to an enlarged prostate gland)
- Urinary retention
- Bowel incontinence
- Diabetes

VOCABULARY

catheter: A hollow, flexible tube that can be inserted into a vessel, organ, or cavity of the body to withdraw or instill fluid, monitor information, and visualize a vessel or cavity.

Signs and Symptoms. Symptoms of cystitis include the following:
- Low-grade fever
- Nocturia, dysuria, urgency, and frequency
- Urinary retention
- Cloudy, bloody, or strong/foul-smelling urine
- Low abdominal pressure or cramping
- With older adults: confusion, mental changes

Diagnostic Procedures. Usually the provider will order a urinalysis and a urine culture and sensitivity. This requires the patient to provide a clean-catch midstream urine sample. You will learn more about urine specimen samples in Chapter 42. The urinalysis will provide information fairly quickly that will help diagnose cystitis. It may take up to 3 days for the culture and sensitivity to identify the organism and then provide information on the best medications to treat the infection. If the urinalysis and culture come back negative for an infection, the provider may do additional tests (e.g., cystoscopy) to try to identify the cause of the symptoms.

Treatment. For bacterial cystitis, antibiotics are used to treat the infection. After starting the antibiotic, the patient's symptoms should improve within a few days. If a patient has a history of repeated infections, the provider may refer the patient to a urologist for more testing. Hospital-acquired bladder infections are usually resistant to the common antibiotics used to treat UTIs. Stronger antibiotics may be given.

Home care treatments may include the following:
- Drinking plenty of liquids and avoiding coffee, alcohol, and soft drinks
- Taking an analgesic, having a sitz bath, or using a heating pad to decrease the discomfort

Prognosis. Cystitis is uncomfortable. When treated, in most cases cystitis will resolve without complications.

Prevention. To decrease the risk of UTIs, keeping hydrated and urinating frequently are recommended. Women can decrease the risk of UTIs by doing the following:
- Wiping from front to back, which prevents bacteria in the anal area from spreading to the urethra
- Taking showers instead of baths
- Urinating after intercourse

End-Stage Renal Disease

End-stage renal disease (ESRD) is also called end-stage kidney disease and kidney failure. ESRD occurs when the kidneys are no longer filtering waste from the blood. Dangerous levels of electrolytes, waste products, and fluids build up in the bloodstream.

More than 660,000 Americans have kidney failure. Over 44% of those patients are between the ages of 45 and 64. The top two causes of ESRD are diabetes mellitus and high blood pressure.

Etiology. End-stage kidney disease is a complication of several diseases:
- Diabetes mellitus with poor glucose control
- Hypertension
- Glomerulonephritis
- Polycystic kidney disease
- Prolonged obstructions or recurrent kidney infections
- Vesicoureteral reflux

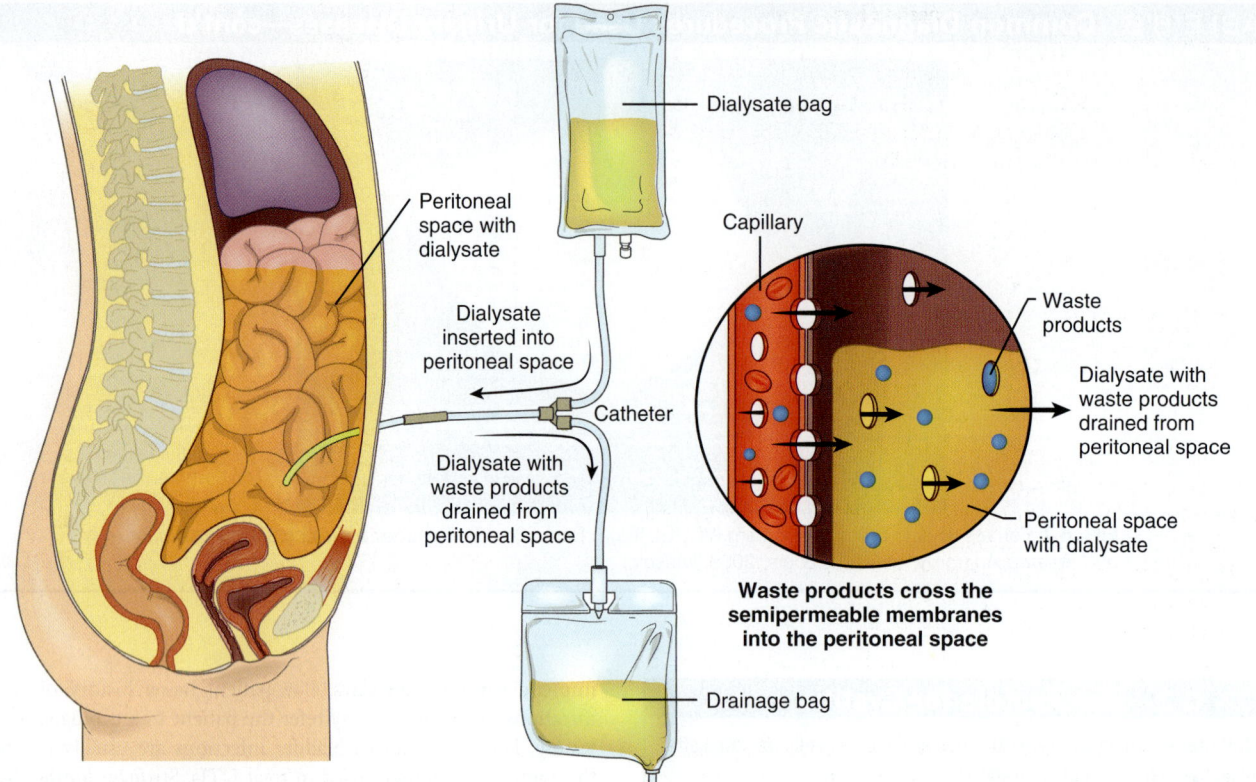

FIG. 6.8 Peritoneal dialysis. (From Proctor D, et al: *Kinn's The Medical Assistant*, ed 13, St. Louis, 2017, Elsevier.)

Additional factors that can increase a person's risk for ESRD include tobacco use, African American descent, gender [male], and being 45 years and older.

Signs and Symptoms. The kidneys can slowly stop functioning over the course of 10 to 20 years before ESRD occurs, and a number of symptoms can signal renal failure:
- Loss of appetite, nausea, and weight loss
- Fatigue, headache, and feeling ill
- Pruritus (proo RAHY tuhs), dry skin, changes in skin color and nails
- Numbness in extremities, twitching, and muscle cramps
- Difficulty concentrating, sleep problems

> **VOCABULARY**
> **pruritus**: Itching.

Diagnostic Procedures. Besides a physical exam, providers will order blood work and a bone density test. The blood work usually includes a complete blood count (CBC), electrolytes (e.g., potassium, sodium, calcium, and magnesium), albumin, and parathyroid hormone. The patient's blood pressure will be monitored closely.

Treatment. ESRD is often treated with dialysis or a kidney transplant. Dialysis works like a kidney by filtering out the waste products, extra fluids, and electrolytes. There are two different types of dialysis:
- *Peritoneal dialysis*: A catheter is surgically placed in the abdomen. The patient can then infuse a special sterile solution through the catheter into the abdomen. The peritoneal membrane is used as a natural filter, and waste from the blood moves into the infused solution. After a few hours, the patient drains the fluid out of the abdomen via the catheter (Fig. 6.8). New fluid is then infused into the abdomen. There may be four to six exchanges of fluid a day. This type of dialysis allows the person to work, travel, or sleep during the process.
- *Hemodialysis*: A vascular access (i.e., catheter, arteriovenous [ahr teer ee oh VEE nuhs] graft, arteriovenous fistula) is placed. Using the vascular access, the patient is hooked up to a dialysis machine. The person's blood flows through the special filter inside of the machine (Fig. 6.9). The filter cleans the blood of waste products

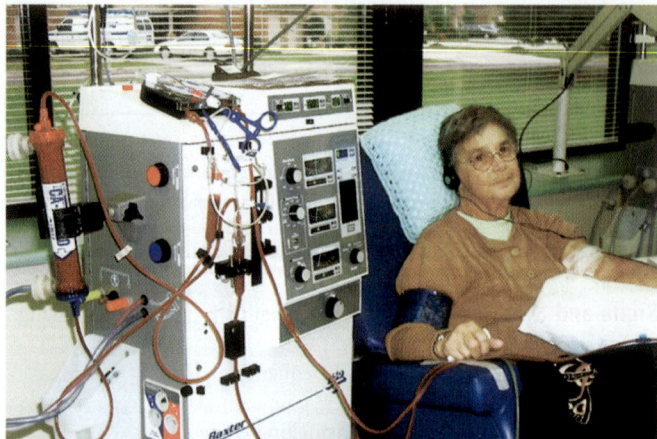

FIG. 6.9 Hemodialysis machine. (From Ignatavicius DD, Workman ML: *Medical-Surgical Nursing: Critical Thinking for Collaborative Care*, ed 6, Philadelphia, 2011, Saunders.)

and extra fluids. Typically, patients need to have hemodialysis three times a week at the dialysis center.

Besides dialysis and kidney transplant, other treatments are available:
- Special diet: low-protein, limiting fluids and electrolytes
- Antihypertensive (an tie hie per TEN siv) medication and supplements (i.e., calcium, iron, and vitamin D)

> ### CRITICAL THINKING 6.7
> With Hannah's experience in the dialysis unit, she learned that many people need to do hemodialysis three times a week for several hours each day. How might this impact a patient's lifestyle?

Prognosis. The prognosis varies. Once the kidneys have been damaged, there is no treatment to reverse the damage. If untreated, ESRD will lead to death. ESRD can lead to additional complications:
- Fluid retention and electrolyte imbalance (e.g., hyperkalemia)
- Anemia and cardiovascular disease
- Weakened bones (increased risk for fractures)
- Central nervous system changes including seizures, confusion, and personality changes

Prevention. Prevention includes prompt monitoring and treatment of conditions that can lead to ESRD. It is important to monitor and treat diabetes mellitus and high blood.

Glomerulonephritis

Several diseases affect kidney functioning by impacting the glomeruli. Glomerulonephritis (gloe MER yuh loe nah FRIE tis) is inflammation of the glomeruli. Damage to the glomeruli can cause protein and red blood cells to leak into the urine. Glomerulonephritis usually has an abrupt onset.

Etiology. The cause is often unknown. It can follow a streptococcal infection.

Signs and Symptoms. Glomerulonephritis can cause the following:
- Changes in the urine: hematuria, cola-colored urine, proteinuria, and oliguria
- Headache and pain over the kidney region
- Puffy eyes, fatigue, and low-grade fever

Diagnostic Procedures. After the physical exam, the provider may order the following:
- Laboratory tests: urinalysis, blood urea nitrogen (BUN), creatinine, erythrocyte sedimentation rate (ESR)

> ### VOCABULARY
> **antihypertensive**: A substance (i.e., medication) that reduces high blood pressure.
> **arteriovenous**: Pertains to the arteries and veins.
> **arteriovenous fistula**: An abnormal joining of an artery and vein.
> **graft**: Tissue taken from one area in the body and inserted into another area or person.
> **hyperkalemia**: High potassium levels in the blood.
> **vascular access**: A surgical procedure that creates a vein to remove and return blood during the hemodialysis procedure.

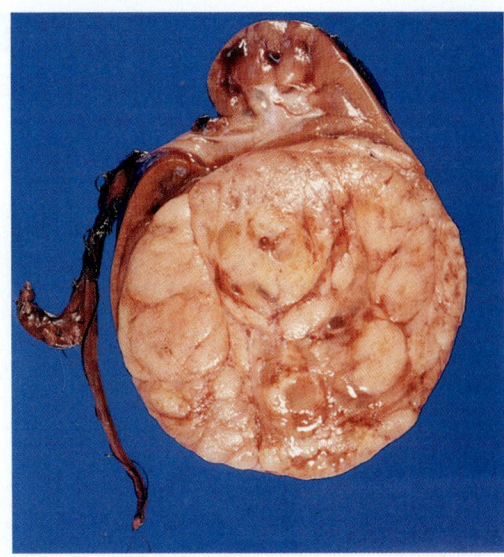

FIG. 6.10 Wilms tumor of the kidney. (From Kumar P, Clark ML: *Kumar and Clark's Clinical Medicine,* ed 7, Philadelphia, 2009, Saunders.)

- Imagining tests: CT scan, x-ray, and ultrasound
- Renal biopsy

Treatment. Treatment is based on the cause of the illness. Possible treatments may include the following:
- Hypertensive and diuretic medications; antibiotics if bacterial related
- Bed rest
- Dietary restrictions: protein, salt, and potassium

Prognosis. Usually the prognosis is good. Symptoms resolve in a few weeks after treatment.

Prevention. Prompt treatment of streptococcal infections is important. For other causes, no preventive measures are known.

Kidney Cancer

Kidney cancer or primary kidney cancer occurs when a cancer starts in the kidney. There are three main types of primary kidney cancer:
- Renal cell carcinoma (RCC) (or renal adenocarcinoma): most common type in adults; forms in the lining of the kidney tubules
- Wilms tumor: accounts for about 95% kidney cancer in children, usually diagnosed when the person is younger than 5 years; occurs in the kidney tissue (Fig. 6.10); improved treatments have increased the survival rate
- Transitional cell cancer: occurs in adults; forms in the ureter and renal pelvis (Fig. 6.11)

Etiology. The cause of kidney cancer is not clear. A mutation occurs in the kidney cells. This can lead to the development of a tumor. See Table 6.6 for the etiology and risk factors for the three common types of kidney cancer.

Signs and Symptoms. With kidney cancer, pain and hematuria can be key symptoms. See Table 6.6 for the symptoms for the three types of kidney cancer.

Diagnostic Procedures. Diagnostic procedures for the three types of kidney cancer are similar (see Table 6.6). During the exam, the provider may identify a kidney mass. Urinalysis and blood work may be done

TABLE 6.6 Common Types of Kidney Cancer

	Renal Cell Carcinoma	Transitional Cell Cancer	Wilms Tumor
Other Names	Renal Adenocarcinoma		Nephroblastoma
Etiology and Risk Factors	Etiology is unclear Risk factors: • Misuse of some pain medications • Obesity • High blood pressure • Smoking • Inherited conditions (i.e., von Hippel-Lindau disease, family history of disease)	Etiology is unclear Risk factors: • Misuse of some pain medications • Smoking cigarettes • Exposure to certain dyes and industrial chemicals	Etiology is unclear Risk factors: • Family history of the disease • African American descent • Congenital abnormalities including aniridia (ane eye RID ee ah), hypospadias (hie poe SPA de as), and undescended testicles
Signs and Symptoms	Hematuria, lump in abdomen, side and back pain (below the ribs), loss of appetite, weight loss, anemia, intermittent fever	Hematuria, back pain, extreme fatigue, weight loss, dysuria	Hematuria, fever, and abdominal pain, mass and swelling
Diagnostic Procedures	Physical exam, CBC, blood chemistry tests, UA, liver function tests, CT, MRI, US, biopsy	Physical exam, CBC, blood chemistry tests, UA, ureteroscopy, IVP, CT, US, MRI, biopsy	Physical exam, CBC, blood chemistry tests, UA, US, CT, MRI
Treatment	Surgery (nephrectomy [neh FREK tah mee]), radiation, chemotherapy, biologic therapy, targeted therapy	Segmental resection of the ureter, nephroureterectomy, chemotherapy, radiation (see Table 6.7)	Surgery (nephrectomy), radiation, chemotherapy
Prognosis	Stage of disease, age and general health of person, location of tumor		Very good with treatment

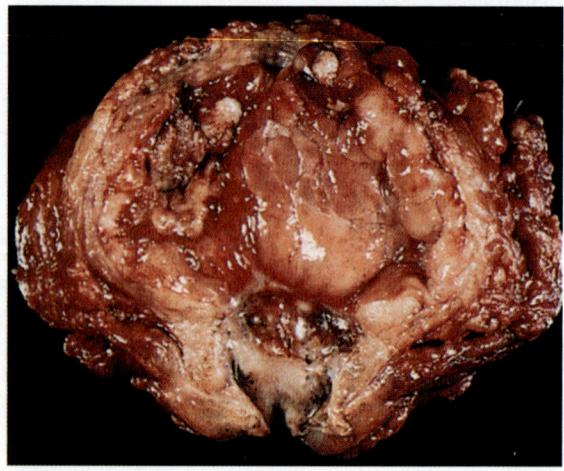

FIG. 6.11 Transitional cell carcinomas of the bladder. (From Damjanov I: *Anderson's Pathology*, ed 10, St. Louis, 2000, Mosby.)

TABLE 6.7 Types of Surgery for Kidney Cancer

Surgery	Description
Partial nephrectomy	Removing the cancer and surrounding tissue; kidney remains functional; used when other kidney has been damaged or removed
Simple nephrectomy	Removal of the kidney
Radical nephrectomy	Removal of the kidney, adrenal gland, surrounding tissue, and local lymph nodes
Nephroureterectomy (nef roe you REE ter ek to mee)	Removal of the kidney and ureter
Segmental resection of the ureter	Removal of the diseased section of the ureter; ureter is then reconnected

to check for hematuria and the person's overall health. Once kidney cancer is diagnosed, imaging tests are done to check for cancer in other parts of the body.

Treatment. Treatment for kidney cancer can involve surgery (Table 6.7). A person can live with just a part of one kidney functioning. If the person does not have any kidney function, dialysis is required. A kidney transplant could also be a treatment option. Radiation and chemotherapy are also treatment options with kidney cancer.

If surgery is not an option, an arterial embolization can be done. A catheter is inserted through an incision. It is passed into the main blood vessel of the kidney. A special gelatin sponge is inserted through the catheter into the blood vessel. This creates a blockage, which then cuts the blood flow to the cancerous area. Cancer cells rely on blood flow for oxygen and nutrients.

Biologic therapy and targeted therapy are also treatment options. Biologic therapy, as already described, boosts the body's natural ability to fight off cancer. Targeted therapy requires the use of drugs that attack cancer cells only. The normal cells remain unharmed, while the medications cause the tumor to shrink.

Clinical trials are examining new treatments:
- New surgical techniques: laser surgery, segmental resection of the disease tissue, fulguration (destroys tissue using an electrical current)
- Regional chemotherapy and regional biologic therapy: medication is administered directly into the organ impacted by cancer

Prognosis. The prognosis of kidney cancer depends on the age and health of the person. It also depends on the stage, type, and location of the tumor. The prognosis can change if the cancer is recurring.

Prevention. Many cases of kidney cancer are attributed to smoking. Stopping smoking can help prevent kidney cancer. Decreasing risk factors is important. This includes limiting chemical exposure, achieving a healthy weight, not misusing pain medication, and controlling hypertension.

Nephrotic Syndrome

Nephrotic (nah FROT ik) syndrome consists of a collection of symptoms that indicate kidney damage. The syndrome is caused by other disorders that eventually lead to kidney tissue destruction. Symptoms can include the following:
- Swelling
- Proteinuria
- Low serum (blood) protein levels
- High cholesterol and triglyceride levels

Etiology. Nephrotic syndrome occurs more often in males than in females. It can impact children, usually 2 to 6 years of age, and adults. Minimal change disease is the most common cause of nephrotic syndrome in children. Membranous glomerulonephritis is the most common cause in adults. Nephrotic syndrome can also occur as the result of cancer, chronic disease (e.g., diabetes, systemic lupus erythematosus), infections, immune and genetic disorders, and with certain drugs.

Signs and Symptoms. The most common sign is swelling of the face, extremities, and abdomen. Additional symptoms can include poor appetite, weight gain, seizures, skin sores, and foamy appearing urine. Blood and urine tests show proteinuria, hyperlipidemia (hie per lip i DEE mee ah), and hypoalbuminemia (hie poh al byoo mi NEE mee ah).

Diagnostic Procedures. Providers will do a physical exam, laboratory testing, and a kidney biopsy. Laboratory work includes the following:
- Blood testing: albumin, blood chemistry tests, BUN, creatinine
- Urine testing: creatinine clearance, urinalysis

Additional testing may be ordered to identify the specific cause of nephrotic syndrome. HIV, hepatitis, and syphilis are just a few of the diseases that could lead to nephrotic syndrome.

Treatment. The treatment goals are to reduce symptoms, delay kidney damage, and prevent additional complications. The following are common treatments for nephrotic syndrome:
- Antihypertensive medications to keep the blood pressure in the normal range
- Corticosteroids to reduce the immune and inflammatory reactions
- Vitamin D supplements
- Anticoagulants (an tee koe AG UE lants) (i.e., heparin or warfarin) to reduce the risk of blood clots
- Antihyperlipidemic (an tie hie per lip i DEE mik) medication to control the cholesterol level
- Diuretic medications to reduce the swelling
- Dietary changes: low-fat, low-cholesterol, low-salt, and low-protein diet

Prognosis. The outcome of necrotic syndrome varies from complete recovery to kidney failure. Those experiencing kidney failure need dialysis and a possible kidney transplant. Additional complications include the following:
- Atherosclerosis, congestive heart failure and pulmonary edema
- Infections
- Chronic kidney diseases
- Hypertension and anemia
- Hypothyroidism

Prevention. Prompt treatment of conditions that lead to necrotic syndrome is important.

Neurogenic Bladder

The central nervous system, nerves that supply the bladder, and muscles work together for bladder control. Damage or disorders that impact the bladder nerves or the central nervous system can cause neurogenic bladder. A person with neurogenic bladder lacks bladder control. The bladder can be overactive or underactive.

The bladder muscles contract uncontrollably with an overactive bladder. This causes urgency and frequency with urination and an inability to control urination. With an underactive bladder, the bladder fills but the person does not have the urge to go. Overfill incontinence (or urine leakage) can occur when the bladder is full.

Etiology. The central nervous system disorders that can cause neurogenic bladder include the following:
- Birth defects (e.g., spina bifida) and cerebral palsy
- Alzheimer disease and brain or spinal cord tumors
- Multiple sclerosis (MS)
- Parkinson disease
- Stroke and spinal cord injury

> **VOCABULARY**
> **aniridia**: A condition in which the iris in the eye is partially formed or fails to form.
> **anticoagulant**: A substance (i.e., medication or chemical) that prevents clotting of blood.
> **antihyperlipidemic**: A substance (i.e., medication) that lowers the lipid levels in the blood.
> **corticosteroids**: A group of steroid hormones produced in the body or given as a medication; some have metabolic functions, and others decrease tissue inflammation. Glucocorticoids and mineralocorticoids are two types.
> **diuretic**: A substance (i.e., medication) that increases the amount of urine produced.
> **hyperlipidemia**: An elevated level of lipids in the blood.
> **hypoalbuminemia**: A decreased level of albumin (protein) in the blood.
> **hypospadias**: A condition in which the urethral opening is on the underside of the penis.
> **intermittent**: Occurring in intervals.
> **nephrectomy**: Surgical removal of a kidney.
> **undescended testicles**: A condition in which one or both testicles do not descend into the scrotum.

Damage and disorders of the bladder nerves can be caused by the following:
- Diabetes
- Syphilis
- Heavy alcohol use
- Neuropathy (nu ROP a thee)
- Nerve damage from pelvic surgery, herniated disk, or spinal canal stenosis

Signs and Symptoms. Neurogenic bladder can cause overactive or underactive bladder activity. With an overactive bladder, a person experiences loss of bladder control. Urgency and frequency to urinate are common.

With an underactive bladder, the bladder fills but the person does not have the urge to go. Incontinence or urine leakage can occur with a full bladder. Problems starting to urinate or completely emptying the bladder can also be experienced.

Diagnostic Procedures. Procedures used to help diagnose neurogenic bladder include the following:
- Postvoid residual volume
- Blood tests to check kidney functioning (i.e., serum creatinine)
- Renal ultrasonography and cystoscopy

Treatment. Treatment is aimed at managing the symptoms of neurogenic bladder. Possible treatments include the following:
- Medications: antimuscarinic (AN tee mus kah RIN ik), anticholinergic (AN tee kol i NER jik), botulinum toxin, GABA supplements, and antiepileptics (Table 6.8)
- Surgical procedures: artificial urinary sphincter, an implanted electronic device to stimulate bladder nerves, and urinary stoma (STOH mah) (urostomy [yoo ROS te mee])
- Additional procedures: Kegel exercises (Box 6.4) and a urinary catheter

Prognosis. If the disorder is diagnosed and treated before kidney damage occurs, the prognosis is good. If kidney damage occurs prior to treatment, there is an increased risk of complications.

Prevention. For most cases of neurogenic bladder, there are no preventive measures. Symptoms of the condition are managed.

CRITICAL THINKING 6.8
Dr. Riney asked Hannah to coach Mrs. Smith on doing Kegel exercises. How might Hannah explain the process of doing Kegels to Mrs. Smith?

VOCABULARY
neuropathy: A nervous system disorder of the peripheral nerves that causes discomfort, numbness, and weakness, especially in the extremities.
stoma: A temporary or permanent surgically created opening used for drainage (i.e., urine, stool).
urostomy: A surgically created opening on the abdominal wall used to drain urine.

TABLE 6.8 Medications Used for Urology Conditions

Classification	Description	Examples
Alpha-blockers	Relax bladder neck and prostate muscles, make it easier to empty the bladder; used to treat urge or overflow incontinence	Tamsulosin (tam SOO loe sin) (Flomax) Terazosin (ter AY zoe sin) Doxazosin (dox ay' zoe sin) (Cardura)
Anticholinergic (AN tee kol i NER jik)	Stimulate the bladder to contract, which helps urination; used to treat overactive bladder and urge incontinence	Bethanechol (be THAN e kole)
Antimuscarinic (AN tee mus kah RIN ik)	Relax bladder muscles and decreases bladder contractions	Oxybutynin (ox i BYOO ti nin) (Ditropan XL) Tolterodine (tole TER a deen) (Detrol) Propantheline (proe PAN the leen)
Beta-3 adrenergic agonist	Relaxes the bladder muscles to prevent urgent, frequent, or uncontrolled urination; used to treat urge incontinence	Mirabegron (mir a BEG ron)

BOX 6.4 Kegel Exercises
Kegel exercises are used to strengthen the pelvic floor muscles. Both males and females can do them. To use the right muscles, pretend you have to urinate but hold it. The muscles you tighten to stop urination help tighten the pelvic floor muscles. Muscles in the vagina (for females), rectum, and bladder should tighten. The muscles in the thighs, buttock, and abdomen should not be tightened. Kegel exercises should be done three times a day.
To perform Kegel exercises:
1. Empty your bladder.
2. You can be sitting or lying down during the exercises.
3. Tighten the pelvic floor muscles ("hold the urine"). Tighten as you count to 8.
4. Relax the muscles as you count to 10.
5. Repeat this sequence 10 times.

Polycystic Kidney Disease
Polycystic (POL ee sis tik) kidney disease (PKD) is an inherited condition. Cysts form in the kidneys, causing the kidneys to become enlarged (Fig. 6.12). A cyst-filled kidney could weigh up to 30 pounds.

Etiology. There are two types of PKD:
- *Autosomal* (aw toe SOE mal) *dominant*: the gene is inherited from one parent and the child will get the disease. Often the parent also has the disease. This is the most common form of PKD and

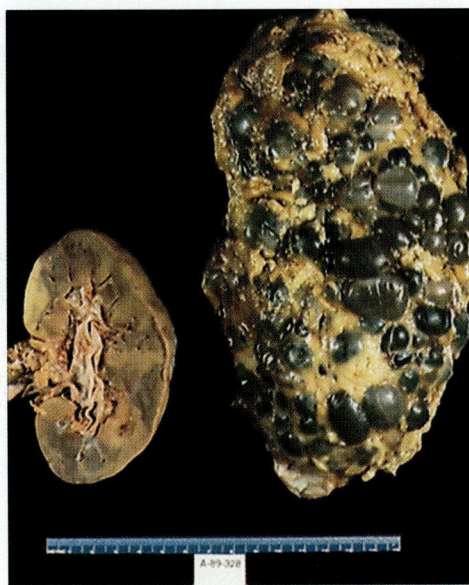

FIG. 6.12 Comparison of a polycystic kidney *(right)* with a normal kidney *(left)*. (From Lewis SM: *Medical-Surgical Nursing: Assessment and Management of Clinical Problems,* ed 8, St. Louis, 2011, Mosby.)

also the most common inherited kidney disorder. It is typically identified between the ages of 30 and 50, though it can occur in childhood.
- *Autosomal recessive*: to get the disease a person must get a copy of the defected gene from both parents.

People with PKD may also have cysts in their liver and pancreas. Aneurysms and diverticula of the colon may also be associated with PKD. Males can have cysts in their testes and tend to have more kidney failure. Women with PKD, hypertension, and who have had three or more pregnancies are also more at risk for kidney failure.

Signs and Symptoms. The symptoms of PKD may include the following:
- Pain in the flank, abdomen, or joints
- Nocturia, hematuria
- Drowsiness
- Nail abnormalities

Diagnostic Procedures. During the physical examination, the following may be found:
- Pain or tenderness over the liver, enlarged liver
- Heart murmur
- High blood pressure

The provider may order a CBC, liver blood tests, and urinalysis (UA). To check for aneurysms, a cerebral angiography may be done. An intravenous pyelogram (IVP), abdominal CT, MRI, and ultrasound (US) may be ordered to check for cysts on the liver and other organs.

Treatment. The treatment goals are to control symptoms and prevent complications. Treatment often includes hypertensive medications, diuretics, and a low-salt diet. PKD can increase the risk of urinary tract infections due to blockages. UTIs should be treated quickly with antibiotics. Surgery to remove one or both kidneys may be required. The patient may also need dialysis or a kidney transplant.

With the chronic nature of this condition, it is important for patients to get support. Sometimes support groups can help the patient and family cope with the disease process.

Prognosis. PKD is a chronic condition that slowly gets worse. Eventually, the person will progress to end-stage kidney failure. Liver disease due to the liver cysts may also occur. Treatment can slow the disease progression and decrease the complications. Complications of PKD include the following:
- Bleeding from the ruptured cysts and anemia
- Kidney disease: end-stage, chronic, stones, UTIs
- Liver failure
- High blood pressure

Prevention. There are no treatments that can prevent the formation of cysts. Treatment can slow the progression of the disease.

Prostate Cancer

Prostate cancer is the second most common cancer among males. About one in seven men will be diagnosed with prostate cancer. The survival rate for prostate cancer is very high, thus most diagnosed do not die of it. With prostate cancer, the gland can also increase in size, obstructing the urethra and causing additional urinary complications.

Etiology. Risk factors for prostate cancer include the following:
- Increasing age: prostate cancer is rare for those younger than 40, but the incidence increases for those older than 60. In the United States, the average age upon diagnosis is 69.
- African Americans: have a greater risk of developing and dying from prostate cancer.
- Family history of prostate cancer: having a brother or father with prostate cancer doubles the risk.

African American descent and family history are also risk factors for aggressive prostate cancer. Additional risk factors for aggressive prostate cancer include the following:
- Obesity, lack of exercise, sedentary lifestyle
- Tall height
- High calcium intake
- Agent Orange exposure (Box 6.5)

> ### CRITICAL THINKING 6.9
> Hannah is rooming Sam Fox, a 40-year-old father of three children. He is 6 feet tall. When Hannah obtains a family history on Sam, she learns that his father, a Vietnam veteran, was just diagnosed with aggressive prostate cancer. What risk factors does Sam have for prostate cancer?

Signs and Symptoms. Prostate cancer tends to be a silent disease in the early stages. It is not until the cancer grows large enough to obstruct

> ### BOX 6.5 Agent Orange
> Agent Orange was an herbicide used by the US military to remove the dense foliage during the Vietnam War. It is presumed that any veteran who served in Vietnam was exposed to Agent Orange. The Veterans Administration has attributed several diseases to Agent Orange. These diseases include diabetes mellitus, Hodgkin disease, multiple myeloma, Parkinson disease, respiratory cancers, and prostate cancers. A 2013 study found that veterans exposed to Agent Orange had a higher risk for developing prostate cancer. They also have a greater risk for aggressive prostate cancer. Screening for prostate cancer is important in veterans exposed to Agent Orange. Male children of veterans with aggressive prostate cancer are at greater risk of developing prostate cancer too.

the urethra that symptoms are noticeable. With advanced prostate cancer, the symptoms can include the following:
- Problems with urination: slow, weak stream; urinating more often, nocturia
- Hematuria, blood in the semen
- Difficulty getting an erection
- Hip pain, back pain
- Loss of bladder or bowel control

Diagnostic Procedures. The *prostate-specific antigen* (PSA) *blood test* is used as a screening tool for prostate cancer. Both normal and cancerous prostate cells make the protein PSA. Often PSA levels increase in the blood with prostate cancer. It is recommended for men to have a baseline PSA test at the age of 40. If the patient has an increased risk, the provider may decide to get a baseline PSA test earlier than age 40. The provider then checks the PSA level over time by comparing it to the baseline level. The reliability of the PSA blood test is debated, but it is the only screening tool available at this time.

The provider completes a *digital rectal exam* (DRE) during the examination (Fig. 6.13). If the DRE is abnormal or the PSA level has increased from the baseline, a needle biopsy of the prostate may be done. If cancer is detected, additional imaging tests will be ordered to determine the extent of cancer.

Treatment. Treatment will be based on the type of prostate cancer. If the cancer is a nonaggressive type, the provider may suggest frequent checks to monitor any signs that the cancer is growing or changing. Other options for early stage and aggressive prostate cancers include the following:
- *Prostatectomy* (pras tah TEK tah mee): a surgery to remove the prostate
- Radiation

Prognosis. The prognosis depends on a number of factors:
- The extent and grade of the tumor: if the cancer has spread to a distant body structure, the prognosis is poor
- Patient's age and health: the age can impact the treatment decisions; more aggressive treatment will be done if the person is younger
- PSA level

Prevention. There are no preventive measures for prostate cancer. However, it is important to reduce risk factors. Some risk factors like age, race, and exposure to Agent Orange cannot be changed. If a person is at risk for prostate cancer, routine screening is important.

Pyelonephritis

Pyelonephritis (PIE ah loe ni frie tis) is a urinary tract infection of one or both of the kidneys. Prompt treatment is required to prevent kidney damage and septicemia (sep tih SEE mee ah). The bacteria can spread to the bloodstream, causing an overwhelming infection that can be life threatening.

> **VOCABULARY**
> **septicemia**: A systemic infection involving pathologic microbes in the blood as a result of an infection that has spread from elsewhere in the body.

Etiology. Like other UTIs, pyelonephritis is caused by a bacterium or virus. The pathogen can move from the bladder to the kidneys, or it can be carried by the bloodstream to the kidneys. Increased risk factors for pyelonephritis include the following:
- Structural defect

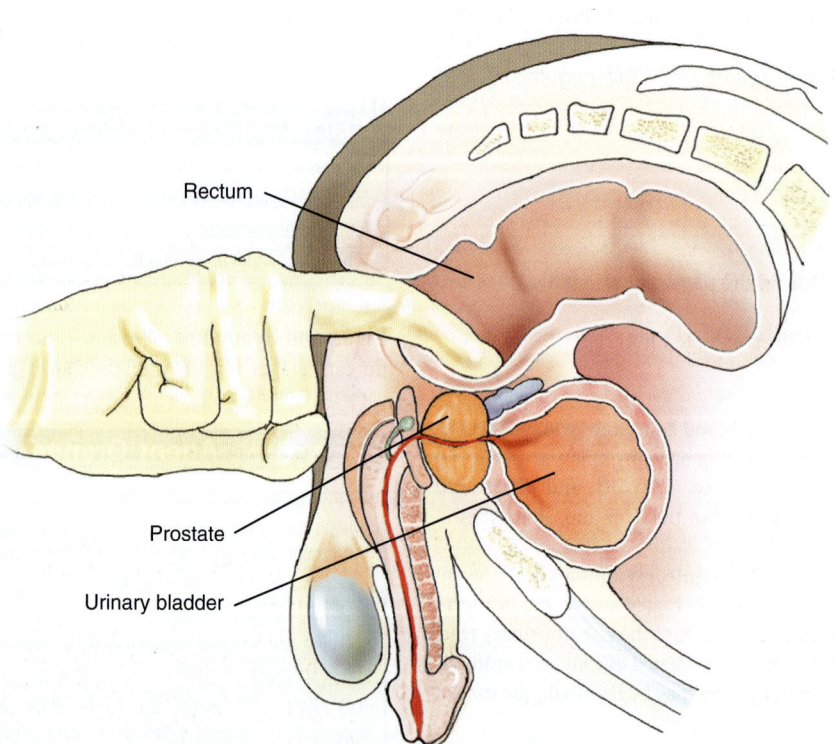

FIG. 6.13 Digital rectal examination to diagnose prostate cancer. (From Shiland B: *Mastering Healthcare Terminology*, ed 5, St. Louis, 2016, Elsevier.)

- Urinary reflux
- Obstruction
- Bladder infection

> **MEDICAL TERMINOLOGY**
> **bacterium** (singular), **bacteria** (plural)
> **-emia**: blood condition
> **septic/o**: infection

Signs and Symptoms. The symptoms of pyelonephritis include the following:
- Fever and chills
- Nausea, vomiting
- Dysuria and frequency
- Low back, side (flank), or groin pain
- Blood in urine, bad smelling urine

The only symptom sometimes seen in infants and young children is the fever. For older adults, confusion and speech difficulties may be present, but other symptoms may not be experienced.

Diagnostic Procedures. After the patient's history has been taken and the physical examination has concluded, the provider will usually order a urinalysis, urine culture, blood culture, and blood work. For the most accurate results, all cultures need to be obtained prior to starting the patient on antibiotics. Additional tests may include the following:
- Ultrasound
- CT scan
- Voiding cystourethrogram
- Digital rectal examination
- Dimercaptosuccinic acid scintigraphy

Treatment. Initially the provider will treat the infection with a broad-spectrum antibiotic. When the blood and urine culture results are known, the provider may have the patient take an antibiotic that is known to kill the pathogen. For severely ill patients, hospitalization, intravenous fluids and antibiotics, and close observation may be required. Repeat cultures may be taken after the antibiotics have been completed to ensure that the infection is gone.

Prognosis. If left untreated, pyelonephritis can have life-threatening complications, including permanent kidney damage and septicemia. With treatment, usually there are no significant complications.

Prevention. Urgent treatment of bladder infections is important to prevent pyelonephritis.

Renal Calculi

Renal **calculi** (KAL kyuh lie) or kidney stones are mineral pebbles that form in the kidney. Small stones may not cause issues. If they grow larger or move into the ureters or renal pelvis, symptoms can occur (Fig. 6.14). If a stone blocks the flow of urine, infection can develop from the backflow of urine. This blockage also can result in **hydronephrosis** (hie droh nuh FROH sis) (Fig. 6.15).

> **VOCABULARY**
> **calculi**: Stones formed in the kidneys, gallbladder, and other parts of the body.
> **hydronephrosis**: A backup of urine that causes dilation of the ureters and calyces; can increase pressure on the nephron units.

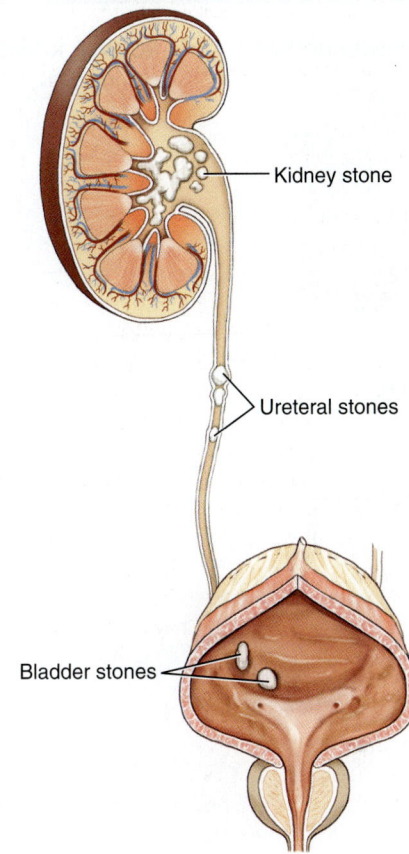

FIG. 6.14 Locations of ureteral calculi. (From Shiland B: *Mastering Healthcare Terminology*, ed 5, St. Louis, 2016, Elsevier.)

Etiology. Renal calculi can occur when high levels of certain minerals collect in the kidney. Common minerals include calcium, oxalate, and uric acid. Calculi can also form if fluid intake is low and the filtrate becomes highly concentrated. The tendency to develop kidney stones runs in families.

Signs and Symptoms. With small stones, the person may not experience symptoms as the stone passes through the urinary tract. With larger stones or stones that cause blockages, symptoms will be experienced. Signs and symptoms of kidney stones include the following:
- Severe constant pain on either side of the lower back
- Urine that smells bad or looks bloody or cloudy
- Dysuria
- Nausea and vomiting
- Fever and chills

Diagnostic Procedures. After the medical history has been taken and the physical exam concluded, urine, blood, and imaging tests are used to diagnose renal calculi. Common tests include the following:
- Urinalysis: can detect blood and minerals in urine; white blood cells and bacteria can indicate an infection
- Blood tests: can indicate high levels of certain minerals that might be causing the stones
- Abdominal x-ray: may be able to show stone, but not all stones are visible based on the size and type of stone

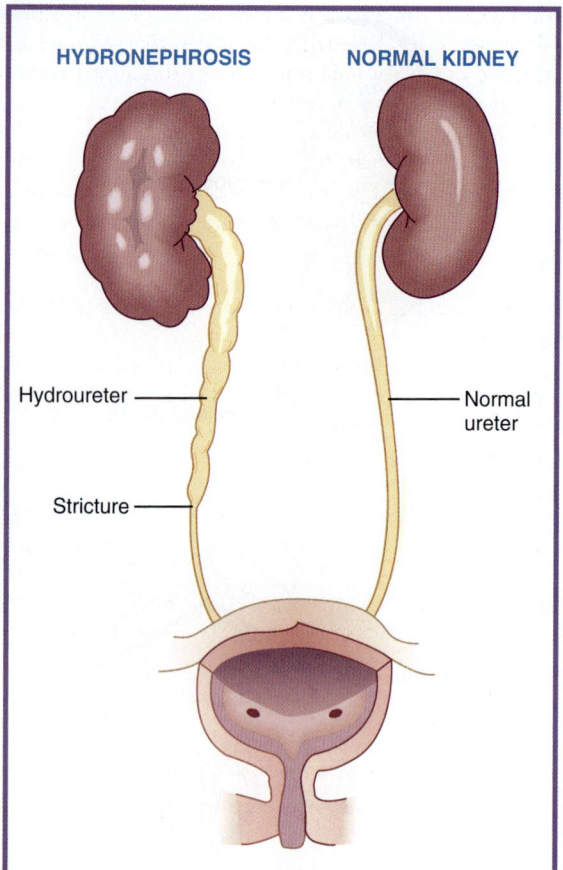

FIG. 6.15 Hydronephrosis. (From Proctor D, et al: *Kinn's The Medical Assistant*, ed 13, St. Louis, 2017, Elsevier.)

TABLE 6.9	Types of Incontinence
Type of Incontinence	Description
Stress incontinence	Leakage of urine from stress on the bladder; caused by obesity, pregnancy, laughing, running, sneezing, coughing, or lifting heavy objects
Urge incontinence	Also called overactive bladder; strong sudden urge (urgency) before the accidental loss of urine.
Overflow incontinence	Most often affects men; the person has difficulty emptying the bladder
Functional incontinence	Caused by a mental or physical disease; leakage occurs before the person can reach the toilet.
Mixed incontinence	Typically impacts females; leakage of urine due to overactive bladder and stress incontinence
Total incontinence	Severest type; constant urine leakage
Bed wetting	Usually seen in children; bladder fills during the night and child does not get up to urinate

CRITICAL THINKING 6.10

Hannah received a call from Zach Backstrom. He stated that he has a kidney stone and wondered if he really needed to strain his urine and have it analyzed in the lab. What might be the benefits to Zach if he continued to strain his urine for the stones?

- CT scan: usually done without contrast, but can use contrast; shows the location and size of the stone

Treatment. Treatment of renal calculi depends on the size, type, and location of the stones. Small stones may pass on their own. Analgesics may be encouraged for the pain and discomfort. Extra fluids are encouraged to flush the stone out. Typically, patients are asked to strain their urine. Kidney stone strainers should be supplied. If the patient finds a stone, it should be placed in a specimen container and be brought to the lab to be analyzed.

If stones are too large to pass or are causing complications, providers will recommend other treatments. *Extracorporeal shock wave lithotripsy* (ESWL) can break up stones in the ureters and kidneys. The shock waves break up the stone, which will then pass without a problem. This is a nonsurgical approach.

Ureteroscopy is a common technique to remove stones. The ureteroscope is threaded up through the bladder and ureter. If the provider sees a stone, it can be removed during the procedure. Sometimes ESWL and ureteroscopy are both done. The stone is broken up before it is removed.

For patients who cannot have ESWL or ureteroscopy due to the stone size or other medical conditions, a surgical procedure can be done to remove the stone. A small incision is made on the lower back and a nephroscope is inserted with other instruments. A *nephrolithotomy* (nef roe lih THOT uh mee) occurs if the stones are removed by the tube. With percutaneous (pur kyoo TAE nee es) nephrolithotripsy (nef roe LITH oe trip see) (PNL), the stones are crushed up and removed using suction.

Prognosis. Kidney stones can usually be removed from the body without causing lasting damage. A stent may be placed in the ureter for a short time to prevent an infection. Patients with a history of renal calculi are at increased risk for developing more stones in the future. Complications of renal calculi include urinary tract infections and kidney damage or scarring.

Prevention. To prevent future stones, dietary changes are recommended. Based on the type of stones experienced, a dietician can help identify foods to limit. For the following stones, these dietary changes are recommended:
- Calcium oxalate stones: reduce sodium, oxalate, and animal protein; consume adequate calcium; oxalate-rich foods include rhubarb, beets, spinach, wheat bran, potato chips, French fries, and nuts.
- Calcium phosphate stones: reduce sodium and animal protein; consume adequate calcium.
- Uric acid stone: reduce animal protein

Urinary Incontinence

Urinary incontinence (in KON tah nens) (UI) is the loss of bladder control causing an accidental loss of urine. There are several types of urinary incontinence (Table 6.9).

Etiology. UI can occur for many reasons, including the following:
- Damage to the nerves that control the bladder
- Weak or overactive bladder muscles
- Diseases that make moving difficult
- Urethral blockages (i.e., from an enlarged prostate)
- Increase in urine volume: diuretics, alcohol, caffeine, and sweeteners can increase the urine volume
- UTI and constipation

Additional conditions that can lead to persistent incontinence include the following:
- Pregnancy, childbirth, and menopause: hormone changes, extra pressure on the bladder, and weakened supportive tissues can lead to UI
- Pelvic surgery: may cause weakening of the pelvic floor muscles
- Prostate diseases: may cause enlargement of the prostate that leads to urinary obstruction
- Aging: with age, the bladder capacity for storing urine decreases
- Obstructions: any conditions that cause an obstruction in the urinary flow
- Neurologic disorders: conditions that limit the nerve signals from the brain to the bladder

Signs and Symptoms. Symptoms include accidental leakage of urine. Based on the type of urinary incontinence, the person may also have the following:
- Urgency
- Constant dribbling and an inability to empty the bladder completely

Diagnostic Procedures. Procedures used to diagnose incontinence include the following:
- Urinalysis: to check for abnormalities
- Bladder diary: record the amount drank, urinated, number of incontinence episodes, and frequency and urgency feelings
- Postvoid residual measurement
- *Urodynamic testing*: bladder is filled with water via a catheter while the bladder pressure is measured
- Cystoscopy, cystogram, and pelvic ultrasound

Treatment. Treatments can vary based on the type of incontinence. Behavior techniques recommended include the following:
- Bladder training: timed delay in urination after feeling the urge
- Double voiding: attempt to empty bladder more completely
- Scheduled toilet trips
- Fluid and diet management to regain control

Kegel exercises and electrical stimulation are used to strengthen pelvic floor muscles. With electrical stimulation, electrodes are inserted into the rectum or vagina and the muscles are stimulated. These treatments can help with stress incontinence.

Medications can also be used as part of the treatment for incontinence. Anticholinergics, mirabegron, alpha-blockers, Botox, and topical estrogen can be used for incontinence (see Table 6.8). Surgical procedures can also be performed to treat certain types of incontinence.

Medical devices can also be used as treatment, including the following:
- *Urethral insert*: a disposable device inserted into the urethra before activities that trigger incontinence
- *Pessary*: a stiff ring inserted into the vagina that holds up the bladder; used for incontinence due to prolapsed bladder
- *Nerve stimulator*: an implanted device that delivers electrical pulses to the nerves that control the bladder

Prognosis. Depending on the type of incontinence, prognoses can vary. The prognosis for incontinence that has been treated is good.

Prevention. Urinary incontinence is not preventable. It is important to decrease the risk factors for incontinence and to do the following:
- Maintain a healthy weight
- Practice Kegel exercises
- Avoid caffeine and alcohol

Additional Urinary System Diseases

Table 6.10 provides information on additional urinary system diseases.

LIFE SPAN CHANGES

At about 10 to 12 weeks after conception, the kidneys start producing urine. While the baby is in utero, the mother's placenta performs most of the kidneys' function until the last few weeks before birth. When babies are born, they have the same number of nephrons as an adult. The nephrons are immature and mature by age 2. A baby's kidneys do

TABLE 6.10 Additional Urinary System Diseases

Disease	Description
Acute tubular necrosis	Rapid destruction of the tubular sections of the nephrons due to blood flow impairment or toxins.
Anterior prolapse	Bulging or dropping of the bladder into the vagina; caused by weakening and stretching of supportive tissues and muscles (Fig. 6.16). Also called cystocele, prolapse, or dropped bladder.
Benign prostatic hyperplasia (BPH)	Benign enlargement of the prostate gland.
Bladder outlet obstruction (BOO)	Blockage at the opening of the bladder or in the urethra.
Diabetes insipidus	Endocrine disorder that causes dehydration and vast quantities of urine to be excreted.
Hydronephrosis	Distention of renal pelvis and calyces due to urinary tract obstruction; caused by a congenital defect or renal calculi.
Interstitial cystitis (IC)	Causes recurring bladder and pelvic region pain and discomfort, frequency, and urgency. Also called painful bladder syndrome (PBS).
Membranous glomerulonephritis	Inflammation occurs in the kidney due to glomerular changes, and large amounts of protein are excreted in the urine. The exact etiology is unknown.
Minimal change disease	Damage occurs to the glomeruli, though the cause is unknown.
Nocturnal enuresis	Bladder fills up during the night and the child is in too deep of a sleep to get up to urinate; can run in families. Also called bed wetting.

Continued

TABLE 6.10 Additional Urinary System Diseases—cont'd

Disease	Description
Peyronie disease (penile curvature)	Scar tissue forms in the penis, causing the penis to curve or bend.
Polycystic kidney disease (PKD)	Inherited disease that causes cysts to form in the kidney.
Prostatitis	Inflammation or swelling of the prostate that can impact urinary flow; can be bacterial or chronic.
Prune belly syndrome (PBS)	Group of genetic birth defects usually occurring in boys; involves: enlarged ureters and bladder, hydronephrosis (kidney swelling), poor development of the abdominal muscles, undescended testicles, and wrinkled skin over the abdomen.
Reflux nephropathy	Urine backflows from the bladder causing kidney damage. Can be due to a ureter defect, obstruction, or swelling.
Ureterocele	End of ureter is malformed and bulges, creating an ureterocele, and may obstruct the ureter or bladder.
Ureteropelvic junction (UPJ) obstruction	Blockage where the ureter joins the kidney, causing kidney swelling.
Urethritis	Inflammation of the urethra due to bacteria, viruses, injury, or chemical sensitivity.
Vesicoureteral (ves ih koe yoo REE tur ul) reflux (VUR)	Urine backs up into the ureter from the bladder due to a malformed or missing valve over the end of the ureter.

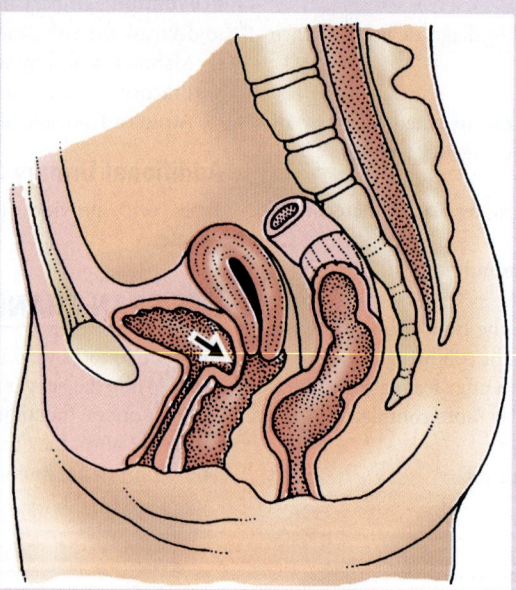

FIG. 6.16 Anterior prolapse. The urinary bladder is displaced downward *(arrow)*, which causes bulging of the anterior vaginal wall. (From Ignatavicius DD, Workman ML: *Medical-Surgical Nursing: Critical Thinking for Collaborative Care,* ed 6, Philadelphia, 2011, Saunders.)

not retain water like adult kidneys do. Thus babies can lose water quickly, especially when they are hot or if they have diarrhea. During childhood, the bladder continues to grow. Bladder control is learned usually between age 2 and 3.

During the adult years, men are more likely to develop kidney stones. This may be attributed to the amount of food men eat. They need to drink more water than women to clear the waste products from the body. Male kidneys also have an increased ability to concentrate urine, a risk factor for kidney stones. Women are at more risk for urinary tract infections than are men. This is attributed to the anatomic differences. Most UTIs are caused by *Escherichia coli,* which is found near the vagina and rectum. The closeness of the urethra to these structures and the shortness of the urethra increase the risk of UTIs.

During pregnancy, the filtration rate increases in women. The number of nephrons remains the same, but the filtration surface increases. This increase allows the kidneys to filter more blood, which is useful with the increased blood flow during pregnancy. In late pregnancy, the bladder may be twice as big. The anatomic and physiologic changes that occur during pregnancy put women at more risk for pyelonephritis at that time.

In older adults, the kidney tissue and number of nephrons are reduced up to 20%. The renal arteries can harden. This causes the kidneys to filter blood slower. The kidneys become less able to regulate water balance. Older adults are at more risk of dehydration when the weather is hot or if they have diarrhea. The bladder wall becomes less stretchy with age. The bladder cannot hold as much urine as before. Bladder muscles weaken. The urethra may be obstructed by an enlarged prostate gland or a prolapse of the bladder or vagina. Older adults are at more risk for chronic kidney disease, UTIs, and incontinence.

CLOSING COMMENTS

When one is working in the ambulatory care field, assisting patients with urinary disorders is common. It is important for the medical assistant to be familiar with the pronunciation and spelling of medical terminology (Tables 6.11, 6.12, and 6.13). Many healthcare providers will use common abbreviations when documenting or talking with other healthcare professionals. It is critical that you know what the abbreviations stand for so that miscommunication does not occur (Table 6.14).

Remember, patients may not be aware of what an abbreviation or a medical term means. It is very important that, when working with patients, medical assistants explain the meaning of commonly used terminology and abbreviations. If patients can understand what is being discussed, they will be more comfortable and adhere to the treatment plan.

In addition to medical terminology and abbreviations, medical assistants need to understand the following:
- The basics of the urinary system (e.g., urinary structures)
- The important roles that the urinary system provides to maintain the homeostasis of the body
- The diseases that impact the urinary system

Having this understanding will help you provide great care to your patients. It will also help you recognize the importance of the different treatments ordered by providers.

TABLE 6.11 Combining and Adjective Forms for Urinary Medical Terminology

Meaning	Combining Form	Adjective Form	Meaning	Combining Form	Adjective Form
artery	arteri/o	arterial	parenchyma	parenchym/o	parenchymal
bladder	cyst/o, vesic/o	cystic, vesical	peritoneum	peritone/o	peritoneal
calyx	calic/o, cali/o, calyc/o	caliceal, calyceal	renal pelvis	pyel/o	
cell	cellul/o	cellular	stroma	strom/o	stromal
cortex	cortic/o	cortical	trigone	trigon/o	trigonal
glomerulus	glomerul/o	glomerular	ureter	ureter/o	ureteral
hilum	hil/o	hilar	urethra	urethr/o	urethral
kidney	nephr/o, ren/o	nephric, renal	urinary meatus	meat/o	meatal
medulla	medull/o	medullary	urine, urinary system	urin/o, ur/o	urinary

From Shiland B: *Mastering Healthcare Terminology*, ed 5, St. Louis, 2016, Elsevier.

TABLE 6.12 Common Prefixes

Prefix	Meaning
extra-	outside
en-	in
par-	beside, near
retro-	backward

From Shiland B: *Mastering Healthcare Terminology*, ed 5, St. Louis, 2016, Elsevier.

TABLE 6.13 Common Suffixes

Suffix	Meaning
-al, -ar, -ic	pertaining to
-ation, -ion	process of

From Shiland B: *Mastering Healthcare Terminology*, ed 5, St. Louis, 2016, Elsevier.

TABLE 6.14 Common Abbreviations Related to Urinary Diseases

Abbreviation	Definition	Abbreviation	Definition
ADH	antidiuretic hormone	GN	glomerulonephritis
ARF	acute renal failure	HD	hemodialysis
BUN	blood urea nitrogen	IVU	intravenous urography
CAPD	continuous ambulatory peritoneal dialysis	KUB	kidney, ureter, and bladder
CCPD	continuous cycling peritoneal dialysis	pH	acidity/alkalinity
CKD	chronic kidney disease	PKD	polycystic kidney disease
CT	computed tomography	SG	specific gravity
DI	diabetes insipidus	TCC	transitional cell carcinoma
DM	diabetes mellitus	UA	urinalysis
ESRD	end-stage renal disease	UTI	urinary tract infection
ESWL	extracorporeal shock wave lithotripsy	VCUG	voiding cystourethrography
GFR	glomerular filtration rate		

From Shiland B: *Mastering Healthcare Terminology*, ed 5, St. Louis, 2016, Elsevier.

CHAPTER REVIEW

The urinary system is composed of two kidneys, two ureters, a bladder, and a urethra. The role of the urinary system is to filter the blood and eliminate the waste through urine. The urine moves down the ureters from the kidneys. The bladder stores to the urine until it is excreted out of the body via the urethra.

Through complex processes the kidney can save or excrete substances, including electrolytes and water. This helps the body maintain homeostasis. The nephrons in the kidney are responsible for filtering the blood and maintaining homeostasis. One end of the nephron is the renal corpuscle, and the rest of the nephron is the tubule. The renal corpuscle includes the glomerulus, which is inside of the Bowman capsule. The pressure of the blood in the glomerulus helps push the substances past the thin walls and into the Bowman capsule. This is the filtration process.

From there, the filtrate moves through the proximal tubule and the Henle loop. During this time, the reabsorption process occurs as substances move from the filtrate back to the blood. Water, glucose, amino acids, urea, and electrolytes (i.e., sodium, chloride, and phosphate) move to the blood. The secretion process also starts as urea moves from the blood to the filtrate to maintain homeostasis. This occurs in the Henle loop. As the filtrate moves farther along the tubule, through the distal tubule and collecting duct, the reabsorption and secretion processes continue. Antidiuretic hormone helps more water to be reabsorbed in these structures. Sodium and chloride are also reabsorbed. The body rids itself of extra substances (e.g., ammonium, potassium, and hydrogen) as the final secretion processes occur. Once the filtrate moves past the collecting ducts, it enters the calyces and renal pelvis. These are extensions of the ureter inside the kidney. The urine then goes into the ureter, bladder, and urethra before it is excreted out of the body.

Urinary diseases were also discussed in this chapter. Common etiologies include age, genetics, and congenital abnormalities, as well as viral, bacterial, and other diseases. Common signs and symptoms of urinary disease include pain, nocturia, dysuria, hematuria, frequency, and urgency. Typical diagnostic tests ordered include digital rectal examination, cystoscopy, ureteroscopy, CT, dimercaptosuccinic acid (DMSA) scan, IVP, postvoid residual urine test, US, voiding cystourethrogram, BUN test, urinalysis, and urine culture. The urinalysis is a CLIA-waived test.

The urinary system changes with age. The kidneys start to function 10 to 12 weeks after conception and mature by age 2. Adult males are more prone to kidney stones, and females are at more risk for UTIs. In older adults, the kidneys become less able to regulate water balance. The bladder muscles weaken, and the urethra can be obstructed by other organs (e.g., the prostate).

SCENARIO WRAP-UP

When Hannah started working with the urology team, she realized she knew very little about the urinary system. She had studied it during her medical assistant program, but she never appreciated what it might be like if her kidneys did not work. She was familiar with kidney cancer and UTIs, but she was amazed at all of the other urinary diseases. As she learned more, she realized that hypertension (high blood pressure) could lead to kidney disease. She also figured out that kidney disease could lead to hypertension.

Looking back over the last weeks, Hannah realized that one of her favorite experiences was working with Mr. Rodgers. He had been on dialysis for the past 5 years and never had a vacation. He wanted to see his new grandson who lived on the East Coast. Hannah found a dialysis unit in the city where he was going to stay. She was able to get him scheduled for 2 weeks' worth of dialysis during his stay. She still can recall Mr. Rodgers' excitement when he realized he could do dialysis while on vacation. He started talking about other trips he was dreaming of taking.

Hannah is excited to continue her work with the urology team. She has learned so much in the short time she has worked with the patients.

7

Reproductive System

LEARNING OBJECTIVES

1. Identify the anatomic location of the major organs of the male and female reproductive systems.
2. Describe the normal function and physiology of the male and female reproductive systems.
3. Discuss diseases and disorders of the reproductive system:
   - Identify the symptoms and etiology for the common pathology related to the male and female reproductive systems.
- Recognize and use terms related to the diagnostic procedures for the male and female reproductive systems.
- Recognize and use the terms related to the therapeutic interventions for the male and female reproductive systems.
4. Compare the structure and function of the male and female reproductive systems across the life span

CHAPTER OUTLINE

1. Opening Scenario, 145
2. You Will Learn, 146
3. Anatomy of the Reproductive System, 146
   a. Male Reproductive System, 146
   b. Female Reproductive System, 147
      i. *Ova and Ovaries, 147*
      ii. *Fallopian Tubes, 147*
      iii. *Uterus, 147*
      iv. *Vagina, 147*
      v. *External Genitalia, 147*
      vi. *Breasts, 147*
4. Physiology of the Reproductive System, 148
   a. Male Reproductive System, 148
   b. Female Reproductive System, 149
      i. *Follicular Phase, 150*
      ii. *Luteal Phase (Secretory Phase), 150*
      iii. *Menstrual Phase, 150*
      iv. *Pregnancy and Delivery, 150*
5. Diseases and Disorders of the Reproductive System, 151
   a. Sexually Transmitted Infections, 151
      i. *Bacterial/Protozoan Sexually Transmitted Infections (Table 7.1), 152*
      ii. *Viral Sexually Transmitted Infections (Table 7.2), 152*
   b. Congenital Disorders of the Male Reproductive System, 152
      i. *Benign Prostatic Hyperplasia, 153*
      ii. *Prostate Cancer, 155*
      iii. *Testicular Cancer, 158*
   c. Cancers of the Female Reproductive System, 158
      i. *Endometriosis, 160*
      ii. *Infections, 161*
      iii. *Additional Female Reproductive System Diseases/Disorders, 161*
6. Life Span Changes, 162
   a. Male Reproductive System, 162
      i. *Pediatrics, 162*
      ii. *Geriatrics, 162*
   b. Female Reproductive System, 162
      i. *Pediatrics, 162*
      ii. *Geriatrics, 162*
7. Closing Comments, 162
8. Chapter Review, 164
9. Scenario Wrap-Up, 165

▶ OPENING SCENARIO

Megan Buhr, CMA (AAMA), is a medical assistant who recently transferred from the urology department to the obstetrics and gynecology department. She is very familiar with the male reproductive system, having spent 5 years working in the urology department, but is less confident about the female reproductive system.

Megan plans to spend some time refreshing her memory of the female reproductive system while comparing it to the male reproductive system, looking at similarities and differences. She knows that sexually transmitted diseases can affect both men and women, but the signs and symptoms can be different. She will work closely with the providers and other team members in her new department and is more than willing to ask questions.

YOU WILL LEARN

1. To recognize and use terms related to the male and female reproductive system.
2. To locate the male and female reproductive system structures.
3. To recognize disease states of the reproductive system, as well as their causes, signs and symptoms, diagnostic processes, treatment, prognoses, and prevention.

ANATOMY OF THE REPRODUCTIVE SYSTEM

Human reproduction requires a male and a female, each of whom contributes half of the genes toward the creation of an embryo. Both male and female anatomy can be divided into two parts:
- *Parenchymal* (puh REN kih mul), or *primary tissue*, which produces sex cells for reproduction
- *Stromal* (STROH mul), or *secondary tissue*, which includes all of the glands, nerves, ducts, and other tissues that serve a supportive function in producing, maintaining, and transmitting these sex cells

Together these types of reproductive tissue, in either sex, are called *genitalia* (jen ih TAIL ee ah). The parenchymal organs that produce the sex cells in both sexes are called **gonads** (GOH nads). The sex cells themselves are called **gametes** (GAM eets) (Box 7.1).

Male Reproductive System

The primary reproductive organs in the male are a pair of **testes** (TESS teez). Each testis is oval in shape and about 4 cm (1.6 inches) long and 2.5 cm (1 inch) wide. The testes are surrounded by a white, fibrous capsule and are suspended together in a sac outside of the body called the *scrotum* (SKROH tum). Testes produce the gametes called **spermatozoa** (spur mat ah ZOH ah).

Spermatozoa are made up of four parts:
- Head: contains the chromosomes
- Acrosome: covers the head and has enzymes to help penetration of the ovum
- Midpiece: contains mitochondria, which provide energy for movement
- Tail [flagellum (flah JEL um)]: used for movement

The spermatozoa are formed in a series of tightly coiled tiny tubes in each testis called the *seminiferous tubules* (sem ih NIFF ur us TOO byools). The formation of sperm (Fig. 7.1) is called *spermatogenesis* (spur mat toh JEN ih sis). The serous membrane that surrounds the front and sides of the testicle is called the *tunica vaginalis testis* (TOON ih kah vaj ih NAL is TESS tis). From the seminiferous tubules, the formed spermatozoa travel to the *epididymis* (eh pih DID ih mis) (plural, *epididymides*), where they mature and are stored. The epididymis is a coiled tube that is almost 6 meters (20 feet) long and rests on top of and behind each testis.

From the epididymis, the spermatozoa move into the *vas deferens* (vas DEH fur ens), also called the *ductus deferens* (DUCK tus DEH fur ens). Each vas deferens is a muscular tunnel about 45 cm (18 inches) long that connects to the base of the epididymis and passes along the side of the testes. Spermatozoa can stay in the vas deferens for several months in an inactive state.

Other anatomic structures found in the male reproductive system include a series of glands that form a fluid that nourishes the sperm. The *seminal vesicles* (SEM ih nul VESS ih kuls), *Cowper* (or *bulbourethral* [bul boh yoo REE thrul]) *glands,* and the *prostate* (PROS tate) *gland* provide fluid either to nourish or to aid in motility and lubrication. The sperm and the fluid together make up a substance called *semen* (SEE men). The *ejaculatory* (ee JACK yoo lah tore ee) *duct* begins where the seminal vesicles join the vas deferens, and this "tube" joins the urethra. The urethra is found within the *penis* (PEE nuss) and transports the semen to the outside of the body. The urethra also transports urine to the outside of the body. The semen exits the body through the tip of the penis, the *glans penis*. Fig. 7.2 shows all of the anatomic structures of the male reproductive system.

CRITICAL THINKING 7.1

To review the anatomy of the male reproductive system, Megan is writing down the process of spermatogenesis, including the all of the structures needed from the formation of the sperm until it leaves the body in semen. Can you do the same?

BOX 7.1 Specialties/Specialists

Andrology (an DROL uh jee) is the study of the male reproductive system, especially in reference to fertility issues. *Urologists* (yoor AW loh jist) treat male urinary and reproductive disorders.

Obstetrics (awb STE triks) is the branch of medicine that deals with pregnancy, labor, and the postpartum period. *Gynecology* (gy neh KAW loh jee) is the study of the female reproductive system. *Obstetricians* (awb steh TRIH shun) are medical doctors who treat women during pregnancy, deliver infants, and follow women through the postpartum period. *Gynecologists* (gy neh KAW loh jist) are medical doctors who diagnose and treat diseases of the female reproductive system. Often times, a provider practices both specialties and is known as an OB/GYN provider.

Midwives are healthcare providers, usually nurses, who assist women through labor and delivery.

Doulas (DOO luh) care for a pregnant mother through labor and delivery or after delivery provides care for the mother and the family after the baby is born.

VOCABULARY

gamete: A mature sexual reproductive cell; spermatozoa or ovum.
gonads: Organs that produce sex cells in both males and females.
spermatozoa (singular, *spermatozoon*): A mature male reproductive cell.
testes (singular, *testis*) or **testicles** (TESS tick kuls): Male gonads.

MEDICAL TERMINOLOGY

-al: pertaining to	**par-**: near
chym/o: juice	**semin/i**: semen
en-: in	**spermat/o**: spermatozoon
epididym/o: epididymis	**spermatozoon** (singular), **spermatozoa** (plural)
-ferous: pertaining to carrying	
-genesis: production	**strom/o**: stroma (supportive tissue)
gonad/o: gonad	**test/o, testicul/o, orchi/o, orchid/o, orch/o**: testis, testicle
gynec/o: female	
-logist: one who specializes in the study of	**testis** (singular), **testes** (plural)
	vas/o: vas deferens, ductus deferens

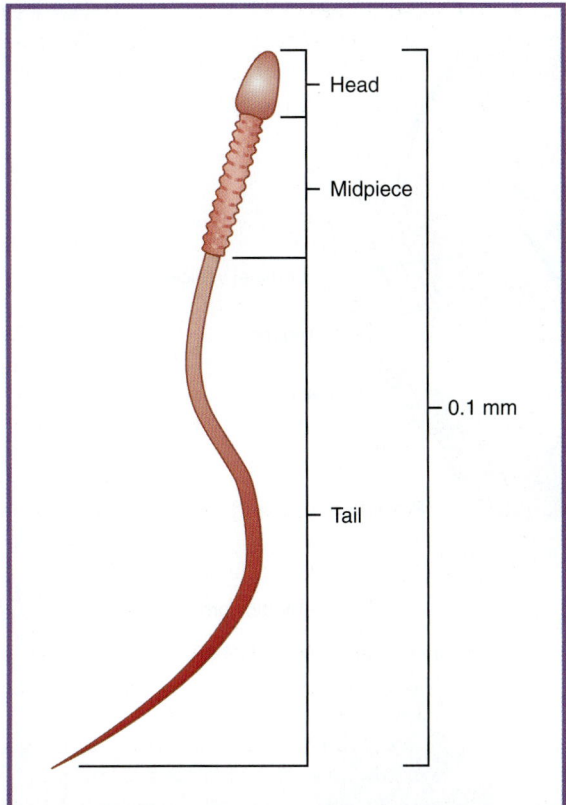

FIG. 7.1 Sperm. (From Proctor D, et al: *Kinn's The Medical Assistant*, ed 13, St. Louis, 2017, Elsevier.)

Female Reproductive System

Ova and Ovaries. In females, the gonads are the *ovaries* (OH vuh reez). They produce *ova*, the female gamete. From *menarche* (meh NAR kee), the first menstrual (MEN stroo al) period, to *menopause* (MEN oh poz), the cessation of menstruation, mature ova are produced. The ovaries are small, almond-shaped, paired organs located on either side of the uterus in the female pelvic cavity. They are attached to the uterus by the ovarian ligaments. The ovaries lie close to the opening of the *fallopian* (fuh LOH pee un) *tubes*, the ducts that convey the ova from the ovaries to the *uterus* (YOO ter us). Fallopian tubes are also called *oviducts* or *uterine tubes*.

Fallopian Tubes. Once the mature ovum has been released, it is drawn into the *fimbriae* (FIM bree ee) (singular, *fimbria*), the feathery ends of the fallopian tube. These tubes are about 1 cm in diameter and about 10 to 12 cm long. The ovum travels down the fallopian tube to the uterus. The fallopian tubes and the ovaries make up what is called the *uterine adnexa* (YOO tuh rin add NECKS ah), or accessory organs, of the uterus.

Uterus. Once the ovum has moved down the fallopian tube, it is secreted into the uterus, or womb. The uterus is a pear-shaped organ that is designed to nurture a developing embryo/fetus. The uterus is composed of three layers:
- Outer layer, called the *perimetrium* (pair ih MEE tree um), or serosa
- Middle or muscle layer, called the *myometrium* (mye oh MEE tree um)
- Lining, called the *endometrium* (en doh MEE tree um)

As a whole, it can be divided into several areas:
- *Corpus* or body: the large central area
- *Fundus* (FUN dus): the raised area at the top of the uterus between the outlets for the fallopian tubes
- *Cervix* (SUR vicks): the narrowed lower area, often referred to as the neck of the uterus; the opening of the cervix is called the *cervical os*

> **CRITICAL THINKING 7.2**
>
> There are many anatomical structures involved in the ovulation process. Can you list them in order, starting with structure that holds the ovum?

Vagina. The *vagina* (vah JY nah) is a 10-cm (4-inch) muscular tube like structure that extends from the uterine cervix to the vulva (the external genitalia). It connects the internal reproductive structures with the external reproductive structures. (Fig. 7.3) The vagina has three purposes:
- Serves as the passageway for endometrium during menstruation
- Receives the penis during intercourse
- Is the birth canal during the delivery of a baby

External Genitalia. The external female genitalia collectively are called the *vulva* (VUL vah); it consists of the following parts:
- *Orifice* (ORE ih fis) or the vaginal opening
- *Hymen* (HYE men) or the membrane covering the opening
- Two folds of skin surrounding the opening:
  - *labia majora* (LAY bee ah muh JOR ah): the larger folds
  - *labia minora* (LAY bee ah min NOR uh): the smaller folds
- *Clitoris* (KLIT uh ris), which is sensitive, erectile tissue
- *Perineum* (pair ih NEE um), which is the area between the opening of the vagina and the anus

The paired glands in the vulva that secrete a mucous lubricant for the vagina are the *Bartholin* (BAR toh lin) *glands*. The *mons pubis* (mons PYOO bis) is a fatty cushion of tissue over the pubic bone (Fig. 7.4).

Breasts. The *breasts*, or *mammary glands*, function to secrete milk. The breast tissue is composed of glandular milk-producing, fatty, and fibrous tissue. The *nipple* of the breast is the *mammary papilla* (MAM

> **MEDICAL TERMINOLOGY**
>
> -arche: beginning
> -ation: process of
> hyster/o, metri/o, metr/o, uter/o: uterus
> men/o, menstru/o: menstruation
> o/o, ov/o, ov/i, ovul/o: ovum, egg
> oophor/o, ovari/o: ovary
> -pause: stop, cease
> salping/o, -salpinx: fallopian tube
> pen/i, phall/o: penis
>
> prostat/o: prostate
> urethr/o: urethra
> vesicul/o: seminal vesicle
> fimbria (singular), fimbriae (plural)
> cervic/o: cervix
> endometri/o: endometrium
> fund/o: fundus
> myometri/o: myometrium
> perimetri/o: perimetrium

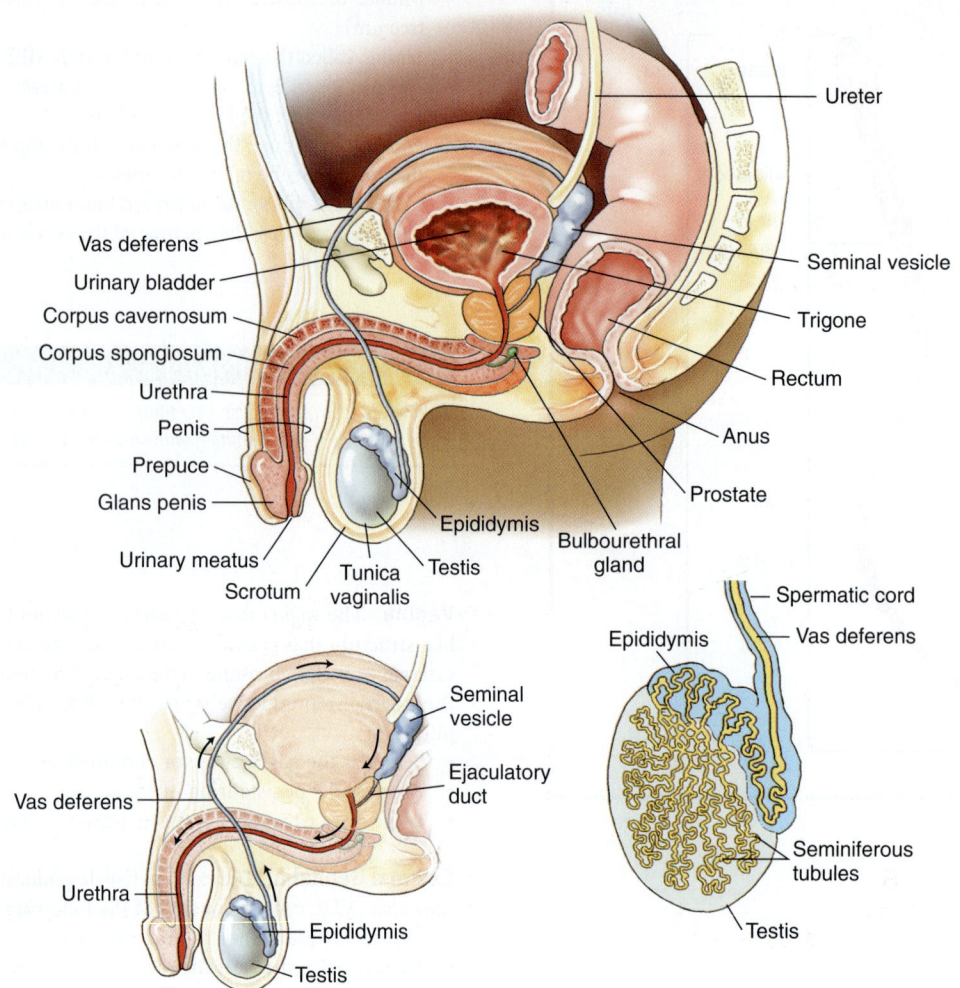

FIG. 7.2 Male reproductive system with insert of sperm production. (From Shiland B: *Mastering Healthcare Terminology*, ed 5, St. Louis, 2016, Elsevier.)

uh ree puh PILL ah), and the darker colored skin surrounding the nipple is the *areola* (ah REE oh lah).

PHYSIOLOGY OF THE REPRODUCTIVE SYSTEM

Male Reproductive System

At **puberty** (PYOO bur tee), the **interstitial** (in ter STIH shal) **cells** in the testicles begin to produce **testosterone** (tess TOSS tur rohn). Testosterone is responsible for the following:

MEDICAL TERMINOLOGY	
areola (singular), **areolae** (plural)	**lact/o, galact/o**: milk
bartholin/o: Bartholin gland	**mamm/o, mast/o**: breast
clitorid/o: clitoris	**papill/o, thel/e**: nipple
colp/o, vagin/o: vagina	**papilla** (singular), **papillae** (plural)
hymen/o: hymen	**perine/o**: perineum
labi/o: labia	**vulv/o, episi/o**: vulva

- Maintaining reproductive structure
- Development of sperm cells
- Development of secondary sex characteristics
  - Deep voice
  - Broad shoulders
  - Narrow hips
  - More body hair

Spermatogenesis starts in the seminiferous tubules where the sperm cells are formed. In addition to testosterone, the process involves *follicle-stimulating hormone* (FALL ih kul) *(FSH)*, secreted by the **pituitary** (pih TOO ih tair ee) **gland**, and promotes the formation of spermatozoa. The pituitary gland also produces *luteinizing* (LOO tin eye zing) *hormone (LH)*, which stimulates the interstitial cells to produce testosterone. Under the influence of these hormones, the sperm cells develop and move in to the epididymis to mature. It is in the epididymis that the spermatozoa develop the ability to move or swim.

To survive and thrive, the sperm are nourished by fluid from a series of glands:
- Seminal vesicles
- Cowper or bulbourethral glands
- Prostate gland

CHAPTER 7 Reproductive System 149

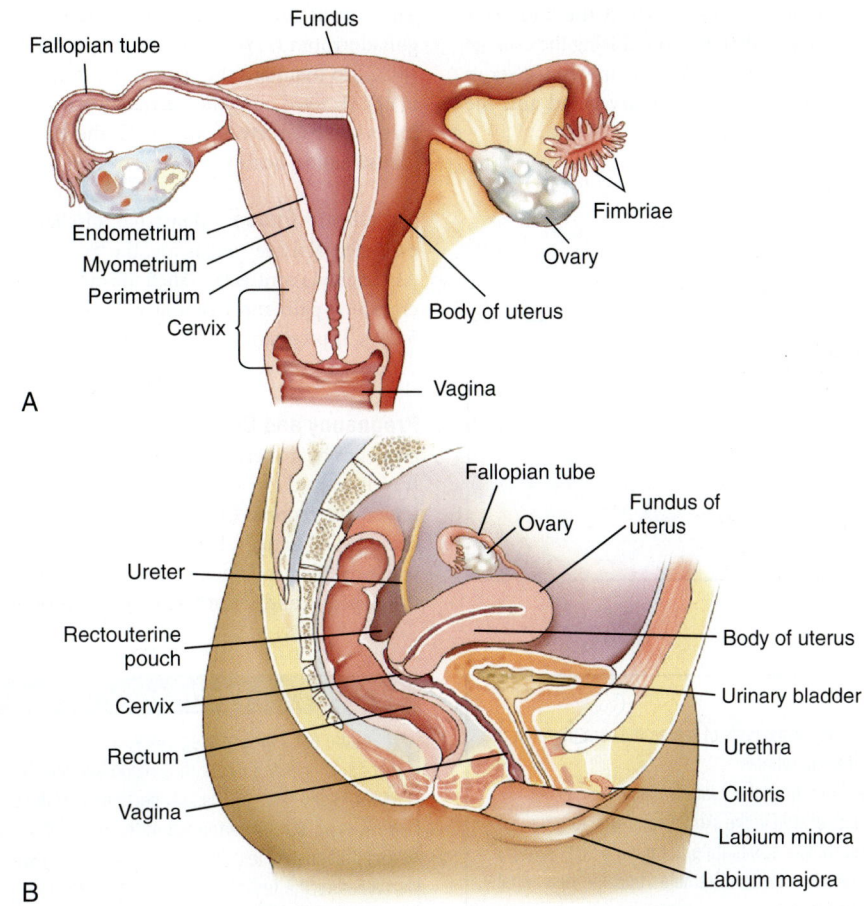

FIG. 7.3 Female reproductive organs. (A) Frontal view. (B) Sagittal view. (From Shiland B: *Mastering Healthcare Terminology*, ed 5, St. Louis, 2016, Elsevier.)

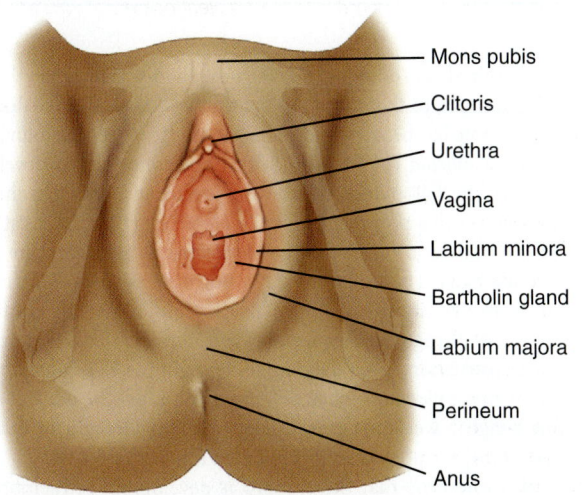

FIG. 7.4 Female external genitalia. (From Shiland B: *Mastering Healthcare Terminology*, ed 5, St. Louis, 2016, Elsevier.)

vascular erectile tissue. There are two columns of *corpora cavernosa* (KORE poor ah kav ur NOH suh) and one of *corpus spongiosum* (KORE puss spun jee OH sum) that fill with blood through the dorsal veins during sexual arousal. During ejaculation, the sperm exit through the enlarged tip of the penis, the *glans penis*. At birth, the glans penis is surrounded by a fold of skin called the *prepuce* (PREE pyoos), or *foreskin*. The removal of this skin is termed *circumcision* (sur kum SIH zhun).

CRITICAL THINKING 7.3

Megan was working with one of her new coworkers, June, who had not worked in an area that dealt with the male reproductive anatomy. June remembered from school that the penis actually had multiple columns, but could not recall what the medical terminology was for each. Can you name the three structures using the correct medical terminology?

The sperm and the fluid together make up a substance called *semen*. The *ejaculatory* (ee JACK yoo lah tore ee) *duct* begins where the seminal vesicles join the vas deferens, and then it joins the urethra. Once the sperm reach the *urethra*, they travel out through the shaft, or body, of the *penis* (PEE nuss), which is composed of three columns of highly

Female Reproductive System

When a girl enters puberty, one of the many changes that occur is *menarche* (meh NAR kee), or the beginning of the menstrual cycle. *Menstruation* (men stroo AA shun) is a normal body process that occurs

in every female. It is the physiologic means by which the body rids itself of the thickened endometrial wall that develops during the average 28-day cycle. The menstrual (MEN stroo uh l) cycle involves a series of events controlled by hormones from the pituitary gland and the ovaries. The cycle is divided into three phases:
- The follicular (fuh LIK yuh ler) phase
- The luteal (LOO tee uh l) phase
- The menstrual phase

> **MEDICAL TERMINOLOGY**
> **a-:** no, not without
> **-al:** pertaining to
> **fet/o:** fetus
> **gravid/o, -gravida, -cyesis:** pregnancy
> **interstiti/o:** spaces between
> **men/o, menstru/o:** menstruation
> **-trophy:** process of nourishment, development

> **VOCABULARY**
> **interstitial cells:** Testosterone-secreting cells of testes that are found in the spaces between the seminiferous tubules.
> **ovulation:** The release of the ovum from the ovarian follicle.
> **pituitary gland:** Endocrine gland located in the skull responsible for producing luteinizing hormone (LH) and follicle-stimulating hormone (FSH).
> **puberty:** The stage of life in which males and females become functionally capable of sexual reproduction.
> **testosterone:** Male sex hormone produced by the interstitial cells in the testes.

Follicular Phase. The follicular phase is also called the proliferative (pruh LIF ruh tiv) phase. The hypothalamus (hy poh THAL ah mus) begins the follicular phase by secreting gonadotropin-releasing (goh nad uh TROH pin) hormone (GnRH). This hormone stimulates the anterior pituitary to release FSH and LH. These hormones mature a graafian follicle (GRAH fee uh n FOL l kuh l) in an ovary that contains an ovum. The mature ovarian follicle secretes estrogen, which stimulates the growth of the endometrium. It takes approximately 9 days for the graafian follicle to ripen and bulge out from the ovarian wall. The ovarian wall becomes thinner as the follicle enlarges until it bursts, releasing the ovum into the abdominal cavity. Expulsion of the ovum ends the follicular phase. The fallopian fimbriae (FIM bree uh) begin their wavelike motion to fan the ovum into the fallopian tube. The rupture spot on the ovary, now called the *corpus luteum (KAWR puh s LOO tee uh m)*, begins to secrete progesterone. Ovulation causes a rise in body temperature, and some women experience cramping and tenderness in the lower abdominal area at this time as a result of the rupture of the graafian follicle.

Luteal Phase (Secretory Phase). The luteal phase is also called the secretory (SEE kreh tor ee) phase. Once ovulation is complete, the luteal phase begins. During this phase, progesterone secreted by the corpus luteum causes extensive growth of the endometrium as it prepares for a possible pregnancy (Box 7.2). If conception occurs, the corpus luteum continues to secrete progesterone until the placenta is well established.

The corpus luteum can secrete progesterone and human chorionic gonadotropin (HYOO muh n kor ee AW nik goh nad oh TROH pin) (hCG) to maintain the pregnancy. If conception does not occur, hCG is not secreted, and the corpus luteum **atrophies**. Without increased levels of progesterone and hCG, the endometrium breaks down, and menstruation begins.

Menstrual Phase. Menstrual discharge is made up of necrotic endometrial tissue, mucus, and the blood from endometrial engorgement. As the uterus contracts to shed the excess tissue, a woman may experience cramping pain and irritability. This phase usually lasts approximately 5 days. If pregnancy does not occur, the endometrium is shed and the process starts over.

Pregnancy and Delivery. Pregnancy begins with the fertilization of an ovum by a spermatozoon, often in the fallopian tube, as the ovum travels toward the uterus (Fig. 7.5). Conception is usually the result of sexual intercourse (also called *copulation* [kop yuh LEY shuh n] or *coitus* [KOH ih tus]). However, other methods of conception are possible if the couple has difficulty conceiving. These methods are discussed in the Diseases and Disorders of the Reproductive System section.

> **BOX 7.2 Pregnancy Tests**
>
> There are two types of pregnancy tests. One is done with a urine sample, and the other one is done with a blood sample. Both tests are looking for hCG levels. Blood tests are usually performed at the provider's office or laboratory. Urine tests can be performed at the provider's office, or the patient may do a home pregnancy test.
> Whether the test is performed at home or at the office, the process is very much the same. A sample of urine is placed on the test stick and then one waits for the results. Some test sticks show a plus sign for a positive test and minus sign for a negative test. Other tests actually display the word *pregnant* for a positive test or *not pregnant* for a negative test.

The fertilized egg, or *zygote* (ZYE gote), divides as it moves through the fallopian tube to the uterus. In the first few days after fertilization, when the zygote has become a solid ball of cells from repeated divisions, it is called a *morula* (MAWR oo luh). As it continues to develop, it moves from the fallopian tube into the uterus and implants into the uterine wall. At this point, it is called a *blastocyst* (BLAS tuh sist).

During implantation, the zygote functions as an endocrine gland by secreting hCG. The function of the hormone is to stop the corpus luteum from deteriorating. The corpus luteum allows the continued production of estrogen and progesterone to support the pregnancy and prevent menstruation. From the third to the eighth week of development, the organism is called an *embryo* (EM bree oh). From the ninth through the thirty-eighth week of development (a normal length for *gestation* [jes TAY shun], or pregnancy), it is called a *fetus* (FEE tus).

At the same time that the embryo is developing, extraembryonic membranes are forming to sustain the pregnancy:
- The *amnion* (AM nee on) and the *chorion* (KORE ee on) form the inner and outer sacs that contain the embryo (Fig. 7.6)
- The fluid that forms inside the amnion is the *amniotic* (am nee AH tick) *fluid*. It cushions the embryo, protects it against temperature changes, and allows it to move.
- The *placenta* (plah SEN tah) is a highly vascular structure that acts as a physical communication between the mother and the embryo.
- The *umbilical* (um BILL ih kul) *cord* is the tissue that connects the embryo to the placenta (and hence to the mother). When the baby

CRITICAL THINKING 7.4

After Megan and June had reviewed the male reproductive anatomy, Megan asked June to help her recall the phases of the menstrual cycle. Write down the different phases of the menstrual cycle and what occurs during each phase.

DISEASES AND DISORDERS OF THE REPRODUCTIVE SYSTEM

There are many diseases and disorders that are related to the male and female reproductive systems. The most common of these are discussed in the following section starting with sexually transmitted infections and moving on to diseases and disorders specific to the male reproductive system and finally to those specific to the female reproductive system.

Sexually Transmitted Infections

Many pathogens cause sexually transmitted infections (STIs), but what they have in common is that all of them are most efficiently transmitted by *sexual contact*. Sexual contact refers to intercourse in addition to any contact between the genitals of one person and the body of another person. No one is immune to these diseases. An individual can be infected with more than one at a time. No cure is available for viral

is delivered, the umbilical cord is cut, and the baby is then dependent on his or her own body for all physiologic processes. The remaining "scar" is the *umbilicus* (um BILL i kus), or navel. The delivery of an infant is termed *parturition* (par tur RIH shun).

If two eggs are released and fertilized, the resulting twins will be termed *fraternal*, because they will be no more or less alike in appearance than brothers or sisters occurring in different pregnancies. If, however, one of the fertilized eggs divides and forms two infants, these are *identical* twins, who share the same appearance and genetic material.

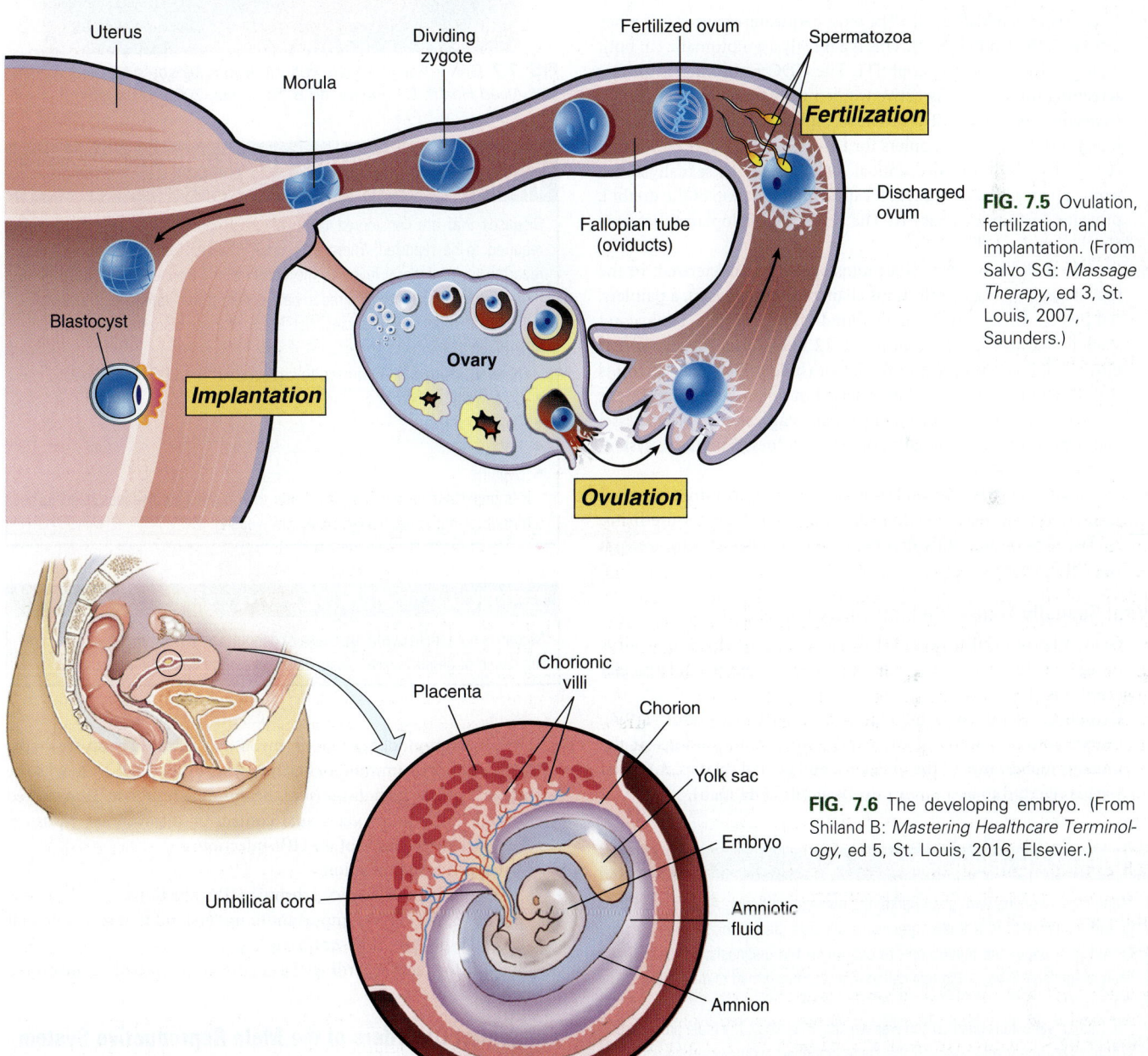

FIG. 7.5 Ovulation, fertilization, and implantation. (From Salvo SG: *Massage Therapy*, ed 3, St. Louis, 2007, Saunders.)

FIG. 7.6 The developing embryo. (From Shiland B: *Mastering Healthcare Terminology*, ed 5, St. Louis, 2016, Elsevier.)

> **MEDICAL TERMINOLOGY**
> **amni/o, amnion/o, -amnios:** amnion
> **chori/o, chorion/o:** chorion
> **nat/o:** birth, born
> **omphal/o, umbilic/o:** umbilicus
> **part/o, -para, -partum, -tocia:** parturition
> **placent/o:** placenta

STIs, such as human immunodeficiency virus (HIV) infection, herpes, and venereal warts. Bacterial infections are increasingly becoming resistant to antibiotic therapy. STIs frequently are asymptomatic in men, although they can cause serious health problems and are infectious regardless of whether symptoms are present.

Bacterial/Protozoan Sexually Transmitted Infections (Table 7.1)

- *Chlamydia* (klah MID ee ah): The most frequently reported infectious disease in the United States. This is a mostly asymptomatic (in both males and females) bacterial STI. The CDC recommends annual screening for all sexually active women who are older than 25.
- *Gonorrhea* (gaw noh REE ah): The second most commonly reported infectious disease. The Centers for Disease Control and Prevention (CDC) has recommended annual screening for all sexually active women who are older than 25. It causes inflammation of the urethra, prostate, rectum, or pharynx. The cervix and fallopian tubes may also be involved (Fig. 7.7).
- *Syphilis* (SIF ih lis): This is a multistage STI characterized, in the first stage, by a highly infectious chancre (SHANG ker), a painless, red pustule (PUS tyool) usually found on the genitals. The second stage is characterized by a rash 2 to 12 weeks after the chancre. If untreated, it can progress to the latent (hidden) stage. A person is still contagious during the latent stage but does not show any signs of having the disease. During the tertiary stage, serious blood vessel and heart problems, mental disorders, blindness, and nerve system problems can occur.
- *Trichomoniasis* (trik oh moh NY ah sis): The most common nonviral sexually transmitted infection. In some men it causes urethritis, epididymitis, or prostatitis. In some women it causes a frothy, greenish vaginal discharge.

Viral Sexually Transmitted Infections (Table 7.2)

- Genital herpes (HER peez) (HSV-2): A form of the herpes virus transmitted through sexual contact causing recurring painful vesicular eruptions (Fig. 7.8).
- Genital warts, human papilloma (pap ih LOH mah) virus (HPV): Causes common warts of the hands and feet and lesions of the mucous membranes of the oral, anal, and genital cavities. A genital wart is referred to as a *condyloma* (kon dih LOH mah).

> **CRITICAL THINKING 7.5**
>
> Megan was working with Jean Burke, the nurse practitioner. A patient came in with complaints of a frothy, greenish discharge. Jean took a sample and looked at it under the microscope to determine the diagnosis. What is the likely diagnosis? What is the test called that was performed to determine the diagnosis?
>
> In Megan's previous position she was working in urology. If a male presented in that department and received the same diagnosis what would his signs/symptoms be?

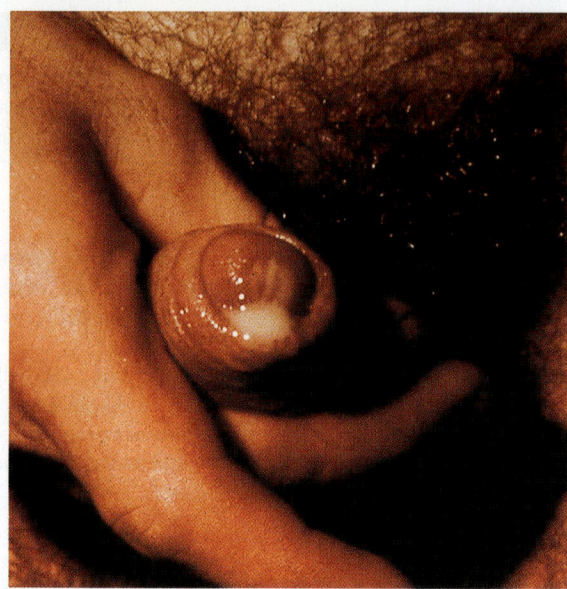

FIG. 7.7 Gonorrhea in a male patient. (From *Mosby's Medical Nursing and Allied Health Dictionary*, ed 8, St. Louis, 2009, Mosby.)

> **BOX 7.3 Reporting of Sexually Transmitted Infections**
>
> Diseases that are considered to be of great public health importance are required to be reported. There are some diseases that are required to be reported at the federal level, to the Centers for Disease Control (CDC), and there are others that are required to be reported at the state level. Most states will have a "reportable diseases" list. Many of those diseases are also on the federal list.
>   There are many STIs that have to be reported. The CDC list includes:
> - Chlamydia trachomatis
> - Gonorrhea
> - HIV
> - Syphilis
>
>   It is important for medical assistants to know which diseases need to be reported for the state in which they are working.

> **CRITICAL THINKING 7.6**
>
> Megan is not familiar with the cause of genital warts. How would you describe the cause of genital warts? Also, how can genital warts be prevented?

- Human immunodeficiency (ih myoo noh deh FIH shun see) virus (HIV)/acquired immunodeficiency syndrome (AIDS): Attacks the helper T cells, which diminishes the immune response. Transmitted through body fluids via sexual contact or intravenous exposure. There are three stages of an HIV infection:
  - Stage 1: acute infection
  - Stage 2: clinical latency (chronic HIV infection)
  - Stage 3: AIDS (It is important to understand that someone that is HIV positive does not have AIDS.)

See Box 7.3 for facts regarding the reporting of sexually transmitted infections.

Congenital Disorders of the Male Reproductive System

Males can be born with a number of conditions that can cause problems with reproductive system. The most common are listed in Table 7.3.

TABLE 7.1 Bacterial/Protozoan Sexually Transmitted Infections

Feature	Chlamydia	Gonorrhea	Syphilis	Trichomoniasis
Etiology	Chlamydia trachomatis (bacterium)	Neisseria gonorrhea (bacterium)	Treponema pallidum (spirochete bacteria)	Trichomonas vaginalis (protozoon)
Signs and symptoms—male	Maybe asymptomatic; Dysuria; Itching and thin watery discharge from penis; Testicular pain	Dysuria and urinary frequency; Thick, cloudy, or bloody discharge from penis	Painless lesion (chancre); Serous discharge from chancre; Lymphadenopathy	Asymptomatic; Itching or irritation inside penis; Burning after urination or ejaculation; Some discharge from penis
Signs and symptoms—female	Asymptomatic; Dysuria; Urinary frequency; Abdominal pain; Increased vaginal discharge	Dysuria; Urinary frequency; Abdominal pain; Increased vaginal discharge	Painless lesion (chancre); Serous discharge from chancre; Lymphadenectomy	Asymptomatic; Urinary frequency, urgency; Dysuria; Frothy yellow-green vaginal discharge; Pruritus
Diagnostic procedures	Testing a first-catch urine specimen (male); Collecting swab specimens from the endocervix or vagina (female); Nucleic acid amplification test (NAAT)	Urethral swab (male); Endocervical swab or vaginal swab (female); Urine specimen (both male and female); NAAT; Gram stain for symptomatic males	Rapid plasma regain (RPR), Venereal Disease Research Laboratory (VDRL), fluorescent treponemal antibody absorption (FTA-ABS)	NAAT; Wet mount preparation of the vaginal discharge examined under a microscope; Culture of discharge; Retest 3 months after treatment
Treatment, medications	Curable with antibiotic therapy; single dose of azithromycin or 1 week of doxycycline	Curable with antibiotic therapy; ceftriaxone, azithromycin, or doxycycline	Penicillin G; if patient is allergic to penicillin, doxycycline or tetracycline	Single dose of metronidazole or tinidazole; partner must be treated
Prognosis	Good with early antibiotic treatment. If untreated or improperly treated: • Male: long term complications are uncommon but may include epididymitis • Female: may cause endometritis, pelvic inflammatory disease (PID), and urethritis	Good with early antibiotic treatment. If untreated or improperly treated: • Male: acute or chronic prostate gland inflammation or testicular infection • Female: may cause sterility, ectopic pregnancy, endometritis, PID, and urethritis	Good with early antibiotic treatment. If untreated or improperly treated: • Both males and females can experience serious blood vessel and heart problems, mental disorders, blindness, nerve system problems • Female: can infect fetus via the placenta, resulting in congenital syphilis	Cure rate is 90% if all sexual partners are treated at the same time. If untreated or improperly treated: • Male: increased risk of getting other STIs • Female: can increase risk of acquiring HIV infection; in pregnant women may cause premature rupture of the membranes
Prevention	Abstinence, limiting of the number of sex partners, male condoms, female condoms, cervical diaphragms (for cervical gonorrhea, chlamydia, and trichomoniasis)			

Benign Prostatic Hyperplasia. As men age, the cells of the prostate gland that surround the urethra can start to reproduce more rapidly, causing the organ to enlarge (hyperplasia [hye per PLEY zhuh]). This nonmalignant process is seen in about half of men over the age of 50 and in more than 90% of men in their 70s and 80s.

Etiology. The enlarged prostate compresses the urethra. The urine is unable to leave the bladder, which can lead to cystitis. This compression leads to much difficulty with urination, causing hesitancy and dribbling.

Signs and symptoms. Signs and symptoms of benign prostatic hyperplasia (BPH) include the following:
- Urinary urgency and frequency
- Difficulty starting urination

VOCABULARY
NAATs: Nucleic acid amplification tests (NAATs) are screening tests for chlamydia trachomatis, Neisseria gonorrhoeae infections, and trichomoniasis. These tests can detect small amounts of DNA or RNA in test samples.

MEDICAL TERMINOLOGY
an-: without
chord/o: cord
crypt/o: hidden
-ism: condition

MEDICAL TERMINOLOGY

epi- : above
hypo-: below
-osis: abnormal condition
-spadias: a rent or tear

CRITICAL THINKING 7.7

A patient brought in her newborn baby boy when she came in for her postpartum visit and he looked very much like a baby who Megan had worked with in her previous position. That baby had a condition where the urethral opening was on the dorsal side of the penis. What is the name of that condition? What is the name of the condition where the urethral opening is on the underside of the penis? What is the treatment for each of those conditions?

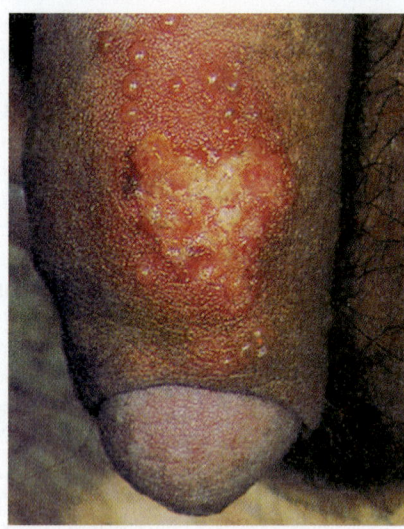

FIG. 7.8 Genital herpes. (From *Mosby's Medical Nursing and Allied Health Dictionary*, ed 8, St. Louis, 2009, Mosby.)

- Unable to empty bladder
- Dribbling
- Hematuria
- Repeated urinary tract infections

Diagnostic procedures. Procedures to diagnose BPH include the following:

- *Digital rectal exam (DRE)*: provider inserts a lubricated, gloved finger in the rectum to palpate the prostate (Fig. 7.12)
- Prostate-specific antigen (PSA) blood test to rule out prostate cancer
- Blood tests to evaluate kidney function
- Biopsy to rule out prostate cancer
- Urinalysis
- Ultrasound
- Cystoscopy

Treatment. Treatments for BPH include the following:
- Medications:

TABLE 7.2 Viral Sexually Transmitted Infections

Feature	Genital Herpes	Genital Warts	Human Immunodeficiency Virus (HIV)/Acquired Immunodeficiency Syndrome (AIDS)
Etiology	Herpes simplex virus-2 (HSV-2)	Human papilloma (pap ih LOH mah) virus (HPV)	Human immunodeficiency virus (HIV)
Signs and symptoms: male Signs and symptoms: female	Painful genital vesicles and ulcers; erythema and pruritus; tingling or shooting pain 1–2 days before outbreak; cycle through episodes	Elevated papillomas on external genitalia; single or cluster of warts	Flulike symptoms, also referred to as acute retroviral syndrome (ARS) or primary HIV infection: Fever Swollen glands Sore throat Rash, muscle and joint aches and pains Headache
Diagnostic procedures		Examination and possible biopsy of warts	Enzyme-linked immunosorbent assay (ELISA); if positive, a Western blot test done to confirm Saliva test Viral load test
Treatment, medications	No cure, but antiviral therapy during episodes shortens duration of lesions; acyclovir, famciclovir, valacyclovir	Topical medications; podofilox solution, imiquimod cream, cryosurgery, electrocautery	Antiretroviral (ART) medications: non-nucleoside reverse transcriptase inhibitors, nucleoside reverse transcriptase inhibitors, protease inhibitors, fusion inhibitors, integrase inhibitors
Prognosis	No cure Antiviral drugs can shorten the duration of the episode	No cure Female: HPV can cause cervical cancer	If HIV is left untreated it will develop into AIDS No cure
Prevention		HPV vaccine; three-dose series	
	Abstinence, limiting of the number of sex partners, male condoms, female condoms		

- Alpha blockers to relax the bladder neck muscles and muscle fibers in the prostate to make urination easier
- 5-alpha reductase inhibitors to shrink the prostate
- A combination of the two
- *Transurethral resection of the prostate (TURP) surgery* (Fig. 7.13): a lighted scope is inserted into the urethra and all but the outer part of the prostate is removed
- *Laser therapy*: a high-energy laser is used to destroy the overgrown prostate tissue

Prognosis and prevention. Most patients see improvement with treatment. If medications are used, the symptoms are reduced but can return if the medications are stopped. There is no way to prevent BPH.

Prostate Cancer. Cancer of the prostate is common in men over age 50 and ranks as the second highest cause of cancer deaths in men, behind lung cancer. Prostate cancer is usually slow growing and initially remains confined to the prostate gland. There are aggressive types of prostate cancer that can spread quickly. Early detection provides the best chance of successful treatment.

Etiology. Prostate cancer starts when the DNA in the cells of the prostate mutate and cause these cells to grow and divide more rapidly than normal cells. Researchers have not determined what causes the mutation of the DNA. They have determined that the following factors can put someone at greater risk for prostate cancer:
- Age: The risk of prostate cancer increases as you age.
- Black race: Black men are at a greater risk for developing prostate cancer, and it is more likely to be aggressive or advanced.
- Family history of prostate or breast cancer: If someone has a family member that has had prostate cancer the risk increases. Also, if there is a family member with the genes that increase the risk of breast cancer or if there is a strong family history of breast cancer, the risk of developing prostate cancer increases.

TABLE 7.3 Congenital Disorders of the Male Reproductive System

Feature	Anorchism (AN or kih zum)	Chordee (KORE dee)	Cryptorchidism (kript OR kid iz um)
Description	Condition of being born without a testicle; may also be an acquired condition due to trauma or disease	Congenital defect resulting in a downward (ventral) curvature of the penis due to a fibrous band (cord) of tissue along the corpus spongiosum; most noticeable during an erection; often associated with hypospadias (Fig. 7.9)	Condition in which the testicles fail to descend into the scrotum before birth; also called cryptorchism (Fig. 7.10)
Treatment	Artificial (prosthetic testicle implants; male hormones (androgens)	Surgery, ideally before the age of 2	May resolve spontaneously; orchiopexy (OR kee oh pek see): repositioning the undescended testicle and suture it within the scrotum

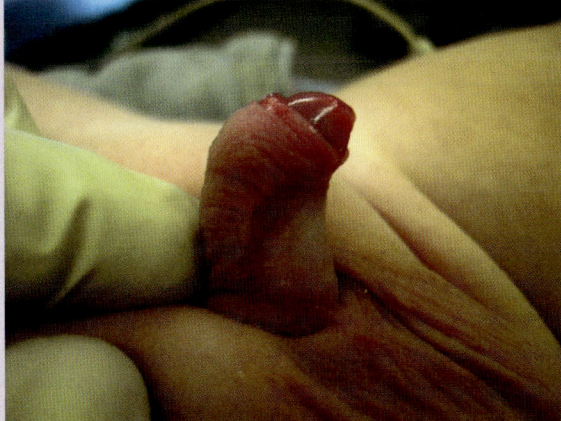

Fig. 7.9 Chordee. (From Shiland B: *Mastering Healthcare Terminology*, ed 5, St. Louis, 2016, Elsevier.)

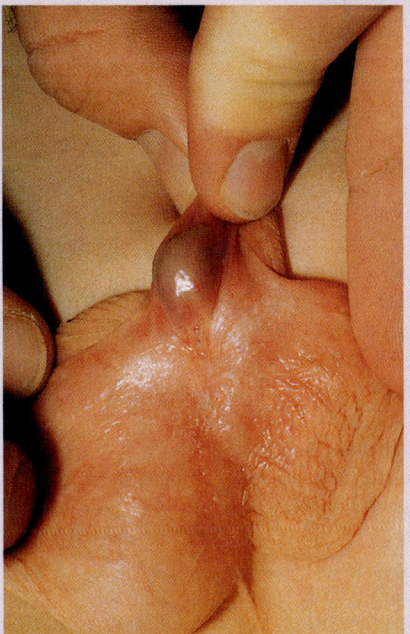

Fig. 7.10 Cryptorchidism. (From Zitelli BJ, Davis HW: *Atlas of Pediatric Physical Diagnosis*, ed 5, St. Louis, 2007, Mosby.)

Continued

TABLE 7.3 Congenital Disorders of the Male Reproductive System—cont'd

Feature	Anorchism (AN or kih zum)	Chordee (KORE dee)	Cryptorchidism (kript OR kid iz um)
Prognosis	Good, with treatment	Good with treatment; if not corrected surgically, may cause problems with sexual function in adulthood	Good
Feature	Epispadias (eh pee SPAY dee ahs)	Hypospadias (hye poh SPAY dee ahs)	Phimosis (fih MOH sis)
Description	Urethral opening on the dorsum (top) of the penis rather than on the tip; also called *hyperspadias*	Urethral opening on the underside of the penis instead of on the tip (Fig. 7.11); may be acquired as a result of the disease process	Congenital condition of tightening of the prepuce around the glans penis so that the foreskin cannot be retracted
Treatment	Surgery to reposition the urethral opening	Surgery to reposition the urethral opening	Steroid ointment applied locally; circumcision
Prognosis	Good	Good	Good

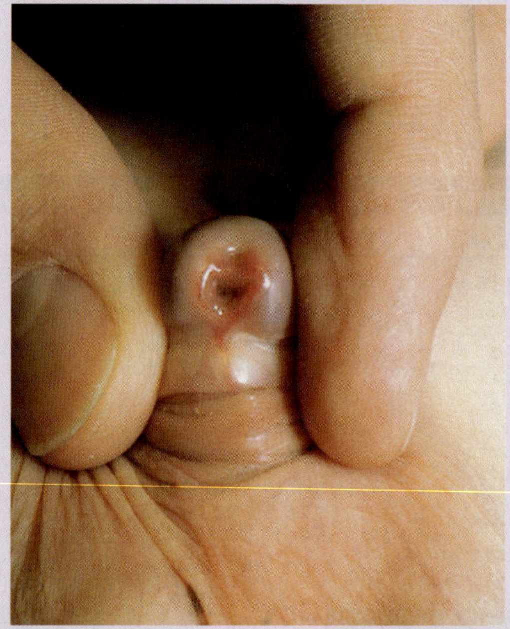

Fig. 7.11 Hypospadius. (From Shiland B: *Mastering Healthcare Terminology*, ed 5, St. Louis, 2016, Elsevier.)

- Obesity: Obese men who are diagnosed with prostate cancer may be more likely to have advanced disease that is more difficult to treat.

Signs and symptoms. In the early stages of prostate cancer, the patient is asymptomatic. Symptoms may not develop until the cancer has spread outside of the prostate gland. When symptoms are present they may include the following:
- Decreased force of the stream of urine
- Weak, dribbling, or interrupted flow of urine
- Blood in the urine or semen
- Frequent urination, especially at night (nocturia)
- Discomfort in the pelvic area
- Bone pain
- Painful ejaculation
- Erectile dysfunction

Diagnostic procedures. The first indication of a problem may come with a routine DRE, when the provider notices a firm or irregular area in the prostate. The primary screening tool for cancer of the prostate is the prostate-specific antigen (PSA) blood test. Blood levels of PSA, a protein produced by the prostate, are elevated with prostatitis, BPH, and cancer of the prostate. The higher the PSA level, the more likely it is that the patient has prostate cancer. However, because the PSA level can be elevated with other disorders, one abnormal screening value is not enough to diagnose cancer. The test should be repeated over time, and if levels continue to rise, further diagnostic studies should be done. If tests indicate cancer, the provider may order a transrectal ultrasound, which involves inserting a small transducer into the rectum to bounce sound waves off the prostate, creating a picture. The ultrasound pictures are used to help pinpoint areas of concern and then a tissue biopsy may be done. If the transrectal ultrasound does not indicate any suspicious areas, the provider takes multiple biopsies (usually eight) from different sections of the prostate gland. Tissue samples are sent to the pathologist for analysis and diagnosis.

If the biopsies show that cancer is present, the provider may order additional imaging tests to determine if the cancer has spread. The additional tests may include those listed here:
- Bone scan
- Ultrasound
- Computerized tomography (CT) scan

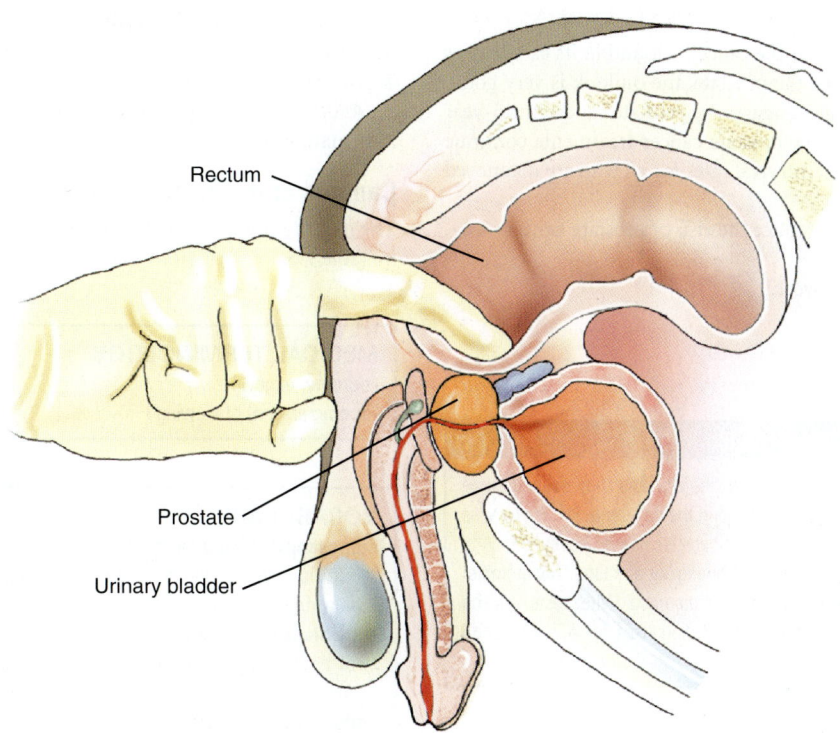

FIG. 7.12 Digital rectal exam (DRE). (From Shiland B: *Mastering Healthcare Terminology*, ed 5, St. Louis, 2016, Elsevier.)

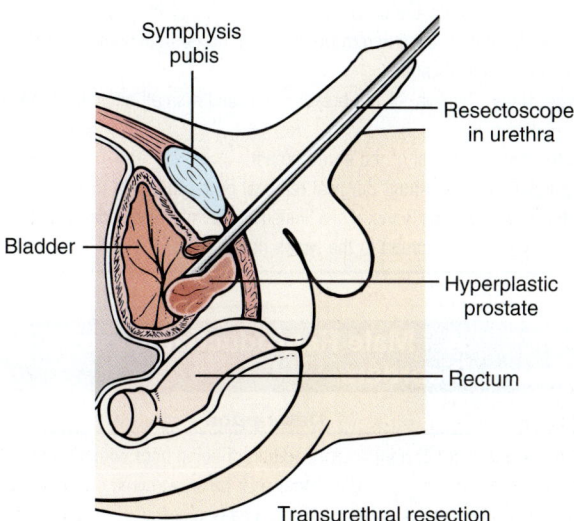

FIG. 7.13 Transurethral resection of the prostate (TURP). (From Shiland B: *Mastering Healthcare Terminology*, ed 5, St. Louis, 2016, Elsevier.)

- Magnetic resonance imaging (MRI)
- Positron emission tomography (PET) scan

Treatment. The treatment plan will depend on how fast the cancer is growing and the patient's overall health. If it is the very early stage prostate cancer, the provider may suggest active surveillance with regular follow-up blood tests, rectal exams, and possibly biopsies.

Radiation therapy is a possible treatment for prostate cancer. There are two options for radiation therapy:
- External beam radiation: The patient lies on a table and the machine moves around the table directing high-powered energy beams to the prostate cancer.
- Brachytherapy: Rice-sized radioactive seeds are implanted in the prostate tissue using a needle guided by ultrasound images. A low dose of radiation is delivered over a long period of time.

The side effects of radiation therapy can include painful urination, frequent urination, urgent urination, loose stools, or pain when passing stools. Erectile dysfunction may also occur.

Hormone therapy is another option for treating prostate cancer. This type of therapy stops the body from producing testosterone. Prostate cancer needs testosterone to grow. If the supply can be cut off, the cancer cells may die or grow more slowly. Hormone therapy options include the following:
- Medications that stop the production of testosterone; luteinizing hormone-releasing hormone (LH-RH) prevent the testicles from getting the message to make testosterone:
  - Leuprolide
  - Goserelin
  - Triptorelin
  - Histrelin
- Medications that block testosterone from reaching the cancer cells; antiandrogens:
  - Bicalutamide
  - Flutamide
  - Nilutamide
- Surgery to remove the testicles (orchidectomy [or kih DECK tuh mee]). This reduces the testosterone levels in the body
- Surgical removal of the whole prostate is another treatment option. A radical prostatectomy (pros thu TECK tuh mee) includes the removal of the prostate and surrounding tissue and a few lymph nodes. This procedure can be accomplished in the following ways:
  - *Suprapubic* (SOO pruh pyoo bik) approach: an incision is made in the lower abdomen
  - *Perineal* (per uh NEE l) approach: an incision is made between the scrotum and the anus

Prognosis and prevention. If the cancer is found in its early stages and has not spread outside of the prostate, the outlook is very good. For those with advanced stage or aggressive prostate cancer, the 5-year survival rate drops significantly. Prostate cancer treatments continue to improve, and so should the survival rates for all who are diagnosed with prostate cancer.

The following are ways to reduce the risk of prostate cancer:
- Eat a healthy diet.
- Exercise most days of the week.
- Maintain a healthy weight.

> **CRITICAL THINKING 7.8**
>
> Megan's provider in OB/GYN was gone for the day and they needed some help in urology, so Megan volunteered to spend the day there. While she was there, Al Neviaser was seen by the urologist because he was having difficulty urinating with only a small amount of urine coming out at a time. The urologist performs a DRE and finds that Al's prostate is enlarged. What tests will the urologist likely order? What are two possible diagnoses for Al's signs and symptoms?

Testicular Cancer. Testicular cancer is the most common cancer in white men 15 to 33 years of age. The cause is unknown, but the primary predisposing factor is cryptorchidism. The patient complains of a mass in either testicle; a heavy sensation in the scrotum accompanied by a sudden collection of fluid; pain in a testicle or in the scrotum, abdomen, or groin; and unexplained fatigue.

Etiology. Many causes of testicular cancer are unknown. However, the known risk factors are listed here:
- Undescended testicle (cryptorchidism)
- Congenital abnormalities
- History of testicular cancer
- White race

Signs and symptoms. The patient usually discovers a lump or swelling in the testicle. There may also be complaints of a heavy sensation in the scrotum accompanied by a sudden collection of fluid; the patient may also experience pain in a testicle, scrotum, abdomen, or groin.

Diagnostic procedures. To determine if a lump is testicular cancer, a provider may order any of the following:
- Ultrasound
- Blood tests measuring testicular cancer markers
  - Alpha fetoprotein (AFP)
  - Beta human chorionic gonadotropin (beta-hCG)
  - Lactate dehydrogenase (LDH)
  - CT scan of the chest abdomen and pelvis
- Biopsy of testicular tissue

Treatment. Testicular cancer can be treated successfully if diagnosed early; the survival rate for stage I testicular cancer is approximately 95%. Unfortunately, because young men may hesitate to go to the provider to report a mass in the testicle, the cancer may have reached an advanced stage before it is diagnosed. In advanced stages, treatment usually involves a combination of orchidectomy, radiation therapy, and chemotherapy.

Prognosis and prevention. The prognosis for those diagnosed with testicular cancer is very good if it is detected early. The prognosis is certainly affected by the stage of the cancer and levels of tumor markers after the tumor has been removed.

There is no way to prevent testicular cancer, but some providers will recommend a regular testicular self-examination (TSE). If a lump is discovered, the patient should contact his provider immediately.

Additional male reproductive system diseases. Table 7.4 provides information on additional male reproductive system diseases.

Cancers of the Female Reproductive System

The most common cancers of the female reproductive system are listed in Table 7.5.

> **MEDICAL TERMINOLOGY**
>
> **-ectomy:** removal
> **-scopy:** process of viewing

> **VOCABULARY**
>
> **colposcopy:** Using a microscope with a light source, the vagina and cervix are visually examined to locate and evaluate abnormal cells. A biopsy of abnormal cells may be taken during this procedure.
> **cone biopsy:** An extensive cervical biopsy during which a cone-shaped wedge of tissue is removed from the cervix and examined under a microscope. Abnormal tissue, along with a small amount of normal tissue, is removed.
> **endocervical curettage:** A small, spoon-shaped instrument (curette) or a thin brush is used to scrape a tissue sample from the cervix.
> **hysterectomy:** Surgical removal of the uterus and cervix. The ovaries and fallopian tubes may also be removed.
> **loop electrosurgical excision procedure (LEEP):** After an anesthetic has been injected into the cervix, a high-frequency electrical current running through a wire is used to remove abnormal tissue from both the cervix and the endocervical canal.
> **lumpectomy:** Removal of the breast tumor and a small amount of the surrounding tissue.
> **mastectomy:** Removal of the entire breast.
> **salpingo-oophorectomy:** Surgical removal of the fallopian tube and ovary.
> **sentinel node biopsy:** Removal of a limited number of lymph nodes to determine if the cancer has spread to the lymph nodes.

TABLE 7.4 Male Reproductive System Diseases/Disorders

Disease	Description
anorchism (AN or kih zum)	Condition of being born without a testicle; may also be an acquired condition due to trauma or disease
erectile (ih REK til) **dysfunction**	Inability to achieve or sustain a penile erection for sexual intercourse; also known as *impotence* (IM poh tense)
gynecomastia (gye neh koh MASS tee ah)	Enlargement of breast tissue in the male; can be just on one side or both sides
hydrocele (HYE droh seel)	Accumulation of fluid in the tunica vaginalis testis
oligospermia (oh lih goh SPUR mee ah)	Condition of temporary or permanent deficiency of sperm in the seminal fluid
priapism (PRY ah piz um)	An abnormally prolonged erection
testicular torsion (tes TICK kyoo lur)	Twisting of a testicle on its spermatic cord, usually caused by trauma
varicocele (VAIR ih koh seel)	Abnormal dilation of the veins of the spermatic cord; can lead to infertility

TABLE 7.5 Cancers of the Female Reproductive System

Feature	Breast Cancer	Cervical Cancer	Ovarian Cancer
Description	Breast cancer is the second leading cause of cancer deaths in women. According to the American Cancer Society, 1 in 8 women have a lifetime risk of developing breast cancer, and 1 in 28 risk of dying from the disease.	Almost all cervical carcinomas are caused by the human papillomavirus (HPV). The first stage of cervical cancer is asymptomatic, but early diagnosis of cervical cellular changes is possible with a Papanicolaou (Pap) test.	Ovarian cancer causes more deaths than any other cancer of the female reproductive system, but it accounts for only about 3% of all cancers in women. Most of the time the cancer has already metastasized before the tumor is diagnosed.
Etiology	It is not known what causes breast cancer. Certain risk factors have been identified: • Being female • Family history of breast cancer • Inherited genes • Radiation exposure • Obesity • Menarche at a younger age • Menopause at an older age • Having your first child at an older age • Having never been pregnant • Postmenopausal hormone therapy • Drinking alcohol	It is not known what causes cervical cancer, but it is known that HPV plays a role. Certain risk factors have been identified: • Many sexual partners • Early sexual activity • Having other STIs • A weak immune system • Smoking	It is not known what causes ovarian cancer. Certain risk factors have been identified: • Age • Inherited gene mutation • Estrogen hormone replacement therapy • Menarche at a young age • Menopause at an older age • Having never been pregnant • Fertility treatment • Smoking • Use of an intrauterine device • Polycystic ovary syndrome

Signs and symptoms	• A breast lump or thickening
	• Change in the size, shape, or appearance of a breast
	• Changes to the skin over the breast, such as dimpling
	• A newly inverted nipple
	• Peeling, scaling, or flaking of the pigmented area of the skin surrounding the nipple (areola) or breast skin
	• Redness or pitting of the skin over the breast
		• Early stages are asymptomatic
		• Advanced stages:
		  • Vaginal bleeding after intercourse, between periods, or after menopause
		  • Watery, bloody vaginal discharge that may be heavy and have a foul odor
		  • Pelvic pain or pain during intercourse
			• Early stages are asymptomatic
			• Advanced stages:
			  • Abdominal bloating
			  • Quickly feeling full when eating
			  • Weight loss
			  • Discomfort in the pelvis area
			  • Changes in bowel habits
			  • A frequent need to urinate

Diagnostic procedures	• Breast exam by provider • Mammogram • Breast ultrasound • Biopsy • Breast magnetic resonance imaging (MRI)	Screening tests: • Pap test • HPV DNA test • Diagnostic test • Punch biopsy • **Endocervical curettage** (en doh SER vih kal kyoo r I TAZH) • **Colposcopy** (kol PAW skoh pee) • **Loop electrosurgical excision procedure (LEEP)**	• Pelvic examination • Ultrasound or CT scan • CA-125 blood test: looks for certain proteins in the blood • Biopsy

Treatment	• **Lumpectomy** (luhm PEK tuh mee)
	• **Mastectomy** (ma STEK tuh mee)
	• **Sentinel node biopsy**
	• Removal of both breasts; some women with cancer in one breast choose to have the other breast removed (contralateral prophylactic [proh fih LAK tic] mastectomy)
	• Radiation therapy
	• Chemotherapy
	• Hormone therapy
	• Surgery or medications to stop hormone production in the ovaries
		• LEEP: this procedure can be diagnostic or may remove all of the cancer cells
		• **Cone biopsy**
		• **Hysterectomy**
		• Radiation
		• Chemotherapy
			• Surgery
			  • Hysterectomy
			  • Unilateral **salpingo-oophorectomy** (sal ping goh oh of or EK toh mee)
			  • Bilateral salpingo-oophorectomy
			• Chemotherapy

Prognosis	If found in the early stages, the prognosis is very good	If found in the early stages, the prognosis is very good	If found in the early stages, the prognosis is very good

Continued

TABLE 7.5 Cancers of the Female Reproductive System—cont'd

Feature	Breast Cancer	Cervical Cancer	Ovarian Cancer
Prevention	• Breast cancer screening such as clinical screenings and mammograms • Become familiar with your breasts • Drink alcohol in moderation • Exercise most days of the week • Limit postmenopausal hormone therapy • Maintain a healthy weight • Choose a healthy diet • Preventive surgery; women with a high risk of breast cancer may choose to have prophylactic mastectomy	• HPV vaccination • Routine Pap tests • Practice safe sex • Do not smoke	There is no way to prevent ovarian cancer; the risk can be lowered by the following: • Use of oral contraceptives • Previous pregnancy • History of breast-feeding • Daily use of aspirin

> **CRITICAL THINKING 7.9**
>
> A patient was seen in the OB/GYN department after there was an abnormal Pap test and Dr. Walden had recommended a LEEP procedure. Megan was wondering why a LEEP was recommended instead of a cone biopsy. Can you explain the difference between the two procedures?

Endometriosis. With endometriosis (en doh mee tree OH sis), functional endometrial tissue is located outside of the uterus. It commonly is found attached to the ovaries, urinary bladder, fallopian tubes, uterosacral ligaments, intestines, and peritoneum.

The endometrial tissue continues to act as it normally would during a menstrual cycle. It will thicken, break down, and bleed just like the endometrium found in the uterus. This can cause inflammation at the implantation site that will recur with each cycle. Scar tissue and **adhesions** (ad HEE zhuns) may form.

Endometriosis can cause infertility and put women at higher risk for ovarian cancer.

> **VOCABULARY**
> **adhesions:** Bands of scar tissue that can bind anatomic structures together.
> **laparoscopy:** A procedure used to visually examine the abdomen.

> **MEDICAL TERMINOLOGY**
> **dys-:** bad, difficult, painful, abnormal
> **lapr/o:** abdomen
> **pareun/o:** sexual intercourse
> **-rrhagia:** bursting forth

Etiology. The exact cause of endometriosis is not known, although there are some possible explanations:
- Retrograde menstruation: the menstrual blood containing endometrial cells flow back through the fallopian tubes instead of leaving the uterus thorough the cervix.
- Endometrial cells are transported through the blood vessels or lymphatic system to other parts of the body.
- Immune system disorder: the immune system does not recognize and destroy the endometrial tissue that is growing outside of the uterus.

Risk factors for endometriosis include the following:
- Never giving birth
- Menarche at a younger age
- Short menstrual cycles
- Low body mass index
- Alcohol consumption
- Family history of endometriosis
- Uterine abnormalities

Signs and symptoms. Common signs and symptoms of endometriosis include the following:
- *Dysmenorrhea* (diss men uh REE ah): painful menstrual flow, cramps
- *Dyspareunia* (dis ph ROO nee ah): painful or difficult intercourse
- Pain with bowel movements or urination
- Excessive bleeding
  - *Menorrhagia* (men or RAH zsa): abnormally heavy menstrual flow or prolonged menstrual periods
  - *Menometrorrhagia* (men oh meh troh RAH zsa): excessive menstrual flow and uterine bleeding other than that caused by menstruation
- Infertility
- Fatigue (fuh TEEG)
- Diarrhea
- Constipation
- Bloating
- Nausea (NAH see ah)

Diagnostic procedures. To diagnose endometriosis, oftentimes an ultrasound will be done. The ultrasound could be done through the abdomen or transvaginally.

Another method of diagnosing endometriosis is a **laparoscopy** (lap ar AW scoh pee). The surgeon will look inside the abdomen for signs of endometriosis.

Treatment. There are two methods for treating endometriosis: medications or surgery.

Medications might include the following:
- Pain medications
  - Over-the-counter medications such as ibuprofen or naproxen sodium

- Hormone therapy
  - Contraceptives: birth control pills, patches, and vaginal rings
  - Gonadatropin (goh nad uh TROH pin)-releasing hormone (GN-RH) agonists and antagonists: block the production of ovarian-stimulating hormones, lowering estrogen levels, and preventing menstruation
  - Progestin (proh JES tin) therapy: a progestin-only contraceptive such as an intrauterine device can stop menstrual periods and also the growth of endometrial implants

  Surgical options might include the following:
- Removal of the endometrial implants; this can be done laparoscopically or through an abdominal incision, and it will preserve the uterus and ovaries
- Hysterectomy: removal of the uterus, cervix, and both ovaries

Prognosis and prevention. Women with endometriosis are at a greater risk for disorders such as systemic lupus erythematosus, Sjögren syndrome, rheumatoid arthritis, and multiple sclerosis. Chronic fatigue syndrome and fibromyalgia are also more common in women with endometriosis.

Infertility often is caused by endometriosis, but if a woman becomes pregnant the endometriosis should not affect the pregnancy.

At this time, there is no way to prevent endometriosis.

Infections. The female genitalia provide an excellent environment for infections to occur. There is moisture, warmth, and plenty of nutrients for the infectious agents to flourish. Table 7.6 covers the most common infections of the female reproductive system.

Additional Female Reproductive System Diseases/Disorders. There are many female reproductive system diseases. Table 7.7 provides information on additional female reproductive diseases. Table 7.8 provides information on pregnancy-related conditions.

TABLE 7.6 Common Infections of the Female Reproductive System

Feature	Candidiasis (kan dih DYE ah sis)	Cervicitis (sur vih SYE tis)	Pelvic Inflammatory Disease
Description	Commonly called a yeast infection. *Candida* organisms are commonly part of the normal flora of the mouth, skin, intestinal tract, and vagina. Overgrowth of the organism can be caused by antibiotic use, high estrogen levels, oral contraceptive use, diabetes mellitus, pregnancy, and immunosuppressive disorders, including acquired immunodeficiency syndrome (AIDS).	Cervicitis is an inflammation of the cervix caused by an invading organism.	PID is any acute or chronic infection of the reproductive system that ascends from the vagina, cervix, uterus, fallopian tubes, and ovaries. These infections may cause the fallopian tubes to fill with pus, and chronic episodes can result in scarring of the fallopian tubes and the formation of adhesions.
Etiology	Candida albicans (fungus)	• Sexually transmitted infections • Allergic reactions • Bacterial overgrowth	• Gonorrhea • Chlamydia • Other bacteria
Signs and symptoms	• Vulvovaginal itching • Dry, bright red vaginal tissue • Odorless, white, "cottage cheese" like vaginal discharge	• Thick, **purulent** (PYOOR yoo lent) discharge with odor • Dysuria • Dyspareunia • Vaginal bleeding after intercourse	• May be asymptomatic • Fever • Abdominal or pelvic pain • Vaginal discharge • Dysuria • Dyspareunia
Diagnostic procedures	• Pelvic examination • Test of vaginal secretions		
Treatment	Antifungal medications; cream, ointments, tablets, and suppositories; some of these treatments may be available over the counter	Treatment may not be needed unless the cervicitis is caused by an STI; then both the patient and her partner must be treated for the STI	• Antibiotics for the patient and her partner • Analgesics
Prognosis	Good if treatment plan is followed	Good if treatment plan is followed	Good if treatment plan is followed; repeated infections can cause infertility
Prevention	• Wear cotton underwear and loose-fitting pants • Avoid tight-fitting underwear, pantyhose, or tights • Immediately change out of wet clothes, such as swimsuits or workout attire • Stay out of hot tubs or very hot baths • Avoid unnecessary antibiotic use	• Use condoms consistently and correctly	• Use condoms consistently and correctly • Early treatment of an STI

TABLE 7.7 Female Reproductive System Diseases

Disease	Description
Amenorrhea (ah men uh REE ah)	Lack of menstrual flow.
Dysfunctional uterine bleeding (DUB)	Abnormal uterine bleeding not caused by a tumor, inflammation, or pregnancy.
Menopause (MEN oh poz)	The cessation of menses.
Ovarian cysts	Benign, fluid-filled sac. Can be either a follicular cyst, which occurs when a follicle does not rupture at ovulation, or a cyst of the corpus luteum, which is caused when it does not continue its transformation.
Polycystic ovary syndrome	Bilateral presence of numerous cysts, caused by a hormonal abnormality leading to the secretion of androgens. Can cause acne, facial hair, and infertility.
Premenstrual dysphoric disorder (PMDD)	Mood disorder that includes depression, irritability, fatigue, changes in appetite or sleep, and difficulty concentrating; occurs 1–2 weeks before the onset of the menstrual flow.
Premenstrual syndrome (PMS)	Poorly understood group of symptoms that occur in some women on a cyclical basis: breast pain, irritability, fluid retention, headache, and a lack of coordination are some of the symptoms.
Tumors fibroid/myoma	Fibroids are smooth muscle tumors of the uterus. They are usually nonpainful growths that may be removed surgically. Theses tumors may also be referred to as myomas.

TABLE 7.8 Pregnancy-Related Conditions

Disease	Description
Abruptio plancentae (ah BRUP she oh plah SEN tee)	Premature separation of the placenta from the uterine wall; may result in a severe hemorrhage that can threaten both infant and maternal lives.
Eclampsia (eh KLAMP see ah)	Extremely serious form of hypertension secondary to pregnancy. Patients are at risk for coma, convulsions, and death.
Hemolytic (hee moh LIT ick) **disease of the newborn (HDN)**	A mother with Rh- blood will develop antibodies to an Rh+ fetus during the first pregnancy. If another pregnancy occurs with an Rh+ fetus, the antibodies can destroy the fetal blood cells.
Hyperemesis gravidarum (hy per EM eh sis grav ih DAIR um)	Excessive vomiting that causes weakness, dehydration, and fluid and electrolyte imbalance.
Placenta previa (plah SEN tah PREE vee ah)	Placenta that is positioned in the uterus so that it covers the opening of the cervix.
Preeclampsia (pree eh KLAMP see ah)	Abnormal condition of pregnancy with unknown cause, marked by hypertension, edema, and proteinuria.
Zika (ZEE kuh) **virus**	A mosquito-borne virus that typically causes a mild fever, rash, and joint pain. The virus can be passed to a fetus and is associated with certain birth defects such as **microcephaly**.

> **MEDICAL TERMINOLOGY**
> **cephal/o**: head
> **micro-**: small
> **-y**: process of; condition

> **CRITICAL THINKING 7.10**
> As Megan was working with more pregnant patients, she was becoming more familiar with the complications that can occur. She was still a bit confused between pre-eclampsia and eclampsia. How would you describe the differences?

LIFE SPAN CHANGES

Male Reproductive System

Pediatrics. Aside from the congenital disorders that a male child may be born with, few male reproductive system disorders are specific to childhood. Seminoma, a cancer of the testicles, is one of the few cancers that can affect youth. Fortunately, early detection makes this cancer almost 100% curable.

Geriatrics. Senior men have some significant disorders. Disorders of the prostate gland are common and are usually accompanied by difficulty with urination because of the location of the prostate around the urethra. Usually benign, this condition also has a malignant form, and prostate cancer is the second greatest cause of cancer deaths.

Erectile disorders, now treatable with a variety of medications on the market, have also emerged as a significant "reason for visit" to the family physician.

Female Reproductive System

Pediatrics. A review of the most recent national statistics for all diagnoses for hospital inpatients who were newborns or children under the age of 17 revealed some surprises. For neonates (28 days old and younger), diagnoses that included complications of delivery were common. Meconium staining and cord entanglement were high on the list. However, for fertile females between the ages of 1 and 17, the delivery of a single live born is second only to hypovolemia for all diagnoses. (Pneumonia and asthma follow closely behind.) Still within the top 50 diagnoses are a large number of complications of delivery.

Geriatrics. Later in life, senior women are seen most often for neoplasms of the breast, uterus, cervix, and ovaries. Breast cancer alone will be diagnosed in one in eight women in their lifetime in the United States.

CLOSING COMMENTS

Understanding the common terms and diseases related to the reproductive system will be helpful for medical assistants in a various areas in ambulatory care. Whether you are working in primary care, urology, or obstetric/gynecology, being familiar with the pronunciation and spelling of the medical terminology associated with this system will be vital (Tables 7.9 through 7.16). Abbreviations are also commonly used in healthcare, and it is important that you know the appropriate abbreviation to use and that you understand the abbreviations found in the healthcare setting.

TABLE 7.9 Combining and Adjective Forms for the Anatomy of the Male Reproductive System

Meaning	Combining Form	Adjective Form
epididymis	epididym/o	epididymal
glans penis	balan/o	balanic
gonad	gonad/o	gonadal
juices	chym/o	chymous
male	andr/o	
penis	pen/i, phall/o	penile, phallic
prepuce, foreskin	preputi/o, posth/o	preputial
prostate	prostat/o	prostatic
scrotum	scrot/o	scrotal
semen	semin/i	seminal
seminal vesicle	vesicul/o	vesicular
spermatozoon	sperm/o, spermat/o	spermatic
steroid	ster/o	steroidal
stroma	strom/o	stromal
testis, testicle	test/o, testicul/o, orchid/o, orch/o	testicular
urethra	urethr/o	urethral
vas deferens, ductus deferens	vas/o	vasal, ductal

From Shiland B: *Mastering Healthcare Terminology*, ed 5, St. Louis, 2016, Elsevier.

TABLE 7.10 Prefixes for the Anatomy of the Male Reproductive System

Prefix	Meaning
en-	in
par-	near

From Shiland B: *Mastering Healthcare Terminology*, ed 5, St. Louis, 2016, Elsevier.

TABLE 7.11 Suffixes for the Anatomy of the Male Reproductive System

Suffix	Meaning
-al, -ous, -ar, -ile, -atic, -ic	pertaining to
-ferous	pertaining to carrying
-genesis	production
-logy	the study of
-one	substance that forms

From Shiland B: *Mastering Healthcare Terminology*, ed 5, St. Louis, 2016, Elsevier.

TABLE 7.12 Abbreviations for the Anatomy of the Male Reproductive System and Sexually Transmitted Infections

Abbreviation	Definition
BPH	benign prostatic hyperplasia/hypertrophy
Bx	biopsy
DRE	digital rectal exam
FTA-ABS	fluorescent treponemal antibody (test)
Gc	gonococcus
GCT	germ cell tumor
GU	genitourinary
HPV	human papillomavirus
HSV-2	herpes simplex virus-2, herpes genitalis
NGU	nongonococcal urethritis
PSA	prostate-specific antigen
STI	sexually transmitted infection
TSE	testicular self-examination
TUIP	transurethral incision of the prostate
TUR	transurethral resection (of the prostate)
TURP	transurethral resection of the prostate
VD	venereal disease
VDRL	Venereal Disease Research Laboratory (test for syphilis)

TABLE 7.13 Combining and Adjective Forms for the Anatomy and Physiology of the Female Reproductive System

Meaning	Combining Form	Adjective Form	Meaning	Combining Form	Adjective Form
amnion	amni/o, amnion/o	amniotic	myometrium	myometri/o	myometrial
Bartholin gland	bartholin/o		nipple	papill/o, thel/e	papillary, thelial
birth, born	nat/o	natal	ovary	oophor/o, ovari/o	ovarian
breast	mamm/o, mast/o	mammary	ovum, egg	ov/o, ov/i, ovul/o, o/o	
cervix	cervic/o	cervical	parturition, delivery	part/o	
chorion	chori/o, chorion/o	chorionic	perimetrium	perimetri/o	perimetrial
clitoris	clitorid/o		perineum	perine/o	perineal
endometrium	endometri/o	endometrial	placenta	placent/o	placental
fallopian tube	salping/o, fallopi/o	salpingeal, fallopian	pregnancy	gravid/o	
female	gynec/o		puerperium	puerper/o	
fetus	fet/o	fetal	rectouterine pouch	culd/o	
fundus	fund/o	fundal	umbilicus, navel	omphal/o, umbilic/o	omphalic, umbilical
hymen	hymen/o	hymenal	uterus	hyster/o, metri/o, metr/o, uter/o	uterine
labia	labi/o	labial			
menstruation, menses	men/o	menstrual	vagina	colp/o, vagin/o	vaginal
milk	lact/o, galact/o	lactic, galactic	vulva	vulv/o, episi/o	vulvar

TABLE 7.14 Prefixes for the Anatomy and Physiology of the Female Reproductive System

Prefix	Meaning
endo-	within
multi-	many
neo-	new
nulli-	none
peri-	surrounding
primi-	first

From Shiland B: *Mastering Healthcare Terminology*, ed 5, St. Louis, 2016, Elsevier.

TABLE 7.15 Suffixes for the Anatomy and Physiology of the Female Reproductive System

Suffix	Meaning
-arche	beginning
-ation	process of
-gravida, -cyesis	pregnancy, gestation
-ic, -al, -ine	pertaining to
-ician, -logist	one who specializes in the study of
-para, -partum, -tocia	delivery, parturition
-pause	stop, cease
-salpinx	fallopian tube
-um	structure

From Shiland B: *Mastering Healthcare Terminology*, ed 5, St. Louis, 2016, Elsevier.

TABLE 7.16 Abbreviations for the Anatomy of the Female Reproductive System

Abbreviation	Definition	Abbreviation	Definition
AFP	alpha fetoprotein (test)	ICSI	intracytoplasmic sperm injection
AI	artificial insemination	IDC	infiltrating ductal carcinoma
BCP	birth control pill	IUD	intrauterine device
CIN	cervical intraepithelial neoplasia	IVF	in vitro fertilization
CS	cesarean section, C-section	LEEP	loop electrocautery excision procedure
CST	contraction stress test	LH	luteinizing hormone
CVS	chorionic villus sampling	LMP	last menstrual period
Cx	cervix	NST	nonstress test
D&C	dilation and curettage	OB	obstetrics
DUB	dysfunctional uterine bleeding	OCP	oral contraceptive pill
ECP	emergency contraceptive pill	PCOS	polycystic ovary syndrome
EDD	estimated delivery date	PID	pelvic inflammatory disease
EOC	epithelial ovarian cancer	PKU	phenylketonuria
ERT	estrogen replacement therapy	PMB	postmenopausal bleeding
FHR	fetal heart rate	PMDD	premenstrual dysphoric disorder
FSH	follicle-stimulating hormone	PMS	premenstrual syndrome
GIFT	gamete intrafallopian transfer	Rh	Rhesus factor
GPA	gravida, para, abortion	TAH-BSO	total abdominal hysterectomy with a bilateral salpingo-oophorectomy
hCG	human chorionic gonadotropin		
hMG	human menopausal gonadotropin	UAE	uterine artery embolization
HRT	hormone replacement therapy	VBAC	vaginal birth after cesarean section
HSG	hysterosalpingography	ZIFT	zygote intrafallopian transfer

As a medical assistant, it is important that you have a basic understanding of the following:
- Basics of both the male and the female reproductive systems
- The diseases that impact the reproductive systems

To provide your patients with the best care, you must understand the various body systems, the diseases that affect them, and the different treatments that a provider may order.

CHAPTER REVIEW

The reproductive system is made up of parenchymal tissue and stromal tissue. The parenchymal tissue produces the sex cells for reproduction, and the stromal tissue includes all of the glands, nerves, ducts, and other tissues that help to produce, maintain, and transmit the sex cells.

The anatomy of the male reproductive system is made up of the testes, which include the seminiferous tubules, epididymis, vas deferens, spermatic cord, seminal vesicles, and Cowper glands; prostate gland; ejaculatory duct; urethra; and the penis.

There are many conditions and disorders related to the reproductive system. STIs can affect both the male and the female reproductive tract. There are bacterial and viral STIs, and the signs and symptoms for a particular STI can be different in a man than in a woman. It is important to know the different signs and symptoms for the most common STIs. In the male reproductive system, BPH and prostate cancer are two common issues. The signs and symptoms are similar, and it is helpful to know what tests are involved to tell the difference between the two.

When discussing the diseases and disorders of the female reproductive tract, there are many to consider. There are various vaginal infections and gynecologic disorders, but you must also consider the possible complications of pregnancy. Familiarity with the most common diseases and disorders is going to allow you to provide the best possible care to your patients.

SCENARIO WRAP-UP

Megan is enjoying her new department and is excited to learn more about the field of obstetrics and gynecology. There are many new diseases, disorders, and treatments to learn about. She is also able to share her expertise in the male reproductive system with her coworkers, who are interested to learn about that area of healthcare and how it relates to the female reproductive system.

8

Blood

LEARNING OBJECTIVES

1. Discuss the constituents of blood.
2. Describe the normal function and physiology of blood.
3. Complete the following related to diseases and disorders of the blood:
   - Identify the common etiology, signs and symptoms, and diagnostic measures of blood diseases.
   - Identify CLIA-waived tests associated with common blood diseases.
   - Describe treatment modalities used for blood diseases.
4. Compare the structure and function of the blood across the life span.

CHAPTER OUTLINE

1. Opening Scenario, 166
2. You Will Learn, 166
3. Introduction to the Blood, 166
4. Anatomy of the Blood, 167
   a. Liquid Portion of Blood, 167
      i. Plasma, 167
      ii. Serum, 168
   b. Formed Elements of Blood, 168
      i. Red Blood Cells, 168
      ii. White Blood Cells, 169
      iii. Thrombocytes, 170
5. Physiology of the Blood, 170
   a. Red Blood Cells: Blood Types, 170
   b. White Blood Cells: Phagocytosis, 172
   c. Platelets: Coagulation and Hemostasis, 172
6. Diseases and Disorders of the Blood, 173
   a. Anemia: Iron Deficiency, 173
   b. Anemia: Sickle-Cell Disease, 175
   c. Hemophilia, 177
   d. Idiopathic Thrombocytopenic Purpura, 178
   e. Infectious Mononucleosis, 179
   f. Leukemias: Acute Lymphocytic, and Acute Myelogenous, 180
   g. Leukemias: Chronic Lymphocytic and Chronic Myelogenous, 181
   h. Thrombophlebitis, 182
   i. Additional Diseases and Disorders of the Blood, 183
7. Life Span Changes, 184
8. Closing Comments, 184
9. Chapter Review, 185
10. Scenario Wrap-Up, 186

▶ OPENING SCENARIO

Lily Hiddleston has been a medical assistant at Walden-Martin Family Medical (WMFM) Clinic for about 2 years. She enjoys working with Dr. James Martin and developing relationships with their patients. One patient Lily truly enjoys is Erma Willis. Erma is an older patient who loves to talk about her grandchildren and shares Lily's love of dogs. Erma is still living independently with her two dogs, Henry and Trapper.

Today Erma is coming in for a late morning appointment. Lily was working the reception desk last week when Erma called in to make an appointment. It seems that she has been feeling a bit tired lately and has been spending more time than usual in her favorite chair. She has had some headaches recently, and sometimes she feels dizzy when she stands up after being in her chair. She said she has not been taking the dogs out for a walk quite as often, and just yesterday she started having a pain in the back of her left leg. Lily is looking forward to seeing Erma today. Maybe she will even see a few new photos of Henry and Trapper!

YOU WILL LEARN

1. To recognize and use terms related to the blood.
2. To locate the structures and cells related to blood.
3. To understand and describe functions of the blood: transportation and protection.
4. To recognize disease states of the blood, as well as their causes, signs and symptoms, diagnostic processes, treatment, prognoses, and prevention.

INTRODUCTION TO THE BLOOD

Homeostasis (hoh mee oh STAY sis) is the term used to describe the internal environment of the body that is compatible with life. It is a steady state that is created by all the body systems working together to provide a consistent and unvarying internal environment. Blood contributes to homeostasis in the following ways:

- Transportation of
  - Gases: oxygen and carbon dioxide
  - Chemical substances such as hormones, nutrients, salts, and waste products of metabolism
  - Cells of the blood
- Protection from
  - Pathogens: white blood cells are part of the immune response, which will be discussed in detail in Chapter 9

CHAPTER 8 Blood

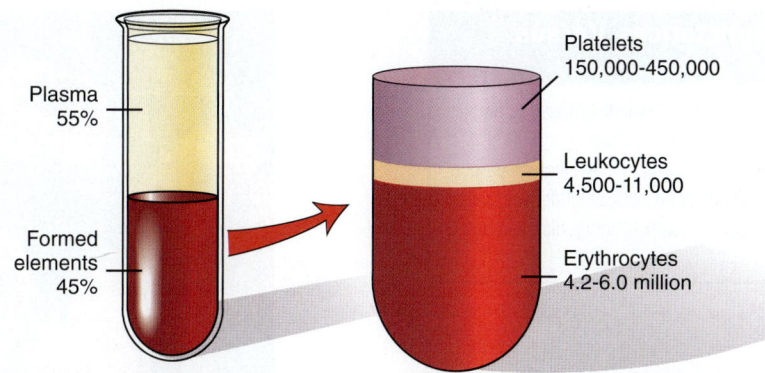

FIG. 8.1 Composition of blood. (From Shiland B: *Mastering Healthcare Terminology*, ed 5, St. Louis, 2016, Elsevier.)

- Blood loss: the process of **coagulation** (koh AG yuh ley shun), or clotting, can stop blood flow when needed
- Regulation of the body's fluid and electrolyte balance, acid-base balance, and body temperature.

Box 8.1 discusses the *hematology* (hem uh TOL uh jee) specialty.

BOX 8.1 Specialty and Specialist

Hematology is the healthcare specialty that deals with most diseases and disorders of the blood and blood-forming organs. A *hematologist* (hem uh TOL uh jist) is a specialist involved in the study, diagnosis, treatment, and prevention of disorders of the blood.

VOCABULARY

carbon dioxide: A colorless, odorless gas (CO_2) that is present in the air we breathe. It is a waste product of cellular respiration and is removed from the body by exhaling via the lungs.
coagulation: The process of changing a liquid into a solid.
oxygen: A colorless, odorless gas (O_2) that makes up about 25% of the air we breathe. It is essential for life and cellular respiration.
pathogen: A disease-causing organism.

MEDICAL TERMINOLOGY

hem/o, hemat/o: blood	**-logy:** the study
home/o: same	**-stasis:** controlling, stopping
-logist: one who studies	

ANATOMY OF THE BLOOD

Because blood plays an important role in the diagnostic process of many diseases and disorders, students need to understand its normal composition. Blood is made up of two components:
- The liquid portion is called *plasma* (PLAZ muh) and makes up about 55% of the total blood volume.
- *Formed elements*, also called blood cells, make up about 45% of the total blood volume (Fig. 8.1). The formed elements freely float in the liquid plasma. This makes blood a suspension.

The following sections present examples of these two components in more depth.

TABLE 8.1 Functions of the Plasma Proteins

Plasma Protein	Function in the Body
Albumin	Most abundant protein in the plasma. The presence of albumin keeps water in the plasma from flowing out of the blood vessels and into the surrounding tissues; this is known as *osmotic pressure*. Manufactured in the liver.
Globulins	Antibodies are a type of globulin that circulate in the plasma and help protect the body from infections from pathogens. Manufactured in the liver.
Clotting factors	Fibrinogen and prothrombin are two proteins that circulate in the plasma and are necessary for proper blood clotting or coagulation. There are other coagulation factors that circulate in the plasma too. Manufactured in the liver.
Complement	A group of enzymes that support antibodies in their battle against pathogens. Manufactured in the liver.

From Shiland B: *Mastering Healthcare Terminology*, ed 5, St. Louis, 2016, Elsevier.

Liquid Portion of Blood

Plasma. *Plasma* is the liquid portion of **whole blood**. Plasma is made up of the following substances:
- Water (90%)
- **Plasma proteins** (albumin, globulin, clotting proteins [e.g., fibrinogen, prothrombin, and **clotting factors**] and complement) (Table 8.1)
- Inorganic substances and **electrolytes** (sodium, calcium, potassium, chloride, magnesium, bicarbonate) (Box 8.2)
- Organic substances (amino acids, glucose, fats, cholesterol, hormones)
- Waste products (urea, uric acid, ammonia, creatinine)

Each dissolved component of plasma serves a specific function in the blood and in the body. Water makes up the bulk of plasma. Water is the **solvent** for all the dissolved substances that travel in the plasma. The plasma proteins each have a unique function (see Table 8.1). Without organic and inorganic substances, individual cells would not be able to work, metabolize, repair, and reproduce. Waste products from cellular metabolism are also dissolved in plasma. Without waste products being transported to the liver, kidneys, and lungs for excretion, the body

> **BOX 8.2 Inorganic Substances Versus Organic Substances**
>
> - *Organic substances* or chemicals contain the element **carbon**. Examples are amino acids, carbohydrates, and fats to name a few.
> - *Inorganic substances* or chemicals do not contain the element carbon. Examples are electrolytes, such as sodium, potassium, chloride, and water. It is that easy—organic substances contain carbon, inorganic substances do not.

> **BOX 8.3 Two Latin Terms**
>
> Two Latin terms are used to describe the difference between a process that take place in the body, *in vivo*, and a process that takes place in the laboratory, *in vitro*. The translation for in vivo means "in life." The translation for in vitro means "in glass."

would become toxic and could not survive. A lot happens in the liquid portion of the blood.

Plasma also maintains a very narrow pH range (7.35–7.45). This precise pH range is necessary to make sure that red blood cells can transport the optimal level of oxygen in the blood. The range also allows needed chemical reactions in the body to continue to work. Most chemical reactions in the body are pH dependent. Without a stable blood pH, homeostasis is unlikely to be maintained.

Serum. Serum (SEER um) is the liquid that remains after blood has formed a **clot**. When blood leaves the body and is no longer moving, it naturally clots. Serum is plasma minus the clotting proteins, fibrinogen and prothrombin. Serum is not normally found in the body, because if all the blood in your body clotted, you would be dead!

Blood outside the body (e.g., in a venipuncture tube) needs to have an **anticoagulant** (an tee koh AG yuh luh nt) added to remain liquid (Box 8.3). If an anticoagulant is not added, the blood will clot. When red blood cells, white blood cells, platelets, and clotting proteins stick together, they form a *clot* (also called a *fibrin clot*). The liquid that remains after a clot has formed is serum. The formation of a fibrin clot and coagulation will be discussed later in the physiology section of this chapter.

Although serum should not be found in the body, in the laboratory it is often a preferred testing sample. *Serology* is the branch of laboratory medicine that studies serum for the presence of antibodies or antigens.

Formed Elements of Blood

The formed elements of blood are composed of three different types of cells:
- *Erythrocytes* (eh RITH roh sites), also called *red blood cells* (RBCs)
- *Leukocytes* (LOO koh sites), also called *white blood cells* (WBCs)
- *Thrombocytes* (THROM boh sites), also called *platelets* (PLATE lets), *clotting cells*, or *cell fragments*

A milliliter of blood has approximately 4.2 million to 6 million RBCs, 4500 to 11,000 WBCs, and 150,000 to 450,000 platelets. The average 150-lb (68-kg) person has approximately 5 L of blood circulating throughout the body.

Red Blood Cells. Erythrocytes have the important function of transporting O_2 and CO_2 throughout the body (Fig. 8.2). The **hemoglobin**

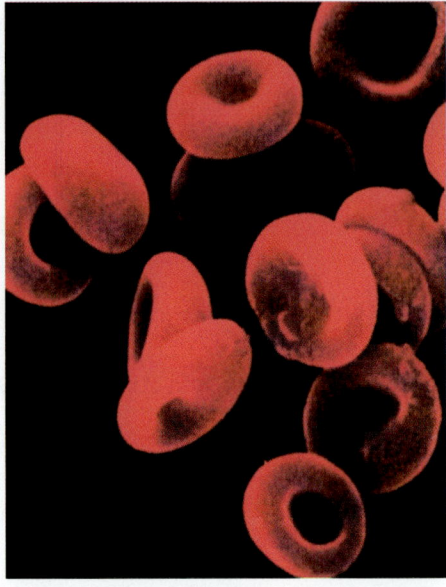

FIG. 8.2 Red blood cells. (From Shiland B: *Mastering Healthcare Terminology*, ed 5, St. Louis, 2016, Elsevier.)

(HEE moh gloh bin) molecule on the RBC is responsible for transporting O_2 and CO_2. Hemoglobin is made up of protein and iron, which is capable of binding and releasing oxygen and carbon dioxide.

> **VOCABULARY**
>
> **anticoagulant:** A chemical substance that keeps blood from clotting.
> **carbon:** A naturally abundant, nonmetallic element that occurs in all organic compounds and can be found in all known forms of life. A pure form of carbon is diamond.
> **clot:** A mass of coagulated blood that is made up of red blood cells, white blood cells, and platelets in a protein (fibrin) mesh. It has a semisolid consistency.
> **clotting factors:** Substances in the blood that interact in sequence to stop bleeding by forming a clot. Examples include prothrombin, fibrinogen, thromboplastin, and calcium.
> **electrolytes:** Inorganic compounds, mainly salts. A major factor in controlling fluid balance within the body.
> **plasma proteins:** Proteins that circulate in the blood and are made in the liver.
> **solvent:** A liquid that can dissolve other substances. An example is water.
> **whole blood:** Plasma and the formed elements of blood in a free-flowing liquid form.

> **MEDICAL TERMINOLOGY**
>
> **-cyte, -cyto:** cell
> **erythr/o:** red
> **leuk/o:** white
> **plasm/o:** plasma
> **ser/o:** serum
> **serum** (singular), **sera** (plural)
> **thromb/o:** clotting, clot

Granulocytes			Agranulocytes	
	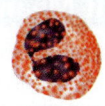	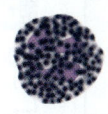	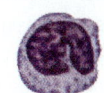	
A. Neutrophil	B. Eosinophil	C. Basophil	D. Monocyte	E. Lymphocyte

FIG. 8.3 White blood cells. (From Proctor D, et al: *Kinn's The Medical Assistant*, ed 13, St. Louis, 2017, Elsevier.)

RBC production is stimulated by a hormone produced in the kidneys called *erythropoietin* (eh rith roh POY uh tin). The formation of RBCs takes place in red bone marrow located in the blood-producing cavities found in bones. (See Chapter 3 for more details.) Stem cells produce immature RBCs that contain a nucleus. As an RBC matures, it loses its nucleus, which shows it is ready to be released into the bloodstream. RBCs also have a unique shape. They are *biconcave*, which means they are shaped like a disk that is squished a bit in the middle. The shape is like a donut, but without a hole in the middle, just a dent. This shape allows the RBC to increase its surface area and carry more O_2 or CO_2 attached to hemoglobin. The biconcave shape also gives RBCs some flexibility, so that the cell is not rigid. This is very helpful because RBCs travel through tiny blood capillaries. The RBCs can bend and twist because of its shape and can pass through tight spots.

Red blood cells have a life span of approximately 120 days. When an RBC is no longer useful, it is broken down into iron and bilirubin. The iron is stored mainly in the liver and is recycled into new RBCs. The bilirubin is further broken down into *bile*, which is excreted by the liver.

White Blood Cells. There are five types of WBCs, each with unique characteristics (Fig. 8.3). The function of white blood cells is to protect the body from invading pathogens. The two main types of white blood cells are *granulocytes* and *agranulocytes*.

Granulocytes. Named for their appearance, *granulocytes* (GRAN yoo loh sites) are WBCs that have granules, or speckles, within the cytoplasm (Box 8.4). They also have a nucleus that is segmented or multilobed. There are three types of granulocytes: *neutrophils, eosinophils, and basophils*. Each has its own role in immunity.

Neutrophils (NOO troh fils) are cells that absorb neither an acidic nor a basic dye in the laboratory, and consequently they are a purplish color. They are *phagocytic* (fag oh si TICK) cells, which means they protect the body by engulfing and then destroying foreign substances. A neutrophil is one of the most aggressive phagocytic cells in the body. Neutrophils are drawn to the site of a pathogen and then destroy the invading pathogen. They often help clean up the infection site, which aids the healing process. Neutrophils can be referred to as polymorphonucleocytes (PMNs), segs, or polys. They are the most abundant white blood cell in the circulation.

Eosinophils (ee oh SIN oh fils) are cells that absorb an acidic dye, which causes the beadlike granules to appear bright pinkish orange. Eosinophils increase in number when the body is defending against allergens and parasites. They are also called *eos* (EE ohs) and make up about 1% of the WBCs in the circulation.

Basophils (BAY soh fils) are cells that absorb a basic (or alkaline) dye, and the granules in the cytoplasm stain a dark bluish color. Especially effective in combating parasites, they release *histamine* (a substance that initiates an inflammatory response) and heparin (an anticoagulant), both of which are instrumental in healing damaged tissue. They are often called *basos* (BAY sohs) and make up 1% or less of the WBCs in the circulation.

Agranulocytes. *Agranulocytes* (a GRAN yoo loh sites) are WBCs that lack granules in the cytoplasm. Another characteristic that distinguishes them from granulocytes is that they are *mononuclear leukocytes*:

BOX 8.4 Granulocytes

Granulocytes are also referred to as *polymorphonucleocytes* (pah lee morf oh NOO klee oh sites), PMNs, polys, or segs. They have poly (many) morpho (shaped) nucleus. Neutrophils are most often referred to with these nicknames because they are the most abundant granulocyte seen in the blood and display a multilobed nucleus.

VOCABULARY

bilirubin: A reddish pigment that results from the breakdown of red blood cells in the liver.
hemoglobin: An oxygen-carrying pigment of red blood cells that contains iron. It gives red blood cells their color and carries oxygen to the cells.
stem cells: Undifferentiated cells that can become specialized cells in the body.
surface area: Total area of the surface of a three-dimensional object. Measured in square units. For example, the surface area of the ball could be 14 cubic millimeters.

CRITICAL THINKING 8.1

Lily calls Erma back to the exam room and completes her vitals. She asks Erma to describe how she has been feeling lately. It seems that she has been a bit tired, has been napping more often, and recently developed a pain in her leg that has her concerned. As Lily notes the information in Erma's medical record, Dr. Martin steps into the exam room. The doctor and Erma talk about how she is feeling, and Dr. Martin orders a capillary puncture and hemoglobin. Lily will collect the sample and run the hemoglobin level so that Dr. Martin will have the information when he comes back to look at Erma's leg and complete the appointment. Why is Erma's hemoglobin level useful information for Dr. Martin to know as they continue her exam?

MEDICAL TERMINOLOGY

bas/o: base	**neutr/o:** neutral
eosin/o: rose colored	**nucle/o:** nucleus
granul/o: little grain	**phag/o:** eat, swallow
-globin: protein substance	**-phil:** attraction
-lysis: breaking down	**-poietin:** forming substance
morph/o: shape	**poly-:** many
myel/o: bone marrow	

> **BOX 8.5 Diapedesis**
>
> WBCs that are moving from the bloodstream into tissue use a process called *diapedesis* (dahy uh pi DEE sis) to get out of the blood capillaries. Diapedesis allows WBCs to move through the capillary walls and into an infection site or into tissue (most frequently lymphatic tissue).

> **BOX 8.6 Two Similar Words, Very Different Meanings**
>
> Do not confuse *hemostasis*, which means "control of blood flow," with *homeostasis*, which means "a steady or constant state."

white blood cells with one nucleus. Granulocytes originate in the bone marrow and mature after entering the lymphatic system. There are two types of agranulocytes: monocytes and lymphocytes.

Monocytes (MON oh sites) are named for their single, large nucleus. Monocytes are the largest phagocytic white blood cells in the blood. Because of their size, they can engulf and destroy larger pathogens and particles. Monocytes are in the bloodstream, but when they leave the bloodstream and take up residence in lymphatic tissue, they transform into *macrophages* (MACK roh fay jehs) (Box 8.5). They get larger but are essentially the same cell. When they are in the blood, they are called monocytes; when they are in lymphatic tissue, they are called macrophages. Monocytes/macrophages are very aggressive phagocytic cells than can destroy pathogens, malignant cells, and tumor cells in the body. Monocytes are also called *monos* (MON ohs).

Lymphocytes (LIM foh sites), also called *lymphs* (limfs), are key cells in the immune response. There are two types of lymphocytes, B cell lymphocytes and T cell lymphocytes. They look the same but they function differently. All lymphocytes recognize pathogens as foreign substances. Once they see something as foreign, they try to destroy it. The foreign substances are called *antigens* (AN tih juns) and could be bacteria, viruses, or other pathogens. B cell lymphocytes produce *antibodies* that inactivate or neutralize antigens. T cell lymphocytes cannot produce antibodies, but they help expose pathogens, making it possible for antibodies to inactivate or neutralize the antigen. The immune response will be described in detail in Chapter 9.

Thrombocytes. *Thrombocytes* are most commonly known as *platelets* (Fig. 8.4). A platelet has an irregular round or oval shape that resembles a small plate. Platelets are formed in the bone marrow from stem cells. They are just a small piece or *fragment* of a much larger cell called a *megakaryocyte* (meg uh KAR ee oh site) that is in the bone marrow. Platelets aid in coagulation, the process of changing a liquid to a solid. When an injury to a blood vessel occurs, platelets rush to the area and *agglutinate* (ah GLOO tih nate), or clump together. This stops or slows the escape of blood. *Hemostasis* is a term that means, control of blood flow (Box 8.6). Hemostasis will be discussed later in this chapter.

> **CRITICAL THINKING 8.2**
>
> Lily asks Erma to follow her to the phlebotomy area. She collects a capillary sample and runs a hemoglobin test. It only takes a few moments. As she is waiting for the results, she checks Erma's finger and makes sure that the bleeding has stopped. Why is it important to check Erma's finger to make sure she is no longer bleeding? What blood cells are involved in the process of blood clotting?

> **MEDICAL TERMINOLOGY**
>
> **a-:** without
> **lymph/o:** lymph
> **mono-:** one

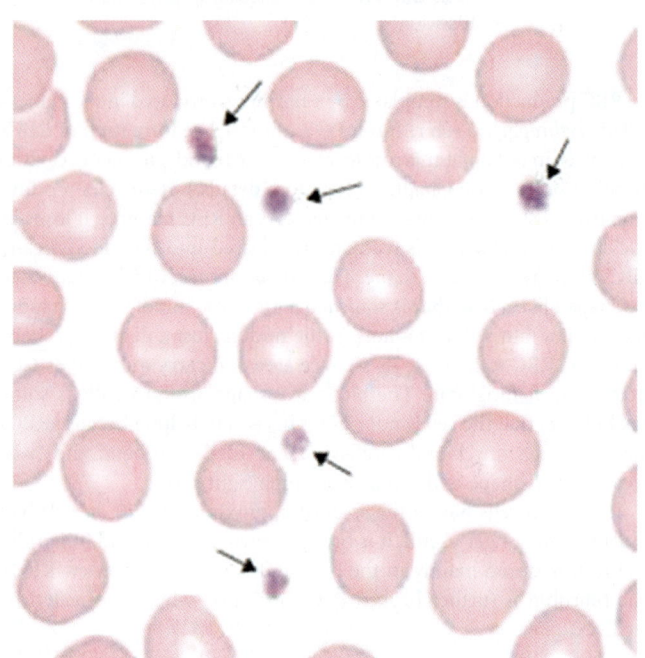

FIG. 8.4 (From *Mosby's Dictionary of Medicine, Nursing, & Health Professions*, ed 8, St. Louis, 2009, Elsevier.)

PHYSIOLOGY OF THE BLOOD

The process of blood formation is called *hematopoiesis* (hee mah toh poy EE sis). All blood cells originate from a single type of cell called a stem cell. The formation of blood takes place in the red bone marrow. Red blood cells, white blood cells, and platelets all start from stem cells, but every blood cell has a unique role in the body.

> **MEDICAL TERMINOLOGY**
>
> **-poiesis:** formation

Red Blood Cells: Blood Types

Human blood is amazing and complex. One aspect of blood that is important is blood typing. Red blood cells can have antigens attached to their cell surface. These antigens are a key factor in blood transfusions. Blood from one person cannot be given to another person without making sure that both **blood types** are compatible. Human blood is one of four different ABO types: A, B, AB, and O (Fig. 8.5). The different blood types are possible due to specific antigens present or absent on the surface of the RBCs and specific antibodies circulating in the plasma.

Antigens are substances that stimulate an immune reaction; they are foreign to the immune system (Box 8.7). In response, the immune system wants to attack the antigens with antibodies. The immune system produces antibodies to neutralize an antigen, making it inactive and unable to cause harm. For each ABO blood type, there is a specific antigen(s) on the surface of the red blood cell. Also, for each ABO blood group, antibodies are **preformed** against the antigen(s) that would be

Blood Type	Antigen (RBC membrane)	Antibody (plasma)	Can receive blood from	Can donate blood to
A (40%)	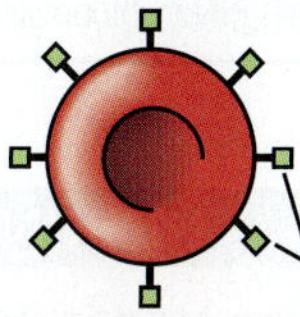 A antigen	Anti-B antibodies	A, O	A, AB
B (10%)	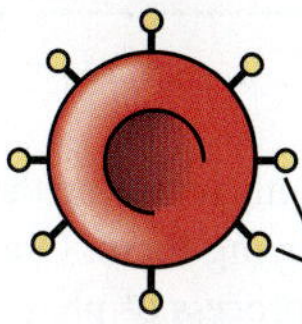 B antigen	Anti-A antibodies	B, O	B, AB
AB (4%)	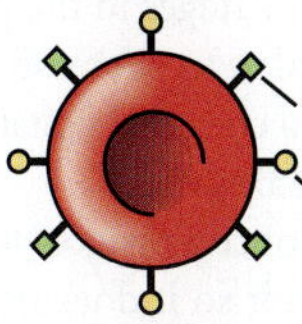 A antigen, B antigen	No antibodies	A, B, AB, O	AB
O (46%)	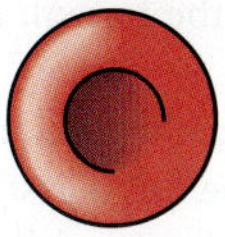 No antigen	Both Anti-A and Anti-B antibodies	O	O, A, B, AB

FIG. 8.5 ABO blood types. (From Herlihy B, Maebius NK: *The Human Body in Health and Illness*, ed 4, Philadelphia, 2011, Saunders.)

> **BOX 8.7 Antibodies and Antigens in the Blood**
>
> Blood antigens are also called *agglutinogens* (ah gloo TIN oh jens) because their presence can cause blood to clump or *agglutinate*. A blood antibody is also called an *agglutinin* (ah GLOO tin nin).

> **BOX 8.8 Rh Factor in Blood Donation**
>
> Rh-positive blood can be given to someone who has Rh-positive blood but *not* to someone who has Rh-negative blood. Rh-negative blood can be given to someone who has Rh-positive or Rh-negative blood.

---

incompatible. See Fig. 8.5 for antigen and antibody combinations for each ABO blood type.

If an individual with type A blood is transfused with type B blood, the anti-B antibodies are ready to attack the B blood cells, because the immune system knows they are foreign. The opposite is also true—if an individual with type B blood is transfused with type A blood, the anti-A antibodies are ready to attack the A blood cells.

Looking at the antigen-antibody reactions for type AB, individuals with type AB blood do not make antibodies because they have both A and B antigens on their RBC surface. This is why type AB blood is the universal recipient: it has no antibodies to attack any other blood type.

Type O blood has no antigens on the RBC surface, so type O blood can be donated to any other ABO blood type. Because type O has no antigens to cause incompatibility, an individual with type O blood is considered the universal donor.

There is another antigen that plays a major role in blood compatibility, the *Rh antigen*. The Rh antigen is also known as Rh factor or D antigen. There is a collection of 47 antigens that act together as a group and are referred to as the Rh antigen or Rh factor. The ABO type is the first factor in blood compatibility, but the Rh factor must be compatible too. Someone who possesses the Rh antigen is said to be Rh-positive. About 85% of the population in the United States is Rh-positive, so that leaves about 15% of the population that is Rh-negative. Why is this important?

Rh antibodies are different than ABO antibodies. Rh antibodies are not preformed like ABO antibodies. Someone must be exposed to the Rh antigen for his or her immune system to produce antibodies. This process is called *sensitization*. The first time an Rh-negative person encounters the Rh antigen is when the immune system becomes sensitized, or recognizes, the Rh antigen as foreign. The first time the contact is made, there is no noticeable reaction by the Rh-negative person. But, any time after sensitization, an Rh-negative recipient will react to the Rh antigen (Box 8.8). The reaction is usually the lysis of red blood cells.

This is very important in pregnancy because a mismatch between the fetus and the mother can cause *hemolytic* (hee moh LIT ick) *disease of the newborn (HDN)* or *erythroblastosis fetalis*. In this disorder, a mother who is Rh-negative and is carrying an Rh-positive fetus will develop antibodies to the Rh-positive blood if fetal blood exposure occurs during a pregnancy. If another pregnancy occurs with a Rh-positive fetus, the

BOX 8.9 Rh Immunoglobulin

RhoGAM is one brand of Rh immunoglobulin (RhIg). It is an injectable drug given to women with Rh-negative blood during pregnancy (28–30 weeks). It is also given after delivery (within 72 hours) if the baby is Rh-positive. RhoGAM binds to any Rh-positive cells that sneak into the mother's bloodstream. RhoGAM binds to the Rh antigen and makes the fetal cells seem invisible to the mother's immune system. RhIg is given to prevent sensitization of an Rh-negative mother to a future Rh-positive pregnancy.

BOX 8.10 Role of the Liver in Coagulation

Most clotting factors are proteins that are produced in the liver. Without a healthy functioning liver, blood will not clot properly.

CRITICAL THINKING 8.3

Why is it so important for a woman to know her blood type, ABO and Rh type?

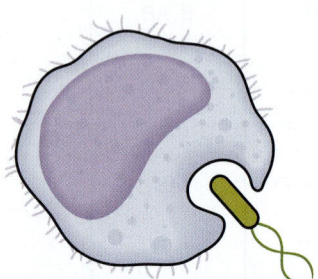

FIG. 8.6 Phagocytosis.

mother's immune system already knows that Rh-positive is foreign and will produce antibodies that cross the placenta and destroy the fetal red blood cells. It is important for women to know if they are Rh-positive or Rh-negative. Providers will order a RhoGAM for Rh-negative women with every pregnancy to safeguard against Rh sensitization (Box 8.9). Rh-negative women may also receive it with an ectopic pregnancy, miscarriage, abortion, or significant vaginal bleeding during pregnancy.

White Blood Cells: Phagocytosis. *Phagocytosis* is the process by which a cell attaches to a microorganism, particle, or other cell then ingests and destroys it (Fig. 8.6). The immune system is an essential and active system in our everyday lives. Unknown to us, the immune system is constantly searching the body for pathogens and foreign objects and then destroying them. One way the immune system protects the body is by the process of phagocytosis.

There are four stages in the process of phagocytosis. Each step must take place in order, to successfully destroy a foreign invader:

- *Chemotaxis*: a chemical signal that alerts phagocytic cells to a potential threat to the body
- *Attachment*: once a phagocyte locates a foreign invader it must attach, or grab onto it so it does not get away
- *Ingestion*: the phagocytes extends its cell membrane to engulf or wrap around the foreign invader and bring it into the phagocytic cell
- *Digestion*: once the foreign invader is inside of the phagocytic cell, enzymes in the cell digest or destroy the invader

White blood cells, especially monocytes/macrophages and neutrophils, are aggressive phagocytic cells. They help protect the body from a variety of dangers through the process of phagocytosis. Some of the substances that are removed from the body by phagocytic cells are the following:

- Pathogens: microorganisms such as bacteria, virus, fungi
- *Senescent cells*: old, dead, dying, or useless cells that are now seen as foreign to the immune system
- Malignant and tumor cells: even though they are part of the person's body, their appearance, function, and chemical makeup identify them as foreign, and the immune system wants to destroy them

Even though this chapter is about the blood, it is important to understand the role of white blood cells in the body. Phagocytosis is one process in the immune system. The immune system will be described in Chapter 9.

Platelets: Coagulation and Hemostasis. The process involved in forming a blood clot is complicated, with many specific chemical reactions and clotting factors involved (Box 8.10). What follows is a simplified version of this process.

It all starts with an injury to a blood vessel. Normally the inside of a blood vessel is very smooth, but when there is an injury, a rough area is created. This starts the process of coagulation.

First, a damaged vessel will **constrict** to slow the flow of blood through the vessel. In response to the injury, platelets become sticky and clump together (*aggregation*). Platelets then stick to the area of injury (*adhesion*). Because of platelet aggregation and adhesion, a *platelet plug* is formed over the injury and platelets release clotting factors, which aid in the process of coagulation. The injured blood vessel tissue also activates clotting factors in the blood plasma. The interaction between the clotting factors works to form *fibrin*, a white, **filamentous**, tough protein strand that creates a netlike structure (Fig. 8.7). The fibrin net traps red blood cells and more platelets to form a blood clot or *thrombus*. This process is called *blot clotting* or *coagulation*. When the body stops the flow of blood through coagulation the process is called *hemostasis*.

VOCABULARY

blood type: A person's blood is categorized based on the presence or absence of specific antigens on the red blood cell's surface. Also known as a blood group. Blood type is inherited and is present before birth.
constrict: To contract or shrink.
filamentous: Composed of or containing filaments or strands of a substance.
lysis: Destruction or break down of cells. Rupture or dissolution.
preformed (antibodies): Antibodies are that formed before being introduced to an antigen. ABO antibodies are preformed.

MEDICAL TERMINOLOGY

agglutin/o: clumping
anti-: against
fibrin/o: fiber substance
-gen: producing
-in: substance
-lytic: pertaining to breaking down
-stasis: stopping, controlling

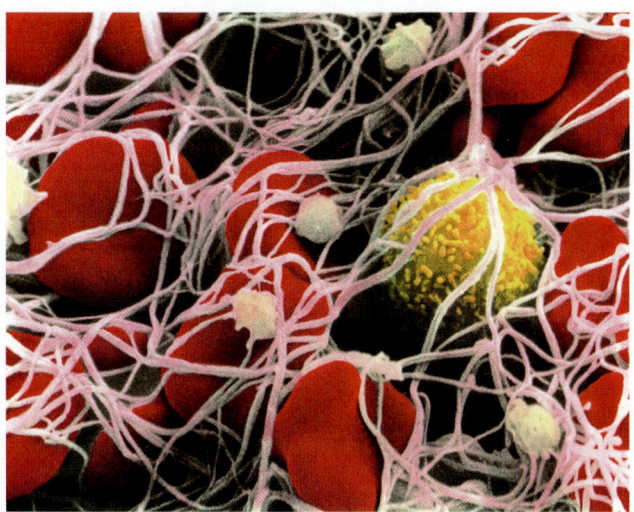

FIG. 8.7 Fibrin clot. (Reprinted with permission of CNRI/Photo Researchers, Inc.)

> **CRITICAL THINKING 8.4**
>
> Dr. Martin went back into the exam room to look at Erma's leg. On the back of her left leg there was a bruised area that was slightly swollen. Dr. Martin observed a few varicose veins around the bruise but did not see anything that made him suspect a blood clot. The area was tender when Dr. Martin touched it, and Erma indicated that this was the spot that was giving her pain. What is another term for a blood clot? In your own words, write a definition for the terms *coagulation* and *hemostasis*. Share your answers with the class.

DISEASES AND DISORDERS OF THE BLOOD

Diseases of the blood are diverse and have many causes. Many factors can be associated with blood diseases, disorders, and infections. These diseases can involve red blood cells, white blood cells, and platelets. Causes of blood diseases and disorders can be infections, structural abnormalities, malignant mutations, and congenital conditions. Common signs and symptoms of blood diseases and disorders include the following:
- Fatigue, pale skin, bleeding gums or nose bleeds, frequent or unexplained bruising
- Pain, weakness, headaches, dizziness, light-headedness
- Swelling of the affected area

Tables 8.2 and 8.3 provide common terminology related to diagnostic laboratory tests and therapeutic interventions.

> **MEDICAL TERMINOLOGY**
>
> -apheresis: removal
> auto-: self
> -fusion: pouring
> homo-: same (species)
> log/o: study
> -ous: pertaining to
> -stasis: stopping, controlling
> trans-: across

Anemia: Iron Deficiency

When the body does not have an adequate supply of iron to make healthy red blood cells, iron deficiency *anemia* can occur. Iron is necessary to produce hemoglobin. Oxygen binds to hemoglobin and is carried to the cells of the body. Without adequate iron intake, the body cannot make red blood cells, and the ability to supply blood to the cells is compromised.

> **VOCABULARY**
>
> **anemia:** A deficiency of hemoglobin in the blood and lack of healthy red blood cells. Can be caused by a nutrient deficiency or an inability to absorb vital nutrients.

Etiology. Iron deficiency anemia occurs when the body does not have enough iron to produce hemoglobin. The causes of iron deficiency include the following:
- An iron-poor diet: inadequate intake of iron through food
- An inability to absorb iron: because of digestive system surgery or malabsorption disorders such as celiac disease
- Blood loss: due to peptic ulcers, intestinal bleeding, or nondigestive chronic blood loss
- Pregnancy: iron stores are used up to produce maternal and fetal red blood cells

Those at risk for developing iron deficiency anemia include the following:
- Women: bleeding during menstruation and iron needs during pregnancy increase iron deficiency risks
- Infants and children: infants born with low birth weight, born prematurely, or who do not get an adequate supply of iron from breast milk or enriched formula; children require healthy foods of adequate nutrition and variety to meet their growth needs
- Vegetarians

Signs and Symptoms. Iron deficiency anemia can have mild signs and symptoms at first, but if the body becomes more deficient in iron, the signs and symptoms can intensify. Iron deficiency anemia signs and symptoms may include the following:
- Fatigue (it may be intense), weakness, pale skin, and brittle nails
- Headache, dizziness, or lightheadedness
- Chest pain, fast heartbeat (tachycardia), or shortness of breath (SOB)
- Cold hands and feet, thick or sore tongue

Complications can occur if iron deficiency anemia becomes severe or goes untreated:
- Heart problems such as rapid or irregular heartbeat. Untreated anemia can lead to an enlarged heart or heart failure.
- Problems during pregnancy. Severe iron deficiency anemia can cause premature births or low birth weight.
- Growth and development can be affected for infants and children. They may also be more susceptible to infections.

Diagnostic Procedures. The provider may recommend the following tests to diagnose iron deficiency anemia:
- Complete blood count, including red blood cell size and color. Red blood cells that lack iron tend to be smaller and paler in color.
- *Hematocrit* (hee MAT uh krit), which is defined as the percentage by volume of red blood cells in a sample of blood after it has been centrifuged (Fig. 8.8). Normal values for men and women are different.
- Hemoglobin. Lower than normal hemoglobin levels indicate anemia.
- Blood ferritin. Ferritin is a protein that helps store iron in the body.

TABLE 8.2 Terms Related to Laboratory Tests

Term	Definition
blood cultures	Blood samples are submitted to grow microorganisms that may be present.
complete blood cell count (CBC)	Twelve tests, including RBC count, WBC count, hemoglobin, hematocrit/packed-cell volume (Hct/PCV), and WBC differential. Some CLIA-waived tests available.
comprehensive metabolic panel (CMP)	Set of blood tests that assess organ function, metabolism, and electrolyte levels. Some CLIA-waived tests available.
Coombs antiglobulin test (koomz an tee GLOB yoo lin)	Blood test to help diagnose HDN, acquired hemolytic anemia, or a transfusion reaction.
differential count	A blood slide is stained and put under a microscope. The laboratory then looks at 100 WBCs, determines WBC type and percentage, and looks at size and shape of RBCs and platelets. Also known as a "diff."
erythrocyte sedimentation rate (ESR) (eh RITH roh syte seh dih men TAY shun)	This test determines the time it takes for mature RBCs to settle out of a blood sample after an anticoagulant is added. An increased ESR indicates inflammation. Some CLIA-waived tests available.
hematocrit/packed-cell volume (Hct/PCV) (hee MAT oh krit)	Measure of the percentage of RBCs in a blood sample. Some CLIA-waived tests available.
hemoglobin (Hgb, Hb) (HEE moh gloh bin)	Measure of iron-containing pigment in RBCs. Some CLIA-waived tests available.
hemoglobin electrophoresis (HEE moh gloh bin ih lek troh fuh REE sis)	A blood test that can separate different types of hemoglobin using an electric current and gel media. Useful for diagnosing hemophilia and thalassemias.
hemoglobin fractionation by high-pressure liquid chromatography (HPLC) (HEE moh gloh bin frak shuh NEY shuh n) (kroh muh TOG ruh fee)	A blood test that can separate different types of hemoglobin by using high-pressure liquid chromatography. Useful for diagnosing hemophilia (hee muh FIL ee uh) and thalassemias (thal uh SEE mee uhs).
hemoglobin isoelectric focusing	A blood test similar to hemoglobin electrophoresis. Useful for diagnosing hemophilia and thalassemias.
iron studies	Testing blood for a variety of iron components. Can be done to diagnose iron deficiency anemia or monitor sickle-cell anemia.
mean corpuscular hemoglobin (MCH) (kor PUS kyoo lur)	Test to measure the average weight of hemoglobin per RBC. Useful in diagnosing anemia.
mean corpuscular hemoglobin concentration (MCHC)	Test to measure the concentration of hemoglobin in RBCs. Useful for measuring a patient's response to anemia treatments.
monospot (MAH noh spot)	A test for infectious mononucleosis. Checks the blood sample for antibodies to the Epstein-Barr virus. Some CLIA-waived tests available.
partial thromboplastin time (PTT) (THROM boh plas tin)	Test of blood plasma to detect coagulation defects. Used to detect hemophilia.
peripheral blood smear	This test is used to confirm RBC, WBC, and platelet counts from a CBC. A blood slide is stained and observed under a microscope. Size, shape, color, and cellular characteristics can be seen.
prothrombin time (PT) (proh THROM bin)	Test that measures the time it takes for blood to clot. Used to determine the cause of unexplained bleeding, to assess levels of blood thinners in blood, and to assess the liver's ability to make clotting factors. Some CLIA-waived tests available.
Schilling test (SHILL ing)	Nuclear medicine test used to diagnose vitamin B_{12} deficiency and pernicious anemia.
white blood cell (WBC) count	Measurement of the number of leukocytes in the blood. Some CLIA-waived tests available.

From Shiland B: *Mastering Healthcare Terminology*, ed 5, St. Louis, 2016, Elsevier.

> **VOCABULARY**
> **centrifuged:** A machine that rotates at high speed and separates substances of different densities by centrifugal force. For example, a tube of blood is separated into plasma/serum, white blood cells, platelets, and red blood cells.

Treatment. Iron deficiency anemia is most frequently treated with iron supplements. Over-the-counter iron tablets can be taken to replace iron stores in the body. For infants and children, a liquid supplement is recommended. To increase the absorption of iron in the supplements, the provider may recommend the following:
- Instead of taking iron supplements with water, take them with orange juice to improve the absorption of iron.
- Do not take iron supplements with food. Taking them on an empty stomach is better, if possible.
- Do not take iron supplements with an antacid because it decreases the absorption of iron.

Treating the cause of iron deficiency is very important. If iron supplements do not improve blood-iron levels, then the anemia may be caused by chronic bleeding or inadequate absorption of iron in the digestive system. Further testing may be recommended. Depending on the cause, anemia treatment may include the following:
- Antibiotics and other medications to treat peptic ulcers
- Oral contraceptives to lighten heavy menstrual flow
- Surgery to remove intestinal polyps or tumors, or uterine fibroids

If iron deficiency is severe, intravenous iron supplementation or blood transfusion can be used to replace iron and hemoglobin quickly.

TABLE 8.3 Terms Related to Blood and Bone Marrow Interventions

Term	Definition
apheresis (aff ur EE sis)	Temporary removal of blood from a donor, in which one or more blood components are removed. The rest of the blood is reinfused into the donor. Examples include *leukapheresis,* removal of WBCs; *plasmapheresis,* removal of plasma; and *plateletpheresis,* removal of platelets.
autologous BMT (ah TALL uh gus)	Harvesting a patient's own healthy bone marrow before treatment, then reintroducing the bone marrow later.
autologous transfusion	Process in which the donor's own blood is removed and stored for future need.
autotransfusion	Process in which the donor is transfused with his or her own blood, after anticoagulation and filtration, from an active bleeding site in cases of major surgery or trauma.
blood transfusion	Intravenous transfer of blood from a donor to a recipient, giving either whole blood or *components* (RBC only, platelets, plasma).
bone marrow transplant (BMT)	The transplantation of bone marrow to stimulate production of normal blood cells.
homologous BMT (hoh MALL uh gus)	Transplantation of healthy bone marrow from a donor to a recipient, to stimulate formation of new blood cells.

From Shiland B: *Mastering Healthcare Terminology,* ed 5, St. Louis, 2016, Elsevier.

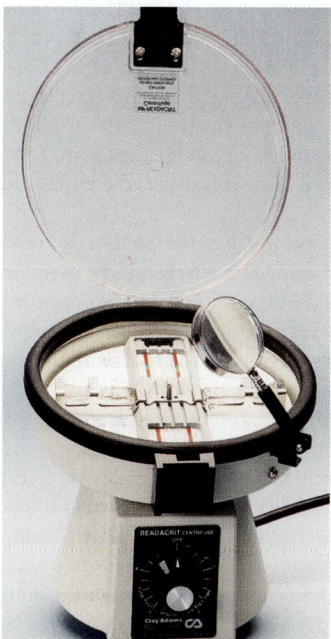

FIG. 8.8 Hematocrit centrifuge. (From Proctor D, et al: *Kinn's The Medical Assistant,* ed 13, St. Louis, 2017, Elsevier.)

Prognosis. Without complications, the prognosis is very good. Iron deficiency anemia with complications is less predictable.

Prevention. To prevent iron deficiency anemia, individuals should start by eating a diet that includes iron-rich foods such as these:
- Red meat, pork, poultry, fish, seafood
- Nonmeat or vegetarian iron-rich foods such as eggs, leafy green vegetables, lentils, soybeans, many nuts and seeds, raisins, dried apricots, peas
- Iron-fortified cereals, bread, pasta

Other ways to prevent iron deficiency anemia include the following:
- Enhance absorption of iron by eating or drinking vitamin C-rich foods at the same time iron-rich foods are eaten
- In infants, give breast milk or iron-fortified formula up to the first year; after 6 months of age, feed with iron-fortified cereals to ensure adequate iron intake

> **CRITICAL THINKING 8.5**
> After Dr. Martin completed his exam, he looked up Erma's hemoglobin results. A normal hemoglobin would be about 11.5 to 14.5 mg/dl. Erma's results were 10.3 mg/dl. Discuss the possible reasons for Erma's low hemoglobin.

Anemia: Sickle-Cell Disease

A normal red blood cell shape is round, biconcave, and flexible. This allows the RBC to easily travel through blood capillaries. Someone who has inherited sickle-cell anemia has RBCs that have a crescent moon or sickle shape. Because sickle-cell RBCs are abnormally shaped, they are rigid and do not carry oxygen as efficiently. They can become stuck or lodged in blood capillaries. When this happens, blood flow can slow down or capillaries can even become blocked. Cells, tissues, or organs may not receive an adequate oxygen supply.

Etiology. In the United States, sickle-cell disease most frequently affects black individuals. An abnormal sickle-cell gene is an inherited condition that follows an *autosomal recessive inheritance* pattern. This means that the mother and the father must both pass on the defective gene for a child to be affected.

If only one parent passes on the sickle-cell gene, that child will have the sickle-cell trait. He or she will have one normal gene and one sickle-cell gene. People who have the sickle-cell trait make normal hemoglobin (hemoglobin A [HbA]) and sickle-cell hemoglobin (hemoglobin S [HbS]). Most of their blood cells will be normal, but some may be sickle cells (Fig. 8.9). People who have the sickle-cell trait generally do not have symptoms. They are carriers of the defective gene, which means they can pass the gene to their children.

Signs and Symptoms. Signs and symptoms of sickle-cell anemia may include some or all of the following:
- Anemia and accompanying fatigue, pale or yellowish skin, and fever.
- Periodic episodes of pain, called *crises*. Pain intensity and duration vary with each crisis. When sickle-shaped RBCs get stuck in blood capillaries, pain develops. Common sites include the chest, joints, abdomen, and bones. If a severe crisis occurs, hospitalization may be necessary. Some individuals may experience chronic pain due to past crisis damage. Bone and joint damage is common.
- Painful swelling of hands and feet.

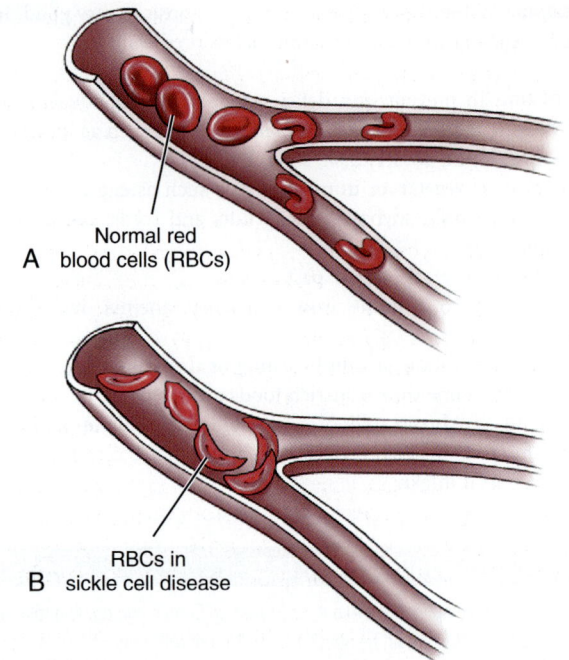

FIG. 8.9 Sickle cells. (From Herlihy B, Maebius NK: *The Human Body in Health and Illness*, ed 4, Philadelphia, 2011, Saunders.)

- Abdominal swelling and frequent infections. Sickle cells can damage the spleen, which is in the abdomen and is involved in the immune system.
- Vision problems and delayed growth.

Sickle-cell anemia crises can lead to many complications, including the following:

- Stroke, organ damage, leg ulcers, and blindness may occur, all because of capillary blockage or lack of blood flow.
- *Acute chest syndrome*, a life-threatening complication that includes chest pain, fever, and difficulty breathing. This may be caused by a lung infection or by blocked capillaries in the lungs.
- *Pulmonary hypertension*, which is high blood pressure that develops in the lungs. This most often affects adults and causes fatigue and shortness of breath. This can be a fatal complication.
- Gallstones may form due to high bilirubin levels in the blood.
- *Priapism*, a painful, long-lasting erection, can occur when sickle cells block the capillaries in the penis. This can lead to impotence.

Diagnostic Procedures. The following tests can be performed to diagnose sickle-cell anemia, specifically looking for hemoglobin S in the blood:

- Hemoglobin electrophoresis
- Hemoglobin fractionation by high-pressure liquid chromatography (HPLC)
- Hemoglobin isoelectric focusing

If testing a child in utero for sickle-cell anemia, *amniotic fluid*, or the fluid surrounding the fetus in the womb, can be sampled and tested at about 14 to 16 weeks into the pregnancy. DNA analysis looks for genetic alterations or mutations, and can tell if the fetus will have the sickle-cell trait or will have sickle-cell anemia.

Once sickle-cell anemia has been diagnosed, the following tests may be performed periodically to monitor the disease:

- Complete blood count (CBC), with a **peripheral blood smear**
- Hemoglobin and hematocrit

BOX 8.11 Hydroxyurea

Hydroxyurea is a medication that works by stimulating the production of fetal hemoglobin, HbF. Fetal hemoglobin is found in newborns and helps prevent sickle-shaped red blood cells from being formed. Hydroxyurea decreases pain and crisis episodes for people with sickle-cell anemia. It may increase the risk of infections and there is concern about long-term use, but for now it has given relief to people with sickle-cell disease.

BOX 8.12 Blood Is a Biologic

Blood is classified as a **biologic product**, or biologic, and can be used to treat disease. The Food and Drug Administration (FDA) is responsible for ensuring that the blood supply is safe for use as a transfusable biologic.

- Blood bilirubin levels
- Iron studies

Treatment. Depending on the frequency and severity of a person's sickle-cell crises, treatment may include the following:

- Medications may include antibiotics and pain relievers. Hydroxyurea is a specific medication that can be taken daily to reduce crises and the need for blood transfusions (Box 8.11).
- Vaccinations may be administered to avoid preventable infections.
- Blood transfusions (Box 8.12) are given to increase the amount of normal hemoglobin in the blood, alleviate anemia, and reduce the risk of complications and crises.
- For persons with significant symptoms or crisis episodes, a **bone marrow transplant** (also called a stem cell transplant) can offer a cure to sickle-cell anemia. This therapy is most frequently done on children 16 years or younger. It carries significant risks, involves lengthy hospital stays, and may result in complications. Complications may lead to rejection of the bone marrow, which may result in death.

Prognosis. People who have the sickle-cell trait have a very good prognosis and may never have any signs or symptoms of the condition.

People who have sickle-cell anemia can experience signs and symptoms that range from relatively mild to life threatening. Proper treatment, ongoing follow up, and patient compliance are all necessary to prevent sickle-cell crisis episodes and complications of the disease.

Prevention. If a person has the sickle-cell trait, seeing a genetic counselor before having children would be useful in determining the risk of having a child with sickle-cell anemia. A person who has sickle-cell anemia cannot prevent the disease but can help prevent situations that may bring on a crisis episode. The following steps may help a person stay healthy and avoid complications:

- Drink plenty of water and do not become dehydrated.
- Avoid temperature extremes and high altitudes.
- Exercise regularly but do not push exercise to extremes.
- Choose a healthy diet that is rich in lean protein and lots of fresh fruits and vegetables. Consider a folic acid or multivitamin supplement.
- Use any over-the-counter medications with caution.

MEDICAL TERMINOLOGY
crisis (singular), **crises** (plural)

> **BOX 8.13 Hemophilia Inheritance**
>
> Genetically a female has two sex chromosomes, one X from the mother and one X from the father. Males also have two sex chromosomes, one X from the mother and one Y from the father. The X chromosome is larger and contains more genetic material, so when a woman carries a genetic trait that is not matched on the Y chromosome, her sons will have the trait she passed on the X chromosome. The different types of hemophilia are inherited a bit differently:
> - Hemophilia A or B is caused by a gene located on the X chromosome. Hemophilia A or B almost always occurs in males and is inherited from mother to son.
> - Hemophilia C is a milder form of hemophilia, with less severe signs and symptoms. The gene for hemophilia C is not located on the X chromosome, so this condition can be passed on to sons and daughters equally.

> **VOCABULARY**
>
> **biologic product:** Also known as a biologic, it is made from a variety of natural resources that can be human, animal, or microorganism based.
> **bone marrow transplant:** A procedure that replaces a person's bone marrow with bone marrow from a healthy donor (such as a sibling). Also called a stem cell transplant.
> **peripheral blood smear:** A thin layer of blood is smeared on a glass microscope slide, then stained. This allows a trained laboratory technician or pathologist to examine various characteristics of the blood cells microscopically.

Hemophilia

Hemophilia is the deficiency of clotting factor VIII (hemophilia A, the most common type), clotting factor IX (hemophilia B), or clotting factor XI (hemophilia C). For blood to clot, platelets and plasma proteins interact to create a fibrin clot. In the case of hemophilia, one of the clotting factors is reduced or missing completely. This means that it takes longer for blood to clot completely.

If a person has hemophilia, blood clotting is not as efficient as it is for someone without hemophilia. Small cuts and scrapes do not pose a significant bleeding risk for most hemophiliacs, but internal bleeding and bleeding into the joints (especially the knees, ankles, and elbows) are causes for concern. Bleeding deep in the body can cause damage to organs, tissues, and joints, and it can be life threatening if not treated appropriately.

Etiology. Hemophilia is most frequently an *inherited recessive condition*. For hemophilia to be passed on to a daughter, both the mother and the father would need to carry the hemophilia gene. For hemophilia to be passed on to a son, only the mother needs to have the hemophilia gene. A mother can be a carrier with no symptoms of the condition and pass it on to her son (Box 8.13).

About 30% of people with hemophilia have no family history of the disease. In these cases, hemophilia is caused by a *genetic mutation*, or a random change in a gene that causes the condition.

Signs and Symptoms. Signs and symptoms for hemophilia depend on the deficiency of the clotting factor. Some people have a reduced amount of clotting factor, whereas others have almost no clotting factor. Signs and symptoms will reflect the lack of clotting factor, which may include the following:
- Prolonged bleeding after an injury or large, deep bruising
- Severe headache, neck pain, or double vision
- Pain, swelling, tightness or bruising in the joints especially after activity or injury
- Longer clotting times after cuts, scrapes, injuries, or after dental work or surgery
- Blood in urine or stool, nosebleeds with no known cause

Complications of moderate to severe hemophilia may include deep internal bleeding, joint damage, and adverse reactions to clotting factor treatments and medications.

Diagnostic Procedures. For people with a family history of hemophilia, genetic testing can be done before a pregnancy to determine the chances of passing on hemophilia. Also, during pregnancy, *in utero* testing can be done to see if hemophilia affects the fetus. A conclusive prenatal diagnosis can only be made with invasive procedures such as *amniocentesis* or *chorionic villus sampling*. Both procedures are risky for the pregnancy, so benefits and risks should be discussed with the provider. Chapter 31 provides additional information on amniocentesis and chorionic villus sampling.

In children and adults, a blood test is done to detect clotting-factor deficiencies. Hemophilia is frequently diagnosed when one is between 9 and 24 months of age. Mild forms of hemophilia may not be recognized or diagnosed until a surgery or invasive dental procedure is performed.

Treatment. Hemophilia cannot currently be cured, but treatments can help manage the disease. Treatment for bleeding incidents will depend on the severity of hemophilia and the severity of the bleed. Treatments may include the following:
- Injection or nasal spray application of the hormone *desmopressin*
- *Infusion* of clotting factor (often, recovered from donated human blood or plasma); repeated infusions may be given if bleeding is severe

To help prevent bleeding incidents, the following treatments may be used to manage hemophilia:
- Regular infusions of desmopressin or clotting factor
- Application of *fibrin sealants*
- Physical therapy to ease pain from damage to joints
- First aid for minor cuts

> **VOCABULARY**
>
> **desmopressin:** A hormone that is injected into a vein (or given as a nasal spray) that may help stimulate a release of more clotting factor in the body to help stop bleeding.
> **fibrin sealants:** Also known as fibrin glue, these topical medications are applied directly to the skin. They are made up of substances that promote blood clotting and long-term healing and can be used for a variety of wounds where stitches, bandages, or staples cannot be used.
> **in utero:** The term means "in the uterus," referring to the fetus' time of development.
> **infusion:** When a medication or treatment is given intravenously, but it needs to be given slowly. May be given through a port, catheter, or peripherally inserted central catheter (PICC) line.

Prognosis. For mild to moderate hemophilia, the prognosis is good for compliant patients. For moderate to severe hemophilia, compliant patients can manage the condition well, but for noncompliant patients or in the case of a severe bleed or injury, the prognosis can be less positive.

Prevention. People with hemophilia should protect themselves from injury and joint damage by doing the following:
- Wear a medical alert bracelet, and let people know he or she has hemophilia.

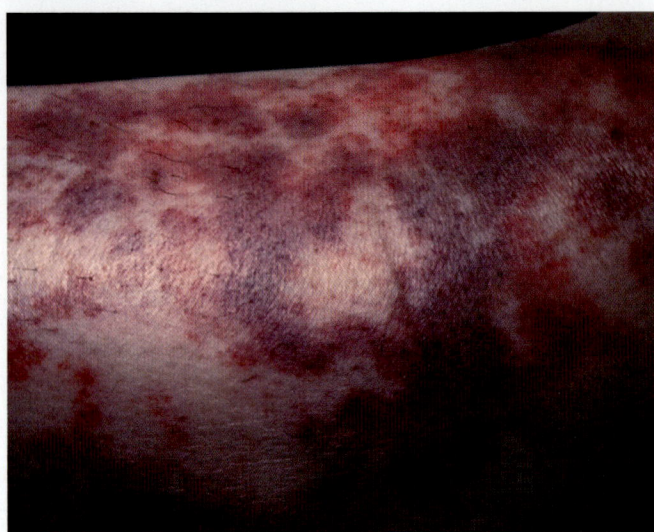

FIG. 8.10 Purpura. (From Bolognia JL: *Dermatology*, ed 2, St. Louis, 2008, Mosby.)

> **MEDICAL TERMINOLOGY**
> **-penia:** deficiency

Signs and Symptoms. Idiopathic thrombocytopenic purpura may be asymptomatic, or it may show the following signs and symptoms:
- Bleeding into the skin that looks like a pinpoint-sized reddish purple or purple brownish spots or rash called a *petechiae* (pi TEE kee uh), often on the lower legs
- Easy or excessive bruising, bleeding gums, or nosebleeds
- Blood in urine or stools, extended bleeding time from cuts, and unusually heavy menstrual flow

An extraordinary complication of ITP is bleeding into the brain, lungs, muscles, or joints. If this happens, it can be fatal and medical intervention should be immediate.

Diagnostic Procedures. Diagnosis of ITP will most likely include the following:
- History and physical exam by a medical provider. History to include any medications and recent viral infections.
- Complete blood count (CBC). ITP will present normal WBC and RBC counts, but an abnormally low platelet count. CLIA-waived test.
- Peripheral blood smear.
- Bone marrow exam. This test may be used to help identify the cause of a low platelet count and rule out causes other than ITP. Bone marrow of a person with ITP should be normal because the platelets are being destroyed in the blood, not in the bone marrow.

Treatment. Children with ITP usually improve without treatment. Mild ITP in adults may only need monitoring for signs and symptoms, and periodic platelet counts. Many adults with ITP will eventually need treatment, as the condition can become chronic or more severe with time. Treatment for ITP may include the following:
- Medications to boost the platelet count.
- Medications to suppress the immune system (short-term only), often a corticosteroid.
- Surgery to remove the spleen (*splenectomy*) if symptoms persist or become worse. This is extremely rare for children.
- If bleeding becomes an emergency, platelet transfusions can be administered and intravenous corticosteroids can be given to treat a crisis.

Prognosis. The prognosis for children is usually very good. The prognosis for adults varies with the severity of the disease.

Prevention. The cause of idiopathic thrombocytopenic purpura is not certain, so prevention is not possible. Once the diagnosis of ITP has been made, there are methods to lessen the chance of a relapse or progression of symptoms, especially in adults:
- Avoid activities that could cause injury. Avoid contact sports or high-impact activities such as martial arts, football, basketball, hockey, or boxing.
- Watch for signs of infection, especially postsplenectomy.
- Use over-the-counter medications sparingly. Avoid NSAIDs, as they can weaken platelet function.
- Drink alcohol only in moderation or not at all. Alcohol reduces the production of platelets in the body.

- Participate in regular, low-impact exercise such as bicycling, walking, or swimming. Contact sports and high impact exercises are not safe for a person with hemophilia.
- Avoid medications that prolong blood clotting, such as nonsteroidal antiinflammatory drugs (NSAIDs) and blood thinners.
- Practice good dental hygiene to prevent tooth decay and possible extractions.
- Wear protective gear to avoid injuries with a fall, such as kneepads, elbow pads, and helmets.

Idiopathic Thrombocytopenic Purpura

Idiopathic thrombocytopenic purpura (id ee uh PATH ik throm boh sahy tuh PEE nick PUR pyoo r uh), or ITP, is also known as immune thrombocytopenia (Fig. 8.10). This condition is a result of an abnormally low number of platelets in the blood, which leads to easy bruising and possibly excessive bleeding. Children can develop ITP after a viral infection and typically improve without treatment. In adults however, ITP may become a long-term condition.

Etiology. The cause of ITP is unknown, but it frequently occurs after a viral infection, especially in children. Scientists feel that a viral infection may trigger the immune system to incorrectly see platelets as foreign. The immune system then destroys the platelets, leaving the person with an abnormally low platelet count.

Platelets help blood clot, and when counts become low the risk of bruising and bleeding increases. If the platelet count drops very low (10,000 cells or fewer/microliter) internal bleeding could occur spontaneously, without injury.

There are a few risk factors for developing ITP:
- Women are more likely to develop ITP than men.
- ITP can develop after a viral infection, especially in children. Viral infections that are associated with ITP are measles, mumps, and respiratory infections.

> **VOCABULARY**
> **idiopathic:** Of unknown cause.
> **purpura:** A rash of purple spots on or under the skin often caused by internal bleeding from small blood vessels.

> **CRITICAL THINKING 8.6**
> Could ITP cause Erma's bruise? Discuss your thoughts with the class. What laboratory test would help diagnose ITP?

Infectious Mononucleosis

Infectious mononucleosis (in FEK shuh s mon uh noo klee OH sis) is also known as mono, or the kissing disease. It is commonly acquired as a child or adolescent. Most children do not show signs and symptoms, or they are very mild. People who acquire the disease in late childhood, adolescence, or young adulthood usually have signs and symptoms. It is generally a mild, self-limiting viral infection, but it can have serious complications such as hepatosplenomegaly.

Mono is passed from person to person via saliva—that's why it can be passed by kissing. It can also be passed by a sneezing, coughing, or by sharing eating or drinking utensils.

Etiology. The most common cause of infectious mononucleosis is the *Epstein-Barr virus (EBV)*, which is a type of herpes virus. Other viruses can also cause mono, but EBV is by far the most common.

EBV is passed from an infected person to a nonimmune person by saliva. Mono is usually a mild viral illness and may be asymptomatic for young children. Most adults have antibodies to EBV by the end of their 20s. Once a person develops antibodies, he or she is considered immune and cannot have mono again. Although the disease is usually mild, some people can develop complications and may become very sick.

Risk factors for acquiring mono include the following:
- Contact with someone who has an active infection
- Kissing, sharing food and drink, sharing eating utensils or toothbrush

Signs and Symptoms. Signs and symptoms of infectious mononucleosis may include the following:
- Fatigue, fever, swollen lymph nodes in the neck and armpits
- Sore throat, perhaps a strep throat that does not get better with antibiotic use
- Swollen tonsils (may obstruct breathing or cause wheezing), headache, skin rash
- Swollen upper abdomen, soft-swollen spleen

EBV has an incubation time of about 4 to 6 weeks for adolescents and young adults. The incubation time may be less for young children. Signs and symptoms usually subside within 2 to 4 weeks. Fatigue and enlarged lymph nodes and spleen may last for 4 to 6 weeks.

Complications of mono may include the following:
- Enlarged spleen and pain in the left upper abdomen; if left untreated, the spleen could rupture. Immediate medical attention is necessary.
- Inflammation of the liver, *hepatitis,* can occur.
- *Jaundice* (JAWN dis), associated with hepatitis, is a yellowing of the skin, mucous membranes, and whites of the eye; indicates a build-up of bilirubin in the blood due to stress on the liver. Medical attention is necessary.
- Anemia and thrombocytopenia can occur with mono.
- Rarely, myocarditis, meningitis, encephalitis, *Guillain-Barre* (gee YAN buh ray) syndrome can occur (Box 8.14).
- Severe complications can take place for someone who is immune compromised, such as a person with HIV/AIDS or on immunosuppressive drugs.

> **BOX 8.14 Guillain-Barre Syndrome**
> Guillain-Barre syndrome is a rare disorder in which the immune system attacks the nerves causing weakness and tingling. It may spread throughout the body and cause paralysis. In its worst form, it is a medical emergency, and a patient needs to be hospitalized for treatment.
> The cause of Guillain-Barre is unknown, but one of the viral infections that can trigger the condition is EBV, the cause of infectious mononucleosis. Most people recover completely from Guillain-Barre.

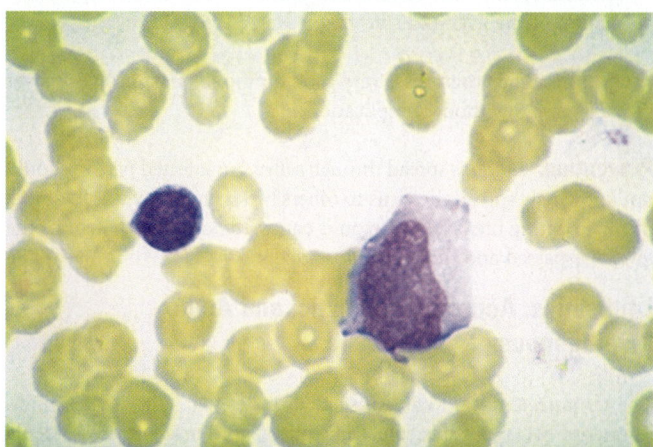

FIG. 8.11 Atypical lymphocytes. (From Thibodeau GA, Patton KT: *Anatomy and Physiology,* ed 7, St. Louis, 2010, Mosby.)

> **VOCABULARY**
> **hepatosplenomegaly:** Inflammation of the liver and spleen. Can be severe.
> **immune:** A condition in which a person has developed protective antibodies against a pathogen and is no longer at risk for acquiring the infection.
> **self-limiting viral infection:** A viral infection that causes signs and symptoms, but after a period of time the person's immune system defeats the infection and the individual is no longer ill. An example is the common cold.

> **MEDICAL TERMINOLOGY**
> **hepat/o:** liver
> **-megaly:** enlargement
> **spleen/o:** spleen

Diagnostic Procedures. If the provider suspects infectious mononucleosis, the following tests may be performed to diagnose the condition:
- History and physical exam to look for swollen lymph nodes, liver, and spleen, fever, and sore throat
- Blood tests including a monospot test to look for antibodies to EBV in the patient blood
- CBC and differential to look for an elevated WBC count and atypical lymphocytes in the blood (Fig. 8.11)

Treatment. Mono is a viral infection, so supportive care should be given. Antibiotics are not necessary and are not useful for viral infections. Lots of rest, fluids (especially water), over-the-counter pain- or fever-reducing medications (not aspirin), and a healthy diet are the best treatments for mono. Within 2 to 4 weeks, the virus should run its course, and most people recover completely.

One more important treatment for mono is to limit activities while symptoms remain. Staying away from school or work, getting extra rest, and limiting physical activities and sports is recommended. The provider should give permission to resume a normal schedule.

Treating the complications of infectious mononucleosis may include the following:
- Sometimes streptococcal throat infections can occur secondary to mono. Antibiotics should be used to treat streptococcal infections.
- If hepatosplenomegaly occurs, the person should seek medical attention. Sometimes corticosteroids are given to reduce the inflammation of the liver and spleen.

Prognosis. The prognosis is very good for mono; most people recover in 2 to 4 weeks without complications.

Prevention. Mono is spread through saliva. An infected person should not knowingly spread the virus to others by kissing or by sharing food, drink, or eating utensils. A person is considered noninfective once the fever has passed and the symptoms are gone.

Leukemias: Acute Lymphocytic, and Acute Myelogenous

The term *acute* refers to a disease or disorder that progresses rapidly. There are two types of acute leukemia: acute lymphocytic leukemia (ALL) and acute *myelogenous* (my uh LOHJ uh nus) leukemia (AML). ALL and AML are cancers of the blood and bone marrow. Bone marrow is a spongy material located inside bones. Bone marrow is where blood cells are produced.

In the case of acute leukemia, the bone marrow creates many white blood cells that cannot function as they should because they are too young to be competent. Acute leukemias have a high WBC count with many immature white blood cells in the blood.

Etiology. Acute leukemias begin with a bone marrow cell that develops errors in its DNA. The errors incorrectly instruct the cell to continue growing and dividing. When this happens, the bone marrow produces immature cells that develop into lymphoblasts or myeloblasts. These immature cells cannot function as they should, but the bone marrow keeps making them. The immature cells are produced so quickly that they crowd out healthy cells.

The cause of DNA mutations is unknown, but some of the risk factors for developing an acute leukemia include the following:
- Previous cancer treatment such as chemotherapy or radiation therapy.
- Exposure to radiation or cancer-causing chemicals.
- Age: Children are most at risk for ALL, but adults over the age of 65 are most at risk for AML.
- Genetics: Men are more likely to develop AML, and people with Down syndrome are more likely to develop AML. Siblings of a person with ALL are more likely to develop the condition.
- Smokers have a higher risk of developing AML because of the chemicals contained in cigarette smoke.

Signs and Symptoms. Signs and symptoms of acute leukemias may include the following:
- Fever, bone pain, weakness, fatigue, or loss of energy
- Frequent infections
- Pale skin, nosebleeds, or bleeding gums
- Shortness of breath
- Swollen lymph nodes in the neck, armpits, abdomen or groin (seen in AML)

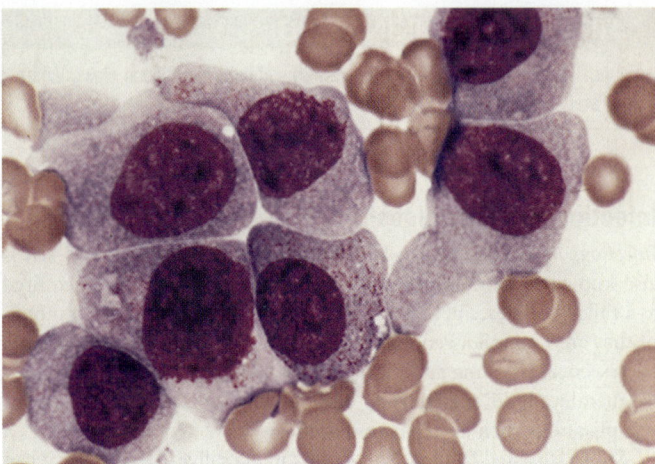

FIG. 8.12 Microscope slide of leukemia. (From Damjanov I: *Anderson's Pathology,* ed 10, St. Louis, 2000, Mosby.)

Many of these signs and symptoms are similar to the flu or a viral infection. If symptoms persist, the person should contact a provider.

Diagnostic Procedures. The provider may recommend the following tests and procedures to diagnose ALL or AML:
- Complete blood count and differential: The provider is looking for the number of white blood cells and their maturity (Fig. 8.12).
- A bone marrow biopsy may be advised.
- Imaging tests such as an x-ray, computerized tomography (CT) scan, or ultrasound scan, may help determine whether cancer has spread to other parts of the body.
- Lumbar puncture, also known as a spinal tap, may be needed to collect a sample of spinal fluid.

Treatment. The provider may recommend the following treatments. The patient age, cancer stage, and general health should be considered with any aggressive treatment.

Treatment for acute leukemia can be separated into two types, each with a different goal:
- *Induction therapy* is designed to kill most of the leukemia cells and to allow normal cell production to resume.
- *Consolidation therapy* is also called postremission therapy and is used to kill any remaining leukemia cells in the body.

Each individual situation is different. Treatment choices and length of treatment should be discussed with the provider. Treatments may include the following:
- Chemotherapy: Medications are used to kill cancer cells. Chemotherapy can be administered intravenously and sometime orally.
- Targeted drug therapy also uses medication that attacks specific irregularities present in cancer cells.
- Radiation therapy uses high-powered radiation beams, such as x-rays, to kill cancer cells.
- Stem cell transplant is used to replace leukemic bone marrow with healthy bone marrow. Before a stem cell transplant can take place, chemotherapy or radiation is used to destroy the leukemic bone marrow. The diseased bone marrow is then replaced with healthy bone marrow from a compatible donor.

Once the bone marrow is producing healthy blood cells, maintenance therapy may be recommended. The goal of maintenance therapy is to prevent leukemia cells from regrowing in the bone marrow. With this type of treatment, therapies are often given at a lower dose spread over a longer period of time.

For some leukemia patients, alternative treatments are used to help with chemotherapy or radiation side effects and to improve a person's outlook through difficult treatment. Some alternative therapies used include the following:
- Meditation, relaxation exercises, aromatherapy
- Acupuncture and massage therapy
- A change of diet to manage the side effects of chemotherapy

Prognosis. Prognosis for any cancer depends on many factors, but the following groups have historically had the following prognoses:
- ALL is the most common type of cancer diagnosed in children, and treatments offer children a good chance for a cure.
- ALL in adults can also occur, but the chance of cure is much lower than for children.
- AML is most commonly diagnosed in adults over the age of 65. The prognosis varies depending on the patient's overall health and the presence of additional chronic conditions.

Prevention. Acute leukemias do not have specific prevention methods, but the following practices are generally healthy for everyone:
- Do not smoke or use alcohol to excess
- Eat a healthy diet, full of whole foods, fresh fruits and vegetables, lean proteins, plenty of fiber, and lots of water to maintain proper hydration.
- Eat the following foods sparingly: sugar and sweets, soda, processed foods, and foods with artificial ingredients.
- Get an appropriate amount of sleep.

Leukemias: Chronic Lymphocytic and Chronic Myelogenous

The term *chronic leukemia* refers to a leukemia that does not progress as rapidly as an acute leukemia. A person may have a chronic leukemia for years before it is even diagnosed. There are two types of chronic leukemia: chronic lymphocytic leukemia (CLL) and chronic myelogenous leukemia (CML). CLL and CML are cancers of the blood and bone marrow.

In the case of chronic leukemia, the bone marrow creates abnormal white blood cells that cannot function as they should. Abnormal cells appear in the bloodstream with chronic leukemia, but the number of abnormal cells increases depending on the stage at diagnosis. Chronic leukemias have a higher than normal WBC count, but it is not as elevated as with an acute leukemia. Chronic leukemias generally occur in older individuals, although they can occur at any age. The occurrence of CML is less common than CLL.

Etiology. CLL begins in the bone marrow, when a DNA error develops in a lymphocytic cell. The abnormal DNA incorrectly instructs lymphocytes to grow and divide abnormally. When this happens, the bone marrow produces lymphocytes that are atypical and do not function properly. Not only are the cells abnormal, but they live longer than normal cells, so they build up in the blood and accumulate in certain organs. When this happens, they may overcrowd the normal productive blood cells.

The development of CML is a bit different. There is a specific abnormality that occurs in people who develop CML. They have a specific chromosomal change that takes place, which causes an abnormal chromosome, called the *Philadelphia chromosome*, to be produced. This changed chromosome is present in 90% of people with CML. Scientists do not know what causes the change, but the abnormal chromosome seems to start the process that becomes CML. Like CLL, the white blood cells with the Philadelphia chromosome do not function as they should and live longer than normal. The abnormal cells increase in number and overcrowd the normal productive blood cells.

The cause of the initial changes for CLL and CML are unknown, but some of the risk factors for developing a chronic leukemia include the following:
- Being over the age of 60.
- CML is more common in males. CLL is more common in whites.
- Previous cancer treatment such as chemotherapy or radiation therapy.
- Exposure to radiation or cancer-causing chemicals (herbicides, insecticides, and Agent Orange).
- A family history of blood and bone cancers increases the risk for CLL in particular.

Signs and Symptoms. Many people with chronic leukemias have few early symptoms. Those who do develop signs and symptoms may experience the following:
- Fatigue, loss of appetite, and weight loss
- Pain in the upper left abdomen and possibly an enlarged spleen (*splenomegaly*)
- Fever and frequent infections
- Night sweats
- CLL only: enlarged but painless lymph nodes
- CML only: bleed more easily (nosebleeds, bruising, and pale skin)

Diagnostic Procedures. Tests and procedures used to diagnose chronic leukemia include the following:
- Physical examination and history
- Complete blood count and differential to look for the number of white blood cells and their maturity
- Bone marrow biopsy
- Imaging tests such as an x-ray or computerized tomography (CT) scan to help determine whether cancer has spread to other parts of the body

Once a diagnosis of chronic leukemia is confirmed and typed (CLL or CML), it is staged. Clarifying the stage is an important detail that determines the proper course of treatment. For chronic leukemia, some very early stages may not need treatment immediately. For later stages, treatment may need to start right away and be more aggressive.

> **VOCABULARY**
> **staged or staging:** The process of determining how much cancer is in the body and where it is located. Staging describes the severity of an individual's cancer.

Treatment.
- The patient's age, cancer stage, and general health should be considered with any aggressive treatment. The provider may recommend the following treatments: Chemotherapy. Medications are used to kill cancer cells. Chemotherapy can be administered intravenously and sometimes orally.
- Targeted drug therapy also uses medication that attacks specific irregularities present in cancer cells.
- Stem cell transplant is used to replace leukemic bone marrow with healthy bone marrow. Before a stem cell transplant can take place, chemotherapy or radiation is used to destroy the leukemic bone marrow. The diseased bone marrow is then replaced with healthy bone marrow from a compatible donor.
- Biologic therapy helps the body use its own immune system to find and destroy cancer cells.

For some leukemia patients, alternative treatments are used to help deal with the side effects of chemotherapy and the stress of continued

medical treatment. Alternative therapies can be helpful in improving a person's outlook through difficult treatment. Alternative therapies used include the following:
- Meditation, relaxation exercises, aromatherapy
- Acupuncture and massage therapy
- A change of diet to manage the side effects of chemotherapy

Because chronic leukemias are seen most frequently in an older population, palliative care may be a patient's choice of treatment.

> **VOCABULARY**
> **palliative care:** Care that focuses on providing relief from the symptoms and stress of a serious, possibly terminal illness. Improving the overall quality of life for the patient and his or her family.

Prognosis. Depending on the type of leukemia, patient age, existing chronic conditions, overall health, and leukemia stage, the prognosis is variable.

Prevention. Chronic leukemias cannot fully be prevented, but maintaining a healthy lifestyle and diet and limiting exposure to radiation and chemicals over the course of a lifetime are probably the best strategies to decrease the risk of developing chronic leukemia.

> **CRITICAL THINKING 8.7**
> Are Erma's signs and symptoms consistent with either acute or chronic leukemia? What laboratory test or tests might Dr. Martin order to help rule out acute or chronic leukemia?

Thrombophlebitis

Thrombophlebitis (throm boe fluh BY tis) is a condition in which the lining of a vein becomes irritated and inflamed, which then causes the formation of a blood clot. Thrombophlebitis is most frequently found in the veins of the legs, but it can also occur in the veins of the arms. Once a blood clot forms, it can block the flow of blood in the vein causing pain, swelling, and discoloration in the affected area (Fig. 8.13).

When the affected vein is near the surface of the skin, the condition is known as *superficial thrombophlebitis*. When the affected vein is deep in muscle tissue, the condition is known as *deep vein thrombosis*, or DVT.

The risk of developing a *pulmonary embolism* (EM buh liz uhm) (PE) is increased with DVT. The deep-vein clot can separate from a vein (Fig. 8.14). The *embolus* (circulating blood clot) can move into the lungs. It can block a pulmonary artery, causing a pulmonary embolism. This condition is a medical emergency and can be fatal.

Etiology. Common causes of thrombophlebitis include the following:
- An injury or trauma to a vein
- Not moving for long periods of time (e.g., bed rest after an illness)
- An inherited blood-clotting disorder

Risk factors for thrombophlebitis increase in the following circumstances:
- The presence of varicose veins, which are the most common cause of superficial thrombophlebitis
- Inactivity for extended periods of time; being bed or wheelchair bound or traveling in a car or plane without adequate breaks for movement
- Being pregnant, having just given birth, using birth control pills, or taking hormone replacement therapy
- Having a pacemaker or a venous catheter used to administer medication, which may irritate the inside of the vein and slow blood flow around the device
- Family history of a blood-clotting disorder or a previous bout of thrombophlebitis
- Having had a stroke, being overweight, obese, having cancer, or smoking

Signs and Symptoms. The signs and symptoms of superficial thrombophlebitis and DVT may include the following:
- Warmth, redness, tenderness, and pain in the affected area
- Swelling of the limb affected

Complications associated with DVT include the following:
- Pulmonary embolism
- Postphlebitic syndrome, also called postthrombotic syndrome, which can cause chronic, disabling pain, swelling, and a feeling of heaviness in the affected area, usually the legs, and can develop any time after experiencing DVT

Diagnostic Procedures. To diagnose thrombophlebitis, the provider will ask questions related to health history and perform a physical exam.

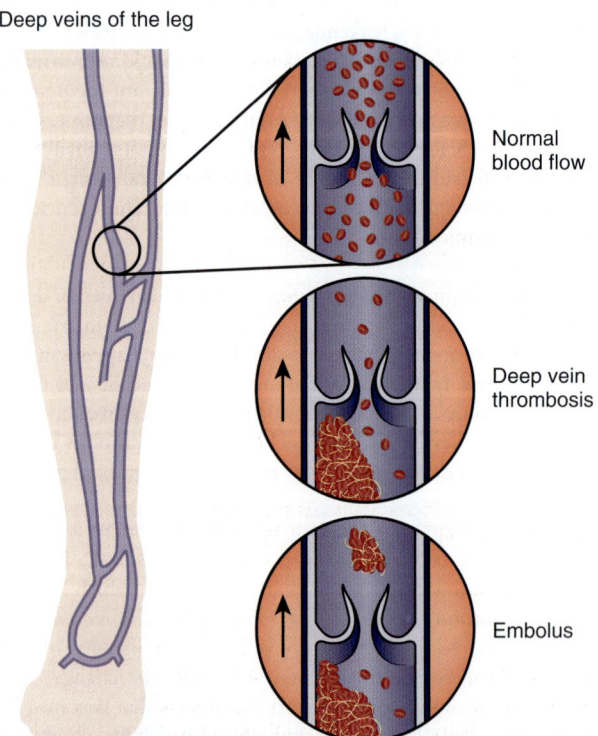

FIG. 8.14 Deep vein thrombosis versus embolus.

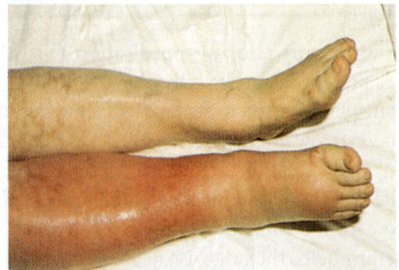

FIG. 8.13 Deep vein thrombosis (DVT). (From Lewis SM: *Medical-Surgical Nursing: Assessment and Management of Clinical Problems*, ed 8, St. Louis, 2011, Mosby.)

Superficial thrombophlebitis may be diagnosed at this point, but normally the following tests are recommended to differentiate between superficial thrombophlebitis and DVT:
- Ultrasound of the affected area: This test can confirm the diagnosis and distinguish between superficial and deep vein thrombosis.
- Blood test for *D dimer*: This test measures D dimer, which is a naturally occurring substance that is released when a blood clot is dissolving in the body. It is not diagnostic for only DVT, but together with ultrasound and the physical exam it may indicate DVT or the need for further testing.

Treatment. Superficial thrombophlebitis generally improves on its own without additional treatment, but if treatment is recommended it may include the following:
- Elevate the affected leg, and apply heat to the affected area
- Use an over-the-counter NSAID medication to help alleviate pain
- Wear compression stockings

For DVT, the provider may also recommend the following treatments:
- Blood-thinning medications may be needed. It is possible with DVT to have an anticoagulant injected into the affected area and then take oral anticoagulants as prescribed by the provider.
- Clot-dissolving medications may be advised. This treatment is called *thrombolysis* and is a common treatment for complicated DVT, including a pulmonary embolus.
- A blood filter can be inserted into the main vein in the abdomen (*vena cava*) to prevent clots in the legs from moving to the lungs. The filter is removed after the clots have dissolved and danger to the patient no longer exists.
- Varicose veins that cause pain or are the site of reoccurring thrombophlebitis can be stripped, or surgically removed.

Prognosis. The prognosis for superficial thrombophlebitis is very good with a compliant patient. Prognosis for uncomplicated DVT is also good, but the prognosis for complicated DVT varies.

Prevention. Prevention of thrombophlebitis may include the following:
- Do not sit for extended periods of time and in the same position. Whether at home or traveling, try to move for at least 5 minutes every hour.
- Take a walk every day. If traveling, walk the aisle of the bus, plane, or train every hour. If traveling by car, stop every hour or two and walk around.
- Wear compression stockings as a preventive measure.
- Move legs regularly when seated; wiggle and flex ankles and knees, and raise legs as room allows. Try to do this every hour for a few minutes.
- Drink plenty of water to avoid dehydration, and wear loose and comfortable clothing.

> **CRITICAL THINKING 8.8**
>
> Are Erma's signs and symptoms consistent with thrombophlebitis? Could it be superficial thrombophlebitis or DVT? Explain your answer.

Additional Diseases and Disorders of the Blood

There are many diseases and disorders of the blood that cannot be presented in detail within this chapter. Tables 8.4 through 8.7 provide brief descriptions of additional complaints, diseases, and disorders.

TABLE 8.4 Terms Related to Red Blood Cells and Deficiency Anemias

Term	Definition
B_{12} deficiency	Insufficient blood levels of vitamin B_{12}, which is essential for RBC maturation. Condition may be caused by inadequate dietary intake, as in some extreme vegetarian diets, or it may result from absence of *intrinsic factor*, a substance in the gastrointestinal (GI) system essential to vitamin B_{12} absorption. Also known as *pernicious* (per NISH uh s) *anemia*.
folate deficiency (FOH late)	Anemia as a result of a lack of folate from dietary, drug-induced, congenital, or other causes.
hypovolemia (hye poh voh LEE me ah)	Deficient volume of circulating blood.
sideropenia (sih dur roh PEE nee ah)	Reduced numbers of healthy RBCs due to chronic blood loss, inadequate iron intake, or unspecified causes. A type of iron deficiency anemia.
polycythemia vera (pah lee sye THEE mee ah VARE ah)	Chronic increase in the number of RBCs and the concentration of hemoglobin.
vitamin deficiency anemia	Occurs when the body does not have enough of the vitamins needed to produce adequate numbers of healthy red blood cells. May result from malabsorption of nutrients.

From Shiland B: *Mastering Healthcare Terminology*, ed 5, St. Louis, 2016, Elsevier.

TABLE 8.5 Terms Related to Aplastic and Hemolytic Anemias

Term	Definition
aplastic anemia (a PLAS tick)	Suppression of bone marrow function leading to a reduction in RBC production; also called hypoplastic anemia
autoimmune acquired hemolytic anemia (hee moh LIT ick)	Anemia caused by the body's destruction of its own RBCs
hemolytic anemia	A group of anemias caused by destruction of RBCs
pancytopenia (pan sye toh PEE nee ah)	Deficiency of all blood cells caused by dysfunctional stem cells
thalassemia (thal ah SEE mee ah)	Group of inherited disorders where anemia is the result of a decreased synthesis of hemoglobin, resulting in decreased production and increased destruction of RBCs

From Shiland B: *Mastering Healthcare Terminology*, ed 5, St. Louis, 2016, Elsevier.

TABLE 8.6 Terms Related to Systemic Infections of the Blood

Term	Definition
septic shock (SEP tick)	Inadequate blood flow caused by an overwhelming infection and low blood pressure. Organs fail and death may occur.
septicemia (sep tih SEE mee ah)	Systemic infection with pathologic microbes in the blood that has spread from somewhere else in the body. The term *sepsis* means "infection."
systemic inflammatory response syndrome (SIRS)	A type of septic shock, SIRS is an inflammatory state affecting the whole body. SIRS can be caused by infection, trauma, ischemia, or inflammation.

From Shiland B: *Mastering Healthcare Terminology*, ed 5, St. Louis, 2016, Elsevier.

TABLE 8.7 Terms Related to Leukocytic Disorders

Term	Definition
leukocytosis (loo koh sye TOH sis)	Abnormal increase in WBCs
leukopenia (loo koh PEE nee ah)	Abnormal decrease in WBCs; also called *leukocytopenia*
neutropenia (noo troh PEE nee ah)	Abnormal decrease in neutrophils due to disease process; formerly called *agranulocytosis* (aye gran yuh loh sahy TOH sis)

From Shiland B: *Mastering Healthcare Terminology*, ed 5, St. Louis, 2016, Elsevier.

LIFE SPAN CHANGES

Childhood diseases and disorders of the blood may include hemolytic disease of the newborn, hemophilia, anemia, infectious mononucleosis, and leukemias.

Adult and geriatric diseases and disorders of the blood may include a variety of conditions. Anemias are common, along with a lack of blood volume (*hypovolemia*), which may be due to internal bleeding, trauma, or a disease process. Hemophilia can be seen throughout a person's lifetime. Thrombophlebitis is seen much more frequently in older adults as mobility becomes an issue. Cancers include leukemia, which can be acute or chronic varieties.

CLOSING COMMENTS

When working in an ambulatory care setting, assisting patients with diseases and disorders of the blood is common. It is important for the medical assistant to understand the content and functions of the blood and the normal values associated with red blood cells, white blood cells, and platelets. Hematology is the specialty that focuses on the blood, but medical assistants working in urgent care and primary care (e.g. pediatrics, internal medicine, and family practice) will see many blood-related diseases and disorders too. Medical terminology related to the blood will be invaluable in your career. Knowing word parts, definitions, and common abbreviations is vital when working with patients and providers (Tables 8.8 through 8.11). The medical assistant should also know the etiologies, signs and symptoms, diagnostic procedures, treatments, prognoses, and prevention of common blood-related diseases, disorders, and traumas.

TABLE 8.8 Combining and Adjective Forms Relating to the Blood

Meaning	Combining Form	Adjective Form	Meaning	Combining Form	Adjective Form
base	bas/o	basal	neutral	neutr/o	neutral
blood	hem/o, hemat/o	hematic	nucleus	nucle/o	nuclear
bone marrow	myel/o		plasma	plasm/o	
clotting, clot	thromb/o	thrombic	red	erythr/o	
clumping	agglutin/o	agglutinous	rosy-colored	eosin/o	
disease	path/o		safety, protection	immun/o	
eat, swallow	phag/o		same	home/o	
fever, fire	pyr/o	pyretic	serum	ser/o	serous
fiber	fibr/o	fibrous	shape	morph/o	morphous
little grain	granul/o	granular	spleen	splen/o	splenic
lymph	lymph/o, lymphat/o	lymphatic	white	leuk/o	

From Shiland B: *Mastering Healthcare Terminology*, ed 5, St. Louis, 2016, Elsevier.

TABLE 8.9 Prefixes Relating to the Blood

Prefix	Meaning	Prefix	Meaning
a-	without	mono-	one
anti-	against	poly-	many
inter-	between	pro-	before
macro-	large		

From Shiland B: *Mastering Healthcare Terminology*, ed 5, St. Louis, 2016, Elsevier.

TABLE 8.10 Suffixes Relating to the Blood

Suffix	Meaning	Suffix	Meaning
-cyte	cell	-lytic	pertaining to breaking down
-exia	condition	-osis	abnormal condition
-gen	producing	-phil	attraction
-globin	protein substance	-poiesis	formation
-in	substance	-poietin	forming substance
-kine	movement	-siderin	iron substance
-leukin	white substance	-stasis	controlling, stopping
-logy	study of	-thrombin	clotting substance
-lysis	breaking down		

From Shiland B: *Mastering Healthcare Terminology*, ed 5, St. Louis, 2016, Elsevier.

TABLE 8.11 Abbreviations

Abbreviation	Definition	Abbreviation	Definition
A, B, AB, O	blood types	Hct	hematocrit
ALL	acute lymphocytic leukemia	HDN	hemolytic disease of the newborn
AML	acute myelogenous leukemia	Hgb	hemoglobin
basos	basophils	Ig	immunoglobulin
BMP	basic metabolic panel	K	potassium
BMT	bone marrow transplant	lymphs	lymphocytes
BUN	blood urea nitrogen	MCH	mean corpuscular hemoglobin
bx	biopsy	MCHC	mean corpuscular hemoglobin concentration
Ca	calcium		
CBC	complete blood cell count	Na	sodium
Cl	chloride	neuts	neutrophils
CLL	chronic lymphocytic leukemia	PCV	packed-cell volume
CML	chronic myelogenous leukemia	plats	platelets, thrombocytes
CMP	comprehensive metabolic panel	PMNs, polys	polymorphonucleocytes
CO_2	carbon dioxide	PT	prothrombin time
diff	differential (WBC count)	PTT	partial thromboplastin time
eosins	eosinophils	RBC	red blood cell (count)
ESR	erythrocyte sedimentation rate	Rh	rhesus
Hb	hemoglobin	WBC	white blood cell (count)

From Shiland B: *Mastering Healthcare Terminology*, ed 5, St. Louis, 2016, Elsevier.

CHAPTER REVIEW

The blood is made up of two main components. Plasma is the liquid portion of blood, and formed elements are suspended in the plasma. The formed elements consist of red blood cells, white blood cells, and platelets. The functions of the blood are to carry oxygen and carbon dioxide via the RBCs, to protect and provide immunity through the WBCs, and to permit blood clotting by the platelets and clotting factors in the plasma.

RBCs have a vital role in the body. They carry oxygen to individual body cells and carry carbon dioxide back to the lungs to be exhaled as a waste gas from the body. Hemoglobin is an iron-containing molecule that gives RBCs their characteristic red color. Hemoglobin is also responsible for transporting oxygen and carbon dioxide. If the body is anemic or if the hemoglobin is ineffective, the body will not get a proper supply of oxygen to cells, tissues, and vital organs.

WBCs are also found in the blood. There are two main categories of WBCs, granulocytes and agranulocytes. The granulocytes are neutrophils, eosinophils, and basophils. The agranulocytes are monocytes and lymphocytes. Each of these five types of white blood cells participates in the immune system. Each has a unique role to play in protecting the body from foreign pathogens.

Platelets are involved in the process of blood clotting or coagulation. They plug leaks or injuries to blood vessels and keep blood in the body. Stopping the flow of blood is referred to as hemostasis.

Many blood diseases and disorders were presented in this chapter. Common signs and symptoms include pain, fatigue, paleness, bleeding, bruising, weakness, headaches, and dizziness. Common etiology includes infection, injury, congenital, and malignancies. Typical diagnostics include physical exam and history, imaging procedures, and laboratory testing. CLIA-waived tests include complete blood count, hemoglobin, hematocrit, and monospot testing.

The diseases related to blood change with age. Infants and children are most at risk for anemias, infections, and congenital conditions. Older adults are at risk for anemias, blood clots or bleeding disorders, and malignancies.

Blood is an amazing substance that affects every cell of the body. Medical assistants should be familiar with blood, how it works, and the normal values for RBCs, WBCs, platelets, and hemoglobin.

SCENARIO WRAP-UP

At the end of Erma's appointment, Dr. Martin discusses her hemoglobin test results and her physical exam. Dr. Martin's initial diagnosis for Erma is mild anemia. Erma's hemoglobin is a bit low, so Dr. Martin has asked Lily to go over some patient education materials with Erma about anemia. Dr. Martin has also ordered iron studies, a vitamin B_{12} level, CBC, and peripheral blood smear with a differential. These tests are aimed at diagnosing the cause of Erma's low hemoglobin.

Dr. Martin and Erma also talk about the bruise on the back of her left leg that has her concerned. One of Erma's friends has DVT, and because she could not see the affected area, Erma was concerned that something serious was happening. Dr. Martin did find a bruise, but he did not find anything that would indicate that Erma had thrombophlebitis. Erma did mention that she had a pretty hard bump to her leg from one of her dogs when they were playing. Dr. Martin has also asked Lily to go through some patient education with Erma concerning how to care for a bruise and signs and symptoms of thrombophlebitis to put Erma's mind at ease.

Lily sits down with Erma and goes through the pamphlets on anemia and thrombophlebitis. They talk about diet choices, the importance of regular exercise, and how great dogs are. Lily asks Erma if she has any questions and asks her to repeat back some of the information they went over. Lily is satisfied that Erma understands the information in the pamphlets and reminds her to call and leave questions for Dr. Martin if she thinks of something later.

Lily enjoys here work at WMFM Clinic. She continues to learn about medical assisting, her chosen career. She also loves the days that she gets to see pictures of a patient's dogs!

9

Lymphatic and Immune Systems

LEARNING OBJECTIVES

1. List the major organs and structures for the lymphatic and immune systems. Also identify the anatomical location of these major organs and structures.
2. Describe the physiology of the lymphatic and immune systems.
3. Differentiate between active and passive immunity.
4. Identify the etiology, signs and symptoms, diagnostic procedures, treatment, prognosis, and prevention of autoimmune diseases and disorders.
5. Identify the etiology, signs and symptoms, diagnostic procedures, treatment, prognosis, and prevention of HIV/AIDS.
6. Identify the etiology, signs and symptoms, diagnostic procedures, treatment, prognosis, and prevention of lymphoma.
7. Identify the etiology, signs and symptoms, diagnostic procedures, treatment, prognosis, and prevention of multiple myeloma. Also identify these factors for other diseases and disorders of the lymphatic and immune systems.
8. Compare the structure and function of the lymphatic and immune systems across the life span. Also, discuss medical terminology related to the lymphatic and immune systems.

CHAPTER OUTLINE

1. Opening Scenario, 187
2. You Will Learn, 187
3. Introduction to the Lymphatic and Immune Systems, 188
4. Anatomy of the Lymphatic and Immune Systems, 188
    a. Flow of Lymphatic Fluid, 188
    b. Organs of the Lymphatic and Immune Systems, 188
    c. Cells of the Immune System, 189
        i. *Granular White Blood Cells, 189*
        ii. *Agranular White Blood Cells, 190*
5. Physiology of the Lymphatic and Immune Systems, 190
    a. Immune System Levels of Defense, 190
        i. *Nonspecific Immunity, 190*
        ii. *Specific Immunity, 191*
    b. Hypersensitivity Reactions, 194
6. Types of Acquired Immunity, 194
    a. Active Immunity, 194
    b. Passive Immunity, 194
7. Diseases and Disorders of the Lymphatic and Immune Systems, 195
    a. Autoimmune Diseases and Disorders, 195
    b. HIV/AIDS, 198
    c. Lymphoma: Hodgkin's and Non-Hodgkin's, 201
    d. Multiple Myeloma, 202
    e. Additional Diseases and Disorders of the Lymphatic and Immune Systems, 203
8. Life Span Changes, 204
9. Closing Comments, 204
10. Chapter Review, 205
11. Scenario Wrap-Up, 206

OPENING SCENARIO

Julia Shaw, CMA (AAMA), is a medical assistant working at Walden-Martin Family Medicine Clinic (WMFM). She is working with Dr. Angela Perez today. Julia enjoys the family practice setting and likes the variety of ages and conditions that she sees each day. Today, Dr. Perez and Julia will see a patient who is new to the clinic. The rest of their appointments are with existing patients. Each day is different. Each day is busy. Each day brings patients who need help and encouragement. Julia is a people person. Helping patients is Julia's passion.

YOU WILL LEARN

- To recognize and use terms related to the lymphatic and immune systems.
- To locate the structures related to the lymphatic and immune systems.
- To understand and describe the functions of the lymphatic and immune systems.
- To recognize disease states of the lymphatic system. This includes their causes, signs and symptoms. diagnostic processes, treatment, prognosis, and prevention.

- To recognize disease states related to immunity, including their causes, signs and symptoms, diagnostic processes, treatment, prognosis, and prevention.

INTRODUCTION TO THE LYMPHATIC AND IMMUNE SYSTEMS

The lymphatic (lim FAT ik) and immune (ih MYOON) systems are two different systems. However, they cooperate and work together to maintain homeostasis (hoh mee uh STEY sis). They also defend the body from foreign pathogens. The cells, tissues, and organs of the lymphatic system and the immune system are almost the same. But the two systems help the body in very different ways. The lymphatic system can be described as mostly structural. It is the physical parts of the two systems. The immune system can be described as mostly functional. The cells of the immune system work to keep the body safe from pathogens (PATH uh juhn). These two systems together make up an amazingly complex and efficient means of maintaining the body's health. Box 9.1 presents the specialty practices and specialists who treat patients with diseases of the lymphatic and immune systems.

BOX 9.1 Specialty and Specialist

Immunology (im yuh NOL uh jee) is the healthcare specialty that deals with many immune- and lymphatic-related diseases and disorders. An *immunologist* (im yuh NOL uh jist) is a specialist involved in the diagnosis, treatment, and prevention of disorders of the immune and lymphatic systems.

Other healthcare specialists who work with the diseases and disorders of the lymphatic and immune systems are cardiologists (kahr dee OL uh jist), otolaryngologists (oh toh lar ing GOL uh jist), rheumatologists (roo muh TOL uh jist), endocrinologists (end oh kruh NOL uh jist), pulmonologists (puhl muh NOL uh jist), and nephrologists (nuh FROL uh jist).

VOCABULARY

debris: The remains of anything broken down or destroyed; ruins, rubble.
lymph: A clear, yellowish fluid containing white blood cells in a liquid similar to plasma. The fluid comes from the tissues of the body and is moved through the lymphatic vessels and the bloodstream.
lymphocytes: A type of white blood cell that has a large, round nucleus that is surrounded by a thin layer of agranular cytoplasm.
macrophages: Large white blood cells that live in the tissues. They engulf foreign particles, microorganisms, and cell debris.
mediastinal: The location separating the right and left thoracic cavities.
microorganisms: Any living organisms of microscopic size. Examples include bacteria, protozoa, fungi, parasites, and helminths. Some definitions include viruses, which are not alive.
monocytes: Large, circulating white blood cells that are formed in the bone marrow. An agranulocyte that can engulf foreign particles, microorganisms, and cell debris.
Peyer patches: Small masses of lymphatic tissue found mostly in the ileum of the small intestine. They are an important part of the immune system, because they monitor intestinal bacteria populations and prevent the growth of pathogenic bacteria in the intestines.

MEDICAL TERMINOLOGY

axill/o: axilla, armpit
cervic/o: neck
inguin/o: groin
lymph/o, lymphat/o: lymph
lymphaden/o: lymph gland
lymphangi/o: lymph vessel
macro-: large
mediastin/o: mediastinum
mono-: one, singular

The lymphatic system is responsible for a number of functions, with the help of the immune system. Lymphatic functions include:
- Cleansing the cellular environment
- Returning proteins and tissue fluids to the blood
- Providing a pathway for the absorption of fats into the bloodstream
- Defending the body against disease

ANATOMY OF THE LYMPHATIC AND IMMUNE SYSTEMS

The lymphatic and immune systems (see Fig. 9.7) are composed of many structures. **Lymph** (limf), or interstitial (in ter STISH uhl) fluid, flows through the lymphatic system, which is composed of these structures:
- lymph vessels, lymph nodes, lymph glands, and lymphoid tissue
- lymph organs: the tonsils (TON suhl), adenoids (AD n oid), vermiform appendix (VUR muh fawrm uh PEN diks), spleen, thymus gland (THAHY muhs), and **Peyer patches** (PEYH urh PACH ehs)

Many of the above structures are shared by the immune system. **Monocytes** (MON uh sahyt) and **lymphocytes** (LIM fuh sahyt) pass from the bloodstream through the blood capillary walls into the spaces between the cells in body tissue. When they pass into the lymph (interstitial fluid) that surrounds cells, they perform their protective functions. Monocytes change into **macrophages** (MACK roh fay jehs). These cells destroy pathogens and collect debris from damaged cells. Lymphocytes are much more complicated. They are essential to the immune response, so they are discussed in a later section of this chapter Once monocytes and lymphocytes pass into the lymphatic capillaries, the fluid is called *lymph* or *lymphatic fluid*.

Flow of Lymphatic Fluid

Lymph moves in one direction. This prevents pathogens from flowing through the entire body. The system filters out the **microorganisms** as the lymph passes through its various capillaries, vessels, and nodes. Lymph travels in the following sequence:
1. From the *interstitial spaces* between the cells.
2. Toward the heart through lymphatic capillaries.
3. To lymphatic vessels, which carry lymph via valves (one-way vessels).
4. To the lymphatic nodes (also called *lymph glands*), which filter the **debris** (duh BREE). These nodes can become enlarged when pathogens are present. Note the major lymph nodes in Fig. 9.7, including the cervical (SUR vi kuhl), axillary (AK suh ler ee), inguinal (ING gwuh nuhl), and **mediastinal** (mee dee a STAHY nuhl) nodes.
5. Then to either the right lymphatic duct or the thoracic (thaw RAS ik) duct. Both of these ducts empty into the superior or inferior venae cava (VEE nuh KAY vuh).
6. Once in the venous (VEE nuhs) blood, the lymph is recycled through the body via the circulatory system.

Organs of the Lymphatic and Immune Systems

The organs of the lymphatic system are the spleen, thymus gland, tonsils (Fig. 9.1), appendix, and Peyer patches (Fig. 9.2).
- The *spleen* is located in the upper left quadrant of the abdomen. It works to filter, store, and produce blood cells. The spleen also removes old or inefficient red blood cells (RBCs) and activates B lymphocytes.
- The *thymus gland* is located in the mediastinum. It is instrumental in the development of T lymphocytes (T cells). T cells play a major role in the immune system.

CHAPTER 9 Lymphatic and Immune Systems

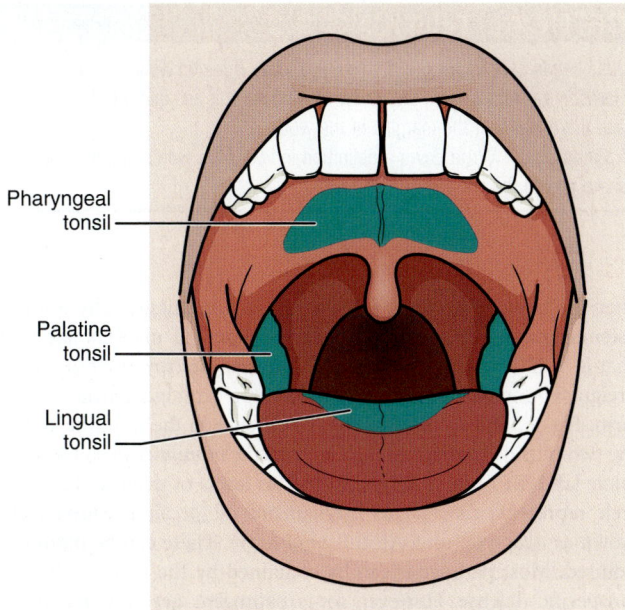

FIG. 9.1 Tonsils.

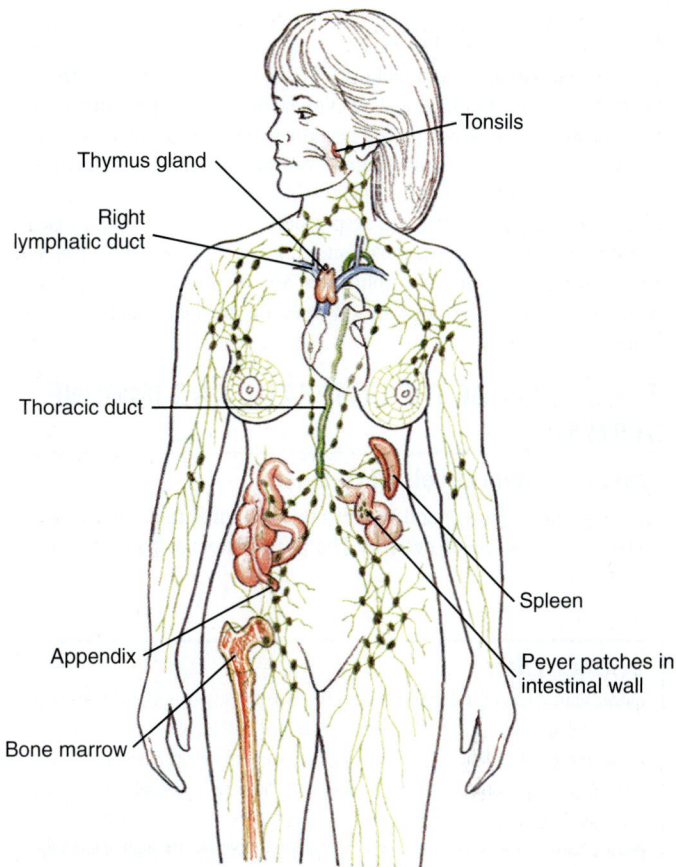

FIG. 9.2 Organs of the lymphatic and immune systems. (From Shiland B: *Mastering Healthcare Terminology*, ed 5, St Louis, 2015, Elsevier.)

- The *tonsils* are lymphatic tissue. There are three types: lingual (LING gwuh l), pharyngeal (fuh RIN jee uhl), and palatine (PAL uh tahyn). The tonsils help protect the entrances to the respiratory and digestive systems.
- The *vermiform appendix* and the *Peyer patches* are lymphoid tissue in the intestines.

> ### CRITICAL THINKING 9.1
> Ryenn Ablesman is an 8-year-old girl who has been having some problems with a recurring sore throat and tonsillitis. Can you name the three types of tonsils in the nasopharynx? Using the medical terminology tables at the end of the chapter, what does the suffix -itis mean?

Cells of the Immune System

The *immune system* is composed of organs, tissues, cells, and chemical messengers. The components of the immune system interact to protect the body from external invaders, and from the body's own internally altered cells. The chemical messengers are *cytokines* (SYE toh kynez). They are secreted by cells of the immune system that direct immune cellular interactions. Most of the cells involved in the lymphatic and immune systems are white blood cells (WBCs). A quick review of the white blood cells may help in the discussion of the immune system.

Granular White Blood Cells

The three types of granular WBCs are the *neutrophils* (NOO truh fil), *eosinophils* (ee uh SIN uh fil), and *basophils* (BEY suh fil) (Box 9.2). They are characterized by their heavily granulated cytoplasm and segmented nuclei. Neutrophils are aggressively *phagocytic*; that is, they engulf and destroy invading pathogens. Unlike RBCs, WBCs are found in both the bloodstream and the tissues. During inflammation (in fluh MEY shuhn), the blood carries neutrophils through blood vessels to the site of injury. Capillary walls become more permeable (PUR mee uh buhl), and the granular cells squeeze through to the site of infection. Once at the site of infection or injury, the neutrophils engulf the invading microorganism. The collection of WBCs, dead WBCs, bacteria, and tissue cells create *pus* (puhs) at the site of infection. Eosinophils are involved in allergies, and basophils play a part in inflammation.

> ### BOX 9.2 Granulocytes
> A little reminder about granulocytes:
> - *Neutrophils* are also called *PMNs*, *segs*, or *polys*. They are very aggressive phagocytic cells!
> - *Eosinophils* are also called *eos*. Basophils are also called *basos*.
> - All three types of granulocyte end in the suffix -phil. Just remember the three -phils!

> ### MEDICAL TERMINOLOGY
> **append/o, appendic/o:** appendix **lymph/o:** lymph
> **cyt/o:** cell **mono-:** one
> **inter-:** between **splen/o:** spleen
> **-kine:** movement **thym/o:** thymus
> **-leukin:** white substance **tonsill/o:** tonsil

Agranular White Blood Cells

The two types of agranular leukocytes (Box 9.3) are the *monocytes* and the *lymphocytes*. They have a clear cytoplasm (no granules) and a solid nucleus. Monocytes are large and become *macrophages* when they enter tissues. Macrophages are also aggressively phagocytic (FAG uh sih tik) cells – that engulf pathogens and debris. Lymphocytes are small cells that have a big job! They are responsible for much of the work in specific immunity (see the next section, Physiology of the Lymphatic and Immune Systems). Lymphocytes are further classified into T lymphocytes and B lymphocytes, depending on their function in the immune response.

PHYSIOLOGY OF THE LYMPHATIC AND IMMUNE SYSTEMS

Immune System Levels of Defense

The best way to understand the immune system is to learn about the body's various levels of defense. The goal of foreign pathogens is to enter the body, reproduce, and damage healthy tissue. The immune system's primary function is to **differentiate** (dif uh REN shee eyt) what is "self" and what is "foreign," and then destroy anything that is foreign. The immune system wants to stop pathogens from causing harm. Fig. 9.3 illustrates the levels of defense in the immune system. The two outside circles represent *nonspecific immunity* (also known as *innate* (ih NEYT) *immunity*) and its two levels of defense. The inner circle represents the various mechanisms of *specific immunity* (also known as *adaptive* (uh DAP tiv) *immunity*). These can be natural or acquired. Most pathogens can be contained by the first two lines of nonspecific defense. However, some pathogens get past nonspecific defenses. These pathogens are met with the third line of defense, or specific immunity.

Nonspecific Immunity

The term *nonspecific immunity* refers to the many ways the body protects itself from pathogens without having to "recognize" them. The first line of defense in nonspecific immunity consists of the following methods of protection.

- *Physical:* Examples include **intact** (in TAKT) skin and mucous membranes. These are physical barriers to pathogens. The skin protects the inside of the body from the outside environment. The sticky mucous membranes at many body openings trap pathogens.
- **Reflexes:** Examples include coughing, sneezing, vomiting, and diarrhea. These actions help get rid of pathogens by forcing them back out of the body.
- *Chemical:* Examples include tears, saliva, and perspiration. These have a slightly acidic pH, which discourages pathogens from entering the body. All these fluids also help wash the pathogens away. In addition, stomach acids and **enzymes** (EN zahym) try to kill pathogens.

> **CRITICAL THINKING 9.2**
>
> Julia needs to change a dressing on a patient's infected wound today. Robert Harrison has an abrasion that became infected. It is red and a little swollen, and there is pus at the margins of the wound.
>
> What is pus? Write down a definition in your own words and be ready to share it with the class.

> **VOCABULARY**
>
> **cytoplasm:** The cell substance that fills the area between the nucleus and the cell membrane. It contains the organelles of the cell.
>
> **inflammation:** A pathology characterized by redness, swelling, pain, tenderness, heat, and disturbed function of an area of the body. Especially a reaction of tissues to injury.
>
> **permeable:** A substance or structure that can be passed through, especially by liquids or gases.

> **BOX 9.3 Agranulocytes**
>
> A little reminder about agranulocytes:
> - *Monocytes* are in the bloodstream, *macrophages* are in the tissues. They are very aggressive phagocytic cells!
> - B lymphocytes and T lymphocytes do not look different. But they function differently. B and T lymphocytes are also called *B cells* and *T cells*.

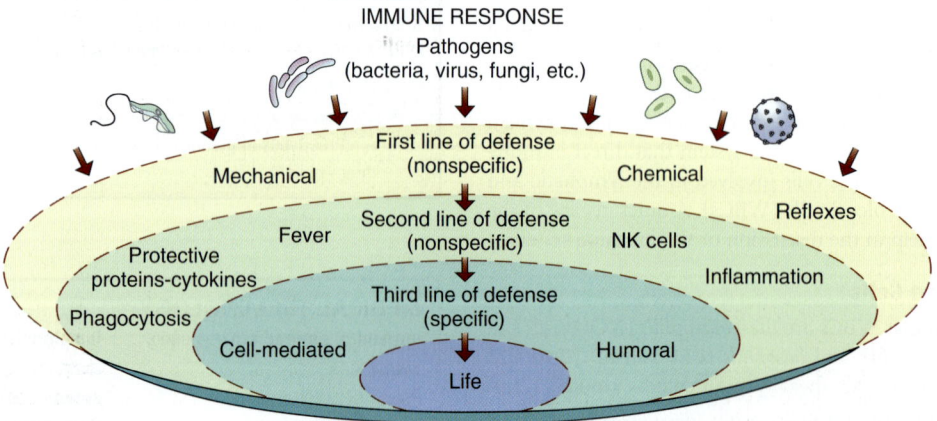

FIG. 9.3 Immune system levels of defense. (From Shiland B: *Mastering healthcare terminology*, ed 5, St Louis, 2015, Elsevier.)

CHAPTER 9 Lymphatic and Immune Systems

> **CRITICAL THINKING 9.3**
> What are the three methods of protection in the first line of defense? Write all three down and briefly describe each one in your own words. Share your answers with your classmates.

> **BOX 9.6 Genetic Immunity**
> An inherited ability to resist certain diseases because of one's species, race, gender, or individual genetic makeup.

> **CRITICAL THINKING 9.4**
> Review the second line of defense in nonspecific immunity. What are the five different chemical or cellular responses discussed in this text? Briefly describe each of the five protective measures. Can you name the characteristic signs and symptoms of inflammation? Write down your answers and share them with the class.

The second line of defense in nonspecific immunity goes to work if the pathogens make it past the first line of defense. The second line of defense uses cellular and chemical responses to destroy the pathogen. The following are the protective measures of the second line of defense.

- *Phagocytosis* (fag oh sye TOH sis): The process of cells engulfing and destroying invaders. Pathogens that make it past the first line of defense and enter the bloodstream may be consumed by neutrophils, monocytes, or macrophages. See Chapter 8 for a description of phagocytosis.
- *Inflammation*: A protective response to irritation or injury. Signs and symptoms of inflammation include heat, swelling, redness, and pain. This process causes immediate **vasoconstriction** (vas oh kuhn STRIK shuhn), followed by an increase in vascular permeability. These conditions provide a good environment for healing. If caused by a pathogen, the inflammation is called an *infection*.
- *Pyrexia* (pye RECK see uh): The medical term for fever. When an infection is present, fever helps protect the infected area. Fever increases the action of phagocytes and reduces the **viability** (vahy uh BIL ih tee) of certain pathogens. Most pathogens love body temperature, so when a fever is present the environment gets too hot and they cannot function as they should.
- *Protective proteins* are part of the second line of defense. These include *interferons* (in tur FEER ons), which disrupt viral **replication** and limit a virus's ability to damage cells. *Complement* proteins (Box 9.4) are inactive in the blood until they encounter bacteria. Meeting bacteria activates complement, enabling it to *lyse* (destroy) the organisms.
- *Natural killer* (NK) cells (Box 9.5) are the last cell type involved in the second line of defense. This special kind of lymphocyte acts nonspecifically to kill cells that have been infected by certain viruses and cancer cells.

Fig. 9.4 presents an overview of nonspecific immunity.

Specific Immunity

Specific immunity is different from nonspecific immunity in several ways:

- Specific immunity means that the immune response is generated against one specific **antigen**. The response will not be effective against any other antigens.
- Specific immunity counts on the immune cells to identify antigens and recognize them if they encounter them again. An antigen can be an infectious agent from outside the body (*exogenous* [ek SOJ uh nuhs]), or it can be a malignant or tumor cell inside the body (*endogenous* [en DOJ uh nuhs]). Both types of antigen are foreign, something that is not normal to the immune system.
- Specific immunity prepares a specific response (**antibody** production) to that unique antigen.
- Specific immunity intensifies with repeated challenges by the same antigen. When the body encounters a known antigen, it can respond more efficiently and react to the antigen quickly.
- Specific immunity may be either genetic (Box 9.6) or acquired.

> **BOX 9.4 Complement**
> Complement is a group of proteins made in the liver. Complement is involved in blood clotting and blood antigen-antibody interactions.

> **BOX 9.5 Natural Killer (NK) Cells**
> Natural killer cells are a type of lymphocyte. They are:
> - derived from stem cells in the bone marrow.
> - concentrated in the liver and lungs.
> - involved in nonspecific immunity and inflammation.
> - capable of destroying targeted cells, such as tumor cells and viral infected cells.
> - *not* phagocytic cells.

> **VOCABULARY**
> **differentiate:** To distinguish one thing from another. To make a distinction between items.
> **enzymes:** Special proteins that speed up a chemical reaction in the body.
> **intact:** Complete or whole. Not altered; unbroken.
> **reflexes:** Movements or processes caused by a reflex response. A reflex is an automatic response. It doesn't require thought.
> **replication:** The production of exact copies of a complex molecule, such as DNA.
> **vasoconstriction:** A contraction of muscles that causes narrowing of the inside tube of a vessel.
> **viability:** The ability to live.

> **MEDICAL TERMINOLOGY**
> **constrict/o:** narrowing, binding
> **cyt/o:** cell
> **endo-:** in, within
> **-exia:** condition
> **exo-:** out, away from
> **-gen:** substance that produces
> **-osis:** abnormal condition
> **-ous:** pertaining to
> **phag/o:** eat, swallow
> **pyr/o:** fever, fire
> **vas/o:** vessel

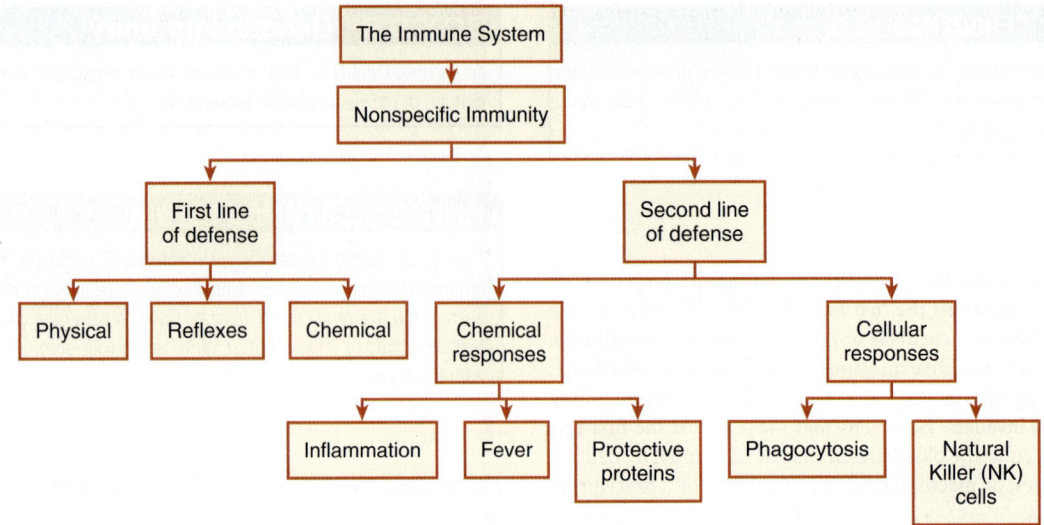

FIG. 9.4 Nonspecific immunity.

BOX 9.7 Five Classes of Immunoglobulins (Ig)

- IgG – most abundant immunoglobulin in the serum. It can cross the placenta from mother to fetus
- IgM – first antibody to be formed in the immune response. It does not cross the placenta, but can be produced by a fetus in utero
- IgA – found mostly in secretions, such as tears, saliva, colostrum (kuh LOS truhm), and the mucous of the respiratory and digestive systems
- IgE – very small amounts in the serum. It is important in the allergy response
- IgD – found on B cell surface. Scientists don't really know what it does yet!

BOX 9.8 T Cells and Antibodies

T cells do not produce antibodies! They are bossy and sometimes tell B cells what to do. They tell B cells to recognize antigens. They tell B cells to produce more antibody or produce less antibody. But one thing T cells do *not* do is produce antibodies themselves.

Antibodies belong to a group of proteins called *immunoglobulins* (Ig) (ih myoo noh GLOB you lins). There are five distinct classes of immunoglobulins: IgG, IgM, IgE, IgA, and IgD (Box 9.7). Each class of immunoglobulin responds to different types of immune challenges, or antigens.

Specific immunity has two different methods of destroying pathogens: humoral immunity and cell-mediated immunity.

Humoral immunity. Humoral immunity, also known as *antibody-mediated immunity*, involves the production of antibodies. B cells are formed from stem cells in the bone marrow. They then migrate to lymph organs (e.g., lymph nodes, spleen), where they multiply and live. B cells are the most important cell in humoral immunity, but T cells and macrophages are also involved in the process. When an antibody combines with an antigen, an antibody-antigen complex is formed.

MEDICAL TERMINOLOGY
-al: pertaining to
humor/o: liquid

CRITICAL THINKING 9.5
Review the five immunoglobulins. Can you make a saying, word, or rhyme that might help you remember them? Share your ideas with the class.

The following steps are a simplified description of the sequence of humoral immunity, an incredibly complex process.
1. An antigen invades a host.
2. The antigen is engulfed and digested by a macrophage.
3. The macrophage presents small protein portions of the antigen to T cells.
4. The T cells become sensitized (SEN sih tahyz) to the antigen (Box 9.8)
5. The T cells send out a chemical signal to B cells. This stimulates the B cells to produce antibodies (this is a process called *activation*).
6. Activated B cells proliferate (pruh LIF uh reyt) and clone (klohn) themselves.
7. Some of the B cell clones rapidly mature into antibody-producing *plasma* (PLAZ muh) *cells*.
8. Plasma cells produce antibodies rapidly and efficiently.

VOCABULARY
antibody: Protein substances produced in the blood or tissues in response to a specific antigen, that destroys or weakens the antigen. Part of the immune system.
antigen: A substance that stimulates the production of an antibody when introduced into the body. Antigens include toxins, bacteria, viruses, and other foreign substances.
colostrum: The first milk secreted by mammals after having given birth. Different from the rest of the milk supply because it contains more protein and is rich in antibodies. Also called *foremilk*.

9. After a few days of rapid antibody production, the plasma cells die. However, even though the plasma cells die, the antibodies remain viable and continue with their work.
10. The B cell clones that don't become plasma cells remain in the immune system as *memory cells*. Memory cells can recognize the same antigen if it ever invades the body again. They also can quickly produce antibodies anytime in the future.

CRITICAL THINKING 9.6
Why are memory cells so important in the immune system? Share your ideas with the class.

Antibodies are amazing structures. They are protein molecules that specifically attach to antigens. They can neutralize toxins or destroy viruses directly. They can combine with larger antigens (e.g., bacteria) to form antibody-antigen complexes. These complexes signal neutrophils to come and destroy them. Neutrophils engulf the complexes and destroy the antigen.

Antibodies can protect the body in many ways. They circulate in the plasma and are present in secretions (i.e., tears, saliva, colostrum), ready to attach to unsuspecting antigens. However, there is one thing antibodies are unable to do – they cannot enter a cell. That can be a problem, because sometimes antigens go inside of host cells. When that happens, antibodies cannot destroy the antigen. This is when cell-mediated immunity takes over.

stem cells: Undifferentiated cells that can become specialized cells in the body.
sensitized: To make reactive to an antigen.
proliferate: To increase in numbers or spread rapidly and often excessively.
clone: To make identical units, cells, or individuals that come from the same parent. Or, an identical unit, cell, or individual made in this way.

Cell-mediated immunity. T cells are formed from stem cells in bone marrow. They then migrate to the thymus, where they mature and learn their role in the immune system. They are the most important cell in cell-mediated immunity. T cells do not produce antibodies, but they can help antibodies do their job. T cells are very effective against intracellular (in truh SEL yuh ler) pathogens (antigens). When an antigen enters a cell, T cells help expose the antigen so that antibodies can destroy it.

The following steps are a simplified description of the sequence of cell-mediated immunity. This is another incredibly complex process.
1. An antigen invades a host.
2. The antigen is engulfed and digested by a macrophage.
3. The macrophage presents small protein portions of the antigen to T cells.
4. A specific type of T cell, called a *cytotoxic* (sahy tuh TOK sik) *T cell*, becomes sensitized to the antigen. Cytotoxic T cells proliferate and clone themselves.
5. Cytotoxic T cells search for cells infected with an antigen. When they find them, they bind (attach) to the infected cell.
6. Cytotoxic T cells discharge enzymes into the antigen-infected cell. Enzymes destroy the cell membrane. The cell dies and exposes the antigens to circulating antibodies. Antibodies combine with the antigens, creating an antigen-antibody complex. This complex can be engulfed by macrophages and destroyed.

BOX 9.9 Different Types of T Cells
Four main types of T cells work in specific immunity. Look at the following list and see how important T cells are to immunity in general.
1. *T helper cells* (T_H), also known as CD4+ T cells. They help in B-cell activation and activation of cytotoxic T cells.
2. *Cytotoxic T cells* (T_C), also known as CD8+ cells. They destroy virus-infected cells and tumor cells. They also can cause damage to or rejection of organ transplants. In addition, they can cause autoimmune diseases.
3. *Memory T cells* rapidly proliferate if an antigen is re-exposed to the body.
4. *Regulatory T cells* (T_{reg}), also known as *suppressor T cells*. They help shut down the immune response when the antigen has been destroyed.

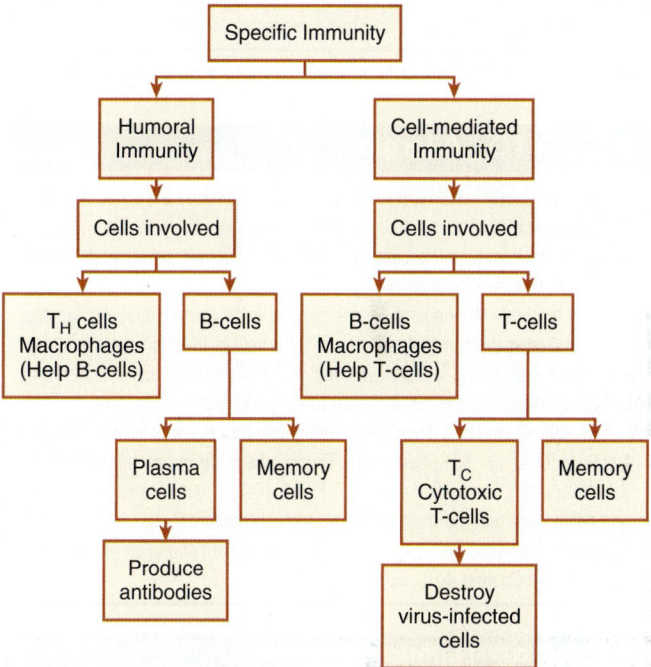

FIG. 9.5 Specific immunity.

7. The T cell clones that don't become cytotoxic T cells remain in the immune system as memory cells. Memory cells can recognize the same antigen if it ever invades the body again. (Box 9.9).

MEDICAL TERMINOLOGY
cyto-: cell
-tox/o: poison

Cell-mediated immunity is particularly well suited to destroying viruses. Viruses must be inside a host cell to reproduce. Cytotoxic T cells destroy a virus once it gets inside of a cell. Cell-mediated immunity helps stop the spread of viral infections within the body. Another job of cell-mediated immunity is to recognize and destroy cancer cells or tumor cells. Even though these cells are part of a person's body, they are not normal. They have changed and are now harming the body. Cell-mediated immunity recognizes malignant (muh LIG nuh nt) changes in cells. It works to destroy them before they cause disease (cancer) or tumors.

Fig. 9.5 presents an overview of specific immunity.

TABLE 9.1 Hypersensitivity Reactions

Type of Hypersensitivity	Reactions	Examples
Type I – immediate hypersensitivity; also called an *allergic reaction*	• Reactions may be local (runny nose, itching eyes). • Reactions can also be systemic (swelling of the airway and tongue). • Anaphylaxis (an uh fuh LAK sis) is the systemic form of immediate hypersensitivity. It can be fatal.	Food allergies, insect venom allergies (bee and wasp stings), latex allergies
Type II	• Antibodies to cell surface antigens are produced	Hemolytic (hee MOL ih tik) disease of the newborn (HDN), blood bank transfusion reactions
Type III	• Antibody-antigen complexes are deposited in tissues of the body	Organ damage with systemic lupus erythematosus (sih STEM ik LOO puhs er uh THEE muh toh sus), glomerulonephritis (gloh mer yuh loh nuh FRAHY tis), rheumatic (roo MAT ik) fever, rheumatoid arthritis
Type IV, also known as *delayed hypersensitivity*	• Allergic reaction appears 24-48 hours after exposure to an antigen	Poison ivy rash, tuberculosis (TB) skin tests, organ transplant rejection

From Shiland B: *Mastering healthcare terminology*, ed 5, St Louis, 2015, Elsevier.

BOX 9.10 Allergies

An allergic reaction is a type I hypersensitivity reaction (see Table 9.1). It is the body responding to an allergic trigger, called an *allergen*. Allergens are harmless environmental substances, but in an allergic reaction, the body overreacts to their presence.

When the body responds to an allergen, immune cells release *histamines, kinins,* and other inflammatory substances. This causes the characteristic allergy symptoms: runny nose, watery eyes, and possibly a rash or hives. Sometimes drugs called *antihistamines,* are used to alleviate allergy symptoms.

If an allergic reaction is severe, it can cause a dangerous condition called anaphylactic shock (see Chapter 40). This can be a life-threatening condition. Sometimes people who know they are highly allergic to a substance will carry an EpiPen with them to treat an anaphylactic reaction.

For more information on allergens and emergency care during an anaphylactic reaction, see Chapter 40.

CRITICAL THINKING 9.7

T cells are very important cells in the immune system. List five ways T cells help protect the body from foreign antigens. Share your thoughts with the class.

Hypersensitivity Reactions

The immune system is quite remarkable. When it works well, it keeps our bodies from harm. When it doesn't work properly, the immune system can harm the body. *Hypersensitivity* (hahy per SEN si tiv ih tee) reactions are an example of the immune system overreacting.

Hypersensitivity is defined as an immune response that causes tissue damage in the host. It is an excessive response to a stimulus or foreign agent. A hypersensitivity reaction does not occur the first time an antigen is encountered. It is when the person encounters the antigen for a second or subsequent exposure that the reaction develops. Chapter 40 covers allergic reactions, which are a type of hypersensitivity reaction. Box 9.10 provides more information on allergies. Table 9.1 presents an overview of hypersensitivity reactions.

CRITICAL THINKING 9.8

- What type of hypersensitivity is hemolytic disease of the newborn (HDN)?
- What type of hypersensitivity is anaphylaxis?
- What type of hypersensitivity is delayed hypersensitivity?

TYPES OF ACQUIRED IMMUNITY

Acquired immunity is classified as active or passive. *Active immunity* requires the body to respond to an antigen, and produce antibodies for protection. *Passive immunity* does not require the body to do anything. In passive immunity, premade antibodies are given to a person. This occurs through transmission from the mother to the fetus or infant, or through an injection of immune globulin..

Active immunity and passive immunity are each categorized as natural immunity or artificial immunity. All four types of acquired immunity describe ways the body has acquired antibodies to specific diseases.

Active Immunity

Active acquired immunity can take either of the following two forms.
- *Natural:* When a person is exposed to an antigen in the natural course of life (e.g., exposure to a cold virus), and he or she naturally goes through the process of antibody development. The person also develops memory cells to protect against a second exposure.
- *Artificial:* When a person is given a vaccination (immunization). Vaccines (vak SEEN s) have antigens that have been altered so that they cannot cause disease. But they still contain the proteins required to stimulate an antibody response. This an intentional exposure to an altered antigen. Examples of vaccines include the diphtheria-tetanus-pertussis (DTP) vaccine, the measles-mumps-rubella (MMR) vaccine, and the varicella vaccine.

Active immunity usually takes a little while for the body to produce antibodies. However, it lasts a person's whole life.

Passive Immunity

Passive acquired immunity can take either of the following two forms.
- *Natural:* When a person takes in antibodies from a natural source. Examples include the passage of antibodies from mother to fetus through the placenta, or from mother to infant through breast milk.
- *Artificial:* When a person is given an injection of immune globin (or immunoglobulins). Immune globulin comes from donated blood plasma that is pooled from many donors. There are several types of immune globulin. Some types are good for just one disease, whereas others cover multiple diseases.

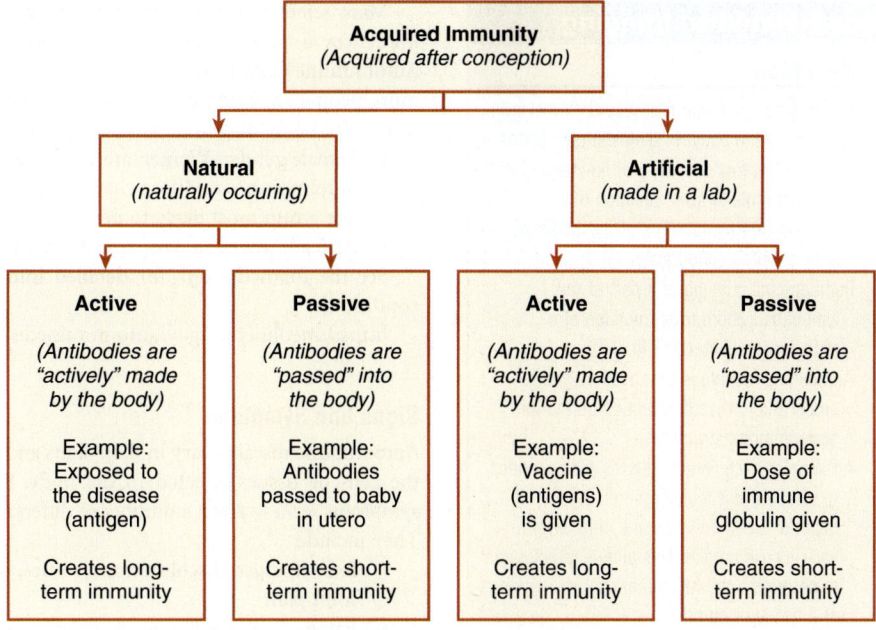

FIG. 9.6 Acquired immunity.

Passive immunity is effective as soon as the antibodies enter the body, but they last only a short time (about 3 months).

Fig. 9.6 helps to explain acquired immunity.

CRITICAL THINKING 9.9

Rich and Jan Dallman have an appointment to see Dr. Perez today. They both want to get the shingles vaccine. Julia prepares their vaccinations and then sits down with Rich and Jan to go over the Vaccine Information Statement (VIS), which discusses the vaccine. What type of immunity is a vaccination, active or passive? Is it natural or artificial? Discuss your answers with the class.

DISEASES AND DISORDERS OF THE LYMPHATIC AND IMMUNE SYSTEMS

Diseases of the lymphatic and immune systems are diverse and have many different causes (Box 9.11). Many factors can be associated with lymphatic and immune system diseases, disorders, and infections. These diseases can involve the cells, tissues, and organs of the lymphatic system or the immune system. Some causes include:
- Microbial infections
- Malignant changes
- Congenital conditions

Tables 9.2 to 9.5 present common diagnostic laboratory tests and therapeutic interventions for lymphatic and immune diseases and disorders.

Autoimmune Diseases and Disorders

Recall that the goal of the immune system is to protect the body from foreign pathogens. The immune system normally can distinguish self from foreign. However, in autoimmune diseases, something goes wrong in the immune system – it begins to attack healthy self cells.

BOX 9.11 Common Signs and Symptoms of Lymphatic and Immune System Diseases and Disorders

Common signs and symptoms of lymphatic and immune system diseases and disorders include:
- Fatigue, joint pain, swollen joints
- Low-grade fever
- Skin changes, discoloration, or rash
- Weight loss

VOCABULARY
microbiome: The total collection of microorganisms, and their genetic material, present on or in the human body or a specific site in the human body.

According to the National Institutes of Health website MedlinePlus (https://medlineplus.gov), there are more than 80 different autoimmune diseases. The common factor among all autoimmune diseases is that a person's own immune system attacks healthy tissues. No matter what the symptoms are, the underlying cause of the disease is an immune system that is not working properly.

Etiology

The cause of autoimmune diseases is a mystery. There are many theories about how the immune system becomes confused. The following is a brief list of suspected causes.
- A viral or bacterial infection that triggers the immune system to attack healthy cells
- Exposure over time to toxins (e.g., chemicals, pesticides, and food additives)
- A weakness in a person's immune system, brought on by stress, past infections, and hormone fluctuations
- An imbalance in the intestinal **microbiome** (mahy kroh BAHY ohm)
- Existing allergies (another type of immune system overreaction)

TABLE 9.2 Terms Related to Imaging

Term	Definition
computed tomography (CT) scan	An imaging technique that records transverse planes of the body for diagnostic purposes.
lymphadenography (lim fad uh NAH gruh fee)	Radiographic (rey dee OH graf ik) imaging of the lymph gland after injection of a radiopaque (rey dee oh PEYK) substance. Also called *lymphography*.
lymphangiography (lim fan jee AH gruh fee)	Radiographic imaging of a part of the lymphatic system after injection of a radiopaque substance (Fig. 9.7).
magnetic resonance imaging (MRI)	An imaging technique that uses magnetic properties to record detailed information about internal structures.
positron emission tomography (PET)	An imaging technique that uses radionuclides to visualize tissues. Measurements can be taken of blood flow, volume, and oxygen and glucose uptake. This allows radiologists to determine the functional characteristics of a tissue or an organ.
splenic arteriography (SPLEH nik ar teer ee AH gruh fee)	Radiographic imaging of the spleen using a contrast medium.
x-ray (radiograph)	An imaging technique that uses electromagnetic radiation to record internal structures. Images can be taken from several different angles, allowing abnormalities to be detected.

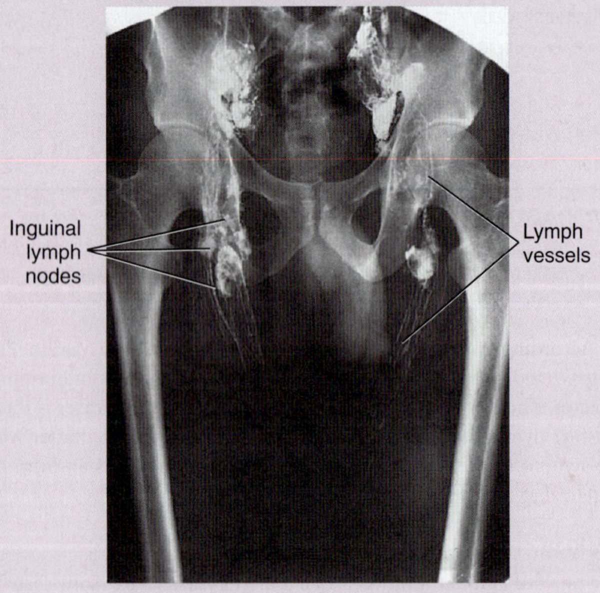

FIG. 9.7 Lymphangiogram of the inguinal region and upper thighs. (From Frank ED, Long BW, Smith BJ: *Merrill's atlas of radiographic positions and radiologic procedures*, ed 12, St Louis, 2012, Mosby.)

From Shiland B: *Mastering healthcare terminology*, ed 5, St Louis, 2015, Elsevier.

Many scientists think that a combination of all these possible causes influences a person's risk of developing an autoimmune disease. Autoimmune diseases are an area of intense scientific research, because more people are being diagnosed with autoimmune conditions. Risk factors for being diagnosed with an autoimmune disease include;

- Female gender: Women are more likely to be diagnosed with an autoimmune condition than men. Women ages 15 to 45 are the age group most likely to develop an autoimmune disease.
- African American, Hispanic American, or Native American race

See the following link for detailed information on autoimmune conditions:

https://medlineplus.gov/autoimmunediseases.html.

Signs and Symptoms

Autoimmune diseases vary in their signs and symptoms, depending on the cells or tissues affected in the body. Some common signs and symptoms seem to affect a number of different autoimmune conditions. They include:

- Skin changes, discolorations, rashes, or lesions
- Joint pain
- Fatigue/malaise, low-grade fever, general ill-feeling

Commonly affected cells or tissues include:

- Joints, muscles, and skin
- Blood vessels, red blood cells
- Connective tissue
- Endocrine glands (i.e., thyroid, pancreas)

Diagnostic Procedures

To diagnose an autoimmune condition, the provider takes a complete history and performs a thorough physical examination. Laboratory tests also are part of the diagnostic process. Diagnostic testing procedures vary, depending on the patient's signs and symptoms (see Table 9.3 for additional information on testing). For most suspected autoimmune conditions, some or all of the following laboratory tests may be ordered.

- *Antinuclear antibody test (ANA)* – A blood test that looks for the presence of antibodies to the nucleus or the organelles of the nucleus. A serum sample is used for this type of test.
- *Autoantibody test* – A blood/serum test that looks for autoantibodies.
- *Complete blood cell count (CBC)* – A blood test. See Chapter 8 and Chapter 44 for more information. Some CLIA–waived tests are available.
- *Comprehensive metabolic panel (CMP)* – A blood test. See Chapter 8 and Chapter 44 for more information. Some CLIA-waived tests are available
- *C-reactive protein (CRP)* – A blood test that measures CRP. CRP is elevated in people with inflammation. Some CLIA-waived tests are available
- *Erythrocyte sedimentation rate (ESR)* – A whole blood test. People with inflammation have elevated values. Some CLIA-waived tests are available.
- *Urinalysis* – See Chapter 42 for more information. Some CLIA-waived tests are available.

The following imaging tests may be ordered.

- Joint and bone x-rays, magnetic resonance imaging (MRI), ultrasound scans. Information on each of these procedures can be found in Chapter 2, and in Table 9.2.

Tissue biopsies also may be requested. See Chapter 2 and Table 9.5 for more information.

CHAPTER 9 Lymphatic and Immune Systems

TABLE 9.3 Terms Related to Laboratory Tests

Term	Definition
AIDS tests – enzyme-linked immunosorbent assay (ELISA), Western blot	Tests to detect the presence of the human immunodeficiency virus (HIV).
allergy testing	A series of tests involving a patch, scratch, or intradermal injection of an attenuated amount of an allergen to test for hypersensitivity (Fig. 9.8). See MAST allergy testing.
antinuclear antibody (ANA) testing	Detects antibodies to the nucleus or parts of the nucleus of cells. A blood sample is used. It is diagnostic for SLE, and it can be positive for other autoimmune diseases.
autoantibody testing	Detects antibodies to many specific cells and tissues of the human body.
complete blood cell count (CBC)	A group of 12 tests. Some of them are a red blood cell count (RBC), a white blood cell count (WBC), hemoglobin (Hb), hematocrit/packed-cell volume (Hct/PCV), and diff (WBC differential). Some Clinical Laboratory Improvement Amendments (CLIA)–waived tests are available.
comprehensive metabolic panel (CMP)	A set of blood tests that assess organ function, metabolism, and electrolyte levels. Some CLIA-waived tests are available.
C-reactive protein (CRP)	CRP is a nonspecific marker for inflammation in the body. CRP is produced in the liver and measured by testing the blood. CRP levels rise in response to inflammation. Some CLIA-waived tests are available.
differential (diff) count	A measure of the different types of WBCs.
erythrocyte sedimentation rate (ESR) (eh RITH roh syte seh dih men TAY shun)	A test that measures the time required for mature RBCs to settle out of a blood sample after an anticoagulant has been added. An increased ESR indicates inflammation. Some CLIA-waived tests available.
MAST allergy testing	Multiple-antigen simultaneous testing (MAST) is a blood test that can examine multiple antigens at the same time. Antihistamines do not affect this blood test. MAST has replaced radioallergosorbent testing (RAST).
urinalysis	Tests different components of the urine. It can help rule out conditions that may cause abdominal pain, such as a urinary tract infection (UTI), kidney stones, and some kidney and liver diseases. Some CLIA-waived tests are available.
white blood cell (WBC) count	Measurement of the number of leukocytes in the blood. An increase may indicate the presence of an infection; a decrease may be caused by radiation or chemotherapy. Some CLIA-waived tests are available.

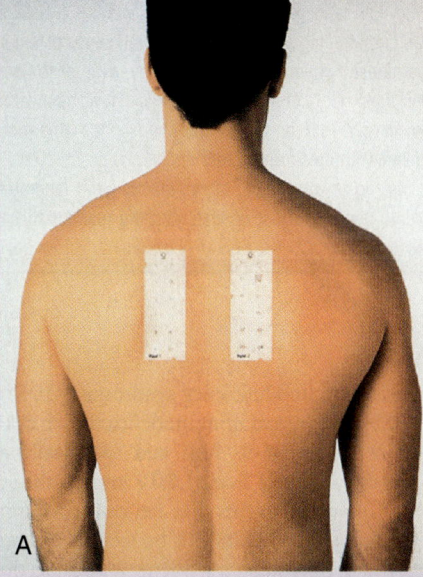 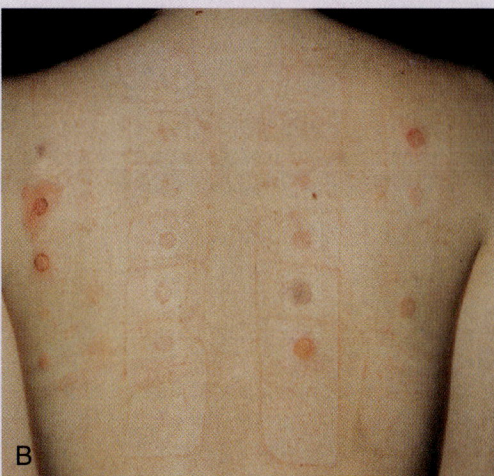

FIG. 9.8 (A) An allergen patch test, saturated with individual allergens, is applied to a patient's back. (B) Positive allergy reactions of varying intensity. (From Habif TP: *Clinical dermatology*, ed 5, St Louis, 2010, Mosby.)

From Shiland B: *Mastering healthcare terminology*, ed 5, St Louis, 2015, Elsevier.

TABLE 9.4 Terms Related to Bone Marrow Interventions

Term	Definition
bone marrow transplantation (BMT)	Transplantation of bone marrow to stimulate production of normal blood cells.
autologous BMT (ah TALL uh gus)	Harvesting of a patient's own healthy bone marrow before treatment for reintroduction later.
homologous BMT (hoh MALL uh gus)	Transplantation of healthy bone marrow from a donor to a recipient to stimulate the formation of new blood cells.

From Shiland B: *Mastering healthcare terminology*, ed 5, St Louis, 2015, Elsevier.

TABLE 9.5 Terms Related to Lymphatic and Immune System Interventions

Term	Definition
adenoidectomy (ad eh noyd ECK tuh mee)	Removal of the adenoids (also called the *pharyngeal* (fuh RIN jee uhl) *tonsils*).
biopsy (bx) of lymphatic structures	Removal of the lymph nodes or lymphoid tissue, for the purpose of diagnosis and/or treatment.
lymphadenectomy (lim fad uh NECK tuh mee)	Removal of a lymph node.
splenectomy (spli NEK tuh mee)	Removal of the spleen.

From Shiland B: *Mastering healthcare terminology*, ed 5, St Louis, 2015, Elsevier.

Treatment

Treatments will vary, depending on the signs and symptoms of the condition, However, common goals of treatment for most autoimmune conditions include:
- Diminishing the signs and symptoms of the condition, and/or reducing their occurrence
- Controlling the autoimmune process
- Maintaining the body's ability to fight disease and infections

Treatments may include:
- Physical therapy, to help with the movement of affected joints, muscles, and bones
- Blood transfusions, if the condition affects blood cells
- A modified diet, to reduce inflammation and boost the immune system with nutrient-dense foods
- Stress reduction, adequate sleep, regular exercise, and avoiding smoking

Medications may include:
- NSAIDs (e.g., ibuprofen) to reduce inflammation
- Prescription corticosteroids to reduce inflammation
- Supplementation to replace substances lacking in the body, examples include: thyroid hormones, insulin, vitamin B12, vitamin D, and others depending on the condition
- Immunosuppressive drugs to reduce the body's immune response

Some alternative therapies that may bring symptom relief include:
- Yoga, massage therapy, and relaxation therapy
- Special diets to reduce inflammation or that remove specific types of proteins from the diet (e.g., gluten-free diet, grain-free diet, elimination of sugar and natural/artificial sweeteners)

Prognosis

The prognosis can vary greatly with autoimmune diseases. Some conditions are relapsing-remitting, but they can become progressive or can cause permanent damage to affected cells and tissues. Some conditions are relatively mild and are not life threatening. Some conditions can be very aggressive and ultimately fatal.

Prevention

Because their cause is unknown (Table 9.6), autoimmune diseases and disorders are hard to prevent. Some practices that may reduce the chances of developing an autoimmune condition include:
- Taking steps to reduce stress
- Getting an adequate amount of sleep
- Refraining from smoking or consuming alcohol to excess
- Eating a healthy, nutrient-rich diet – lots of fruits and vegetables, high fiber, good protein sources, very few processed foods, very low sugar or sweetener intake, and reduced food additives and colorants
- Getting adequate exercise
- Reducing toxin exposures wherever possible

CRITICAL THINKING 9.10

Laney Sharma is a new patient to the Walden-Martin Family Medical Clinic. Laney is in her late 30s. She is married, has three children, and works full time. She is in good overall health. She has a busy schedule, but lately she has been feeling more tired than usual. Laney comments to Dr. Perez that she just doesn't seem to have any energy, even at the beginning of the day! She has been very cold lately, her wrists have been achy, and she has a faint, pinkish red rash on one of her cheekbones. She just wants to see if any of these symptoms are related.

Looking at Laney's list of symptoms, what laboratory tests might Dr. Perez order? Share your list of tests and the reasons for choosing them with your classmates.

HIV/AIDS

Acquired immunodeficiency syndrome (AIDS) is a chronic condition caused by the human immunodeficiency virus (HIV). HIV attacks the immune system of its host and specifically damages the CD4+ T lymphocytes (helper T cells). HIV impairs the immune system's ability to fight infectious agents that can cause disease.

Currently, HIV/AIDS can be treated but not cured. And without proper and consistent treatment, it is a life-threatening disease. The treatment for HIV/AIDS that is available now slows the progression of the disease and allows a person to live a relatively normal life.

Etiology

HIV is the causative agent of AIDS. HIV is a blood-borne virus that can be transmitted through sexual contact, through a sharps exposure (e.g., needlestick), or from mother to child during pregnancy or childbirth.

The following are risk factors for acquiring HIV:
- Having *unprotected sex* (unprotected sex is having sex without using a new latex or polyurethane condom at every exposure)

TABLE 9.6 Common Autoimmune Conditions

Condition	Overview of Condition, Signs and Symptoms
Hyperthyroidism (hahy per THAHY roi diz uhm) or *Graves' disease*	An overactive thyroid gland. Overproduction of thyroid hormones. **Symptoms include:** anxiety/nervousness, weight loss, heat sensitivity, an enlarged thyroid gland (goiter), bulging eyes, *exophthalmos*, fatigue, rapid or irregular heartbeat.
Hypothyroidism (hahy puh THAHY roi diz uhm) or *Hashimoto thyroiditis* (HAH shee moh toh THAHY roi di tihs)	An underactive thyroid gland. Underproduction of thyroid hormones. **Symptoms include:** cold sensitivity, fatigue/achiness/tenderness, dry skin, weight loss, muscle weakness, elevated blood cholesterol, enlarged thyroid gland (goiter), thinning hair, slow heart rate, depression.
Type 1 diabetes	The pancreas produces little or no *insulin*. Insulin allows glucose to enter cells to produce energy. **Symptoms include:** high blood sugar, increased thirst, frequent urination, extreme hunger, weight loss, fatigue, weakness, blurred vision.
Multiple sclerosis (MUHL tuh puh l skli ROH sis)	Breaking down and scarring of the protective covering of the nerves (*myelin sheath*). This causes problems with nerves communicating with the brain. It can cause permanent nerve damage. **Symptoms include**: numbness, weakness or tingling in limbs, vision disturbances, prolonged double vision, slurred speech, unsteady walking, fatigue, dizziness. Symptoms may come and go at first, but then may become progressive.
Rheumatoid arthritis (ROO muh toid)	A chronic inflammatory disorder of the joints. It may also affect a wide variety of systems in the body. **Symptoms include**: joint pain, stiffness; warm, tender joints, especially in the morning; fatigue, low-grade fever, weight loss. *See more detail in Chapter 3.*
Systemic lupus erythematosus (SLE)	A chronic inflammatory disease that may affect the skin, joints, kidneys, blood cells, brain, heart, and lungs. **Symptoms include:** fatigue, fever, joint pain/stiffness, butterfly-shaped rash on the face that covers the cheeks and bridge of the nose (Fig. 9.9), chest pain, shortness of breath, dry eyes, cognitive issues.
Sjögren syndrome (SHO greh n)	An inflammatory condition of the tear ducts and salivary glands. Symptoms may be seen alone, but the disorder commonly accompanies rheumatoid arthritis and SLE. **Symptoms include:** dry eyes and mouth; the joints, thyroid gland, kidneys, liver, lungs, skin, and nerves also can be affected.
Celiac disease (SEE lee ak)	An immune reaction set off by the presence of gluten (found in wheat, barley, and rye). Gluten damages the lining of the small intestines. **Symptoms include:** diarrhea, fatigue, weight loss, bloating, abdominal pain, iron-deficiency anemia, osteoporosis, itchy skin, mouth ulcers, headache, nervous system damage (painful or tingling hands and feet), joint pain. *See more detail in Chapter 5.*
Vitiligo (vit l AHY goh)	A skin condition in which the immune system destroys the pigment-producing cells of the skin or hair. It can be patchy throughout the body or localized in one area. **Symptoms include:** patchy loss of skin color (Fig. 9.10); premature whitening of the hair, eyelashes, eyebrows, or beard; loss of color on the inside of the mouth and nose; loss or change of color in the *retina* of the eye (lining of the inside of the eye).

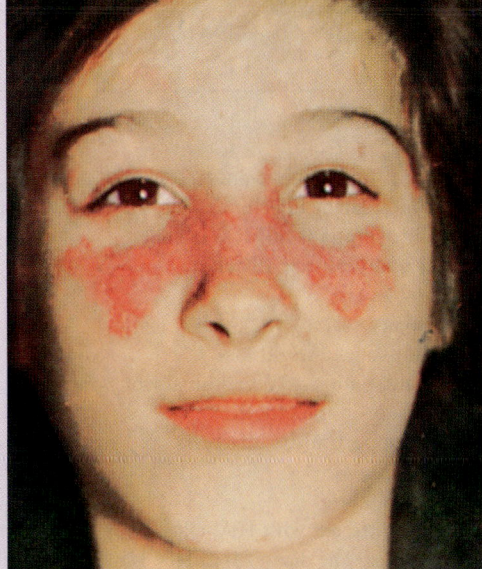

FIG. 9.9 Butterfly rash of systemic lupus erythematosus (SLE). (Modified from Kliegman RM et al: *Nelson textbook of pediatrics*, ed 18, Philadelphia, 2007, Saunders.)

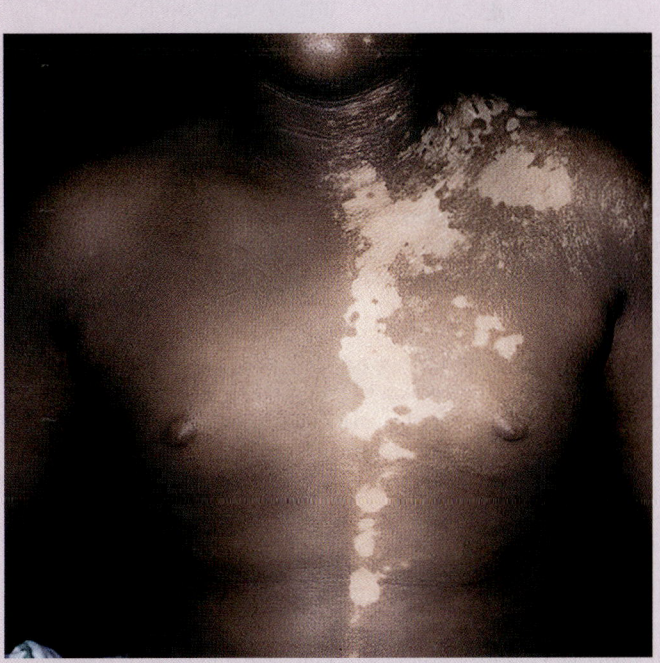

FIG. 9.10 Vitiligo. (From Shiland B: *Mastering healthcare terminology*, ed 5, St Louis, 2017, Elsevier.)

Continued

TABLE 9.6 Common Autoimmune Conditions—cont'd

Condition	Overview of Condition, Signs and Symptoms
Psoriasis (suh RAHY uh sis)	A skin condition in which skin cells are produced quickly. This leads to areas of thick, scaly, red-pink/silver patches of skin. **Symptoms include:** red-pink patches of skin with silvery scales; dry, cracked skin that may bleed; itching-burning sore skin; thickened and pitted fingernails or toenails; swollen-stiff joints. *See more detail in Chapter 4.*
Alopecia areata (al uh PEE shee uh AHR ee ah ta)	Excessive hair loss. It may be on any part of the body, and it may be patchy. **Symptoms include:** often seen as patchy-circular bald spots (Fig. 9.11), loosening of hair, full-body hair loss.
Myasthenia gravis (mahy uh s THEE nee uh GRAW vihs)	Weakness and rapid fatigue of any voluntary muscles, commonly in the face, throat, and neck. **Symptoms include:** drooping of one or both eyelids; double vision; trouble speaking, swallowing, and chewing; limited facial expressions.
Scleroderma (skleer uh DUR muh)	A hardening and tightening of the skin and connective tissues. In some people it may affect only the skin. In others it may affect the skin and internal organs (i.e., systemic) and can be fatal. **Symptoms include:** hardened and tight skin; intolerance to cold temperatures, especially in the fingers and toes; digestive system issues; heart, lung, or kidney problems.
Polymyositis (pohl ee MAHY oh sih tis)	An inflammatory condition that causes weakness on both sides of the body. It makes it difficult to climb stairs, lift objects overhead, and stand up from a seated position. **Symptoms include:** weakness in muscles close to the core of the body: the hips, thighs, shoulders, (upper) arms, and neck. It may become difficult to swallow or to breathe properly.
Mixed connective tissue disorder	A combination of a number of autoimmune conditions (e.g., SLE, scleroderma, polymyositis). It has a combination of symptoms. **Symptoms include:** general pain, fatigue, cold intolerance (especially in the hands and feet), swollen fingers or hands, muscle and joint pain, a reddish brown rash over the knuckles of the hands.

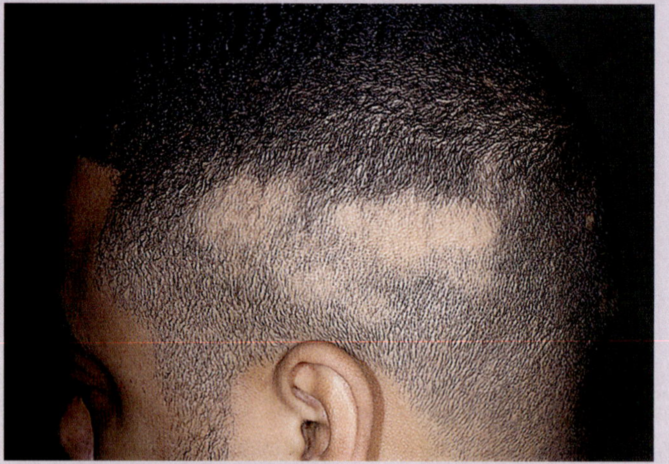

FIG. 9.11 Alopecia. (From Callen JP, Greer KE, Saller AS, et al: *Color Atlas of Dermatology*, ed 2, Philadelphia, 2000, Saunders.)

From Shiland B: *Mastering healthcare terminology*, ed 5, St Louis, 2015, Elsevier.

- Using intravenous drugs, especially if sharing needles
- Having another sexually transmitted infection (STI)
- Uncircumcised man (circumcised men have a lower chance of acquiring HIV)

Signs and Symptoms

A primary HIV infection occurs when a person is first exposed to the virus. Signs and symptoms of primary HIV include:

- Flu-like symptoms (fever, fatigue)
- Swollen lymph nodes, especially in the neck
- Diarrhea, weight loss

After the initial infection with HIV, the virus becomes *latent* (shows no signs or symptoms). During this time, the person will test positive on an HIV blood test; However, he or she does not show signs or symptoms of the infection. HIV can remain latent for up to 10 years. But many HIV-positive people move into symptomatic HIV within several years.

If an HIV-positive person is not treated with antiviral drugs, HIV will change from a latent infection to an active one, and progress to AIDS. Signs and symptoms of AIDS include:

- Chronic and persistent diarrhea
- Recurring fevers
- Night sweats, soaking wet
- Profound fatigue, weight loss
- Skin rashes, bumps, and continual white patches or lesions on the tongue or in the mouth
- Repeated opportunistic infections

Diagnostic Procedures

Most individuals infected with HIV take about 12 weeks to produce anti-HIV antibodies. The diagnosis of HIV is made by testing a blood sample or a saliva sample for anti-HIV antibodies. Newer generation testing can also detect a protein made by the HIV virus shortly after infection. This gives a quick diagnosis after exposure to the antigen.

CLIA-waived kits are available for home use, but their results should be confirmed by laboratory tests. Confirmatory tests include the enzyme-linked immunosorbent assay (ELISA) and Western blot testing (see Table 9.3).

Treatment

HIV infection is not a curable disease, but a regimen of antiviral medications is available to control the virus. Five different drug classes can be used to control HIV. Most providers recommend using three drugs from at least two different drug classes. This helps to keep the virus from becoming resistant to a single drug. All HIV drugs block the virus from entering the CD4+ T lymphocytes, but in different ways.

HIV treatment should include additional methods of staying healthy. The drug treatments can be difficult, and they have many side effects. Staying healthy and keeping the immune system healthy is an important overall goal for each patient. In addition to medications, HIV-positive individuals should include the following in their treatment plan.
- Eating healthy, nutrient-rich foods
- Getting adequate sleep, exercise, and relaxation (to reduce stress)
- Avoiding foods that can cause food-borne illnesses, because these illnesses can be serious in HIV-positive individuals. Examples of food to avoid include raw or unpasteurized dairy products, raw eggs, and seafood. Do not eat undercooked meat – cook it until it is well done.
- Staying up-to-date on immunizations. However, do not get vaccines that use live viruses.
- Taking care when handling pets. Some pets can carry organisms or parasites that can cause serious infections in an HIV-positive individual. Care should be taken around cats, reptiles, and birds in particular. Always wash hands thoroughly after handling pets or cleaning out litter boxes.

Prognosis

HIV-positive individuals who comply with their medication regimen can live productive and full lives. Many HIV-positive patients who began anti-HIV medications 25 years ago are still healthy. Compliance and taking good care of the immune system are important to living with HIV. The infection is treated as a chronic condition. It can be controlled and managed with proper medication and lifestyle changes.

Prevention

The following recommendations can help prevent individuals from acquiring or spreading the HIV virus.
- Use a new condom every time you have anal or vaginal sex. Women can use a female condom. Protection should be used during oral sex, too.
- Tell any sexual partners that you have HIV.
- Use clean, one-use disposable needles if you inject drugs. Do not share needles under any circumstances.
- If you are pregnant, get immediate medical care.
- Consider male circumcision. Scientific evidence has shown that men who are circumcised have a reduced risk of acquiring HIV.
- Consider taking pre-exposure prophylaxis (PrEP). It can reduce the risk of sexually transmitted HIV infections in high-risk groups. Consult a provider for information on PrEP medications.

Lymphoma: Hodgkin's and Non-Hodgkin's

Lymphoma is a cancer of the lymphatic and immune systems. Lymphocytes, a type of white blood cell, mutate and reproduce rapidly in lymphoma. The overproduced, diseased lymphocytes crowd out healthy WBCs. This causes the patient to be more susceptible to infections.

There are two main types of lymphoma:
- Hodgkin's lymphoma is also called *Hodgkin disease*. It is characterized by the presence of Reed-Sternberg cells in the blood. This type of cell is specific to Hodgkin lymphoma.
- Non-Hodgkin's lymphoma is a collection of all other lymphatic cancers that are not Hodgkin's lymphomas. This type is the more common of the two lymphomas. It is the sixth most common type of cancer in the United States.

Etiology

The cause of lymphomas is not well understood or obvious in most cases. There isn't a direct link to any one event, chemical exposure, or genetic mutation that can predict the development of a lymphoma. However, some factors may increase a person's risk of developing this type of cancer.

Risk factors for developing Hodgkin's lymphoma are:
- *Family history of lymphoma.* If a close relative has had any type of lymphoma, it increases the risk a person can develop the disease.
- *Age.* Hodgkin's lymphoma is seen most frequently in people between the ages of 15 and 30, and then again after the age of 55.
- *Male gender.* Males have lymphoma a little more frequently than females.
- *Having had an Epstein-Barr (EBV) infection.* EBV primarily causes infectious mononucleosis (mono).

Risk factors for developing non-Hodgkin's lymphoma are as follows:
- *Age.* Non-Hodgkin's lymphoma can occur at any age, but a person's risk of developing it increases with age. It is most common after age 60.
- *Therapy/medication that suppresses the immune system.* These individuals have a greater risk of developing lymphoma.
- *Having had certain infections.* Examples include EBV, which primarily causes infectious mononucleosis (mono), HIV, or *Helicobacter pylori*, which causes stomach and intestinal ulcers.
- *Chemical exposure.* Pesticide and insecticide exposure can contribute to a person's risk of developing lymphoma.

Signs and Symptoms

Signs and symptoms of both Hodgkin's lymphoma and non-Hodgkin's lymphoma include:
- Painless swelling of lymph nodes, especially in the neck, armpits, or groin
- Fatigue, fever and chills, night sweats
- Unexplained weight loss

Additional symptoms that are more common with Hodgkin's lymphoma are itching and an increased sensitivity to alcohol. Some people even find that they feel pain in lymph nodes after consuming alcohol.

Additional symptoms that are more common with non-Hodgkin's lymphoma are abdominal swelling and/or pain, trouble breathing, coughing, or chest pain.

Diagnostic Procedures

For both types of lymphoma, the diagnostic process is the same. The following diagnostic tools will be used to diagnose lymphoma and to determine the type a person has.
- The provider will perform a physical exam. He or she will specifically look for enlarged and nontender lymph nodes, liver, and spleen.
- Blood and urine tests will be done to rule out other possible disease conditions and infections.
  - Blood tests would likely include a complete blood cell count (CBC) and differential and a comprehensive metabolic panel (CMP). Some CLIA-waived tests are available.
  - Urinalysis. Some CLIA-waived tests are available.

- Imaging tests – x-ray films or computed tomography (CT), magnetic resonance imaging (MRI), or positron emission tomography (PET) scans – may be done to locate and/or visualize affected lymph nodes and tumors. See Chapter 2 and Table 9.2 for more information on imaging tests.
- Lymph node, tissue, and/or bone marrow biopsy may be done. By removing a sample of lymph node, tissue, or bone marrow to be analyzed, the provider can make an accurate diagnosis about the type of lymphoma present and the stage of the disease. Staging a cancer is important because it affects the treatment plan the provider will recommend. See Chapter 2 for more information on biopsies and cancer staging.

Treatment

Treatment depends on the type and stage of the lymphoma. Not all lymphomas are treated. Some slowly progressing types of non-Hodgkin's lymphoma may not be treated. Instead, they are monitored to make sure they are not progressing.

Depending on the type and stage of the lymphoma, treatment may include:
- Chemotherapy – A drug treatment that uses medication to kill lymphoma cells. It can be used together with radiation therapy.
- Radiation therapy – The use of high-energy x-rays to kill lymphoma cells. It can be used together with chemotherapy.
- Stem cell transplantation – Also known as a *bone marrow transplant*. This treatment is used to replace diseased bone marrow with healthy stem cells. Stem cells can then repopulate the bone marrow with healthy cells.
- Targeted cancer therapy – This treatment is often used if other treatments have not been successful, or if lymphoma has recurred. This type of medication is designed to target specific weaknesses in cancer cells.
- Biologic therapy – The use of specific drugs that enhance the patient's immune system, helping it to destroy lymphoma cells.

Follow-up visits will be required throughout treatment and beyond. Periodic checkups will be required to monitor treatment and the patient's post-treatment status.

Prognosis

For any cancer, the prognosis is best the earlier the cancer is found. With many effective treatments, people are surviving cancer and living many years after being diagnosed with the disease.

Prevention

There are no specific preventive measures for lymphoma. General strategies include a healthy diet rich in vegetables, fruits, lean proteins, and high fiber. In addition, getting sufficient sleep and regular exercise, reducing stress, and a low toxin exposure are helpful in maintaining health.

Multiple Myeloma

Multiple myeloma is a cancer of white blood cells called plasma cells. Plasma cells are a type of B lymphocyte that produce antibodies to help fight infection. In multiple myeloma, plasma cells reproduce so much that they crowd out healthy blood cells. The malignant plasma cells don't produce antibodies. Instead, they produce an abnormal protein (M protein) that can cause kidney damage.

This condition is called *multiple myeloma* because the tumors are found in many or multiple bones. If it occurs in only one bone or area, the tumor is referred to as a *plasmacytoma*.

Etiology

The cause of multiple myeloma is unknown, or *idiopathic*. But for most people, multiple myeloma starts out as monoclonal gammopathy of undetermined significance (MGUS). People with MGUS also produce M protein, but at such a low level it does not harm the body.

Risk factors for developing multiple myeloma include:
- *Age.* Most people with multiple myeloma are diagnosed after the age of 60.
- *Male gender.* Men are more likely to develop multiple myeloma than women.
- *Race.* Blacks are more likely to develop multiple myeloma than whites.
- *History of MGUS.* This makes developing multiple myeloma more likely.

Signs and Symptoms

Signs and symptoms of multiple myeloma may be subtle at first. There may be no symptoms at all in the beginning. Noticeable signs and symptoms include:
- Bone pain, especially in the spine, chest, or hips
- Anemia
- Loss of kidney function, excessive thirst
- Nausea, loss of appetite, weight loss, constipation, and fatigue
- Frequent infections
- Weakness or numbness in the legs
- Mental confusion

Diagnostic Procedures

The following tests may be used to help diagnose multiple myeloma.
- Blood tests, which may include:
  - CBC and differential
  - Tests for the presence of M protein and beta-2 microglobulin protein, to help determine the aggressiveness of the myeloma
  - CMP, which includes kidney and liver function tests
- Urinalysis (some CLIA tests are available). Also specific tests for M protein in the urine (called *Bence Jones proteins*).
- Bone marrow biopsy and examination of cells.
- Imaging tests, which may include x-ray films and MRI, CT, and PET scans. See Chapter 2 and Table 9.2 for more information on imaging tests.

At diagnosis, multiple myeloma will be staged, and a treatment plan will be based on the staged diagnosis. See Chapter 2 for more information on cancer staging.

Treatment

Treatment for asymptomatic multiple myeloma, MGUS, may not be needed. The provider will want to watch the condition and run periodic blood and urine tests to monitor signs of activity.

Treatment for multiple myeloma includes:
- Targeted cancer therapy – This treatment is designed to target specific weaknesses in myeloma cancer cells in order to kill the cells.
- Biologic therapy – Specific drugs are used to enhance the patient's immune system to help destroy myeloma cells.
- Chemotherapy – A drug treatment that uses medication to kill rapidly growing myeloma cells. High-dose chemotherapy is often given before a stem cell transplant
- Stem cell transplant – Also known as a *bone marrow transplant*. This treatment is used to replace diseased bone marrow with

healthy stem cells. Stem cells can then repopulate the bone marrow with healthy cells.
- Radiation therapy – The use of high-energy x-rays to kill rapidly growing myeloma cells. In multiple myeloma, radiation therapy may be used to shrink a plasmacytoma, especially if it is causing pain or destroying bone tissue.

Follow-up treatment is needed for any form of multiple myeloma. Blood and urine tests are ordered periodically to assess treatment or monitor the patient's health.

Prognosis

For any cancer, the prognosis is best the earlier the cancer is found. With many effective treatments, people are surviving cancer and living many years after being diagnosed.

Prevention

There are no specific preventive measures for multiple myeloma. General strategies include a healthy diet rich in vegetables, fruits, lean proteins, and high fiber. Also, getting sufficient sleep and regular exercise, reducing stress, and a low toxin exposure are helpful in maintaining health.

Additional Diseases and Disorders of the Lymphatic and Immune Systems

There are many other diseases and disorders of the lymphatic and immune systems. See Tables 9.7 and 9.8 for additional conditions that may be of interest.

TABLE 9.7 Terms Related to Lymphatic Disorders

Term	Definition
edema (eh DEE muh)	An abnormal accumulation of fluid in the interstitial spaces of tissues.
hypersplenism (hye purr SPLEE niz um)	Increased function of the spleen, resulting in hemolysis.
lymphadenitis (lim fad uh NYE tis)	Inflammation of a lymph node.
lymphadenopathy (lim fad uh NOP puh thee)	A disease of the lymph nodes or vessels. It may be localized or generalized.
lymphangitis (lim fan JYE tis)	Inflammation of lymph vessels.
lymphedema (lim fuh DEE muh)	The accumulation of lymphatic fluid. This results in swelling caused by obstruction, removal, or hypoplasia of lymph vessels. (Fig. 9.12).
lymphocytopenia (lim foh sye toh PEE nee ah)	A deficiency of lymphocytes. It can be caused by infectious mononucleosis, malignancy, nutritional deficiency, or a hematologic disorder.
lymphocytosis (lim foh sye TOH sis)	An abnormal increase in lymphocytes.
infectious mononucleosis (mon uh nook lee OH sis)	A disease marked by an increase in the number of mononuclear cells (monocytes and lymphocytes) in the blood. It is caused by the Epstein-Barr virus (EBV), and it can result in *splenomegaly* (enlarged spleen) (Fig. 9.13). See Chapter 8 for more detail on this condition.

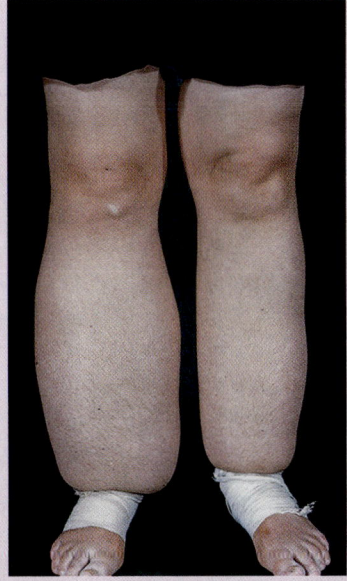

FIG. 9.12 Lymphedema. The patient had to bind her feet so that she could wear shoes. (From Black JM, Hawks JH, Keene A: *Medical surgical nursing: clinical management for positive outcomes*, ed 8, Philadelphia, 2009, Saunders.)

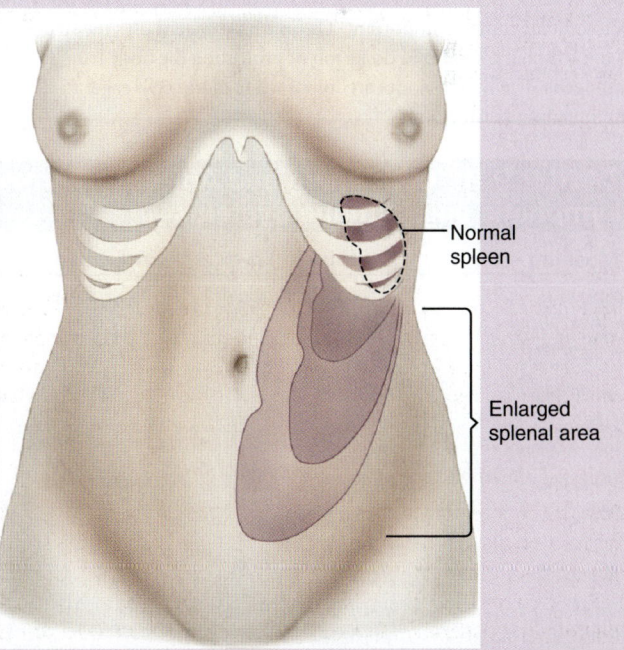

FIG. 9.13 Splenomegaly. (From Shiland B: *Mastering healthcare terminology*, ed 5, St Louis, 2017, Elsevier.)

From Shiland B: *Mastering healthcare terminology*, ed 5, St Louis, 2015, Elsevier.

TABLE 9.8 Terms Related to Malignant and Benign Neoplasms

Term	Definition
acute lymphocytic leukemia (ALL) (limf oh SIH tick loo KEE mee ah)	A cancer characterized by the uncontrolled proliferation of immature lymphocytes. It is the most common type of leukemia seen in individuals under age 19. Also called *acute lymphoblastic leukemia*. See Chapter 8 for more detail on this condition.
acute myelogenous leukemia (AML) (mye ah LAJ en us loo KEE mee ah)	A rapidly progressive form of leukemia that develops from immature bone marrow stem cells. See Chapter 8 for more detail on this condition.
chronic lymphocytic leukemia (CLL) (limf oh SIH tick loo KEE me ah)	A slowly progressive form of leukemia in which immature lymphocytes proliferate. It occurs most frequently in middle-aged and older adults. It rarely occurs in children. See Chapter 8 for more detail on this condition.
chronic myelogenous leukemia (CML) (mye ah LAJ en us loo KEE me ah)	A slowly progressive form of leukemia in which immature bone marrow cells proliferate. Like CLL, CML occurs most frequently in middle-aged and older adults. It rarely occurs in children. See Chapter 8 for more detail on this condition.
thymoma, malignant (thigh MOH mah)	A rare malignancy of the thymus gland that is particularly invasive. Unlike its benign form, it is not associated with autoimmune disorders. Also called *thymic carcinoma*.
thymoma, benign (thigh MOH mah)	A noncancerous tumor of epithelial origin. It is often associated with myasthenia gravis.

From Shiland B: *Mastering healthcare terminology*, ed 5, St Louis, 2015, Elsevier.

LIFE SPAN CHANGES

Childhood disorders of the lymphatic and immune systems include:
- hypersensitivities or allergies to foods, pollen, or pet dander
- childhood leukemias or lymphomas
- the development of autoimmune disease in late adolescence.

Unlike children, adults and seniors will have a host of diagnoses from this chapter on their medical charts. Autoimmune diseases are most common in young adulthood to middle age. Cancers of these systems also appear in significant numbers. Non-Hodgkin's lymphoma and AML account for thousands of hospitalizations every year. Multiple myeloma is most frequently diagnosed after age 60.

CLOSING COMMENTS

The lymphatic and immune systems are intertwined and are hard to separate. They share organs and cells, but their functions are different. The lymphatic system is a collection system for interstitial fluids of the body. It is the system that helps filter out debris. Keeping the body free from cellular clutter is important. The immune system uses the structures of the lymphatic system to do its job of protecting the body from foreign pathogens. The lymph nodes are full of white blood cells eager to destroy any invading pathogen.

These two systems, working together, are a wonderful example of cooperation and efficiency. Our bodies would not function well without the support and protection of the lymphatic and immune systems. See Tables 9.9 to 9.12 for medical terminology related to the lymphatic and immune systems.

TABLE 9.9 Combining and Adjective Forms for the Anatomy and Physiology of the Lymphatic and Immune Systems

Meaning	Combining Form	Adjective Form	Meaning	Combining Form	Adjective Form
appendix	append/o, appendic/o	appendicular	neck	cervic/o	cervical
axilla, armpit	axill/o	axillary	neutral	neutr/o	neutral
bone marrow	myel/o		nucleus	nucle/o	nuclear
clumping	agglutin/o	agglutinous	plasma	plasm/o	
disease	path/o		rosy-colored	eosin/o	
eat, swallow	phag/o		safety, protection	immun/o	
fever, fire	pyr/o	pyretic	same	home/o	
fiber	fibr/o	fibrous	serum	ser/o	serous
groin	inguin/o	inguinal	shape	morph/o	morphous
little grain	granul/o	granular	spleen	splen/o	splenic
lymph	lymph/o, lymphat/o	lymphatic	thymus	thym/o	thymic
lymph gland (node)	lymphaden/o		tonsil	tonsill/o	tonsillar
lymph vessel	lymphangi/o	lymphangial	white	leuk/o	
mediastinum	mediastin/o	mediastinal			

From Shiland B: *Mastering healthcare terminology*, ed 5, St Louis, 2015, Elsevier.

TABLE 9.10 Prefixes for the Anatomy and Physiology of the Lymphatic and Immune Systems

Prefix	Meaning	Prefix	Meaning
a-	without	mono-	one
anti-	against	poly-	many
inter-	between	pro-	before
macro-	large		

From Shiland B: *Mastering healthcare terminology*, ed 5, St Louis, 2015, Elsevier.

TABLE 9.11 Suffixes for the Anatomy and Physiology of the Lymphatic and Immune Systems

Suffix	Meaning	Suffix	Meaning
-cyte	cell	-leukin	white substance
-exia	condition	-logy	study of
-gen	producing	-lysis	breaking down
-globin	protein substance	-lytic	pertaining to breaking down
-in	substance	-osis	abnormal condition
-kine	movement	-phil	attraction

From Shiland B: *Mastering healthcare terminology*, ed 5, St Louis, 2015, Elsevier.

TABLE 9.12 Abbreviations

Abbreviation	Definition	Abbreviation	Definition
AIDS	acquired immunodeficiency syndrome	EBV	Epstein-Barr virus
ALL	acute lymphocytic leukemia	eosins	eosinophils
AML	acute myelogenous leukemia	ESR	erythrocyte sedimentation rate
ANA	antinuclear antibody	HDN	hemolytic disease of the newborn
basos	basophils	HIV	human immunodeficiency virus
BMT	bone marrow transplant	Ig	immunoglobulin
bx	biopsy	lymphs	lymphocytes
Ca	calcium	neuts	neutrophils
CBC	complete blood cell count	NK	natural killer (cells)
Cl	chloride	PMNs, polys	polymorphonucleocytes
CLL	chronic lymphocytic leukemia	RBC	red blood cell (count)
CML	chronic myelogenous leukemia	Rh	Rhesus
CMP	comprehensive metabolic panel	SIRS	systemic immune response syndrome
CO_2	carbon dioxide	WBC	white blood cell (count)
diff	differential (WBC count)		

From Shiland B: *Mastering healthcare terminology*, ed 5, St Louis, 2015, Elsevier.

CHAPTER REVIEW

The chapter covered two systems, the lymphatic system and the immune system. The two systems share structures, such as the lymph nodes, spleen, tonsils, thymus, appendix, and Peyer patches. The cells of the immune system live and work in the lymphatic system and structures. The immune system is made up of WBCs, which protect the body from foreign antigens (pathogens) that can cause harm.

There are two groups of WBCs in the immune system: granulocytes and agranulocytes. Both types of cells are important, but they have different functions within the system. Granulocytes are neutrophils, eosinophils, and basophils. Neutrophils are aggressive phagocytic cells in the immune system that work as part of nonspecific immunity. Neutrophils are involved in the process of inflammation, and work very hard to keep pathogens from causing harm in the body. Eosinophils are involved in protecting the body from parasites. Basophils are involved in inflammation and the response to allergens.

Agranular WBCs are monocytes and lymphocytes. Monocytes are an interesting cell. When they are in the bloodstream, they are called *monocytes*; however, when they slip out of the bloodstream and into tissues, they are called *macrophages*. Macrophages are very aggressive phagocytic cells, and they play an important role in specific immunity. There are two types of lymphocytes involved in specific immunity: B cells and T cells. These cells look the same, but their functions are quite different.

The immune system is divided into levels of defense. The first line of defense is made up of barriers that try to keep out pathogens. There are physical barriers (skin and mucous membranes), reflex barriers (e.g., coughing and sneezing), and chemical barriers (tears, saliva, and perspiration). These barriers exist to keep pathogens out of the body. But if pathogens do get past the first line of defense, there is the second line of defense waiting.

The second line of defense is another series of cellular and chemical responses designed to destroy pathogens before they can cause harm to the body. Examples of the second line of defense are fever production, protective proteins, inflammation, phagocytosis, and NK cells. These protective mechanisms try to keep pathogens out of the body. But if they do get past the second line of defense, there is still the third line of defense, or the specific immune response.

The third line of defense is specific. It attacks each pathogen individually and tries to destroy it before it has a chance to cause disease in the body. There are two parts of specific immunity: humoral immunity (or antibody-mediated immunity) and cell-mediated immunity. B cells are the most active cell in humoral immunity. B cells that clone and mature into plasma cells are the only cell in the body that can produce antibodies. Antibodies can attach or connect to antigens. When they do that, they either destroy the antigen or make it incapable of causing disease. B cells are helped in humoral immunity by T cells and macrophages. One thing antibodies cannot do is enter a cell – this is when cell-mediated immunity takes over. T cells are the most active cell in cell-mediated immunity. They are helped by B cells and macrophages, but T cells do most of the work. T cells can destroy antigen-infected cells. They can destroy intracellular pathogens. So even if a pathogen tries to hide from an antibody, T cells can destroy pathogen-infected cells.

The immune system is a very complex system of cells and chemical substances. The parts of this system are all working to keep the human body safe from pathogens. The reactions of the immune system usually work efficiently. But sometimes this system may overreact. Hypersensitivity reactions are an overreaction by the immune system. There are four types of hypersensitivity reactions:
- Type I is immediate hypersensitivity, or an allergic reaction, which includes anaphylaxis.
- Type II is cell-surface reactions, which include hemolytic disease of the newborn (HDN).
- Type III is antigen-antibody complexes that are deposited in tissues, which includes glomerulonephritis.
- Type IV is delayed hypersensitivity, which includes contact dermatitis and TB skin sensitivity reactions.

Immunity is further divided into active and passive immunity. Active immunity requires the body to react to an antigen. Passive immunity is given to a person, but does not require a response. Active and passive immunity can also be natural or artificial.

Many disease states were covered in the chapter. Autoimmune diseases are somewhat of a mystery. Scientists debate their cause. But all autoimmune diseases damage a person's own tissues and harm the body. HIV/AIDS was also covered in the diseases of the lymphatic and immune systems, along with lymphomas and multiple myeloma.

SCENARIO WRAP-UP

Dr. Perez orders a number of laboratory tests to help diagnose Laney's condition. She has ordered a complete blood cell count (CBC), erythrocyte sedimentation rate (ESR), comprehensive metabolic panel (CMP), C-reactive protein, and urinalysis. Dr. Perez is confident that the lab test results will help her focus her efforts to find the cause of Laney's condition.

Julia enjoys working with Dr. Perez. She feels like they work as a good team. Julia has often thought about how fortunate she is to work in a job that she loves, with co-workers who appreciate her talents and effort. There are very few slow days at the clinic, but she likes it that way. Helping people is Julia's passion, and she has a great opportunity to do just that at the Walden-Martin Family Medicine Clinic!

10

Cardiovascular System

LEARNING OBJECTIVES

1. List the major organs of the cardiovascular system, and identify the anatomic location of major cardiovascular system organs.
2. Describe the normal function and physiology of the cardiovascular system.
3. Discuss the diseases and disorders related to the cardiovascular system:
   - Identify the common signs and symptoms of cardiovascular diseases.
   - Identify the common etiology of cardiovascular diseases.
   - Describe diagnostic measures used for cardiovascular diseases.
   - Identify CLIA-waived tests associated with common cardiovascular diseases.
   - Describe treatment modalities used for cardiovascular diseases.
4. Compare the structure and function of the cardiovascular system across the life span.

CHAPTER OUTLINE

1. Opening Scenario, 207
2. You Will Learn, 207
3. Anatomy of the Cardiovascular System, 208
   a. Blood Vessels, 208
   b. The Heart, 209
      i. *Heart Chambers, 209*
      ii. *Heart Valves, 209*
      iii. *Heartbeat, 209*
   c. Blood Flow, 211
      i. *Pulmonary and Systemic Circulations, 211*
      ii. *Coronary Circulation, 213*
      iii. *Hepatic Portal Circulation, 213*
      iv. *Fetal Circulation, 214*
4. Physiology of the Cardiovascular System, 215
   a. Conduction System, 215
      i. *Cardiac Muscle, 215*
      ii. *Conduction System Structures, 215*
      iii. *States of Cardiac Cell, 216*
      iv. *Conduction System and Blood Flow, 216*
      v. *Conduction System and the Nervous System, 217*
   b. Blood Pressure, 217
      i. *Blood Volume, 217*
      ii. *Strength of Ventricular Contractions, 217*
      iii. *Resistance to Blood Flow, 217*
5. Diseases and Disorders of the Cardiovascular System, 217
   a. Arrhythmias, 224
   b. Atherosclerosis–Related Diseases, 225
   c. Cardiomyopathy, 225
   d. Congenital Heart Defects, 226
   e. Congestive Heart Failure, 228
   f. Deep Vein Thrombosis, 228
   g. Heart Valve Diseases, 229
   h. Hypertension, 229
   i. Myocardial Infarction, 231
   j. Postural Orthostatic Tachycardia Syndrome, 232
   k. Shock, 233
   l. Additional Cardiovascular System Diseases, 235
6. Life Span Changes, 235
7. Closing Comments, 235
8. Chapter Review, 236
9. Scenario Wrap-Up, 237

▶ OPENING SCENARIO

Rebecca White is a certified medical assistant at Walden-Martin Family Medical (WMFM) Clinic. She was hired 8 months ago. She works with several family practice providers at the clinic. Many of the patients she works with have cardiovascular diseases. High blood pressure or hypertension seems to be the most common cardiovascular disease seen in her patients.

During her first few months at the clinic, Rebecca spent a lot of time learning about cardiovascular diseases, diagnostic procedures, and treatments. She found out that learning the cardiovascular system takes time, but she is proud of how much she has learned over the months.

Rebecca's supervisor approached her and asked her to mentor a medical assistant student, Lizzy, for her practicum experience. Rebecca is excited about the opportunity, but she is a bit nervous to teach someone else about her job.

YOU WILL LEARN

1. To recognize and use terms related to the cardiovascular system.
2. To locate the cardiovascular system structures.
3. To understand and describe the process of the conduction system.
4. To understand and describe factors that impact blood pressure.

5. To recognize disease states of the cardiovascular system: the cause, signs and symptoms, diagnostic process, treatment, prognosis, and prevention.

ANATOMY OF THE CARDIOVASCULAR SYSTEM

The *cardiovascular* (kar dee oh VAS kyoo lur) *system* is also called the *circulatory* (sir kue lah TORE ee) *system*. The cardiovascular system brings oxygen (O_2), nutrients, water, and other substances (e.g., salts and hormones) to the body's cells. It also carries waste products (e.g., metabolic waste and carbon dioxide [CO_2]) away from the cells to be excreted.

The cardiovascular system is a closed system that includes the following:
- Blood vessels, consisting of arteries, arterioles, capillaries, venules, and veins that act as pipes to carry the blood around the body
- A heart, which pumps the blood
- Blood, which contains the nutrients for the cells and the waste products to be excreted

Blood was described in depth in Chapter 8, so the focus of this chapter is the other cardiovascular structures. Cellular injury and death of the cells will occur if the system malfunctions and critical substances are withheld from the cells (Box 10.1).

> **MEDICAL TERMINOLOGY**
> **-ar:** pertaining to
> **cardi/o, coron/o, cordi/o:** heart
> **-logy:** study of
> **vascul/o, angi/o, vas/o:** vessel

Blood Vessels

Blood vessels create a "pipeline" for blood to move out to the body and back to the heart. Blood vessels differ in their role, structure, and size (see Fig. 10.1).

- *Arteries* (AR tur reez): strong, stretchy, thick-walled vessels that carry blood from the heart. They are made to withstand the pressure of the blood being pumped out from the heart. Arteries are involved with maintaining the blood pressure.
- *Arterioles* (ar TEER ee olez): smaller arteries that move blood to the capillaries and also involved with maintaining the blood pressure.
- *Capillaries* (CAP ih lair eez): thin-walled vessels that allow for exchange of oxygen, nutrients, waste products, and other substances between the blood and cells. The diameter of the capillaries is so tiny that only one blood cell can pass through at a time.
- *Venules* (VEEN yools): collect blood from capillaries and begin the return journey to the heart.
- *Veins* (vayns): collect blood from the venules and return blood to the heart. Medium to large veins have valves, which help keep blood moving in one direction. The skeletal muscle contractions help move the blood toward the heart. Vessel walls are thinner and less rigid than arteries (see Table 10.1). Veins hold about 70% of the blood supply at any one time.

> **BOX 10.1 Specialty and Specialist**
>
> Cardiology (kar DEE ol oh jee) is the healthcare specialty that deals with cardiovascular disorders. A cardiologist (kar DEE ol oh jist) is a specialist involved in the diagnosis, treatment, and prevention of disorders of the cardiovascular system.

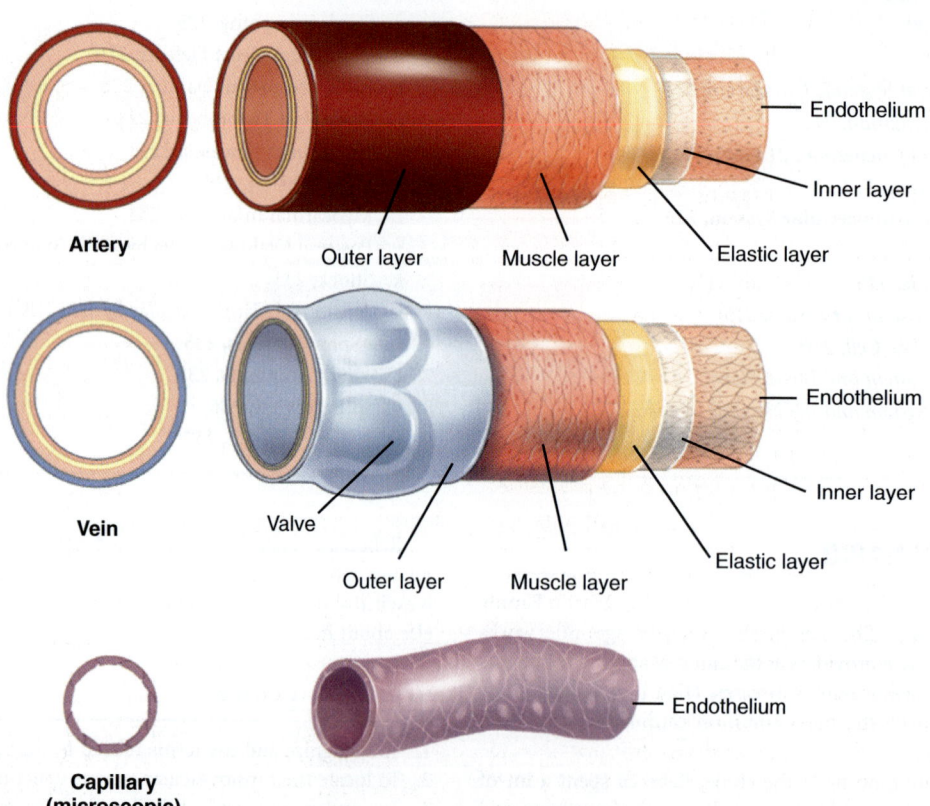

FIG. 10.1 Differences among arteries, veins, and capillaries. (From Shiland B: *Mastering Healthcare Terminology*, ed 5, St. Louis, 2016, Elsevier.)

TABLE 10.1 Comparison Between the Walls of the Arteries and Veins

Layers of the Walls	Arteries	Veins
Tunica intima (inner layer)	Contains epithelium and elastic-like fibers	Some contain valves to prevent backflow of blood
Tunica media (middle layer)	Thick layer of smooth muscles regulated by the autonomic nervous system that constricts or dilates vessels to maintain blood pressure	Contains smooth muscles; thin layer
Tunica externa (outer layer)	Made of connective tissue	Thickest layer and made of connective tissue

Fig. 10.2 shows the principal arteries and veins of the body. It is important to learn the location and names of these vessels:
- The *radial artery* by the wrist is used to take the pulse. (See Fig. 10.3 for pulse points in the body.)
- The *carotid artery* in the neck is used to check for a heartbeat in an unresponsive adult.
- The *median cubital vein* in the arm is commonly used for phlebotomy.

The Heart

The heart is a complex muscular organ that pumps blood around the body. A person's heart is about the size of his or her fist. It is located in the mediastinum (mee dee uh STY num) of the thoracic cavity, slightly left of the midline. The *apex* (pointed tip) of the heart rests just above the diaphragm. The area of the chest wall anterior to the heart and lower thorax is referred to as the *precordium* (pree KORE dee um).

Heart Chambers. The heart has two sets of chambers. The two upper chambers are called *atria* (A tree uh). The atria are smaller chambers with thinner walls. The right atrium receives blood from the body, and the left atrium receives blood from the lungs. The second set of chambers is referred to as the *ventricles* (VEN trih kuls). These larger lower chambers have thick muscular walls, which help as they pump blood to the body and the lungs. The ventricles are known as the left ventricle and the right ventricle (Fig. 10.4).

The *septum* (SEP tum) is the thick muscular wall that divides the heart into a right and left section. The *interatrial* (in ter A tree uhl) *septum* is the wall that separates the left and right atria. The *interventricular* (in ter ven TRICK yoo lur) *septum* divides the right and left ventricles.

The heart wall is composed of three layers:
- *Endocardium* (en doh KAR dee um): the inner thin endothelial layer that lines the chambers and valves.
- *Myocardium* (mye oh KAR dee um): the middle and thickest layer of the heart, composed of cardiac muscles.
- *Epicardium* (eh pee KAR dee um) or *visceral* (VIS uh rul) *pericardium* (pare ee KAR dee um): the outer layer that covers the heart. A space separates the epicardium from the *parietal* (puh RYE uh tul) *pericardium*, which loosely covers the heart like a sac. The two layers of pericardium are serous membranes, which means they are moist. As the heart beats, the two layers rub against each other. The moisture between the layers decreases the amount of friction.

Heart Valves. The heart has valves between the chambers and the arteries. The valves allow the blood to flow in one direction. Valves are *competent* if they open and close properly, letting through or holding back an expected amount of blood. The heart has two sets of valves: atrioventricular (AV) valves and semilunar (SL) valves.

An AV valve is found between each atrium and ventricle. The AV valve opens to allow blood to flow into the ventricle. It closes when the ventricle contracts to prevent backflow of blood into the atrium. The AV valves open and close with the help of the papillary muscles. **Chordae tendineae** (KOR dee ten DIN ee ee) attach the muscle to the valve. The AV valves can be described as follows:
- *Bicuspid* (bye KUSS pid) or *mitral* (MYE trul) *valve*: between the left atrium and left ventricle; made up of two cusps or flaps (see Fig. 10.4)
- *Tricuspid* (try KUSS pid) *valve*: between the right atrium and right ventricle; made up of 3 cusps or flaps

The SL valves are found between the ventricles and the arteries leading out of the heart. The SL valves allow blood to flow out of the heart and prevent the backflow of blood into the ventricles. The valves are created by flaps from the pulmonary artery and aorta (AE ore tah). The SL valves can be described as follows:
- *Pulmonary valve*: between the right ventricle and the pulmonary artery
- *Aortic* (AE ore tik) *valve*: between the left ventricle and the aorta

Heartbeat. A provider listens to the heart sounds with a stethoscope. The normal sound is a *lub dup*. The *lub* sound occurs from the AV valves closing as the ventricles contract. This is a lower pitch, longer sound, which is followed by a pause. The *dup* sound occurs from the closing of the SL valves. With **incompetent valves**, the provider might hear additional abnormal noises.

CRITICAL THINKING 10.1

Lizzy, the medical assistant student, asks Rebecca how she can remember the chambers and valves of the heart. What is a way to remember the chambers and the names of the valves in the heart? (Be creative.)

VOCABULARY

chordae tendineae: Cordlike tendons that attach the papillary muscle to the heart valve.
incompetent valves: valves do not close completely and blood leaks backward into the prior chamber; also called "leaky valves"

MEDICAL TERMINOLOGY

apic/o: apex	**pariet/o**: parietal
arteri/o, arter/o: artery	**pericardi/o**: pericardium
arteriol/o: arteriole	**pre-**: before
atri/o: atrium	**sept/o**: septum, wall
atrium (singular), **atria** (plural)	**septum** (singular), **septa** (plural)
capillar/o: capillary	**-um**: structure
chorda tendinea (singular), **chordae tendineae** (plural)	**valvul/o**: valve
	ven/o, phleb/o: vein
endocardi/o: endocardium	**venul/o**: venule
epi-: above, on top of	**ventricul/o**: ventricle
myocardi/o: myocardium	**viscer/o**: visceral

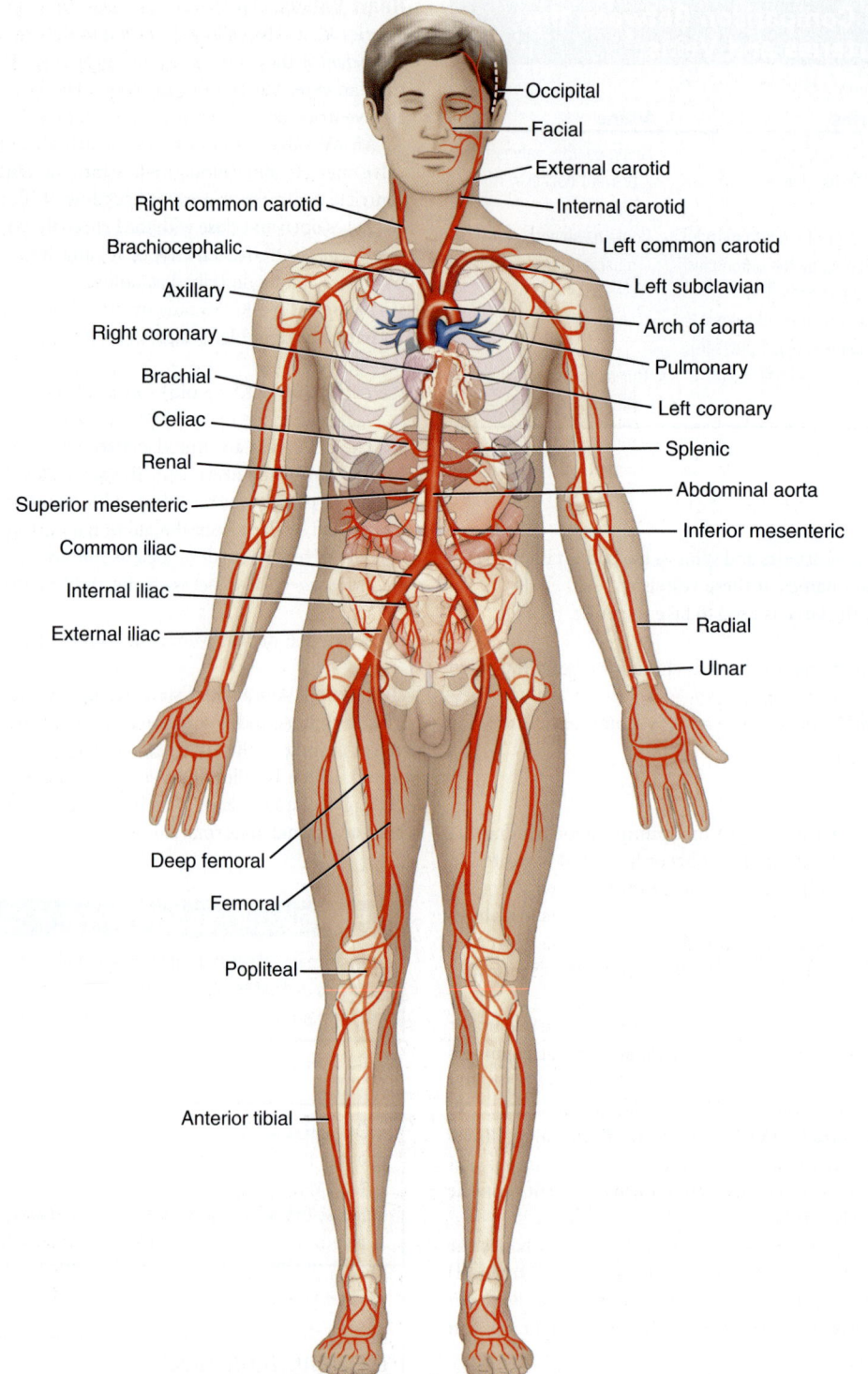

FIG. 10.2 (A) Principal arteries of the body. (From Shiland B: *Mastering Healthcare Terminology*, ed 5, St. Louis, 2016, Elsevier.)

CHAPTER 10 Cardiovascular System

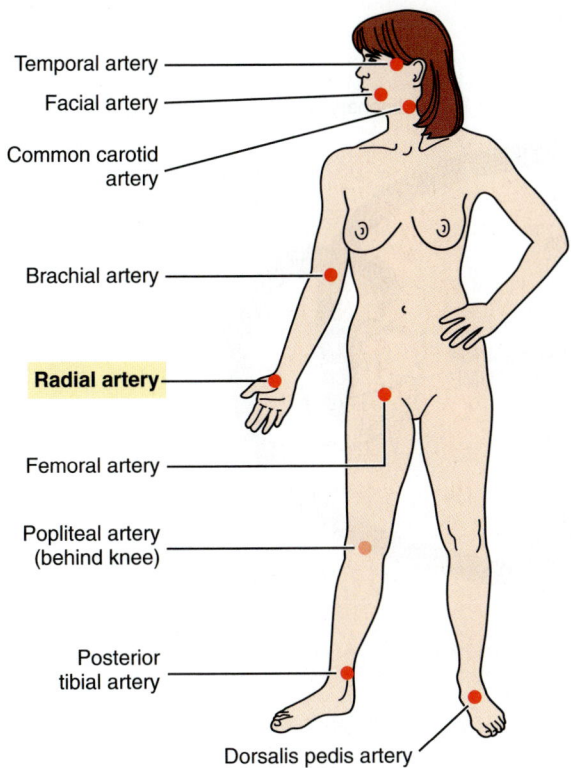

FIG. 10.3 Pulse points in the body. (From Shiland B: *Mastering Healthcare Terminology*, ed 5, St. Louis, 2016, Elsevier.)

A complete heartbeat or *cardiac cycle* can be divided into the diastole (di AS toe lee) and systole (SIS toe lee) phases. During the *diastole* phase, the heart is at rest and the atria fill with blood. The *systole* phase occurs when the heart is contracting.

Blood Flow

The body has several types of blood flow pathways or circulations. The heart, being a double pump, sends blood in two different directions, resulting in two major circulatory pathways:
- *Pulmonary circulation*: deoxygenated blood is pumped from the right side of the heart to the lungs, gas exchange occurs, and oxygenated blood returns to the heart.
- *Systemic circulation*: oxygenated blood is pumped from the left side of heart and moves through the body. Oxygen, nutrients, and other substances are brought to the cells while the blood picks up waste products. The deoxygenated blood returns to the heart (Fig. 10.5).

Because these two pathways are so closely tied, we will examine them together. Besides the two major circulations, we will examine the coronary circulation, or the blood flow through the heart tissues. The final circulation that will be discussed is the fetal circulation or the blood flow of an unborn baby.

Pulmonary and Systemic Circulations. Pulmonary circulation begins as the blood returns from the body. The superior vena cava (VEE nuh KAY vuh) and the inferior vena cava bring **deoxygenated** (dee OCK sih juh nay tid) blood from the body to the right atrium. As the atria contract, the blood from the right atrium passes the tricuspid

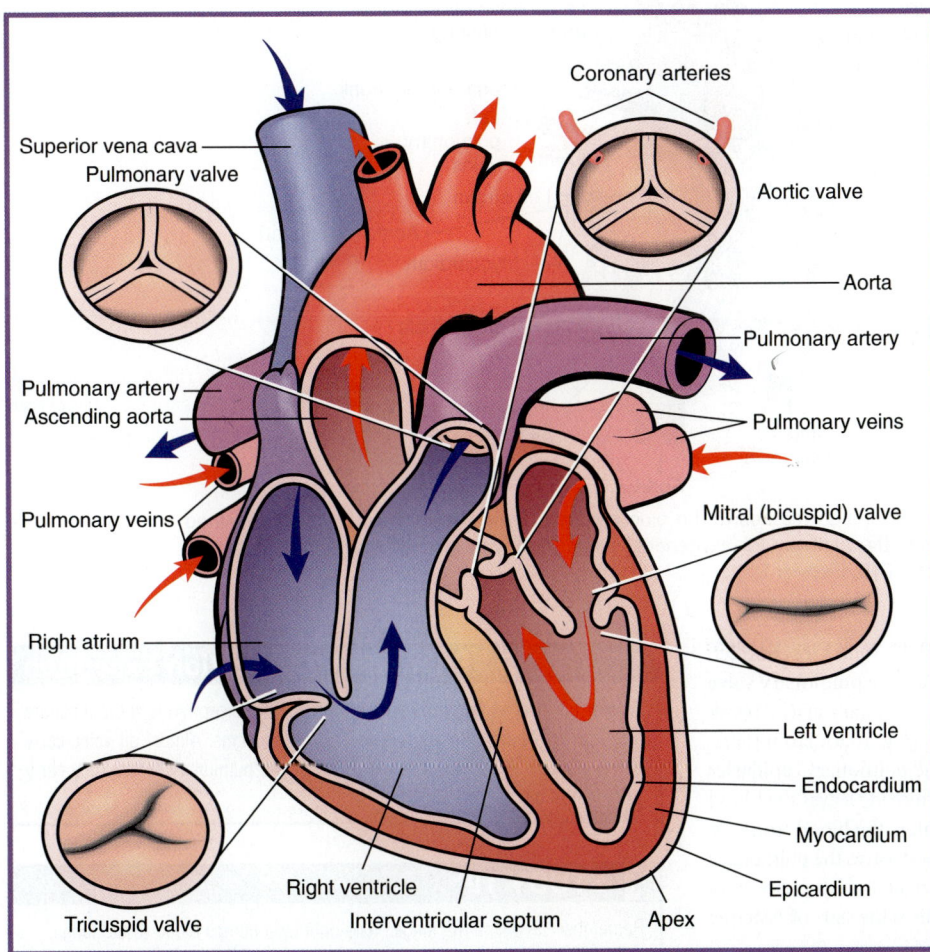

FIG. 10.4 Chambers and valves of the heart. (From Damjanov I: *Pathology for the Health-Related Professions*, ed 4, St. Louis, 2012, Saunders.)

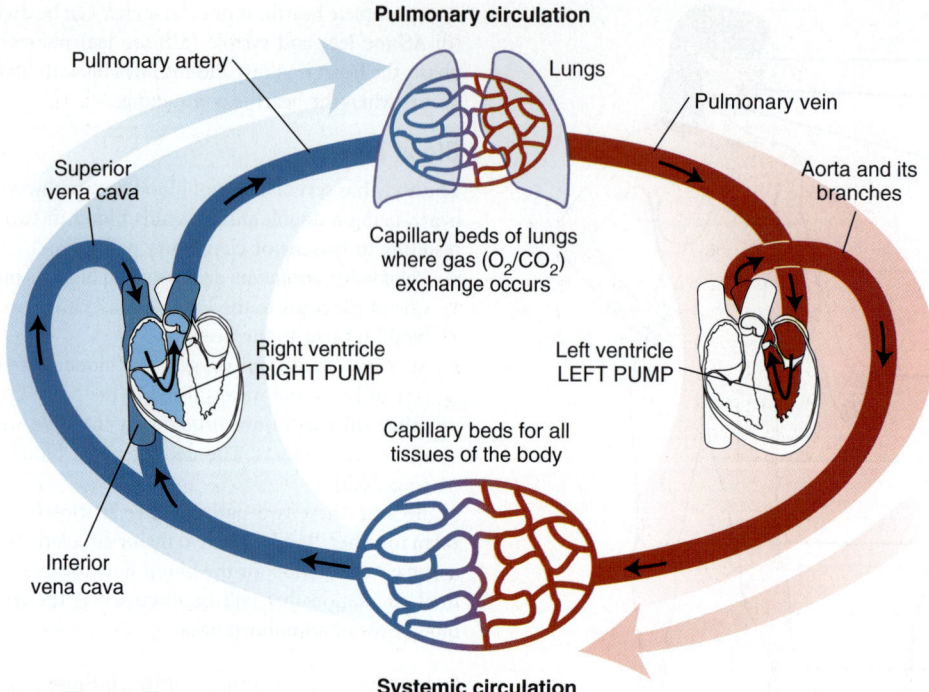

FIG. 10.5 Pulmonary and systemic circulation. (From Shiland B: *Mastering Healthcare Terminology*, ed 5, St. Louis, 2016, Elsevier.)

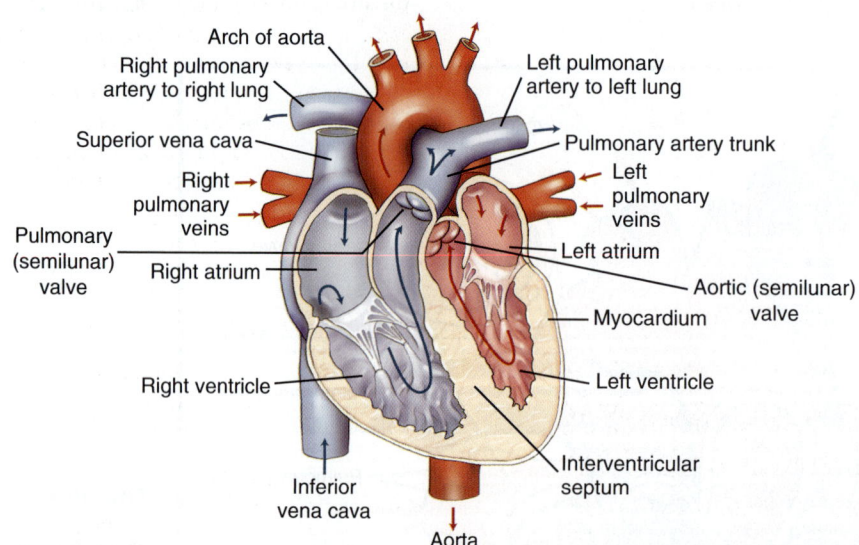

FIG. 10.6 Route of the blood through the heart. The blue represents the pathway for the deoxygenated blood, and the red represents the pathway for oxygenated blood. (From Shiland B: *Mastering Healthcare Terminology*, ed 5, St. Louis, 2016, Elsevier.)

valve and empties into the right ventricle. When the ventricles contract, the blood in the right ventricle is pushed out past the pulmonary valve and enters the pulmonary artery trunk. The pulmonary artery trunk splits into the right and left pulmonary arteries (Fig. 10.6). From there, the blood moves into the arterioles and then the pulmonary capillaries in the lungs. The gas exchange occurs. Carbon dioxide leaves the blood and enters the lungs to be expelled. Oxygen enters the blood from the lungs. The oxygenated (OCK sih juh nay tid) blood leaves the pulmonary capillaries and enters the pulmonary veins. The right and left pulmonary veins bring the blood back to the left atrium. This is the start of systemic circulation (Box 10.2).

BOX 10.2 Pulmonary Circulation Exception

Almost all arteries carry oxygenated blood. The exception is the pulmonary arteries. They carry deoxygenated blood to the lungs. Almost all veins carry deoxygenated blood, with the exception of the pulmonary veins. They carry oxygenated blood to the heart.

STUDY TIP

Remember: "Right to the lungs." The right side pumps blood to the lungs.

CHAPTER 10 Cardiovascular System

> **VOCABULARY**
> **deoxygenated**: Oxygen deficient; oxygen was removed.

> **CRITICAL THINKING 10.2**
> Rebecca is helping Lizzy review the blood flow through the body. She tells Lizzy to explain the blood flow through the pulmonary and systemic circulations, starting with the blood returning from the body. How should Lizzy answer her?

When the atria are full of blood, they contract. The oxygenated blood in the left atrium moves past the bicuspid or mitral valve and empties into the left ventricle. When the ventricles contract, the blood in the left ventricle moves out of the heart, passing the aortic valve, and empties in to the aorta. From here, the blood will move through the body before it returns to the heart. Blood from the head, neck, and upper extremities empties into the superior vena cava before returning to the right atrium. Blood from the lower body empties into the inferior vena cava before returning to the right atrium. Refer to Fig. 10.7 for the pathway of oxygenated and deoxygenated blood.

Coronary Circulation. The heart has its own blood vessels that support the tissues. The right and left coronary (KORE ih nair ee) arteries are the first branches off of the ascending aorta (a ORE tuh) (Fig. 10.8). The coronary arteries bring nutrients and oxygen to the heart tissue. The blood moves from the arteries to the capillaries in the myocardium. From there, the blood moves into the coronary veins. The coronary veins remove the waste products from the heart tissue. Blood from the coronary veins drains into the coronary sinus, which opens into the right atrium.

Coronary arteries have an important role of maintaining the myocardium. If a branch of the coronary artery gets blocked, a person will experience a heart attack. The tissue supplied by the blocked artery will be deprived of oxygen and nutrients. More information will be discussed about coronary arteries in the Diseases and Disorders of the Cardiovascular System section of this chapter.

Hepatic Portal Circulation. In most cases, veins leaving an abdominal organ empty blood into the inferior vena cava as it heads to the heart. Veins from the spleen, gallbladder, pancreas, stomach, and intestines take an alternative route. Veins from these organs dump the blood into the hepatic portal vein, which takes the blood to the liver. In the liver, the blood moves through capillaries as it is filtered. Eventually, the blood drains into the hepatic veins before emptying into the inferior vena cava.

The liver has a special role in filtering the blood and metabolizing or breaking down substances. The hepatic portal system has many advantages:
- The **glucose** absorbed can be filtered and stored in the liver as glycogen. It will later be added back to the blood when the glucose levels are low.
- Toxic substances like alcohol or medications can be partially filtered before moving to the rest of the body.

> **VOCABULARY**
> **glucose**: A simple sugar that is absorbed by the intestines and found in the blood; used by cells for energy, and extra is stored in the liver as glycogen.

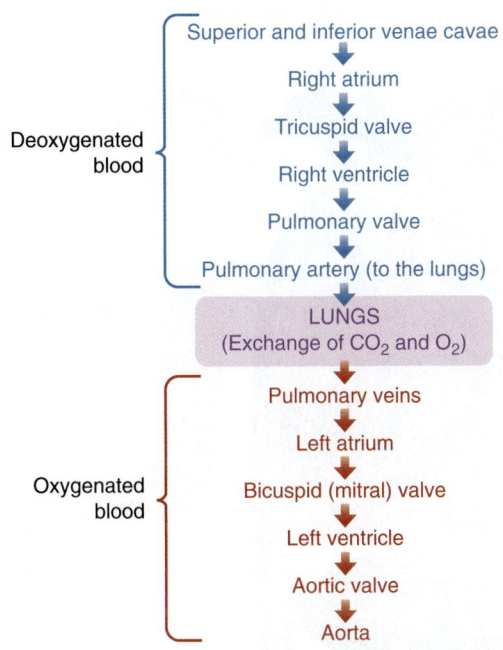

FIG. 10.7 Oxygenated/deoxygenated status. (From Shiland B: *Mastering Healthcare Terminology*, ed 5, St. Louis, 2016, Elsevier.)

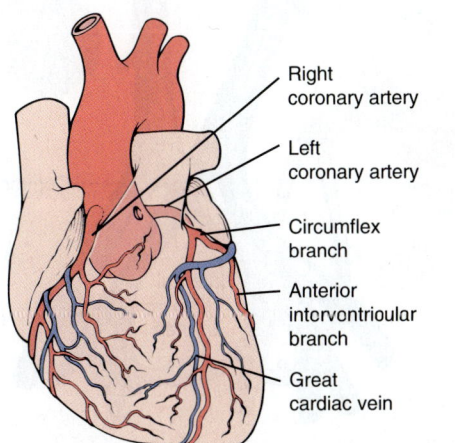
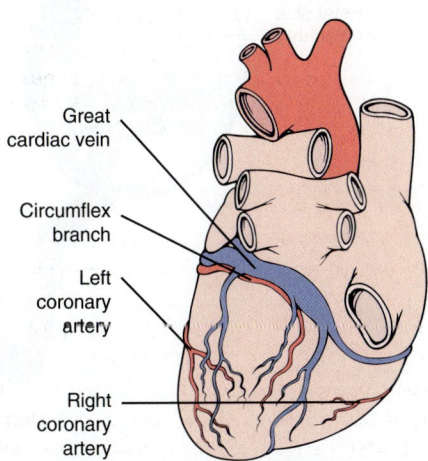

FIG. 10.8 Coronary arteries. (From Frazier MS, et al: *Essentials of Human Diseases and Conditions*, ed 5, St. Louis, 2013, Saunders.)

Fetal Circulation. Prior to birth, the baby is called a *fetus*. The fetal circulation differs from what we have discussed so far in this chapter. Before birth, the baby's lungs, gastrointestinal tract, and kidneys are not functioning like they will after birth. Toward the end of pregnancy, babies "practice" breathing, as they breathe in the amniotic fluid. No gas exchange occurs. Babies also urinate, but the waste products in their blood are being removed by their mothers' blood. Nutrients are being passed through the blood from the mother. Let's examine the differences with fetal circulation.

During the early weeks of pregnancy, the placenta (reproductive organ) begins to grow. It attaches to the mother's uterus and connects to the growing baby via the umbilical cord. The umbilical cord contains two umbilical arteries and one umbilical vein. The arteries carry the fetal blood to the placenta. The umbilical vein carries oxygen and nutrient-rich blood to the baby. The waste, oxygen, and nutrient exchange occurs in the placenta. There is a very thin wall separating the fetal blood from the mother's blood. There is no mixing of the two different blood supplies, though substances can pass between the separating wall. Oxygen and nutrients move from the mother's bloodstream to the fetal blood. Waste products (i.e., carbon dioxide) move from the fetal blood to the mother's blood.

Other structures that are unique to the growing baby include the following:

- *Ductus venosus* (DUK tus vee NOE sus): shifts the majority of the blood from the umbilical vein and empties it into the inferior vena cava (Fig. 10.9). This structure helps the blood bypass the immature liver. After birth, with the lack of blood flow from the umbilical vein, the ductus venosus constricts. Within 1 to 3 months from birth, it is permanently sealed.
- *Foramen ovale* (FOR ae men oh VAL ee): a small flaplike opening in the interatrial septum that allows blood to move from the right atrium to the left atrium. This allows most of the blood to bypass the immature lungs. After birth, the flap opening is forced closed with the pressure of the blood pumping in the heart. During infancy, the flap should seal permanently.
- *Ductus arteriosus* (DUK tus are TEER ee oh sus): a short vessel that connects the pulmonary artery with the aorta. About 90% of the blood in the pulmonary artery is redirected to the aorta,

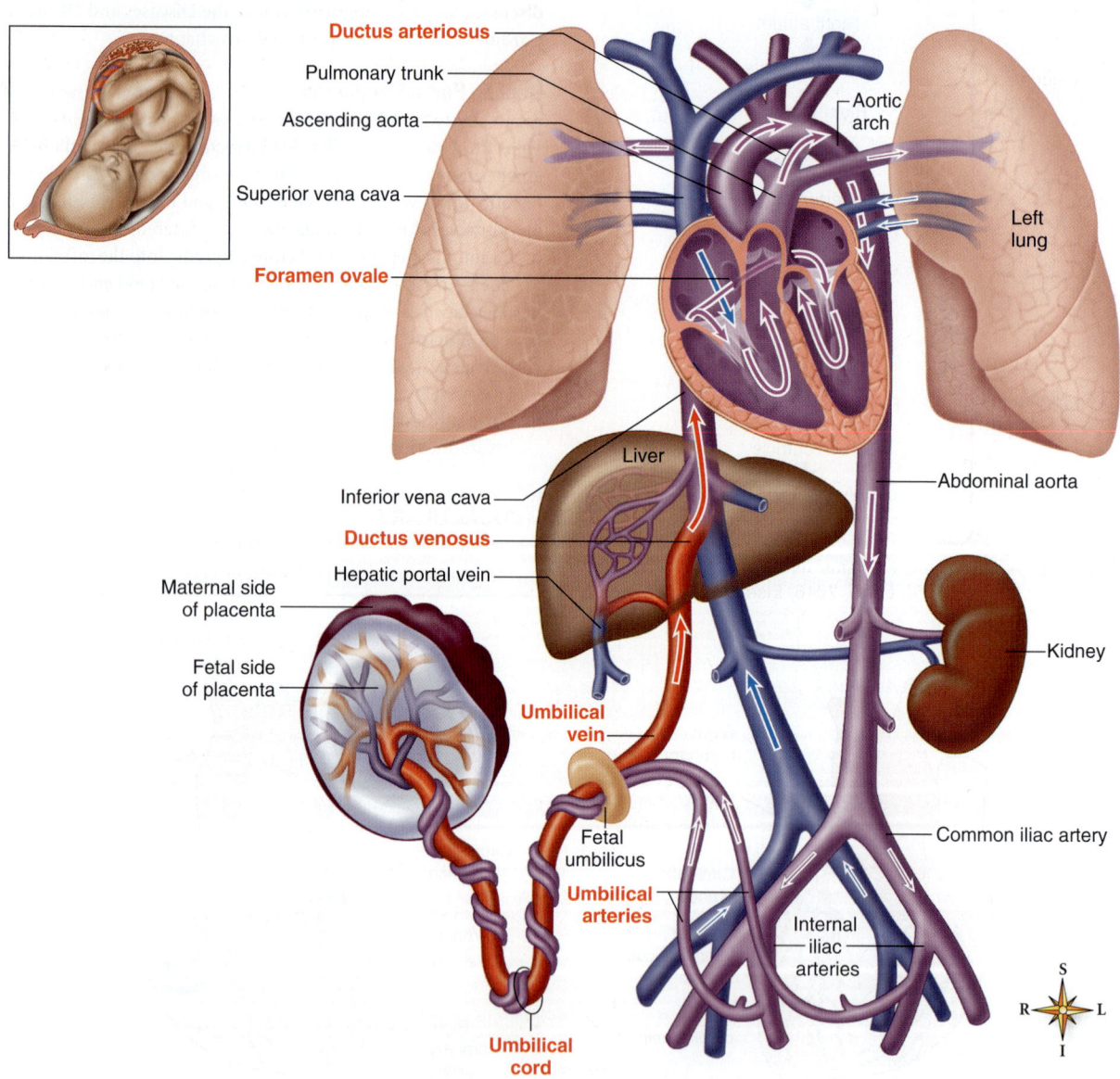

FIG. 10.9 Fetal circulation. (From Patton KT, Thibodeau G: *The Human Body in Health and Disease*, ed 6, St. Louis, 2014, Mosby.)

bypassing the immature lungs. Usually it closes at birth or shortly after.

At birth, when a baby takes his or her first breath and the umbilical cord is cut, these special structures are no longer needed. With the first breath, more pressure is caused in the cardiovascular system. This helps with the closure of the foramen ovale. With the cutting of the umbilical cord, the remaining structures (ductus venosus, ductus arteriosus, and umbilical vessels) collapse.

PHYSIOLOGY OF THE CARDIOVASCULAR SYSTEM

We will examine two major topics that relate to the physiology of the cardiovascular system. These include the conduction system of the heart and the factors that impact blood pressure.

Conduction System

To explain the conduction system, we will first describe the characteristics of the cardiac muscle and the three states they must undergo for each impulse. We will discuss the conduction system, and lastly we will tie the conduction system into the blood volume.

Cardiac Muscle. There are two kinds of cardiac cells, electrical or conduction system cells and myocardial cells. The electrical cells are found in the conduction system. They have three unique characteristics:
- *Automaticity*: the cells create and discharge the electrical impulse
- *Excitability*: the cells respond to the electrical impulse
- *Conductivity*: the cells transmit electrical impulses to other cells

The myocardial cells are found in the myocardium. They can shorten and lengthen their fibers for contraction (called *contractility*). The fibers made from the myocardial cells can contract for prolong periods of time without fatigue and use less adenosine triphosphate (ATP) than other muscles. These features are beneficial for the heart.

Cardiac muscle fibers are electrically linked together, forming one unit. A myocardial cell forms a strong, electrical connection to the next cells through special junctions called intercalated disks. The intercalated disks are responsible for cell-to-cell communication that is required for coordinated muscle contraction. The intercalated disks help the muscle fibers form one unit that contracts all at once instead of a little at a time. The "one unit" approach is important, as the atrial chambers need to contract together and then the ventricles contract at about the same time.

Conduction System Structures. As previously stated, the electrical cells make up the conduction system of the heart. These cells are found throughout the myocardium. They can respond to and transmit electronic impulses to neighboring cells. The conduction system is composed of five structures (Fig. 10.10):

1. *Sinoatrial* (SIE noe ae tree el) (SA) *node:* It is located in the posterior, superior wall of the right atrium. The SA node is called the "pacemaker of the heart." This is because the electrical cells in the SA node generate the impulse that starts the heartbeat. When the SA node discharges the impulse, it travels in many directions through the

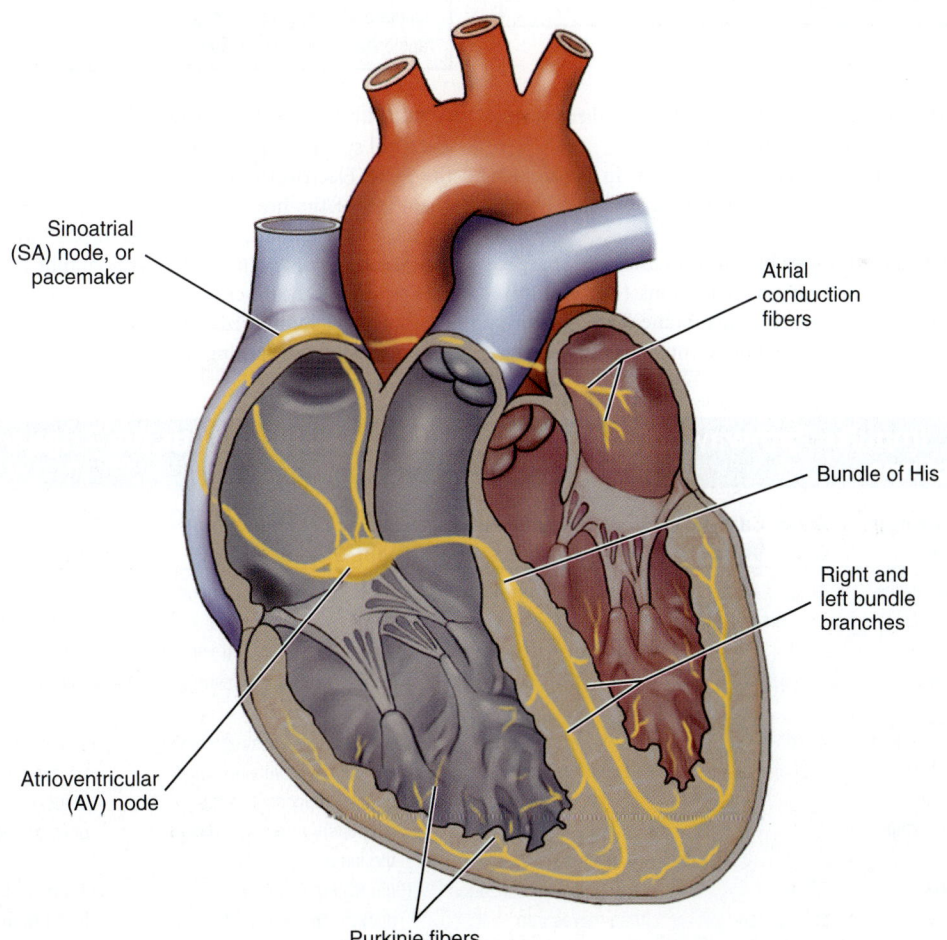

FIG. 10.10 Electrical conduction pathway of the heart. (From Shiland B: *Mastering Healthcare Terminology*, ed 5, St. Louis, 2016, Elsevier.)

heart muscle. The impulse also moves quickly across special bands of tissue called *internodal tracts*. The Bachmann bundle, a specialized internodal tract, takes the impulse to the left atrium. Other internodal tracts take the impulse quickly to the atrioventricular (AV) node. The impulse moving through the atrial chambers triggers the chambers to contract.

2. *Atrioventricular* (AE tree oh ven trik yah lar) (AV) *node*: The AV node is located at the base of the interatrial septum. When the impulse reaches the AV node, it moves very slowly through the node.
3. *Bundle of His* (his) (or called *atrioventricular [AV] bundle*): The Bundle of His is located in the upper interventricular septum. When the impulse leaves the AV node, it moves to the Bundle of His.
4. *Right and left bundle branches*: The bundle branches are located in the lower interventricular septum. After the impulse passes through the Bundle of His, it enters the right and left bundle branches. The right bundle branch brings the impulse to the right ventricle. The left bundle branch brings the impulse to the left ventricle.
5. *Purkinje* (pur KIN jee) *fibers*: The bundle branches split into many Purkinje fibers. Purkinje fibers transmit the impulse quickly and efficiently to the ventricular myocardial cells. This causes the ventricular chambers to contract.

CRITICAL THINKING 10.3

Rebecca is helping Lizzy review the conduction system of the heart. To see what Lizzy can remember, Rebecca has her write down the five conduction system structures. What should Lizzy write down? What might be a creative way to remember these structures in order?

States of Cardiac Cell. The cardiac cells cycle through three states or steps in the same sequence for each impulse:
1. *Polarized state*: Before the impulse hits the cells, they are in a polarized state. There is no electrical activity during the polarized state. Think of this as the "waiting" stage.
2. *Depolarized state*: When the impulse hits the cells, the cells' charges change. This is due to the movement of the ions (e.g., sodium, potassium, and calcium) across the cells' membrane. The change of the cells' charges allows the impulse to move through the cell causing *action potential*, also called depolarization. Electrical activity can be recorded on an electrocardiogram (ECG) when the cells are in the depolarized state. ECGs are discussed in Chapter 39.
3. *Repolarized state*: After the impulse passes over the cell, the ions move back to their original location. This causes the cell's charge to change. This recovery phase is called the repolarized state. Electrical activity (less than the depolarized state) can be recorded on an ECG during the repolarized state.

CRITICAL THINKING 10.4

Lizzy struggles with remembering what occurs with polarization, depolarization, and repolarization. Rebecca encourages her to keep the definitions simple, maybe using one to two words to summarize what is occurring. How might Lizzy define each of these words?

When discussing the three states and the chambers impacted, the chamber (atrial, ventricular) comes before the state:
- Atrial polarization
- Ventricular depolarization
- Ventricular repolarization

This terminology will be used as we examine the blood flow and the conduction system together. In Chapter 39, we will revisit these terms.

STUDY TIP

Summarize these three stages as follows:
polarized: "waiting" stage
depolarized: "discharge" stage
repolarized: "recovery" stage

Conduction System and Blood Flow. The conduction system is the electrical system in the heart. As already mentioned, it is recorded on the ECG. Electrical impulses from the conduction system cause the chambers of the heart to contract. This contraction is a mechanical action, and, as a result, blood moves through the heart. The mechanical action can be seen with an echocardiography (eck oh kar dee AH gruh fee), which will be described later in this chapter.

Table 10.2 summarizes an impulse's path through the conduction system and the resulting mechanical action with the blood flow

TABLE 10.2 Impulse Pathway Through the Conduction System With the Triggered Mechanical Actions

Impulse Moving Through Conduction System	Atrial Cardiac Cells' State	Ventricular Cardiac Cells' State	MECHANICAL ACTION TRIGGERED BY IMPULSE	
			Right Side of Heart	Left Side of Heart
SA node (pacemaker) generates the impulse, which travels to the AV node	Atrial depolarization	Ventricular polarization	Right atrium contracts; blood passes the tricuspid valves and empties into the right ventricle	Left atrium contracts; blood passes the bicuspid valves and empties into the left ventricle
Impulse moves slowly through AV node			Allows the atrial chambers to finish contracting	
Impulse leaves the AV node and moves to the bundle of His, to the right and left bundle branches, and to the Purkinje fibers	Atrial repolarization	Ventricular depolarization	Right ventricle contracts; blood passes the pulmonary valve before emptying into the pulmonary artery as it heads to the lungs	Left ventricle contracts; blood passes the aortic valve before emptying into the aorta as it goes to the body
(The impulse is now done.)	Atrial polarization	Ventricular repolarization (then moves into ventricular polarization)	Right atrium fills with deoxygenated blood from the body via the inferior vena cava and the superior vena cava	Left atrium fills with oxygenated blood from the lungs via the pulmonary vein

movement. Notice that the atrial chamber state is always one step ahead of the ventricular chambers.

Conduction System and the Nervous System. Cardiac muscle is different than other muscles in the body. The heart is controlled by the autonomic nervous system and the heart's own conduction system. When the heart rate needs to change to meet the demands of the body, the autonomic nervous system automatically kicks in. You will learn more about the autonomic nervous system in Chapter 12.

Blood Pressure

About one in every three American adults has high blood pressure. This means that many of the patients seen in an ambulatory care center may be diagnosed with high blood pressure, or *hypertension* (hye pur TEN shun). More information on hypertension will be provided later in the chapter. On the flip side, low blood pressure, or *hypotension,* can be life threatening in some cases.

The pressure of the blood is highest in the arteries and lowest in the veins. Thus we measure arterial blood pressure. *Blood pressure* (BP) can be defined as the resulting force of blood against the walls of the arteries. Two measurements are taken during the cardiac cycle:
- *Systole* (SIS toh lee) or the contractive phase; systolic pressure is measured when the heart is contracting and pumping out the blood.
- *Diastole* (dye AS toh lee) or the relaxation phase; diastolic pressure is measured when the heart is resting between contractions.

You will learn more about the procedure to take blood pressures in Chapter 29. This section addresses the factors that can influence blood pressure.

Blood Volume. Blood volume, or the amount of circulating blood, has a direct influence on blood pressure. The greater the blood volume, the more force it makes on the arterial walls. If the blood volume is low, less force or pressure will be on the arterial walls. Think of a garden hose attached to a faucet. If you turn on the faucet to the maximum level, there will be a lot of water pressure in the hose. If you turn on the faucet to get a trickle, then there is very little water pressure in the hose.

Let's briefly exam the factors that increase and decrease blood volume. The blood volume can be raised by the following:
- Blood, plasma, and fluid (intravenous [IV]) transfusions
- Increased sodium intake (because water follows sodium, more water will be drawn into the bloodstream due to the elevated sodium levels)

Fluid volume can decrease due to *hemorrhage* (HEM ahr ij) (bleeding), dehydration, and diuretic (DIE ah ret ik) medications. Diuretics help pull water and sodium from the blood, thus lowering blood volume.

Strength of Ventricular Contractions. The left ventricle pumps blood to the body. The greater the force of the contraction, the more blood is pumped into the arteries. This increases the blood pressure. If the left ventricular contraction is weak, less blood is pumped out of the heart and thus the blood pressure is lower. Digoxin is a medication that decreases the heart rate and strengthens the contractions of the heart.

With heart disease, tests are done to check how the left ventricle is functioning. The *stroke volume* is the amount of blood that is pushed out of the left ventricle compared with the total volume of blood that filled the ventricle. It is a measure of the ejection fraction of the cardiac output. As heart disease occurs, the stroke volume can decrease.

Resistance to Blood Flow. Any factor that increases the resistance for blood to flow through the arteries will increase the blood pressure. Factors that increase resistance include the size of the *lumen* (inner opening) of the arteries, the elasticity of the arterial walls, and the *viscosity* (thickness) of the blood.

The *peripheral resistance* of blood vessels refers to the size of the lumen and the amount of blood flowing through it. The smaller the vessel's lumen, the greater the resistance to blood flow, thus increasing blood pressure. Several dynamics lead to decreased lumen size, including the following:
- *Plaque* (plak) (waxy substance) builds up in the arteries and hardens over time. This buildup narrows the arteries and causes higher blood pressure.
- Smoking.
- Constriction of smooth muscles causing vasoconstriction (VAE zoe kon strik shahn). Several medications, including benazepril, lisinopril, and losartan, relax smooth muscles, thus decreasing blood pressure.

Another factor that increases blood flow resistance is the loss of vessel elasticity. The inner layer of an artery contains elastic-like fibers that allow the vessel to expand and contract. Arteries dilate as the blood is pumped out of the heart and narrow between heartbeats to help maintain blood pressure. Increasing age and plaque buildup decrease the elasticity of the vessels. To understand the effect of plaque on the vessels, think of dried glue on a balloon. The dried glue prevents that section of the balloon from expanding. The plaque is like the dried glue. It prevents the walls from expanding.

Lastly, the viscosity (thickness) of blood influences the resistance of blood flow. As the viscosity of the blood increases, so does the resistance, and the blood pressure rises. The thickness of blood increases when more blood cells are present (e.g., **polycythemia** [pol ee sie THEE mee ah], blood transfusion).

> **VOCABULARY**
>
> **polycythemia**: A condition caused by an abnormally large number of red blood cells (RBCs) in the blood.

In summary, blood pressure can be influenced by blood volume, the strength of ventricular contractions, and the resistance of blood flow. Resistance can be increased by the following:
- Narrowed lumen (e.g., due to plaque, smoking, and vasoconstriction)
- Loss of vessel elasticity due to aging and plaque
- Increased viscosity of the blood

> **CRITICAL THINKING 10.5**
>
> With many of their patients having high blood pressure, Rebecca wants to make sure Lizzy understands the factors that impact blood pressure. She asks Lizzy to summarize factors that increase blood pressure. How might Lizzy respond?

DISEASES AND DISORDERS OF THE CARDIOVASCULAR SYSTEM

Cardiovascular diseases are conditions that impact heart or the blood vessels. Common cardiovascular signs and symptoms are listed in Table 10.3. Common cardiovascular diagnostic tests are listed in Table 10.4. Commonly used cardiovascular treatment procedures are listed in Table 10.5.

Text continued on p. 224

TABLE 10.3 Common Cardiovascular Signs and Symptoms

Term	Word Origin	Definition
Angina pectoris (an JYE nuh PECK tore us)	pector/o chest -is structure	Paroxysmal (PAR ahk siz ehm) chest pain that is often accompanied by shortness of breath (SOB) and a sensation of impending doom.
Bradycardia (brad dee KAR dee ah)	brady- slow -cardia heart condition	Slow heartbeat with ventricular contractions less than 60 bpm (beats per minute).
Bruit (BROO ee)		Abnormal sound heard when an artery is listened to with a stethoscope or Doppler (Fig. 10.11). Usually a blowing or swishing sound, higher pitched than a murmur.
Cardiodynia (kar dee oh DIN ee uh)	cardi/o heart -dynia pain	Heart pain that may be described as atypical or ischemic. *Atypical pain* is a stabbing or burning pain that is variable in location and intensity and unrelated to exertion. *Ischemic* (i SKEE mic) *pain* is a pressing, squeezing, or weightlike cardiac pain caused by decreased blood supply that usually lasts only minutes. *Precordial pain* is pain in the area over the heart. Also called *cardialgia* (KAHR dee al jah).
Cardiomegaly (kar dee oh MEG uh lee)	cardi/o heart -megaly enlargement	Enlargement of the heart.
Claudication (klah dih KAY shun)		Cramplike pains in the calves caused by poor circulation in the leg muscles.
Cyanosis (sye uh NOH sis)	cyan/o blue -osis abnormal condition	A bluish or grayish discoloration of skin, nail beds, or lips caused by a lack of oxygen in the blood.
Diaphoresis (dye uh foh REE sis)		Profuse secretion of sweat.
Dyspnea (DISP nee uh)	dys- difficult -pnea breathing	Difficult or painful breathing; dyspnea on exertion (DOE) occurs when effort is expended.
Edema (eh DEE muh)		Abnormal accumulation of fluid in interstitial spaces of tissues.
Emesis (EM uh sis)	emesis to vomit	Forcible or involuntary emptying of the stomach through the mouth; vomit.
Ischemia (i SKEE mee ah)	isch/o to hold back -emia blood condition	Lack of blood in a body part due to a blockage or functional constriction.
Murmur		Abnormal heart sound heard during systole, diastole, or both, which may be described as a gentle blowing, fluttering, or humming sound.
Nausea (NAH zsa)		Sensation that accompanies the urge to vomit but does not always lead to vomiting.
Orthopnea (or THOP nee uh)	orth/o straight, upright -pnea breathing	Condition in which a person must sit or stand to breathe comfortably.
Pallor (PAL ur)		Paleness of skin or mucous membranes. On darker pigmented skin, it may be noted on the inner surfaces of the lower eyelids or the nail beds.
Palpitations (pal pih TAY shuns)		Pounding or racing of the heart, such that the patient is aware of his or her heartbeat.
Pulmonary congestion	pulmon/o lung -ary pertaining to	Excessive amount of blood in the pulmonary vessels. Usually associated with heart failure (HF).
Shortness of breath (SOB)		Breathlessness, air hunger.
Syncope (SING kuh pee)		Fainting, loss of consciousness.

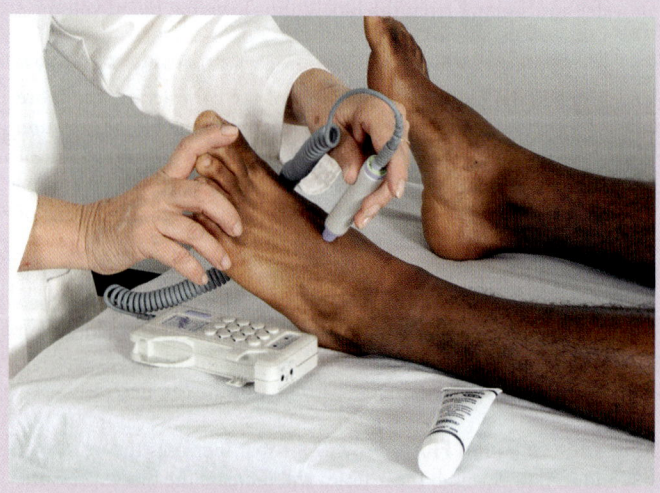

FIG. 10.11 Using a Doppler to check the pulse. (From Jarvis C: *Physical Examination and Health Assessment*, ed 7, St. Louis, 2016, Saunders.)

TABLE 10.3 Common Cardiovascular Signs and Symptoms—cont'd

Term	Word Origin	Definition
Tachycardia (tack ee KAR dee ah)	**tachy-** rapid **-cardia** heart condition	Rapid heartbeat, more than 100 bpm (beats per minute).
Thrill		Fine vibration felt by the examiner on palpation.
Venous distention	**ven/o** vein **-ous** pertaining to	Enlarged or swollen veins.

TABLE 10.4 Common Diagnostic Procedures Used for Cardiovascular Diseases

Done by/Type of Test	Procedure	Description
Provider during the exam	Heart sounds	Provider uses a stethoscope to listen to (or auscultates) the heart sounds.
Medical assistant	Blood pressure	A measure of the systolic over the diastolic pressure. The instrument used is a *sphygmomanometer* (sfig MOE mah nom i tur).
	Electrocardiography (ECG, EKG) (ee leck troh kar dee AH gruf ee)	Recording of electrical impulses of the heart as wave deflections on an instrument called an *electrocardiograph*. The record, or recording, is called an *electrocardiogram*.
	Holter monitor (HOLE tur)	Portable electrocardiograph that is worn to record the reaction of the heart to daily activities (Fig. 10.12).
Imagining procedures	Angiocardiography (an jee oh kar dee AH gruh fee)	Injection of a radiopaque substance during cardiac catheterization for the purpose of imaging the heart and related structures. Also called coronary angiography (KORE ih nair ee an jee AH gruh fee).
	Cardiac catheterization (KAR dee ack kath ih tur ih ZAY shun)	Threading of a catheter (thin tube) into the heart under fluoroscopic guidance to collect diagnostic information about structures in the heart, coronary arteries, and great vessels; also used to aid in treatment of coronary artery disease (CAD), congenital abnormalities, and heart failure (Fig. 10.13).
	Digital subtraction angiography (DSA) (an jee AH gruh fee)	Digital imaging process wherein contrast images are used to "subtract" the noncontrast image of surrounding structures, leaving only a clear image of blood vessels (Fig. 10.14).
	Echocardiography (ECHO) (eck oh kar dee AH gruh fee)	Use of ultrasonic waves directed through the heart to study the structure and motion of the heart (Fig. 10.15). *Transesophageal echocardiography* (TEE) images the heart through a transducer introduced into the esophagus.
	Magnetic resonance imaging (MRI)	Computerized imaging that uses radiofrequency pulses in a magnetic field to detect damaged areas and areas of blood flow.
	MUGA scan (MOO guh)	Multiple-gated acquisition scan is a noninvasive method of imaging a beating heart by tagging RBCs with a radioactive substance. A gamma camera captures the outline of the chambers of the heart as the blood passes through them.

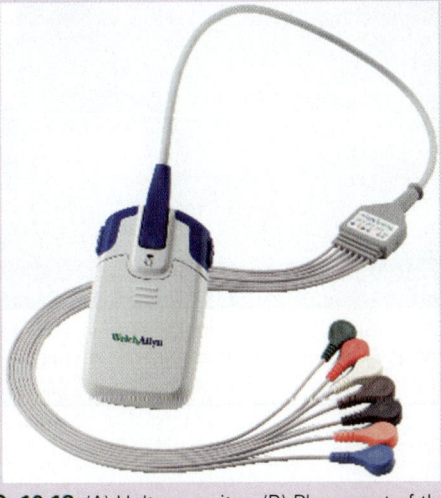 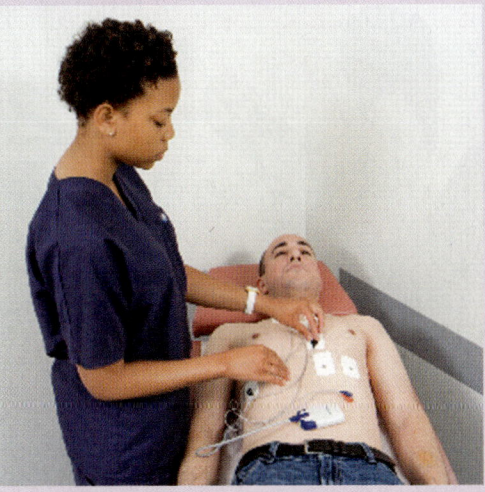

FIG. 10.12 (A) Holter monitor. (B) Placement of the leads on the chest. (From Young AP, Proctor DB: *Kinn's The Medical Assistant*, ed 11, Philadelphia, 2011, Saunders.)

Continued

TABLE 10.4 Common Diagnostic Procedures Used for Cardiovascular Diseases—cont'd

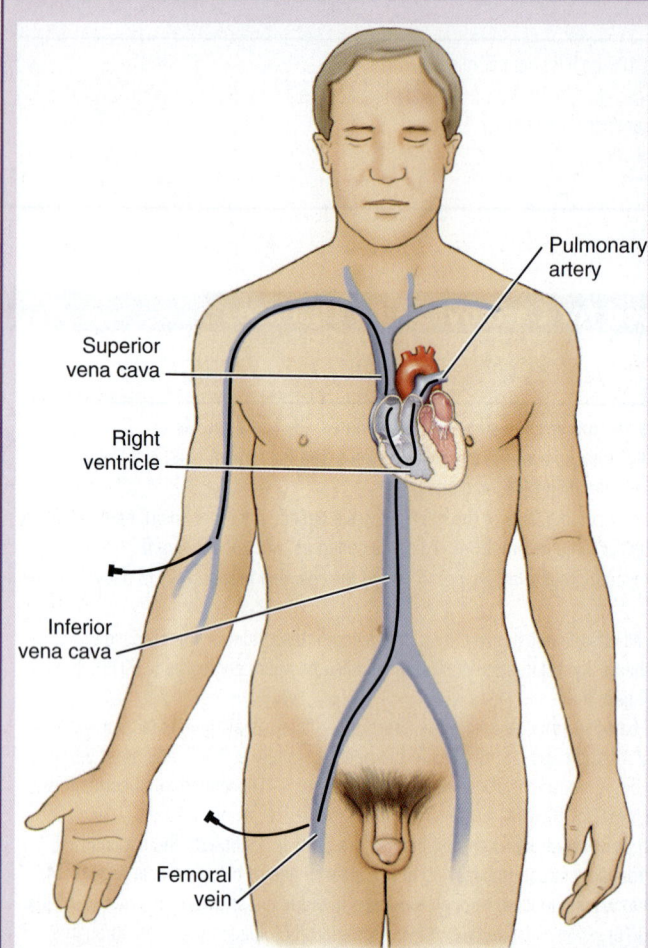

FIG. 10.13 Right-sided heart catheterization. The catheter is inserted into the femoral or brachial vein and advanced through the vena cava through the right side of the heart and then into the pulmonary artery. (From Shiland B: *Mastering Healthcare Terminology*, ed 5, St. Louis, 2016, Elsevier.)

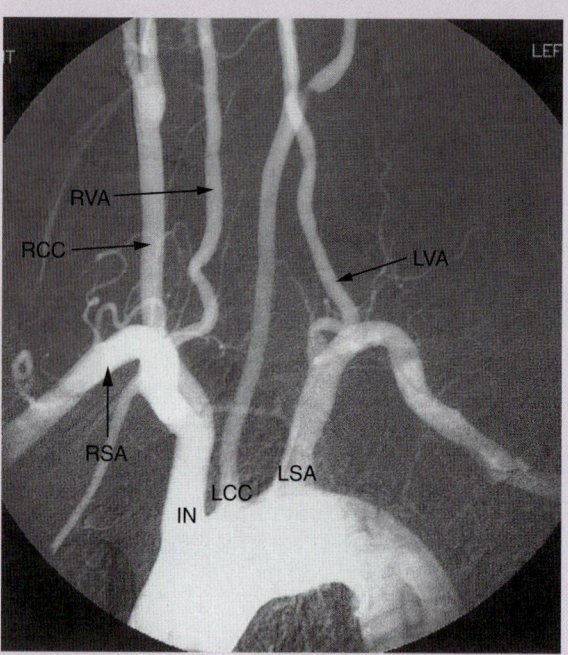

FIG. 10.14 Digital subtraction image of the aorta. (From Frank ED, Long BW, Smith BJ: *Merrill's Atlas of Radiographic Positions and Radiologic Procedures*, ed 12, St. Louis, 2012, Mosby.)

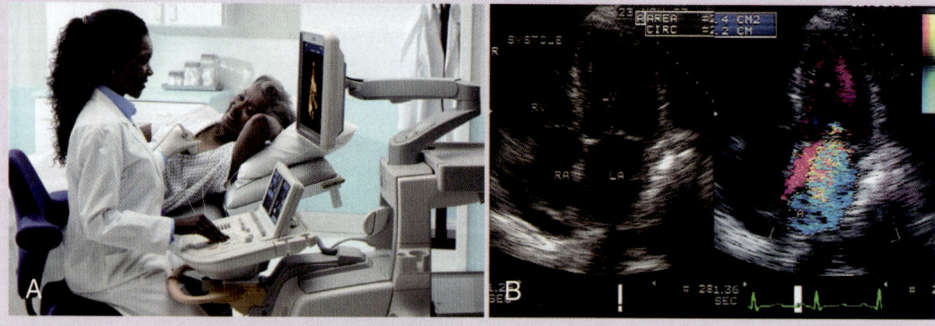

FIG. 10.15 (A) Person undergoing echocardiography (ECHO). (B) Color Doppler image of the heart. (From Frank ED, Long BW, Smith BJ: *Merrill's Atlas of Radiographic Positions and Radiologic Procedures*, ed 12, St. Louis, 2012, Mosby.)

TABLE 10.4 Common Diagnostic Procedures Used for Cardiovascular Diseases—cont'd

Done by/Type of Test	Procedure	Description
	Myocardial perfusion imaging (mye oh KAR dee ul pur FYOO zhun)	Use of radionuclide to diagnose CAD, valvular or congenital heart disease, and cardiomyopathy.
	Phlebography (fleh BAH gruh fee)	X-ray imaging of a vein after the introduction of a contrast dye.
	Positron emission tomography (PET) (POZ ih tron ee MIH shun toh MAH gruh fee)	Computerized nuclear medicine procedure that uses inhaled or injected radioactive substances to help identify how much a patient will benefit from revascularization procedures.
	Swan-Ganz catheter (swann ganz)	Long, thin cardiac catheter with a tiny balloon at the tip that is fed into the femoral artery near the groin and extended up to the left ventricle. Used to determine left ventricular function by measuring pulmonary capillary pressure.
Other tests	Exercise stress test (EST)	Tests the electrical activity of the heart during exercise on a treadmill; may include the use of radioactive substance. Also called an *exercise electrocardiogram*.
Medical laboratory	CLIA-waived tests	Cholesterol testing: for heart disease. Prothrombin testing: for anticoagulant therapy and heart disease.
	Cardiac enzymes test	Blood test that measures the amount of cardiac enzymes characteristically released during a heart attack (myocardial infarction); determines the amount of lactate dehydrogenase (LDH) and creatine phosphokinase (CPK) in the blood.
	Lipid profile	Blood test to measure the lipids (cholesterol and triglycerides) in the circulating blood (see a sample lipid profile in Table 10.5).

TABLE 10.5 Commonly Used Cardiovascular Treatment Procedures

Term	Word Origin	Definition
angioplasty (AN gee oh plas tee)	**angi/o** vessel **-plasty** surgical repair	Reconstruction of blood vessels damaged by disease or injury, often performed by inflating a balloon within a vessel at the site of narrowing to restore blood flow. A stent can also be placed (Fig. 10.16).
atherectomy (ath uh RECK tuh mee)	**ather/o** fat, plaque **-ectomy** removal	Removal of plaque from the coronary artery (or other arteries) through a catheter with a rotating shaver or a laser.
automatic implantable cardioverter-defibrillator (AICD)		A device that is implanted in the chest to monitor the heartbeat and correct it if needed (speed it up or slow it down).
Cardiac ablation (uh BLAY shun)		Destruction of abnormal cardiac electrical pathways causing arrhythmias. To destroy the tissue, radiofrequency catheter ablation (RFCA) uses heat energy, and cryoablation uses very cold temperatures.
cardiac defibrillator (dee FIB ruh lay tur)		Either external or implantable device that provides an electric shock to the heart to restore a normal sinus rhythm.
cardiac pacemaker		Small, battery-operated device that helps the heart beat in a regular rhythm; can be either internal (permanent) or external (temporary) (Fig. 10.18).
cardiopulmonary resuscitation (CPR) (kar dee oh PULL muh nare ee reh suss ih TAY shun)	**cardi/o** heart **pulmon/o** lung **-ary** pertaining to	Manual external cardiac massage and artificial respiration used to restart the heartbeat and breathing of a patient.
cardioversion		Pharmacologic or electrical procedure to restore a fast or irregular heartbeat to a normal sinus rhythm. In electrical cardioversion, the heart is given low-energy shocks using a cardioverter.
carotid endarterectomy (kuh RAH tid en dar tur ECK tuh mee)	**end-** within **arter/o** artery **-ectomy** removal	Removal of the atheromatous plaque lining the carotid artery to increase blood flow and leave a smooth surface. Done to prevent thrombotic occlusions (Fig. 10.17).
commissurotomy (kom ih shur AH tuh mee)	**commissur/o** connection **-tomy** incision	Surgical division of a fibrous band or ring connecting corresponding parts of a body structure. Commonly performed to separate the thickened, adherent leaves of a narrowed or hardening mitral valve.
coronary artery bypass graft (CABG)	**coron/o** heart, crown **-ary** pertaining to	Open-heart surgery in which a piece of a blood vessel from another location is grafted onto one of the coronary arteries to reroute blood around a blockage (Fig. 10.19).
endovenous laser ablation (EVLT) (ah BLAY shun)	**endo-** within **ven/o** vein **-ous** pertaining to	Thermal destruction of varicose veins using laser fibers within a vein.

Continued

TABLE 10.5 Commonly Used Cardiovascular Treatment Procedures—cont'd

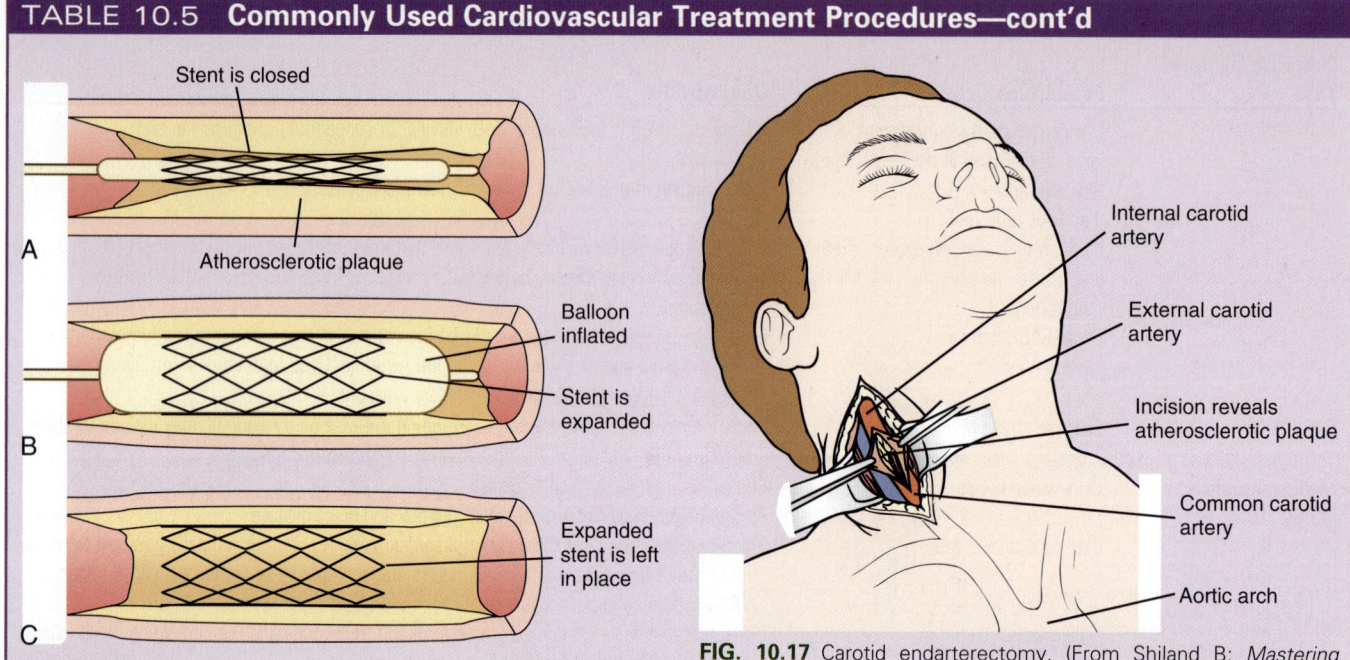

FIG. 10.16 Angioplasty with stent placement. (From LaFleur Brooks M: *Exploring Medical Language*, ed 9, St. Louis, 2014, Mosby.)

FIG. 10.17 Carotid endarterectomy. (From Shiland B: *Mastering Healthcare Terminology*, ed 5, St. Louis, 2016, Elsevier.)

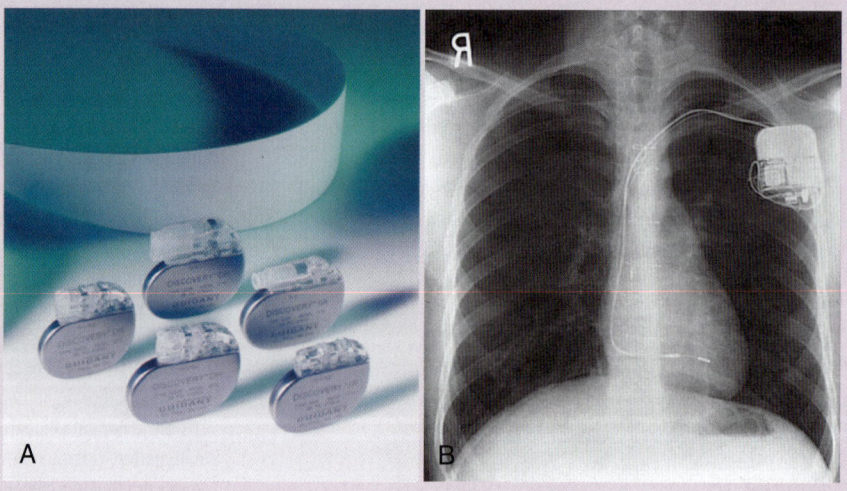

FIG. 10.18 (A) Pacemakers. (B) Chest x-ray of a patient with a permanent implanted pacemaker. (From Frank ED, Long BW, Smith BJ: *Merrill's Atlas of Radiographic Positions and Radiologic Procedures,* ed 12, St. Louis, 2012, Mosby.)

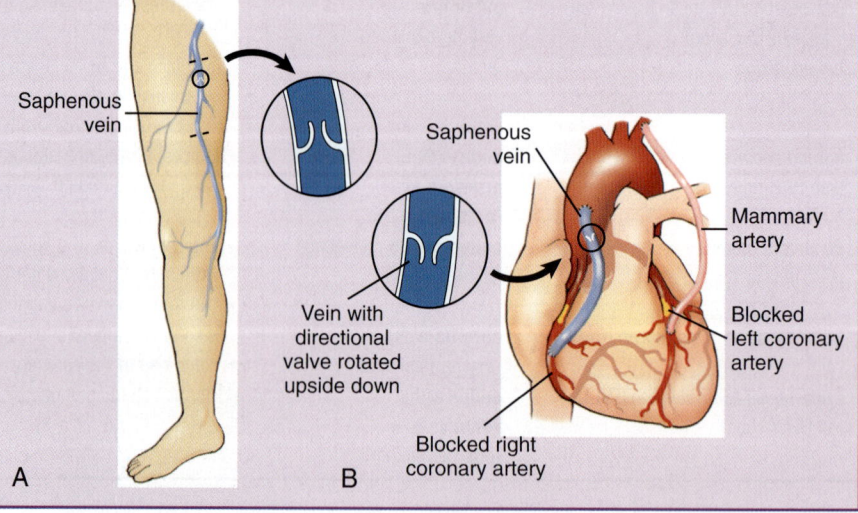

FIG. 10.19 Coronary artery bypass graft (CABG). (A) A section of vein is harvested from the right leg. (B) The harvested vein is anastomosed (surgically connected) to bypass a right coronary artery blockage. Bypass of the left coronary artery with a mammary artery. (From Shiland B: *Mastering Healthcare Terminology*, ed 5, St. Louis, 2016, Elsevier.)

TABLE 10.5 Commonly Used Cardiovascular Treatment Procedures—cont'd

Term	Word Origin	Definition
extracorporeal circulation (ECC) (ecks truh kore PORE ee ul)	**extra-** outside **corpor/o** body **-eal** pertaining to	Use of a cardiopulmonary machine to do the work of the heart during open-heart procedures.
heart transplantation		Removal of a diseased heart and transplantation of a donor heart when cardiac disease can no longer be treated by any other means.
hemorrhoidectomy (hem uh royd ECK tuh mee)	**hemorrhoid/o** hemorrhoids **-ectomy** removal	Excision of *hemorrhoids* (HEM uh royd) (swollen, inflamed veins in the lower rectum and anus from pregnancy or straining with a bowel movement).
left ventricular assist device (LVAD)		Mechanical pump device that assists a patient's weakened heart by pulling blood from the left ventricle into the pump and then ejecting it out into the aorta. LVADs may be used on patients awaiting a transplant.
minimally invasive direct coronary artery bypass (MIDCAB)		Surgical procedure in which a minimal incision is made over the blocked coronary artery. An artery from the chest wall is used as the bypass.
percutaneous transluminal coronary angioplasty (PTCA) (pur kyoo TAY nee us trans LOO mih nul KOR in nare ee AN jee oh plas tee)	**per-** through **cutane/o** skin **-ous** pertaining to **trans-** across **lumin/o** lumen **-al** pertaining to **coron/o** heart, crown **-ary** pertaining to **angi/o** vessel **-plasty** surgical repair	A catheter is threaded into the coronary artery affected by atherosclerotic heart disease. The balloon at the tip of the catheter is inflated and deflated to compress the plaque against the wall of the artery and increase blood flow. *Stents,* wire mesh tubes, are placed in the arteries and used to prop them open after the angioplasty.
pericardiocentesis (pair ee kar dee oh sen TEE sis)	**pericardi/o** pericardium **-centesis** surgical puncture	Aspiration of fluid from the pericardium used to treat cardiac tamponade (Fig. 10.20).
phlebectomy (fleh BECK tuh mee)	**phleb/o** vein **-ectomy** removal	Removal of a vein.
port-access coronary artery bypass (PACAB)		Procedure in which the heart is stopped and bypass surgery is accomplished through small incisions in the chest.
sclerotherapy (skleh roh THAIR uh pee)	**scler/o** hard **-therapy** treatment	Injection of chemical solution into varicosities to cause inflammation, resulting in an obliteration of the lining of the vein; blood flow then is rerouted through adjoining vessels. *Microsclerotherapy* is a treatment to remove spider veins.
thromboendarterectomy (TEA) (throm boh en dar tur ECK tuh mee)	**thromb/o** clot, clotting **end-** within **arter/o** artery **-ectomy** removal	Removal of a blood clot along with part of the lining of the obstructed artery.
transmyocardial revascularization (TMR) (trans mye oh KAR dee ul ree vas kyoo lair ih ZAY shun)	**trans-** through **myocardi/o** myocardium **-al** pertaining to **re-** again **vascul/o** vessel **-ization** process	Procedure used to relieve severe angina in a patient who cannot tolerate a CABG or PTCA. A laser is used to make a series of holes in the heart tissue in the hope of increasing blood flow by stimulating new blood vessels to grow (*angiogenesis*).
valvuloplasty (VAL vyoo loh plas tee)	**valvul/o** valve **-plasty** surgical repair	Repair of a stenosed heart valve with the use of a balloon-tipped catheter.

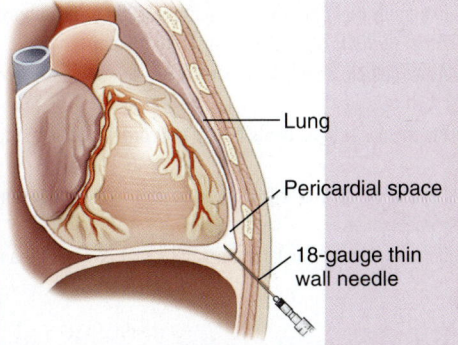 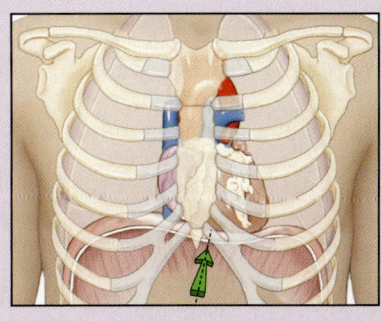

FIG. 10.20 Pericardiocentesis for aspiration of pericardial fluid. (From Shiland B: *Mastering Healthcare Terminology,* ed 5, St. Louis, 2016, Elsevier.)

> **CRITICAL THINKING 10.6**
> To see if Lizzy understands the difference between an ECG and an ECHO, Rebecca asks her to describe what each test shows. What might be Lizzy's answer?

Arrhythmias

An *arrhythmia* (ah RITH mee ah) means the heart rate or rhythm is abnormal. The heart rate may be too fast (*tachycardia*) or too slow (*bradycardia*), or the rhythm may be irregular. The most common arrhythmia is *atrial fibrillation* (Table 10.6). This means the rate is fast and the rhythm is irregular. Table 10.6 lists terms and definitions related to arrhythmias.

Arrhythmias are caused by an issue with the heart's conduction system. Arrhythmias happen when extra beats occur, electrical impulses are blocked or slowed, or electrical impulses take different pathways through the heart. Arrhythmias can be harmless, a sign of a heart disease, or life threatening.

Etiology. Arrhythmias can be caused by the following:
- Diseases like heart attacks, congenital heart defects, heart failure, enlarged heart, and thyroid problems
- Stress and substances (i.e., alcohol, caffeine, nicotine)
- Medications (i.e., stimulants, antidepressants) and abnormal levels of electrolytes (i.e., potassium)

Signs and Symptoms. Arrhythmias may come and go or always be present. Signs and symptoms of arrhythmias include the following:
- Fast or slow heart rate
- Irregular, skipping, or uneven heart beats
- Lightheadedness, dizziness, shortness of breath
- Paleness, chest pain, sweating

Diagnostic Procedures. The provider will listen to the heart with a stethoscope. An ECG is usually the first test done. Heart monitoring devices (e.g., Holter monitor and an event monitor) provide ECG monitoring over days to weeks. Other tests ordered may include an echocardiography, a coronary angiography, and an *electrophysiology study* (EPS). An EPS provides an in-depth study of the heart's electrical system.

Treatment. Treatment depends on the severity of the arrhythmia. Treatments include the following:
- Defibrillation or cardioversion, which shocks the heart into a normal rhythm
- Implanting a pacemaker to help establish a normal rate and rhythm
- Antiarrhythmic medications
- Cardiac ablation and an implantable cardiac defibrillator

Prognosis. The prognosis can vary based on the type of arrhythmia and any additional heart diseases present.

Prevention. For some arrhythmias, there are no preventive measures. For others, following a healthy lifestyle can decrease coronary artery disease.

TABLE 10.6 Terms Related to Cardiac Arrhythmias

Term	Word Origin	Definition
arrhythmia (ah RITH mee ah)	**a-** without **rhythm/o** rhythm **-ia** condition	Abnormal variation from the normal heartbeat rhythm. Also called *dysrhythmia* (dis RITH mee ah).
atrioventricular (AV) block (a tree oh ven TRICK yoo lur)	**atri/o** atrium **ventricul/o** ventricle **-ar** pertaining to	Partial or complete heart block that is the result of a lack of electrical communication between the atria and the ventricles. Also termed *heart block*.
bundle branch block (BBB)		Incomplete electrical conduction in the bundle branches, either left or right.
ectopic beats (eck TOP ick)	**ec-** out of **top/o** place **-ic** pertaining to	Heartbeats that occur outside of a normal rhythm.
fibrillation (fibrill LAY shun)		Extremely rapid and irregular contractions (300 to 600 bpm) occurring with or without an underlying cardiovascular disorder, such as coronary artery disease (CAD). Atrial fibrillations (AFs) are the most common type of cardiac arrhythmia. Ventricular fibrillation can be fatal.
flutter		Extremely rapid but regular heartbeat (250 to 350 bpm). *Atrial flutter* is a rapid, regular atrial rhythm.
premature atrial contractions (PACs)	**atri/o** atrium **-al** pertaining to	Atrial ectopic beats (AEBs) that are irregular contractions of the atria.
premature ventricular contractions (PVCs)	**ventricul/o** ventricle **-ar** pertaining to	Ventricular ectopic beats (VEBs) that are irregular contractions of the ventricles.
sick sinus syndrome (SSS)		Any abnormality of the sinus node that may include the necessity of an implantable pacemaker.
ventricular tachycardia (ven TRICK yoo lur tack ee KAR dee ah)	**ventricul/o** ventricle **-ar** pertaining to **tachy-** rapid **-cardia** heart condition	Condition of ventricular contractions that are more than 100 bpm.

(From Shiland B: *Mastering Healthcare Terminology*, ed 5, St. Louis, 2016, Elsevier.)

Atherosclerosis–Related Diseases

Atherosclerosis is a condition in which plaque or atheromas (ath uh ROH mahs) build up in the arteries. An *atheroma* is a waxy lesion of cholesterol, fat, calcium, cells, and other substances that builds up on the inner wall of an artery. Over time, the waxy plaque becomes larger, thus narrowing the artery. The plaque can prevent the arteries from properly constricting and dilating. Several diseases can result from plaque building. See Table 10.7 for atherosclerosis-related diseases.

At times, small cracks in the vessel wall can occur, causing a *thrombus* (blood clot) to form over the atheroma. The thrombus can partially or completely occlude the vessel. If a section of the thrombus breaks away and travels in the bloodstream, this is an embolus (EM boh lus) (Fig. 10.21). More information regarding the risk of an embolus will be discussed later in the chapter.

Etiology. The cause of atherosclerosis is unknown. Studies have shown that it can develop in childhood and get worse with age. Risk factors for atherosclerosis include smoking, an unhealthy diet, lack of physical activity, high blood pressure, unhealthy cholesterol levels, and uncontrolled diabetes mellitus.

Signs and Symptoms. The signs and symptoms depend on which arteries are affected by the plaque. In many cases, no symptoms are felt until the artery is severely narrowed or blocked. See Table 10.7 for the signs and symptoms for the different diseases.

Diagnostic Procedures. Diagnostic procedures include blood tests to check the cholesterol, glucose, and protein levels. Additional tests include ECG, echocardiography, chest x-ray, CT scan, angiography, and a stress test.

Treatment. The goals of treatment are to lower the risk of blood clot formation, prevent diseases, and widen the affected arteries. Heart-healthy lifestyle changes will be encouraged. This means exercise, a healthy diet, building stress coping and management skills, maintaining a healthy weight, and smoking cessation. Medications that lower cholesterol levels may be used. Percutaneous coronary intervention, coronary artery bypass grafting (CABG), or a carotid endarterectomy may also be performed.

Prognosis. The prognosis can vary. It depends on the severity of the disease and if other conditions (e.g., stroke, heart attack) occur.

Prevention. Heart-healthy eating, physical activity, quitting smoking, and maintaining a healthy weight are ways to decrease the risk of atherosclerosis.

> **CRITICAL THINKING 10.7**
>
> Lizzy is working with Ken Thomas, a patient. He asks her about plaque in the arteries and what can happen if a person has a lot of plaque. How might Lizzy answer Ken's questions?

Cardiomyopathy

With cardiomyopathy (kar dee oh mye AH puh thee), the heart muscle becomes abnormal. It may become thin and weakened, enlarged and thick, or rigid. As the disease worsens, the heart becomes less efficient pumping blood and maintaining a normal electrical rhythm. Cardiomyopathy can lead to arrhythmias, heart failure, edema, and heart valve problems.

Etiology. There are many types of cardiomyopathy. Some types of cardiomyopathy develop over time due to other diseases. Some types are inherited. In many cases, the cause of the cardiomyopathy is not known. This disease can impact people of all ages.

Major risk factors for cardiomyopathy include the following:
- Diabetes mellitus, metabolic diseases, or severe obesity
- Diseases that cause heart damage (e.g., heart attack, coronary heart disease)
- A family history of cardiomyopathy
- Long-term alcoholism
- Long-term hypertension (high blood pressure)

Signs and Symptoms. Some people may never have symptoms, whereas others do not experience symptoms during the early stages of the disease. As the condition worsens, a person may experience the following:
- Shortness of breath, especially after activity
- Swelling of the legs, feet, ankles, and abdomen
- Swelling of the neck veins
- Fatigue

Diagnostic Procedures. The provider obtains a history and performs an examination. Abnormal heart sounds and lung sounds might be heard with a stethoscope. A heart murmur may be present. Crackling in the lungs may indicate fluid in the lungs. Swelling can also be seen,

TABLE 10.7   Atherosclerosis-Related Diseases

Disease	Description	Signs and Symptoms
Carotid artery disease	Plaque builds up in the carotid arteries and may lead to a stroke.	Sudden weakness or paralysis (inability to move), numbness, confusion, problems speaking or seeing, dizziness, and other symptoms of a stroke
Coronary heart disease (CHD) or coronary artery disease (CAD)	Plaque builds up in the coronary arteries. Can lead to *angina* (chest pain) or *myocardial infarction* (heart attack). Also known as ischemic heart disease.	Angina; pain in the shoulder, arm, neck, jaw or back; indigestion, shortness of breath, arrhythmias
Coronary microvascular disease (MVD)	Plaque builds up in the tiny coronary arteries damaging the vessel walls.	Angina, shortness of breath, fatigue, lack of energy, sleep problems
Peripheral artery disease (PAD)	Plaque builds up in the large arteries of the legs, arms, and pelvis.	Numbness, pain, and life-threatening infections
Chronic kidney disease	Plaque builds up in the renal arteries and can cause kidney damage.	Tiredness, loss of appetite, nausea, swelling of hands or feet, numbness, changes in amount urine

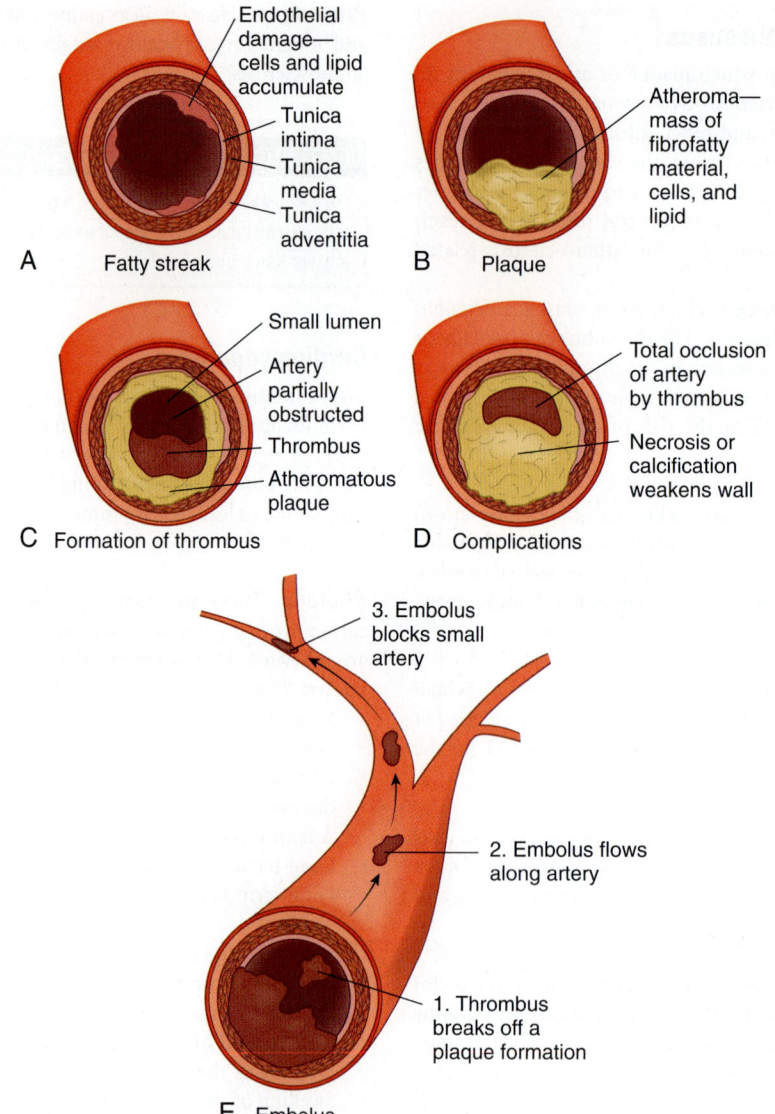

FIG. 10.21 Development of an atheroma, leading to arterial occlusion. (From Proctor D, et al: *Kinn's The Medical Assistant*, ed 13, St. Louis, 2017, Elsevier.)

as mentioned in the prior section. A chest x-ray, an ECG, an echocardiography, and a stress test may be ordered. Further procedures may include a cardiac catheterization, coronary angiography, or a myocardial biopsy.

Treatment. Treatments depend on the severity of the condition. Treatments may include the following:
- Lifestyle changes: heart-healthy diet, healthy weight, stress management, and smoking cessation
- Medications
  - Antiarrhythmics to prevent arrhythmias
  - Antihypertensives to keep the blood pressure at a normal level
  - Anticoagulants to prevent blood clots
  - Diuretics to remove extra sodium and water from the body
  - Beta-blockers to lower the heart rate
- Surgery to treat the damaged heart area and to increase blood flow; heart transplant
- Pacemaker to prompt a normal heartbeat

Prognosis. The outcome of cardiomyopathy depends on the severity and type of disease. Some people do not experience symptoms and need no treatments. For others, it may cause death.

Prevention. Genetic forms of cardiomyopathy cannot be prevented. For other forms, it is important to treat diseases that can lead to cardiomyopathy. Leading a healthy lifestyle will also help prevent cardiomyopathy.

Congenital Heart Defects

There are numerous congenital heart defects. See Table 10.8 for descriptions of some of the common defects. Depending on the type and severity of the defect, the newly born baby may require immediate surgery.

> **MEDICAL TERMINOLOGY**
> **tetra-:** four

CHAPTER 10 Cardiovascular System

TABLE 10.8 Congenital Heart Defects

Congenital Heart Defects	Description
Atrial septal defect (ASD)	A hole in the interatrial septum allows oxygen rich blood from the left atrium to flow into the right atrium. May not have many symptoms. Hole may close on its own or with surgery.
Atrioventricular septal defect	Holes are between the right and left chambers, and the valves are malformed. Surgery is required to patch holes.
Coarctation of the aorta (koh ark TEY shun)	Narrowing of the aorta resulting in blood back, flowing into the left ventricle, high blood pressure, and weakened pulses in the legs (Fig. 10.22). Surgery or balloon angioplasty can correct the condition.
Dextro-transposition of the great arteries (d-TGA) (DECKS tro trans poh ZI shun)	The pulmonary artery and the aorta are switched. Oxygen-rich blood is pumped back to the lungs and the deoxygenated blood is pumped back to the body. Requires emergency surgery.
Hypoplastic left heart syndrome (hi puh PLAS tik)	Structures on the left side of the heart are not correctly developed. Treated with medications and surgery to improve blood flow.
Patent foramen ovale (PFO)	Foramen ovale does not close during infancy. It remains open or *patent*. May not have any symptoms and may not require treatment
Patent ductus arteriosus (PDA)	Ductus arteriosus does not close soon after birth, causing too much blood to move into the pulmonary circulation. A heart murmur may be the only sign.
Pulmonary atresia (PULL mun airy ah TREE sha)	Pulmonary valve does not form and blood cannot flow to the lungs. Requires immediate surgery after birth to improve blood flow to the lungs.
Tetralogy of Fallot (TOF) (te tral uh jee of Fal oh)	Consists of four major conditions: ventricular septal defect, pulmonary stenosis, defective aortic valve, and ventricular hypertrophy (Fig. 10.23). Requires immediate surgery.
Ventricular septal defect (VSD)	Septal wall is not fully developed between the ventricles causing a hole. Blood tends to flow from the left ventricle into the right ventricle, stressing the pulmonary system.

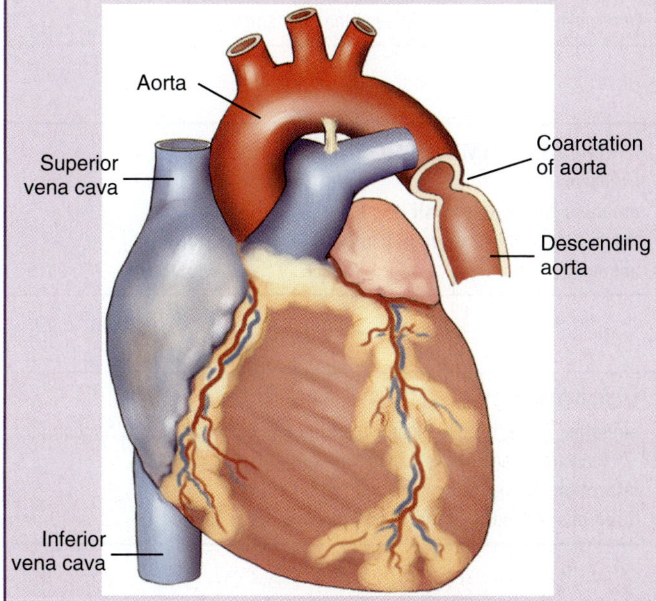

FIG. 10.22 Coarctation of the aorta. (From Shiland B: *Mastering Healthcare Terminology*, ed 5, St. Louis, 2016, Elsevier.)

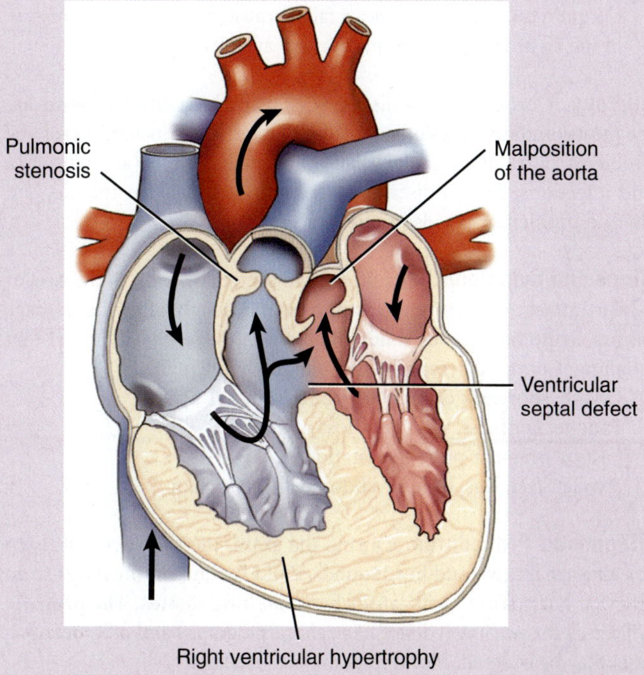

FIG. 10.23 Tetralogy of Fallot. (From Shiland B: *Mastering Healthcare Terminology*, ed 5, St. Louis, 2016, Elsevier.)

Etiology. The cause of these congenital defects may be genetic, chromosomal, or unknown.

Signs and Symptoms. The signs and symptoms of the defect will depend on its type and severity. For some, there are no symptoms and the person may not realize the condition exists until adulthood. Other defects may cause the baby to have the following conditions:
- *Cyanosis* (blue-tinted nails or lips), increased respiration rate, breathing difficulties
- Difficulty feeding, tiredness with feeding, weight loss
- Abnormal heart murmur
- Sweating with feeding or crying

Diagnostic Procedures. Some of the defects may be identified during the pregnancy. Fetal echocardiography can be used on unborn babies to detect cardiac abnormalities. After birth, echocardiography, pulse oximetry, ECG, and chest x-rays may be performed to help diagnose the defect.

Treatment. Treatment for congenital heart defects depends on the type and severity of the defect. Some holes may close on their own, whereas others may require surgery to patch them. Some defects will be monitored, but no treatment will be required. Life-threatening defects will require emergency surgery after birth and follow-up through childhood.

Prognosis. Prognosis depends on the type and severity of the defect. For some, surgery corrects the problem. For other defects, multiple surgeries may be required.

Prevention. None known.

Congestive Heart Failure

Congestive heart failure (CHF) is also known as heart failure. It occurs when the heart does not efficiently pump blood. Blood backs up behind the failing pump (side of the heart). Systolic heart failure occurs when the heart muscle cannot pump the blood out of the heart. Diastolic heart failure occurs when the chamber muscle is stiff and does not completely fill up with blood. Heart failure can impact one or both sides of the heart. Types of heart failure include the following:
- Right-sided heart failure: fluid may back up into the body, causing swelling in the legs, feet, and abdomen
- Left-side heart failure: fluid may back up into the lungs, causing shortness of breath and abnormal lung sounds
- Cor pulmonale: right-side heart failure caused by high blood pressure in the right ventricle and pulmonary arteries

Etiology. Coronary artery disease (CAD) and high blood pressure are the most common causes of heart failure. Other causes include congenital problems, heart attack, faulty valves, abnormal rhythms (arrhythmias), and infections. Several diseases (i.e., emphysema, severe anemia, and thyroid problems) can also cause heart failure.

Signs and Symptoms. Symptoms can occur slowly or, in the case of a heart attack, the symptoms can appear suddenly after the damage occurs. Symptoms can be different based on the side of the heart that is failing. Common symptoms include the following:
- Cough, shortness of breath with reclining or activity
- Fatigue, faintness, weakness, loss of appetite
- Fast or irregular pulse, palpitations
- Swollen feet, legs, liver, or abdomen; weight gain

Diagnostic Procedures. During the exam, the provider will listen for abnormal heart and lung sounds. Fluid buildup in the lungs from left-side heart failure will cause abnormal lung sounds. The provider will check for swelling (edema). An echocardiography and other imaging tests may be ordered. Blood tests may be ordered.

Treatment. Home care will include monitoring weight. An increase in weight may be a sign of fluid retention. Dietary changes including limiting cholesterol, salt, and fluids may be encouraged. Medications used to treat CHF can include diuretics, antihypertensives, and digoxin to strengthen the heart muscle. Additional treatments may include the following:
- Surgery to repair weakened structures
- A pacemaker to help heart rate and contraction
- An implantable defibrillator to correct abnormal heart rhythms
- A heart transplant

Prognosis. Treatment can help control CHF. Because it is a chronic disease, it will get worse over time.

Prevention. Healthy living and taking steps to reduce the risk of heart disease can prevent CHF.

Deep Vein Thrombosis

Deep vein thrombosis (thrahm BOW sis) (DVT) or thrombophlebitis occurs when a blood clot (**thrombus**) forms in a vein deep in the body. As the blood flow slows or pools, the blood thickens and a clot forms in the vessel. A thrombus can also form over an atheroma, as discussed in prior section. DVTs usually occur in the lower leg and thigh. They can also occur in the arms and pelvis. DVTs can occur at any age, but they most commonly occur in people over the age of 60.

DVT is a serious condition. If the clot breaks away from the vessel wall, it can travel through the bloodstream. This is called an **embolus** (EM boh lus). An embolus can block an artery. If this occurs in the brain, it causes a cerebrovascular (seh ree broh VAS kyoo lur) accident (also called a CVA or stroke). If an embolus blocks a pulmonary artery, it is called a pulmonary embolism (EM boh li zehm) (PE). If the embolus blocks a coronary artery, it will cause a myocardial **infarction** (mye oh KAR dee ul in FARCK shun) (also called an MI or heart attack).

> ### CRITICAL THINKING 10.8
> Lizzy is preparing for a national exam. She is struggling to remember the difference between an embolus and a thrombus. What is a creative way to remember the differences between the two terms?

> ### MEDICAL TERMINOLOGY
> **cerebr/o**: cerebrum
> **embolus** (singular), **emboli** (plural)
> **thrombus** (singular), **thrombi** (plural)
> **vascul/o**: vessel

> ### VOCABULARY
> **embolus**: An air bubble, blood clot, or foreign body that travels through the bloodstream and blocks a blood vessel.
> **infarction**: Tissue death.
> **thrombus**: A blood clot that blocks the flow of blood.

Etiology. Blood clots can form when the vein's inner lining and valves are damaged (Fig. 10.24). Surgery, injuries, inflammation, and immune responses can cause damage to the lining. Blood clots can also occur when the blood flow is slow from a lack of activity or motion. Lastly, clots can form if the blood is thicker (increased viscosity) or at higher risk for clotting. Estrogen, birth control pills, and inherited conditions can cause an increased risk for clotting.

Other risk factors for DVTs include the following:
- A family history of blood clots
- Medical conditions: pregnancy or up to 6 months after delivery, pelvis and leg fractures, bed rest, polycythemia, surgery, indwelling catheter in the blood vessel, lupus, and cancer
- Smoking, obesity

Signs and Symptoms. With DVT usually affecting the leg, symptoms include leg pain, swelling, warmth, and redness (Fig. 10.25).

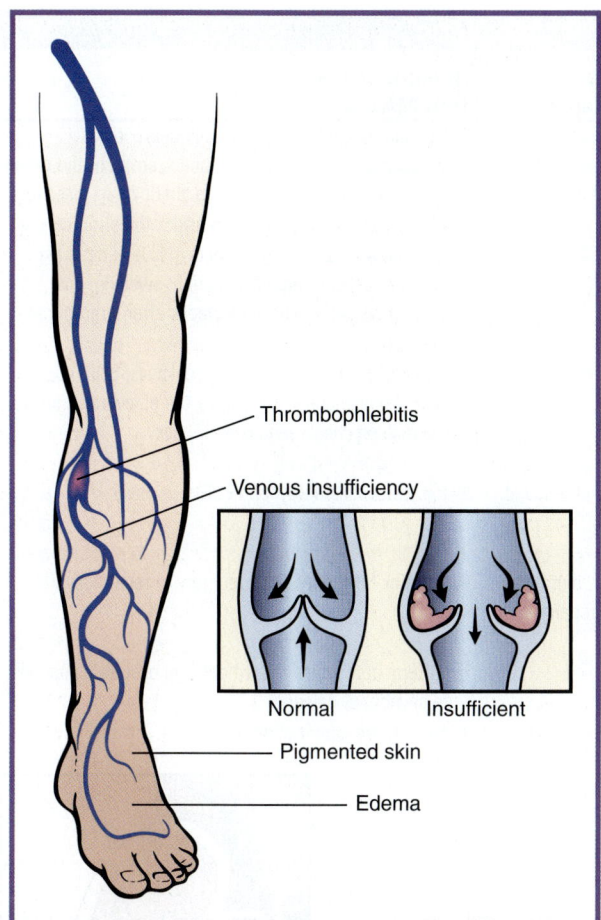

FIG. 10.24 Deep vein thrombosis or thrombophlebitis. (From Damjanov I: *Pathology for the Health-Related Professions*, ed 4, St. Louis, 2012, Saunders.)

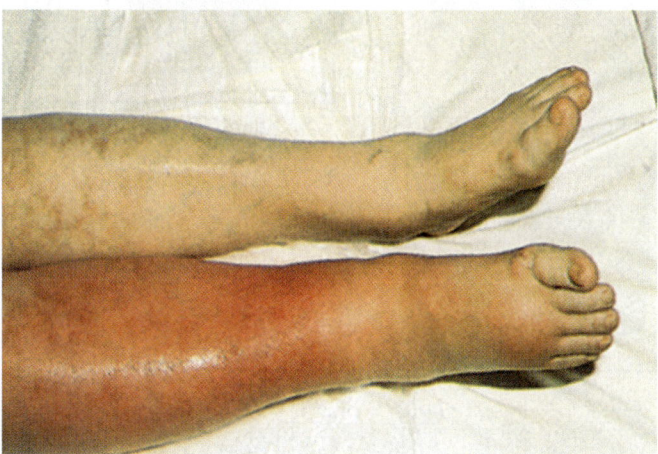

FIG. 10.25 Deep vein thrombosis (DVT). (From Lewis SM: *Medical-Surgical Nursing: Assessment and Management of Clinical Problems*, ed 8, St. Louis, 2011, Mosby.)

Diagnostic Procedures. The provider will do a history and an exam. Additional diagnostic procedures include the following:
- Ultrasound of the affected area
- Blood tests: D-dimer blood test, antithrombin levels, and complete blood count (CBC); other blood tests may be ordered to identify additional causes for the DVT

Treatment. The goals of treatment are to prevent any additional clots and to prevent the current clot from getting larger. Anticoagulant medications, such as heparin and warfarin, will help prevent the RBCs from sticking together and forming a clot. Additional treatments may include compression stockings on the legs and, in rare cases, surgery to remove the clot.

Prognosis. Usually, the prognosis is good. The condition may return. Postphlebitic syndrome may occur and cause long-term pain and swelling. Blood clots in the thigh are at more risk for causing pulmonary embolus.

Prevention. To prevent DVTs, it is important to wear compression stockings if prescribed. Move legs during periods of inactivity. Take prescribed anticoagulant medications. Do not smoke.

Heart Valve Diseases

There are several types of heart valve disease:
- *Stenosis* (sten OH sis): occurs when the valve flaps are stiff or fused together, thus narrowing the valve. The heart may need to work harder to push blood through the smaller opening. Any of the four valves can be stenotic causing the following:
  - Tricuspid stenosis
  - Pulmonic stenosis
  - Aortic stenosis
  - Mitral stenosis
- *Insufficiency*: also called regurgitation or incompetence. The valve does not close completely, and blood leaks backward across the valve into the prior chamber. Depending on the valve impacted, the condition is as follows:
  - Tricuspid regurgitation
  - Pulmonary regurgitation
  - Aortic regurgitation
  - Mitral regurgitation

Table 10.9 describes several Valvular Diseases.

Hypertension

Hypertension (hye pur TEN shun) (HTN) is high blood pressure. Blood pressure (BP) is the force of the blood pushing against the artery wall.

There are three types of hypertension:
- *Primary hypertension* (essential hypertension): the most common type with no identifiable cause; develops with age
- *Secondary hypertension*: high blood pressure is caused by another disease condition or medication; if the disease is treated or the medication is removed, the high blood pressure resolves
- *Malignant hypertension*: very high blood pressure that causes organ damage

MEDICAL TERMINOLOGY
hyper-: excessive
-ion: process of
-itis: inflammation
-lapse: fall
pro-: forward
stenosis: narrowing
tens/o: stretching

TABLE 10.9 Valvular Diseases

Disease	Aortic regurgitation (a OR tick ree gur jih TAY shun)	Mitral valve prolapse (MYE trul valv PRO laps)	Rheumatic fever (roo MAT ik)
Description	Aortic valve does not close tightly; blood backs up into the left ventricle; common in males 30–60 years old	Protrusion of one or both cusps of the mitral valve back into the left atrium during ventricular systole (Fig. 10.26)	Inflammatory reaction affecting the heart valves (valvulitis), causing swelling and scarring of the valves; permanent damage leads to rheumatic heart disease
Etiology	Many conditions cause this disease including high blood pressure, syphilis, congenital problem, and endocarditis	Congenital, genetic	Antibodies made by the body to attack the streptococcal infection start attacking the body tissues (joints and heart valves) causing inflammation, swelling, and scarring; usually occurs 2–4 weeks after strep throat infection
Signs and Symptoms	No-to-slowly developing symptoms; bounding pulse, angina, fainting, fatigue, palpitations, shortness of breath (SOB), and swelling of feet	Palpitations, SOB, cough, fatigue, dizzy, anxiety, migraines, chest discomfort	Fever, joint pain, stomach pain, weakness, SOB, nodules (small bumps) under the skin by the elbows and knees, and rash on chest, abdomen, or back
Diagnostic Procedures	Aortic angiography, echocardiography, left heart catheterization, MRI, and transthoracic echocardiography	Echocardiography, Doppler ultrasound, chest x-ray, ECG	Blood tests, chest x-ray, and ECG
Treatment	Reduce blood pressure through medications; regular echocardiography; surgery to replace valve	Medications (beta blockers, diuretics, vasodilators), surgery to repair or replace valve	Antibiotics for the infection, surgery to repair valve
Prognosis	Surgery can cure symptoms	Good prognosis	Long-term antibiotics if valve damage occurred; depends on severity of damage
Prevention	Control blood pressure	No preventive measures are known	Immediate treatment of strep throat

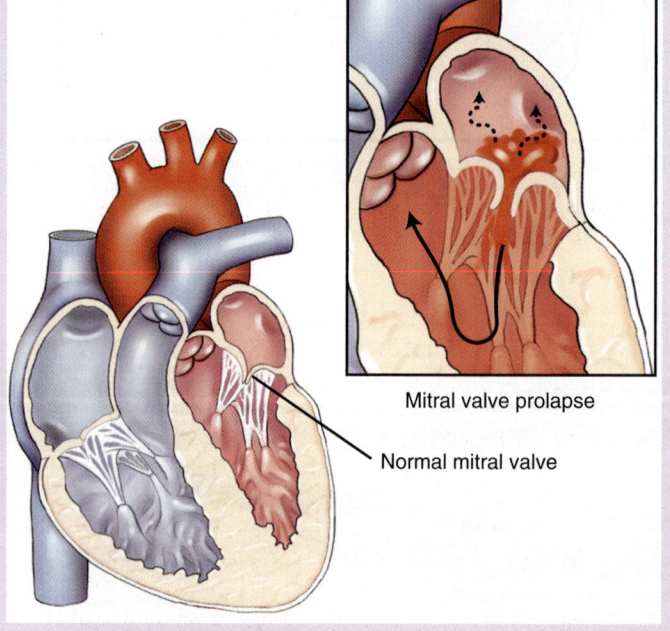

FIG. 10.26 Mitral valve prolapse (MVP). (From Shiland B: *Mastering Healthcare Terminology*, ed 5, St. Louis, 2016, Elsevier.)

Etiology. Hypertension has many causes:
- Genetics: hypertension tends to run in families.
- Environmental factors: high sodium diet, alcohol, smoking, lack of exercise, obesity, and some medications can lead to hypertension.
- Kidney fluid and salt balances: the kidney regulates the electrolyte and water balance in the body. Kidney disease can lead to increased blood volume, which leads to hypertension.
- Renin-angiotensin-aldosterone system: a complex system that makes angiotensin, which constricts blood vessels. It also makes aldosterone, which affects kidney function and leads to increased blood volume. Both can cause hypertension.
- Sympathetic nervous system: involved with blood pressure regulation.
- Changes in blood vessels: loss of elasticity in the walls can lead to hypertension.

> **VOCABULARY**
> **valvulitis**: An Inflammatory condition of a valve caused most commonly by rheumatic fever, bacterial endocarditis, or syphilis; results in valve stenosis and obstructed blood flow.

TABLE 10.10 Blood Pressure Stages for Adults

Categories	Systolic		Diastolic
Normal blood pressure	less than 120 mmHg		less than 80 mmHg
Elevated	120-129 mmHg	AND	less than 80 mmHg
Hypertension Stage 1	130-139 mmHg	OR	80-89 mmHg
Hypertension Stage 2	at least 140 mmHg	OR	at least 90 mmHg
Hypertensive Crisis	over 180 mmHg	AND/OR	over 120 mmHg

TABLE 10.11 Medication Categories Used to Treat Hypertension

Actions to Decrease Blood Pressure	Medication Category
Helps kidneys pull extra water and sodium from the blood, thus decreasing blood volume	Diuretics ("water pills")
Relax blood vessels, which reduces blood pressure	Angiotensin II receptor blockers (ARBs)
	Angiotensin converting enzyme (ACE) inhibitors
	Calcium channel blockers (CCBs)
	Alpha-blockers

Signs and Symptoms. High blood pressure has no symptoms. The only sign is a high blood pressure reading. Hypertension can cause serious problems including stroke, heart attack, heart failure, and kidney failure.

Diagnostic Procedures. Blood pressure is measured and recorded as two numbers. The top number is the systolic pressure, or the blood pressure during a heartbeat. The bottom number is the diastolic pressure, or the blood pressure when the heart rests. Blood pressure is measured in millimeters of mercury (mm Hg). Table 10.10 lists the stages of blood pressure.

Treatment. The goals of treatment are to bring the blood pressure down to the normal level and prevent other diseases from occurring. Typically, treatment involves many factors including medications and lifestyle changes. See Table 10.11 for categories of medications used to help relax the blood vessels or reduce the blood volume. Both actions decrease blood pressure. Lifestyle changes include establishing a healthy diet (low-salt diet, heart-healthy diet), maintaining a healthy weight, stopping smoking, being physically active, limiting alcohol intake, and developing healthy strategies to cope with stress.

Prognosis. The prognosis depends on the type of hypertension and other diseases present. For instance, kidney disease causes hypertension. Following the treatment plan and frequent blood pressure monitoring can lead to a better prognosis.

Prevention. Healthy lifestyle habits can help prevent hypertension. Regular medical care can identify hypertension in the early stages and prevent additional complications.

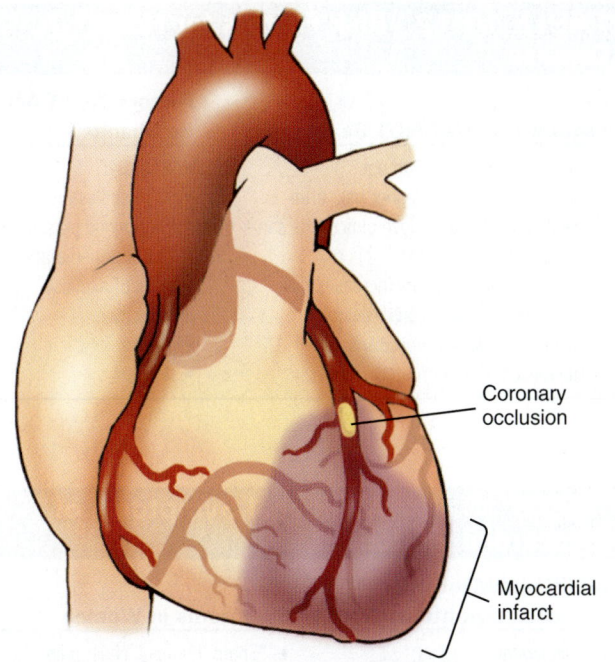

FIG. 10.27 Myocardial infarction. (From Shiland B: *Mastering Healthcare Terminology*, ed 5, St. Louis, 2016, Elsevier.)

Myocardial Infarction

Myocardial infarction is also known as an MI or heart attack. More than 1 million people in the United States have an MI a year, and about half of them die as a result. Without immediate help, permanent heart damage or death can occur.

With a myocardial infarction, the blood flow is limited or blocked. When the heart muscle cells do not receive the amount oxygen each cell requires, they soon die off.

Etiology. A blood clot in a coronary artery is the cause of most myocardial infarctions. Remember, the coronary arteries bring nutrients and oxygen to the heart muscle. If a blockage occurs, heart cells in that part of the muscle serviced by the coronary artery can die.

Plaque can build up in the coronary arteries. A heart attack can result when the following occurs:
- A tear occurs in the plaque causing a clot to form. The clot can partially or totally block the artery (Fig. 10.27). This is the most common cause of MIs.
- Plaque slowly builds up and narrows the inside of the coronary artery.

Table 10.12 lists the risk factors for heart disease.

Signs and Symptoms. The most common warning symptoms of MIs include the following:
- *Angina pectoris* (an JYE nuh PECK tore us) (chest pain): may also be described as mild or severe heaviness, squeezing, pressure, or heartburn (Fig. 10.28); pain may be constant or intermittent (comes and goes)
- Upper body discomfort or pain in one or both arms, shoulders, neck, jaw, upper part of the abdomen
- Shortness of breath with activity or rest

Table 10.13 lists additional symptoms of an MI. Females can experience different symptoms than males. See Table 10.13 for the more common female symptoms.

TABLE 10.12 Risk Factors for Heart Disease

Factors That CANNOT Be Changed	Factors That CAN Be Changed
• Age: risk increases with age • Gender: males have higher risk; after menopause females have almost the same risk as males • Genetics: family history increases risk • Race: African Americans, Mexican Americans, Native Americans, and Hawaiians have a greater risk	• Smoking • High cholesterol • High blood pressure • Uncontrolled diabetes • Lack of exercise • Obesity • Stress • Alcohol

TABLE 10.13 Additional Symptoms of Myocardial Infarctions

Additional Myocardial Infarction Symptoms	Symptoms in Women
• Cold sweat • Tiredness without a reason • Nausea and vomiting • Dizziness, light-headedness • Angina (chest pain) is different than the person's normal pain • Arrhythmia, palpitations	• "Sharp, burning" chest pain • More commonly experience neck, jaw, throat, or abdomen pain • Back pain • Two-thirds have no symptoms

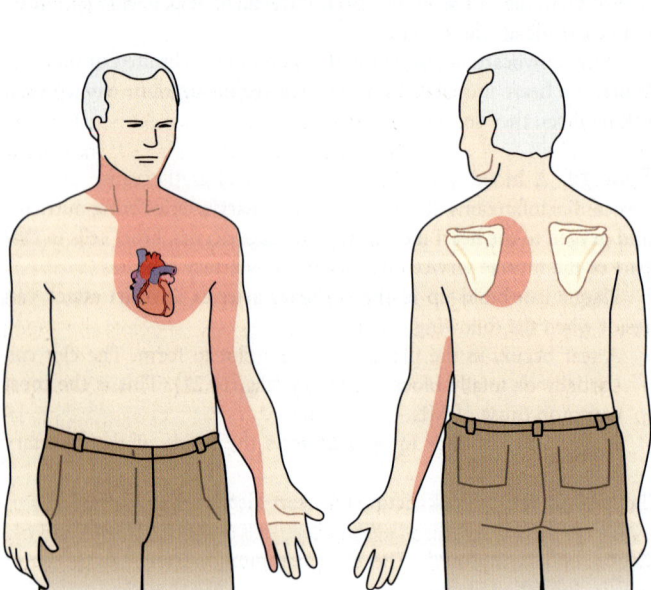

FIG. 10.28 Common sites of pain in angina pectoris. (From Shiland B: *Mastering Healthcare Terminology*, ed 5, St. Louis, 2016, Elsevier.)

MEDICAL TERMINOLOGY
pector/o: chest
-is: structure

Diagnostic Procedures. Diagnostic tests for an MI include an ECG and blood tests (i.e., troponin, creatine kinase [CK], creatine kinase -MB [CK-MB], and serum myoglobin tests). CK-MB is an enzyme found in the heart muscle cell. Within hours of a heart attack, the CK-MB level increases in the blood. It peaks within 12-24 hours and returns to normal by 48-72 hours. The blood tests may be repeated over time to look for changes. An angiocardiography may be done to study the coronary blood flow and to identify blockages.

Treatment. Immediate treatment involves the following:
- Chewing aspirin to prevent additional clots
- Nitroglycerin to dilate the coronary arteries and help increase the oxygen to the heart muscle
- Oxygen therapy

As soon as the diagnosis is determined, thrombolytic medications (also called "clot busters") are given. These medications help the body's natural process of dissolving blood clots. Percutaneous coronary intervention may be done to open the coronary artery. Medications, lifestyle changes, and cardiac rehabilitation may also be done.

> **CRITICAL THINKING 10.9**
>
> Rebecca reviews the chest pain protocol with Lizzy. It states that patients with chest pain need to chew an aspirin. Nitroglycerin and oxygen must also be administered to the patient. Rebecca asks Lizzy why is aspirin, nitroglycerin, and oxygen important if a person is experiencing chest pain. How might Lizzy answer this question?

Prognosis. The prognosis varies. It depends on the time frame from the attack to the medical intervention. It also depends on the location of the blockage and the extent of damage.

Prevention. To prevent MIs, it is important to reduce the risk factors for heart disease. See Table 10.12 for risk factors that can be changed. These should be targeted to prevent heart disease.

Postural Orthostatic Tachycardia Syndrome

Postural orthostatic tachycardia syndrome (POTS) is estimated to affect 1 million to 3 million Americans. It can occur at any age and with either gender, though it most commonly affects females between 15 and 50 years of age.

POTS is a syndrome because it has a group of symptoms that are commonly seen together. This syndrome is considered a dysautonomia, an abnormal condition of the autonomic nervous system (ANS). The ANS does not control the blood pressure or heart rate when standing up. Orthostatic hypotension (hye poh TEN shun) and tachycardia (high heart rate) are seen. Orthostatic (postural) hypotension occurs when there is a decrease in blood pressure within 3 minutes of standing up. The systolic blood pressure drops 20 or more mm Hg, and the diastolic blood pressure decreases 10 or more mm Hg.

> **VOCABULARY**
> **orthostatic (postural) hypotension:** A temporary fall in blood pressure that occurs when a person rapidly changes from a recumbent position to a standing position.

Etiology. Many times, providers cannot identify the underlying cause of a person's POTS. Researchers have identified many diseases that are known to cause or are associated with POTS. These diseases and conditions include autoimmune diseases, diabetes, infections (mononucleosis, Epstein-Barr virus, Lyme disease), multiple sclerosis, trauma, and vitamin deficiencies.

Signs and Symptoms. The symptoms can vary. Commonly the person has *hypovolemia* (low blood volume). As the person stands, the blood pools in the abdomen and legs. A drop in blood pressure (*orthostatic hypotension*) with standing is seen. Other symptoms include the following:
- Fatigue, exercise intolerance, nausea, headaches, and poor concentration
- Lightheadedness, blurred vision, *syncope* (fainting), heart palpitations, chest pain, and shortness of breath
- Cold or painful extremities (fingers and toes)
- Fainting with blood draws (phlebotomy) or deep breathing

Sometimes the symptoms are mild and do not interfere with daily activity. Others experience significant symptoms that interfere with eating, moving, bathing, and working. About 25% of patients with POTS are disabled and cannot work.

> **CRITICAL THINKING 10.10**
>
> Rebecca and Lizzy are working with a patient who has been diagnosed with POTS. Having never heard of POTS, Rebecca asks the patient to explain about the disease. The patient explains that her blood volume is low. She needs to consume a lot of sodium and water to maintain the blood volume. The patient states that she has problems with blood draws and faints. Rebecca thanks the patient for her explanation. Why is it important for medical assistants to listen to their patients about their special needs?

Diagnostic Procedures. Diagnostic testing for POTS includes the following:
- *Orthostatic vital signs*: blood pressure and heart rate are obtained as the patient reclines, sits, and stands. In many cases, the blood pressure drops and the heart rate increases.
- *Tilt table test*: a patient is strapped to a table; gradually the table is tilted into the upright position and the patient is monitored to see the effects of the position changes.

Treatment. Treatment can vary. Medicines to regulate the heart rate and blood pressure may be prescribed. Lifestyle changes are encouraged, including the following:
- Drinking plenty of fluids (2–3 L per day) and eating the prescribed amount of salt to maintain the blood volume
- Reclined exercises (e.g., rowing, recumbent bicycling) to help tone the muscles and limit the pooling of blood
- Healthy diet and in some cases a low-carbohydrate, high-protein diet
- Compression stockings to prevent pooling of blood in the legs

Prognosis. Currently there is no cure for POTS. Following the prescribed lifestyle changes and taking the medication can limit the symptoms.

Prevention. There are no known preventive measures.

Shock

Shock occurs when there is not enough blood and oxygen getting to the organs and tissues. It causes very low blood pressure.

TABLE 10.14 Types and Causes of Shock

Type of Shock	Description and Etiology
Anaphylactic	Severe allergic reaction; caused from exposure to an allergen (e.g., insect bites/stings, food allergy, drug allergy).
Cardiogenic	The damaged heart cannot pump blood effectively; caused by a heart attack, arrhythmias, pulmonary embolism, or congestive heart failure
Hypovolemic	Excessive loss of blood or body fluids from internal or external hemorrhage (bleeding); severe dehydration, burns, vomiting, or diarrhea
Neurogenic	Peripheral vessels dilate due to a neurologic injury or disorder (e.g., spinal cord injury)
Septic	Overwhelming infection; caused from bacteria, fungi, and rarely viruses.

Shock usually happens with a serious injury and can be life threatening.

Etiology. There are several types of shock. See Table 10.14 for the types of shock and the causes of shock.

Signs and Symptoms. Signs and symptoms of shock include the following:
- Weak rapid pulse and rapid shallow respirations
- Changes in the level of consciousness: confusion, lack of alertness, loss of consciousness
- Dizziness, lightheadedness, or faintness
- Sweaty, pale skin; cool hands and feet; bluish lips and fingernails
- Decreased or no urine output

Diagnostic Procedure. Shock is diagnosed based on the history, exam, and vital signs of the patient. If time allows, additional testing may be done to identify the cause. Treatment for shock may occur before the cause is identified.

Treatment. Immediate treatment is necessary to save the person's life. If outside of a medical facility, 911 should be called immediately. Lay the person down with the feet elevated 12 inches above the head (if no head or spine injuries or broken bones are suspected). Monitor breathing and heart rate until help arrives.

The goals of medical treatment include increasing the cardiac output and blood pressure with medications and IV blood and fluids. Additional treatments will address the cause of the shock.

Prognosis. The prognosis depends on the type of shock, the underlying cause, and the amount of blood volume lost. With cases of milder degrees of shock, the prognosis is good. Severe cases of shock have a poor prognosis.

Prevention. Immediate treatment of conditions that might lead to shock is important. Early first aid is important.

> **MEDICAL TERMINOLOGY**
>
> **hypo-**: below, deficient
> **myx/o**: mucus
> **-sarcoma**: connective tissue cancer

TABLE 10.15 Additional Cardiovascular Diseases

Disease	Description
Aneurysm (AN yoo rizz um)	Bulging of the blood vessel wall (Fig. 10.29). Commonly seen in the aorta (aortic aneurysm). If rupture occurs, can cause a stroke (if in the brain) or can be deadly (if an aortic aneurysm). Causes include congenital conditions, acquired weakness, arteriosclerosis, trauma, infection, or inflammation.
Angiosarcoma (an jee oh sar KOH mah)	Rare cancer of the cells that line the blood vessels. Also called a *hemangiosarcoma* (hee man jee oh sar KOH mah).
Arteriosclerosis (ar teer ee oh sklah ROH sis)	Disease in which the arterial walls become thickened and lose their elasticity.
Atrial myxoma (A tree uhl mick SOH mah)	Benign growth usually occurring on the interatrial septum.
Buerger disease	Arteries and veins in extremities can swell up and clots can occur. Blood supply can be cut off. If severe, may require amputation of toes and fingers.
Cardiac myxosarcoma (mick soh sar KOH mah)	Rare cancer of the heart usually originating in the left atria.
Cardiac tamponade (tam pon ADE)	Compression of the heart caused by fluid in the pericardial sac.
Endocarditis (en doh kar DYE tis)	Also called infective endocarditis (IE), a condition in which the inner lining of the heart is inflamed. Bacterial endocarditis is most common. It can damage valves and be life threatening.
Esophageal varices (eh sof uh JEE ul VARE ih seez)	Varicose veins that appear at the lower end of the esophagus as a result of portal hypertension; they are superficial and may cause ulceration and bleeding.
Familial dilated cardiomyopathy	Genetic condition; a wall of one of the chambers becomes thin and weakened leading to an inefficiency with pumping the blood.
Marfan syndrome	A genetic condition that affects the connective tissues throughout the body. In terms of cardiovascular issues, they can have weakening of the aorta that can lead to a rupture. Heart valves can be incompetent, causing heart murmurs.
Metabolic syndrome	A group of factors that increase a person's risk for heart disease, diabetes, and stroke. Having three of the five risk factors leads to the diagnosis: large waistline, high triglyceride level, low high-density lipoprotein (HDL) cholesterol level, high blood pressure, and high fasting blood sugar.
Pericarditis (pair ee kar DYE tis)	Inflammation of the sac surrounding the heart with the possibility of *pericardial effusion* (the escape of blood into the pericardium).
Peripheral vascular disease (PVD) (puh RIFF uh rul VAS kyoo lur)	Any vascular disorder limited to the extremities; may affect not only the arteries and veins but also the lymphatics.
Raynaud phenomenon (ray NODE)	Small arteries in the fingers and toes may twitch or cramp with cold temperatures. Causes limited blood supply in the area, making skin look white or bluish and feeling cold. Unknown cause (*idiopathic*). Also called Raynaud disease or Raynaud syndrome.
Varicose veins (VARE ih kose)	Elongated, dilated superficial veins (varices) with incompetent valves that permit reverse blood flow. Usually seen on the legs.
Vasculitis (vas kyoo LYE tis)	Inflammation of the blood vessels.

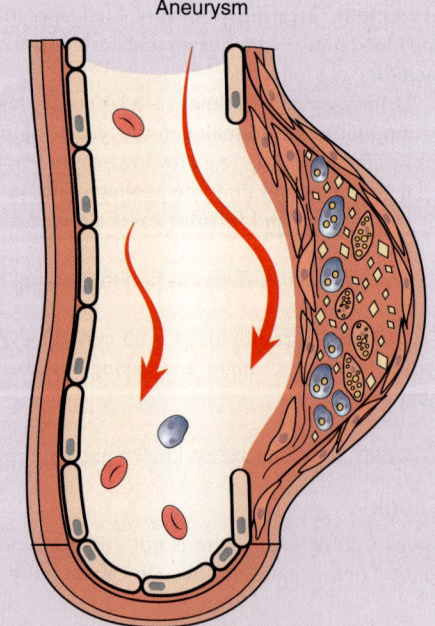

FIG. 10.29 Aneurysm caused by weakening of the vessel wall. (From Damjanov I: *Pathology for the Health-Related Professions*, ed 4, St. Louis, 2012, Saunders.)

Additional Cardiovascular System Diseases

There are many cardiovascular diseases. Table 10.15 provides a brief description of additional cardiovascular diseases.

LIFE SPAN CHANGES

An unborn child receives oxygen and nutrients from the mother's blood through the placenta. As described earlier in this chapter, the ductus venosus, ductus arteriosus, foramen ovale, and the umbilical vessels are special structures that help with fetal circulation. After birth, these structures are no longer necessary.

As a child grows and matures, the heart rate decreases. The systemic vascular resistance increases with age. This means that the resistance for blood flow increases and thus the blood pressure increases with age.

During pregnancy, the mother's cardiovascular system undergoes changes:
- Cardiac output (amount of blood pushed out of the heart in 1 minute) increases.
- Extracellular fluid volume increases, thus the blood volume is more.
- Total peripheral resistance decreases, thus decreasing the blood pressure.
- Blood flow to various organs increases.

TABLE 10.16 Cardiovascular Changes With Age

Heart Changes	Blood Vessel Changes
• SA node (pacemaker) loses some cells, thus the heart rate can be slower. • The left ventricle may increase in size, thus decreasing the amount of blood that it can hold. • Normal ECG changes can occur with age. • Valves can become thicker and stiffer, causing a heart murmur.	• *Baroreceptors* in the carotid arteries and aorta detect changes in blood pressure. They help maintain a fairly constant blood pressure with position changes. With age, the baroreceptors become less sensitive making older people more at risk for orthostatic hypotension when moving positions. • Arterial walls become stiffer, thus increasing blood pressure.

- As the pregnancy progresses into the third trimester, the blood pressure increases.

As a person ages, the heart and blood vessels undergo changes. Table 10.16 describes the changes to the heart and blood vessels with age.

CLOSING COMMENTS

Working with patients who have cardiovascular disorders is common in ambulatory care. It is important for the medical assistant to be accurate with the pronunciation and spelling of medical terminology (Tables 10.17, 10.18, and 10.19). It is also important to understand the meaning of common abbreviations (Table 10.20).

If an abbreviation relates to a patient's condition, diagnostic test, or treatment, the medical assistant must make sure the patient is aware of the meaning of the abbreviation. Clear and accurate communication is important between patients and healthcare staff.

Besides medical terminology and abbreviations, medical assistants need to understand the following:

TABLE 10.17 Combining and Adjective Forms for Cardiovascular Medical Terminology

Meaning	Combining Form	Adjective Form	Meaning	Combining Form	Adjective Form
aorta	aort/o	aortic	pull	tract/o	
apex	apic/o	apical	rhythm	rhythm/o	rhythmic
arteriole	arteriol/o		septum, wall	sept/o	septal
artery	arteri/o, arter/o	arterial	sinus	sin/o	
atrium	atri/o	atrial	system	system/o	systemic
carbon dioxide	capn/o		valve	valvul/o	valvular
endocardium	endocardi/o	endocardial	vein	ven/o, phleb/o	venous
epicardium	epicardi/o	epicardial	ventricle	ventricul/o	ventricular
heart	cardi/o, coron/o, cordi/o	cardiac, coronary, cordial	venule	venul/o	
lung	pulmon/o, pneum/o, pneumat/o	pulmonary, pneumatic	vessel	vascul/o, angi/o, vas/o	vascular
myocardium	myocardi/o	myocardial	viscera	viscer/o	visceral
oxygen	ox/i, ox/o		wall	pariet/o	parietal
pericardium	pericardi/o	pericardial			

From Shiland B: *Mastering Healthcare Terminology*, ed 5, St. Louis, 2016, Elsevier.

TABLE 10.18 Common Prefixes

Prefix	Meaning
a-	without
con-	together
e-	out
pre-	before

From Shiland B: *Mastering Healthcare Terminology*, ed 5, St. Louis, 2016, Elsevier.

TABLE 10.19 Common Suffixes

Suffix	Meaning
-ar, -ary, -ic, -al	pertaining to
-ia	condition
-ion	process of
-logy	study of
-um	structure

From Shiland B: *Mastering Healthcare Terminology*, ed 5, St. Louis, 2016, Elsevier.

TABLE 10.20 Common Abbreviations Related to Cardiovascular System

Abbreviation	Definition	Abbreviation	Definition
AEB	atrial ectopic beat	EVLT	endovenous laser ablation
AF	atrial fibrillation	HF	heart failure
AICD	automatic implantable cardiac-defibrillator	HTN	hypertension
AS	aortic stenosis	LVAD	left ventricular assist device
ASD	atrial septal defect	MI	myocardial infarction
ASHD	arteriosclerotic heart disease	MIDCAB	minimally invasive direct coronary artery bypass
BP	blood pressure	MR	mitral regurgitation
bpm	beats per minute	MS	mitral stenosis
CABG	coronary artery bypass graft	MVP	mitral valve prolapse
CAD	coronary artery disease	O_2	oxygen
Cath	(cardiac) catheterization	PDA	patent ductus arteriosus
CHF	congestive heart failure	PTCA	percutaneous transluminal coronary angioplasty
CO_2	carbon dioxide	PVD	peripheral vascular disease
CPK	creatine phosphokinase	RFCA	radiofrequency catheter ablation
CV	cardiovascular	SA	sinoatrial
DOE	dyspnea on exertion	SK	streptokinase
DSA	digital subtraction angiography	SOB	shortness of breath
DVT	deep vein thrombosis	TEA	thromboendarterectomy
ECC	extracorporeal circulation	TEE	transesophageal echocardiography
ECG, EKG	electrocardiography, electrocardiogram	TS	tricuspid stenosis
ECHO	echocardiography	VSD	ventricular septal defect
EST	exercise stress test		

- Basics of the cardiovascular system including the structures and functions of the structures
- Importance of the heart's conduction system
- Factors that impact blood pressure
- Diseases that impact the cardiovascular system

Having this understanding will help you provide great care to your patients. It will also help you recognize the importance of different treatments ordered by the providers.

CHAPTER REVIEW

The cardiovascular system consists of blood vessels, a heart, and blood. The cardiovascular system brings oxygen (O_2), nutrients, water, and other substances (e.g., salts and hormones) to the body's cells. It also carries waste products (e.g., metabolic waste, carbon dioxide [CO_2]) away from the cells to be excreted. The heart has two sets of chambers (atria and ventricles) and two sets of valves. The AV valves are between the atria and ventricles. The SL valves are between the ventricles and the arteries leading out of the heart.

The pulmonary circulation takes deoxygenated blood from the right side of the heart to the lungs. Blood returns from the lungs and empties into the left atrium. Blood from the left side of the heart is pumped to the body, which is the systemic circulation. The coronary circulation provides oxygen and nutrients to the heart muscle. The hepatic portal circulation allows blood from the spleen, gallbladder, pancreas, stomach, and intestines to be taken directly to the liver, where it is filtered. The filtered blood then is returned to the inferior vena cava. The last circulation system is fetal circulation, which is found in unborn babies. This system allows oxygen and nutrients to move from the mother's bloodstream to the baby's blood. Fetal circulation is no longer needed at birth.

The conduction system is the heart's electrical system. It is composed of the SA node (the pacemaker), the AV node, the bundle of His, right and left bundle branches, and the Purkinje fibers. An electrical impulse is required for the heart muscle to contract. With each cardiac cycle, blood is moved from the atria to the ventricles and then out of the heart.

Blood pressure is influenced by several factors including blood volume, the strength of ventricular contractions, and the resistance to blood flow. The size of the lumen of the arteries, the elasticity of the arterial walls, and the viscosity of the blood impact the resistance to blood flow. The higher the resistance, the higher the blood pressure.

Many cardiovascular diseases were discussed in the chapter. A common etiology includes unhealthy habits (high-cholesterol diets, high-sodium diets, lack of exercise, smoking, and being overweight), congenital problems, and infection. Common signs and symptoms of cardiovascular diseases impact the heart rate and rhythm and the respiration status. Many symptoms can be related to the lack of adequate blood flow to tissues. Typical diagnostic tests ordered include blood pressure reading, ECG, many imaging procedures, and several blood tests. Several CLIA-waived tests are available for diagnosing and monitoring cardiovascular diseases. These include cholesterol testing and prothrombin testing.

The cardiovascular system changes with age. After birth, the fetal circulation structures are no longer used. Older adults have changes in their heart and blood vessels. Cardiovascular diseases are more common with advanced age.

SCENARIO WRAP-UP

As the weeks followed, Lizzy became more independent in the practicum. She was very excited to interview for a medical assistant position in a cardiology department in a nearby city. During her last day with Rebecca, they celebrated her completion of her practicum. Lizzy shared that she was offered the medical assistant position, which she accepted.

In the weeks that followed Lizzy's last day, Rebecca thought about all the information she shared with Lizzy. She realized that she too had learned a lot from the practicum experience and found that she really enjoyed mentoring students. Rebecca planned on talking with her supervisor about future opportunities to mentor students in the department.

11 Respiratory System

LEARNING OBJECTIVES

1. List the major organs of the respiratory system and identify the anatomical location of major respiratory system organs.
2. Describe the normal function and physiology of the respiratory system.
3. Discuss the diseases and disorders related to the respiratory system. Also:
   - Identify the common signs and symptoms of respiratory diseases.
   - Identify the common etiology of respiratory diseases.
   - Describe diagnostic measures used for the respiratory diseases.
   - Identify CLIA-waived tests associated with common respiratory diseases.
   - Describe treatment modalities used for respiratory diseases.
4. Compare the structure and function of the respiratory system across the life span.

CHAPTER OUTLINE

1. Opening Scenario, 238
2. You Will Learn, 238
3. Anatomy of the Respiratory System, 238
   a. Upper Respiratory Tract, 239
   b. Lower Respiratory Tract, 240
4. Physiology of the Respiratory System, 242
   a. Ventilation, 242
      i. Inspiration, 242
      ii. Expiration, 242
   b. Acid-Base Balance, 242
5. Diseases of the Respiratory System, 242
   a. Asthma, 245
   b. Bronchitis, Acute, 246
   c. Chronic Obstructive Pulmonary Disease, 247
   d. Cystic Fibrosis, 248
   e. Infectious Mononucleosis, 249
   f. Lung Cancer, 249
   g. Pneumonia, 251
   h. Pulmonary Embolism, 251
   i. Pulmonary Tuberculosis, 252
   j. Respiratory Syncytial Virus Pneumonia, 252
   k. Respiratory Tract Diseases, Lower, 253
   l. Respiratory Tract Diseases, Upper, 253
   m. Additional Respiratory System Diseases, 253
6. Life Span Changes, 258
7. Closing Comments, 258
8. Chapter Review, 259

 OPENING SCENARIO

Renee Thomas, CMA (AAMA), was hired 6 months ago as a certified medical assistant. She assists the specialists who hold outreach clinics at Walden-Martin Family Medical (WMFM) Clinic. On Tuesdays the pulmonologist from a local larger city comes for a pulmonary outreach clinic. The pulmonologist brings his own equipment and one medical assistant, John, to the outreach clinic.

Renee's job is to help the pulmonology medicine team, because she knows the WMFM clinic and the local community resources. Renee studied the anatomy and physiology of the respiratory system during her medical assistant training. She learned about common diseases, but she found that she has a lot more to learn. Besides obtaining patients' vital signs and medical histories, Renee does a pulse oximetry measurement on most of her patients. She has observed John performing a spirometry test, which she will learn to do in the future.

In her work with the pulmonologist and John, Renee sees patients with many interesting respiratory diseases. She continues to learn from her work with the specialist and the patients.

YOU WILL LEARN

- To recognize and use terms related to the respiratory system.
- To locate the upper and lower respiratory system structures.
- To understand and describe the ventilation process.
- To recognize disease states of the upper and lower respiratory tract. This includes the causes, signs and symptoms, diagnostic processes, treatment, prognosis, and prevention.

ANATOMY OF THE RESPIRATORY SYSTEM

The respiratory system is divided into the upper respiratory tract and the lower respiratory tract. Each section has specific structures and

CHAPTER 11 Respiratory System

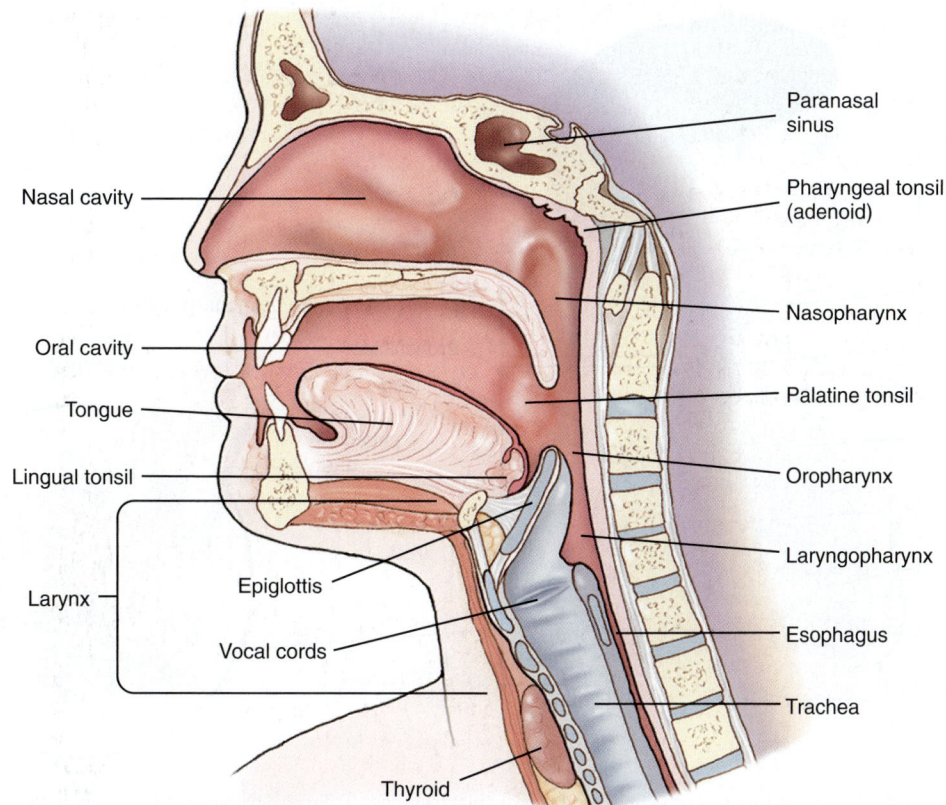

FIG. 11.1 The upper respiratory system. (From Shiland B: *Mastering Healthcare Terminology*, ed 5, St Louis, 2016, Mosby.)

> **BOX 11.1 Specialty and Specialist**
>
> Pulmonology (PULL mun ahl ah jee) is the healthcare specialty that deals with respiratory disorders. A pulmonologist (PULL mun ahl ah jist) is a specialist involved in the diagnosis, treatment, and prevention of disorders of the respiratory system.

functions. The upper respiratory tract structures are considered passageways for the air, whereas the lower respiratory tract structures are involved in gas exchange (Box 11.1).

Upper Respiratory Tract

The upper respiratory tract is composed of structures from the nose to the larynx. These organs are located outside of the chest cavity. The main functions of the upper respiratory tract include:
- warming and cleaning the inspired air.
- serving as a passageway for air.
- providing the sense of smell.

Air can enter through the mouth, but the majority enters the nose. Air enters through the two nares (NAIR eez) (nostrils) in the nose. The nasal septum (NAY zul SEP tum) separates the nares. The air then moves into the nasal cavity. The surface capillaries, mucous membrane, and cilia (SEE lee uh) (small hairs) found in the nasal cavity clean, warm, and moisten the air. The cilia continually move in a wavelike motion to push mucus and debris out of the respiratory tract. Receptors for smelling are in the nasal cavity. The nasal cavity is connected to the paranasal sinuses (pair uh NAY zul SYE nus suhs). The four pairs of paranasal sinuses are named for the bone they are found in:
- Maxillary
- Frontal
- Sphenoid
- Ethmoid

> **VOCABULARY**
>
> **paranasal sinuses**: Hollow, air-filled cavities in the skull and facial bones. They lighten the weight of the skull and increase the tone, or resonance, of speech.

Air continues to travel into the nasopharynx (NAY zoh fair inks), which is the part of the throat (pharynx) behind the nasal cavity (Fig. 11.1). The eustachian (yoo STAY shun) tubes and the pharyngeal tonsils (fur IN jee ul TAHN suls) are found in this area. The eustachian tube connects the middle ear to the nasopharynx. It equalizes the pressure in the ear with the air pressure outside of the body. The pharyngeal tonsils, or adenoids (AD uh noyds), are lymphatic tissue that help protect against pathogens.

After the nasopharynx, air enters the oropharynx (or oh FAIR inks), which is posterior to the mouth (see Fig. 11.1). Because the oropharynx is involved in passing air from the nasopharynx to the laryngopharynx, it is part of the respiratory system. The oropharynx is also part of the digestive system. It receives food from the mouth and passes it to the esophagus. The palatine tonsils (PAL ah tyne TAHN suls), which are lymphatic tissue, are found in this area. The lingual tonsil, located on the posterior aspect of the tongue, also serves a protective function.

After the oropharynx, air enters the laryngopharynx (luh ring goh FAIR inks) and then the larynx (LAIR inks), or voice box (see Fig. 11.1). The epiglottis (eh pee GLOT is) is a flap of cartilage at the opening to the larynx. The epiglottis closes off the trachea (TRAY kee uh) during swallowing so that food goes into the esophagus. As air passes back out

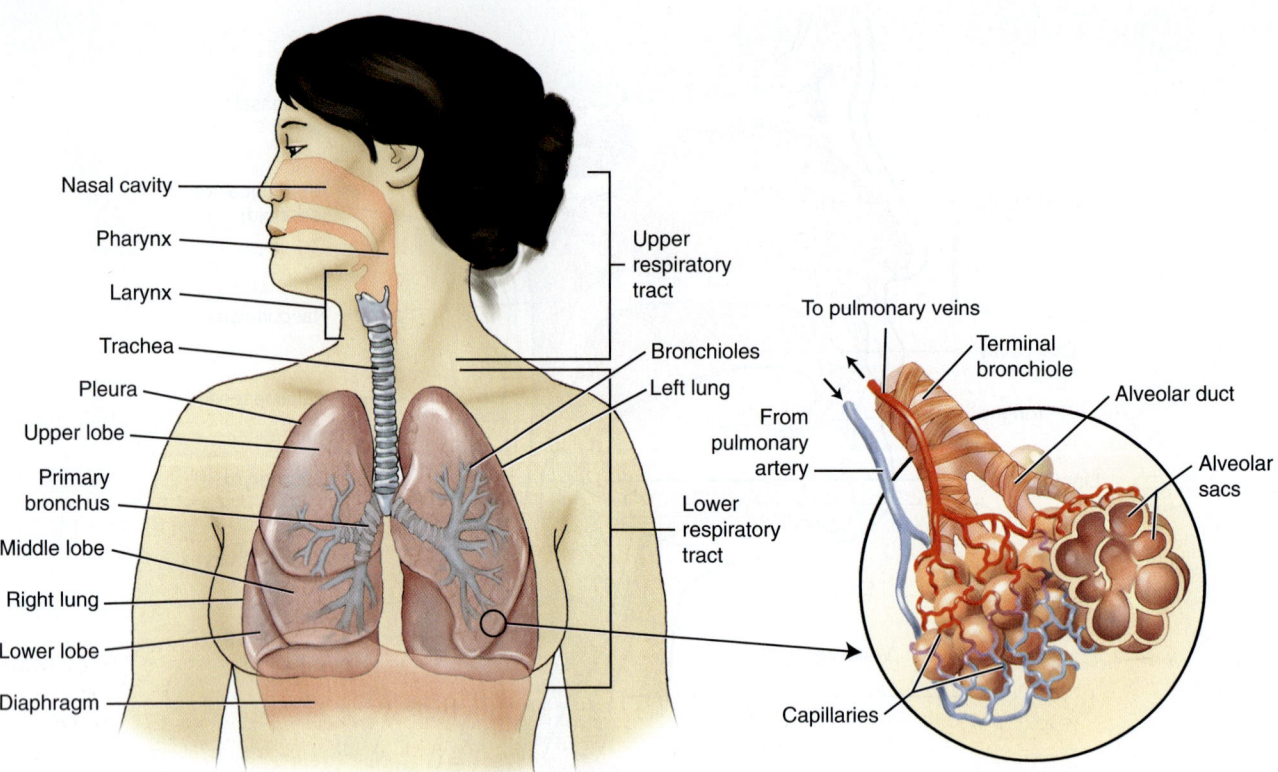

FIG. 11.2 The respiratory system showing the bronchial tree *(inset)*. (From Shiland B: *Mastering healthcare terminology*, ed 5, St Louis, 2016, Mosby.)

through the opening of the larynx, the vocal cords, which are paired bands of cartilaginous tissue, vibrate to produce speech.

MEDICAL TERMINOLOGY	
adenoid/o: adenoid	**muc/o:** mucus
epiglott/o: epiglottis	**nas/o, rhin/o:** nose
salping/o: eustachian tube	**pharyng/o:** pharynx
laryng/o: larynx	**sinus/o, sin/o:** sinus
or/o: mouth	**tonsill/o:** tonsils

Lower Respiratory Tract

The lower respiratory tract consists of the trachea, bronchial tubes, and lungs (Fig. 11.2). These structures are also lined with mucous membranes and cilia. When dust and foreign particles accumulate in the cilia, the coughing reflex is initiated. These defense mechanisms help remove pathogens from the respiratory tract. Cigarette smoke and other air pollutants slow the action of the cilia and damage the mucous membrane lining.

C-shaped cartilaginous rings surround the trachea (windpipe). These rings hold the trachea open, regardless of changes in air pressure. The trachea lies in the space between the lungs, called the *mediastinum* (mee dee uh STY num). Air travels from the larynx through the trachea, and then the trachea branches into the right and left bronchi (BRONG kee) (Fig. 11.3). The right bronchus is wider than the left bronchus. It accommodates the larger right lung lobes.

The bronchi divide into smaller branches, called *bronchioles* (BRONG kee ohls). These bronchioles end in microscopic ducts capped by air sacs, called *alveoli* (al VEE oh lye). Each thin-walled alveolus is

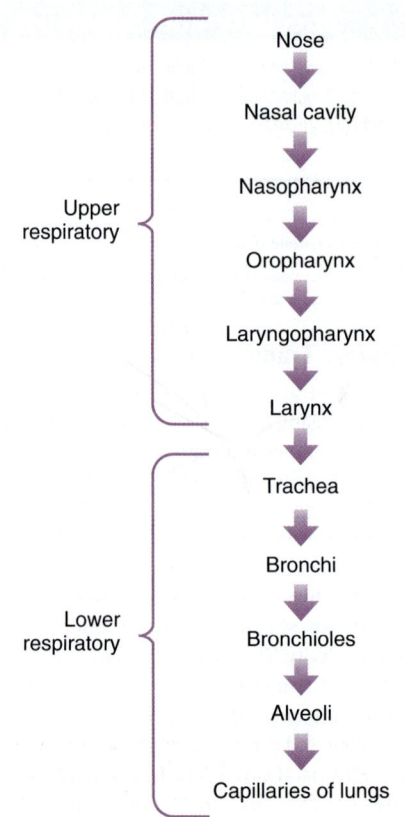

FIG. 11.3 The order in which air passes through the respiratory system. (From Shiland B: *Mastering healthcare terminology*, ed 5, St Louis, 2016, Mosby.)

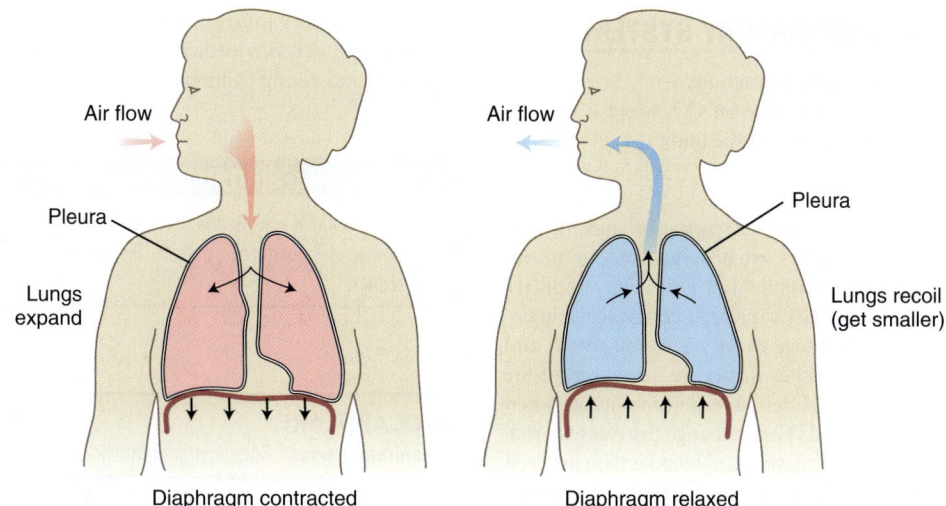

FIG. 11.4 Inspiration and expiration. (From Shiland B: *Mastering healthcare terminology*, ed 5, St Louis, 2016, Mosby.)

in contact with a blood capillary. This contact between the two structures allows the exchange of gases. It is at this point that oxygen (O_2) from the expired air moves across the one-cell membrane into the blood cells. Carbon dioxide (CO_2) moves in the other direction, from the blood into the air to be expired. Each alveolus is coated with a substance called **surfactant** (sur FACK tunt), which keeps it from collapsing. Without surfactant, the alveoli stick together during exhalation and deflate. Inhalation becomes more difficult, and less O_2 is able to move into the bloodstream. This condition is life threatening. Babies born before 37 to 39 weeks are at risk for not having enough surfactant.

> ### CRITICAL THINKING 11.1
> Renee works with patients of all ages in the pulmonary outreach clinic. Today Pedro Gomez, an elementary school student, comes in with his mother. He is there for a check-up on his asthma. As Renee is rooming him, Pedro mentions that he is learning about the respiratory system in school. He asks Renee to tell him all the structures, from the nose to the lungs, in order. Renee agrees to his request. What does she say? (What would be your answer to Pedro's request?)

The bronchial tree and alveoli are the major structures in the right and left lungs. The lungs are soft and spongy because of the air sacs that make up most of their mass. They hang in the right and left sides of the chest, separated by the pericardial sac, which contains the heart. Each lung is composed of sections called *lobes*. The right lung consists of three lobes, whereas the left has only two. The abbreviations for the lobes of the lungs are: RUL (right upper lobe), RML (right middle lobe), RLL (right lower lobe), LUL (left upper lobe), and LLL (left lower lobe).

Because each lobe has its own bronchus and blood supply, the removal of one lobe (lobectomy) results in little or no damage to the rest of the lung. The left lung is longer and narrower. It has a distinct indentation in its center, known as the *cardiac notch*. This is where the left ventricle of the heart is located and where an apical pulse is heard.

Each lung is also enclosed by a double-folded, serous membrane called the *pleura* (PLOOR uh). The side of the membrane closest to the lungs is the *visceral pleura* (VIH sur ul PLOOR ah). The side that lines the inner surface of the rib cage is the *parietal pleura* (puh RYE uh tul PLOOR ah). Small amounts of pleural fluid fill the space between the two membranes and provide lubrication for the movement of the lungs during inhalation and exhalation.

The muscles responsible for normal, quiet respiration are the **diaphragm** (DYE uh fram) and the **intercostal** (in tur KOS tul) **muscles**. On **inspiration**, the diaphragm is pulled down as it contracts, and the intercostal muscles expand, pulling air into the lungs (Fig. 11.4). On **expiration**, the diaphragm relaxes and moves upward, pushing air out of the lungs.

> ### VOCABULARY
> **diaphragm**: A broad, dome-shaped muscle used for breathing. It separates the thoracic and abdominopelvic cavities.
> **expiration**: Exhaling; movement of waste gases from the alveoli into the atmosphere.
> **inspiration**: Inhaling; movement of O_2 from the atmosphere into the alveoli.
> **intercostal muscles**: Muscles located between the ribs that help with quiet respiration.
> **surfactant**: A mixture of protein and fats that lines the alveoli and prevents the tissues from sticking together and collapsing during exhalation.

> ### MEDICAL TERMINOLOGY
> **alveol/o**: alveolus
> **alveolus** (singular), **alveoli** (plural)
> **bronch/o, bronchi/o**: bronchus
> **bronchiol/o**: bronchiole
> **bronchus** (singular), **bronchi** (plural)
> **diaphragm/o, diaphragmat/o, phren/o**: diaphragm
> **lob/o, lobul/o**: lobe
> **mediastin/o**: mediastinum
> **pariet/o**: wall
> **pleur/o**: pleura
> **pleura** (singular), **pleurae** (plural)
> **pneumon/o, pulmon/o, pneum/o**: lung
> **thorac/o, steth/o, pector/o**: chest
> **trache/o**: trachea
> **viscer/o**: viscera

PHYSIOLOGY OF THE RESPIRATORY SYSTEM

The respiratory system has two primary functions:
- To exchange O_2 from the atmosphere for CO_2 waste
- To maintain the acid-base balance in the body

Ventilation

There are two types of respiration: external respiration and internal respiration. External respiration occurs when oxygenated air moves into the alveoli. Surrounding each alveolus is a pulmonary capillary network. The alveoli and the pulmonary capillaries are made of single-celled walls. This allows the O_2 to move easily across the alveoli and capillaries into the blood. CO_2 and other wastes are forced out of the capillaries and move into the alveoli. Internal respiration occurs when O_2 is exchanged for CO_2 in the blood. This exchange provides O_2-rich blood that is returned to the heart. The oxygenated blood is then pumped throughout the body. The CO_2 and other waste materials are excreted with exhalation. Ventilation is the process involved in this gaseous exchange.

Inspiration. A healthy person breathes when the blood CO_2 level increases. A person with chronic obstructive pulmonary disease (COPD) has a constantly elevated blood CO_2 level. At some point, the body no longer uses the elevated blood CO_2 level as a trigger to breathe. A secondary system kicks in. Breathing is triggered by a decreased blood O_2 level.

> **CRITICAL THINKING 11.2**
> Renee sees many patients with COPD using oxygen constantly. She realizes that the amount of oxygen is much lower than the amount providers give to ill "healthy" patients. Confused, she asks John why patients with COPD do not get the "typical dose" of oxygen. What might be John's response to her question?

When the breathing trigger is activated, it signals the medulla oblongata (the respiratory center) in the brainstem. The respiratory center causes a stimulus (i.e., signal) to be carried by the phrenic nerve to the diaphragm. When the diaphragm receives the signal, it flattens out and pulls downward. At the same moment, the intercostal muscles between the ribs contract. This causes the ribs to move outward and the chest cavity to enlarge. This movement causes the lungs to expand and increase their volume. The greater the contraction, the deeper the inhalation and the greater the air volume.

When individuals are experiencing respiratory distress, they are unable to move enough air into the lungs. To help move additional air into their lungs, they use accessory muscles. Accessory muscles are muscles in the neck, abdomen, and back that assist in breathing. To identify whether a person is using the accessory muscles, expose the chest and look for chest retractions with breathing. With intercostal retractions, the chest tissue in between the ribs is indrawn or pulled in during breathing. Upper airway obstructions can cause:
- suprasternal retractions (sucking in of the skin just above the sternum)
- supraclavicular retractions (sucking in of the skin just above the clavicle)

Lower airway obstructions can cause:
- substernal retractions (sucking in of the abdomen just below the sternum)
- subcostal retractions (sucking in of the abdomen just below the ribs)

Using accessory muscles to breathe can tire a person. This can lead to *respiratory arrest*, a medical emergency. Typically, this occurs quicker in infants and young children.

> **CRITICAL THINKING 11.3**
> The pulmonologist asks Renee to review the signs of respiratory distress with the mother of an asthmatic patient. Discuss what Renee should review with the mother.

> **VOCABULARY**
> **respiratory arrest**: Stoppage of breathing.

Expiration. The second half of ventilation is expiration. Once inspiration is complete, the diaphragm and intercostal muscles relax. This causes the diaphragm to move upward into the thoracic cavity and the ribs to move inward. This movement reduces the lung capacity and forces air out of the lungs. Typically, expiration requires very little energy. However, with some conditions (e.g., asthma and emphysema), the person has difficulty getting air out of the lungs. The accessory muscles are needed to help with complete exhalation.

Acid-Base Balance

The body attempts to keep the pH between 7.35 and 7.45. The respiratory system has an important role in the acid-base balance. It regulates the amount of CO_2 in our blood. CO_2 in the blood can combine with water to form the buffer bicarbonate. If a person *hyperventilates* (breathes rapidly), the CO_2 and bicarbonate levels in the blood decrease. This causes the pH of the body to rise, resulting in *respiratory alkalosis* (al kah LOW sis). This can be seen in patients with anxiety or an acute asthma attack. If hypoventilation occurs, the CO_2 in the blood increases (*hypercapnia* [hie per KAP nee ah]), and *respiratory acidosis* can occur. Respiratory alkalosis and respiratory acidosis are both life-threatening disorders if the underlying causes are not corrected.

DISEASES OF THE RESPIRATORY SYSTEM

Many diseases affect the respiratory system. The following sections describe in detail some of the more common diseases you will see in the ambulatory care setting. Table 11.1 defines terms related to respiratory symptoms.

Often providers describe what they hear in the lungs when a patient has a respiratory condition. Table 11.2 describes common abnormal lung sounds. Common diagnostic procedures used to help diagnose respiratory diseases are listed in Table 11.3.

> **CRITICAL THINKING 11.4**
> Renee needs to collect sputum from a patient who needs a sputum culture. Renee tells the patient that she needs the sputum to come from the lungs. The patient asks why she can't just use "spit" from his mouth. How might Renee respond?

TABLE 11.1 Terms Related to Respiratory Symptoms

Term	Word Origin	Definition
aphonia (ah FOH nee ah)	a- without; phon/o sound; -ia condition	Loss of ability to produce sounds.
apnea (AP nee ah)	a- without; -pnea breathing	Abnormal, periodic cessation of breathing.
bradypnea (brad IP nee ah)	brady- slow; -pnea breathing	Abnormally slow breathing.
Cheyne-Stokes respiration (shayne stokes)		Deep, rapid breathing followed by a period of apnea.
clubbing		Abnormal enlargement of the distal phalanges (fingers and toes) associated with cyanotic heart disease or advanced chronic pulmonary disease. Results from diminished oxygen (O_2) in the blood.
cyanosis (sye uh NOH sis)	cyan/o blue; -osis abnormal condition	Lack of O_2 in the blood, seen as bluish or grayish discoloration of the skin, nail beds, and/or lips.
dysphonia (dis FOH nee ah)	dys- difficult; phon/o sound; -ia condition	Difficulty making sounds.
dyspnea (DISP nee ah)	dys- difficult; -pnea breathing	Difficult and/or painful breathing.
epistaxis (ep ih STACK sis)	epi- above, upon; -staxis dripping, trickling	Nosebleed. Also called *rhinorrhagia*.
eupnea (YOOP nee ah)	eu- healthy, normal; -pnea breathing	Good, normal breathing.
hemoptysis (heh MOP tih sis)	hem/o blood; -ptysis spitting	Coughing up blood or blood-stained sputum.
hypercapnia (hye pur KAP nee ah)	hyper- excessive; capn/o carbon dioxide; -ia condition	Condition of excessive carbon dioxide (CO_2) in the blood.
hyperpnea (hye PURP nee ah)	hyper- excessive; -pnea breathing	Excessively deep breathing.
hyperventilation (hye pur ven tih LAY shun)	hyper- excessive	Abnormally increased breathing.
hypopnea (hye POP nee ah)	hypo- deficient; -pnea breathing	Extremely shallow breathing.
hypoxemia (hye pock SEE mee ah)	hypo- deficient; ox/o oxygen; -emia blood condition	Condition of deficient O_2 in the blood.
hypoxia (hye pock SEE ah)	hypo- deficient; ox/o oxygen; -ia condition	Condition of deficient O_2 in the tissues.
orthopnea (or THOP nee ah)	orth/o straight; -pnea breathing	Condition of difficult breathing unless in an upright position.
pleurodynia (ploor oh DIN ee ah)	pleur/o pleura; -dynia pain	Pain in the chest caused by inflammation of the intercostal muscles.
pyrexia (pye RECK see ah)	pyr/o fire; -exia condition	Fever.
rhinorrhea (rye noh REE ah)	rhin/o nose; -rrhea discharge	Discharge from the nose.
shortness of breath (SOB)		Breathlessness; air hunger.
sputum (SPYOO tum)		Mucus coughed up from the lungs and expectorated through the mouth. If abnormal, it may be described as to its amount, color, or odor.
tachypnea (tack ip NEE ah)	tachy- fast; -pnea breathing	Rapid, shallow breathing.
thoracodynia (thor uh koh DIN ee ah)	thorac/o chest; -dynia pain	Chest pain.

(From Shiland B: *Mastering healthcare terminology*, ed 5, St Louis, 2016, Mosby.)

TABLE 11.2 Terms Related to Abnormal Lung Sounds

Term	Definition
friction sounds	Sounds made by dry surfaces rubbing together.
hiccup (HICK up)	Sound produced by the involuntary contraction of the diaphragm, followed by rapid closure of the glottis. Also called *hiccough*.
rales (rayls)	An abnormal lung sound heard on auscultation, characterized by discontinuous bubbling noises. Also called *crackles*.
rhonchi (RON kye)	An abnormal rumbling sound heard on auscultation, caused by blockage of the airways by secretions or muscle contractions.
stridor (STRY dur)	High-pitched inspiratory sounds from the larynx; a sign of upper airway obstruction.
tympany, chest (TIM puh nee)	A low-pitched, resonant sound from the chest.
wheezing (WHEE zeeng)	A whistling sound made during breathing.

TABLE 11.3 Common Diagnostic Procedures for Respiratory Diseases

Performed by/Test Type	Procedure	Description
Provider during the exam	Lung sounds	The provider uses a stethoscope to listen to (or auscultates) the lung sounds as the patient inhales and exhales.
Medical assistant	Peak flow monitor	A handheld device that measures the exhaled air. It can also be used at home (Fig. 11.5 and 11.6).
	Pulse oximetry (ok SIM e tree)	A noninvasive test used to measure the oxygen saturation of the blood (Fig. 11.7).
	Spirometry test (spi ROM e tree)	Measures the volume of inhaled and exhaled air, and the time required for each. (Fig. 11.8).
Endoscopy	Bronchoscopy (bron KOS ko pee)	The insertion of an instrument (bronchoscope) through the mouth to visualize the trachea and bronchi.

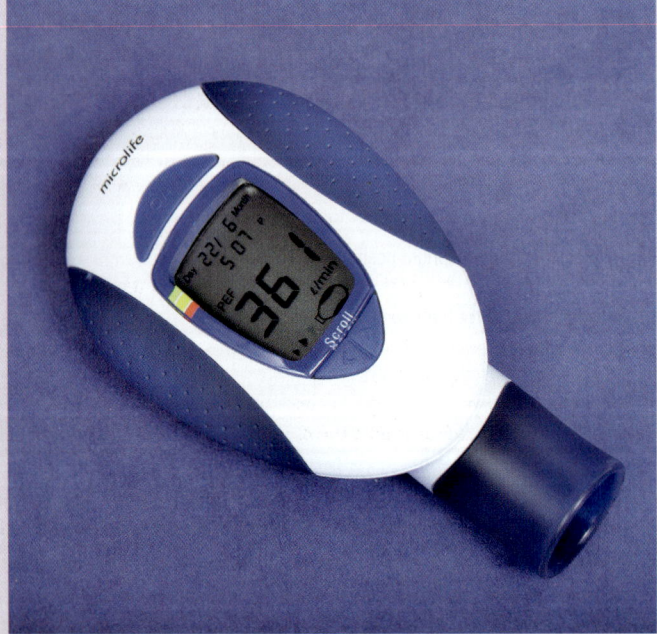

FIG. 11.5 Digital peak flow meter. (From Proctor D, et al: *Kinn's the medical assistant*, ed 13, St Louis, 2017, Elsevier.)

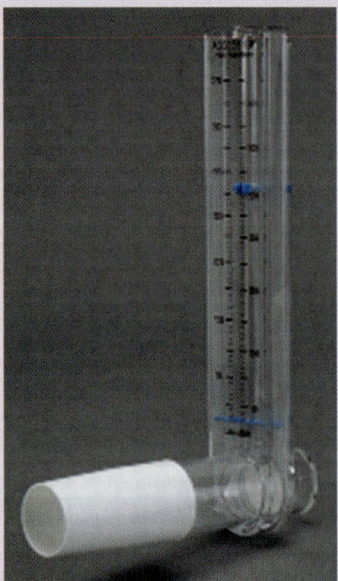

FIG. 11.6 Peak flow meter. (From Young AP, Proctor DB: *Kinn's the medical assistant*, ed 11, Philadelphia, 2011, Saunders.)

TABLE 11.3 Common Diagnostic Procedures for Respiratory Diseases—cont'd

Performed by/Test Type	Procedure	Description
Imaging procedures	Chest x-rays (CXRs)	Images taken from several directions, which provide a good outline of the heart and lungs. Abnormal air "pockets," fluid, and tumors can be seen on chest x-rays.
	Computed tomography (CT)	An imaging technique that can provide more information than chest x-rays.
	Magnetic resonance imaging (MRI)	An imaging technique that can provide more information than chest x-rays.
	Lung ventilation/perfusion scan (VQ scan)	A procedure in which a radioisotope substance is inhaled and also injected; then a special x-ray scanner creates a picture of the blood flow and airflow in the lungs.
	Pulmonary angiography (an jee AH gruh fee)	A procedure in which a catheter is inserted into the pulmonary blood vessels. Dye is injected, and x-ray pictures show the blood flow through the pulmonary vessels
Medical laboratory	CLIA-waived tests	• *Legionella* Urinary Antigen Test – for legionnaires' disease • Mono test – for infectious mononucleosis • Influenza A & B test – for influenza • Rapid strep A test – for strep throat • RSV test – for respiratory syncytial virus pneumonia
	Arterial blood gas (ABG)	A test in which a blood specimen is collected from the artery in the wrist, and the pH of the blood, carbon dioxide (CO_2) and oxygen (O_2) content are measured.
	Sputum cytology (sye TALL uh jee)	A test in which sputum is collected and examined under a microscope for abnormal cells.
	Sputum culture	A test in which sputum is collected and analyzed in the lab for bacterial growth over a period of days.

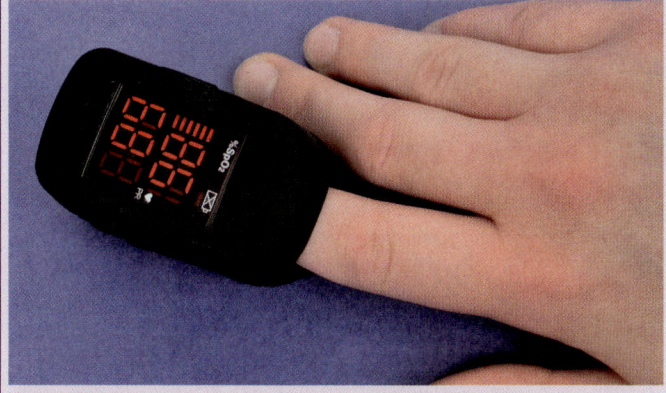

FIG. 11.7 Pulse oximeter. (From Proctor D, et al: *Kinn's The Medical Assistant*, ed 13, St Louis, 2017, Elsevier.)

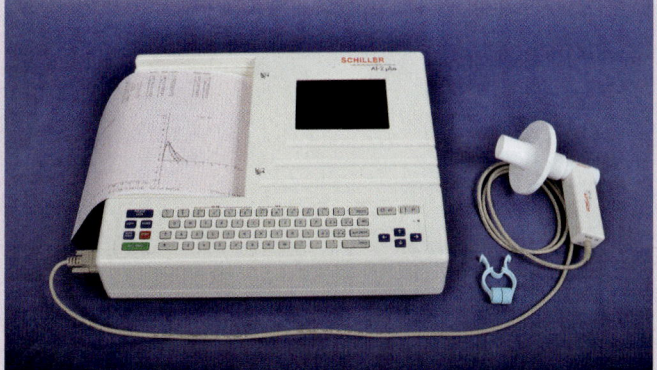

FIG. 11.8 Spirometer. (From Proctor D, et al: *Kinn's The Medical Assistant*, ed 13, St Louis, 2017, Elsevier.)

CLIA, Clinical Laboratory Improvement Amendments.

Asthma

Asthma (AZ muh) is a chronic disease that affects the airway. Bronchospasms and airway swelling narrow the passageway. Mucus in the lungs clogs the airway (Fig. 11.9). Getting air into and out of the lungs becomes harder. The frequency of asthma episodes can vary. Severe asthma attacks are life threatening and require immediate emergency care.

Etiology. Many different things can trigger an asthma episode. Common triggers include:
- Allergens (pollen, mold spores, pet dander, tobacco smoke, dust mites, cockroaches, and wood smoke, in addition to food, environmental, and medication allergens, such as nuts and latex)
- Environmental causes (chemical gases or fumes, dust, high humidity, and cold, dry air)
- Strong emotional states
- Strenuous physical exercise

Signs and Symptoms. Asthma symptoms can vary in type and frequency. Typical symptoms include:
- Shortness of breath or breathlessness
- Chest tightness or pain
- Coughing or wheezing attacks
- Early morning or nighttime coughing

Diagnostic Procedures. A complete medical history and a physical examination are important when diagnosing asthma. Diagnostic procedures typically used include:
- Peak flow monitoring
- Pulse oximetry
- Spirometry test

Treatment. Treatment for asthma is based on the severity of the disease. Asthma medications can be taken orally or inhaled. The medications taken can be grouped as long-term control or quick-relief medications (Table 11.4). Long-term control medications are usually taken

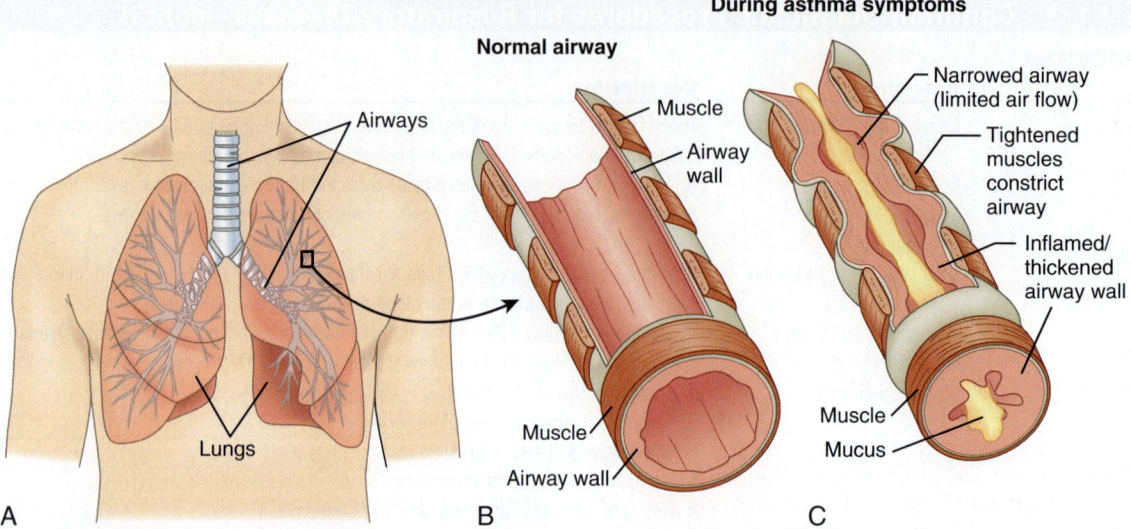

FIG. 11.9 Inflammation and bronchospasm. (From Proctor D, et al: *Kinn's The Medical Assistant*, ed 13, St Louis, 2017, Elsevier.)

TABLE 11.4	Asthma Medications
Long-Term Asthma Control Medications	**Quick-Relief Asthma Medications**
• Inhaled **corticosteroids**: fluticasone, budesonide, beclomethasone, and mometasone • Leukotriene modifiers: montelukast, zafirlukast, and zileuton • Long-acting beta agonist: salmeterol and formoterol • Combination inhalers: fluticasone-salmeterol, budesonide-formoterol, and formoterol-mometasone	• Short-acting beta agonists metered-dose inhalers (MDIs): albuterol and levalbuterol • Oral and intravenous corticosteroids

TABLE 11.5	Asthma Action Plan	
Zone	**Symptoms**	**Action to Take**
Green Zone – Doing Well	No asthma symptoms; peak flow is more than 80% of normal peak flow	Take prescribed long-term control medications
Yellow Zone – Asthma is getting worse	Asthma symptoms are present, or waking at night, or can't do usual activities, or peak flow is 50%–79% of normal peak flow.	Add quick-relief medication to the Green Zone medication. Continue to monitor. Contact provider if not improving.
Red Zone – Medical Alert	Very short of breath, or quick-relief medications have not helped, or peak flow is less than 50% of best peak flow.	Take short-acting beta agonist medication and/or oral steroid. Contact the provider immediately.

Adapted from National Institutes of Health. Asthma Action Plan. https://www.nhlbi.nih.gov/files/docs/public/lung/asthma_actplan.pdf. Accessed January 2, 2017.

daily. Quick-relief medications are usually taken during the asthma episode. They provide rapid, short-term relief. If the quick-relief medications do not reduce the episode, immediate emergency care is required.

Many providers recommend home use of peak flow monitors to monitor lung volume. These monitors measure the amount of air exhaled. The provider can set up an Asthma Action Plan (Table 11.5).

> **VOCABULARY**
>
> **corticosteroids:** A group of steroid hormones produced in the body or given as a medication. Some have metabolic functions, and others reduce tissue inflammation. Glucocorticoids and mineralocorticoids are two types.

Prognosis. The prognosis for asthma depends on the person's ability to stop the asthma episodes. The more controlled the asthma, the better the prognosis. Asthmatic symptoms may disappear as a child grows older. In some children the symptoms may disappear temporarily, only to return. Children with severe asthma may never outgrow it.

Prevention. Preventing asthma episodes from occurring is the best prevention. It is important to avoid triggers and to use the prescribed medication. If an episode starts, early detection and treatment are important. Allergy shots can help by reducing the immune system's reaction to allergens.

Bronchitis, Acute

Bronchitis (bron KIE tis) is an inflammation of the lining of the bronchial tubes. The bronchial tubes become irritated and swollen, narrowing the airway. Excessive mucus is produced, leading to increased coughing.

CRITICAL THINKING 11.5

Renee is working with an adult patient newly diagnosed with asthma. She has just explained how to use a peak flow monitor at home, and she and the patient have identified the patient's "normal" peak flow volume. As Renee explains the Asthma Action Plan the pulmonologist has ordered, the patient begins to look confused. He asks, "Why can't I just call or come in if I don't feel good? Why do I need to bother with the Asthma Action Plan?" What might be the benefits of using the Asthma Action Plan for the patient? How should Renee respond to the patient?

Bronchitis is classified as acute or chronic. We will focus on acute bronchitis in this section. Chronic bronchitis will be addressed in the section on COPD.

Etiology. Acute bronchitis is usually caused by a lower respiratory viral infection. Viral conditions. such as the common cold, influenza, and *pertussis* (whooping cough), can also cause acute bronchitis. In rare cases a bacterial infection causes the disease. In addition, breathing in irritants or inhaling food or vomit can cause acute bronchitis.

Signs and Symptoms. Symptoms of acute bronchitis include:
- a dry, hacking cough that can turn into a *productive cough*.
- a low-grade fever.
- fatigue and weakness.

> **VOCABULARY**
> **productive cough**: A cough that produces phlegm or mucus.

Diagnostic Procedures. After obtaining a medical history and performing an examination, the provider may order a chest x-ray. Pulse oximetry may also be performed.

Treatment. In most cases, acute bronchitis is viral, so no antibiotics are prescribed. At-home treatment may consist of:
- reducing the inhalation of irritants, such as smoke.
- using cough drops and a humidifier to soothe a dry throat.
- drinking plenty of fluids and getting adequate rest.
- using over-the-counter medications for the fever and body aches.

Prognosis. Acute bronchitis usually resolves in 2 to 3 weeks. A complication of acute bronchitis is bacterial pneumonia.

Prevention. To prevent acute bronchitis, it is important to limit your exposure to inhaled irritants.
- Use a mask when working with chemicals or paints that might irritate your lungs.
- Quit smoking and avoid breathing in secondhand smoke (Boxes 11.2 and 11.3).
- Get a yearly influenza vaccination.
- Practice good hand washing and disinfect surfaces. Also, cough and sneeze into tissues, which will help minimize infections that can lead to acute bronchitis.

Chronic Obstructive Pulmonary Disease

More than 11 million people in the United States have the disabling disease COPD. It is the third leading cause of death in the United States. But this condition is both treatable and preventable.

BOX 11.2 Health Risks Associated With Smoking and Smokeless Tobacco

Tobacco smoke contains more than 7000 chemicals. Of these, 250 are harmful, and at least 69 can cause cancer. It is estimated that 1 in 5 deaths are related to smoking. According to the Centers for Disease Control and Prevention (CDC), smokers are more likely to develop heart disease, lung cancer, and strokes. Smoking can cause the following effects.

- *Respiratory system*: pneumonia, chronic obstructive pulmonary disease, tuberculosis, asthma, and cancer of the trachea, bronchus, and lung
- *Nervous system:* stroke
- *Cardiovascular system*: aortic aneurysm, early abdominal aortic atherosclerosis in young adults, coronary heart disease, atherosclerotic peripheral vascular disease, and acute myeloid leukemia
- *Sensory system*: blindness, cataracts, age-related macular degeneration
- *Digestive system*: orofacial clefts (congenital defect from maternal smoking), periodontitis, and oropharynx, larynx, esophagus, stomach, liver, and colorectal cancers
- *Endocrine system*: type 2 diabetes mellitus and pancreatic cancer
- *Musculoskeletal system*: hip fractures, rheumatoid arthritis
- *Urinary system*: cancer of the bladder, kidney, and ureters
- *Immune system*: immune function issues
- *Reproductive system*: women – reproductive effects (e.g., reduced fertility), ectopic pregnancy, and cervical cancer; men – erectile dysfunction

Secondhand smoke causes lung cancer, strokes, low-birth-weight babies, and heart disease. Children exposed to secondhand smoke have an increased risk of sudden infant death syndrome (SIDS), ear infections, bronchitis, pneumonia, colds, and asthma.

The CDC reports that at least 28 cancer-causing chemicals have been found in smokeless tobacco (e.g., chew and dip). Smokeless tobacco can cause cancer of the mouth, pancreas, and esophagus.

Advantages of quitting:
- Blood pressure and heart rate begin to return to normal.
- Within a few hours, carbon monoxide levels in the blood decline.
- Within a few weeks, circulation improves and abnormal respiratory systems (e.g., cough, wheezing) decrease.
- One year after quitting smoking, the cardiovascular risks decrease sharply.
- Two to 5 years after quitting, the risk for stroke returns to a nonsmoker's level.
- Five years after quitting, the risk of cancer of the esophagus, bladder, throat, and mouth is cut in half.
- Ten years after quitting, the lung cancer risk decreases by 50%.

Available resources to quit:
- Websites, such as https://smokefree.gov
- National Cancer Institute (NCI) Smoking Quitline: 1-877-44U-QUIT (1-877-448-7848)
- Local resources
- Medications can also be helpful. These should be discussed with the healthcare provider.

Centers for Disease Control and Prevention (CDC). https://www.cdc.gov/tobacco/infographics/health-effects/index.htm#smoking-risks. Accessed July 29, 2017.

COPD develops slowly, making it hard to breathe. It includes two conditions:
- Emphysema (em fi SEE mah): Thinning and eventual destruction of the alveoli. This usually accompanies chronic bronchitis.
- Chronic bronchitis: Inflammation of the bronchial tubes, excessive production of mucus, and diminished activity of the cilia.

BOX 11.3 E-Cigarettes

E-cigarettes heat liquids to form an aerosol that is then inhaled. Many people call this "vaping." The liquids typically contain nicotine, flavorings, and other additives. E-cigarettes are considered tobacco products because they contain nicotine that comes from tobacco. The nicotine makes e-cigarettes addictive. The additives can pose health risks.

U.S. Surgeon General. Know the risks. https://e-cigarettes.surgeongeneral.gov/. Accessed July 29, 2017.

BOX 11.4 Alpha-1 Antitrypsin Deficiency

Alpha-1 antitrypsin (AAT) deficiency is a rare inherited disorder that can increase a person's risk for developing lung disease and liver disease. The onset of lung disease occurs at a younger age than normal (around 30 to 40 years of age).

AAT is a protein in the blood and lungs. It protects the lungs from chronic obstructive pulmonary disease (COPD). Sometimes a person may not make enough of this protein, or the AAT that is made is abnormal. Genetic testing is available to determine a person's risk. There is no cure for AAT deficiency, although the lung disease can be managed.

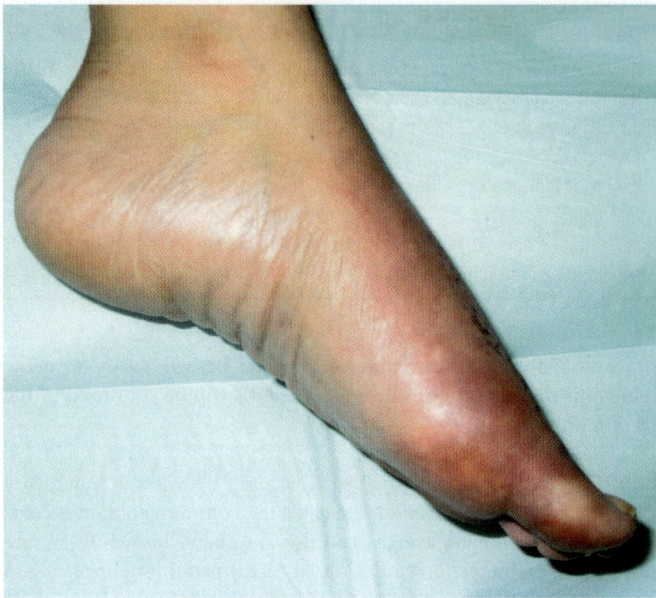

FIG. 11.10 Cyanosis of the lower foot and great toe. (From Shiland B: *Mastering Healthcare Terminology*, ed 5, St Louis, 2016, Mosby.)

Etiology. The main cause of COPD is smoking tobacco. Other causes include secondhand smoke, air pollution, dust, and chemical fumes. COPD can also be caused by an alpha-1 antitrypsin (AAT) deficiency (Box 11.4).

Signs and Symptoms. The symptoms of COPD often appear after damage has already been done to the lungs. With chronic bronchitis, a long-term, daily productive cough is seen. Additional symptoms of COPD include:
- Shortness of breath, chest tightness, breathlessness, wheezing
- Cyanosis of the lips and nail beds (Fig. 11.10)
- Lack of energy, fatigue
- Frequent respiratory infections

Diagnostic Procedures. The provider will obtain a medical history and perform an examination. Listening to the lungs with a stethoscope is part of the examination. Additional diagnostic tests include:
- Lung function tests: spirometry and pulse oximetry
- Chest x-ray or chest computed tomography (CT) scan
- Arterial blood gas test, which can indicate the severity of the COPD

CRITICAL THINKING 11.6

Renee is working with a patient who needs to have a pulse oximetry measurement. The patient asks Renee what this test shows. Thinking back to what you have learned already in this chapter, how should Renee answer the patient?

Treatment. There is no cure for COPD. The goals of treatment include slowing the disease progression and allowing the person to stay as active as possible. Treatments include:
- Quitting smoking and avoiding secondhand smoke
- Adequate nutrition
- Using **bronchodilators** and a bronchodilator-corticosteroid combination to reduce the inflammation.
- Vaccinations (influenza, pneumococcal)
- Low-level oxygen therapy

With severe COPD, surgical options may be considered:
- Lung volume reduction surgery (removal of damaged lung tissue)
- Lung transplantation

VOCABULARY

bronchodilators: A category of medication that relaxes smooth muscle contractions in the bronchioles to improve lung ventilation.

Prognosis. COPD is a chronic disease with symptoms that worsen over time. Any additional lower respiratory disease, such as influenza, can suddenly worsen the symptoms of COPD.

Prevention. To prevent COPD, stop smoking and reduce other lung irritants. This includes secondhand smoke, chemical fumes, and paint fumes. Use a protective mask when working around substances that can irritate the lungs.

Cystic Fibrosis

Cystic fibrosis (CF) (SIS tik fie BROE sis) is a life-threatening, congenital disease. Mucus builds up in the lungs, pancreas, and other organs. The mucus blocks the airways and increases the risk of infections. In the pancreas, the mucus interrupts the release of digestive enzymes used to break down food.

More than 30,000 people in the United States have cystic fibrosis. Half of them are age 18 or younger. All states require newborn screening tests for cystic fibrosis. With improvements in treatments, people with CF can live, work, and play with a much greater quality of life than in the past. Enzyme supplementation, respiratory drugs, and antibiotics have improved the prognosis in the past 25 years.

Etiology. Cystic fibrosis is a genetic disease. Each parent gives one copy of a specific gene to the child. As a result, the child gets two copies of a specific gene. If one of the copies is defective, the person will be a carrier of that disease. If both copies are defective, the person will have the disease (Box 11.5).

> ### BOX 11.5 What Are the Odds?
> If both parents are carriers of a defective cystic fibrosis (CF) gene, what is the chance for each child?
> - 50% chance the child will be a carrier of the defective CF gene
> - 25% chance the child will have cystic fibrosis
> - 25% chance the child will not be a carrier or will not have the disease

Signs and Symptoms. The signs and symptoms of CF depend on the severity of the disease. Symptoms include:
- Higher than normal levels of salt in the sweat
- A persistent cough that produces a thick, sticky sputum
- Breathlessness, shortness of breath, wheezing
- Frequent lung infections
- Foul-smelling, greasy stools
- Poor growth and weight gain
- Intestinal blockage, severe constipation
- Electrolyte imbalances

Diagnostic Procedures. To diagnose cystic fibrosis one of the following can be done:
- Two positive sweat tests (the tests must be performed on different days)
- Genetic testing, to detect two defective genes (for CF), and one positive sweat test

Treatment. There is no cure for CF. Treatment centers on reducing the complications and symptoms. Treatment can include:
- Antibiotics for lung infections
- Antiinflammatory medications to reduce the swelling in the lungs
- Mucus-thinning medications to help clear the lungs of mucus
- Bronchodilators to relax the airway muscles
- Chest physical therapy and vest therapy (vibrating vest) to help loosen mucus
- Oral pancreatic enzymes to help with digestion
- O_2 therapy
- Surgical options (bowel surgery for blockages, lung transplantation)

Prognosis. Cystic fibrosis is chronic and worsens over time. Chronic infections, pneumothorax, nutritional deficiencies, intestinal obstructions, diabetes, and acute respiratory failure (ARF) can occur.

Prevention. CF is a genetic disorder and cannot be prevented.

Infectious Mononucleosis

Infectious mononucleosis (also called "mono" and the "kissing disease") is a contagious disease. It is commonly seen in teens and young adults.

Etiology. Infectious mononucleosis is usually caused by the Epstein-Barr virus (EBV), although other viruses also can cause it. The virus is spread through body fluids, especially saliva. Blood from blood transfusions and semen are additional ways the virus can spread. Of those infected with EBV, about 25% will develop infectious mononucleosis.

Signs and Symptoms. In individuals who get infectious mononucleosis, the symptoms appear about 4 to 6 weeks after infection with EBV. Symptoms can include:
- Extreme fatigue, fever
- Sore throat, achiness
- Rash
- Swollen lymph nodes in the neck and axilla area.
- Swollen liver and/or spleen

Diagnostic Procedures. Many times infectious mononucleosis is diagnosed based on a person's medical history and the physical exam. In addition, providers may order a complete blood count (CBC), liver function tests, and a CLIA–waived mono test.

Treatment. Treatment usually includes keeping hydrated by drinking plenty of fluids, getting adequate rest, and taking over-the-counter medications for the discomfort and fever. Many providers will also encourage patients not to take part in any contact sports or similar activities that may increase the risk of rupturing an enlarged spleen.

Prognosis. Usually the symptoms diminish in 2 to 4 weeks, but for some it may take months for the symptoms to resolve.

Prevention. The best prevention against mononucleosis is not to kiss or share drinks, food, or toothbrushes with a person who has the disease.

> ### CRITICAL THINKING 11.7
> Renee is working with Julia Berkley, who has just been diagnosed with infectious mononucleosis. Julia tells Renee, "I heard that mononucleosis is called the 'kissing disease.' Why is that?" Thinking of what you have learned about infectious mononucleosis, how might Renee answer this question?

Lung Cancer

There are two main types of lung cancer, non–small cell and small cell. Non–small cell lung cancer is more prevalent. Lung cancer leads the cancer-related deaths in the United States.

Etiology. The leading cause of lung cancer is cigarette smoking. The longer a person has smoked and the more a person has smoked can increase the risk of lung cancer. High exposure levels of asbestos, radiation, and pollution can also increase a person's risk for lung cancer.

Signs and Symptoms. Common symptoms of lung cancer include:
- A chronic, worsening cough with hemoptysis
- Constant chest pain
- Wheezing, breathlessness, shortness of breath
- Fatigue, loss of appetite, weight loss
- Swelling of the face and hands
- More frequent episodes of pneumonia, bronchitis, or other lung infections
- Clubbing (KLUH bing) (Fig. 11.11)

> **VOCABULARY**
> **clubbing**: Abnormal enlargement of the distal phalanges (fingers and toes) associated with cyanotic heart disease or advanced chronic pulmonary disease.

Diagnostic Procedures. Tests used to diagnose lung cancer include:
- Chest x-rays and a chest CT scan
- Sputum cytology
- Bronchoscopy and biopsy of lung tissue (Fig. 11.12)

Treatment. Treatment for lung cancer is based on the person's health, the stage of the disease, and the person's preferences. Treatments can include:
- Chemotherapy and radiation therapy
- Targeted drug therapy
- Surgery (Table 11.6 and Fig. 11.13)

It is important for the person to learn how to cope with the shortness of breath and remain as active as possible. Learning to cope with cancer and its treatments is also important. In addition, some alternative approaches are encouraged, including acupuncture, yoga, massage, and meditation.

Prognosis. Currently there is no cure for lung cancer. The prognosis is based on the severity of the disease and the effectiveness of the treatments. A person who is diagnosed with an early stage of lung cancer has a longer life expectancy than someone who is diagnosed with late-stage lung cancer.

Prevention. To reduce your risk of lung cancer, stop smoking. Limiting inhalation of lung irritants (e.g., secondhand smoke, chemical fumes, and radon), exercise, and eating a healthy diet will also help reduce your risk.

TABLE 11.6	Common Surgical Options for Lung Cancer
Surgical Option	**Description**
Wedge resection	Removal of a small portion of the lung tissue. It includes the tumor and the healthy tissue on the edge of the tumor.
Segmental resection	Removal of a larger portion or segment of the lung
Lobectomy	Removal of a lobe of the lung
Pneumonectomy	Removal of the entire lung

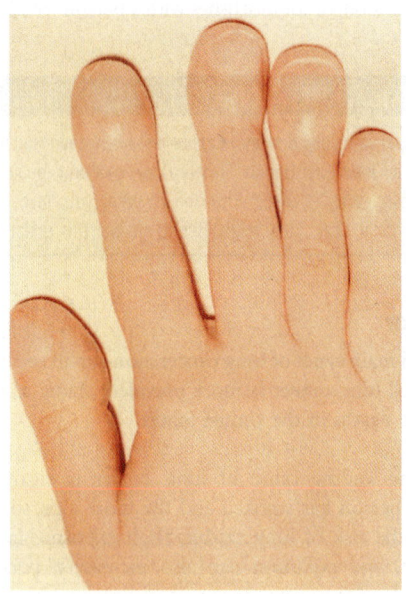

FIG. 11.11 Clubbing. (From Frowen P, et al: *Neale's disorders of the Foot*, ed 8, Oxford, 2010, Churchill Livingstone.)

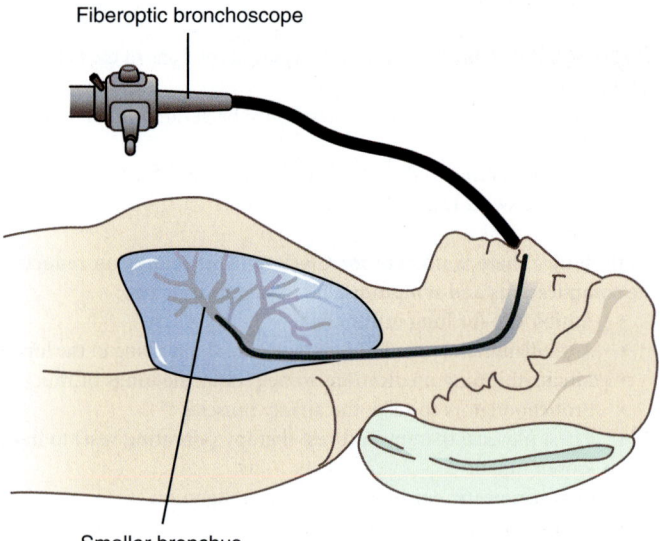

FIG. 11.12 Bronchoscopy. (From Shiland B: *Mastering healthcare terminology*, ed 5, St Louis, 2016, Mosby.)

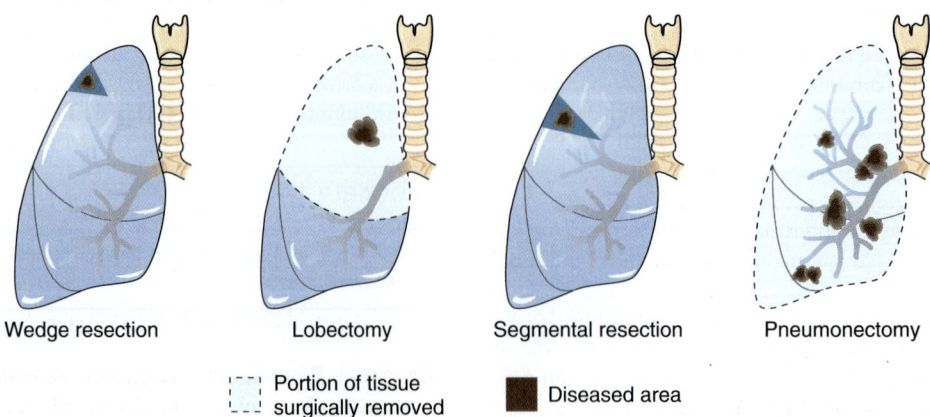

FIG. 11.13 Pulmonary resections. (From Shiland B: *Mastering healthcare terminology*, ed 5, St Louis, 2016, Mosby.)

Pneumonia

Pneumonia (noo MOAN yah) is an infection of the lungs. It may affect one or both lungs. The alveoli fill with fluid or pus. Those most at risk include:
- Young children and the elderly (over 65 years of age)
- People who smoke
- Those with one or more chronic illnesses

The severity of pneumonia can range from mild to life threatening. In the United States, about 1 million people have pneumonia a year, and about 50,000 people die from the disease. Adults are at most risk. Globally, it is the leading infectious disease killer of children under age 5.

> **CRITICAL THINKING 11.8**
>
> Renee is rooming Carl Bowden. He is here today for a recheck appointment. He was diagnosed 10 days ago with pneumonia. As Renee is gathering a history on Carl, he tells her that he has smoked 2 packs a day for the past 30 years. He also states that he has had pneumonia six times over the past 2 years. He asks Renee if smoking might have something to do with that. Thinking back to the respiratory structures and functions you have learned in this chapter, how might Renee answer his question?

Etiology. Pneumonia can be caused by many different pathogens, including:
- Bacteria (Streptococcus pneumoniae)
- Viruses (influenza and respiratory syncytial virus)
- Fungi

Various chemicals can also cause pneumonia. If a person has viral pneumonia, there is also a risk of getting bacterial pneumonia.

Signs and Symptoms. Symptoms of pneumonia can vary based on the severity of the illness. Typical symptoms include:
- High fever, chills
- Productive cough, shortness of breath
- Chest pain with breathing or coughing
- Low appetite, fatigue
- Confusion in the elderly

Diagnostic Procedures. Providers will listen to a patient's lungs for abnormal sounds. Chest x-rays, a CBC, sputum culture, and pulse oximetry are typical diagnostic procedures used to check for pneumonia.

Treatment. Treatment for pneumonia is based on the type of pneumonia a person has. Common treatments include:
- Antibiotics for bacterial pneumonia
- Antiviral medications for viral pneumonia
- Drinking plenty of fluids and getting rest
- Over-the-counter **antipyretics** (an tie pie RET ik) and **analgesics** (an ahl JEE ziks) (e.g., ibuprofen and acetaminophen)

Using over-the-counter cough medications may be discouraged. Coughing is a natural reflex to help clear the lungs. However, if coughing affects a person's sleep, the provider may recommend taking medication.

Prognosis. Within a week, typically older children and younger adults return to normal. It can take weeks for older adults to feel better. Pneumonia can cause many complications, including respiratory failure and sepsis. If complications occur, the prognosis may not be as good.

> **BOX 11.6 Vaccines That Lower Pneumonia Risk**
> - *Haemophilus influenzae* type b (Hib)
> - Pneumococcal
> - Influenza (flu)
> - Measles (MMR)
> - Pertussis (DTaP, TDaP)
> - Varicella (chickenpox)

Prevention. To lower the risk of getting pneumonia, stay current on your vaccinations (Box 11.6). Reducing the risk of infection is also important. Washing your hands frequently, disinfecting surfaces, and coughing or sneezing into your elbow or into a tissue are important.

> **VOCABULARY**
> **analgesics**: A category of medication used to relieve pain.
> **antipyretics**: A category of medication used to reduce a fever.
> **pulmonary hypertension**: High blood pressure that affects the pulmonary system (pulmonary arteries and the right side of the heart).

Pulmonary Embolism

Pulmonary embolism (PE) is a condition in which one of the pulmonary arteries is blocked. PE is a medical emergency and can be life threatening. Due to the blockage:
- blood flow may be interrupted to that section of the lung. This can lead to **pulmonary hypertension**.
- oxygen can be limited to other body organs.

Etiology. Often PE is a complication of deep vein thrombosis (DVT). Blood clots form in the veins, usually in the legs. Some of the clots break off and travel through the bloodstream. Eventually, the clot blocks a pulmonary artery.
Risk factors for PE include:
- Current or past DVT
- Being bedridden, having surgery
- Breaking a bone
- Pregnancy
- Chronic illness (stroke, hypertension, chronic heart disease, obesity)
- Smoking
- The use of birth control pills or hormone therapy pills

Signs and Symptoms. Signs and symptoms of pulmonary embolism include:
- Problems breathing or unexplained shortness of breath
- Chest pain
- Coughing or coughing up blood
- Arrhythmia
- Lightheadedness, fainting, rapid breathing and pulse

Diagnostic Procedures. Besides a medical history and physical examination, the provider may order the following diagnostic procedures:
- Ultrasound: to detect DVT in the legs
- CT scan with contrast: to detect PE or DVT

- Lung ventilation/perfusion scan (VQ scan)
- Pulmonary angiography
- Chest x-ray and chest magnetic resonance imaging (MRI)
- Echocardiography and electrocardiogram (ECG)

Treatment. The goals of treatment include preventing more clots or larger clots from forming. Treatment includes:
- *Anticoagulants*: "blood thinners" (e.g., warfarin [Coumadin] and heparin) help stop the clots from forming.
- *Thrombolytics*: medications that break up the clot. These are used in emergencies. Thrombolytics can be delivered by a catheter to the site of the clot.
- Compression stockings: to help prevent blood from pooling and clotting in the legs.

Prognosis. The prognosis depends on the size of the PE and the length of time before treatment is initiated. If the clot is large or many clots develop in the lungs, death can occur.

Prevention. If a person has a history of DVTs, it is important to follow the treatment plan of medications and compression stockings to prevent future clot development.

Pulmonary Tuberculosis

Pulmonary tuberculosis (TB) (too bur kyoo LOH sis) is caused by bacteria that can affect the lungs. There are two TB-related conditions: latent TB infection and TB disease (Table 11.7).

Etiology. Tuberculosis is caused by Mycobacterium tuberculosis, which is spread through the air. A person with TB disease can spread it by coughing, sneezing, singing, or talking. Individuals at risk for TB include:
- Anyone who has lived in a country where TB is prevalent
- Anyone in frequent close contact with someone with TB disease
- Those working in health care, a homeless shelter, or a prison
- Those living in a nursing home, prison, or homeless shelter
- People who have latent TB infection and a weakened immune system – TB can become active under these conditions.

Signs and Symptoms. TB disease in the lungs can cause a bad cough that lasts 3 or more weeks, pain in the chest, and blood in the sputum. Other symptoms include:
- Weakness
- No appetite and weight loss
- Chills, fever, and night sweats

Diagnostic Procedures. Initially, the person is tested with either a Mantoux tuberculin skin test (TST) (also known as a purified protein derivative [PPD] test) or a TB blood test (e.g., QuantiFERON-TB Gold [QFT], T-SPOT.TB). If the test is positive, then the person will have additional testing to determine if it is latent TB infection or TB disease. Additional testing includes chest x-rays and sputum cultures.

Treatment. For TB disease, isoniazid, rifampin, ethambutol, or pyrazinamide may be prescribed. For latent TB infections, isoniazid or rifapentine may be prescribed. The medication treatment may last up to 9 months.

Prognosis. Most people recover from pulmonary TB with treatment. Symptoms usually improve within 2 to 3 weeks after starting the medication. With the length of treatment, **adherence** to the treatment plan is important to prevent drug-resistant TB. At times TB maybe reactivated, or latent TB infection can lead to TB disease. This is seen more in the elderly, in infants, and in people with weakened immune systems due to disease or medications.

TABLE 11.7 Comparison of Latent TB Infection and TB Disease

	Latent TB Infection	TB Disease
Signs/Symptoms	None; doesn't feel sick	Has signs and symptoms; feels sick
Spreads Disease to Others?	Cannot spread tuberculosis (TB) bacteria to others	May spread TB bacteria to others
Test Results	Skin test or blood test indicates TB infection. Chest x-ray is normal, and sputum smear/culture is negative.	Skin test or blood test indicates TB infection. Chest x-ray is abnormal, and sputum smear/culture is positive.
Treatment	Needs treatment to prevent TB disease	Needs treatment to treat disease
Prognosis	Often latent TB infections do not turn into TB disease, but a weakened immune system can increase the risk of TB disease.	With treatment, symptoms tend to diminish within 2-3 weeks.

> **VOCABULARY**
> **adherence:** The act of sticking to something.

Prevention. In some countries, people receive bacille Calmette-Guérin (BCG) vaccine to prevent TB. Anyone who has received a BCG vaccine will always have a positive TB skin test. However, the TB blood test will be unaffected by a prior BCG immunization. (See Chapter 38). BCG vaccine is not generally recommended in the United States. The best prevention is to stay away from those with TB disease. If a person is exposed to tuberculosis, prompt testing and treatment will prevent the spread of the disease.

Respiratory Syncytial Virus Pneumonia

Respiratory syncytial (sin SISH uhl) virus (RSV) produces upper respiratory "cold" symptoms in healthy older children and adults. For young children and adults with medical problems, it can cause pneumonia and severe breathing problems.

> **CRITICAL THINKING 11.9**
> Renee is confused about the two different types of tuberculosis (TB). She asks John to summarize the difference between latent TB infection and TB disease. How might John answer this question?

Etiology. RSV spreads by coughing or sneezing. The virus can survive for several hours on infected surfaces. Typical outbreaks of RSV occur in winter and early spring.

Signs and Symptoms. RSV can cause nasal congestion, low-grade fevers, a runny nose, and a mild cough. Complications can include a barking cough from swelling near the vocal cords, high fevers, wheezing, apnea, cyanosis, and difficulty breathing.

Diagnostic Procedures. The provider will check the lungs for wheezing and other abnormal lung sounds. Additional diagnostic procedures include:
- Pulse oximetry
- Chest x-rays
- Laboratory tests: blood tests to check for infection; a CLIA–waived RSV test; and viral cultures of the respiratory secretions from the nose

Treatment. Treatment consists of over-the-counter medication (acetaminophen [Tylenol]) for the fever and plenty of fluids to prevent dehydration. People with severe cases of RSV are hospitalized. Supplemental oxygen, albuterol breathing treatments, and epinephrine (inhaled) may also be given.

Prognosis. By age 2, most children have been infected with RSV. The symptoms of RSV usually resolve in 8 days, and the prognosis is good.

Prevention. Steps to preventing RSV include:
- Frequent hand washing
- Covering your mouth when coughing
- Disinfecting surfaces
- Staying home
- Avoiding those with RSV, if possible

> **VOCABULARY**
> **decongestants**: A category of medication used for nasal congestion.
> **pharyngitis**: Inflammation or infection of the pharynx, usually causing symptoms of a sore throat.
> **pleural effusion**: Abnormal accumulation of fluid in the intrapleural space around the lungs.
> **thoracentesis**: Aspiration of a fluid from the pleural cavity.

Respiratory Tract Diseases, Lower

Lower respiratory tract diseases affect the lungs and trachea. Table 11.8 covers additional lower respiratory diseases.

Respiratory Tract Diseases, Upper

Upper respiratory tract diseases affect the respiratory tract structures above the chest. Table 11.9 covers additional upper respiratory tract diseases.

Additional Respiratory System Diseases

There are many respiratory diseases. Table 11.10 provides a brief description of additional common respiratory diseases.

Text continued on p. 258

TABLE 11.8 Lower Respiratory Tract Diseases

Disease	Croup (croop)	Influenza (in floo EN zah)	Pertussis (pur TUSS is)	Pleurisy (PLOOR ih see)	Pneumothorax (noo moh THOR acks)
Description	Inflammation of the trachea and larynx	Acute infectious disease of the respiratory tract; also called *flu*	Bacterial infection of the respiratory tract, marked by a characteristic high-pitched "whoop"; also called *whooping cough*	Infection of the pleura	Air or gas in the pleural space, causing the lung to collapse (Fig. 11.14)
Etiology	Variety of viruses, including influenza	Influenza viruses; spread by droplets from coughing or sneezing	*Bordetella pertussis* (bacteria); very contagious, spread by coughing or sneezing	Bacteria, fungus, parasites, or viruses; also caused by inhaled toxins	Rupturing of a small blister on the lung's surface; trauma; may occur secondary to other respiratory conditions
Signs and Symptoms	Harsh, bark-like cough; hoarseness, fever, inspiratory stridor	Fever, cough, sore throat, muscle aches, headaches, fatigue, cough	Early stage (lasts 1-2 weeks): runny nose, low-grade fever, mild cough, apnea in babies Later stage (symptoms may last over 10 weeks): fits of many, rapid coughs, followed by a whooping sound, vomiting, and exhaustion	Stabbing pain, especially with inspiration, cough, fever, chills, and dyspnea	Sudden, sharp pleuritic pain that increases with movement, breathing, or coughing; shortness of breath, cyanosis, rapid pulse, respiratory distress

Continued

TABLE 11.8 Lower Respiratory Tract Diseases—cont'd

Disease	Croup (croop)	Influenza (in floo EN zah)	Pertussis (pur TUSS is)	Pleurisy (PLOOR ih see)	Pneumothorax (noo moh THOR acks)
Diagnostic Procedures	Cultures to identify causative organism; neck and chest x-ray	History and physical, nasopharyngeal swab, and rapid influenza diagnostic tests (CLIA waived)	History of cold, physical exam, nasopharyngeal specimen culture, PCR (rapid test)	Pleural friction rub is heard over the lung field, chest x-ray, ultrasound, CT scan	Decreased breathe sounds heard over the collapsed lung field, chest x-ray, CT scan, pulse oximetry, and arterial blood gases
Treatment and Follow-Up	Antipyretics, humidifier, bed rest, increase fluid intake, sitting may help child breathe easier. In severe cases, hospitalization with antibiotic and oxygen therapy.	Bed rest, increased fluids, antiviral medications, analgesics	Antibiotics, stay home, good hand washing, humidifier	Analgesics, antiinflammatory agents, bed rest, **thoracentesis** (thor ack sen TEE sis)	Treatment depends on cause of collapse; bed rest and monitoring of vital signs, chest tube, surgical procedures to remove a portion of the pleura (*pleurectomy*)
Prognosis	Good with treatment. Symptoms usually resolve in a few days.	Depends on severity. Complications can occur, including pneumonia, asthma, heart conditions, and death.	Complications can include death in young children and tissue injury from coughing and pneumonia.	Good, although **pleural effusion** (PLOOR ul eh FYOO zhun) may occur.	Good with treatment. Spontaneous pneumothorax may recur.
Prevention	Prompt treatment of respiratory tract infections	Yearly influenza vaccine	Pertussis vaccine (DTaP, TDaP)	Early treatment of respiratory illnesses	After spontaneous pneumothorax, refrain from extreme atmospheric pressure changes

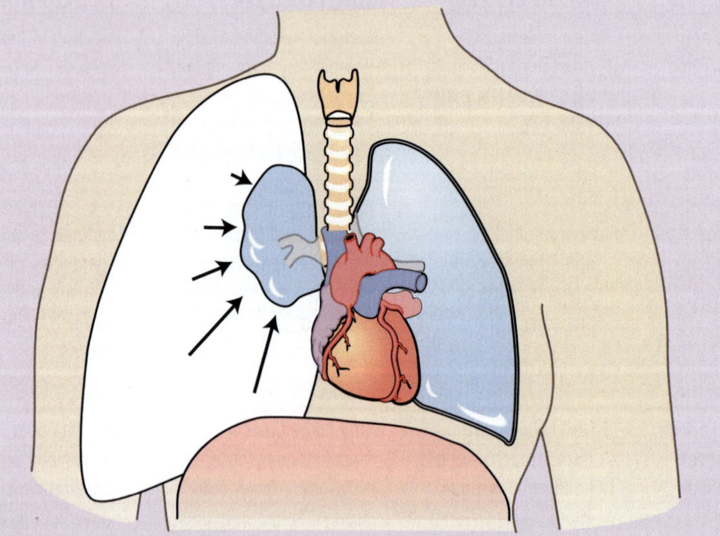

FIG. 11.14 Pneumothorax. The lung collapses as air gathers in the pleural space. (From Shiland B: *Mastering healthcare terminology*, ed 5, St Louis, 2016, Mosby.)

CLIA, Clinical Laboratory Improvement Amendments; *CT*, computed tomography; *PCR*, polymerase chain reaction.

TABLE 11.9 Upper Respiratory Tract Diseases

Disease	Epiglottitis (eh pee glah TYE tis)	Laryngitis (lair in JYE tis)	Sinusitis (sye nuh SYE tis)	Strep throat (strep)
Description	Life-threatening inflammation of the epiglottis (Fig. 11.15)	Inflammation of the voice box (larynx)	Inflammation of the sinuses	Highly contagious bacterial infection of the throat.
Etiology	*Haemophilus influenzae* type b, *Streptococcus pneumoniae*, or viruses (herpes simplex, varicella-zoster)	Overuse, irritation, or infection	Structural abnormalities or a cold may cause mucus to pool and pathogens to grow	Group A streptococcal bacteria are highly contagious. They spread by airborne droplets and by sharing food.
Signs and Symptoms	High fever, **pharyngitis** (fair in JYE tis), stridor, cyanosis, drooling, difficulty breathing and swallowing, hoarseness	Hoarseness, weakened (or loss of) voice, tickling sensation, sore or dry throat, dry cough	Fever, weakness, fatigue, nasal and sinus congestion, cough, bad breath or loss of smell	Rash, nausea and vomiting, fever, headache, painful swallowing, sore throat, tiny red spots at the back of the mouth
Diagnostic Procedures	Viewing the back of the throat during exam, blood/throat cultures, CBC, neck x-ray	History and physical exam. For chronic problems, laryngoscopy, biopsy.	History and physical exam, x-rays	History and physical, rapid antigen test (CLIA waived), throat culture
Treatment and Follow-Up	Hospitalization, humidified oxygen, antibiotics, corticosteroids	Antibiotics, corticosteroids, increase fluid intake, rest voice, breathe moist air	Antibiotics, decongestants, analgesics, heating pads, saline nasal sprays, vaporizers	Antibiotics, stay home until on antibiotics for 24 hours, analgesics
Prognosis	Good with proper care	Acute: lasts 2-3 weeks	Most cases resolve with home care and medication. If repeated cases occur, additional checking should be done for abnormalities.	Good if treated quickly. Can lead to additional infections (sinuses, skin, blood) and inflammatory reactions (scarlet fever, rheumatic fever, poststreptococcal glomerulonephritis).
Prevention	Hib vaccine	Avoid inhaled irritants	Avoid irritants, individuals with colds; practice good hand washing	

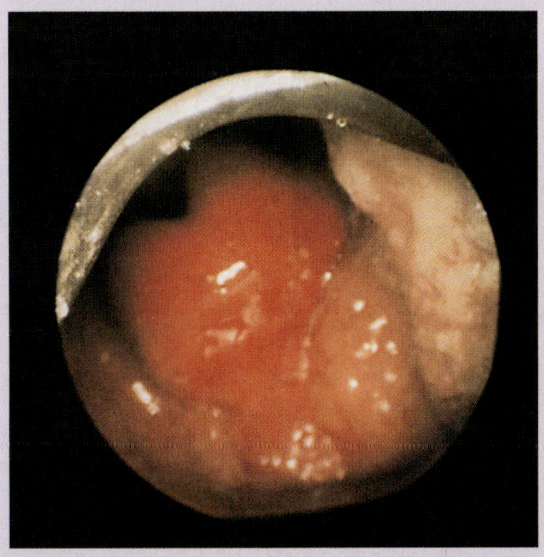

FIG. 11.15 Epiglottitis. The epiglottis is red and swollen. (From Shiland B: *Mastering healthcare terminology*, ed 5, St Louis, 2016, Mosby.)

CBC, Complete blood count; *CLIA*, Clinical Laboratory Improvement Amendments; *Hib*, *Haemophilus influenze* type b

TABLE 11.10 Additional Respiratory System Diseases

Disease	Description
Acute respiratory failure (ARF)	A sudden inability of the respiratory system to provide oxygen (O_2) and/or remove carbon dioxide (CO_2) from the blood.
Adult respiratory distress syndrome (ARDS)	Life-threatening condition causing severe pulmonary congestion, hypoxemia, and acute respiratory distress.
Allergic rhinitis (rye NYE tis)	Inflammation of the nasal mucosa, caused by an environmental allergen. Also called *hay fever*.
Anosmia (an OZ mee ah)	Loss of the sense of smell.
Anthracosis (an thrah KO sis)	Loss of lung capacity caused by an accumulation of coal dust in the lungs; also called *black lung disease* or *coal workers' pneumoconiosis* (CWP).
Asbestosis (as bes TOE iss)	Loss of lung capacity, caused by an accumulation of asbestos in the lungs.
Atelectasis (at ih LECK tuh sis)	Collapse of lung tissue or an entire lung.
Avian flu	Results from transmission of the avian influenza virus to humans, causing a life-threatening condition. Also called *bird flu*.
Bronchiectasis (brong kee ECK tuh sis)	Chronic dilation of the bronchi. Symptoms include dyspnea, expectoration of foul-smelling sputum, and coughing.
Bronchiolitis (brong kee oh LYE tis)	Viral inflammation of the bronchioles. It is more common in children younger than 18 months.
Bronchitis (bron KIE tis)	Inflammation of the bronchi. It may be acute or chronic.
Deviated septum (DEE vee a tid SEP tum)	Nasal septum that is not on the midline, causing one of the nares to be smaller than the other.
Diphtheria (diff THEER ee ah)	Bacterial respiratory infection, characterized by a sore throat, fever, and headache.
Epistaxis (ep ih STACK sis)	Nosebleed.
Flail chest (flale)	Unstable chest wall, resulting from fracture (breaking) of the ribs and/or sternum. (Fig. 11.16).
Hemothorax (hee moh THOR acks)	Accumulation of blood in the pleural cavity (between the lung and the chest wall) (Fig. 11.17).
Histoplasmosis (his toe plaz MOE sis)	Fungal disease of the lungs, caused by inhalation of *Histoplasma capsulatum*. *H. capsulatum* is found in soil and dust contaminated with bird or bat droppings.

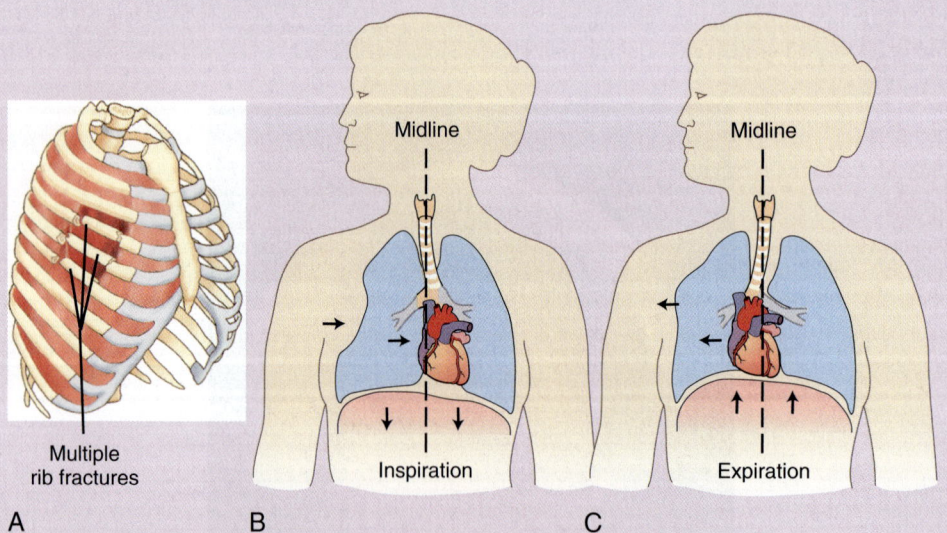

FIG. 11.16 Flail Chest. (A) Fractured rib sections are unattached to the rest of the chest wall. (B) On inspiration, the flail segment of the ribs is sucked inward, causing the lung to shift inward. (C) On expiration, the flail segment of the ribs bellows outward, causing the lung to shift outward. Air moves back and forth between the lungs instead of through the upper airway. (From Shiland B: *Mastering healthcare terminology*, ed 5, St Louis, 2016, Mosby.)

TABLE 11.10 Additional Respiratory System Diseases—cont'd

Disease	Description
Influenza A (H1N1) infection (in floo EN zah)	Results from transmission of the novel influenza A (H1N1) virus to humans, causing influenza symptoms, diarrhea, and vomiting. Also called *swine flu*.
Laryngeal cancer (lah rin JEE ahl)	Malignant tumors in the larynx, usually caused by squamous cell carcinomas.
Legionnaires' disease (lee jon NARES)	Bacterial pneumonia caused by *Legionella* bacteria. These bacteria are found in lakes, streams, water tanks, hot tubs, and air conditioners.
Nasal polyps (PAWL ups)	Benign, teardrop-shaped growths in the sinuses and nose. They are often linked to allergies and asthma.
Nasopharyngeal carcinoma (NAE zoe fah RIN jee ahl kar sah NOE mah)	Malignant tumors in the pharynx, which can be related to diet or to the Epstein-Barr virus. They cause a mass in the neck, nasal obstruction, epistaxis, and serous otitis media (middle ear infection).
Obstructive sleep apnea (OSA) (APP nee ah)	Condition caused by narrowed or blocked airways, which become blocked when muscles relax during sleep. This results in apnea, loud snoring, and snort and gasp episodes.
Pharyngitis (fair in JYE tis)	Inflammation or infection of the pharynx, usually causing the symptoms of a sore throat.
Pulmonary abscess (PULL mun nair ee AB ses)	Localized collection of infectious material in the lungs.
Pulmonary edema (PULL mun nair ee eh DEE mah)	Accumulation of fluid in the lung tissue, caused by the inability of the heart to pump blood. It is often present in congestive heart failure.
Pyothorax (pye oh THOR acks)	Pus in the pleural cavity. Also called *empyema*.
Respiratory distress syndrome	Results from lack of surfactant in the lungs, which causes the alveoli to deflate. This is a life-threatening disease usually seen in premature infants.
Rhinomycosis (rye noh mye KOH sis)	Abnormal condition of fungus in the nose.
Sarcoidosis (sar koi DOE sis)	Condition that causes lesions to form in the lungs and chest lymph nodes. It can lead to chronic illness and organ damage. Its origin is unknown.
Severe acute respiratory syndrome (SARS)	Viral respiratory disorder, caused by a coronavirus. It usually results in pneumonia.
Silicosis (sil ih KOH sis)	Loss of lung capacity, caused by an accumulation of glass dust in the lungs.
Tonsillitis (TON sah lie tis)	Inflammation of the tonsils.
Upper respiratory tract infection	Inflammation and/or infection of the upper respiratory structures. Known as the common cold.

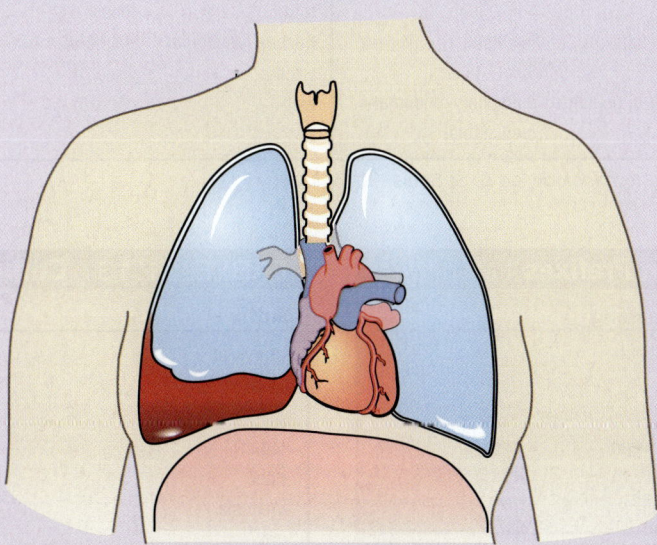

FIG. 11.17 Hemothorax. Blood below the right lung causes the lung to collapse. (From Shiland B: *Mastering healthcare terminology*, ed 5, St Louis, 2016, Mosby.)

LIFE SPAN CHANGES

Infants have a narrow airway. Their trachea is short and softer than that of an adult. If their necks are overextended, their airways can collapse. Infants tend to breathe through their noses. Respiratory illnesses that cause nasal congestion can make breathing difficult in infants. Infants are abdominal breathers and have immature respiratory muscles. Fatigue with breathing difficulties can set in quickly. With a disproportionately larger tongue and epiglottis, infants and young children are at risk for airway obstruction.

Around age 20 to 25, the lungs reach maturity. By age 35, lung function starts to decline. People who smoke can increase the aging in their lungs. As a person ages, the following respiratory system changes occur:
- Chest wall and thoracic spine deformities cause increased work of breathing.
- Diaphragm grows weaker, leading to decreased ability to inhale and exhale.
- Decrease in respiratory muscles causes the coughing reflex to be less effective.
- Decrease in tissue elasticity leads to inability to keep the airway completely open.
- Alveoli lose their shape and become baggy – these changes can allow air to be trapped in the lungs. This leads to a decrease in gas exchange and the lung capacity.

Pneumonia, asthma, and acute bronchitis are some of the most common reasons for hospitalization in children. Older people are at higher risk of getting pneumonia. Many providers will encourage older adults to keep their immunizations updated and to get the yearly influenza vaccine. COPD, lung cancer, and respiratory failure are also seen more in the elderly.

CLOSING COMMENTS

When you work in an ambulatory care setting, assisting patients with respiratory diseases is common. It is important for the medical assistant to understand the anatomical structures of this system and the physiology. Understanding the respiratory-related medical terminology, including the word parts, definitions, and common abbreviations, is vital when working with patients and providers (Tables 11.11 to 11.14). The medical assistant should also know the etiology, signs and symptoms, diagnostic procedures, treatments, prognosis, and prevention of common respiratory diseases.

TABLE 11.11 Combining and Adjective Forms for Respiratory Medical Terminology

Meaning	Combining Form	Adjective Form	Meaning	Combining Form	Adjective Form
adenoid	adenoid/o	adenoidal	mouth	or/o, stomat/o	oral
air	pneum/o, aer/o	pneumatic	mucus	muc/o	mucous
alveolus	alveol/o	alveolar	nose	nas/o, rhin/o	nasal, rhinal
bronchiole	bronchiol/o	bronchiolar	oxygen	ox/i, ox/o	
bronchus	bronch/o, bronchi/o	bronchial	pharynx (throat)	pharyng/o	pharyngeal
carbon dioxide	capn/o		pleura	pleur/o	pleural
chest	steth/o, thorac/o, pector/o	thoracic, pectoral	rib	cost/o	costal
diaphragm	diaphragm/o, diaphragmat/o, phren/o	diaphragmatic	septum, wall	sept/o	septal
			sinus	sinus/o, sin/o	
epiglottis	epiglott/o		to breathe	spir/o, hal/o	
eustachian tube	salping/o	salpingeal	tonsil	tonsill/o	tonsillar
larynx (voice box)	laryng/o	laryngeal	trachea (windpipe)	trache/o	tracheal
lobe	lob/o, lobul/o	lobar, lobular	viscera	viscer/o	visceral
lung	pulmon/o, pneumon/o, pneum/o	pulmonary, pneumatic	wall	pariet/o	parietal
mediastinum	mediastin/o	mediastinal			

(From Shiland B: *Mastering healthcare terminology*, ed 5, St Louis, 2016, Mosby.)

TABLE 11.12 Common Prefixes

Prefix	Meaning
a-	without
ex-	out
in-	in
inter-	between
para-	near
re-	again

(From Shiland B: *Mastering healthcare terminology*, ed 5, St Louis, 2016, Mosby.)

TABLE 11.13 Common Suffixes

Suffix	Meaning
-atory, -al	pertaining to
-ation	process of
-itis	inflammation
-logist	one who specializes in the study of
-pnea	breathing
-stenosis	narrowing
-um	structure

(From Shiland B: *Mastering healthcare terminology*, ed 5, St Louis, 2016, Mosby.)

TABLE 11.14 Common Abbreviations Related to Respiratory Diseases

Abbreviation	Definition	Abbreviation	Definition
ABG	arterial blood gas	O_2	oxygen
ARF	acute respiratory failure	OSA	obstructive sleep apnea
CF	cystic fibrosis	PPD	purified protein derivative
CO_2	carbon dioxide	QFT	QuantiFERON-TB Gold test
COPD	chronic obstructive pulmonary disease	RLL	right lower lobe (of the lung)
CPAP	continuous positive airway pressure	RML	right middle lobe (of the lung)
CT	computed tomography	RSV	respiratory syncytial virus
CXR	chest x-ray	RUL	right upper lobe (of the lung)
LLL	left lower lobe (of the lung)	SOB	shortness of breath
LUL	left upper lobe (of the lung)	TB	tuberculosis
MDI	metered dose inhaler	URI	upper respiratory infection
MRI	magnetic resonance imaging		

(From Shiland B: *Mastering healthcare terminology*, ed 5, St Louis, 2016, Mosby.)

CHAPTER REVIEW

The respiratory system is divided into the upper and lower tracts. The main functions of the respiratory system are bringing oxygen to the blood and removing waste products (CO_2) from the body. In healthy individuals, an increase in blood carbon dioxide levels triggers breathing. The respiratory center is triggered, and a message is sent via the phrenic nerve to the diaphragm. The diaphragm pulls downward while the intercostal muscles contract, causing lung expansion. Once the diaphragm and intercostal muscles relax, the diaphragm moves upward and the ribs move inward. This movement reduces the lung capacity and forces air to be exhaled.

Many respiratory diseases were discussed in this chapter. Common etiologies include:
- Allergies, smoking, and environmental irritants
- Viral or bacterial infections
- Structural changes

Common signs and symptoms of respiratory diseases affect the breathing and can cause abnormal lung sounds. Typical diagnostic tests ordered include:
- Peak flow monitoring, pulse oximetry, and spirometry
- Imaging procedures
- Laboratory tests (e.g., sputum cytology, sputum culture, arterial blood gas, and CLIA-waived tests [strep throat, legionnaires' disease, influenza, respiratory syncytial virus, and infectious mononucleosis])

The respiratory system changes with age. Infants and children are at risk for obstructions, pneumonia, acute bronchitis, and asthma. Older adults have many changes in the respiratory structures and have an increased risk for pneumonia.

SCENARIO WRAP-UP

As Renee works with John, she realizes she has a lot more to learn. Pulmonary disease is common. Renee decides to research the diseases she encounters every week. She feels that to be professional, it is important to be up-to-date on the latest information. She likes to be confident in her skills and knowledge. This helps when patients have questions about diseases, procedures, or treatments.

Renee looks forward to her weekly pulmonary experiences. She is confident in rooming patients, performing pulse oximetry, and gathering sputum specimens. She is excited about learning how to do peak flows and spirometry tests in the coming weeks.

12

Nervous System and Mental Health

LEARNING OBJECTIVES

1. List the major organs of the nervous system. Also, identify the anatomical location of these major nervous system organs.
2. Describe the normal function of the central nervous system.
3. Discuss the peripheral nervous system, including the cranial nerves.
4. Discuss the autonomic nervous system, including both the sympathetic and the parasympathetic nervous systems.
5. Describe the physiology of mental and behavioral health, including mental and behavioral health terminology, substance-related disorders, mood disorders, and personality disorders.
6. Identify the common signs, symptoms, and etiology of nervous system diseases.
7. Discuss the etiology, signs and symptoms, diagnostic procedures, treatment, prognosis, and prevention of cerebrovascular accidents.
8. Discuss the etiology, signs and symptoms, diagnostic procedures, treatment, prognosis, and prevention of epilepsy.
9. Discuss the etiology, signs and symptoms, diagnostic procedures, treatment, prognosis, and prevention of Parkinson's disease. Also, discuss additional diseases and disorders of the nervous system.
10. Discuss diagnostic procedures related to mental and behavioral health.
11. Discuss the etiology, signs and symptoms, diagnostic procedures, treatment, prognosis, and prevention of Alzheimer's disease, dementia, depressive disorders, and additional diseases and disorders related to mental and behavioral health.
12. Compare the structure and function of the nervous system, in addition to mental and behavioral health, across the life span.

CHAPTER OUTLINE

1. **Opening Scenario,** 261
2. **You Will Learn,** 261
3. **Introduction to the Nervous System,** 261
4. **Anatomy of the Nervous System,** 261
    a. Organization of the Nervous System, 261
    b. Cells of the Nervous System, 262
        i. *Neurons,* 262
        ii. *Neuroglia,* 263
5. **Central Nervous System,** 265
    a. Brain, 265
        i. *Cerebrum,* 265
        ii. *Cerebellum,* 266
        iii. *Diencephalon,* 266
    b. Brainstem, 266
    c. Spinal Cord, 266
        i. *Meninges,* 266
6. **Peripheral Nervous System,** 267
7. **Autonomic Nervous System,** 269
    a. Sympathetic Nervous System, 269
    b. Parasympathetic Nervous System, 270
8. **Physiology of Mental and Behavioral Health,** 270
    a. Mental and Behavioral Health Terminology, 271
    b. Substance-Related Disorders, 271
    c. Mood Disorders, 271
    d. Personality Disorders, 271
9. **Diseases and Disorders of the Nervous System,** 271
    a. Cerebrovascular Accident, 272
    b. Epilepsy, 274
    c. Parkinson's disease, 275
    d. Additional Diseases and Disorders of the Nervous System, 279
10. **Diseases and Disorders of Mental and Behavioral Health,** 279
    a. Diagnostic Procedures, 279
        i. *Mental Status Examination,* 279
        ii. *Laboratory Tests,* 283
        iii. *Imaging,* 283
        iv. *Psychological Testing,* 283
    b. Alzheimer's Disease and Dementia, 285
    c. Depressive Disorders, 287
    d. Additional Diseases and Disorders Related to Mental and Behavioral Health, 288
11. **Life Span Changes,** 288
12. **Closing Comments,** 293
13. **Chapter Review,** 293
14. **Scenario Wrap-Up,** 294

CHAPTER 12 Nervous System and Mental Health

▶ OPENING SCENARIO

Tia Rochester, CMA (AAMA), is a medical assistant at Walden-Martin Family Medicine (WMFM) Clinic. This is Tia's fourth week on the job. She recently graduated from a medical assisting program and passed her certification exam 5 days after graduation. She started working at WMFM shortly after she passed her exam. It has been a whirlwind few weeks. Tia likes the clinic and enjoys her co-workers and patients. This morning, Tia will be helping with a patient she has not met before, Elaine Pope Graham.

Elaine is 64 years old and in good overall health. She does not smoke or drink to excess. She likes to cook for herself and her husband, and she loves to try new recipes. She likes to walk in the local mall for exercise, and she loves to clean! Elaine is in for a physical, but she is also scheduled for some extra time because she wants to talk to the doctor about some symptoms that have been bothering her. She will be seeing Dr. Kahn today.

YOU WILL LEARN

- To recognize and use terms related to the nervous system.
- To locate the nervous system structures.
- To understand and describe the functions of the nervous system, which are to communicate, cooperate, and regulate body functions in order to maintain homeostasis.
- To recognize disease states of the nervous system. Also, their causes, signs and symptoms, diagnostic processes, treatment, prognosis, and prevention.
- To understand the role of the DSM-5 and the definitions of mental and behavioral health.
- To recognize and use terms related to the pathology of mental and behavioral health.
- To recognize and use terms related to the diagnostic procedures for mental and behavioral health.
- To recognize and use terms related to the therapeutic interventions for mental and behavioral health.

INTRODUCTION TO THE NERVOUS SYSTEM

The *nervous system* is a complex system that plays a major role in homeostasis (hoh mee oh STAY sis). The nervous system works in partnership with the endocrine system to help the body respond to its internal and external environments. This effort is responsible for communication and control throughout the body. There are three main functions of the nervous system:

- Collecting information about the external and internal environments (sensing)
- Processing this information and making decisions about action (interpreting)
- Directing the body to put into action the decisions made (acting)

For example, the sensory function begins with a *stimulus* (e.g., the uncomfortable pinch of a tight shoe). That information travels to the brain, where it is *interpreted*. The return message is sent to *react to the stimulus* (e.g., remove the shoe) (Box 12.1).

ANATOMY OF THE NERVOUS SYSTEM

Organization of the Nervous System

To carry out its functions, the nervous system is divided into two main subsystems. Fig. 12.1 shows a schematic of the divisions of the nervous system. The *central nervous system* (CNS) is composed of the brain and the spinal cord. It is the only site of nerve cells called *interneurons* (in tur NOOR ons), which connect sensory and motor neurons. The *peripheral* (puh RIF er uhl) *nervous system* (PNS) is composed of the nerves that extend from the brain and spinal cord to the tissues of the body. These are organized into 12 pairs of cranial (KREY nee uhl) nerves and 31 pairs of spinal nerves. The PNS is further divided into voluntary and involuntary nerves, which may be afferent (AF er uh nt) (or sensory), carrying impulses to the brain and spinal cord, or *efferent* (EF er uh nt) (or motor), carrying impulses from the brain and spinal cord to an organ, gland, or muscle.

MEDICAL TERMINOLOGY
home/o: same
inter-: between
-logy: study of
neur/o: nerve
-on: structure
somat/o: body
-stasis: stopping, controlling

BOX 12.1 Specialty and Specialist

Neurology (noo ROL uh jee) is the healthcare specialty that studies the nerves, especially their role in communication to and from the brain. It is also the study of the diseases and disorders of the nervous system. A *neurologist* (noo ROL uh jist) is a specialist involved in the diagnosis, treatment, and prevention of nervous system diseases and disorders.

Psychiatry (sih KAHY uh tree) is the healthcare specialty that studies the brain and its effects on the body. It is the study of the diseases and disorders of the nervous system as they affect the brain and behavior. A *psychiatrist* (sih KAHY uh trist) is a medical doctor who specializes in the diagnosis, treatment, and prevention of mental health diseases and disorders. A *psychologist* (sahy KOL uh jist) is a healthcare provider trained and educated to perform psychological research, testing, and therapy.

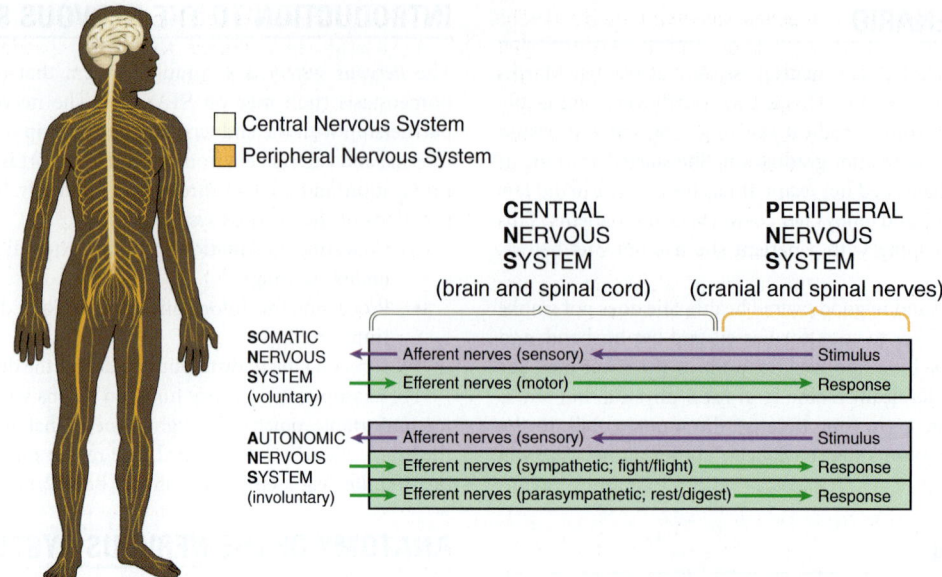

FIG. 12.1 The nervous system. Afferent nerves carry nervous impulses from a stimulus toward the central nervous system (CNS). Efferent nerves carry the impulse away from the CNS to effect a response to the stimulus. (From Shiland B: *Mastering healthcare terminology*, ed 5, St Louis, 2016, Elsevier.)

PNS nerves are further categorized into two subsystems:
- *Somatic* (soh MAT ick) *system:* This system is voluntary. The nerves collect information from and return instructions to the skin, muscles, and joints.
- *Autonomic* (ah toh NAH mick) *system:* This system is mostly involuntary. These nerves collect sensory information from the internal environment (organs and glands) and send it to the CNS. The return instructions come through motor impulses from the CNS to involuntary muscles, organs, and glands.

> ### ✱ STUDY TIP
> In the nervous system, *efferent* means to carry away from the brain, and *afferent* means to carry toward the brain.

Cells of the Nervous System

The nervous system is made up of two types of cells (Box 12.2):
- *neurons* (NOO R ons), the cells that carry out the work of the nervous system
- *glia* (GLEE uh), the cells that provide a supportive function to the neurons

Neurons. The basic unit of the nervous system is the nerve cell, or neuron (Fig. 12.2). Not all neurons are the same, but they all have features in common. *Dendrites* (DEN drytes) are branching projections that extend from the cell body. Dendrites receive nerve impulses and carry them to the cell body, which is the control center of the cell. From the cell body, the impulse moves away along the *axon* (AX on). The axon is a slender, elongated projection that carries the nervous impulse away from the cell and toward the next neuron.

> ### BOX 12.2 Names for Cells
> Neurons may be referred to parenchymal (puh RENG kuh muhl) cells, and glia cells may be referred to as stromal (STROH muhl) cells, or neuroglia.

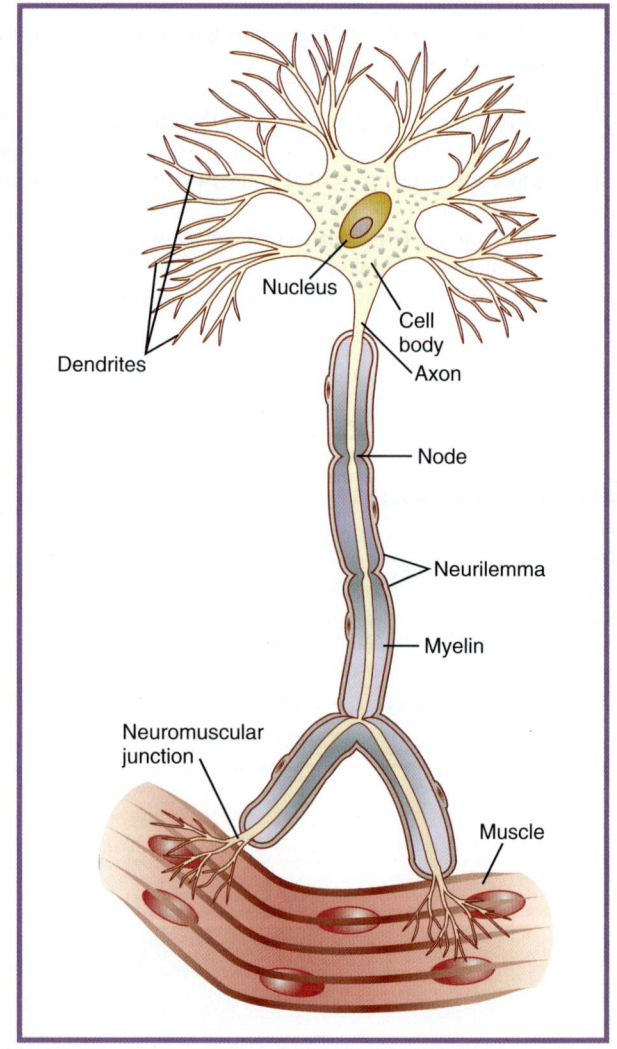

FIG. 12.2 The neuron. (From Proctor D, Niedzwiecki B: *Kinn's the medical assistant*, ed 13, St Louis, 2017, Elsevier.)

A nerve impulse is also called an *action potential* (Box 12.3). The transfer of the action potential begins as an electrical impulse that travels down an axon of one neuron. It then becomes a chemical impulse while moving across the *synapse* (SIN aps) to the dendrite of another neuron (Fig. 12.3) A synapse is the gap between two neurons. The transfer of impulses from the end of one neuron to the dendrites of another is enhanced by chemical **neurotransmitters** (noo roh TRANS mit ers) found in the synapse. Neurotransmitters (Box 12.4) bind to specific receptor sites on the dendrites of the next neuron or the **target tissue**. Messages move throughout the entire nervous system in this manner. Impulses in the neuron are electrical; the impulses become chemical as a neurotransmitter is released at each synapse. The action potentials become electrical again as they are picked up by the next dendrites of another neuron or by the target tissue.

Neuroglia. Supportive cells of the nervous system are called *glia*, or *neuroglia* (noo RAH glee ah) cells. Glial cells care for and support neurons throughout the body. These specialized cells perform specific functions within the nervous system. The list below explains the different types of neuroglia.

- *Schwann cells* (shwahn) form the **myelin** (MAHY uh lin) **sheath** that covers the axons of peripheral nerves.
- *Astrocytes* (AS truh sahyt) in the CNS help form the *blood-brain barrier* (BBB), which closely regulates what substances enter the brain tissue. Oxygen, water, and glucose molecules easily pass into the brain. Many chemicals and drugs are prevented from moving into brain tissue.
- *Microglia* (mahy kroh GLEE uh) are smaller than astrocytes and live in the CNS. If brain tissue is inflamed or damaged, microglia grow larger and move around. They hunt for microorganisms or debris to engulf and destroy.
- *Oligodendrocytes* (oh li goh DEN druh sahyt) also live in the CNS. They help hold nerve fibers together. They also produce the myelin sheath that surrounds the nerve fibers in the brain and spinal cord.

> **VOCABULARY**
> **myelin sheath:** A protective insulation, formed by Schwann cells, that covers PNS nerve axons. It helps with the transmission of nerve impulses.
> **neurotransmitter:** A chemical that helps a nerve cell communicate with another nerve cell or muscle.
> **target tissue:** The destination, or intended tissue of the nervous impulse (e.g., a muscle).

> **MEDICAL TERMINOLOGY**
> **astr/o:** star   **-glia:** glue
> **-cyte:** cell   **micro-:** small
> **dendr/o:** dendrite   **oligo-:** scant

> **CRITICAL THINKING 12.1**
> What type of cell produces the myelin sheath that surrounds some nerve axons?

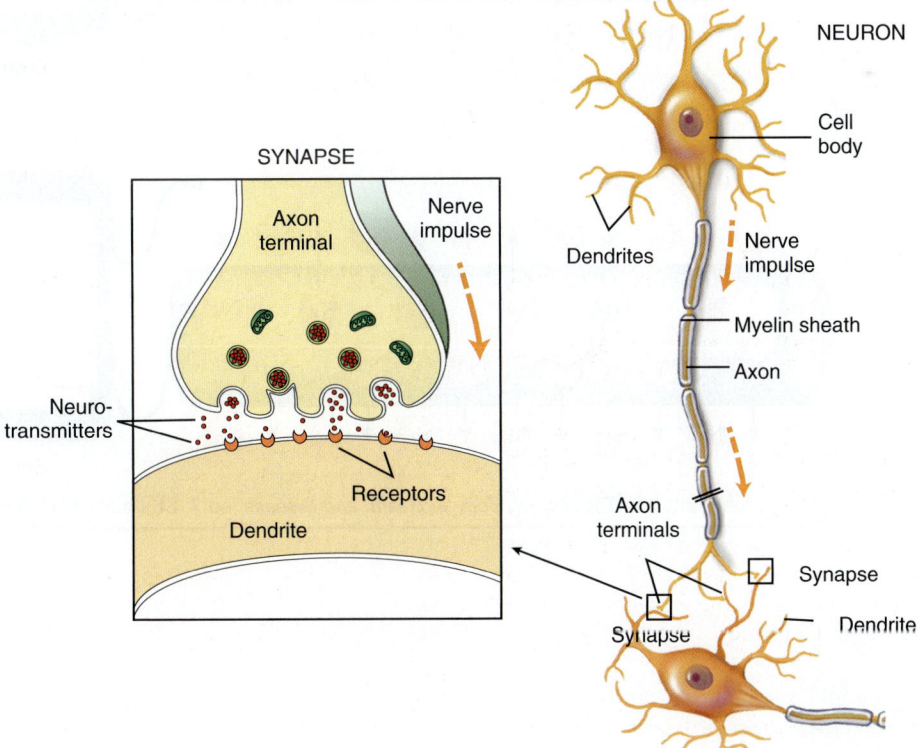

FIG. 12.3 Neuron and synapse *(inset)*. (From Seidel HM, Ball JW, Dains JE, et al: *Mosby's guide to physical examination,* ed 7, St Louis, 2011, Mosby.)

BOX 12.3   Action Potential

An action potential (Fig. 12.4) is a self-propagating wave of electrical impulse that travels along the surface of a neuron membrane. An action potential proceeds in the following steps:

1. A stimulus, (e.g., pressure, temperature, sound wave) starts an impulse.
2. The resting nerve cell has a slightly positive charge (due to sodium ions) on the outside of the cell membrane, and a negative charge inside the cell. This state is called *polarization* (poh ler uh ZEY shuh n).
3. When a section of the membrane is stimulated, the positively charged ions on the outside of the cell enter the nerve cell. This changes the outside charge to a negative charge. This state is called *depolarization* (dee poh ler uh ZEY shuh n).
4. Almost immediately after the impulse passes, the positively charged ions move outside the nerve cells again. This returns the outside charge to a positive charge. This state is called *repolarization* (ree poh ler uh ZEY shuh n).
5. Once everything changes back, the cell is at rest again, and the cycle continues.

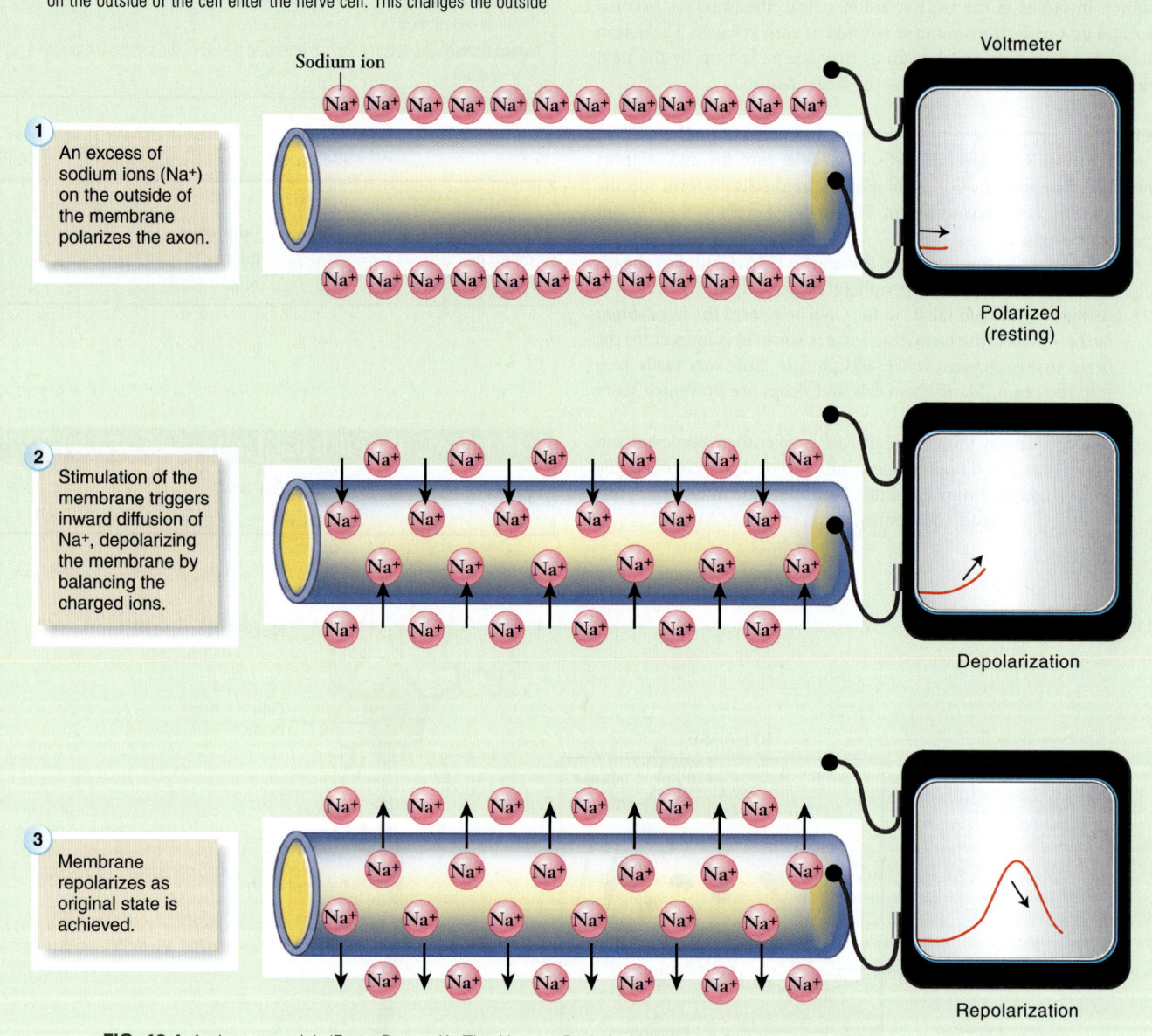

FIG. 12.4 Action potential. (From Patton K: *The Human Body in Health and Disease*, ed 7, St. Louis, 2018, Elsevier.)

BOX 12.4 Neurotransmitters

Examples of neurotransmitters include:
- epinephrine (ep uh NEF rin) and norepinephrine (nohr ep uh NEF rin)
- dopamine (DOH puh meen)
- serotonin (ser uh TOH nin)
- endorphins (en DAWR fins) and enkephalins (en KEF uh lins)

STUDY TIP

The acronym BBB can stand either for blood-brain barrier, or for bundle branch block, a cardiac condition.

THE CENTRAL NERVOUS SYSTEM

The brain and spinal cord make up the CNS. The brain is enclosed inside the skull. The spinal cord is a bundle of nervous tissue that extends from the **brainstem** at the base of the brain. The spinal cord exits the skull at the **foramen magnum** (fuh REY muh n MAG nuh m). It is about 17 inches long and runs inside the spinal canal, which is in the center of the spinal column.

VOCABULARY

brainstem: The part of the brain that is continuous with the top of the spinal cord. It is made up of the medulla oblongata, pons, and midbrain. The brainstem is concerned with reflexes and vital functions of the body, such as respiration, heartbeat, and swallowing.

foramen magnum: A large opening in the base of the skull. It forms a passageway for the spinal cord.

Brain

The brain is one of the most complex organs of the body. It is divided into four parts: the *cerebrum* (suh REE brum), the *cerebellum* (sair ih BELL um), the *diencephalon* (dye en SEF fuh lon), and the *brainstem* (Fig. 12.5).

MEDICAL TERMINOLOGY
encephal/o: brain
cerebr/o: cerebrum
cerebell/o: cerebellum

Cerebrum. The largest portion of the brain, the cerebrum, is divided into two halves, or *hemispheres* (HEM ih sfeers). The surfaces of the hemispheres are covered with gray matter and are called the *cerebral cortex* (suh REE bruh l KAWR teks). The right hemisphere usually controls artistic functions, such as drawing, rhythm, and picture memory. The left hemisphere controls verbal functions, such as reading, writing, speaking, and mathematical calculations. The two halves of the brain are connected by the *corpus callosum* (KAWR puh s kuh LOH suh m). This bundle of nerve tissue facilitates communication between the two sides of the brain. The cerebral cortex is arranged into folds that look like ridges and valleys. The valleys are referred to as *sulci* (SULL sye), and the ridges are *gyri* (JYE rye) (Fig. 12.6).

The cerebrum is further divided into sections called *lobes*, each of which has its own functions:
- The *frontal lobe* contains the functions of speech and the motor area that controls voluntary movement on the opposite side of the body.
- The *temporal* (TEM pur rul) *lobe* contains the hearing and smell functions of the brain.
- The *parietal* (puh RYE uh tul) *lobe* controls the sensations of touch and taste.
- The *occipital* (ock SIP ih tul) *lobe* is responsible for vision.

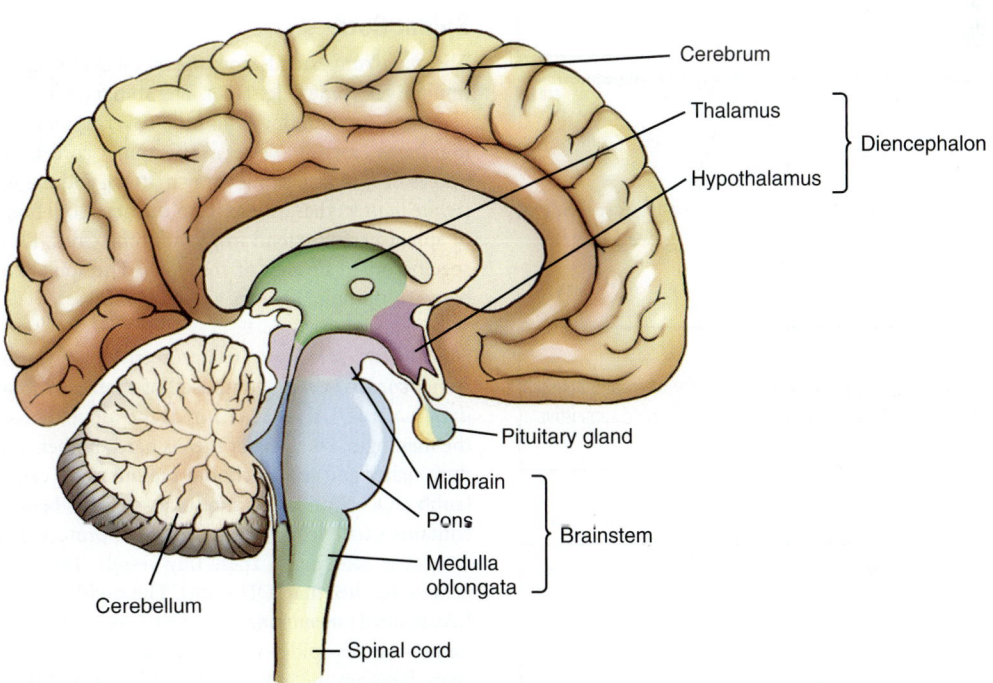

FIG. 12.5 The brain. (From Shiland B: *Mastering healthcare terminology*, ed 5, St Louis, 2015, Elsevier.)

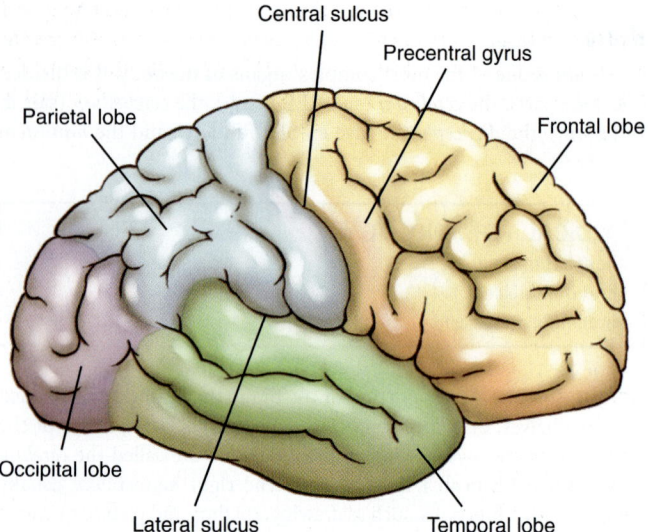

FIG. 12.6 The cerebrum. (From Shiland B: *Mastering healthcare terminology*, ed 5, St Louis, 2015, Elsevier.)

Cerebellum. The cerebellum is located below the occipital lobe of the cerebrum. It coordinates equilibrium (ee kwih LIB ree uh m) or balance, posture, and muscle coordination.

Diencephalon. The *diencephalon* is composed of the *thalamus* (THAL uh mus) and the structure below it, the *hypothalamus* (HYE poh thal uh mus). The thalamus is responsible for relaying sensory information to the cerebral cortex. It also translates some sensory information into sensations of pain, temperature, and touch. The hypothalamus controls the autonomic (aw tuh NOM ik) nervous system (ANS). In this role, it regulates the endocrine system, and manages body temperature, sleep, and appetite to maintain homeostasis.

CRITICAL THINKING 12.2

Tia has roomed Elaine and has taken vital signs. She is asking Elaine the set of questions necessary to help prepare the electronic medical record for Dr. Kahn. One question has Elaine thinking a bit, Tia asked if she has felt unsteady or unable to balance properly. Elaine answers that she does feel unsteady from time to time.

What part of the brain is involved in maintaining balance? Share your thoughts with the class.

Brainstem

The brainstem connects the cerebral hemispheres to the spinal cord. It is composed of three main parts: the *midbrain*, the *pons* (ponz), and the *medulla oblongata* (muh DOO lah ob lon GAH tah). The midbrain connects the pons and cerebellum with the hemispheres of the cerebrum. It is the site of reflex centers for eye and head movements in response to visual and auditory (AW dih tawr ee) stimuli. The second part of the brainstem, the pons, serves as a bridge between the medulla oblongata and the cerebrum. The lowest part of the brainstem, the medulla oblongata, regulates the heart rate, blood pressure, and breathing (see Fig. 12.5).

Spinal Cord

The *spinal cord* extends from the medulla oblongata to about the second lumbar vertebrae (Fig. 12.7). The spinal cord is protected by the bony vertebrae surrounding it and the coverings unique to the CNS, called meninges (meh NIN jeez). The spinal cord is composed of the cell bodies of motor neurons (gray matter), and the myelin-covered axons (*white matter*) that extend from the nerve cell bodies. Thirty-one pairs of spinal nerves extend from the spinal cord. Each nerve stimulates a specific organ or area of the body. The spinal cord carries messages between the spinal nerves and the brain.

Meninges. Meninges are a protective covering around the brain and spinal cord. They are composed of three membranes (Fig. 12.8). The *dura mater* (DUR ah MAY tur) is the tough, fibrous, outer covering of the meninges. Dura mater means hard mother. The space between the dura mater and the arachnoid membrane is called the *subdural space* (suhb DOO R uhl). The subdural space lies below the dura mater and contains small veins that are not well protected. Trauma to the head can cause bleeding of these tiny vessels. This may lead to a *subdural hematoma* (hee ma TOH muh). The middle layer is the *arachnoid* (uh RACK noyd) *membrane*. It is a thin, delicate membrane that takes its name from its spider-web appearance. The *subarachnoid space* is the space between the arachnoid membrane and the pia mater. The subarachnoid space contains cerebrospinal (suh ree broh SPAHYN uhl)

BOX 12.5 Brain Injuries

The Centers for Disease Control and Prevention (CDC) has developed a free, downloadable tool kit, "Heads Up: Brain Injury in Your Practice," which is available at the following website: http://www.cdc.gov/headsup/index.html. It provides practical, easy-to-use clinical tools for assessing and managing head injuries. Medical assistants should be knowledgeable about the potentially serious damage that can occur with concussions and the importance of early diagnosis. Information on the website includes:
- A booklet for physicians with information on the diagnosis and management of mild traumatic brain injury (MTBI) or concussion
- A patient assessment tool (Acute Concussion Evaluation [ACE])
- A care plan to help guide a patient's recovery
- Fact sheets in English and Spanish on preventing concussion
- A palm card for on-field management of sports-related concussion (ideal for education of coaches)

Centers for Disease Control and Prevention. Heads Up. Accessed July 31, 2017. http://www.cdc.gov/headsup/index.html.

Box 12.5 presents information from the Centers for Disease Control and Prevention (CDC) about assessing and managing head injuries.

VOCABULARY
gray matter: Brownish gray nerve tissue, especially in the brain and spinal cord. It is made up of nerve cell bodies, their dendrites, and some supportive tissue.

MEDICAL TERMINOLOGY
cortic/o: cortex
gyrus (singular), **gyri** (plural)
lob/o: lobe
sulcus (singular), **sulci** (plural)

CHAPTER 12 Nervous System and Mental Health

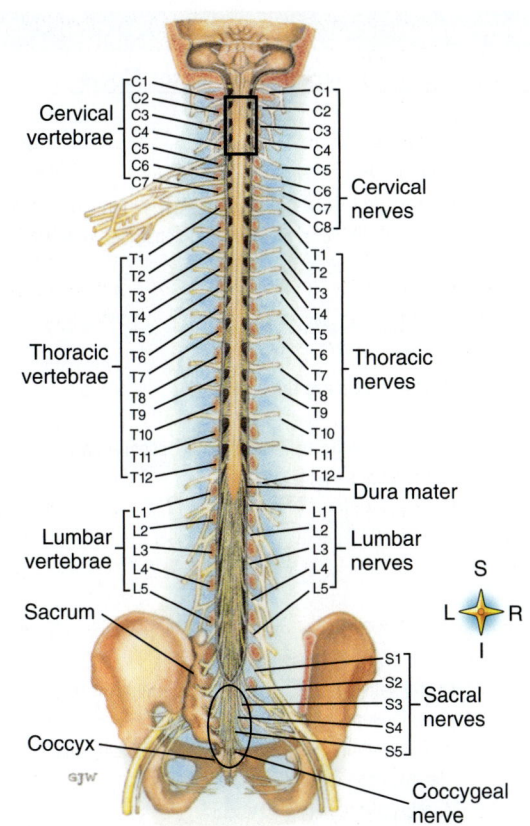

FIG. 12.7 The spinal cord, showing the spinal nerves. (From Vidic B, Suarez FR: *Photographic Atlas of the Human Body,* St Louis, 1984, Mosby.)

fluid (CSF). CSF circulates continuously around the brain and spinal cord to supply nutrients and remove waste products. CSF is also present in cavities in the brain called **ventricles** (VEN tri kuh ls). Finally, the inner most layer is the *pia mater* (PEE uh MAY tur). It is a thin, highly vascular membrane. Pia mater means soft mother.

> **VOCABULARY**
> **meninges:** The three membranes covering the brain and spinal cord.
> **cerebrospinal fluid:** A clear fluid that fills the ventricles of the brain, covers the surface of the brain and spinal cord, and subarachnoid space. It lubricates the tissues and cushions them from shock and injury.
> **ventricles:** A series of connecting cavities in the brain.

> **MEDICAL TERMINOLOGY**
> **cord/o, chord/o, myel/o:** spinal cord
> **mening/o, meningi/o:** meninges
> **dur/o:** dura mater
> **ventricul/o:** ventricle

THE PERIPHERAL NERVOUS SYSTEM

The peripheral nervous system is made up of the nerves that exit the brain or spinal cord. The peripheral nerves exiting the brain directly through the skull are called *cranial* (KREY nee uhl) *nerves*. Cranial nerves originate from the underside of the brain and relay information to and from the sensory organs and muscles of the face and neck (Table 12.1). Some cranial nerves are motor nerves. Others are sensory nerves. And some nerves can be both.

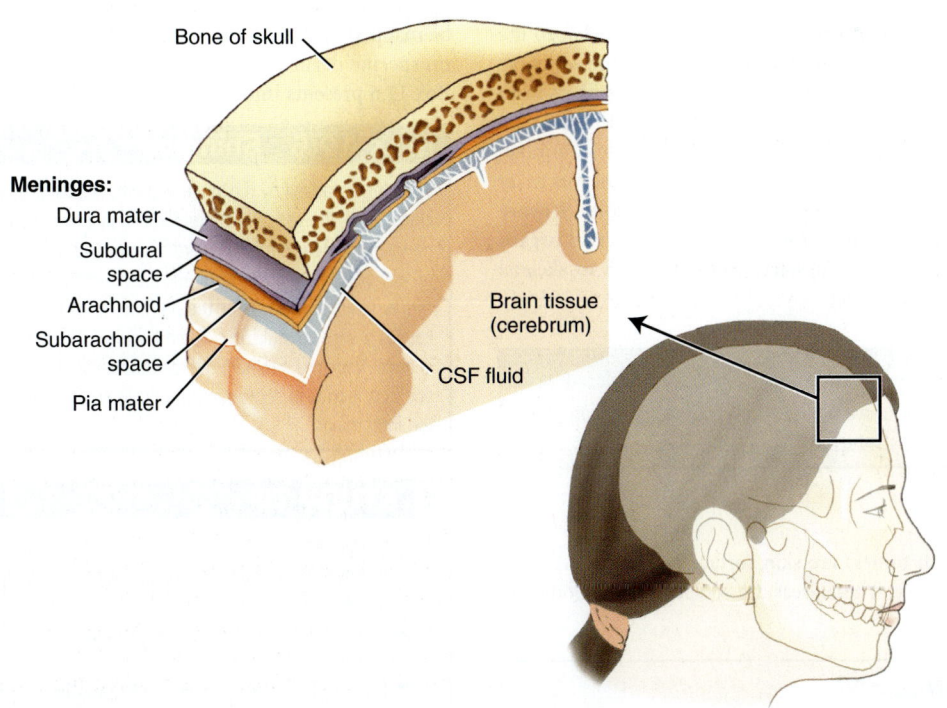

FIG. 12.8 The meninges. (From Shiland B: *Mastering healthcare terminology,* ed 5, St Louis, 2015, Elsevier.)

TABLE 12.1 Cranial Nerves

Number	Name	Origin of Sensory Fibers	Effector Innervated by Motor Fibers
I	Olfactory (ol FAK tuh ree)	Olfactory epithelium of the nose (smell)	None
II	Optic	Retina of the eye (vision)	None
III	Oculomotor (ok yuh loh MOH ter)	Proprioceptors* of eyeball muscles (proh pree uh SEP ter)	Muscles that move the eyeball; muscles that change the shape of the lens; muscles that constrict the pupil
IV	Trochlear (TROK lee er)	Proprioceptors of eyeball muscles	Muscles that move the eyeball
V	Trigeminal (trahy JEM uh nl)	Teeth and skin of face	Some muscles used in chewing
VI	Abducens (ab DOO senz)	Proprioceptors of eyeball muscles	Muscles that move the eyeball
VII	Facial	Taste buds of the anterior part of the tongue	Muscles used for facial expression; submaxillary and sublingual salivary glands
VIII	Vestibulocochlear (auditory) (VES tib yoo loh KOK lee awr)		None
	Vestibular branch (VES tib yoo lahr)	Semicircular canals of the inner ear (senses of movement, balance, and rotation)	
	Cochlear branch (KOK lee awr)	Cochlea of the inner ear (hearing)	
IX	Glossopharyngeal (glos oh fuh RIN jee uhl)	Taste buds of the posterior third of the tongue and the lining of the pharynx	Parotid salivary gland; muscles of the pharynx used in swallowing
X	Vagus (VEY guh s)	Nerve endings in many of the internal organs (e.g., lungs, stomach, aorta, larynx)	Parasympathetic fibers to the heart, stomach, small intestine, larynx, esophagus, and other organs
XI	Spinal accessory	Muscles of the shoulder	Muscles of the neck and shoulder
XII	Hypoglossal (HAHY poh glos uhl)	Muscles of the tongue	Muscles of the tongue

*Proprioceptors are receptors located in muscles, tendons, or joints that provide information about body position and movement.
From Shiland B: *Mastering healthcare terminology*, ed 5, St Louis, 2015, Elsevier.

The *spinal nerves* exit the spinal canal through spaces between the vertebrae. Spinal nerves closely mimic the organization of the vertebrae and provide stimulation to the rest of the body. If the nerve fibers from several spinal nerves form a network, it is called a *plexus* (PLECK sus). Spinal nerves are named by their location (cervical, thoracic, lumbar, sacral, and coccygeal) and by number (Fig. 12.9). Spinal nerves carry information to and from the brain through the spinal cord. Sensory fibers in these nerves carry stimuli from the skin and internal organs to the CNS. Motor fibers carry messages from the CNS to skeletal muscles, causing them to contract.

CRITICAL THINKING 12.3

Which cranial nerves help to move the eye or eyeball? List and share them with a classmate. Are your lists the same?

Dermatomes (DUR mah tomes) are skin surface areas supplied by a single afferent spinal nerve. These areas are so specific, the body can be mapped by dermatomes (Fig. 12.10). Shingles, for example, appears on specific dermatomes based on which nerve the virus has infected. Box 12.6 presents information on shingles.

BOX 12.6 Shingles

Shingles is caused by the same virus that causes chickenpox. If you have had chickenpox, the varicella-zoster virus is inactive in your body. The virus lies in nerve tissue near the spinal cord and brain until it is revived. It can re-emerge on any part of the body. But it most commonly infects the side of the body at the curve of the ribs, near the hairline, or at the back of the neck. Shingles causes a very painful rash. Some people experience pain long after the rash is gone. Vaccines can help reduce the risk of shingles. Treatment is available and is effective in shortening the duration of shingles if it is started early in the infection.

STUDY TIP

The term *dermatome* can be used in more than one way.
1. It is used to describe the skin surface supplied by a single afferent spinal nerve.
2. It is used to describe an instrument that cuts thin slices of skin for grafting.
3. It is used to indicate a layer of tissue in early fetal development that becomes the dermal layers of the skin.

Always look at the context of the sentence for a clue to the word's meaning!

MEDICAL TERMINOLOGY
dermat/o: skin
-tome: instrument used to cut

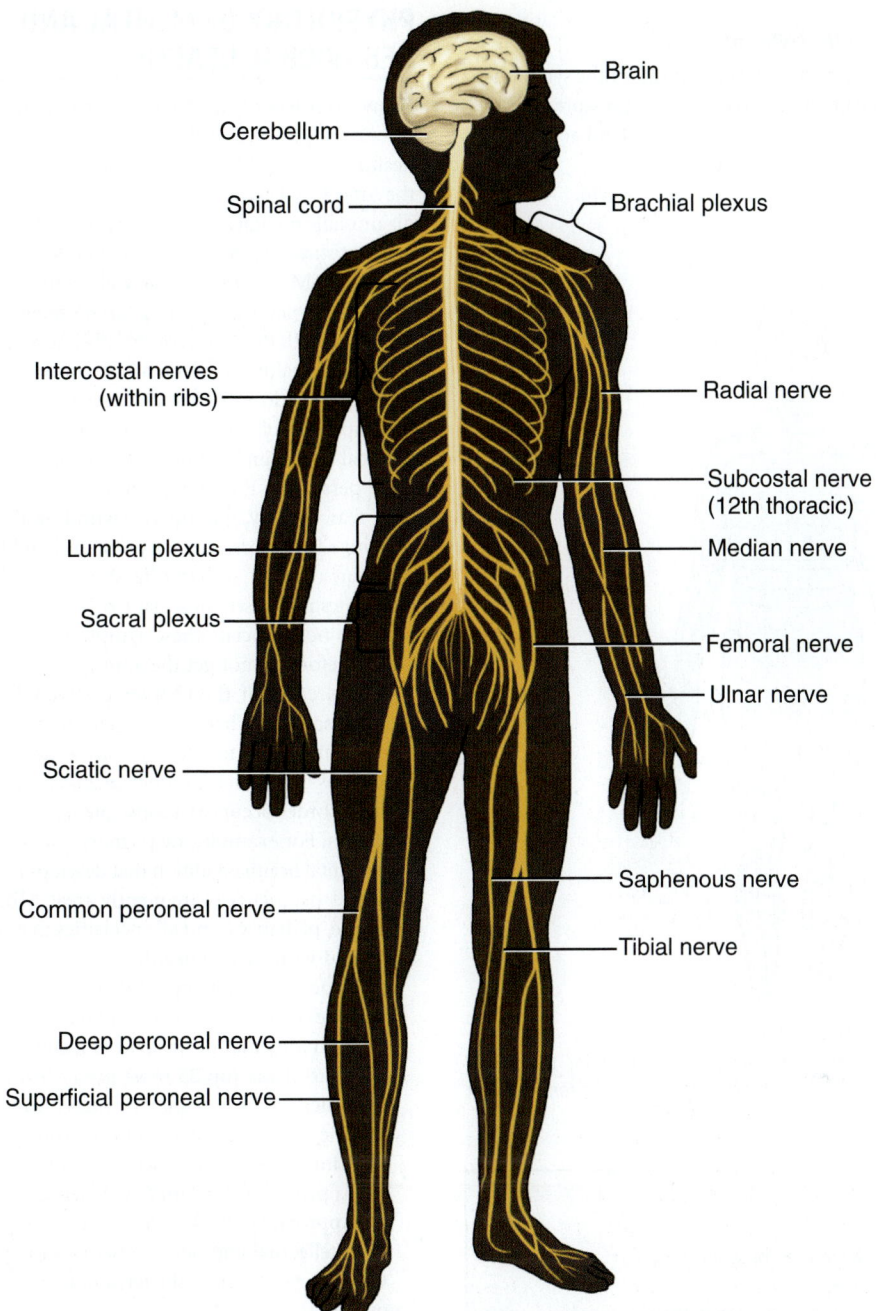

FIG. 12.9 Spinal nerves. (From Shiland B: *Mastering healthcare terminology*, ed 5, St Louis, 2015, Elsevier.)

THE AUTONOMIC NERVOUS SYSTEM

The autonomic nervous system consists of nerves that regulate involuntary function. The ANS is an automatic system that regulates body functions such as breathing, heart rate, sweating, circulation, and digestion. It also controls the actions of muscles in blood vessel walls, organs, and glands. The motor portion of this system is further divided into the sympathetic (sim puh THET ik) nervous system and the parasympathetic (par uh sim puh THET ik) nervous system. These two opposing systems help maintain homeostasis throughout the body systems.

Sympathetic Nervous System

The *sympathetic nervous system* can produce a "fight or flight" response. This is the part of the nervous system that helps the individual respond to perceived stress. It speeds up the heart rate, raises blood glucose levels, raises blood pressure, slows the digestive system, and widens the bronchioles, allowing more oxygen to enter the body quickly. It also stimulates the adrenal glands to increase their secretions.

CRITICAL THINKING 12.4

It is important to know the differences between the sympathetic and parasympathetic nervous systems. List three characteristics of each, and compare your list with a neighboring classmate. Do your lists agree?

Parasympathetic Nervous System

The *parasympathetic nervous system* does the opposite of the sympathetic nervous system. It slows the heart rate, lowers blood pressure, increases digestive functions, and reduces adrenal and sweat gland activity. This is sometimes called the "rest and digest" system.

Fig. 12.11 presents a flow chart of the nervous system.

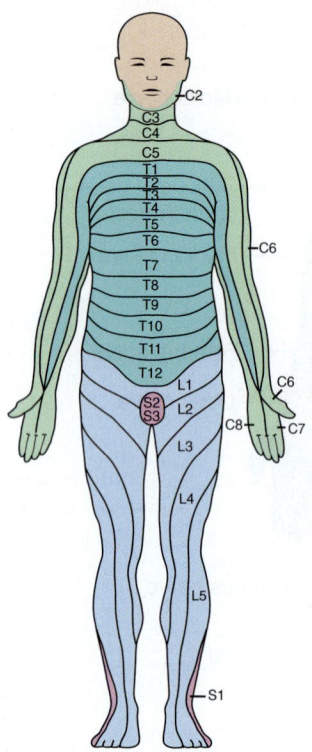

FIG. 12.10 Dermatomes. Each dermatome is named for the spinal nerve that serves it. (From Shiland B: *Mastering healthcare terminology*, ed 5, St Louis, 2015, Elsevier.)

MEDICAL TERMINOLOGY
iatr/o: treatment
logist: one who specializes in the study of
psych/o, thym/o, phren/o: mind

PHYSIOLOGY OF MENTAL AND BEHAVIORAL HEALTH

Many disorders of the body systems are described by their abnormal laboratory, physical, or clinical findings. However, mental and behavioral health disorders (MBHDs) are not as easily defined. In the United States, the American Psychiatric Association (APA) publishes the official list of diagnosable mental and behavioral disorders in a manual, the *Diagnostic and Statistical Manual of Mental Disorders*. The manual is now in its fifth edition (DSM-5). This revision will eventually result in a closer alignment with the *International Statistical Classification of Diseases and Health-related Problems*, 10th Revision, commonly known as the ICD-10.

Mental health disorders can be caused by a number of factors, alone or in combination. These include changes in brain chemicals, hereditary makeup, psychological disposition, and life experiences. Emotional and physical symptoms can occur for no apparent reason, and they can be quite persistent. Emotional symptoms may include panic, apprehension, fear, anxiety, nightmares, withdrawal, flashbacks, and ritualized repetitive behaviors, such as constant hand washing. Possible physical symptoms include tachycardia, shortness of breath, sleep disturbances, gastrointestinal upset, muscular tension, and cold, clammy hands. Patients often do not associate these symptoms with a mental health disorder and therefore do not get the appropriate diagnosis and treatment.

This section of the chapter is devoted to mental and behavioral health disorders. There is no anatomy for mental health, other than the structure of the nervous system. Some mental and behavioral health conditions are related to other primary disease states, and the mental health disorder occurs as a consequence or complication of the primary condition. For example, the primary diagnosis is terminal brain cancer – the mental health condition that develops may be depression. Psychologists and psychiatrists frequently treat MBHDs. Providers in family medicine, pediatrics, and all specialties may also treat some conditions associated with mental health.

Consider the following information:
- One of every 4 American adults and children has been diagnosed with a mental or behavioral health condition.
- Four of the top 25 most prescribed medications in the United States are for a mental or behavioral health disorder.
- The fourth most common diagnostic category for inpatient admissions is substance-related mental disorders.
- Approximately 40 million Americans are diagnosed with anxiety.
- Approximately 8 million Americans are classified as having intellectual and developmental disabilities.

Given these statistics, the terminology related to MBHDs cannot be ignored.

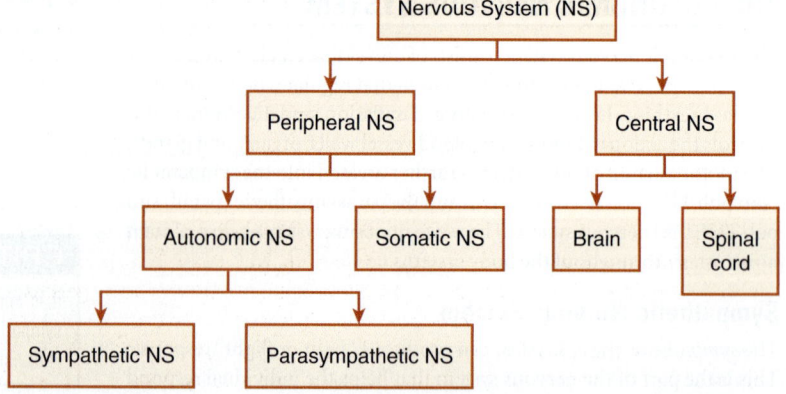

FIG. 12.11 Nervous system flow chart.

Mental and Behavioral Health Terminology

Mental health may be defined as a relative state of mind in which a person who is healthy is able to cope with and adjust to the recurrent stresses of everyday living in a culturally acceptable way. *Mental illness* may be generally defined as a functional impairment that substantially interferes with or limits one or more major life activities for a significant period of time.

> **STUDY TIP**
>
> *Psychiatry*, the treatment of mental disorders, is different from *physiatry*, the treatment of physical disorders.

The term *behavioral health* reflects an integration of the outdated concept of the separate nature of the body (physical health/illness) and the mind (mental health/illness). Advances in research continually acknowledge the roles of culture, environment, and spirituality in influencing physical and behavioral health. The use of the term *behavior* refers to observable, measurable activities that may be used to evaluate the progress of treatment.

As have previous chapters, this chapter examines disorders that result when an individual has a **maladaptive** (mal uh DAP tiv) response to his or her environment (internal or external). However, even though some mental illnesses have *organic causes* (i.e., causes in which neurotransmitters and other known brain functions play a role), there is often no mental anatomy to be tested. Instead, behavioral health is a complex interaction of an individual's emotional, physical, mental, and behavioral processes in an environment that includes cultural and spiritual influences.

> **VOCABULARY**
> **maladaptive:** Unacceptably adapted, or adapting poorly to a situation or purpose.

> **CRITICAL THINKING 12.5**
>
> Why is it so important for a medical assistant to be aware of mental and behavioral health issues? Discuss as a class. What types of behavior should be noted or passed on to the provider?

Substance-Related Disorders

A rapidly increasing group of disorders is substance-related disorders. These include abuse of a number of substances, including alcohol, opioids, cannabinoids, sedatives or hypnotics, cocaine, stimulants (including caffeine), hallucinogens, tobacco, and volatile solvents (inhalants). Classifications for substance abuse include psychotic, amnesiac, and late-onset disorders. It is important to be aware that addiction is not a character flaw. Rather, addiction has a neurologic basis – the effects of specific drugs are localized to equally specific areas of the brain.

An individual is considered an *abuser* if he or she uses substances in ways that threaten health or impair social or economic functioning. Levels of abuse vary (Table 12.2).

Mood Disorders

Patients with mood disorders, also called *affective* (AF ek tiv) *disorders*, show a disturbance of affect ranging from depression (dih PRESH uh n) (with or without associated anxiety) to elation (ih LEY shuh n). The mood change is usually accompanied by a change in the overall level of activity. Most of the other symptoms are either secondary to, or easily understood in the context of, the change in mood and activity. Most of these disorders tend to be recurrent, and the onset of individual episodes can often be related to stressful events or situations (Table 12.3).

Personality Disorders

Personality disorders have several common characteristics, including long-standing, inflexible, dysfunctional behavior patterns and personality traits that result in an inability to function successfully in society. These characteristics are not caused by stress, and affected patients have very little to no insight into their disorder (Table 12.4).

DISEASES AND DISORDERS OF THE NERVOUS SYSTEM

Diseases of the nervous systems are diverse and have many different causes (Box 12.7). Many factors can be associated with nervous system diseases, disorders, and infections. These diseases can involve the cells, tissues, and organs of the nervous system. Causes of nervous system diseases and disorders can be:

- Microbial infections
- Malignant changes
- Congenital conditions

TABLE 12.2 Terms Related to Substance Abuse

Term	Definition
acute intoxication	Episode of behavioral disturbance following ingestion of alcohol or psychotropic drugs
delirium tremens (DTs) (deh LEER ee um TREM uns)	Acute and sometimes fatal delirium induced by the cessation of ingesting excessive amounts of alcohol over a long period
dependence syndrome	Difficulty in controlling use of a drug
harmful use	Pattern of drug use that causes damage to health
tolerance	State in which the body becomes accustomed to the substances ingested. Therefore, the user requires greater amounts to create the desired effect.
withdrawal state	Group of symptoms that occur during cessation of the use of a regularly taken drug

From Shiland B: *Mastering healthcare terminology*, ed 5, St Louis, 2015, Elsevier.

TABLE 12.3 Terms Related to Moods

Term	Definition
affect	Caused by or expressing emotion or feeling. An emotion or emotional perception or attitude.
anxiety	Anticipation of impending danger and dread accompanied by restlessness, tension, tachycardia, and breathing difficulty not associated with an apparent stimulus.
dysphoria (dis FOR ree ah)	Generalized negative mood characterized by depression.
elation	A feeling or state of great joy or gladness.
euphoria (yoo FOR ree ah)	Exaggerated sense of physical and emotional well-being not based on reality, disproportionate to the cause, or inappropriate to the situation.
euthymia (yoo THIGH mee ah)	Normal range of moods and emotions.

From Shiland B: *Mastering healthcare terminology*, ed 5, St Louis, 2015, Elsevier.

TABLE 12.4 Terms Related to Personality Disorders

Term	Definition
delirium (dih LEER ree um)	Condition of confused, unfocused, irrational agitation. In mental disorders, agitation and confusion may also be accompanied by a more intense disorientation, incoherence, or fear, and illusions, hallucinations, and delusions.
delusion (dih LOO zhun)	Persistent belief in a demonstrable untruth or a provable inaccurate perception despite clear evidence to the contrary.
hallucination (hah loo sih NAY shun)	Any unreal sensory perception that occurs with no external cause.
illusion (ill LOO zhun)	Inaccurate sensory perception based on a real stimulus. Examples include mirages and interpreting music or wind as voices.
psychosis (sye KOH sis)	Disassociation with, or impaired perception of, reality. It may be accompanied by hallucinations, delusions, incoherence, akathisia, and/or disorganized behavior.

From Shiland B: *Mastering healthcare terminology*, ed 5, St Louis, 2015, Elsevier.

BOX 12.7 Common Signs and Symptoms of Nervous System Diseases and Disorders

- Recurrent headache, a change in sleep patterns
- Periodic memory loss, difficulty speaking or finding the right word
- Numbness, tingling, frequently dropping items
- Visual disturbances, abrupt changes in vision
- Confusion or disorientation, loss of consciousness

Tables 12.5 to 12.11 present information on common diagnostic imaging, laboratory testing, and therapeutic interventions for nervous system diseases and disorders.

CRITICAL THINKING 12.6

As Elaine talks to Dr. Kahn, she complains that she seems to walk a bit slower than she used to and just doesn't seem to have the same bounce in her step. Elaine wonders if something is wrong with her legs. Dr. Kahn decides to do a gait assessment rating.

Define gait assessment rating. Why do you think Dr. Kahn decided to do this assessment with Elaine? Discuss with your class.

Cerebrovascular Accident

A cerebrovascular accident (CVA) (seh ree broh VAS kyoo lur) can also be called a *stroke*. Stroke is the fifth leading cause of death in the United States. Each year about 795,000 people have a stroke, which is about 1 person every 40 seconds.

A stroke is a medical emergency, because blood flow to the brain has stopped. With no oxygen, the brain cells die very quickly. There are two types of stroke:

- *Ischemic stroke:* An artery in the brain is blocked by an embolus (EM bah lus) or thrombus (THROM bus). The blockage can be caused by a clot (e.g., blood) or by the build up of plaque. This is the most common type of stroke. (Box 12.8 presents information on TIAs.)
- *Hemorrhagic stroke:* A blood vessel bursts (aneurysm [AN yoo rizz um]) in the brain. Blood builds up, damaging the brain tissue.

BOX 12.8 TIAs

Transient ischemic attacks (TIAs), also called *ministrokes,* occur when the blood supply to a part of the brain is inadequate. This causes *ischemia* for a short period. TIAs cause the same symptoms as a stroke, but they generally disappear in about an hour. Symptoms can include numbness or weakness in the face, limbs, or on one side of the body. Confusion, difficulty talking or understanding speech, vision abnormalities, difficulty walking, and loss of coordination may all occur.

These episodes may occur in the days, weeks, or months before a stroke. Patients and their families should understand that any strokelike symptom should be taken seriously. Anyone experiencing TIA symptoms should be seen by a provider within 1 hour of the onset of the symptoms.

Etiology. High blood pressure, smoking, and high cholesterol are leading causes of stroke. Risk factors for strokes include:

- *Race:* Native Americans, Alaska Natives, and African Americans are more likely to have a stroke.
- *Age:* The risk increases with age, but strokes can occur at any age. Ten percent of children with sickle cell disease suffer a stroke.

Signs and Symptoms. The symptoms of a stroke depend on the part of the brain injured. Symptoms are sudden and include:

- Numbness or weakness of the face, leg, or arm
- Difficulty seeing in one or both eyes
- Difficulty speaking, forming coherent sentences, or understanding speech; or, confusion
- Problems walking, loss of balance or coordination
- Severe headache or dizziness

See Chapter 40, for more information. The memory aid FAST is important if you suspect a person is having a stroke.

Diagnostic Procedures. If a stroke is suspected, quick and thorough observation and testing needs to be done. The provider will rule out other conditions, such as a drug reaction or possible brain tumor. He or she then must determine what type of stroke the patient has had.

Testing during stroke determination may include the following:
- Physical examination: This will include:
    - questions about symptoms the patient has experienced
    - questions about the types of medications the patient is currently taking
    - personal and family history
    - blood pressure check
    - using a stethoscope to listen to the heart and carotid arteries of the neck
    - an ophthalmic check
- Blood tests: These may include blood sugar levels and blood clotting tests.
- Imaging tests: These may include a computed tomography (CT) scan, magnetic resonance imaging (MRI), cerebral angiogram, and echocardiogram. (Table 12.5 presents more information about imaging tests)

TABLE 12.5 Terms Related to Imaging Techniques

Term	Definition
brain scan	Nuclear medicine procedure involving intravenous injection of radioisotopes to localize and identify intracranial masses, lesions, tumors, or infarcts. Photography is done by a scintillator or scanner.
cerebral angiography	X-ray of the cerebral arteries, including the internal carotids, taken after the injection of a contrast medium (Fig. 12.12). Also called *cerebral arteriography*.
computed tomography (CT) scan	Transverse sections of the central nervous system (CNS) are imaged, sometimes after the injection of a contrast medium (unless bleeding is suspected). Used to diagnose strokes, edema, tumors, and hemorrhage resulting from trauma.
echoencephalography (eh koh en seh fah LAH gruh fee)	Sonographic exam of the brain, usually done only on newborns because sound waves do not readily penetrate mature bone.
magnetic resonance imaging (MRI)	Medical imaging that uses radiofrequency pulses in a powerful magnetic field. *Magnetic resonance angiography (MRA)* is imaging of the carotid arteries using injected contrast agents.
myelography (mye eh LAH gruh fee)	X-ray of the spinal canal after the introduction of a radiopaque substance.
positron emission tomography (PET)	Use of radionuclides to visualize brain function. Measurements can be taken of blood flow, volume, and oxygen and glucose uptake, enabling radiologists to determine the functional characteristics of specific parts of the brain (Fig. 12.13). PET scans are used to assist in the diagnosis of Alzheimer's disease (AD) and stroke.
single-photon emission computed tomography (SPECT)	Imaging technique involving injection of a radioactive sugar substance that is metabolized by the brain, which is then scanned for abnormalities.

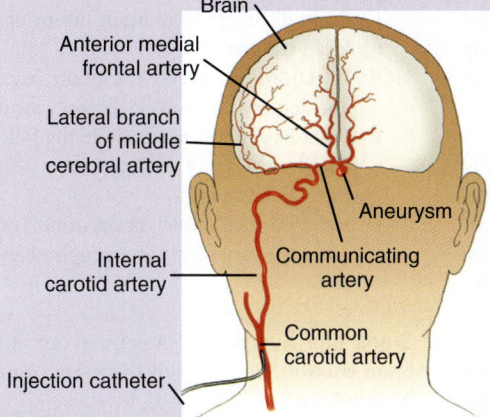
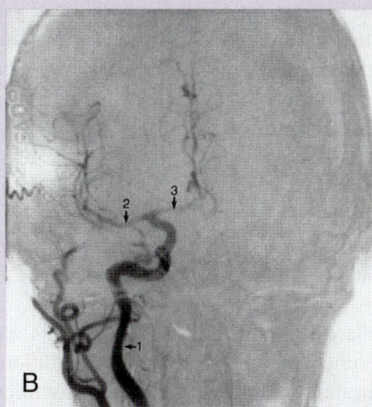

FIG. 12.12 Cerebral angiography. (A) Insertion of dye through a catheter in the common carotid artery outlines the vessels of the brain. (B) Angiogram showing vessels: *1*, Internal carotid artery; *2*, middle cerebral artery; *3*, middle meningeal artery. (**A** from Shiland B: *Mastering healthcare terminology*, ed 5, St Louis, 2015, Elsevier; **B** from Black JM, Hawks JH, Keene A: *Medical surgical nursing: clinical management for positive outcomes*, ed 8, Philadelphia, 2009, Saunders.)

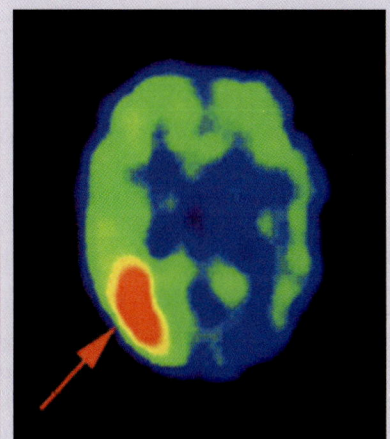

FIG. 12.13 Positron emission tomography (PET) scan of the brain of a 6-month-old male with seizures, demonstrating focal area. (From Shiland B: *Mastering healthcare terminology*, ed 5, St Louis, 2015, Elsevier.)

From Shiland B: *Mastering healthcare terminology*, ed 5, St Louis, 2015, Elsevier.

- Carotid ultrasound: This scan can reveal fatty deposits (known as plaques) in the arteries and show the flow of blood through the vessel.

See Chapter 2 for more information about imaging tests.

Treatment. Treatment begins immediately with medication, depending on the type of stroke.
- *Ischemic stroke:* The focus is on dissolving the clot that is causing the stroke.
  - Aspirin may be given orally to prevent blood clots from forming.
  - Tissue plasminogen activator (TPA) can be given intravenously to break down existing clots that may be blocking blood flow in the brain. It should be given intravenously within 4.5 hours of the start of symptoms. TPA also can be administered directly into the brain through a catheter.
- *Hemorrhagic stroke:* The focus is on stopping the bleeding in the brain and controlling the pressure in the brain.
  - Medications may be given to help stop bleeding in the brain and lower the pressure in the brain.
  - Once the bleeding has stopped, supportive care is given while the body absorbs the blood and heals from the bleed.
  - Surgical repair of vessels may be necessary with this type of stroke.

After emergency care is complete, the patient will be assessed for physical and mental function. The goal of post-stroke care is to help the patient gain strength and function so that he or she can be as independent as possible. Additional therapies may include:
- Physical, occupational, and speech therapy
- A change in diet, as recommended by a dietitian
- The provider may prescribe an anticoagulant or antiplatelet medication, depending on the type of stroke.
- A social worker or case manager may oversee the patient's progress and recommend additional rehabilitation activities to the primary provider.

Follow-up care, as rehabilitation progresses, is likely until the patient has recovered. If some functions cannot be regained, additional care will be required. Medication monitoring may also continue after rehabilitation is complete.

Prognosis. For many patients, full recovery from a stroke is very possible. The sooner the person is treated after symptoms of a stroke start, the more likely the recovery. Severe strokes can damage physical and mental functions and can be fatal.

Prevention. Many tactics for preventing stroke are also useful in maintaining good heart health. Some healthful strategies include the following:
- Control high blood pressure
- Lower blood cholesterol and monitor fat intake in your diet
- Stop smoking and drink alcohol only in moderation
- Control diabetes by controlling blood sugar levels
- Eat a diet rich in vegetables, fruits, and lean protein, and high in fiber
- Maintain a healthy weight and exercise regularly

> **CRITICAL THINKING 12.7**
>
> Elaine and Dr. Kahn continue to talk about some symptoms that have been bothering her. She has noticed that her left hand trembles. When she sits and watches TV at night, it is the most obvious. When she is tired or in a hurry, it seems to bother her more.
> Dr. Kahn takes Elaine's hands and examines them. He can feel her left hand tremble. Why would a trembling hand be significant?

Epilepsy

Epilepsy is a neurologic condition in which electrical activity suddenly increases in one or more parts of the brain. There are three major groups of seizures:
- *Generalized onset seizure*: Affects both sides of the brain at the same time. It includes several types of seizures (e.g., tonic-clonic and absent). Symptoms may include jerking, rigid or twitching muscles, and staring spells.
- *Focal onset seizure*: Affects one area of the brain. This term replaces the partial seizure terminology. The two subgroups of focal onset seizures are aware seizures and impaired awareness seizures. If the person is awake and alert during the seizure, it is a focal onset aware seizure. If the person is confused during the seizure, it is a focal onset impaired awareness seizure (formerly called a complex partial seizure).
- *Unknown onset seizure*: the beginning of the seizure is unknown.

Etiology. The cause of epilepsy can arise from a variety of sources, but some of the most common causes are:
- Genetic predisposition
- Brain disorders (e.g., brain tumor or the effects of a stroke)
- Head trauma
- Infection that affects the brain (e.g., meningitis, encephalitis, and acquired immunodeficiency syndrome [AIDS])

Risk factors for epilepsy include the following:
- Family history of epilepsy, or a personal history of a seizure during childhood
- Head injuries, stroke, brain tumor, or vascular disease
- Age – the very young and people older than age 60 are at greatest risk

Signs and Symptoms. A seizure can affect any function that the brain controls, but some of the more common signs and symptoms include:
- Confusion and/or disorientation
- Staring for periods of time, loss of awareness
- Jerking, random movements of the arms and legs
- Loss of consciousness, loss of alertness

Because the signs and symptoms of a seizure can cause loss of function in any part of the body, complications can be dangerous. Complications could include:
- Falls and other physical accidents
- Drowning, if a seizure happens while the person is in water
- Car (or any moving vehicle) accident
- Emotional and mental health issues (e.g., anxiety and depression)

Diagnostic Procedures. The following tests and procedures are likely done to aid in the diagnosis of epilepsy:
- Physical examination
- Neurologic examination
- Laboratory tests: These may include a complete blood count (CBC), testing for infectious diseases (Lyme, syphilis, human immunodeficiency virus [HIV], meningitis, encephalitis). Table 12.6 presents more information on laboratory testing.
- Imaging tests: Electroencephalogram (EEG), CT scan, MRI, positron emission tomography (PET) scan, single-photon emission computed tomography (SPECT) scan. Table 12.5 and Chapter 2, present more information on imaging.

TABLE 12.6 Terms Related to Laboratory Tests

Term	Definition
Blood alcohol testing	Testing to determine the level of alcohol in the blood
complete blood cell count (CBC)	Twelve tests, including red blood cell (RBC) count, white blood cell (WBC) count, hemoglobin (Hb), hematocrit/packed-cell volume (Hct/PCV), and diff (WBC differential). Some Clinical Laboratory Improvement Amendments (CLIA)–waived tests are available.
comprehensive metabolic panel (CMP)	Set of blood tests that assess organ function, metabolism, and electrolyte levels. Some CLIA-waived tests are available.
differential (diff) count	Measure of the different types of WBCs
erythrocyte sedimentation rate (ESR) (eh RITH roh syte seh dih men TAY shun)	Measurement of the time required for mature RBCs to settle out of a blood sample after an anticoagulant is added. An increased ESR indicates inflammation. Some CLIA-waived tests are available.
human chorionic gonadotropin (hCG) – urine or serum (KOHR ee on ick goh nad uh TROH pin)	hCG testing is routinely used to screen for a pregnancy. This test may be used to rule out pregnancy as it relates to abdominal pain and the digestive system. CLIA-waived test (urine only) is available.
human immunodeficiency virus (HIV) testing	Tests to detect the presence of HIV. Some CLIA-waived tests are available.
syphilis testing	Performed to rule out tertiary syphilis as a cause of neurologic or mental health and behavioral diseases and disorders
thyroid function tests	Blood tests done to assess T_3, T_4, and calcitonin. They may be used to evaluate abnormalities of thyroid function. Some CLIA-waived tests are available.
urinalysis	Tests different components of urine. It can help rule out conditions that may cause abdominal pain, such as a urinary tract infection (UTI), kidney stones, and some kidney and liver diseases. Some CLIA-waived tests are available.
urine drugs of abuse screening test	Urine multidrug screening tests are available to test for up to 10 different drugs of abuse simultaneously. Drugs tested may include a combination of the following substances: amphetamines, barbiturates, benzodiazepines, cocaine, morphine, methadone, phencyclidine (PCP), tricyclic antidepressants, marijuana (THC), ecstasy, methamphetamines, oxycodone, and opiates. Some CLIA-waived tests are available.
white blood cell (WBC) count	Measurement of the number of leukocytes in the blood. An increase may indicate the presence of an infection; a decrease may be caused by radiation or chemotherapy. Some CLIA-waived tests are available.

From Shiland B: *Mastering healthcare terminology*, ed 5, St Louis, 2015, Elsevier.

Treatment. The most common treatments are:
- Medications: Some individuals can take one antiseizure medication, whereas other people may need to combine medications to become seizure free. Antiseizure medications are known as *anticonvulsants*.
- Surgery: Surgery is most successful when seizures affect a well-defined part of the brain.
- Vagus nerve stimulation: A small device, similar to a heart pacemaker, is implanted in the chest. The device sends electrical energy to the brain and the vagus nerve. The nerve stimulation reduces the occurrence of seizures.
- Ketogenic diet: A strict high-fat, very-low-carbohydrate diet has been shown to reduce seizures. In a ketogenic diet, fats, rather than carbohydrates, are used for energy.

Patient follow-up is needed on a regular basis to check medication levels and evaluate any changes in the type or frequency of seizures.

Prognosis. As with almost any condition, a patient who follows the treatment regimen, takes medications as directed, and maintains a healthy lifestyle will have a good prognosis. Care must be taken with epilepsy to not participate in activities that could be dangerous if a seizure occurred.

Prevention. Prevention of epileptic seizures is easiest when a person understands the condition and adjusts his or her lifestyle to remain safe. Sometimes seizures cannot be eliminated, so putting safeguards in place is necessary. Preventive measures include keeping the patient safe. These would include:
- Correctly taking medications as directed
- Getting adequate sleep, maintaining a healthy diet, getting regular exercise, and reducing stress as much as possible
- Wearing a medical alert bracelet or necklace
- Having a support network in place

Parkinson's Disease

Parkinson's disease (PD) is a progressive neurologic condition that affects movement, muscle control, and balance. It develops gradually and progresses to significant physical and often mental impairment. Patients with PD do not produce enough *dopamine* in the brain. Dopamine is a neurotransmitter, or chemical messenger. Without enough dopamine, the brain cells that control muscle movement and coordination do not function properly, and the patient develops the major symptoms of PD. Dopamine is also important for efficient processing of information. Without dopamine, problems occur in memory, concentration, and organization of thought.

Etiology. The cause of PD is unknown, but scientists think that genetic and environmental factors may work together to cause PD. Environmental factors may activate the process of PD in people who are genetically predisposed to the condition. Exposure to herbicides and pesticides may be one environmental factor that sets off PD in susceptible individuals.

TABLE 12.7 Terms Related to Electrodiagnostic Procedures

Term	Definition
electroencephalography (EEG) (ee leck troh en seff fah LAH gruh fee)	Recording of the electrical activity of the brain. It may be used in the diagnosis of epilepsy, infection, and coma (Fig. 12.14). The resultant record is called an *electrocardiogram*.
evoked potential (EP) (ee VOHKT)	Electrical response from the brainstem or cerebral cortex that is produced in response to specific stimuli. This results in a distinctive pattern on an EEG.
multiple sleep latency test (MSLT)	Test that consists of a series of short, daytime naps in the sleep lab to measure daytime sleepiness and how fast the patient falls asleep. It is used to diagnose or rule out narcolepsy.
nerve conduction test	Test of the functioning of peripheral nerves. Conduction time (impulse travel) through a nerve is measured after a stimulus is applied. The test is used to diagnose polyneuropathies.
polysomnography (PSG) (pah lee som NAH gruh fee)	Measurement and recording of a number of functions while the patient is asleep (e.g., cardiac, muscular, brain, ocular, and respiratory functions). It is most often used to diagnose sleep apnea.

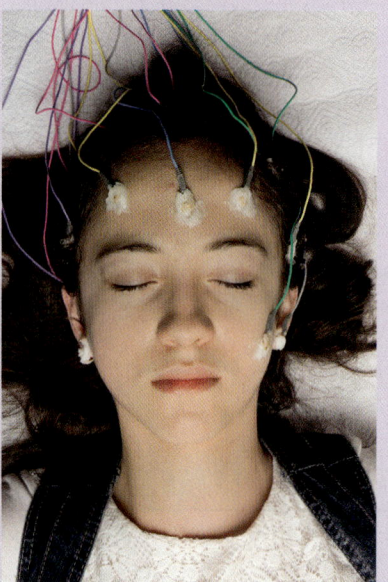

FIG. 12.14 Electroencephalography (EEG). (From Shiland B: *Mastering healthcare terminology*, ed 5, St Louis, 2015, Elsevier.)

From Shiland B: *Mastering healthcare terminology*, ed 5, St Louis, 2015, Elsevier.

Risk factors may include:
- *Age.* People over age 60 are at greatest risk of developing PD.
- *Genetic makeup.* People with a close relative with PD have a slightly higher risk of developing the disease.
- *Exposure to toxins.* Exposure to herbicides and pesticides may put a person at increased risk of developing PD.
- *Male gender.* Men are more likely than women to develop PD.

Signs and Symptoms. The signs and symptoms of Parkinson's disease are different for each person. They are usually mild at the beginning. Common signs and symptoms include:
- Tremors, which frequently start in the fingers or hand, even while at rest. A characteristic thumb and index finger tremor is known as a pill-rolling tremor.
- Slowed movement (bradykinesia) and shuffling when walking.
- Stiff muscles that limit range of motion and may be painful.
- Slightly stooped posture and diminished balance control.
- Speech that becomes quieter or slurred. Some people pause frequently, which slows down their conversations.
- Loss of affect; as a result, people with PD don't smile, frown, or seemed excited. They develop a flat affect. Box 12.9 presents more information about affect.

BOX 12.9 Affects

Affects are observable demonstrations of emotion that can be described in terms of quality, range, and appropriateness. The following list defines the most significant affects encountered in behavioral health and some neurologic conditions:

- **blunted:** Moderately reduced range of affect.
- **flat:** The diminishment or loss of emotional expression. It sometimes is observed in schizophrenia, intellectual and developmental disabilities, some depressive disorders, and Parkinson's disease (PD).
- **labile:** Multiple, abrupt changes in affect. These are seen in certain types of schizophrenia and bipolar disorder (BD).
- **full/wide range of affect:** Generally appropriate emotional response.

Diagnostic Procedures. No single specific test can be used to diagnose Parkinson's disease. Most frequently a neurologist who specializes in movement disorders will make the diagnosis. It is based on the medical history and signs and symptoms, in addition to a physical and neurologic exam.

Blood tests may be ordered to rule out other conditions. Imaging tests are not very useful for diagnosing PD. Some providers may prescribe

TABLE 12.8 Terms Related to Other Diagnostic Tests

Term	Definition
activities of daily living (ADLs)	An ADL assessment may be used to evaluate a patient's ability to live independently after an illness or event (e.g., a cerebrovascular accident [CVA])
Babinski's reflex (bah BIN skee)	In normal conditions, the dorsiflexion of the great toe when the plantar surface of the sole is stimulated. *Babinski's sign* is the loss or diminution of the Achilles tendon reflex, seen in sciatica.
cerebrospinal fluid (CSF) analysis	Examination of fluid from the central nervous system (CNS) to detect pathogens and abnormalities. It is useful in the diagnosis of hemorrhages, tumors, and various diseases.
deep tendon reflex (DTR)	Assessment of an automatic motor response by striking a tendon. It is useful in the diagnosis of stroke.
gait assessment rating scale (GARS)	Inventory of 16 aspects of gait (how one walks) to determine abnormalities. It may be used as one method to evaluate cerebellar function.
lumbar puncture (LP)	Aspiration of CSF from the lumbar subarachnoid space. A needle is inserted between two lumbar vertebrae to withdraw the fluid for diagnostic purposes. Also called a *spinal tap* (Fig. 12.15).
neuroendoscopy (noor oh en DOSS kuh pee)	Use of a fiberoptic camera to visualize neural structures. It is used to place a shunt in hydrocephalic patients.

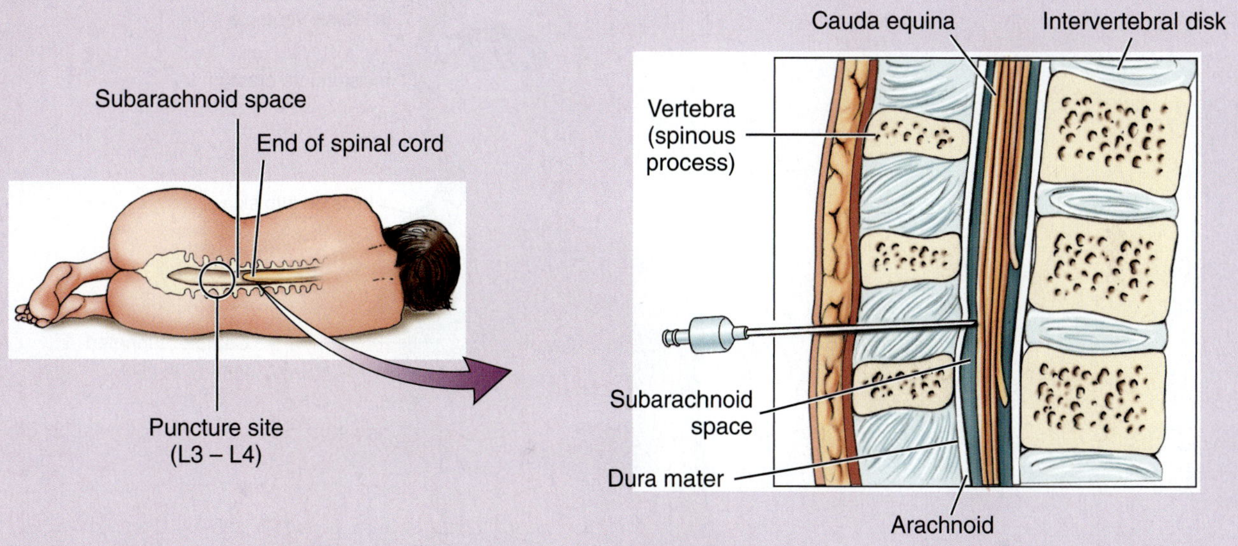

FIG. 12.15 Lumbar puncture (LP). (From Shiland B: *Mastering healthcare terminology*, ed 5, St Louis, 2015, Elsevier.)

From Shiland B: *Mastering healthcare terminology*, ed 5, St Louis, 2015, Elsevier.

---

a low dose of carbidopa-levodopa, a medication that alleviates the symptoms of PD by replacing lost dopamine. If the symptoms improve while the patient takes carbidopa-levodopa for a period of time, the diagnosis of PD is confirmed.

Treatment. Treatments for Parkinson's disease include some or all of the following:
- Medication: Carbidopa-levodopa to prescribed to replace the lost dopamine in the brain. The drug is usually taken orally. It is given in small doses at first, and then increased doses as the disease progresses. Carbidopa-levodopa can also be given through a feeding tube as a gel for people who have an unpredictable response to the oral medication. Other medications can be added to help preserve brain dopamine, control involuntary movements, and diminish limb tremors as the disease progresses.
- Surgical procedures: Deep brain stimulation (DBS). DBS requires surgical implantation of electrodes in the brain. The electrodes are connected to a generator that is implanted under the skin of the patient's chest. The generator sends electrical impulses to the brain and lessens PD symptoms. DBS is useful for patients who have unpredictable responses to medication. It does not stop the progression of the disease.
- Additional treatments, such as the following, may help PD patients:
  - Healthy diet that is high in fiber. PD patients are prone to constipation.
  - Regular exercise to maintain movement, balance, and range of motion
  - Occupational therapy to help with daily living tasks
  - Learning strategies to avoid falls
  - Massage therapy, tai chi, and yoga, which all increase strength, balance, and movement
  - Music, art, and pet therapy, which are activities that raise a person's mood, help them to relax, and increase movement in an enjoyable way

Follow-up office visits should be expected, especially as PD symptoms progress.

Prognosis. PD is a progressive disease. There is no cure, and it does not get better. Medications may alleviate symptoms, but the disease will progress and affect everyday life more and more with each passing

TABLE 12.9 Terms Related to Brain and Skull Interventions

Term	Definitions
craniectomy (kray nee ECK tuh mee)	Removal of part of the skull
craniotomy (kray nee AH tuh mee)	Incision into the skull as a surgical approach or to relieve intracranial pressure. Also called *trephination* (treff fin NAY shun).
stereotaxic radiosurgery (stair ee oh TACK sick)	Surgery using radio waves to localize structures within 3D space
ventriculoperitoneal shunt (ven trick yoo loh pair ih tuh nee uhl)	A tube used to drain fluid from brain ventricles into the abdominal cavity (Fig. 12.16).
ventriculostomy, endoscopic	A new opening, made between the third ventricle and the subarachnoid space, to relieve pressure and to treat one type of hydrocephalus

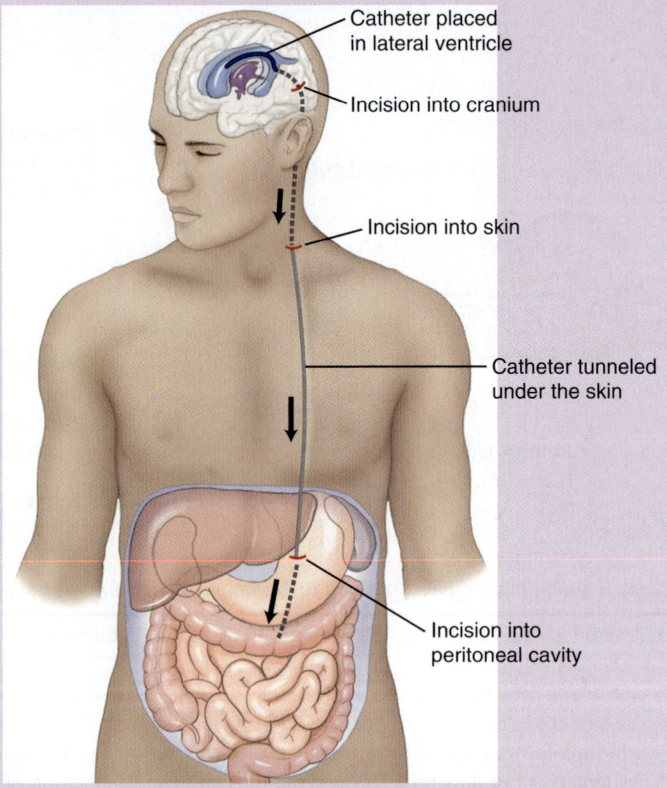

FIG. 12.16 Ventriculoperitoneal shunt. (From Shiland B: *Mastering healthcare terminology*, ed 5, St Louis, 2015, Elsevier.)

From Shiland B: *Mastering healthcare terminology*, ed 5, St Louis, 2015, Elsevier.

year. As with any long-term condition, compliance with the treatment plan, taking care not to fall, and having a good support system in place improve a patient's ability to cope with a chronic, progressive disease.

Prevention. Some research has shown that caffeine helps reduce the risk of developing PD. Caffeine is found in coffee, tea, and cola soft drinks. Also, reduced exposure to herbicides and pesticides may be beneficial.

CRITICAL THINKING 12.8

Dr. Kahn and Elaine are finishing her physical exam. Dr. Kahn has observed a few other things during the exam. Elaine also mentioned that she gets stiff through her back and hips when she cleans and does yard work. Dr. Kahn noticed that she walks with a slightly stiff, bent forward posture. Also, she doesn't pick up her feet, but rather shuffles.

Are these observations significant? What additional testing might Dr. Kahn order to help diagnose Elaine's condition?

CHAPTER 12 Nervous System and Mental Health

TABLE 12.10 Terms Related to General Interventions

Term	Definition
microsurgery	Surgery in which magnification is used to aid the repair of delicate tissues
neurectomy (noo RECK tuh mee)	Excision of part or all of a nerve
neurolysis (noo RAH lih sis)	Destruction of a nerve
neuroplasty (NOO roh plas tee)	Surgical repair of a nerve
neurorrhaphy (noo ROAR ah fee)	Suture of a severed nerve
neurotomy (noo RAH tuh mee)	Incision of a nerve
vagotomy (vay GAH tuh mee)	Cutting of a branch of the vagus nerve to reduce the secretion of gastric acid (Fig. 12.17)

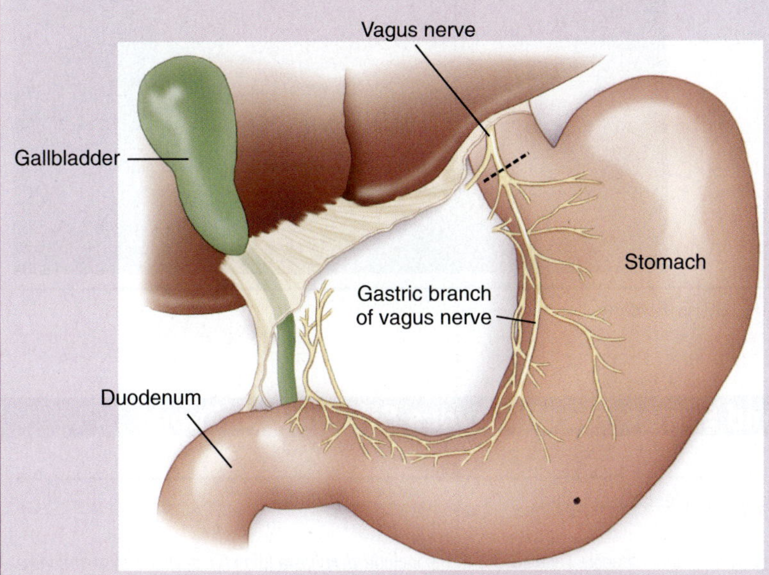

FIG. 12.17 Vagotomy. (From Shiland B: *Mastering healthcare terminology*, ed 5, St Louis, 2015, Elsevier.)

From Shiland B: *Mastering healthcare terminology*, ed 5, St Louis, 2015, Elsevier.

Additional Diseases and Disorders of the Nervous System

Many other diseases and disorders affect the nervous system. Tables 12.12 to 12.22 present additional conditions that may be of interest.

DISEASES AND DISORDERS OF MENTAL AND BEHAVIORAL HEALTH

Diseases and disorders of mental and behavioral health are diverse and have many different causes (Box 12.14). Many factors can be associated with mental and behavioral health diseases and disorders. These diseases can involve the cells, tissues, and organs of the nervous system. Mental and behavioral diseases and disorders can arise from:
- Genetic predisposition
- Abuse, trauma, head injury, or drug/alcohol addiction
- Malignant changes or infections

Tables 12.23 and 12.24 present common diagnostic imaging, laboratory testing, and therapeutic interventions for nervous system diseases and disorders.

Diagnostic Procedures

Behavioral diagnoses must take into account underlying healthcare abnormalities that may cause or influence a patient's mental health. Some of the common laboratory and imaging procedures are mentioned here, along with procedures that are traditionally considered to be psychological.

Mental Status Examination. A diagnostic procedure to determine a patient's current mental state. It includes assessment of the patient's appearance, affect, thought processes, cognitive function, insight, and judgment.

Text continued on p. 283

TABLE 12.11 Terms Related to Pain Management

Term	Definition
cordotomy (kore DAH tuh mee)	Incision of the spinal cord to relieve pain. Also spelled *chordotomy*
nerve block	Use of anesthesia to prevent sensory nerve impulses from reaching the central nervous system (CNS)
rhizotomy (rye ZAH tuh mee)	Resection of the dorsal root of a spinal nerve to relieve pain
sympathectomy (sim puh THECK tuh mee)	Surgical interruption of part of the sympathetic pathways for the relief of chronic pain or to promote vasodilation
transcutaneous electrical nerve stimulation (TENS)	Method of pain control achieved by the application of electrical impulses to the skin (Fig. 12.18)

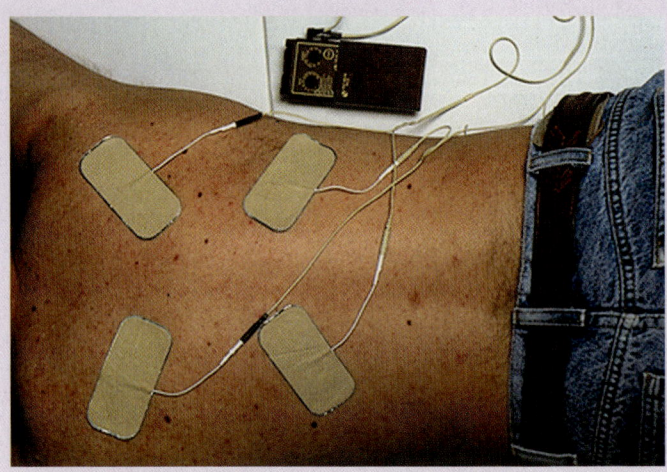

FIG. 12.18 Transcutaneous electrical nerve stimulation (TENS) treatment. (From Lewis SM: *Medical-surgical nursing: assessment and management of clinical problems*, ed 8, St Louis, 2011, Mosby.)

From Shiland B: *Mastering healthcare terminology*, ed 5, St Louis, 2015, Elsevier.

TABLE 12.12 Terms Related to Signs and Symptoms of Nervous System Conditions

Term	Definition
amnesia (am NEE zsa)	Loss of memory caused by brain damage or severe emotional trauma
aphasia (ah FAY zsa)	Lack or impairment of the ability to form or understand speech. Less severe forms include *dysphasia* (dis FAY zsa) and *dysarthria* (dis AR three ah). Dysarthria is difficulty in the articulation (pronunciation) of speech.
athetosis (ath uh TOH sis)	Continuous, involuntary, slow, writhing movement of the extremities
aura (OR uh)	Premonition; a sensation of light or warmth that may precede an epileptic seizure or the onset of some types of headache
dysphagia (dis FAY zsa)	Condition of difficulty with swallowing
dyssomnia (dih SAHM nee ah)	Disorders of the sleep-wake cycles. *Insomnia* is the inability to sleep or stay asleep. *Hypersomnia* is excessive depth or length of sleep, which may be accompanied by daytime sleepiness.
fasciculation (fah sick yoo LAY shun)	Involuntary contraction of small, local muscles
gait, abnormal	Disorder in the manner of walking. An example is *ataxia* (uh TACK see uh), a lack of muscular coordination, as in cerebral palsy (CP).
hypokinesia (hye poh kih NEE sza)	Decrease in normal movement. It may be due to paralysis.
neuralgia (noor AL jah)	Nerve pain. If it is described as a "burning pain," it is called *causalgia*.
paresthesia (pair uhs THEE zsa)	Feeling of prickling, burning, or numbness
seizure (SEE zhur)	Neuromuscular reaction to abnormal electrical activity within the brain. Causes include fever or epilepsy, a recurring seizure disorder. Also called *convulsions*.
spasm (SPAZ um)	Involuntary muscle contraction of sudden onset. Examples are hiccoughs, tics, and stuttering.

TABLE 12.12 Terms Related to Signs and Symptoms of Nervous System Conditions—cont'd

Term	Definition
syncope (SINK oh pee)	Fainting. A *vasovagal* (VAS soh VAY gul) *attack* is a form of syncope that results from abrupt emotional stress involving the vagus nerve's effect on blood vessels.
tremors (TREH murs)	Rhythmic, quivering, purposeless skeletal muscle movements seen in some elderly individuals and in patients with various neurodegenerative disorders.
vertigo (VUR tih goh)	Dizziness; an abnormal sensation of movement (either of oneself moving, or of objects moving around oneself) when there is no such movement.

From Shiland B: *Mastering healthcare terminology*, ed 5, St Louis, 2015, Elsevier.

TABLE 12.13 Terms Related to Learning and Perceptual Difficulties

Term	Definition
acalculia (ay kal KYOO lee ah)	Inability to perform mathematical calculations
ageusia (ah GOO zsa)	Absence of the ability to taste. *Parageusia* (pair ah GOO zsa) is an abnormal sense of taste or a bad taste in the mouth.
agnosia (ag NOH zsa)	Inability to recognize objects visually, auditorily, or with other senses
agraphia (a GRAFF ee ah)	Inability to write
anosmia (an NAHS mee ah)	Lack of sense of smell
apraxia (ah PRACK see ah)	Inability to perform purposeful movements or to use objects appropriately
dyslexia (dis LECK see ah)	Inability or difficulty with reading and/or writing

From Shiland B: *Mastering healthcare terminology*, ed 5, St Louis, 2015, Elsevier.

TABLE 12.14 Terms Related to Congenital Disorders

Term	Definition
cerebral palsy (CP) (SAIR uh brul PAWL zee)	Motor function disorder that results from a permanent, nonprogressive brain defect or lesion caused perinatally. Neural deficits may include paralysis, ataxia, athetosis, seizures, and/or impairment of sensory functions.
Huntington's chorea (koh REE ah)	Inherited disorder that manifests itself in adulthood as a progressive loss of neural control, uncontrollable jerking movements, and dementia.
hydrocephalus (hye droh SEFF uh lus)	Condition of abnormal accumulation of fluid in the ventricles of the brain. It may or may not result in impaired intelligence and developmental disabilities (Fig. 12.19). Although usually diagnosed in babies, it may also occur in adults as a result of stroke, trauma, or infection.

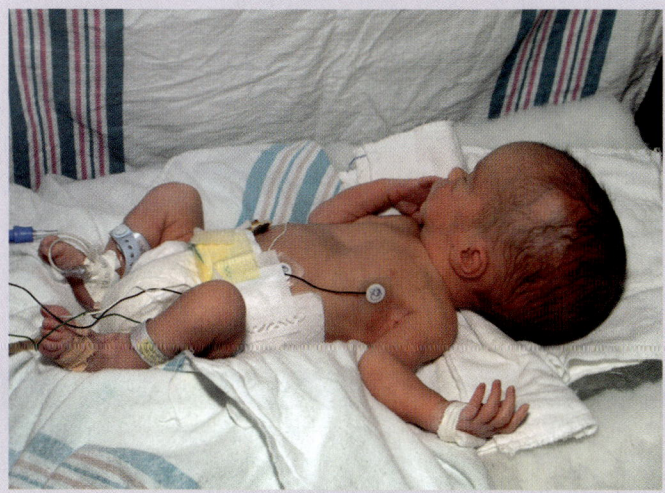

FIG. 12.19 Hydrocephalus. (From Kliegman R, Stanton BF, St. Geme JW, et al: *Nelson textbook of pediatrics*, ed 19, St Louis, 2011, Saunders.)

Continued

TABLE 12.14 Terms Related to Congenital Disorders—cont'd

Term	Definition
spina bifida (SPY nah BIFF uh dah)	Condition in which the spinal column has an abnormal opening that allows protrusion of the meninges and/or spinal cord. This is called a *meningocele* (meh NIN goh seel) (meninges only) or a *meningomyelocele* (meh nin goh MYE eh loh seel) (meninges and spinal cord) (Fig. 12.20). *Spina bifida occulta* is a congenital malformation of the bony spinal canal without involvement of the spinal cord (*occulta* means "hidden").
Tay-Sachs disease (tay sacks)	Inherited disease that occurs mainly in people of Eastern European Jewish origin. It is caused by an enzyme deficiency, that results in deterioration of the central nervous system (CNS).

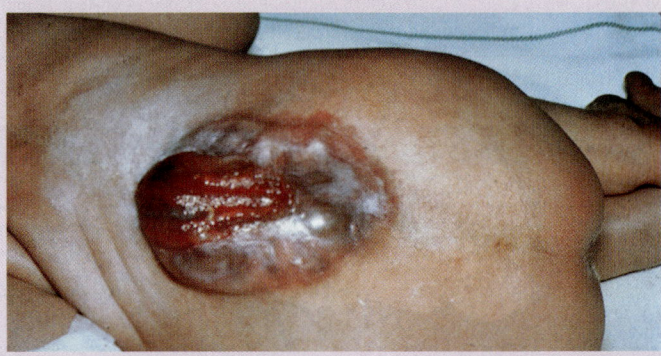

FIG. 12.20 Meningomyelocele. (Courtesy of Dr. Christine L. Williams, MD. From Zitelli BJ, Davis HW: *Atlas of Pediatric Physical Diagnosis*, ed 5, St Louis, 2007, Mosby.)

From Shiland B: *Mastering healthcare terminology*, ed 5, St Louis, 2015, Elsevier.

TABLE 12.15 Terms Related to Traumatic Conditions

Term	Definition
coma (KOH mah)	Deep, prolonged unconsciousness from which the patient cannot be aroused. It is usually the result of a head injury, neurologic disease, acute hydrocephalus, intoxication, or metabolic abnormalities.
concussion (kun KUH shun)	Serious head injury characterized by one or more of the following: loss of consciousness, amnesia, seizures, or a change in mental status. Box 12.10 presents the signs of a concussion.
contusion, cerebral (kun TOO zhun)	Head injury of sufficient force to bruise the brain. Bruising of the brain often involves the brain surface and causes extravasation of blood without rupture of the pia-arachnoid. It is often associated with a concussion.
hematoma (hee muh TOH mah)	Localized collection of blood, usually clotted, in an organ, tissue, or space, due to a break in the wall of a blood vessel (Fig. 12.21). A *subdural hematoma* is an accumulation of blood in the subdural space. An *epidural hematoma* is an accumulation of blood in the epidural space.
herniated intervertebral disk (HIVD)	Displacement of an intervertebral disk, causing it to press on a nerve. This results in pain and/or numbness.

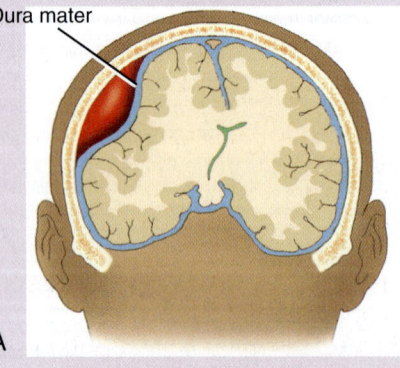 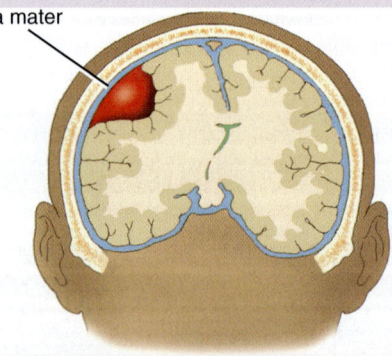

FIG. 12.21 (A) Epidural hematoma. (B) Subdural hematoma. (From Damjanov I: *Pathology: a color atlas*, St Louis, 2000, Mosby.)

From Shiland B: *Mastering healthcare terminology*, ed 5, St Louis, 2015, Elsevier.

BOX 12.10 Signs of a Concussion

A possible concussion should be taken very seriously. Signs and symptoms of a concussion that occur seconds to minutes after a head injury include:

- Possible loss of consciousness
- Difficulty focusing, with slowed responses, slurred speech, confusion, disorientation, or amnesia
- Nausea and vomiting, headache, or blurred vision

The patient should be seen immediately if he or she reports any of the following signs and symptoms days or weeks after a head injury:

- Persistent headache, vertigo (dizziness), seizures
- Inability to concentrate, repeated problems with memory, sleep problems
- Nausea or vomiting (especially if vomiting is projectile)
- Unusual anger, irritability, anxiety, or depression

CHAPTER 12 Nervous System and Mental Health

TABLE 12.16 Terms Related to Degenerative Disorders

Term	Definition
amyotrophic lateral sclerosis (ALS) (ay mye oh TROH fick LAT ur ul sklih ROH sis)	Degenerative, fatal disease of the motor neurons. The patient shows progressive muscle weakness and atrophy; also called *Lou Gehrig's disease*. Box 12.11 presents additional information on ALS.
Guillain-Barré syndrome (GEE on bar AY)	Autoimmune disorder of acute polyneuritis. It produces profound *myasthenia* (muscle weakness) that may lead to paralysis.
multiple sclerosis (MS) (skleh ROH sis)	Neurodegenerative autoimmune disease. It involves destruction of the myelin sheaths on the central nervous system (CNS) neurons (demyelination). These areas are abnormally replaced by gradual accumulation of hardened plaques. The disease may be progressive or may show remissions and relapses.
trigeminal neuralgia (try JEM ih nuhl noo RAL jun)	Disorder of cranial nerve V (trigemina) characterized by stabbing pain that radiates along the nerve. Also called *tic douloureux* or *prosopalgia* (Fig. 12.22).

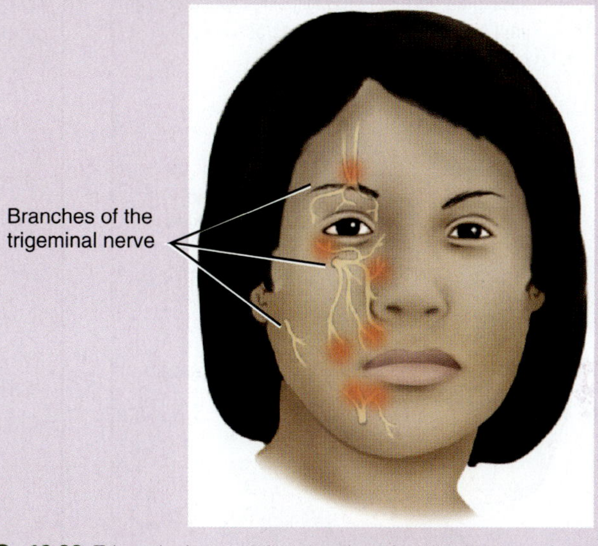

FIG. 12.22 Trigeminal neuralgia, showing the distribution of trigger zones. (From Shiland B: *Mastering healthcare terminology*, ed 5, St Louis, 2015, Elsevier.)

From Shiland B: *Mastering healthcare terminology*, ed 5, St Louis, 2015, Elsevier.

BOX 12.11 ALS

Amyotrophic lateral sclerosis (ALS), or Lou Gehrig's disease, is a rapidly progressing, fatal neurologic disease. ALS destroys the motor neurons responsible for voluntary muscle control. Without stimulation from motor neurons, muscles cannot function and gradually weaken and **atrophy** (A truh fee). The cause is unknown. The disease is more common among white males 60 to 69 years of age. The diagnosis is based on the signs and symptoms, and on a series of tests to rule out other diseases.

As the disease progresses, the patient has difficulty with speech, chewing, swallowing, and breathing. In most cases the disease does not affect a person's personality, memory, or ability to see, smell, taste, hear, or recognize touch. There is no cure for ALS. Most treatments are **palliative** (PAL ee ey tiv). Death from failure of the respiratory muscles usually occurs within 3 to 5 years after the onset of symptoms.

VOCABULARY

atrophy: Wasting away, degeneration from disuse.
palliative care: Care that is focused on providing relief from the symptoms and stress of a serious, possibly terminal illness. The goal is to improve the overall quality of life for the patient and his or her family.

Laboratory Tests. See Table 12.6 for laboratory testing information.

Imaging. See Table 12.5 for diagnostic imaging information.

Psychological Testing

- *Bender Gestalt Test:* A test of visual-motor and spatial abilities. It is useful for children and adults.
- *Draw-a-Person (DAP) Test:* An analysis of a patient's drawings of male and female individuals. It is used to assess personality.
- *Minnesota Multiphasic Personality Inventory (MMPI):* An assessment of personality characteristics through a battery of forced-choice questions.
- *Rorschach inkblot test:* A projective test using inkblots to determine the patient's ability to integrate intellectual and emotional factors into his or her perception of the environment (Fig. 12.27).
- *Thematic Apperception Test (TAT):* A test in which patients are asked to make up stories about the pictures they are shown. This may provide information about a patient's interpersonal relationships, fantasies, needs, conflicts, and defenses.
- *Wechsler Adult Intelligence Scale (WAIS):* A measure of verbal IQ, performance IQ, and full-scale IQ.

TABLE 12.17 Terms Related to Nondegenerative Disorders

Term	Definition
Bell's palsy (PALL zee)	Paralysis of the facial nerve. The cause is unknown, and the condition usually resolves on its own within 6 months Box 12.12 presents additional information on Bell's palsy (Fig. 12.23).
narcolepsy (NAR koh lep see)	Disorder characterized by sudden attacks of sleep
Tourette's syndrome (tur ETT)	Disorder characterized by facial grimaces, tics, involuntary arm and shoulder movements, and involuntary vocalizations, including *coprolalia* (kop pro LAYL yah), the use of vulgar, obscene, or sacrilegious language.

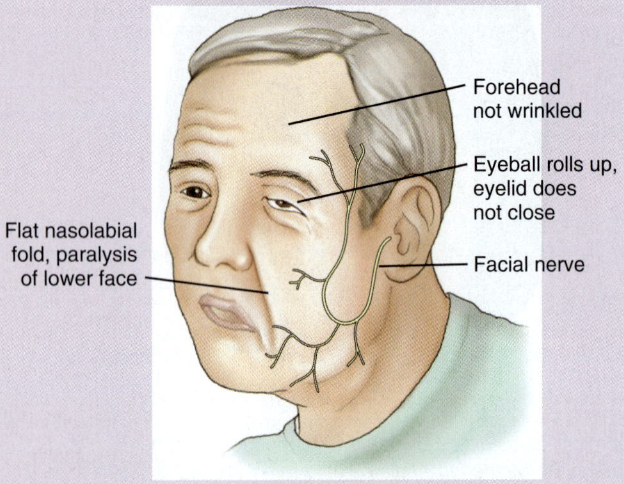

FIG. 12.23 The facial characteristics of Bell's palsy. (From Shiland B: *Mastering healthcare terminology*, ed 5, St Louis, 2015, Elsevier.)

From Shiland B: *Mastering healthcare terminology*, ed 5, St Louis, 2015, Elsevier.

BOX 12.12 Bell's Palsy

Bell's palsy is a temporary facial paralysis. It results from inflammation and edema of cranial nerve VII. This is often caused by an infection (e.g., herpes simplex virus, Epstein-Barr virus, Lyme disease). The condition occurs suddenly, and symptoms reach their peak within 48 hours. The disorder usually subsides spontaneously over several weeks to months. Symptoms range from mild weakness to complete paralysis on the affected side. The patient can experience facial twitching, eyelid drooping, excessive tearing of the affected eye, and drooping of the mouth. The antiviral drug acyclovir may be prescribed, in addition to corticosteroids to reduce the inflammation.

TABLE 12.18 Terms Related to Infectious Diseases and Inflammations

Term	Definition
encephalitis (en seff uh LYE tis)	Inflammation of the brain. It is most frequently caused by a virus transmitted by an infected mosquito.
meningitis (men in JYE tis)	Any infection or inflammation of the membranes covering the brain and spinal cord. It is most commonly due to viral infection, although more severe strains are bacterial or fungal in nature.
neuritis (noo RYE tis)	Inflammation of the nerves
poliomyelitis (poh lee oh mye uh LYE tiss)	Inflammation of the gray matter of the spinal cord that is caused by a poliovirus. Severe forms cause paralysis.
polyneuritis (pahl ee noo RYE tis)	Inflammation of several peripheral nerves
radiculitis (rad ick kyoo LYE tis)	Inflammation of the root of a spinal nerve
sciatica (sye AT ick kah)	Inflammation of the sciatic nerve. Symptoms include pain and tenderness along the path of the nerve through the thigh and leg (Fig. 12.24).

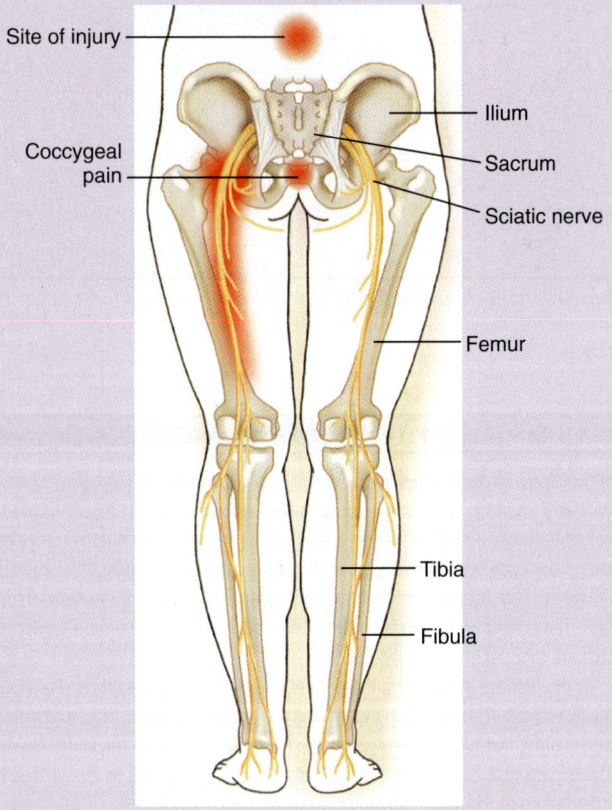

FIG. 12.24 Sciatica. (From Shiland B: *Mastering healthcare terminology*, ed 5, St Louis, 2015, Elsevier.)

From Shiland B: *Mastering healthcare terminology*, ed 5, St Louis, 2015, Elsevier.

TABLE 12.19 Terms Related to Vascular Disorders

Term	Meaning
migraine headache (MYE grain)	Headache of vascular origin. It may be classified as migraine with aura or migraine without aura. Box 12.13 presents more information on migraine headache.

From Shiland B: *Mastering healthcare terminology*, ed 5, St Louis, 2015, Elsevier.

BOX 12.13 Migraine Headache

Migraine headaches can be completely incapacitating. They frequently are associated with other symptoms, such as nausea, vomiting, visual disturbances, and throbbing pain on one side of the head. The signs and symptoms of migraine headaches differ from one individual to another. The patient may experience an *aura* before the onset of the headache. An aura often consists of a visual disturbance, such as dark lines or spots within the visual field or a flash of light.

Medical science has not yet discovered the underlying cause of migraines. Individuals who suffer from migraine headaches report many different triggers. They can include changes in estrogen levels, certain foods (alcohol, chocolate, aspartame, monosodium glutamate [MSG] and caffeine), elevated stress levels, altered sleep patterns, and changes in the weather. The diagnosis is established from a complete medical history. An electroencephalogram (EEG), computed tomography (CT) scan, or magnetic resonance imaging (MRI) may be performed to rule out other causes of the headaches.

Drugs used to treat migraines include nonsteroidal antiinflammatory drugs (NSAIDs) and triptans, such as sumatriptan (Imitrex). These drugs must be taken at the start of the headache to be effective. Other medications recommended for prevention of migraines include beta blockers and antidepressants. Other treatments include biofeedback techniques and elimination diets to identify foods that trigger migraines.

Alzheimer's Disease and Other Forms of Dementia

The term *dementia* encompasses a group of disorders that damage brain cells and cause profound changes in a person's ability to think, remember, and function. Alzheimer's disease (AD) is the most common form of dementia. AD slowly robs individuals of their memories and the ability to control their own bodies.

Etiology. The cause of Alzheimer's disease is not clear, but scientists believe it is the result of a combination of environmental factors, genetic factors, and lifestyle factors over the course of a person's life. A very small percentage of people have a genetic mutation that almost ensures they will develop the disease.

AD kills brain cells. As a result, the brain shrinks in size. There are many fewer functioning cells in the brain, and the cells that remain do not seem to function as efficiently as normal, healthy brain cells. There are also two abnormalities in the brains of Alzheimer patients:
- *Tangles:* The brain has its own transportation system, which brings nutrients and other vital substances to the nerve cells. The system is made up of a protein called *tau*. In AD, the tau protein is abnormally shaped and tangled. Because of these tangles, the brain transport system doesn't work.

TABLE 12.20 Terms Related to Paralytic Conditions

Term	Meaning
diplegia (dye PLEE jee ah)	Paralysis of the same body part on both sides of the body
hemiparesis (hem mee pah REE sis)	Muscular weakness or slight paralysis on the left or right side of the body
hemiplegia (hem mee PLEE jee ah)	Paralysis on the left or right side of the body (Fig. 12.25)
monoparesis (mah noh pah REE sis)	Weakness or slight paralysis of one limb on the left or right side of the body
monoplegia (mah noh PLEE jee ah)	Paralysis of one limb on the left or right side of the body
paraparesis (pair uh pah REE sis)	Slight paralysis of the lower limbs and trunk
paraplegia (pair uh PLEE jee ah)	Paralysis of the lower limbs and trunk (see Fig. 12.25)
quadriparesis (kwah drih pah REE sis)	Weakness or slight paralysis of the arms, legs, and trunk
quadriplegia (kwah drih PLEE jee ah)	Paralysis of the arms, legs, and trunk (see Fig. 12.25)

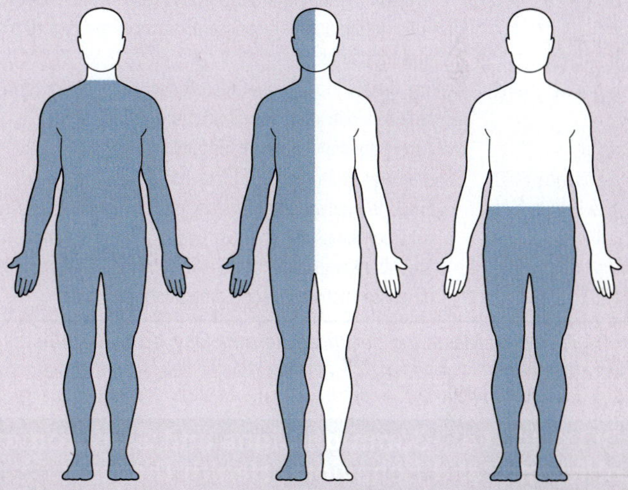

FIG. 12.25 Types of paralysis. (From Shiland B: *Mastering healthcare terminology*, ed 5, St Louis, 2015, Elsevier.)

From Shiland B: *Mastering healthcare terminology*, ed 5, St Louis, 2015, Elsevier.

TABLE 12.21 Terms Related to Benign Neoplasms

Term	Meaning
meningioma (meh nin jee OH mah)	Slow growing, usually benign tumor of the meninges. Although benign, it may cause problems because of its size and/or location
neurofibroma (noor oh fye BROH mah)	Benign fibrous tumors composed of nervous tissue
neuroma (noor OH mah)	Benign tumor of the nerves

From Shiland B: *Mastering healthcare terminology*, ed 5, St Louis, 2015, Elsevier.

TABLE 12.22 Terms Related to Malignant Neoplasms

Term	Definition
astrocytoma (as troh sye TOH mah)	Tumor that arises from star-shaped glial cells. It is malignant in higher grades. A grade IV astrocytoma is referred to as a *glioblastoma multiforme*, which is the most common primary brain cancer.
medulloblastoma (med yoo loh blass TOH mah)	Tumor arising from embryonic tissue in the cerebellum. It is most commonly seen in children.
neuroblastoma (noor oh blass TOH mah)	Highly malignant tumor that arises either from the autonomic nervous system (ANS) or from the adrenal medulla. It usually affects children younger than 10 years of age.

From Shiland B: *Mastering healthcare terminology*, ed 5, St Louis, 2015, Elsevier.

TABLE 12.23 Terms Related to Psychotherapy

Term	Definition
behavioral therapy	Therapeutic attempt to alter an undesired behavior by substituting a new response or set of responses to a given stimulus.
cognitive therapy	Wide variety of treatment techniques that attempt to help the individual alter inaccurate or unhealthy perceptions and patterns of thinking.
psychoanalysis (sye koh uh NAL ih sis)	Behavioral treatment developed initially by Sigmund Freud to analyze and treat any dysfunctional effects of unconscious factors on a patient's mental state. This therapy uses techniques that include analysis of defense mechanisms and dream interpretation.

From Shiland B: *Mastering healthcare terminology*, ed 5, St Louis, 2015, Elsevier.

BOX 12.14 Common Signs and Symptoms of Mental and Behavioral Health Diseases and Disorders

- Sadness, hopelessness, irritability, feelings of fear and anxiety
- Memory loss, difficulty speaking or finding the right word, confusion or disorientation
- Change in appetite, sleep patterns, or social engagement
- Loss of motivation, loss of enjoyment in life
- Visual disturbances, hearing voices, hallucinations

TABLE 12.24 Terms Related to Other Therapeutic Methods

Term	Definition
detoxification (dee tock sih fih KAY shun)	Removal of a chemical substance (drug or alcohol) as an initial step in the treatment of a chemically dependent individual.
electroconvulsive therapy (ECT) (ee leck troh kun VUHL siv)	Method of inducing convulsions to treat affective disorders in patients who have been resistant or unresponsive to drug therapy.
hypnosis (hip NOH sis)	Induction of an altered state of consciousness to change an unwanted behavior or emotional response.
light therapy	Exposure of the body to light waves to treat patients with depression due to seasonal fluctuations (Fig. 12.26).
narcosynthesis (nar koh SIN thih sis)	Use of intravenous barbiturates to elicit repressed memories or thoughts.
pharmacotherapy	Use of medication to affect behavior and/or emotions.

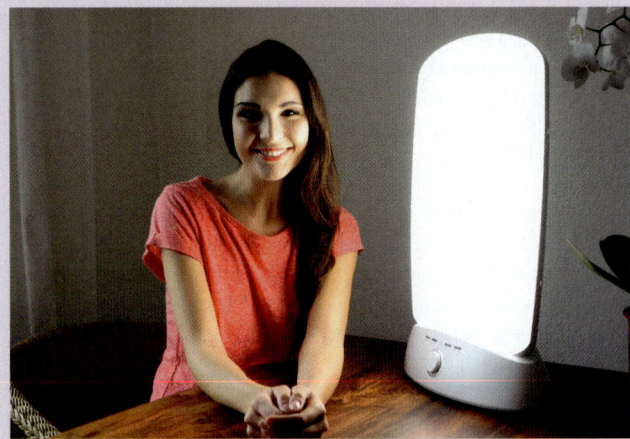

FIG. 12.26 Broad-spectrum fluorescent lamps, such as the one shown here, are used in daily therapy sessions from autumn into spring for individuals with seasonal affective disorder (SAD). (From Rocky89/iStock/Thinkstock.)

- *Plaques:* These are protein clumps or clusters that seem to inhibit cell-to-cell contact or communication within the brain. Scientists don't know exactly how plaques kill brain cells, but somehow their presence leads to cell death.

Risk factors for AD include the following:
- Older age: The disease is most common after age 65.
- Past head injuries or trauma
- Lifestyle and overall health: People who are sedentary, obese, smoke, have high blood pressure, high blood cholesterol, and uncontrolled type 2 diabetes, and who eat a poor diet have a higher risk of developing Alzheimer's disease
- Female gender: Women are more likely to develop the disease than men.

Signs and Symptoms. At first people with AD may be mildly confused or forgetful. They have trouble forming thoughts, thinking of words, or organizing something. As the disease progresses, the symptoms become clearer.

Mild symptoms include:
- Repeating questions, forgetting appointments, misplacing items around the house
- Having trouble finding words to describe something, having trouble concentrating

As AD progresses, symptoms may include:
- Not remembering having asked a question or having had a conversation
- Getting lost in familiar places (e.g., neighborhood, house, or city)
- Forgetting names of family members and friends
- Confusion and frustration when attempting to do two tasks at one time (e.g., cooking a meal while talking to a family member)
- Having trouble with numbers and simple math

As AD becomes advanced, symptoms include:
- Mood swings, personality changes, frustration, and irritability
- Loss of facial affect (Box 12.9)
- Social withdrawal, depression, isolation
- Inability to take care of daily tasks, such as grooming, dressing and undresssing, cooking, reading, recognizing family and friends, eating, and bathing; also loss of bowel/ bladder control and ability to swallow

Diagnostic Procedures. No one specific test can diagnose Alzheimer's disease. The provider will look at a number of factors to make the diagnosis. Testing will likely include:
- A physical exam, to check the person's overall health
- A neurologic exam, to check coordination, reflexes, balance, and memory
- Laboratory tests, which may include a comprehensive metabolic profile, to rule out other causes and deficiencies
- Imaging tests, which may include MRI, a CT scan, and a PET scan. (See Table 12.5 and Chapter 2 present more information on imaging.)

Treatment. Medications are available that can help, especially in the early stages of the disease. Examples include donepezil (Aricept) and memantine (Namenda). Sometimes antidepressants and antianxiety medications are used to help alleviate symptoms, but they must be used with caution.

Creating a living area where the person feels safe and comfortable is very important. As the disease progresses, the person must have a living space that protects him or her from falling or harm. Helping the person with daily schedules and reminders will limit frustrations.

Other measures to help ensure comfort and safety include:
- Installing safety rails in the living space and bathroom
- Getting rid of clutter, excess furniture, and throw rugs
- Encouraging daily exercise and fresh air
- Keeping photos in the living area to help remind the person of loved ones
- Providing highly nutritious meals (i.e., lots of veggies, fruits, and good-quality protein)
- Reminding the person to drink water and juice. Sometimes people forget to get enough fluids, and this may lead to constipation or dehydration. Beverages with caffeine should be avoided.

Regular follow-up visits to the provider may be required.

Prognosis. AD is a slowly progressive condition. It will not get better. However, thoughtful preparations and a good support system can help the patient have a good quality of life as long as possible.

Prevention. Avoiding the risk factors mentioned previously may help prevent AD. Other strategies to prevent AD and other types of dementia include:
- regular exercise
- maintaining good cardiovascular health
- healthy diet rich in vegetables, fruits, and high-quality protein
- staying mentally active and socially connected

Depressive Disorders

Depression is a mood disorder that causes feelings of sadness, or lack of interest in things that would normally be pleasant. Depression is typically characterized by its degree (minimal, moderate, or severe) or occurrence (single episode, recurrent, or persistent). Patients show dysphoria (dis FAWR ee uh), a reduction of energy, and a decrease in activity. Symptoms include anhedonia (an hee DOH nee uh), lack of ability to concentrate, and fatigue. The person may experience *parasomnia*s (abnormal sleep patterns), diminished appetite, and loss of self-esteem.

Etiology. The causes of depression can vary, and they can change with time. In many mental disorders, more than one cause or factor may be involved. Factors that may affect the development of depression include:
- Brain chemistry – this has an effect on mood stability.
- Hormones – the change in body hormones is seen as a possible cause of depression.
- Genetic susceptibility – if a person's close relatives have depression, he or she is more likely to develop it, too.

Risk factors for depression include:
- Close relatives with depression
- Traumatic and stressful events, either recent or in the past (e.g., abuse, death of a loved one, a difficult relationship or break up, loss of a job, and financial difficulties)
- A history of anxiety, eating disorders, or posttraumatic stress disorder
- Abuse of drugs or alcohol
- A serious chronic illness (e.g., cancer, chronic pain, or terminal illness)
- A person who has low self-esteem and/or is self-critical, pessimistic, and easily overwhelmed

Signs and Symptoms. Depression has many signs and symptoms, including some or all of the following:
- Feeling sad, hopeless, weepy, or empty
- No interest in activities that used to be fun and enjoyable
- Easily frustrated or angry
- Change in sleep habits
- Anxiety, restlessness, irritability
- Loss of appetite and weight loss, or increased appetite and weight gain
- Tired, slow, lacking energy; every task seems to require a lot of effort to complete
- Thoughts of death or suicide, or an attempted suicide
- Physical pain (e.g., headaches, backaches, stomach aches or nausea)

> **CRITICAL THINKING 12.9**
>
> Dr. Kahn tells Elaine he must leave the room for a few minutes. He asks her to wait, because he will be back to talk with her about her concerns. Tia steps back into the exam room and asks Elaine if she would like a magazine while she waits. Elaine seems a bit flustered, so Tia asks if she can help. Elaine says that she cannot find a note card she made with questions for Dr. Kahn. She had it in her jacket pocket, but cannot find it now. Tia sees a note card on the exam desk in the room and asks Elaine if that is her card. "Yes, it is," replies Elaine. "I seem to misplace everything these days!"
> Can memory issues be significant? Should Tia mention this to Dr. Kahn?

Signs and symptoms can affect the person's everyday life and interfere with work, relationships, and social activities.

Diagnostic Procedures. Like many mental health conditions, depression cannot be diagnosed with a simple blood test. It can be a complicated diagnosis. Providers will base their diagnosis on the following tests and procedures:

- Physical examination: Depression can be related to physical or mental health problems (e.g., premenstrual syndrome [PMS], bipolar disorder)
- Laboratory tests: These may include a CBC, thyroid function tests, comprehensive metabolic panel (CMP), syphilis testing, and testing for drugs of abuse (see Table 12.6).
- Psychiatric assessment: The provider may ask questions about the patient's state of mind, feelings, interpersonal and social behaviors, and current medications. Patients may also be asked to fill out one or more personality profiles or questionnaires to help with the assessment. (For additional information on methods of mental health assessment, see Diagnostic Procedures, under the section Diseases and Disorders of Mental and Behavioral Health, earlier in this chapter.)
- *Diagnostic and Statistical Manual of Mental Disorders* (DSM-5): A manual used to help diagnose mental and behavioral disorders. It is published by the American Psychiatric Association.

There are many types of depression, with different causes and possible treatments. An accurate diagnosis is important to proper treatment and a positive outcome for the patient.

Treatment. A combination of medication and psychotherapy is the most common treatment for depression. Some types of mild depression may require only medication. Some types of severe depression may require hospitalization or involvement in an outpatient program until symptoms get better.

Medication may include:

- Selective serotonin reuptake inhibitors (SSRIs): These drugs are considered a starting point for medication because they are well tolerated, safer, and have fewer side effects. Examples include fluoxetine (Prozac), paroxetine (Paxil), and sertraline (Zoloft).
- Serotonin-norepinephrine reuptake inhibitors (SNRIs): For example, duloxetine (Cymbalta).
- Tricyclic antidepressants (TCAs): These medications have more side effects, and the side effects can be more severe. Examples include imipramine (Tofranil), nortriptyline (Pamelor), and desipramine (Norpramin).

The provider will work with the patient to find the safest medication that helps alleviate symptoms. Sometimes medications are combined to achieve the desired effect. All antidepressants are required by the Food and Drug Administration (FDA) to be labeled with warnings of increased thoughts of suicide. Patients should be monitored by family and friends for worsening signs of depression and an increased risk for suicide.

Psychotherapy may also be part of a patient's treatment. Talking about issues with other people or healthcare providers can be very useful in resolving feelings of depression. One-on-one or group sessions can both be helpful. Psychiatrists, psychologists, family therapists, and support groups can all help a person deal with mental health issues. Many types of therapy are available. Talking with a therapist about programs, support groups, and non–traditional delivery therapies may be very helpful in meeting an individual's needs.

As with all healthcare issues, self-care is very important. The patient must take time to eat, sleep, and exercise regularly for his or her overall good health. Also, relaxation techniques, massage therapy, music, or art therapy, in addition to continued social engagement, can help to ease depression.

Follow-up care is necessary for any mental health issue. Medication adjustments, therapy sessions, and office visits are part of depression care.

Prognosis. Most depression patients do find relief, but sadly, not all patients do. Patients who comply with and maintain their treatment plan generally do better than patients who are not compliant. Patients who do the best are those who have a good system of support and pursue social engagement. Isolation makes dealing with depression even harder.

Prevention. Preventive measures can be taken to avoid depression. The following strategies can help reduce the risk of depression:

- Take active steps to control stress in all areas of your life and relationships
- Maintain a social support group and use it, especially when you're feeling overwhelmed or sad, or you're suffering a recent loss
- Don't wait to seek treatment. See a provider as early as signs and symptoms appear.
- Be diligent about self-care. Learn how to cope with disappointment and loss. Talk to people you care about, and don't become isolated.

The CDC has a number of suicide prevention resources listed on its website: https://www.cdc.gov/violenceprevention/suicide/prevention.html.

Additional Diseases and Disorders Related to Mental and Behavioral Health

There are many other diseases and disorders related to mental and behavioral health. Tables 12.25 to 12.38 present additional terms and conditions related to mental and behavioral health that may be of interest.

LIFE SPAN CHANGES

Nervous system. Most neurologic disorders involving children are congenital ones. Cerebral palsy is usually the result of birth trauma. Tay-Sachs is an inherited condition. Hydrocephalus (hye droh SEFF uh lus) may be detected on an ultrasound before delivery, and intrauterine prenatal procedures can be done to lessen the effects of the disorder. It should be noted that hydrocephalus may occur in adults after trauma or disease, although this is rare. Spina bifida is yet another congenital disorder that may be detected before birth through prenatal testing. Two pathologic conditions that are not congenital but that are a concern to parents are viral and bacterial meningitis. Viral meningitis is less severe and usually resolves without treatment. Bacterial meningitis can be fatal. *Haemophilus influenzae,* type b (HEE mohf uh lis in floo EN zuh), or Hib, causes meningitis. A vaccine for Hib is available and recommended.

Mental and behavioral health. In addition to the disorders first diagnosed in childhood – autism spectrum disorder, ADHD, conduct disorders, and intellectual and developmental disorders – more and more children are being diagnosed with depressive disorders, substance abuse, and eating disorders.

Nervous system disorders. The two major neurologic disorders of concern as we age are cerebrovascular disease and Alzheimer's disease. Cerebrovascular disease manifests itself in two forms: ministrokes (TIAs) and strokes (CVAs). AD causes a progressive cognitive mental deterioration. It is estimated that by age 65, 1 in 10 individuals will be diagnosed with AD. By age 85, more than half of the population will be diagnosed with the disease.

Mental and behavioral health disorders. Seniors can experience disorders associated with depression and anxiety, along with those caused by dementia.

TABLE 12.25 Terms Related to General Symptoms

Term	Definition
akathisia (ack uh THEE zsa)	Inability to remain calm, still, and free of anxiety
amnesia (am NEE zsa)	Inability to remember either isolated parts of the past, or one's entire past. It may be caused by brain damage or severe emotional trauma.
catatonia (kat tah TOH nee ah)	Paralysis or immobility from psychological or emotional rather than physical causes
confabulation (kon fab byoo LAY shun)	Effort to conceal a gap in memory by fabricating detailed, often believable stories. It is associated with alcohol abuse.
defense mechanism	Unconscious mechanism for psychological coping, adjustment, or self-preservation in the face of stress or a threat. Examples include *denial* of an unpleasant situation or condition and *projection* of intolerable aspects onto another individual.
dementia (dih MEN shah)	Mental disorder in which the individual experiences a progressive loss of memory, personality alterations, confusion, loss of touch with reality, and *stupor* (seeming unawareness of, and disconnection with, one's surroundings).
echolalia (eh koh LAYL yuh)	Repetition of words or phrases spoken by others
libido (lih BEE doh)	Normal psychological impulse drive associated with sensuality, expressions of desire, or creativity. Abnormality occurs only when such drives are excessively heightened or depressed.
somnambulism (som NAM byoo liz um)	Sleepwalking

From Shiland B: *Mastering healthcare terminology*, ed 5, St Louis, 2015, Elsevier.

TABLE 12.26 Terms Related to Disorders Usually First Diagnosed in Childhood

Term	Definition
attention deficit/ hyperactivity disorder (ADHD)	Series of syndromes that includes impulsiveness, inability to concentrate, and short attention span
conduct disorder	Any of a number of disorders characterized by patterns of persistent aggressive and defiant behaviors. *Oppositional defiant disorder (ODD),* an example of a conduct disorder, is characterized by hostile, disobedient behavior.
intellectual and developmental disabilities	Condition of subaverage intellectual ability, with impairments in social and educational functioning. The intelligence quotient (IQ) is a measure of an individual's intellectual functioning compared with the general population. DSM-5 refers to this condition as *intellectual disability* (ID), but the renaming has caused debate. *Mild ID:* IQ range of 50 to 69; learning difficulties result *Moderate ID:* IQ range of 35 to 49; support needed to function in society *Severe ID:* IQ of 20 to 34; continuous need for support to live in society *Profound ID:* IQ less than 20; severe self-care limitations
autism spectrum disorder (ASD) (ah TISS um)	Group of developmental delay disorders characterized by impairment of communication skills and social interactions (including delayed language acquisition), and repetitive behaviors.

From Shiland B: *Mastering healthcare terminology*, ed 5, St Louis, 2015, Elsevier.

TABLE 12.27 Terms Related to Mood Disorders

Term	Definition
bipolar disorder (BD), BP (bye POH lur)	Disorder characterized by swings between an elevation of mood, increased energy and activity (hypomania and mania), and a lowering of mood and decreased energy and activity (depression).
cyclothymia (sye kloh THIGH mee ah)	Disorder characterized by recurring episodes of mild elation and depression that are not severe enough to warrant a diagnosis of BD.
dysthymia (dis THIGH mee ah)	Mild, chronic depression of mood that lasts for years but is not severe enough to justify a diagnosis of depression.
persistent mood disorders	Group of long-term, cyclic mood disorders in which the majority of the individual episodes are not sufficiently severe to warrant being described as hypomanic or mild depressive episodes.
seasonal affective disorder (SAD)	Weather-induced depression resulting from decreased exposure to sunlight in autumn and winter.

From Shiland B: *Mastering healthcare terminology*, ed 5, St Louis, 2015, Elsevier.

TABLE 12.28 Terms Related to Personality Disorders

Term	Definition
borderline personality disorder	Disorder characterized by impulsive, unpredictable mood and self-image, resulting in unstable interpersonal relationships and a tendency to see and respond to others as unwaveringly good or evil.
dissocial personality disorder	Disorder in which the patient shows a complete lack of interest in social obligations, to the extreme of showing antipathy for other individuals. Patients frustrate easily, are quick to display aggression, show a tendency to blame others, and do not change their behavior even after punishment. Also called *dyssocial personality disorder*.
paranoid personality disorder	State in which the individual exhibits inappropriately suspicious thinking, self-importance, a lack of ability to forgive perceived insults, and an extreme sense of personal rights.
schizoid personality disorder	Condition in which the patient withdraws into a fantasy world with little need for social interaction. Most patients have a limited capacity to experience pleasure or to express their feelings.
schizophrenia	Disorders characterized by fundamental distortions of thinking and perception, coupled with affects that are inappropriate or blunted (see Fig. 12.27).
acute and transient psychotic disorders	Group of disorders characterized by the acute onset (2 weeks or less) of psychotic symptoms (e.g., delusions, hallucinations, and perceptual disturbances) and by the severe disruption of ordinary behavior. The condition is not severe enough to justify a diagnosis of delirium. It may be associated with acute stress.
persistent delusional disorders	Variety of disorders in which long-standing delusions constitute the only clinical characteristic.

From Shiland B: *Mastering healthcare terminology*, ed 5, St Louis, 2015, Elsevier.

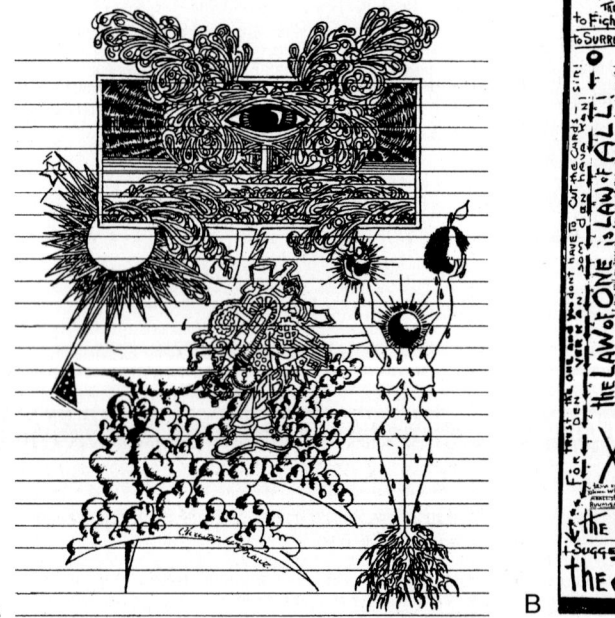
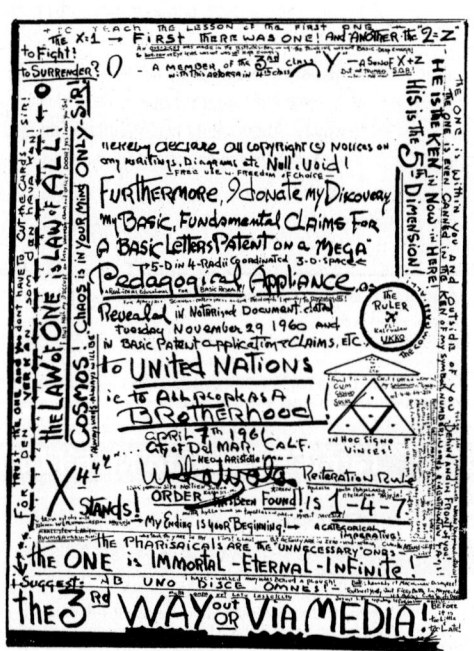

FIG. 12.27 (A) Drawing by a delusional patient with schizophrenia. (B) This drawing by a patient with schizophrenia demonstrates thought disorder. (From Stuart GW, Laraia MT: *Principles and practice of psychiatric nursing*, ed 9, St Louis, 2009, Mosby.)

TABLE 12.29 Terms Related to Anxiety Disorders

Term	Definition
acrophobia (ack roh FOH bee ah)	Fear of heights
agoraphobia (ah gore uh FOH bee ah)	Fear of leaving home and entering crowded places
anthropophobia (an throh poh FOH bee ah)	Fear of scrutiny by other people; also called *social phobia*
claustrophobia (klos troh FOH bee ah)	Fear of enclosed spaces
generalized anxiety disorder (GAD)	One of the most common diagnoses assigned, but not specific to any particular situation or circumstance. Symptoms may include persistent nervousness, trembling, muscular tension, sweating, lightheadedness, palpitations, dizziness, and epigastric discomfort.
obsessive-compulsive disorder (OCD)	Recurrent, distressing, and unavoidable preoccupations or irresistible drives to perform specific rituals (e.g., constantly checking locks, excessive hand washing) that the patient feels will prevent some harmful event.
panic disorder (PD)	Recurrent, unpredictable attacks of severe anxiety (panic) that are not restricted to any particular situation. Symptoms may include vertigo, chest pain, and heart palpitations.
posttraumatic stress disorder (PTSD)	Extended emotional response to a traumatic event. Symptoms may include flashbacks, recurring nightmares, anhedonia, insomnia, hypervigilance, anxiety, depression, suicidal thoughts, and emotional blunting.

From Shiland B: *Mastering healthcare terminology*, ed 5, St Louis, 2015, Elsevier.

TABLE 12.30 Terms Related to Adjustment and Coping Disorders

Term	Definition
adjustment disorder	Disorder that tends to manifest during periods of stressful life changes (e.g., divorce, death, relocation, job loss). Symptoms include anxiety, impaired coping mechanisms, social dysfunction, and a reduced ability to perform normal daily activities.
dissociative identity disorder	Maladaptive coping with severe stress by developing one or more separate personalities. A less severe form, *dissociative disorder* or *dissociative reaction*, results in identity confusion accompanied by amnesia, a dreamlike state, and somnambulism.
somatoform disorder (soh MAT toh form)	Any disorder that has unfounded physical complaints by the patient, despite medical assurance that no physiologic problem exists. One type of somatoform disorder is *illness anxiety disorder*, which is a preoccupation with the possibility of having one or more serious and progressive physical disorders.

From Shiland B: *Mastering healthcare terminology*, ed 5, St Louis, 2015, Elsevier.

TABLE 12.31 Terms Related to Eating Disorders

Term	Definition
anorexia nervosa (an oh RECKS see ah nur VOH sah)	Prolonged refusal to eat adequate amounts of food and an altered perception of what constitutes a normal minimum body weight. These are caused by an intense fear of becoming obese. The condition primarily affects adolescent females; emaciation and amenorrhea result (Fig. 12.28).
bulimia nervosa (boo LIM ee ah nur VOH sah)	Eating disorder in which the individual eats large quantities of food and then purges the body through self-induced vomiting or inappropriate use of laxatives.

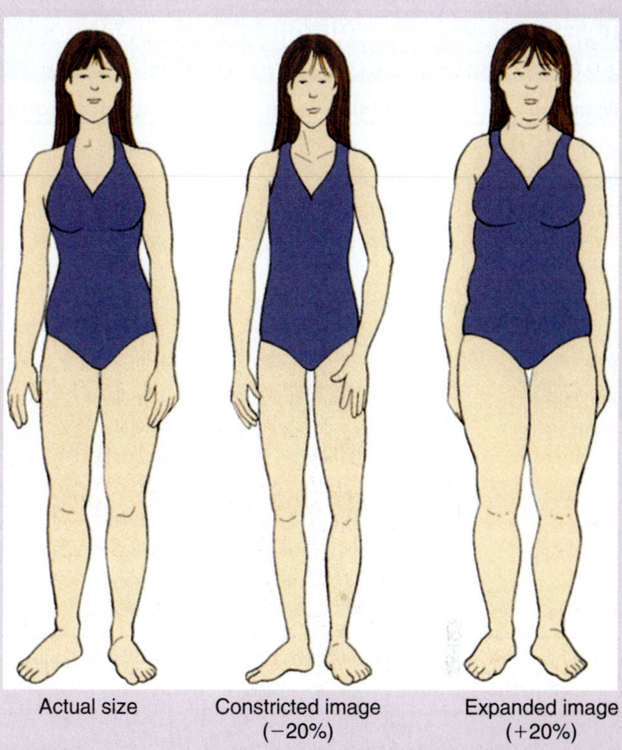

FIG. 12.28 The perception of body shape and size can be evaluated with the use of special computer drawing programs. These programs allow a subject to distort (increase or decrease) the width of an actual picture of a person's body by as much as 20%. Individuals with anorexia consistently adjusted their own body picture to a size 20% larger than its true form. This suggests that they have a major problem with the perception of self-image. (From Stuart GW, Laraia MT: *Principles and practice of psychiatric nursing*, ed 9, St Louis, 2009, Mosby.)

Actual size — Constricted image (−20%) — Expanded image (+20%)

From Shiland B: *Mastering healthcare terminology*, ed 5, St Louis, 2015, Elsevier.

TABLE 12.32 Terms Related to Habit and Impulse Disorders

Term	Definition
kleptomania (klep toh MAY nee ah)	Uncontrollable impulse to steal
pyromania (pye roh MAY nee ah)	Uncontrollable impulse to set fires
trichotillomania (trick oh till oh MAY nee ah)	Uncontrollable impulse to pull one's hair out by the roots

From Shiland B: *Mastering healthcare terminology*, ed 5, St Louis, 2015, Elsevier.

TABLE 12.33 Combining and Adjective Forms for the Nervous System

Meaning	Combining Form	Adjective Form
body	somat/o	somatic
brain	encephal/o	
cerebellum	cerebell/o	cerebellar
cerebrum	cerebr/o	cerebral
cortex	cortic/o	cortical
dendrite	dendr/o	dendritic
dura mater	dur/o	dural
lobe	lob/o	lobular, lobar
meninges	mening/o, meningi/o	meningeal
nerve	neur/o	neural
nerve root	rhiz/o, radicul/o	radicular
same	home/o	
skin	dermat/o	dermatic
spinal cord	cord/o, chord/o, myel/o	cordal, chordal
star	astr/o	astral
ventricle	ventricul/o	ventricular

From Shiland B: *Mastering healthcare terminology*, ed 5, St Louis, 2015, Elsevier.

TABLE 12.34 Suffixes for the Nervous System

Suffix	Meaning
-cyte	cell
-glia	glue
-logy	study of
-on	structure
-stasis	stopping, controlling
-tome	instrument used to cut

From Shiland B: *Mastering healthcare terminology*, ed 5, St Louis, 2015, Elsevier.

TABLE 12.35 Abbreviations for the Nervous System

Abbreviation	Definition
AD	Alzheimer's disease
ADL	activity of daily living
ALS	amyotrophic lateral sclerosis
ANS	autonomic nervous system
BBB	blood-brain barrier
C1-C8	cervical nerves
CNS	central nervous system
CP	cerebral palsy
CSF	cerebrospinal fluid
CT scan	computerized tomography scan
CVA	cerebrovascular accident
DTR	deep tendon reflex
EEG	electroencephalogram, electroencephalography
EP	evoked potential
GARS	gait assessment rating scale
HIVD	herniated intervertebral disk
L1-L5	lumbar nerves
LP	lumbar puncture
MRI	magnetic resonance imaging
MS	multiple sclerosis
MSLT	multiple sleep latency test
PD	Parkinson's disease
PET scan	positron emission tomography scan
PNS	peripheral nervous system
PSG	polysomnography
S1-S5	sacral nerves
SNS	somatic nervous system
SPECT	single-photon emission computed tomography
T1-T12	thoracic nerves
TENS	transcutaneous electrical nerve stimulation
TIA	transient ischemia

From Shiland B: *Mastering healthcare terminology*, ed 5, St Louis, 2015, Elsevier.

TABLE 12.36 Combining and Adjective Forms for Mental and Behavioral Health

Meaning	Combining Form	Adjective Form
attraction	phil/o	
mind	psych/o, thym/o, phren/o	psychic, thymic
treatment	iatr/o	

From Shiland B: *Mastering healthcare terminology*, ed 5, St Louis, 2015, Elsevier.

TABLE 12.37 Suffixes for Mental and Behavioral Health

Suffix	Meaning
-ia, -ism	condition
-iatrist	one who specializes in treatment
-mania	condition of madness
-phobia	condition of fear

From Shiland B: *Mastering healthcare terminology*, ed 5, St Louis, 2015, Elsevier.

TABLE 12.38 Abbreviations for Mental and Behavioral Health

Abbreviation	Definition
ADHD	attention deficit/hyperactivity disorder
APA	American Psychiatric Association
ASD	autism spectrum disorder
BD, BP	bipolar disorder
DAP	Draw-a-Person (Test)
DSM	Diagnostic and Statistical Manual of Mental Disorders
DTs	delirium tremens
ECT	electroconvulsive therapy
GAD	generalized anxiety disorder
ICD	International Classification of Diseases
IQ	intelligence quotient
MMPI	Minnesota Multiphasic Personality Inventory
MR	mental retardation
OCD	obsessive-compulsive disorder
ODD	oppositional defiant disorder
PD	panic disorder
PTSD	posttraumatic stress disorder
SAD	seasonal affective disorder
SSRI	selective serotonin reuptake inhibitor
TAT	Thematic Apperception Test
WAIS	Wechsler Adult Intelligence Scale

From Shiland B: *Mastering healthcare terminology*, ed 5, St Louis, 2015, Elsevier.

CLOSING COMMENTS

The nervous system is the major communication and control system in the human body. It influences and regulates all mental activity, including thought, learning, and memory. Along with the endocrine system, it is responsible for regulating body systems to maintain homeostasis. Through its many receptors, the nervous system constantly monitors what is happening inside the body.

When the nervous system becomes damaged or diseased, signs and symptoms can appear in all body systems. Motor activity can become erratic, or a person's activity level can decline to the point where the individual becomes unable to communicate or function normally.

As a medical assistant, you should always observe, listen, and report to the provider any changes you notice in a patient's behavior. Even signs and symptoms that may seem minor can give the provider a needed clue to the proper diagnosis.

CHAPTER REVIEW

Our chapter on the nervous system is packed with information. The nervous system is a complex system with many structures to learn. We started out with the anatomy of the nervous system. The central nervous system is composed of the brain and spinal cord. The peripheral nervous system is composed of all the nerves that extend from the brain and the spinal cord to the tissues of the body. There are 12 pairs of cranial nerves and 31 pairs of spinal nerves. The PNS is further divided into the somatic system and the autonomic system. The somatic system is voluntary. It collects information from the skin, muscles, and joints. The autonomic system is mostly involuntary. It collects information from the internal organs and glands and sends it on to the brain. Instructions return from the brain for the affected muscles, organs, and glands.

The cells of the nervous system are the neuron and neuroglia. The neuron is responsible for communicating information to and from the brain to maintain homeostasis. The neuroglia help support the functions of the neurons. Neurons are made up of three parts: dendrites, cell body, and axons. Dendrites receive nerve impulses and carry them to the cell body, which is the control center of the cell. From the cell body, the impulse moves away along the axon, a slender, elongated projection that carries the impulse toward the next neuron.

A nerve impulse is called an action potential. It is an electrical impulse that travels down the axon of one neuron, crosses the synapse between nerve cells, and arrives at the dendrite of another neuron. The impulse is passed across the synapse by a chemical messenger called a neurotransmitter. Messages move through the nervous system in this fashion until they reach the target tissue.

The brain is made up of four different parts: the cerebrum, the cerebellum, the diencephalon, and the brainstem. The cerebrum is the largest part of the brain. It is responsible for higher order thinking. Because of our developed cerebrum, we can think, draw, write, sing, dance, and perform any number of complex tasks. The cerebrum

EXCEPTIONAL CUSTOMER SERVICE

The ability to think critically is an important part of exceptional customer service. An essential component of critical thinking is the ability to question patients logically, and then listen carefully to their answers. We must always be on the alert for any personal bias that may prevent us from delivering respectful patient care. This is especially true for interacting with patients who have been diagnosed with mental and behavioral disorders. The medical assistant's ability to conduct a professional and respectful patient history shows his or her professionalism. Using appropriate interpersonal communication skills lays the groundwork for the client's care in the provider's office.

---

is further divided into the frontal lobe, temporal lobe, parietal lobe, and occipital lobe. Each area of the cerebrum has specialized functions.

The cerebellum is just below the cerebrum at the back of the brain. It controls balance, posture, and muscle coordination. The diencephalon is composed of the thalamus and hypothalamus. The thalamus is responsible for relaying sensory information to the cerebrum, and for translating some sensory information into sensations of pain, temperature, and touch. The hypothalamus controls the ANS, regulates the endocrine system, and manages body temperature, sleep, and appetite to maintain homeostasis.

The brainstem is composed of three main parts: midbrain, pons, and medulla oblongata. The midbrain is the reflex center for eye and head movements in response to visual and auditory stimuli. The pons serves as a bridge between the medulla oblongata and the cerebrum. The lowest part of the brainstem, the medulla oblongata, regulates the heart rate, blood pressure, and breathing.

The spinal cord extends from the medulla oblongata to the second lumbar vertebra. The spinal cord is protected by the bony vertebrae surrounding it and the coverings unique to the CNS, called meninges. The spinal cord is composed of the cell bodies of motor neurons (gray matter), and the myelin-covered axons (white matter) that extend from the nerve cell bodies. Spinal nerves come out from the spinal cord, and each nerve stimulates a specific organ or area of the body.

The PNS is made up of cranial and spinal nerves. Cranial nerves originate from the underside of the brain. They relay information to and from the sensory organs and muscles of the face and neck. The spinal nerves exit the spinal canal through spaces between the vertebrae. Spinal nerves closely mimic the organization of the vertebrae and provide stimulation to the rest of the body. Spinal nerves carry information to and from the brain through the spinal cord.

The ANS consists of nerves that regulate involuntary function. The ANS is an automatic system that regulates body functions such as breathing, heart rate, sweating, circulation, and digestion. It also controls the actions of muscles in blood vessel walls, organs, and glands. The motor portion of this system is further divided into the sympathetic nervous system and the parasympathetic nervous system. These two opposing systems help maintain homeostasis throughout the body systems. The sympathetic nervous system can produce a fight-or-flight response. This is the part of the nervous system that helps the individual respond to perceived stress. The parasympathetic nervous system does the opposite; it is sometimes called the rest-and-digest system.

In the physiology section of this chapter, we talked about mental and behavioral health. Mental health disorders can be caused by a number of factors, alone or in combination. These factors include changes in brain chemicals, hereditary makeup, psychological disposition, and life experiences. Emotional and physical symptoms can occur for no apparent reason and can be quite persistent. However, even though some mental illnesses have organic causes, in which neurotransmitters and other known brain functions play a role, there is often no mental anatomy to be tested. Instead, behavioral health is a complex interaction involving an individual's emotional, physical, mental, and behavioral processes in an environment that includes cultural and spiritual influences.

In this chapter we discussed nervous system diseases and disorder. We also discussed mental and behavioral diseases and disorders. The chapter discussed a large number of conditions, but those covered in depth were cerebrovascular accidents (strokes), epilepsy, Parkinson's disease, Alzheimer's disease, and depressive disorders. Many other diseases, disorders, and conditions were briefly explained in tables at the end of the chapter.

SCENARIO WRAP-UP

Dr. Kahn and Elaine had a wonderful chat as they worked through Elaine's physical. He learned a lot about her and enjoyed their conversation. He also had a chance not only to talk with Elaine, but also to observe her and assess her walk, speech, hand tremor, and muscle flexibility. He listened to her concerns. He has ordered a few routine laboratory tests as part of her physical, including a CBC, a lipid profile, and a urinalysis.

Dr. Kahn suspects that Elaine's lab work will come back normal. But he would like her to see a specialist, a neurologist. Dr. Kahn suspects that Elaine may have a condition that is affecting her nerves. He wants her to see a specialist and get a neurologic work-up and diagnosis. Dr. Kahn calls Tia into the exam room and asks her to help Elaine set up an appointment through the neurology clinic in town. Elaine seems a little nervous. But she is relieved that Dr. Kahn and Tia have taken such good care of her today, and that they have spent extra time listening to her concerns.

Tia talks to Dr. Kahn at the end of the day. They enjoyed the appointment with Elaine. Tia was able to set up an appointment with the neurologist for 2 weeks from today. Dr. Kahn and Tia hope that Elaine can get a clear diagnosis after that appointment. Dr. Kahn doesn't say anything to Tia, but he suspects that Elaine has Parkinson's disease.

13

Sensory System

LEARNING OBJECTIVES

1. Discuss the anatomy of the eye, list the major structures of the eye, and identify the anatomic location of the major structures of the eye.
2. Discuss the anatomy of the ear, list the major structures of the ear, and identify the anatomic location of the major structures of the ear.
3. Describe the normal function and physiology of the eye.
4. Describe the normal function and physiology of the ear.
5. Complete the following related to the diseases and disorders of the eye:
   - Identify the common etiology, signs and symptoms, and diagnostic measures of diseases and disorders related to the eye.
   - Identify CLIA-waived tests associated with common eye diseases and disorders.
   - Describe treatment modalities used for eye diseases and disorders.
6. Complete the following related to the diseases and disorders of the ear:
   - Identify the common etiology, signs and symptoms, and diagnostic measures of diseases and disorders related to the ear.
   - Identify CLIA-waived tests associated with common ear diseases and disorders.
   - Describe treatment modalities used for ear diseases and disorders.
7. Compare the structure and function of the sensory system across the life span.

CHAPTER OUTLINE

1. Opening Scenario, 295
2. You Will Learn, 295
3. Introduction to the Special Senses, 296
4. **Anatomy of the Eye, 296**
   a. Ocular Adnexa, 296
   b. Eyeball, 297
5. **Anatomy of the Ear, 299**
   a. Outer (External) Ear, 299
   b. Middle Ear, 299
   c. Inner Ear, 300
6. Physiology of the Eye, 301
7. Physiology of the Ear, 301
8. **Diseases and Disorders of the Eyes and Ears, 301**
9. **Diseases and Disorders of the Eye, 309**
   a. Cataract, 309
   b. Glaucoma, 310
   c. Macular Degeneration, 311
10. **Diseases and Disorders of the Ear, 313**
    a. Ménière Disease, 313
    b. Otosclerosis, 314
    c. Presbycusis, 314
11. Additional Diseases and Disorders of the Eyes and Ears, 315
12. Life Span Changes, 315
13. Closing Comments, 321
14. Chapter Review, 322
15. Scenario Wrap-Up, 323

▶ OPENING SCENARIO

Rosie Tran-Moore, a certified medical assistant (CMA) through the American Association of Medical Assistants (AAMA), has been working at Walden-Martin Family Medicine (WMFM) Clinic for about 3 years. She really enjoys the variety of patients she sees at the clinic. She is working with Dr. Julie Walden today.

One of the things Rosie likes about a family practice clinic is the different ages of the patients. They see young children, adolescents, middle-aged adults, and some older adult patients. They also see an assortment of health conditions too. It reminds Rosie to stay up-to-date with her continuing education units (CEUs). She knows she needs to stay current with technology and procedures so that she can provide the best care for her patients.

YOU WILL LEARN

1. To recognize and use terms related to the special senses.
2. To locate the structures of the special senses.
3. To understand and describe the functions of the special senses: sight, hearing, and balance.
4. To recognize disease states of the eyes and ears, as well as their causes, signs and symptoms, diagnostic processes, treatment, prognoses, and prevention.

> **BOX 13.1 Specialties/Specialists**
>
> *Ophthalmology* (of thuh l-MOL uh jee) is the healthcare specialty that diagnoses, treats, and helps prevent most eye-related diseases and disorders. An *ophthalmologist* (of thuh l-MOL uh jist) is a healthcare specialist in this field. An *optometrist* (op TOM ih trist) is a healthcare professional who measures and evaluates vision and prescribes corrective solutions as needed. Although glasses and contact lenses used to be the only options to correct vision, corrective surgery is now an accepted practice.
> *Audiology* (aw dee OL uh jee) is the healthcare specialty that diagnoses and treats hearing loss and the diseases and disorders or the ear related to hearing. An *audiologist* (aw dee OL uh jist) is a healthcare specialist in this field.
> *Otorhinolaryngology* (oh toh rahy noh lar ing GOL uh jee) is the healthcare specialty that diagnoses and treats disorders of the ears, nose, and throat (ENT). The specialist is an *otorhinolaryngologist* (oh toh rahy nol lar ing GOL uh jist).

> **BOX 13.2 Smell and Taste**
>
> The *olfactory* (ol FAK tuh ree) sense is the sense of smell. The receptors for smell are in the upper part of the nasal cavity.
> The sense of smell is very sensitive, but it can easily become fatigued. When you enter a room you may smell a scent or odor, but within a few minutes you may not notice it any more. That is sensory fatigue.
> The *gustatory* (GUHS tuh tawr ee) sense is the sense of taste. There are five tastes: sweet, sour, bitter, salty, and umami or savory. Eating something sweet at the end of a meal helps the brain form a memory of a meal.

INTRODUCTION TO THE SPECIAL SENSES

A medical assistant is responsible for performing a wide variety of procedures in an *ophthalmologic* (of thuh l-MOL uh jik) or *otorhinolaryngologic* (oh toh rahy noh lar ing GOL uh jik) practice (Box 13.1). First, the medical assistant must be familiar with the normal anatomy and physiology of the eyes, ears, nose, and throat. Learning the fundamental procedures gives you a good knowledge base on which to build advanced techniques.

There are two categories of senses in the body. There are general senses and special senses. The general senses have receptors scattered throughout the body and gather information through all areas of the body. These are the general senses:
- Touch
- Pressure
- Temperature
- Pain

The special senses have receptors that are concentrated in one area. Each of the special senses has a complex organ with receptors to gather stimuli and send the information to the brain for interpretation. The special senses include the following:

- Vision
- Hearing
- Equilibrium (balance)
- Taste
- Smell

Senses allow us to experience our environment and then act on our perceptions. They also give the body information that can protect us from harm. This chapter covers the eyes, ears, and equilibrium. See Box 13.2 for a brief description of the special senses of smell and taste.

ANATOMY OF THE EYE

The eye can be divided into the *ocular adnexa* (OK yuh ler ad NEK suh), the structures that surround and support the function of the eyeball, and the structures of the eye itself.

Ocular Adnexa

Each of our paired eyes is encased in a protective, bony socket called the *orbit*. Our **binocular** (buh NOK yuh ler) vision sends two slightly different images to the brain that produce depth of vision. Within the orbit, a cushion of fatty tissue protects the eyeball. Only about one-sixth of the eye lies outside the orbit. The eyelid helps protect the eye from trauma. The eyebrows help keep irritants out of the eyes. The eyelashes line the margins of the eyelids and help trap foreign particles (Fig. 13.1).

The *conjunctiva* (kun jungk TYE vuh) is a thin mucous membrane that lines the eyelid. It covers the outside of the eyeball except for the most central portion. The *cornea* (KOR nee uh) covers the center of the eye. The mucus secreted from the conjunctiva helps keep the eye moist. The eye blinks about every 2 to 3 seconds. Blinking causes the *lacrimal* (LAK ruh muhl) gland, located in the superior outer portion of the upper eyelid, to secrete tears. Tears move across the eyes, cleansing and moistening the surface of the eye. Tears drain into the lacrimal canals in the medial corner of the eye. The tears then drain into the nasal cavity through the *nasolacrimal* (ney zoh LAK ruh muhl) duct. This is why when a person cries, the excess tears ultimately empty into the nose, producing a watery nasal discharge.

> **VOCABULARY**
> **binocular:** Involving, relating, or seeing with both eyes.

> **MEDICAL TERMINOLOGY**
> **-ar:** pertaining to
> **audi/o, acous/o:** hearing
> **bi-, bin-:** two
> **laryng/o:** throat
> **-logy:** study of
> **ocul/o, ophthalm/o:** eye
> **ocul/o:** eye
> **opt/o, optic/o:** vision
> **orbit/o:** orbit
> **ot/o:** ear
> **rhin/o:** nose

> **CRITICAL THINKING 13.1**
>
> Last night Rosie was completing a CEU regarding the senses. Can you list the general senses and special senses? Can you think of a phrase or saying that may help you remember special and general senses? Share your ideas with the class.

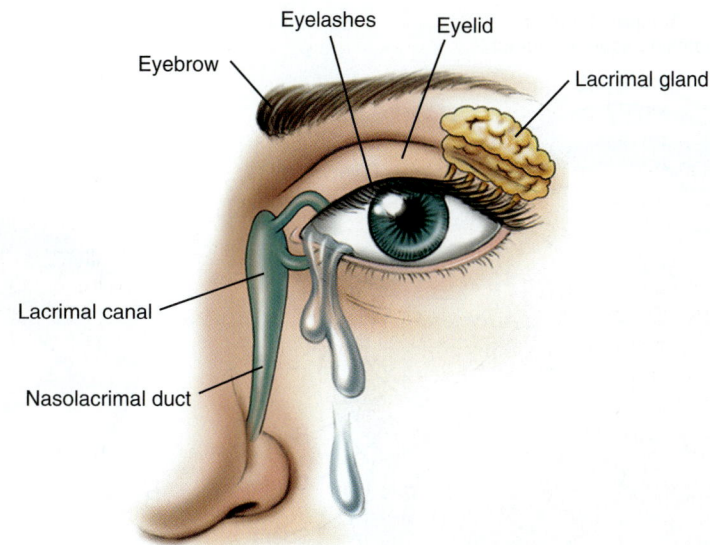

FIG. 13.1 Ocular adnexa. (From Herlihy B, Maebius NK: *The Human Body in Health and Illness*, ed 4, Philadelphia, 2011, Saunders.)

> **BOX 13.3 Corneal Transplants**
>
> The cornea was one of the first tissues to be transplanted in the human body. Corneal transplants are now common. Long-term success after corneal implant surgery is excellent.

> **BOX 13.4 Uvea**
>
> The *uvea* is the middle, highly vascularized layer of the eye. It includes the following structures: the iris, the ciliary body, and the choroid.

> **BOX 13.5 Albinism**
>
> People who have **albinism** (AL buh niz uhm) will have reddish pink eyes. They lack pigment in their skin and in the iris of the eye. Their eyes appear pink or red because without a normally colored iris, the blood vessels inside the eye show through the iris.

The *extraocular* (eck strah OCK yoo lur) muscles attach the eyeball to the orbit and move the eyes. There are six skeletal muscles that help move the eyeball: four *rectus* (straight) and two *oblique* (diagonal) muscles.

Eyeball

The eyeball consists of three layers. The outermost layer is made up of the white, opaque *sclera* (SKLAIR uh) and the transparent cornea. The sclera is a tough, fibrous lining that protects the entire eyeball lying within the orbit. It is also known as the white of the eye. The transparent cornea covers the exposed one-sixth of the eyeball (Box 13.3). The cornea acts like a window that allows light to enter the eye. The cornea also *refracts*, or bends the direction of light rays, after they enter the eye (Fig. 13.2).

The middle layer is made up of the *choroid* (KOR oyd), the *iris* (EYE ris), and the *ciliary* (SILL ih air ee) body (Box 13.4). The iris is the colored portion of the eye (Box 13.5). It is doughnut shaped, with the opening of the *pupil* in the center. The iris contains muscles that regulate the size of the pupil depending on the intensity of light. It becomes smaller in bright light and opens wider in dim light. The ciliary body contains both the ciliary muscle, which regulates the shape of the lens, and the ciliary processes, which secrete *aqueous* (AY kwee us) *humor*. The choroid is the posterior portion of the middle layer of the eye. It is the eye's **vascular** (VAS kyuh ler) layer. It contains many blood vessels that supply nutrients to the outer layers of the *retina* (RET in uh). The choroid also has a brown pigment that absorbs excess light rays that could interfere with vision.

> **MEDICAL TERMINOLOGY**
> **-al:** pertaining to
> **blephar/o, palpebr/o:** eyelid
> **conjunctiv/o:** conjunctiva
> **conjunctiva** (singular), **conjunctivae** (plural)
> **corne/o, kerat/o:** cornea
> **dacryoaden/o:** lacrimal gland
> **extra-:** outside
> **lacrim/o, dacry/o:** tears
> **nas/o:** nose
> **ocul/o:** eye
> **scler/o:** sclera

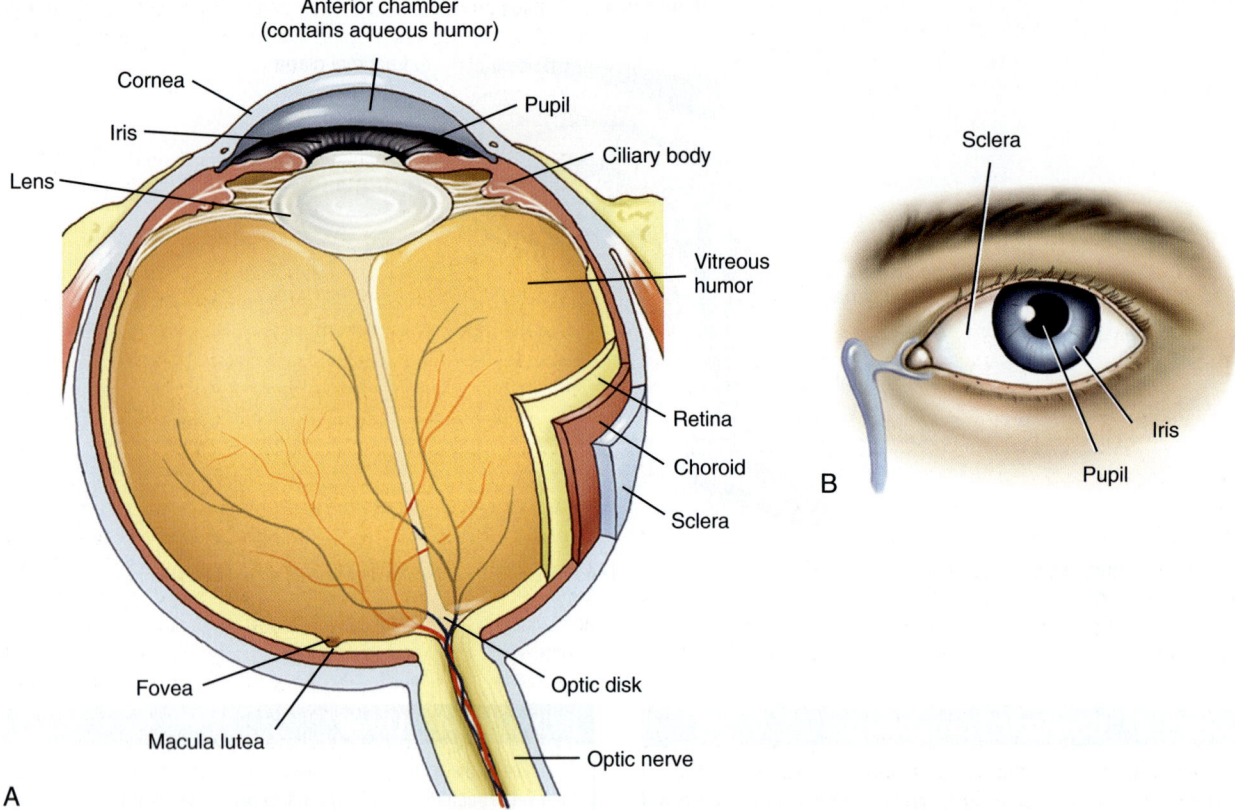

FIG. 13.2 (A) The eyeball viewed from above. (B) Anterior view of the eyeball. (From Shiland: *Mastering Healthcare Terminology*, ed 5, St. Louis, 2016, Elsevier.)

VOCABULARY
albinism: A condition that leaves a person with pale skin, light or white hair, and red or pinkish eyes. Caused by a genetic inability to produce the pigment melanin.
blind spot: A small area on the retina that is insensitive to light. Where the optic nerve joins the retina.
vascular: Having (blood) vessels that conduct or circulate liquids (blood).

MEDICAL TERMINOLOGY
aque/o: water
choroid/o: choroid
cycl/o: ciliary body
ir/o, irid/o: iris
iris (singular), **irides** (plural)
macul/o: macula lutea
papill/o: optic disk
pupill/o, core/o, cor/o: pupil
retin/o: retina
scler/o: hard
vascul/o: blood vessel

BOX 13.6 Rods
Rods sense light with the help of a light-sensitive pigment called rhodopsin. The body needs vitamin A to produce rhodopsin.

CRITICAL THINKING 13.2
It has been a few years since Rosie took her certification exam, so a review of the anatomy of the eye and ear was a good refresher. What structure in the eye helps regulate the shape of the lens? What structure in the eye has a brown color and is highly vascular?

The inner layer of the eye includes the retina in the posterior portion and the lens in the anterior portion. The delicate tissue of the retina is composed of light-sensitive neurons called rods and cones. *Rods* are highly sensitive to light and can function in dim light (Box 13.6). *Cones* function in bright light and detect color. Rods and cones convert light into nerve impulses. These impulses travel through the optic nerve to the brain, where they are converted into images.

During daylight, the area of the retina where light rays focus is called the *macula lutea* (MACK yoo lah LOO tee uh). The *fovea* (FOH vee uh) *centralis* is an area within the macula that only contains cones and provides the sharpest image. There is a natural **blind spot** in our vision where the *optic disk* is located. The optic disk is where the optic nerve leaves the retina to travel to the brain. There are no light receptors in the optic disk.

> **CRITICAL THINKING 13.3**
> There are two types of photoreceptors on the retina. Can you name them both? Which receptor detects color? Which receptor functions in dim light?

The lens is a transparent, **biconvex** (bahy KON veks) body that helps focus light after it passes through the cornea. The lens and the ciliary body divide the eye into two cavities. The posterior cavity, which is between the lens and the retina, contains the transparent, gel-like *vitreous* (VIT ree us) *humor*. The vitreous humor maintains the shape of the posterior eyeball. The anterior cavity, between the cornea and the lens, is filled with aqueous humor, which is continuously produced by the ciliary processes. Aqueous humor helps maintain normal pressure within the eye and provides nutrients to the lens and the cornea (see Fig. 13.2).

The pupil is the dark area in the center of the iris where the light continues its progress through to the lens. The lens is an **avascular** (ahy VAS kyuh ler) structure made of protein and covered by an elastic capsule. It is held in place by the thin strands of muscle that make up the ciliary body. The fluid produced by the capillaries of the ciliary body is called the aqueous humor. It nourishes the cornea, gives shape to the anterior eye, and maintains an optimum *intraocular* (in truh OK yuh ler) *pressure* (IOP). It normally drains through tiny veins called the *canals of Schlemm*. The aqueous humor circulates in both the anterior chamber (between the cornea and the iris) and the posterior chamber (behind the iris and in front of the lens). Between the lens and the retina is the vitreous humor, which holds the choroid membrane against the retina to ensure an adequate blood supply. The choroid is the vascular membrane between the sclera and the retina. Any damage to the retina has the potential to cause partial or complete blindness. The retina is the neurologic center of vision.

> **STUDY TIP**
> The lens of the eye flattens to adjust to something seen at a distance, or it thickens for close vision. The process by which the lens flattens or thickens its shape is called *accommodation*.

ANATOMY OF THE EAR

The visible portion of the ear is only a small part of the actual organ of hearing. Most of the sensory structure lies hidden in the *temporal* (TEM per uhl) bone. The ear is divided into the outer, middle, and inner ear (Fig. 13.3).

Outer (External) Ear

The outer ear consists of the *auricle* (ORE ick kul), or *pinna* (PIN nuh). This is the fleshy part of the ear that can be seen on the side of the head. The next structure is the external *auditory* (AH dih tor ee) canal, the tube that extends from the auricle in to the *tympanic* (tim PAN ick) *membrane* (eardrum).

The auricle collects sound waves and sends them down the auditory canal. The skin that lines the auditory canal contains numerous hair follicles and many nerve endings. Earwax, or *cerumen* (sih ROO men), is secreted by modified sweat glands within the external auditory canal. Both the hair and the waxy cerumen help prevent foreign objects from reaching the eardrum. The canal has a slightly curved-shape and is approximately 1-inch (2.5-cm) long.

Middle Ear

The middle ear is an air-filled cavity that contains three tiny bones called the *ossicles* (AH sick kuls). The ossicles are named for their shapes:
- *Malleus* (MAL ee us) or hammer
- *Incus* (ING kus) or anvil
- *Stapes* (STAY peez) or stirrup

Tiny ligaments link these three tiny bones to form a bridge from the tympanic membrane to the inner ear. The ossicles transmit sound to the inner ear through the movement of the stapes. Within the middle ear is an opening for the *eustachian* (yuh STAHY shuh n) tube. This is a connection between the ears and the throat. This connection helps equalize pressure within the middle ear. Without equalized pressure in the ear, hearing would not be possible. The tympanic membrane is a thin, disk-shaped tissue that seals off the outer ear from the middle ear. Sound waves conducted through the external auditory canal hit the tympanic membrane and cause it to vibrate. The vibrations are picked up by the three ossicles and are changed from air-conducted sound waves to bone-conducted sound waves. The ossicles transmit the bone-conducted sound waves through the middle ear to the *oval window*. The oval window is a membrane that connects the middle ear and the inner ear. At the oval window, the sound waves move into the fluids of the inner ear. The fluid motion excites receptors, changing the

> **CRITICAL THINKING 13.4**
> Nathan Jorgenson, age 3, has an appointment with Dr. Walden because he has a cut on his ear. He fell onto a sprinkler while he was playing in the yard with his sister. The sprinkler cut his ear, and his mother brought him in to see if he might need stitches. Rosie cleaned up the wound, and now Nathan's mother is holding a gauze in place until Dr. Walden can see Nathan.
> What is the name of the outer ear? What is the function of the outer ear? Answer these questions in your own words.

> **VOCABULARY**
> **avascular:** Not supplied or associated with blood vessels.
> **biconvex:** Having two outward-curving surfaces on a lens.

> **MEDICAL TERMINOLOGY**
> **bi-:** two
> **cerumin/o:** cerumen, earwax
> **lens** (singular), **lenses** (plural)
> **ot/o, aur/o, auricul/o:** ear
> **phak/o, phac/o:** lens
> **tympan/o, myring/o:** eardrum
> **vitre/o:** vitreous humor

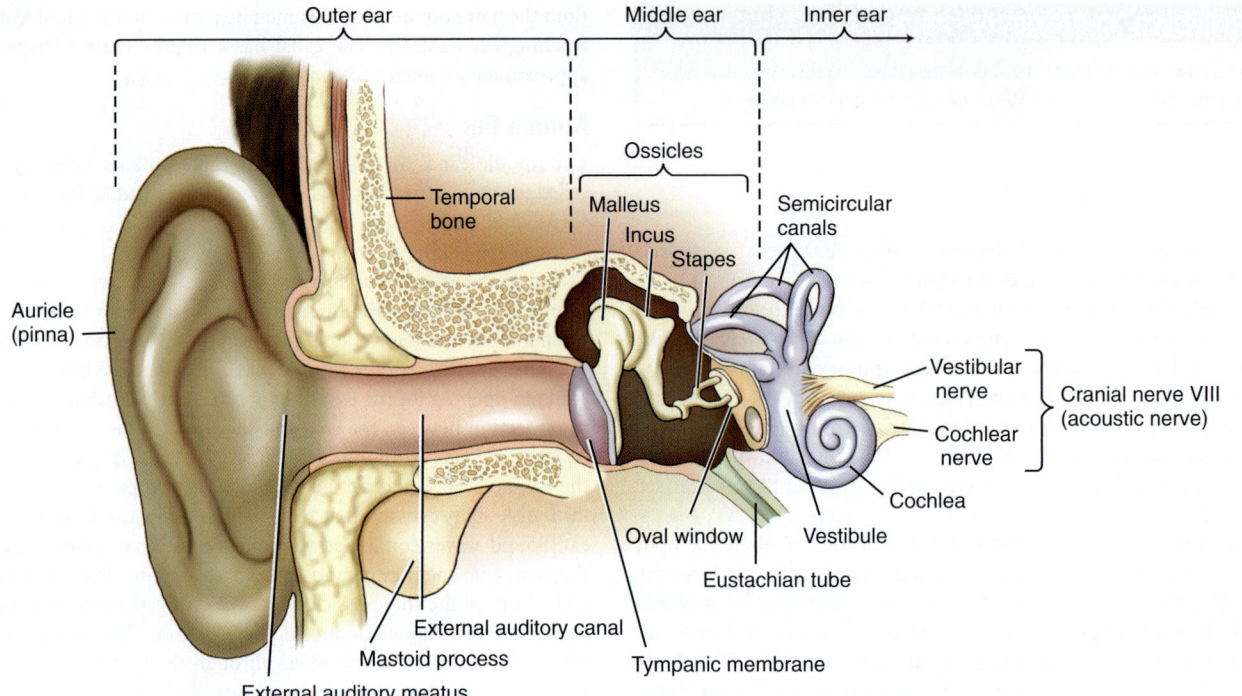

FIG. 13.3 Anatomy of the ear. (From Shiland: *Mastering Healthcare Terminology*, ed 5, St. Louis, 2016, Elsevier.)

bone-conducted sound into **sensorineural** (sen suh ree NOOR uhl) impulses.

MEDICAL TERMINOLOGY

audi/o, acous/o: hearing
cochle/o: cochlea
-ic: pertaining to
labyrinth/o: labyrinth, inner ear
ossicul/o: ossicle
pharyng/o: pharynx
salping/o: eustachian tube or fallopian tube
staped/o: stapes
tympan/o: eardrum
vestibul/o: vestibule

VOCABULARY

dynamic equilibrium: Relating to balance when moving at an angle or rotating.
equilibrium: A state of rest or balance due to the equal action of opposing forces.
sensorineural: Involving the sensory nerves, especially as they affect hearing.
static equilibrium: Relating to balance when moving in a straight line.

CRITICAL THINKING 13.5

Rosie's CEU also covered the anatomy of the ear. Can you name the three ossicles of the middle ear?

Inner Ear

Once sound is conducted to the oval window, it is transmitted to a structure called the *labyrinth* (LAB uh rinth), or the inner ear. The inner ear is divided into the *cochlea* (KAH klee ah) and the *semicircular* (SEM ih sur kuh lahr) canals, which are joined by the *vestibule* (VES tih byool). The semicircular canals and vestibule function to maintain **equilibrium** (ee kwuh LIB ree uh m). The cochlea is responsible for the sense of hearing.

The *organ of Corti* (KAWR tee), which contains the receptors for sound, is located within the cochlea. It is made up of hairlike sensory cells surrounded by sensory nerve fibers that form the cochlear branch of the eighth cranial nerve. Sound impulses cause the hairs to bend and rub against the nerve fibers, which initiate stimuli to travel through the cochlear nerve into the brain for sound interpretation.

The semicircular canals are responsible for evaluating the position of the head in relation to the pull of gravity. The three canals are positioned at right angles to one another, on different planes. When the head turns rapidly, these fluid-filled canals must rapidly adjust and send the information to the central nervous system (CNS). The CNS then interprets the information and initiates the desired response to maintain balance. The semicircular canals detect **dynamic** (dahy NAM ik) **equilibrium**. Within the vestibule, two saclike structures function to establish the body's **static** (STAT ik) **equilibrium**. With repetitive or excessive stimulation to the equilibrium receptors, some people become nauseated and may vomit. This condition is known as *motion sensitivity* or *motion sickness*.

TABLE 13.1 Functions of the Major Structures of the Eye

Structure	Function
Sclera	External protection
Cornea	Light refraction
Choroid	Blood supply
Iris	Light absorption and regulation of pupil width
Ciliary body	Secretion of vitreous fluid; changes the shape of the lens
Lens	Light refraction
Retinal layer	Light receptor that transforms optic signals into nerve impulses
Rods	Distinguish light from dark and perceive shape and movement
Cones	Color vision
Central fovea	Area of sharpest vision
Macula lutea	Center of the retina; contains the fovea centralis, the area of most highly acute vision
External ocular muscles	Move the eyeball
Optic nerve	One of a pair of nerves that transmit visual stimuli to (cranial nerve II) the brain
Lacrimal glands	Produce tears
Eyelid	Protects eye

Modified from Damjanov I: *Pathology for the Health-Related Professions*, Philadelphia, 1996, Saunders.

CRITICAL THINKING 13.6

Can you define the term *equilibrium* in your own words?

PHYSIOLOGY OF THE EYE

Here is a brief overview of how vision takes place:
- Vision requires light and depends on the proper functioning of all parts of the eye (Table 13.1).
- A visual impulse begins with the passage of light through the cornea, where the light is refracted or bent.
- Then it passes through the aqueous humor and the pupil into the lens.
- The ciliary muscle adjusts the curvature of the lens to refract the light rays again so that they pass onto the retina.
- Focused light triggers the photoreceptor cells called rods and cones.
- Light energy is converted into an electrical impulse.
- The electrical impulse is sent through the optic nerve to the **visual cortex** (KOHR teh x) of the **occipital** (OK sih puh tohl) **lobe** of the brain.
- The brain interprets the light impulses, and a picture is created that we perceive as sight.
- When this process does not work as it should, a person can experience refractive errors in vision. Box 13.7 explains refractive errors.

PHYSIOLOGY OF THE EAR

Here is a brief overview of how hearing takes place:
- The organ of Corti, which contains the receptors for sound, is located within the cochlea of the inner ear.
- It is made up of hairlike sensory cells surrounded by sensory nerve fibers that form the cochlear branch of the eighth cranial nerve.
- Sound impulses cause the hairs to bend and rub against the nerve fibers.
- The movement initiates an auditory impulse, which travels through the cochlear nerve onto the eighth cranial nerve.
- The eighth cranial nerve transmits the auditory impulse to the **medulla oblongata** (muh DUHL uh ob lawng GAH tuh).
- The impulses then travel to the **thalamus** (THAL uh muh s) and on to the **auditory cortex** of the temporal lobe of the brain.
- The brain then interprets the auditory impulse into **audible** (AW duh buh l) sound and speech patterns.
- When this process does not work as it should, a person can suffer hearing loss. Box 13.8 explains hearing loss. Box 13.9 explains how hearing loss is tested.

DISEASES AND DISORDERS OF THE EYES AND EARS

Diseases of the eye and ear are diverse and have many causes. Many factors can be associated with eye and ear diseases and disorders. These diseases can involve the cells, tissues, and structures of the eye and ear. Eye and ear diseases and disorders have a variety of causes:
- Microbial infections
- Malignant changes
- Congenital conditions

Please see Tables 13.2 to 13.9, which refer to common diagnostic testing and therapeutic interventions for eye and ear diseases and disorders.

STUDY TIP

Common signs and symptoms of eye and ear diseases and disorders include the following:
- Changed vision, blurry vision, pain
- Dizziness, headaches
- Hearing changes

Text continued on p. 309

VOCABULARY

audible: Capable of being heard.
auditory cortex: The region of the cerebral cortex that receives auditory data.
medulla oblongata: The lowest part of the brain, continuous with the top of the spinal cord.
occipital lobe: The lobe of the brain located at the back of the skull below the parietal lobe.
thalamus: The middle part of the brain through which sensory impulses pass to reach the cerebral cortex.
visual cortex: The portion of the cerebral cortex of the brain that receives and processes impulses from the optic nerve.

BOX 13.7 Refractive Errors

Four major types of refractive errors result when the eye is unable to focus light effectively on the retina. Defects in the shape of the eyeball can cause a refractive error. Most refractive errors can be corrected with corrective lenses, contacts, or surgery (Fig. 13.4).

- *Hyperopia* (hahy per OH pee uh) (farsightedness). When light enters the eye, and focuses behind the retina, a person has *hyperopia*. This disorder occurs when the eyeball is too short from the anterior to the posterior wall. An individual with hyperopia has difficulty seeing objects that are close.
- *Myopia* (mahy OH pee uh) (nearsightedness). *Myopia* occurs when light rays entering the eye focus in front of the retina. This causes objects at a distance to appear blurry and dull. Objects viewed at reading or working level are seen clearly. This disorder occurs when the eyeball is too long from front to back. An individual with myopia has difficulty seeing objects that are far away, or distant.
- *Astigmatism* (uh STIG muh tiz uhm). *Astigmatism* occurs when light rays entering the eye are focused irregularly. This usually occurs because the cornea or the lens is not smooth but has an irregular shape. It is like attempting to focus on objects seen through a wavy piece of window glass.
- *Presbyopia* (prez bee OH pee uh). As people age, the lens of the eye becomes less flexible, and the ciliary muscles weaken. When this happens, changing the point of focus from distance to near becomes difficult. This is called *presbyopia*. The condition results in difficulty seeing at reading level. People frequently notice a change in their vision in their early 40s.

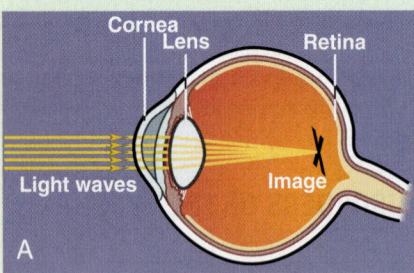 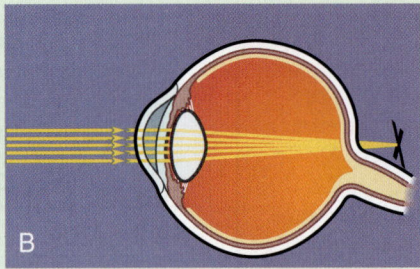 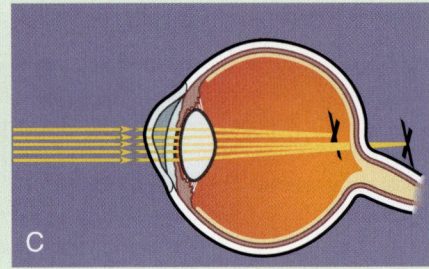

FIG. 13.4 Refraction errors. A-Myopia, B-Hyperopia, C-Astigmatism. (From Herlihy B, Maebius NK: *The Human Body in Health and Illness*, ed 4, Philadelphia, 2011, Saunders.)

BOX 13.8 Hearing Loss

Hearing Loss

Two problems result in hearing loss: a conduction problem and a sensorineural impairment. Some individuals have both conditions.

Conductive (kuh n DUHK tiv) *hearing loss* is caused by a problem that starts in the external or middle ear and prevents sound vibrations by the following:
- An inability to pass through the external auditory canal
- Limiting the movement of the tympanic membrane
- Interfering with the movement of bone-conducted sound in the middle ear

Patients with conductive hearing loss receive the greatest benefit from a hearing aid.

Sensorineural (sen suh ree NOO R uhl) *hearing loss* results from an abnormality of the organ of Corti or auditory nerve. Sensorineural hearing loss causes include the following:
- Viral infection (e.g., rubella, influenza, herpes)
- Head trauma
- Certain **ototoxic** (oh tuh TOK sik) medications
- Prolonged exposure to loud noise (repetitive noise in the workplace or loud music)

Presbycusis (prez buh KYOO sis) is progressive sensorineural deafness associated with aging. This is caused by a reduction in the number of receptor cells in the organ of Corti. See more information on presbycusis in the disease section of this chapter.

If the sensorineural hearing loss cannot be improved by hearing aids, an option is surgically inserting *cochlear implants*. These are complex devices that use electrical impulses to stimulate the auditory nerve. The brain then interprets the nerve impulses as sound. Cochlear implants bypass damaged portions of the ear and directly stimulate the auditory nerve. The implants do not create normal hearing but provide increased sound for a person with profound or complete hearing loss.

Mixed hearing loss is a combination of conductive and sensory deafness. This type of loss can result from tumors, toxic levels of certain medications, hereditary factors, and stroke.

VOCABULARY

ototoxic: A medicine or substance capable of damaging cranial nerve VIII or the organs of hearing and balance.

CHAPTER 13 Sensory System 303

BOX 13.9 Audiometric Testing

An *audiometric* (aw dee OH met rik) test may be done in an otology or family practice and is performed by medical assistants who have received additional training. *Audiometry* (aw dee OM i tree) measures the lowest intensity of sound an individual can hear (Fig. 13.5).

Testing can be performed as a traditional manual hearing test or an automated test. To start testing, the patient places headphones over the ears. In the automatic mode, the patient is prompted to press a hand button as soon as he or she hears a tone. The advantages of automated testing are as follows:
- Voice prompts available in multiple languages
- Testing requires less time to complete
- The medical assistant can watch the progress on the audiometer's LCD screen

Each ear is tested by delivering a single frequency at a specific intensity, starting with low-frequency tones and going up to very high frequencies. Patients are asked to signal when they hear a sound. The results are printed on a graph, called an *audiogram* (AW dee uh gram), or the medical assistant charts the results on a graph sheet (Fig. 13.6). An adult with normal hearing can hear tone frequencies below 25 decibels, and children with normal hearing can hear tones below 15 decibels.

If initial screening indicates a hearing deficit, the provider may recommend an appointment with an audiologist for audiometric evaluation. The evaluation consists of a battery of tests and assesses the level of hearing impairment. The assessment includes testing the frequency, intensity, and audibility of sound. This process takes approximately 1 hour.

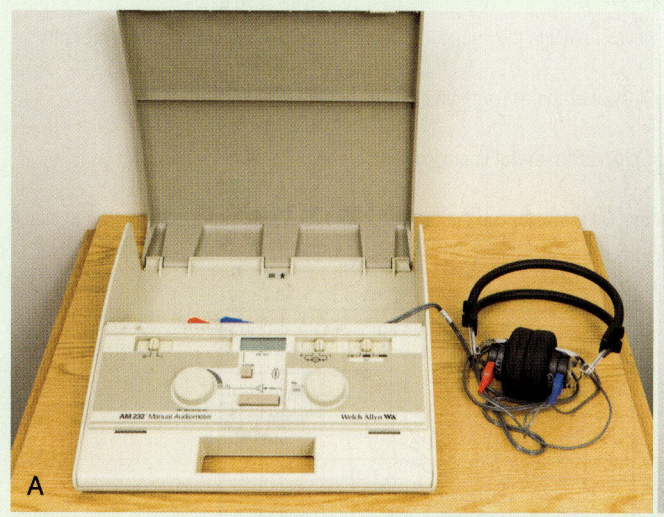
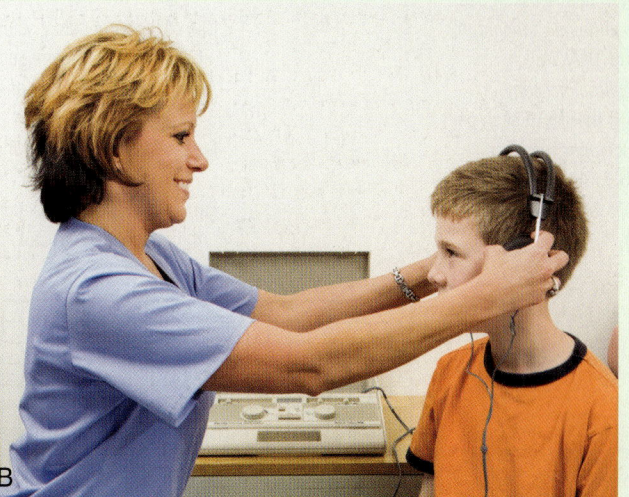

FIG. 13.5 Audiometric testing. (From Proctor D, et al: *Kinn's The Medical Assistant*, ed 13, St. Louis, 2017, Elsevier.)

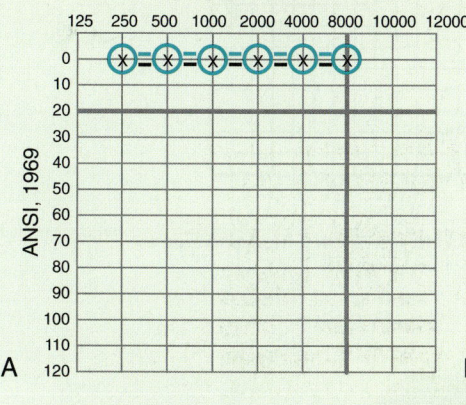
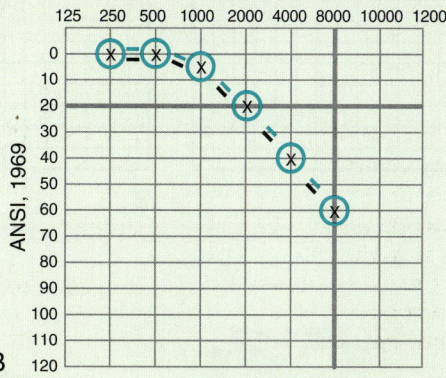
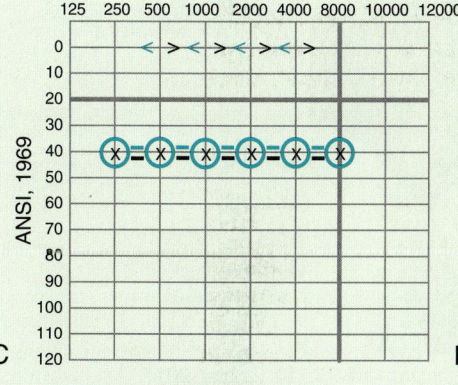
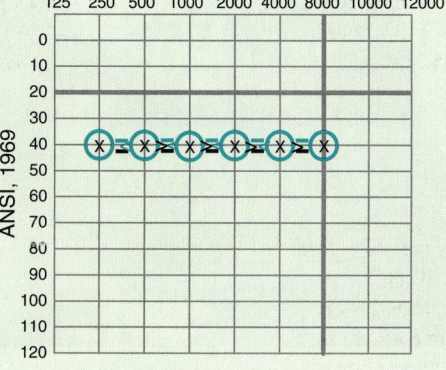

FIG. 13.6 Audiograms. (From Black JM, Hawks JH, Keene A: *Medical Surgical Nursing: Clinical Management for Positive Outcomes,* ed 8, Philadelphia, 2009, Saunders.)

Air conduction left = x
Air conduction right = ○
Bone conduction left = >
Bone conduction right = <

TABLE 13.2 Terms Related to Eye Diagnostic Procedures

Term	Definition
amsler grid (AMZ lur)	Test to assess central vision and to help diagnose age-related macular degeneration (Fig. 13.7).
diopters (DYE op turs)	Measurement that quantifies refraction errors, including the amount of nearsightedness (– number), farsightedness (+ number), and astigmatism.
fluorescein angiography (FLOO reh seen an jee AH gruh fee)	Procedure to confirm retinal disease. Injection of a fluorescein dye into the eye and use of a camera to record the vessels of the retina.
fluorescein staining (FLOO reh seen)	Dye dropped into the eyes that allows differential staining of abnormalities of the cornea.
gonioscopy (goh nee AH skuh pee)	Used to diagnose glaucoma and to inspect ocular movement.
ophthalmic sonography (off THALL mick)	Use of high-frequency sound waves to image the interior of the eye when cloudiness of the lens prevents other imaging techniques.
ophthalmoscopy (off thal MAH skuh pee)	Any visual examination of the interior of the eye with an ophthalmoscope.
Schirmer tear test (SHURR mur)	Determines the amount of tear production; useful in diagnosing dry eye (xerophthalmia).
slit lamp examination	Part of a routine eye examination. Used to examine the layers of the eye. Medications may be used to dilate the pupils (mydriatics), numb the eye (anesthetics), or dye the eye (fluorescein staining) (Fig. 13.8).

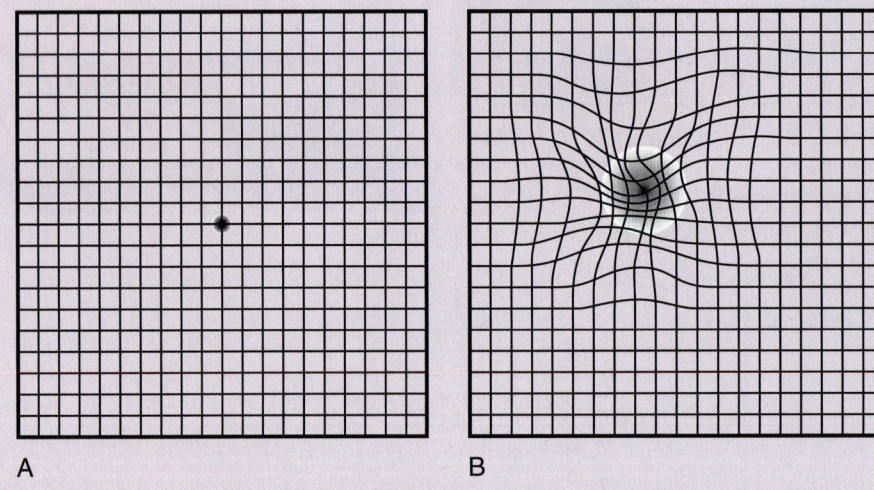

FIG. 13.7 Amsler grid. (From Miller RG, Ashar B, Sisson SD: *The Johns Hopkins Internal Medicine Board Review 2010-2011*, ed 3, Philadelphia, 2010, Mosby.)

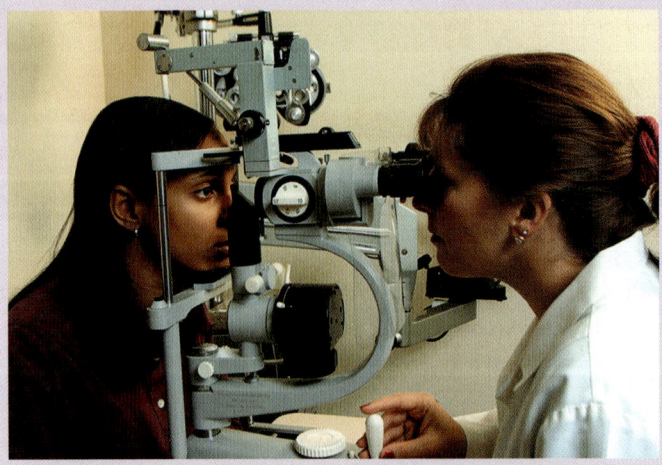

FIG. 13.8 Slit lamp. (From Proctor D, et al: *Kinn's The Medical Assistant*, ed 13, St. Louis, 2017, Elsevier.)

TABLE 13.2 Terms Related to Eye Diagnostic Procedures—cont'd

Term	Definition
tonometry (toh NAH meh tree)	Measurement of IOP. Used in the diagnosis of glaucoma. In Goldmann tonometry, the eye is numbed and measurements are taken directly on the eye. In air-puff tonometry, a puff of air is blown onto the cornea.
visual acuity (VA) assessment (ah KYOO ih tee)	Test of the sharpness of vision; also called the *Snellen test*. Normal vision is 20/20. The top figure is the number of feet the examinee is standing from the Snellen chart (Fig. 13.9); the bottom figure is the number of feet a normal person would be from the chart and still be able to read the letters. If the result is 20/40, the highest line that the individual can read is what a person with normal vision can read at 40 feet.
visual field (VF) test	Determines the area of physical space visible to an individual. A normal VF is 65 degrees upward, 75 degrees downward, 60 degrees inward, and 90 degrees outward.

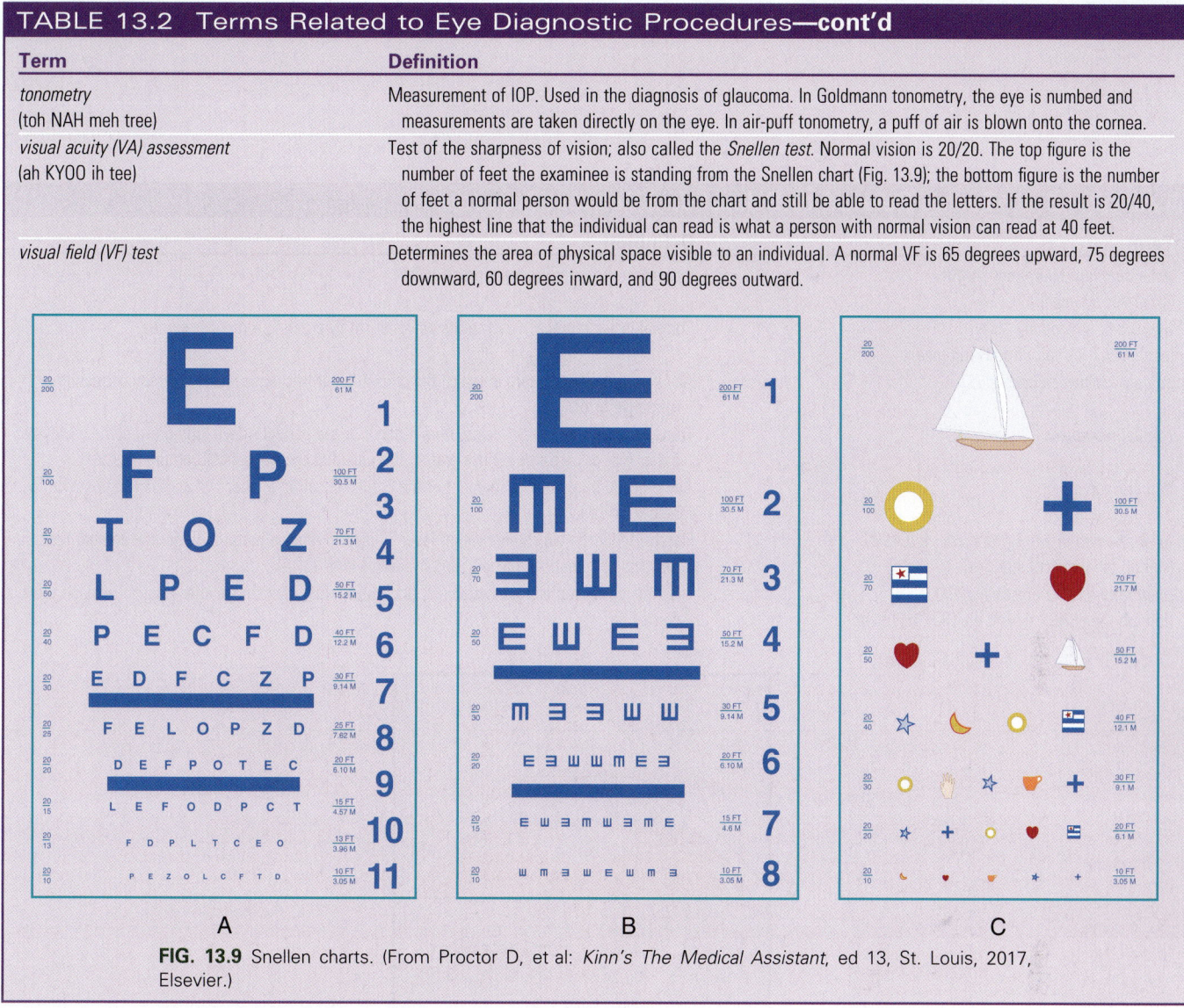

FIG. 13.9 Snellen charts. (From Proctor D, et al: *Kinn's The Medical Assistant*, ed 13, St. Louis, 2017, Elsevier.)

From Shiland B: *Mastering Healthcare Terminology*, ed 5, St. Louis, 2016, Elsevier.

TABLE 13.3 Terms Related to Interventions of the Eyeball and Adnexa

Term	Definition
blepharoplasty (BLEFF or uh plas tee)	Surgical repair of the eyelids; may be done to correct blepharoptosis or blepharochalasis
blepharorrhaphy (BLEFF ar oh rah fee)	Suture of the eyelids
dacryocystorhinostomy (dak ree oh sis toh rye NOSS tuh mee)	Creation of an opening between the tear sac and the nose
enucleation of the eye (eh noo klee AY shun)	Removal of the entire eyeball
evisceration of the eye (eh vis uh RAY shun)	Removal of the contents of the eyeball, leaving the outer coat (the sclera) intact
exenteration of the eye (eck sen tur RAY shun)	Removal of the entire contents of the orbit

From Shiland B: *Mastering Healthcare Terminology*, ed 5, St. Louis, 2016, Elsevier.

TABLE 13.4 Terms Related to Scleral and Corneal Procedures

Term	Definition
anterior ciliary sclerotomy (ACS) (sklair AH tuh mee)	Incision in the sclera to treat presbyopia.
astigmatic keratotomy (AK) (as tig MAT ick kair uh TAH tuh mee)	Corneal incision process that treats astigmatism by creating a rounder cornea.
corneal incision procedure	Any keratotomy procedure in which the cornea is cut to change shape, thereby correcting a refractive error.
corneal transplant	Transplantation of corneal tissue from a donor or the patient's own (autograft) cornea. May be either full- or partial-thickness grafts; also called *keratoplasty* (KAIR uh toh plas tee).
flap procedure	Any procedure in which a segment of the cornea is cut as a means of access to the structures below (LASIK).
laser-assisted in-situ keratomileusis (LASIK) (kair uh toh mih LOO sis)	Flap procedure in which an excimer laser is used to remove material under the corneal flap. Corrects astigmatism, myopia, and hyperopia (Fig. 13.10).
photorefractive keratectomy (PRK) (foh toh ree FRACK tiv kair uh TECK tuh mee)	Treatment for astigmatism, hyperopia, and myopia that uses an excimer laser to reshape the cornea.

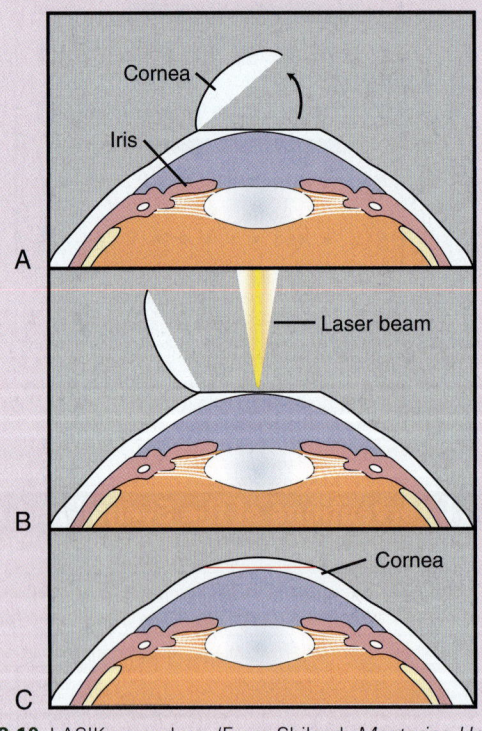

FIG. 13.10 LASIK procedure. (From Shiland: *Mastering Healthcare Terminology*, ed 5, St. Louis, 2016, Elsevier.)

From Shiland B: *Mastering Healthcare Terminology*, ed 5, St. Louis, 2016, Elsevier.

TABLE 13.5 Terms Related to Lens Interventions

Term	Definition
cataract extraction	Removal of the lens to treat cataracts. May be *intracapsular cataract extraction (ICCE)*, in which the entire lens and capsule are removed, or *extracapsular cataract extraction (ECCE)*, in which the lens capsule is left in place (Fig. 13.11).
intraocular lenses (IOLs) (in truh OK yuh ler)	Use of an artificial lens implanted behind the iris and in front of the natural abnormal lens to treat myopia and hyperopia. Also called *implantable contact lenses (ICLs)*.
phacoemulsification and aspiration of cataract (fay koh ee mull sih fih KAY shun)	Vision correction done through the destruction and removal of the contents of the capsule. Contents are broken into small pieces and removed by suction.

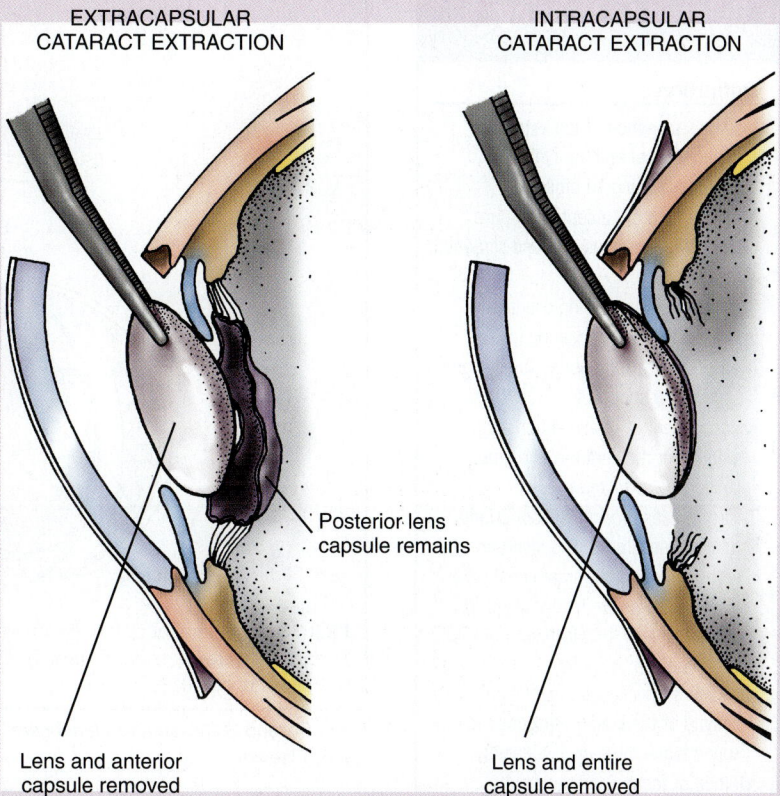

FIG. 13.11 Cataract extraction. (From Ignatavicius DD, Workman ML: *Medical-Surgical Nursing: Critical Thinking for Collaborative Care*, ed 6, Philadelphia, 2011, Saunders.)

From Shiland B: *Mastering Healthcare Terminology*, ed 5, St. Louis, 2016, Elsevier.

TABLE 13.6 Terms Related to Iris Interventions

Term	Definition
coreoplasty (KORE ee oh plas tee)	Surgical repair to form an artificial pupil.
goniotomy (goh nee AH tuh mee)	Incision of the Schlemm canal to correct glaucoma. Provides an exit for the aqueous humor.
laser peripheral iridotomy (puh RIF er uhl ir ih DOT uh mee)	A provider creates a small hole in the iris using a laser. This allows fluid to flow out through the iris, which will relieve the pressure in the eye.
trabeculotomy (truh beck kyoo LAH tuh mee)	Incision of the orbital network of the eye to promote intraocular circulation and decrease IOP.

From Shiland B: *Mastering Healthcare Terminology*, ed 5, St. Louis, 2016, Elsevier.

TABLE 13.8 Terms Related to Hearing Tests

Term	Definition
otoscopy (oh TAH skuh pee)	Visual examination of the external auditory canal and the tympanic membrane using an otoscope
pure tone audiometry (ah dee AH meh tree)	Measurement of perception of pure tones with extraneous sound screened out
Rinne tuning fork test (RIH nuh)	Method of distinguishing conductive from sensorineural hearing loss
speech audiometry	Measurement of the ability to hear and understand speech
tympanometry (tim pan NAH muh tree)	Measurement of the condition and mobility of the eardrum; the graph is called a *tympanogram*
Universal Newborn Hearing Screening (UNHS) test	Test that uses *otoacoustic emissions (OAEs)* measured by the insertion of a probe into the baby's ear canal, and *auditory brainstem response (ABR)*, which involves the placement of four electrodes on the baby's head to measure the change in electrical activity of the brain in response to sound while the baby is sleeping
Weber tuning fork test (WEB ur)	Method of testing auditory acuity

From Shiland B: *Mastering Healthcare Terminology*, ed 5, St. Louis, 2016, Elsevier.

TABLE 13.7 Terms Related to Retina Interventions

Term	Definition
retinal photocoagulation (RET in ul foh toh koh agg yoo LAY shun)	Destruction of retinal lesions using light rays to solidify tissue.
scleral buckling (SKLAIR ul BUCK ling)	Reattachment of the retina with a cryoprobe and a silicone sponge. The procedure pushes the sclera in toward the retinal scar. Includes the removal of fluid from the subretinal space (Fig. 13.12).
vitrectomy (vi TREK tuh mee)	Removal of part or all of the vitreous humor.

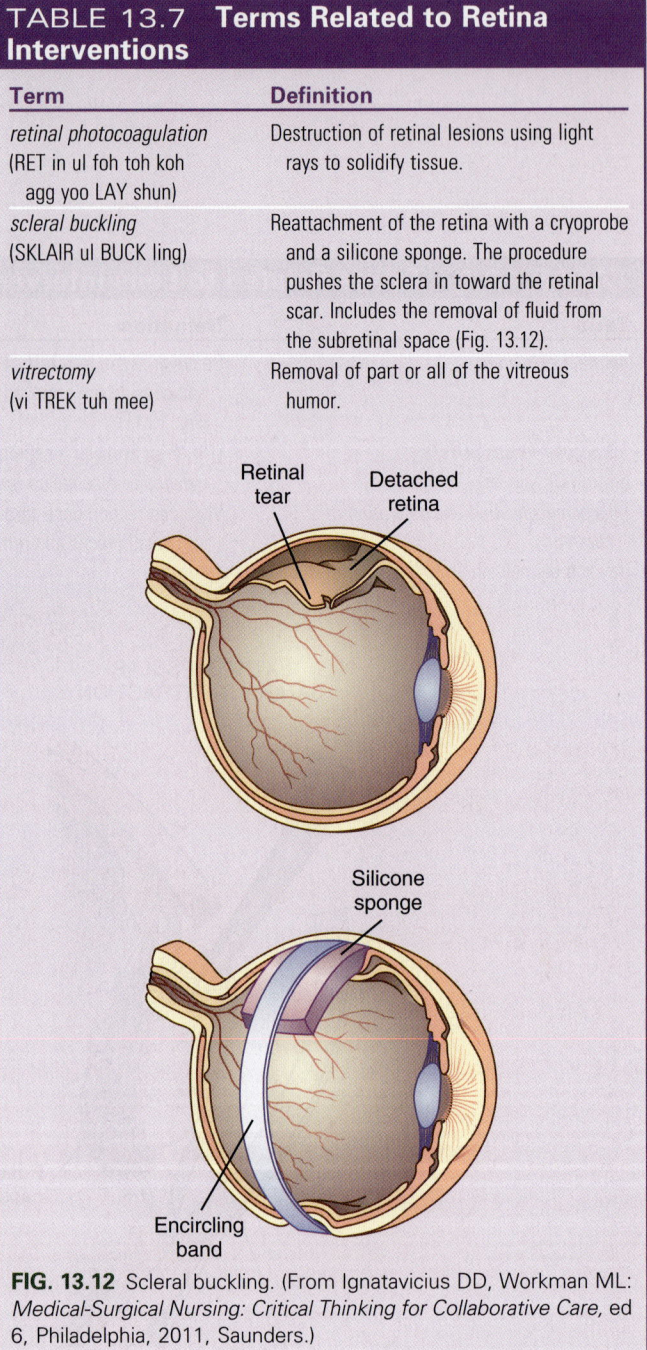

FIG. 13.12 Scleral buckling. (From Ignatavicius DD, Workman ML: *Medical-Surgical Nursing: Critical Thinking for Collaborative Care*, ed 6, Philadelphia, 2011, Saunders.)

From Shiland B: *Mastering Healthcare Terminology*, ed 5, St. Louis, 2016, Elsevier.

TABLE 13.9 Terms Related to Therapeutic Interventions of the Ear

Term	Definition
cochlear implant (KAH klee ur)	Implanted device that assists those with hearing loss by electrically stimulating the cochlea (Fig. 13.13).
hearing aid	Electronic device that amplifies sound.
mastoidectomy (mass toyd ECK tuh mee)	Removal of the mastoid process, usually to treat intractable mastoiditis.
otoplasty (OH toh plas tee)	Surgical or plastic repair and/or reconstruction of the external ear.
stapedectomy (stay puh DECK tuh mee)	Removal of the third ossicle, the stapes, from the middle ear. Done to correct otosclerosis.
tympanoplasty (TIM pan oh plas tee)	Surgical repair of the eardrum, with or without ossicles reconstruction. Some patients may require a prosthesis (an artificial replacement) for one or more of the ossicles.
tympanostomy (tim pan AH stuh mee)	Surgical creation of an opening through the eardrum to promote drainage and/or allow the introduction of artificial tubes to maintain the opening (Fig. 13.14); also called a *myringostomy* (mir ring AH stuh mee).
tympanotomy (tim pan AH tuh mee)	Incision of an eardrum; also called a *myringotomy* (mir ring AH tuh mee).

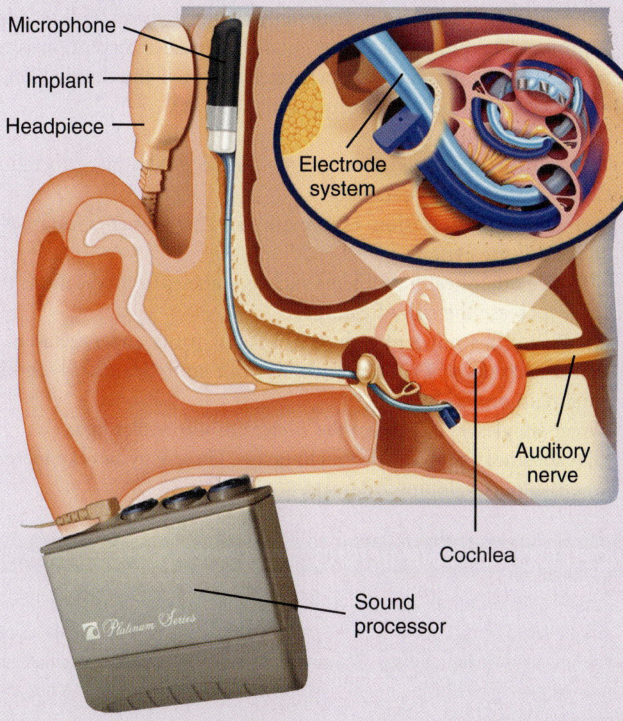

FIG. 13.13 Cochlear implant. (From Shiland: *Mastering Healthcare Terminology*, ed 5, St. Louis, 2016, Elsevier.)

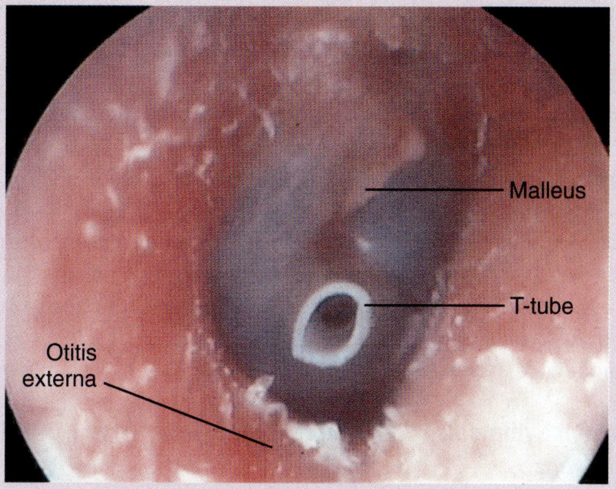

FIG. 13.14 Tympanostomy tube in place. (From Swartz MH: *Textbook of Physical Diagnosis*, ed 7, Philadelphia, 2014, Saunders.)

From Shiland B: *Mastering Healthcare Terminology*, ed 5, St. Louis, 2016, Elsevier.

DISEASES AND DISORDERS OF THE EYE

Cataract

A *cataract* (KAT uh rakt) is a cloudy or opaque area in the normally clear lens of the eye. The cloudiness blocks the passage of light into the retina, causing impaired vision. A cataract scatters light as it passes through the lens, preventing a sharply defined image from reaching the retina. This results in blurred and dimmed vision (Fig. 13.15).

A patient may need a brighter reading light or may hold objects closer to the eyes for better viewing. Continued clouding of the lens may cause **diplopia** (dih PLOH pee uh). Patients with cataracts report difficulty with night vision (*nyctalopia* [nik tl OH pee uh]). They see halo images around lights and have increased sensitivity to glare. If left untreated, cataracts ultimately can lead to blindness.

> **VOCABULARY**
> **diplopia:** A pathologic condition of vision where a single object is seen as two. Double vision.

Etiology. Most cataracts develop slowly and progressively because of natural aging of the lens of the eye. Generally, cataracts occur after age 60. Cataracts may result from injury to the eye, exposure to extreme

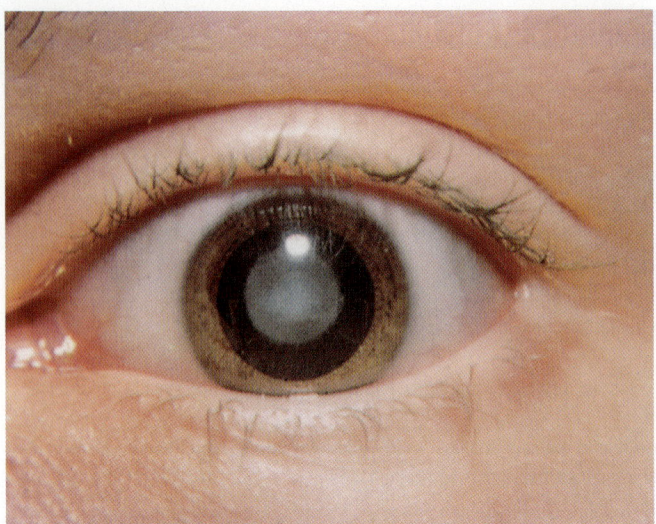

FIG. 13.15 Cataract. (From Black JM, Hawks JH, Keene A: *Medical Surgical Nursing: Clinical Management for Positive Outcomes*, ed 8, Philadelphia, 2009, Saunders.)

heat or radiation, or inherited factors. With advanced cataracts, the pupil of the eye appears white or gray.

Risk factors for developing cataracts include the following:
- Increasing age
- Diabetes, high blood pressure, obesity, unprotected exposure to sunlight
- Previous eye surgery, injury, inflammation, or prolonged use of corticosteroids
- Smoking or excessive alcohol consumption

Signs and Symptoms. Signs and symptoms of cataracts may include the following:
- Clouded, blurry, dim vision
- Sensitivity to light and glare, difficulty with night vision or night driving, seeing "halos" around lights
- Double vision, especially in just one eye
- Brighter lights needed for reading, and fading or yellowing of colors

When a cataract is first forming and is small, it may not disturb vision. But as it increases in size, vision loss will increase and become more noticeable.

Diagnostic Procedures. When the patient's vision becomes distorted or appears to be deteriorating, the provider should include the following procedures for diagnosis:
- A visual acuity test. This should be done to get an idea of a person's overall ability to see.
- A *slit-lamp* examination. This allows the provider to examine the structures at the front of the eye using a combination of a low-power microscope and high-intensity light. The light shines into the eye as a slit beam. (See Table 13.2 and Fig. 13.8.)
- An examination of the retina. Medication is dropped into the eye to dilate (make bigger) the pupil. This makes it easier for the provider to examine the retina.

Diagnostic procedures for cataracts are most often performed by an ophthalmologist.

Treatment. The symptoms of early cataracts may be improved with new eyeglasses, brighter lighting, and antiglare sunglasses. If these measures do not help, surgical removal of the lens is the only effective treatment.

Surgery is performed as an outpatient procedure in a clinic or hospital. After the eye has been numbed with a local anesthetic, the clouded lens is removed. Then an artificial intraocular lens (IOL) is positioned in the same place as the natural lens. The procedure usually takes 15 minutes, and the patient typically can leave the facility after 1 hour. Vision gradually improves and stabilizes within about 2 to 6 weeks. Once vision stabilizes, the patient should be fitted with new corrective lenses to match the improved vision. (See Table 13.4 and Fig. 13.10.)

Patients should be aware that they will not be able to drive until cleared by the ophthalmologist and that they may need help at home until their vision is clear. As with any surgical procedure, there is always a risk of infection or bleeding. Cataract surgery also has a risk of *retinal detachment*. This is when the retina pulls away from its normal position at the back of the eye. Follow-up appointments may be necessary for the first month.

Prognosis. The prognosis for cataracts is good if surgical intervention is done once the cataract has noticeably changed vision. Full recovery is common. The prognosis is not good if surgical intervention is not completed once the cataract has changed vision. If the clouded lens is not replaced, blindness can occur.

Prevention. The following measures can be put in place to reduce the risks of developing cataracts:
- Schedule regular vision examinations. The sooner a cataract is detected, the better.
- Manage other health problems such as diabetes or medications that may increase the risk of cataracts.
- Eat a healthy, nutrient-rich diet. Lots of fruits and vegetables of varying colors will supply the body with antioxidants, which help maintain eye health.
- Wear sunglasses to protect the eyes from ultraviolet light.
- Do not smoke or drink alcohol to excess. These activities can increase the risk of developing cataracts.

> ### CRITICAL THINKING 13.7
> Jason Van den Hooval, age 63, has an appointment today to have his blood drawn. While he is chatting with the phlebotomist, he mentions that his vision is a little blurry in his right eye. He was wondering if Dr. Walden had a moment to look at it today. Rosie brings Jason back to an exam room and preps the room for Dr. Walden.
> Dr. Walden looks at both of Jason's eyes and does see an area that is a little cloudy. What might Dr. Walden be seeing? What specialty provider could she refer Jason to?

Glaucoma

One of the most common and serious eye disorders is a group of diseases known as *glaucoma*. Glaucoma is characterized by increased intraocular pressure (IOP), which damages the optic nerve. If glaucoma is not treated, it can cause blindness. It rarely occurs in people younger than age 40 and usually is seen in individuals older than age 60. Glaucoma is one of the leading causes of blindness among African Americans. It is estimated that more than 3 million Americans have glaucoma, but only half of those know they have it.

Etiology. Glaucoma is the result of damage to the optic nerve. The nerve damage is usually related to an increased pressure in the eye.

What causes the increased pressure is still unknown. Glaucoma can run in families, so heredity can be an influence.

In the eye, the ciliary body constantly produces aqueous humor, which should circulate freely between the anterior and posterior chambers of the eye. Eventually the fluid should empty into the general circulation. A healthy eye is filled with fluid to maintain the shape of the eyeball. In those with glaucoma, over time fluid builds up. This results in increased pressure in the eye, which affects the blood supply to the retina and optic nerve. There are two main types of glaucoma: open-angle glaucoma and angle-closure glaucoma.

Risk factors for developing glaucoma include the following:
- Having high intraocular pressure
- Being over age 60, having a family history of glaucoma
- Being African American or Hispanic
- Having other medical conditions such as diabetes, heart disease, high blood pressure, or sickle cell anemia
- Having had eye surgery or injury in the past

Signs and Symptoms. Patients can have chronic open-angle glaucoma for a long time before symptoms occur. Early detection through regular eye exams that include IOP measurements is important to prevent permanent vision loss. Signs and symptoms of chronic glaucoma include the following:
- The need to change eyeglass prescriptions frequently
- A loss of peripheral vision (often called "tunnel vision")
- Mild headaches
- Impaired adaptation to the dark

Acute closed-angle glaucoma has more obvious symptoms:
- Severe pain and headaches
- Inflammation, sensitivity to light, and seeing halos around lights

If left untreated, acute glaucoma can cause permanent blindness in a matter of days (Fig. 13.16).

Diagnostic Procedures. The provider should review the patient's medical history and perform a comprehensive eye exam. They may perform the following tests in addition to a regular eye exam:
- *Tonometry*, measuring the intraocular pressure (IOP) of the eye; see Table 13.2
- Testing the optic nerve for damage
- *Visual field test* (VFT), checking for areas of vision loss; see Table 13.2
- *Gonioscopy*, inspecting the drainage angle of the eye; see Table 13.2
- Measuring corneal thickness

Treatment. Once damage is done to the optic nerve, it cannot be reversed. Preventing damage to the optic nerve is the goal of glaucoma treatment. Lowering pressure in the eye will help to prevent damage. Regular checkups and eye exams are part of the treatment plan. Also, eyedrops that help improve fluid drainage or decrease the volume of fluid in the eyes will help to decrease eye pressure and slow the progression of the disease. There are a number of different eyedrops that can be prescribed, but all of them work to decrease intraocular pressure.

In addition to eyedrops, oral medications may be prescribed. Laser surgery, filtering surgery, and drainage tubes may be used to help lower eye pressure in chronic glaucoma. See Table 13.6 for additional information on glaucoma procedures.

In closed-angle glaucoma, medications to lower IOP are prescribed so that surgery can be performed to create a channel for aqueous fluid to circulate. This is a medical emergency because the pressure must be relieved within a few hours or permanent vision damage occurs. A procedure called a laser peripheral iridotomy may be performed. See Table 13.6 for additional information.

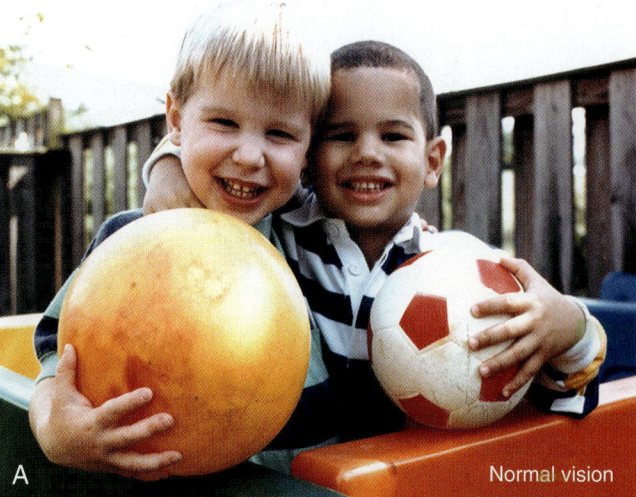

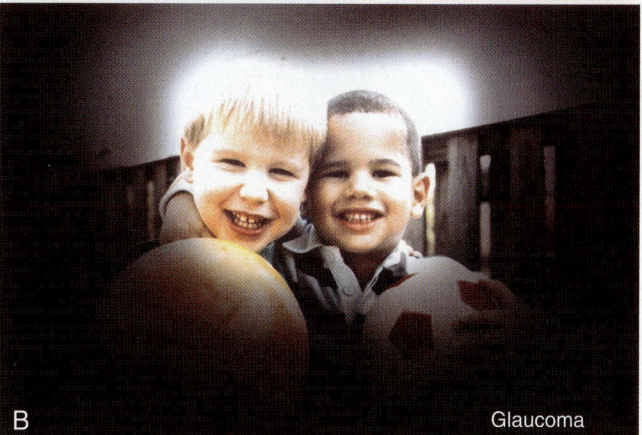

FIG. 13.16 Glaucoma. (From the National Eye Institute: *Age-Related Macular Degeneration: What You Should Know*, Bethesda, MD, National Institutes of Health.)

Prognosis. With proper treatment, patient compliance, and early detection, the prognosis for chronic glaucoma is very good. For acute glaucoma, immediate treatment is necessary to maintain eyesight. Without immediate treatment, the prognosis for maintaining sight is poor.

Prevention. Preventing high eye pressure and slowing the progression of glaucoma is the goal. The following behaviors can help with the prevention and treatment of glaucoma:
- Eat a healthy diet, rich in nutrients. Lots of fruits and vegetables of a various colors will help maintain eye health.
- Exercise safely and within the proper level of fitness. Contact the provider before starting an exercise program.
- Limit caffeine, but drink fluids throughout the day.
- Sleeping with the head slightly elevated (about 20 degrees) to reduce eye pressure.
- Take all prescribed medications as directed by the provider.
- Relaxation therapies may be effective in handling stress.

Macular Degeneration

The *macula lutea* is the part of the retina near the optic nerve, and it defines the center of the field of vision. Macular degeneration is progressive deterioration of the macula lutea, which causes loss of central vision. The patient can see only the edges of the visual field (Fig. 13.17).

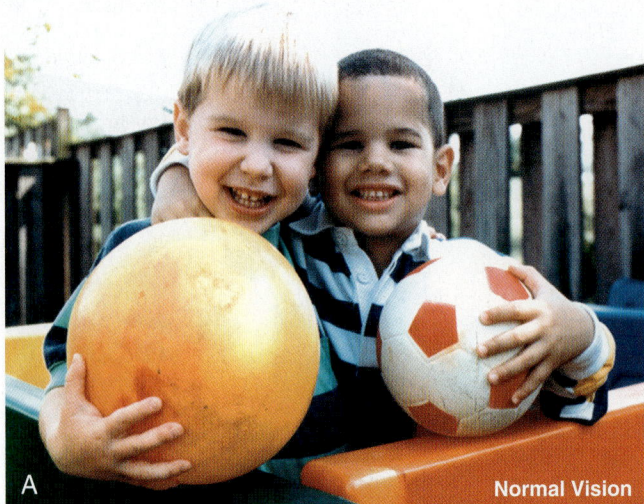
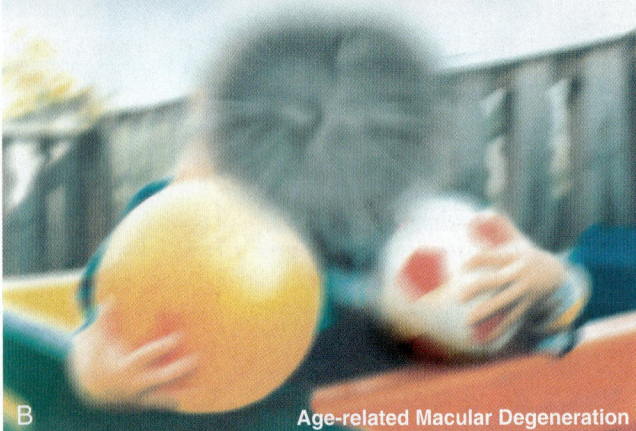

FIG. 13.17 Macular degeneration. (From the National Eye Institute: *Age-Related Macular Degeneration: What You Should Know*, Bethesda, MD, National Institutes of Health.)

The condition affects more than 10 million Americans and is a leading cause of blindness in persons older than 50.

Etiology. Two types of macular degeneration can occur. The dry form accounts for most cases; it is painless and develops slowly, affecting sharp vision over time, so that reading and other activities that require fine, detailed vision become impossible. Dry macular degeneration is caused by the breakdown of light-sensitive cells in the region of the macula.

Wet macular degeneration causes severe vision loss and has a rapid onset and progression. Wet macular degeneration is seen when new blood vessels behind the retina form and then leak blood and fluid into the macula.

The cause of both dry and wet macular degeneration is unknown. The wet condition develops in people who have had the dry form of the disease.

Risk factors for developing macular degeneration include the following:
- Age. It is most common in people over 65 years old.
- Race. Macular degeneration is more common in Caucasians than in any other race.
- Cigarette smoking or being around cigarette smoke significantly increases the risk of macular degeneration.
- A family history of the disease, obesity, and existing cardiovascular disease can also increase risk.

Signs and Symptoms. Symptoms of *dry* macular degeneration develop over time with no associated pain. Other signs and symptoms may include the following:
- Visual changes, including straight lines that seem bent, loss of central vision in one or both eyes
- Need for brighter light when reading or performing tasks, difficulty adapting to low light, increased blurriness when reading
- Fading of bright colors, less contrast in colors
- Difficulty identifying faces or detail

Symptoms of *wet* macular degeneration develop quickly and progress rapidly. Other signs and symptoms may include the following:
- Visual changes, including straight lines that seem bent, loss of central vision in one or both eyes
- A distinct blurry spot or blind spot in the field of vision
- Rapid onset of symptoms and rapid progression of symptoms
- An overall dimness in vision
- Fading of bright colors, less contrast in colors

Diagnostic Procedures. The provider will review medical history and complete a comprehensive eye exam. To confirm macular degeneration, the provider may do several additional tests:
- Examination of the back of the eye. Pupils will be dilated and the retina of the eye is examined. The provider is looking for fluid, blood, or a speckled area caused by *drusen*. Drusen are small, yellowish deposits that form under the retina of the eye.
- Testing for central vision loss using an Amsler's grid. See Table 13.2 and Fig. 13.7 for more information
- Fluorescein angiography. (See Table 13.2.)
- Optical coherence tomography. This imaging test is used to detail cross sections of the retina. It distinguishes areas of thickening, thinning, or swelling of the retina. This test is often used to observe a patient's reaction to macular degeneration treatment.

Treatment. Treatment for macular degeneration is designed to help slow the progression of the disease, preserve existing vision, and possibly recover some lost vision.

Dry macular degeneration treatments may include the following:
- Low-vision rehabilitation. Macular degeneration does not affect peripheral vision, just central vision. Patients with dry macular degeneration may find benefits in working with a low-vision rehabilitation specialist or occupational therapist who may be able to help patients adapt to their changing vision
- Antioxidant-rich foods may contribute to eye health. Fruits and vegetables of varying colors are high in antioxidants—the more color, the more antioxidants. Supplements for lutein, zeaxanthin, zinc, and omega-3 fatty acids may be useful. Also, protein-rich foods contain zinc.

Wet macular degeneration treatments may include the following:
- Medications to stop the growth of new blood vessels. Examples are bevacizumab (Avastin), ranibizumab (Lucentis), and aflibercept (Eylea). These medications are injected directly into the eye about every 4 weeks to be beneficial. Some partial recovery of vision as blood vessels shrink is possible.
- Photodynamic therapy. A medication is injected into a vein in the arm, which passes into the blood vessels in the eye. A special focused laser is shined onto the abnormal vessels in the eye and the vessel closes, which stops leakage behind the retina. This may improve vision and delay the progression of vision loss.

- Photocoagulation. Lasers are used to seal abnormal blood vessels, which stops leakage. May slow the progression of vision loss.
- Low-vision rehabilitation. Macular degeneration does not affect peripheral vision, just central vision. Patients with dry macular degeneration may find benefits in working with a low-vision rehabilitation specialist or occupational therapist who may be able to help patients adapt to their changing vision.
- For persons with intermediate or advanced macular degeneration, high-level supplements of vitamin C, vitamin E, zinc, and copper may reduce the risk of vision loss. This is not effective for dry macular degeneration.

Prognosis. Prognosis for wet macular degeneration is not as good as it is for dry macular degeneration. Compliance with treatment gives the best chance for a better outcome. Both wet and dry macular degeneration may lead to vision loss. Wet has a poorer prognosis for vision loss.

Prevention. The following actions may reduce the chances of developing dry or wet macular degeneration or for preventing additional vision loss:
- Have routine eye exams.
- Manage any existing or chronic medical conditions.
- Do not smoke or drink alcohol to excess.
- Maintain a healthy weight and exercise regularly.
- Choose a diet rich in fruits and vegetables, and eat fish regularly.
- Supplement with vitamin C, vitamin E, zinc, and copper only if directed to do so by the provider.

> **CRITICAL THINKING 13.8**
>
> Bruce Bartlet, age 53, has an appointment with Dr. Walden today. He is in for a routine physical, but he has several questions written down for the doctor. He was recently diagnosed with dry macular degeneration. After Rosie rooms Bruce, she takes his vital signs and asks if he has any questions for the doctor. Bruce asks Rosie, "Is there anything I can do to help prevent this condition from getting worse?" Rosie mentions that there is a patient education pamphlet on macular degeneration that she can get for him. He can look through it until the doctor comes in.
> What preventative measures might be included in a patient education brochure for macular degeneration? Write out a list of possible preventative measures.

DISEASES AND DISORDERS OF THE EAR

Meniere Disease

Meniere disease is a disorder of the inner ear. It is characterized by vertigo, tinnitus, progressive hearing loss, and sometimes a feeling of pressure or fullness in the ear. It usually only affects one ear. See Table 13.21 (presented later in the chapter) for definitions of vertigo and tinnitus.

Etiology. The cause of Meniere disease is not well understood. The inner ear of persons with this condition seems to have an abnormal amount of fluid (endolymph). What causes the excess fluid is not known. Some research indicates possible causes could be the following:
- Abnormal anatomy of the inner ear, genetic predisposition
- Possible autoimmune reaction, allergies, or viral infection
- Head trauma, migraines

Risk factors for Meniere disease include the following:
- Preexisting autoimmune disorders
- Allergies
- Head or ear trauma

Signs and Symptoms. Signs and symptoms for Meniere disease include the following:
- Episodes of vertigo (dizziness). Episodes may last for minutes or hours. Vertigo may cause nausea and vomiting.
- Tinnitus. A constant perceived ringing, buzzing, clicking, roaring, or whistling sound in the ear without an external stimulus
- Progressive hearing loss. It may fluctuate in the beginning, but some hearing loss does become permanent
- Feeling of pressure or fullness in the ear or on the affected side of the head.

Signs and symptoms can come and go but rarely disappear permanently. Because vertigo can happen at any time, the unpredictability can be stressful. Some hearing loss does become permanent. Frequent vertigo can cause fatigue, anxiety, and depression. Vertigo can also cause people to lose their balance, fall, or have an accident while driving.

Diagnostic Procedures. Diagnostic procedures for Meniere disease may include the following:
- A physical exam and detailed health history.
- Two confirmed episodes of vertigo, which last at least 20 minutes but not longer than 24 hours.
- Hearing loss confirmed by audiometry (hearing test). Most Meniere patients have low-frequency hearing loss or hearing loss with a combination of low and high frequencies. Mid frequencies are usually normal.
- Tinnitus and possibly pressure/feeling of fullness in the ear.
- Magnetic resonance imaging (MRI) to rule out other conditions such as a brain tumor or multiple sclerosis (MS).
- Specific tests and procedures may be used to evaluate the function of the inner ear.

Treatment. Meniere disease has no cure, but there are treatments that can reduce signs and symptoms and the frequency of vertigo. Treatments include the following:
- Motion sickness medications, antinausea medication, and diuretics
- Following a low-sodium (salt) diet
- A hearing aid for the affected ear
- Balance rehabilitative therapy

These treatments are most commonly used, but for individuals who have frequent or debilitating vertigo, more aggressive treatments may be used:
- Steroid medications.
- Gentamicin (an antibiotic) injections to damage the balance structure in the affected ear. This procedure can further damage hearing in the affected ear.
- Surgery to destroy the affected inner ear (labyrinthectomy).
- Surgery to cut the vestibular nerve that leads from the ear to the brain. This often corrects vertigo and preserves hearing in the affected ear.

Lifestyle changes that can positively affect Meniere disease include a low-salt diet and stress management. A high-salt diet and stress can bring on vertigo attacks and make tinnitus more noticeable.

Follow-up visits are likely because Meniere is a chronic condition. Medication changes, hearing checkups, and possible balance therapy visits may be necessary.

Prognosis. Generally, the prognosis is good for Meniere disease. The compliant patient that eats a low-salt diet and reduces stress will likely have the fewest complications. Some patients with frequent vertigo that is not affected by diet and medication may have to participate in more aggressive therapies and surgery.

Prevention. Since the cause for Meniere disease is unknown, prevention is difficult. Eating a healthy diet that is low in sodium, reducing stress, getting adequate sleep, and exercising regularly will always be helpful to overall health.

Otosclerosis

Otosclerosis is a condition in which the ossicles of the middle ear (malleolus, incus, and stapes) become fused and act as a single unit instead of individual bones. This restricts the movement of the ossicles and results in conductive hearing loss. Another variation of otosclerosis only involves the stapes. Development of bone around the oval window can result in immobility or stiffening of the stapes to the oval window. This results in progressive conductive hearing loss.

Etiology. The cause of otosclerosis seems to be a combination of genetic and viral involvement. If one parent carries the gene, a child has a 50% chance of inheriting the gene. But some research suggests that only if a person with the gene is exposed to certain viruses will he or she develop otosclerosis.

Risk factors for developing otosclerosis include the following:
- Having an inherited gene that predisposes a person to otosclerosis.
- Having close family members with the condition, especially parents.
- Being female. Females are twice as likely to develop the condition as men.
- Being pregnant or having been pregnant. Otosclerosis can worsen during a pregnancy or shortly after the birth of a child, suggesting the condition may be affected by hormone fluctuations.
- Caucasian and Asian women are more likely to develop the condition.
- Having a viral infection that may start the development of otosclerosis. Viruses may include German measles, perhaps some members of the herpes family of viruses, and unknown additional infectious viral agents.

Signs and Symptoms. Signs and symptoms of otosclerosis include the following:
- Progressive conductive hearing loss that may begin age 10 to 30 years. It is most commonly diagnosed in persons who are between 25 and 45 years old.
- About 10% to 15% of persons with otosclerosis may experience dizziness.
- Some patients may experience tinnitus.

Diagnostic Procedures. Diagnosis of otosclerosis is usually made with a combination of procedures, which may include the following:
- Patient and family medical history
- Physical examination including examination of the middle ear
- Audiometry (hearing test) (see Box 13.9)
- Tympanometry to look for a stiffening of the ossicles (see Table 13.8)

Treatment. Treatment of otosclerosis includes the following:
- Hearing aids are used to amplify sound.
- If hearing impairment cannot be adequately treated with hearing aids, a surgical procedure called a stapedectomy (partial removal of the stapes and implantation of a prosthetic device) can be performed. The procedure helps restore movement to the ossicles and can restore conductive hearing loss. Stapedectomy may also improve tinnitus.
- If stapedectomy is unsuccessful, cochlear implants are another option to restore hearing.

Prognosis. The prognosis is generally good, and treatments for conductive hearing loss are most often helpful in amplifying or restoring hearing.

Prevention. There is no effective way to prevent otosclerosis.

> **CRITICAL THINKING 13.9**
>
> Rosie is reviewing the anatomy of the ear before she finishes her CEU tonight. She is looking at a poster of ear anatomy in one of the exam rooms. Where is the oval window? Look back at Fig. 13.3. Locate the oval window, cochlea, vestibule, and semicircular canals.

Presbycusis

Presbycusis is age-related hearing loss. By the age of 65, about 30% of people have some hearing loss. By the age of 75, that number jumps to 50%. Age-related hearing loss affects both ears equally and most often happens gradually over a number of years.

Etiology. Several factors may contribute to presbycusis:
- High blood pressure, diabetes, ototoxic drugs, or chemotherapy
- Long-term exposure to loud noises (or noise-induced hearing loss)
- Abnormalities in the tympanic membrane (eardrum)
- Otosclerosis

The factors that contribute to presbycusis can also be considered influences that put a person at risk for developing the condition.

Signs and Symptoms. Signs and symptoms of presbycusis include the following:
- A gradual loss of hearing as a person ages
- The inability to hear clearly in a conversation or room where more than one person is talking
- The inability to understand a conversation or hear the full range of sound in music

Diagnostic Procedures. Diagnostic procedures for presbycusis include the following:
- Complete health history, physical examination, and examination of the middle ear to rule out other conditions.
- Audiometry (hearing test)

Treatment. Treatments for presbycusis include the following:
- Hearing aids can be used to amplify sound.
- If hearing loss is severe, cochlear implants may be recommended.
- Bone-anchored hearing systems. A hearing system that bypasses the middle ear, captures sound waves and converts them to vibrations which are transferred through your skull bones to the inner ear. The inner ear then processes the vibrations onto the brain.
- Assisted listening devices can be employed, such as amplifying devices for telephones, cell phones, and smart phone and tablet apps.
- Lip reading can help the hearing-impaired follow conversations in a small group.

Periodic follow-up with a provider may be needed. Yearly hearing tests are recommended.

Prognosis. The prognosis is good for patients with presbycusis. Using hearing aids and other assistive devices can compensate for lost hearing. Remaining socially engaged and not becoming isolated is important for a person's overall health and well-being.

Prevention. Presbycusis really cannot be prevented, but noise-induced hearing loss (which often contributes to presbycusis) can be prevented.

The following measures can be taken to reduce the risk of noise-induced hearing loss:
- Avoid loud noises if possible.
- Wear hearing protection if loud noises cannot be avoided. Use earplugs or earmuffs to protect hearing.

ADDITIONAL DISEASES AND DISORDERS OF THE EYES AND EARS

There are many other diseases and disorders of the eyes and ears. See Tables 13.10 through 13.26 for additional conditions that may be of interest.

> ### CRITICAL THINKING 13.10
>
> Lael Greenwood, is 10 years old and will be seeing Dr. Walden today for a routine physical. Before he sees the doctor, Lael is going to have his vision checked. Rosie will screen his vision by asking him to read the eye chart. They will also be doing an Ishihara color vision test.
>
> Can you explain the Ishihara color vision test in your own words? Why is it important to screen for color blindness? Share your answers with your classmates.

LIFE SPAN CHANGES

In children, the most prevalent disorder of the eyes is conjunctivitis (commonly known as pinkeye), which accounts for a large number of pediatric visits. Because it is highly contagious, entire classrooms may be infected because of one student's infection. Most newborns receive erythromycin shortly after birth. This has significantly reduced the number of cases of ophthalmia neonatorum conjunctivitis, which is usually due to gonorrhea or a chlamydial infection.

Age-related macular degeneration (ARMD) and cataracts are the most common causes of blindness in older adults. Although there are several successful procedures to treat cataracts, currently there are no treatments to cure ARMD. Diabetic retinopathy is the most common cause of blindness, but it may also occur much earlier in life. Presbyopia is a visual disorder that usually accompanies aging and results in farsightedness.

Few babies are born with a hearing loss. The Universal Newborn Hearing Screening (UNHS) test is a means to detect deafness in infancy. Once an infant has been diagnosed, the parents can plan for future treatments and determine how to best handle the condition. Otitis media (OM) is the most frequently diagnosed childhood ear disease.

In adults, hearing loss that may accompany the aging process is termed *presbycusis*.

Text continued on p. 321

TABLE 13.10 Terms Related to Eyelid Disorders

Term	Definition
blepharedema (bleff ah ruh DEE mah)	Swelling of the eyelid
blepharitis (bleff ah RYE tis)	Inflammation of the eyelid
blepharochalasis (bleff ah roh KAL luh sis)	Hypertrophy of the skin of the eyelid
blepharoptosis (bleff ah rop TOH sis)	Drooping of the upper eyelid
ectropion (eck TROH pee on)	Turning outward (*eversion*) of the eyelid, exposing the conjunctiva (Fig. 13.18)
entropion (en TROH pee on)	Turning inward of the eyelid toward the eye (Fig. 13.19)

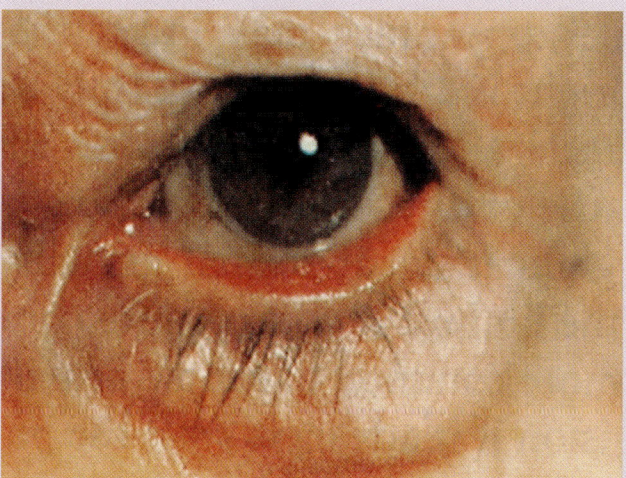

FIG. 13.18 Ectropion of the lower lid. (From Seidel HM, Ball JW, Dains JE, et al: *Mosby's Guide to Physical Examination*, ed 7, St. Louis, 2011, Mosby.)

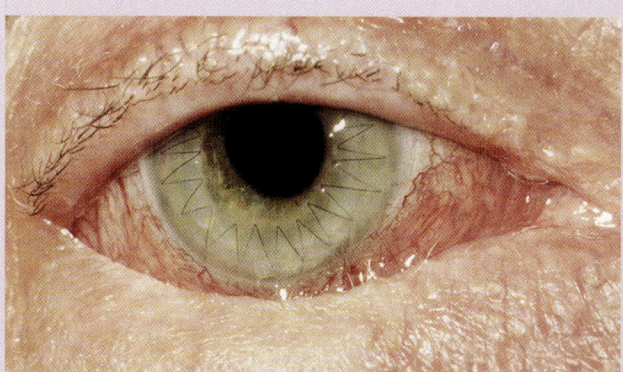

FIG. 13.19 Entropion of the lower lid. (From Sorrentino SA: *Assisting With Patient Care*, ed 2, St. Louis, 2004, Mosby.)

From Shiland B: *Mastering Healthcare Terminology*, ed 5, St. Louis, 2016, Elsevier.

TABLE 13.11　Terms Related to Eyelash Disorders

Term	Definition
chalazion (kuh LAY zee on)	Hardened swelling of a meibomian gland resulting from a blockage; also called *meibomian cyst* (Fig. 13.20)
hordeolum (hor DEE uh lum)	*Stye*; infection of one of the sebaceous glands of an eyelash (Fig. 13.21)

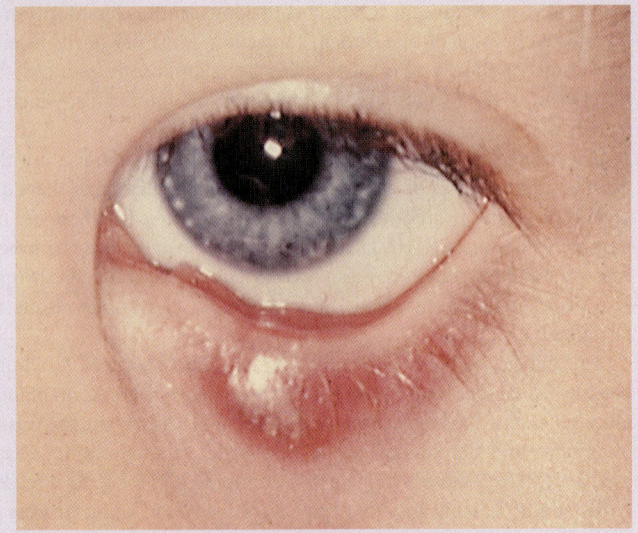

FIG. 13.20 Chalazion. (From Zitelli BJ, Davis HW: *Atlas of Pediatric Physical Diagnosis*, ed 5, St. Louis, 2007, Mosby.)

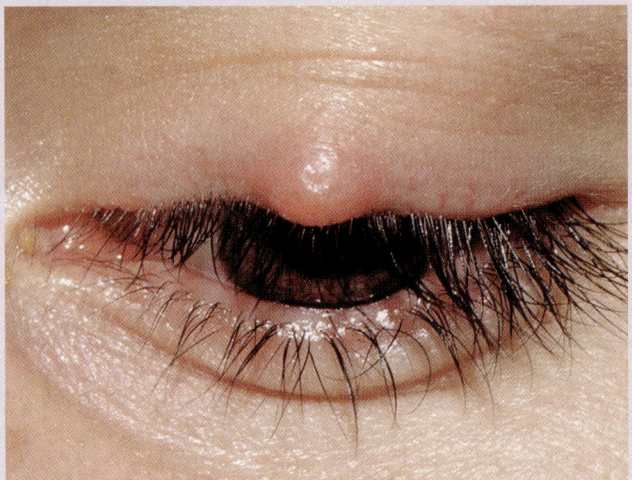

FIG. 13.21 Hordeolum. (From Seidel HM, Ball JW, Dains JE, et al: *Mosby's Guide to Physical Examination,* ed 7, St. Louis, 2011, Mosby.)

From Shiland B: *Mastering Healthcare Terminology*, ed 5, St. Louis, 2016, Elsevier.

TABLE 13.12　Terms Related to Tear Gland Disorders

Term	Definition
dacryoadenitis (dack ree oh add eh NYE tis)	Inflammation of a lacrimal gland
dacryocystitis (dack ree oh sis TYE tis)	Inflammation of a lacrimal sac (Fig. 13.22)
epiphora (eh PIFF or ah)	Overflow of tears; excessive lacrimation
xerophthalmia (zeer off THAL mee ah)	Dry eye; lack of adequate tear production to lubricate the eye; usually the result of vitamin A deficiency

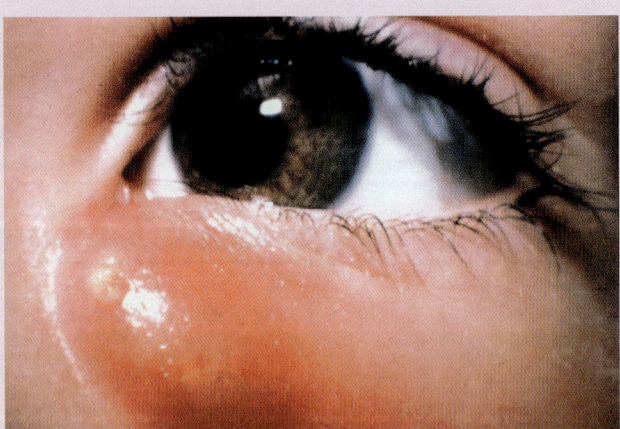

FIG. 13.22 Dacryocystitis. (From Marx J, Hockberger R, Walls R: *Rosen's Emergency Medicine*, ed 7, Philadelphia, 2010, Saunders.)

From Shiland B: *Mastering Healthcare Terminology*, ed 5, St. Louis, 2016, Elsevier.

TABLE 13.13　Terms Related to Conjunctiva Disorders

Term	Definition
conjunctivitis (kun junk tih VYE tis)	Inflammation of the conjunctiva, commonly known as *pinkeye*, a highly contagious disorder (Fig. 13.23).
ophthalmia neonatorum (off THAL mee uh nee oh nay TORE um)	Severe, purulent conjunctivitis in the newborn, usually due to gonorrheal or chlamydial infection. Routine introduction of an antibiotic ophthalmic ointment (erythromycin) prevents most cases.

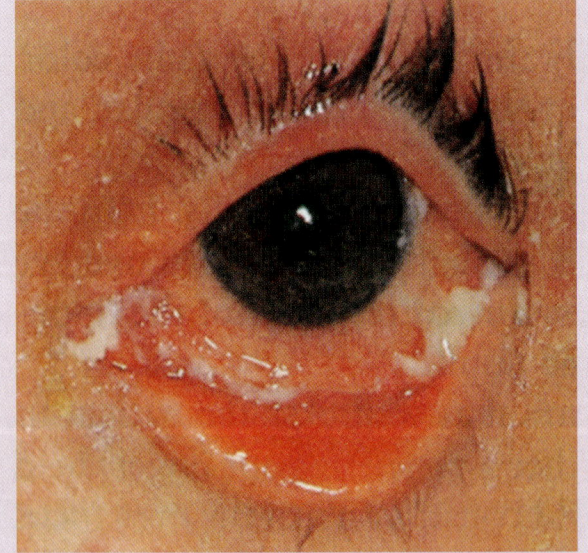

FIG. 13.23 Acute purulent conjunctivitis. (From Shiland: *Mastering Healthcare Terminology*, ed 5, St. Louis, 2016, Elsevier.)

From Shiland B: *Mastering Healthcare Terminology*, ed 5, St. Louis, 2016, Elsevier.

TABLE 13.14 Terms Related to Eye Muscle and Orbital Disorders

Term	Definition
amblyopia (am blee OH pee ah)	Dull or dim vision due to disuse.
diplopia (dih PLOH pee ah)	Double vision. *Emmetropia* (EM, Em) means normal vision.
esotropia (eh soh TROH pee ah)	Turning inward of one or both eyes (Fig. 13.24).
exophthalmia (eck soff THAL mee ah)	Protrusion of the eyeball from its orbit; may be congenital or the result of an endocrine disorder.
exotropia (eck so TROH pee ah)	Turning outward of one or both eyes (Fig. 13.25).
photophobia (foh toh FOH bee ah)	Extreme sensitivity to light. The suffix *-phobia* here means "aversion," not fear.
strabismus (struh BIZ muh s)	General term for a lack of coordination between the eyes, usually due to a muscle weakness or paralysis. Sometimes called a "squint," which refers to the patient's effort to correct the disorder.

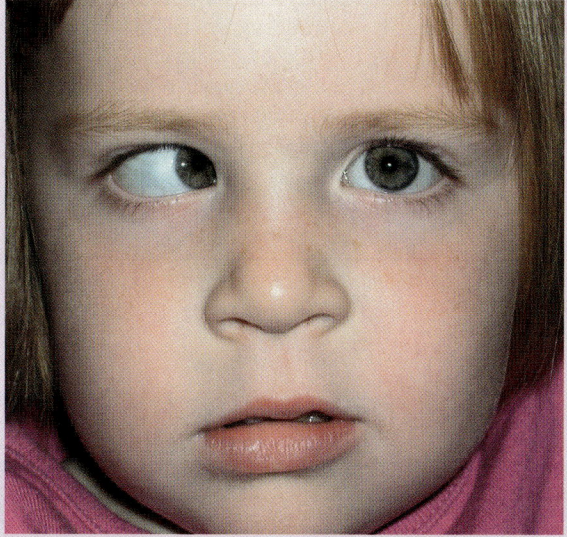

FIG. 13.24 Esotropia. (From Shiland B: *Medical Terminology & Anatomy for ICD-10 Coding*, St. Louis, 2012, Mosby.)

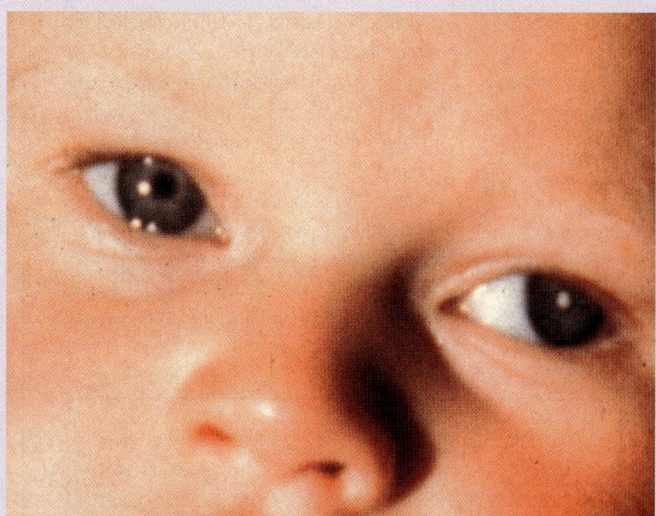

FIG. 13.25 Exotropia in left eye. (From Kanski J, Bowling B: *Clinical Ophthalmology*, ed 7, London, 2011, Saunders.)

From Shiland B: *Mastering Healthcare Terminology*, ed 5, St. Louis, 2016, Elsevier.

TABLE 13.15 Terms Related to Sclera Disorders

Term	Definition
corneal ulcer (KORE nee uhl UHL sur)	Trauma to the outer covering of the eye, resulting in an abrasion
keratitis (kair uh TYE tis)	Inflammation of the cornea

From Shiland B: *Mastering Healthcare Terminology*, ed 5, St. Louis, 2016, Elsevier.

TABLE 13.16 Terms Related to Uvea Disorders

Term	Definition
anisocoria (an nye soh KORE ee ah)	Condition of unequally sized pupils, sometimes due to pressure on the optic nerve because of trauma or lesion (Fig. 13.26)
hyphema (hye FEE mah)	Blood in the anterior chamber of the eye because of hemorrhage due to trauma
uveitis (yoo vee EYE tis)	Inflammation of the iris, ciliary body, and choroids, also known as the *uvea*

FIG. 13.26 Anisocoria. (From Albert D: *Albert & Jakobiec's Principles and Practice of Ophthalmology*, ed 3, London, 2008, Saunders.)

From Shiland B: *Mastering Healthcare Terminology*, ed 5, St. Louis, 2016, Elsevier.

TABLE 13.17 Terms Related to Lens and Retina Disorders

Term	Definition
achromatopsia (ah kroh mah TOP see ah)	Impairment of color vision. Inability to distinguish between certain colors because of abnormalities of the photopigments produced in the retina. Also called *color blindness*. See Box 13.10 for information on testing for color blindness.
diabetic retinopathy (dye ah BET ick ret in OP ah thee)	Damage of the retina due to diabetes; the leading cause of blindness (Fig. 13.27). Classified according to stages from mild, nonproliferative diabetic retinopathy (NPDR) to proliferative diabetic retinopathy (PDR).
hemianopsia (hem ee an NOP see ah)	Loss of half the visual field (VF), often as the result of a cerebrovascular accident.
nyctalopia (nick tuh LOH pee ah)	Inability to see well in dim light. May be due to a vitamin A deficiency, retinitis pigmentosa, or choroidoretinitis.
retinal tear, retinal detachment	Separation of the retina from the choroid layer. May be due to trauma, inflammation of the interior of the eye, or aging. A hole in the retina allows fluid from the vitreous humor to leak between the two layers.
retinitis pigmentosa (ret in EYE tis pig men TOH sah)	Hereditary, degenerative disease marked by nyctalopia and a progressive loss of the VF.
scotoma (skoh TOH mah)	Area of decreased vision in the VF. Commonly called a *blind spot*.

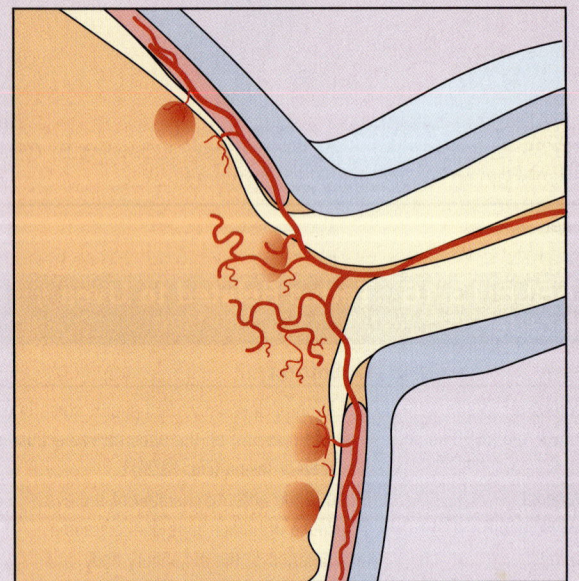

FIG. 13.27 Diabetic retinopathy. (From Shiland: *Mastering Healthcare Terminology*, ed 5, St. Louis, 2016, Elsevier.)

From Shiland B: *Mastering Healthcare Terminology*, ed 5, St. Louis, 2016, Elsevier

BOX 13.10 Color Blindness Testing
Ishihara Color Vision Test

Defects in color vision are classified as congenital or acquired. Congenital defects are caused by an inherited color vision defect and are found most often in males. Acquired defects are caused by eye injury or disease. The Ishihara test is a simple, convenient, and accurate procedure that detects total color blindness and red-green color blindness. (See Chapter 30 for a detailed procedure). The test assesses the perception of primary colors and shades of colors.

TABLE 13.18 Terms Related to Optic Nerve Disorders

Term	Definition
nystagmus (nye STAG mus)	Involuntary, back-and-forth eye movements due to a disorder of the labyrinth of the ear and/or parts of the nervous system associated with rhythmic eye movements
optic neuritis (OP tick nyoo RYE tis)	Inflammation of the optic nerve resulting in blindness; often mentioned as a predecessor to the development of multiple sclerosis

From Shiland B: *Mastering Healthcare Terminology*, ed 5, St. Louis, 2016, Elsevier.

TABLE 13.19 Term Related to Benign Neoplasms

Term	Definition
choroidal hemangioma (koh ROY dul hee man jee OH mah)	Tumor of the blood vessel layer under the retina (the choroid layer); may cause visual loss or retinal detachment

From Shiland B: *Mastering Healthcare Terminology*, ed 5, St. Louis, 2016, Elsevier.

TABLE 13.20 Terms Related to Malignant Neoplasms

Term	Definition
intraocular melanoma (in trah AHK yoo lur mell uh NOH mah)	Malignant tumor of the choroid, ciliary body, or iris that usually occurs in individuals in their 50s or 60s (Fig. 13.28)
retinoblastoma (ret noh bla STOH muh)	An inherited condition present at birth that arises from embryonic retinal cells (Fig. 13.29)

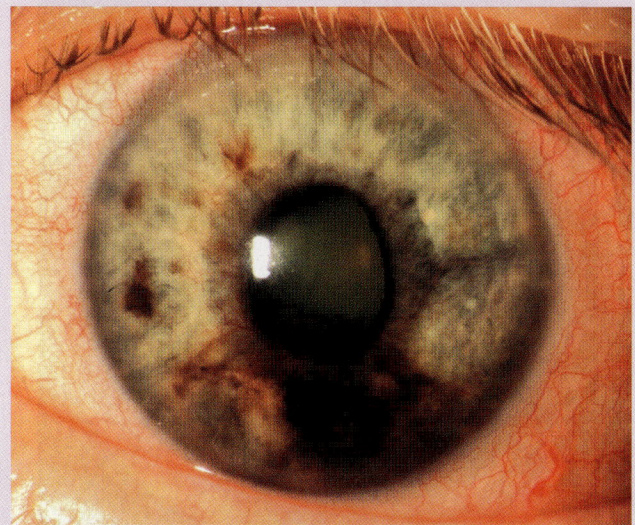

FIG. 13.28 Intraocular melanoma. (From Nguyen Q, Rodrigues EB, Farah ME, et al: *Retinal Pharmacotherapy*, London, 2010, Saunders.)

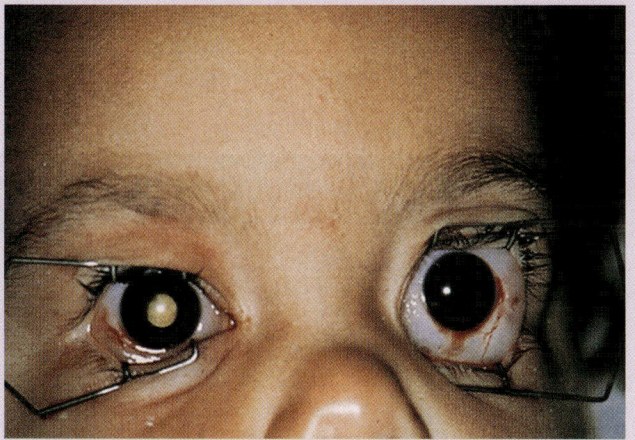

FIG. 13.29 Retinoblastoma. (From Damjanov I: *Anderson's Pathology*, ed 10, St. Louis, 2000, Mosby.)

From Shiland B: *Mastering Healthcare Terminology*, ed 5, St. Louis, 2016, Elsevier.

TABLE 13.21 Terms Related to Symptomatic Disorders of the Ear

Term	Definition
otalgia (oh TAL juh)	Earache, pain in the ear; also called *otodynia* (oh toh DIN nee ah)
otorrhea (oh tuh REE ah)	Discharge from the auditory canal; may be serous, bloody, or purulent
tinnitus (tin EYE tis)	Abnormal sound heard in one or both ears caused by trauma or disease; may be a ringing, buzzing, or jingling
vertigo (VUR tih goh)	Dizziness; abnormal sensation of movement when there is none, either of one's self moving or of objects moving around oneself; may be caused by middle ear infections or the toxic effects of alcohol, sunstroke, and certain medications

From Shiland B: *Mastering Healthcare Terminology*, ed 5, St. Louis, 2016, Elsevier.

TABLE 13.22 Terms Related to Outer Ear Disorders

Term	Definition
impacted cerumen (sur ROO mun)	Blockage of the external auditory canal with cerumen
macrotia (mah KROH sha)	Condition of abnormally large auricles
microtia (mye KROH sha)	Condition of abnormally small auricles
otitis externa (oh TYE tis eck STER nah)	Inflammation of the outer ear and ear canal; also called *swimmer's ear*

From Shiland B: *Mastering Healthcare Terminology*, ed 5, St. Louis, 2016, Elsevier.

TABLE 13.23 Terms Related to Middle Ear Disorders

Term	Definition
cholesteatoma (koh less tee ah TOH mah)	Cystic mass composed of epithelial cells and cholesterol. Mass may occlude middle ear and destroy adjacent bones.
infectious myringitis (meer in JYE tis)	Inflammation of the eardrum due to a bacterial or viral infection.
mastoiditis (mass toy DYE tis)	Inflammation of the mastoid process of the temporal bone (Fig. 13.30).
otitis media (OM) (oh TYE tis MEE dee ah)	Inflammation of the middle ear. *Suppurative OM* is characterized by a pus-filled fluid. *Secretory OM* is characterized by clear fluid discharge (Fig. 13.31).

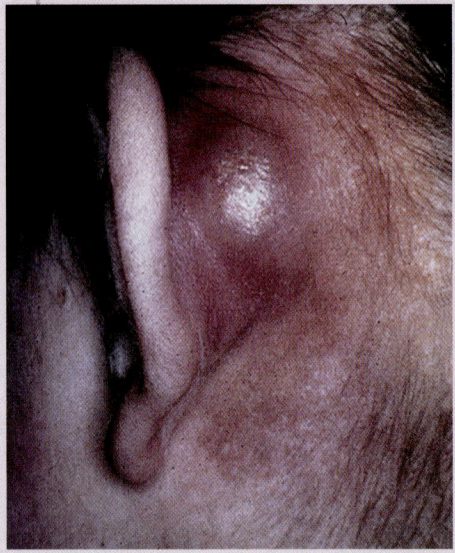

FIG. 13.30 Mastoiditis. (From Stone DR, Gorbach SL: *Atlas of Infectious Diseases*, Philadelphia, 2000, Saunders.)

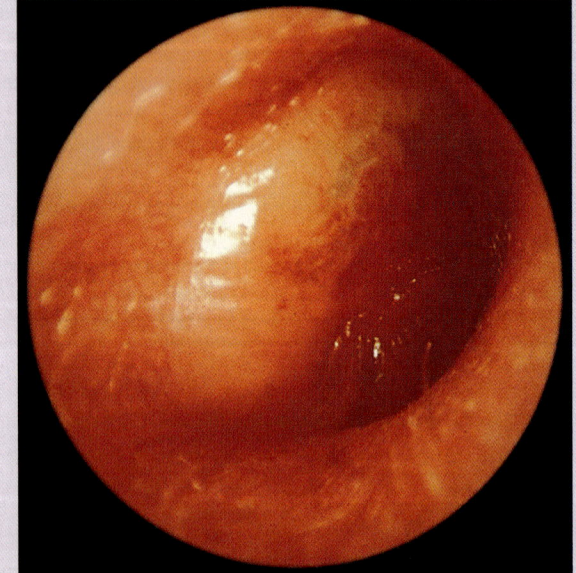

FIG. 13.31 Otitis media. (Courtesy of Dr. Michael Hawke, MD. From Zitelli BJ, Davis HW: *Atlas of Pediatric Physical Diagnosis*, ed 5, St Louis, 2007, Mosby.)

From Shiland B: *Mastering Healthcare Terminology*, ed 5, St. Louis, 2016, Elsevier.

TABLE 13.24 Terms Related to Inner Ear Disorders

Term	Definition
labyrinthitis (lab uh rinth EYE tis)	Inflammation of the inner ear that may be due to infection or trauma; symptoms may include vertigo, nausea, and nystagmus
ruptured tympanic membrane (TM)	Tear (perforation) of the eardrum due to trauma or disease process (Fig. 13.32)

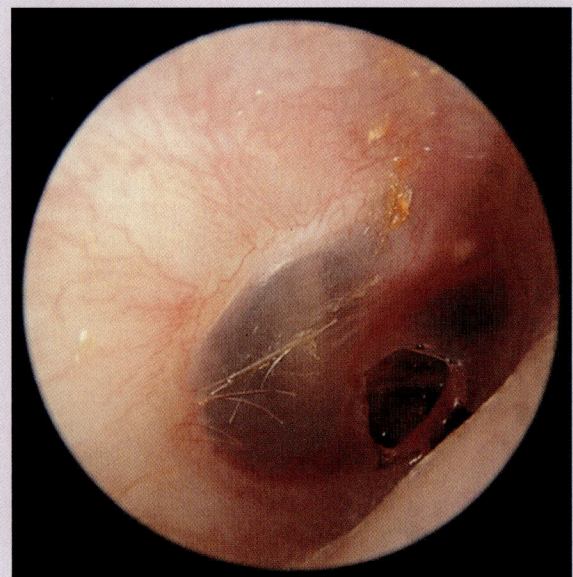

FIG. 13.32 Ruptured tympanic membrane. (Courtesy of Dr. Michael Hawke, MD. From Zitelli BJ, Davis HW: *Atlas of Pediatric Physical Diagnosis*, ed 5, St Louis, 2007, Mosby.)

From Shiland B: *Mastering Healthcare Terminology*, ed 5, St. Louis, 2016, Elsevier.

TABLE 13.25 Terms Related to Hearing Loss Disorders

Term	Definition
anacusis (an uh KYOO sis)	General term for hearing loss or deafness
conductive hearing loss	Hearing loss resulting from damage to or malformation of the middle or outer ear
paracusis (pair uh KYOO sis)	Abnormality of hearing

From Shiland B: *Mastering Healthcare Terminology*, ed 5, St. Louis, 2016, Elsevier.

TABLE 13.26 Terms Related to Benign Neoplasms

Term	Definition
acoustic neuroma (ah KOO stik noo ROH mah)	A benign tumor of the eighth cranial nerve (vestibulocochlear) that causes tinnitus, vertigo, and hearing loss; also called *vestibular schwannoma*
ceruminoma (si ROO muh noh mah)	A benign adenoma of the glands that produce earwax

From Shiland B: *Mastering Healthcare Terminology*, ed 5, St. Louis, 2016, Elsevier.

CLOSING COMMENTS

Patients with vision or hearing impairment face serious challenges. For these patients, the medical assistant must use good listening skills and appropriate nonverbal communication to convey empathy and understanding. Patient education may have to be adapted to meet the special needs of these patients. A person with a vision loss benefits from large-print forms and handouts, increased lighting, and verbal rather than written instructions to reinforce learning. For an individual with a hearing deficit, printed instructions, demonstrations of how to manage treatments, or sign language interpretation should be available to ensure accurate communication. Including family members in the patient's treatment plan and offering referrals to appropriate community or professional resources may be very beneficial to a patient with sensory loss. Each patient must be assessed individually to determine the type of adaptation that he or she needs.

An important part of patient education for those administering eye medications at home is stressing the need to maintain the sterility of the medication. Patients or family members must be taught how to apply the medication while preventing trauma to the eye and contamination of the applicator. Patients administering ear treatments also must understand how to apply the medication.

The eyes and ears are complicated and wonderful sensory organs. Sight and sound add so much to our everyday lives. See Tables 13.27 through 13.32 for medical terminology related to the eyes and ears.

EXCEPTIONAL CUSTOMER SERVICE

Diminished sight or hearing may render a patient seriously impaired. To prevent accidents and office injuries, always ask sight- or hearing-impaired patients whether they require assistance. When you escort the patient to an examination room, offer your arm and tell the patient the approximate distance you will be walking. If the patient is to have an examination that involves local anesthesia or eyedrops that dilate the pupil, be sure the patient has recovered, has sunglasses, and that someone is available to drive the patient home before allowing him or her to leave the facility.

TABLE 13.27 Combining and Adjective Forms for the Anatomy and Physiology of the Eye

Meaning	Combining Form	Adjective Form	Meaning	Combining Form	Adjective Form
canthus	canth/o	canthal	macula lutea	macul/o	macular
choroid	choroid/o	choroidal	optic disk	papill/o	papillary
ciliary body	cycl/o	cyclic	orbit	orbit/o	orbital
conjunctiva	conjunctiv/o	conjunctival	pupil	pupill/o, core/o, cor/o	pupillary
cornea	corne/o, kerat/o	corneal, keratic	retina	retin/o	retinal
eye	ocul/o, ophthalm/o	ocular, ophthalmic	sclera	scler/o	scleral
eyelid	blephar/o, palpebr/o	palpebral	tears	lacrim/o, dacry/o	lacrimal
iris	ir/o, irid/o	iridic	uvea	uve/o	uveal
lacrimal gland	dacryoaden/o	dacryoadenal	vision	opt/o, optic/o	optic, optical
lacrimal sac	dacryocyst/o	dacryocystic	vitreous humor	vitre/o, vitr/o	vitreous
lens	phak/o, phac/o				

From Shiland B: *Mastering Healthcare Terminology*, ed 5, St. Louis, 2016, Elsevier.

TABLE 13.28 Prefixes for Anatomy of the Eye

Prefix	Meaning
bin-	two
extra-	outside
supra-	above

From Shiland B: *Mastering Healthcare Terminology*, ed 5, St. Louis, 2016, Elsevier.

TABLE 13.29 Abbreviations for the Eye

Abbreviation	Meaning	Abbreviation	Meaning
Acc	accommodation	IOL	intraocular lens
ACS	anterior ciliary sclerotomy	IOP	intraocular pressure
AK	astigmatic keratotomy	LASIK	laser-assisted in-situ keratomileusis
ARMD, AMD	age-related macular degeneration	MY	myopia
Astigm, As, Ast	astigmatism	NPDR	nonproliferative diabetic retinopathy
ECCE	extracapsular cataract extraction	Ophth	ophthalmology
EM, Em	emmetropia	PDR	proliferative diabetic retinopathy
EOM	extraocular movements	PRK	photorefractive keratectomy
ICCE	intracapsular cataract extraction	VA	visual acuity
ICL	implantable contact lens	VF	visual field

From Shiland B: *Mastering Healthcare Terminology*, ed 5, St. Louis, 2016, Elsevier.

TABLE 13.30 Combining and Adjective Forms for the Anatomy and Physiology of the Ear

Meaning	Combining Form	Adjective Form	Meaning	Combining Form	Adjective Form
cerumen, earwax	cerumin/o	ceruminous	lymph	lymph/o, lymphat/o	lymphatic
cochlea	cochle/o	cochlear	macula	macul/o	macular
ear	ot/o, aur/o, auricul/o	otic, aural, auricular	mastoid process	mastoid/o	mastoidal
eardrum	tympan/o, myring/o	tympanic	meatus	meat/o	meatal
eustachian tube	salping/o	salpingeal	ossicle	ossicul/o	ossicular
hearing	audi/o, acous/o	acoustic	stapes	staped/o	stapedial
labyrinth, inner ear	labyrinth/o	labyrinthine	vestibule	vestibul/o	vestibular

From Shiland B: *Mastering Healthcare Terminology*, ed 5, St. Louis, 2016, Elsevier.

TABLE 13.31 Prefixes for Anatomy of the Ear

Prefix	Meaning
endo-	within
peri-	surrounding

From Shiland B: *Mastering Healthcare Terminology*, ed 5, St. Louis, 2016, Elsevier.

TABLE 13.32 Abbreviations for the Ear

Abbreviation	Meaning	Abbreviation	Meaning
ABR	auditory brainstem response	OM	otitis media
ASL	American sign language	oto	otology
ENT	ear, nose, throat	TM	tympanic membrane
OAE	otoacoustic emission	UNHS	Universal Newborn Hearing Screening test

From Shiland B: *Mastering Healthcare Terminology*, ed 5, St. Louis, 2016, Elsevier.

CHAPTER REVIEW

The senses are divided into general senses and special senses. The general senses have receptors spread throughout the body. General senses are pressure, temperature, pain, and touch. The special senses have complex organs that have specific receptors for that sense. Special senses are vision, hearing, equilibrium, taste, and smell. This chapter covered two of the special senses in detail: vision (the eyes) and hearing/equilibrium (the ears).

The anatomy of the eye was discussed in detail. The eye is made up of the ocular adnexa (the supporting structures around the eye) and the eyeball. The ocular adnexa is composed of the following:

- The bony orbit or socket that surrounds the eye
- The eyebrows, eyelashes, and eyelids
- The conjunctiva that lines the eyelid
- Lacrimal glands, canals, and duct (which produce and drain tears)

The eyeball is what we think of as the eye, the structure that detects light and sends signals to the brain. The brain then processes the information into a visual picture we recognize as sight.

The eyeball consists of three layers. The outermost layer is made up of the following:

- The sclera, or white of the eye, and the cornea, the clear window that lets light enter the eye. The cornea also helps refract or bend light.

The middle layer of the eye is made up of the following:

- The choroid, the iris, and the ciliary body. These three structures together are known as the uvea.
- The iris is the colored part of the eye with an opening in the center called the pupil. The iris is a muscle that regulates the size of the pupil. The iris regulates the amount of light that enters the eye.
- The ciliary body changes the space of the lens.
- The choroid is the back portion of the middle layer. It is highly vascular and contains many blood vessels that supply nutrients to the retina. The choroid has a brown color, which helps absorb excess light that could interfere with vision.

The inner layer of the eye is made up of the following:

- The biconvex lens in the front of the eye lets light into the eye.
- The retina is in the back of the eye. It has many photoreceptors, known as rods and cones, on its surface.
- Rods are sensitive to light; cones can detect color.
- The vitreous humor is a gel-like substance that gives the eyeball its shape
- The macula lutea and fovea centralis are areas with large numbers of photoreceptors. Light is focused toward these areas for sharp vision.
- The optic disk is an area that has no photoreceptors. The optic disk is where the optic nerve leaves the retina.

Together rods and cones detect light and convert it into neurologic impulses. The impulses travel along the optic nerve to the brain. The brain then converts the impulses to visual images.

The ear is the second sensory organ that we discussed in detail. The ear is made up of three sections: the outer ear, the middle ear, and the inner ear. The outer ear is composed of three structures:
- Auricle or pinna, the outer ear that we see on the side of the head
- External auditory canal, which leads sound waves captured by the auricle inside the ear
- Tympanic membrane or eardrum, which vibrates when sound waves meet it

The outer ear collects sound waves and focuses them to the tympanic membrane. The middle ear is a space inside the temporal bone that houses three small bones called ossicles:
- Malleus, or hammer
- Incus, or anvil
- Stapes, or stirrup

These tiny bones are connected to each other and form a bridge from the tympanic membrane to the inner ear. One other structure that is connected to, but is not part of, the middle ear is the eustachian tube.

The ossicles transmit sound to the inner ear through the movement of the stapes. The oval window is a membrane that connects the middle ear to the inner ear. At the oval window, sound waves move into the fluids of the inner ear. The inner ear is composed of the following structures:
- The cochlea contains the organ of Corti, which contains the receptors for sound. The receptors are tiny hairlike structures that are surrounded by sensory nerve fibers. The movement of the receptors creates a sound impulse that is carried by the cochlear nerve to the brain, where it is interpreted and is sensed as sound.
- The semicircular canals, which sense dynamic equilibrium.
- The vestibule, which senses static equilibrium.

The ear is a complex organ that not only senses sound but also senses and helps maintain our sense of balance.

Sometimes the senses of sight and sound are impaired. We discussed several conditions that affect sight and hearing. For the eyes, we discussed refractive errors. These are not really diseases, but they are certainly structural differences that make seeing difficult without the aid of glasses, contact lenses, or corrective surgery. The four refractive errors discussed are as follows:
- Myopia, or nearsightedness
- Hyperopia, or farsightedness
- Astigmatism, or an irregular shaped cornea or lens
- Presbyopia, which is an inflexibility of the lens and weakened ciliary muscles that come with aging

Regarding the sense of hearing, we discussed certain impairments that can make it difficult to hear without the help of a hearing aid or cochlear implant. The two types of hearing impairment discussed are as follows:
- Conductive hearing loss, caused by problems in the outer or middle ear that prevent sound vibrations from entering the ear.
- Sensorineural hearing loss, caused by an abnormality of the organ of Corti or the auditory nerve. Presbycusis is a progressive sensorineural hearing loss associated with aging.

Hearing loss can often be reduced or hearing can be recaptured with the use of hearing aids or cochlear implants. These devices may not be able to completely restore lost hearing, but they can improve hearing and quality of life.

Many sensory diseases and disorders were presented in the chapter. Common signs and symptoms include altered vision or hearing, pain, headaches, and dizziness. Common etiology includes infections, autoimmune conditions, anatomic changes, or malignancies. Typical diagnostics include physical exam and history, vision or hearing examinations, imaging procedures, and laboratory testing.

The sensory system changes with age. Infants and children are most at risk for infections and anatomic abnormalities. Older adults are at risk for some infections, but loss of function is more common. Older adults experience cataracts, loss of vision, and loss of hearing due to aging known as presbycusis.

SCENARIO WRAP-UP

Rosie and Dr. Walden have had a busy day. Rosie reflects on her day and just has to smile. She is glad she has been working on CEUs to maintain her certification. She feels it is important to stay current with changing practices. She also is glad that her current CEU was a review of eye and ear anatomy. It is good to look back and remember details that you learned in school. She does not work in a specialty clinic, so she needs to remind herself of the anatomy terms that she may not use every day. Striving to be the best for the patients is Rosie's motivation for staying current.

14

Endocrine System

LEARNING OBJECTIVES

1. Discuss the anatomy of the endocrine system, list the major organs for the endocrine system, and identify the anatomic location of major endocrine system organs.
2. Describe the normal function and physiology of the endocrine system.
3. Complete the following related to the endocrine system diseases and disorders:
   - Identify the common etiology, signs and symptoms, and diagnostic measures of endocrine diseases.
   - Identify CLIA-waived tests associated with common endocrine diseases.
   - Describe treatment modalities used for endocrine diseases.
4. Compare the structure and function of the endocrine system across the life span.

CHAPTER OUTLINE

1. Opening Scenario, 324
2. You Will Learn, 324
3. Introduction to the Endocrine System, 325
4. Anatomy of the Endocrine System, 325
    a. Pituitary Gland, 325
    b. Thyroid Gland, 326
    c. Parathyroid Glands, 327
    d. Adrenal Glands, 327
    e. Pancreas, 328
    f. Thymus Gland, 328
    g. Gonads, Ovaries, and Testes, 329
    h. Pineal Gland, 329
5. Physiology of the Endocrine System, 329
    a. Mechanisms of Hormone Regulation, 329
    b. Target Cells, 329
    c. Hormone Action, 329
        i. Nonsteroid Hormones, 329
        ii. Steroid Hormones, 329
    d. Prostaglandins, 329
6. Diseases and Disorders of the Endocrine System, 330
    a. Pituitary Gland Diseases, 330
        i. *Diabetes Insipidus, 330*
    b. Thyroid Gland Diseases, 332
        i. *Hyperthyroidism, 332*
        ii. *Hypothyroidism, 333*
    c. Adrenal Gland Diseases, 333
        i. *Addison Disease, 335*
        ii. *Cushing Disease, 335*
    d. Pancreatic Diseases, 336
        i. *Diabetes Mellitus: Type 1 and Type 2, 337*
        ii. *Gestational Diabetes, 337*
7. Life Span Changes, 339
8. Closing Comments, 339
9. Chapter Review, 340
10. Scenario Wrap-Up, 341

OPENING SCENARIO

Lexie England, a certified medical assistant (CMA) through the American Association of Medical Assistants (AAMA), has worked at the Walden-Martin Family Medicine (WMFM) Clinic for just over 14 years. She has gotten a lot of experience with different people, providers, and disease conditions. Lexie has noticed that the number of patients at the clinic with type 2 diabetes has grown steadily over the years. She has seen patients do well and be compliant, and she has seen the complications for patients who have not been compliant.

Lexie is excited because one of the local endocrinologists, Dr. Samir Afrose, is going to be at the clinic for the afternoon. Dr. Afrose and Dr. Perez have several type 2 diabetes patients who will be in for joint consultation appointments. Then after clinic hours, the staff and Drs. Afrose and Perez are going to have a discussion on type 2 diabetes and patient adherence to treatment plans. It is going to be a full day.

YOU WILL LEARN

1. To recognize and use terms related to the endocrine system.
2. To locate the endocrine system structures.
3. To understand and describe the functions of the endocrine system; the goal of the endocrine system is hormone regulation that in turn maintains homeostasis.
4. To recognize disease states of the endocrine system, as well as their causes, signs and symptoms, diagnostic processes, treatment, prognoses, and prevention.

CHAPTER 14 Endocrine System

INTRODUCTION TO THE ENDOCRINE SYSTEM

The *endocrine* (EN duh krin) *system* is composed of ductless glands that secrete chemical messengers, called *hormones* (HAWR mohn s), directly into the bloodstream. Hormones travel through the body transferring information from one group of cells to another. Through this chemical message system, hormones regulate many body functions, including the following:
- Metabolism and growth
- Mood
- Sexual maturity and reproduction
- Water and **electrolyte** (ih LEK truh lahyt) balance

Hormone levels vary and can be affected by outside factors, such as illness and stress. See Fig. 14.1 for an illustration showing endocrine gland locations. Box 14.1 briefly describes the specialty of endocrinology.

ANATOMY OF THE ENDOCRINE SYSTEM

The glands of the endocrine system are as follows:
- *Hypothalamus* (hahy puh THAL uh muh s)
- *Pituitary* (pih TOO ih tare ree) gland
- *Pineal* (PAHY nee uhl) gland
- *Thyroid* (THAHY roid) gland
- *Parathyroid* (par uh THAHY roid) glands
- *Thymus* (THAHY muh s)
- *Pancreas* (PAN kree uhs)
- *Adrenal* (uh DREEN l) glands
- *Reproductive* (ree pruh DUHK tiv) glands (i.e., the ovaries and the testes)

The *hypothalamus*, located in the middle of the brain, is the major connection between the nervous and endocrine systems (Box 14.2). The hypothalamus controls the action of the *pituitary gland*, a pea-sized gland located just below the hypothalamus. The pituitary often is called the "master gland" because it secretes hormones that regulate multiple endocrine glands.

Pituitary Gland

The pituitary gland, is a tiny gland that is called the master gland because it controls other endocrine glands (Box 14.3). It is composed of anterior and posterior lobes, each having their own functions and hormones. The anterior lobe regulates the functions of the thyroid, adrenals, and reproductive glands. The anterior lobe secretes hormones in response to stimulation by the hypothalamus. The hypothalamus secretes hormones that cause the anterior pituitary to release or to inhibit the release of specific hormones. The anterior lobe affects many other endocrine glands in the body (Fig. 14.2 and Table 14.1).

> **VOCABULARY**
> **electrolyte:** An inorganic compound, usually a salt. A major factor in controlling fluid balance within the body.

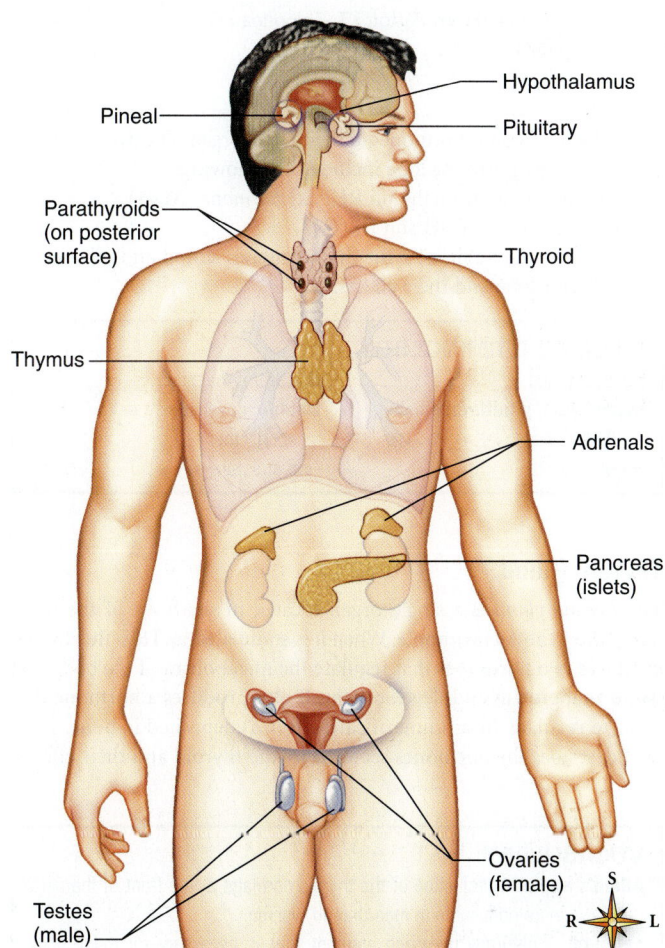

FIG. 14.1 Location of the endocrine glands. (From Patton KT, Thibodeau GA: *Anatomy and Physiology*, ed 9, St. Louis, 2016, Mosby.)

> **MEDICAL TERMINOLOGY**
> **-crine, crin/o:** to secrete
> **endo-:** within
> **-logy:** study of
> **hypo:** deficient, below, less than normal, under
> **pan:** all
> **para:** near, beside, abnormal, apart from

> **BOX 14.1 Specialty and Specialist**
> *Endocrinology* (en doh kruh NOL uh jee) is the healthcare specialty that studies the glands, hormones, and hormonal effects on the body. It also studies the diseases and disorders of the endocrine system. An *endocrinologist* (en doh kruh NOL uh jist) is a specialist involved in the diagnosis, treatment, and prevention of endocrine diseases and disorders.

> **BOX 14.2 Endocrine–Nervous System Connection**
> The nervous system and endocrine system perform similar functions in the body: communication and maintaining homeostasis. The nervous system communicates quickly through nerve impulses and delivers rapid response control to maintain homeostasis. The endocrine system communicates slowly through hormones and delivers longer-lasting control to maintain homeostasis. The body needs both types of communication and both types of control.

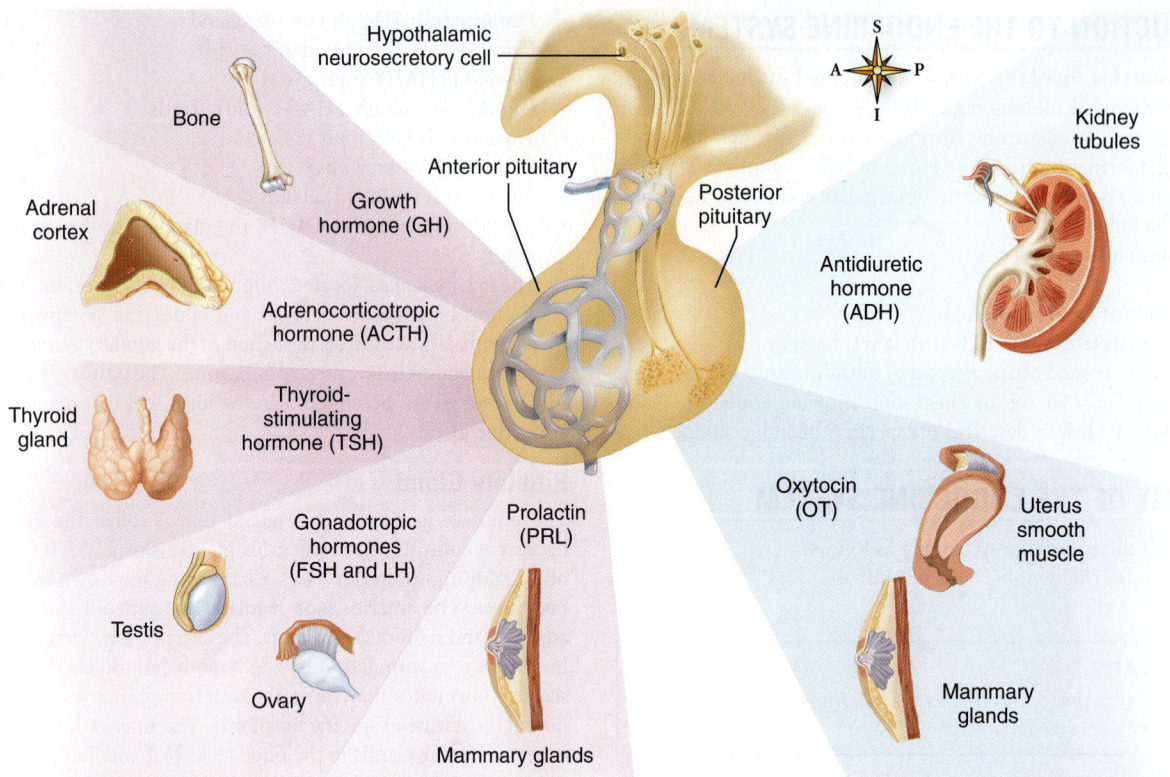

FIG. 14.2 Anterior and posterior pituitary hormones and the target organs. (From Patton KT, Thibodeau GA: *The Human Body in Health and Disease,* ed 6, St. Louis, 2014, Mosby.)

BOX 14.3 Pituitary Gland

The pituitary gland is also known as the *hypophysis* (hye POFF ih sis). The anterior pituitary is also known as the *adenohypophysis* (add uh noh hye POFF ih sis). The posterior pituitary is also known as the *neurohypophysis* (noo roh hahy POF uh sis).

STUDY TIP

- Luteinizing hormone (LH) is secreted in females and males. Some sources call LH in males *interstitial cell stimulating hormone (ICSH)*. They are the same hormones, just named differently for males.
- Growth hormone (GH) is also called human growth hormone (hGH) or somatotropin hormone (STH)—three names for the same hormone.

CRITICAL THINKING 14.1

What gland is referred to as the *master gland*? Why is it called that? Write down your answer, and be willing to share your thoughts with the class.

The posterior lobe of the pituitary gland is composed of nervous tissue. It does not produce hormones, but it stores hormones produced by the hypothalamus. The hormones are transported from the hypothalamus to the posterior lobe directly through the tissue connecting the organs. The posterior lobe stores the hormones until it gets a signal from the hypothalamus. Once the posterior lobe receives the signal, it releases the hormones from storage and into the blood supply. The blood then carries the hormones to their target organ. The two hormones released by the posterior lobe include the following:
- *Antidiuretic* (an tee dahy uh RET ik) *hormone* (ADH)
- *Oxytocin* (ok sih TOH suh n) (OT)

See Fig. 14.2 and Table 14.2 for the hormones stored and released by the posterior lobe and their effects.

MEDICAL TERMINOLOGY

aden/o: gland
hypophys/o, pituitar/o: pituitary gland
lob/o: lobe
thalam/o: thalamus
troph/o: development or nourishment
-us: structure

Thyroid Gland

The *thyroid gland* is a single organ located in the front of the neck, right below the **Adam's apple**. When it is stimulated by TSH, the thyroid produces two hormones that regulate the metabolism of the body and its normal growth and development. It also produces a hormone that helps to regulate the amount of **calcium** (Ca) deposited in bone. Table 14.3 describes the hormones secreted by the thyroid and their effects.

VOCABULARY

Adam's apple: A projection of the thyroid cartilage at the front of the neck that is more noticeable in men than in women.
calcium: A naturally occurring element that is necessary for many body functions, including strong bones and teeth, proper blood clotting, nerve conduction, and muscle contractions.

TABLE 14.1 Anterior Pituitary Hormones and Their Effects

Anterior Pituitary Hormone	Effect
adrenocorticotropic hormone (ACTH) (uh DREE noh kawr ti koh TROP ik)	Stimulates the adrenal cortex to release steroids (e.g., cortisol).
follicle-stimulating hormone (FSH)	*Females:* Stimulates the development of ova up to maturity (ovulation) and stimulates maturing ova to secrete estrogen. *Males:* Stimulates the seminiferous tubules to grow and form sperm.
growth hormone (GH)	Stimulates growth of long bones and skeletal muscle. Converts proteins to glucose, increasing blood glucose levels.
luteinizing hormone (LH) (LOO tee nahyz ing)	*Females:* Stimulates ova to mature, stimulates ovulation, stimulates the secretion of estrogen, and stimulates the development of the corpus luteum and the production of progesterone. *Males:* Stimulates interstitial cells in the testes to develop and secrete testosterone
prolactin (PRL) (proh LAK tin)	Stimulates breast development during pregnancy and milk production after delivery.
thyroid-stimulating hormone (TSH)	Stimulates the thyroid to release T3 and T4. (See the section on the thyroid in this chapter for more information.)

From Shiland B: *Mastering Healthcare Terminology*, ed 5, St. Louis, 2016, Elsevier.

TABLE 14.2 Posterior Pituitary Hormones and Their Effects

Posterior Pituitary Hormone	Effect
antidiuretic hormone (ADH) (also called vasopressin)	Stimulates the kidneys to reabsorb water and return it to circulation. It is also a vasoconstrictor, which increases the blood pressure.
oxytocin (OT)	Stimulates the uterine muscles to contract during delivery. Also stimulates the muscles surrounding the mammary ducts to contract, releasing milk.

From Shiland B: *Mastering Healthcare Terminology*, ed 5, St. Louis, 2016, Elsevier.

TABLE 14.3 Thyroid Gland Hormones and Their Effects

Thyroid Gland Hormone	Effect
calcitonin (kal sih TOH nin)	Promotes the retention of calcium in the bones and lowers blood calcium levels. (Works against parathyroid hormone.)
thyroxine (T_4) (thahy ROK seen) (also called Tetraiodothyronine)	Increases cell metabolism.
triiodothyronine (T_3) (trahy ahy oh doh THAHY ruh neen)	Increases cell metabolism.

From Shiland B: *Mastering Healthcare Terminology*, ed 5, St. Louis, 2016, Elsevier.

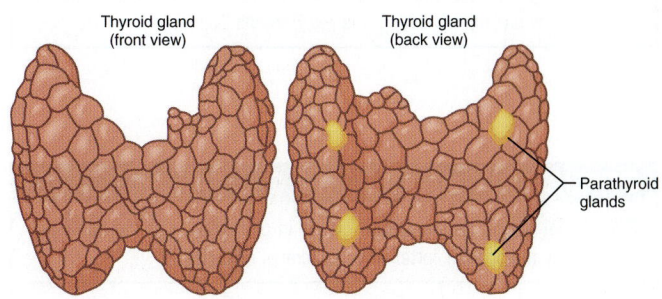

FIG. 14.3 Parathyroid gland.

Parathyroid Glands

The *parathyroid glands* are four small glands located on the back surface of the thyroid gland (Fig. 14.3). They secrete *parathyroid hormone* (PTH) in response to low levels of calcium in the blood. When low calcium is detected, PTH increases blood calcium by releasing calcium from bone. The kidneys and the digestive system also reabsorb calcium. PTH is inhibited by high blood calcium levels. PTH increases blood calcium when needed.

Adrenal Glands

On top of each kidney are the adrenal glands, which are triangular glands consisting of an outer layer, called the *adrenal cortex* (uh DREE nul KORE tecks), and an inner body, called the *adrenal medulla* (uh DREE nul muh DOO lah). The adrenal cortex secretes hormones that influence a wide range of bodily functions (Table 14.4). The adrenal medulla produces hormones that activate the body's reaction to stress (Table 14.5).

> **MEDICAL TERMINOLOGY**
> **calc/o:** calcium
> **parathyroid/o:** parathyroid gland
> **thyr/o, thyroid/o:** thyroid gland

TABLE 14.4 Adrenal Cortex Hormones and Their Effects

Adrenal Cortex Hormones	Effect
glucocorticoids (e.g., cortisol, cortisone) (gloo koh KAWR ti koid)	Respond to stress. Regulate carbohydrate, protein, and fat metabolism. Increase blood glucose levels; have anti-inflammatory properties.
mineralocorticoids (e.g., aldosterone) (min er uh loh KAWR ti koid)	Promote sodium retention in the kidneys. Regulate blood volume, blood pressure, and electrolytes.
sex hormones (e.g., androgen)	Stimulate the growth of pubic and axillary hair in boys and girls.

From Shiland B: *Mastering Healthcare Terminology*, ed 5, St. Louis, 2016, Elsevier.

TABLE 14.5 Adrenal Medulla Hormones and Their Effects

Adrenal Medulla Hormones	Effect
epinephrine (also called adrenaline)	Sustains the flight-or-fight response to stress in the body. Acts as a neurotransmitter in the nervous system. Increases blood pressure and heart rate. Dilates the bronchioles. Increases blood glucose levels.
norepinephrine (also called noradrenaline)	Sustains the flight-or-fight response to stress in the body. Acts as a neurotransmitter in the nervous system.

From Shiland B: *Mastering Healthcare Terminology*, ed 5, St. Louis, 2016, Elsevier.

> **STUDY TIP**
>
> The adrenal glands, are also called the suprarenal (soo pruh REEN l) glands. *Supra-* means on "top or above," and *ren/o* means "kidney."

> **CRITICAL THINKING 14.2**
>
> The adrenal glands are really two glands in one organ. List the hormones produced by the adrenal cortex and the adrenal medulla.

> **VOCABULARY**
>
> **exocrine:** A glandular secretion released through a duct.
> **fatty acids:** Result when fats are broken down; used by the body for energy and tissue development.
> **ketones:** This class of organic compounds is a by-product of fatty acid metabolism. An example of a ketone is acetone.
> **mediastinum:** The space in the thoracic cavity that lies between the lungs, containing the heart, trachea, and esophagus.
> **stem cells:** Undifferentiated cells that can become specialized cells in the body.
> **T cells:** T cells are formed from stem cells in bone marrow and then migrate to the thymus where they mature and learn their role in the immune system. They are effective against intracellular pathogens.

> **MEDICAL TERMINOLOGY**
>
> **adren/o:** adrenal gland
> **-al:** pertaining to
> **cortic/o:** cortex
> **-crine:** to secrete
> **exo-:** outward
> **gluc/o, glyc/o:** glucose, sugar
> **ket/o, keton/o:** ketone
> **medull/o:** medulla
> **-oma:** tumor, mass
> **pancreat/o:** pancreas
> **ren/o:** kidney
> **supra-:** above
> **thym/o:** thymus gland

Pancreas

The *pancreas* is located inferior and posterior to the stomach in the abdomen. It is a gland with both exocrine (EK suh krin) and endocrine functions. The exocrine function is to release digestive enzymes through a duct into the small intestines. The endocrine function is to release hormones into the bloodstream. Hormones are produced in special cells called *islets of Langerhans* (EYE lets of LANG gur hahnz). The pancreas contains two types of islets of Langerhans cells: alpha and beta cells. The hormones, glucagon (gloo kuh gon) and insulin (IN suh lin), are produced in the islet cells.

The function of glucagon and insulin is to regulate the level of glucose in the blood. Glucagon is produced in alpha islets of Langerhans cells. Glucagon stimulates the liver to make glucose by:
- Converting the stored glycogen to glucose
- Breaking down fatty acids and amino acids into glucose

The glucose is released into the blood, increasing the blood glucose level. Insulin is produced in beta islets of Langerhans cells. Insulin decreases blood glucose when levels are high. Insulin is needed to transport glucose out of the bloodstream and into cells. Glucose is used for energy inside the cells. In the absence of glucose in the cells, proteins and fats are broken down, causing excessive fatty acids and ketones in the blood. Normally, these hormones regulate glucose levels through the metabolism of fats, carbohydrates, and proteins.

> **CRITICAL THINKING 14.3**
>
> The pancreas is involved in the digestive system (it releases enzymes into the small intestine; see Chapter 5 to review) and in the endocrine system (it secretes insulin and glucagon). Which substances are released into ducts? Which substances are released directly into the blood? Define *endocrine* and *exocrine* in your own words.

Thymus Gland

The *thymus gland* is in the mediastinum (mee dee a STAHY nuh m) above the heart. It releases a hormone called *thymosin* (THAHY moh sin). This hormone stimulates the production of T cells in the bone marrow from stem cells. Thymosin also helps T cells mature and become active in the immune system. See Chapter 9 for more details.

> **CRITICAL THINKING 14.4**
> What is the function of the thymus gland?

Gonads, Ovaries, and Testes

The **gonads** produce sex hormones. The male gonads are the *testes* (TES teez). They secrete *testosterone* (tes TOS tuh rohn), which does the following:
- Regulates the development of male secondary sexual characteristics (e.g., voice changes, growth of facial and pubic hair)
- Promotes the production of sperm

The female gonads are the *ovaries* (OH vuh REEs).

They produce eggs (ova) and secrete the hormones estrogen and progesterone which include the following functions:
- Regulate the development of female secondary sex characteristics
- Regulate menstruation
- Maintain a pregnancy

> **VOCABULARY**
> **gonads:** Organs that produce sex cells in both males and females.

> **MEDICAL TERMINOLOGY**
> **gonad/o:** gonads

Pineal Gland

The *pineal* (PIN ee uhl) *gland* is located deep within the brain and secretes the hormone *melatonin* (mel uh TOH nin). Melatonin helps regulate waking and sleeping patterns and may affect seasonal reactions to the availability of sunlight.

> **CRITICAL THINKING 14.5**
> What is the function of melatonin in the body?

PHYSIOLOGY OF THE ENDOCRINE SYSTEM

Mechanisms of Hormone Regulation

The goal of hormone regulation is to maintain **homeostasis** (hoh mee uh STEY sis). A few **mechanisms** regulate hormone secretion, including the following:
- Nervous stimulation
- Endocrine control
- Feedback systems

An example of *nervous system regulation* of the endocrine function is the release of adrenaline from the adrenal medulla in response to stimulation from the sympathetic nervous system during a stressful event.

An example of *endocrine control regulation* of the endocrine function is when a hormone from one gland (TSH from the anterior pituitary) stimulates the release of a hormone from another gland (the thyroid secretes T_3 and T_4 in response.)

An example of *feedback system regulation* of the endocrine function is when an imbalance activates an endocrine gland and then acts to correct the imbalance by stopping the hormone secretion process. The most common feedback system is a **negative feedback** system. For example, a negative feedback system using the parathyroid gland is as follows:

> **BOX 14.4 Why Is It Important to Know How Hormones Work?**
>
> Knowing the differences between steroid and nonsteroid hormones and how they work is important. Endocrine disorders are often complex and difficult to treat. Knowing how the messengers in the system function will help scientists discover ways to possibly treat the system when it does not work.

- If the calcium blood level falls below normal, the parathyroid glands are stimulated to release PTH.
- PTH increases blood calcium levels by stimulating the absorption of calcium from the intestines or by chemically breaking down bone to release stored calcium into the blood.
- The change in the blood calcium level is detected by the parathyroid gland, which then stops production of PTH.

Target Cells

Each hormone released into the bloodstream has specific *target cells* for action. The target cells have **receptors** (rih SEP ter s) that attract only certain hormones. The cell membrane only lets selected hormones pass into the cell and affect cellular action.

Hormone Action

There are two categories of hormones, nonsteroid hormones and steroid hormones. All hormones are messengers, but how they deliver their message is where they differ (Box 14.4). Both hormone categories work to maintain body homeostasis.

Nonsteroid Hormones. *Nonsteroid hormones* are made up of protein or amino acids. They are chemical messengers that work in the following way:
- Nonsteroid hormone attaches to a target cell membrane.
- Another molecule takes the message from the nonsteroid hormone and carries it to the target cell **nucleus** (NOO klee uh s) or **organelle** (awr guh NEL).
- The target cell nucleus or organelle then puts the message into action in the cell.

Steroid Hormones. *Steroid hormones* are small *lipid-soluble* (fat-soluble) molecules. They are also chemical messengers that bring information to target cells:
- Steroid hormones attach to a target cell membrane and then pass directly into the target cell.
- Once inside the target cell, steroid hormones travel directly to the nucleus of the cell.
- They enter the nucleus and bind to a receptor site, which creates a hormone-receptor site complex.
- The complex communicates its message with DNA in the nucleus.
- DNA then tells the cell how to put the hormone's message into action.

Prostaglandins

Prostaglandins (pros tuh GLAN din s) (PGs), also known as tissue hormones, are substances found in many body tissues. PGs are produced in tissues and **diffuse** (dih FYOOZ) only a short distance to affect cells in their local area. They help regulate processes such as respiration, blood pressure, digestive system secretions, and reproductive functions. They are powerful molecules that are made locally and act locally.

BOX 14.5 Common Signs and Symptoms of Endocrine System Diseases and Disorders

Common signs and symptoms of endocrine system diseases and disorders include the following:
- Fatigue, muscle weakness or stiffness
- Joint pain, swelling, or inflammation
- Changes in food or water consumption
- Weight gain or weight loss without trying to adjust weight
- Nervousness, irritability, anxiety, change in sleep patterns, depression, mood changes
- Changes in skin, hair, or nails
- Changes in blood pressure, heart rate, or respirations

VOCABULARY

diffuse: To spread, scatter, disperse, or move.
homeostasis: The internal environment of the body that is compatible with life. A steady state that is created by all the body systems working together to provide a consistent and unvarying internal environment.
mechanism: A sequence of steps that allow something to be produced or a purpose to be accomplished.
negative feedback: An output or response that affects the input of a system.
nucleus: A specialized portion of a cell that is encased in a membrane and directs growth, metabolism, and reproduction of the cell.
organelle: A structure within a cell that performs a specific function.
receptors: Structures or sites on or in a cell that bind with substances such as hormones, antigens, or drugs.

CRITICAL THINKING 14.6

In your own words define the term *prostaglandin*. Write out the answer, and be willing to share your thoughts with the class.

TABLE 14.6 Terms Related to Laboratory Tests

Term	Definition
A1c	Measure of average blood glucose during a 3-month time span. Used to monitor response to diabetes treatment. Also called *glycosylated hemoglobin* or *HbA1c*. Some CLIA-waived tests available.
fasting blood glucose (FBG)	The amount of glucose present is used to measure the body's ability to break down and use glucose; 100 to 125 mg/dL = prediabetes; more than 126 mg/dL = diabetes. Some CLIA-waived tests available.
glucometer (gloo KAH muh tur)	An instrument for measurement of blood sugar. Some CLIA-waived tests available.
hormone tests	Measure the amount of ADH, cortisol, GH, or PTH in the blood.
oral glucose tolerance test (OGTT)	Blood test to measure the body's response to a concentrated glucose solution. Values used to consider normal may vary by laboratory. Generally, 140 mg/dL or lower is normal. May be used to diagnose DM or gestational diabetes.
radioimmunoassay (RIA) studies (ray dee oh ih myoo noh AHS say)	Nuclear medicine tests used to tag and detect hormones in the blood.
thyroid function tests (TFTs)	Blood tests done to assess T_3, T_4, and calcitonin. May be used to evaluate abnormalities of thyroid function. Some CLIA-waived tests available.
total calcium	Measures the amount of calcium in the blood. Results may be used to assess parathyroid function, calcium metabolism, or cancerous conditions.
urinalysis (UA) (yoor in AL ih sis)	Physical, chemical, and microscopic examination of urine. Some CLIA-waived tests available.
urine glucose	Used as a screen for or to monitor DM; a urine specimen is tested for the presence of glucose. Some CLIA-waived tests available.
urine ketones (KEE tones)	Test to detect presence of ketones in a urine specimen; may indicate DM or hyperthyroidism. Some CLIA-waived tests available.

From Shiland B: *Mastering Healthcare Terminology*, ed 5, St. Louis, 2016, Elsevier.

DISEASES AND DISORDERS OF THE ENDOCRINE SYSTEM

Faulty secretion of any hormone, whether too much or too little, can cause health problems for patients. The goal of treatment is either to control the hypersecretion of hormones or to replace hormones that are not being secreted at therapeutic levels. See Box 14.5 for common signs and symptoms of endocrine diseases and disorders. Tables 14.6 to 14.8 refer to common diagnostic testing and therapeutic interventions for the endocrine system diseases and disorders.

Most of the pathology of the endocrine system is the result of either *hyper-* (too much) or *hypo-* (too little) hormonal secretion. Developmental issues also play a role in determining when the malfunction occurs and what the results will be. See Table 14.9 for terminology related to signs and symptoms of endocrine system disorders.

Pituitary Gland Diseases

Many hormones are secreted by the anterior and posterior pituitary glands. Table 14.10 describes pituitary gland disorders. *Diabetes insipidus* (dye ah BEE teez in SIP ih dus) is discussed in more detail in the next section.

Diabetes Insipidus. Diabetes insipidus (DI) (dye ah BEE teez in SIP ih dus) is a rare condition that occurs when the hypothalamus and/or posterior pituitary do not produce or release adequate amounts of antidiuretic hormone (ADH), also known as vasopressin.

Etiology. A tumor, trauma, pituitary surgery, or a lack of blood supply to the pituitary gland can cause a lack of ADH. Diabetes insipidus can also occur if there is an inadequate response to ADH in the renal tubules in the nephrons. This can be caused by kidney disease or the side effects of certain medications. Diabetes insipidus can be genetic and is more common in males.

Signs and symptoms. Diabetes insipidus usually has an acute onset and is potentially fatal if not treated. The patient presents with a variety of signs and symptoms:

CHAPTER 14 Endocrine System

TABLE 14.7 Terms Related to Imaging

Term	Definition
computed tomography (CT) scan	May be used to test for bone density in hypoparathyroidism and the size of the adrenal glands in Addison's disease.
magnetic resonance imaging (MRI)	May be used to examine changes in the size of soft tissues (for example, the pituitary, pancreas, or hypothalamus).
radioactive iodine uptake (RAIU) scan	May be used to test thyroid function by measuring the gland's ability to concentrate and retain iodine. Useful to test for hyperthyroidism.
radiography	X-rays are done to examine suspected endocrine changes that affect the density or thickness of bone; also, may reveal underlying causes of an endocrine disorder.
ultrasound (US) (also called sonography)	Used to visualize the pancreas, guide biopsies of the thyroid gland, and discern solid and fluid-filled cysts.

From Shiland B: *Mastering Healthcare Terminology*, ed 5, St. Louis, 2016, Elsevier.

TABLE 14.8 Terms Related to Excisions

Term	Definition
adrenalectomy (uh dree nuh LECK tuh mee)	Bilateral removal of the adrenal glands to reduce excess hormone secretion.
hypophysectomy (hye poff uh SECK tuh mee)	Excision of the pituitary gland; usually done to remove a pituitary tumor.
pancreatectomy (pan kree uh TECK tuh mee)	Excision of all or part of the pancreas to remove a tumor or to treat an intractable inflammation of the pancreas.
pancreatoduodenectomy (pan kree ah toh doo ah den ECK tuh mee)	Excision of the head of the pancreas together with the duodenum; used to treat pancreatic cancer. Also called *Whipple procedure.*
parathyroidectomy (pair uh thigh roy DECK tuh mee)	Removal of the parathyroid gland, usually to treat hyperparathyroidism.
thyroidectomy (thahy roi DEK tuh mee)	Partial or total removal of the thyroid gland to treat hyperthyroidism that does not respond to medication. A partial thyroidectomy results in a regrowth of the gland with normal function. If cancer is detected, a total thyroidectomy is performed.

From Shiland B: *Mastering Healthcare Terminology*, ed 5, St. Louis, 2016, Elsevier.

- Polydipsia, polyuria, nocturia (frequent urination at night), and very dilute urine
- Trouble sleeping, fussiness, irritability
- Fever, vomiting, diarrhea, hypotension (low blood pressure)
- Delayed growth and weight loss in children

TABLE 14.9 Terms Related to Signs and Symptoms of Endocrine Disorders

Term	Definition
exophthalmia (eck soff THAL mee ah)	Protrusion of eyeballs from their orbits.
glucosuria (gloo koh SOOR ee ah)	Presence of glucose in the urine. May indicate diabetes mellitus (DM). Also called *glycosuria.*
goiter (GOY tur)	Enlargement of the thyroid gland, not due to a tumor.
hypocalcemia (hye poh kal SEE mee ah)	Condition of deficient calcium (Ca) in the blood. The opposite is *hypercalcemia*—excessive calcium in the blood.
hypoglycemia (hye poh gly SEE mee ah)	Condition of deficient sugar in the blood. The opposite is *hyperglycemia*—excessive sugar in the blood.
hypokalemia (hye poh kuh LEE mee ah)	Condition of deficient potassium (K) in the blood. The opposite is *hyperkalemia*—excessive potassium in the blood.
hyponatremia (hye poh nuh TREE mee ah)	Condition of deficient sodium (Na) in the blood. The opposite is *hypernatremia*—excessive sodium in the blood.
ketoacidosis (kee toh ass ih DOH sis)	Excessive number of ketone acids in the bloodstream.
ketonuria (kee toh NOOR ee ah)	Presence of ketones in urine.
paresthesia (pair uh STHEE zsa)	Abnormal sensation, such as prickling.
polydipsia (pah lee DIP see ah)	Condition of excessive thirst.
polyphagia (pah lee FAY jee ah)	Condition of excessive appetite.
polyuria (pah lee YOO ree ah)	Condition of excessive urination.
tetany (TET uh nee)	Continuous muscle spasms.

From Shiland B: *Mastering Healthcare Terminology*, ed 5, St. Louis, 2016, Elsevier.

- Complications may occur such as hypernatremia (high blood sodium levels), severe dehydration, electrolyte imbalance, and low blood pressure. DI can be fatal if not adequately treated.

Diagnostic procedures. Diagnostic tests may include the following:
- Urinalysis and blood tests (e.g., electrolytes [sodium]).
- Water deprivation test: water is withheld for a period of time and the patient's weight, urine output, and urine concentration are monitored.
- Imaging tests: MRI to scan for pituitary abnormalities.

Treatment. Treatment depends on the cause. The patient may need to take an ADH synthetic hormone medication (desmopressin). If the kidneys are not responding to the ADH, the patient may need to take a diuretic. The diuretic helps the body excrete water and sodium. Prognosis.

Prognosis. Patients responding to the treatments do well. It is important to take the medication and prevent dehydration. It is important to wear a medic alert bracelet or necklace and carry a wallet medic alert card.

Prevention. There is no way to prevent diabetes insipidus.

> **CRITICAL THINKING 14.7**
>
> Is diabetes insipidus a disease that is associated with the hormones of the pancreas? What hormone is involved in diabetes insipidus? Does it affect blood sugar? Write out a brief description of diabetes insipidus in your own words. Share your thoughts with the class.

Thyroid Gland Diseases

The thyroid gland is responsible for setting and maintaining the body's metabolism. Thyroid diseases cause hypersecretion or hyposecretion of thyroid hormone. Initially, some diseases may cause hypersecretion, but later stages of the disease may cause hyposecretion of thyroid hormone. Table 14.11 describes thyroid diseases. Hyperthyroidism and hypothyroidism are described in depth in the following sections.

Hyperthyroidism. When too much thyroid hormone is produced, *hyperthyroidism* occurs.

Etiology. The most common cause of hyperthyroidism is an autoimmune disorder called Graves disease. Thyroid nodules, pituitary disorders and tumors, and thyroiditis are also causes of hyperthyroidism (Table 14.11).

Risk factors include a family history of thyroid disorders and having an existing autoimmune disease. Hyperthyroidism is more common in women.

Signs and symptoms. Common signs and symptoms of hyperthyroidism include the following:
- Fatigue, muscle weakness
- Weight loss, even with adequate food intake and an increased appetite
- Difficulty sleeping, restlessness, irritability, nervousness, anxiety
- Rapid heart rate, irregular heart rate, pounding heart in chest (palpitations)
- More frequent bowel movements
- Sensitivity to heat, increased sweating
- *Exophthalmia*, which is red, swollen, protruding eyes
- Changes in menstrual cycle
- *Thyrotoxicosis* (thahy roh tok si KOH sis) or thyroid storm, a life-threatening condition that causes fever, and increased pulse, respiration, and blood pressure. A medical emergency.

TABLE 14.10 Pituitary Gland Disorders

Gland	Hormone	Condition	Definition
Anterior pituitary	Growth hormone, hypersecretion		Occurs after normal growth has finished (e.g., during adulthood). Leads to an enlargement of the extremities (hands and feet), jaw, nose, and forehead (Fig. 14.4). Also causes an excessive overgrowth of soft tissue. Usually caused by an adenoma of the pituitary gland. Treatment includes surgery and radiation to reduce the size of the pituitary gland.
		gigantism (jye GAN tiz um)	Occurs during childhood, leading to excessive growth (Fig. 14.5). Treatment includes surgery and radiation to reduce the size of the pituitary gland.
	Growth hormone, hyposecretion	*dwarfism*	Occurs during childhood, leading to smaller than normal body frame size (Fig. 14.6). Treated with injections of growth hormone during childhood.
	Prolactin, hypersecretion	*prolactinoma* (pro lack tih NOH mah)	Most common type of pituitary tumor. Women: Causes abnormal lactation and impacts the menstrual cycle. Men: Causes impotence.
	Prolactin, hyposecretion		Women: Unable to maintain breast milk production.
	All hormones, hyposecretion	*panhypopituitarism* (pan hye poh pih TOO ih tur iz um)	Destruction of or deficiency of the entire anterior lobe. Most common in women. Causes hypotension, weight loss, weakness, and loss of libido.

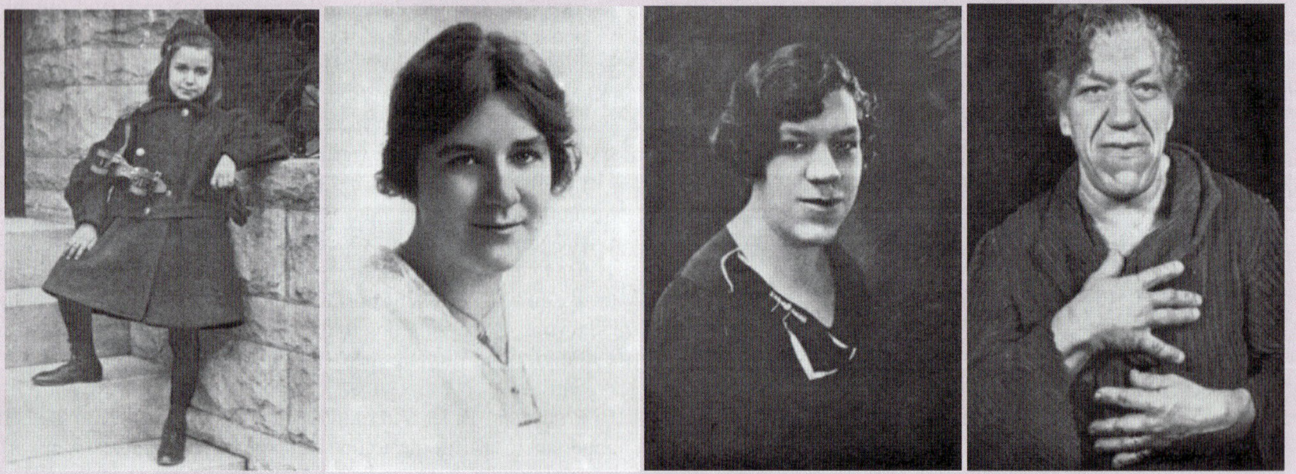

FIG. 14.4 Acromegaly. (From Ignatavicius DD, Workman ML: *Medical-Surgical Nursing: Critical Thinking for Collaborative Care*, ed 6, Philadelphia, 2011, Saunders.)

TABLE 14.10 Pituitary Gland Disorders—cont'd

Gland	Hormone	Condition	Definition
Posterior pituitary	Antidiuretic hormone (ADH), hypersecretion	*syndrome of inappropriate antidiuretic hormone (SIADH)*	Causes inability to produce and secrete dilute urine. Water retention, hyponatremia, and weight gain are seen.
	Antidiuretic hormone (ADH), hyposecretion	*Diabetes Insipidus*	Causes the patient to excrete large quantities of diluted urine.

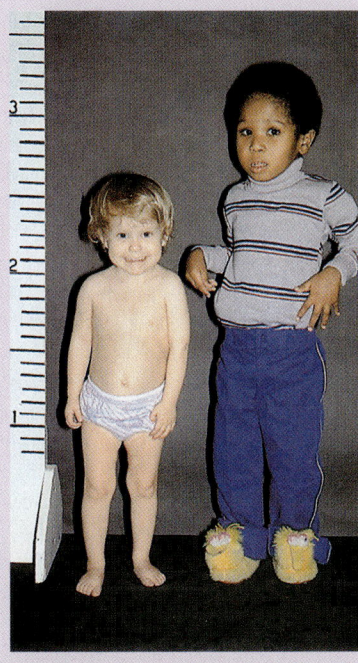

FIG. 14.6 The normal 3½-year-old boy is in the 50th percentile for height. The short 3-year-old girl exhibits the characteristic "kewpie doll" appearance, suggesting a diagnosis of growth hormone deficiency (GHD). (From Zitelli BJ, Davis HW: *Atlas of Pediatric Physical Diagnosis*, ed 5, St. Louis, 2007, Mosby.)

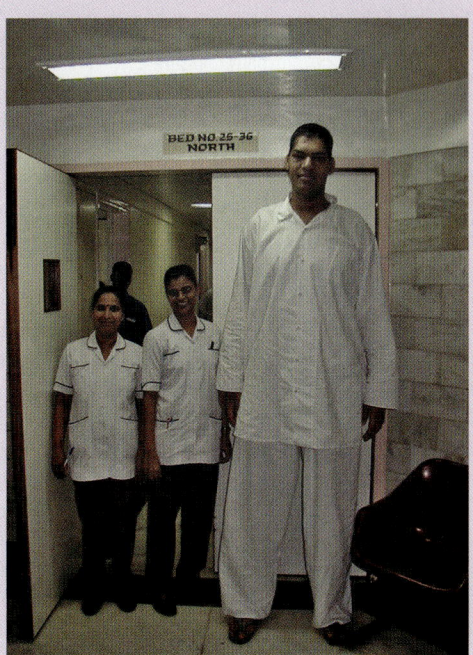

FIG. 14.5 Gigantism. (From Sainani GS, Joshi VR, Sainani RG: *Manual of Clinical & Practical Medicine*, New Delhi, 2010, Elsevier India.)

Diagnostic procedures. The provider will obtain a medical history and perform a physical. Thyroid function tests and a radioactive iodine uptake (RAIU) scan may be ordered.

Treatment. Treatment for hyperthyroidism includes radioactive iodine therapy to shrink the thyroid. Antithyroid medications, such as methimazole (Tapazole), may be ordered. The patient may also have a thyroidectomy.

Prognosis. Typically, treatment interventions help to achieve a normal thyroid hormone level in the body. Lifelong follow-up may be recommended.

Prevention. There is no way to prevent hyperthyroidism.

Hypothyroidism. When too little thyroid hormone is produced, *hypothyroidism* occurs.

Etiology. Hypothyroidism can occur after thyroidectomy and radiation therapy. Table 14.11 describes additional conditions that cause hypothyroidism. Risk factors for hypothyroidism include the following:
- Having an existing autoimmune disease
- Being a woman older than 60 years
- Having a family history of hypothyroidism
- Having been pregnant or delivered a baby within the previous 6 months

Signs and symptoms. With hypothyroidism, the metabolism slows down, resulting in the following signs and symptoms:
- Fatigue, muscle weakness, tenderness, aches, stiffness
- Constipation, weight gain
- Dry skin, sensitivity to cold, thinning hair
- Slowed heart rate, hoarseness, depression
- Elevated blood cholesterol

Diagnostic procedures. The provider will obtain a medical history and perform a physical. Thyroid function tests and a thyroid ultrasound scan may be ordered.

Treatment. The patient needs to take lifelong daily synthetic thyroid hormone (e.g., levothyroxine [Levothroid, Synthroid]).

Prognosis. Typically, treatment interventions help to achieve a normal thyroid hormone level in the body. Lifelong follow-up is required.

Prevention. There is no way to prevent hypothyroidism.

Adrenal Gland Diseases

Adrenal gland diseases are described in Table 14.12. The most common diseases are Addison's disease and Cushing's disease. These are described in more detail in the coming sections.

TABLE 14.11 Conditions That Cause Hyperthyroidism and Hypothyroidism

Condition	Thyroid Function	Description
Simple goiter (GOY ter)	Hyperthyroidism or hypothyroidism	Simple enlargement of the thyroid gland, causing swelling in the neck (Fig. 14.7). Usually not malignant. Can be caused from iodine deficiency, immune disorders, infections, medications, and other thyroid conditions. More common in people over 40, women, and those with a family history of goiters. Depending on the symptoms, may be treated with potassium iodide or thyroid hormone.
Thyroid nodule	Hyperthyroidism or hypothyroidism	A growth in the thyroid gland. Can be benign or malignant. More common in women. Causes neck enlargement, pain, hoarseness, problems swallowing. Treatment may consist of monitoring, surgery, and thyroid hormone if hypothyroidism is occurring.
Thyroiditis (THY roi DIE tis)	Hyperthyroidism or hypothyroidism	Inflammation of the thyroid. Several types of thyroiditis. Can be an autoimmune condition or caused from a virus, bacteria, or medication. For several types, the patient may start with hyperthyroidism symptoms and then have hypothyroidism symptoms. Treatment depends on the symptoms and type.
Thyroid carcinoma	Hyperthyroidism or hypothyroidism	The most common types of thyroid carcinoma are follicular and papillary. Both have high 5-year survival rates. Women are three times more at risk for thyroid cancer. Causes a hard, painless lump in the thyroid gland. May cause hoarseness and enlargement of the neck. Treatment depends on the type of cancer; may include surgery, chemotherapy, radiation, and thyroid hormone.
Graves disease	Hyperthyroidism	Autoimmune disease that results in hypersecretion of the thyroid hormone. Most common cause of hyperthyroidism. Causes heat intolerance, heart palpitations, weight loss, and nervousness. Can cause Graves eye disease or Graves ophthalmopathy (e.g., bulging of the eyes [exophthalmia], double vision, light sensitivity, and irritation).
Cretinism (KREET n IZ ehm)	Hypothyroidism	Occurs during infancy and childhood. Leads to low metabolic rate, stunned growth and sexual development, and cognitive deficits. Treated with thyroid hormone.
Myxedema (MIK si DEE mah)	Hypothyroidism	Occurs during adolescence and adulthood. Symptoms include menorrhagia; dry, scaly skin with no perspiration. Weakness, fatigue, bloating, facial puffiness, cold intolerance, and cognition issues. Treated with thyroid hormone.
Hashimoto thyroiditis	Hypothyroidism	A chronic immune system disease that attacks the thyroid gland. Often occurs in middle-age females. Occurs slowly, leading to difficulty thinking, dry skin, goiter, fatigue, hair loss, cold intolerance, mild weight gain, and irregular periods. Treatment may include thyroid medication.

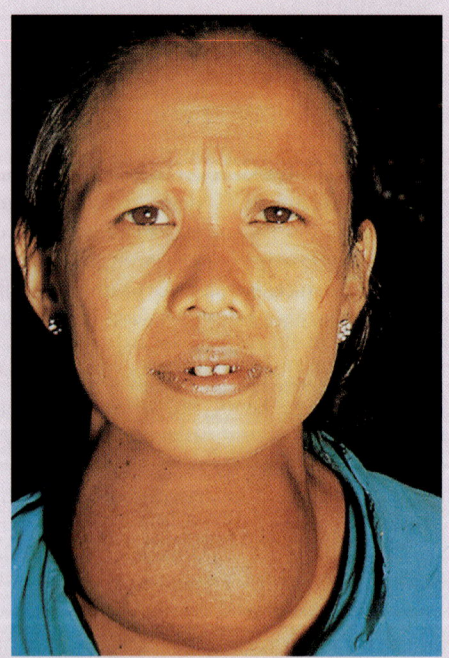

FIG. 14.7 Goiter. (From Thibodeau GA, Patton KT: *The Human Body in Health and Disease,* ed 5, St. Louis, 2010, Mosby.)

TABLE 14.12 Adrenal Gland Diseases

Gland	Hormone	Condition	Definition
Adrenal cortex	Cortisol, hypersecretion	Cushing disease	Malfunction of the cortex, leading to many symptoms, including weight gain, decrease healing of wounds, depression, and impaired growth.
	Cortisol, hyposecretion	Addison disease	Malfunction of the cortex, leading to many symptoms, including low back pain, low blood pressure, and electrolyte imbalance.
Adrenal medulla	Epinephrine and norepinephrine, hypersecretion	Pheochromocytoma (fee oh kroh mah sye TOH mah)	Usually benign tumor that causes headache, palpitation, sweating, hyperglycemia, flushing, nausea, vomiting, and syncope. Condition can lead to hypertension (high blood pressure), arrhythmias, and heart failure.

Addison Disease. *Addison* (ADD ih sun) disease is a malfunction of the adrenal cortex. Adrenal insufficiency (hyposecretion) of cortisol is called *Addison disease*.

Etiology. Addison disease is most frequently caused by an autoimmune reaction that damages the adrenal cortex, which secretes cortisol. Other causes include tuberculosis and disease or damage to the adrenal glands or the pituitary gland.

Addison disease can be acute or chronic. Acute Addison disease may be called *Addisonian crisis*, a condition marked by life-threatening symptoms. A crisis can be brought on by stressful situations, infections, minor illness, or surgery.

Signs and symptoms. Acute Addison disease may have the following signs and symptoms:
- Pain in the lower back, abdomen, or legs
- Severe vomiting and diarrhea, dehydration, and low blood pressure
- Loss of consciousness
- High blood potassium (*hyperkalemia*) and low blood sodium (*hyponatremia*)

Chronic Addison disease may have the following signs and symptoms:
- Irritability, extreme fatigue, weight loss, lack of appetite, craving for salt
- Darkening of the skin (*hyperpigmentation*) (Fig. 14.8)
- Hypotension, fainting, nausea, diarrhea, vomiting
- Low blood sugar (*hypoglycemia*)
- Muscle pain, depression, body hair loss

Diagnostic procedures. Addison disease can be difficult to diagnose and to determine the proper cause. Common diagnostic tests include the following:
- Blood tests: to measure cortisol levels, sodium, potassium, ACTH, and to detect antibodies associated with autoimmune Addison's disease.
- Adrenocorticotropic (ACTH) stimulation test: the blood cortisol level is measured. Then the patient is injected with synthetic ACTH and the blood cortisol level is measured again. If the adrenal gland is damaged, cortisol levels after ACTH stimulation will still be low or absent.
- Imaging tests: computed tomography (CT) scan or magnetic resonance imaging (MRI) scan.

Treatment. Addisonian crisis treatment requires immediate administration of an intravenous saline and dextrose solution with corticosteroids. Additional treatments for Addison disease include the following:
- Replacement of cortisol with the long-term daily administration of glucocorticoids (e.g., prednisone)
- Replacement of aldosterone with fludrocortisone
- Intake of an adequate amount of sodium and fluids to maintain normal blood pressure

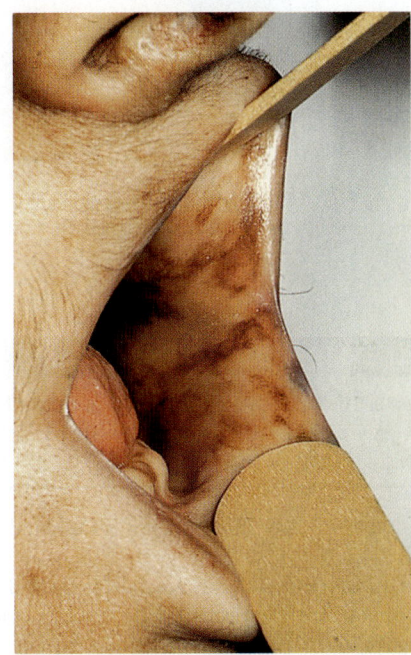

FIG. 14.8 Hyperpigmentation of the buccal (cheek) membranes caused by Addison disease. (From Thibodeau GA, Patton KT: *The Human Body in Health and Disease*, ed 5, St. Louis, 2010, Mosby.)

- A diet high in complex carbohydrates and protein
- Periodic checks of sodium and potassium levels

Prognosis. Addison disease can be difficult to diagnose and may pose complications. Patients who adhere to the treatment plans have a better prognosis.

Prevention. There is no way to prevent Addison disease.

Cushing Disease. *Cushing* (CUSH ing) disease is a malfunction of the adrenal cortex. An overactive adrenal cortex secretes increased levels of cortisol.

Etiology. Cushing disease is caused by several conditions, which include the following:
- A benign pituitary tumor, which causes the release of excessive amounts of ACTH.
- Primary adrenal gland disease. The most common is a noncancerous tumor of the adrenal cortex, called an adrenal adenoma.
- An ectopic (ek TOP ik) ACTH-secreting tumor. A tumor develops in an organ that does not secrete ACTH, but the tumor begins to secrete ACTH for an unknown reason. Malignant or benign tumors of the lungs, pancreas, thyroid, or thymus can secrete ACTH.
- Taking long-term corticosteroids for medical reasons, such as organ transplantation, severe asthma, or rheumatoid arthritis.

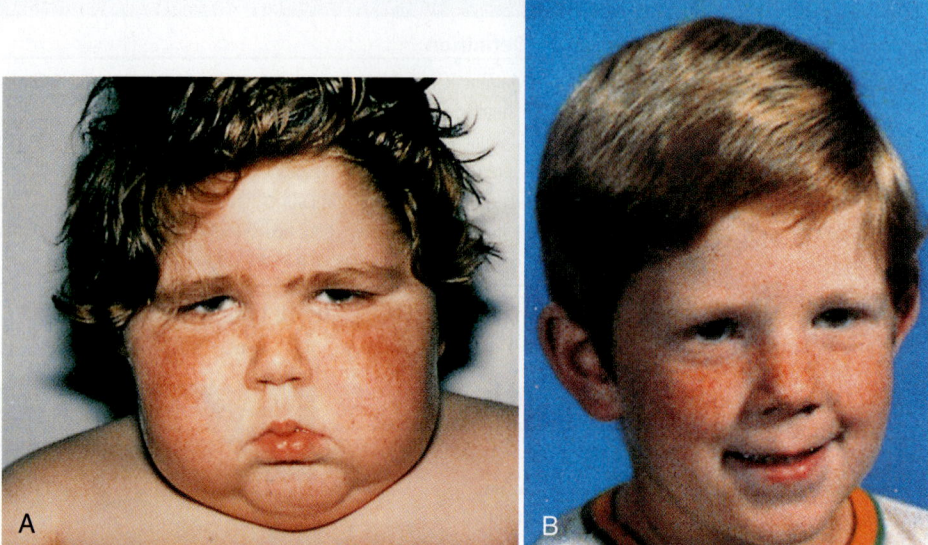

FIG. 14.9 Cushing disease. (A) First diagnosed. (B) After 4 months of treatment. (From Shiland B: *Mastering Healthcare Terminology*, ed 5, St. Louis, 2016, Elsevier.)

CRITICAL THINKING 14.8

Addison disease and Cushing disease are caused by an improperly functioning adrenal gland. Write down the differences between the two diseases. What hormone is involved in both diseases?

Signs and symptoms. Signs and symptoms of Cushing disease include the following:
- High blood pressure; weight gain, especially in the abdomen, upper back, face (moon face), and between the shoulder blades (buffalo hump) (Fig. 14.9).
- Pink or purple stretch marks on the abdomen, thighs, breasts, and arms; fragile, thin skin that bruises easily
- Infections, slow-healing wounds, acne
- Severe fatigue, muscle weakness, headaches
- Depression, anxiety, irritability, loss of emotional control, difficulty thinking clearly
- In children: slowed or impaired growth
- In women: thicker or more noticeable facial and body hair (*hirsutism* [HUR soo tiz um] or *hypertrichosis*) (Fig. 14.10)
- In men: decreased libido (lih BEE doh) and fertility

VOCABULARY
ectopic: Occurring in an abnormal position or place. Displaced.
libido: Sexual drive or instinct.

Diagnostic procedures. It can be difficult to diagnose Cushing disease and to determine the proper cause. Common diagnostic procedures include the following:
- Blood tests: to measure cortisol levels
- Urine tests: to measure cortisol levels; may recommend a 24-hour urine sample; most accurately determines urine cortisol levels
- Saliva test: for cortisol levels.
- ACTH stimulation test
- Imaging tests: CT scan or MRI scan

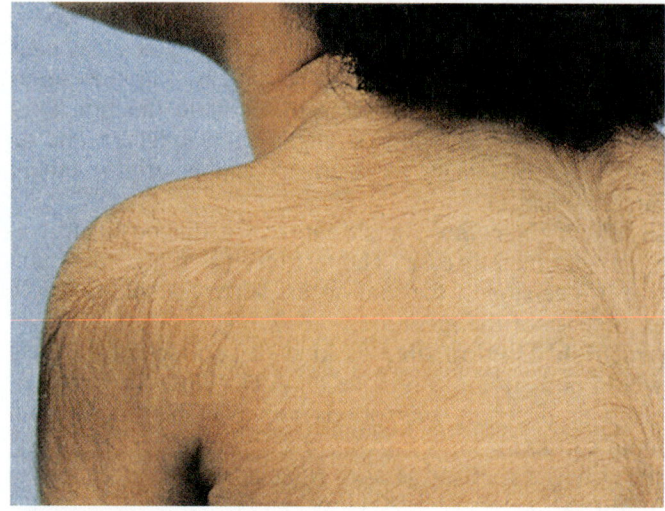

FIG. 14.10 Hirsutism. (From *Mosby's Medical Nursing and Allied Health Dictionary*, ed 8, St. Louis, 2009, Mosby.)

Treatment. Treatment depends on the cause of the disorder and may include the following:
- Medication to control cortisol levels
- Radiation therapy to reduce the size of a tumor
- Surgery to remove the tumor

Prognosis. Cushing disease may pose complications that include bone loss (osteoporosis), type 2 diabetes, frequent infections, and loss of muscle mass and strength. Patients who adhere to the treatment plans have a better prognosis than those who do not.

Prevention. There is no way to prevent Cushing disease.

Pancreatic Diseases

Pancreatic diseases are described in Table 14.13. *Diabetes mellitus* (dahy uh BEE tis MEL i tuhs) (DM) is the most common pancreatic disease. Diabetes mellitus is a group of metabolic disorders characterized by an inadequate production of insulin, a resistance to insulin, or a

TABLE 14.13 Pancreatic Diseases

Condition	Description
Type 1 diabetes mellitus	Condition resulting from a total lack of insulin production. Requires insulin injections. Previously called insulin-dependent diabetes mellitus (IDDM) or juvenile diabetes.
Type 2 diabetes mellitus	Condition resulting from deficient insulin productions. Insulin is being produced, but the body does not respond to it. Previously called non–insulin-dependent diabetes mellitus (NIDDM) or adult-onset diabetes.
Prediabetes	A condition in which the blood glucose level is higher than normal, but not high enough for a diagnosis of type 2 diabetes.
Gestational diabetes	Insulin resistance acquired during pregnancy.
Hyperinsulinism (hye pur IN suh lin iz um)	Hypersecretion of insulin; seen in some newborns of diabetic mothers. Causes severe hypoglycemia.
Islet cell carcinoma (EYE let)	Also called *pancreatic cancer*; fourth leading cause of cancer death in the United States. Treated with a Whipple procedure (pancreatoduodenectomy).

TABLE 14.14 Relationship Between the A1c and Average Plasma Glucose Levels

A_{1c} (%)	Average Plasma Glucose (mg/dL)
4	65
5	97
6	126
7	154
8	183
9	212
10	240
11	269
12	298
13	326

NIH, http://www.niddk.nih.gov/health-information/health-topics/diagnostic-tests/a1c-test-diabetes/Pages/index.aspx#14.

Diagnostic procedures. The following diagnostic results suggest diabetes:

- Glycated hemoglobin (A1c) test, 6.5% or greater on two separate samples (Table 14.14)
- Fasting blood sugar test, 126 mg/dL on two separate samples (see Table 14.14)
- Oral glucose tolerance testing
- Random blood sugar test, no matter when a person ate last, with a value of 200 mg/dL or greater and diabetes symptoms

Treatment. For all types of diabetes, it is important to do the following:

- Monitor blood sugar and prevent hypoglycemia and hyperglycemia (Table 14.15).
- Maintain a healthy whole-food diet rich in vegetables, fruits, lean protein, good fats, and high fiber; avoid processed foods, sugary foods, and sweetened drinks.
- Exercise regularly and maintain a healthy weight.

Besides these suggestions, patients with type 1 diabetes need to take insulin injections or use an insulin pump. Insulin intake must balance with the carbohydrates consumed and with the person's exercise. Maintaining a normal blood glucose level is important.

Patients with type 2 diabetes take oral or injectable antihyperglycemic medications. Some patients may take insulin. Bariatric surgery may be recommended for people with a body mass index (BMI) of 35 or greater.

Prognosis. Patients who maintain blood glucose levels as close to the norm as possible prevent additional complications. The American Diabetes Association recommends blood glucose levels between 70 and 130 mg/dL before meals, below 180 mg/dL 2 hours after starting a meal, and an A1cb level below 7%. Uncontrolled DM will cause the progressive destruction of small blood vessels that may lead to complications (Box 14.6).

Prevention. There is no way to prevent type 1 diabetes. The best way to prevent type 2 diabetes is to maintain an ideal weight, exercise regularly, and eat a healthful diet rich in vegetables, fruits, lean protein, good fats, and high fiber. It is important to avoid processed foods, sugary foods, and sweetened drinks.

Gestational Diabetes. Insulin resistance acquired during pregnancy is gestational diabetes. This condition usually resolves after delivery.

Etiology. Gestational diabetes is thought to be caused by the hormones produced by the placenta. Pregnancy changes in the body cause

combination of both. The following sections will discuss type 1, type 2, and gestational diabetes.

Diabetes Mellitus: Type 1 and Type 2. Diabetes mellitus can result in excessive amounts of glucose in the blood or urine. DM is a common chronic condition seen in people of all ages.

Etiology. Type 1 diabetes is an autoimmune disorder in which the insulin production by the beta cells of the pancreas is severely impaired or destroyed. Risk factors include a family history, genetics, and age. Typically, type 1 is a rapid-onset disease affecting people younger than 25 years of age.

Type 2 diabetes has a complicated connection with obesity, lifestyle factors, genetic predisposition, and an individual's health history. Risk factors for type 2 include the following:

- Being overweight, fat distribution mostly around the abdomen; a sedentary lifestyle
- Already having prediabetes
- Having a close relative who has type 2 diabetes
- Being older than 45 years, though due to obesity, young adults and adolescents are also affected
- Being black, Hispanic, Native American, or Asian, as these groups have higher risk than the white population

Signs and symptoms. Common signs and symptoms for types 1 and 2 diabetes include the following:

- Polydipsia, polyuria, polyphagia, weight loss, and fatigue.
- Blurred vision, frequent infections, slow-healing wounds

Additional symptoms that occur with type 1 diabetes include bedwetting with the polyuria, mood changes, and irritability.

TABLE 14.15 Hypoglycemia and Hyperglycemia

	Hypoglycemia	Hyperglycemia
Definition	Blood glucose level is below 70 mg/dL	Blood glucose levels rising as high as 300 to 750 mg/dL
Why does it occur?	Imbalance between insulin and the blood glucose. Too little glucose is in the blood because the individual: • Took too much insulin • Didn't eat enough carbohydrates • Did too much physical activity • Drank alcohol (may occur up to 2 days after drinking)	Imbalance between insulin and the blood glucose. Too much glucose is in the blood because the individual: • Took too little insulin • Ate too many carbohydrates • Is ill, has an infection, trauma, or surgery. • Used an illegal drug (e.g., cocaine, Ecstasy)
Symptoms	Hypoglycemia • Double or blurry vision • Fast pulse, palpitations • Irritable, aggressive, nervous • Headache, unclear thinking • Shaking, tired • Sweaty, cold skin • Hunger • Insulin shock (also called severe hypoglycemia or insulin reaction): • Disorientation, unconsciousness • Seizures • Shock • Diabetic coma and death	Hyperglycemia • Thirsty, hungry, stomach pain • Nausea (NAH zsa), vomiting • Frequent urination • Fatigue • Shortness of breath • Very dry mouth • Rapid pulse • Diabetic ketoacidosis (DKA) (also called severe hyperglycemia) • Fruity odor on breath • Diabetic coma and death
Treatment	If conscious and able to swallow, give 4 oz of fruit juice or regular (nondiet) soda or 3 glucose tablets. For an unconscious adult patient, glucagon (GLUE kah gon) injection is given to increase blood glucose levels.	Insulin is needed. For DKA, intravenous (IV) fluids, insulin, and electrolytes are needed.

BOX 14.6 Complications of Diabetes Mellitus

- Nerve damage (neuropathy)
- Heart and blood vessel disease
- Kidney damage (nephropathy)
- Eye damage (diabetic retinopathy, blindness)
- Skin, mouth, and foot infections; slow-healing infections
- Pregnancy complications

the cells to use insulin less effectively. This is called insulin resistance. Risk factors for gestational diabetes include the following:

- Being a woman who is 25 years or older
- Having a history of existing prediabetes or gestational diabetes, or having a family history of type 2 diabetes
- Being overweight before the pregnancy with a BMI of 30 or greater
- Being black, Hispanic, Native American, or Asian

Signs and symptoms. There are no distinct signs and symptoms of gestational diabetes.

Diagnostic procedures. Pregnant women are tested for gestational diabetes between weeks 24 and 28 of pregnancy. An oral glucose tolerance test is done.

Treatment. Treatment for gestational diabetes includes the following:

- Eating a healthful diet rich in vegetables, fruits, lean protein, good fats, and high fiber; avoiding processed foods, sugary foods, and sweetened drinks
- Monitoring blood sugar
- Exercising regularly and maintaining a healthy weight
- Taking insulin injections if ordered to maintain proper blood glucose levels
- Closely observing fetal development; if delivery does not occur by the due date, labor is induced

Prognosis. Gestational diabetes usually resolves after the delivery. Possible complications for the mother include hypertension (high blood pressure), **preeclampsia** (pree i KLAMP see uh), and a greater risk of type 2 diabetes in the future.

Possible complications for the baby include a large birth weight (more than 9 pounds), preterm birth, and respiratory distress. The baby could develop either *hypoglycemia* or type 2 diabetes.

VOCABULARY
preeclampsia: A form of toxemia during pregnancy, characterized by high blood pressure, fluid retention, and protein in the urine. May progress to eclampsia.

Prevention. There is no way to prevent gestational diabetes. To decrease the risk, the woman should enter pregnancy at an ideal weight and exercise regularly. It is also important to eat a healthful diet rich in vegetables, fruits, lean protein, good fats, and high fiber. She should avoid processed foods, sugary foods, and sweetened drinks.

CRITICAL THINKING 14.9
What is the cause of type 1 diabetes? What is the cause of type 2 diabetes? What are some unique characteristics of gestational diabetes? Be ready to share your thoughts with the class.

> ### CRITICAL THINKING 14.10
>
> Lexie escorted Mr. Ironside into an exam room after he had his blood drawn. Mr. Ironside has type 2 diabetes (he was diagnosed 2 months ago) and has not been able to bring down his blood sugar with diet and exercise. He is seeing Drs. Afrose and Perez today.
>
> Lexie takes Mr. Ironside's vital signs and prepares the room for the doctors. She notices the blood glucose on Mr. Ironside is posted from the lab. Lexie asks Mr. Ironside if he has any questions for the doctors, and he says he does. Mr. Ironside wants to know why his hands and feet are tingly a lot. He said he watches his diet but still has trouble with his blood sugars. Lexie notices that his fasting blood glucose is at 155 mg/dL.
>
> Is Mr. Ironside's blood sugar in the normal range? What is the normal range for a fasting blood sugar?

LIFE SPAN CHANGES

A few endocrine disorders affect children. Congenitally, growth hormone deficiency and gigantism cause extremes in height. Children usually develop type 1 diabetes at a young age, between birth and 25 years of age. Cushing disease (overactive adrenal cortex) can also be seen in children.

Often more severe symptoms of endocrine system disorders are seen in adults or in older adults. Diabetes mellitus is seen in any age group, but it is most likely to occur in adults over the age of 30 years. The consequences and complications of diabetes mellitus are seen most frequently in older adults. Uncontrolled diabetes can lead to amputations, blindness, kidney problems, and infections, which severely limit a senior's independence and mobility.

> ### CRITICAL THINKING 14.11
>
> Drs. Afrose and Perez join Mr. Ironside in the exam room. They talk about blood sugar numbers and why Mr. Ironside's is still high. He says he does not like to exercise much, and he really does not have 2 hours a day to go to the gym. He also says that he loves his sweet tea but he has changed from sweetening his tea with sugar to sweetening it with honey. Because honey is a natural sweetener, he thought that was a better choice.
>
> What information has Mr. Ironside given the doctors that might help them understand his elevated blood sugar? What changes can Mr. Ironside make to improve his blood sugar numbers? Be willing to share your thoughts with the class.

CLOSING COMMENTS

Because the management of endocrine disorders can be complicated, the medical assistant must make sure the patient understands procedures for at-home treatment. By demonstrating a given procedure in the office, the medical assistant can provide necessary patient education, as well as answer any questions the patient may have. Visual materials and procedure cards are helpful because they can be taken home and used as a reminder. If the patient is taking medication, the medical assistant should do the following:
- Review the dosage schedule with the individual.
- Discuss the purpose of the treatment.
- Answer any questions the patient may have.

As always, if the medical assistant is uncertain of any procedures or information, she or he should ask the provider for assistance before explaining the information to the patient.

An important part of becoming a professional medical assistant is to be familiar with the medical terminology and abbreviations related to the endocrine system (Tables 14.16 through 14.19). Being professional also means a person is committed to lifelong learning. Diabetes mellitus is the most common endocrine system disease. Regardless of where you work as a medical assistant, you will end up caring for patients with diabetes and interacting with their families on some level. Diabetes researchers are constantly discovering more information about the disease. You must commit to continually learning about diabetes so that you are prepared to care for patients with this serious disorder.

> ### EXCEPTIONAL CUSTOMER SERVICE
>
> **Additional Thoughts on Patient Education for Diabetics**
>
> Patient education should be documented completely to establish legal proof that the information was shared with the patient. The following suggestions can help ensure the patient's welfare and promote risk management:
> - Advise patients that a Medic Alert bracelet with their diagnosis and medication information is an important safeguard.
> - Patients must take medication as prescribed, following the directions for dosage, route of administration, and storage.
> - Patients should be alert for possible side effects.
> - Patients newly diagnosed with diabetes should not drive until blood sugar has stabilized. Patients also should be warned about possible visual impairment from the disease.
> - Remember that you are always representing your profession and provider, and respond to each situation accordingly.
> - Ask for assistance or further information if you feel unprepared to perform a procedure or give accurate information.

TABLE 14.16 Combining and Adjective Forms for the Anatomy and Physiology of the Endocrine System

Meaning	Combining Form	Adjective Form	Meaning	Combining Form	Adjective Form
adrenal gland	adren/o, adrenal/o	adrenal	medulla	medull/o	medullary
calcium	calc/o		pancreas	pancreat/o	pancreatic
cortex	cortic/o	cortical	parathyroid gland	parathyroid/o	parathyroidal
gland	aden/o		pituitary gland	hypophys/o, pituitar/o	hypophyseal
glucose, sugar	gluc/o, glyc/o, glucos/o		thalamus	thalam/o	thalamic
gonads	gonad/o	gonadal	thymus gland	thym/o	thymic
ketone	ket/o, keton/o		thyroid gland	thyr/o, thyroid/o	thyroidal
kidney	ren/o, nephr/o	renal	to secrete	crin/o	
lobe	lob/o	lobar	turning	trop/o	tropic

From Shiland B: *Mastering Healthcare Terminology*, ed 5, St. Louis, 2016, Elsevier.

TABLE 14.17 Prefixes for the Anatomy of the Endocrine System

Prefix	Meaning
endo-	within
exo-	outward
hypo-	under
supra-	above

From Shiland B: *Mastering Healthcare Terminology*, ed 5, St. Louis, 2016, Elsevier.

TABLE 14.18 Suffixes for the Anatomy of the Endocrine System

Suffix	Meaning
-al	pertaining to
-crine	to secrete
-logy	study of
-us, -is	structure

From Shiland B: *Mastering Healthcare Terminology*, ed 5, St. Louis, 2016, Elsevier.

TABLE 14.19 Abbreviations for the Endocrine System

Abbreviation	Meaning	Abbreviation	Meaning
A1c	average glucose level	NIDDM	non–insulin-dependent diabetes mellitus
ACTH	adrenocorticotropic hormone	OGTT	oral glucose tolerance test
ADH	antidiuretic hormone	OT	oxytocin
Ca	calcium	PGH	pituitary growth hormone
DI	diabetes insipidus	PRL	prolactin
FBS	fasting blood sugar	PTH	parathyroid hormone
FPG	fasting plasma glucose	RAIU	radioactive iodine uptake (scan)
FSH	follicle-stimulating hormone	RIA	radioimmunoassay
GH	growth hormone	SIADH	syndrome of inappropriate antidiuretic hormone
GHD	growth hormone deficiency	STH	somatotropic hormone
hGH	human growth hormone	T_3	triiodothyronine
ICSH	interstitial cell-stimulating hormone	T_4	thyroxine
IDDM	insulin-dependent diabetes mellitus	TFT	thyroid function test
K	potassium	TSH	thyroid-stimulating hormone
LH	luteinizing hormone	UA	urinalysis
Na	sodium		

From Shiland B: *Mastering Healthcare Terminology*, ed 5, St. Louis, 2016, Elsevier.

CHAPTER REVIEW

The endocrine system is composed of ductless glands that secrete chemical messengers, called hormones, directly into the bloodstream. Hormones travel through the body transferring information from one group of cells to another. Through this chemical message system, hormones regulate many body functions, including the following:
- Metabolism and growth
- Mood
- Sexual maturity and reproduction
- Water and electrolyte balance

Hormone levels vary and can be affected by outside factors, such as illness and stress.

The glands of the endocrine system are the pituitary gland, thyroid gland, parathyroid gland, adrenal gland, pancreas, thymus, gonads (ovaries and testes), and pineal gland. Each gland secretes unique hormones with defined target cells as their receptors. Once target cells receive the message from a hormone, they start making the needed changes in the cell. The endocrine system is not a quick-acting system. The changes made throughout the body may take time, but they are often long-lasting changes that help maintain homeostasis.

The pituitary gland is often described as the master gland. The pituitary gland is made up of an anterior and posterior lobe. Hormones produced in the anterior pituitary gland affect other glands. Some of the hormones produced in the anterior pituitary gland are adrenocorticotropic hormone (ACTH), thyroid-stimulating hormone (TSH), follicle-stimulating hormone (FSH), luteinizing hormone (LH), prolactin, and growth hormone (GH). The posterior pituitary does not produce any hormones, but it stores hormones that are made in the hypothalamus. The posterior pituitary releases the hormones once it receives a signal from the hypothalamus. Hormones stored and released in the posterior pituitary are antidiuretic hormone (ADH) and oxytocin.

The thyroid and parathyroid glands are located on the anterior portion of the neck, just below the Adam's apple. The thyroid gland produces three hormones: triiodothyronine (T_3), thyroxine (T_4), and calcitonin. T_3 and T_4 help regulate growth and metabolism, whereas calcitonin lowers the blood calcium level and direct calcium to be stored in the bones. The parathyroid glands are four little glands located on the posterior side of the thyroid gland. The parathyroid produces one hormone called parathyroid hormone (PTH). It is responsible for raising blood calcium levels by signaling the bones to release calcium into the bloodstream.

The adrenal glands also have two separate glands within the structure, the adrenal cortex and medulla. The adrenal cortex produces mineralocorticoids (aldosterone), glucocorticoids (cortisol), and sex hormones (androgens). The adrenal medulla produces epinephrine and norepinephrine.

The pancreas is an endocrine and exocrine gland. As an endocrine gland, it produces insulin and glucagon, two hormones with opposite functions. Insulin lowers blood sugar and glucagon raises blood sugar. Insulin is a hormone that most people know about because it is lacking or nonfunctional in people who have diabetes mellitus.

The thymus, gonads, and pineal glands all contribute to the endocrine system too. The thymus produces thymosin, which helps T-cell lymphocytes to mature and work in cell-mediated immunity. The gonads (ovaries and testes) produce sex hormones: estrogen and progesterone in females and testosterone in males. The pineal gland produces melatonin, which helps regulate the wake-sleep cycle. In the physiology of the endocrine system, we discussed the mechanisms of hormone regulation, target cells, hormone actions (steroid and nonsteroid hormones), and prostaglandins.

The diseases of the endocrine system are most frequently conditions that exist because of hyper- or hyposecretion of the affected hormone. Diseases covered included Addison disease; Cushing disease; diabetes insipidus; diabetes mellitus types 1, 2, and gestational; hyperthyroidism; hypothyroidism; and additional diseases. The changes in the endocrine system across the life span included diabetes mellitus, a disease that affects a growing number of people in the United States and worldwide.

The endocrine system is complex and fascinating. It is made up of glands and hormones that are just trying to maintain body homeostasis.

SCENARIO WRAP-UP

Drs. Perez and Afrose ask Lexie to join them in the exam room as they talk about blood sugar control with Mr. Ironside. The doctors explain to Mr. Ironside that exercising does not have to be 2 hours a day and that he does not have to go to the gym. He can take a brisk 15- to 20-minute walk in the morning or at lunch and another 15- to 20-minute brisk walk before or after dinner. Moving is important. They stress the importance of making it part of his daily routine.

The doctors also talk about his sweet tea. Sugar and honey are both sweeteners that will raise his blood sugar. Mr. Ironside does admit that he drinks sweet tea for lunch and throughout the afternoon most days. Sometimes he even has sweet tea and crackers for breakfast as he drives to work.

It has been a good discussion with Mr. Ironside. Learning how to eat and exercise is part of the adjustment needed to manage diabetes.

Dr. Perez also looks at Mr. Ironside's electronic medical record and notices that he has canceled appointments with a nutritionist twice. The doctors leave Mr. Ironside with Lexie to go over some patient education brochures about type 2 diabetes. As they finish looking at the information, Lexie also points out several websites and apps listed in the brochures. Mr. Ironside loves technology, so he is excited about tracking his food intake and exercise on his smart phone. Lexie walks Mr. Ironside out to the reception area where he is going to schedule an appointment with the nutritionist. He says that he will go to the appointment this time and that he is going to work on managing his diabetes from now on.

Lexie finishes her day and gathers with her colleagues to see what Drs. Perez and Afrose say in their discussion today. She wonders if Mr. Ironside is going for a walk tonight?

15

Professionalism in Healthcare

LEARNING OBJECTIVES

1. Do the following related to characteristics of professional medical assistants:
   - Describe characteristics of professional medical assistants.
   - Discuss examples of diversity. Include cultural, social, and ethnic examples.
   - Explain how to demonstrate respect for individual diversity, including gender, race, religion, age, economic status, and appearance.
2. Discuss the appropriate professional appearance of a medical assistant.
3. Describe professionalism as a team member. Also, define a patient-centered medical home (PCMH).
4. Discuss continuing education for medical assistants, including how to achieve a credential.
5. Explain barriers to professionalism.
6. Identify types of nonverbal communication.
7. Do the following related to verbal communication:
   - Identify types and styles of verbal communication.
   - Recognize the elements of oral communication using a sender-receiver process.
   - Describe the behaviors seen in passive, aggressive, passive-aggressive, manipulative, and assertive communicators.
   - Identify barriers to communication, and techniques for overcoming communication barriers.
   - Describe the impact of the Americans with Disabilities Act Amendments Act (ADAAA) on communication barriers in healthcare.
   - Describe how Erikson's psychosocial development stages and Kübler-Ross's stages of grief and dying relate to communication and behavior.
8. Discuss how Maslow's hierarchy of needs relates to communication and behavior.
9. Differentiate between adaptive and nonadaptive coping mechanisms. Also, discuss coping mechanisms.

CHAPTER OUTLINE

1. **Opening Scenario, 343**
2. **You Will Learn, 343**
3. **Introduction, 343**
   a. Customer Service, 343
4. **Professionalism, 343**
   a. Characteristics of Professional Medical Assistants, 343
      i. *Courtesy and Respect, 344*
      ii. *Empathy and Compassion, 344*
      iii. *Tact and Diplomacy, 344*
      iv. *Respect for Individual Diversity, 344*
      v. *Honesty, Dependability, and Responsibility, 344*
      vi. *Personal Boundaries with Communication, 345*
   b. Professional Appearance, 345
   c. Professionalism as a Team Member, 346
      i. *Work Ethic and Punctuality, 347*
      ii. *Cooperation and Willingness to Help, 347*
      iii. *Prioritizing and Time Management Skills, 348*
      iv. *Responding to Criticism, 349*
      v. *Problem Solving and Chain of Command, 349*
   d. Continuing Education, 349
      i. *Achieving a Credential, 349*
   e. Barriers to Professionalism, 350
      i. *Personal Problems and "Baggage", 350*
      ii. *Gossip, 350*
      iii. *Personal Communication, 350*
5. **Nonverbal Communication, 350**
   a. Physical Boundaries, 351
   b. Nonverbal Communication Delivery Factors, 352
   c. Cultural Differences, 352
6. **Verbal Communication, 353**
   a. Communication Cycle, 353
   b. Written Communication, 353
   c. Oral Communication, 353
      i. *Styles of Oral Communication, 353*
   d. Therapeutic Communication, 354
      i. *Active Listening, 354*
      ii. *Other Therapeutic Communication Techniques, 355*
   e. Barriers to Communication, 355
      i. *Age and Disease Status Barriers, 355*
7. **Understanding Behavior, 357**
   a. Maslow's Hierarchy of Needs, 357
   b. Defense Mechanisms, 358
   c. Coping Mechanisms, 358
8. **Closing Comments, 359**
9. **Chapter Review, 360**

CHAPTER 15 Professionalism in Healthcare

OPENING SCENARIO

Christi Michelson is a newly hired medical assistant at Walden-Martin Family Medicine (WMFM) Clinic. She graduated from the local community college last month. She is currently in her probationary period at WMFM Clinic. Christi has orientation for 1 month, and her probationary period will last for 3 months. Over the next 3 months, she must pass a national certification exam. At the end of 3 months, she will have an evaluation. If the evaluation is positive, she will continue in her position.

Christi is very excited with her first healthcare job. In the past, she has worked as a waitress and a sales clerk. These jobs have helped her learn customer service skills, which she is now using in her current position. Christi is finding that the professionalism at WMFM Clinic is much different than at her previous jobs. She now has a dress code that she must follow. Christi is learning the clinic's customer service policies and procedures. She was surprised to learn that her customers include not only the patients, but also her coworkers. She is learning new communication skills. Christi is excited to continue learning more skills to help her provide the best patient care possible.

YOU WILL LEARN

- To recognize characteristics of professional medical assistants.
- To describe how to show respect for individual diversity.
- To identify types of nonverbal communication.
- To identify styles and types of verbal communication.
- To recognize communication barriers and identify techniques to overcome barriers.
- To recognize why people behave the way they do.

INTRODUCTION

A medical assistant is a multiskilled healthcare professional. A healthcare professional:
- has high ethical standards.
- displays **integrity**.
- completes work accurately and in a timely fashion.

It is important for successful professionals to show professionalism. *Professionalism* is having a courteous, **conscientious**, and respectful approach. This approach is used during all interactions and situations in the workplace. Our patients and coworkers expect professional behavior. Patients base much of their trust and confidence in those who show professionalism.

In this chapter, we will start by describing customer service and its importance to the healthcare facility. Customer service closely relates to professional behaviors. One must be professional to provide exceptional customer service. We will explore professional characteristics as they relate to patients and team members. We will examine nonverbal and verbal communication. Therapeutic communication and active listening will be discussed, because they are critical to working with patients. We will examine the reasons people behave the way they do. These are all important topics for a medical assistant.

Customer Service

In healthcare today, many of our patients have the ability to choose where they go to seek care. Healthcare is a business. The ambulatory care facility needs to attract and retain patients to remain open and for you to have a job. Two of the quickest ways to lose patients are to treat them poorly and to act in an unprofessional manner. Happy patients will tend to tell others about their experiences. Great customer service leads to a successful healthcare facility and allows growth.

To understand customer service, we first need to know who our customers are. A *customer* is one who purchases goods or services. A customer can also be a person whom you deal with in the work environment. By that definition, we can see that patients are our customers. They choose our ambulatory care facility to seek healthcare services. They (or their insurance company) pay for the services provided. Patients are considered *external customers,* or people we do business with who are "outside" (i.e., not employed by) the healthcare facility. Other external customers include medical equipment and supply vendors and pharmaceutical representatives.

The second part of the customer definition relates to internal customers, or people whom you deal with in the work environment. These are individuals we interact with inside the facility. They include our coworkers, employees in other departments, and the administrative staff. Both internal and external customers are important for the success of the healthcare facility.

Customer service is whatever we do for our customers to improve their experience at our healthcare facility. People may have different ideas about how they should be treated during their interactions. Our goal is to provide *customer satisfaction,* or a sense of contentment with the interaction. Typically, the more we get to know the customer, the better we can provide customer service. This might not always be possible. For instance, a new patient comes for an appointment. If you are at the reception desk, you do not have a lot of time to get to know the patient. The most important things for you to do are:
- Be considerate and treat the patient as you would want to be treated
- Look and act professional

As you read subsequent chapters, customer service tips will be provided. It is important to use these tips as you interact with patients.

> **CRITICAL THINKING 15.1**
>
> During Christi's orientation, she learned about customer service and customer satisfaction. In your own words, how would you define both of these phrases?

PROFESSIONALISM

Medical assistants represent the healthcare facility. They are viewed as an extension of the provider and the facility. How they act is a direct reflection on the facility and provider. If a medical assistant is rude to a patient, the patient will think that the provider is rude. The perceived quality of care will be negative. Medical assistants must always display professionalism. This includes their attitude, appearance, and behavior. Regardless of the situation, they must always act professionally.

Characteristics of Professional Medical Assistants

Medical assistants must have professional *characteristics*, or distinguishing traits. You will start developing these traits while in school. You will put them into practice during practicum. They will follow you into your first job. If a student is unprofessional during practicum, it will be difficult to get a job. That behavior may be **detrimental** to the medical assistant's professional career.

> **VOCABULARY**
> **conscientious**: Meticulous, careful.
> **detrimental:** Harmful.
> **integrity**: Adhering to ethical standards or right conduct standards.

Courtesy and Respect. Courtesy, respect, and dignity often come together when discussing professionalism. *Courtesy* is having good manners or being polite. Courteous behavior is polite, open, and welcoming. *Respect* means to show consideration or appreciation for another person. *Dignity* (DIG ni tee) is the inherent worth or state of being worthy of respect.

We show our patients dignity by treating all patients the way we would want to be treated. It does not matter if the patient has bad body odor or is dressed in tattered clothes. The patient is a person worthy of respect. Patients expect to be treated as individuals who matter. They want to be respected, and not be treated as an annoyance or a medical condition. How can the medical assistant treat others with courtesy and respect?

- Make patients feel welcome and respected. A pleasant greeting and eye contact should be the first things patients experience. Thanking patients at the end of the visit is also important.
- Display positive nonverbal behaviors. Use a calm tone of voice, eye contact when appropriate, and provide privacy for patients. Maintain patient confidentiality.
- Learn about other cultures in your area. When working with patients from those cultures, make sure to avoid gestures, words, and behaviors that could be perceived as disrespectful. (This is discussed later in the chapter.)
- Always use proper grammar, without slang words. Explain medical treatments and conditions in simple lay language. If you need to use a medical word, explain it to the patient.

Empathy and Compassion. It is important that professional medical assistants demonstrate empathy and compassion to their patients. Empathy, sympathy, and compassion can easily be confused. *Empathy* (EM pah thee) is the ability to understand another's perspective, experiences, or motivations. We can share another's emotional state. Empathy differs from sympathy. *Sympathy* is feeling sorrow or concern for what the other person has gone through. *Compassion* means we have a deep awareness of the suffering of another and wish to ease it.

Tact and Diplomacy. Tact and diplomacy are extremely valuable traits in healthcare professionals. Being *tactful* means being acutely sensitive to what is proper and appropriate when interacting with others. A tactful person has the ability to speak or act without offending others. Being *diplomatic* means using tact and sensitivity when interacting with others. The medical assistant must be sensitive to the needs of others.

How can a medical assistant use these traits when communicating with others?

- Consistently be polite and honest during your communication. Show sensitivity to others through your communication and behaviors.
- Recognize the needs and rights of others. Attempt to reach a mutually beneficial resolution to the problem.
- Assess your personal response to the situation. Your personal beliefs and biases should not prevent you from interacting diplomatically and tactfully with others.

> **CRITICAL THINKING 15.2**
>
> During Christi's orientation, she learned about the importance of courtesy, respect, empathy, compassion, tact, and diplomacy. Select three of these words and share with a peer examples of how a medical assistant could display these traits.

Respect for Individual Diversity. Medical assistants work with diverse populations. Your patients will come from different backgrounds. *Diversity* describes the differences and similarities in identity, perspective, and points of view among people. Table 15.1 describes different types of diversity. It is important for a medical assistant to understand the different types of diversity. Table 15.2 describes specific diversities that we may encounter with patients and coworkers.

It is important to be open and nonjudgmental when working with patients and coworkers who are different than ourselves. Be aware and accepting of other cultural differences. Be aware of your own cultural values. What preconceived ideas do you have of other diverse groups? How might your biases affect the care you provide to those in different groups?

It is important to educate yourself about other groups. Get to know their customs and practices. Culture can affect healthcare. It can influence how people describe their symptoms, when healthcare is sought, and how treatment plans are followed. For instance, people in some cultures eat traditional foods high in sodium. This could be an issue if a person has high blood pressure or kidney disease. Understanding and accepting the differences represented by your patients will help you provide the best care possible for them.

Honesty, Dependability, and Responsibility. *Honest* means to be sincere and upright. *Dependable* is the same as trustworthy. *Responsible*

TABLE 15.1 Types of Diversity

Type	Description	Example
Nationality	Pertains to the country where the person was born and holds citizenship.	John was born in Mexico and moved to the United Stated. He became a U.S. citizen.
Race	A group of people that has the same physical characteristics (e.g., skin color).	Even though John was born in Mexico, his mother is Mongolian (Japanese descent) and his father is Caucasian.
Cultural	General customs, norms, values, and beliefs held by a group of people.	John has adapted to the U.S. culture. He likes to be on time for appointments. Even though he grew up in a large family (six children), he is comfortable with having two or three children.
Ethnic	A group of people who share a common ancestry, culture, religion, traditions, nationality, language, etc.	John states he is Mexican. Growing up he learned his family's Mexican traditions. He plans to share these with his children someday. He values his family and respects his grandparents and parents.
Social	All the ways a person is different from others (e.g., lifestyle, religion, tastes, and preferences).	John does not drink alcohol or smoke. He exercises in the gym each day. He likes to visit art museums and learn about history.

TABLE 15.2 Diversity in Specific Factors

Factor	Discussion
Language	Some people are fluent in more than one language. For others, English is not their primary language. It is important to be sensitive to and respectful of language differences. Using resources (e.g., translated materials, an interpreter) can also show respect to patients.
Age	There are many stereotypes about age. For instance, the older generation may not be college educated, but may have "street smarts." The younger generation may be more comfortable with computers and digital devices. It is important not to stereotype a person because of his or her age. Ask, never assume anything!
Religion	There is a wide range of belief systems in this country. There are also different degrees of religious observations in the workplace. Some patients may refuse certain medical treatments based on their religion. Be sensitive to patients who refuse medical care or want to involve their shaman or healer in their care.
Economic status	Our patients may be from a variety of economic backgrounds. Some patients may be very wealthy and can afford to pay for healthcare without insurance. Other patients may rely on food banks and charities to get by. Be sensitive and respectful if your patient doesn't have the financial means to pay for healthcare services. Help the patient seek resources for medications, transportation, and food.
Gender	There are many stereotypes attributed to gender. We need to make sure we don't stereotype our patients and peers. Some of our patients may identify as a gender other than their birth gender. We need to respect their choices and be sensitive to any issues that arise.
Appearance	Our patients' appearances can greatly vary. If you work in a farming community, patients may come to appointments in their work clothes and smell of the barn. With the popularity of piercings, tattoos, and hair dye, we can see a variety of differences in our patients. We need to move beyond the patient's appearance and provide exceptional patient care.

is defined as being trusted or depended upon. These are three traits that are valuable for employers to have in employees. Professional medical assistants should be honest, dependable, and responsible. When given a task, they should complete it accurately, on time, and to the best of their ability. If they make an error, they should be upfront about it. Patient safety is the number one priority. Any mistake in patient care needs to be reported immediately to the provider and to the supervisor. Dependability and honesty are critical components in earning the trust and respect of others. How can medical assistants perform their duties using these three characteristics?

- Be honest and straightforward when interacting with others.
- Accept responsibility for your mistakes. Determine how to prevent them in the future.
- Follow through on your promises.
- Complete your work to the best of your abilities. Complete it on time.

Personal Boundaries With Communication. When we are talking with family and friends, the topics of our conversations can vary greatly. We can discuss many different things. When we are in the healthcare environment, we need to remember that certain topics are inappropriate. Discussions regarding relationships, politics, religion, and other such topics are not appropriate for the workplace.

Besides what we talk about, we also need to consider the phrases or words we use. Many people swear or use words that are insulting or degrading to others. Some people routinely use religious names (e.g., God) when they are surprised or upset. For some people, religious names have sacred meaning. When you say these names in their presence, it can be offensive. We need to ensure our language is professional.

The relationship between the medical assistant and the patient needs to be professional. It cannot be a dual relationship, where the medical assistant also becomes a friend to the patient. When working with patients, we need to keep our lives personal. It is not appropriate for the medical assistant to:

- Share personal issues, struggles, life stories, or other personal intimate information
- Contact the patient outside of the work environment
- Befriend the patient on social media
- Engage in a flirty or romantic relationship with the patient.
- Gossip and share what happens in the workplace with patients and others.

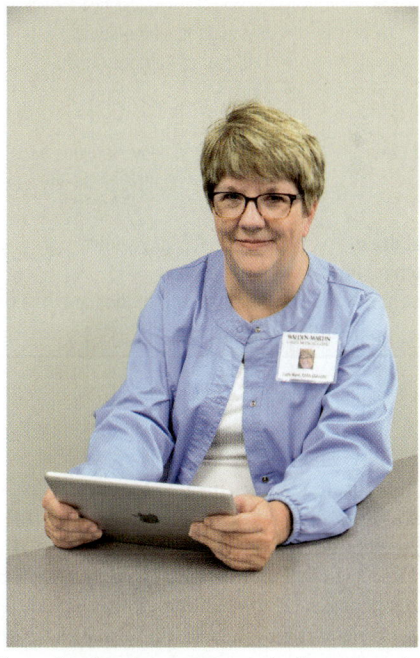

FIG. 15.1 A professional appearance is important for a medical assistant.

CRITICAL THINKING 15.3

During Christi's orientation, she shadowed Grace, another medical assistant. Grace has a personality that always makes the patients comfortable. She follows up with patients and does what she promised to do. Christi could see how much the provider trusted Grace. What kind of traits did Grace demonstrate to Christi?

Professional Appearance

Most ambulatory healthcare facilities have dress codes for employees. Medical assistants are usually required to wear scrubs, along with the facility's nametag (and a photo) clearly visible (Fig. 15.1). Table 15.3 provides a typical dress code. Dress codes will vary by facility. Some communities are more conservative and thus the dress codes reflect this.

TABLE 15.3 Typical Dress Code for Medical Assistants

Dress Code	Professional	Unprofessional	Comments
Uniform: scrubs and white shoes	• Scrubs must be clean, pressed (ironed), and fit properly. • Scrub pants must be hemmed to the appropriate length. • Closed-toed shoes must be white and clean.	• Dirty, wrinkled, ripped scrubs • Scrub pants dragging on the floor • Scruffy, dirty shoes • Open shoes (sandals), fabric shoes	• Shoes need to protect your feet. Cloth and open-toed shoes provide very little protection. • Pants dragging on floors pick up and transfer bacteria.
Hair	• Natural colors; clean and styled • Long hair must be tied back	• Unnatural colors; dirty, messy hair • Hair in face or hanging down	• Hair hanging in front can interfere with patient care, spread bacteria, and get caught in equipment.
Fingernails	• Cut short, unpolished	• Long, polished, artificial nails	• Bacteria can multiply and grow under long, artificial, and/or polished nails.
Cosmetics and body odors	• Professional makeup • No odors on the body	• Over use of makeup • Wearing perfume, cologne, etc. • Smelling like a cigarette • Body odor (from not bathing)	• Too much makeup can look unprofessional. • Smells like perfumes, colognes, or cigarettes can trigger allergies in others. • Offensive body odor is unprofessional because we are in patients' intimate/personal space.
Jewelry	• Wedding band (no stones) • One pair of earrings (studs) • Watch	• Rings with stones • Multiple earrings on each ear • Necklaces, bracelets • Lanyards	• Bacteria can accumulate in rings and bracelets. • Necklaces and lanyards can be choking hazards if grabbed by a patient.
Tattoos and body piercings	• Tattoos and body piercings must follow the healthcare facility's policy	• Not following the healthcare facility's policy	• In conservative communities, body piercings and tattoos may be perceived as unprofessional.
Professional dress (street clothes) for special events	• Blouse, top, or sweater • Dress pants • Dress or skirt (to the top of the knee) • Dress shoes	• Low-cut tops; sheer tops • Jeans, ripped pants, exercise clothes • Flip-flops, tennis shoes • Mini skirts	• Clothes should look professional; should not be ripped or casual in appearance.

Typically, healthcare facilities include terms such as "modest" and "business attire" in describing their dress codes. The rule of thumb is to make sure the employee does not expose too much at the neckline, the abdomen, and below the waist when bending and raising the arms. Business attire is not casual clothes. Casual clothes include jeans, T-shirts, shorts, exercise/sports clothing, and so on. Business attire is considered dressier, more professional, than casual clothes.

> ### CRITICAL THINKING 15.4
> Rosie, a business office employee at the clinic, is allowed to dress in business attire. She interacts with patients who have questions about their bill. Describe how Rosie should dress.

Professionalism as a Team Member

A *team* is a group of people organized for work or a specific purpose. In the healthcare setting, usually the team consists of the employees working in the same department. A broader definition could include all the employees at the facility. A *team member* is loyal to the group and works well with the other people in the group (Fig. 15.2). As a member, the medical assistant must help the team function. To do this,

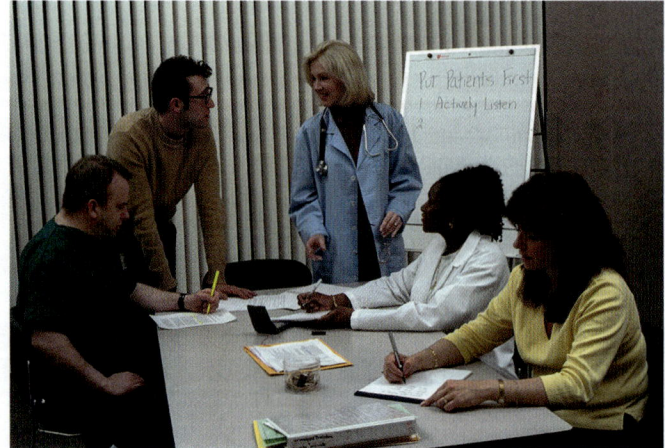

FIG. 15.2 Teamwork is a vital part of the medical profession. All staff members must work together to care for the patient and perform required duties in the healthcare facility. (From Proctor D, Niedzwiecki B: *Kinn's the medical assistant*, ed 13, St Louis, 2017, Elsevier.)

it is important to know the roles of the different team members. Tables 15.4 to 15.6 describe various healthcare professionals found in ambulatory care facilities.

To be a valuable team member, it is important to have several qualities. Work ethic, punctuality, cooperation, and the willingness to help are

TABLE 15.4 Ambulatory Allied Health Occupations

Title (Credential)	Job Description
Diagnostic cardiac sonographer or vascular technologist (DCS, DVT)	Trained and certified to perform noninvasive tests (e.g., echocardiographs and electrocardiographs) to help diagnose cardiac and vascular diseases.
Diagnostic medical sonographer (RDMS)	Trained and certified to use medical ultrasound, which can aid the diagnosis of a variety of conditions and diseases; also monitors fetal development.
Electroneurodiagnostic technologist (REEG-T)	Records and studies the electrical activity of the brain and nervous system.
Health information management professional (RHIA, RHIT)	Provides expert assistance in the management of health information.
Medical assistant (CMA, RMA, CCMA, CMAA)	Performs both administrative and clinical procedures and duties; a multiskilled health professional.
Nuclear medicine technologist (RT)	Performs nuclear diagnostic tests, which helps in the diagnosis of diseases.
Certified ophthalmic assistant (COA); **Certified ophthalmic technician** (COT)	Assists an ophthalmologist in providing eye care.
Pharmacy technician (CPhT)	Supervised by a pharmacist; assists in preparing medications based on prescriptions.
Surgical technologist (ST, CST)	Helps prepare patients for surgery and assists surgeon during the surgery.

TABLE 15.5 Licensed Healthcare Professions

Title	Job Description
Audiologist (aw dee OL oh jist) (CCC-A)	Assesses individuals with hearing loss, balance issues, and neural problems.
Certified nurse midwife (CMN)	RN with additional training and certification; provides prenatal, labor/delivery, and gynecologic care.
Licensed practical or vocational nurse (LPN, LVN)	A nurse who has been trained to assess and care for patients in a variety of environments; has less education than a registered nurse.
Medical technologist (MT)	Performs tests on blood, body fluids, and other types of specimens to assist the provider in arriving at a diagnosis.
Nurse anesthetist (NA)	RN with additional training and certification; provides pain management during surgical procedures.
Nurse practitioner (NP)	RN with additional training and certification; provides direct patient care and can diagnose and treat patients (write prescriptions).
Occupational therapist (OT)	Assists patients with physical disabilities to learn daily skills so they can be as independent as possible
Physical therapist (PT)	Assists patients in regaining mobility and strength.
Physician assistant (PA)	Provides direct patient care services under the supervision of a licensed physician; can diagnose and treat patients (write prescriptions).
Radiology technician (RT)	Performs medical imaging procedures (e.g., CT, MRI, x-rays).
Registered dietitian (RD)	Trained in nutrition; provides a dietary education to patients.
Registered nurse (RN)	A nurse who has been trained to assess and care for patients in a variety of environments.
Respiratory therapist (RT)	Performs diagnostic tests that measure lung capacity.

important traits in a team member. It takes all members working together to make an effective and productive team. When a member "drops the ball," others must step in and do extra work (Boxes 15.1 and 15.2).

Work Ethic and Punctuality. A *work ethic* is composed of sets of values based on hard work and diligence. The medical assistant should always display *initiative* (i NISH eh tiv) and be *reliable*. People with a good worth ethic arrive on time, are rarely absent, and always perform to the best of their ability. Coworkers become frustrated if another employee consistently arrives late or is absent. This forces the coworkers to take on additional duties, and it may prevent them from completing their own work. One missing employee can disrupt the entire day. Phones may not be answered promptly. Patients may have to wait longer for appointments. Lunch breaks may be shortened to allow all the work to be done. All employees should know and follow the attendance policies of the facility as outlined in the policies and procedures manual.

Most new hires have a probationary period that may last 30 to 90 days. Excessive absences or *tardiness* (being late) will negatively affect the employee. It may be grounds for *termination* (job loss). If the medical assistant must be absent or tardy, the supervisor must be notified prior to the start time. Make sure to follow the office policy. All employees

> **VOCABULARY**
> **initiative**: The ability to start a task and energetically complete it.
> **reliable**: Dependable, able to be trusted.

> **CRITICAL THINKING 15.5**
> Christi tends to arrive at the clinic with about 1 minute to spare. She realizes that she needs to change her habits and arrive about 10 minutes before her start time. This would give her a little "cushion" if traffic is slow. If you were Christi, what strategies could you use to make sure to get to the healthcare facility 10 minutes before the start time?

must be *punctual* (on time) every day. Providers and patients alike expect this reliability.

Cooperation and Willingness to Help. Each team member must be willing to cooperate and help others on the team. It is not uncommon that one team member might be very busy or handling an emergency. Other team members must be willing to step up and lend a helping hand. For instance, a medical assistant may be tied up caring for a very sick patient. Other patients who have appointments are waiting to be

TABLE 15.6 Examples of Medical Specialties

Practitioner's Title (Specialty)	Description
Allergist (AL ahr jist) (Allergy)	Physician who specializes in the diagnosis and treatment of diseases or conditions caused by allergies.
Anesthesiologist (AN is thee zee ol ah jist) (Anesthesiology)	Physician who provides pain relief and pain management during surgical procedures; also treats patients with chronic pain.
Colorectal surgeon (Colon and rectal surgery)	Surgeon who specializes in the diagnosis and treatment of intestinal conditions.
Dermatologist (DUR mah tol ah jee) (Dermatology)	Physician who specializes in skin disorders.
Emergency physician (Emergency medicine)	Specially trained physician who assesses and treats patients in emergency conditions (emergency departments).
Family practice physician (Family medicine)	Physicians that provide comprehensive primary care from infants through the elderly.
Surgeon (SUR jen) (General surgery)	Perform surgical procedures to correct deformities and injuries or treat diseases.
Medical geneticist (juh NET i sist) (Genetics)	Physicians specially trained to treat patients with genetically linked diseases.
Internist (in TUR nist) (Internal medicine)	Physicians that provide comprehensive primary care to adults.
Neurosurgeon (NOOR oh sur jen) (Neurologic surgery)	Specially trained surgeons that provide surgical care for patients with nervous systems conditions.
Obstetrician/gynecologist (OB stri trish uhn)/(GIE ni KOL uh jist) (Obstetrics and gynecology)	Obstetricians are physicians that provide care to women during and immediately after pregnancy. Gynecologists are physicians that provide reproductive care to females.
Ophthalmologist (OF thahl mol uh jist) (Ophthalmology)	Ophthalmologists diagnose, treat, and provide comprehensive care for the eye and its supporting structures. These physicians also offer vision services, including corrective lenses.
Otolaryngologist (O toe lar ing GOL uh gee) (Otolaryngology)	Specially trained physicians that medically and surgically treat diseases of the ear, nose, and throat (ENT).
Pathologist (pa THOL uh jee) (Pathology)	Physicians that study the cause and development of disease.
Pediatrician (PEE dee ah trish ahn) (Pediatrics)	Physicians that provide comprehensive primary care to children.
Physiatrist (FIZ ee at rist) (Physical medicine and rehabilitation)	Physician that specializes in physical medicine, which includes treating patients with musculoskeletal disabilities.
Plastic surgeon (Plastic surgery)	Specially trained surgeon who perform reconstructive cosmetic surgery.
Psychiatrist (si KIE ah trist) (Psychiatry)	Physician who specializes in the diagnosis and treatment of people with mental, emotional, or behavioral disorders.
Radiologist (RAE de ol uh ist) (Radiology)	Physician who specializes in the diagnosis and treatment of conditions using medical imaging procedures (e.g., CT, MRI, x-rays).
Thoracic surgeon (thah RAS ik) (Thoracic surgery)	Surgeon that specializes in the operative treatment of the chest and chest wall, lungs, heart, heart valves, and respiratory passages.
Urologist (yoo ROL ah jist) (Urology)	Physician that specializes in the treatment of urinary tract diseases.

seen. One of the other team members needs to help room the patients (e.g., take their vital signs and histories for the provider). This is how the department can provide exceptional customer service. Team members watch out for each other. If someone is getting behind, others help out.

Through cooperation, the team is more productive. Team members have greater job satisfaction. When members cooperate and work together, there is a great sense of communication and understanding in a team. Most importantly, the patients are cared for, and great customer service is provided.

Prioritizing and Time Management Skills. Prioritizing duties and using time management skills are critical for the success of medical assistants. *Prioritizing* means to arrange and complete duties in the order of most importance. *Time management strategies* are methods that maximize personal efficiencies and prioritize tasks. This means that we are to use our time efficiently and concentrate on the most important duties first. To do this, we must first prioritize our duties. We must arrange our schedules to ensure that these duties can be performed. The first way to improve time management is to plan the tasks that need to be done that day. Take 10 minutes to write down the tasks for the day. This helps ensure the tasks get done. Make sure to reference the list throughout the day to keep on track. Don't schedule too much to do each day, so that it is impossible to get everything done. Keep the list manageable. You need to build in some extra time in case of emergencies or urgent issues that come up. The key to managing time is prioritizing.

BOX 15.1 Patient-Centered Medical Home

Many healthcare facilities are adopting the patient-centered medical home (PCMH) model of healthcare. This model has an impact on the makeup of the healthcare team and also on reimbursement. This box will focus on the makeup of the healthcare team.

The goal of the PCMH is to improve patient care and reduce costs. The patient is the key player on the PCMH team. This is a model that responds to each patient's unique needs and preferences. It is used in primary care settings, such as family practice, internal medicine, and pediatrics.

With the PCMH model there is, of course, a provider involved, and a nurse or medical assistant who works with that provider. Most of us are familiar with this setup. In addition to those individuals, there is a Registered Nurse Care Coordinator (RNCC) and a pharmacist.

The RNCC helps the patient work his or her way through the healthcare system, make informed healthcare decisions, and find the healthcare resources he or she needs. The RNCC will contact patients after a visit to the emergency department, urgent care, or hospitalization to make sure the patients have everything they need. The RNCC may also have regular contact with a patient regarding wellness issues. This care coordinator may call to check on weight loss progress, blood pressure readings, and diabetic diets, to name a few such issues.

A pharmacist is part of the PCMH. The pharmacist helps patients manage medications and educates patients on possible medication side effects. The pharmacist is on staff at the healthcare facility rather than at the pharmacy.

The patient is actively involved in his or her own healthcare when the PCHM model is used. Steps are taken to ensure that patients receive the care and services they need from their healthcare team.

BOX 15.2 Huddles at the Start of the Day

Huddles are becoming more popular at the start of the day in ambulatory care. The purpose of huddles is to communicate important information to all team members, from the administrative staff to the clinical staff and providers. Huddles are quick meetings that help communicate the care needs of the patients being seen that day.

Prior to the huddle, a medical assistant reviews the patients' records, identifying missing information, preventive care required, and chronic disease management needs. These details are shared at the huddle. This information helps the providers, medical assistants, and other team members to be aware of the patients' needs. If the provider is busy, the medical assistant can work with the patient to obtain missing information and arrange preventive care.

Huddles help the staff members support each other. They also provide supervisors an opportunity to communicate quick messages on staffing issues, policy changes, and upcoming events.

When prioritizing your tasks, use a code system to indicate when they need to be done. For instance:
- Use an "M" for tasks that *must* be done that day.
- Use an "S" for tasks that *should* be done that day.
- Use a "C" for tasks that *could* be done if time permits.

Once the tasks have been divided into these categories, they can be further classified in each section. For instance, if category *M* has six tasks, they can be numbered in the order they should be performed. The same process is completed with the tasks in categories *S* and *C*. As the tasks are completed, they are checked off. At the end of each day, create a new "to do" list for the next day so that nothing important is forgotten.

CRITICAL THINKING 15.6

Christi needs to practice her time management skills. Using the system described, make your "to do" list. Use M, S, and C to categorize your activities.

Responding to Criticism. As we work, we are evaluated by others. It may be informal or formal for a job evaluation. We learn from others' feedback on our performance. This criticism can be hard to take. It threatens our confidence and self-esteem. We need to realize the value of the feedback. It will help us improve our skills and refine our professional skills. When a person gives us feedback or criticism, it is important to take it as a professional. Becoming defensive or blaming others, is not professional. This type of behavior will be a negative reflection on you.

Problem Solving and Chain of Command. When you are working as part of a team, it is important to understand how to solve differences with other members. Typically, it is best to talk with the person with whom you are having an issue. Try not to use statements that accuse the other person. Refrain from using sentences that start with "You are…" Try to remove the emotion from the situation if you can. Use more "I feel…" statements. If your attempt to resolve the situation is unsuccessful, then it is usually recommended that you talk with the supervisor.

If the issue is related to theft, confidentiality, or harassment, you may need to follow the chain of command in the healthcare facility. Usually, you need to start with your supervisor or the person you report to. Then the next step is the supervisor of your supervisor, and so on. Most employee handbooks discuss the facility's chain of command.

Continuing Education

As a professional medical assistant, it is important to stay current (up-to-date) with the newest medications, treatments, and diagnostic tests. Education beyond your medical assistant degree is considered continuing education. Most healthcare professionals need to do continuing education to renew their certification or license. There are many opportunities for continuing education. These include:
- Reading professional journals and reputable health websites
- On-the-job educational conferences
- Local, state, and national medical assistant conferences

Typically, additional continuing education opportunities exist if a medical assistant is a member of an organization. Popular medical assistant professional organizations include:
- American Association of Medical Assistants (AAMA) (*www.aama-ntl.org*)
- American Medical Technologist (AMT) (*https://www.americanmedtech.org*)

Achieving a Credential. Medical assistants have several options if they choose to become credentialed. Being a credentialed medical assistant has certain benefits:
- Credentialed medical assistants have had to pass a national standardized exam. Passing the exam indicates that they have the knowledge to perform the medical assistant's duties.
- Some employers require the credential prior to hiring or within a few months after hiring.
- Some employers will pay more if a person has achieved a medical assistant credential.

There are several national agencies that will provide credentials to medical assistants upon successful completion of their exam. Table 15.7 presents some of the more common medical assistant credentials. It is

TABLE 15.7 Credentialing Agencies for Medical Assistants

Agency/Website	Credential	Recertification Methods
American Association of Medical Assistants (AAMA) http://www.aama-ntl.org	Certified Medical Assistant (CMA [AAMA])	Recertify every 5 years either by exam or by earning 60 continuing education points. Specific points must be achieved in the three content areas. At least 30 points must be from AAMA-approved continuing education units (CEUs).
American Medical Technologist (AMT) https://www.americanmedtech.org	Registered Medical Assistant (RMA)	Recertify every 3 years either by exam or by completing specific activities.
National Healthcareer Association (NHA) https://www.nhanow.com	Clinical Medical Assistant (CCMA) Medical Administrative Assistant (CMAA)	Recertify every 2 years either by exam or by earning 10 continuing education credits.
National Center for Competency Testing (NCCT) https://www.ncctinc.com	Medical Assistant (NCMA)	Recertify every year either by exam or by completing 14 contact hours of continuing education.

important for graduating medical assistants to research whether credentials are preferred or required by the local employers. It is also important to identify which credential is most wanted by local employers. Your instructors are also excellent resources if you have additional questions on credentials for medical assistants.

Barriers to Professionalism

At times it is not easy to be a professional. Sometimes patients and coworkers try our patience. It can be difficult to maintain a professional attitude in these cases. Some of the obstructions to professional behavior are discussed in this section.

Personal Problems and "Baggage". We all have a personal life. Sometimes things happen in our lives before we go to work. It is important that we push these issues aside and focus on our job. If we carry this "baggage" to work, it can interfere with our ability to do our job. We may be tempted to make personal calls, check emails, and so on. This takes time away from our job, and our focus is not on our job. If the "baggage" is so important and concerning, the medical assistant needs to speak with the supervisor. It might not be appropriate to be working, if one cannot concentrate on the job at hand. The patient must be the prime concern of all the employees in the healthcare facility.

Gossip. *Gossip* is casual or idle chat (rumors) about other people and their business. Many times, the "discussion" is based on someone's opinion and not fact. Most people enjoy working in an environment in which employees cooperate and get along with each other. Rumors and gossip can cause problems with employee morale. They can affect how a team functions. A medical assistant should refuse to participate in the rumor mill (Fig. 15.3). Attempting to be cordial and friendly to everyone at work is important. Supervisors regard those who gossip or spread rumors as unprofessional and untrustworthy. You should always avoid passing along work-related rumors to patients and family members.

Personal Communication. Making personal phone calls and checking personal emails should not be done during work time. Only emergency calls can be taken. Many healthcare facilities require cell phones to be silenced and out of sight during the workday. Because most phones have cameras, facility administrators are concerned about unlawful pictures being taken. Many healthcare computer networks block certain nonhealthcare websites (e.g., social media sites). Table 15.8 describes acceptable and unacceptable activities for digital communication devices and online activities.

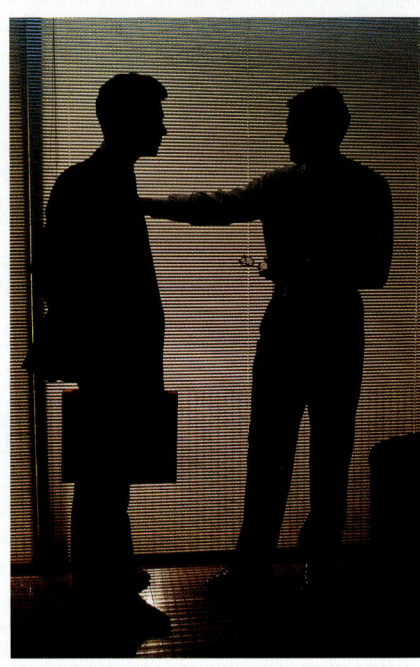

FIG. 15.3 Gossip and rumors have no place in the medical profession. Avoid employees who participate in this type of activity. (From Proctor D, Niedzwiecki B: *Kinn's the medical assistant*, ed 13, St Louis, 2017, Elsevier.)

> **CRITICAL THINKING 15.7**
>
> Christi loves her phone. But she learned very quickly that her phone was to be turned off and put away during work hours. Explain why having cell phones out and turned on can create issues in the healthcare facility.

NONVERBAL COMMUNICATION

Communication is the exchange of information, feelings, and thoughts between two or more people using spoken words or other methods. What we say and how we say something directly affects how the other person perceives the message. It is important to communicate effectively. We need to communicate in a manner that is clear, concise, and easy to understand. This helps the message to be understood by the other person.

TABLE 15.8 Using Digital Communication Devices and Online Activities in Healthcare Facilities

	Acceptable, Professional	Unacceptable, Unprofessional
Phone calls/text messages	• Emergency calls only • Turn off or silence ringer • Make personal calls only on break time	• Frequent checking for calls received • Making personal calls • Have phone out and visible when working with patients • Taking pictures
Personal emails and social media	• Do not open, read, or post	• Sending and reading personal emails • Viewing social media postings
Online	• Work-related web-related activity	• Shopping, gaming, nonwork websites

Nonverbal communication includes body language and expressive behaviors. More communication occurs nonverbally than verbally. Experts agree that nonverbal communication greatly exceeds verbal communication. It is important that the verbal communication match the perceived nonverbal message.

Think of a time when you were talking with a person, and that person did something that left a greater impression on you than the verbal message did. Nonverbal communication is powerful. In healthcare, we use nonverbal communication to show acceptance and understanding. We want to appear positive and open with others. In turn, we read others' nonverbal behaviors as we interpret what is being said. Table 15.9 describes both positive and negative nonverbal behaviors.

> **VOCABULARY**
> **poised:** Having a confident composure.

Physical Boundaries

Besides the nonverbal behaviors listed in Table 15.9, we need to discuss the importance of personal space and physical boundaries. We all have a personal space, or "bubble," around us. We may be uncomfortable and on guard if someone we don't know well gets into our personal

TABLE 15.9 Positive and Negative Nonverbal Behaviors

Nonverbal Behaviors	Positive and Open	Negative and Closed (Interpreted as or Means)
Position	Be at the level of the other person; angled toward the other person (Fig. 15.4)	Being at a higher level (looking down on the person); leaning backward (disinterest); direct face to face (confrontational, intimate)
Arms	Arms at the side	Arms are crossed (discomfort, defensive, disagree); hands behind back (secretive, mistrustful); clenched fists (anger, aggressive)
Posture	Poised	Poor or slumped posture (poor self-worth, lack of confidence, unwillingness, lack of interest, less knowledgeable, unreliable); stiff, immobile (uncomfortable)
Facial expression	Smile	Rolling eyes, yawning (boredom); frowning (sadness, disagree, anger) (Fig. 15.5)
Gestures	Small gestures	Overuse of hands (nervousness, excitement)
Touch	Light touch on hand, appropriate touch	Inappropriate touching or hugging (makes the person feel uncomfortable or violated)
Eye contact	Movement of eyes, blinking	Staring at the person (makes it awkward); avoiding eye contact (low-self-esteem, low confidence, and dishonesty)
Mannerisms	Focus on person; do not fidget or be impatient	Looking at watch, phone, or clock (bored, anxious, impatient)

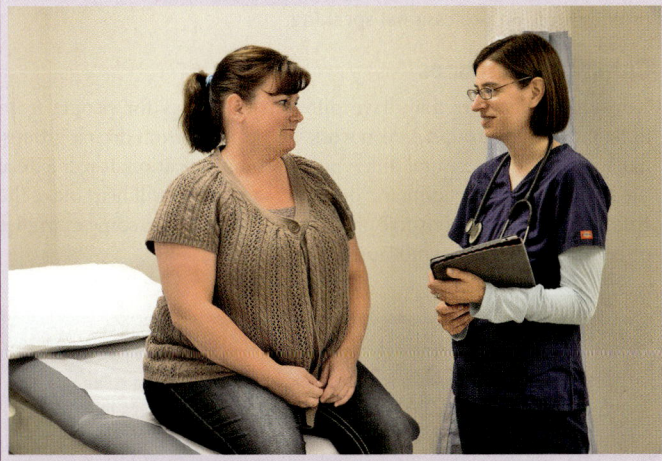

FIG 15.4 The medical assistant's position should be at the level of the patient. (From Proctor D, Niedzwiecki B: *Kinn's the medical assistant,* ed 13, St Louis, 2017, Elsevier.)

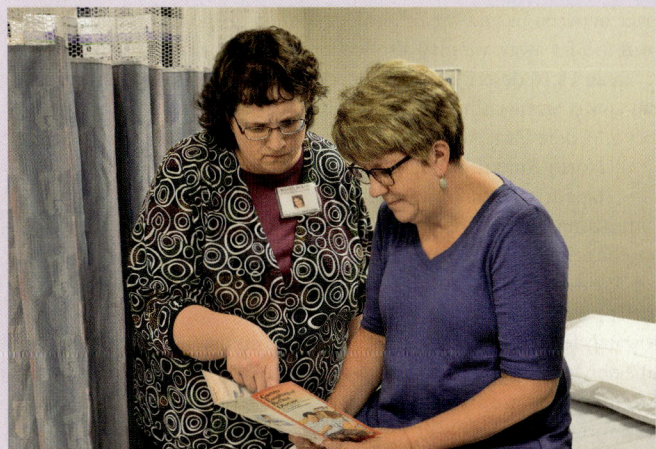

FIG 15.5 Frowning can be interpreted in many ways.

TABLE 15.10 Different Types of Space

Space	Distance	Personal Life	Healthcare
Intimate or personal	0–1.5 feet	Used with close family and friends; intimacy, hugs	Used for procedures, personal care; electrocardiograms (ECGs), wound care, vital signs
Casual person	1.5–4 feet	Used with conversations with friends, minimal touching	Used when talking with patients (e.g., history taking)
Social-business	4–12 feet	Used in business transactions, socializing with acquaintances	Used for business tasks (e.g., reception desk, billing questions)
Public space	>12 feet	Used in activities in public	Used with group events

TABLE 15.11 Nonverbal Communication Delivery Factors

Nonverbal Delivery Factors	Definition	Professional Tips
Rate	Refers to the speed at which the speaker talks	Use a moderate rate. If the rate is too fast, the message may be missed. If the rate is too slow, it may be perceived as more negative by the receiver.
Clarity	Refers to the quality of the voice	Use a clear voice when talking with others. Muffled, mumbling, or unclear speech can create inaccuracies with the message.
Volume	Refers to the loudness of the speaker's voice	Use a moderate volume. If too loud, it may be perceived as yelling, and if too soft, the message may be missed. In healthcare, we need to keep information confidential. So using a loud voice can violate the patient's privacy.
Pitch	Refers to the highness and lowness of the voice	Using a varying pitch, or inflections, helps a person to emphasize important points. It is important to have a rhythm in your voice to help the receiver understand what is important.
Tone	Refers to the emotion in the voice	Use an accepting or a neutral tone in healthcare. An angry tone can cause the receiver to misinterpret the message and/or also become angry.
Pauses	Refers to a period of not talking	Using pauses helps the receiver absorb the message. Limit verbalized pauses (e.g., "ah," "umm," and "er").
Intonation	Refers to the melodic pattern or the pitch variation	With statements, we usually use a medium intonation and finish the sentence on a lower pitch. Finishing the statement on a higher pitch usually indicates a question. Using correct intonation will help the correct message to be received.
Vocabulary	Refers to the word choice used	Using precise words helps the message to be correctly received. Incorrect use of words may create a negative impression of the speaker. It is important to use words that the receiver understands. If medical terminology, slang, or generational terms are used, the message may not be understood.
Grammatical structure	Refers to the sentence structure	Using incorrect grammatical sentence structure can create a negative impression of the speaker.
Pronunciation	Refers to how the word is said	Using the correct pronunciation will help ensure the correct message will be received. Incorrect pronunciation of a word (e.g., medication name) may lead to inaccuracies with the message.

space. We may take a step back or move back in a chair to increase the space between us and the other person. If someone is communicating from too far away, we may also feel uncomfortable.

Table 15.10 describes the different types of spaces and how we use that space. Some cultures have different casual personal distances:
- Middle East: About 1 foot
- North American and Western European: About 1.5 feet
- Japanese culture: About 3 feet

It is important to realize that as healthcare professionals, we move into the personal or intimate space of patients many times while providing care. We need to respect this space. We need to be aware of our grooming, our appearance, and our habits. When working with others, we need to watch for clues regarding the person's comfort level with distance. A person who needs more space may move backward. Leaning, shifting, or moving forward shows the person wants to decrease the distance. It is important to recognize the physical space boundaries.

Nonverbal Communication Delivery Factors

Nonverbal communication delivery factors include how the message was delivered by the sender. This helps create the context of the message. Table 15.11 lists the nonverbal communication delivery factors and provides tips on professional speaking.

Cultural Differences

Nonverbal behaviors may have different meanings for people from different cultural groups. As you work with patients from diverse groups, make sure to learn cultural differences in communication. It will reduce the likelihood of offending the other person. It also will help make the patient's experience a positive one. Table 15.12 provides some examples of cultural differences with nonverbal behaviors.

CRITICAL THINKING 15.8

Christi had heard that people from the Hmong and Vietnamese culture do not like others commenting on their children. They fear the words might be overheard by a spirit who might try to harm the children. Christi mentioned this to a coworker. The coworker doesn't believe in this. Do they need to worry about belief when working with patients from the Hmong and Vietnamese culture? Explain your answer.

CHAPTER 15 Professionalism in Healthcare

TABLE 15.12 Cultural Differences in Nonverbal Behaviors

Nonverbal Behaviors	Cultural Differences
Eye contact	Hispanics, Asians, Native Americans, and Middle Easterners: eye contact is considered rude and offensive. Females: may avoid eye contact with males so it is not perceived as a sign of sexual interest.
Touch	Asians and Middle Easterners: the head is a sacred part of the body; it is considered offensive to pat the head. Middle Easterners: left hand is reserved for bodily hygiene; it is inappropriate to use that hand to touch others or transfer objects. Muslims: inappropriate to touch a person of the opposite gender. Latin Americans and Eastern Europeans: very comfortable with touching others, even new acquaintances.

Gestures	Some cultures:
	    Using the "come here" finger/hand gesture is used with dogs and considered offensive.
	    Pointing with one finger is considered very rude.
	Asians and Indians: use the whole hand to point at something or someone.
	Venezuelans: use their lips to point; finger pointing is impolite.

Winking	Some Latin American cultures consider winking a romantic or a sexual invitation. Nigerians wink at children to indicate they should leave the room. Chinese consider winking rude.
Posture	Many cultures: consider poor posture disrespectful.
Personal space	Latin Americans and Middle Easterners stand quite close to those they don't know. Muslim males (even providers) cannot be too close to females.

If you are interacting with a person from another cultural group, and you are unfamiliar with it, try following these tips:
- Follow the other person's lead in terms of nonverbal behaviors and personal space.
- Use gestures cautiously.
- Remember that facial expressions can be misinterpreted (e.g., grimacing with pain may not be acceptable in some cultures, whereas other cultures "encourage" it).
- Lack of eye contact maybe be related to nervousness or the culture. It is not due to fear or dishonesty.

VERBAL COMMUNICATION

Verbal communication can be defined as words used either orally or in written form. Medical assistants use verbal communication all the time. We will explore the process of communication. Written and oral communication will be discussed.

Communication Cycle

The communication cycle is a way to describe the communication process (Fig. 15.6). A breakdown of any part of the cycle can lead to a message being misunderstood. The communication cycle proceeds as follows:
- **Sender creates the MESSAGE:** The person with a message is called the *sender*. The sender must organize his or her thoughts and communicate a clear, concise, easy to understand message.
- **Receiver DECODES the message:** The person getting the message is the *receiver*. This person must decode or translate the message based on personal factors and subjective perceptions. If the message was correctly translated within the context of the message sent, then it matches the message the sender sent. If the message was incorrectly translated, then the receiver develops a different perception of the message than what the sender intended.
- **Receiver creates FEEDBACK:** The receiver then provides feedback based on the perceived message.
- **Sender DECODES feedback:** The sender gets the feedback message. Again, the feedback must be decoded correctly for the communication to be accurate

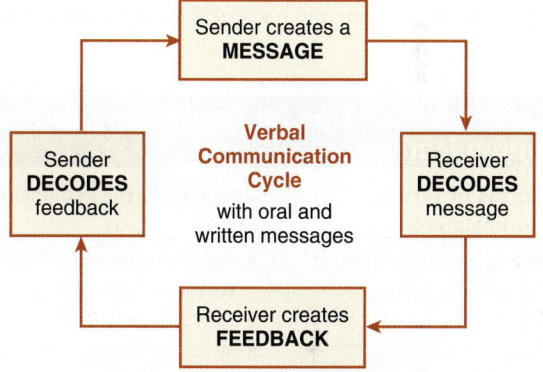

FIG. 15.6 Verbal communication cycle.

As indicated in Fig. 15.6, the verbal communication cycle exists with written and oral messages. We will exam both types of verbal communication.

Written Communication

Written communication is a type of verbal communication. We create written messages for the receiver. Written communication includes:
- Written messages (e.g., phone messages)
- Letters and emails
- Online information and media (e.g., informational flyer)

Table 15.13 provides tips for composing written communication. Chapter 21 provides additional information on composing professional letters and emails.

Oral Communication

Oral communication is a type of verbal communication. Oral communication means we talk with others and we listen to others. In the ambulatory care environment, oral communication occurs in person, over the phone, and using remote devices (e.g., webcams).

Styles of Oral Communication. Besides the types of communication, we need to discuss the styles of communication. How a person

communicates affects his or her interaction with another person. There are five main styles of communication.
- *Passive communicators*: Avoid expressing feelings or opinions, fail to exert themselves, allow others to infringe on their rights, and tend to speak softly. They may feel depressed, resentful, or anxious because life seems out of their control.
- *Aggressive communicators*: Try to dominate others; have low frustration tolerance, criticize and attack others, have poor listening skills, and use "you" statements. This can cause them to be alienated or feared by others.
- *Passive-aggressive communicators*: Deny problems; do not confront problems or people, appear to be cooperative, but plan subtle sabotage or disruptions. They may become alienated from others and feel powerless.
- *Manipulative communicators*: Cunning and controlling of others. Use others to get what they want. Can cause others to feel sorry for them or guilty.
- *Assertive communicators*: Clearly state their needs and wants. They use "I" statements and listen without interrupting. They are relaxed, use good eye contact, feel connected with others, and stand up for their rights. They feel in control of their lives and are mature enough to address issues.

It is important that healthcare professionals understand each type. We should also evaluate our own communication style. What style do we use? Identifying how you communicate is an important part of your professionalism journey. A healthcare professional needs to communicate in an assertive manner. This is the healthy form of communication. It leads to better team dynamics.

As you learn about these styles, think about the people you interact with. How do they communicate? How do you feel when you interact with them? Table 15.14 reviews the nonverbal communication behaviors for each communication style. It also identifies common feelings others may have when interacting with such a person.

CRITICAL THINKING 15.9
Of the five communication styles, which one should Christi use at work? Explain your answer.

Therapeutic Communication

Therapeutic communication is a process of communicating with patients and family members in healthcare. It is an interactive relationship that conveys acceptance and respect without judging or blaming. It encourages healthcare professionals to build **rapport** (ra PORE) with patients. When that bond develops and grows, patients are more comfortable when expressing their feelings, ideas, and concerns. Thus, therapeutic communication techniques are helpful in building the relationship with the patient. Active listening and other therapeutic communication techniques will be described in the following sections.

VOCABULARY
rapport: A relationship of harmony and accord between the patient and the healthcare professional.

Active Listening. Active listening is the most important therapeutic communication technique. This skill takes time to master. Active listening means we fully concentrate on what is being said and how it is said. This is different from passively hearing what the speaker is saying and being distracted by our own thoughts.

When a person is actively listening, the speaker can easily see it. The listener shows interest by verbal messages, such as "Yes." The listener also shows interest through nonverbal messages. As discussed earlier, nonverbal messages include eye contact, nodding your head, body position, and facial features (Fig. 15.7). Box 15.3 lists characteristics of a good listener. Showing interest at this level will encourage the speaker to be more at ease. Communication between the two people will be more open, honest, and clear.

TABLE 15.13 Tips for Composing Written Communication

All Forms of Written Communication	Specifically for Professional Emails
• Draft the message and then read what you have written. Make sure the message is clear, concise, easy to understand, and provides the message you intended. • Check the grammar, spelling, punctuation, and sentence structure. • Make sure to address the message to the correct receiver.	• Add a few meaningful words in the subject line. • Start with a courteous greeting. • Write out all words. • Write in complete sentences. Capitalize the first letter of the first word and end the statement with the correct punctuation. • Do not use all-capital letters. It is viewed as shouting at the receiver.

TABLE 15.14 Communication Styles

Communication Style	Nonverbal Communication Behaviors	Others' Feelings with this Behavior
Passive	Soft voice, head down, fidgets, no eye contact. "Victim mentality."	Exasperated and frustrated. Feel they can take advantage of the person.
Aggressive	Low voice; big, sharp, and fast gestures. Glare and frown. Invade others' personal space intentionally.	Hurt, fearful, afraid, humiliated, and resentful. Loss of respect for the person.
Passive-aggressive	Sugary sweet voice and often look sweet and innocent. Often in others' personal space and touch others to pretend to be warm and friendly.	Confused, angry, and hurtful with the "two-faced" personality of the person.
Manipulative	Patronizing voice, uses high pitch.	Angry, resentful, guilty, and frustrated with being manipulated.
Assertive	Medium pitch, speed, and volume of voice; good eye contact. Open posture and respectful of others.	Can trust individual. Know the person can handle criticism and accept compliments.

Other Therapeutic Communication Techniques. When you are working with patients and family members, several therapeutic communication techniques can be used. It is critical that we understand the message correctly. We need to make sure patients know we are listening. We also need to check that we understand the message. Assuming what someone means or feels can lead to miscommunication. Therapeutic communication techniques are detailed in Table 15.15.

Barriers to Communication

Effective communication is critical for compassionate, quality patient care. Medical assistants must understand barriers that prevent patients from understanding communication or communicating clearly with others. Taking steps to overcome these barriers will help promote effective communication. Table 15.16 discusses common barriers and ways to overcome barriers.

Overcoming communication barriers is more than just providing great patient care. Healthcare providers are legally required to provide ways to overcome communication barriers. This legal requirement comes from:

- Civil Rights Act: All providers that accept federal funds for the healthcare provided must ensure equal access to services.
- Americans with Disabilities Act (ADA): All healthcare providers must provide free effective communication to patients (and companions) with disabilities.
- Americans with Disabilities Act Amendments Act (ADAAA): Expanded the definition of disabilities established in the ADA.

Ways that providers can meet their federal obligations for accommodating patients with communication disabilities include:

- Provide a qualified medical interpreter free of charge to the patient. This can be done by having an interpreter available to the patient or by using online interpretation services during the visit. The interpreter may be present for the visit, available over the phone, or via videoconferencing. Table 15.17 describes types of interpreters used in healthcare.
- Informational and educational materials should be translated into the primary languages of the patients seen in the ambulatory care facility.
- Provide large-print materials.
- Write out instructions.

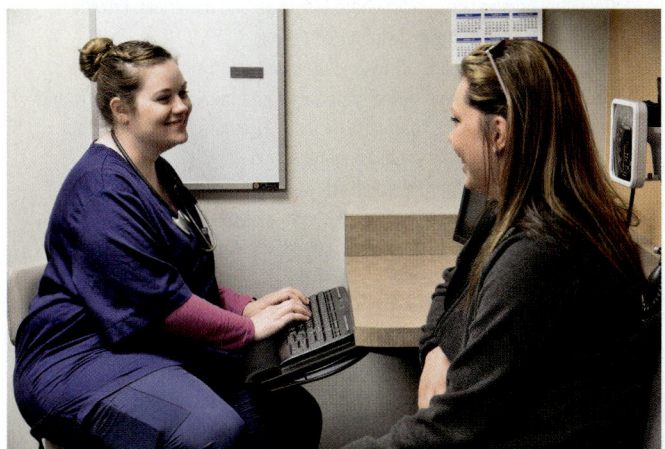

FIG. 15.7 Nonverbal communication (e.g., eye contact and a smile) is important when working with patients. (From Proctor D, Niedzwiecki B: *Kinn's the medical assistant*, ed 13, St Louis, 2017, Elsevier.)

Age and Disease Status Barriers. Besides the barriers listed in Table 15.16, the person's age and disease status may be barriers to communication. Let's first examine the barriers related to age. We communicate differently with a 3-year-old child than with a 30-year-old adult. Understanding the developmental stages will help us as we interact with others.

Erik Erikson, a psychoanalyst, described the emotional, physical, and psychological stages of human development. He stated that a person in each stage had a specific development task to complete. Understanding the task or goal of each stage helps healthcare professionals communicate more effectively with patients. Table 15.18 presents the developmental stages, goals of each stage, and communication tips for healthcare professionals.

BOX 15.3 Characteristics of a Good Listener

- Remain nonjudgmental and neutral.
- Refrain from interrupting with a comment or question.
- Allow for periods of silence.
- Smile and nod your head to show you are listening to the message.
- Use appropriate eye contact so the speaker is not intimidated.
- Lean slightly forward or sideways toward the speaker.
- Avoid distractions (e.g., fidgeting, looking at the clock, doodling).

TABLE 15.15 Therapeutic Communication Techniques

Techniques	Definition	Feedback to Speaker
Reflection	Putting words to the person's emotional reaction, which acknowledges the person's feelings. Also helps to check what the person is feeling instead of just assuming. Shows **empathy** and helps build **rapport**.	Reflect what you think was said. For example: "It sounds like you are feeling scared…" or "I understand you are having trouble with…" or "You feel that…"
Restatement or paraphrasing	Rewording or rephrasing a statement to check the meaning and interpretation. Also shows you are listening and understanding the speaker.	Don't repeat the person's exact words. Use phrases such as, "What I'm hearing is…" or "It sounds like you are saying…" Refrain from using "I know what you mean."
Neutral	Encourages the speaker to continue and conveys you are interested and listening to the message.	Use phrases like: "Uh huh," "I see," "That is very interesting."
Silence	Allows time to gather thoughts and answer questions.	Can be uncomfortable to some people. Allows time to think about what was said.
Clarification	Allows the listener to get additional information.	Using statements such as, "Can you clarify…" and "Do you mean…"
Summarizing	Allows the listener to recap and review what was said.	Using a statement such as, "If I understand how you feel about this situation…"

TABLE 15.16 Barriers to Communication and Ways to Overcome the Barriers

Type of Barrier	Patient Barriers	Ways to Overcome Barriers
Environmental distractions	Noise, lack of privacy, temperature	Provide privacy for patients. Talk with patients in a quiet room with the door closed. Make sure the room temperature is comfortable.
Internal distractions	Hunger, pain, anger, tiredness	Help make the patient comfortable. Provide food and drink if available. Administer pain medications as ordered.
Visually impaired	Unable to see written communication	Use audio recordings, screen magnifiers, large-print materials, and screen reader software.
Hearing impaired	Unable to hear verbal communication	Use print materials and written instructions. Use videos with captions. Have text telephones (TTYs) available. Use a sign language interpreter.
Intellectual disability	Unable to understand what is being said; may be functioning at a lower age level	Use "functioning age"–appropriate language and materials. Provide information also to the guardian/caregiver.
Illiterate	Unable to read or write	Use pictures and models. Draw pictures and using simple language.
Non-English speaking	English is not the patient's primary language; lack of understanding of medical terminology	Use translators and translated materials. Limit medical terminology and define medical terms that must be used. Use culturally appropriate materials and visuals (pictures, graphs, and models).
Emotional distractions	Fear and anxiety related to being judged by the healthcare professional; inability to explain personal feelings; angry or distraught patients may not hear what is said or may not be able to communicate effectively	Provide a warm, caring environment. Make sure your body language (nonverbal behaviors) is consistent with an open, caring manner. Gain the person's trust. Keep voice at normal level; raising voice can increase the person's anger (Fig. 15.8)

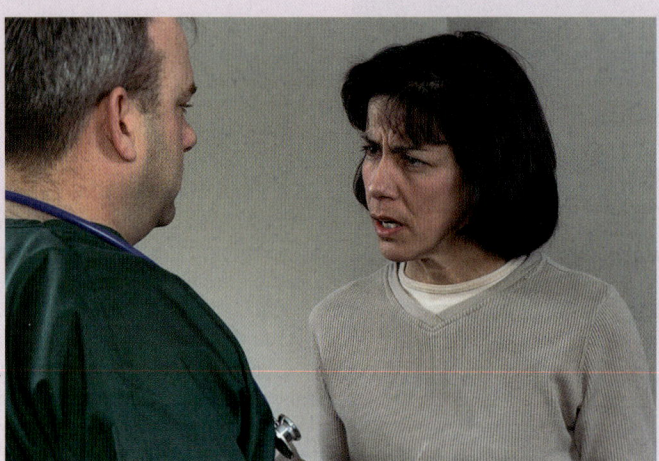

FIG 15.8 Remain calm, even if a patient becomes verbally aggressive. Attempt to calm the person by listening and expressing empathy whenever possible. (From Proctor D, Niedzwiecki B: *Kinn's the medical assistant*, ed 13, St Louis, 2017, Elsevier.)

TABLE 15.17 Types of Interpreters

Type	Description
Sign language interpreter	Uses American Sign Language or Signed English.
Oral interpreter	Silently mouths speech to the hearing-impaired patient. Uses gestures.
Cued-speech interpreter	Does everything an oral interpreter does. Also uses a hand code to stand for each speech sound.
Qualified medical interpreter	Interprets between the healthcare provider and the non-English or limited English speaking patient. (Using a family member to interpret can be risky, because the message may be changed. There is no guarantee the family member is translating exactly what the provider states.)

A person's disease status also can affect communication. For instance, think about these scenarios:
- Jim was just notified by his provider that he may only have 3 months to live. Jim has been healthy until the last few weeks, when he started to feel very ill.
- Rose was just informed that she has diabetes mellitus. She needs to take medication, change her diet, and exercise.

If you were Jim or Rose, how would you feel? Could you understand and remember a lot of new information after hearing the diagnosis? Could you even converse normally with others or would you be "blown away"? Would you deny the diagnosis?

Elizabeth Kübler-Ross studied people's reactions to dying. She found that people experienced similar stages as they came to terms with the situation. Over the years, these stages have been applied to grief. They

TABLE 15.18 Erikson's Psychosocial Development Stages

Erikson's Psychosocial Development Stages	Goals of Stage	Communication Tips
Trust versus Mistrust (age range: 0–1.5 years [infancy])	Must develop trust, with the ability to mistrust should the need arise.	Use calm, soothing voice, hold child securely. Loud voices and noises can startle child.
Autonomy versus Shame and Doubt (age range: 1.5–3 years [toddler])	Must explore and manipulate things in their "world" to develop autonomy and self-esteem.	Use simple language. Allow child to touch and explore objects. Allow child to play and make choices.
Initiative versus Guilt (age range: 3–6 years [preschool])	Encouraged to try new activities. Must assume responsibilities and learn new skills. Will make child feel purposeful and increase self-esteem.	Use short, simple sentences. Encourage questions. Use imitation, play, and role-playing.
Industry versus Inferiority (age range: 6–12 years [school age])	Must seek to finish tasks. Recognition for accomplishments is important.	Use engaging simple tools to communicate information (DVDs, gaming software, pamphlets). Encourage discussion and questions.
Identity versus Role Confusion (age range: 12–18 years [adolescence])	To know who you are as a person and how you fit into the world around you. Creates a meaningful self-image.	Provide privacy and independence. Encourage responsible decision making. Encourage discussion and questions.
Intimacy versus Isolation (age range: 18–25 years [young adult])	Can vary. Develops friendships; takes on commitments.	Identify motivating factors and use them as needed during communication. Realize person may be juggling a lot of obligations.
Generativity versus Stagnation (age range: about 25–60 years [middle adulthood])	Achieve a balance between the concern for the next generation (having a family) and being self-absorbed.	
Ego Integrity versus Despair (age range: 60 and older [late adulthood])	Reflect on one's life and come to terms with it, instead of regretting the past.	Communicate with dignity and respect. Limit slang and "generational" terms. Use simpler language. Speak clearly. Allow time to respond.

TABLE 15.19 Stages of Grief and Dying

Stage	Description
Denial	Refuses to accept the fact (e.g., diagnosis or prognosis). Defense mechanism that allows the person to ignore what is happening.
Anger	Can be directed at self or others.
Bargaining	Attempts to bargain with the higher power the person believes in (e.g., God).
Depression	Feels sad, fearful, and uncertain. May not participate in normal activities. Distances self from others.
Acceptance	Has come to terms with situation.

can relate to patients who are informed of a chronic or terminal illness. Family and friends of the ill person can also experience these stages. Not everyone progresses through the stages at the same time, nor does everyone get to the final stage. Table 15.19 describes the stages of grief and dying.

When you are communicating with those with a terminal or chronic illness, it is important to understand that they are working through these stages. Remember, the emotions they display may not be related to you. They may be related to the grief the patient is dealing with. For instance, a terminally ill patient yells at the receptionist. He is upset about his wait time, although it was under 5 minutes. His emotions may relate more to his stage of grieving than to his wait time. It is important that we provide a supportive accepting, environment. We should be empathetic to these patients.

UNDERSTANDING BEHAVIOR

Throughout this chapter, we have discussed professional behaviors and the appropriate way a medical assistant should behave. As healthcare professionals, it is important we understand why our patients and peers behave the way they do. Why do they make the choices they make? What is important to them? Many times, their behaviors relate to their needs, defense mechanisms, and coping skills. By understanding these factors, we can interact more effectively with others.

Maslow's Hierarchy of Needs

In 1943 psychologist Abraham Maslow proposed the **hierarchy** of needs. This is a motivational theory that depicts five levels of needs. Years later, he expanded the theory to include eight levels of needs. Maslow believed that our human needs can be categorized into these eight levels. Each level must be satisfied before we can move up to the next level. These levels are often depicted as a triangle (Fig. 15.9).

The "Deficiency" needs consist of the four bottom levels. They are considered the coping behaviors. We must fulfill these needs to cope with life and survival. We all have similar needs, but when they are not met, it motivates us to get them met. Fulfillment of these needs leads to instant short-term gratification. For example, when we are thirsty, we find water to drink. We are satisfied for the moment but will be thirsty a short time later.

The top four levels are "Growth" needs. These levels relate to making ourselves a better person or being all that we can be. Achieving these levels brings long-lasting happiness. The happiness is more meaningful than the gratification achieved from meeting the lower level needs.

> **VOCABULARY**
> **hierarchy**: Things arranged in order or rank.

Let's review the needs, starting at the bottom and working toward the top level.
1. **Physiological needs**: These include air, food, drink, shelter, warmth, oxygen, sleep, and so on. We need these things to survive. For instance, when we are hungry, we look for food.

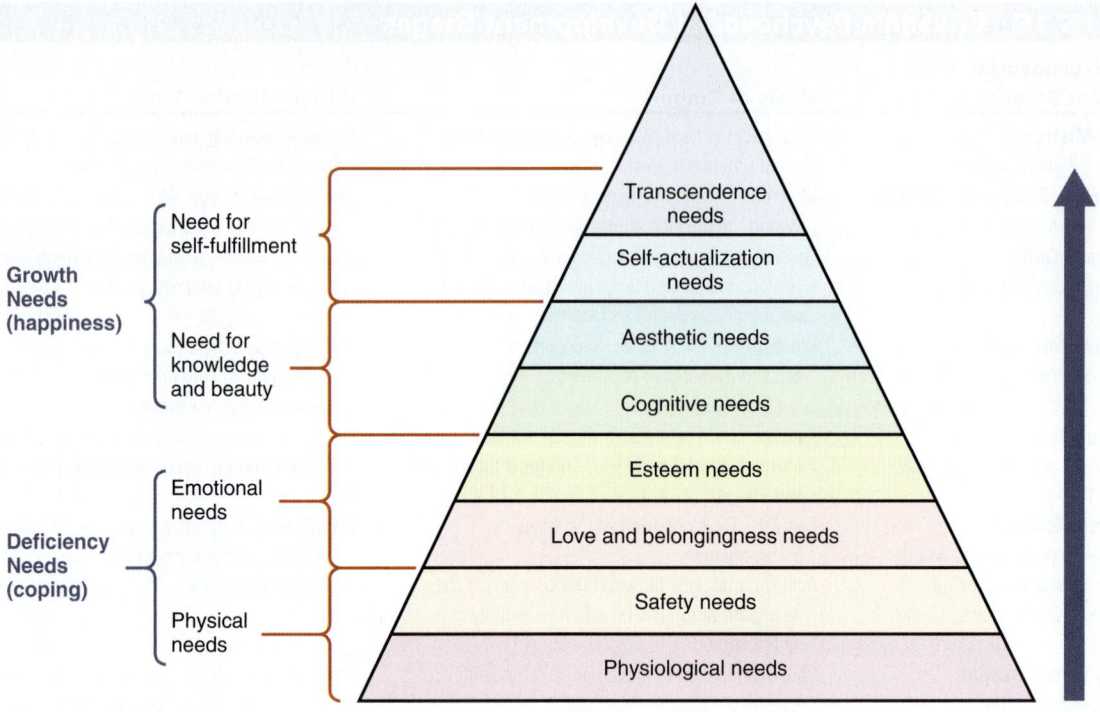

FIG. 15.9 Maslow's Hierarchy of Needs.

2. **Safety needs**: These include protection from the elements, security, order, law, stability, and so forth. These needs relate to keeping us safe and secure. Unmet safety needs can lead to fear, stress, and anxiety. Some examples of meeting safety needs include:
   - Staying in a job that one really dislikes for the security of the paycheck
   - Staying in an abusive relationship, because it is familiar
   - Getting the brakes on your car fixed
3. **Love and belongingness needs**: These include friendship, intimacy, acceptance in a group, and receiving and giving affection and love. We need to be accepted by others. Unmet needs in this level can lead to feelings of isolation, loneliness, and depression. A person may feel anxious about going out in social situations if this need is not met.
4. **Esteem needs**: These include our self-esteem, achievement, mastery of skills, independence, status, prestige, and so on. Our needs relate to our reputation and what we think of ourselves. It's important to remember the saying, "People who matter don't judge, people who judge don't matter." The only thing we have total control over is what we think of ourselves. Some examples of how people attempt to meet this level include:
   - Buying the latest electronic devices to "show off" to others
   - Fishing for complements
   - Cutting down others to make oneself feel better
5. **Cognitive needs**: These include knowledge, curiosity, understanding, and exploration. We are driven to learn more about something.
6. **Aesthetic needs**: We appreciate and search for beauty, balance, symmetry, form, etc. Some people find true happiness when they create music, paint a picture, take a picture, or explore nature. Think of how relaxing it is to be at a beach, enjoying the sound of the water and the feeling of nature.
7. **Self-actualization needs**: We need to realize our potential, seek self-fulfillment, and experience personal growth.
8. **Transcendence needs**: We meet these by helping others achieve their very best, or self-actualization. This requires that we give of our time and talent to help others meet their needs.

Maslow believed that only a few people ever achieve the top levels of the hierarchy. He believed that when people did something bad (e.g., steal, put others down), they were motivated to meet their own needs. The method used to meet needs could be unhealthy or dysfunctional. It is important for medical assistants to realize that people meet their own needs in different ways. Their ways may be different and wrong by our standards. We still need to respect our patients and provide the best possible care.

Defense Mechanisms

Defense mechanisms are unconscious mental processes that protect people from anxiety, loss, conflict, or shame. We use defense mechanisms and so do our patients and peers. People use defense mechanisms to protect themselves from situations or information they cannot manage psychologically.

Defense mechanisms may hide a variety of thoughts or feelings, including anger, fear, sadness, despair, and helplessness. A patient who uses defense mechanisms can be very difficult to deal with. If medical assistants are aware of a patient's needs for psychological protection, they may be able to find a way to provide excellent care for the patient. There are many types of defense mechanisms. Table 15.20 describes several of the more common behaviors using patient and peer situations.

Coping Mechanisms

Stress is a condition that causes physical and/or emotional tension. Stress can be positive (e.g., learning a new job) or negative (e.g., dealing with a love one's terminal illness). We use coping mechanisms when we are stressed. *Coping mechanisms* are behavioral and psychological strategies used to deal with or minimize stressful events. Two types include:

TABLE 15.20 Common Defense Mechanisms

Defense Mechanism	Description	Example
Denial	The person completely rejects the information.	"I couldn't possibly have breast cancer. You must be mistaken."
Repression	The person simply forgets something that is bad or hurtful.	"I wasn't driving the car that killed my best friend."
Regression	The person reverts to an old, usually immature behavior to express her feelings.	Perhaps instead of discussing the diagnosis and the need for treatment, she just storms out of the room and slams the door shut.
Displacement	The person transfers the emotion toward one person to another person or thing.	After being reprimanded by her supervisor, the person goes home and screams at her children.
Projection	The person accuses someone else of having the feelings that he or she has.	A patient is angry about the diagnosis. She may say, "You don't have to lose your temper about this," even though the medical assistant's demeanor is completely professional.
Suppression	The person is consciously aware of the information or feeling but refuses to admit it.	"I don't think the test is accurate. My mammograms are always normal."
Splitting	The person views another person as all bad or all good and not a mixture of good and bad traits.	An abused patient may say, "He is a good husband and father."
Reaction formation	The person expresses his feelings as the opposite of what he really feels.	A patient is angry at the medical assistant for insisting that a biopsy be scheduled. He expresses the opposite emotion: "I appreciate your trying to help me, but I just can't come to the hospital that day."
Rationalization	The person comes up with various explanations to justify her response.	"I think the results are wrong. I didn't follow the directions for the tests like I should have, and besides, there's no history of breast cancer in my family."

- Adaptive (healthy) coping mechanisms: Improve our functioning level and reduce our stress level.
- Maladaptive (unhealthy) coping mechanisms: Reduce the feelings associated with stress for a short time, but they do not decrease the actual stressor and can lead to future problems.

Table 15.21 lists the adaptive and maladaptive coping mechanisms. Understanding the different types of coping mechanisms is important in our own lives and in our role as a healthcare professional. We may have times when we are stressed and tend to use more maladaptive coping mechanisms. It's important for our health and wellbeing to use more adaptive strategies. Our patients and coworkers are not immune to stress. They will also be using different coping mechanisms. Our role is to encourage the use of healthy coping mechanisms and provide resources for these strategies.

TABLE 15.21 Adaptive and Maladaptive Coping Mechanisms

Adaptive Coping Mechanisms	Maladaptive Coping Mechanisms
- Eat healthy, well-balance meals - Exercise - Drink water - Get plenty of sleep - Take breaks when you feel stressed - Talk and share with others - Get help when you need it	- Hostility, aggression, manipulation - Recognition-seeking - Passive-aggressive behavior - Compliance, dependence - Social withdrawal, isolation - Denial, fantasy - Drugs and alcohol use - Gambling, shopping, risk-taking behaviors

CRITICAL THINKING 15.10

Christi is starting to exercise after work each night. She found that it helps her deal with the stress of the day. What coping mechanisms do you use when you are stressed? Are they adaptive or maladaptive coping mechanisms?

CLOSING COMMENTS

Providing exceptional customer service is a necessity for healthcare professionals. The medical assistant needs to remember that both coworkers and patients are customers. By being professional and communicating effectively, the medical assistant can provide great customer service to patients and coworkers.

Understanding other's behaviors and what influences behaviors can take time. It is important to evaluate our own behaviors. By understanding ourselves better, we may have an easier time becoming more professional and striving to make ourselves better!

EXCEPTIONAL CUSTOMER SERVICE

To provide exceptional customer service, medical assistants need to:
- Remember that patients, family members, and coworkers are all customers
- Be professional in behavior and appearance
- Consider cultural differences when using nonverbal communication
- Prepare clear, concise verbal communication (written and oral)
- Use therapeutic communication, including active listening

To help promote professionalism when you first meet a patient, it is important to GIVE:
- **G**reet the patient.
- **I**dentify yourself.
- **V**erify the patient's identity by asking for the person's full name and date of birth.
- **E**xplain the procedure to be performed in a manner that is understood by the patient.

CHAPTER REVIEW

Customer service is strongly linked to professionalism in the healthcare team. The professional medical assistant should be courteous, respectful, empathetic, compassionate, tactful, and diplomatic. It is important for the professional medical assistant to be respectful of individual diversity. Honesty, dependability, and responsibility are other important character traits. Professional appearance and being a true team member are important. A medical assistant's work ethic, punctuality, cooperation, and problem-solving skills are important to the healthcare team.

Communication is also an important aspect of customer service and professionalism. This chapter discussed the importance of nonverbal communication and cultural differences. Verbal communication includes written and oral communication. Verbal delivery factors and styles of oral communication are very important when working with peers and patients. Therapeutic communication is used in healthcare, and active listening is critical.

Maslow described what motivates people. His theory helps describe behaviors of individuals as they cope with the world or strive for happiness. Understanding defense and coping mechanisms commonly used by patients and coworkers is also important. Medical assistants need to be empathic and understanding while working with patients.

SCENARIO WRAP-UP

Christi is enjoying her orientation. She is nervous about her upcoming evaluation, but she knows that she is improving her professionalism. She is now arriving 10 to 15 minutes before the start time. That gives her time to put her things away and wash her hands before starting. She has no issues with the dress code. It is becoming a habit. In addition, she is learning some great communication techniques to use with patients.

Christi feels she is becoming more professional not only with the patients, but also with her team. She really wants to be the best medical assistant she can be. She wants to be dependable and trustworthy. She is already starting to read up on the Hmong and Mexican cultures, because a high percentage of her patients come from those two backgrounds. Christi is also studying to take her CMA (AAMA) exam. She is enjoying working at the clinic.

16

Legal Basics

LEARNING OBJECTIVES

1. Discuss the balance of power in the United States, including the three branches of government. Also, list and describe the four types of laws.
2. Compare criminal and civil law as they apply to the practicing medical assistant.
3. Discuss intentional torts, and define the following terms: negligence, malpractice, scope of practice, arbitration, mediation, deposition, subpoena. Also, describe the 4 Ds of negligence.
4. Discuss the different types of professional insurance.
5. Describe the patient-provider relationship, and define the following terms: patient incompetence, emancipated minor, mature minor, *respondeat superior*, and breach of contract.
6. Define the following medical legal terms related to consent: implied consent, expressed consent, and informed consent.
7. Summarize the Patient's Bill of Rights and apply it as it relates to: choice of treatment, consent for treatment, and refusal of treatment.
8. Discuss licensure, scope of practice, and disciplinary action as they apply to healthcare providers and practice requirements. Also, using an internet search, locate a medical assistant's legal scope of practice in a particular state.
9. Discuss certification, registration, and accreditation for medical assistants.

CHAPTER OUTLINE

1. **Opening Scenario, 361**
2. **You Will Learn, 362**
3. **Introduction to the Law, 362**
4. **Sources of Law, 362**
   a. Balance of Power, 362
   b. Types of Laws, 362
5. **Criminal and Civil Law, 362**
   a. Criminal Law, 362
   b. Civil Law, 363
6. **Tort Law, 363**
   a. Intentional Torts, 363
   b. Negligent Torts, 364
      i. Defenses to Liability, 366
      ii. Proving Malpractice, 366
      iii. Damages, 368
      iv. Professional Insurance, 368
7. **Contracts, 369**
   a. Provider-Patient Relationship, 370
   b. Breach of Contract, 370
8. **Consent, 371**
   a. Doctrine of Informed Consent, 371
9. **Patient's Bill of Rights, 372**
10. **Practice Requirements, 372**
    a. Practice Acts and State Boards, 377
       i. Licensure, 377
       ii. Scope of Practice, 377
       iii. Disciplinary Action, 377
    b. Certification and Registration, 378
    c. Accreditation, 378
11. **Closing Comments, 379**
12. **Chapter Review, 379**

▶ OPENING SCENARIO

Daniela Garcia was just hired as a part-time float receptionist at Walden-Martin Family Medical (WMFM) Clinic. As a float receptionist, she will be working with many different coworkers and providers. Besides working, Daniela is enrolled in a medical assistant program at the local community college. She is just starting a law and ethics course. The first part of the course explains legal concepts.

Daniela learned about the government in high school, but she has never been in a courtroom, nor witnessed court proceedings. Learning about law concepts is very different from her other courses. Many of her classmates didn't realize that medical assistants need to learn about legal concepts and laws. Daniela hopes that she can relate what she does in the clinic to what she is learning in her course. She finds concepts are easier to remember if she can apply them to real world situations.

Bella, a new certified medical assistant (CMA), has offered to help Daniela study for her law course. Bella stated that she enjoyed learning about law and its importance in healthcare. Daniela is considering asking her for help on their breaks. Studying with another person also helps her retain and understand the concepts.

UNIT 2 Professional Medical Assistant

YOU WILL LEARN

- To describe the different sources of law.
- To explain the differences between criminal and civil law.
- To describe intentional torts and negligent torts.
- To explain the requirements for a legal contract.
- To describe expressed, implied, and informed consent.
- To describe the difference between the provider's and the medical assistant's scope of practice and practice requirements.

INTRODUCTION TO THE LAW

In the United States, the number of lawsuits has increased over the years. Working in a **litigious** (LI ti jehs) society requires that we know how to protect ourselves against lawsuits. This is the reason that medical assistants need to learn about the law. To avoid the risk of lawsuits, medical assistants need to practice within the guidelines of the law.

SOURCES OF LAW

Law is a custom or practice of a community. It is a rule of conduct or action prescribed or formally recognized as enforceable by a controlling authority. Law is the system by which society gives order to our lives.

The United States has both federal and state laws. The U.S. Constitution is the supreme law of the United States (Fig. 16.1). Each state has a constitution that is the supreme law of that state. State laws cannot conflict with the U.S. Constitution. In the following sections, we will examine the makeup of the federal and state government and the sources of law.

Balance of Power

The federal government was designed to allow for a balance of power. The three branches of government share power so that no one branch is more powerful than any other. Table 16.1 describes the three branches of the federal government. The states also have three branches of government.

When members of Congress or the state houses want new legislation, a bill is brought forward. After much debate, the bill will either die or be passed and become an *act* or *statute*. The act or statute is now part of the laws for the state or country. (The terms "act" and "statute" are used interchangeably. Most of the time you will hear the word "act" in the name of a specific law; statute is used more to refer to the contents of the actual law.)

On the local level, an *ordinance* is a piece of legislation passed by a municipality or local government. A city ordinance to ban smoking from restaurants is an example of local legislation.

Types of Laws

There are four types of laws:

- *Constitutional law*: Derived from the federal and state constitutions, which give power to federal and state governments. Examples of constitutional law include prohibiting slavery (based on an 1865 constitutional amendment) and the power to tax.
- *Case law*: Derived from legal **precedents** and **common law**. Common law originated in England and was used by the colonists.
- *Regulatory* and *administrative law*: Concerns the procedures, regulations, and rules of federal, state, and local governmental administrative agencies. Examples include: zoning boards, licensing agencies, the Social Security Administration, and unemployment commissions.
- *Statutory law:* Refers to the laws enacted by the state and federal legislatures. An example is the speed limits set by the state legislature.

CRIMINAL AND CIVIL LAW

Laws can be divided into two main categories:

- *Substantive law*: Laws that determine rights and obligations of people derived from common law and statutes. Substantive laws include criminal, civil, military, and international law.
- *Procedural law*: Laws that all parties (courts, officers, and lawyers) must follow when investigating and prosecuting unlawful acts. With criminal law, procedural law ensures that a person receives due process under the U.S. Constitution.

We will examine criminal and civil law in depth as they relate to healthcare.

Criminal Law

Criminal laws are statutes that define actions or *omissions* (lack of actions) that threaten and/or harm public safety and welfare. These actions or omissions are prohibited by the government and are called *crimes*. Criminal law can be summarized as crimes against the state (or government). When criminal cases are brought to court, the **plaintiff** (PLAIN tif) is the government. The **defendant** (dih FEN dant) is the person or party charged with the offense.

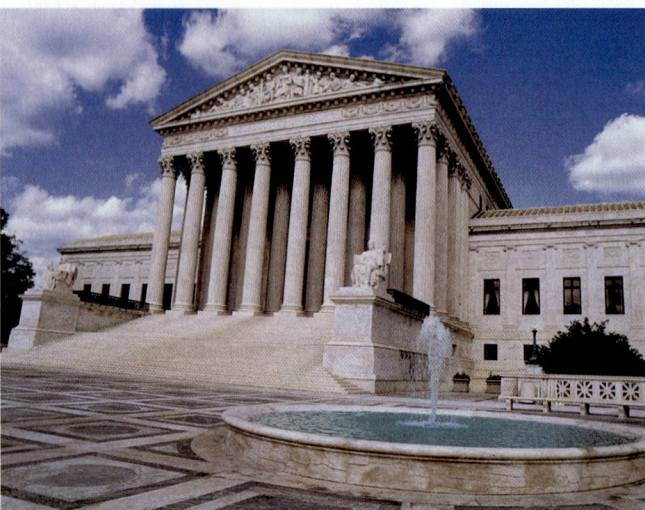

FIG. 16.1 The U.S. Supreme Court. The Supreme Court decides cases that involve the interpretation of the U.S. Constitution. (From Proctor D, Niedzwiecki B: *Kinn's the medical assistant*, ed 13, St Louis, 2017, Elsevier.)

> **VOCABULARY**
> **common law**: Unwritten laws that come from judicial decisions based on societal traditions and customs.
> **litigious**: Prone to lawsuits.
> **precedent**: A prior court decision that serves as a model for similar legal cases in the future.

TABLE 16.1 Branches of the Federal and State Governments

Branch	Federal Government	State Government
Legislative	*Made Up Of:* • Two houses of Congress (Senate and House of Representatives). Members of the houses are elected by eligible voters from the state they represent. *Roles:* • Makes new federal laws • Can impeach the President or remove judges from office for misconduct • Must approve: all appointments for judges, budget spending, and treaties • Can override the President's veto of a bill by a ⅔ vote	*Made Up Of:* • Most states have two houses, although the names can differ. Officials are elected. *Roles:* • Introduce legislation to become new state laws • Can impeach state officials for misconduct • Must approve state budget • Can override the governor's veto and amend the state constitution
Executive	*Made Up Of:* • President of the United States administers this branch *Roles:* • Can issue *executive orders* that become law without the approval of Congress • Creates a budget • Appoints judges • Carries out laws • Makes treaties with other nations • Can veto bills from Congress	*Made Up Of:* • Headed by the elected governor; each state has a different executive organizational structure. *Roles:* • Creates a budget • Carries out laws • Can veto bills from state houses • Issues executive orders • Appoints state court judges (in most states)
Judicial	*Made Up Of:* • Supreme Court, which has nine justices *Roles:* • Interpret laws according to the U.S. Constitution • Determine if laws from Congress and executive actions are constitutional	*Made Up Of:* • State supreme court *Roles:* • Interpret laws according to the state constitution • Hear cases from lower courts • Determine if state laws are constitutional

Criminal offenses can vary in severity from traffic violations to murders. In most states criminal offenses are classified as *misdemeanors* (mis di MEE ners) and *felonies* (FEL uh nees). (Table 16.2).

CRITICAL THINKING BOX 16.1

Bella and Daniela are reviewing criminal law concepts during lunch break. Bella asks Daniela how criminal law would apply to medical assistants. How might Daniela respond? Discuss your response with a peer.

Civil Law

Civil laws protect and define private rights. An individual or institution can sue another person, institution (business), or the government in a civil matter (Table 16.3). Civil laws govern disputes related to contracts, property, family law, and personal injury. Common civil disputes involve contract issues, divorce, child custody, product liability (LIE ah bil i tee), and accidents. There are many branches of civil law. Table 16.4 describes the four most significant types of civil law. The following sections will address **tort** (torte) law and contract law.

TORT LAW

Tort law enforces rules that we have in our society. If these rules are violated, then an individual can sue another individual, institution (business), or government. There are two types of torts that will be discussed: intentional torts and negligent torts (unintentional torts).

Intentional Torts

With an intentional tort, the plaintiff must prove the defendant had specific intent to perform the action that caused the injury. The focus is not on whether the harm was intended, but if the action was intended.

VOCABULARY

damages: Monetary settlement the defendant pays the plaintiff in a civil case for loss or injury.
declaratory judgment: A court judgment that defines the legal rights of the parties involved.
defendant: An individual or business against whom a lawsuit is filed.
injunction: A court order by which an individual or institution is required to perform or restrain from performing a certain act.
liability: State of being liable or responsible for something.
plaintiff: An individual or party who brings the suit to court.
tort: A civil wrongdoing that causes harm to a person or property, excludes breach of contract.
tortfeasor: An individual who committed the tort.

TABLE 16.2 Misdemeanors and Felonies

	Misdemeanor	Felony
Description	Lesser criminal offense	Serious criminal offense; classified by degree, with first degree being the most serious.
Examples of crimes	• Assault • Battery • False imprisonment • Perjury • Shoplifting • Most cases of operating while intoxicated (OWI) and operating under the influence (OUI)	• Murder • Kidnapping • Robbery • Embezzlement • Rape • Arson • Sodomy • Mayhem • Larceny • Burglary • Manslaughter • Treason
Punishable by	Substantial fine and possible jail time under 1 year. (*Jails* are usually operated by local law enforcement and are used for short-term stays.)	Substantial fine and prison time over 1 year. (*Prisons* are usually operated by the state or federal government and are for long-term stays.)
Possible post-conviction consequences	• Appears on the person's criminal record	• Appears on the person's criminal record • May lose the right to vote and own firearms • May have difficulty obtaining a job, especially in healthcare

TABLE 16.3 Criminal Law Compared to Civil Law

	Criminal Law	Civil Law
Plaintiff	State or federal government	Victim (individual or institution) of the wrongdoing
Defendant	Person or party accused of the criminal complaint or charge	Wrongdoer (also called **tortfeasor** [TORTE fee zahr] with tort law); could be a business, individual, or the government
Wrong act against	Wrongful act against the government (state or federal)	Wrongful acts against an individual or an institution (business)
Offense/wrong called	Crime	Tort, breach of contract (depends on the type of civil law)
Attorney	Defendant entitled to an attorney. The state must provide an attorney if the defendant can't afford one.	Defendant must pay for the attorney or defend himself or herself.
Court	Tried in criminal court system; almost always involves a trial by jury.	Tried in a civil court system; may not involve a jury. Cases are typically decided by the judge.
Standard of proof	Must prove beyond a reasonable doubt.	The preponderance of evidence (more than likely it occurred)
Consequence	Substantial fine and prison time	**Damages**, **injunction** (in JUNGK shahn), **declaratory judgment**
Healthcare example	A medical assistant determines a patient should have a specific medication and gives the patient the medication without a provider's order, thus practicing medicine.	A medical assistant changes a sterile dressing per a provider's order, but does the procedure incorrectly. The wound develops an infection, and the patient subsequently dies.

TABLE 16.4 Types of Civil Law

Types of Civil Law	Description
Tort law	Applies when one person, business, or the government does a wrongdoing to an individual that causes injury or property damage. Includes intentional tort, negligence, and strict liability (strict duty to ensure safety of manufactured products).
Contract law	Applies to agreements between two or more individuals or parties.
Property law	Applies to personal property (e.g., copyrights, stocks, animals, physical goods) and real property (e.g., land, mineral rights).
Family law	Applies to marriage, divorce, annulment, child custody and support, birth, and adoption.

Many intentional torts are also criminal in nature. The defendant may be prosecuted in both a civil court and a criminal court for the action. Table 16.5 defines a list of common intentional torts. Box 16.1 provides a legal example of a defamation suit.

CRITICAL THINKING BOX 16.2

Bella and Daniela are reviewing civil law concepts after work. Bella asks Daniela how civil law would apply to medical assistants. How might Daniela respond? Discuss your response with a peer.

Negligent Torts

Negligent torts are more common in healthcare because they are unintentional. (Negligent torts may also be called *unintentional torts*.) The harm that is caused by **negligence** (NEG li juhns) is the result of a person's carelessness. Negligence results when a person's conduct falls below the standard of behavior expected of a reasonable person in the same situation.

TABLE 16.5 Common Intentional Torts

Intentional Tort	Definition	Example in Healthcare
Assault	Intentional threat to do harm or acting in a manner that causes another to fear bodily harm.	Threatening a child to behave or you would give him a "shot."
Battery	Intentional harmful or offensive contact with another that was unconsented. Only proof of unconsented contact is required; proof of harm is not required.	Giving a child a vaccination without consent from the parent or guardian.
False imprisonment	Intentional restraint of another individual without consent or reason	Using restraints to keep a patient in a wheelchair without significant reason.
Fraud	Deceiving (lying) to a person or party for monetary gain.	Billing an insurance company for services not provided to the patient.
Defamation	Intentionally saying something false about another person, which causes harm. Written defamation is *libel*. Spoken defamation is *slander*.	Posting lies about a coworker on a social media site that could cause harm to that person. (Another example is provided in Box 16.1.)
Invasion of privacy	Disclosing private facts without the consent of the individual or intrusion into a person's personal life.	Telling a family member or friend about a patient who was seen in your department. (Breaching confidentiality of patient health records.)

TABLE 16.6 Classification of Negligent Acts

Classification	Definition	Healthcare Example
Malfeasance (mal FEE zahns)	Performance of an unlawful, wrongful act	A medical assistant determines that a patient needs pain medication and gives a large dose without a provider order. The patient dies from the overdose. (It is illegal for the medical assistant to practice medicine [prescribe the medication], and the dose was wrong.)
Misfeasance (mis FEE zahns)	Improper performance of a lawful act, that causes damage or injury	A medical assistant gives an injection ordered by the provider. The injection is given in the wrong location, and the patient has lifelong pain.
Nonfeasance (non FEE zahns)	Failure to act when one had a legal duty to act	After a patient is given an injection, the patient starts to have a reaction. The medical assistant fails to act and notify the provider. The medical assistant sends the patient home, and the patient later dies.

BOX 16.1 Legal Example: Defamation Suit

According to the complaint: In 2013 in Fairfax, Virginia, the plaintiff was to have a colonoscopy. He was told he could be groggy afterwards and was concerned about recalling post-procedure instructions. Prior to the procedure, he set his mobile phone to record the post-procedure instructions. His clothing and phone ended up in the operating suite with him during the procedure. His phone recorded the entire procedure. While the plaintiff was unconscious, the doctors and medical assistant joked that he had syphilis and tuberculosis that caused a penile rash. The defendants mocked the patient for a variety of reasons and then discussed how to avoid the patient when he woke up. The medical assistant attempted to mislead the plaintiff. She indicated falsely that the physician spoke to him after surgery, but the patient must not have remembered. The plaintiff and his wife discovered the recording on their way home.

The jury awarded the plaintiff $50,000 in compensatory damages for defamation for the provider's remarks about each disease. He was also awarded $200,000 for overall medical malpractice and $200,000 in punitive damages.

D.B. v Ingham et al., 2013-16811, (2015, Fairfax Circuit Court)

BOX 16.2 Legal Example: Malpractice Case

In October 2007 in Syracuse New York, Tina Holstein (31 years old) delivered her third child at Community General Hospital. After the delivery, she began vomiting, and the nurse administered an intramuscular (IM) injection. Ms. Holstein sued the hospital and the nurse who administered the injection, alleging malpractice. She claimed she had permanent injury of her sciatic nerve because the nurse failed to properly administer the IM injection. The case against the nurse was dropped, but the jury found the hospital liable for the injury. Ms. Holstein was awarded $1.69 million.

Holstein v. Community General Hospital Greater Syracuse, 17 N.Y.3d 948 (2011). https://www.leagle.com/decision/innyco20111122672

VOCABULARY
negligence: Conduct not expected of a reasonably prudent person acting under similar circumstances; it falls below the standards of behavior established by law for the protection of others against unreasonable risk of harm.

The *reasonable person standard* applies reasonable behavior as an objective test to measure another's actions or lack of actions. The accused person's actions or lack of actions are measured against what a reasonable person would or would not do in the same situation. The accused person is negligent if his or her actions or lack of actions do not measure up to the reasonable person standard. Negligent acts can be classified as malfeasance, misfeasance, and nonfeasance (Table 16.6).

Malpractice (mal PRAK tis) is a type of negligence that applies to professionals. Medical malpractice occurs when a healthcare professional's performance falls below the professional minimum standard of care and thus causes harm to the plaintiff (Box 16.2). *Standard of care* refers to the level and type of care an ordinary, prudent healthcare professional, having the same training and experience in a similar practice, would have provided under a similar situation.

CRITICAL THINKING BOX 16.3

Bella asks Daniela to describe negligence and malpractice in her own words. How might Daniela respond?

The standard of care takes into account the accused person's skills and knowledge. It also considers the environment. For instance, the care provided by Dr. Walden, a family practice doctor practicing in a midsize Midwestern city, would be compared to a family practice doctor who practiced in a similar-sized city in the same geographic location. It would be unfair to compare Dr. Walden's family practice to a large family practice located on the East Coast. The resources available to the providers could be different.

Medical assistants need to be aware of the standard of care. If medical assistants identify themselves as nurses to patients, they may be held to the standard of care (including the educational level) of a nurse. If medical assistants practice beyond their scope of practice, they may be held to the higher standard of care. Also, medical assistants who are nationally certified may be held to a higher level than those who are not certified. It is important for credentialed medical assistants to pursue continuing education to keep updated and current in their practice. Scope of practice will be discussed later in the chapter.

CRITICAL THINKING BOX 16.4

Daniela asks Bella why medical assistants can't call themselves nurses. How might Bella address this question? How might scope of practice relate to the question?

Defenses to Liability. When the defendant's attorney accepts a case, a defense (di FENS) is planned for the lawsuit. There are three main defenses used for lawsuits:
- *Technical defense*: The attorney will review the case and if possible try to get the case dismissed based on a legal technicality. Table 16.7 describes legal technicalities used to dismiss cases.
- *Denial defense*: When absolutely none of the facts are true, this defense can be used. However, if any of the facts are true, then denial cannot be used.
- *Affirmative defense*: The defendant admits wrongdoing. The defendant's attorney introduces facts that support the defendant's conduct. If the defense is successful, it will reduce the defendant's legal liability. Table 16.8 describes common affirmative defenses.

VOCABULARY
defense: A strategy used by the defendant to avoid liability in a lawsuit.
malpractice: A type of negligence in which a licensed professional fails to provide the standard of care, causing harm to a person.
res judicata: Latin for "a thing decided." Once a case has been decided by the court, it cannot be litigated again.
scope of practice: Range of responsibilities and practice guidelines that determine the boundaries within which a healthcare worker practices.

TABLE 16.7 Common Legal Technicalities That Can Be Used as Technical Defenses

Technicality	Description
Statute of limitations	The length of time legal action can be taken after an event has occurred. When the time has expired, the court will reject the claim or lawsuit. Statute of limitations vary from state to state (see Box 16.3 for additional details).
Good Samaritan law	These laws vary in each state, with some states providing protection if the provider acts "in good faith." For Good Samaritan protection: • A person must provide treatment in a true emergency. • Care must be provided outside of a place with necessary medical equipment. • The provider cannot bill the patient for the care provided.
Release of tortfeasor	The plaintiff signed a release to give up the right to sue the defendant (tortfeasor) in the future, in exchange for a monetary compensation. If this release is signed, any future lawsuits from the plaintiff will be dismissed.
res judicata (RAZE JOO di kah tah)	Latin for "a thing decided." If a case has already been decided by the court, the plaintiff cannot bring a similar suit against the defendant in the future.

BOX 16.3 Statute of Limitations

The statute of limitations for medical malpractice varies by states. Typically, it is 2 to 5 years, with exceptions. In most states the "clock" starts when the patient "reasonably should have known" the malpractice occurred. For instance, if a patient awoke after surgery to find that the operation had been performed on the wrong leg, the clock would start then. In some cases, patients don't realize the malpractice occurred for months to years after the event. With the "Discovery Rule," the malpractice needs to be discovered (the patient "reasonably should have known") before the "clock starts" on the statute of limitations. The statute of limitations for children greatly varies; some states use age 8, whereas others use age 18.

CRITICAL THINKING BOX 16.5

Daniela is studying affirmative defenses. She asks Bella if she has any study tips for remembering the different affirmative defenses. How might Bella answer? Share your answer with a peer.

Proving Malpractice. When a plaintiff sues the defendant, the defendant can attempt to settle outside of court or go to trial. *Alternative dispute resolution* (ADR) is the process of settling disputes outside of litigation. This process is usually cheaper and quicker than going to trial. Two types of alternative dispute resolution are arbitration (AHR bi trae shuhn) and mediation (MEE dee ae shuhn). Both ADR procedures involve a neutral third party who hears both sides. With mediation, the mediator facilitates an agreement that is acceptable to both parties. With arbitration, the arbitrator listens to both sides and makes the final decision. In arbitration the decision of the arbitrator is *legally binding* (or a legal obligation).

TABLE 16.8 Common Affirmative Defenses

Affirmative Defense	Description
Contributory negligence	The plaintiff's actions or lack of actions caused the injury. In other words, had the plaintiff used ordinary care, the injury would not have occurred. The plaintiff's carelessness (e.g., ignoring warnings or safety rules, inattention) caused the injury. (In many states contributory negligence has been replaced by comparative negligence).
Comparative negligence	The plaintiff's action or lack of action caused the injury to a certain percent. The damages to the plaintiff are calculated based on the percent the defendant was responsible.
Assumption of risk	The defendant can show evidence that the plaintiff had actual, subjective knowledge of the risks involved and the plaintiff consented to proceed with the activity (see Box 16.4). Informed consent is critical for this defense. (Informed consent will be discussed later in the chapter.)
Limited or no harm	The defendant claims the plaintiff suffered no or little harm; much less than what the plaintiff claims.
Intervening cause	The defendant acknowledges the plaintiff suffered injuries due to defendant's negligence, but the injury was made worse by the plaintiff's actions following the situation.

BOX 16.4 Legal Example: Assumption of Risk

The plaintiff was being treated for bronchitis. Following his clinic visit, a coughing episode caused him to black out and hit his head at home. Upon returning to the clinic a few weeks later for a follow-up visit on the bronchitis, a medical assistant took the plaintiff into the examination room. The medical assistant instructed the plaintiff to sit on the exam table while his vital signs were obtained. The plaintiff mentioned to the medical assistant that he had fainted twice as a result of coughing episodes. After the medical assistant left to get the physician, the plaintiff had a coughing episode, fainted, and fell to the floor. He sustained injuries because of the fall.

The plaintiff sued the clinic and the medical assistant, alleging that the medical assistant was negligent for failing to move him to another location upon learning about his fainting episodes. The defendants moved for a summary judgment. They stated that an assumption of risk defense applied. The plaintiff could have chosen to sit on one of the two chairs present in the room, but he did not. The court agreed. The plaintiff appealed, and the Georgia Court of Appeals unanimously sided with the trial court's ruling. The defendants proved the plaintiff had knowledge of the danger, understood the risks associated with the danger, and exposed himself to the danger. The plaintiff lost the case.

Watson v. Regional First Care, Inc., No. A15A1708, Ga. App. (February 19, 2016). https://www.leagle.com/decision/ingaco20160219174

With civil litigation, either party or the judge can move for a summary judgment. A *summary judgment* is a process that can be used if there are no disputes about the facts in the case. This process speeds up cases. It allows a judgment to be made based on the facts. With a summary judgment, there is no trial.

If the disputing parties decide to take the lawsuit to court, a specific process must be followed (Box 16.5). When a medical negligence suit is brought to court, four elements must be proven for malpractice to be found. These elements are the 4 *D*s of negligence: duty, dereliction, damages, and direct cause. Let's examine the 4 *D*s of negligence.

- *Duty of care*: The healthcare professional has a legal obligation to the patient. Many times, the duty of care comes from the provider-patient relationship. This will be examined in more depth later in the chapter.
- *Dereliction* (DER uh lik shuhn): The healthcare professional breaches (violated) the duty of care to the patient. In other words, the professional did not follow through with the duty to the patient.
- *Damages*: The patient suffers a legally recognized injury. Examples of such an injury include physical pain, mental anguish, additional medical bills, and loss of work/earning capacity.
- *Direct cause*: The breach of duty of care (the negligent act or lack of action) directly causes the patient's injury.

The plaintiff's attorney is responsible for proving each of these four elements. In many cases, medical experts are hired by attorneys to be expert witnesses. These expert witnesses help establish the standard of care and some of the 4 *D*s. If one of the elements is not proven, malpractice will not be found. For instance, if the provider performed below the standard of care, but the patient did not suffer any harm, malpractice cannot be found.

CRITICAL THINKING BOX 16.6

Daniela struggles with remembering the 4 *D*s of negligence. Be creative and work with a peer. How might a person remember the 4 *D*s of negligence?

VOCABULARY

arbitration: The process in which conflicting parties in a dispute submit their differences to a court-appointed person (arbitrator), who submits a legally binding decision.
deposition: A sworn testimony made before a court-appointed officer; it is used in the discovery process and may be used in the trial.
expert witnesses: People who are educated and knowledgeable in the area of concern; they testify in court and provide an expert opinion on the topic of concern.
fact witnesses: People who observed the situation and testify in court about the facts of the case.
mediation: The process of facilitating conflicting parties to make an agreement, settlement, or compromise.
interrogatory: Written or oral questions that must be answered under oath.
subpoena: A court order requiring a person to appear in court at a specific time to testify in a legal case.
subpoena duces tecum: A legal document commanding a person to bring a piece of evidence (such as the plaintiff's health record) to court.

BOX 16.5 Stages of a Civil Lawsuit

1. **Pre-filing phase:** The situation occurs, and the patient seeks the advice of a civil attorney. After reviewing the person's story, the medical record, and other documents, the attorney accepts the case.
2. **Initial pleading phase:**
   - The plaintiff's attorney files a complaint with the clerk of the court. The complaint includes the patient's version of the situation and the damages (amount of money) sought from the defendant.
   - The clerk of the court issues a summons to the defendant. The summons outlines the complaint and damages and states a deadline for a response.
   - The defense attorney files an answer or motion with the court. The answer provides the court with the defendant's version of the situation. (If the deadline is missed, the defendant may be responsible for the damages.)
3. **Discovery phase:**
   - Both sides exchange information and gather evidence to support their side in court.
   - A *subpoena* (suh PEE nuh) is issued for the healthcare professionals involved in the case. They may be required to go to court or to attend a *deposition* (dep ah ZISH uhn). They may also be required to complete an *interrogatory* (IN tah rog ah TOOR ee). Failure to comply with a deposition or subpoena will result in a *contempt of court* charge. The person may be fined or imprisoned.
   - A *subpoena duces tecum* (suh PEE nuh DOO seez TEE kuhm) may also be issued.
4. **Post discovery phase:**
   - The judge may meet with both attorneys to discuss the case.
   - The plaintiff may drop the case if not enough evidence was available to make the case.
   - The defendant may settle the lawsuit by "making a deal" so it doesn't move to trial.
5. **Trial phase:** The case is heard by the judge and/or jury. A jury is selected. *Expert witnesses* and *fact witnesses* are questioned and cross-examined by the opposing attorney (see Fig. 16.2). Closing arguments are made, and the jury retires to make a decision. The verdict is read to the court, and the judge enters the judgment.
6. **Appeals phase:** Post-trial motions are filed. An appeal to a higher court may be made.

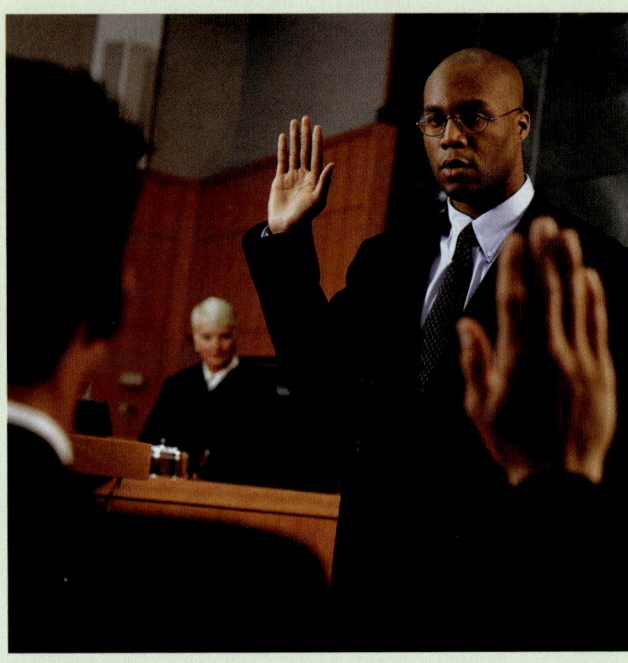

FIG. 16.2 Witnesses must be credible and must tell the truth on the stand in court to avoid charges of perjury. (From Proctor D, Niedzwiecki B: *Kinn's the medical assistant*, ed 13, St Louis, 2017, Elsevier.)

CRITICAL THINKING BOX 16.7

Bella is helping Daniela study for a law exam. She asks Daniela to describe the differences between the following sets of terms. How might Daniela respond?
- Subpoena and subpoena duces tecum
- Fact witness and expert witness

In a case in which there was obvious negligence, the doctrine *res ipsa loquitur* (RASE ipsah low kwah tuhr) may apply. *Res ipsa loquitur* is Latin for "the thing speaks for itself." The *res ipsa loquitur* doctrine may be used for:
- Cases that involve an object being left in the patient's body during a surgery
- Cases that involve an operation on the wrong extremity

The evidence shows that the plaintiff did not cause the injury. The defendant caused the injury as a result of negligence. The defendant breached the duty to the plaintiff.

VOCABULARY
res ipsa loquitur. Latin term meaning "the thing speaks for itself."

Damages. The defendant may need to pay damages when the plaintiff wins a civil suit. Damages are a monetary settlement. There are several types of damages:

- *Punitive damages:* Vast payment meant to punish the defendant.
- *Nominal damages:* Very small settlement because the plaintiff's injury was slight.
- *Compensatory damages:* A settlement for losses suffered. Losses can be related to loss of income, property damage, and medical care.
- *General damages:* A settlement for emotional pain and anguish, loss of future earning power, and so on. Often sought with compensatory damages.
- *Special damages:* A settlement for a specific dollar amount that directly relates to medical bills.

Professional Insurance. Many people are familiar with car insurance and home owner's insurance. When a person becomes a professional, the risk of being sued increases. Having insurance (to protect oneself in case of civil damages) is important. Providers, nurses, and in some cases medical assistants, purchase annual insurance policies. Ambulatory healthcare facilities also must carry insurance. It is important for medical assistants to understand the types of insurance available.

The person or company purchasing the insurance policy is called the *insured*. The insured pays a specific amount of money to the insurance company. This payment is called a *premium*. The insurance company is the *insurer*. The insurer agrees to compensate the insured for specific losses covered in the insurance contract or policy. When the insurer (insurance company) pays the plaintiff, the

TABLE 16.9 Five Elements Required for Legally-Binding Contracts

Element	Description	Provider-Patient Example
Offer	Made by one party.	A family practice physician advertises complete physicals for $150.
Acceptance	A second party agrees to the offer.	After seeing the advertisement, a patient calls to make an appointment.
Consideration	Each party exchanges something of value.	The physician gives a physical exam, and the patient pays $150.
Legal subject matter	The consideration must be legal.	The board-certified physician can legally perform physical exams. The payment is legal tender (money).
Competency and capacity	A person entering a contract must have the legal capacity to be held liable for the contract obligation. If one or both parties is underage (a **minor**) or shows signs of **incompetence** (in KOM pi tahns), intoxication, or acting under the influence of drugs, this would invalidate a contract. An **emancipated minor** can enter into contracts (see Box 16.6).	Both the physician and the patient are adults with the capacity to understand the contract.

plaintiff is known as the *third party*. The following are different types of insurance.

- *Liability insurance*: Provides protection from claims of injuries or damage to people or property. It can be referred to as third-party coverage because it covers claims from a party other than the insured. Different types of liability insurance include:
  - *Professional liability insurance*: A type of liability coverage used by professionals to protect them against liability suits incurred because of errors and omissions while performing their professional services.
  - *Medical malpractice insurance*: A type of professional liability insurance. Protects healthcare professionals from liability related to wrongful practices resulting in injury, expense, and property damages. It also covers the cost of defending lawsuits.
  - *General liability* or *commercial liability insurance*: A type of liability coverage purchased by companies. It protects businesses from lawsuits for property loss and bodily injury from nonemployees.
- *Personal injury insurance*: A type of liability coverage that protects against claims related to harm other than bodily injury. Coverage can be for invasion of privacy, slander, imprisonment, and so on.

When purchasing a policy, it is important to understand the types of policies.

- *Claims-made policy*: An insurance policy that covers claims made during the policy year. For example: if a provider has a claims-made policy for the current year, any claims that come in this year will be covered.
- *Occurrence policy*: An insurance policy that covers claims for wrongful acts that occurred during the policy year. For example, if a provider has an occurrence policy for the current year, any wrongful acts that occur this year will be covered when the claims are filed in future years.
- *Nose coverage*: A limited-term policy purchased from the new carrier the provider is joining. The policy covers the provider between the end of the prior policy and the start of next policy. Nose coverage can also be referred to as *retroactive* or *prior acts coverage*.
- *Tail coverage*: A limited-term policy purchased from the insurance carrier that the provider is leaving. The policy covers the provider until the new policy starts. A person would need only nose or tail coverage, but not both.

BOX 16.6 Emancipated Minors

Conditions for Emancipation
Must be at least 16 years of age in most states and usually must meet one of the following:
- Married
- In the U.S. military
- Living on his or her own and managing own money

Benefits of Emancipation
- Can be a party in a contract (e.g., rent housing, purchase agreements)
- Can sue
- Can keep earned income and apply for public benefits
- May make all healthcare decisions regarding himself or herself

CONTRACTS

Most people are aware of contracts. We sign contracts for cell phone plans, rental properties, and payment plans. We also have contracts in healthcare. The healthcare facility's business manager signs contracts for equipment and building rental, service agreements, and so on. The most common contract is the provider-patient contract.

A *contract* is an agreement between two parties. For a contract to be legally binding, five elements must be present; these elements are explained in Table 16.9. Contracts can either be:

- *Implied contract*: The parties have agreed to the terms of the contract through their actions and behaviors. The provider-patient relationship is an implied contract (Fig. 16.3).
- *Expressed contract*: The parties have specifically stated the terms of the contract in writing, orally, or both.

Specific types of contracts must be in writing to avoid fraud. These types of contracts are outlines in each state's *statute of frauds*. Statutes of fraud vary slightly, but all indicate that contracts need to be in writing and signed by both parties. Contracts that need to be in writing include:

- Contracts that are property related – real estate sales, real estate leases for longer than 1 year, and transfer of property upon the owner's death.
- Agreements to pay another's debt

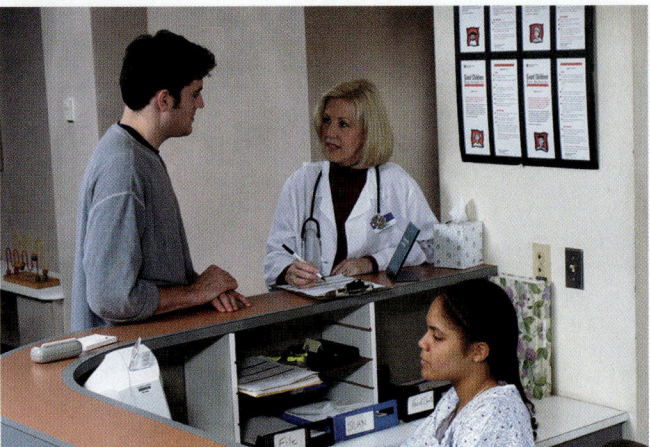

FIG. 16.3 The provider-patient relationship is built on a strong foundation of trust, but it also is a contractual relationship. (From Proctor D, Niedzwiecki B: *Kinn's the medical assistant*, ed 13, St Louis, 2017, Elsevier.)

- Contracts that last longer than 1 year or last longer than the life of an individual
- Contracts over a certain amount of money (varies by state)

Provider-Patient Relationship

The contract that is established between the provider and the patient is legally binding. The patient accepts the provider's offer when a patient makes an appointment to see the provider. This means the provider has a duty to see, diagnose, and treat the patient. The patient has the responsibility to follow the provider's recommendations and pay the bill.

As indicated earlier, duty to the patient is one of the 4 *D*s in proving malpractice. The duty to the patient is established during the initial visit of the patient. From that time onward, the provider has a duty to the patient. Both parties can terminate the contract or relationship. A patient can terminate the contract at any time. The patient may no longer need the provider's services. The patient may decide to use another provider.

The provider must follow the legal process to terminate the contract. Table 16.10 lists reasons providers terminate the patient relationship or contract. A provider can be charged with **patient abandonment** if he or she simply stops providing care to the patient. To prevent abandonment allegations, the provider must follow the correct legal steps to terminate the provider-patient relationship. Table 16.10 lists the steps the provider needs to follow to terminate the contract or relationship with the patient.

There are many situations in which allegations of patient abandonment may occur, including:
- Failing to follow up with the patient. If a patient calls or emails the provider or facility, follow-up with the patient must be made in a reasonable period of time.
- Failing to have another provider cover the practice during vacations or when the facility is closed.
- Discharging a patient without proper instructions.

The medical assistant has an important role in ensuring that the patient is not abandoned. Typically, the medical assistant is responsible for answering patient calls and emails in a timely manner. Documentation in the patient's health record must reflect all communication with the patient.

TABLE 16.10 Terminating the Provider-Patient Relationship

Reasons Providers Terminate Provider-Patient Relationship	Steps to Terminate Provider-Patient Relationship
• Retirement or moving • Patient isn't paying for the services provided • Patient isn't following or is noncompliant with the provider's treatment plan • Patient's behavior (e.g., rude, abusive, drug seeking, not showing up for appointments,)	• Provider must notify the patient in writing of the withdrawal of care. • A date must be indicated for the termination. There must be an adequate period of coverage to allow the patient to find another provider. Fifteen to 30 days is usually recommended. • The termination letter should be sent as a certified letter with return receipt requested. • A copy of the letter and the return receipt need to be placed or scanned into the patient's health record. • Scheduling staff should be notified of the termination date, so no appointments are made after that date.

If the medical assistant does not follow up with the patient, allegations of abandonment can be brought against the medical assistant and the provider. *Respondeat superior* is a common-law doctrine that means "let the master answer." The doctrine means that the employer/provider is **liable** for actions that the employee did or didn't do within the scope of employment. This means that the medical assistant's actions affect the employer and the provider. The medical assistant's actions or lack of actions can lead to malpractice allegations for the provider.

Breach of Contract

A *breach of contract* occurs when the terms of the contract are not fulfilled by one party without a legitimate legal reason. The breach can occur when the terms are not met by the stated deadline. It can also happen when the terms are not met or performed. An allegation of a breach of contract can lead to a lawsuit. The injured party attempts to

VOCABULARY

emancipated minor: A minor who has been granted emancipation by the court; the minor can assume the rights and responsibilities of adulthood.
incompetence: The state of being incompetent or lacking the ability to manage personal affairs due to mental deficiency; an appointed guardian or conservator manages these people's affairs.
liable: Legally responsible or obligated.
minor: One who has not reached adulthood; usually age 18 or 21, depending on the jurisdiction.
patient abandonment: A form of medical malpractice, also called *negligent termination*; the provider ends the provider-patient relationship without reasonable or adequate notification.
***respondeat supe*rior**: A legal doctrine meaning "let the master answer"; the employer/provider is legally responsible for the wrongful actions or lack of actions of employees if done within the scope of employment.

force the contract terms to be met or to receive compensation for financial loss caused by the breach.

In the healthcare field, a breach of contract can occur with the provider-patient relationship. Breach of contract may occur with improper termination and abandonment situations. Breach of contract may also occur with the business side of the facility, including:
- Business contracts (e.g., leases for equipment)
- Payment contracts with patients

CONSENT

Consent means one party voluntarily agrees with another party's proposition or plan. In healthcare, several types of consent are used.
- *Implied consent*: Consent that is inferred based on signs, actions, or conduct of the patient rather than oral communication (using words). For instance, the medical assistant asks a patient if he can obtain a blood pressure reading. The patient removes her arm from her jacket sleeve and extends it towards the medical assistant.
- *Expressed consent*: Consent that is given either by the spoken or written word. For example, the medical assistant asks the patient where she would like her pain medication injection. The patient states she wants the injection in her upper right arm. The medical assistant gave the patient a choice, and the patient expressed her consent by stating her choice.
- *Informed consent*: A legal process that ensures the patient or guardian understands the treatment and gives consent for the treatment. With informed consent, the provider must educate the patient on the treatment before the patient signs the consent form. More information on the Doctrine of Informed Consent is given in the following section.

CRITICAL THINKING BOX 16.8

Daniela is studying consents. How might you define implied, expressed, and informed consents in your own words?

Doctrine of Informed Consent

With many medical procedures and treatments, informed consent is required (Box 16.7). The provider, not the medical assistant, has a duty to provide information to the patient or guardian. The provider must educate the patient on the treatment options. Once the information is given, the patient or guardian makes an informed decision regarding treatment. Informed consent requirements may vary slightly from state to state. The requirements are usually described in the state's medical practice act. For an informed consent to occur, seven elements must be present:

1. The patient or guardian is competent to understand and decide.

BOX 16.7 Reasons for Informed Consent

- Surgical procedures; may include minor surgery done in ambulatory care facilities
- Complex procedures and tests (e.g., endoscopy, biopsy, exercise or nuclear stress test)
- High-risk medications
- Participating in a research study
- Most vaccines
- Cancer treatment (e.g., radiation, chemotherapy)
- Some medical laboratory testing

2. The patient or guardian voluntarily decides to agree to or refuse the treatment.
3. The patient or guardian understands the diagnosis and reason for treatment.
4. The patient or guardian understands the proposed treatment and the risks of the treatment.
5. The patient or guardian understands the alternative treatments available and the risks of the treatments.
6. The patient or guardian understands the risks if treatment is delayed or not done.
7. The patient or guardian signs a treatment consent form.

Adults of sound mind can give informed consent. Married minors, minor parents, emancipated minors, and **mature minors** can also give informed consent (Box 16.8). Patients who cannot legally give informed consent are listed in Box 16.9.

VOCABULARY
mature minor: A person under the age of adulthood who demonstrates the maturity to make a personal healthcare decision and can give informed consent for treatment.

CRITICAL THINKING BOX 16.9

Daniela is trying to distinguish between a mature minor and an emancipated minor. How would you describe each? What rights would each have in terms of healthcare?

In special situations, such as abortion, sterilization procedures, and human immunodeficiency virus (HIV) testing, each state has specific restrictions. Box 16.10 lists possible state restrictions for abortions. Currently, with abortions, the father of the fetus has no rights. No state requires the father to give consent or to be told about the abortion. For sterilization procedures, states may have waiting periods between signing the consent form and the procedure. The patient may have

BOX 16.8 Mature Minor

Many states address the Mature Minor Doctrine in their statutes. The definition of a mature minor and restrictions vary from state to state. Differences can be based on:
- A specific age (e.g., 14, 16) or no age when one can be considered a mature minor
- The availability of the parent
- The medical concern or treatment

BOX 16.9 Patients Who Cannot Legally Give Informed Consent

- Patients under the influence of alcohol or drugs
- Patients medicated with a preoperative medication that may affect their understanding (e.g., a sedative)
- A minor
- A patient who is mentally incompetent
- A patient who speaks little to no English. (An interpreter must be used for the patient to give informed consent. The interpreter will translate the information from the provider, questions from the patient, and the information on the consent form. It is important to document in the health record that an interpreter was used.)

> **BOX 16.10 Types of State Restrictions for Abortions**
>
> - Must be performed by a licensed physician
> - Mandated counseling on the possible link between abortion and breast cancer, the fetus (unborn baby) feels pain, and/or long-term mental health consequences
> - Required waiting period (often 24 hours) between the counseling and performing an abortion
> - Parent involved for pregnant minor
> - Must be performed in a hospital after a certain gestational age.
> - Gestational limits (abortion is prohibited after a certain point in the pregnancy)

> **BOX 16.11 Information on the Informed Consent Forms**
>
> - Patient's name, date of birth, health record number
> - Name of hospital or facility
> - Name of provider(s) performing treatment(s)
> - Risks and benefits of the treatment(s)
> - Alternative treatment(s) and risks
> - Risk if treatment(s) is delayed or not done
> - Statement indicating the treatment was explained to the patient or guardian
> - Signature of patient or guardian
> - Signature and name of person who explained the treatment options
> - Signature of the witness
> - Date and time consent form was completed

to be an adult. For HIV testing, the Centers for Disease Control and Prevention (CDC) recommends that a general consent for medical care form be completed prior to HIV testing. Most states have specific language in the statutes regarding consent and counseling for HIV testing.

In many states, the patient's written consent is required to take a video or picture of the patient. Pictures are taken to show before and after images. These pictures are added to the patient's electronic chart.

The medical assistant may need to prepare the informed consent form. Box 16.11 lists information that should be on the informed consent form. The medical assistant may also need to sign the form as a witness to the signature of the patient. It is important to ask patients before they sign the form if the provider discussed the treatment and if they have any questions. If patients have questions, let the provider know. After all the questions have been answered, then the informed consent form can be signed. Do not have the patient sign if he or she:

- does not understand the treatment.
- cannot legally give consent.
- has questions.

PATIENT'S BILL OF RIGHTS

Congress has attempted to create laws effecting a patient's "bill of rights" related to patient care and services, but none of the proposed bills has passed. The Affordable Care Act's Patient's Bill of Rights focuses on rights related to insurance. With no federal laws to follow, the American Hospital Association created a patient's bill of rights for its members. Since then, many healthcare facilities have created their own patient's bill of rights. Many agencies title theirs as "Patient's Rights and Responsibilities" (Fig. 16.4).

A medical assistant is likely to encounter a situation in which a choice of treatments is given to a patient (Procedure 16.1). It is important that the provider discuss the treatment choices with the patient. If the medical assistant is involved, it is important to find out if the patient has any questions. Questions need to be answered before a decision is made. It is important to be respectful and professional during the discussion. Do not attempt to sway the patient in one direction. If the patient selects the treatment that was not the provider's top choice, it is important to respect the patient's decision. The medical assistant should relay the information to the provider.

A medical assistant should know how to handle the situation if a patient refuses a procedure or treatment (see Procedure 16.1). It is important to follow the facility's policy and procedure in such a situation. Most times the following applies when a patient refuses treatment or procedures:

- Show sensitivity to the patient's rights by being respectful and professional. Remember, it is the right of the patient to refuse.
- Ask the patient if he or she has questions regarding the procedure. If so, let the provider know.
- Notify the provider of the refusal.
- Document the refusal in the health record. Make sure to include which provider was notified.

For example: the medical assistant is given an order to administer a vaccine and prepares the medication. However, when the medical assistant enters the exam room, the patient states that she has decided against being vaccinated. The medical assistant should be respectful of the patient's decision and let the provider know. The refusal of the medication is noted in the patient's health record.

> **CRITICAL THINKING BOX 16.10**
>
> Bella is working with Daniela on the Patient's Bill of Rights. Bella asks Daniela to summarize these rights. What might Daniela say?

> **CRITICAL THINKING BOX 16.11**
>
> Daniela asks Bella how much a medical assistant really uses the Patient's Bill of Rights. Bella provides this scenario for Daniela: Mrs. Ella Jones, a new patient to the practice, comes in for her 28-week pregnancy check. After the provider examines her, he comes out and gives you an order for the patient. You are to give the patient RhoGAM, because she has Rh-negative blood. This is a standard practice with mothers who have Rh-negative blood. You prepare the medication and go to the exam room. You explain to Mrs. Jones what the provider ordered. She asks, " Is RhoGAM a blood product?" and you reply that it is. She refuses it, explaining that she is a Jehovah's Witness and can't accept blood products. Bella asks Daniela, "Keeping in mind the Patient's Bill of Rights, how might a medical assistant demonstrate sensitivity to Mrs. Jones' rights in this situation"? How might Daniela answer? Discuss your answer with a peer.

PRACTICE REQUIREMENTS

Many healthcare professionals are required to complete an educational program before they can work in healthcare. Upon completion, they usually must pass an exam before practicing. This section will discuss the practice requirements and scope of practice of physicians, advanced practice professionals, and other healthcare professionals (Table 16.11).

Text continued on p. 377

WALDEN-MARTIN
FAMILY MEDICAL CLINIC
1234 ANYSTREET | ANYTOWN, ANYSTATE 12345
PHONE 123-123-1234 | FAX 123-123-5678

Patient Bill of Rights
RIGHTS

1. **Medical Care and Dental Care.** The right to quality care consistent with available resources and accepted standards. The right to refuse treatment to the extent permitted by law and Government regulations, and to be informed of refusal consequences. When concerned about care received, the right to request review of care adequacy.
2. **Respectful Treatment.** The right to considerate and respectful care, with recognition of personal dignity.
3. **Privacy and Confidentiality.** The right, within law and military regulations, to privacy and confidentiality concerning medical care.
4. **Identity.** The right to know, at all times, the identity, professional status, and professional credentials of health care personnel, as well as the name of the health care provider primarily responsible for his or her care.
5. **Explanation of Care.** The right to an explanation concerning diagnosis, treatment, procedures, and prognosis of illness in terms the patient can understand. When it is not medically advisable to give such information to the patient, information should be provided to appropriate family members or, in their absence, another appropriate person.
6. **Informed Consent.** The right to be advised in non-clinical terms of information (significant complications, risks, benefits, and alternative treatments) needed to make knowledgeable decisions on treatment consent or refusal.
7. **Research Projects.** The right to be advised if the facility proposes to perform research associated with care. The right to refuse to participate in any research projects.
8. **Safe Environment.** The right to care and treatment in a safe environment.
9. **Medical Treatment Facility (MTF) or Dental Treatment Facility (DTF) Rules and Regulations.** The right to be informed of facility conduct rules and regulations. The patient should be informed about smoking rules and should expect compliance with those rules from other individuals. Patients are entitled to information about the MTF or DTF mechanism for the initiation, review, and resolution of patient complaints.

RESPONSIBILITIES

1. **Providing Information.** The responsibility to provide, to the best of his or her knowledge, accurate and complete information about complaints, past illness, hospitalizations, medications, and other matters relating to his or her health. A patient has the responsibility to let his or her primary health care provider know whether he or she understands the treatment and what is expected of him or her.
2. **Respect and Consideration.** The responsibility for being considerate of the rights of other patients and MTF and DTF health care personnel and for assistance in the control of noise, smoking, and the number of visitors. The patient is responsible for being respectful of the property of other persons and of the facility.
3. **Compliance with Medical Care.** The responsibility for complying with medical and nursing treatment plans, including follow-up care, recommended by health care providers. This includes keeping appointments on time and notifying the MTF or DTF when appointments cannot be kept.
4. **Medical Records.** The responsibility for ensuring that medical records are promptly returned to the medical facility for appropriate filing and maintenance when records are transported by the patients for the purpose of medical appointment or consultation, etc. All medical records documenting care provided by any MTF or DTF are the property of the U.S. Government.
5. **MTF and DTF Rules and Regulations.** The responsibility for following the MTF and DTF rules and regulations affecting patient care conduct. Regulations regarding smoking should be followed by all patients.
6. **Reporting of Patient Complaints.** The responsibility for helping the MTF or DTF commander provide the best possible care to all beneficiaries. Patients' recommendations, questions, or complaints should be reported to the patient contact representative.

FIG. 16.4 Patient's Bill of Rights.

PROCEDURE 16.1 Apply the Patient's Bill of Rights

Tasks
Apply the patient's bill of rights in scenarios related to choice of treatment, consent for treatment, and refusal of treatment.

Scenario 1 (Choice of Treatment)
Julia Berkley (DOB 07/05/1992) saw Dr. Angela Perez during her entire pregnancy. Julia is experiencing some complications. Dr. Perez explained the choices Julia had for delivery. She stated that, with the complications, a cesarean delivery (C-section) may be the best option. Because you are working with Dr. Perez, you prepare the consent form for the C-section. You go into the exam room to have Julia sign the consent form. As you discuss the form, Julia tells you that she is fearful of a C-section and wants a vaginal delivery.

Scenario 2 (Consent for Treatment)
Ken Thomas (DOB 10/25/61) sees Jean Burke, N.P., before leaving on a week-long trip out of the country. He is leaving in 3 days and wants a hepatitis A vaccine injection. The area he is traveling to has a high risk for hepatitis A. Ms. Burke orders immune globulin for Ken. You prepare the injection and enter the exam room. As you are telling Ken about the side effects of the medication, he asks, "What is immune globulin?" You reply that it is a sterile medication made of antibodies from blood. Ken states that he is a Jehovah's Witness and cannot receive blood products.

Scenario 3 (Refusal of Treatment)
Aaron Jackson (DOB 10/17/2011) is brought in by his mother for his well-child checkup. His records indicate that he is due for his first varicella vaccine injection. You bring the Chickenpox Vaccine VIS (vaccine information statement) and the Vaccine Authorization form to the exam room. As you start to discuss the vaccine, Aaron's mother, Patricia, interrupts you and tells you she is not interested in having Aaron get his chickenpox vaccination.

Equipment and Supplies
- Patient health records
- Patient's Bill of Rights (see Fig. 16.4)
- General Procedure Consent form (Fig. 16.5)
- Chickenpox VIS (available at https://www.cdc.gov)
- Vaccine Authorization form (Fig. 16.6)

Continued

PROCEDURE 16.1 Apply the Patient's Bill of Rights—cont'd

Procedural Steps

1. Review the Patient's Bill of Rights. Apply the Patient's Bill of Rights as you role-play each of the three scenarios.
   Purpose: A medical assistant needs to be knowledgeable about the facility's Patient's Bill of Rights.
2. Using Scenario 1, role-play the situation with a peer. You are the medical assistant. Demonstrate how a medical assistant should handle the situation. Apply the Patient's Bill of Rights to the situation by remembering the rights of the patient.
   a. Show sensitivity to the patient by being respectful and professional. Be open and accepting in your verbal and nonverbal body language.
   Purpose: Being open and accepting shows the patient sensitivity and respect. The medical assistant should never show any mannerisms that would pressure the patient into making a choice that isn't what he or she wants.
   b. Ask the patient if she has any questions about the procedures. Let the provider know if the patient has questions.
   Purpose: All patient questions need to be addressed before the patient can make an informed decision on the treatment.
   c. Ask the patient what she would like to do. Based on her answer, follow-up as necessary.
   Purpose: If the patient wants a C-section, then the consent form should be completed. If the patient wants a vaginal delivery, then no consent form will be needed unless indicated by state laws.
   d. Using the health record, document the patient's decision and the name of the provider notified.
   Purpose: Documenting the patient's refusal of treatment is important legally. It is also important that the medical assistant document that the provider was informed of the decision.

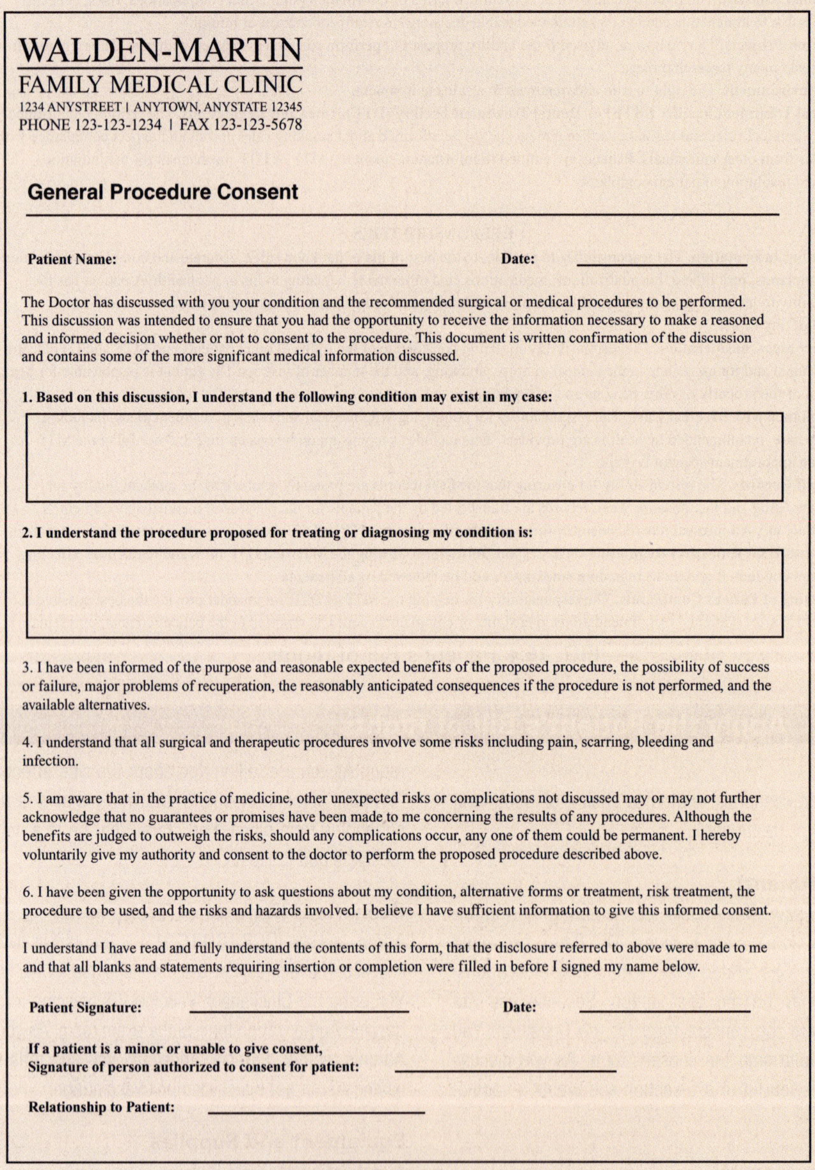
WALDEN-MARTIN
FAMILY MEDICAL CLINIC
1234 ANYSTREET | ANYTOWN, ANYSTATE 12345
PHONE 123-123-1234 | FAX 123-123-5678

General Procedure Consent

Patient Name: ____________ **Date:** ____________

The Doctor has discussed with you your condition and the recommended surgical or medical procedures to be performed. This discussion was intended to ensure that you had the opportunity to receive the information necessary to make a reasoned and informed decision whether or not to consent to the procedure. This document is written confirmation of the discussion and contains some of the more significant medical information discussed.

1. Based on this discussion, I understand the following condition may exist in my case:

2. I understand the procedure proposed for treating or diagnosing my condition is:

3. I have been informed of the purpose and reasonable expected benefits of the proposed procedure, the possibility of success or failure, major problems of recuperation, the reasonably anticipated consequences if the procedure is not performed, and the available alternatives.

4. I understand that all surgical and therapeutic procedures involve some risks including pain, scarring, bleeding and infection.

5. I am aware that in the practice of medicine, other unexpected risks or complications not discussed may or may not further acknowledge that no guarantees or promises have been made to me concerning the results of any procedures. Although the benefits are judged to outweigh the risks, should any complications occur, any one of them could be permanent. I hereby voluntarily give my authority and consent to the doctor to perform the proposed procedure described above.

6. I have been given the opportunity to ask questions about my condition, alternative forms or treatment, risk treatment, the procedure to be used, and the risks and hazards involved. I believe I have sufficient information to give this informed consent.

I understand I have read and fully understand the contents of this form, that the disclosure referred to above were made to me and that all blanks and statements requiring insertion or completion were filled in before I signed my name below.

Patient Signature: ____________ **Date:** ____________

If a patient is a minor or unable to give consent,
Signature of person authorized to consent for patient: ____________

Relationship to Patient: ____________

FIG. 16.5 General Procedure Consent Form.

CHAPTER 16 Legal Basics

PROCEDURE 16.1 Apply the Patient's Bill of Rights—cont'd

3. Using Scenario 2, role-play the situation with a peer. You are the medical assistant. Demonstrate how a medical assistant should handle the situation. Apply the Patient's Bill of Rights to the situation by remembering the rights of the patient.
   a. Show sensitivity to the patient regarding his rights to refuse. Be respectful and professional. Be open and accepting in your verbal and nonverbal body language. Be accepting of his beliefs and his refusal.

   Purpose: Being open and accepting shows the patient sensitivity and respect. The medical assistant should never show any mannerisms that would pressure the patient into making a choice that isn't what he or she wants. The patient has a right to make decisions that follow his religious beliefs.

   b. When the patient refuses the medication, be respectful in your body language and words. Notify the provider.

   Purpose: It is important to be respectful of the patient's decision and notify the provider of the refusal.

   c. Using the health record, document the patient's decision and the name of the provider notified.

   Purpose: Documenting the patient's refusal of treatment is important legally. It is also important that the medical assistant document that the provider was informed of the decision.

4. Using Scenario 3, role-play the situation with a peer. You are the medical assistant. Demonstrate how a medical assistant should handle the situation. Apply the Patient's Bill of Rights to the situation by remembering the rights of the patient.
   a. Show sensitivity to the mother of the patient by being respectful and professional. Be open and accepting in your verbal and nonverbal body language.

   Purpose: Being open and accepting shows the family member and the patient sensitivity and respect. The medical assistant should never show any mannerisms that would pressure the patient or guardian into making a choice that isn't what he or she wants.

WALDEN-MARTIN
FAMILY MEDICAL CLINIC
1234 ANYSTREET | ANYTOWN, ANYSTATE 12345
PHONE 123-123-1234 | FAX 123-123-5678

Vaccine Authorization

Last Name: _____   First Name: _____
Date of Birth: _____   Sex: ☐ Male ☐ Female

Please answer the following questions:

Question	Yes	No	Unknown
1. Are you sick or do you have a high fever today? (if yes, you should not receive vaccine)	☐	☐	☐
2. Are you allergic to chicken, eggs, or egg products?	☐	☐	☐
3. Have you ever has an allergic reaction to an injection?	☐	☐	☐
4. Are you pregnant, or think you may be?	☐	☐	☐
5. Do you have a blood clotting disorder or are you taking blood thinning medication?	☐	☐	☐

CONSENT AND RELEASE STATEMENT

I, THE UNDERSIGNED, WISH TO RECEIVE A _____ VACCINE. I CONSENT TO THE VACCINATION BEING GIVEN TO ME. I HAVE READ THE PROVIDED INFORMATION OR HAVE HAD SUCH EXPLAINED TO ME. I UNDERSTAND THE RISKS AND BENEFITS OF THIS VACCINE. I HAVE HAD AN OPPORTUNITY TO ASK QUESTIONS WHICH HAVE BEEN ANSWERED TO MY SATISFACTION. I HEREBY REQUEST THAT THE VACCINE BE GIVEN TO ME OR TO THE PERSON NAMED ABOVE FOR WHOM I AM AUTHORIZED TO MAKE THIS REQUEST.

Signature: _____   Date: _____

FIG. 16.6 Vaccine Authorization Form.

Continued

PROCEDURE 16.1   Apply the Patient's Bill of Rights—cont'd

b. Ask the mother if she has any questions about the vaccine. Let the provider know if the mother has questions.
Purpose: All patient and parent/guardian questions need to be addressed before an informed decision can be made on the treatment.
c. Ask the mother what she would like to do. Based on her answer, follow-up as necessary.
Purpose: If the parent/guardian consents to the vaccination, the Vaccine Authorization Form must be completed. If the parent/guardian refuses, the provider needs to be notified.

d. Using the health record, document the patient's decision and the name of the provider notified.
Purpose: Documenting the patient's refusal of treatment is important legally. It is also important that the medical assistant document that the provider was informed of the decision.

TABLE 16.11   Physicians, Advanced Practice Professionals, and Other Healthcare Professionals

Title	Scope of Practice	Education	Credential and License
Physicians			
Doctor of Medicine (MD)	Trained in all areas of medicine to diagnose, treat, and prescribe medications; more focus on symptoms experienced by patient.	Beyond a bachelor's degree, must complete 4 years of medical school and 2–4 years of residency. Additional years of training may be required for specialties.	Must pass all three parts of the United States Medical Licensing Examination (USMLE). Must obtain state license to practice.
Doctor of Osteopathy (DO)	Trained in all areas of medicine, like MD. Specially trained in the nervous and musculoskeletal systems and their influence on health and disease.		
Advanced Practice Professionals			
Physician Assistant (PA)	Diagnose, treat, and prescribe medication; may specialize. Supervised by physician.	Must complete a 3-year PA program beyond a bachelor's degree.	Physician Assistant–Certified (PA-C) after passing the national exam. Must obtain state license to practice.
Advanced Practice Registered Nurse (APRN)		Must complete a master's degree beyond registered nurse training.	Must pass the national certification (ser ti fi KAE shun) exam. Must obtain state license to practice.
Clinical Nurse Specialist (CNS)	Diagnose and treat patients. Many work in hospital and community settings.		
Nurse Practitioner (NP)	Diagnose, treat, and prescribe medication; may specialize. Depending on state law, can be more independent than a PA.		
Certified Nurse Midwife (CNM)	Provide prenatal and postpartum care; deliver babies.		
Certified Registered Nurse Anesthetist (CRNA)	Give anesthesia and related care to patients in surgery and for outpatient procedures.		
Other Healthcare Professionals			
Registered Nurse (RN)	Work in a wide range of positions, including clinical and administrative; perform more advanced assessments, patient care, and treatments than LPNs.	Have 2–4 years of education.	Must pass a licensure exam to practice.
Licensed Practical Nurse (LPN)	Work in long-term care, ambulatory care, and hospital settings; perform basic patient assessments, patient care, and treatments.	Have 1 year of education.	Must pass a licensure exam to practice.
Medical Assistant (MA)	Primarily work in ambulatory care settings. Perform administrative, clinical, and waived laboratory testing under the supervision of a provider.	Varies from about 8 to 24 months; may get a diploma or an associate degree.	National certification exam is optional.

> **MEDICAL TERMINOLOGY**
>
> **oste/o**: bone
> **-pathy**: disease process
> **pre-**: before
> **nat/o**: birth, born
> **-al**: pertaining to
> **post-**: after
> **-partum**: delivery

Practice Acts and State Boards

The Tenth Amendment of the U.S. Constitution empowers each state to establish laws that protect the health and safety of that state's citizens. Each state has passed laws and regulations that govern the practice of medicine. These laws and regulations are in a state statute called the *Medical Practice Act*. The Medical Practice Act also outlines the responsibility of the state medical board.

Each state's medical board issues licenses to practice medicine. The board also investigates complaints and disciplines members who violate the law. The state medical board creates policies related to the practice of medicine. Other healthcare professionals (i.e., nurses) have Practice Acts and state boards with similar roles.

Licensure. Many healthcare professionals must have a state license before they begin their practice. The **licensure** (LIE sen shur) process allows the state board to ensure that the healthcare professional meets the education and training requirements. Passing the state licensing exam is a requirement for the license. Once a person gets a license, it needs to be renewed, about every 1 to 2 years. Besides the renewal fee, many state boards require evidence of continuing education.

If a healthcare professional is already licensed in one state, there are different methods of obtaining a license in additional states (Table 16.12). In 2015 the Interstate Medical Licensure Compact was created. This compact helped create a streamlined pathway for physicians to get licensure in multiple states. With the changes in healthcare, more rural care is provided by **telemedicine** (TEL i med i sin), and more physicians are becoming **locum tenens** (LOE kuhm TEE nenz). With these changes, the need for licensure from multiple states has increased. To be eligible for licensure through the Compact process, physicians need to meet several requirements. Eligible physicians can select the Compact member states where they would like to practice. Once the verification process has been completed, the physician will get a full, unrestricted license to practice medicine in those states.

> **VOCABULARY**
>
> **licensure**: A mandatory process established by state law that ensures a person has met the legal standards for practicing an occupation in that state.
> **telemedicine**: The use of telecommunication technology to provide healthcare services to patients at a distance; it is usually used in rural communities.
> **locum tenens**: Latin for "to substitute for"; physicians or advance practice professionals who temporarily contracted to provide healthcare services when a facility has a vacancy, vacation, or a leave of absence.

Scope of Practice. The *scope of practice* for an occupation defines the procedures, actions, and processes that individuals are permitted to perform. A state board determines the scope of practice for that state's specific occupation. In some cases, the medical state board oversees the scope of practice of other healthcare occupations. If healthcare professionals practice beyond their scope of practice, they risk being sued for malpractice (Box 16.12).

The scope of practice for physicians is similar across the states. Physicians diagnose, treat, prevent, or monitor disease conditions. The scope of practice differs between specialties. For instance, a family practice physician cannot perform heart surgery.

For medical assistants, the scope of practice laws vary by state. Box 16.13 provides a list of common medical assistant duties. Some states allow medical assistants to perform injections. Some states do not allow medical assistants to give certain types of injectable medications or to calculate the medication amount. It is important for you to know the legal scope of practice in your state (Procedure 16.2).

Disciplinary Action. The state boards have an obligation to the public to protect consumers. To do this, state boards take disciplinary action against licensed professionals for felony convictions and

TABLE 16.12 Methods to Obtain a License

Method	Description
Licensing exam	Passing the state's licensing exam and meeting the requirements
Endorsement (en DOORS ment)	A state board grants a license to a person who is currently licensed in another state that has the same or stricter standards.
Reciprocity (RES i pros i tee)	A state has a written agreement with another state to recognize licenses issued by that state without additional review of the person's credentials.

> **BOX 16.12 Legal Example: Scope of Practice**
>
> An obstetrician-gynecologist performed a procedure on a patient in her office. A few days after the procedure, the patient had increased pain that radiated along her side to her back. The patient called the office and spoke to a medical assistant. She mentioned the increase in pain, bleeding, and changes in her bowel movement. The medical assistant thought she had a urinary tract infection, so she asked the patient if she had any of the typical symptoms. The medical assistant did not talk to the provider about the patient's pain or bleeding because she did not think the complaints were serious enough. The medical assistant did not ask more questions about the pain or bleeding. The medical assistant told the patient her symptoms could be normal and advised her to take 800 mg of ibuprofen. (The medical assistant had been instructed by the providers to advise patients to take ibuprofen, 800 mg, every 8 hours as needed, for any sort of abdominal or back pain.) Later the patient was admitted to the intensive care unit, had to undergo a hysterectomy, and later died. Two months after the procedure, the patient's antibiotic prescription was found at the front desk. (The front desk staff had failed to give the patient the prescription after the procedure.)
>
> The plaintiff sued for damages for the doctors' professional negligence (malpractice) and the clinic for the medical assistant and front desk staff's negligence. After a 16-day trial, the jury returned a verdict for the defense. The plaintiff appealed. The appeals court ruled that the complaint was ordinary negligence and not medical malpractice. The appeals court also stated that the plaintiff could sue the clinic and medical assistant. The jury would have to decide if the medical assistant had practiced medicine without a license.

Wong v. Chappell, No. 333 Ga. App. 422, (2015). https://www.leagle.com/decision/ingaco20150713164

BOX 16.13 Typical Duties of a Medical Assistant

- Obtain and record patient history and personal information
- Obtain and record vital signs (blood pressure, pulse, respiration rate), height, and weight
- Assist the provider during physical exams
- Administer oral, injectable, and inhaled medications as directed by provider and as permitted by state law
- Obtain blood samples for laboratory tests
- Perform waived laboratory tests
- Schedule patients for appointments
- Perform receptionist duties
- Bill patients for services

BOX 16.14 Examples of Unprofessional Conduct for Physicians

- Substance and alcohol abuse
- Neglect of a patient
- Sexual misconduct
- Not meeting the accepted standard of care
- Dishonesty when obtaining a license or failing to meet the continuing education requirement
- Convicted of a felony or fraud
- Inadequate record keeping
- Delegating others to practice medicine

PROCEDURE 16.2 Locate the Medical Assistant's Legal Scope of Practice

Tasks
Search online to locate the legal scope of practice for a medical assistant practicing in your state. Summarize the scope of practice.

Equipment and Supplies
- Computer and printer with word processing software and internet access

Procedural Steps
1. Using the internet, search for the medical assistant's scope of practice in your state. Read the scope of practice for your state.
   Purpose: Scope of practice information is available online.
2. Using the word processing software, create a short paper summarizing the medical assistant's scope of practice. Address the following points:
   a. Can medical assistants give injections? If so, what type of injections?
   b. Can medical assistants give oral, topical, and/or inhaled medications?
   c. Can medical assistants calculate drug dosages?
   d. What is the medical assistant's role with prescriptions?
   e. Describe additional duties that a medical assistant can legally perform in your state.
   f. Include the website address(es) you used for this paper.
   Note: If your instructor does not provide you with different guidelines for the paper, follow these. Create at least a one-page paper, using double line spacing and a 10–12 pt font. Margins should be 1 inch for all sides.
   Purpose: Summarizing the scope of practice will help identify the duties a medical assistant can legally perform in your state.
3. After completing the paper, proofread the paper. Use correct spelling, punctuation, sentence structure, and capitalization. Make any changes required. Based on your instructor's directions, submit the paper to the instructor.
   Purpose: Proofreading helps to identify mistakes.

unprofessional, improper, or incompetent practice. Box 16.14 lists examples of unprofessional conduct for physicians. The following are some of the disciplinary actions state boards can take against healthcare professionals:

- *License revoked*: License is terminated, and the person can no longer practice in that occupation in the state.
- *License suspended*: Person cannot practice in that occupation for a specific period of time.
- *License surrendered*: Person voluntarily gives up license.
- *Probation*: Person's license is monitored for a specific period of time.
- *Reprimand*: Person is sent a warning or letter of concern.

Certification and Registration

For some healthcare professional occupations, certification or registry is available. *Certification* (ser ti fi KAE shun) is a voluntary process indicating that a person has met predetermined criteria. The certification is granted by a nongovernmental agency, such as a national association. Most certifications require educational preparation and passing the certification exam. Medical assistants can obtain a certification. For advanced practice professionals, many state boards require certification before the professional can apply for a license. Ongoing certification requirements vary by state. In many states, the ongoing certification is voluntary.

Some healthcare occupations have registration. People working in a specific occupation have their name entered into an official registry. To become registered, a person must meet requirements. These may include educational training, passing a registry exam, participating in continuing education, and conditions of that registry.

Accreditation

Accreditation differs from licensure and certification. *Accreditation* (ah KRED i tae shun) is a recognition granted by a specific organization to educational, healthcare, or managed care organizations that have demonstrated compliance with standards. Common accreditation organizations include:

- The Joint Commission: Accredits ambulatory care facilities, hospitals, behavioral healthcare facilities, home healthcare agencies, and laboratory services.
- National Committee for Quality Assurance (NCQA): Accredits health plans (i.e., managed care plans).
- College of American Pathologists (CAP) Laboratory Accreditation Program: Accredits medical laboratories.
- Commission on Accreditation of Allied Health Education Programs (CAAHEP): Accredits specific allied health programs, including medical assisting.
- Accrediting Bureau of Health Education Schools (ABHES): Accredits both schools and specific allied health programs, including medical assisting.

There are advantages to being accredited. Students from accredited medical assisting programs can take specific certification examinations. Agencies that have Joint Commission accreditation gain the community's confidence in the quality and safety of the care provided. The accreditation is recognized by insurance companies and may reduce liability insurance costs.

CLOSING COMMENTS

Learning about concepts of law is important for all healthcare professionals. With the increase in lawsuits through the years, healthcare professionals must practice within their scope of practice and ensure that patients have no grounds for lawsuits.

The medical assistant is trained to perform administrative, patient care, and waived laboratory skills. With this wide range of duties, it is critical that the medical assistant always remember to work within the boundaries of the law. Two examples of situations that can lead to lawsuits are *not* following up with patients who called the facility, and *not* getting consent before giving a child a vaccination. The medical assistant is not exempt from being named in lawsuits. Strategies to reduce the risk of lawsuits include:

- Respecting and communicating professionally with patients
- Working within one's scope of practice
- Accurately and concisely documenting all patient encounters
- Following the facility's policies and procedures

EXCEPTIONAL CUSTOMER SERVICE

One of the key elements to providing customer service is respecting the patient. The medical assistant may not understand why a patient refuses a test, procedure, or treatment. Some patients do not share their thoughts on such matters. Other patients may cite a personal belief or a religious belief. As a medical assistant, you might not agree with the patient's ideas or beliefs. To provide exceptional customer service, a medical assistant must be sensitive to the patient's rights. This means the medical assistant must be respectful of the patient's right to refuse and must notify the provider. It is not the time for the medical assistant to:

- pressure the patient into changing the refusal.
- gossip with peers about the patient's refusal.
- make fun of the patient.

Being professional and sensitive means the medical assistant respects patients and their right to refuse.

CHAPTER REVIEW

This chapter discussed the balance of power in the state and federal governments. Types of law, including criminal and civil laws, were explained. The plaintiff in criminal cases is the government. Criminal offenses are classified as misdemeanors and felonies. The plaintiff in civil cases is an individual. The plaintiff can sue the government, businesses, and individuals. When the plaintiff wins a civil suit, damages may be awarded. Intentional torts and negligent torts can occur in healthcare. It is important that all healthcare professionals make sure their actions and behaviors do not lead to intentional or negligent torts.

In healthcare cases, the defense lawyer may use different defenses. Using a legal defense, a legal technicality (e.g., the statute of limitations), can lead to dismissal of a case. Denial and affirmative defenses may also be used.

The court process was discussed, along with the two types of alternative dispute resolution. Arbitration leads to a binding decision, whereas mediation does not.

In malpractice cases, the 4 *D*s of negligence need to be proven: duty of care, dereliction, damages, and direct cause. If one of these is not proven, malpractice has not occurred. Professional liability insurance can be purchased by providers (and other healthcare professionals) to help protect against lawsuit settlements.

The provider has a unique relationship with patients. This provider-patient relationship is a contract. It is important that the staff's and the provider's actions do not lead to a breach of contract.

The following consents were discussed:
- *Implied consent*: Consent that is inferred based on signs, actions, or conduct of the patient rather than oral communication (using words).
- *Expressed consent*: Consent that is given either by the spoken or written word.
- *Informed consent*: A legal process that ensures that the patient or guardian understands the treatment and gives consent for the treatment.

The licensure process allows a state board to ensure that a healthcare professional meets the education and training requirements. Providers and other licensed healthcare professionals have several options for obtaining a secondary license to practice in another state.

The scope of practice for an occupation defines the procedures, actions, and processes that individuals in that occupation are permitted to perform. A state board determines the scope of practice for that state's specific occupation.

The state boards can take disciplinary actions against licensed professionals for felony convictions and unprofessional, improper, or incompetent practice.

SCENARIO WRAP-UP

Daniela enjoyed working with Bella as she studied for her midterm exam in her law class. She found that Bella had unique ways of remembering and explaining concepts. These methods helped Daniela. Daniela knew it was important for her to understand the concepts because they might appear on her national certification test.

Daniela now understands the legal importance of answering patients' calls and returning them. She knows this is important to prevent abandonment suits from patients. Daniela encourages her peers to return calls in a timely manner and has talked with her supervisor about strategies to make the reception desk more efficient.

Thanks to Bella's help, Daniela also realizes the importance of the Patient's Bill of Rights to patients and to every healthcare professional. These rights must be upheld and respected. Medical assistants and other healthcare professionals must be sensitive when patients refuse tests, treatments, and procedures. Daniela is looking forward to studying more about the healthcare laws and learning how they affect her job.

17 Healthcare Laws

LEARNING OBJECTIVES

1. Describe components of the Health Information Portability and Accountability Act (HIPAA); apply HIPAA rules in regard to privacy and the release of information.
2. Describe the Health Information Technology for Economic and Clinical Health (HITECH) Act.
3. Describe the Genetic Information Nondiscrimination Act of 2008 (GINA), as well as drug laws such as the Food, Drug, and Cosmetic Act and the Controlled Substances Act.
4. Describe the Patient Protection and Affordable Care Act, the Clinical Laboratory Improvement Amendments (CLIA), the Occupational Safety and Health Act, and the Needlestick Safety and Prevention Act.
5. Define the Good Samaritan Act(s), and discuss laws for end-of-life issues.
6. Describe compliance with public health statutes related to communicable diseases, as well as perform such compliance.
7. Describe compliance with public health statutes related to wounds of violence, abuse, neglect, and exploitation.
8. Describe compliance with reporting vaccination issues.
9. Discuss how compliance programs work, examine common compliance concerns in healthcare, follow protocol in reporting an illegal activity, and correctly complete an incident report.

CHAPTER OUTLINE

1. **Opening Scenario, 380**
2. **You Will Learn, 381**
3. **Introduction to Law, 381**
4. **Privacy and Confidentiality, 381**
   a. Health Insurance Portability and Accountability Act, 381
      i. *Privacy Rule, 382*
      ii. *Security Rule, 386*
   b. Health Information Technology for Economic and Clinical Health Act, 386
   c. Genetic Information Nondiscrimination Act, 387
5. **Additional Healthcare Laws and Regulations, 387**
   a. Drug Laws, 388
      i. *Food, Drug, and Cosmetic Act, 388*
      ii. *Controlled Substances Act, 388*
   b. Insurance Law, 388
      i. *Patient Protection and Affordable Care Act, 388*
   c. Medical Laboratory Regulations, 388
      i. *Clinical Laboratory Improvement Amendments, 388*
   d. Workplace Safety Laws, 389
      i. *Occupational Safety and Health Act, 389*
      ii. *Needlestick Safety and Prevention Act, 389*
   e. Good Samaritan Laws, 390
   f. Laws for End-of-Life Issues, 390
6. **Compliance Reporting, 391**
   a. Compliance With Public Health Statutes, 391
      i. *Reportable Diseases, 391*
      ii. *Wounds of Violence, 391*
      iii. *Child Abuse, Neglect, and Exploitation, 391*
      iv. *Adult Abuse, Neglect, and Exploitation, 392*
   b. Reporting Vaccination Issues, 393
   c. Compliance Programs, 393
      i. *Financial Concerns, 393*
      ii. *Employment Concerns, 394*
      iii. *Environmental Safety Concerns, 396*
      iv. *Patient Safety Concerns, 396*
7. **Closing Comments, 399**
8. **Chapter Review, 399**
9. **Scenario Wrap-Up, 399**

▶ OPENING SCENARIO

Daniela Garcia was recently hired as a part-time float receptionist at Walden-Martin Family Medical (WMFM) Clinic. She works with many coworkers and providers. Daniela is attending the medical assistant program at the local community college. She is currently taking a law and ethics course. She has learned about the basic law concepts. She is now learning about the healthcare laws.

Many of Daniela's friends find law and ethics to be less exciting than other courses. Daniela disagrees with them. She sees the value in learning about laws that impact healthcare. She realizes it will make her a better medical assistant.

The WMFM clinic administration created the policies and procedures to follow the federal and state laws. Daniela has already started to see how compliance with laws impacts what she does as a receptionist. She understands the importance of following the clinic's policies and

CHAPTER 17 Healthcare Laws

procedures. Daniela realizes that by not complying with laws, she puts her job in jeopardy. It can also raise many issues for the facility, including fines from governmental agencies. Daniela is excited to continue learning about healthcare laws.

YOU WILL LEARN

1. To describe the Health Insurance and Portability and Accountability Act, related terminology, the Privacy Rule, and the Security Rule.
2. To explain the impact of the Health Information Technology for Economic and Clinical Health Act.
3. To describe additional healthcare laws and regulations that impact ambulatory care.
4. To explain the provider's role and compliance with public health statutes.
5. To describe compliance programs including financial, employment, and environmental safety concerns.

INTRODUCTION TO LAW

In this chapter, we discuss federal and state laws that impact healthcare. Typically, a few people are the "experts" on healthcare laws in an ambulatory care setting. They work with management to create policies and procedures that follow the laws:
- *Policies* are written principles that provide goals for the employees and the facility. For instance, a policy statement may indicate that patient confidentiality is protected at all times.
- *Procedures* are step-by-step directions. They provide a consistent and repetitive approach to accomplish the goal. For instance, there might be a procedure on how to update patient information while protecting the patient's privacy.

Following the laws is important. Not only does it safeguard patients, it also protects employees and the facility. Facilities that do not comply with laws can be fined and have additional penalties imposed by governmental agencies. Therefore medical assistants need to be knowledgeable about healthcare laws.

PRIVACY AND CONFIDENTIALITY

Privacy (PRI vah see) means being free from unwanted intrusion. Privacy was one of the principles our country was built on. The word *privacy* does not appear in the Constitution. Privacy elements appear in the amendments (Box 17.1). An *invasion of privacy* is the disclosing private facts without consent of the individual. An invasion of privacy is an intentional tort.

Confidentiality (KON fi den shee ahl i tee) is a legally protected right of patients. Healthcare professionals have the duty not to disclose medical, financial, and insurance information unless authorized by the patient. Information is shared during the provider-patient relationship, so creating a trusting relationship is critical (Fig. 17.1). The patient shares sensitive, personal information with the provider, which needs to remain confidential. It cannot be discussed outside of the provider-patient relationship.

All states have laws regarding confidentiality. If the state law is stricter than the federal law, then the state law takes **precedence** (PRES i duhns). This concept is known as *state preemption*. We will examine the federal laws that relate to privacy and confidentiality in the following sections.

Health Insurance Portability and Accountability Act

With the anticipated changes in healthcare technology (e.g., the **electronic health record [EHR]**), Congress passed the Health Insurance Portability and Accountability Act of 1996 (HIPAA). The U.S. Department of Health and Human Services (HHS) is the agency responsible for developing the specific requirements of the law. The HHS Office for Civil Rights (OCR) enforces HIPAA.

Before HIPAA, the billing and payment processes were slow. Nationwide, insurance companies used many different **coding systems**. The coding systems were used to provide information on disease and treatments for payment purposes. It took months for facilities to receive insurance payments for services provided to patients. Paper transactions and paper checks were commonly used.

One of the goals of HIPAA was to simplify the electronic exchange of information. All health plans, **claims clearinghouses**, and healthcare facilities needed to be consistent with their electronic exchange of information. This meant they all needed to use the same coding systems. They also needed to follow the same requirements for the electronic exchange of information. Today, this is called *administrative simplification*.

VOCABULARY

claims clearinghouse: An organization that accepts the claim data from the provider, reformats the data to meet the specifications outlined by the insurance plan, and submits the claim.

coding system: A system designed to use characters (i.e., numbers and letters) to represent something like a medical procedure or a disease.

electronic health record (EHR): An electronic record conforms to nationally recognized standards and contains health-related information about a specific patient. It can be created, managed, and consulted by authorized clinicians and staff from more than one healthcare organization.

precedence: Followed first.

BOX 17.1 Amendments Related to Privacy

- Amendment 1: Freedom of religion, speech, and the press (allows the right to peaceably assemble)
- Amendment 2: Freedom from housing soldiers unless owner consents
- Amendment 4: Freedom from unreasonable searches and seizure (need a supported probable cause before a house and property can be searched and seized)
- Amendment 5: Protection of rights to life, liberty, and property
- Amendment 14: Freedom from being deprived from life, liberty, or property without due process of law

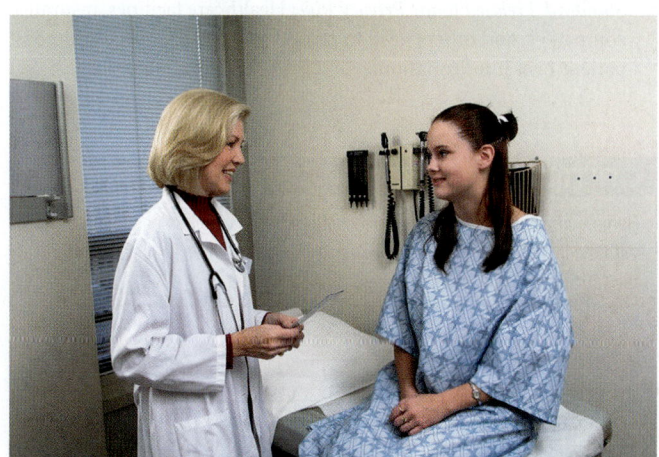

FIG. 17.1 Patient confidentiality is the most important trust that exists between the patient and the provider. (From Proctor D, et al: *Kinn's The Medical Assistant*, ed 13, St. Louis, 2017, Elsevier.)

BOX 17.2 HIPAA Terminology

- *Covered entities*: Healthcare providers, health (insurance) plans, and *claims clearinghouse* that transmit protected health information electronically (Box 17.3).
- *Protected health information* (PHI): Individually identifiable health information stored or transmitted by covered entities or business associates. Includes verbal, paper, or electronic information.
- *Business associate*: A person or business that provides a service to a covered entity that involves access to PHI. Examples include legal, billing, and management services; accreditation agencies; consulting firms; and claims processing organizations.
- *Permission*: A reason for releasing or disclosing patient information under HIPAA.
- *De-identify:* To remove all direct patient identifiers from the PHI information. In other words, this is the process to remove anything that can link the information back to a specific person. This process can create the limited data set (Table 17.1).
- *Limited data set*: PHI that has had all of the direct patient identifiers removed. This would include the name, contact information, Social Security number, and so on. The only information left would be health information (see Table 17.1).

BOX 17.3 Examples of Covered Entities Under HIPAA

- Providers (medical doctors, doctors of osteopathic medicine, nurse practitioners, physician assistants, etc.)
- Dentists
- Chiropractors
- Psychologists
- Nursing homes
- Pharmacies
- Ambulatory care facilities (e.g., clinics)
- Health insurance companies
- Government insurance programs (Medicare, Medicaid)
- Health maintenance organizations (HMOs)
- Claims clearinghouses
- Billing services

TABLE 17.1 Example of Protected Health Information (PHI) Under HIPAA Grouped by Direct Patient Identifiers and De-Identified Information

Examples of Direct Patient Identifiers	Examples of Limited Data Set Information
Personal demographic information (name, date of birth, address, phone number, Social Security number)	Physical or mental health conditions
	Test results
	Medications currently taking
Payment and insurance information	Allergies

The goal is to reduce clerical burden and increase **electronic transaction** adoption.

With the increased electronic transactions, HIPAA also contained provisions for the privacy and security of the patients' information. Primary provisions of the law were stated in four standards:

- *Standard 1 related to transactions and code sets:* HHS adopted standard transactions for the electronic exchange of administrative healthcare information. This included insurance claims, payment, and insurance eligibility information. The goal was to speed up the process of identifying insurance benefits, submitting insurance claims, and receiving payment. Standard 1 also included mandating universal coding systems. Processes become more efficient with everyone using the same coding systems.
  - The *Current Procedural Terminology* (CPT) is used to code procedures and services.
  - The *International Classification of Diseases* (ICD) is used to code diseases and disorders.
- *Standard 2 related to the Privacy Rule*: Healthcare facilities, insurance companies, and others need to protect written, electronic, and oral patient health information.
- *Standard 3 related to the Security Rule*: Healthcare facilities, insurance companies, and others need to protect the patient information that is electronically stored and transmitted.
- *Standard 4 related to unique identifiers:*
  - *National Provider Identifier (NPI)*: Each covered healthcare provider has a unique identification number that is used for financial and administrative transactions. The NPI is a 10-digit number.
  - *Health Plan Identifier (HPI)*: Each health plan has a unique identifier.
  - *Employer Identification Number (EIN)*: Each employer has a unique identifier issued by the Internal Revenue Services.

In addition to these provisions, HIPAA focused on insurance portability. HIPAA allows extra opportunities to enroll in health insurance plans. For instance, a person can request special enrollment if there is a loss in coverage from another policy. HIPAA prohibited enrollment discrimination based on a person's health history or genetics.

Box 17.2 describes HIPAA-related terminology. It is important to have a good understanding of these terms when studying HIPAA.

Privacy Rule. The HIPAA Privacy Rule has created national standards that protect health records and other patient information. The Privacy Rule's main purpose is to define and limit the situations in which a patient's information can be used or disclosed. The rule also describes the patients' rights over their information. Patients have the right to do the following:

- Examine their health information.
- Obtain a copy of their health records.
- Request corrections to be made if information is incorrect.

CRITICAL THINKING 17.1

Daniela is working with Bella, a medical assistant who has been helping her with the law course. They are reviewing HIPAA. Bella asks Daniela to describe the four HIPAA standards. How might Daniela respond?

VOCABULARY

electronic transaction: The electronic exchange of information between two agencies to accomplish financial or administrative healthcare activities.

TABLE 17.2 Permissions Not Requiring Written Patient Authorization

Permission	Description
To the individual	A covered entity can disclose PHI to the patient. If you want a copy of your health record, you can get it without completing a written authorization (record release form) (Box 17.5).
Treatment, payment, and healthcare operations (TPO)	• Treatment relates to when the covered entity discloses PHI when coordinating or managing healthcare. For instance, you do not need to sign a written authorization for your provider to send a prescription to a pharmacy. • Payment relates to activities related to payment or reimbursement for services. For instance, if you were not paying your bill, the healthcare facility might turn your account over to a collection agency. They would not need a written authorization from you to disclose your information. • Healthcare operations relate to the financial, legal, quality improvement, and administrative activities that healthcare facilities need to do to run and support their business.
Uses and disclosures with opportunity to agree or object	The patient can give informal permission when asked outright or can be given an opportunity to agree or object. For example, a patient comes into the exam room with a friend. You ask the patient if she wants the friend to remain. The patient can say yes or no.
Incidental use and disclosure	We need to take reasonable precautions so patient information is not overheard or seen by others. The Privacy Rule does not require that we get written authorization for incidental disclosures. For instance, you take precautions but you are overheard discussing patient PHI on the phone. There is no need for you to get a written authorization from the patient on the phone for the incidental disclosure.
Public interest and benefit activities	PHI can be released when required by law, law enforcement, and for public health activities. PHI can also be released for research, organ and tissue donation, and for workers' compensation. Funeral directors, coroners, and medical examiners can also obtain PHI.
Limited data set	The direct patient identifiers are removed from the PHI. The remaining information can be used for research, public health purposes, and healthcare operations.

BOX 17.4 Legal Example: HIPAA Settlement for Lack of Business Associate Agreement

In 2015 the HHS Office for Civil Rights (OCR) investigated the Center for Children's Digestive Health (CCDH). CCDH failed to obtain a written signed business associate agreement with Filefax. CCDH disclosed the PHI of at least 10,728 patients to Filefax. In 2017 CCDH paid the HHS $31,000 to settle the potential violations and agreed to implement a corrective action plan.

From https://www.hhs.gov/sites/default/files/ra_cap_ccdh.pdf.

BOX 17.5 Patients and Their Health Information

It is understood that the contents of the health record belong to the patient. The physical part of the record belongs to the facility or provider. Patients own the contents and can request a copy of their own record at any time. There are state laws that regulate the release. In most cases, the patient can get a copy and can be told of his or her health information immediately. The following examples illustrate cases in when patients cannot get their information immediately:

When a provider is treating a patient for emotional or mental conditions, the provider can exercise professional judgment to determine if the records should be released to the patient. This is known as the *doctrine of professional discretion*. The provider may feel that if the patient saw the records, more harm than good would result. For instance, you are obtaining a weight on a patient with an eating disorder. The provider's policy is that you do not share the weight with the patient. The provider makes the decision if the weight is shared. For some patients, a weight gain may harm their current success.

Another situation when patients cannot get health information immediately when requested relates to diagnostic tests. In the ambulatory care setting, patients have diagnostic tests done all the time. The provider must review the results before the results are given to the patient. After reviewing the results, the provider instructs the medical assistant what to tell the patient. The medical assistant contacts the patient and discusses what the provider stated. After the call, the medical assistant documents the call in the patient's health record.

Covered entities must comply with the Privacy Rule. They must safeguard all patient information. Covered entities must ensure that business associates also keep protected health information (PHI) private. A written agreement detailing how the business associate will safeguard the PHI must be signed. Cover entities cannot give PHI to business associates until the agreement has been signed (Box 17.4). Only PHI required for the job of the business associates can be given.

The Privacy Rule lists *permissions* or reasons that the health information can be released. Table 17.2 describes the permissions that do not require written authorization from the patient to release PHI. The only permission that requires written authorization from patients is disclosing the PHI to a third party. Examples of this type of disclosure may include the following:

- The patient wants another person to be told information.
- The patient wants the records transferred to another facility, such as the following:
  - A life insurance company
  - An employer for the preemployment health requirements
  - Another healthcare facility (patients request release because they are switching providers)
  - The patient's lawyer

In both situations, the patient must sign a form allowing the information to be released. In some agencies, a *disclosure authorization form* (also called authorization to disclose form) must be completed before information can be shared with another person. The patient must complete a *record release form* before the records can be transferred. The form names can differ from facility to facility. To make things more interesting, some facilities combine the forms into one document and may call it release of information authorization or something similar.

The forms typically require the patient to indicate the information to be released/disclosed. The form must include the patient's name and the date of the request. The person or facility disclosing the information and receiving the information must be indicated. The form must include an expiration date. The forms also include a statement to notify patients of their right to revoke the release.

> **STUDY TIP**
>
> Remember that *permission* is a reason for release. In HIPAA, it does not mean the patient gives permission for the release.

Disclosure authorization process. When patients request their information to be given to another person (e.g., family member, friend), the medical assistants can help. They can assist patients in completing the disclosure authorization form (Fig. 17.2). Once completed, this form must be added to the patient's health record.

When a person calls requesting information on a current patient, the medical assistant should first ask the caller's name. The medical assistant must check to see if the caller is listed on the patient's disclosure authorization form (Procedure 17.1). If that caller's name appears, then, per the facility's policy, the medical assistant can release information about the patient. If the caller's name is not on the form, the medical assistant

- Cannot release the patient's information
- Cannot even acknowledge that person is a patient of the facility

Applying HIPAA rules is important when protecting a patient's privacy.

In some facilities, the patient comes up with a code word or number. This is entered into the patient's record. The patient gives this code to family members. When they call the staff and give the code, the staff member can provide an update on the patient. It is understood that the patient gives consent to anyone that received the code. This helps to settle the issue of who is really calling requesting information. The code system may be seen more in the ambulatory surgical departments.

WALDEN-MARTIN
FAMILY MEDICAL CLINIC
1234 ANYSTREET | ANYTOWN, ANYSTATE 12345
PHONE 123-123-1234 | FAX 123-123-5678

Disclosure Authorization

Full Name: _____ Date of Birth: _____

I hereby authorize _____ to use or disclose my protected health information related to _____

to _____

Representative's Address:

Purpose:

- I understand that I may inspect or copy the protected health information described by this authorization.
- I understand that, at any time, this authorization may be revoked, when the office that receives this authorization receives a written revocation, although that revocation will not be effective as to the disclosure of records whose release I have previously authorized, or where other action has been taken in reliance on an authorization I have signed. I understand that my health care and the payment for my health care will not be affected if I refuse to sign this form.
- I understand that information used or disclosed, pursuant to this authorization, could be subject to re-disclosure by the recipient and, if so, may not be subject to federal or state law protecting its confidentiality.

Signature of individual or Representative: _____
Date: _____

Authority or Relationship to Individual, if Representative: _____

This authorization will expire on: _____ If no date or event is stated, the expiration date will be six years from the date of this authorization.

The subject of this authorization shall receive a copy of this authorization, when signed.

FIG. 17.2 Disclosure authorization form.

CHAPTER 17 Healthcare Laws

PROCEDURE 17.1 Protecting a Patient's Privacy

Tasks
Apply HIPAA rules, and protect a patient's privacy. Demonstrate sensitivity to a patient and his rights.

Scenario
Ken Thomas (DOB 10/25/61) saw nurse practitioner Jean Burke this past week. He was diagnosed with acute leukemia after several tests. You work with Ms. Burke and was involved with arranging Ken's tests. Today, Ken's adult child, Alex Thomas, calls you. Alex wants to know what is going on with Ken. You look at Ken's health record and see that Alex is not on the disclosure authorization form or a medical records release form. Per the facility's policy, for information to be given to a patient's family, a disclosure authorization form must be completed.

Later Ken calls and asks why you did not update Alex on his condition. He sounds upset while he is talking with you.

Equipment and Supplies
- Patient record
- Disclosure authorization form (electronic or paper) (see Fig. 17.2)

Procedural Steps

1. Using the scenario, role-play the situation with a peer. You are the medical assistant and just realized that Alex is not on the release form. Be professional and respectful as you apply HIPAA to the situation
   Purpose: As a professional, you need to follow the law and yet be professional and respectful.

2. Inform Alex that his name is not on a disclosure authorization form. Discuss the purpose of the disclosure authorization form.
   Purpose: The patient must sign a disclosure authorization form and indicate who can be given information. If a person wants information but is not listed on the form, legally the medical assistant cannot give any information.

3. Explain to Alex how you would be able to give him information. Encourage Alex to talk with his father about the situation.
   Purpose: The medical assistant can only give information if the person's name is on the release form.

4. When Ken calls, be professional and respectful as you hear his complaints. Keep your voice even and do not raise the volume.
   Purpose: The release form needs to indicate where the records are being sent.

5. Inform Ken that you understand his frustration. Be sensitive to his feelings and his rights. Explain why you could not give information to Alex.
   Purpose: Having the patient understand that you could not legally give the information to Alex is important. Speaking in a sensitive, respectful tone may help Ken feel less frustrated with the situation.

6. Discuss with Ken how you could prepare the disclosure authorization form. Make plans for how Ken would sign the form.
   Purpose: Helping to come up with a solution to achieve the patient's wishes is important to solving Ken's frustration.

7. Document the phone calls with Alex and Ken. Describe the facts and the plan to complete the release form.
   Purpose: All phone calls with patients or related to patients should be documented. This provides an ongoing log of what occurs with the patient and can be helpful in a court of law should something come up.

BOX 17.6 Psychotherapy Notes

Under HIPAA, psychotherapy notes are treated with higher levels of confidentiality. Psychotherapy notes include the patient-provider details from mental health treatment either from private, group, or family therapy. Psychotherapy notes include the following:
- What the patient stated during the session
- The provider's analysis of the patient's statements and the situation

Items not part of the psychotherapy notes are not held at a higher level of confidentiality. These items include the following:
- Prescriptions
- Start and stop times of sessions
- Types and frequency of treatment
- Results of clinical tests

Psychotherapy notes need to be stored separately from the patient health record. If electronic, the access to the psychotherapy notes is limited to those healthcare professionals who work in the mental health area. When a patient completes a general release of medical records form, psychotherapy notes are not released. It takes special permission from the patient to release psychotherapy notes.

CRITICAL THINKING 17.2

Daniela and Bella are reviewing HIPAA concepts. They start to discuss local news and a case where a medical assistant snaps a picture of a patient's record and posts it to a popular social media site. Bella asks Daniela what this act violated. How would you answer this question? Why are employee cell phones a risk in the healthcare setting?

Record release process. Patients must complete, date, and sign a (medical) records release form for their records to be transferred to another facility (Fig. 17.3, Procedure 17.2). No records, including images and videos, can be released without the completed form. Release forms may specifically address the release of videos and images. With these forms, patients must indicate they want these to be release. If that is not done, then the videos and images are not released.

Parts of the patient's record are held at a higher level of confidentiality:
- Psychotherapy notes (Box 17.6)
- Substance abuse information (Box 17.7)
- Human immunodeficiency virus (HIV) information (see Box 17.7)

Some facilities use a special records release forms for these records. Other facilities address these topics in a special area on their record release forms. The patient must specifically request this information to be released. If not requested, then this information is not released.

BOX 17.7 Substance Abuse and HIV Content

Drug and alcohol substance abuse and HIV content in patient records are held at a higher level of confidentiality. There are many federal and state laws that relate to the privacy of these records. State preemption applies with these privacy laws.

The Alcohol and Drug Abuse Patient Records Privacy Law is one example. It is enforced by a division of HHS. This law restricts the release and use of patient records that include substance use diagnoses and services.

WALDEN-MARTIN
FAMILY MEDICAL CLINIC
1234 ANYSTREET | ANYTOWN, ANYSTATE 12345
PHONE 123-123-1234 | FAX 123-123-5678

Medical Records Release

Patient Name: ____________ Date of Birth: ____________
SSN: ____________ Phone: ____________
Address:

I, ____________ authorize ____________
to disclose/release the following information (check all applicable):

- ☐ All Records
- ☐ Abstract/Summary
- ☐ Laboratory/pathology records
- ☐ Pharmacy/prescription records
- ☐ X-ray/radiology records
- ☐ Other
- ☐ Billing records

**Note: If these records contain any information from previous providers or information about HIV/AIDS status, cancer diagnosis, drug alcohol abuse, or sexually transmitted disease, you are hereby authorizing disclosure of this information. A copy of this signed authorization must be given to the individual.*

These records are for services provided on the following date(s): ____________

Please send the records listed above to (use additional sheets if necessary):

Name: ____________ Phone: ____________
Address: Fax: ____________

The information may be used/disclosed for each of the following purposes:

- ☐ At patient's request
- ☐ For employment purposes
- ☐ For patient's health care
- ☐ Other
- ☐ For payment/insurance

This authorization shall expire no later than: ______ or upon the following event ______, and may not be valid for greater than one year from the date of signature for medical records.

I understand that after the custodian of records discloses my health information, it may no longer be protected by federal privacy laws. I understand that this authorization is voluntary and I may refuse to sign this authorization which will not affect my ability to obtain treatment; receive payment; or eligibility for benefits unless allowed by law. By signing below I represent and warrant that I have authority to sign this document and authorize the use or disclosure of protected health information and that there are no claims or orders that would prohibit, limit, or otherwise restrict my ability to authorize the use or disclosure of this protected health information.

Patient signature (or patient's personal representative) ____________ Date ____________

Printed name of patient representative ____________ Representative's authority to sign for patient *(i.e. parent, guardian, power of attorney, executor)* ____________

FIG. 17.3 Medical records release form.

Security Rule. HIPAA's Security Rule addresses the national standards used to protect electronic protected health information (e-PHI). This rule covers the records that are created, used, received, and maintained by the covered entities. Safeguards important to ensure the security of the e-PHI include the following:

- *Administrative safeguards*: The security officer is responsible for creating and carrying out security policies and procedures. Potential risks to the e-PHI must be identified. Steps must be taken to prevent any issues. Cyber attackers pose a huge risk to network security (Box 17.8).
- *Physical safeguards*: Facility, workstation, and device security must be implemented. A security officer must create procedures for the proper use of workstations and e-PHI.
- *Technical safeguards*: Only authorized employees should have access to e-PHI. Safeguards include audits to track activities of users with the e-PHI. They also include safeguards to prevent improper alteration, destruction, or transmission of e-PHI.

BOX 17.8 Legal Example: Cyber Attackers Breach Insurer's Database

In 2015 Anthem Inc., the second largest insurer in the United States, announced that cyber attackers breached its database. The PHI for almost 80 million people (e.g., names, birthdays, social security numbers, addresses, employment information, and email addresses) was compromised. Anthem agreed to pay $115 million to settle the class-action lawsuit.

BOX 17.9 Legal Example: HIPAA Settlement for Inappropriate PHI Access

In 2012 Memorial Healthcare System (MHS) submitted a breach report to HHS indicating that two of its employees inappropriately accessed PHI potentially impacting 80,000 patients. Several months later MHS notified HHS of another 12 users that inappropriately accessed PHI, which potentially impacted another 105,646 individuals. As a result, some of the PHI was sold and fraudulent tax returns were filed. In 2017 MHS paid the HHS $5.5 million to settle the potential violations and agreed to implement a corrective action plan.

From https://www.hhs.gov/sites/default/files/memorial-ra-cap.pdf.

Chapter 21 provides additional information on network security procedures. It is important for the medical assistant to follow the facility's electronic security procedures. Many facilities have policies to keep passwords confidential. Downloading personal documents puts the computer network at risk and thus is not allowed. Audit trails monitor who is looking at which patient's chart (Box 17.9). If the medical assistant is not working with a specific patient, then the patient's record should not be accessed. Violating this rule will cause the medical assistant to breach the patient's confidentiality and security. Many healthcare professionals, from providers to medical assistants, have breached confidentiality. They have lost their jobs and licenses or certifications. Many have also been fined.

Health Information Technology for Economic and Clinical Health Act

One of the issues with HIPAA was the limited enforcement and penalties. In 2009, as part of the American Recovery and Reinvestment Act, the Health Information Technology for Economic and Clinic Health (HITECH) Act was enacted. HITECH is enforced by the HHS Office for Civil Rights (OCR). The HITECH Act contains provisions that increased the enforcement of the privacy and security of electronic transmission and health information. HITECH modified HIPAA in the following ways:

- Made business associates directly liable for compliance to HIPAA.
- Prohibited the sale of PHI without the patient's authorization.
- Created a tiered violation category that included unknowing, reasonable cause, willful neglect–corrected, and willful neglected–uncorrected. Violation penalties go from $100 for each "unknowing" violation to $1.5 million per calendar year. The greater the violation, the greater the penalty amount. Individuals, healthcare agencies, and business associations could be penalized and fined.
- **Breach** notification requirements were increased. Individuals must be notified of the breach via mail or email. If the facility does not have up-to-date contact information for 10 or more patients, then a notice must be posted on the company's website for at least 90 days. If more than 500 individuals were impacted, then the media

VOCABULARY

breach: Disclosure of protected health information, without a reason or permission, which compromises the security or privacy of the information.

PROCEDURE 17.2 Completing a Release of Record Form for a Release of Information

Tasks
Apply HIPAA rules, and complete a release of record form for a release of information.

Scenario
Aaron Jackson was seen at Walden Hospital for a high fever. You need to help Aaron's mother complete a record release form so his record from the emergency department visit can be sent to the clinic. She needs to request all records from the visit on the first of this month. The clinic information is on the form. The release shall expire in 1 month.

Aaron's Information	Walden Hospital's Information
Date of birth: 10/17/2011	Address:
Social Security number: 164-72-4618	Walden Hospital
Address:	123 Healing Way
555 McArthur Avenue	Anywhere, AL 12345-1234
Anytown, AL 12345-1234	Phone: (123) 814-4563
Phone: (123) 814-7844	Fax: (123) 814-6544
Mother: Patricia Jackson	

Equipment and Supplies
- Records release form (electronic or paper) (see Fig. 17.3)
- Patient record

Procedural Steps

1. Using the medical record release form, insert the patient information (see Fig. 17.3). Add the patient's name, date of birth, and social security number (SSN). Include the current address and phone number that is found in the patient record. If an electronic form is used, select the correct patient and the fields will auto-populate.
   Purpose: The patient's information is required on the form. The patient name, date of birth, and SSN are direct identifiers, which will also help the hospital identify the correct patient.
2. Complete the parts of the form that specify who authorizes the release and who is to release the information.
   Purpose: Depending on state law and the facility's policy, the mother's name or the child's name may be the party authorizing the release. The hospital is the party who will release the information.
3. Check the box(es) of the information that needs to be released. If required, write in what other records need to be released.
   Purpose: Depending on state law and the facility's policy, the "Other" location might be where substance abuse and HIV records can be specifically requested. Other forms have a specific section for the release of substance abuse and HIV records.
4. Add the date of the visit. Add the name and contact information for the facility where the records need to be sent.
   Purpose: The release form needs to indicate where the records are being sent.
5. Indicate how the released information will be used.
   Purpose: This information tells the releasing facility what the information will be used for. In this situation, the provider is requesting the information for healthcare purposes.
6. Indicate when the authorization should expire. Proofread the form for accuracy. If using an electronic form, save the form to the patient's record. Print the form so the mother can sign.
   Purpose: In some situations, this may be an ongoing release. For example, the patient may get weekly blood tests at a local clinic and the results need to be sent to the patient's specialist.
7. During a role-play with the patient's mother, explain what the provider is requesting. Ensure she can understand and read English. Have the mother read the form.
   Purpose: To be legal, the mother must understand what she is signing. If she does not understand English, you will need to have a translator available to help in this situation.
8. Ask the mother if she has any questions. Answer any questions, and then explain where she needs to sign if she agrees with the documentation.
   Purpose: By answering questions, you can help her understand the release process. It is important to make sure she is agreement with the form before she signs. After the mother has signed, the form will be faxed to the hospital. The signed form should be filed in the patient's record or scanned and uploaded in to the electronic health record.

BOX 17.10 Breaches Affecting 500 or More People

As required by the HITECH Act, the Secretary for the HHS Office for Civil Rights must maintain a list of PHI breaches that affects 500 or more individuals. This list can be found at https://ocrportal.hhs.gov/ocr/breach/breach_report.jsf.
The most common types of breaches include the following:
- Cyber hacking into servers
- Theft of laptops, servers, and other computer hardware
- Improper disposal of PHI

CRITICAL THINKING 17.3

Daniela and Bella are reviewing HITECH. Daniela asks Bella why it is important for large breaches to be posted on the OCR website. How would you answer this question as an employee? How would you answer as a patient of a facility that had a posting on the OCR website?

and the OCR secretary must be notified. A list of breaches reported are published on the OCR website (Box 17.10).

It is important for the medical assistant to be aware of the importance of keeping the PHI secure. Any breaches or loss/theft of computers must be reported immediately to the facility's security officer.

Genetic Information Nondiscrimination Act

The Genetic Information Nondiscrimination Act (GINA) became law in 2008. It modified HIPAA and increased the protection for individuals. GINA prohibits genetic discrimination in health coverage and employment.

ADDITIONAL HEALTHCARE LAWS AND REGULATIONS

This section presents additional laws that impact healthcare. Throughout the textbook, these laws and others will be discussed in more depth. This chapter introduces the more common laws that impact ambulatory healthcare.

Drug Laws

Food, Drug, and Cosmetic Act. In 1906, the Food and Drug Act became law. It prohibited the misbranding of food and drugs. It was replaced in 1938 by the Food, Drug, and Cosmetic Act, which is still enforced today. The Food and Drug Administration (FDA) enforces the act. The FDA is responsible for the safety, effectiveness, security, and quality of drugs, cosmetics, and food. Box 17.11 provides a list of areas the FDA oversees. When you see recalls of food, cosmetics, or medications, the FDA is involved with the process.

The www.fda.gov website provides useful information for the healthcare facility. The website is the resource for information and recalls on the areas overseen by the FDA. Many times the medical assistant is responsible for maintaining the stock medications and equipment in the department. Any medications or medical devices recalled need to be removed immediately and not used. The providers should be notified of recalls.

Controlled Substances Act. The Controlled Substances Act (part of the Comprehensive Drug Abuse Prevention and Control Act of 1970) is a federal law. The U.S. Drug Enforcement Agency (DEA) enforces the law. The DEA oversees the manufacturing, importation, possession, use, and distribution of certain drugs and chemicals. The DEA handles both illegal and legal drugs. The Controlled Substance Act has five schedules of medications. These schedules are arranged from the greatest to least abuse potential (Table 17.3). State statutes also address procedures related to scheduled medications. Some scheduled medication prescriptions are handled differently. It is important for the medical assistant to be aware of the schedule of medications.

> **BOX 17.11 Areas Overseen by the Food and Drug Administration**
>
> - Human drugs
> - Veterinary drugs
> - Vaccines
> - Biologic products (e.g., blood components)
> - Medical devices
> - Food supply
> - Cosmetics
> - Dietary supplies
> - Products that give off radiation

Each provider prescribing scheduled medications needs to have a unique DEA number. The DEA number needs to be renewed every 3 years. The medical assistant may need to assist the provider in renewing or obtaining a DEA number. This can be done at the DEA website (www.deadiversion.usdoj.gov).

Insurance Law

Patient Protection and Affordable Care Act. The Patient Protection and Affordable Care Act is commonly known as the Affordable Care Act. This federal statute was signed into law in 2010. The goal of the law was to provide Americans with affordable health insurance. It also attempted to reform the healthcare system and decrease healthcare spending. A few of the reforms include the following:

- Insurance coverage of preventive services and immunizations.
- People with preexisting health conditions could not be dropped or charged more for insurance.
- Dependents can stay on their parent's insurance plan until age 26.
- Large businesses have to provide insurance to full-time workers. Small businesses were eligible for tax credits to help offer insurance coverage to their employees.
- Physician Payments Sunshine Act (PPSA) (part of law): Increase the transparency between providers, teaching hospitals, and manufacturers of medical products (e.g., drugs and medical devices). The manufacturers must report any payments and transfers of value (e.g., gifts, meals) to the Open Payments Program by the Centers for Medicare and Medicaid Services (CMS).

Medical Laboratory Regulations

Clinical Laboratory Improvement Amendments. Congress passed the Clinical Laboratory Improvement Amendments (CLIA) in 1988. CLIA establishes quality standards and regulates laboratory testing. The quality standards focus on accuracy, reliability, and timeliness of test results. The federal agencies involved with administering CLIA are listed in Table 17.4.

All agencies providing clinical laboratory services, including ambulatory care laboratories, must meet the CLIA requirements. The laboratories must have a CLIA certificate to operate and must be certified by the state. Smaller ambulatory care laboratories have one of the following certificates:

- Certificate of Waiver: allows the facility to perform waived tests. *Waived tests* are simple and accurate with little risk for error if done correctly; a urine pregnancy test is a waived test.

TABLE 17.3 Schedules of Drugs, Substances, or Chemicals

Schedule	Psychological and Physical Dependence	Examples
I	Highest potential for abuse; drugs with no currently accepted medical use	• *Examples:* Heroin, lysergic acid diethylamide (LSD), ecstasy
II/IIN (C–II)	High level of abuse and can lead to severe psychological or physical dependence	• *Schedule II narcotics:* oxycodone (OxyContin, Percocet), fentanyl (Duragesic), codeine, morphine • *Schedule IIN stimulants:* amphetamine (Adderall), methamphetamine (Desoxyn), methylphenidate (Concerta, Ritalin LA)
III/III N (C–III)	Moderate to low physical dependence or high psychological dependence	• *Schedule III narcotics:* acetaminophen with Codeine (Tylenol #2 or #3), buprenorphine (Suboxone) • *Schedule III N non-narcotics:* ketamine, anabolic steroids (e.g., Depo-Testosterone)
IV (C–IV)	Low potential for abuse relative to substances in schedule III	• *Schedule IV:* alprazolam (Xanax), clonazepam (Klonopin), diazepam (Valium), lorazepam (Ativan)
V (C-V)	Lowest potential for abuse relative to substances listed in schedule IV; contains limited quantities of certain narcotics	• *Schedule V substances:* Robitussin AC, ezogabine (Potiga)

- Certificate for Provider-Performed Microscopy Procedures (PPMP): allows the provider to perform only specific microscopy procedures and waived tests.

Additional certificates are obtained by larger laboratories. These laboratories perform more complex tests.

TABLE 17.4 Federal Agencies Involved With Administering CLIA

Federal Agency	Role With CLIA
The Food and Drug Administration (FDA)	Oversees the medical laboratory tests. Categorizes the tests based on the complexity: waived, moderate, or high complexity. High complexity laboratories can perform more tests than waived complexity laboratories.
Center for Medicare and Medicaid Services (CMS)	Inspects laboratories and issues certificates. Enforces compliance with regulations.
Centers for Disease Control and Prevention (CDC)	Develops standards and laboratory practice guidelines. Develops professional information and resources (Box 17.12).

BOX 17.12 Role of the Centers for Disease Control and Prevention

The Centers for Disease Control and Prevention (CDC) is a division of HHS. The CDC focuses on disease control and prevention, environmental health, and health promotion. Its overall mission is to improve the health of the people in the United States. The CDC website (www.cdc.gov) is a helpful resource for health and disease topics.

Workplace Safety Laws

Occupational Safety and Health Act. Occupational Safety and Health Act of 1970 (OSH Act) created and is enforced by the Occupational Safety and Health Administration (OSHA). Based on this act, OSHA sets workplace standards and conducts inspections to ensure employee safety. Employers must comply with all of OSHA's regulations. Table 17.5 addresses the OSHA standards in healthcare.

VOCABULARY

egress: Leaving a place; exit route.

CRITICAL THINKING 17.4

Daniela is reading about OSHA. She thinks back to what she has heard about OSHA in other businesses. What have you heard about OSHA and other businesses? Is OSHA's role in that company similar to its role in healthcare? Explain.

Needlestick Safety and Prevention Act. The Needlestick Safety and Prevention Act was signed into law in 2000. The goal of the act was to decrease the risk of healthcare workers' exposure to bloodborne diseases. The act required OSHA to update its Bloodborne Pathogens Standard. The revised standards apply to all employees with anticipated occupational exposure to blood or other potentially infectious materials (OPIM). The impacts of this act include the following:

- Healthcare workers must use safer medical devices. For example, many needles can be capped with a special safety device after use (Fig. 17.4).
- The Exposure Control Plan must include a sharps injury log documenting all instances of injuries from sharps (e.g., used needles, blades).
- Used needles, blades, and other sharps must be put in sharps disposal containers (Fig. 17.5).

TABLE 17.5 OSHA Standards Related to Healthcare

Standard	Summary	Examples of Workplace Application
Blood-borne pathogens	Protects healthcare workers against the hazards caused by blood-borne pathogens.	Exposure control plans, universal precautions, safety needles, personal protective equipment, hepatitis B vaccination, and record keeping.
Hazard communication	Requires employers to provide information about the chemical hazards in the workplace. The *General Duty Clause* states that any equipment that can pose a health danger must be considered a hazard.	All chemicals are labeled. Safety data sheets (SDS) must be available for each chemical in the workplace. Employees must be trained on how to handle the chemical hazards in the workplace.
Occupational exposure to hazardous chemicals in laboratories	Also called the "laboratory standard." Specifies the requirements of a chemical hygiene plan (CHP).	The CHP is a written program that includes the policies, procedures, and responsibilities that protect employees from hazardous chemicals. The CHP describes the appropriate handling of chemicals in the laboratory.
Ionizing radiation	Addresses the protections needed when working with ionizing radiation (i.e., x-rays).	Posted signs where x-rays are taken. Employees wear personal radiation monitors to detect radiation amounts. X-ray rooms are built with protected areas for the employee. Limited x-ray exposure if the employee is pregnant.
Nonionizing radiation	Addresses the protections needed in place when working with nonionizing radiation (i.e., lasers).	Signs need to be posted on the door of rooms where lasers are being used. Appropriate eye protection must be worn at all times for both the patient and the employees. Goal is to prevent blindness, retinal burns, and eye damage due to the radiation.
Means of egress (E gress)	Addresses the exit routes in a building.	Employers are responsible for having appropriate building exit routes. Routes are posted. Exits are unlocked and clear in case of emergency.

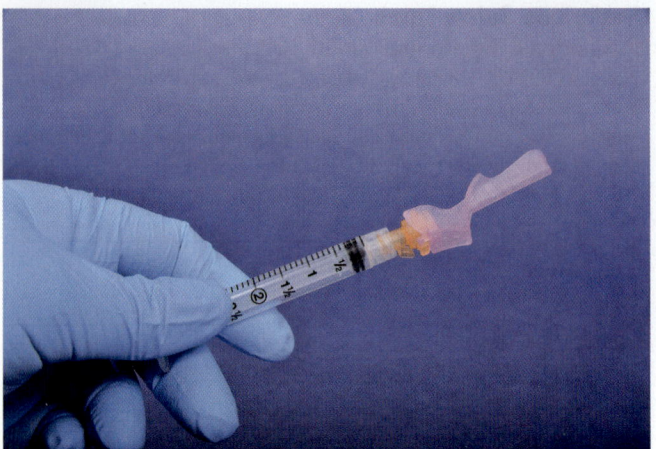

FIG. 17.4 A safety needle device. (From Proctor D, et al: *Kinn's The Medical Assistant*, ed 13, St. Louis, 2017, Elsevier.)

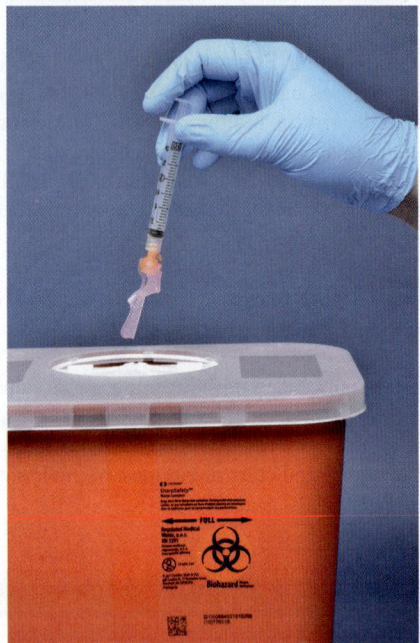

FIG. 17.5 Used needles need to be placed in a biohazard sharps container.

- Personal protective equipment (PPE) (i.e., gloves, mask, and gown) must be worn if there is a risk of blood or body fluid exposure (Fig. 17.6).

Good Samaritan Laws

Good Samaritan laws are state laws that provide legal protection for those assisting an injured person during an emergency. If possible, the injured person needs to agree to the help. The person responding must meet the following criteria:
- Not be paid for the care given.
- Act reasonably exercising the same professional standard of care within the limitations of the situation.
- Not act negligently or recklessly; such action makes the responder liable for damages.

The Good Samaritan law does not mean you cannot be sued. In some states, healthcare professionals who do not assist another person in an emergency can be held liable. It is important to be aware of your state's Good Samaritan law. Do you as a medical assistant have an obligation to stop and provide first aid?

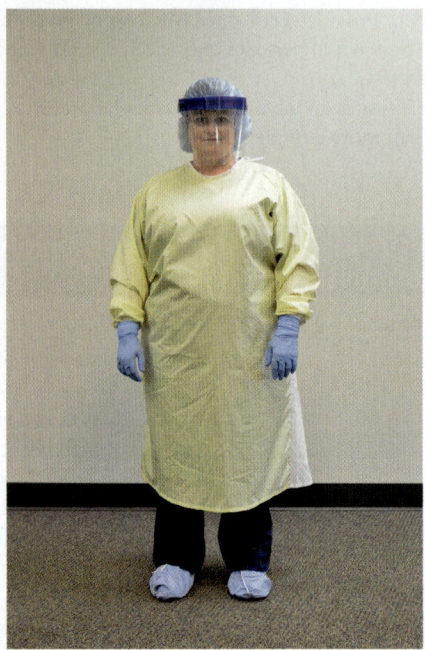

FIG. 17.6 Personal protective equipment. (From Proctor D, et al: *Kinn's The Medical Assistant*, ed 13, St. Louis, 2017, Elsevier.)

TABLE 17.6 Acts That Relate to End-of-Life Issues

Act	Description
Patient Self-Determination Act	Requires most healthcare institutions to inform patients of their rights to make decisions and the facility's policies respecting advance directives
Uniform Determination of Death Act (UDDA)	Served as a guide for state lawmakers to create their own laws that define death
Uniform Anatomical Gift Act (UAGA)	Purpose of the act was to make organ donation easier for people
National Organ Transplant Act (NOTA)	Established the Organ Procurement and Transplant Network (OPTN) and also established a national registry for organ matching

CRITICAL THINKING 17.5

Daniela is reviewing Good Samaritan laws. How might she describe these laws in terms of importance during an emergency situation?

Laws for End-of-Life Issues

A medical assistant should be aware of laws that relate to end-of-life issues. Table 17.6 provides a brief description of acts that relate to advance directives, organ donation, and determining death. These acts will be discussed in depth in Chapter 18.

VOCABULARY

advance directives: Written instructions about healthcare decisions in case a person is unable to make them.

BOX 17.13 Reportable Cases per State Statutes

- Births and deaths
- Specific diseases
- Sexually transmitted infections
- Specific injuries related to violence
- Abuse, neglect, and exploitation

COMPLIANCE REPORTING

Healthcare agencies and employees are required to comply with all federal and state laws and regulations. There are several areas of compliance that the healthcare facility must focus on. Administrators must have policies and procedures in place for employees to report issues. Reports need to be followed up on. Documentation may need to be done for federal or state agencies regarding compliance issues. Healthcare providers also need to report specific diseases, injuries, and issues with vaccines. We will focus on compliance that occurs in ambulatory care facilities.

Compliance With Public Health Statutes

Public health statutes exist in each state to help promote the health of the residents. According to these statutes, healthcare providers have a responsibility to report specific information to various authorities (Box 17.13). We examine these closer in the following sections.

Per the HIPAA permission "public interest and benefit activities," PHI can be released when required by law, law enforcement, and for public health activities. For the mandatory reporting situations based on state statutes, the provider can release PHI without the patient's authorization.

Reportable Diseases. Reportable diseases are communicable diseases that have a significant public health impact. When a provider diagnoses a reportable disease, the state's public health department must be notified. This notification process is called disease reporting. Each state has statutes that address disease reporting. Lists of reportable diseases and reporting requirements are typically available on the state's public health department website.

If the disease is an urgent public health concern, reporting must be done immediately, usually by phone or fax. Less urgent communicable diseases may be reported electronically, by mail or fax (Table 17.7). The provider usually has up to 3 days to file the report. For HIV and AIDS, the provider may need to mail the paperwork to increase confidentiality. Disease reporting procedures and regulations may vary by state. The medical assistant should be aware of the state's disease reporting process. The provider may ask the medical assistant to contact the public health department regarding a new reportable disease case (Procedure 17.3).

Wounds of Violence. Most state statutes require healthcare providers to report cases of violence. Statutes vary from state to state. Typically, reportable cases include wounds from gunshots; stabbing; specific types of burns; and nonaccidental knife, axe, or sharp pointed instruments. The medical assistant should be aware of the state's statutes for reporting wounds of violence. In some cases, the medical assistant may need to

CRITICAL THINKING 17.6

Daniela is learning about public health statutes and reporting obligations of providers. Why is it important for the public health services to be notified about specific diseases?

TABLE 17.7 Examples of Reportable Diseases

Level	Disease Examples	
Urgent reporting	Hepatitis A Food or water disease outbreaks Pertussis (whooping cough)	Measles Plague Tuberculosis
Less urgent reporting	Sexually transmitted infections Hepatitis B, C, D, and E Legionellosis Lyme disease Malaria	Mumps Meningitis, bacterial Tetanus Toxic shock syndrome Varicella (chickenpox)
Highly confidential reporting	Acquired immune deficiency syndrome (AIDS) Human immunodeficiency virus (HIV) infection	

Note: Level titles and diseases may vary by state.

CRITICAL THINKING 17.7

Daniela is learning about public health statutes and the reporting obligations of providers. Why is it important for the law enforcement to be notified about cases of violence?

assist the provider in preparing documents for law enforcement for such cases.

Child Abuse, Neglect, and Exploitation. The Federal Child Abuse Prevention and Treatment Act (CAPTA) aided the states as state statutes were drafted. The act was updated by the CAPTA Reauthorization Act of 2010. This updated act defined child abuse and neglect as follows:
1. Any recent act or failure to act on the part of a parent or caretaker which results in death, serious physical or emotional harm, sexual abuse, or exploitation (EK sploi tae shahn); or
2. An act or failure to act which presents an imminent risk of serious harm.

These definitions set the minimum standard for describing child abuse and neglect. States typically address child maltreatment in both the civil and criminal statutes.

All states and territories require child maltreatment to be reported. Most states mandate specific professionals to report any child maltreatment (Box 17.14). Some states require anyone who suspects child abuse or neglect to report the situation (Table 17.8). Mandatory reporters need to provide the facts. They do not have to prove that abuse or neglect occurred. Most state statutes do not consider abuse and neglect information as privileged communication between the patient and

VOCABULARY
abuse: An action that purposely harms another person.
communicable diseases: Diseases spread from person to person by either direct contact or indirect contact (i.e., insects).
exploitation: The act of using another person for one's own advantage.
neglect: Failure to provide proper attention or care to another person.
privileged communication: Communication that cannot be disclosed without authorization of the person involved; includes provider-patient and lawyer-client communications.

PROCEDURE 17.3 Perform Disease Reporting

Tasks
Research the state's disease reporting public health statutes and complete the disease reporting paperwork based on public health statutes.

Scenario
Nurse practitioner (NP) Jean Burke received the test results from Ken Thomas. He tested positive for gonorrhea. She wants you to file the report with the public health department. Here is the information from his health record and the clinic. For any missing information, follow the instructor's directions, or make it up if no directions were provided.

Patient Information	Provider and Lab Information	Health Record Information
Ken Thomas 398 Larkin Avenue Anytown, AL 12345-1234 Anycounty k.thomas@anytown.mail **Phone:** (123) 784-1118 **DOB:** 10/25/61 **Race:** Multiple races **Ethnicity:** Unknown **Marital status:** Single, living with Sandy Brown, who was not treated	**Provider:** Jean Burke, NP Walden-Martin Family Medical Clinic 1234 Anystreet Anytown, AL 12345-1234 **Phone:** (123) 123-1234 **Fax:** (123) 123-5678 **Lab:** Walden-Martin Family Medical Clinic Lab	**Diagnosis:** Gonorrhea **Symptoms:** Started 5 days ago, greenish discharge from penis, burning with urination **Test:** Urine specimen was collected yesterday; gonorrhea nucleic acid amplification test (NAAT) test done yesterday, results are positive **Treatment:** Patient treated today with ceftriaxone 250 mg intramuscular (IM) single dose and azithromycin 1 g orally single dose

Equipment and Supplies
- Computer with internet access and printer
- Patient record (see table with information)
- Black pen

Procedural Steps

1. Using the Internet, search for the disease reporting procedure in your state's public health department or similar facility. Read the procedure.
   Purpose: A medical assistant needs to be aware of the disease reporting procedure for the state.
2. Identify which form is required based on the patient's diagnosis. Print the form.
   Purpose: Some department of health service agencies may have several forms available on the website. It is important to use the correct form. Gonorrhea is a sexually transmitted infection.
3. Use a black pen to complete the form. Neatly complete the patient's demographic information section using the information from the health record.
   Purpose: All forms require the patient's name and contact information.
4. Complete the diagnosis, symptoms, testing, and treatment information.
   Purpose: The public health department needs information on the diagnosis, symptoms, test results, and the treatment provided.
5. Complete the rest of the form. Review the form for accuracy. Make any changes required before submitting the form to the instructor.
   Purpose: The form must be accurate and complete before sending it to the public health department.
   Note: After performing the disease reporting, the medical assistant needs to document the activity in the patient's health record.

BOX 17.14 Mandatory Reporters for Child Maltreatment

- School personnel
- Social workers
- Healthcare providers, nurses, and other professionals
- Mental health professionals
- Child care providers
- Medical examiners or coroners
- Law enforcement officers

---

the provider. This allows the provider to report the information (and thus protect the maltreated child). The medical assistant should be aware of the state statutes regarding child maltreatment. The Child Welfare Information Gateway website (www.childwelfare.gov) can be used as a resource for state reporting information.

The Unborn Victims of Violence Act was signed into law by Congress in 2004. This act protects unborn babies from acts of violence. Prior to this act, unborn babies harmed or killed due to violence were not considered victims. This act considers unborn babies who are harmed or killed during certain acts of violence to be victims, and charges could be brought forth.

Adult Abuse, Neglect, and Exploitation. In 1965 the Older Americans Act was signed into law. The purpose of the act was to maintain the rights and dignity of the older person. It also created the Administration on Aging. Since then, several federal laws have been created to help fund federal programs.

Abuse, neglect, and exploitation of older adults and *dependent adults* are dealt with in state statutes. All states have the following:
- Adult or elder protective services statutes that provide the reporting and investigating procedures for elder abuse in the state
- Statutes that establish a Long-Term Care Ombudsman Program that advocates for the safety and rights of long-term care facility residents
- General criminal statutes on fraud, sexual assault, battery, and other abuses that can relate to elder abuse

CRITICAL THINKING 17.8

Daniela is learning about child abuse and neglect. How might she describe the difference between abuse and neglect? Why is this information important for medical assistants to be aware of?

VOCABULARY

dependent adults: People between the ages of 18 and 64 who have a mental or physical impairment that prevents them from doing normal activities or from protecting themselves.

TABLE 17.8 Types of Child Neglect and Abuse		
Child Maltreatment		**Description**
Neglect	Physical	Failure to provide adequate nutrition, clothing, shelter, and hygiene. Child has poor growth and hygiene and may hide food for later.
	Educational	Failure to enroll child in school or to home-school child. Child may have a poor school attendance record.
	Medical	Failure to provide needed care for injury, impairment, or illness. Child may have untreated injuries. May see developmental delays from lack of therapy to help with impairment.
Abuse	Physical	Bruises, fractures, or burns that are unexplained or do not match the explanation given; untreated dental or medical problems.
	Sexual	Sexual behaviors inappropriate for child's age; sexually transmitted infections, genital pain and bruising, bleeding.
	Emotional	Delayed emotional development, loss of self-confidence, social withdrawal, headaches, depression, poor school performance.

Some states require financial institutions (banks) to report suspected financial abuse or exploitation of older adults.

The state statute will dictate who are mandated reporters, when to report, and how to report the situation. Many ambulatory healthcare facilities are screening older adults to identify those that do not feel safe in their living conditions. If the medical assistant suspects abuse, neglect, or exploitation of an older person, it is important to bring it to the provider's attention. Typically, the provider is a mandated reporter under state law. If the provider suspects neglect, abuse, or exploitation, then a report needs to be filed.

State statutes on domestic violence and abuse vary. In some cases, the reporting for injuries caused from violence covers some domestic abuse situations. Some states have mandatory reporting for domestic violence. It is recommended that providers talk to the victim of the domestic violence. They should inform them when it must be reported. In states where domestic violence is not a mandatory reporting situation, providers can encourage the victim to report the situation. Safe houses are also available in many areas for victims. Having information on local resources for domestic abuse is important in the ambulatory care setting. Providing the information in restrooms is very common. Typically, that might be the only location where the abuser does not follow the victim. It is important to remember that both men and women can be victims of domestic abuse.

Reporting Vaccination Issues

When a healthcare provider orders a vaccine to be given to a child, the medical assistant must provide the parent or guardian with a Vaccine Information Statement (VIS). This document reviews the reasons and risks for the vaccine. Prior to giving the vaccine, the medical assistant must have the parent or guardian sign a consent form allowing the administration of the immunization.

If a patient is having an unusual side effect from a vaccine, the provider might need to file a report to the Vaccine Adverse Event Reporting System (VAERS). Patients and families can also file a report. The VAERS is a national surveillance program that monitors vaccine safety. It collects information on unusual vaccine side effects. VAERS is co-sponsored by the Centers for Disease Control and Prevention (CDC) and FDA.

In 1986 the National Childhood Vaccine Injury Act was passed. It created the National Vaccine Injury Compensation Program (VICP). This program provides compensation for children injured by childhood vaccines. The VICP lifts the burden of lawsuits from the vaccine manufacturers and healthcare providers. The VIS contains information about the VICP for patients' families.

Compliance Programs

A compliance program or corporate compliance is a program within a business that detects and prevents violations of state and federal laws. An effective compliance program helps protect the organization from fines and lawsuits. Most compliance programs have reporting mechanisms (i.e., a toll-free number or website) where employees can report suspected violations, suspected illegal activity, fraud, abuse, safety issues, and noncompliance issues. It is important that employees can report issues without fear of **retaliation** (re TAL ee shahn) and **retribution** (RET rah byou shahn). Many times reports can be submitted anonymously.

If a medical assistant needs to report a situation, it is important to follow the healthcare facility's policies and procedures. Different reporting pathways are seen in ambulatory care settings:

- If the facility has a compliance reporting procedure: a report can be filed through the compliance reporting mechanisms available to the employee.
- If the facility does not have a compliance reporting procedure: the employee may need to report the situation using the chain-of-command. This means the employee must report the issue to the supervisor. If the supervisor was involved with the situation, then the employee must report the issue to the supervisor's supervisor.
- For employment or conflict-of-interest issues: some agencies require the employee to contact the human resource supervisor.

In the following sections, we will examine the more common compliance concerns in healthcare.

Financial Concerns. Financial concerns relate to financial and property theft, identify theft, conflict of interest, and fraud. Theft can be of drugs, equipment, supplies, or money. *Identify theft* occurs when someone sells or uses another person's personal information for financial gain. In healthcare, medical identify theft occurs. When a person poses as another person during a healthcare visit, this is considered medical identify theft, because the wrong person's insurance is getting billed for the services. To prevent medical identity theft, many agencies are doing the following:

- Requiring photo identification during the check-in process for visits and services.
- Taking the patient's picture, which is uploaded to the electronic health record for future reference

> **VOCABULARY**
> **retaliation:** Getting back at others for something they did to you.
> **retribution:** Punishment inflicted on someone as vengeance for a wrong or criminal act; the act of taking revenge.

> **BOX 17.15 Legal Example: False Claim Act Violations**
>
> The lawsuit alleged that Berkeley Heart Lab Inc. paid kickbacks to physicians and patients to use the company for blood testing. The kickbacks were disguised as "processing and handling" fees. Patients received kickbacks in the form of waived copayments, which they were legally required to pay for the services provided. The government also alleged that unnecessary cardiovascular tests were being charged to Medicare and TRICARE programs. Quest acquired Berkeley in 2011 and ended the practice of kickbacks. In 2017 Quest Diagnostics Inc. agreed to pay $6 million to resolve a lawsuit by the United States.

From United States ex rel. Mayes v. Berkeley HeartLab Inc., et al., Case No. 9:11-cv-01593-RMG (D.S.C.) Consolidated with U.S. EX REL. LUTZ v. BERKELEY HEARTLAB, INC. See: https://www.leagle.com/leaglesearch?all=paid+kickbacks+to+physicians+and+patients+to+use+the+company+for+blood+testing&pty=Berkeley

Conflict of interest relates to any financial interest, personal or professional activity, or obligation that impacts a person's objectivity when performing the job. For instance, a provider owns stock in a pharmaceutical company. This provider then prescribes medications made by that company. The provider is benefiting from patients purchasing medications from that company.

Fraud is a deceitful action that causes another to give up something of value. Healthcare fraud is prevalent. Some experts have concluded that Medicare fraud totals more than $60 billion a year. Examples of healthcare fraud include the following:

- Providers and agencies bill for services that did not occur (Box 17.15).
- Information is falsified for payment.
- Services are overcharged.
- Medical identification theft occurs.

The list of fraud examples is long. The Office of Inspector General of the HHS oversees fighting fraud and abuse in governmental programs. Table 17.9 describes federal laws that address fraud in healthcare.

A medical assistant should be aware of the laws related to fraud and conflict of interest. If violations or illegal activities are noticed in the workplace, the medical assistant should follow the reporting procedures outlined in the facility's compliance program (Procedure 17.4). Conflicts of interest need to be reported immediately to the human resources supervisor or to your supervisor.

> **CRITICAL THINKING 17.9**
>
> Daniela and Bella are studying compliance. They start to discuss the importance of declaring a conflict of interest. Describe why being upfront and notifying administration/human resources about a conflict of interest is important in healthcare.

Employment Concerns. Employment concerns relate to *discrimination* (di SKRIM eh nae shahn), *harassment* (HAR ahs ment), retaliation and retribution, and unfair employment practices. Most medical assistant positions are considered *employment-at-will*. This means that the employer can end employment at any time for any reason. Many states recognize this concept. It also means the employee can quit at any time

> **VOCABULARY**
>
> **discrimination**: Unfair treatment of another person based on the person's age, gender (sex), ethnicity, sexual orientation, disability, marital status, or other selective factors.
>
> **harassment**: The continued, unwanted, and annoying actions done to another person.

TABLE 17.9 Laws Related to Fraud and Conflict of Interest

Laws	Description
Federal Anti-Kickback Law	Since 1972, prohibits intentionally receiving or giving anything of value to get referrals or generate federal healthcare program business.
False Claims Act	Originally signed into law during the American Civil War in 1863. It was revised in 2010. Prohibits a person from submitting false or fraudulent Medicare or Medicaid claims for payment. Under this act, a person can bring a civil suit on behalf of the government when he or she finds others sending false claims to the government for payment. The individual can receive part of the settlement (see Box 17.15).
Stark Law (or also called the Physician Self-Referral Law)	Became law in 1989 and became effective in 1992. Several revisions have occurred since then. Prohibits a healthcare provider from referring a Medicare patient for services to a facility in which the provider or the provider's immediate family has a financial relationship.
The Healthcare Fraud Statute	Originated in 1996 and revised in 2010. Prohibits intentionally defrauding any healthcare benefit program.

> **BOX 17.16 Legal Example: Wrongful Termination and Invasion of Privacy**
>
> The plaintiff was a security guard at Children's Hospital. He was involved in an accident while on the job. He was examined at the emergency department, given a painkiller, and released. There was no record of intoxication or impairment. The next day while recovering at home he was called to the hospital to submit to a drug test. The test was positive for hydrocodone and the hospital terminated him based on its drug-free workplace policy. He was an employee for 18 years and had a clean record with no work-related accidents or drug abuse issues. The plaintiff sued the hospital for wrongful termination, invasion of privacy, and defamation. The case went through mediation and the hospital offered $40,000 to settle. With no resolution, the case was brought to trial. After deliberation, the 12-member jury came back with 12–0 decision for the plaintiff. He was awarded $385,050 for past and future economic loss and $650,000 for past and future emotional distress. The total verdict for the plaintiff was $1,035,050.

From Mckinley Nou v. Children's Hospital Central California, (October 16, 2014) Fresno Superior Court, Case Number: 12-CECG-02169.

for any reason, though giving a 2-week notice is considered professional. Most jobs are considered employment-at-will.

Employers cannot fire an employee for an illegal reason. The employer needs to have a *just cause* or legal reason for firing an employee. Legal reasons could include terminations due to cutbacks in staffing or an employee's behavioral issues. A terminated employee may have an opportunity to sue if wrongful termination occurred. *Wrongful termination* means that the employer did not have just cause for firing the employee (Box 17.16). For instance, an employee reported that fraud was occurring in the billing department at the facility. The facility then is under investigation for the fraud. The supervisor fires the **whistleblower**. Federal and state laws protect the whistleblower from retaliation and retribution (Box 17.17).

Many federal laws regulate issues regarding employment (Table 17.10). State laws also protect the employees in different areas. For instance, state workers' compensation laws protect employees that are injured on the job. The employee may collect money to cover lost wages, medical expenses, and retraining.

> **VOCABULARY**
> **whistleblower:** A person (usually an employee) who reports a violation of the law within the organization. The person reports the information to the public or to a person in authority.

> **BOX 17.17 Legal Example: Whistleblower Retaliation**
>
> According to the complaint, psychologist Melody Jo Samuelson was hired by Napa State Hospital in California. For 2 years she received good reviews, and then she testified in a case where she alleged that a patient had been improperly assessed as competent to stand trial. In court she indicated the hospital did not use adequate methods to analyze patients. She complained that the hospital immediately retaliated against her, and she was fired from her job. She appealed her firing and filed a whistleblower retaliation complaint. She was reinstated but the retaliation continued she stated. She claimed anxiety and depression as a result of the situation. She was awarded $1 million.

From Samuelson v. California Department of Mental Health, et. al., No. 26-57631 (N.D.Cal. Feb. 20, 2014). https://www.leagle.com/decision/incaco20161121002; https://www.leagle.com/decision/incaco20161114006; https://www.leagle.com/decision/incaco20161114010

PROCEDURE 17.4 Report Illegal Activity

Task
Report an illegal activity in the healthcare setting following proper protocol.

Scenario
Today you witness a coworker, Sally Brown taking medical samples from the supply cabinet. You see her sticking them in her purse. She sees you and states, "This was the same medication I had to pay $200 for the last time I was sick. I don't see why we need to pay for medications when we have samples that we give free to patients. We should be able to use them also." You know the facility's professional policy prohibits taking medical samples from the sample cabinet for personal reasons.

Facility's Compliance Reporting Protocol
Walden-Martin Family Medical Clinic's Compliance Program has a phone number and email address for employees to report suspected violations, suspected illegal activity, fraud, abuse, theft, and workplace safety concerns. Concerns can be left on the voice mail or emailed without fear of retribution or retaliation. Please include as many details as possible, including dates, names, and the situation.

Any employee who seeks retribution or retaliation against another employee for reporting an offense needs to be aware of criminal penalties for such actions.

Equipment and Supplies
- Computer with email and internet access or phone
- Instructor's email address or voice mail phone number
- Pen and paper
- Facility's compliance reporting protocol (see box above)

Procedural Steps
1. Read the facility's corporate compliance reporting protocol.
   Purpose: Prior to reporting an illegal action, the medical assistant needs to identify the facility's protocol or the reporting chain of command. (Chain of command usually begins with your supervisor, then the supervisor of your supervisor, and so on. It is recommended you start with the lowest level that you feel comfortable with.)
2. Using the paper and pen, write down the facts of what you witnessed.
   Purpose: Writing down the facts soon after the situation will help you to remember the details.
3. Using the paper and pen, compose the message you want to email or leave on the voice mail for the compliance office.
   Purpose: Composing a message will help you organize your thoughts and leave an accurate message.
4. Proofread the message and make any changes required. Make sure to include the date, names of people involved, and the details of the situation.
   Purpose: It is important to have an accurate, complete message for the compliance office. Proofreading helps to ensure the message is accurate.
5. Using your email or phone, send a message to the corporate compliance office. Use the email address or phone number provided by your instructor.
   Purpose: To complete the reporting process, the medical assistant must contact the corporate compliance office or the required supervisor if following the chain of command.

TABLE 17.10 Federal Laws Related to Employment

Type of Law	Law	Description
Discrimination in Employment Practices	National Labor Relations Act	Also called the Wagner Act of 1935. Gave the right to most workers to organize or join a union.
	Title VII of the Civil Rights Act of 1964 (Title VII)	Prohibits employment discrimination based on color, race, gender, religion, or national origin (Box 17.18).
	Age Discrimination in Employment Act of 1967 (ADEA)	Revised several times. Protects applications and employers 40 years and older from discrimination. Includes hiring, promotion, termination, and compensation practices.
	Rehabilitation Act of 1973	Prohibits discrimination in employment practices based on physical or mental disabilities. Applies to federal employers or employers that are federal contractors (provide services to the federal government) (Box 17.19).
	Pregnancy Discrimination Act of 1978	Amended Title VII of the Civil Rights Act of 1964. Prohibits gender discrimination based on pregnancy.
	Title I and Title V of the Americans with Disabilities Act of 1990 (ADA)	Prohibits employment discrimination against qualified persons with disabilities. Box 17.20 describes the latest amendment to ADA.
	Genetic Information Nondiscrimination Act of 2008 (GINA)	Prohibits employment discrimination based on the person's genetic information.
	Civil Rights Act of 1991	Provides punitive damages in cases of intentional employment discrimination.

Continued

TABLE 17.10 Federal Laws Related to Employment—cont'd

Type of Law	Law	Description
Related to hours, pay, and leave	Federal Insurance Contributions Act of 1935 (FICA)	Created a payroll tax that requires a deduction from a person's paycheck. The withheld amount and an employer contribution fund the Social Security program and a portion of Medicare.
	Fair Labor Standards Act of 1938	Prohibits child labor. Also provides overtime pay and a minimum wage.
	Equal Pay Act of 1963 (EPA)	Protects against gender-based wage discrimination. Equal pay for both men and women who are performing the same job at the same organization.
	Employee Retirement Income Security Act of 1974 (ERISA)	Sets minimum standards for pension and health plans in private industry and protects individuals in these plans.
	Family Medical Leave Act (FMLA) of 1991	Provides unpaid leave time for maternity, adoption, or caring for ill family members.

A medical assistant should be aware of the employment laws. If violations are noticed in the workplace, the medical assistant should follow the reporting procedures outlined in the facility's compliance program. If no program exists, then it is important to discuss the issues with the person responsible for the human resources duties.

Environmental Safety Concerns. Compliance reporting also relates to environmental safety violations. Offenses can be violations of local, state, or federal regulations. The unsafe activities or practices may cause hazardous conditions that impact the health or safety of employees, patients, and others. If you recall, OSHA is involved with creating a safe environment for employees. Any situation that risks the safety of employees or patients must be reported immediately. Box 17.21 discusses how an employee can file a complaint with OSHA.

When a person is injured or equipment malfunctions, most ambulatory care facilities require an incident report to be completed (Box 17.22). Incident reports are communication tools used by risk management teams. *Risk management* involves techniques used to reduce or eliminate accidental loss to the healthcare facility. It involves identifying, assessing, and controlling risks. Risks can relate to financial issues, legal liabilities, accidents, and electronic data security threats.

Patient Safety Concerns. Patient safety concerns are of utmost importance in healthcare facilities. Even with careful practices, patients can be harmed. A patient can fall. The wrong medication may be given to the patient. The wrong procedure may be done. All issues of safety can lead to potential liability for injuries that result.

If a medical assistant is involved in a situation in which a person is harmed, it is important to do the following:
- Immediately notify the provider. This is especially important if the wrong medication was given to the patient. The provider must identify what steps need to be taken.
- Arrange to have the person seen by a provider immediately. The provider can assess the extent of the injuries and provide the required treatment. Information on the injuries and treatment will then be documented in the health record should future litigation occur.
- Complete the incident report (Procedure 17.5). The employee witnessing the situation should be the person completing the report if possible. The incident report communicates what occurred and provides information should future litigation occur.

BOX 17.18 Illegal Interview Questions

To prevent legal issues related to hiring practices, healthcare facilities need to stay away from specific topics during the interview process. Asking questions related to these topics can put the facility at risk for discrimination lawsuits. Illegal and legal topics are listed here.

Topic	Examples of Illegal Questions	Examples of Legal Questions
Birthplace, ancestry, or national origin	When did you move to the United States?	Are you eligible to work in this state?
Marital status, children, or pregnancy	Who will look after your child when he is born?	Are you able to work an 8 a.m. to 5 p.m. schedule?
Physical disability, health or medical history	What medications are you on?	Can you perform the essential job functions of a medical assistant with or without reasonable accommodation?
Religion or religious days observed	Where do you attend church services?	Can you work on weekends?
Age, race, ethnicity, gender, or color	How old are you?	Are you 18 or older? (or whatever the minimum age is for the facility)
Criminal records	Have you ever been arrested?	Have you ever been convicted of a crime?

- Notify the department supervisor. The supervisor can follow up with the patient. Many agencies do not charge the injured patient for the services provided. If the wrong medication is given, many agencies do not charge for the medication and services provided.
- Notify state or federal government agencies regarding the injury. Some states have medical error reporting systems in place. OSHA requires agencies to record all work-related needlestick injuries and cuts from sharp objects that are contaminated with another person's blood or other potentially infectious material. The case must be reported on the OSHA 300 Log.

BOX 17.19 Americans With Disabilities Act and the Rehabilitation Act of 1973 in Healthcare

People with disabilities have a right to accessible healthcare. The Americans With Disabilities Act (ADA) prohibits discrimination against individuals with disabilities in everyday activities including getting healthcare. The Rehabilitation Act of 1973 prohibits discrimination against individuals with disabilities in services that receive federal financial assistance, including healthcare services. These laws require that healthcare agencies make their services accessible to people with disabilities.

Examples of how these laws impact ambulatory care facilities:
- Patients in wheelchairs: These patients need to be moved to exam tables when the exam requires the patient to be lying. Lifts and low exam tables are available to help in these situations. Patients with disabilities cannot be denied care on the grounds that accessible medical equipment is not available.
- Patients with disabilities: If a patient has an interpreter or companion, it is important that the healthcare provider focus on the patient.
- Exam table location: Patients must have a minimum of 30 inches by 48 inches of clear space adjacent to the exam table and the accessible route out of the room. This allows individuals in wheelchairs to approach the table and be able to transfer onto it. An adjustable-height exam table should be available.
- Accessible scales: Special wheelchair scales and in-floor scales (built into the floor) are needed for patients with limited-to-no mobility.

BOX 17.20 ADA Amendments Act of 2008

The ADA Amendments Act of 2008 is also known as ADA Amendment Act and ADAAA. The original ADA narrowly defined disability. The ADA Amendment Act expanded the meaning and interpretation of the definition of disability. People with cancer, diabetes, attention deficit hyperactivity disorder, learning disabilities, and epilepsy are now included. This should ensure that individuals with disabilities receive protection under the law.

BOX 17.21 How to File a Complaint With OSHA

The Occupational Safety and Health Act of 1970 gives employees the right to file a complaint with OSHA. Employees can request an OSHA inspection if they believe their workplace has safety hazards. The employee filing the report does not need to be knowledgeable about the OSHA regulations. OSHA will keep the reporting person's information confidential.

To report a safety and health issue, the employee can file an electronic form, fax or mail a report to the local OSHA office, or call the local OSHA office. Specific information and forms are available at https://www.osha.gov.

BOX 17.22 Incident Reports

An incident report is an internal document that needs to be completed whenever an unexpected event occurs. The purposes of the incident report are to gather information about the situation in case of a future lawsuit and to communicate issues for risk management procedures. The medical assistant should remember these points about incident reports:
- Complete an incident report for patient complaints, medication errors, medical device malfunctions, and any injury.
- Complete the incident report clearly and accurately in pen or electronically. List the facts. Do not speculate or draw conclusions.
- Make sure to complete it by the end of the day the situation occurred.
- Do not mention the incident report in the patient's health record. If it is mentioned, a lawyer may request a copy of the report.

PROCEDURE 17.5   Complete Incident Report

Task
Complete an incident report form for a medication error.

Scenario
Johnny Parker (DOB 06/15/10) was seen by nurse practitioner Jean Burke for a well child visit. Johnny is off schedule with his hepatitis B vaccine series, and today he is to get his last hepatitis B booster. You (a medical assistant) prepare the medication and give the injection in his right deltoid muscle. Later in the day you realize that hepatitis B was out of stock for 1 week. You must have given a hepatitis A booster to Johnny. You realized that you failed to read the label three times during preparation of the medication. You reported the mistake to Jean Burke and your supervisor. Your supervisor called Lisa Parker, Johnny's mother. They will come back next week for the hepatitis B vaccine. You need to complete the incident report.

Equipment and Supplies
- Incident report form (Fig. 17.7) and black pen or computer with an internet connection and SimChart for the Medical Office (SCMO)

Procedural Steps
1. *SCMO method:* Access SCMO and enter the Simulation Playground. If a popup window appears, select "Return to previous session with saved patient information" and click Start. On the Calendar screen, click on the Form Repository icon. Click on Office Forms on the left Info Panel and select Incident Report. *For both methods:* Accurately complete the information from the date down to the reason for the patient's visit.
   Purpose: It is important to have the accurate information regarding the date, time, location, incident type, and the reason for the visit. Giving the background information will help the reader understand what occurred.
2. *For both methods:* Specify the incident description, immediate action and outcome, and contributing factors, and fill in the prevention boxes. Provide as much detail as possible. Be honest and concise with your facts.
   Purpose: It is important to give a clear, concise, and honest description of what occurred. It is hard to admit fault, but doing so shows your professionalism in the situation.

WALDEN-MARTIN
FAMILY MEDICAL CLINIC
1234 ANYSTREET | ANYTOWN, ANYSTATE 12345
PHONE 123-123-1234 | FAX 123-123-5678

Incident Report

Date: _____   Time: _____

Incident Type: ☐ Staff   ☐ Patient   ☐ Visitor   ☐ Equipment/Property

Witness: ☐ Staff   ☐ Patient   ☐ Visitor

Department: _____   Exact Location: _____

Medical Team: _____

Patient Reason for Visit: _____   Medication Incident: ☐ Yes ☐ No

Incident Description: [   ]   Immediate Actions and Outcome: [   ]

Contributing Factors: [   ]   Prevention: [   ]

Next of kin / guardian notified / patient?   ☐ Yes ☐ No ☐ N/A   Medical staff notified? ☐ Yes ☐ No ☐ N/A

Reported By: _____   Position: _____

Contact Phone Number: _____

Other Persons Involved: _____   Position: _____

Contact Phone Number: _____

Medical Report (Document patient's assessment and list investigations and treatments):
_____

Provider: _____   Designation: _____

Provider Signature: _____   Date/Time: _____

FIG. 17.7 Incident report form.

PROCEDURE 17.5 Complete Incident Report—cont'd

3. *For both methods:* Complete the reported by, position, and contact phone number sections. Your information should be in these fields. Make up a contact phone number.
   Purpose: It is important to have accurate information in these fields so that if people have questions, they can contact you.
4. *For both methods:* Complete the other persons involved, position, and contact phone number sections. Jean Burke's information should be in these fields. Make up her contact phone number.

   Purpose: Having additional people listed on the form helps if questions arise about the situation. The rest of the form from the Medical Report field to the end needs to be completed by the provider.
5. *For both methods:* Review the form for accuracy. Make any changes required before submitting the form to the instructor. (*For the SCMO method:* Save or print the form based on your instructor's directions.)
   Purpose: It is important to proofread the form to ensure it is accurate and complete.

CLOSING COMMENTS

During a busy day in an ambulatory care facility, the medical assistant performs many administrative and clinical tasks. It is important for the medical assistant to perform these tasks following the facility's policies and procedures. Remember that these policies and procedures are created so that staff complies with the state and federal laws. Should a medical assistant feel that a task conflicts with a law, the medical assistant should talk with the supervisor.

CHAPTER REVIEW

Throughout this chapter, we discussed laws related to privacy and confidentiality. HIPAA is a complex law that influences healthcare. The medical assistant has an important role in complying with the Privacy Rule and the Security Rule (see the box titled "Exceptional Customer Service"). It is important to keep PHI confidential. Medical assistants can only access health records of patients with whom they are working. Browsing random patient records or looking up a family member's health information are HIPAA violations.

Additional laws that impact healthcare were also discussed. The FDA enforces the Food, Drug, and Cosmetic Act. It ensures that medications on the market are safe for the public. The DEA enforces the Controlled Substances Act. The Occupational Safety and Health Act and OSHA focus on keeping the workplace safe for employees. Acts related to end-of-life issues encourage organ donation and advance directives.

Compliance reporting is important for providers. They need to ensure that specific communicable diseases are reported to the public health department. Wounds of violence need to be reported to law enforcement agencies. Healthcare providers are mandatory reporters for child abuse, neglect, and exploitation. The reporting laws vary for adults, but in many states elder abuse needs to be reported.

Many healthcare agencies have developed compliance programs. Employees are asked to report suspicious behaviors. In turn, many times the facility then needs to file reports with governmental agencies for noncompliance issues. The medical assistant has important duties in the healthcare setting that help the provider fulfill obligated responsibilities. The medical assistant as an employee also has a responsibility to comply with laws and report suspicious behaviors. Knowing the healthcare laws is important for a medical assistant.

EXCEPTIONAL CUSTOMER SERVICE

When working with older patients, questions on record release and disclosure authorization forms can be common. Years ago such forms did not exist. Today patients may feel they have to complete forms for everything. Make sure to take time to explain why it is important to have the forms completed. Remember that some of the older patients may have difficulty reading the forms. Some may not be able to hear as well as they used to. Take time and communicate clearly and slowly with the older patients. Use simple phrases when answering their questions. If possible, help complete whatever information you can. Be patient and respectful during your interaction with patients.

SCENARIO WRAP-UP

Daniela has learned a lot about healthcare-related laws. Not only did she learn about laws that healthcare professionals must follow, she also learned about employment laws. One of Daniela's assignments for her course was to identify three risks of HIPAA violations. Daniela and Bella talked about the assignment and the risks in their department.

Unattended computers that were open to the electronic health record were problems. This is especially a risk in the patient examination rooms, as each room is equipped with a personal computer for documenting. Daniela also mentioned conversations about patients in the medical assistant station. Sometimes she hears medical assistants discussing a patient that came in. She feels uncomfortable about those conversations and ensures she does not take part in them.

Cell phones in the workplace and frequent use of social media sites during work hours can be risks. Bella mentioned that she heard several stories of employees being terminated. The employees posted patient-related photos and information on social media sites. Bella and Daniela admit they work hard to prevent HIPAA violations. They do not ever want to be named in a lawsuit for such violations.

18 Healthcare Ethics

LEARNING OBJECTIVES

1. Do the following related to ethics:
   - Define ethics and morals.
   - Differentiate between personal and professional ethics.
   - Identify the effect of personal morals on professional performance.
   - Recognize the impact personal ethics and morals have on the delivery of healthcare.
   - Develop a plan for separation of personal and professional ethics.
2. List and describe the principles of healthcare ethics.
3. Demonstrate appropriate responses to ethical issues involving genetics.
4. Demonstrate appropriate responses to ethical issues involving reproductive issues.
5. Demonstrate appropriate responses to ethical issues involving childhood issues.
6. Demonstrate appropriate responses to ethical issues involving end-of-life issues. Also, discuss the following:
   - Discuss the theories of Elizabeth Kübler-Ross.
   - Define the Patient Self Determination Act.
   - Define advance directives, living will, medical durable power of attorney, and healthcare proxy.
7. Demonstrate appropriate responses to ethical issues involving organ donation issues, and define the Uniform Anatomical Gift Act.

CHAPTER OUTLINE

1. Opening Scenario, 400
2. You Will Learn, 401
3. Introduction to Ethics, 401
4. Personal and Professional Ethics, 401
   a. Personal Ethics, 401
   b. Professional Ethics, 401
      i. *Code of Ethics for Medical Assistants, 402*
   c. Separation Plan, 402
      i. *Creating a Plan, 403*
5. Principles of Healthcare Ethics, 403
   a. Autonomy, 404
   b. Nonmaleficence, 404
   c. Beneficence, 404
   d. Justice, 404
6. Ethical Issues, 404
   a. Genetics Issues, 404
      i. *Cloning, 405*
      ii. *Genetic Engineering, 405*
   b. Reproductive Issues, 406
      i. *Assisted Reproductive Technology, 406*
      ii. *Abortion, 406*
   c. Childhood Issues, 407
      i. *Adoption, 407*
      ii. *Safe Haven Infant Protection Laws, 407*
      iii. *Confidential Healthcare for Minors, 407*
   d. End-of-Life Issues, 408
      i. *Patient Self-Determination Act, 408*
      ii. *Uniform Determination of Death Act, 409*
      iii. *Withholding or Withdrawing Life-Sustaining Treatment, 410*
      iv. *Euthanasia, 410*
   e. Organ Donation Issues, 410
      i. *Uniform Anatomical Gift Act, 410*
      ii. *National Organ Transplant Act, 410*
      iii. *Xenotransplantation, 411*
7. Closing Comments, 411
8. Chapter Review, 411
9. Scenario Wrap-Up, 411

OPENING SCENARIO

Daniela Garcia was just hired as a part-time float receptionist at Walden-Martin Family Medical (WMFM) Clinic. As a float receptionist, she will be working with many coworkers and providers. Besides working, Daniela is also attending the local community college for medical assisting. She is currently taking a law and ethics course.

Daniela has completed the law part of the course. She is starting the ethics unit. Daniela grew up in a conservative family. They lived in a very small town in the Midwest. She has since relocated and finds that some of the beliefs she held as a teen are now changing as she encounters more life challenges. As she studies various topics, she has also found that what she believed to be true when she was younger is not actually true. Daniela is very interested to continue to learn about ethics.

CHAPTER 18 Healthcare Ethics

YOU WILL LEARN

1. To describe personal and professional ethics.
2. To create a plan to separate personal and professional ethics.
3. To state the four principles of healthcare ethics.
4. To examine ethical issues related to genetics, reproductive, childhood, end-of-life, and organ donation issues.

INTRODUCTION TO ETHICS

As you move into healthcare, you may be faced with situations in which you do not agree with a person's decision. As a healthcare professional, you need to respect a patient's decision whether or not you agree with it.

This chapter examines ethics (ETH iks). Ethical issues are different from legal issues. What may be legal may not be ethical. Personal ethics and its impact on professional performance will be discussed. Professional ethics differs from personal ethics. This topic is explored, along with how to handle the differences. Common ethical issues in healthcare are examined. End-of-life issues, including advance directives, are also discussed.

PERSONAL AND PROFESSIONAL ETHICS

Personal Ethics

Personal ethics includes an individual's honesty, fairness, commitment, integrity, and accountability. It also includes doing what one considers to be correct.

Our morals (MORE ahls) tell us what is right and wrong. Our moral compass develops as we grow. Our first lessons on right and wrong come from our parents/guardians. Our socialization and background shape our morals. For instance, if your parents instilled in you the importance of always being on time, you may grow up feeling that a person should always be on time. You may feel others are in error if they are late for an event. As we grow, our morals may change if our beliefs change. Our morals impact how we conduct ourselves or, in other words, our personal ethics.

Our personal morals impact our professional performance. If people believe in being on time, this characteristic will transfer to the work environment. The employees will be on time for work. Being timely when rooming patients will be important to the employees. Having patients wait for long periods of time in the reception area will be challenging to accept. Personal ethics that align with professional characteristics will positively impact one's professional performance.

Our personal morals may also negatively impact our professional performance. Let's say a person grew up without grandparents or older adults in the family. That person may view older people as not being as knowledgeable as the younger generations. If a medical assistant had this belief, imagine how that might impact his or her professional performance. That person may not respect an older adult. An older adult may be viewed as being useless, no longer important, not as smart, and a lesser individual. This will impact how the medical assistant would treat an older patient. As professionals, we cannot let our personal morals negatively impact the care that we provide to patients.

> **CRITICAL THINKING 18.1**
>
> Daniela was working on her ethics assignment on break at the clinic. She thought about her personal ethics. She decided that some of her personal ethics would benefit her in a job. She realizes that some of her personal morals may negatively impact the care she provides to patients. She realizes that she needs to explore these morals and make some personal decisions.
>
> Think about your personal ethics and morals. What will positively influence your professional performance? What personal morals will negatively impact your professional performance?

Professional Ethics

Professional ethics are codes of conduct stated by an employer or professional association (Table 18.1). Many employers state how employees need to conduct themselves in the workplace. This information can usually be found in the employee handbook.

Many healthcare professional associations have published professional ethics for their members. These are called codes of ethics. A *code of ethics* is a set of rules about good and bad behavior. If a member or employee violates a professional ethic, the association or agency will discipline the person. We will examine the codes for physicians and medical assistants.

Code of ethics for physicians. One of the most famous and oldest codes of ethics is the Hippocratic oath. The original oath has been around for longer than 2000 years. Hippocrates, often called the father of medicine, is credited for the oath. The oath is a code of ethics for physicians. Over the years, the code has been modernized (Fig. 18.1).

In 1847 the American Medical Association (AMA) adopted its Code of Medical Ethics. The code lists the values that physicians commit themselves to as they practice medicine. The AMA's current Code of Medical Ethics is available on its website (www.ama-assn.org). The code is a living document. This means that as medicine and technology changes, the code is updated by the members. Key themes in the code include the following:

- Physicians should provide competent care and continue learning.
- Physicians should respect human dignity and rights.

TABLE 18.1 Differences Between Personal and Professional Ethics

	Personal Ethics	Professional Ethics
Definition	Individual's code of conduct	Codes of conduct stated by an employer or professional association
Ability to Change	Individuals can change their own personal ethics	Individuals cannot change and must comply; only changed by employer or professional association
Accountability	On the individual	On the members and organization

---

VOCABULARY

ethics: Rules of conduct.
morals: Internal principles that distinguish between right and wrong.
personal ethics: An individual's code of conduct.

> *I swear to fulfill, to the best of my ability and judgment, this covenant:*
>
> I will respect the hard-won scientific gains of those physicians in whose steps I walk, and gladly share such knowledge as is mine with those who are to follow.
>
> I will apply, for the benefit of the sick, all measures [that] are required, avoiding those twin traps of overtreatment and therapeutic nihilism.
>
> I will remember that there is art to medicine as well as science, and that warmth, sympathy, and understanding may outweigh the surgeon's knife or the chemist's drug.
>
> I will not be ashamed to say "I know not," nor will I fail to call in my colleagues when the skills of another are needed for a patient's recovery.
>
> I will respect the privacy of my patients, for their problems are not disclosed to me that the world may know. Most especially must I tread with care in matters of life and death. If it is given me to save a life, all thanks. But it may also be within my power to take a life; this awesome responsibility must be faced with great humbleness and awareness of my own frailty. Above all, I must not play at God.
>
> I will remember that I do not treat a fever chart, a cancerous growth, but a sick human being, whose illness may affect the person's family and economic stability. My responsibility includes these related problems, if I am to care adequately for the sick.
>
> I will prevent disease whenever I can, for prevention is preferable to cure.
>
> I will remember that I remain a member of society, with special obligations to all my fellow human beings, those sound of mind and body as well as the infirm.
>
> If I do not violate this oath, may I enjoy life and art, respected while I live and remembered with affection thereafter. May I always act so as to preserve the finest traditions of my calling and may I long experience the joy of healing those who seek my help.
>
> *Written in 1964 by Louis Lasagna, Academic Dean of the School of Medicine at Tufts University, and used in many medical schools today.*

FIG. 18.1 Modern version of the Hippocratic oath. (From Proctor D, et al: *Kinn's The Medical Assistant*, ed 13, St. Louis, 2017, Elsevier.)

- Physicians should follow the laws, be professional, and uphold the standard of the medical profession.
- Physicians should contribute to the welfare of the community.

The Council of Ethical and Judicial Affairs (CEJA) is one of the councils within the AMA. CEJA analyzes ethical issues in healthcare. The council develops ethical policies and recommendations. These recommendations, along with the Code of Medical Ethics, are used by physicians to guide their practice. CEJA promotes AMA members to adhere to the Code of Medical Ethics.

Code of Ethics for Medical Assistants. The American Association of Medical Assistants (AAMA) developed a code of ethics that provides the principles of ethical and moral conduct for the profession (Box 18.1). The Medical Assisting Creed by the AAMA is a statement of beliefs for the profession (Box 18.2). The Medical Assisting Creed supports the code of ethics.

It is important for the medical assistant to follow the code and creed. The care provided to others must reflect respect for that person. The medical assistant is legally and ethically obligated to keep patient information confidential. Continual learning is critical. The medical assistant must provide the best care possible and uphold the standard of the profession.

> **CRITICAL THINKING 18.2**
>
> Daniela read the AMA Code of Medical Ethics and the AAMA Medical Assisting Code of Ethics. She notices some similarities between the codes. What similarities do you notice between the two codes?

> **BOX 18.1 Medical Assisting Code of Ethics**
>
> Members of AAMA dedicated to the conscientious pursuit of their profession, and thus desiring to merit the high regard of the entire medical profession and the respect of the general public which they serve, do pledge themselves to strive always to:
>
> A. Render service with full respect for the dignity of humanity.
> B. Respect confidential information obtained through employment unless legally authorized or required by responsible performance of duty to divulge such information.
> C. Uphold the honor and high principles of the profession and accept its disciplines.
> D. Seek to continually improve the knowledge and skills of medical assistants for the benefit of patients and professional colleagues.
> E. Participate in additional service activities aimed toward improving the health and well-being of the community.
>
> From the American Association of Medical Assistants, http://www.aama-ntl.org/about/overview#.WSDywmjytPY.

Separation Plan

Sometimes an individual's personal ethics clashes with professional ethics. It is important to take steps to separate one's personal ethics from professional ethics.

Let's examine a few situations that might impact a medical assistant. Imagine if a medical assistant has personal beliefs that vaccines are not needed and harm individuals. This medical assistant obtains a job in a pediatric department. She is required to give vaccines numerous times a day. In this situation, her personal ethics would clash with her

PROCEDURE 18.1 Developing an Ethics Separation Plan

Task
To develop a plan for separating personal and professional ethics.

Scenario
You are working at Walden-Martin Family Medical (WMFM) Clinic. Your provider sees many children, including teens. New state laws allow confidential healthcare for minors. The agency has now adopted policies and procedures to allow providers to see teens 16 years and older without parental consent. The teens can be seen for sexually transmitted infections (STIs) and reproductive issues (including birth control). All health records related to these visits are confidential, meaning parents cannot be told about their child's visit.

Your personal belief is that parents should always be allowed to know what is occurring with their children. They are responsible for the child until age 18 and they pay the bills. You also believe that children under 18 are too young to be in an intimate relationship with others. This type of relationship should be only for adults in a committed relationship. You do not believe in birth control.

Equipment and Supplies
- Paper and pen
- Medical Assisting Code of Ethics (see Box 18.1)

Procedural Steps
1. Read the code of ethics for medical assistants. Write down key themes or phrases.
   Purpose: Medical assistants need to follow the code of ethics for the medical assistant professional.
2. Using the scenario, write down the professional ethics involved in the situation.
   Purpose: Medical assistants need to follow the laws and agency's policies and procedures. The procedures indicate how the healthcare professional needs to perform duties.
3. Using the scenario, write down the personal ethics involved in the situation.
   Purpose: Medical assistants need to identify their personal ethics. They need to be honest when analyzing how they think and feel about different scenarios that may occur in healthcare. Understanding one's biases is the first step in ensuring that respectful, ethical care is provided to all patients.
4. Compare the lists. Identify the personal ethics that conflict with the code of ethics and the professional ethics of the agency.
   Purpose: Medical assistants must identify areas where their personal ethics conflict with the code of ethics and the professional ethics of the agency. Medical assistants need to follow the professional ethics. Personal ethics should not supersede professional ethics.
5. For each area of conflict, create a plan on how you will separate your personal and professional ethics. Remember, as a professional, you need to follow the professional ethics of the agency and the profession. Address how you will handle the situation and what would be your options if you were in the situation.
   Purpose: Medical assistants must create a plan and be aware of how they will handle situations that conflict with their personal ethics. This might mean they need to find another job. They may need to rethink their biases. Learning more about a bias can help a person identify errors in his or her thinking.
6. Describe how the personal ethics and morals in this scenario would impact the patient care.
   Purpose: It is important that medical assistants recognize the impact personal ethics and morals have on the delivery of healthcare.

BOX 18.2 Medical Assisting Creed of the AAMA

- I believe in the principles and purposes of the profession of medical assisting.
- I endeavor to be more effective.
- I aspire to render greater service.
- I protect the confidence entrusted to me.
- I am dedicated to the care and well-being of all people.
- I am loyal to my employer.
- I am true to the ethics of my profession.
- I am strengthened by compassion, courage, and faith.

From the American Association of Medical Assistants, http://www.aama-ntl.org/about/overview#.WSDywmjytPY.

professional ethics. She would be professionally obligated to give the vaccines to patients. She could not share her antivaccine beliefs with patients. Due to the clash of ethics, it might be a stressful job for her.

In another situation, a medical assistant believes that everything that can be done should be done when someone is dying. Professional ethics mandate that each person has a right to make end-of-life decisions. Legally and ethically, the medical assistant must follow what the patient decides. The medical assistant cannot put pressure on the patient to change his or her decision.

Creating a Plan. As you complete your medical assistant courses, it is important to evaluate if your personal ethics conflict with the medical assistant code of ethics.

- Are there groups of people with whom you have issues? Maybe you do not believe in their behaviors, actions, or ideas based on your morals.
- Do you have preconceived ideas about people with differing ethnicities, sexual preferences, or specific diseases?

If you identified conflicts, how might you provide respectful care to these people? Honestly, think about your biases. How would you approach a situation if it involved your bias? Remember, the professional code of ethics supersedes your personal code. You need to follow the professional ethics of your agency and profession (Procedure 18.1).

Before a medical assistant starts applying for positions, it is important to evaluate if personal ethics will clash with the professional ethics of an agency. If a person does not believe in vaccinations, then working in a department that gives vaccinations would not be a good job choice. If a person does not believe in abortions, then working in an agency that does abortions would not be a good choice.

CRITICAL THINKING 18.3

Daniela decided to create a plan to separate her personal ethics from her professional ethics. Think about your personal ethics. What steps might you take to change your personal morals so that they better align with your professional ethics? What might you do to deal with the personal ethics that conflict with the professional ethics?

PRINCIPLES OF HEALTHCARE ETHICS

Healthcare professionals have an ethical duty to their patients. Four ethical principles summarize this ethical duty. These principles include *autonomy* (ah TON eh mee), *nonmaleficence* (non mah LEF i sens), *beneficence* (be NEF i sens), and *justice*. Technically all four of these principles should have equal weight in ethical decisions. Many times autonomy overshadows the other three principles.

Besides healthcare professionals, **bioethicists** (BYE oh eth i sists) also use the principles of healthcare ethics. They apply these principles when they evaluate medical technology and procedures. Are the new technology advances ethical? Are these procedures ethical?

We will examine the four ethical principles. Ethical actions to meet the principles will be discussed for both the provider and the medical assistant.

Autonomy

Autonomy is the freedom to determine one's own actions and decisions. Patients have the right to make their own healthcare decisions. Providers need to tell patients of the risks and benefits of different procedures (informed consent). After being told what may be most successful, the patients can make their own decisions. The patient's decision-making process should be free from pressure or interference from others. Healthcare professionals must respect and honor the patient's decision.

The medical assistant must protect patients' privacy. It is important to respect the uniqueness, dignity, and decisions of others. This includes patients, families, and coworkers. You must also maintain your own dignity and self-respect (Box 18.3).

> ### CRITICAL THINKING 18.4
> When Daniela learned about the autonomy principle and the role of the medical assistant, it reminded her of healthcare laws that she learned about. What healthcare laws address autonomy and the healthcare professional's role?

Nonmaleficence

Nonmaleficence means to do no harm. Healthcare professionals are obligated to not inflict intentional harm to patients. By providing the appropriate standard of care, we can decrease the risk of negligence. It is important to provide competent care to patients for both legal and ethical reasons.

The medical assistant must prevent harm to others—this means to intervene when a patient is at risk (e.g., falling). It is important to make sure the environment is both physically and psychologically safe for others and that safety hazards are reported and corrected. For instance, malfunctioning equipment must never be used until fixed. Hazardous chemicals and sharps (needles) must be unavailable to patients. The medical assistant must also provide safe and competent care to all patients.

Beneficence

Beneficence means to do good. For healthcare professionals, this means promoting health in patients and assisting patients to recover from illness. Promoting health with ambulatory care patients is an important role for medical assistants. With the current focus on prevention of diseases, medical assistants help providers by identifying the immunizations and screening tests their patients need.

Justice

Justice means to treat patients fairly and give them what is due to them. This means that patients in similar situations should receive the same services and treatments.

The medical assistant must provide equal respect and courtesy to all people. Regardless of the person's color, sexual preference, nationality, religion, and health history, every person must be treated respectfully. It is important that medical assistants think about their biases. Do you really feel everyone is equal? Is there any group of individuals whose ideas you do not agree with? Understanding one's biases is important. If we do not identify our biases, there is a tendency to treat others differently. As healthcare professionals, we are obligated to treat everyone equally and with respect.

ETHICAL ISSUES

There are many ethical issues in healthcare. As technology and medicine evolve, additional ethical issues arise. We will examine common ethical issues, and the CEJA's recommendation will also be explained.

Genetics Issues

Each person is made up of 46 **chromosomes** (KROE mah somes), 23 from each parent. *Genes (jeens)* are the basic units of heredity or the instructions on how our bodies should develop and function. Genes provide the differences among us and the similarities in families. From genes we get our physical appearance, as well as our susceptibility to disease. During the process of conception and subsequent cell division, an extra chromosome (or a change in the chromosome structure) may occur. Types of genetic diseases include the following:
- *Monogenic* (MON ah jen ik) disorder: a defective gene is inherited from one or both parents. Huntington disease, *cystic fibrosis* (SIS tik fie BROE sis), and sickle cell anemia are examples of monogenic disorders.
- Chromosomal disorder: an abnormal number of chromosomes or a change in the chromosomal structure causes diseases such as *Klinefelter* (KLINE fel ter) *syndrome* and Turner syndrome.

With the advances in technology, a lot of research has occurred with cloning, genetic engineering, and gene therapy. Along with the advancements come ethical issues and questions. We will explore cloning and genetic engineering advancements and related ethical issues.

> ### BOX 18.3 Maintaining Your Dignity and Self-Respect
> - Help to make others around you look good without minimizing yourself. Do this by being supportive and helpful to your team members.
> - Refrain from being negative and whining.
> - Be assertive, not aggressive, when standing up for your rights (e.g., adequate work environment, hours, and pay).
> - Collaborate and cooperate with coworkers. Do not be afraid to stand up for what is right and fair.
> - Avoid bringing personal issues into the workplace.

> ### VOCABULARY
> **bioethicists:** People who study the ethical effect of biomedical advances (e.g., drugs and genetic engineering).
> **chromosomes:** Rod-shaped structures found in the cell's nucleus; they contain genetic information.

Cloning. *Cloning* is the process of creating a genetically identical biologic entity. A clone is the copy, which has the same genetic makeup as the original entity. Researchers have cloned genes, cells, tissues, and organisms. Dolly, the sheep, was the first mammal cloned. Since then, at least eight different mammals have been cloned, including horses and pigs. Advocates for human cloning discuss the need for organ transplants. Opponents for human cloning address the rights of the clone.

Genetic Engineering. *Genetic engineering* is the manipulation of genetic material in cells to change *hereditary* (he RED i tare ee) traits or produce a specific result. Genetic engineering is used in many areas, including agriculture and medicine. For instance, a lot of corn and soybeans are genetically modified to resist disease and insects. These foods may be labeled as genetically modified organisms (GMOs). In medicine, insulin, human growth hormone, and drugs are genetically engineered. We will focus on genetic engineering in medicine.

A *genome* (jee NOME) is the entire genetic makeup of an organism. The Human Genome Project, a 13-year international project, mapped the human genome. The entire human genome contains about 30,000 genes. The goal of the project was to gain information that will eventually lead to the prevention and treatment of many diseases. *Genomic* (jee NOE mik) *medicine* resulted from the Human Genome Project. Genomic medicine is an emerging branch of medicine involved with using patients' genomic information as part of their clinical care. Genetic testing, pharmacogenetics, and stem cell transplants are important advances in genomic medicine. Gene therapy is currently being researched.

Genetic testing. Genetic testing can identify issues with a person's chromosomes, genes, or proteins. More than 1000 genetic tests are available. Table 18.2 summarizes the different categories of genetic testing. The results of genetic tests can indicate if a person has or may develop a genetic condition. Box 18.4 provides the CEJA's opinions on genetic testing.

TABLE 18.2 Types of Genetic Testing

Types of Genetic Testing	Description
Newborn screening	All states have newborn screening procedures to identify genetic disorders that can be treated early in life.
Diagnostic testing	Used to diagnose a specific genetic or chromosomal condition. Testing can occur prior to birth or after. Not all genetic conditions have diagnostic tests.
Carrier testing	Used to determine if a person is carrying one copy of a gene mutation. Two copies of a gene mutation (one from each parent) can result in a genetic disorder in a child.
Prenatal testing	Used to detect genetic or chromosomal issues with a fetus (unborn baby).
Preimplantation testing	Used to detect genetic issues in embryos that were created using assisted reproductive technology, which will be explained later in the chapter.
Predictive and presymptomatic testing	Used to detect gene mutations associated with specific disorders that occur after birth. Usually done when a patient has a family member with a genetic disorder and the patient wants to see if he or she has it also.
Forensic testing	Used to identify crime or catastrophe victims, identify or rule out crime suspects, or establish biologic relationships between people (e.g., paternity).

> **CRITICAL THINKING 18.5**
>
> When Daniela learned about genetic testing, she remembered hearing about how people could trace their relatives. She also had heard about forensic testing while watching crime drama shows. What types of genetic testing were you familiar with?

> **BOX 18.4 CEJA's Opinions on Genetic Testing**
>
> The impact of genetics on diseases is complex. Understanding genetic counseling and helping the patient to understand the results requires special skill from the provider. Genetic testing is most important when it makes a meaningful impact on the person's health. The provider ordering genetic testing should have the appropriate knowledge and expertise to counsel the patient on the findings and implications. Providers must keep genetic testing information confidential.

Pharmacogenetics. *Pharmacogenomics* (FAR mah koe jah NOE miks) is a branch of pharmacology that studies the genetic factors that influence a person's response to a medication. Based on a person's genome, pharmacogenomics can determine if a specific therapy will be effective. More than 100 medications approved by the U.S. Food and Drug Administration (FDA) already have pharmacogenomics information available. Some of these medications include analgesics, antivirals, cardiovascular drugs, and anticancer drugs.

Stem cell transplants. Stem cells can *differentiate* (DIF uh REN shee ate). This means they can develop into specialized cells (e.g., muscle, blood, or brain cells). They can *self-renew* or make copies of themselves. The new cell can remain as a stem cell or turn into a specialized cell. Depending on where the stem cells are located, they may be constantly repairing and replacing damaged tissue (e.g., intestinal tract). In other locations like the heart, they only divide under special situations.

There are two main categories of stem cells: adult and *embryonic* (EM bree on ik). Table 18.3 describes both types of stem cells. Stem cell research has been going on since the 1960s. New technology has helped advance the research. Many researchers are excited about the potential of stem cells. Cord blood stem cell transplants have been used to treat more than 75 diseases, including cancers, anemias, metabolic disorders, and immune system disorders.

Although both types of stem cell research have ethical issues, embryonic stem cell research has greater ethical issues. Harvesting stem cells from an embryo would mean destroying the embryo. For those believing life begins at the moment of conception, this means a life is lost.

Gene therapy. Gene therapy is currently an experimental technique that uses genes to prevent or treat diseases. With this procedure, a gene is inserted into a patient's cell. The hopes are that the new gene might do the following:

- Replace a mutated gene
- Prevent the mutated gene from functioning
- Help fight the disease

TABLE 18.3 Types of Stem Cells

	Adult Stem Cells	Embryonic Stem Cells
Derived From	Found in infants through adults; found in many organs and tissues including the brain, bone marrow, blood, skin, heart, teeth, testis, liver, blood vessel, and skeletal muscles. Umbilical cord blood also contains adult stem cells.	Taken from a 4- to 5-day old human *embryo* (EM bree oh)
What Types of Cells Can They Become?	Thought to be limited; could become cell types similar to their tissue of origin. Scientists have found a way to "reprogram" some types of adult stem cells so they act like embryonic cells.	Can become all cell types
Advantages	Thought to cause less rejection issues with transplants if a person's own stem cells are used.	Easy to grow in a laboratory setting
Ethical Issue	Risks involved with adult stem cell use are still being evaluated.	For those believing life begins at the moment of conception, removing stem cells from an embryo would mean killing a person

Gene or genome editing is a specific gene therapy. This technique can remove, add, or alter sections of the gene. With new technology emerging in this area, ethical issues have also arisen. Genome editing of somatic (soe MAT ik) cells would only impact the individual. This treatment has already been used and is considered ethical. Genome editing of germline cells can cause issues that may impact future generations. Genome editing of germline cells raises ethical concerns and is illegal in the United States.

> **VOCABULARY**
> **germline cells**: Sperm and egg cells.
> **somatic cells**: Nonreproductive cells; they do not include sperm and egg cells.

Reproductive Issues

Assisted Reproductive Technology. *Infertility* is the inability to get pregnant after 1 year of unprotected intercourse (sex). Infertility can affect both males and females. There are many causes of infertility. With advances in technology, assisted reproductive technology (ART) has allowed many couples to have children. Assisted reproductive technology includes all procedures that involve the handling of the eggs, sperm, or embryos. Table 18.4 lists common assisted reproductive technologies.

One of the complications of ART is multiple births. An ethical issue can arise if the success of the pregnancy may be hindered by the number of fetuses (unborn babies). If this situation occurs, the provider must inform the patient of the risks with multiple births. Box 18.5 provides the CEJA's opinions on assisted reproductive technology.

Abortion. *Elective abortion* is the deliberate termination of a pregnancy. Abortions can be done through medications and medical procedures. Abortions raise many ethical questions and concerns. Some feel that women have the right to determine what occurs with their bodies and babies have no rights until they are born. Others feel that from the moment of conception, babies have rights.

The advancement of technology has impacted abortions. With greater technology, complex testing and treatments can occur. Surgery on unborn babies can treat health issues that in the past caused death or elected abortions. Advanced testing can diagnose issues sooner. For instance, imaging tests provide clearer pictures of unborn babies. In cases where diagnostic tests indicate major abnormalities, providers discuss the worst-case scenarios with the parents and include termination as part of informed consent. Box 18.6 provides the CEJA's opinion on abortion.

TABLE 18.4 Procedures for Infertility

Types of Procedures	Description
In vitro fertilization	Involves removing egg cells from a female's ovaries. The egg cells are fertilized with sperm cells outside of the body. The fertilized egg is then implanted in the uterus for pregnancy.
Intrauterine insemination (IUI) (IN truh YOU tuh rin in sem uh NAY shun)	Also called artificial insemination. Specially prepared sperm is placed into a woman's uterus using a long, narrow tube (like a straw). The woman's partner's sperm or a donor's sperm can be used.
Surrogacy (SUHR ah gah see)	A woman carries and gives birth for another couple. A legal contract should be in place to protect all parties. • Traditional or partial surrogacy: sperm is from the father and the egg is from the surrogate. • Gestational or full surrogacy: sperm and egg can come from the intended parents or be donated. The surrogate is not related to the baby.

BOX 18.5 CEJA's Opinions on Assisted Reproductive Technology

Providers that offer assisted reproductive services should provide accurate advertising of their services. They need to provide all information including success rates and costs so patients can make an informed decision. Prospective donors need to be tested for infectious disease agents and genetic disease. Donors need to provide informed consent.

PROCEDURE 18.2 Demonstrate Appropriate Response to Ethical Issues

Tasks
Identify ethical issues and demonstrate appropriate and professional responses. Recognize the impact personal ethics and morals have on the delivery of healthcare.

Scenario 1
You are working at Walden-Martin Family Medical (WMFM) Clinic. You are responsible for collecting payments from patients. Mr. Smythe, who is visually impaired, paid for his visit in cash. He gives you a $500 for a $402 bill. You make change and give him a receipt. At the end of the day, you notice that you have $60 more than what you should have and some of the bills were mixed up in the cashbox. You realize you gave Mr. Smythe the incorrect amount of money.

Scenario 2
You are setting up a laceration repair tray for Dr. Martin to use. As you are preparing the sterile equipment, one of the instruments gets contaminated. You know Dr. Martin urgently needs the tray. You do nothing about the contamination, which you realize can cause an infection. You finish setting up the tray.

Equipment and Supplies
- Paper and pen

Procedural Steps
1. Read both scenarios. Identify and write down the ethical issues involved.
   Purpose: It is important to identify the issues as the first step in responding to ethical situations.
2. With a peer, role-play scenario #1. Your peer should be the supervisor in this scenario. Demonstrate a professional and appropriate ethical response to this situation.
   a. Explain the situation to the supervisor.
   b. Describe how you felt the error occurred and who received the incorrect change.
   c. Explain how you would like to handle the situation and correct the error.
   Purpose: It is important that medical assistant acts professional and ethically when a mistake is discovered.
3. With a peer, role-play scenario #2. Your peer should be the provider in this scenario. During the role-play, demonstrate a professional and appropriate ethical response to this situation.
   Purpose: It is important that medical assistant acts ethically and notifies the provider when an error is made.
4. In a written response, discuss the potential implication to the patient's health related to not reporting or correcting the error.
   Purpose: It is important that medical assistant realizes how unethical actions impact patient care.

BOX 18.6 CEJA's Opinion on Abortion

Providers are not prohibited from performing an abortion in situations where it does not violate the law.

BOX 18.7 CEJA's Opinions on Parental Refusal of Treatments

Providers are encouraged to seek consultation with **ethics committees** in the following situations:
- The parent or guardian refuses treatment for a reversible life-threatening condition
- There are disagreements about the minor's best interest

The provider should only ask the courts to resolve the disagreement as the last option.

Childhood Issues

In most cases, parents of minor children must authorize or decline treatment. In some cases, the state may need to provide the parental authority. *Parens patriae* (PAR enz PA tree ee) is Latin for "father of the country." This doctrine gives the courts the power to make decisions for people who cannot. Many times this doctrine is used for children or people who are incompetent. It can be used when the parent or parents refuse healthcare for the child. The court may take over the parental rights and make decisions for the child.

There have been situations where parents refuse procedures or treatments for their children based on religious or personal beliefs. One of the more common situations in ambulatory care is the refusal of vaccinations (Procedure 18.2). It is important for the medical assistant to respect the patient's bill of rights. If the patient provides a reason for the refusal, the medical assistant should let the provider know. The provider should also be told of the refusal, so other procedures or treatments can be discussed if needed. Box 18.7 provides the CEJA's opinion on parental refusal of treatments for minors.

> **VOCABULARY**
> **ethics committee:** A committee composed of members from a variety of disciplines that analyzes ethical issues.

Adoption. Federal and state laws govern adoption. In healthcare, we run into adoption fairly often. Our patients may be adopted and do not know their family medical history. We need to be understanding of their situation. We may also work with pregnant women who are planning to give up their babies. Again, these are situations where medical assistants need to be sensitive and understanding. Table 18.5 describes the types of adoptions.

Safe Haven Infant Protection Laws. Safe haven infant protection laws allow a person to give up an unwanted infant anonymously. The goal is to protect unwanted babies from abuse or death. The person is not prosecuted if
- The infant is not abused
- The infant is left at a designated location as indicated by the state law
- The infant is within the age limit as indicated by the state law

The designated locations vary by state. They may include hospitals, emergency departments, fire and police stations, and child welfare agencies. The age of the child varies. A few states allow children up to 1 year of age. Opponents of the safe haven laws voice concerns for fathers' rights and the lack of family medical history obtained. Supporters state these laws save babies by providing a safe drop-off location and no questions asked.

Confidential Healthcare for Minors. Providers have an ethical duty to promote decision making in minor patients to the degree of the child's ability. Providers have a responsibility to protect the confidentiality of minor patients, within certain limits. We see this in the ambulatory care setting, when parents wait in the reception area while minor children

TABLE 18.5 Types of Adoption

Type of Adoption	Description
Adopting through an agency	Private and public adoption agencies are regulated by the state and must be licensed to place children with adoptive parents. Public agencies usually place abandoned, orphaned, or abused children who are wards of the state.
Adopting independently	The birth parents and the adoptive parents have an arrangement. Some states do not allow this type of adoption.
Adopting through identification	Adoptive parents and birth parents work with an adoption agency to complete the adoption process.
Adopting internationally	Adoptive parents work with an international adoption agency to adopt a child from another country. International adoption agencies must be certified by the State Department.
Relative adoptions	Relatives of a child adopt the child.
Closed adoptions	There is no contact between the adoptive parents and the birth parents.
Open adoptions	Adoptive parents meet and may stay in contact with birth parents.

TABLE 18.6 Stages of Grief and Dying

Stage	Description
Denial	Person refuses to accept the diagnosis or prognosis. Defense mechanism that protects people from being overwhelmed. Disbelief and numbness may occur.
Anger	Person's anger can be directed at self or others. May blame others.
Bargaining	Person attempts to bargain with the higher power the person believes in (i.e., God).
Depression	Person feels sadness, fear, and uncertainty. Crying and depression may occur. Person may not participate in normal activities; distance self from others.
Acceptance	Person has come to terms with the situation.

(usually teens) have their physical exams. Many providers feel that the minor's answers to questions on safety, sex, drugs, and alcohol may be more truthful without the presence of parents.

In some states, laws permit unemancipated minors to request and receive confidential services. These services must relate to contraception, pregnancy testing, prenatal care, and delivery services. Additional services can include prevention and treatment of sexually transmitted infections (STIs), substance use disorders, and mental illness. Box 18.8 provides the CEJA's opinion on confidential healthcare for minors.

> **CRITICAL THINKING 18.6**
>
> On break one afternoon, Daniela was talking to Jan, a medical assistant. She asked Jan how she handles parents who want to find out confidential information on their children. How might you professionally and respectfully handle a phone call from a parent who is requesting confidential information on her or his child?

End-of-Life Issues

With the changes in healthcare and technology, more treatment options exist today to prolong a person's life. Ventilators assist the breathing process, and feeding tubes provide nutrition. Medications and defibrillators can help restart the heart. Legislation exists at the state and federal levels to help address the death and dying issues. There are also many ethical questions that surround end-of-life issues.

It may sound like end-of-life issues are only addressed in the hospital. End-of-life issues also impact ambulatory care. Medical assistants may accompany providers in skilled nursing facilities (nursing homes) visits. Medical assistants provide ambulatory care to patients who have terminal illnesses (Box 18.9).

Working with patients who have a terminal illness can be emotionally challenging. It is important for the medical assistant to remember that patients and families go through the grieving process. Table 18.6 provides the stages of grief and dying by Elizabeth Kübler-Ross. Not everyone goes through all five stages. They may not go through the stages in the order listed on the table. Some people may switch back and forth between the stages. Various behaviors may be seen during the grieving process (Box 18.10).

> **BOX 18.8 CEJA's Opinions on Confidential Healthcare for Minors**
>
> - When the law does not grant minor decision-making authority for healthcare, the provider should do the following:
>   - Involve the parent or guardian in situations where it is necessary to prevent harm to the patient or others.
>   - Involve the parent or guardian if the provider does not feel it will impact the patient's health.
> - Explore reasons why the minor does not want the involvement of the parent or guardian.
> - Inform the minor that parents may learn of the treatment through insurance statements.
> - Protect the confidentiality of the information from the minor, keeping within ethical and legal standards.

> **BOX 18.9 Palliative Medicine and Hospice Care**
>
> It is not uncommon for the medical assistant to process a referral for hospice care for a patient. The medical assistant should know the differences between *palliative* (PAL ee ah tiv) medicine and *hospice* (HOS pis) care.
>
> *Palliative* means to help relieve the symptoms of a serious illness. Palliative medicine is a subspecialty. The providers offer palliative care to patients who are seriously ill. Palliative care can be provided to any patient regardless of age. The disease may be curable, chronic, or life threatening. Palliative care focuses on the entire person. It does not provide a cure, just helps to reduce the symptoms.
>
> *Hospice* is a type of palliative care for people who have about 6 months or less to live. The goal of hospice care is to allow patients who are dying to have dignity, comfort, and peace. Hospice programs not only work with the patient but also the family. Hospice care can be provided in the hospital, skilled nursing facility (nursing home), hospice center, and at home.

Patient Self-Determination Act. The Patient Self-Determination Act (PSDA) became law in 1990. This act requires most healthcare institutions at the time of admission to do the following:

- Provide patients with a written document of their rights to make decisions and the facility's policies respecting advance directives.
- Ask patients if they have advance directives, and document the response in the health record.

Healthcare agencies must provide advance directive training to their staff. Staff cannot discriminate against patients that have or do not have

BOX 18.10 Possible Grief Responses

- Sadness
- Anger and guilt
- Denial and confusion
- Numbness
- Helplessness
- Fatigue
- Social isolation
- Loneliness
- Nightmares
- Difficulty concentrating
- Crying
- Sleep changes
- Appetite changes

BOX 18.11 CEJA's Opinions on Advance Care Planning

- Providers should discuss advance care planning with all patients regardless of health status or age.
- Providers should explain advance directives and document in the health record information about advance care planning.
- Providers should review the advance care planning periodically with the patients.

BOX 18.12 CEJA's Opinions on Advance Directives

- Providers should identify if patients have advance directives, including a healthcare proxy.
- Providers must respect the wishes of the patient's surrogate and help the surrogate understand the patient's wishes in the advance directives.
- If a patient lacks advance directives and is unable to communicate, the provider should seek assistance from the ethics committee.

TABLE 18.7 Typical Types of Advance Directives

Advance Directives	Description
Living will	Provides instructions about life-sustaining medical treatment to be administered or withheld when the patient has a terminal condition.
Medical durable power of attorney	May be known by other names. Similar to a living will but includes all healthcare decisions. It lasts as long as the person is not able to make decisions. Can be used when the situation is not terminal. Names a healthcare proxy and can include healthcare wishes.
Healthcare proxy	Also called healthcare agent or surrogate. A competent adult can appoint a person (called a proxy or agent) to make healthcare decisions in the event he or she is unable to do so.
Organ donation	Indicates if a person wants to donate organs.
Do not resuscitate (DNR)	Indicates if the person refuses cardiopulmonary resuscitation (CPR) if he or she stops breathing or has no pulse.

BOX 18.13 Additional Topics on Advance Directive Forms

- Life-sustaining treatments (e.g., drugs, machines, medical procedures, feeding tubes)
- Desires if permanently unconscious
- Desires with terminal condition
- Mental health treatment
- Admission to nursing home
- Unconscious and pregnant
- Pain relief
- Additional desires

BOX 18.14 Physician Orders for Life-Sustaining Treatment (POLST)

Physician Orders for Life-Sustaining Treatment (POLST) can be known by similar names across the United States. It is promoted to work with advance directives. When a person is diagnosed with advanced illness or frailty, having a POLST may be recommended. The POLST is a one-page physician order sheet that indicates the care a person should receive. It should be based on the advance directives and the person's wishes.

For some people POLST is concerning. The POLST can supersede a person's advance directives. Keep in mind that the POLST is a limited document, and some forms state that the healthcare staff should follow the orders listed before contacting the provider. Opponents to POLST encourage patients to refuse it. They cite that the provider should be contacted when the patient's condition changes and the advance directives in its entirety can be followed, not the summarized version listed in the POLST.

---

advance directives. Box 18.11 provides the CEJA's opinion on advance care planning.

If patients present advance directive paperwork, the medical assistant needs to ensure it gets into the health record. It is not uncommon for medical assistants to provide advance directive information to patients. The medical assistant must also be familiar with the different types of advance directives.

Advance directives. *Advance directives* are written instructions about healthcare decisions, should a person be unable to make them. Advance directives are not just for older adults to complete. It is important for everyone to consider completing advance directives. Once completed, advance directives can be modified in the future. It is important that local healthcare agencies have a copy of your advance directive paperwork. Box 18.12 provides the CEJA's opinions on advance directives.

Today most states have a multiple-page document for people to complete. The document can be found online or at healthcare agencies. The document may be called advance directives, durable power of attorney for healthcare, or something similar. It replaces multiple documents of the past. Generally, the advance directives document contains sections for the different types of advance directives (Table 18.7). The document can also include additional topics (Box 18.13). Remember, each state has its own advance directives form for residents to complete. Box 18.14 discusses the Physician Orders for Life-Sustaining Treatment (POLST), which is promoted to work with advance directives.

Uniform Determination of Death Act. The Uniform Determination of Death Act (UDDA) was drafted in 1981. It served as a guide for state lawmakers to create their own laws. The act provided a definition of death. A person may legally be declared dead if one of the following two events occurs:

- Irreversible cessation of circulatory and respiratory functions
- Irreversible cessation of all functions of the entire brain, including the brainstem

VOCABULARY
cessation: Bringing to an end.

> **BOX 18.15 CEJA's Opinions on Withholding or Withdrawing Life-Sustaining Treatment**
>
> Providers should identify the patient's wishes early in the treatment. Should providers have questions regarding life-sustaining treatments, they should do the following:
> - Review the patient's advance directives.
> - Support decisions of the patient or surrogate.
> - Seek advice from an ethics committee.

TABLE 18.8 Types of Euthanasia

Type	Description
Active euthanasia	Killing the person using an active means like an injection.
Passive euthanasia	Withholding a lifesaving treatment (e.g., feeding tube) and letting the person die.
Voluntary euthanasia	The patient consents to the action.
Involuntary euthanasia	The patient does not consent to the action. Patients may be unconscious or unable to communicate their wishes.
Self-administered euthanasia	The patient kills himself or herself.
Other-administered euthanasia	Another person kills the patient.
Assisted suicide	The patient kills himself or herself with the assistance of another person (e.g., physician-assisted suicide).

> **BOX 18.16 CEJA's Opinions on Physician-Assisted Suicide and Euthanasia**
>
> Physician-assisted suicide is against the fundamental nature of the healer role of the provider. Providers must respond to the patient's needs at the end of life. They should respect patient autonomy and provide effective communication and emotional support. Providers need to make the patients comfortable and provide adequate pain medications.

> **BOX 18.17 Organ Donation Needs**
>
> - More than 118,000 people in the United States need a lifesaving organ transplant.
> - Six people are added to the national transplant waiting list every hour.
> - On average, 22 people die each day while waiting for a transplant.
> - There continues to be a gap between the supply of donated organs and the demand. More people need organs than are available.
>
> From https://optn.transplant.hrsa.gov.

> **BOX 18.18 Organ and Tissue That Can Be Donated**
>
> - Kidneys
> - Liver
> - Lungs
> - Heart
> - Pancreas
> - Intestines
> - Hands
> - Faces
> - Corneas and eyes
> - Heart valves
> - Skin
> - Bones
> - Tendons
> - Bone marrow
> - Cord blood stem cells
> - Blood
> - Platelets

This act provided an accepted definition of death. Most states have adopted the exact wording of the UDDA. Some states have added additional regulations to their laws.

Withholding or Withdrawing Life-Sustaining Treatment. Withholding or withdrawing treatments that extend the life of a person can be emotional for the patient and family. This situation can also be ethically challenging for healthcare providers. It is important to remember that patients have the right to decline medical intervention. They can also determine when the intervention should be stopped. If the patient cannot make these decisions, it is up to the patient's surrogate. Box 18.15 provides the CEJA's opinion on withholding or withdrawing life-sustaining treatment.

Euthanasia. *Euthanasia* (YOU thah nae zhah) is the act of killing a person who is suffering from an incurable disease. It can also be called "mercy killing" because it is ending the patient's suffering. Table 18.8 describes the different types of euthanasia.

Physician-assisted suicide occurs when the provider makes available the means for a patient to end his or her life. The means can be sleeping pills in lethal doses or some other medication that impacts the breathing or heartbeat. The provider is also aware that the patient wants to commit suicide. Most states make physician-assisted euthanasia illegal. Only six states have legalized physician-assisted euthanasia.

Proponents state that terminally ill patients have a right to end their suffering when they want to. Opponents state providers have a moral responsibility to keep their patients alive. Box 18.16 provides the CEJA's opinion on physician-assisted suicide and euthanasia.

Organ Donation Issues

Each year more names are added to the organ donation list. The gap between available organs and those needing organs is increasing (Box 18.17). There continues to be a great need for organ and tissue donations (Box 18.18). Some organs and cells can be donated by living donors. Blood, a part of a liver, and a kidney are just some examples. Other organs and tissues can be donated upon the death of a person. A driver's license or an advance directive can communicate your wishes for a donation upon your death. We will examine laws and ethical recommendations related to organ donation.

Uniform Anatomical Gift Act. The Uniform Anatomical Gift Act (UAGA) was enacted in 1968. All 50 states have adopted this law. The purpose of the act was to make it easier for people to donate organs. This act has been revised several times over the years. States enacted the UAGA, but differences existed between states. In 2006 the UAGA was revised to provide uniformity in organ and tissue donations across the nation. The 2006 revisions include the following:
- Clarified who can make donation decision for the patient
- Strengthened language on protecting the patient's decision on donating or not donating organs
- Established standards for donor registries, which will help match donors to recipients

Box 18.19 provides the CEJA's opinion on organ transplantation from deceased donors.

National Organ Transplant Act. The National Organ Transplant Act (NOTA) was passed by Congress in 1984. The act established the

> **BOX 18.19 CEJA's Opinions on Organ Transplantation from Deceased Donors**
>
> Providers should do the following:
> - Avoid conflicts of interest and ensure that no members of the transplant team are involved with pronouncing the patient dead.
> - Ensure the death is pronounced using accepted clinical and ethical standards.
> - Ensure the transplant procedures are done by knowledgeable providers.
> - Ensure the prospective recipient of the donor is fully informed about the procedure.

Organ Procurement and Transplant Network (OPTN) to be run by contract by the secretary of Health and Human Services. The act established a national registry for organ matching. NOTA also made it a criminal action to exchange organs for transplant for something of value (i.e., money).

Xenotransplantation. With the lack of available organs and tissues, researchers are studying the use of nonhuman tissue and organs. *Xenotransplantation* (ZEN oh trans plan tay shahn) is any procedure where nonhuman cells, tissues, or organs are implanted or infused into a person.

Currently, pigs are the animals of choice for xenotransplants. Their organs are about the same size as humans and they breed quickly. Pig heart valves are already being used to treat human heart valve issues.

CLOSING COMMENTS

All healthcare professionals need to provide ethical, respectful care to all patients. Professional ethics guide healthcare employees on how to be ethical in their role. A medical assistant should be aware of the medical assisting code of ethics and the healthcare facility's professional ethics. The medical assistant needs to practice these professional ethics in every patient situation.

It is important for the medical assistant to continue to learn about healthcare advances. New procedures, treatments, and medications are continually impacting patient care. As technology advances and healthcare changes, the medical assistant needs to remain updated on the ethical issues that surround the changes. Following the professional code of ethics, as well as learning the CEJA's opinion on the new advances, will help guide the medical assistant's practice.

> **EXCEPTIONAL CUSTOMER SERVICE**
>
> As mentioned in prior chapters, one of the key elements to providing customer service is respecting the patient. When working with ethical situations, it is important for the medical assistant to remember the Patient Bill of Rights. Patients have the right to refuse treatment. They have the right to make their own decisions. Their decisions may not be our decisions in that situation, but we need to do what they want. It is important to respect patients and ensure their dignity during beginning-of-life issues through end-of-life issues.

CHAPTER REVIEW

Personal ethics are individual choices and are impacted by one's morals. Professional ethics are created by associations for members to follow. They are also created by employers for employees to follow. A medical assistant must create a plan to separate personal and professional ethics, if they conflict.

There are four ethical principles in healthcare:
- Autonomy: the freedom to determine one's own actions and decisions
- Nonmaleficence: to do no harm
- Beneficence: to do good
- Justice: to treat patients fairly and give them what is due to them

These four principles need to be considered equally when evaluating ethical issues. The medical assistant has related responsibilities for each of these principles.

There are many ethical issues in healthcare. This chapter presented a brief description of some of them:

- Genetics issues, including cloning and genetic engineering (genetic testing, pharmacogenetics, stem cell transplants, and gene therapy)
- Reproductive issues, involving assisted reproductive technology (ART) that helps with infertility and abortions
- Childhood issues, including adoption, safe haven infant protection laws, and confidential healthcare for minors
- End-of-life issues, involving the Patient Self-Determination Act, advance directives, the Uniform Determination of Death Act, withholding or withdrawing life-sustaining treatment, and euthanasia
- Organ donation issues including the Uniform Anatomical Gift Act, the National Organ Transplant Act, and xenotransplantation

The CEJA has opinions on many healthcare ethical issues. It is important for the medical assistant to be familiar with these opinions.

SCENARIO WRAP-UP

Daniela has completed the ethics unit in her law and ethics course. She is excited to be done with the course. What she has learned in the ethics unit has helped her to stop and think about why she believes what she believes. She is realizing that some of her values and morals were built on information that was old or inaccurate. She needs to do some research to verify the information. Daniela feels that as she continues to learn and gain experience, her moral compass may change in the future. She hopes that this will help her to provide the best possible care to her patients.

19

The Health Record

LEARNING OBJECTIVES

1. List and describe the types of medical records.
2. State several reasons accurate health records are important.
3. Differentiate between subjective and objective information.
4. Register a new patient in the practice management software.
5. Explain who owns the health record.
6. Distinguish between an electronic health record (EHR) and an electronic medical record (EMR).
7. Discuss the Health Information Technology for the Economic and Clinical Health Act, and explain meaningful use as it applies to an EHR.
8. Explore the capabilities of an electronic health record system, and upload documents to the EHR.
9. Discuss the importance of nonverbal communication with patients when an EHR system is used.
10. Explain the importance of data backup.
11. Differentiate among active, inactive, and closed medical records.
12. Discuss requests for medical information and how to release health record information.
13. Identify methods of organizing the patient's medical record based on (a) the problem-oriented medical record and (b) the source-oriented medical record.
14. Discuss how to document in an electronic and paper health record, as well as how to make corrections and alterations to health records.
15. Discuss the processes of dictation and transcription.
16. Identify equipment and supplies needed to create an efficient paper health records management system.
17. Describe filing indexing rules.
18. Discuss the pros and cons of various filing methods, as well as how to file patient health records correctly.
19. Discuss the proper way to organize files.

CHAPTER OUTLINE

1. Opening Scenario, 413
2. You Will Learn, 413
3. Introduction, 413
4. Types of Records, 413
5. Importance of Accurate Health Records, 414
6. Contents of the Health Record, 414
    a. Subjective Information, 414
        i. *Personal Demographics, 414*
        ii. *Past Health, Family, and Social History, 414*
    b. Objective Information, 418
        i. *Vital Signs and Anthropometric Measurements, 418*
        ii. *Findings and Laboratory and Radiology Reports, 418*
        iii. *Diagnosis, 418*
        iv. *Treatment Prescribed and Progress Notes, 418*
    c. The Medical Assistant's Role, 418
7. Ownership of the Health Record, 419
8. Technologic Terms in Health Information, 419
9. Health Information Technology for the Economic and Clinical Health Act (HITECH Act) and Meaningful Use, 420
10. Capabilities of Electronic Health Record Systems, 420
11. Maintaining a Connection With the Patient When Using the Electronic Health Record, 422
12. Backup Systems for the Electronic Health Record, 424
13. Retention and Destruction of Health Records, 424
14. Releasing Health Record Information, 425
15. Organization of the Health Record, 425
    a. Source-Oriented Records, 425
    b. Problem-Oriented Records, 425
16. Documenting in an Electronic Health Record, 428
17. Documenting in a Paper Health Record, 428
18. Making Corrections and Alterations to Health Records, 428
19. Dictation and Transcription, 429
    a. Voice Recognition Software, 429
20. Creating an Efficient Paper Health Records Management System, 430
    a. Filing Equipment, 430
        i. *Drawer Files, 430*
        ii. *Horizontal Shelf Files, 430*
        iii. *Rotary Circular Files, 430*
        iv. *Compactable Files, 431*
        v. *Automated Files, 431*
        vi. *Card Files, 431*
    b. Filing Supplies, 431
        i. *Divider Guides, 431*
        ii. *Out Guides, 431*
        iii. *File Folders, 431*
        iv. *Labels, 431*
21. Indexing Rules, 432
22. Filing Methods, 432
    a. Alphabetic Filing, 432
    b. Numeric Filing, 433

c. Subject Filing, 434
d. Color Coding, 435
   i. *Alphabetic Color Coding,* 435
   ii. *Numeric Color Coding,* 435
23. Organization of Files, 435
    a. Health-Related Correspondence, 435
    b. General Correspondence, 435
    c. Practice Management Files, 435
    d. Miscellaneous Files, 435
    e. Tickler or Follow-Up Files, 436
    f. Transitory or Temporary File, 436
24. Closing Comments, 436
25. Chapter Review, 436
26. Scenario Wrap-Up, 437

OPENING SCENARIO

Susan Beezler has just begun her career in the medical assisting profession. In the morning, she attends medical assisting school, and in the afternoon, she works part-time for Walden-Martin Family Medical (WMFM) Clinic as a record assistant. Susan is eager to learn about healthcare and looks forward to taking on more responsibility at the office.

Dr. David Kahn is a new provider that has recently joined WMFM. Dr. Kahn has enjoyed working with Susan and feels that her energy will be just what his patients need. He has taken a professional interest in Susan and often lets her assist him with patients when her other duties allow.

Susan knows that although she is a beginner in the office, she will gain trust from her supervisors and patients as long as she projects a teachable attitude. The office has recently converted to an electronic records system but is still using paper records as well. Susan uses the information she learned in school about both types of health records. She cheerfully performs filing and even does some transcription for Dr. Kahn. The other staff members are pleased with her willingness to perform the most mundane tasks.

Susan enjoys sharing her experiences with her classmates. She is the only student currently working in the medical field, and the others ask her lots of questions about the "real world" of medical assisting. She is careful not to breach patient confidentiality; she discusses situations only in general terms, never mentioning any patients' names.

Susan feels a great sense of pride in knowing that she is already a member of the healthcare team and is able to contribute to the lives of her patients.

YOU WILL LEARN

1. To define and apply subjective information.
2. To define and apply objective information.
3. To understand the impact of the Health Information Technology for the Economic and Clinical Health (HITECH) Act on health records.
4. To maintain a connection with the patient when using an electronic health record.
5. To back up an electronic health record using different methods.
6. To apply the correct procedures for destroying records.
7. To document the health record.
8. To determine the equipment and supplies needed for a paper record system.
9. To apply the indexing rules for alphabetic and numeric filing systems.

INTRODUCTION

Health records can be found in two different formats, electronic and paper. Most healthcare facilities have switched to the **electronic health record (EHR)** format. EHRs offer a number of benefits:

- Easy storage of patient information
- Accessibility to multiple users at the same time
- A more efficient claim submission process

The U.S. federal government has also offered financial incentives for providers to implement EHRs. Although most providers are using EHRs, some still use paper records and others use a combination of both electronic and paper. When a provider is making the switch to an EHR, he or she may decide to keep the patient's previous records in the paper format and just use the electronic format moving forward. Some providers may decide to scan the past 3 to 5 years of the paper record into the electronic record. Whatever the scenario the healthcare facility has chosen, it is important for the medical assistant to understand both systems and to be able to perform well with either one.

TYPES OF RECORDS

Paper health records have been shown to be much less efficient than an EHR. In most cases, only one person at a time can use the paper record. It is fairly common for information to be filed in the incorrect record. The entire record also can be misfiled. Gathering data for research and **quality control** is more challenging. Data are difficult to share in facilities with multiple departments or locations. The paper-based record is good for documentation of patient care, but it is not nearly as useful in other capacities.

With an EHR, multiple users can access the record at the same time. There are fewer errors because handwritten notes do not have to be interpreted. Most EHRs link the clinical information needed for billing purposes. An EHR also includes practice management capabilities that allow for patient scheduling and the generation of reports needed for research and quality control.

> **VOCABULARY**
>
> **electronic health record (EHR):** An electronic record conforms to nationally recognized standards and contains health-related information about a specific patient. It can be created, managed, and consulted by authorized clinicians and staff from more than one healthcare organization.
>
> **quality control:** A process to ensure the reliability of test results, often using manufactured samples with known values.

> **CRITICAL THINKING 19.1**
>
> Some of Dr. Khans' patients are concerned that computer-based health records may not be completely private. They are worried that unauthorized individuals could access their information on the computer and do them harm. Should patients be allowed to decide whether their records are kept on computer or on paper? Why or why not?

IMPORTANCE OF ACCURATE HEALTH RECORDS

Health records are kept for five basic reasons:
- To provide the best possible medical care for the patient. The provider examines the patient and enters the findings in the patient's health record. These findings are clues to the diagnosis. The provider may order many types of tests to confirm the clinical findings. As the reports of these tests come in, the findings fall into place, much like the pieces of a jigsaw puzzle. With these data, the provider can prescribe treatment and form an opinion about the patient's **prognosis** (prog NOH sis). The health record provides a complete history of all the care given to the patient.
- To provide critical information for others. By reading through the record and discovering the methods used to treat the patient, healthcare professionals can provide **continuity of care**. Each provider knows what services have been provided and can continue the care, even from one facility to another.
  - For example, when a patient is transferred from a hospital to a skilled nursing facility, the information from the patient's hospital record helps the nursing facility staff to better care for the patient. When patients move from place to place or caregivers change, copies of the pertinent information should move with the patient to provide this continuity of care.
- To provide legal protection for those who provided care to the patient. A well-documented health record is excellent proof that certain procedures were performed or that medical advice was given. An accurate record is the foundation for a legal defense in cases of medical professional liability. This is one reason that it is critical to write legibly in the paper record when documenting exactly what happened to the patient and the provider's response. Remember, if it is not documented, it did not happen.
- To provide statistical information that is helpful to researchers. The patient's record provides information about medications taken and the reactions to them. Health records may be used to evaluate the effectiveness of certain kinds of treatment or to determine the **incidence** (IN si duh ns) of a given disease. Providers often take part in drug studies that track adverse reactions and side effects. The effects of various treatments and procedures also can be tracked and statistics gathered from patients' records. When tracking statistical information the patient-specific data are removed. This information may result in a new outlook on some phases of medicine and can lead to revised techniques and treatments. The statistical data from health records also are valuable in the preparation of scientific papers, books, and lectures.
- To provide support for claims reimbursement, which is required by most insurance companies.

CONTENTS OF THE HEALTH RECORD

The patient's health record is the most important record in a healthcare facility. For completeness, each patient's record should contain **subjective information** provided by the patient and **objective information** obtained by the provider and staff of the healthcare facility. If all entries are complete, the health record will stand the test of time. No branch of medicine is exempt from the need to keep patient health records.

Subjective Information

Personal Demographics. The patient's health record begins with routine personal data, which the patient usually supplies on the first visit when the health record is established. Most patients are required to complete a patient information form (Fig. 19.1, Box 19.1, and Procedure 19.1).

Past Health, Family, and Social History. Information regarding a patient's past health, family, and social history is often obtained by having the patient complete a questionnaire. The medical assistant may review the form for completeness, and he or she may need to clarify any questions or missing information with the patient before the patient is seen by the provider. The provider will also add information provided during the patient interview. The responses furnish information about the following:
- Any past illnesses (including injuries or physical defects, whether congenital or acquired)
- Hospitalizations or surgeries the patient has had (Fig. 19.2)
- Patient's daily health habits

Stickers can be used on the front of paper health records to indicate allergies, advance directives, and other information (Fig. 19.3). In an EHR, there will be alerts that may appear as a pop-up window when the record is accessed that will indicate that the patient has allergies, that immunizations are due, or that there is no advance directive on file. These are useful for helping the health professional keep important facts about the patient in the forefront of the mind while treating the individual.

VOCABULARY

continuity of care: The smooth continuation of care from one provider to another. This allows the patient to receive the most benefit and with no interruption or duplication of care.
incidence: How often something happens.
objective information: Data obtained through physical examination, through laboratory and diagnostic testing, and by measurable information.
prognosis: The likely outcome of a disease, including chance of recovery.
subjective information: Data or information obtained from the patient, including the patient's feelings, perceptions, and concerns; obtained through interview or questions.

BOX 19.1 Basic Details Found on a Patient Information Form

- Patient's full name, spelled correctly
- Names of parents/guardians if the patient is a child or legally incompetent
- Patient's gender
- Date of birth
- Marital status
- Name of spouse if married
- Home address, telephone number, and email address
- Occupation
- Name of employer
- Business address and telephone number
- Employment information for spouse
- Healthcare insurance information
- Source of referral
- Social Security number

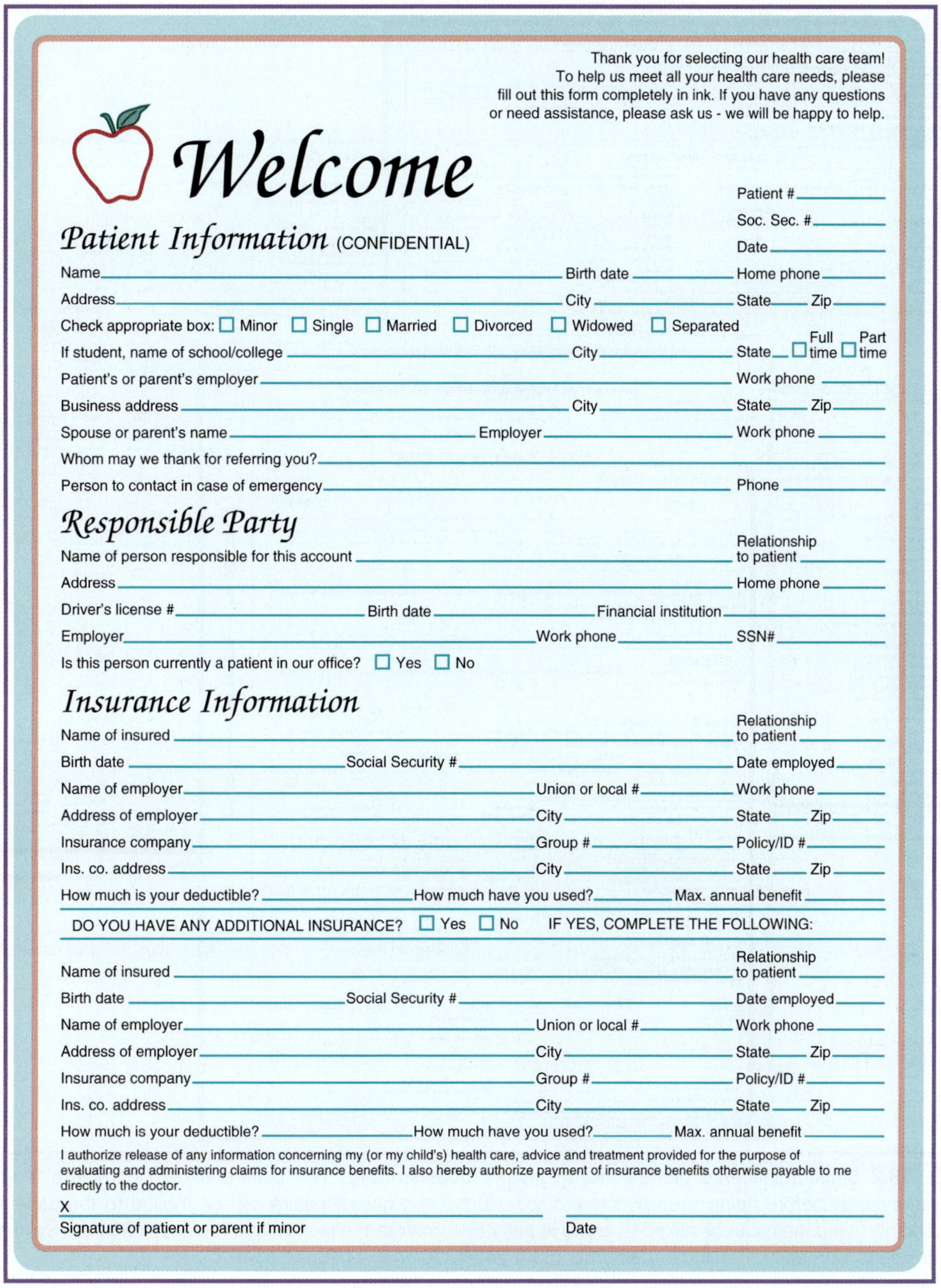
Thank you for selecting our health care team!
To help us meet all your health care needs, please fill out this form completely in ink. If you have any questions or need assistance, please ask us - we will be happy to help.

Welcome

Patient #
Soc. Sec. #
Date

Patient Information (CONFIDENTIAL)

Name Birth date Home phone
Address City State Zip
Check appropriate box: ☐ Minor ☐ Single ☐ Married ☐ Divorced ☐ Widowed ☐ Separated
If student, name of school/college City State ☐ Full time ☐ Part time
Patient's or parent's employer Work phone
Business address City State Zip
Spouse or parent's name Employer Work phone
Whom may we thank for referring you?
Person to contact in case of emergency Phone

Responsible Party

Name of person responsible for this account Relationship to patient
Address Home phone
Driver's license # Birth date Financial institution
Employer Work phone SSN#
Is this person currently a patient in our office? ☐ Yes ☐ No

Insurance Information

Name of insured Relationship to patient
Birth date Social Security # Date employed
Name of employer Union or local # Work phone
Address of employer City State Zip
Insurance company Group # Policy/ID #
Ins. co. address City State Zip
How much is your deductible? How much have you used? Max. annual benefit
DO YOU HAVE ANY ADDITIONAL INSURANCE? ☐ Yes ☐ No IF YES, COMPLETE THE FOLLOWING:
Name of insured Relationship to patient
Birth date Social Security # Date employed
Name of employer Union or local # Work phone
Address of employer City State Zip
Insurance company Group # Policy/ID #
Ins. co. address City State Zip
How much is your deductible? How much have you used? Max. annual benefit

I authorize release of any information concerning my (or my child's) health care, advice and treatment provided for the purpose of evaluating and administering claims for insurance benefits. I also hereby authorize payment of insurance benefits otherwise payable to me directly to the doctor.

X
Signature of patient or parent if minor Date

FIG. 19.1 The patient information form provides all of the information the medical assistant needs to construct the patient's record. (From Proctor D, et al: *Kinn's The Medical Assistant*, ed 13, St. Louis, 2017, Elsevier.)

Past health history. The patient's health history includes information about the following:

- Previous illnesses/injuries (including childhood illnesses such as chickenpox or measles)
- Previous hospitalizations
- Previous surgeries

The dates that these occurred will need to be documented, as well as any complications that may have arisen. The provider needs to be aware of this information because it could affect the patient's current condition.

Family history. The family history includes the following:

- The physical condition of the various members of the patient's family
- Any illnesses or diseases individual members may have had
- Causes of death of various family members

This information is important because certain diseases may have a **hereditary** pattern. Most providers are interested in the immediate family members: parents, grandparents, siblings, and children.

Social history. The social history includes information about the patient's lifestyle, such as the following:

- Living situation
- Marital status
- Employment
- Tobacco use
- Alcohol and drug use

VOCABULARY

hereditary: Passed from parents to offspring through the genes.

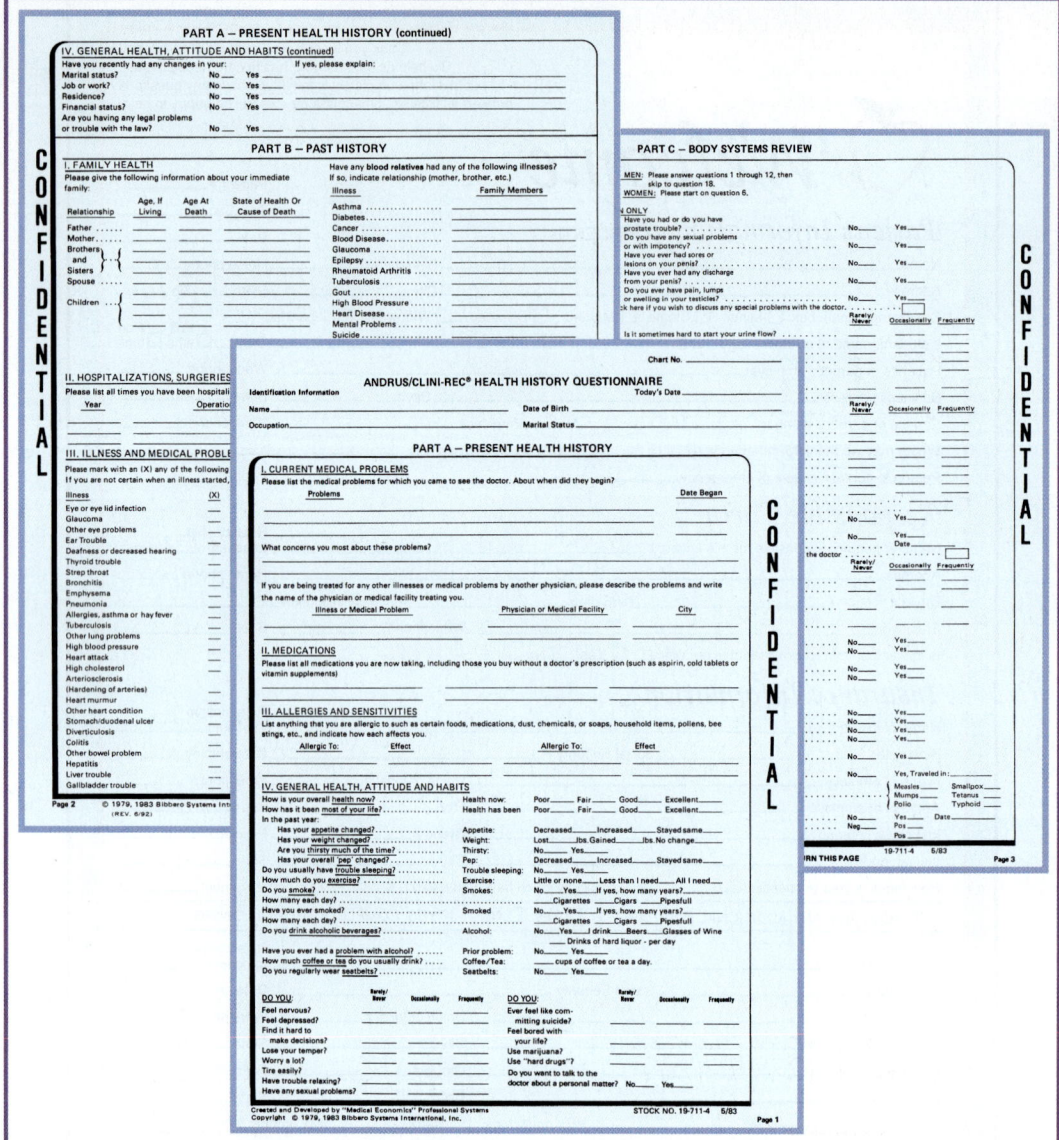

FIG. 19.2 Self-administered general health history questionnaire. The patient should complete lengthy questionnaires before being seen by the provider. Either the questionnaire can be mailed to the patient in advance or the patient can be asked to come in early to complete the paperwork. (Courtesy Bibbero Systems, An InHealth Company, Petaluma, California (800) 242-2376, www.bibbero.com)

- Exercise
- Nutrition

All of these factors can have an impact on a patient's overall health and also help to highlight risk factors.

Chief complaint. The chief complaint is a concise account of the patient's symptoms, explained in the patient's own words. It should include the following:

- The nature, location, frequency, and duration of pain, if any
- When the patient first noticed the symptoms
- Treatments the patient may have tried before seeing the provider and whether or not they helped with the symptoms; when the last dose was taken
- Whether the patient has had the same or a similar condition in the past
- Other medical treatment received for the same condition in the past

CRITICAL THINKING BOX 19.2

While taking a patient's medical history, Susan asks about his social history. She asks whether he drinks alcohol. The patient immediately becomes defensive and accuses Susan of getting too personal about his affairs. How might Susan explain her reasons for asking these questions? What options are available if the patient refuses to discuss his social history with Susan? Could this opposition to questions about the social history raise suspicion in Susan's mind? What might she suspect?

VOCABULARY

concise: Using as few words as possible to express the message.

PROCEDURE 19.1 Register a New Patient Using the Practice Management Software

Task
Register a new patient using the practice management software, prepare a Notice of Privacy Practices (NPP) form and a disclosure authorization form for the new patient, and document this in the electronic health record (EHR).

Equipment and Supplies
- Computer with SimChart for the Medical Office or practice management and EHR software
- Completed patient registration form
- Scanner

Procedural Steps

1. Obtain the new patient's completed registration form. Log into the practice management software.
Purpose: The registration form will provide the information needed to create the new record in the practice management system.
2. Using the patient's last and first names and date of birth, search the database for the patient.
Purpose: To help ensure the integrity of the practice management and EHR systems, a search for the new patient's name must always be done before registering that person. This prevents a double record from being created if the patient had been entered into the database at an earlier time.
3. If the database does not contain the patient's name, add a new patient and enter the patient's demographics from the completed registration form.
Purpose: This will create the patient's record in the practice management system.
4. Verify that the information entered is correct and that all fields are completed before saving the data.
Purpose: Errors during the registration process can affect the communication with the patient (e.g., if a wrong address or email is entered) or can affect billing (e.g., if the incorrect insurance information is added). Accuracy is extremely important when entering the patient's information.
Note: The software will generate a health record number for the patient.
5. Using the EHR software, prepare and print a copy of the NPP and a disclosure authorization form for the new patient. The disclosure authorization form should indicate that the information will be disclosed to the patient's insurance company.
Purpose: Before the medical office can release patient information to the insurance company, the patient has to give consent in writing.
Scenario Update: The patient received both documents and signed the disclosure authorization form.
6. Using the EHR, document that the patient received a copy of the NPP and signed the disclosure authorization form. Scan the disclosure authorization form, and upload it into the EHR.
Purpose: Documentation in the health record provides a legal record of what was done or communicated to the patient.
7. Log out of the software upon completion of the procedure.
Purpose: Logging into and out of the software helps to protect the integrity of the data saved in the software and prevents unauthorized people from viewing the information.

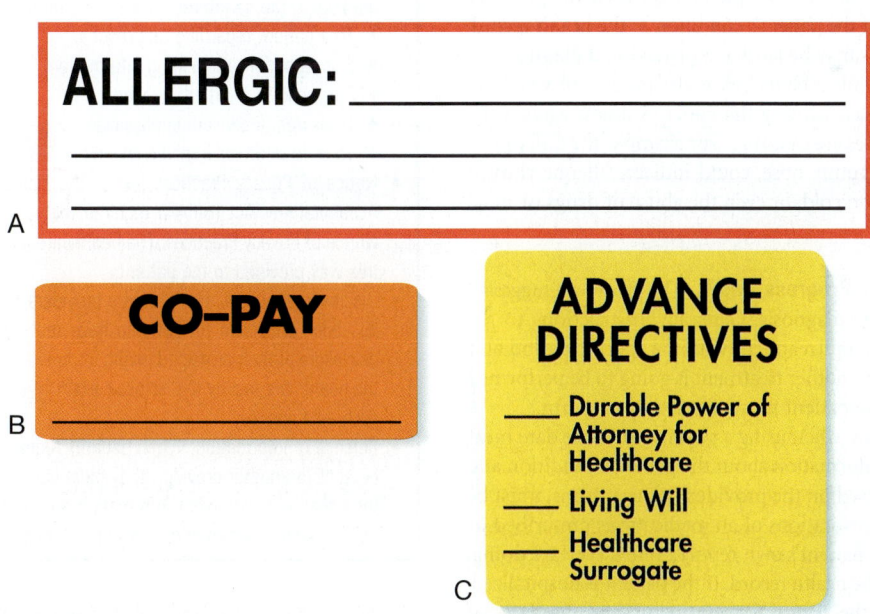

FIG. 19.3 Record stickers. Information on stickers on the outside of the record allows the provider and medical staff to see important information about the patient quickly. (Courtesy Bibbero Systems, An InHealth Company, Petaluma, California (800) 242-2376, www.bibbero.com)

Most healthcare facilities use a pain scale to determine the severity of the patient's discomfort. The medical assistant might ask, "How bad is your pain on a scale of 1 to 10, with 1 being almost no pain and 10 being the worst pain you've ever experienced?" The pain scale or wording used in individual facilities should be documented in the office policy and procedures manual and followed by the medical assistant.

Objective Information

Objective findings, sometimes referred to as *signs*, are findings that can be observed and measured. They can include vital signs, measurements, and observations made by the medical assistant and findings from the provider's examination of the patient.

Vital Signs and Anthropometric Measurements. The medical assistant's responsibilities include taking the patient's
- Vital signs (i.e., temperature, pulse, respirations, blood pressure, pulse oximetry)
- Height and weight

These measurements are documented in the patient's health record, and the provider uses them in his or her assessment. If the medical assistant observes other signs such as a rash, this would also be documented in the patient's health record and brought to the provider's attention.

Findings and Laboratory and Radiology Reports. After the provider has examined the patient, the physical findings are documented in the health record. The results of other tests or requests for these tests are then documented. If the tests were done elsewhere, the report would be attached to the paper record. When an EHR is being used, the separate sheet may be scanned so that it is in an electronic format and can be added to the patient's EHR.

Diagnosis. Based on all the evidence provided in the patient's history, the provider's examination, and any supplementary tests, the provider notes his or her diagnosis of the patient's condition in the health record. If some doubt remains, this may be labeled a **provisional diagnosis**. A *differential diagnosis* (dahy uh g NOH sis) is the process of weighing the probability of one disease causing the patient's illness against the probability that other diseases are causative. For example, the differential diagnosis of rhinitis, or a runny nose, could indicate allergic rhinitis (i.e., hay fever), the common cold, or even the abuse of drugs or nasal decongestants.

Treatment Prescribed and Progress Notes. The provider's suggested treatment is listed after the diagnosis. Generally, instructions to the patient to return for follow-up treatment within a specific period also are noted here. If surgery or another treatment is going to be performed during the current visit, the patient must sign a consent form.

On each **subsequent** visit, when using a paper record, the date must be entered on the record; information about the patient's condition and the results of treatment, based on the provider's observations, must be added to the health record. Notations of all medications prescribed or instructions given, and the patient's own report of how they are doing, should be documented in the health record. If the patient is hospitalized, the name of the hospital, the reason for admission, and the dates of admission and discharge are documented. Much of this information can be obtained from the hospital discharge summary (Box 19.2).

The Medical Assistant's Role

It is important to ensure patient privacy when documenting the health record. If you are interviewing the patient to obtain history information, do it where others cannot hear the patient's answers. If privacy is not possible, the patient should be given a form to fill out. The information can be transferred to the permanent record later. When privacy is available, the medical assistant may ask the patient questions and document the answers directly into the health record. This allows you to become better acquainted with the patient while completing the necessary records. It can also ensure that the patient understands the meaning of all of the questions.

If new patients must complete a lengthy form, there are several options:
- The form can be mailed to the patient. The accompanying letter can request that it be completed and returned to the provider before the appointment.
- If the record is electronic, the patient may access his or her record through a **patient portal**. Using this method, the information is documented directly into the EHR system. It is then reviewed by the medical assistant and provider during the office visit.
- Another option with an EHR is for the patient to complete a paper form and the medical assistant enters the information into the EHR while reviewing the form with the patient.

The medical assistant may document the patient's chief complaint. The provider will question the patient in more detail. Many providers write their own entries in the record in longhand if a paper record is used. Some may document the findings directly into the computer if an electronic record is used. Others may dictate the material directly into the EHR. Another option is for a medical assistant or scribe (Box 19.3) to document the provider's findings. A final option is for the provider to use a recording device. If the material is dictated and

---

BOX 19.2 Additional Information Found in the Health Record

- Correspondence: Copies of any letters that are written regarding the patient are kept in the health record. Example letters could include the following:
  - To a patient regarding test results
  - From a patient requesting information
  - Response to a patient question
  - To or from a consulting physician
  - To or from an insurance company
- Notice of Privacy Practices (NPP): The Health Insurance Portability and Accountability Act (HIPAA) requires that the patient is provided with a Notice of Privacy Practices. The healthcare facility needs to document that this was provided to the patient.
- Disclosures: HIPAA also requires providers to track who the information has been disclosed to. Patients have the right to be notified about the disclosure of their protected health information (PHI). Patients can authorize the healthcare facility to disclose certain information to specific individuals, such as a spouse.
- Release of information: When patients request their health information to be sent to another provider, they must complete a release of information form that specifies what information and to whom it is being disclosed. This release of information form must be kept in the health record.

VOCABULARY

patient portal: A secure online website that gives patients 24-hour access to personal health information using a user name and password.

provisional diagnosis: A temporary diagnosis made before all test results have been received.

subsequent: Occurring later or after.

> **BOX 19.3 Use of a Medical Scribe**
>
> Many patients feel that providers are spending more time interacting with the computer than with them. This has led to the development of the medical scribe role. The Joint Commission defines a medical scribe as an unlicensed individual hired to enter information into the electronic health record (EHR) or chart at the direction of a physician or licensed independent practitioner.
>
> A scribe's responsibilities could include the following:
> - Assisting the provider in navigating the EHR
> - Entering information into the EHR as directed by the provider
>   - History of the present illness
>   - Review of systems
>   - Vital signs
>   - Lab results
>   - Diagnostic imaging results
>   - Progress notes
>   - Care plans
>   - Medication lists
> - Locating information within the EHR for provider review (laboratory and test results)
> - Responding to patient requests for information as directed by the physician

TABLE 19.1 Electronic Health Record Versus Electronic Medical Record

Electronic Health Record (EHR)	Electronic Medical Record (EMR)
Electronic record of health-related information about a patient	An electronic record of health-related information about an individual
Conforms to nationally recognized *interoperability* standards	An electronic version of a paper record
Can be created, managed, and consulted by authorized clinicians and staff from more than one healthcare organization	Can be created, gathered, managed, and consulted by authorized clinicians and staff within a single healthcare organization

transcribed, the provider should verify each entry. The provider must initial the entry before it is entered into the patient's record. For a record to be admissible as evidence in court, the person dictating or writing the entries must be able to verify that they were true and correct at the time they were written. The best indication of this is the provider's signature or initials on the typed entry. In an EHR, the provider's electronic signature is proof of the accuracy of the entries.

A medical scribe should have an understanding of medical terminology, excellent computer skills, and a strong attention to detail. It is important for medical scribes to understand that they are not obtaining the information from the patient. Their role is to document the information from the provider and enter the information into the EHR, per the provider's instructions.

Healthcare facilities that have hired scribes have found that both the patients and providers are more satisfied with patient encounters. These providers can establish better relationships with patients because they are able to spend their time with face-to-face interaction rather than interacting with computer.

OWNERSHIP OF THE HEALTH RECORD

Who owns the health record? Patients often assume that because the information in the health record is about them, ownership of the record is rightfully theirs. However, the owner of the physical health record is the provider or medical facility, often called the "maker," that initiated and developed the record. The patient has the right of access to the information within the record but does not own the physical record or other documents pertaining to the record. The patient has a **vested** interest and therefore has the right to demand confidentiality of all information placed in the record.

The actual paper health record should never leave the medical facility where it originated. Even the provider should refrain from taking the record from the office to the hospital or nursing facility. If information from the record is needed, copies can be made, and progress notes can be written on site and placed into the original record later. This is not an issue with an EHR because multiple users can access the record at the same time. Patients' paper records should be kept in a locked room or locked filing cabinets when the office is closed. EHRs must be protected from unauthorized access. Regulations defined in the Health Insurance Portability and Accountability Act (HIPAA) state that each user must have a unique user name and password; individual access is determined by the system administrator.

Written health records must be legible. Each record should be written as if the provider and staff expect it to eventually be involved in a lawsuit; therefore every word must be legible to an average reader years after it is written. The record can help the provider prove that he or she treated a patient in a competent manner. It can also prove that the patient was not given competent care. Every person on staff at the provider's office is responsible for writing legibly in every health record.

EHRs eliminate the issue of legibility in the record, but it is just as important to be sure that all patient care is documented in the electronic record. If care is not documented, this will leave the healthcare facility open to potential lawsuits and can affect patient care. In addition, if services are not documented, they cannot be billed.

> **VOCABULARY**
>
> **vested:** Granted or endowed with a particular authority, right, or property; to have a special interest in.

> **CRITICAL THINKING BOX 19.3**
>
> On Susan's third day at work, a man comes into the office and demands to see his mother's health record. Susan accesses the record and sees that the mother has not granted permission for information to be given to her son. What should Susan do in this situation? Are there any viable reasons the son should have access to his mother's medical information?

TECHNOLOGIC TERMS IN HEALTH INFORMATION

There is some confusion regarding the acronyms *EHR* and *EMR* (for electronic medical record). These acronyms have been used interchangeably for many years. The Office of the National Coordinator for Health Information Technology (ONC) has established definitions for EHR and EMR that are easy to understand. Table 19.1 shows the definitions of EHR and EMR.

EMR is being used less and less as the federal regulations regarding electronic records have been established. There is a significant push toward having all electronic records meet the definition of an EHR. There are many advantages to having an electronic record system that can be accessed from more than one healthcare organization. The continuity of patient care is much more easily established when all providers have access to the same records regardless of what organization they are working for. There should be less running of duplicate tests and procedures, which will help reduce the cost of providing healthcare.

A *personal health record (PHR)* is defined by the ONC as an electronic record of health-related information about an individual that conforms to nationally recognized interoperability standards and that can be drawn from multiple sources but that is managed, shared, and controlled by the individual. There are several ways that a PHR can be created. Some health insurance companies offer PHRs for those who they insure, some employers offer it as a service for their employees, and some healthcare facilities offer it to their patients. It is important to remember that the patient maintains a PHR. The information from an EHR does not automatically transfer to a PHR.

Another way for patients to access their healthcare information is through a patient portal. Patient portals allow patients to access their actual EHRs. At any time, a patient can view progress notes, laboratory results, medications, or immunizations. Many patient portal systems also allow for the following:
- Communication between the patient and the provider
- Ability to complete forms online
- Ability to request prescription refills
- Ability to schedule appointments

By establishing effective patient portals, healthcare facilities can meet some of the meaningful use requirements.

HIPAA uses the term *protected health information (PHI)*, which is any information about health status, the provision of healthcare, or payment for healthcare that can be linked to an individual patient. HIPAA requires that all PHI be protected. This applies to the following:
- EHRs
- EMRs
- PHRs
- Patient portals

HEALTH INFORMATION TECHNOLOGY FOR THE ECONOMIC AND CLINICAL HEALTH ACT (HITECH ACT) AND MEANINGFUL USE

The HITECH Act provides financial incentives for the meaningful use of certified EHR technology to achieve health and efficiency goals. It was part of the American Recovery and Reinvestment Act to promote the adoption and meaningful use of health information technology. Remember, HIPAA was created in large part to simplify administrative processes by using electronic devices. *Meaningful use* means that providers must show that they are using EHR technology in ways that can be measured significantly in quality and quantity. If providers meet the meaningful use requirements, they will qualify for incentive payments. Three main components of meaningful use can be identified, including the following:
- Use of certified EHR technology in a meaningful manner, such as e-prescribing
- Use of certified EHR technology for electronic exchange of health information to improve the quality of healthcare
- Use of certified EHR technology to submit clinical quality reports, procedure and diagnosis codes, surveys, and other measures

Providers can expect reductions in the amounts they are paid from Medicare and Medicaid if they are not in compliance. Remember, the computer system in the medical office must be more than a tool for data recall to be considered an EHR system; the provider must use the system for tasks, at a minimum, such as e-prescribing and computerized physician/provider order entry (CPOE).

> **VOCABULARY**
> **compliance:** Meeting the standards and regulations of the practice's established policies and procedures. Can also mean cooperation.
> **computerized physician/provider order entry (CPOE):** The process of entering medication orders or other provider instructions into the electronic health record.
> **e-prescribing:** The use of electronic software to communicate with pharmacies and send prescribing information. It takes the place of writing a prescription by hand and giving it to a patient; most new or refill prescriptions can be submitted electronically, cutting down on fraud and errors.
> **interoperability:** The ability to work with other systems.
> **parameters:** A rule that controls how something should be done; guidelines or boundaries.

> ### CRITICAL THINKING 19.4
> Some of the patients who visit Dr. Kahn and Dr. Martin have expressed concern that electronic health records (EHRs) may not be private enough and that their health information will be "floating around on the Internet." They are worried that unauthorized individuals could somehow access their information on the computer and do them harm. How might Susan alleviate the patients' fears about their records being available on the Internet? What disadvantages with regard to confidentiality are associated with the EHR?

CAPABILITIES OF ELECTRONIC HEALTH RECORD SYSTEMS

The EHR system can perform a multitude of tasks, saving time and money in the provider's office (Fig. 19.4). The following are some of the features of a typical EHR system.
- *Specialty software.* Patient data are captured and processed into a system that is specialty specific. The terminology and patient care treatments are compatible with the provider's specialty. However, additional features can allow the provider to include terminology from other specialties.
- *Appointment scheduler.* The appointment scheduler (Fig. 19.5) allows the staff to do the following:
  - Track and schedule appointments
  - Create the schedule matrix
  - Account for recurring time blocks

The appointments can be merged into specific types with default times so that lengthy procedures are not scheduled in short appointment blocks. The scheduler features also allow various search parameters; if a patient calls because he or she cannot remember the appointment time, a search can be initiated using the following:
- Date
- Provider's name
- Patient's name
- Keywords

- *Appointment reminder and confirmation.* The system can be programmed to automatically remind patients with a confirmation call. The staff can record the message to be sent, and patients are prompted to choose options, such as "Press 1" to confirm or reschedule appointments.
- *Prescription writer.* The EHR system can produce electronic prescriptions, which can be printed and given to patients or automatically

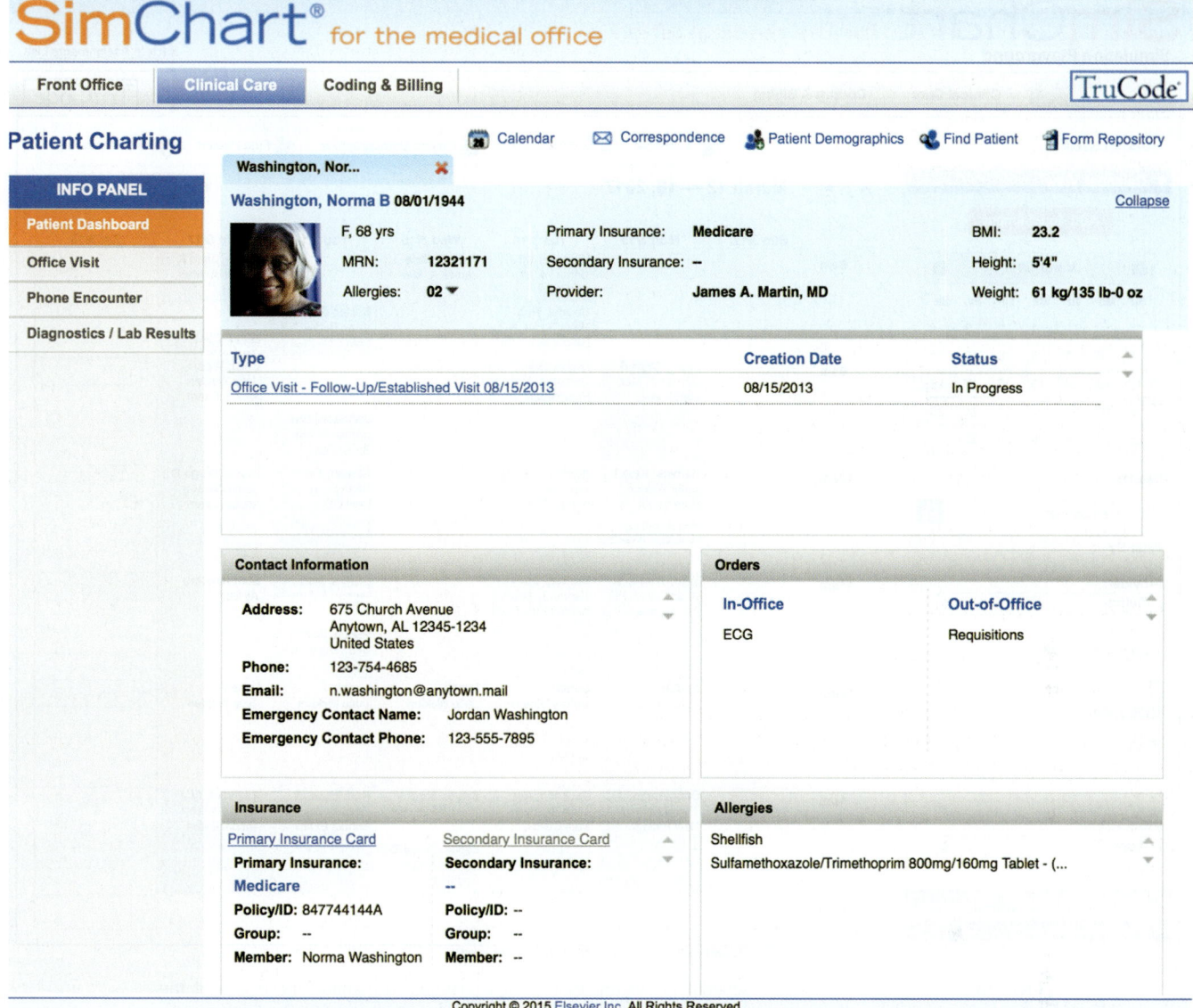

FIG. 19.4 The electronic health record (EHR) can perform numerous tasks, in addition to displaying personal information about the patient. This allows the provider and medical assistants to interact with patients and provide better service. (From Proctor D, et al: *Kinn's The Medical Assistant*, ed 13, St. Louis, 2017, Elsevier.)

submitted to a pharmacy. Lists can be created with the provider's most common drug choices and dosages. An allergy function can be linked to the patient's list of allergies and alert the provider to an issue. The system can also generate a patient information sheet on new prescriptions.

- *Medical billing system.* The EHR billing system can manage all of the practice's billing and accounting systems. The system also can interface with clearinghouses for electronic claims submission and tracking. Reports can be generated that provide accurate details of the financial state of the practice at certain intervals or whenever requested.
- *Charge capture.* The charge capture functions can store lists of billing codes such as the following:
  - International Classification of Diseases (ICD)
  - Current Procedural Terminology (CPT)
  - Charges for procedures, supplies, and laboratory tests
  - Alerts can let the user know when a certain charge does not match a diagnosis code—for instance, a blood glucose done for a sore throat; in such cases, the software alerts the user and helps prevent errors that can lead to a denial of insurance claims
- *Eligibility verification.* EHR billing systems can perform online verification of insurance eligibility and can capture demographic data.
- *Referral management.* In the case of a referral or consultation, information can be shared with another provider electronically. The patient does not have to obtain copies of the record and then bring them to the new provider. This also eliminates the cost of making copies and is faster and more efficient than copying and mailing patient records.

> **VOCABULARY**
> **interface:** An interconnection between systems.

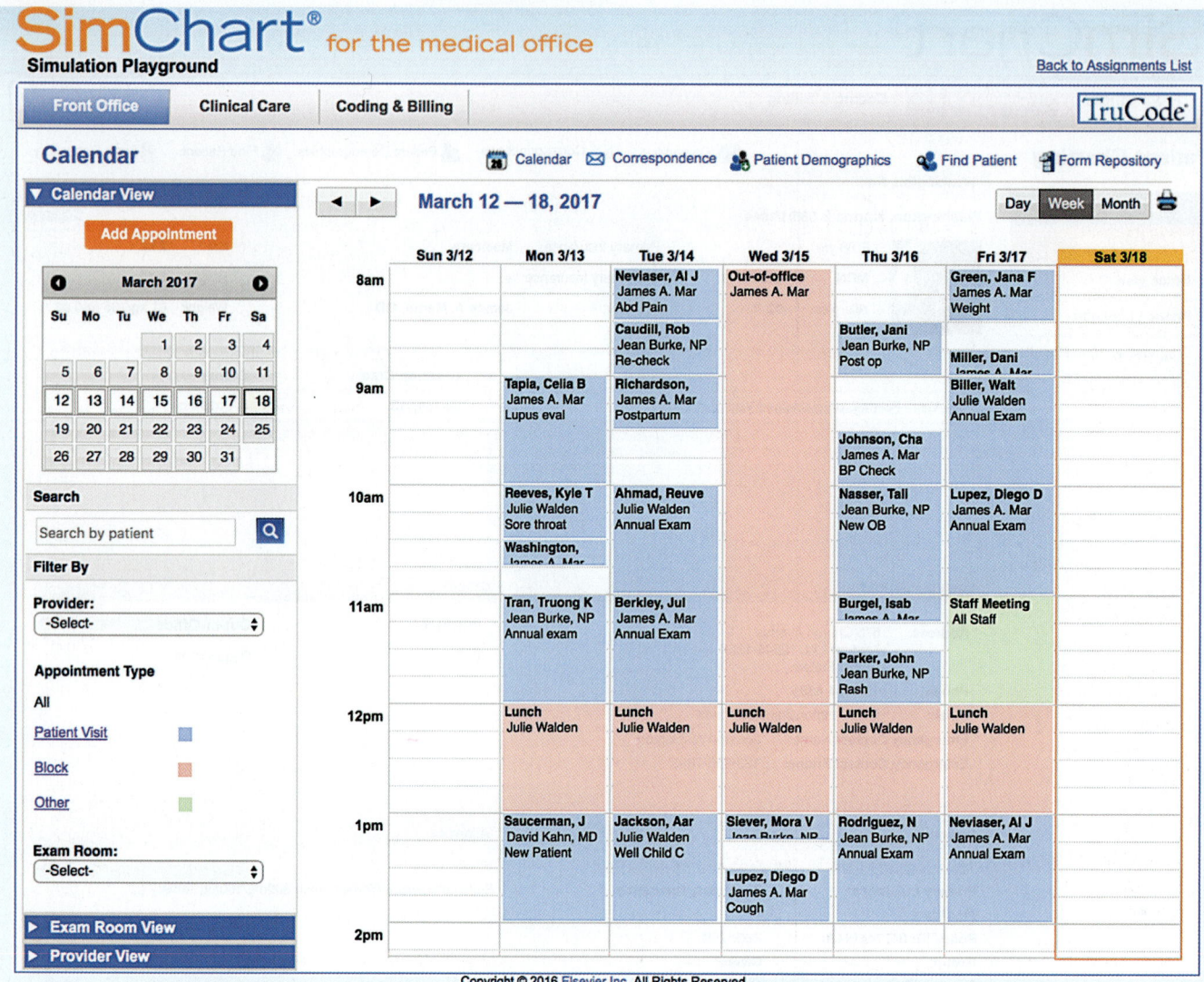

FIG. 19.5 The EHR usually has a scheduling system that can be changed to manage the needs of the provider and office staff. (From Proctor D, et al: *Kinn's The Medical Assistant*, ed 13, St. Louis, 2017, Elsevier.)

- *Laboratory order integration.* The laboratory order integration feature allows the user to interact with outside laboratories. The EHR can receive and post laboratory results to patients' records. Tests can be ordered from the provider's laptop, tablet, or smart phone. Results can be transmitted by fax, scan, or email and uploaded directly into the patient's record (Procedure 19.2).

CRITICAL THINKING 19.5

Jennifer, the office manager, has noticed that Susan seems overwhelmed in the training classes for the EHR system used by the clinic. During a break, Jennifer asks Susan whether she is having any specific problems with the training classes. She also asks for Susan's input on the system. Susan says that she just prefers clinical work and that her typing skills are a little "rusty." She is determined to do her best to learn the system and asks if she could have extra practice time. How might Jennifer respond to Susan's comments? What can Susan do to overcome her issues with the EHR system?

MAINTAINING A CONNECTION WITH THE PATIENT WHEN USING THE ELECTRONIC HEALTH RECORD

Many patients are required to choose a primary care provider (PCP) to be referred to a specialist. They also have the option of changing the PCP or specialist. The patient may decide to change providers simply because he or she does not feel comfortable with that particular provider.

Because the change process is relatively easy, the healthcare facility should strive to provide excellent care and service to its patients. If the care begins to seem impersonal, patients may feel a strong desire to change providers. Patients are consumers of healthcare services, and they expect quality healthcare and service.

When using the EHR, the medical assistant must make sure that his or her nonverbal communication sends the right message to the patient. Eye contact is essential (Fig. 19.6). If the medical assistant constantly looks at the electronic device, the patient feels left out of the process. Make eye contact with the patient while asking questions,

PROCEDURE 19.2 Upload Documents to the Electronic Health Record

Task
Scan paper records and upload digital files to the EHR.

Equipment and Supplies
- Scanner
- Computer with SimChart for the Medical Office or EHR software
- Patient's laboratory and radiology reports

Scenario
A new patient brings in a laboratory report and a radiology report that he would like to have added to his EHR. You need to scan in the original documents and upload them to the EHR.

Procedural Steps
1. Obtain the patient's name and date of birth if not on the reports.
Purpose: You will need the patient's name and date of birth to find the patient's EHR.
2. Using a scanner that is connected to the computer, scan each document, creating an individual digital image for each one.
Purpose: The reports should be scanned separately and not combined to create one file. Each type of report must be uploaded separately to the correct location in the EHR.
3. Locate the files of the two scanned images in the computer drive. Open the files to ensure the images are clear.
Purpose: When scanning and uploading documents to the EHR, it is crucial that the image of the document is clear and can be easily read by the provider. If the image is blurred, rescan the document.
4. In the EHR, search for the patient, using the patient's last and first names. Verify the patient's date of birth.
Purpose: Before uploading to or documenting in the EHR, it is critical to verify that the correct record is opened.
5. Locate the window to upload diagnostic/laboratory results, and add a new result. Enter the date of the test. Select the correct type of result. Browse for the image file of the laboratory file and attach it. Save the information. Select the option to add a new result, and repeat the steps to upload the second report. Verify that both documents were uploaded correctly.
Purpose: Errors during the upload may affect the ability to see the files. Verifying at the time of the upload will help ensure providers can see the results in the future.

PROCEDURE 19.3 Protect the Integrity of the Medical Record

Task
Protect the integrity of the medical record.

Scenario
You are mentoring a medical assistant student, who is in practicum. You notice the student routinely does not sign out of the electronic health record before leaving the desk. The facility's policy is to sign out or lock the computer before leaving it.

Directions
Role-play the scenario with a peer, who plays the student. You, the medical assistant, must explain to the "student" the facility's policy. Also address the hazards of not protecting the medical record. If the student does not change his/her behavior, you will need to address the situation with the department supervisor.

Procedural Steps
1. Professionally and respectfully discuss the situation with the student.
2. Inform the student about the facility's policy and the hazards of not protecting the electronic health record.
3. Provide the student with strategies to protect the electronic health record.
4. Inform the student what will occur if he/she does not protect the electronic record.

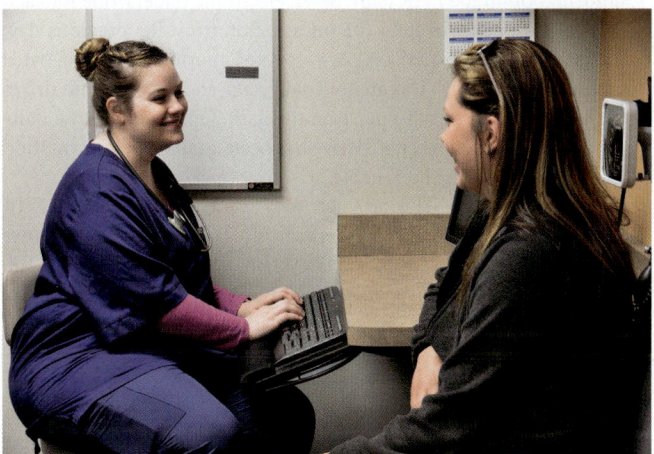

FIG. 19.6 The medical assistant must make eye contact with the patient when using an EHR. (From Proctor D, et al: *Kinn's The Medical Assistant*, ed 13, St. Louis, 2017, Elsevier.)

and look at the screen only when needed to enter information. Do not shield the device from the patient's view when entering information. This can give the impression you are hiding something from the patient. Although patients may not understand anything they see on the screen, they will feel more at ease if their information is not hidden from them. Also, modify your position so that the patient feels like a part of the information process. Just as sitting in a chair across from a supervisor's desk can be intimidating, the patient may feel the same emotions sitting across from a medical assistant entering information into the EHR. Sit next to or at an angle to the patient to support the impression that those in the healthcare facility and the patient are partners in the healthcare plan.

Because patients have the right to make decisions in most aspects of their healthcare plans, offer choices wherever possible. Never expect patients to make quick decisions about their care. They may want to consult family members or give some thought to important medical decisions. The medical assistant needs to allow the patient time to think unless the patient is faced with a critical, time-sensitive decision. Providers often assume that patients will automatically follow their instructions or orders; however, some patients prefer some time to consider their options. Always follow up and make note of any wait time the patient requests, notify the provider, and enter that information into the EHR. Make sure timely communication is done with the patient and that any additional orders that need to be put in place are completed. The many features of the EHR allow the medical assistant to be efficient and highly competent if he or she is willing to make an extra effort to master the EHR system.

Also, make sure patients understand all instructions given to them regarding test procedures or preparation for procedures. Most EHRs can print an instruction sheet, which the medical assistant can review with the patient. The customer service aspect of patient care is even more important when the facility uses an EHR system (Procedure 19.3).

> ### CRITICAL THINKING 19.6
>
> Jennifer walks behind Susan's desk and notices that she is looking at the progress notes on a patient who was recently arrested and indicted for child abuse. The case has been in the newspaper and on television consistently for several weeks. Jennifer asks Susan why she has accessed that record. Susan hesitates and then says she must have entered the wrong patient ID number. Does Susan's explanation sound convincing? Why is Jennifer concerned about Susan looking at the patient's record? Just because the individual is a patient at the clinic, does that mean any employee has the right to look at the patient's EHR?

BACKUP SYSTEMS FOR THE ELECTRONIC HEALTH RECORD

Even the best or most expensive EHR system cannot function without power. If a natural disaster occurs and the provider's office is without electricity for several days or weeks, the provider must have a backup system to protect the information contained in the EHR. HIPAA requires that the facility adopt a backup and recovery plan that includes daily offsite software backup for the EHR system. Several options are available for data preservation and backup:

- *External hard drive.* An external hard drive connects to the main computer, and with fairly simple programming it can copy the information in the EHR daily. Seven electronic folders, one for each day of the week, can hold the information from the previous day; these folders are replaced with new, updated information at designated periods. CDs and DVDs can hold daily data, and some thumb drives have enough capacity to perform this task. Once a habit of a daily backup to the external hard drive has been established, the method is relatively simple and reliable.
- *Full server backup.* The provider may want to back up the EHR system on a dedicated server, which is a large-capacity computer set aside specifically for the EHR system. With these servers, a full backup should be performed monthly. Many large medical facilities and hospitals have one or more dedicated servers for the EHR system.
- *Online backup system.* An online backup system can be used, usually for a subscription fee. Although the cost may be higher than for some other methods, online systems are easy to use because there is no external drive to carry and no CD or thumb drive to put through the process of downloading data. However, time investment is involved, because the process of contacting the company that offers the service and then downloading all the data takes several hours. Also, the initial download can take quite a while. Even so, an online system is stable and reliable.

All of these backup methods require an alternative power source in case of a disaster that interrupts electrical service. Remember that backup systems are not effective if the data are stored at the medical facility and the disaster happens at or affects that physical address. Information technology professionals usually recommend using two of these three methods for the best protection. The system must be protected from theft and unauthorized use, just like the onsite system.

Medical assistants should keep their paper health records skills sharp in case the EHR system is down for an extended period. Always have a supply of the most commonly used forms in a paper format available for use in such instances. When the EHR system comes back up, these paper forms can be scanned into the patients' EHRs.

RETENTION AND DESTRUCTION OF HEALTH RECORDS

In most medical offices, records are classified in three ways:
- *Active:* records of patients currently receiving treatment
- *Inactive:* records of patients whom the provider has not seen for 6 months or longer
- *Closed:* records of patients who have died, moved away, or otherwise terminated their relationship with the provider

The process of moving a file from active to inactive status is called *purging*. An EHR system can be set up to automatically move the inactive records to another server so that processing time will not be slowed down, but the records are still readily accessible if the patient returns to the healthcare facility. Closed EHRs are also separated from the active records and are typically stored elsewhere. They may be placed on CDs, computer hard drives, or maintained in inactive cloud space by the EHR vendor.

As with EHRs, paper health records are also classified as active, inactive, and closed. A paper record system must have a system established for regular transfer of files from active to inactive status or possibly destruction. The expansion of records and the file space available can influence the transfer period. Records for patients currently hospitalized may be kept in a special section for quick reference and then placed in the regular active file when the patient is discharged from the hospital. In a surgical practice, the record frequently includes the specific date on which the patient is discharged from the provider's care, and the notation is made on the record, "Return prn" (from the Latin *pro re nata,* "as the occasion arises" or "when needed"). This record may safely be placed in the inactive file.

Most medical facilities use a year sticker on the file folder that indicates the last year the patient visited the clinic. If the file has a sticker showing that the patient's last visit was in 2016, and he or she presents to the clinic on January 5, 2018, a 2018 sticker should be placed over the one that indicates 2016. These stickers often are included with color-coded filing systems. The medical assistant can easily look at a group of files and see which ones need to be changed to inactive or closed status.

According to the American Medical Association (AMA) Council on Ethical and Judicial Affairs, providers have an obligation to retain patient records whether they are paper or electronic. Currently, no nationwide standard rule exists for establishing a records **retention schedule**.

Medical considerations are the primary basis for deciding how long to retain health records. For example, operative notes and chemotherapy records should always be part of the patient's health record. The laws regarding the retention of health records vary from state to state, and many governmental programs have their own guidelines for specific records retention. When no rules specify the retention of health records, the best course is to keep the records for 10 years. However, for minors, the facility should keep the records until the minor reaches the **age of majority** plus the statute of limitations.

> ### VOCABULARY
>
> **age of majority:** The age at which the law recognizes a person to be an adult; it varies by state.
>
> **retention schedule:** A method or plan for retaining or keeping health records and for their movement from active to inactive to closed.

It is best to know the state requirements related to health records retention and follow those guidelines. The office policy manual should address records retention pertaining to the state where the practice exists.

The records of any patient covered by Medicare or Medicaid must be kept at least 10 years. The HIPAA privacy rule does not include requirements for the retention of health records. However, the privacy rule does require that appropriate administrative, technical, and physical safeguards be applied so that the privacy of health records is maintained.

Some providers refuse to destroy or discard old records. Storage is less of an issue with EHRs as they take up much less physical space. Always refer to state laws when discarding health records.

Before old records are destroyed, patients should be given an opportunity to claim a copy of the records or have them sent to another provider. The medical facility should keep a master list of all records that have been destroyed. To legally destroy an EHR, the record, including the backup record, has to be overwritten using utility software.

RELEASING HEALTH RECORD INFORMATION

The healthcare facility must be extremely careful when releasing any type of medical information. The patient must sign a release for information to be given to any third party.

Requests for medical information should be made in writing (Fig. 19.7). HIPAA has designated that specific information must be included on the release of information form:
- Who is releasing the information
- Who the information is being released to
- What specific information is to be released
- An expiration date for the release

Accepting a faxed request for medical information or a faxed release of information from a patient is unwise. Even requests from the patient's attorney or insurance companies must be cleared by the patient for them to obtain information.

If a provider is involved in a liability suit, there will be a required exchange of information. As both parties to a lawsuit begin to prepare their cases, they enter the discovery process. Each side must disclose the pertinent facts of the case that may influence the final outcome of that case. On each occasion that information is needed from the provider, a separate request must be sent. Because the patient signs this request form, it serves as a release.

Most offices charge a fee to print or copy health records, whether it is a per-page charge or a per-record fee. If the records are sent electronically, no fee is charged. Follow the steps in the policy and procedures manual for the release of records. Some providers designate the office manager to handle requests for records releases.

Pay particular attention to records release requests involving a minor. In most cases, the parent or legal guardian is entitled to read through the patient's health records; however, according to the U.S. Department of Health and Human Services (HHS), there are three situations in which the parent may not be legally entitled to review the records of his or her minor child:
- When the minor is the one who consents to care and the parent is not required to also consent to care under state law
- When the minor obtains medical care at the direction of a court or a person authorized by the court
- When the minor, parent, and provider all agree that the doctor and minor patient can have a private, confidential relationship

If the provider believes that the minor might be in an abusive situation or that the parent or legal guardian may be harming the patient, the provider is required, both legally and ethically, to report the abuse.

Sometimes patients want to look at their own records. They certainly have a right to see this information, but some patients may not understand the terminology used in the record. A staff member should always remain with a patient who is looking at his or her health record. Remember, the original health record should never leave the medical facility. Always follow office policy when releasing health records.

When a release is presented to the office, provide only the records requested in the release. Do not provide information that is not requested. The patient must specify that substance abuse, mental health, or human immunodeficiency virus (HIV) records are to be released. Remember that the patient ultimately decides whether a record can be released. If any question arises about what is to be released, consult the office manager or the provider.

ORGANIZATION OF THE HEALTH RECORD

Source-Oriented Records

The traditional patient record is a source-oriented record (SOR). Observations and data are cataloged according to their source:
- Provider (progress notes)
- Laboratory
- Radiology
- Hospital
- Consultations

Forms and progress notes are filed in **reverse chronologic order** and in separate sections of the record according to the type of form or service rendered (e.g., all laboratory reports together, all x-ray reports together, and so on). Reverse chronologic order is used so that the provider and staff members do not have to search to the bottom of the record to find a recent laboratory report or a test.

Problem-Oriented Records

The problem-oriented medical record (POR) is a departure from the traditional system of keeping patient records. The POR is a method of recording data in a problem-solving system. This system is divided into four components:
- The *database* includes the chief complaint, present illness, patient profile, review of systems, physical examination, and laboratory reports.
- The *problem list* is a numbered, titled list of every problem the patient has that requires management or workup. This may include social and demographic troubles in addition to strictly medical or surgical ones.
- The *treatment plan* includes management, additional workups needed, and therapy. Each plan is titled and numbered with respect to the problem.
- The *progress notes* include structured notes that are numbered to correspond with each problem number.

Several companies have developed file folders for organizing patient data according to the POR. The problem list (Fig. 19.8) is placed at the front of the record. Special sections are provided for current major and chronic diagnoses/health problems and for inactive major or chronic

> **VOCABULARY**
> **reverse chronologic order:** The most recent item is on top and oldest item is last.

Central Texas Dermatology Clinic • 102 Westlake Drive • Austin, Texas 78746
AUTHORIZATION TO DISCLOSE HEALTH INFORMATION

I hereby authorize the use or disclosure of information from the medical record of:
Patient Name: _____ Date of Birth: _____
Social Security# _____ Daytime Phone: _____

I authorize the following individual or organization to disclose the above named individual's health information:
_____ Address: _____

This information may be disclosed TO and used by the following individual or organization:
_____ Address: _____

Please release the following:
____ Progress Notes   ____ Pathology Reports   ____ Lab Reports   ____ Any and all Records
____ Other Diagnostic reports (specify _____
____ Other (specify) _____
   Including Information (if applicable) pertaining to:
     ____ Mental Health   ____ Drug/Alcohol   ____ HIV/AIDS   ____ Communicable Treatment

Purpose or Need for Disclosure:
____ Continued Patient Care   ____ Personal Use
____ Attorney/Legal   ____ Insurance Claim/Application
____ Disability Determination   ____ Other(specify) _____

I understand that the information in my health record may include information relating to sexually transmitted disease, acquired immunodeficiency syndrome (AIDS), or human immunodeficiency virus (HIV). It may also include information about behavioral or mental health services, and treatment for alcohol and drug abuse.

I understand that the information released is for the specific purpose stated above. Any other use of this information without the written consent of the patient is prohibited.

I understand that I have the right to revoke this authorization at any time. I understand that if I revoke this authorization I must do so in writing and present my written revocation to the individual or organization releasing information. I understand that the revocation will not apply to information already released in response to this authorization. I understand that the revocation will not apply to my insurance company when the law provides my insurer the right to contest a claim under my policy. Unless otherwise revoked, this authorization will expire on following date, event or condition: _____

If I fail to specify an expiration date, event or condition, this authorization will expire in six months.

I understand that authorizing the disclosure of this health information is voluntary. I can refuse to sign the authorization. I need not sign this form in order to ensure treatment. I understand that I may inspect or copy the information to be used or disclosed, as provided in CFR 164.524. I understand that any disclosure of information carries with it the potential for an unauthorized re-disclosure and the information may not be protected by federal confidentiality rules. If I have questions about disclosure of my health information, I can contact Theresa Farren at 512-327-7779.

_____   _____
Signature of Patient or Legal Representative   Date

_____   _____
Relationship to Patient (If Legal Representative)   Witness

COMPLETE ONLY IF INFORMATION IS TO BE RELEASED DIRECTLY TO PATIENT:
I understand that my medical record may contain reports, test results, and notes that only a physician can interpret. I understand and have been advised that I should contact my physician regarding the entries made in my medical record to prevent my misunderstanding of the information contained in these entries. I will not hold Central Texas Dermatology liable for any misinterpretation of the information in my medical record as a result of not contacting my physician for the correct interpretation.

_____   _____
Signature of Patient or Legal Representative   Date

_____   _____
Relationship to Patient (If Legal Representative)   Witness

Dr. review/signature/date _____
Date request completed _____ # of pages copied _____
Staff Signature _____
PHI Log completed _____

FIG. 19.7 Authorization to release health records. All requests for health records should be in writing, and the request should be kept in the patient's health record. (From Proctor D, et al: *Kinn's The Medical Assistant*, ed 13, St. Louis, 2017, Elsevier.)

MASTER PROBLEM LIST
For use of this form, see AR 40-66; the proponent agency is the Office of The Surgeon General

MAJOR PROBLEMS

PROBLEM NUMBER	DATE ONSET	DATE ENTERED	PROBLEM	DATE RESOLVED
1.				
2.				
3.				
4.				
5.				
6.				
7.				
8.				
9.				
10.				
11.				
12.				

TEMPORARY (MINOR) PROBLEMS

PROBLEM LETTER	PROBLEM	DATES OF OCCURRENCES
A.		
B.		
C.		
D.		
E.		
F.		
G.		
H.		

PATIENT'S IDENTIFICATION (Use mechanical imprint if available; for typed or written entries give: Name, SSN, Unit, Sex, Birthdate, and Duty Phone)

SUMMARY OF PROBLEMS, ALLERGIES, MEDICATIONS, SURGERIES AND TRAUMAS:

NOTE: DO NOT DISCARD FROM CHART

FIG. 19.8 A problem list designed for a problem-oriented record (POR). (From Proctor D, et al: *Kinn's The Medical Assistant*, ed 13, St. Louis, 2017, Elsevier.)

diagnosis/health problems. Progress notes usually follow the SOAP approach. SOAP is an acronym for the following:
- *Subjective* impressions or patient reports
- *Objective* clinical evidence or observations
- *Assessment* or diagnosis
- *Plans* for further studies, treatment, or management

Some medical offices also use an E in the record to represent *evaluation*; others include E for *education* and R for *response*. The education notation shows that the patient was educated about his or her condition or given a patient information sheet. The response section is used to record an assessment of the patient's understanding of and possible compliance with the treatment plan.

The POR has the advantage of creating order and organization of the information added to a patient's health record. The records are more easily reviewed, and the likelihood of overlooking a problem is greatly reduced. The SOAP method forces a rational approach to the patient's problems and assists in forming a logical, orderly plan of patient care (Fig. 19.9). The POR is especially helpful in clinics, group practices, and hospitals, where more than one person must be able to find essential information in the record.

> ### CRITICAL THINKING 19.7
> Susan learned about SOAP documentation in school and is eager to use it in her new job. Dr. Kahn is seeing a patient who reports to Susan that she has had nausea and vomiting for the past 3 days. Susan obtains a weight of 132.5 pounds, temperature (T) 101.2°F tympanically, pulse (P) 94 beats/min, respiration (R) 14 breaths/min, and blood pressure (BP) 122/84 mm Hg in the right arm. What information would be documented in the Subjective field? What information would be documented in the Objective field? Who would document information in the Assessment field?

FIG. 19.9 SOAP progress notes. The SOAP method keeps information organized and in a logical sequence. An actual progress note would include the provider's or medical assistant's signature or initials after this entry. (Courtesy Bibbero Systems, An InHealth Company, Petaluma, California (800) 242-2376, www.bibbero.com)

DOCUMENTING IN AN ELECTRONIC HEALTH RECORD

Documentation in an EHR involves using radio buttons, drop-down menus, and free-text boxes. The radio buttons and drop-down menus allow for standardization of the content in the EHR, and the free-text boxes allow for the documentation of the unique circumstance found with each patient (Fig. 19.10). It is important to carefully review the choices made with the radio buttons and drop-down menus. Information documented using the free-text boxes should be proofread before submitting.

DOCUMENTING IN A PAPER HEALTH RECORD

When documenting in a paper health record, the entry will always start with the date in the MM/DD/YYYY format. The date will be followed by the time. This may be written in standard or military time. If standard time is used, it must be followed by a.m. or p.m. (e.g., 2:00 p.m.). If military time is used, it is in a four-digit format without a colon (e.g., 1400). All entries must be written in black or blue ink, following the format designated by the healthcare facility. Documentation should be in the order in which the steps were completed. If a temperature, pulse, and respiration (TPR) measurement is done, it would be documented in the "O" or Objective section of the SOAP note starting with temperature, then pulse, and, lastly, respirations.

MAKING CORRECTIONS AND ALTERATIONS TO HEALTH RECORDS

Sometimes corrections must be made to health records. The first step is to verify the proper procedure for making corrections in the facility's policy and procedures manual. Some providers prefer a specific method for correcting errors in the health record. Erasing, using correction fluid, or any other type of **obliteration** (uh blit uh REY shun) is never acceptable. To correct a handwritten entry:

1. Draw a line through the error.
2. Insert the correction above or immediately after the error in a spot where it can be read clearly.
3. If indicated by the policy and procedures manual, write "Error" or "Err." in the margin.
4. The person making the correction should write his or her initials or signature and the date below the correction. Follow the format indicated in the policy and procedures manual (Fig. 19.11).

> **VOCABULARY**
> **obliteration:** To remove or destroy all traces of; do away with; destroy completely.

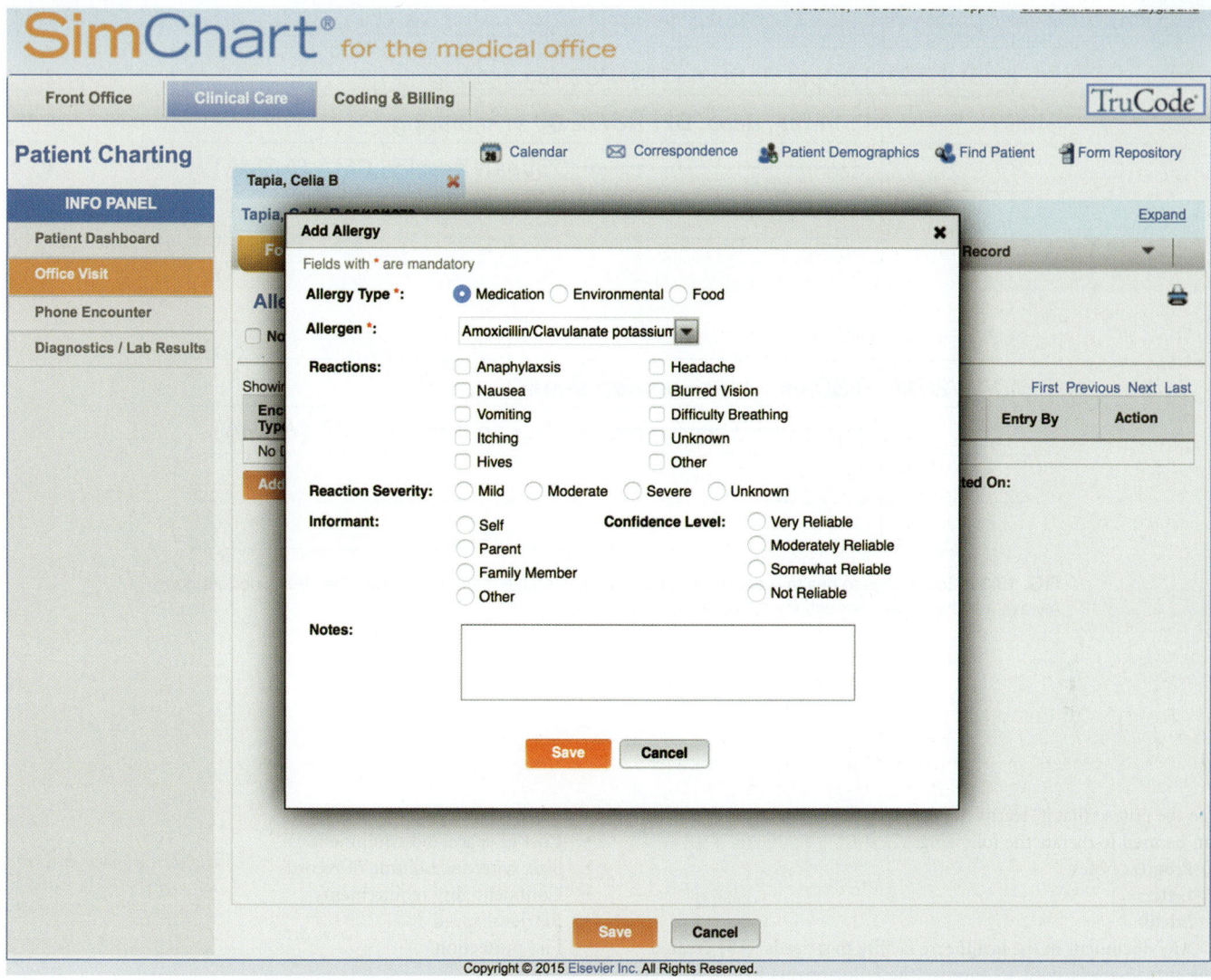

FIG. 19.10 Documentation in an EHR is done using radio buttons, drop-down menus, and free-text boxes. (From Proctor D, et al: *Kinn's The Medical Assistant*, ed 13, St. Louis, 2017, Elsevier.)

Errors made while using the computer are corrected in the usual way. However, an error discovered in an entry at a later date is corrected in the same manner as for a handwritten entry. This is sometimes called an *addendum*. Never attempt to alter health records without using this specific correction procedure, because this alteration of records may indicate a fraudulent attempt to cover up a mistake made by a staff member or the provider. Do not hide errors. If the error could, in any way, affect the patient's health and well-being, it must be brought to the provider's attention immediately. An EHR system will track the changes made within the record.

DICTATION AND TRANSCRIPTION

With the increased use of EHRs and voice recognition software, there is decreased need for transcription. If dictation is still done in the healthcare facility, the administrative medical assistant may find that transcribing the dictation is a job she or he will sometimes perform. Transcription can be done from handwritten notes or, more likely, from machine dictation. Smooth operation of the facility may depend on the timely, accurate performance of assigned responsibilities, such as record documentation and the preparation of special reports. Accuracy and speed are the primary requirements, along with a strong grasp of medical terminology, anatomy, and physiology.

Dictation may be done using a machine transcription unit or a portable transcription unit. Many healthcare facilities now use a system that is accessed by telephone; the provider calls the system using passwords or access codes and records the information for the health record while speaking into the telephone. Later, employees transcribe the information into the health record. The provider must acknowledge and initial all transcripts before they are placed in the health record.

Voice Recognition Software

Some healthcare facilities use voice recognition software for transcription. When first installed, the software requires the user to say several sentences

> **VOCABULARY**
> **dictation:** To say something aloud for another person to write down.
> **transcription:** To make a written copy of dictated material.

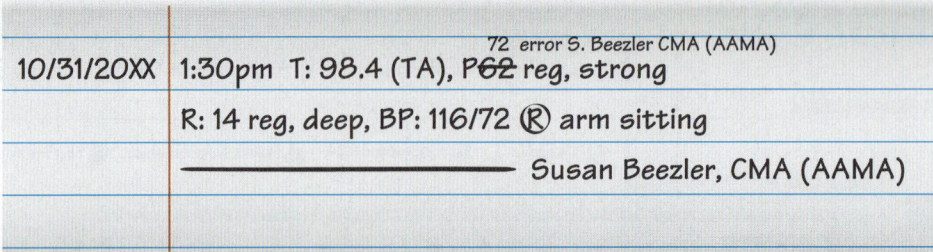

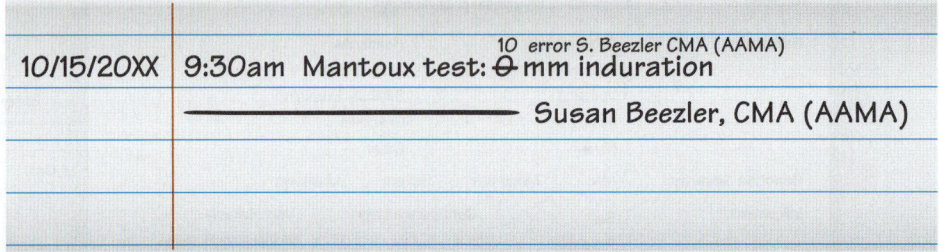

FIG. 19.11 Corrections to health records must be done in a legible manner and must be clearly understood. Always initial and date corrections to paper health records.

into the unit so that it "learns" to recognize the user's voice. The system can be used to dictate the following:
- Progress notes
- Letters
- Emails
- Any document in the healthcare facility that needs to be created

The provider will need to approve these documents before they are permanently attached to the patient's record. Some systems have an authentication component that allows a type of electronic signature, such as those needed for hospital record dictation.

CREATING AN EFFICIENT PAPER HEALTH RECORDS MANAGEMENT SYSTEM

The paper health records management system should provide an easy method of retrieving information. The files should be organized in an orderly fashion. The information must be documented accurately, and corrections should be made and documented properly. The wording in the record should be easily understood and grammatically correct. An efficient method of adding documents to the record must be established so that the provider always has the most up-to-date information. Above all, the health records management system must work for the individual facility.

Filing Equipment

For years, the traditional filing system involved a vertical, four-drawer steel filing cabinet, used with manila folders with the patient's name on the tab. The most popular system today is color coding on open horizontal shelves. Rotary, lateral, compactable, and automated files also are available. Some records are kept in card or tray files. Several factors should be considered when selecting filing equipment:
- Office space availability
- Structural considerations
- Cost of space and equipment
- Size, type, and volume of records
- Confidentiality requirements
- Retrieval speed
- Fire protection
- Cost

Drawer Files. Drawer files should be full suspension; they should roll easily, close securely, and be equipped with a locking device. The best cabinets have a center trough at the bottom of each drawer with a rod for holding divider guides. A drawback of the vertical four-drawer files is that only one person can use a file cabinet at a time. Also, filing is slower, because the drawer must be opened and closed each time a file is pulled or filed.

File cabinets are heavy and can tip over, causing serious damage or injury unless reasonable care is taken. Open only one file drawer at a time, and close it when the filing has been completed. A drawer left even slightly open can injure a passerby.

Horizontal Shelf Files. Shelf files should have doors that lock to protect the contents. A popular type of shelf file has doors that slide back into the cabinet; the door from a lower shelf may be pulled out and used for workspace. Open shelf units hold files sideways and can go higher on the wall because no drawers need to be pulled out (Fig. 19.12). File retrieval is faster, because several individuals can work simultaneously.

Rotary Circular Files. Rotary circular files can hold a large volume of records. They save space and clerical motion. The files revolve easily; some have push-button controls. Several people can work at one rotary file and use records at the same time. One disadvantage is that they afford less privacy and protection than files that can be closed and locked.

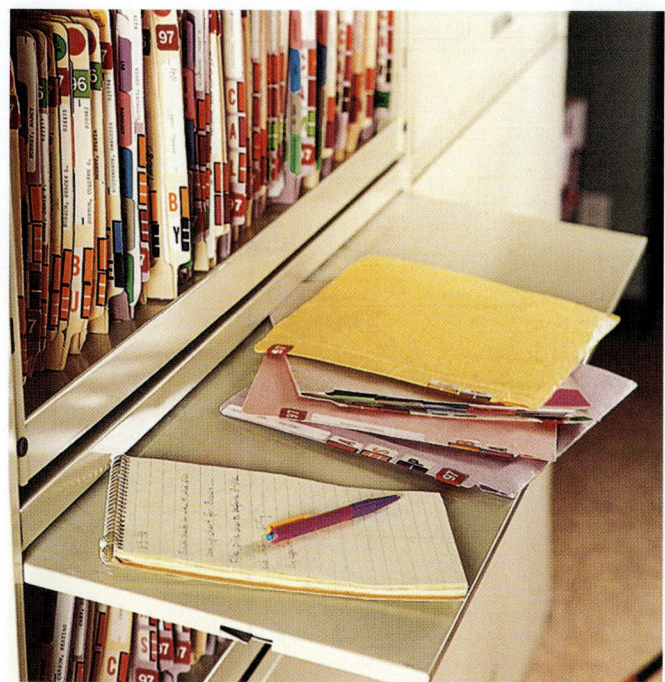

FIG. 19.12 Open shelf filing is an efficient method, especially for color coding filing systems. The shelf door often can be used as a workspace. (From Proctor D, et al: *Kinn's The Medical Assistant*, ed 13, St. Louis, 2017, Elsevier.)

Compactable Files. An office with little space and a great volume of records might use compactable files, which are a variation of open shelf files. The files are mounted on tracks in the floor, and the units slide along the tracks so that access is gained to the needed records. One drawback is that not all records are available at the same time.

Automated Files. Automated files are initially very expensive, and they also require more maintenance than other types of filing equipment. They are likely to be found only in large facilities, such as clinics or hospitals. These files bring the record to the operator instead of the operator going to the record. When the operator presses a button indicating the appropriate shelf, the shelf automatically moves into position in front of the operator for record retrieval. The automated or power file is fast and can store large numbers of records in a small amount of space. However, only one person can use the unit at one time.

Card Files. Almost every office has some occasion to use a card file. This may be for patient ledgers, a patient index, a library index, an index of surgical tray setups, telephone numbers, or numerous other records. A good-quality steel box or tray is a sound investment.

Filing Supplies

Divider Guides. Each file drawer or shelf should be equipped with plenty of dividers or guides. Some authorities recommend one guide for approximately each $1\frac{1}{2}$ inch of material, or every eight to 10 folders. Guides should be of good-quality heavy cardstock or strong plastic. Less-well-constructed guides soon become bent and frayed and have to be replaced. Divider guides have a protruding tab, which may be an integral part of the card or may be made of metal or plastic. The guides reduce the area of search and serve as supports for the folders. They are available in single, third, or fifth cut (i.e., one, three, or five different positions).

Out Guides. Out guides are made of heavyweight cardboard or plastic and are used to replace a folder that has been temporarily removed (Fig. 19.13). They may also have a large pocket to hold any filing that may come in while the folder is out. They should be of a distinctive color for quick detection. This makes refiling simpler and alerts the file clerk that a file is missing. Several colors may be used, each color designating the temporary location of the file. The out guide may have lines for recording information, or it may have a plastic pocket for inserting an information card.

File Folders. Most records to be filed are placed in covers or tabbed folders. The most commonly used is a general purpose, third-cut manila folder that may be expanded to three-quarters of an inch. These are available with a double-thickness, reinforced tab, which greatly extends the life of the folder. Folders kept in drawers have tabs at the top; those kept on shelves have tabs at the side. Many folder styles are available for special purposes.

Hanging, or suspension, folders are made of heavy stock and hang on metal rods from side to side in a drawer. They can be used only with file cabinets equipped with suspension equipment.

Binder folders have fasteners that are used to bind papers in the folder. These offer some security for the papers, but filing the materials is time consuming.

The number of papers that will fit in one folder depends on the thickness of the papers and the capacity of the folder. Near the bottom edge of most folders are one or more score marks, which should be used as the contents of the folders expand. Papers should never protrude from the folder edges, and they should always be inserted with their tops to the left. When papers start to ride up in any folder, the folder is overloaded.

Labels. The label is a necessary filing and finding device. Use labels to identify each shelf, drawer, divider guide, and folder. A label on the drawer or shelf identifies the nature of its contents. It should also indicate the range (i.e., alphabetic, numeric, or chronologic) of the material filed in that space.

The label on the divider guide identifies the range of folder headings following that divider guide up to the next divider (e.g., Ba-Bo). The label on the folder identifies the contents of that folder only, such as the following:
- The name of the patient
- Subject matter of correspondence
- A business topic

Label a folder when a new patient is seen, existing folders are full, or materials need to be transferred within the filing system.

Labels are available in almost any size, shape, or color to meet the individual needs of any facility. Visit an office supply website and review the catalogs to find the best product to meet the needs of the facility.

A narrow label applied to the front of the folder tab is the easiest to use and is satisfactory for folders kept in a drawer file. Labels for shelf filing should be identifiable from both front and back. Always type the label before separating it from the roll or protective sheet. Type the caption on the label in indexing order (Procedure 19.4).

VOCABULARY

out guides: Sturdy cardboard or plastic file-sized cards used to replace a folder temporarily removed from the filing space.
caption: A heading, title, or subtitle under which records are filed.

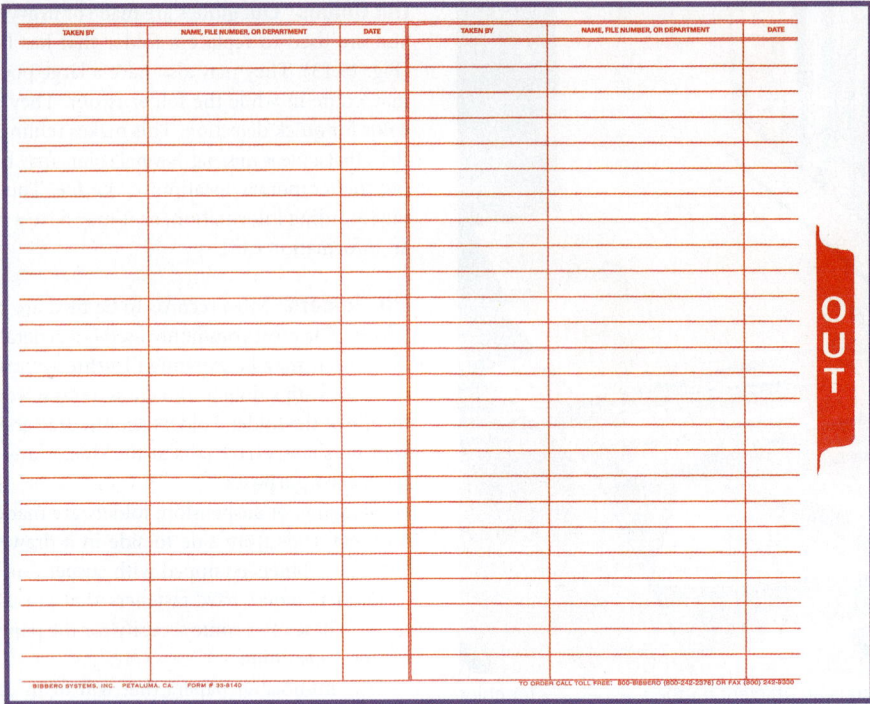

FIG. 19.13 Out guides allow tracking of a file not in its proper location by providing information on the location of the file. (Courtesy Bibbero Systems, An InHealth Company, Petaluma, California (800) 242-2376, www.bibbero.com)

INDEXING RULES

Indexing rules (Table 19.2) are standardized and based on current business practices. The Association of Records Managers and Administrators takes an active part in updating these rules. Some establishments adopt variations of these basic rules to accommodate their needs. In any case, the practices need to be consistent within the system:

1. Last names are considered first in filing; then the given name (first name), second; and the middle name or initial, third. Compare the names beginning with the first letter of the name. When a letter is different in the two names, that letter determines the order of filing.
2. Initials precede a name beginning with the same letter. This illustrates the librarian's rule, "Nothing comes before something."
3. With hyphenated personal names, the hyphenated elements, whether first name, middle name, or surname, are considered to be one unit.
4. The apostrophe is disregarded in filing.
5. When indexing a foreign name in which you cannot distinguish between the first and last names, index each part of the name in the order in which it is written. If you can make the distinction, use the last name as the first indexing unit.
6. Names with prefixes are filed in the usual alphabetic order, with the prefix considered part of the name.
7. Abbreviated parts of a name are indexed as written if that person generally uses that form.
8. Mac and Mc are filed in their regular place in the alphabet. If the files have a great many names beginning with Mac or Mc, some offices file them as a separate letter of the alphabet for convenience.
9. The name of a married woman who has taken her husband's last name is indexed by her legal name (her husband's surname, her given name, and her middle name or maiden surname). There should be a cross-reference, such as an out guide placed where her maiden name falls directing you to her new name.
10. When followed by a complete name, titles may be used as the last filing unit if needed to distinguish the name from another, identical name. Titles without complete names are considered the first indexing unit.
11. Terms of seniority or professional or academic degrees are used only to distinguish the name from an identical name.
12. Articles (e.g., the, a) are disregarded in indexing.

FILING METHODS

The three basic filing methods used in healthcare facilities are as follows:
- Alphabetic by name
- Numeric
- Subject

Patients' records are filed either alphabetically by name or by one of several numeric methods. Subject filing is used for business records, correspondence, and topical materials.

Alphabetic Filing

Alphabetic filing by name is the oldest, simplest, and most commonly used system. It is the system of choice for filing patients' records in most small providers' offices.

The alphabetic system of filing is traditional and simple to set up, requiring only a file cabinet or shelf, folders, and some divider guides (Procedure 19.5). It is a **direct filing system** in that the person filing

---

VOCABULARY

alphabetic filing: Any system that arranges names or topics according to the sequence of the letters in the alphabet.

direct filing system: A filing system in which materials can be located without consulting another source of reference.

PROCEDURE 19.4 Create and Organize a Patient's Paper Health Record

Task
Create a paper health record for a new patient. Organize health record documents in a paper health record.

Equipment and Supplies
- End tab file folder
- Completed patient registration form
- Divider sheets with different color labels (4)
- Progress note sheet (1)
- Name label
- Color-coding labels (first two letters of last name and first letter of first name)
- Year label
- Allergy label
- Black pen or computer with word processing software to process labels
- Health record documents (i.e., prior records, laboratory reports)
- Hole punch

Procedural Steps

1. Obtain the patient's first and last name.
Purpose: To customize the record for the patient, the first and last name will be required.
2. Neatly write or word-process the patient's name on the name label. Left-justify the last name, followed by a comma, the first name, middle initial and a period (e.g., Smith, Mary J.).
Purpose: The label should be easy to read. The last name always comes before the first name.
3. Adhere the name label to the bottom left side of the record tab. When you hold the record by the main fold in your left hand, the writing should be easy to read. (For directional purposes, assume the record main fold is on the left and the tab is at the bottom.)
Purpose: Placing the labels in correct position will make it easier to find the information needed.
4. Put the color-coding labels on the bottom right edge of the folder. Start by placing the first letter of the last name at the farthest right edge. Working left, place the second letter of the last name, then the first letter of the first name, and lastly the year label. The year label should be close to the name label.
Purpose: When the folders are in the file cabinet, they are sorted by the colored labels, starting with the top label (first letter of the last name), followed by the second and remaining labels.
5. Place the allergy label on the front of the record. If allergies are known, clearly write the allergy on the label in red ink.
Purpose: Allergies need to be clearly identified on medical records.
6. Place the divider labels on the record divider sheets, if they come separately. Ensure the labels on the divider sheets are staggered so they do not overlap. Print the name of the section on the front and back of the label. The print should be easy to read when the record is held by the main fold. (Suggested names for dividers: Progress Notes, Laboratory, Correspondence, and Miscellaneous.)
Purpose: Placing divider labels on the divider sheets in a staggered pattern allows the provider to easily see all sections of the health record.
7. Using the prongs on the left-hand side of the record, secure the registration form.
Purpose: The registration form should be in an easy-to-find location in the record.
8. Using the prongs on the right-hand side of the record, secure the index dividers with a progress note sheet under the progress note tab.
Purpose: The provider will need the progress note sheet to document data regarding the visit.
Scenario: The patient authorized his or her prior provider to send health records to your agency. You need to organize these records within the paper health record.
9. Verify the name and the date of birth on the health records, and ensure they match the information on the health record.
Purpose: Before organizing and filing documents in a patient's health record, it is critical to ensure the health record is for the correct patient.
10. Open the prongs on the right side of the record, and carefully remove the record to the point at which the documents need to be inserted. For the documents being inserted, punch holes in the proper location. Insert the papers into the record, and then reassemble the remaining part of the record. Continue to do this until all the documents are filed within the health record.
Purpose: Documents need to be placed in the correct location in the record so the provider can easily find information.

---

needs to know only the name to find the desired file. Alphabetic filing does have some drawbacks:
- The correct spelling of the name must be known.
- As the number of files increases, more space is needed for each section of the alphabet. This results in periodic shifting of folders to allow for expansion.
- As the files expand, more time is required for filing or retrieving each folder because of the greater number of folders involved in the search. The time can be greatly reduced by color coding.

Numeric Filing

Practically every large clinic or hospital uses some form of **numeric filing**, combined with color and shelf filing. Management consultants differ in their recommendations; some recommend numeric filing only if more than 5000 to 10,000 records are involved. Others recommend nothing but numeric filing. Numeric filing is an *indirect filing system*, or one that requires use of an alphabetic cross-reference to find a given file. Some object to this added step and overlook the advantages of numeric filing:
- It allows unlimited expansion without periodic shifting of folders, and shelves are usually evenly filed.
- It provides additional confidentiality to the record.
- It saves time in retrieving and filing records quickly. One knows immediately that the number 978 falls between 977 and 979. By contrast, an alphabetic system, even with color coding, requires a longer search to locate the exact spot.

Several types of numeric filing systems can be used:
- In a straight, or consecutive, numeric system, patients are given consecutive numbers as they first start using the practice. This is the simplest numeric system and works well for files of up to 10,000 records. It is time consuming, and the chance for error is greater, when documents with five or more digits are filed. Filing activity is greatest at the end of the numeric series.
- In a terminal digit system, patients also are assigned consecutive numbers, but the digits in the number usually are separated into groups

> **VOCABULARY**
> **numeric filing:** The filing of records, correspondence, or cards by number.

TABLE 19.2 Applying Indexing Rules

Indexing Rule	Name	Unit 1	Unit 2	Unit 3
1	Robert F. Grinch	Grinch	Robert	F.
	R. Frank Grumman	Grumman	R.	Frank
2	J. Orville Smith	Smith	J.	Orville
	Jason O. Smith	Smith	Jason	O.
3	M. L. Saint-Vickery	Saint-Vickery	M.	L.
	Marie-Louise Taylor	Taylor	Marielouise	
4	Charles S. Anderson	Anderson	Charles	S.
	Anderson's Surgical Supply	Andersons	Surgical	Supply
5	Ah Hop Akee	Akee	Ah	Hop
6	Alice Delaney	Delaney	Alice	
	Chester K. DeLong	Delong	Chester	K.
7	Michael St. John	Stjohn	Michael	
8	Helen M. Maag	Maag	Helen	M.
	Frederick Mabry	Mabry	Frederick	
	James E. MacDonald	Macdonald	James	E.
9	Mrs. John L. Doe (Mary Jones)	Doe	Mary	Jones (Mrs. John L.)
10	Prof. John J. Breck	Breck	John	J. (Prof.)
	Madame Sylvia	Madame	Sylvia	
	Sister Mary Catherine	Sister	Mary	Catherine
	Theodore Wilson, MD	Wilson	Theodore (MD)	
11	Lawrence W. Jones, Jr.	Jones	Lawrence	W. (Jr.)
	Lawrence W. Jones, Sr.	Jones	Lawrence	W. (Sr.)
12	The Moore Clinic	Moore	Clinic (The)	

PROCEDURE 19.5 File Patient Health Records

Task
File patient health records using two different filing systems: the alphabetic system and the numeric system.

Equipment and Supplies
- Paper health records using the alphabetic filing system
- Paper health records using the numeric filing system
- File boxes or file cabinet

Scenario
The agency utilizes the alphabetic system. You need to file health records in the correct location.

Procedural Steps
1. Using alphabetic guidelines, place the records to be filed in alphabetic order.
   Purpose: Placing the records in alphabetic order before filing in the box or cabinet will make the filing process more efficient.
2. Using the file box or file cabinet, locate the correct spot for the first file.
   Purpose: It is important place the record in the correct spot so that others can locate the record.
3. Place the health record in the correct location. Continue these filing steps until all the health records are filed.
4. Using numeric guidelines, place the records to be filed in numeric order.
   Purpose: Placing the records in numeric order before filing in the box or cabinet will make the filing process more efficient.
5. Using the file box or file cabinet, locate the correct spot for the first file.
   Purpose: It is important place the record in the correct spot so that others can locate the record.
6. Place the health record in the correct location. Continue these filing steps until all the health records are filed.

of twos or threes and are read in groups from right to left instead of from left to right. The records are filed backward in groups. For example, all files ending in 00 are grouped together first, then those ending in 01, and so on. Next the files are grouped by their middle digits so that the 00 22s come before the 01 22s. Finally, the files are arranged by their first digits, so that 01 00 22 precedes 02 00 22.
- Middle-digit filing begins with the middle digits, followed by the first digit, and finally by the terminal digits. Numeric filing requires more training, but once the system has been mastered, fewer errors occur than with alphabetic filing.

CRITICAL THINKING 19.8
Susan is unsure whether alphabetic or numeric filing is best in the healthcare facility. What are some advantages and disadvantages of each method?

Subject Filing
Subject filing can be either alphabetic or **alphanumeric** (e.g., A 1-3, B 1-1, B 1-2, and so on) and is used for general correspondence. The main difficulty with subject filing is indexing, or classifying—that is, deciding where to file a document. Many papers require *cross-referencing*. An example would be if you had a subject folder for Laboratory Supplies and the same organization provides you with your General Medical Supplies; there should be a notation in the Laboratory Supplies folder stating "See Also General Medical Supplies," and vice versa. All correspondence

VOCABULARY
alphanumeric: Describes systems made up of combinations of letters and numbers.

dealing with a particular subject is filed together. The papers in the folders are filed chronologically with the most recent on top. The subject headings are placed on the tabs of the folders and filed alphabetically.

Color Coding

When a color-coding system is used, both filing and finding files is easier, and misfiling of folders is kept to a minimum. The use of color visually restricts the area of search for a specific record. A misfiled record is easily spotted even from a distance of several feet. In color coding, a specific color is selected to identify each letter of the alphabet. Any selection of colors may be used, and the division of the alphabet is determined by one's own needs. However, studies have shown that the frequency with which different letters occur varies widely.

Alphabetic Color Coding. As medicine continues to consolidate into larger facilities with more patients in one system, the filing of patients' records becomes more complicated, and color coding becomes more useful. Several color-coding systems use two sets of 13 colors: one set for letters A to M, and a second set of the same colors on a different background for letters N to Z.

Many ready-made systems are available for use. Self-adhesive, colored letter blocks with either two or three letters in the specific colors are supplied in rolls. The color blocks with the appropriate letter are placed on the index tab of the folder, along with the patient's full name. The letters are in pairs so that they can be seen from either side of the record. Strong, easily differentiated colors are used, creating a band of color in the files that makes spotting out-of-place folders easy (Fig. 19.14).

Numeric Color Coding. Color coding is also used in numeric filing. Numbers 0 through 9 are each assigned a different color. In a terminal digit filing system, the colors for the last two numbers are affixed to the tab. If the number 1 is red and 5 is yellow, all files with numbers ending in 15 have a red and yellow band. Usually a predetermined section of the number is color-coded (Box 19.4).

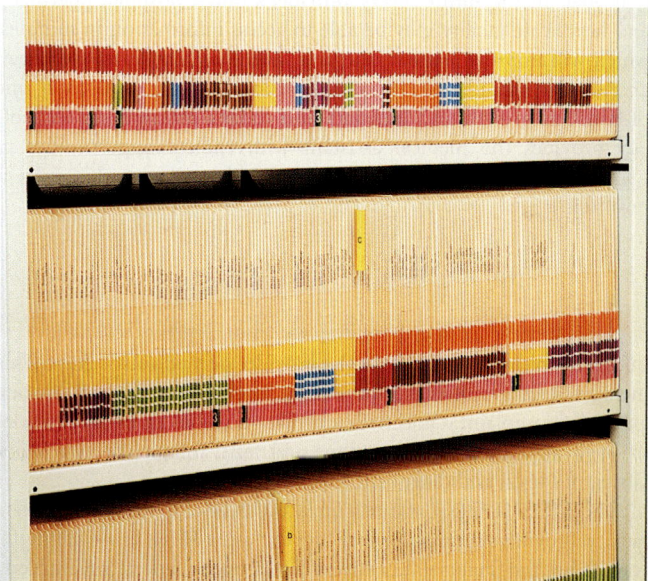

FIG. 19.14 With color coding of patients' records, a misplaced file is easily spotted. (Courtesy Bibbero Systems, An InHealth Company, Petaluma, CA (800) 242-2376 • www.bibbero.com)

ORGANIZATION OF FILES

Providers find studying a disorganized patient record very difficult. Some systematic method must be followed in placing items in the patient folder. From the filing standpoint, it should be emphasized that when a patient record is not in actual use, it should be in only one place—the filing cabinet or on the shelf. Many precious hours can be wasted searching for misplaced or lost records that were carelessly left unfiled.

The patient's full name, in indexing order, should be typed on a label and the label attached to the folder tab. A strip of transparent tape can be placed on the label to prevent smudging. The patient's full name should also be typed on each sheet in the folder. Some of the types of records common to the healthcare setting, other than patient records, include health-related correspondence, general correspondence, practice management files, miscellaneous files, and tickler or follow-up files.

Health-Related Correspondence

Correspondence pertaining to patients' health should be filed in the patient's health record. Other medical correspondence should be filed in a subject file.

General Correspondence

The provider's office operates as both a business and a professional service. Correspondence of a general nature pertaining to the operation of the office is part of the business side of the practice. Usually, a special drawer or shelf is set aside for the general correspondence. The correspondence is indexed according to subject matter or the names of the correspondents. The guides in a subject file may appear in one, two, or three positions, depending on the number of headings, subheadings, and subdivisions.

Practice Management Files

Of course, the most active financial record is the patient ledger. In facilities that still use a manual system, this is a card or vertical tray file, and the accounts are arranged alphabetically by name. At least two divisions are used: active accounts and paid accounts.

Miscellaneous Files

Papers that do not warrant an individual folder are placed in a miscellaneous folder. In that folder, all papers relating to one subject or with one correspondent are kept together in chronologic order, with the most recent on top, and then filed alphabetically with other miscellaneous material. Related materials may be stapled together. Never use paper

---

BOX 19.4 Other Color-Coding Applications

Color can work in many other ways for the efficient healthcare facility. Small tabs in a variety of colors can be used to identify certain types of insured patients and other specific information. For example, a red tab over the edge of the folder may identify a patient on Medicare; a blue tab may identify a Medicaid patient; a green tab may identify a workers' compensation patient; matching tabs may be attached to the insured's ledger card; research cases may be identified by a special color tab; and brightly colored labels on the outside of a patient's record can indicate certain health conditions, such as drug allergies. In a partnership practice, a different color folder or label may identify each provider's patients. Color also can be used to differentiate dates: one color for each month or year.

The use of color in filing is limited only by the imagination. One word of caution: Every person in the facility who uses the files must know the key to the coding, and the key should also be written in the facility's policy and procedures manual.

clips for this purpose. When as many as five papers accumulate with one correspondent or subject, a separate folder should be prepared. Other business files include records of income and expenses, financial statements, income and payroll tax records, canceled checks, and insurance policies. These papers may be filed chronologically.

Tickler or Follow-Up Files

The most frequently used follow-up method is a *tickler file*, so called because it tickles the memory that something needs to be done or followed up on a particular date. The tickler file is always in a chronologic arrangement. In its simplest form, it consists of notations on the daily calendar. If information, such as an x-ray report or laboratory report, is expected about a patient with an appointment to come in, the medical assistant might make a note on the calendar or tickler file a day ahead to check on whether the report has arrived.

The tickler file can be a part of a computerized health record system or could be as simple as an email sent to oneself. Many people put reminders on their cell phones using an application (app) specially designed for memos and reminders. The tickler file could also be a card file; 12 guides, one for each month, are placed at the front of the cabinet, container, or other object used to hold the folders. Notations of actions to be taken are placed behind the guides for specific days of the current month. Notations for future months are placed behind the guide for that month. To be effective, the tickler file must be checked first thing each day.

The tickler file can be used in many ways. It is a useful reminder of recurring events, such as payments, meetings, and so forth. On the last day of each month, all the notations from behind the next month's guide are distributed among the daily numbered guides, and the guide for the month just completed is placed at the back of the file.

> **VOCABULARY**
> **tickler file:** A chronologic file used as a reminder that something must be dealt with on a certain date.

> **CRITICAL THINKING 19.9**
> Susan is responsible for checking the tickler file daily. What types of documents and duties might she find inside these files?

Transitory or Temporary File

Many papers are kept longer than necessary because no arrangement is made for separating those with a limited usefulness. This situation can be prevented by having a transitory or temporary file. For example, if a medical assistant writes a letter requesting a reprint of the new patient brochure, the file copy is placed in the transitory folder until the reprint is received. When the reprint is received, the file copy is destroyed. The transitory file is used for materials with no permanent value. The paper may be marked with a "T" and then destroyed when the action is completed.

> **EXCEPTIONAL CUSTOMER SERVICE**
> Patients worry about the security of their information, particularly about who can access it. Lawsuits are often filed when patients discover that an unauthorized person has accessed their protected health information. The medical assistant should listen to a patient's concerns and explain the safety procedures that apply to the EHR in language the patient can understand. Some facilities prepare a brochure to explain the conversion process to the patient and the advantages of the EHR system.
>
> The medical assistant should expect hesitation and even reluctance from patients who are concerned about the privacy of their health information. Patients are concerned about lack of control over who views their records. Be prepared to answer their questions about the safety of their records as related to the EHR. The medical assistant must know how the EHR is protected and what security measures are in place to be able to reassure the patients that their records are protected at all times.

CLOSING COMMENTS

Just as in every aspect of the medical profession, advances in health records management are occurring rapidly, allowing providers and other caregivers to perform their duties more efficiently and accurately. A medical assistant must constantly be willing to learn and to adapt to changes arising from legislation and technologic advances. Computers have become generally accepted as a means of recording health information.

A primary goal of all healthcare facilities is to provide efficient, high-quality patient care. The EHR system can help the staff reach that goal. In the future, every provider's office, hospital, pharmacy, and healthcare facility may be able to access information in minutes, which will improve patient care and save lives. Stay abreast of news and articles related to EHR systems. The healthcare industry is one of constant growth and learning, and today's information technology provides the medical assistant with endless opportunities to make that growth rewarding and applicable to her or his current position.

CHAPTER REVIEW

Having a good understanding of how both paper records and electronic records work is important for all medical assistants. Knowing how a paper record is organized is helpful when you have to find something in that record that was not scanned into the EHR. If the EHR system goes down, you will need to know how to document on a paper form. That form will later be scanned into the EHR. If your organization already has a fully functioning EHR, you should know how to document all of the patient care and related activities.

Content in the health record can be divided into two categories: subjective and objective. Subjective information is generally the information that a patient tells the provider or medical assistant. This includes demographics, health history, family history, social history, and chief complaint. Objective information comes from the provider or medical assistant's observations and tests, things like vital signs, laboratory tests, and diagnostic imaging.

The HITECH Act significantly impacts the use of EHRs in a healthcare facility. Providers must show that they are using EHRs in a meaningful way. To get the financial incentives offered by the federal government, the healthcare facility must show the following:

- The EHR is being used for e-prescribing and other benefits for patients.

CHAPTER 19 The Health Record

- The EHR is being used to electronically exchange health information to improve the quality of healthcare.
- EHR data are being used to improve the quality of care.

Both paper and electronic records can be set up as either a SOR or a POR. Understanding how each of those record systems works will allow you to work more efficiently in each one. In a SOR, the content is organized by its source. Lab test results will be filed/found in the Laboratory section of the record. Discharge summaries will be filed/found in the Hospital section of the record. A POR record has four components:

- Database
- Problem list
- Treatment plan
- Progress notes
  - SOAP approach
    Subjective
    Objective
    Assessment
    Plan

When creating a paper health records system, a number of supplies will be needed. The first decision is what type of storage system will be used. It could be a drawer type file or a horizontal shelf file. Larger organizations may consider a compact file system or an automated file system. In addition to the storage system, there are supplies needed to set up the actual patient records, including file folders, labels, and out guides.

In all offices, there will be a need to file paper documents, even if an EHR is being used for patient information. There are personnel records, tax records, and general correspondence that will need to be filed. A number of filing methods could be used:

- Alphabetic
- Numeric
- Subject

Color coding can help to keep all track of information in all of the filing methods.

SCENARIO WRAP-UP

Susan looks forward to attending her medical assisting classes each day and works diligently to perform to the best of her ability in the classroom. She strives to do well on each procedure check-off and each examination she completes. Her instructors provide excellent feedback and appreciate her contributions to the class.

Susan has the attitude that everything she is allowed to do in the healthcare facility is a learning tool. She regularly asks for additional responsibilities and is always ready to assist a coworker. Dr. Kahn has recognized that she has the desire to learn, and he gives her many opportunities to glean more knowledge through the everyday activities in the office.

Although she is new to the medical profession, Susan learns quickly and thinks logically. She knows the rules and regulations on patient confidentiality and is always careful about the information she provides to those who request it. She is never hesitant about asking her office manager for guidance if she is unsure about any aspect of her duties. Susan is understanding and respectful when patients are concerned about their privacy. Her confidence and warm personality play a role in the trust she earns from the patients at the clinic.

Susan is willing to admit when she has made an error and has sought advice from Dr. Kahn and her office manager when an error needed correction. Although filing is not one of her favorite duties, she can be counted on to do her best while completing this important task. She realizes that filing is critical because the documents in the patient's health record direct the care provided to the patient. An abnormal laboratory report that is missing can make a crucial difference in the patient's care. She takes pride in her work, and she is efficient and accurate where health records are concerned. When she is faced with a new task, she considers it a learning experience and asks for help if she is not completely sure about the way to handle a situation.

Susan's coworkers are supportive and always willing to help her as she learns to be the best medical assistant she can be. Her future as a professional medical assistant certainly holds opportunity and chances for advancement. Just as important, patients trust her. She has alleviated patients' concerns about EHRs by taking the time to explain privacy policies and exactly what information will be accessible to third parties. This trust also gives patients the confidence to reveal personal information and to know that it will be held in the strictest confidence, not just by Susan, but by each employee in the provider's office.

20

Telephone Techniques and Scheduling

LEARNING OBJECTIVES

1. Identify the features found on a multiple-line telephone system, explain the uses of each feature, and discuss how a multiple-line telephone system can be used effectively in a healthcare facility.
2. Discuss the effective use of the telephone, summarize active listening skills, and demonstrate professional telephone techniques.
3. Discuss how to efficiently manage telephone calls in a healthcare facility, document telephone messages accurately, and report relevant information concisely and accurately.
4. Discuss various types of incoming calls, both typical and atypical.
5. Explain how to handle difficult calls, including angry callers.
6. Discuss typical outgoing calls, as well as how to utilize directory assistance.
7. Describe how answering services and automatic call routing systems are used in a healthcare facility.
8. Describe scheduling guidelines, recognize office policies and protocols for handling appointments, and keep patient and provider needs in mind when scheduling appointments.
9. Discuss how to create and establish the appointment matrix.
10. Discuss the advantages of computerized appointment scheduling, and explain how self-scheduling can reduce the number of calls to the medical office.
11. Describe the legality of the appointment scheduling system.
12. List and discuss the different types of appointment scheduling.
13. Discuss how to best handle telephone scheduling. Describe how to schedule a new patient as well as an established patient.
14. Discuss how to schedule inpatient surgeries, outpatient and inpatient procedure appointments, outside visits, pharmaceutical representatives, and salespeople.
15. Describe how to deal with late patients, rescheduling appointments, emergency situations, patients without appointments, and no-show patients.
16. List and describe various ways to increase appointment show rates.
17. Describe how to handle patient cancellations and delays.

CHAPTER OUTLINE

1. **Opening Scenario,** 439
2. **You Will Learn,** 439
3. **Introduction,** 439
4. **Telephone Techniques,** 440
    a. Telephone Equipment, 440
        i. *Multiple-Line Telephone,* 440
        ii. *Headset,* 440
        iii. *Features,* 440
        iv. *Cell Phones,* 442
    b. Effective Use of the Telephone, 442
        i. *Active Listening,* 442
        ii. *Developing a Pleasing Telephone Personality,* 442
    c. Managing Telephone Calls, 443
        i. *Thinking Ahead,* 443
        ii. *Confidentiality,* 444
        iii. *Answering Promptly,* 444
        iv. *Identifying the Facility,* 444
        v. *Identifying the Caller,* 444
        vi. *Screening Incoming Calls,* 444
        vii. *Getting the Information the Provider Needs,* 445
        viii. *Placing Callers on Hold,* 445
        ix. *Transferring a Call,* 445
        x. *Taking a Message,* 445
        xi. *Taking Action on Telephone Messages,* 446
        xii. *Retaining Records of Telephone Messages,* 446
    d. Typical Incoming Calls, 447
        i. *Requests for Prescription Refills,* 447
        ii. *Requests for Directions,* 447
        iii. *Radiology and Laboratory Reports,* 448
        iv. *Progress Reports From Patients,* 448
        v. *Inquiries About Bills,* 448
        vi. *Inquiries About Fees,* 449
        vii. *Requests for Assistance With Insurance,* 449
        viii. *Non-Patient–Related Calls,* 449
    e. Special Incoming Calls, 449
        i. *Patients Who Refuse to Discuss Symptoms,* 449
        ii. *Requests for Test Results,* 449
        iii. *Requests for Information From Third Parties,* 450
        iv. *Complaints About Care or Fees,* 450
        v. *Calls From Staff Members' Families or Friends,* 450
    f. Handling Difficult Calls, 450
        i. *Angry Callers,* 450
        ii. *Unauthorized Inquiry Calls,* 450
        iii. *Callers Who Have Difficulty Communicating,* 450
    g. Typical Outgoing Calls, 451
        i. *Time Zones,* 451
        ii. *Long-Distance Calling,* 451

h. Using Directory Assistance, 452
i. Telephone Services, 452
   i. *Answering Services, 452*
   ii. *Automatic Call Routing, 452*
5. **Scheduling Appointments, 452**
   j. Establishing the Appointment Schedule, 452
      i. *Patient Needs, 453*
      ii. *Provider Preferences and Habits, 453*
   k. Creating the Appointment Matrix, 453
      i. *Establishing Guidelines for Appointment Scheduling, 453*
      ii. *Available Facilities, 454*
   l. Methods of Scheduling Appointments, 454
      i. *Computerized Scheduling, 454*
      ii. *Appointment Book Scheduling, 455*
      iii. *Self-Scheduling, 455*
   m. Legality of the Appointment Scheduling System, 456
   n. Types of Appointment Scheduling, 456
      i. *Time-Specified (Stream) Scheduling, 456*
      ii. *Wave Scheduling, 456*
      iii. *Modified Wave Scheduling, 456*
      iv. *Double-Booking, 457*
      v. *Open Office Hours, 457*
      vi. *Grouping Procedures, 457*
   o. Telephone Scheduling, 457
   p. Scheduling Appointments for New Patients, 457
   q. Scheduling Appointments for Established Patients, 459
      i. *In Person, 459*
      ii. *By Telephone, 459*
   r. Scheduling Other Types of Appointments, 459
      i. *Inpatient Surgeries, 461*
      ii. *Outpatient and Inpatient Procedure Appointments, 461*
      iii. *Outside Visits, 461*
      iv. *Pharmaceutical Representatives, 461*
      v. *Salespeople, 463*
   s. Special Circumstances, 463
      i. *Late Patients, 463*
      ii. *Rescheduling Appointments, 463*
      iii. *Emergency Situations, 464*
      iv. *Patients Without Appointments, 464*
   t. Failed Appointments, 464
      i. *No-Show Policy, 464*
   u. Increasing Appointment Show Rates, 464
      i. *Automated Call Routing, 464*
      ii. *Appointment Cards, 464*
      iii. *Confirmation Calls, 464*
      iv. *Email Reminders, 465*
      v. *Mailed Reminders, 465*
   v. Handling Cancellations and Delays, 465
      i. *When the Patient Cancels, 465*
      ii. *When the Provider Is Delayed, 466*
      iii. *When the Provider Is Called to an Emergency, 466*
      iv. *When the Provider Is Ill or Out of Town, 466*
6. **Closing Comments, 466**
7. **Chapter Review, 466**
8. **Scenario Wrap-Up, 467**

OPENING SCENARIO

Ashlynn McDowell, a recent graduate of a medical assisting program, has begun her first position as a receptionist in at Walden-Martin Family Medical (WMFM) Clinic. Ashlynn is determined to perform to the best of her abilities. However, she has never held a job in a professional office. She knows that she needs to practice all of the skills she learned in school to be an effective receptionist.

WMFM is customer service oriented and wants its patients to feel cared for and special. Ashlynn is anxious to build trust with the patients and to offer them help with the problems they encounter that fall within her realm of responsibility.

WMFM recently purchased computer software that allows Ashlynn to record telephone messages on the computer, and these messages are automatically routed both to an inbox for the provider and as an entry in the patient's health record. Although the system is new to everyone in the office, Ashlynn is determined to become proficient in its use as quickly as possible.

She knows that she must speak clearly and distinctly and that she must be adept at following up. She must be organized and think quickly and creatively. She plans to dress professionally each day so that she projects the right image to patients.

When scheduling appointments, Ashlynn wants to ensure that the healthcare facility remains on schedule throughout the day with minimal wait time for the patients and providers. She leaves a little time in the morning and afternoon for emergency appointments. The healthcare facility uses an automatic call routing system to contact patients to confirm appointments in advance, which increases the show rate.

Ashlynn will strive to be the type of employee who has a willingness to learn, an ability to adapt, and a heart full of compassion for the patient. She is a team player who sincerely wants to cooperate with other staff members who might need her help.

All of the providers at WMFM are pleased that they have found such an eager person to add to the staff, and they will assist and guide Ashlynn as she learns how to make the patients feel like part of the clinic's family. Ashlynn's self-esteem has increased because she feels she is making a great contribution to healthcare.

YOU WILL LEARN

1. To recognize the features of a multiple-line telephone system.
2. To apply active learning principles when communicating with patients.
3. To manage various types of incoming and outgoing calls.
4. To set up the appointment matrix.
5. To differentiate among the various types of appointment scheduling.
6. To schedule patient appointments and procedures.

INTRODUCTION

In this chapter we look at how a medical assistant uses the telephone. That means that we will explore the equipment and features of a business telephone system. The telephone is one of the most important pieces of equipment in a healthcare facility (Fig. 20.1). It is used to communicate with patients, other healthcare organizations, and suppliers. It would be difficult to run an office without a telephone. It is often the first

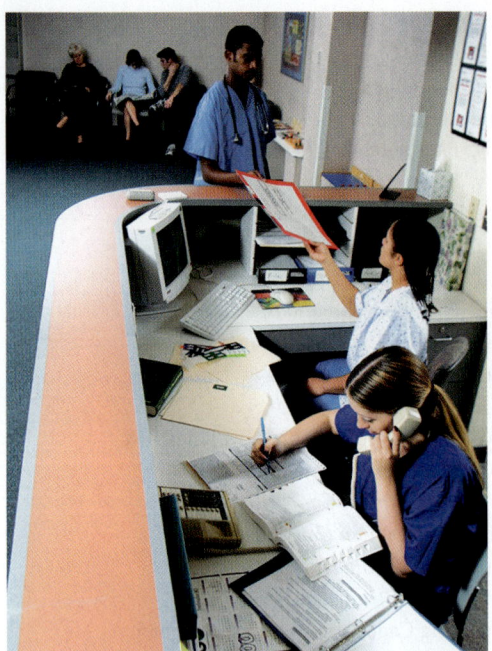

FIG. 20.1 The telephone plays a vital role in the success of the medical practice. (From Proctor D, et al: *Kinn's The Medical Assistant*, ed 13, St. Louis, 2017, Elsevier.)

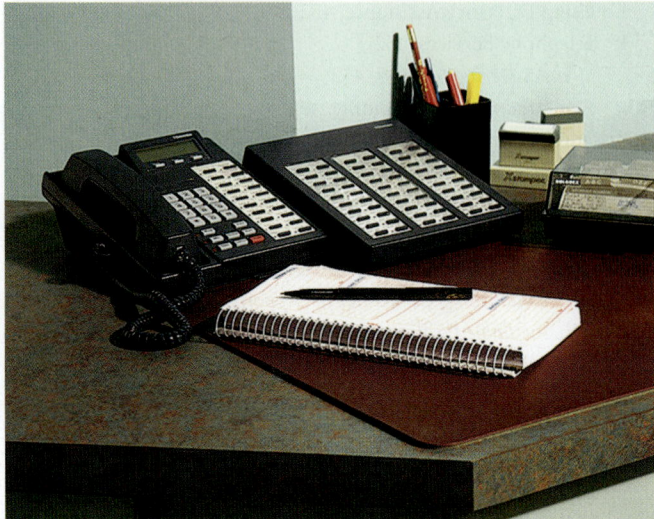

FIG. 20.2 Multiple-line telephones allow numerous calls to come into the office at once. Each call deserves the same kind of attention and care from the medical assistant. (From Proctor D, et al: *Kinn's The Medical Assistant*, ed 13, St. Louis, 2017, Elsevier.)

point of contact with patients, and this is an opportunity to make an outstanding first impression. Developing good telephone techniques will make you a valuable asset to your employer.

We will also look at how an appointment schedule is set up, as well as how to schedule various appointments. Frequently, appointments are scheduled over the telephone, so you will be using the techniques learned in the first part of the chapter. Appointments can also be scheduled in person or even through the facility's web portal. We will also be discussing how to handle missed appointments and how to prevent them from happening.

TELEPHONE TECHNIQUES

Let's start by getting familiar with the equipment used. Then we will move on to how to handle the different types of calls that can be received by the healthcare facility. Finally, we will discuss outgoing calls.

Telephone Equipment

Multiple-Line Telephone. Being familiar with a **multiple-line telephone system** (Fig. 20.2) is a must for medical assistants. Even the smallest healthcare facility has at least two telephone lines so that patients rarely get a busy signal when they try to contact the office. The multiple-line telephone has a button for each line. The button flashes when a call comes in on that line. The button also flashes, although in a different rhythm, when a caller is on hold on that line. This can serve as a reminder for the medical assistant to check back with the caller to see whether he or she would like to remain on hold or leave a message.

The multiple-line telephone also allows you to transfer calls and possibly to set up conference calls, which involve two or more callers. You should be familiar with the multiple-line telephone system used in your healthcare practice.

Headset. Most business telephones have a handset that can be used to answer the telephone. However, the medical assistant who most frequently answers the telephone may want to think about using a *headset* instead (Fig. 20.3). Use of a headset can improve your **ergonomics** (ur guh NOM iks) and help prevent neck strain. Also, having a headset frees your hands to use the computer or take a message.

A headset is a combination earphone and microphone that is attached to the telephone by a cord or is wireless. You can adjust the volume in the earpiece, and you may be able to adjust the sound level of your voice through the microphone for callers who may have difficulty hearing. Bluetooth, a type of short-range wireless technology, allows you to be more mobile while on the telephone. Because this type of headset is not as visible, people may not be aware that you are on the telephone and may start a conversation with you. You should politely indicate that you are on the telephone and you will respond to the person when you can. Some healthcare facilities have a light system that indicates to patients that you are on the phone and you will be with them when the call is complete. Also, many headsets can be muted so that you can speak with someone without the caller hearing you.

Features. Most multiple-line business telephones have many features that allow you to perform a number of different tasks in the healthcare facility. Table 20.1 describes those features and their applications.

CRITICAL THINKING 20.1

Ashlynn hears an employee using the speakerphone function to talk about a patient with another employee. How should she handle this situation? To whom, if anyone, should Ashlynn report this activity? What problems might arise if this type of conversation is overheard?

VOCABULARY

ergonomics: An applied science concerned with designing and arranging things, needed to do your job, in an efficient and safe way.

multiple-line telephone system: A business telephone system that allows for more than one telephone line.

CHAPTER 20 Telephone Techniques and Scheduling

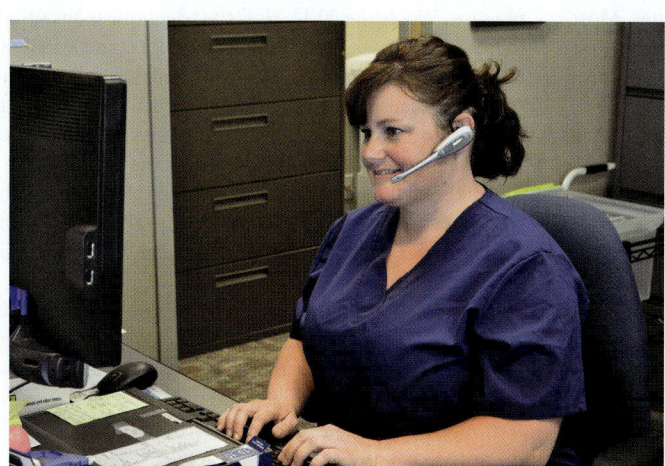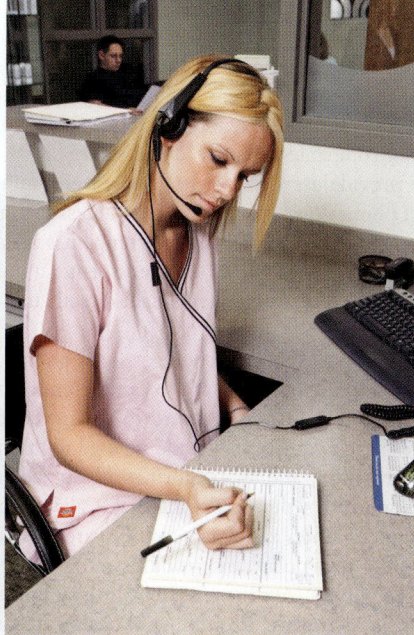

FIG. 20.3 A headset allows the medical assistant to keep the hands free, whereas using the telephone is better ergonomically. (From Proctor D, et al: *Kinn's The Medical Assistant*, ed 13, St. Louis, 2017, Elsevier.)

TABLE 20.1 Telephone Features

Feature	Function	Application
Speakerphone	A telephone with a speaker and a microphone; it can be used without having to pick up and hold the handset. Generally, a button on the telephone is labeled "speaker" (or is indicated with an icon). Once you push it, you can hang up the handset.	Can be useful if you need to have more than two people on the call using the same phone. You should always inform the caller that you will be putting him or her on speakerphone, and let the person know who else will be listening in. You must also be aware of protecting patient information when using a speakerphone. The speakerphone function should not be used in areas such as the patient check-in area or anywhere a conversation can be overheard. The door or reception window should be closed so that no one just walking by can overhear the conversation.
Conference calls	Allow you to have multiple people on the call from different locations.	The person starting the call calls one person, puts that person on hold, and continues the sequence until all parties are on the call. Conference calls can be used when the healthcare facility has more than one location and people from all the locations must be involved in a conversation. For example, a committee may want to discuss policies and procedures for the practice. It is a much better use of time to set up a conference call than to have many people travel to one location.
Voice mail	An electronic system that allows messages from telephone callers to be recorded and stored.	Allows the caller to hear a recorded message that may also provide information about what to do in case of an emergency. Like an answering machine, voice mail records a caller's message, which can later be retrieved. You can keep patients happy by answering voice mail messages quickly.
Call forwarding	Allows the user to automatically send calls to another number, such as an answering service.	If the medical assistant is going to be busy with a patient, the calls can be forwarded to another employee until the task is completed. This prevents the user from missing important calls when away from the main telephone.
Intercom	A two-way communication system with a microphone and loudspeaker at each station. This feature allows for two-way communication, but it does not require you to pick up the handset or use a headset.	This type of communication is not confidential. It can be used to notify staff members of an emergency or to ask the provider to come out of the exam room.

Cell Phones. Considered a luxury item in the very early 2000s, cell (or cellular) phones have become commonplace. Many people no longer have a landline because of the expenses of having two phones, and the cell phone usually is the better buy for the money. Several of the more popular cell phone companies offer free long-distance calls in the United States and may provide users free night and weekend minutes. Most of today's smart phones even allow the user to access the internet and check email on the telephone. Cell phone companies usually offer a text messaging service, which allows the user to enter a message with cell phone keys or by voice, which then is sent directly to a cell phone number.

Many people have a personal cell phone or smart phone. It is a great way to be accessible at all times, but it also can present some issues in a healthcare facility, particularly in regard to patient confidentiality. Most cell phones have a camera that could be used to take pictures of confidential information, and that information can be transmitted quickly to someone else or put on the internet. Calls can be made or taken at inappropriate times and may affect the care of patients. Most healthcare facilities have a policy that prohibits employees from having their personal cell phones with them during working hours.

We have seen an increase in the number of healthcare facilities that are supplying cell phones to their providers. The communication process is improved with the provider use of cell phones. There is ready access to patient information needed for collaboration and care coordination. The provider's cell phone number should never be given out to patients without the provider's permission.

Effective Use of the Telephone

Active Listening. It may seem odd to be discussing listening before speaking in this chapter, but listening well is just as important as speaking well when it comes to communicating on the telephone. When you are on the telephone, you have fewer nonverbal cues to help you determine the message. Therefore it is important that you use good listening skills. When you use active listening skills (Box 20.1), your patients realize that you think they are important and that you respect the message they are communicating to you, whether you are on the telephone or face to face (Box 20.2).

Developing a Pleasing Telephone Personality. Each time a medical assistant answers the telephone, he or she is representing the healthcare practice (Procedure 20.1). How the telephone is answered can influence the caller's impression of the whole office and whether this is where the person wants to be treated. When patients call the healthcare facility, they should hear a friendly yet professional voice. Just as active listening is an important skill to have when receiving the message, a pleasing telephone personality helps when sending the message.

Although it may seem silly, you should always smile when you answer the telephone. The physical act of smiling affects how your words sound. It is as if your caller can hear you smile, and you have created a positive impression.

It is also important to be aware of nonverbal communication that occurs during a telephone conversation. Be aware of your tone of voice. Is it helping to send the message that you want to send? Your callers can tell if you are preoccupied and not focused on the current conversation. You should vary the **pitch** of your voice and avoid speaking in a **monotone**.

Enunciation (in nuhn see EY shuh n) is crucial when speaking on the telephone. You should speak clearly and distinctly so that the caller can understand what you are saying. Many letters of the alphabet sound similar on the telephone, such as B, P, T, and F and S. You may need to clarify with the caller by saying, "That is B as in bravo" (Box 20.3).

VOCABULARY
enunciation: The use of articulate, clear sounds when speaking.
monotone: A succession of syllables, words, or sentences spoken in an unvaried key or pitch.
pitch: The depth of a tone or sound; a distinctive quality of sound.

BOX 20.1 Active Listening

- Be present in the moment.
- Focus solely on the conversation.
- Do not interrupt.
- Do not start forming your response before the person has finished speaking.
- Confirm what the speaker has said, and ask if your interpretation is correct.
- Always be respectful and professional.

Active listening involves:
- Listening to what the speaker is saying
- Interpreting what the message is
- Restating what the speaker said to make sure that you received the intended message

For example, you receive a telephone call from a distraught mother. Using active listening skills, you pick up on the nonverbal cues (see Box 20.2), such as her tone of voice and rate of speech. You can tell she is upset. The mother states that her child has been very sick for the past several days, and nothing she has done has helped with the fever her child has had for 2 days. Your response should be to restate what you heard: the child has been ill with a fever for the past 2 days, and nothing she has tried has brought the fever down. This gives the caller the opportunity to correct any misinformation or to confirm that the information is correct. If it is correct, you should follow the healthcare practice's procedures for handling this situation; most likely, you will schedule an appointment for that same day.

BOX 20.2 Nonvisual/Nonverbal Communication

- Tone of voice
- Speed of speech
- Pitch
- Volume
- Enunciation
- Pausing or hesitation

BOX 20.3 Phonetic Alphabet

A	Alpha	N	November
B	Bravo	O	Oscar
C	Charlie	P	Papa
D	Delta	Q	Quebec
E	Echo	R	Romeo
F	Foxtrot	S	Sierra
G	Golf	T	Tango
H	Hotel	U	Uniform
I	India	V	Victor
J	Juliet	W	Whiskey
K	Kilo	X	X-ray
L	Lima	Y	Yankee
M	Mike	Z	Zulu

CHAPTER 20 Telephone Techniques and Scheduling

PROCEDURE 20.1 Demonstrate Professional Telephone Techniques

Task
Answer the telephone in a provider's office in a professional manner, and respond to a request for action.

Equipment and Supplies
- Telephone
- Pen or pencil
- Appointment book or EHR with appointment scheduling abilities
- Computer
- Notepad

Scenario
Charles Johnson (DOB: 3/3/1958), an established patient of Dr. Martin, has called to schedule an appointment to have his blood pressure checked. This will be a follow-up appointment that is 15 minutes long. He is requesting that the appointment be on a Friday during his lunchtime between 11 a.m. and 12 p.m.

Procedural Steps

1. Demonstrate telephone techniques by answering the telephone by the third ring.
   Purpose: To convey interest in the caller by answering promptly. This makes a positive impression.
2. Speak distinctly with a pleasant tone and expression, at a moderate rate, and with sufficient volume for the person to understand every word.
   Purpose: Proper enunciation will help the patient to understand.
3. Identify the office or provider and yourself.
   Purpose: To assure the caller that the correct number has been reached and to identify the staff member.
4. Verify the caller's identity, and if using an electronic health record, bring the patient's health record to the computer's active screen.
   Purpose: To confirm the origin of the call.
5. Screen the call if necessary.
   Purpose: To determine whether the caller has an emergency and needs immediate attention or referral to a hospital emergency department.
6. Apply active listening skills to assess whether the caller is distressed or agitated and to determine the concern to be addressed.
   Purpose: To make sure the medical assistant hears and understands the message being sent by the patient and to show that the patient has the medical assistant's full attention.
7. Determine the needs of the caller and provide the requested information or service if possible. Provide the caller with excellent customer service. Be as helpful as possible. Check the appointment schedule, and determine the first Friday with an opening available between 11 a.m. and 12 p.m.
   Purpose: To allow the medical assistant to handle many calls and conserve the provider's and staff members' time and energy.
8. Obtain sufficient patient information to schedule the appointment, including the patient's full name, DOB, insurance information, and preferred contact method. Repeat the date and time of the appointment to ensure that the patient has the correct information.
   Purpose: Obtaining the correct patient information ensures that the correct patient record will be pulled (if paper records are used) for the appointment. In an EHR, the appointment will be attached to the correct patient record.
9. Terminate the call in a pleasant manner and replace the receiver gently, always allowing the caller to hang up first.
   Purpose: To promote good public relations, provide excellent customer service, and ensure that the caller has no further questions.

It is important to always be courteous and *tactful*. Think about the words you will use before actually speaking them. For those of us working in a healthcare facility, it is easy to integrate medical terminology into our conversations. However, we must be careful not to use medical *jargon* when speaking with patients, because this makes the message more difficult for them to understand. For example, if you are giving a male patient preprocedural instructions, advise him that he must not eat or drink anything for 12 hours before the procedure; do not tell him he should "stay NPO" (nothing by mouth).

Medical terminology and abbreviations can be considered jargon.

To create a pleasant, friendly, and professional image of the healthcare facility, you must give the caller your full attention. Do not become distracted by other things going on around you. In addition, you should never eat, chew gum, or drink when on the telephone. Use a normal volume and tone of voice, and speak directly into the mouthpiece. Be sure to speak at a moderate rate of speed, because speaking too quickly makes it difficult for the caller to understand you.

VOCABULARY
jargon: The vocabulary of a particular profession as opposed to common, everyday terms.
tactful: The quality of having a sense of what to do or say to maintain good relations with others or to prevent offense.

CRITICAL THINKING 20.2
Ashlynn has a tendency to speak quickly in her normal conversations. How will she need to adjust when answering phones in the healthcare facility? She also is a friendly person and enjoys talking on the phone. What precautions should she take so that this does not become an issue on the job?

Managing Telephone Calls

Thinking Ahead. Whether you are answering incoming calls or placing outgoing calls, it is important to be completely prepared. Before you start answering calls, make sure you have all the supplies needed to do your job:
- Access to a computer (if your office documents telephone messages electronically) or a paper message form
- Working pens
- A watch or clock to record the time

You should be sure to have the healthcare facility's telephone screening guidelines available. Many offices also keep a list of commonly used telephone numbers. This list usually includes poison control, other emergency numbers, community resources to which patients can be referred, and so on.

For outgoing calls, have all the information you need, such as the following:
- Patient's health record
- Telephone number of the person you will be calling
- List of questions
- Notepad and a pen to make notes during the conversation.

Confidentiality. All communication in a healthcare facility must maintain patient confidentiality. When using the telephone, you must be aware of what is going on around you and who may be able to overhear your conversation. If patient-sensitive information will be discussed, place the call in an area where others cannot hear, especially other patients. Be careful when using a speakerphone because the sound can travel farther than you might think. Someone might overhear private medical information. This is a violation of the law, specifically the Health Insurance Portability and Accountability Act (HIPAA).

Answering Promptly. Telephone contact is often the first interaction with a patient. If the person's call is not answered promptly, this can create a negative impression before he or she even talks to someone. It is important that a call be answered within three rings. To accomplish this, you may need to do the following:
- Interrupt the call you are on by asking if you can place the person on hold for a moment.
- Answer the second call; if it is not an emergency, ask that person if you may place him or her on hold.
- Return to the first caller.

An incoming call should never be answered with "Please hold." You should always find out the reason for the call before placing the person on hold. If it is an emergency, the second call is handled promptly, before you return to the first call. If it is not an emergency, you should always ask if you can place the person on hold and wait for an answer before pushing the hold button. If the person refuses to be placed on hold, determine the reason why and assure the caller that you will return to his or her call quickly.

The medical assistant who routinely answers the telephone should know how to activate emergency medical services (EMS) in his or her area. Generally, this means dialing 911. You may need to make this call for a patient who has called the healthcare facility and is now unable to contact EMS on her or his own. If your phone system allows it, you can set up a conference call that includes the patient, EMS, and yourself. It is important to get a telephone number where the caller can be reached, just in case you get disconnected. It also is important to keep the patient or caregiver on the line while contacting EMS.

Identifying the Facility. When answering incoming telephone calls, the medical assistant should do the following:
- Identify the facility.
- State his or her name.
- Follow with an offer of help.

For example, you could begin by saying, "Good morning, Walden-Martin Family Medical Clinic. This is Ashlynn. How may I help you?" Medical assistants must always follow the policy of the healthcare facility when answering incoming calls. Speaking slowly and smoothly, with good enunciation, ensures that your callers understand whom they have reached.

Identifying the Caller. If the caller does not offer a name, the medical assistant should ask, "May I ask who is calling?" It can be helpful to write down the caller's name and try to use it at least three times during the conversation, if it does not compromise patient confidentiality. This helps to make a strong connection and assures the patient that he or she has been identified correctly.

Occasionally callers refuse to identify themselves to the medical assistant and insist that they speak with the provider. You must be clear and state in a professional manner that you cannot connect the caller to the provider without knowing who the caller is. The caller may be a sales representative, and salespeople know that if they identify themselves, they will not get the opportunity to talk with the provider. When it becomes clear that the caller will not give a name but still insists on speaking with the provider, you can tell the person that the provider is busy with patients and offer to take a message. If the caller cannot leave a name for the message, then he or she may want to write a letter and mark it Personal. Most people do not want to wait for a response to a letter and will then give you their names so that you can take a message.

Screening Incoming Calls. Most healthcare facilities expect the medical assistant answering the telephone to *screen* the calls. You must determine which calls should be routed directly to the provider, which to the triage (tree AHZH) area, and which to the billing office. The provider, office manager, and staff members who will be answering the telephone should work together to develop policies for screening calls.

The first step in call screening is to determine who the caller is and the nature of the call. If the call is from a patient with a question about a statement that he or she just received in the mail, the call can be transferred to the billing office. If the call involves determining whether a patient should be seen that day, it can be transferred to the triage area. If the caller asks to speak directly to the provider, the situation can become more complicated, and healthcare facility policies should be created to address these cases.

Healthcare facility policies often state that calls from other providers are put through immediately. If that is not possible, assure the caller that the provider will return the call as soon as possible. Some providers may also ask that calls be put through immediately for certain family members. If the provider does not want to take the call, the medical assistant must tactfully tell the caller that the provider cannot be disturbed at this time.

Screening policies should also address how calls should be handled when the provider is out of the office. If the provider is to be out of the office for an extended period (e.g., for a conference or vacation), another provider is usually designated to handle calls. It should be explained that the provider is out of the office, but another provider is taking the calls. If the call is not an emergency, take a message, and the designated provider can return the call.

If a call is an emergency, the policies for handling emergency calls apply. Many emergency calls require judgment on the part of the person answering the telephone in the medical practice. Good judgment comes from experience and proper training by the provider. It is important to know what a real emergency is, as well as how such calls should be handled. The person answering the telephone should determine whether the call is truly life threatening. If so, never hang up the telephone until an ambulance reaches the patient or other help arrives. When necessary, ask another staff member to call 911 while remaining on the line with the patient. Emergency calls may include the following conditions or symptoms:
- Chest pain
- Profuse bleeding
- Severe allergic reactions
- Cessation of breathing
- Injuries resulting in loss of consciousness
- Broken bones

VOCABULARY

emergency: An unexpected, life-threatening situation that requires immediate action.

triage: To sort out and classify the injured; used in the military and emergency settings to determine the priority of a patient to be treated.

An **urgent** call may be an adult patient with a fever over 102° F (38.9° C), an animal bite, or an increasingly painful ear infection. Emergency calls are life threatening, whereas an urgent call requires prompt attention but is not life threatening. In the case of emergencies, often the provider instructs the patient to go straight to the closest hospital emergency department instead of the office. In an urgent situation, the patient will be given an appointment on the same day. Policies and procedures manuals should indicate the action to take in emergency situations. When in doubt, always ask the office manager or the provider.

If the provider is in, the call may need to be transferred to him or her immediately. All offices should have a written plan of action for the times the provider is not physically present in the office. These policies should include typical questions to ask the caller to determine if the situation is a true emergency. Here are some examples:
- At what telephone number can you be reached?
- Where are you located?
- What are the chief symptoms?
- When did they start?
- Has this happened before?
- Are you alone?
- Do you have transportation?

Getting the Information the Provider Needs. As the medical assistant gains experience and better knows the provider, he or she begins to have a sense of the questions the provider will have for patients who call the facility. For example, the provider is usually interested in the following:
- How long the patient has had symptoms
- What makes the symptoms better or worse
- What remedies have been tried
- What has worked and not worked

If the patient complains of painful urination, the medical assistant should ask about pain in the back or blood in the urine. One way to learn about questions to ask is to carefully listen to the provider as he or she questions patients about their symptoms. This can help you learn more about signs and symptoms and enable you to better assist the provider.

Remember to always be "patient with your patients." Those who call the healthcare facility for help are almost never at their best. When feeling ill, people often are short tempered and even display poor manners. Some can be verbally abusive. Treat patients as if they were family members, and they will recognize care and compassion in the medical facility.

If the provider is unavailable for only part of the day, take a message and inform the caller that the provider currently is out of the office but will return calls when he or she returns. It is important to give the caller the time frame in which the provider will be returning calls so that the patient does not waste time sitting by the phone while waiting for the call. Stress that the time frame is approximate because emergencies cannot be predicted. If the caller is unavailable when the provider usually returns calls, ask when would be a convenient time and let the caller know you will try to work with that time frame.

Screening calls is an important task for medical assistants who answer the telephone. It can keep the healthcare facility running on schedule and ensure that calls that need to get to the provider do so immediately.

> **VOCABULARY**
> **urgent:** An acute situation that requires immediate attention but is not life threatening.

Placing Callers on Hold. When working with a multiple-line telephone, it is not uncommon for more than one call to come in at a time. If you are on one call and another line rings you should do the following:
- Put the first call on hold.
- Answer the second call.
- Determine if it is an emergency or not.
  - If it is an emergency, follow the emergency call procedures.
  - If it is not an emergency, ask if you can place them on hold.
- Return to the first call.

The medical assistant should always ask before placing a caller on hold. If it has been determined through the screening process that this is a call that does not need to be put through to the provider right away (or if the call needs to be transferred to someone else in the healthcare facility and that person is not immediately available), you should ask if the caller would like to be put on hold, or if he or she would prefer to be called back. If you know that the person with whom the caller needs to speak may be busy for quite a while, inform the caller of that. If the caller still wants to wait, check back periodically to make sure the caller wants to remain on hold. No longer than 1 minute should pass before you check back with the caller. When you return to the call, you can use a statement such as "Thank you for waiting. Would you like to continue to hold, or should I take a message?"

Minimizing the wait for the caller shows concern, and freeing up the telephone lines is important for other people trying to contact the healthcare facility.

Transferring a Call. During the screening process, the medical assistant may determine that the call should be transferred to the provider or to another person in the facility. Consider the following example: Ms. Fields calls your office because she has a billing question. You should ask Ms. Fields' permission before placing her on hold, and wait for a response. It is also helpful to give Ms. Fields the name and extension of the person to whom you will be transferring her call (if it is not the provider). This way, if Ms. Fields happens to get disconnected, she will have that information when she calls back. Once you have Ms. Fields' permission to put her on hold, contact the person to whom the call is being transferred. In this case, that is Mr. Lewis in the billing department. Tell Mr. Lewis who is calling and the reason for the call; this allows Mr. Lewis to be prepared to help Ms. Fields when the connection is made. Mr. Lewis may ask for a moment to pull up information before you put Ms. Fields' call through. You should stay on the line to introduce Ms. Fields to Mr. Lewis and to make sure the connection is made. If Mr. Lewis is unavailable, ask Ms. Fields if she would like to be connected to his voice mail. Some callers may prefer that you take a message in written form and bring it to the proper person.

Medical assistants who answer telephone calls must know who does what in the healthcare facility. An organizational chart with telephone extensions can be helpful, but it must be kept up to date so that calls can be transferred successfully.

Taking a Message. Telephone messages are an important part of patient care (Procedure 20.2). The messages may be taken in a handwritten or an electronic format. The patient relies on the medical assistant to deliver the message to a provider or the appropriate person, who can make a decision (then or later). This response is then communicated back to the patient without interrupting the flow of patients through the healthcare facility. You should be sure to let the caller know when to expect a call back; for example, explain that the provider usually returns calls between 3 and 4 p.m.

Whether the message is taken in a handwritten or an electronic format, the information needed for a complete message is the same:

PROCEDURE 20.2 Document Telephone Messages and Report Relevant Information Concisely and Accurately

Task
Take an accurate telephone message and follow up on the caller's requests.

Equipment and Supplies
- Telephone
- Computer or
- Message pad
- Pen or pencil
- Health record

Scenario
Norma Washington (DOB: 8/1/1944), an established patient of Dr. Martin, has called to report her blood pressure (BP) readings, which she has been taking at home. Dr. Martin had made a change in her medication and wanted her to monitor her BP at home for 3 days and call in with the results. She has taken her blood pressure in the morning and in the evening for the past 3 days, with the following results:

Day 1: 144/92 in the a.m., 156/94 in the p.m.
Day 2: 136/84 in the a.m., 142/86 in the p.m.
Day 3: 132/80 in the a.m., 138/82 in the p.m.

Procedural Steps

1. Demonstrate telephone techniques by answering the telephone using the guidelines presented in Procedure 20.1.
Purpose: To answer promptly and courteously, which conveys interest in the caller and promotes good customer service.
2. Take the phone message (either on a message pad or by data entry into the computer), and obtain the following information:
   - Name of the person to whom the call is directed
   - Name of the person calling
   - Caller's telephone number
   - Reason for the call
   - Action to be taken
   - Date and time of the call
   - Initials of the person taking the call

Purpose: To have accurate information, which allows the staff member or provider to address the caller's issues quickly and efficiently.

3. Apply active listening skills, and repeat the information to the caller after recording the message.
Purpose: To verify that all the information was recorded accurately.
4. End the call, and wait for the caller to hang up first.
5. Document the telephone call with all pertinent information in the patient's health record.
Purpose: To ensure that the patient's health record is kept up to date.
6. Deliver the phone message to the appropriate person.
7. Follow up on important messages.
Purpose: To make sure important issues are addressed in a timely manner.
8. If using paper messaging, keep old message books for future reference. Carbonless copies allow the facility to keep a permanent record of phone messages. If using an electronic system, the message will be saved to the patient's record automatically.
Purpose: To have a permanent source of messages in case the information is needed after the paper message has been discarded. This can also serve as a telephone log.
9. File pertinent phone messages in the patient's health record. Make sure to close the computer record after the documentation has been done.
Purpose: To keep a permanent record of important information in the patient's chart.

---

1. The name of the person calling
2. The name of the person to whom the call is directed
3. The caller's daytime, evening, or cell phone number
4. The reason for the call, including the telephone number of the caller's pharmacy if a medication is requested
5. The action to be taken
6. The date and time of the call
7. The initials of the person who took the call

Messages taken on paper. Many types of message pads or books are available (Fig. 20.4). Many are pressure-sensitive, making a copy of the message and serving as a telephone call log. The original is given to the person the message is for and the medical assistant will have a copy to use for follow-up. Having legible handwriting is a must when taking a manual, handwritten message.

Messages recorded electronically. Most electronic health record (EHR) systems can be used to record telephone messages (Fig. 20.5). The EHR automatically saves a copy of the message to the patient's health record and sends the message to the provider. The provider can either call the patient directly or give the medical assistant directions to respond to the patient. The electronic system may also be able to do the following:

- Flag a message
- Indicate its urgency or that it requires a call back
- Note that a prescription refill has been requested

Taking Action on Telephone Messages. The message process is not complete until the necessary action has been taken. If a handwritten system is used, use an identifying mark to indicate a message that requires action. If an electronic system is used, check periodically during the day to be sure you do not have to complete the response to the message, such as calling the patient back or contacting the pharmacy. For risk-management purposes, the healthcare facility should have a policy on the documentation of telephone messages and the specific information that must be included. Medical assistants should become familiar with that policy.

Retaining Records of Telephone Messages. If a handwritten system is used for recording telephone messages, the healthcare facility must establish a policy on how to keep telephone message records. If the message relates to patient care, a copy of the message should be added to the patient's health record. If the health record is electronic, this may mean scanning in a copy of the paper message and attaching it to the EHR. The copy in the message book usually is retained for the same period that the statute of limitations runs for medical professional liability cases.

If an electronic system is used, the message is automatically saved to the patient's record, along with the response to the message. The message record can show the following:

- Whether the patient contacted the office
- If the office responded to that contact
- What the response was

All of these are key points if a medical professional liability case is brought against the provider. In addition, accurate telephone records can ensure quality patient care and customer service.

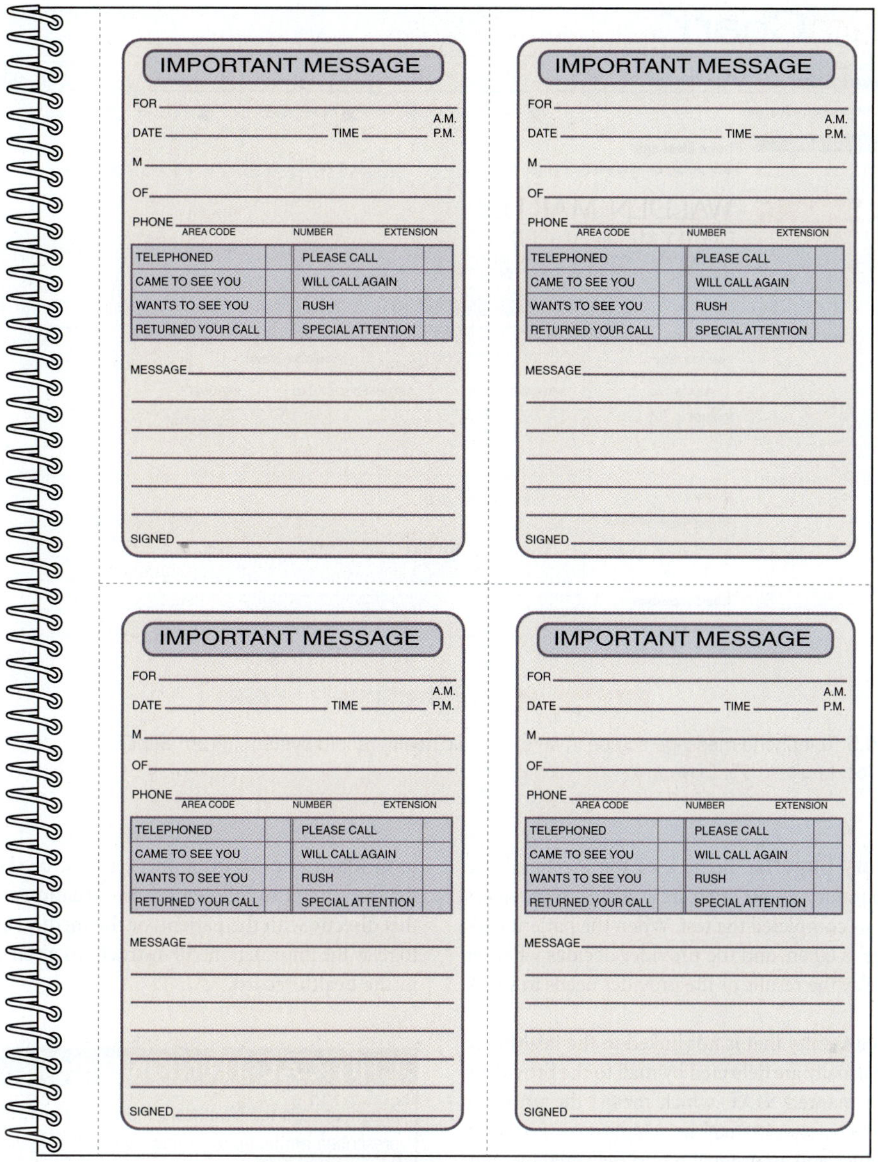

FIG. 20.4 Telephone message forms.

Typical Incoming Calls

Handling incoming calls is often the responsibility of the medical assistant. You can handle many calls directly, but some will require the assistance of others. Knowing how to respond to the different types of calls will make you a valuable asset to the healthcare facility.

Requests for Prescription Refills.
Patients will often call the healthcare facility when they need a prescription refilled. It could be that there were no refills on the original prescription or that they have used all of the refills. Patients must provide the following information when requesting a prescription refill:
- Medication name
- Dosage
- How many pills are taken in a day
- Any issues with the medication
- Whether they want to use a pharmacy mail-order service or pick up the prescription
- Pharmacy address and phone number

It is important for a medical assistant to be familiar with the common medication names and the abbreviations used in a prescription. Using the correct spelling of the medication is very important. See Appendix C for abbreviations and Appendix D for the most common medications and their spelling.

Requests for Directions.
Each office should have a clear set of written directions that can be read to a caller who wants to know how to get to the office. Prepare the directions from various points in the area—for instance, one set for a patient coming from the north and another for a patient coming from the south. Place these directions close to the telephone so that all employees can find them easily. Not all employees live close to the clinic or are familiar with the area; therefore the written set of directions will be helpful both to staff members and to patients. Put a map on the office website, and direct patients there for printable directions. Never simply suggest that callers refer to an internet map when they ask for directions.

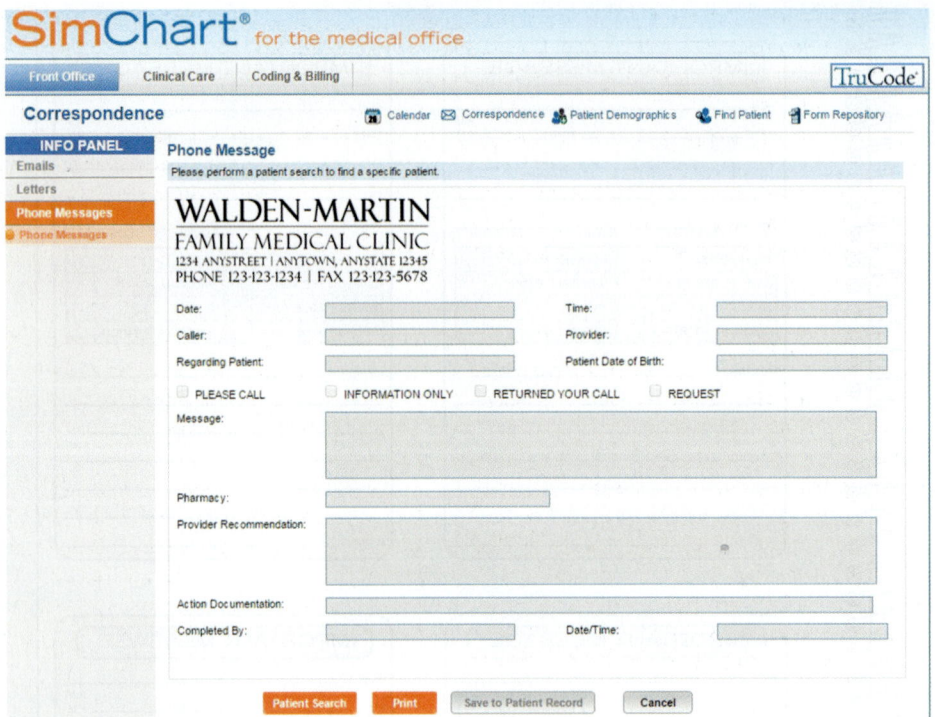

FIG. 20.5 Telephone message screen in an electronic health record system. (From *SimChart for the Medical Office*, St. Louis, 2015, Elsevier.)

Radiology and Laboratory Reports. Because of the increased use of EHRs, radiology and laboratory results often are available to providers as soon as the technician has completed the test. When the patient calls for those results, a message is taken, and the provider decides whether the medical assistant can relay the results or the provider needs to speak to the patient directly.

When tests are done at a facility that is not linked to the healthcare facility's EHR, the findings usually are delivered by mail to the provider's office. If the test has been marked STAT, which means the provider wants the results immediately, reports may be telephoned, faxed, or emailed to the provider's office and an original report delivered by mail.

> **VOCABULARY**
> **STAT:** The medical abbreviation for the Latin term *statum*, meaning immediately; at this moment.

It is helpful to have blank laboratory results forms available that list the various tests, with their normal values, so that you can easily and accurately document results telephoned to the healthcare facility. This can save time, and you can be assured that the test name is spelled correctly. You should repeat the results you have been given to make sure you have written them down correctly. This report must be documented in the patient's health record and given to the provider for review.

Progress Reports From Patients. Providers sometimes ask patients to telephone the office to report on their condition a few days after the office visit. The medical assistant can take such calls and relay the information to the provider. Assure the patient that you will inform the provider of the call. The report should be documented in the health record. The provider should always be informed immediately about unsatisfactory progress reports, and he or she should give instructions for the patient to follow in those situations. The provider may discuss this directly with the patient, or the medical assistant may be instructed to relay the information. All instructions given should also be documented in the health record.

> **CRITICAL THINKING 20.3**
> A patient calls the healthcare facility to report that she has been taking her prescribed antibiotic for 3 days and still does not feel any better. She says she might even feel worse. She asks Ashlynn if she should stop taking the pills. How should Ashlynn respond to this patient? What actions should Ashlynn take in response to this telephone call? What should Ashlynn document in the patient's record?

Inquiries About Bills. A patient may ask to speak with the provider about a recent bill. Ask the caller to hold for a moment while you access the account information from the computer or paper files. If you find nothing irregular in the account, return to the telephone and say, "I have your account in front of me now. Perhaps I can answer your question." Most likely the caller will have a simple inquiry (e.g., whether the insurance company has paid its portion), or the person may want to delay making a payment until the next month. Not all patients realize that the medical assistant usually makes such decisions and is the best person with whom to discuss these matters. If the healthcare facility uses an external billing service, you may need to provide the caller with that agency's telephone number. When an external billing service is used, that telephone number is often shown on the patient's statement. When necessary, document the patient's call in the EHR or in the physical record, such as noting that the patient promised to pay on a certain date.

A patient may have questions about a statement that came in the mail. If another employee handles billing matters, tell the patient that the call will be transferred to the billing office. If you are responsible for billing, politely ask the patient to hold the line while you access the account. When returning to the call, thank the patient for waiting and carefully explain the charges. If an error has occurred, apologize and say that a corrected statement will be sent out at once. Always remember to thank the patient for calling. If patients are properly advised about charges at the time services are rendered, the number of these calls can be reduced considerably.

Inquiries About Fees. Fees vary widely in each healthcare facility, and quoting an exact fee before the provider sees the patient can be difficult. However, patients should be given a good estimate, especially on the first visit. Asking a patient to just appear at the office without having any idea of the cost is unreasonable. Discuss with the provider or office manager what range should be quoted to the patient. Your quote should include the statement that the fees vary depending on the patient's condition as well as any tests the provider might order. Most healthcare facilities require patients to pay the health insurance copayment (or copay) on the day service is provided. The caller should be informed of this policy. If fees are regularly discussed on the telephone, a suggested script should be included in the policies and procedures manual.

Requests for Assistance With Insurance. In the ever-changing world of health insurance, patients are often confused about their coverage, how payment is determined, and what they are financially responsible for when it comes to their bill from the healthcare facility. A solid understanding of the basics of health insurance, including managed care, allows you to answer patient questions about insurance. If the question is beyond your knowledge, you should know to whom to transfer the call so that the patient can get an answer.

Questions about participating providers. Patients may call the office to inquire whether the provider is a participating provider with their insurance plan or managed care organization. A list of the insurance plans that the provider has a contract with should be readily available to the medical assistant who answers the telephone. This is important because insurance benefits vary widely for patients based on whether they see a participating provider or a nonparticipating provider. A claim may even be denied if the provider is not a participant for the patient's insurance company.

Requests for referrals. Primary care providers are often asked for referrals to specialists. If the provider has furnished the medical assistant with a list of providers for this purpose, these inquiries may be handled without consulting the provider, unless the patient's insurance plan requires a written referral. However, the provider should always be informed of such requests. Referrals should also be documented in the patient's health record.

Some managed care organizations require a provider referral before a patient may see a specialist. This referral should come from the provider unless he or she has authorized automatic referrals. Most providers require the patient to come in for an office visit to discuss the referral. Afterward, a staff member completes the referral process. There is often a form that must be completed and sent to the insurance company. This process may also be done electronically. A managed care organization may offer the option of using its website to enter the referral information and then electronically forwarding the information to the new provider. Handle these calls as quickly as possible so that the patient may make an appointment to see the referral provider.

Non-Patient–Related Calls. Not all calls concern patients. Calls may come from the accountant about banking procedures, office supplies, or office maintenance. Most of these calls can be handled by the medical assistant or referred to the appropriate person. For some of these calls, the medical assistant may need to gather additional information and return the call.

Pharmaceutical representatives and salespeople will often call and ask to speak to the provider. A message should be taken that includes what product they want to talk to the provider about. The provider may decide to return these calls or ask that an appointment be scheduled to talk about the new product. It is also possible that the provider will ask the office manager to talk to the salesperson.

Special Incoming Calls

Patients Who Refuse to Discuss Symptoms. Sometimes patients have symptoms that they are embarrassed about. They may ask to speak only to the provider. The medical assistant should let the patient know that it will help the provider to know what the patient's concern is before returning the call. It is important to remain courteous to all patients. If the patient refuses to discuss any symptoms, follow the healthcare facility's procedures, which may include suggesting that the patient make an appointment with the provider to discuss the problem in person.

Requests for Test Results. It is the responsibility of the provider to notify the patient of test results, especially if they are abnormal. Often a patient is told to call the healthcare facility for test results. When a patient calls for the results, make sure of the following:
- The test results are back from the laboratory
- The provider has seen them and has given you permission to communicate the results before sharing them with the patient

If specified in the office policy, the medical assistant can give test results to the patient. Patients do not always understand that the medical assistant cannot give out information without the provider's permission. If the results are unfavorable, the provider should be the one to inform the patient and give further instructions. This call must be handled tactfully. Otherwise, the patient may feel as if the staff is hiding information.

Most providers prefer that medical assistants give only normal test results to patients. However, the medical assistant may give abnormal test results if authorized by the provider. For example, when a patient has an abnormal Pap test result, the medical assistant usually is the person who calls the patient with the result and further instructions from the provider. If the patient has any questions about the test result, she must be referred to the provider. The medical assistant needs good communication skills to relay information like this without crossing the line of practicing medicine without a license.

The best policy for dealing with more serious abnormal test results is to schedule an appointment for the patient to see the provider. These results are best relayed in person instead of on the telephone.

Patients who call the office for test results must be identified before the results are given. Some offices use a special code that is written in

---

VOCABULARY

copayment (copay): A set dollar amount that the policy holder must pay for each visit.

participating provider: A physician or other healthcare provider who enters into a contract with a specific insurance company or program and by doing so agrees to abide by certain rules and regulations set forth by that particular insurance company.

the patient's health record, and knowledge of this code or password gives the person access to the information. Other offices may use the patient's date of birth or other information that is known only to the patient and has been shared with the healthcare facility. You should always use at least two different methods of identifying patients.

Medical assistants must know and follow federal regulations and the laws in their state regarding the release of any information to someone other than the patient. It is important to note that this includes information about a minor. Make sure the right individual is on the line before offering results by verifying the patient's name and date of birth. It is considered a breach of confidentiality and of the Privacy Rules of HIPAA if the patient is not identified correctly and information is released to the wrong individual.

Requests for Information From Third Parties. The patient must give permission before any information is given to third-party callers such as the following:
- Insurance companies
- Attorneys
- Relatives
- Neighbors
- Employers
- Any other third party

HIPAA is specific about the information that should be included in the release of information form. The patient must specify who can receive the information and exactly what information can be released. The release of information form must also include an expiration date. The medical assistant must carefully review the patient's form before releasing any information to third parties.

Complaints About Care or Fees. A medical assistant may be able to offer an acceptable explanation to a patient who complains about the charged fee. Often the patient simply does not understand a charge, and the medical assistant can provide help by reviewing the bill. If a patient seems angry, offer to pull the health record, research the problem, and, if needed, discuss it with the provider. Four magic words often calm the angry patient: "Let me help you." This reassures the patient that someone is willing to talk about the problem. However, if you are unable to calm down the patient easily, the provider or office manager may prefer to talk to the patient directly.

When callers complain, do not attempt to blame someone else, and never argue with the patient. Find the source of the problem, and then present options to the caller as to how the situation can be resolved. Remember to treat callers in the same manner that you would wish to be treated. A complaint may seem small and insignificant to the office staff, but it may be a serious issue to the patient. Provide good customer service to patients, and complaints will be few and far between.

Calls From Staff Members' Families or Friends. Personal calls can tie up the telephone lines. Sometimes a call is necessary in emergencies, but staff members should never monopolize the telephone for personal business and conversations. Patient emergency calls could be coming through, and the lines must be clear. Keep personal calls to an absolute minimum.

Handling Difficult Calls

Angry Callers. No matter how efficient the medical assistant is on the telephone or how well liked the provider might be, sooner or later an angry caller will be on the phone. The anger may have a real cause, or the caller's irritation may have resulted from a misunderstanding. Handling such calls is a real challenge. First, take the needed actions, even if it is to say that the matter will be discussed with the provider as soon as possible and that the patient will be called back later. If answers are not readily available, a friendly promise that the situation is important and that every attempt will be made to find the answer quickly usually calms the angry feelings.

The medical assistant may find that lowering his or her tone of voice and volume of speech may force the angry caller to do the same. This method does not always work, but it usually is true that when dealing with an angry person, calm promotes calm. Some patients may misread this method and become even angrier, thinking that their complaint is not being taken seriously. The ability to get along with others is critical when dealing with angry people. The more skilled the medical assistant becomes, the better able he or she is to deal with multiple types of personalities.

Always avoid getting angry or defensive in response to an angry caller, and try to get to the root of the real problem. Express interest and understanding, take careful notes, and follow through with the problem to the most appropriate resolution. Never "pass the buck" by saying, "That's not my job" or "I am not the person who filed that insurance claim." No matter whose fault the problem is, it is best to deal with it and find a solution instead of placing blame. It is important to respond to the patient when you said you would, even if the call is to tell him or her that you need a bit more time to work on the problem. Keeping the patient in the loop shows that you want to come up with a solution.

> **CRITICAL THINKING 20.4**
>
> An angry caller raises his voice at Ashlynn over an issue that happened before she began to work at WMFM. She suggests that he speak with the office manager, but he refuses and continues to berate Ashlynn. What choices does Ashlynn have in this situation? Should she simply hang up on the patient? How can the call be handled diplomatically?

Unauthorized Inquiry Calls. Some people will call the provider's office requesting information to which they are not entitled. These callers must be told politely but firmly that such information cannot be given to them because of privacy laws. Demanding callers should be referred to the office manager or provider.

Callers Who Have Difficulty Communicating. Occasionally calls come into the office from patients or family members who have difficulty with the English language. The medical assistant must use listening skills to make sure that he or she has understood the caller.

If a certain language is common in the area, the healthcare facility should consider hiring a medical assistant who is **bilingual** (bahy LING gwuh l). Some patients speak English but have a heavy accent, so you should listen carefully and ask questions to be sure you have understood the person correctly.

Many resources are available to help with translation:
- A translator who would be available to help with telephone calls and patient visits in the office
- Online services that offer translation assistance

If the healthcare facility has a number of patients who speak a particular language other than English, it would be helpful to have commonly used phrases available in that language, especially the phrases that would refer the patient to the translation service the healthcare facility uses.

> **VOCABULARY**
> **bilingual:** The ability to communicate effectively in two languages.

Some providers may have patients who are deaf or hard of hearing. These patients may use a *relay system* to communicate with healthcare facilities over the telephone. Some relay systems have the patient use a keyboard to enter the information, which is passed on to an operator. The operator then calls the office and reads the information to you; your response is then typed back to the patient. Newer technology uses an online *captioned* telephone service, much like closed captioning for television. Many smart phones can be equipped with a translation app, which can be used assist the caller. You should be familiar with the way this system works so that you can professionally participate in these conversations.

Typical Outgoing Calls

Most outgoing calls in the healthcare facility are in response to incoming calls. The same rules for courtesy and diction apply to calls made from the healthcare facility to patients, other individuals, and businesses.

It is helpful to plan outgoing calls in advance. For instance, if the medical assistant is placing an order for office supplies, a list should be made that includes the product, the item number, the price, and the quantity needed. Questions about the various products ordered should be noted so that they can be asked while on the telephone with the supplier.

Some medical assistants find it helpful to make all outgoing calls at once, when possible. This way the calls can be made one after another, and if a call back is necessary, the medical assistant is likely to still be by the telephone. Organizing calls increases office efficiency.

Never be rude to an individual on the telephone. Remember to treat those on the other end of the telephone as you would wish to be treated. Do not forget that you represent the provider and must behave in a professional manner at all times.

Time Zones. When making outgoing calls, keep time zones in mind, especially when calling patients. If you are trying to contact a patient who is spending the winter somewhere else, you should place that call at an appropriate time for the patient. If you are trying to get information from an insurance company, you should call when someone is available to answer your questions. The continental United States is divided into four standard time zones: Pacific, Mountain, Central, and Eastern (Fig. 20.6). When it is noon Pacific time, it is 3 p.m. Eastern time. If you will be calling from San Francisco to a business or professional office in New York, plan to make the call no later than 1 p.m. When it is 2 p.m. on the West Coast, it is 5 p.m. on the East Coast.

Long-Distance Calling. Long-distance calls are simple to place, usually inexpensive, and efficient. When information is needed in a hurry, using

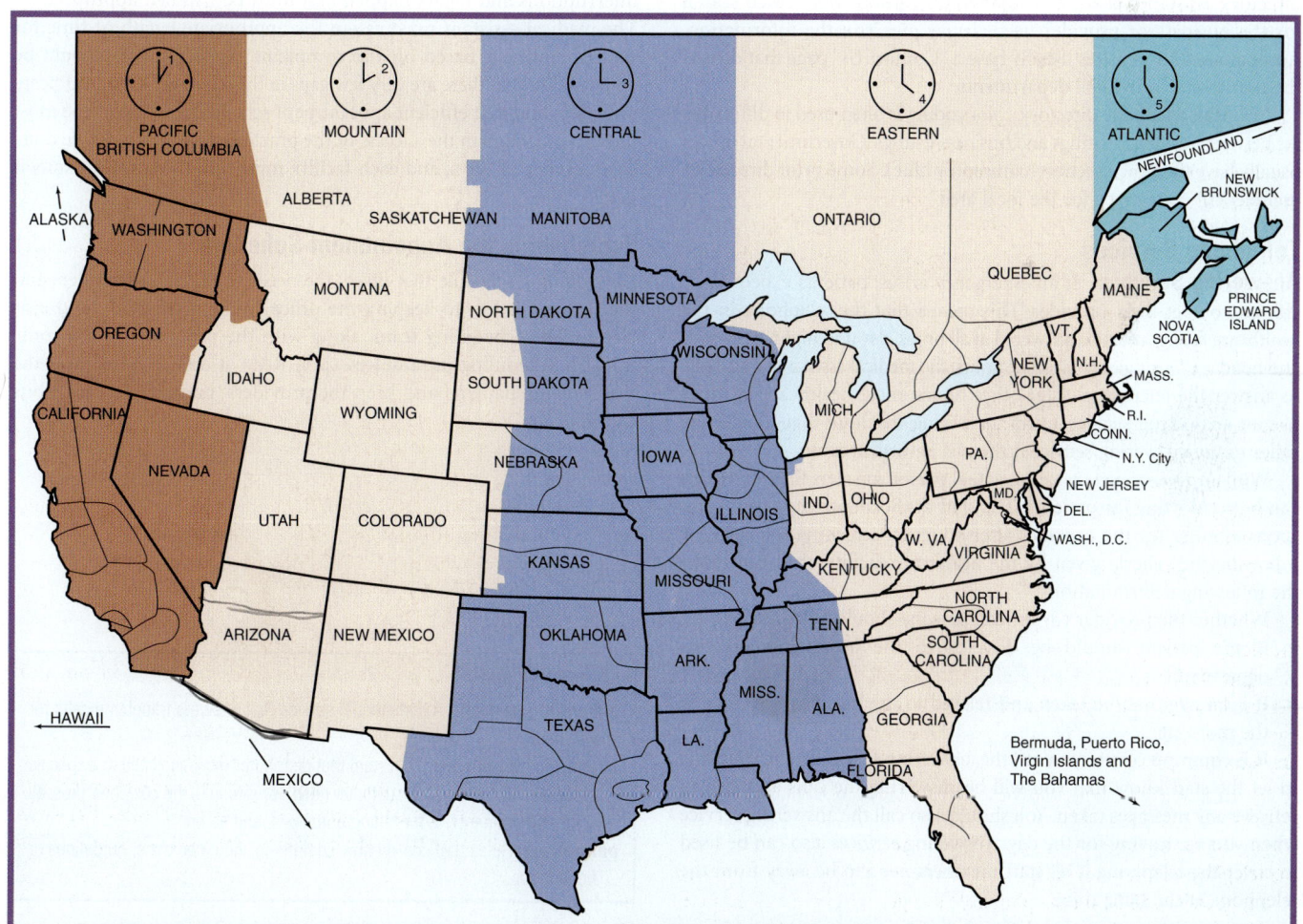

FIG. 20.6 Time zones across the United States. (From Proctor D, et al: *Kinn's The Medical Assistant*, ed 13, St. Louis, 2017, Elsevier.)

the telephone is much quicker than written communication. There can be an additional charge for long-distance calls. Check with the telephone service provider to determine what those charges might be. Some internet services, such as Skype or magicJack, allow the user to call long distance, and sometimes even internationally, through the computer with no long-distance charges.

Using Directory Assistance

Before placing a telephone call, have the correct number ready. If you do not have the number, you may access local directory assistance by calling 411. For long-distance numbers, you can access directory assistance by doing the following:
- Dialing 1
- Followed by the area code of the party you want to call
- Followed by 555-1212

Directory assistance is now an automated service in many regions. You will be asked for the name of the city and person you are calling. Often a fee is charged for using directory assistance, so, whenever possible, look for the telephone number using free sources.

A telephone directory would be one such free source. This directory is a list of those who have telephones, their telephone numbers, and, in most cases, their addresses. Yellow Pages contain listings for businesses. Directories are found on the internet and in print format.

The internet makes searching for telephone numbers much easier. Try to find telephone numbers through websites such as www.yellowpages.com or www.whitepages.com, or use a printed telephone book to avoid directory assistance charges on the monthly phone bill. A web search for the business or provider needed may give you the information. Companies with websites usually have a "Contact Us" page that directs the user to the individual departments.

In a print telephone directory, color coding is often used to differentiate between residence listings and business listings. Governmental offices usually have their own section (commonly blue). Some print directories include ZIP code maps for the local area.

Telephone Services

Answering Services. If an emergency arises, patients expect to be able to contact their provider. This means that the telephone in the healthcare facility must be answered at all times, day and night, weekends and holidays. During normal office hours, the medical assistant is available to answer the telephone. After office hours, most healthcare facilities use an answering service or an answering machine that directs the caller to the answering service if there is an urgent issue.

With an answering service, an actual person answers the call, which can be comforting for patients. The staff at the answering service can act as a buffer for the provider after hours by screening the calls. By following the criteria given by the healthcare facility, they can make the following determinations:
- Whether the provider (or on-call person) should be contacted
- If the patient should be directed to the hospital emergency department
- If a message can be taken and relayed to the healthcare facility in the morning

It is common courtesy to call the answering service in the morning to let the staff know that you will be answering the calls and also to retrieve any messages taken. You should also call the answering service when you are leaving for the day. Answering services also can be used to cover the telephone if all staff members need to be away from the telephone at the same time.

Automatic Call Routing. Many healthcare facilities have started using an automatic call routing system. The caller is given a menu of choices; he or she then presses a number on the telephone keypad to direct the call to the correct department. This can be an efficient way to handle a large volume of calls, but it can also be frustrating for some patients, especially older adults who may have trouble hearing and remembering the options. Some of the frustration can be minimized by providing a number option that connects the caller with a person (e.g., "Press 0"), who can then transfer the call to the appropriate department.

SCHEDULING APPOINTMENTS

The provider's time is one of the most valuable assets of a medical practice. The person responsible for scheduling the provider's time must have certain capabilities:
- Understand the practice
- Be familiar with the working habits and preferences of the provider (or providers)
- Have clear guidelines for time management in the practice

Appointment scheduling is the process that determines the following:
- Which patients the provider sees
- The dates and times of appointments
- How much time is given to each patient based on the complaint and the provider's availability

Scheduling appointments involves the understanding that unexpected interruptions and delays happen and must be handled appropriately. The medical assistant must assign the appropriate length of time for the appointment based on the complaint. Appointments should be scheduled so that there are very few gaps in the schedule. Most healthcare providers find that efficient appointment scheduling is one of the most important factors in the success of the practice. Scheduling can be done in a number of ways, and each facility must find the way that suits it best.

Establishing the Appointment Schedule

Developing a schedule that meets the needs of both the providers and the patients is key to keeping the office running smoothly and efficiently. The scheduling team, along with the provider, should come up with scheduling parameters (puh RAM it ers) to both meet the needs of the patients and keep the providers' preferences and habits in mind.

> **VOCABULARY**
> **answering service:** A commercial service that answers telephone calls for its clients.
> **automatic call routing:** A system that distributes incoming calls to a specific group or person based on customer need; for example, the customer presses 1 for appointments, 2 for billing questions, and so on.
> **parameters:** Rules that control how something should be done; guidelines or boundaries.

Patient Needs. Consider the demographics of the patients when determining office hours and appointment times. The staff should answer the following questions:
- Is the office in a busy metropolitan area or a rural community?
- What types of patients are seen? Are they of a specific age or gender? Do they have common diagnoses? Is the provider a general practitioner?
- Do most of the patients served need evening and weekend appointments?

Knowing when the providers need to be available for patients is one of the factors to be considered when creating the patient schedule.

Provider Preferences and Habits. Consider the preferences and habits of the providers in the practice before establishing and implementing a scheduling plan. Ask the following questions:
- Does the provider become restless if the reception room is not packed with waiting patients?
- Does the provider worry if even one patient is kept waiting?
- Is the provider careful about being in the facility when patient appointments are scheduled to begin?
- Is the provider habitually late?
- Does the provider move easily from one patient to another?
- Does the provider require a "break time" after a few patients?
- Would the provider rather see fewer patients and spend more time with each one or schedule more patients each day?

All of these preferences and habits become an integral (IN ti gruh l) part of the scheduling process. Keep in mind that the provider cannot spend every moment of the day with patients. The provider also has telephone calls to make and receive, reports to examine and dictate, meetings to attend, mail to answer, and many other business responsibilities. An experienced staff can handle many but not all of these tasks.

Next, the office hours and the length of appointment time intervals need to be determined. Keeping in mind patients' needs and the provider's preferences and habits, decide what would be the shortest time possible for an appointment. Most healthcare facilities use 10- or 15-minute time intervals for the appointment schedule. Paper-based appointment books with various time intervals can be purchased. A computerized appointment system can also be set to the specific time interval that has been decided on. A computerized system can be customized for different providers, so that one provider could have 10-minute time slots and another could have 15-minute time slots. If an appointment, such as a complete physical, needs longer than 15 minutes, multiple time slots are used to cover that appointment. Once the minimum time period has been set, then the appointment matrix can be established.

Creating the Appointment Matrix

Setting up the appointment matrix (Procedure 20.3) involves blocking out the times when the provider is not available to see patients (Fig. 20.7):
- Lunchtime
- Hospital rounds
- Conferences
- Vacation

In a paper-based appointment book, the matrix is usually established for 6 months at a time. In a computerized system, the matrix can be set up indefinitely.

Establishing Guidelines for Appointment Scheduling.

The first step in setting up the schedule matrix is to decide the length of the shortest office visit type. This visit type would usually be for a follow-up or recheck appointment for an established patient. Other specific appointment types should then be determined. Appointments fall into general categories:
- Follow-up or recheck
- Wellness examination
- Complete physical examination
- Urgent visit
- New patient visit
- Comprehensive visit

Each category has a specific amount of time assigned to it; for example, a follow-up or recheck appointment could be 10 to 15 minutes, and a comprehensive visit could be 30 to 40 minutes. The providers and scheduling team should work together to come up with these time periods to ensure that the office runs smoothly and efficiently.

If it is decided that a complete physical examination should be scheduled for 30 minutes, yet the provider routinely spends 45 minutes with the patient for a complete physical, then the scheduling guidelines need to be adjusted. Well-planned scheduling and sticking to that schedule allow the provider to do more than run in and out of examination rooms with little time for the patient to talk with the provider. There will be a bit of trial and error when developing the priorities for the appointment schedule.

Some providers need prompting to end the patient visit and move to the next patient. If there is a medical assistant in the examination room, he or she can help the provider remain on schedule by letting the provider know that the end of the appointment time is near. They may work out some type of signal, such as a hand gesture or phrase. A pager may be used when the medical assistant is not in room with the provider. When the provider's pager vibrates he or she will know that it is time to wind things up with that patient. The clinical medical assistant and the administrative medical assistant must work together to keep the healthcare facility running smoothly and efficiently.

> ### CRITICAL THINKING 20.5
> Ashlynn has noticed that Dr. Walden is taking a little longer with patients than normal and that she is consistently running behind schedule by approximately 5 to 15 minutes. How can Ashlynn help fix this situation?
> Discuss ways of approaching the provider when he or she is the cause of the delays in the schedule. What opening remarks can the medical assistant use to start the discussion in a positive way?

> ### VOCABULARY
> **demographics:** Statistical data of a population. In healthcare this includes the patient's name, address, date of birth, employment, and other details.
> **follow-up appointment:** An appointment type used when a patient needs to see the provider after a condition should have been resolved or to monitor an ongoing condition, such as hypertension. Also known as a **recheck appointment**.
> **integral:** Essential; being an indispensable part of a whole.
> **interval:** Space of time between events.
> **matrix:** The environment where something is created or takes shape; a base on which to build.

PROCEDURE 20.3 Establish the Appointment Matrix

Task
Establish the matrix of the appointment schedule.

Equipment and Supplies
- Appointment book or computer with scheduling software
- Office procedure manual (optional)
- Black pen, pencil, and highlighters
- Calendar

Scenario
You have been asked to set up the schedule matrix for Dr. Julie Walden, Dr. James Martin, and Dr. Angela Perez. Block off the following times in the appointment schedule:

Dr. Julie Walden
- Lunch: daily from 11:30 a.m. to 12:30 p.m.
- Hospital rounds: Mondays and Wednesdays from 8 a.m. to 9 a.m.

Dr. James Martin
- Lunch: daily from 12 p.m. to 1 p.m.
- Hospital rounds: Tuesdays and Thursdays from 8 a.m. to 9 a.m.

Dr. Angela Perez
- Lunch: daily from 12:30 p.m. to 1:30 p.m.
- Hospital rounds: Fridays from 8 a.m. to 9 a.m.

Procedural Steps

1. Using the calendar, determine when the office is not open (e.g., holidays, weekends, evenings). If using the appointment book and a black pen, draw an X through the times the office is not open. If using the scheduling software, block the times the office is not open.
   Purpose: Blocking the closed times of the office prevents patients from being scheduled when the office is closed.

2. Identify the times each provider is not available. If using the appointment book, write in the providers' names on each column and then draw an X through their unavailable times. If using the scheduling software, select each provider and block the times the provider is unavailable.
   Purpose: Many providers do rounds in the hospital or long-term care facilities and cannot see patients in the clinic during those times. Providers also attend meetings and conferences during the workday. These events, along with vacations and lunchtimes, should be blocked on their schedules.

3. Using the office procedure manual or providers' preferences, determine when each provider performs certain types of examinations. In the appointment book, indicate these examinations either by writing the examination times or by highlighting the examination times. Follow the office's procedure on indicating these examination times in the appointment book. When using scheduling software, set up the times for the examinations or use the highlighting feature if available.
   Purpose: Some providers perform a variety of examinations. It can be more time efficient to have the same types of examinations on the same day. For instance, a provider in a women's health department may perform both gynecologic and prenatal examinations. The provider may prefer to set aside certain days to do prenatal examinations and other days to do gynecologic examinations.

4. Using the office procedure manual or the list of providers' preferences and availability, identify other times to block on the scheduling matrix. Some providers require catch-up times, and these time slots are blocked. Some medical facilities save appointment times for same-day appointments. When saving time blocks for same-day appointments, make sure to use pencil so it can be erased and the patient's information entered on the day of the appointment. For the scheduling software, block those times when patients cannot be booked and indicate the times for the same-day appointments.
   Purpose: Allowing appointment times to be saved for same-day appointments provides the opportunity for the provider to see a patient who needs to get in immediately and prevents the patient from being turned away or double-booked.

Available Facilities. Another factor to keep in mind when scheduling appointments is the availability of facilities needed for a specific appointment type. Getting a patient into the office at a time when no room or equipment are available for the services needed is a waste of the patient's time. For example, suppose that a healthcare facility with two providers has only one room that can be used for minor surgery. Do not schedule two patients needing minor surgery for the same day and time, even if both doctors could be available. If the healthcare facility has only one electrocardiograph, do not book two electrocardiograms (ECGs) at the same time. As the medical assistant gains **proficiency** (pruh FISH uh n see) in scheduling, it becomes easier to match the patient needs with the available facilities. Major equipment frequently used, or a certain room with such equipment, may need its own scheduling column in the appointment book or software system.

Methods of Scheduling Appointments

The two most common methods of appointment scheduling are as follows:
- Computerized scheduling
- Appointment book or paper-based scheduling

Each has advantages and disadvantages. The healthcare facility should weigh the benefits and choose the method that best suits the provider and the staff.

Computerized Scheduling. The computer has replaced the appointment book in many practices. **Practice management software** ranges from relatively simple programs that merely display available and scheduled times to more sophisticated systems that perform several other functions. To gain the greatest benefit from the software, information such as the following should be entered:
- Length and type of appointment required
- Patient's day or time preferences

The computer can select the best appointment time based on that information.

A computerized scheduling system also has the ability to search for future appointments. For example, when a patient calls and asks about a previously scheduled appointment, the system can search by his or her name to find the time and date. Computerized scheduling allows multiple users to access the schedule at the same time, minimizing the wait time for patients.

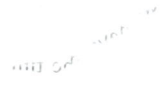

VOCABULARY
practice management software: A type of software that allows the user to enter demographic information, schedule appointments, maintain lists of insurance payers, perform billing tasks, and generate reports.
proficiency: Skilled as a result of training or practice.

CHAPTER 20   Telephone Techniques and Scheduling   455

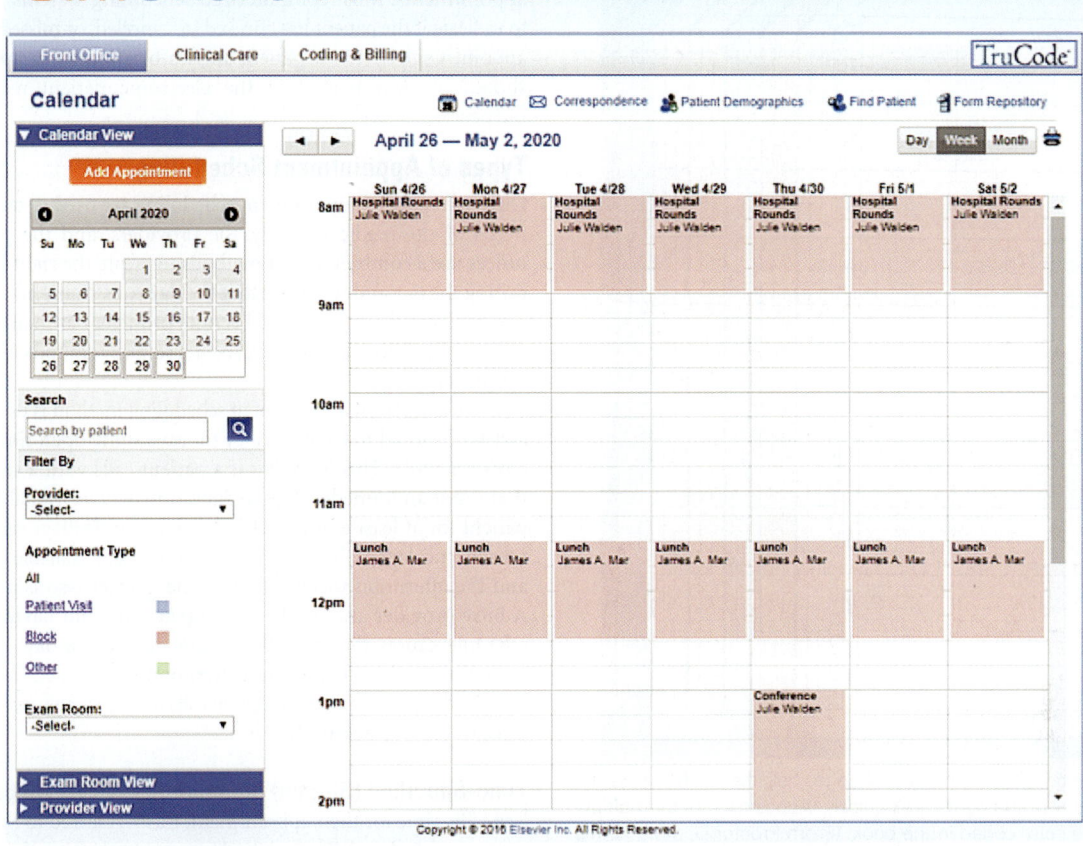

FIG. 20.7 Schedule matrix showing provider availability. (From *SimChart for the Medical Office*, St. Louis, 2015, Elsevier.)

Another advantage of computerized schedules is the reports that can be generated. A hard copy of the provider's daily schedule can be created showing the following information:
- Patients' names
- Telephone numbers
- Reason for the visit

Some healthcare facilities print these out, and others use them on screen. Healthcare facilities must have scheduling procedures to follow when the technology is down.

Appointment Book Scheduling. Office suppliers carry a variety of appointment book styles. Some appointment books show an entire week at a glance; many are color coded, with a special color used for each day of the week (Fig. 20.8). This is very helpful when the provider asks the patient to return, for instance, in 2 weeks. If Wednesdays are colored yellow, the medical assistant can flip quickly to the correct day 2 weeks later and schedule the appointment. Multiple columns may be available to correspond with the number of doctors in a group practice, and the time can be divided according to their preferences.

Self-Scheduling. Allowing patients to schedule their own appointments using the Internet and the healthcare facility's website is becoming much more common. The patient is given limited access to the schedule, so that they see only the available appointment times, not the blocks for patients who have been scheduled.

Software is available that allows the patient to self-schedule through secure links to the provider's appointment book. The software or internet site for the healthcare facility should give the patient guidelines as to the amount of time needed for certain appointments or should allow only a certain length of time to be self-scheduled, such as 15 minutes. These systems reduce the number of calls and are available to the patient 24 hours a day. Some also send an automatic email reminder to the patient the day before the appointment, requesting a reply to confirm. These systems are less frustrating to patients, who do not have to wait on hold to speak to the person who does scheduling for the healthcare facility. However, lengthy or complicated appointments should be scheduled through the staff.

Although this type of system for making appointments appeals to most technologically savvy people, some patients may not be comfortable using it. It does require minimal skills and internet access. Others may object to online scheduling because they do not want their names anywhere on the internet. This is a valid concern, and the facility should allow these patients to schedule over the telephone. If this system is employed, some allowance must be made for patients who choose not to use it.

> **CRITICAL THINKING 20.6**
>
> The software used at WMFM allows patients to self-schedule. Ashlynn has heard about patient self-scheduling and would like to try this method in the office, but Dr. Martin is concerned that his patients will miss the personal contact and is not sold on the idea. What can Ashlynn say to convince Dr. Martin to try this new, timesaving method of scheduling? What challenges might the use of this system bring?

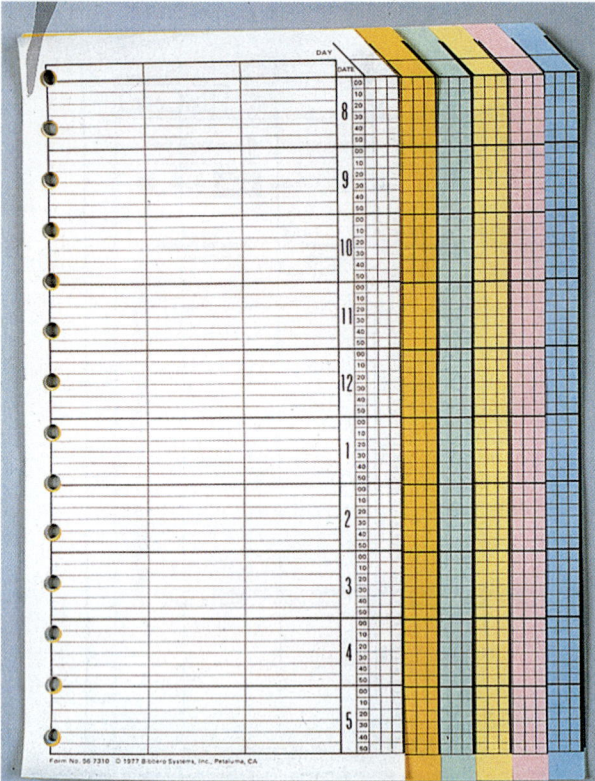

FIG. 20.8 Color-coded appointment book pages help the medical assistant flip to the right day of the right week quickly. Appointments for multiple providers can be color coded in the book. (From Proctor D, et al: *Kinn's The Medical Assistant*, ed 13, St. Louis, 2017, Elsevier.)

Legality of the Appointment Scheduling System

Because the paper-based appointment book can be used as a legal record, it must be accurate and maintained so that it provides correct information about the patients at the healthcare facility. Patients are expected to follow the provider's orders; this includes keeping appointments. If a patient does not show up for an appointment or cancels it and does not reschedule, documentation of this fact should be placed in the patient's health record. If a patient reschedules an appointment and subsequently keeps it, there is no need to document that it was rescheduled.

Pens are permanent, and the appointment book can become illegible if a number of patients change or cancel their appointments. To make changes to an appointment book easier, pencil should be used. The information in the book includes the patient's name and a phone number where the patient can be reached. Some healthcare facilities list the reason for the appointment, but most note only the name and phone number. Listing the reason for the visit is not necessary if the medical assistant references the time needed for the appointment and blocks off that amount of time. Because the appointment book could be evidence as a legal record, it should be kept for the number of years that constitute the statute of limitations in that individual state. If the appointment book is discarded, its contents should be shredded to protect patient privacy. Although the appointment book can be used as a legal record, actual medical records are more likely to be used in matters of litigation. Because *progress notes* are dated, a copy of the medical record shows all pertinent information about the patient's adherence to the provider's orders, including the appointments with the provider.

Computerized scheduling systems can also be used to track patient appointments. Most computerized scheduling systems allow the user to indicate if the patient has checked in, canceled, or missed the scheduled appointment. When a patient misses or cancels an appointment, it should be documented in the electronic patient record for legal purposes.

Types of Appointment Scheduling

Different types of appointment scheduling are used to meet the various needs of the medical facility, the providers, and the patients. Some offices use a combination of methods to create the right mix of activity during the day and to ensure that the day runs smoothly and efficiently. The medical assistant should become proficient at managing appointments. The following section presents several methods of appointment scheduling.

No matter what appointment scheduling method is used, the medical assistant should make it a policy to leave some open time during each day's schedule. This is so that if a patient calls with a special problem that is not an immediate emergency, time will be available to book the patient for at least a brief visit. Mondays and Fridays generally are the most hectic days of the week. Keeping a time slot available in the morning and the afternoon specifically for emergencies also is a wise practice. A busy provider always fills these open slots, and having them in the schedule causes the least *disruption* during the day. If possible, set aside time in the morning and afternoon for a break. Even 15 minutes can give the provider time to return calls from patients, verify prescription calls, or answer questions.

Time-Specified (Stream) Scheduling. When each patient is given a specific time for their appointment, this is referred to as *time-specified* or *stream scheduling*. This method keeps a steady flow of patients moving through the office. This is the most common type of scheduling used in healthcare facilities. Studies have shown that providers can see more patients with less pressure when patient appointments are scheduled for a specific time slot. The medical assistant who is scheduling patients using this method should know the amount of time needed for each appointment type and keep time slots available for urgent visits.

Wave Scheduling. Wave scheduling is an attempt to create flexibility within each hour. Wave scheduling assumes that the actual time needed for all the patients seen will average out over the course of the day. Instead of scheduling patients at each 15-minute interval, wave scheduling has three patients in the office at the same time. They are then seen in the order of their arrival. This way, one person's late arrival does not disrupt the entire schedule.

Modified Wave Scheduling. The wave schedule can be modified in several ways. For example, one method is to have two patients scheduled to come in at 10 a.m. and a third at 10:30 a.m. This hourly cycle is repeated throughout the day. In another version, patients are scheduled to arrive at given intervals during the first half of the hour, and none

---

VOCABULARY

disruption: An unexpected event that throws a plan into disorder; an interruption that prevents a system or process from continuing as usual or as expected.

progress notes: Documentation in the medical record to track the patient's condition and progress.

are scheduled to arrive during the second half of the hour. This would allow time for urgent or walk-in patients to be seen.

Double-Booking. Booking two patients to come in at the same time is sometimes used to work in a patient with an acute illness or injury when there are no open appointments. This works out best if one of the patients needs laboratory work or another procedure done before seeing the provider. The provider can see one of the patients while the other one is being prepared.

Open Office Hours. With the open office hours method, the facility is open at given hours, and the patients are told that they can come in at any time. This type of system is often used in an urgent care setting. Patients are then seen in the order in which they arrive, although patients with urgent conditions may be seen ahead of those who arrived before them.

The open office hours system can have many disadvantages. The office may already be crowded when the provider arrives, resulting in an extremely long wait for some patients. Patients may arrive in waves throughout the day, which causes parts of the day to be very busy and other parts to be slow. This makes accomplishing other office duties difficult. Without planning, the facilities and staff can be overburdened.

> **CRITICAL THINKING 20.7**
>
> Dr. Walden would like to implement evening appointments one night each week and open the office every other Saturday morning. She feels this will better serve her patients with children who have difficulty making daytime appointments. If this is her primary goal, should other types of patients be seen during these time slots? Why or why not?

Grouping Procedures. Grouping, or categorizing, of procedures is another method of scheduling that appeals to many providers. For instance, an internist might reserve all morning appointments for complete physical examinations, or a pediatrician might keep that time for well-baby visits. A surgeon might devote 1 day each week to seeing only referral patients. Obstetricians often schedule pregnant patients on different days from gynecology patients. The providers and staff can experiment with different groupings until the plan that works best for the practice eventually becomes obvious. In applying a grouping system of appointments, the medical assistant may find it helpful to color code the sections of the appointment book reserved for specific procedures.

Telephone Scheduling

A pleasant manner and a willingness to help are just as important on the telephone as when meeting patients face to face. This is especially true when making appointments. The telephone contact may be the patient's first impression of the facility. Often the way the appointment scheduling process is handled makes more of an impression than the convenience of the appointment time.

Be especially considerate if the time requested for an appointment is not available. Briefly explain why, and offer a different date and time. Comply with the patient's wishes as much as possible, and do not show annoyance if the patient does not understand the scheduling process. Most people, however, understand the need for a well-managed office and are willing to cooperate.

Many offices offer the patient a choice when scheduling the appointment and let the patient decide which option is best for him or her. For example, the following dialog might take place during the scheduling call:

Medical assistant:	"Mrs. Thomas, Dr. Stern is available to see you in the office next Tuesday or Wednesday, January 6 or 7. Which day is better for you?"
Patient:	"I will be working on Wednesday, so I would like to come in on Tuesday."
Medical assistant:	"Do you prefer a morning or afternoon appointment?"
Patient:	"The afternoon is best for me."
Medical assistant:	"Great. Would 1:30 or 3:30 be a better time?"
Patient:	"I can be there at 1:30."
Medical assistant:	"Then Dr. Stern will see you at 1:30 next Tuesday, January 6. Thank you for calling, Mrs. Thomas. We'll see you then!"

These small courtesies give patients the feeling that they control their time. Always repeat the time to reinforce the appointment and do not hesitate to ask the patient if he or she has a pen ready to jot down the time and date. While repeating the information to the patient, check the appointment book or computer screen to ensure that it was posted correctly. When scheduling appointments over the telephone, it is not possible to give the patient a reminder card for the appointment. Be sure to ask if the patient would like a telephone, email, or text message reminder of the appointment.

Write legibly when using an appointment book. These records could be called into court, and the medical assistant must be able to read his or her own writing if asked to testify. The patient's daytime telephone number should be recorded for every appointment scheduled. The appointment may need to be canceled or the schedule rearranged in a hurry, and precious minutes can be saved if the telephone number is handy. Cell phone numbers also are quite useful for quickly tracking down a patient.

Scheduling Appointments for New Patients

Arranging the first appointment for a new patient requires time and attention to detail (Procedure 20.4). This encounter provides the first impression of the healthcare facility and may set the tone for all subsequent visits. Tact, courtesy, and professionalism are extremely important. You will need to obtain information about the *chief* complaint (why the patient needs the appointment). This information will be used to determine how much time to allow for the visit. The provider may also expect the medical assistant to give general instructions to patients being seen for specific complaints. For example, the patient may be required to be fasting for certain laboratory tests to be performed. Patient demographic information should be collected during the conversation, including the type of insurance the patient has. Some insurance carriers restrict which providers can be used.

After the necessary information has been collected, offer the patient the first available appointment. Whenever possible, offer a choice between two dates and times. Ask the patient to arrive 15 minutes before the scheduled appointment time to complete any necessary paperwork. Also ask whether he or she knows how to get to the healthcare facility or offer the physical address for those who use a GPS or an internet direction website like MapQuest. Tell the patient whether any special parking conveniences are available and whether the healthcare facility provides a token or parking validation. The patient's options for the first payment should also be discussed. If payment is expected at the

PROCEDURE 20.4 Schedule a New Patient

Task
Schedule a new patient for a first office visit and identify the urgency of the visit using established priorities.

Equipment and Supplies
- Appointment book or computer with scheduling software
- Scheduling and screening guidelines
- Pencil

Role-Play Scenario
Patricia Black, a new patient, calls. She just moved to the area, and her asthma has flared up over the past 24 hours. Her albuterol inhaler is empty, and she needs a new prescription for it. She states that she is doing okay, but without the albuterol she knows it will get worse within the next few days. According to your screening guidelines, she needs to be seen today, and scheduling guidelines indicate she needs a 45-minute appointment.

Procedural Steps
1. Obtain the patient's demographic information (e.g., full name, birth date, address, and telephone number). Write this information down or enter it into the scheduling software. Verify the information.

   Purpose: It is important to verify the information. If you have difficulty hearing the patient, use a system to verify the spelling (e.g., "A" as in "Alpha").

2. Determine whether the patient was referred by another provider.

   Purpose: You may need to request additional information from the referring provider, and your provider will want to send a consultation report.

3. Determine the patient's chief complaint and when the first symptoms occurred. Utilize the scheduling and screening guidelines as needed.

   Purpose: You must know the amount of time that will be required for the visit and how quickly the patient needs to be seen based on the chief complaint.

4. Search the appointment book or scheduling software for the first suitable appointment time and an alternate time. Offer the patient a choice of these dates and times. Be open to alternative times if the patient cannot make the initial options you gave. Provide additional appointment options as needed.

   Purpose: Providing the patient with a choice of dates and times and additional options as needed demonstrates sensitivity when managing appointments. It is an important customer service technique (see the figure).

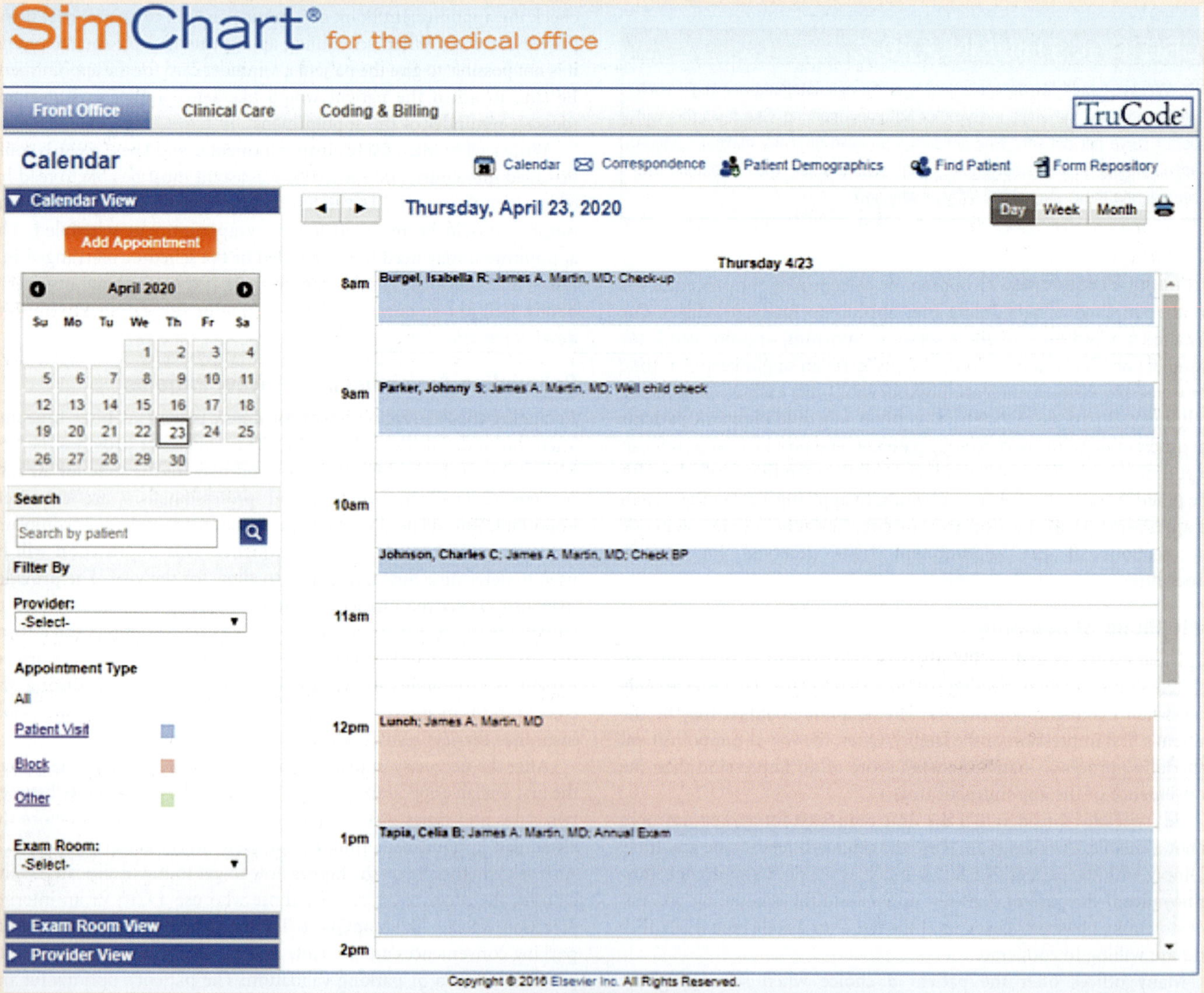

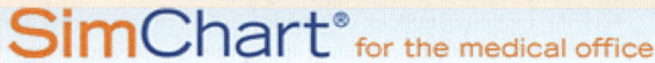

CHAPTER 20 Telephone Techniques and Scheduling

PROCEDURE 20.4 Schedule a New Patient—cont'd

5. Enter the mutually agreeable time into the schedule. Enter the patient's name, telephone number, and add *NP* for new patient.

   Purpose: The *NP* in the appointment book indicates that this is a new patient. Having the phone number available increases your efficiency if you need to contact the patient.

6. Obtain the patient's insurance information. If new patients are expected to pay at the time of the visit, explain this financial arrangement when making the appointment.

   Purpose: Obtaining the patient's insurance information now ensures that the patient is seeing a provider covered by his or her insurance carrier. By explaining the payment policy before the appointment, the patient can come to the appointment prepared to pay.

7. Provide the patient with directions to the healthcare facility and parking instructions if needed.

   Note: Many facilities will email or mail new-patient paperwork to the patient, who is instructed to complete the forms ahead of time and bring them to the appointment.

8. Before ending the call, ask if the patient has any questions. Reinforce the date and time of the appointment. Politely and professionally end the call, making sure to thank the patient for calling.

   Purpose: It is important to restate the appointment time and date to ensure the patient knows the correct information before ending the call.

   Note: For legal and safety reasons, many healthcare practices encourage patients with urgent same-day appointments to seek emergency care immediately if the condition worsens before the appointment time.

---

time of service, inform the patient. The staff should expect patient concerns about the amount of the first bill and should address this issue before the appointment so that there are no surprises or misunderstandings. Before ending the conversation, repeat the appointment date and time, and thank the patient for calling.

Some healthcare facilities mail an information packet/brochure to new patients, especially if the appointment is several days away. With the patient's permission and email address, this information can also be sent via the internet. An ideal tool to use to deliver this information is a new patient brochure (see Chapter 22). This brochure can be printed with graphics and images to promote a professional impression of the healthcare facility. In addition to the brochure, the packet could include a health history form, the **Notice of Privacy Practices (NPP)**, and release of information form (to obtain records from the patient's previous provider).

If another provider has referred the patient, the medical assistant may need to call the referring provider's office to obtain additional information before the patient's appointment. This information should be printed out and given to the attending provider before the patient arrives. Remember to send a thank you note to anyone who refers a patient to the facility.

Often, the medical assistant will need to conduct **preauthorization** or **precertification** to determine whether a patient is eligible for treatment or for certain procedures. The office manager must make certain that these procedures are being done and assigns these duties to a specific person. More about preauthorization and precertification is included in Chapter 26.

Scheduling Appointments for Established Patients

In Person. Most return appointments for **established patients** are scheduled when the patient is leaving the healthcare facility. A good policy is to have all patients stop by the appointment desk to check out before leaving in case any information is needed from the patient or any outside scheduling must be done. The patient's health record can be reviewed to see whether the provider ordered any laboratory tests or procedures, and these can be scheduled and discussed with the patient. When making a return appointment, follow the same procedures as for scheduling any appointment by phone, offering the patient choices in the day and time slots (Procedure 20.5). If a certain time the patient specifically requests is not available, offer two other choices. Always give the patient an appointment card and any necessary instructions, along with a bright smile. Never forget to provide excellent customer service.

By Telephone. When scheduling an appointment over the telephone, the medical assistant usually only needs to determine when the patient must return and to find a suitable time in the schedule. Established patients do not usually need directions and parking information, unless the office has recently moved. The patient's address, telephone number, and insurance should always be verified and any changes documented in the health record. If an email address or cell phone number is not on file, obtain one to have a quick, easy way to notify the patient of appointments and other events.

Scheduling Other Types of Appointments

The medical assistant may also schedule services other than appointments at the healthcare facility, and these will appear on the appointment schedule. This includes the following:

- Surgeries the provider will perform at a hospital or other facility
- Consultations
- Outside appointments and meetings
- House calls (if the provider makes them)

The provider also must have time to get from one location to another, so driving time must be considered when arranging all appointments.

VOCABULARY

established patient: A patient who has been treated by the healthcare provider within the past 3 years.

Notice of Privacy Practices (NPP): A written document describing the healthcare facility's privacy practices. The patient must be provided with the NPP and sign an acknowledgment of receipt.

preauthorization: A process required by some insurance carriers in which the provider obtains permission to perform certain procedures or services or refers a patient to a specialist.

precertification: The process of determining if a procedure or service is covered by the insurance plan and what the reimbursement is for that procedure or service.

460 UNIT 3　Administrative Ambulatory Care

PROCEDURE 20.5　Schedule an Established Patient

Task
Manage the provider's schedule by scheduling appointments for an established patient, and handling rescheduling and a no-show appointment.

Equipment and Supplies
- Appointment book or computer with scheduling software
- Scheduling guidelines
- Pencil, red pen
- Reminder card
- Patient's health record

Role-Play Scenario
Celia Tapia has just finished seeing Dr. Martin and is checking out at your desk. You see that she needs to schedule a follow-up appointment in 2 weeks. The scheduling guidelines indicate a follow-up appointment is 15 minutes long.

Procedural Steps
1. Obtain the patient's name and information, purpose of the visit, provider to be seen, and any scheduling preferences. If using the scheduling software, enter the patient's name and DOB. Verify the correct patient is selected.

Purpose: To schedule an appointment, the patient's information is required, along with the provider to be seen and the type of appointment required. Knowing any scheduling preferences or limitations will help you efficiently find an acceptable appointment time for the patient.

2. Identify the length of the appointment by using the scheduling guidelines.

Purpose: Depending on the appointment type, each provider may require a different length of time for that appointment. Ensuring you schedule the appropriate amount of time will facilitate the flow of patients on that day.

3. Search the appointment book or scheduling software for the first suitable appointment time and an alternate time. Offer the patient a choice of these dates and times. Be open to alternative times if the patient cannot make the initial options you gave. Provide additional appointment options as needed.

Purpose: Providing the patient with a choice of dates and times and additional options as needed helps to demonstrate sensitivity when managing appointments. It is an important customer service technique (see the figure).

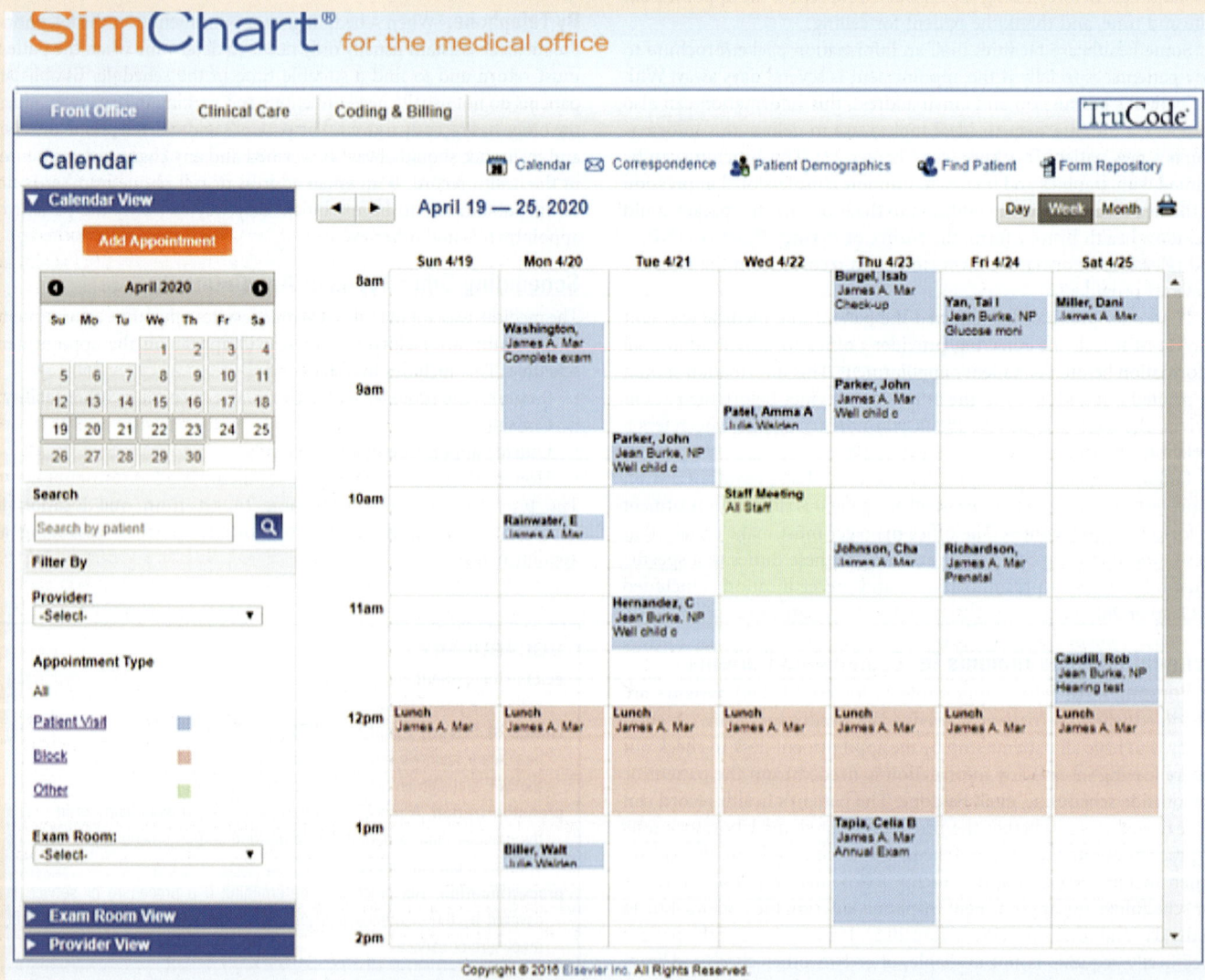

PROCEDURE 20.5 Schedule an Established Patient—cont'd

4. Using a pencil, write the patient's name and phone number in the appointment book, and block out the correct amount of time. Add any other relevant information per the facility's procedures. If using the scheduling software, create the appointment per the facility's guidelines.
   Purpose: Adding the patient's phone number to the appointment book will help save time if the patient needs to be contacted. Using a pencil to write down the information in the book allows it to be erased if the patient cancels or reschedules for another time.
5. Complete the appointment reminder card, and ensure the date and time on the card matches the appointment time. Give the card to the patient.
   Purpose: Appointment reminder cards help patients remember when their appointments are and decreases the number of no-show appointments.

Continuation of Scenario
Later that day, Celica Tapia calls and says she needs to reschedule her appointment for the next day at the same time.

6. When a patient calls to reschedule an appointment, follow steps 1 through 4. When the new appointment is made, make sure to erase the old appointment from the appointment log. With the scheduling software, ensure the old appointment time is removed from the schedule. Repeat the appointment date and time to the patient.
   Note: It is important to erase the old appointment so the patient is not expected on two different days. Erasing or deleting the old appointment opens up that time for another patient.

Continuation of Scenario
Celia Tapia no-shows for her follow-up appointment.

7. In the appointment book, using red pen, indicate the patient no-showed. Using the patient's health record, document that the patient failed to show for the follow-up examination with the provider. In an electronic system, change the appointment status to no-show, and ensure that it is documented in the health record.
   Purpose: For legal purposes, the healthcare facility must keep a record of patients who no-show for appointments. By indicating it in the appointment book and in the health record, the practice is covered if any issues should arise. Some medical practices have procedures that include contacting the patient regarding the no-show appointment and finding out the reason. This is then also charted in the health record.

Always provide the facility with the following critical information when scheduling admission or treatments in other facilities:
- Patient's name, address, phone numbers (both home and cell)
- Social Security number
- Insurance information
- Email address
- Procedures that are to be performed
- Patient allergies
- Admitting diagnosis
- Provider orders

Some facilities require a history form before admission. The patient will be required to bring a form of picture identification, such as a state driver's license, and his or her insurance card.

Inpatient Surgeries. When scheduling a surgery, provide all necessary information and state any special requests the provider may have, such as the following:
- The amount of blood to have available for the patient
- A specific anesthesiologist
- An assistant surgeon
- Specific instruments

The facility may want the patient's insurance information and certainly will want a phone number so that the patient can be contacted before the surgery if necessary. Make sure all of this information is available before placing the call.

Outpatient and Inpatient Procedure Appointments. A medical assistant is often asked to arrange laboratory or radiography appointments for patients. Before calling the facility to schedule the appointment, be sure all necessary information is available. Inform the patient of the time and place of the appointment, relay any special instructions, and then note these arrangements in the patient's health record. Some offices make a reminder call to the patient or send a reminder email or text message.

Outpatient testing is common because most providers do not have extensive x-ray or laboratory equipment in their offices. Magnetic resonance imaging (MRI), computed tomography (CT) scans, numerous x-ray evaluations, sonography, and simple blood tests all may need to be scheduled (Procedure 20.6). See Chapter 2 for information on these tests. Provide the patient with the name, address, and phone number of the facility where the tests will be done.

Some patients may require a series of appointments (e.g., at weekly intervals). Try to set up these appointments on the same day each week at the same time of day. This reduces the risk of the patient forgetting an appointment.

In some cases, the medical assistant may be responsible for scheduling inpatient admissions or inpatient surgical procedures. This is similar to scheduling outpatient testing, but the medical assistant coordinates with a hospital rather than an outside facility, and it should also be documented in the patient's health record.

It is often the medical assistant's responsibility to provide the patient with any special instructions for the procedure or test that is going to be performed. The patient should be provided with written instructions as well. A patient undergoing general anesthesia will need to fast for approximately 12 hours before the procedure. If medications are to be taken the morning of the procedure, the patient may take them with a small sip of water. The provider will instruct the patient about which medications to take. The patient should also be instructed to leave valuables at home. If it is an outpatient procedure and will require sedation, the patient should be instructed to have someone drive him or her home.

Outside Visits. If the provider regularly makes house calls or visits patients in skilled nursing facilities, a special block of time must be reserved in the appointment schedule. There has been an increase in the number of providers who are making house calls again, especially if they have an older adult patient base that includes seniors who are still living independently. The provider needs demographic information, such as addresses, room numbers, and the best route to each home or facility. Remember to allow for travel time.

There are a number of other situations that may have to be added to the schedule, sometimes without much advance warning. Handle these situations with care and courtesy.

Pharmaceutical Representatives. Representatives from drug companies are frequent visitors to healthcare facilities. They are well

PROCEDURE 20.6   Schedule a Patient Procedure

Task
Schedule a patient for a procedure within the time frame needed by the provider, confirm with the patient, and issue all required instructions.

Equipment and Supplies
- Provider's order detailing the procedure required
- Computer with order entry software (optional)
- Name, address, and telephone number of the facility where the procedure will take place
- Patient's demographic and insurance information
- Patient's health record
- Procedure preparation instructions
- Telephone
- Consent form (if required for procedure)

Role-Play Scenario
Monique Jones has just seen Dr. Walden and is checking out at your desk. She gives you an order from the provider that states she needs to have a magnetic resonance image (MRI) of her left ankle within a week. The radiology department in your facility performs MRIs.

Procedural Steps
1. Obtain an oral or written order from the provider for the exact procedure to be performed.

Purpose: For you to schedule the procedure, you will need an order from the provider for the procedure to be performed.

2. Gather the patient's demographic and insurance information. If using an electronic health record, verify you have the correct patient.

Note: For some procedures and diagnostic tests, precertifications or preauthorizations need to be completed before scheduling the patient. This process will be discussed in a later chapter.

3. Determine the patient's availability within the time frame granted by the provider for the procedure (see the figure).

Purpose: Make sure the patient will be able to comply with the arrangements for the test.

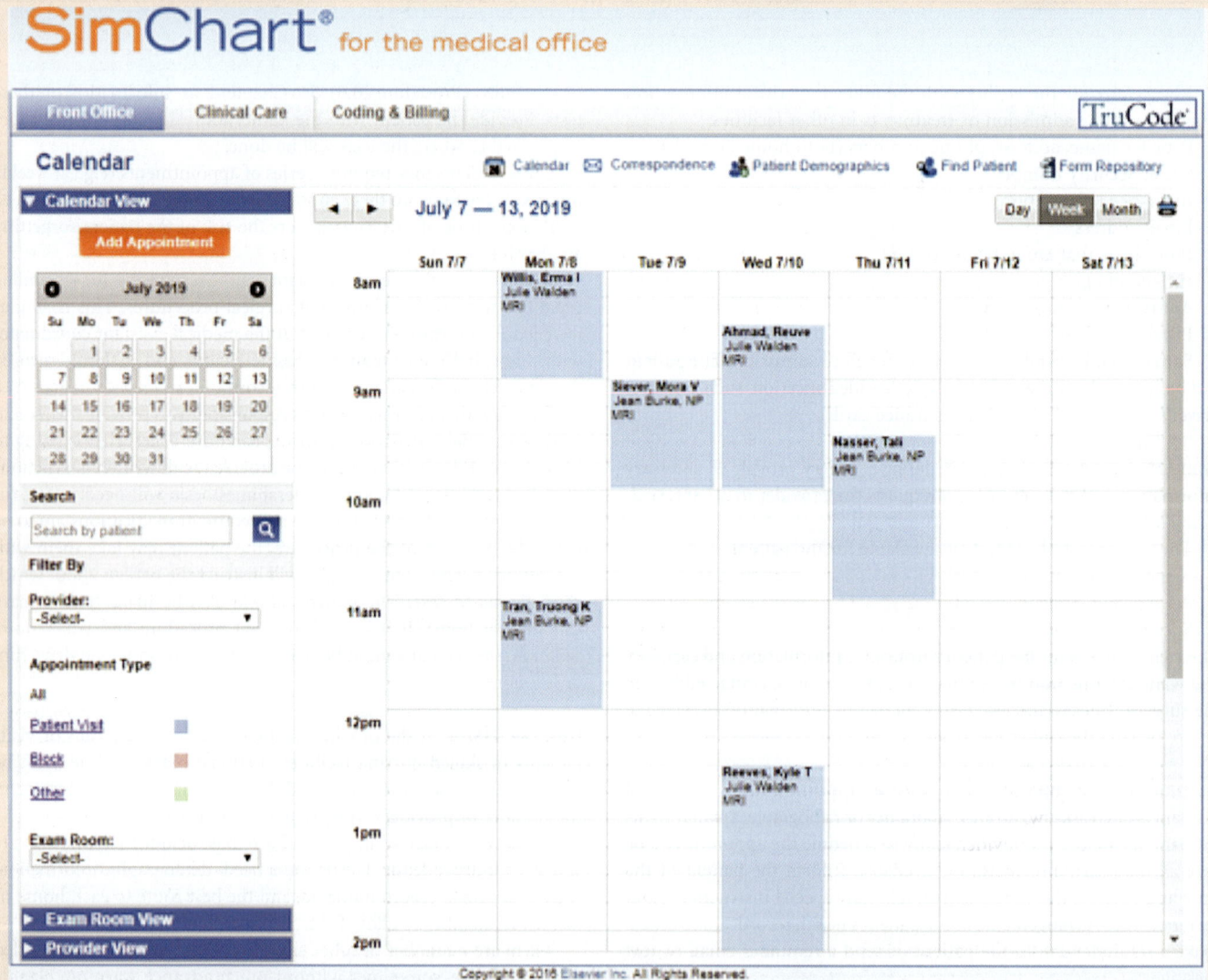

> **PROCEDURE 20.6 Schedule a Patient Procedure—cont'd**
>
> 4. Contact the diagnostic facility, and schedule the patient's procedure. If you are using a computerized provider order entry (CPOE) system and your facility performs the procedure, you also need to enter the order using the CPOE system.
>   - Provide the patient's diagnosis and provider's exact order, including the name of the procedure and the time frame.
>   - Establish the date and time for the procedure.
>   - Give the patient's name, age, address, telephone number, and insurance information (i.e., insurance policy numbers, precertification information, and addresses for filing claims).
>   - Determine any special instructions for the patient or special anesthesia requirements.
>   - Notify the facility of any urgency for test results.
>
>   **Purpose:** Schedule the procedure, and provide needed information.
>
> 5. Notify the patient of the arrangements and provide the information in a written format.
>   - Give the name, address, and telephone number of the diagnostic facility.
>   - Specify the date and time to report for the procedure.
>   - Give instructions on preparation for the test (e.g., eating restrictions, fluids, medications, enemas).
>   - If using another facility, the patient will need to bring a form of picture identification and the insurance card.
>   - If not using a CPOE system, explain whether the patient needs to pick up orders or whether the order will be sent to the facility in advance.
>   - Ask if the patient has any questions, and answer the questions.
>
>   **Purpose:** Make sure the patient understands the necessary preparations and the importance of keeping the appointment. Providing the patient with written instructions reinforces what was discussed and gives the patient a reference for the information.
>
> 6. If a consent form is required for the procedure, ensure the provider has reviewed the form with the patient and the patient has signed the consent form. The diagnostic facility may require a copy of the consent form before performing the procedure. The consent form should be scanned and uploaded into the electronic health record or placed in the paper record.
>
>   **Purpose:** The consent form is used to make sure the patient understands the risks, benefits, and alternatives to the procedure.
>
> 7. Document the details of the scheduled procedure in the patient's health record. If applicable, create a reminder to check on the procedure results after the appointment date.
>
>   **Purpose:** Document that the procedure was scheduled. It is legally important to show that what was ordered was scheduled. Creating a reminder for you to check up on the results of the procedure is also important in assisting the provider. The information can be listed something like this: 2/27/20XX Patient scheduled for colonoscopy on 3/10/20XX 8 a.m. at Anytown Hospital. Patient preparation instructions given, and patient verbalized understanding.

trained and bring the provider valuable information on new drugs. The medical assistant is often expected to screen these visitors and turn away those whose products would not be used in that practice. If the representative or the pharmaceutical company is unknown to the office, ask for a business card and then check with the provider. The provider will decide whether to see the representative. Many healthcare facilities are limiting and even eliminating visits from pharmaceutical representative due to the Physician Payments Sunshine Act (part of the Affordable Care Act).

Pharmaceutical representatives will often bring samples of the medications that they are going to talk to the provider about. It is important for the medical assistant to understand the policies and procedures for the handling and dispensing of the samples. Most healthcare facilities require that these samples are stored in a locked cabinet or closet and are given to patients only with provider approval.

Specialists usually limit their visits with pharmaceutical representatives to their line of practice. The medical assistant, together with the provider, can prepare a list of the representatives with whom the provider is willing to spend time. The medical assistant can say whether the provider will be available that day and give an estimate of the waiting time or suggest a later time at which the representative may return. The representative then can decide whether to wait or return later. Pharmaceutical representatives are usually quite understanding and cooperative and are willing to wait patiently for a long time for just a brief visit with the provider. In turn, the medical assistant should treat the representative with courtesy, showing as much cooperation as possible.

Salespeople. Salespeople from medical, surgical, and office supply houses stop regularly at healthcare facilities. Sometimes they want to see the provider, but the office manager or the medical assistant in charge of ordering supplies can usually handle these visits.

Unsolicited salespeople can sometimes present a problem in the professional office. If the provider does not want to see such callers, the medical assistant must firmly but tactfully send them away. Suggest that they leave their literature and cards for the provider to study, and say that the provider will contact them if further information is desired.

Special Circumstances

Late Patients. Every medical practice has a few patients who are habitually late for appointments. This seems to be a problem for which no cure has been found. Emergencies and small delays can happen to anyone, but a patient who constantly arrives late can put a strain on the practice. Such patients can be booked as the last appointment of the day. Then, if closing time arrives before the patient does, the staff has no obligation to wait and other patients have not been inconvenienced. Some medical assistants tell the patient to come in 30 minutes before the scheduled appointment time. Make an effort to work with patients who have occasional difficulties arriving on time, but do not allow the schedule to be constantly disrupted by late patients.

> **CRITICAL THINKING 20.8**
>
> Seth Jones is always late for his appointments. How might Ashlynn approach him about this issue? What can Ashlynn do to assist Mr. Jones so that he arrives for appointments on time?

Rescheduling Appointments. Changes sometimes must be made to the appointment schedule. Unexpected conflicts might come up that force a patient to change the appointment time. When rescheduling an appointment, make sure the first appointment is removed from the appointment book, and then set the new appointment. Otherwise, the patient will be expected in the office on 2 days, and time will be wasted with calls and follow-up, only to discover that the appointment was rescheduled. Most computerized scheduling systems will allow the medical assistant to open the appointment and change the date and time or to cut and paste the appointment into the new date and time.

Emergency Situations. Periodically, emergency or urgent calls come into the office, and an appointment needs to be scheduled. To some extent, all calls that come in go through a screening process to evaluate the need to see the provider, and emergencies are prioritized. Screening is an extremely important function that requires experience, knowledge of signs and symptoms, and tact.

Emergencies may involve emotional crises in addition to the more obvious physical problems. Patients with emergencies and those who are acutely ill should be seen the same day. The urgency of the call initially can be determined by having a list of questions prepared for reference. The provider should help with this list; he or she should determine what is considered an emergency or urgent. The patient may need to be referred directly to a hospital emergency department, or the provider may want to see the patient that day in the office. If patients are unable to get themselves to the hospital, the medical assistant may need to contact the emergency medical services in your area. Remember to keep the patient on the phone until emergency medical technicians (EMTs) or other help arrives at the patient's location. Never place an emergency call on hold. Always obtain the name, phone number, and location at the start of the call so that the patient can be found if he or she loses consciousness or is disconnected.

Patients Without Appointments. The provider and scheduling team should come up with a policy for patients without appointments, also referred to as walk-in patients. A patient who requires immediate attention will most likely be fit into the schedule. If the patient does not need immediate care, an appointment scheduled for a later time may be the answer. Be sure to follow established office policy.

Failed Appointments

Why do patients fail to keep appointments? Some are simply forgetful. Once this tendency is detected in a patient, form the habit of telephoning or emailing a reminder the day before the appointment. Automated call routing offers the patient the option of canceling an appointment and can be programmed to keep calling until the patient responds and confirms or cancels the appointment.

A patient who has been asked for payment may stay away because of an inability to pay for medical services. Do not make the mistake of classifying such patients as "deadbeats." Many have every desire to pay, but they cannot afford to and feel embarrassed about their situation, so they avoid their appointments.

Patients may also fail to keep appointments because they are in a state of denial about their condition. For instance, if a patient recently tested positive for the human immunodeficiency virus (HIV), he or she may avoid appointments because going to see the provider forces the patient to face the reality of the disease. Take special care with such patients, and if denial is suspected, discuss this with the provider, who may want to refer the patient for counseling.

It is important to determine the reason for failed appointments and to do whatever is possible to remedy the situation. Telephone the patient to make sure no misunderstanding has occurred. If the patient's health requires ongoing care, the provider may write a letter explaining this to the patient. Send the letter by certified mail with return receipt requested. A copy of the letter needs to be added to the patient's medical record for legal protection.

For legal purposes, failed appointments need to be documented in the patient's health record and the appointment schedule. A patient may try to claim abandonment, when he or she has actually been the one to miss the appointments.

No-Show Policy. Some patients may not realize the importance of keeping their appointments. The patient who does not arrive for a scheduled appointment or reschedule it is called a no-show. A busy practice must have a specific policy on appointment no-shows and must enforce it effectively. The first time a patient fails to show, note that fact on the health record or ledger card. The second time, warn the patient, and if a third no-show occurs, consider dropping the patient by using the customary methods that provide legal protection for the provider. Another option is to only allow the patient to schedule for same-day appointments.

The provider may wish to charge patients for not showing up for the appointment. Be understanding whenever possible, but do not let a patient take advantage of the provider's time. The office policy manual must state that patients may be charged for missed appointments, and this should be explained to new patients when their first appointment is made. Because the time slot was scheduled and the provider was ready and available to treat the patient, it is ethical to charge the patient for missing an appointment, especially if he or she did not call to cancel or reschedule. Many providers do not press this issue, but it is an available tool if needed.

Increasing Appointment Show Rates

Everyone benefits from a full schedule of kept appointments. Appointment show rates can be increased in several ways.

Automated Call Routing. As mentioned earlier, automated call reminders can contact patients scheduled for appointments. The patient is asked to press a certain key on the phone to confirm the appointment and a different key to cancel the appointment. This same tool can be used to send messages to patients (e.g., a reminder that it is the time of year to get a flu vaccination), to introduce a new provider at the office, or to announce the availability of a new procedure. The provider can even record the call so that it sounds more personal. These systems can also be set up to send text messages to remind patients of their upcoming appointments.

Appointment Cards. Most healthcare facilities use appointment cards to remind patients of scheduled appointments and to eliminate misunderstandings about dates and times (Fig. 20.9). Make a habit of reaching for an appointment card while writing an entry in the appointment book or scheduling it on the computer. After the date and time have been written on the card, double-check with the book/computer to make sure the entries agree.

Confirmation Calls. Patients who have made appointments in advance may appreciate a confirmation call to remind them that they have a time set aside to see the provider. Always note the phone number the patient prefers the office to use for such calls. Many individuals have home phone, cell phone, and work phone numbers; however, they may want calls from the provider to go only to their home phone. Highlight the preferred phone number in the medical record, or indicate it on

---

VOCABULARY

no-show: When a patient fails to keep an appointment without giving advance notice.

screening: A system for examining and separating into different groups; in the healthcare facility, it means determining the severity of a patient's illness and prioritizing appointments based on that severity.

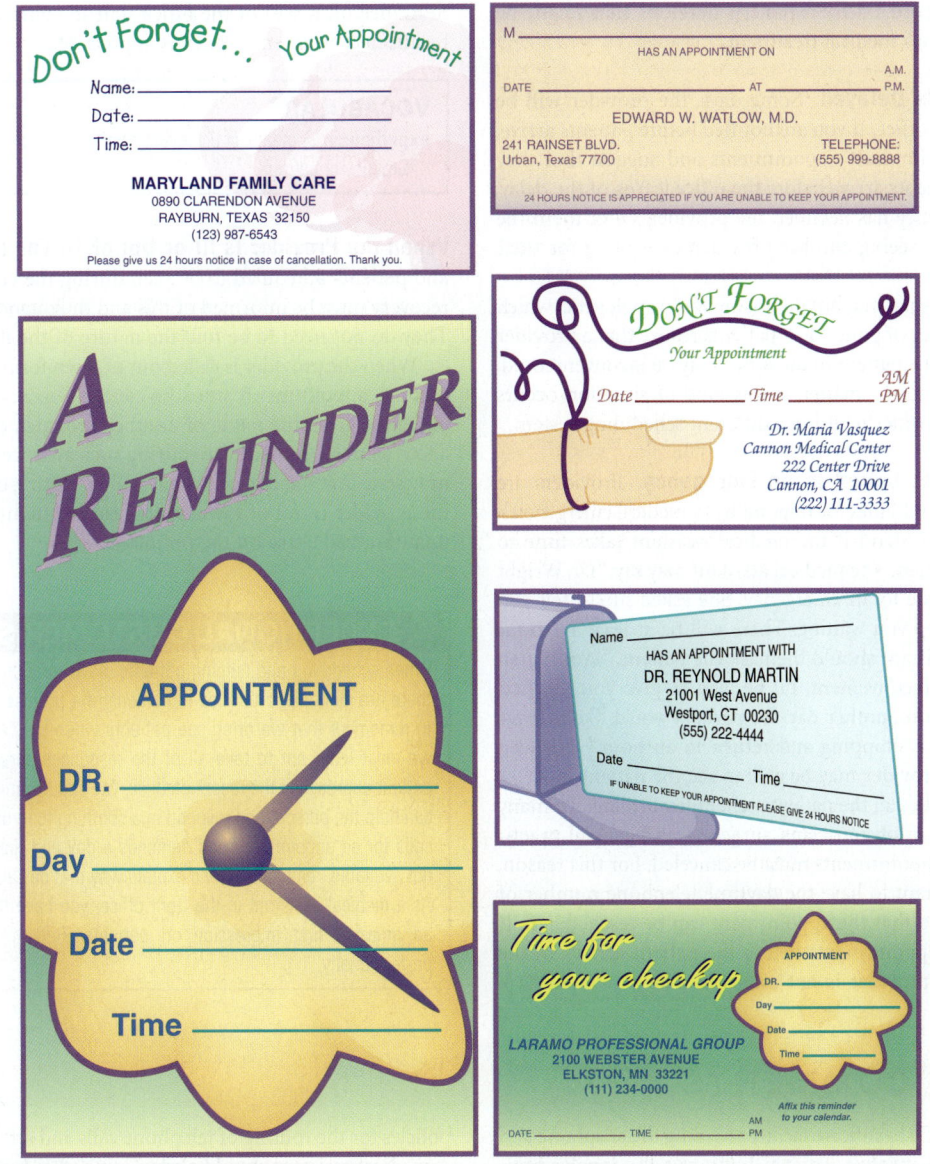

FIG. 20.9 Examples of appointment reminder cards. (From Proctor D, et al: *Kinn's The Medical Assistant,* ed 13, St. Louis, 2017, Elsevier.)

the computer. The office must use caution in making calls to patients because of the significance of privacy guidelines and standards. Some offices may want to prepare a release form on which patients grant the office staff permission to contact them. Many providers insist that messages left on voice mail not mention the term "doctor" or "doctor's office" for confidentiality reasons. The medical assistant might say, "This is Pam at Robert Welch's office confirming your appointment tomorrow at 2 p.m. Please call us if you cannot make the appointment. Our number is 555-212-0909. Thank you!"

If the patient has signed the privacy policy and the policy states that messages from the provider's office may be left at certain numbers, the office certainly can leave messages at that number and mention that the call is from the healthcare facility. Still, it is a good idea to have an established policy on leaving messages that does not breach the patient's confidentiality.

Email Reminders. Many computer scheduling programs can send an email to patients the day before an appointment to remind them of it. This is a great timesaver for the office staff, because no time is taken to perform this duty other than the original scheduling of the appointment.

Mailed Reminders. The office staff may mail reminder letters to patients. This method is a bit time consuming with a paper-based appointment system but worth the effort if the patients show up for their appointments. Computer scheduling systems can be set up to generate the reminder letters for scheduled appointments and also to remind patients that they are due for their annual physical or influenza vaccination.

Handling Cancellations and Delays

When the Patient Cancels. Cancellations occur in every healthcare facility. To minimize the impact of cancellations, keep a list of patients with future appointments who would like to come in sooner. The medical assistant can begin calling those patients to try to get one of them in to fill the available opening. Each cancellation should be noted in the medical record, along with a reason for the cancellation. If the patient simply reschedules an appointment, a notation does not need to be made in the health record unless a pattern develops that might be significant to the patient's medical treatment.

When the Provider Is Delayed. Some days, the provider will be delayed in reaching the office. If you are notified before patients arrive, start calling patients with early appointments and suggest that they come later. If some patients arrive before the office learns of the delay, explain that an emergency has detained the provider. Offer them the option of rescheduling, seeing another provider, or waiting for their provider.

Show concern for the patient, but do not be overly apologetic, which might imply some degree of guilt. Most patients realize that a provider has certain priorities. The patient in the office may be inconvenienced, but it is not a "life or death" matter. If this kind of situation occurs frequently, however, consider devising a different scheduling system.

When the Provider Is Called to an Emergency. Providers are conscious of their responsibilities for responding to medical emergencies, and most patients understand if the medical assistant takes time to explain what has happened. The medical assistant may say, "Dr. Wright has been called away due to an emergency. She asked me to tell you she is very sorry to keep you waiting. There will be at least a 1-hour delay." The medical assistant should then ask the patient, "Would you like to wait? If that is inconvenient, I'll be glad to give you the first available appointment on another day. Or perhaps you'd like to have some coffee or do some shopping and return in an hour." It is also possible that another provider may be able to see the patient.

As quickly as possible, call the patients scheduled for later. In many offices, especially those of obstetricians, surgeons, and general practitioners, a whole day's appointments must be canceled. For this reason, it is particularly important to have the daytime telephone number of each patient available so that the appointment can be rescheduled. If at all possible, cancel appointments before the patient arrives in the office to find that the provider is not available. The *expediency* (ik SPEE dee uh n see) of the office staff in contacting patients who will be affected by an emergency is appreciated.

> **VOCABULARY**
> **expediency:** A means of achieving a particular end, as in a situation requiring urgency or caution.

When the Provider Is Ill or Out of Town. Providers get sick, too, and patients scheduled to be seen during the course of the provider's recovery must be informed of this and their appointments rescheduled. They do not need to be told the nature of the illness.

When the provider is called out of town for personal or professional reasons, appointments must be canceled or rescheduled. Usually, the patient is given the name of another provider, or possibly a choice of a few, who will provide care during such absences. For security reasons, only state that the doctor is unavailable. Stating over the telephone that the provider is out of town could lead to attempted burglary or other unauthorized entry on the premises.

> **EXCEPTIONAL CUSTOMER SERVICE**
> When scheduling and helping patients move through the healthcare facility, there are many opportunities to demonstrate professionalism. It is important to remember that we often see patients when they are not at their best, so we must learn not to take all of the responses personally. When an angry patient approaches the reception desk, you should smile politely, ask how you can help the person, and respond in a soothing tone of voice. When a patient calls for an appointment and demands a day and time when the provider is not available, remain calm and explain why that day and time is not an option. As a medical assistant in the front office, you have the opportunity to make an amazing first impression on patients. Remember to always behave professionally.

CLOSING COMMENTS

Two major activities in the healthcare facility are using the telephone and scheduling. Usually, this involves patients, but it can also involve nonpatients. In either situation, it is important to follow the organization's policies for the routing of telephone calls and scheduling appointments. A medical assistant should always remember to treat calls to the office as if it were one of their own family members on the line.

CHAPTER REVIEW

In this chapter, we started out with a discussion about telephone equipment and the features that a medical assistant needs to be aware of when using a multiple-line telephone. Whether you are working in the administrative or clinical area, you will be using the telephone to communicate with others. Having a good understanding of the features will make this part of your job much easier.

When answering the telephone, it is also important to use excellent listening skills. You do not have the visual cues that you would if you were face to face with the caller. Your listening skills will help you gather the necessary information.

A wide variety of calls come into a healthcare facility. You should know the policies for handling all types of calls. This includes knowing who can receive information about a patient, how to accurately record laboratory results, how to handle an angry caller, and what resources are available for callers who have difficulty communicating.

An important medical assistant responsibility is to handle the appointment schedule. You may even be in charge of setting up the appointment matrix. Meeting the patient needs and provider preferences can be a challenging job. Having an efficient scheduling system is key to keeping the healthcare facility on track timewise. The patients and the providers will be much happier with a schedule that runs smoothly.

SCENARIO WRAP-UP

Ashlynn is quickly becoming a part of the team at WMFM and is developing into a well-liked asset to the staff. She has learned to slow down when speaking on the phone and to adjust her volume and pitch, depending on the patient with whom she is speaking. Although she tends to be talkative, she is balancing just the right amount of friendly chatter with the business at hand. She does this by offering a pleasant greeting to callers, getting to the point of the call, then being affable before ending the call. By expressing her concern and asking how she can be of help to the patients, Ashlynn shows them that she sincerely cares about their problems. She is careful about her tone of voice, realizing that patients may take her comments the wrong way if she does not treat them in a cordial manner.

Ashlynn takes care when she speaks to patients and others on the phone so that she does not breach confidentiality in any way. She has become comfortable with the way she is expected to answer the telephone. The pace of her speech and the wording are now a habit. Ashlynn is determined to maintain a professional relationship with all the people related to her work environment. She is now adept at handling calls from angry patients and can maintain control with even the most aggressive callers. She leaves callers on hold for a minimum of time and reassures them frequently that she is tending to their situation. By treating callers as she would want to be treated, Ashlynn reduces frustration, and she feels that the office is more efficient at handling the large volume of calls that come in each day.

When it comes to scheduling, Ashlynn is flexible and can change the order of the patients seen, if needed, to maximize the use of time and facilities in the office. Because she is so cheerful and friendly, patients do not seem to mind when she asks for their cooperation. She keeps current phone numbers and cell phone information so that she can notify a patient quickly if the providers are running behind schedule. Ashlynn's proficiency on the computer is also an asset, and she makes frequent use of email to take care of patient problems or rescheduling requests.

Ashlynn contributes to the efficiency of the healthcare facility by constantly refining her knowledge about her job. She pays attention to the times during the day that do not run as smoothly as others, evaluates the problems at those times, and then corrects them. She also keeps the schedule moving by communicating with the clinical medical assistants, keeping them informed about arriving patients and those who have come early or are running late. She can quickly adjust and substitute a patient who already has arrived. Ashlynn has learned how to manipulate the schedule to accommodate an emergency. She knows that by making minor adjustments and keeping the waiting patients informed, the staff can handle any emergency.

All medical assistants need to develop skills in flexibility. Establishing a system that works and using it correctly makes patients and staff members more content with their experience in the healthcare facility.

21

Technology and Written Communication

LEARNING OBJECTIVES

1. List and discuss parts of personal computer hardware.
2. Describe how to maintain computer hardware and identify principles of ergonomics.
3. Discuss software used in the ambulatory care center, describe the importance of computer network privacy and security, and discuss the continual technology advances in healthcare.
4. Recognize elements of fundamental writing skills.
5. List the parts of a professional letter.
6. List and discuss different types of business letter formats. Compose a professional business letter.
7. Discuss letter templates, how to prepare a letter for delivery, memorandums, professional emails, and faxed communication. Compose a professional email.

CHAPTER OUTLINE

1. Opening Scenario, 468
2. You Will Learn, 469
3. Introduction, 469
4. Electronic Technology in the Ambulatory Care Center, 469
   a. Personal Computer Hardware, 469
      i. *Input Devices*, 469
      ii. *Output Devices*, 472
      iii. *Internal Components*, 472
      iv. *Secondary Storage Devices*, 473
      v. *Network and internet Access Devices*, 473
   b. Maintaining Computer Hardware, 474
   c. Computer Workstation Ergonomics, 475
   d. Software Used in the Ambulatory Care Center, 475
   e. Computer Network Privacy and Security, 476
   f. Continual Technology Advances in Healthcare, 478
5. Fundamentals of Written Communication, 480
   a. Parts of Speech, 480
   b. Appropriate Use of Words, 480
   c. Capitalization, Numbers, and Punctuation, 480
6. Written Correspondence, 482
   a. Parts of a Professional Letter, 482
      i. *Sender's Address*, 482
      ii. *Date*, 482
      iii. *Inside Address*, 482
      iv. *Reference Line*, 482
      v. *Salutation*, 482
      vi. *Subject Line*, 483
      vii. *Body of the Letter*, 484
      viii. *Closing*, 484
      ix. *Signature Block*, 484
      x. *End Notations*, 484
      xi. *Continuation Pages*, 484
   b. Business Letter Formats, 484
      i. *Full Block Letter Format*, 484
      ii. *Modified Block Letter Format*, 485
      iii. *Semi–Block Letter Format*, 485
   c. Letter Templates, 485
   d. Preparing the Letter for Delivery, 486
      i. *Postage*, 487
   e. Memorandums, 488
   f. Professional Emails, 488
   g. Faxed Communication, 490
7. Closing Comments, 491
8. Chapter Review, 492
9. Scenario Wrap-Up, 492

▶ OPENING SCENARIO

Christiana was a medical assistant at Walden-Martin Family Medical (WMFM) Clinic. She had been working as a clinical medical assistant for 5 years. She helped with diagnostic tests and treatment procedures. Christiana enjoyed providing patient care, but she wanted to use more of the administrative skills she learned. She is organized and enjoys challenges and technology. When a front office position opened up, Christiana moved into the administrative role. She is now the lead administrative medical assistant. Her role involves answering phones, scheduling appointments, greeting patients, and processing correspondence to patients. She is also responsible for reviewing the clinic's emails. Patients are encouraged to use email to communicate with Dr. Kahn. Christiana has seen the number of daily emails increase. She answers those that pertain to appointments. Other emails are forwarded to Dr. Kahn or to his clinical medical assistant. Besides performing her administrative duties, Christiana is now responsible for the clinic's computer system. She is excited to continue to learn the administrative role and the computer system.

CHAPTER 21 Technology and Written Communication

YOU WILL LEARN

1. To describe common hardware and software used in the ambulatory care facility.
2. To discuss how to have an ergonomically correct workstation.
3. To describe computer network security procedures.
4. To compose a professional letter and email.
5. To describe common postal services used in the ambulatory care facility.

INTRODUCTION

When technology was first used in healthcare, it was used in the business departments. Computer *software* was used for the following actions:
- Billing and accounting procedures
- Registration processes
- Scheduling

With the advent of computer technology, what used to take hours to do, now takes minutes. Data are collected once, entered, and used for many purposes. Computer software increases accuracy and efficiency, as well as saves money.

When *electronic health records (EHRs)* were introduced, agencies implemented software to increase the accuracy and efficiency of patient care. The federal government provided financial incentives to use EHRs instead of paper medical records. Currently healthcare workers use "smart" devices for quicker access to information to provide better patient care.

Communication has also changed over the years. Many people have moved from writing letters to sending emails and text messages. Social *media* (ME de ah) sites have gained popularity. Many of these changes have affected the ambulatory care environment. Patients use emails and text messages to contact their providers. To help ensure confidentiality, administrators have created tighter network security procedures. Restrictions on employee social media postings have also been added.

Today, medical assistants must be more computer savvy than ever before to meet technologic demands. They must follow procedures to safeguard the privacy and security of patients' records. The need for correct grammar, punctuation, and word use is greater than ever as medical assistants communicate using letters and electronic technology.

> **CRITICAL THINKING 21.1**
>
> Christiana answers emails from patients. How might her responses differ from her personal emails to her family and friends?

ELECTRONIC TECHNOLOGY IN THE AMBULATORY CARE CENTER

Many clinics are using electronic technology in both administrative and patient care areas. Paper medical charts are being replaced with EHRs. Technology has increased the efficiency of the office environment. It has made patient information and resources quickly accessible to healthcare staff. Medical assistants need to learn and use computers and technology.

Personal Computer Hardware

A personal computer (PC) is a single-user electronic data processing device. Table 21.1 describes common types of personal computers. The PC accepts, stores, and processes data. After processing the information, it generates the data output in a specific form.

The personal computer is a system unit. All other forms of physical equipment used with the PC are called peripheral devices. The PC and peripheral devices are *hardware*. Computer hardware can be divided into the following categories: input devices, *output devices*, internal components, *secondary storage devices*, and network and internet access devices. The following sections describe these categories.

> **CRITICAL THINKING 21.2**
>
> When Christiana transitioned into the administrative role, Dr. Kahn hired Michaela as the new clinical medical assistant. Recently the healthcare facility switched from using desktop computers to tablet computers when working with patients in the exam rooms. How might Christiana's experience using the desktop computer in the exam rooms be different from Michaela's use of the tablet computer? Thinking of the patient's perception, which technology might a patient prefer the medical assistant to use? Why?

Input Devices. An *input device* is any peripheral hardware that allows the user to provide data to the computer. Many types of input devices are available on the market. This discussion focuses on those typically used in the ambulatory care setting. Common input devices include keyboards, mice and other pointing devices, touchscreens, webcams, microphones, scanners, and signature pads.

Keyboards are the most common input devices. The QWERTY keyboard is the standard keyboard for computers. (Q-W-E-R-T-Y are the first six letters, from left to right, just below the number keys on the keyboard.) A wide variety of keyboards are available, including standard, internet, wireless, and ergonomic. Keyboards may have special keys that perform the same functionality as the buttons on Web pages. Numeric keypads are also a feature on many keyboards. Ergonomic keyboards reduce repetitive strain injuries by minimizing muscle strain. These keyboards allow the user's hands to be in a natural position when typing. The two most common ergonomic

> **VOCABULARY**
>
> **electronic health record (EHR):** An electronic record that conforms to nationally recognized standards and contains health-related information about a specific patient. It can be created, managed, and consulted by authorized clinicians and staff from more than one healthcare organization.
> **hardware:** Physical equipment of the computer system required for communication and data processing functions.
> **media:** Types of communication (e.g., social media sites); with computers, the term refers to data storage devices.
> **output device:** Computer hardware that displays the processed data from the computer (e.g., monitors and printers).
> **secondary storage devices:** Media (e.g., jump drive, flash drive, hard drive) capable of permanently storing data until they are replaced or deleted by the user.
> **software:** A set of electronic instructions to operate and perform different computer tasks.

UNIT 3 Administrative Ambulatory Care

TABLE 21.1 Types of Personal Computers

Type of Personal Computer	Description	Use in Healthcare
Desktop computer	Larger unit, designed for use on a desk (Fig. 21.1)	Used by employees who primarily perform word processing, data entry, and business tasks (scheduling, bookkeeping, and billing)
Laptop computer	Thin, lightweight portable PC with a keyboard; may include a touchscreen panel (Fig. 21.2). Also called notebook PC	Used by providers and medical assistants in patient exam rooms and at workstations.
Tablet computer	Thin, lightweight portable PC that functions with a touchscreen (Fig. 21.3) (most popular operating systems include Android and iOS)	

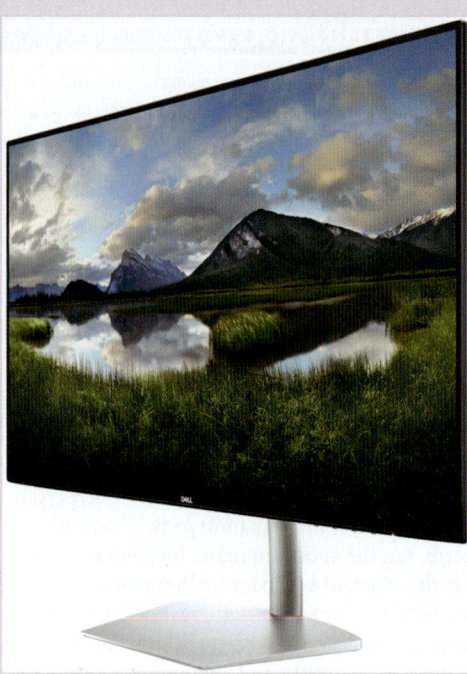

FIG. 21.1 Many healthcare employees, including receptionists, clinical medical assistants, and providers, use desktop computers. The monitors for desktop computers have become larger and thinner over the years. (Courtesy Dell, Round Rock, Texas.)

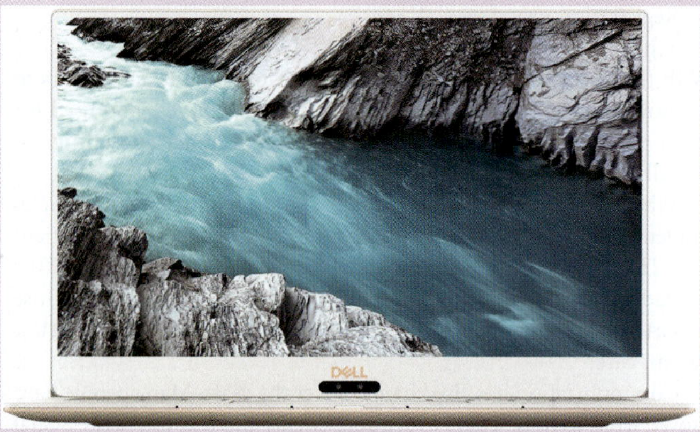

FIG. 21.2 Laptop computers are available in thinner, lighter-weight models with more functionality than older models. (Courtesy Dell, Round Rock, Texas.)

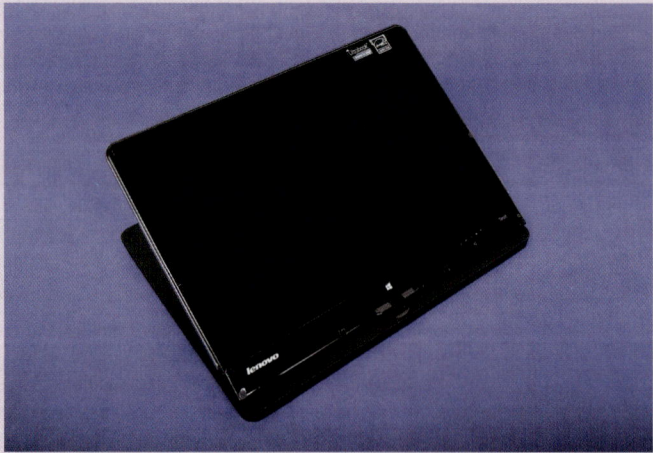

FIG. 21.3 Tablet computers and other new computers have touchscreen panels that allow users to easily enter data. (From Proctor D, et al: *Kinn's The Medical Assistant*, ed 13, St. Louis, 2017, Elsevier.)

CHAPTER 21 Technology and Written Communication

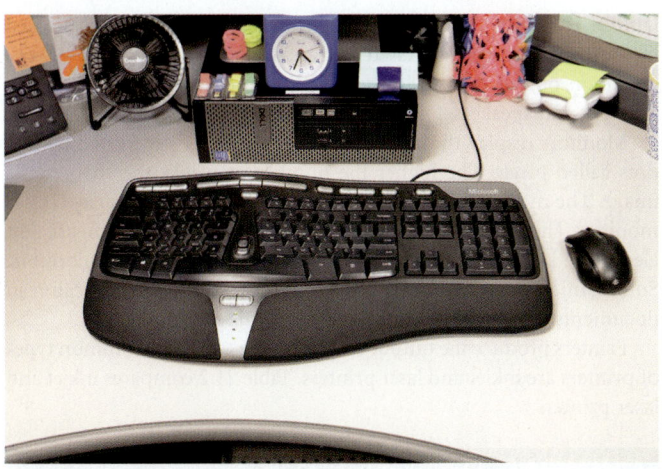

FIG. 21.4 Ergonomic keyboards have different appearances, yet they all reduce repetitive strain injuries. (From Proctor D, et al: *Kinn's The Medical Assistant*, ed 13, St. Louis, 2017, Elsevier.)

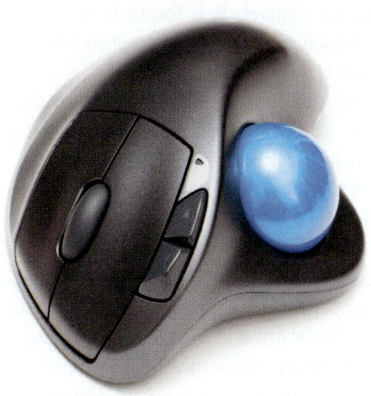

FIG. 21.5 A trackball mouse uses a large ball to control the movement of the cursor/pointer. (From Proctor D, et al: *Kinn's The Medical Assistant*, ed 13, St. Louis, 2017, Elsevier.)

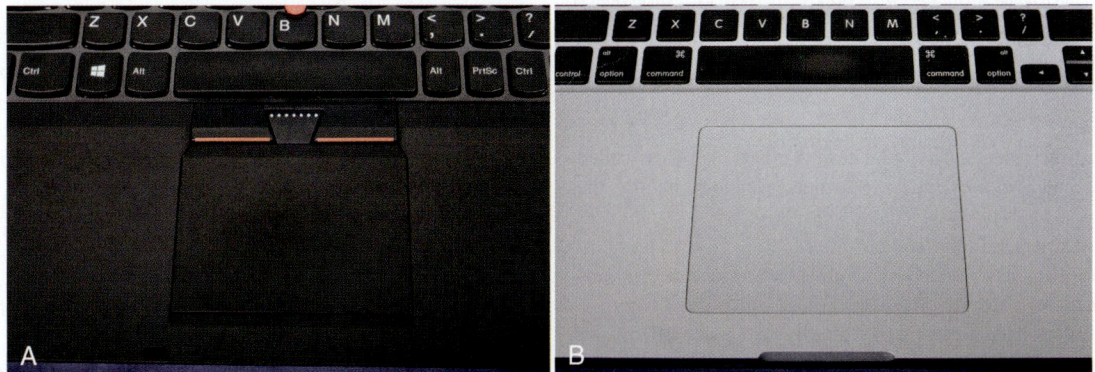

FIG. 21.6 A touchpad is built into a computer, and its functions are like those of a mouse, although different touchpads may have different functions. For example, the device in part A has a left and right click button, whereas the device in part B does not. (From Proctor D, et al: *Kinn's The Medical Assistant*, ed 13, St. Louis, 2017, Elsevier.)

keyboards are the split-key models and the waved or curved key layout (Fig. 21.4).

> **CRITICAL THINKING 21.3**
>
> Christiana's keyboard looks different from Dr. Kahn's keyboard in his office. Why might Christiana have a different keyboard?

Keyboards typically have the following categories of keys:
- *Typing*: include the numeric and alphabetic keys used for typing.
- *Numeric*: numeric keypads in the same position as calculators.
- *Function*: the 12 keys at the top of the keyboard. Each key has a specific purpose. Some software programs allow the function keys to be programmed to complete a specific function.
- *Control*: allow movement of the cursor and the screen; include Home, End, Insert, Delete, Page Up, Page Down, Control, Escape, Alternate, and four arrow keys.
- *Special purpose*: include Enter, Shift, Caps Lock, Num Lock, Space Bar, Print Screen, and Tab keys.

The mouse is one of the most common input devices. It makes screen navigation much simpler than using the keyboard. A mouse is a palm-sized box with a laser sensor that tracks the movement of the user's hand. It sends those messages back to the computer. The mouse is used to move the pointer (cursor) on the screen. The mouse may have left and right buttons with a wheel in between to help with cursor/pointer navigation and functionality. With a trackball mouse, the user moves the enlarged ball on the top of the mouse to control the pointer (Fig. 21.5).

Touchpads are becoming more popular on laptops. They are touch sensitive. Touchpads move the pointer based on the user's finger movements. The functionality of touchpads can vary. Some have left- and right-click buttons like those on a mouse (Fig. 21.6). Other touchpads have a finger tap or click sequence for the left- and right-click action.

A touchscreen is different from a touchpad. A touchscreen allows a person to interact with the computer by touching the display screen with a finger or **stylus** (STI luhs). Touchscreens can vary, which means the compatible stylus can vary:
- *Resistive touchscreen*: responds to the touch of almost anything that can generate pressure (e.g., finger, plastic stylus, rubber-tip stylus). These screens are found in many handheld electronic devices.

> **VOCABULARY**
>
> **stylus**: A pen-shaped device with a variety of tips that is used on touchscreens to write, draw, or input commands.

- *Capacitive* (kah PAS i tiv) *touchscreen*: responds to the electrical characteristics of a finger. It is found in smart phones and other electronic devices. It requires a specialized stylus that has more surface area in the point.
- *Surface acoustic* (ah KOO stik) *wave touchscreen*: responds to an inaudible wave of sound that is created on the screen from a finger. It is common in kiosks and on ordering screens. A stylus with a rubber or soft tip the size of a pencil eraser is required.

Wireless webcams and microphones are becoming more popular. Providers can use webcams, microphones, and internet video chat software to see patients who are at a distance from the healthcare facility. The remote diagnosis and treatment of patients using technology is called *telemedicine*. Webcams and microphones are also used for meetings and continuing education opportunities. Microphones can be used for dictating notes into a patient's health record. Voice recognition software provides instant transcription into the patient's record.

CRITICAL THINKING 21.4

Dr. Kahn works with a home health agency. Patients and nurses can communicate with him using the internet, microphones, and webcams. How does this technology benefit the patients?

Scanners convert images to digital text through a process called *optical character recognition* (OCR). Scanners available include the following:
- Handheld scanners scan bar codes.
- Sheet-fed scanners may be stand-alone units or may include duplicating and faxing features.
- Flatbed scanners have a glass panel on which the documents are placed for scanning.

Scanners in the healthcare setting have become more popular since the use of EHRs has increased. Old medical records are scanned, and the images are uploaded into the patient's EHR. Receptionists use small, sheet-fed scanners to scan insurance cards when patients check in for appointments. The insurance card images are then uploaded into the patient's record and referenced for billing activities.

In the ambulatory care setting, signature pads are used in the reception area (Fig. 21.7). Patients need to sign several documents, including Authorization for Release of Medical Information, consent forms, and the Notice of Privacy Practices. Patients sign the signature pad. The signature is then imported into the EHR as part of the patient's permanent health record.

Output Devices. The data entered into the computer are processed by the computer. The processed data are displayed using *output devices*. Common output devices in the healthcare setting include monitors, printers, and speakers.

Monitors display the output as images. Images are created by tiny dots called *pixels*. The higher the number of pixels, the sharper the image. The most common monitor is the liquid crystal display (LCD) monitor. These monitors are easier on the eyes. They also use less electricity. LCD monitors are smaller and lighter than older monitors. Some clinics use LCD monitors in the reception area. Patients can read documents on the monitor before signing the signature pad.

Printers produce the output on paper. The two most common types of printers are inkjet and laser printers. Table 21.2 compares inkjet and laser printers.

CRITICAL THINKING 21.5

Christiana frequently prints documents, including billing statements, appointment reminders, and receipts for payment. What type of printer might be the most economical to use in the reception area? Why?

Speakers for electronic devices come in all shapes and sizes. Typically, speakers are built into the devices used (e.g., monitor, laptop, and tablet).

Internal Components. For desktop personal computers, the internal components are found in the tower or case. Table 21.3 briefly describes internal computer components (Box 21.1).

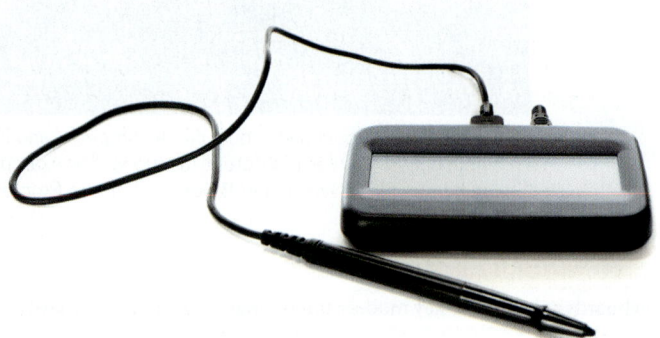

FIG. 21.7 Signature pads allow patients' signatures to be imported into the electronic health record or practice management software. (From Proctor D, et al: *Kinn's The Medical Assistant*, ed 13, St. Louis, 2017, Elsevier.)

TABLE 21.2 Inkjet and Laser Printers

	Inkjet Printer	Laser Printer
How Does It Work	Create images by spraying small drops of ink on the paper	Uses a laser, electrical charges, and toner to produce images on paper
Advantages	• Create high-quality printing • Inexpensive to purchase	• High-speed printing, high-quality output, and quality graphics • Support of many fonts and font sizes • Toner cartridges are changed less often compared with inkjet printers
Disadvantages	• Slower to print a document compared with a laser printer • Frequent need to replace ink cartridges gets expensive	• Initial cost of printer is higher

TABLE 21.3 Internal Components of a Desktop Personal Computer

Internal Component		Description	Role
Central processing unit (CPU)		Processor or "brains" of the computer; sits on the motherboard	Interprets and executes commands from the software (program)
Motherboard		Platform	Attachment point for all internal computer parts
Primary memory	Read-only memory (ROM)	Contains read-only memory that has hardwire instructions	Used when the computer boots up or starts the system diagnostic checks
	Cache memory	Provides temporary use of information; contains data and instructions for opened programs	Allows programs to operate more quickly and efficiently
	Random access memory (RAM)	Working memory lost if power is turned off	Main memory of the computer; required for the computer to operate (see Box 21.1)
Hard drive		"Hard drive" or C drive of computer; includes the hard disk drive (HDD) and the hard drive as one unit	Read and writes on the hard disk; provides the largest amount of permanent storage for the computer
Optical drive		Saves data on removable storage devices	Read or read and write (save) data on optical discs (compact discs [CDs], digital versatile/video discs [DVDs], and Blu-Ray discs [BDs])
Sound card		Also called audio card or audio adapter	Allows audio information to be sent to speakers or headphones
Video card		Also called graphic card or video adapter	Allows the computer to send graphic information to output devices (monitor or projectors)
Universal serial bus (USB) port		Most common type of connector device that allows hardware to be plugged into the computer	Allow hardware to connect to the computer

BOX 21.1 RAM

Before installing new software, make sure the computer has the required random-access memory (RAM). *RAM* (ramm) is the computer memory used for loading and running programs. If there is not enough RAM for the program, the computer must go to the hard drive to read the data, which is a slower process.

Secondary Storage Devices. A secondary storage device, or medium, is capable of permanently storing data. With many types, the user can write over the existing data or delete the data. These devices can be considered removable, internal (such as the hard drive previously discussed), or external. The computer needs a secondary storage device to allow the user to save data. Without a storage device, the computer would be considered a **dumb terminal**. Dumb terminals provide the user access to software, the network, or the internet. They do not allow the user to save data to the C drive of the computer.

The types of computer storage devices are categorized as magnetic, optical, and flash. Table 21.4 provides descriptions and examples of storage devices. The use of cloud storage is becoming more popular. Cloud storage is also called file sharing or online storage. It allows computer files to be stored using the internet and a third-party service. To get started, an individual signs up with a cloud storage service. Many companies allow free minimal storage. Others charge monthly fees or fees based on storage size. After signing up, individuals use the internet to send computer files to the service company's **data servers**. The files are copied onto many servers in various locations. This is called *redundancy*. It allows the information to be accessible even if one site goes down and needs repairs. With internet access and a password, an individual has access to the files anytime and can share the files with others.

The capacity of storage devices also must be considered. The storage capacity is measured in bytes. A byte is usually considered a character, such as a number, letter, or symbol. To simplify communication, the storage size is often estimated. For instance, 1024 bytes might be stated as 1000 bytes. Over the years, the size of storage devices has increased. The cost of storage has also decreased (Table 21.5). Flash drives range in size. Some now can hold more than 250 gigabytes (GB), or 268,435,456,000 bytes.

Network and Internet Access Devices. The computers and output devices are usually all connected to the facility's network. This can be called the *local area network* (LAN). The local area network can span one building or multiple buildings. Some healthcare agencies have clinics at a distance. They may have *wide area network* (WAN) technology, which consists of two or more LANs. LAN and WAN technology can

CRITICAL THINKING 21.6

Christiana would like to have a small patient education space in the reception area. She would like to have a computer with internet access for patients so they can access health information. Christiana knows that cost is a factor in a small healthcare facility. The computer would have to be reasonable and reliable. What technology options might she propose to Dr. Kahn?

VOCABULARY

data server: Computer hardware and software that perform data analysis, storage, and archiving; also called a *database server*.
dumb terminal: A personal computer that does not contain a hard drive and allows the user only limited functions, including access to software, the network, or the internet.

TABLE 21.4 Data Storage Devices

Device	Description	Examples
Magnetic storage device	One of the oldest types of storage; uses magnetic technology to read and write data to the device	Internal hard drive, portable hard drive
Optical storage device	Uses lasers and lights to read and write data onto optical storage devices: • Recordable only: only allows data to be saved once to the disc (example: CD-R disc) • Read/write (RW): allows data to be saved, rewritten (resaved), and deleted (example: CD-RW) many times	Blu-Ray disc (BD), compact disc (CD), digital versatile/video disc (DVD)
Flash memory device	Portable devices that have become cheaper and have larger storage capacity over the years; connects to the USB port in the computer (Fig. 21.8)	Jump drive (also called USB flash, data stick, pen drive, keychain drive, travel drive, or thumb drive), memory card, memory stick, solid-state disk or drive (SSD)

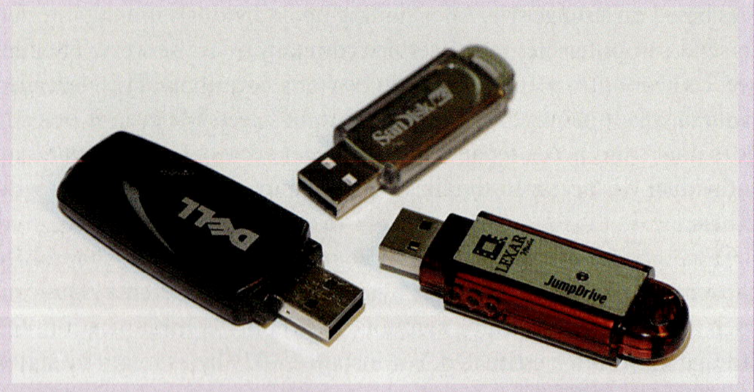

FIG. 21.8 Jump drives, known by many different names, allow users to store documents and files for use on other computers. (From Proctor D, et al: *Kinn's The Medical Assistant*, ed 13, St. Louis, 2017, Elsevier.)

TABLE 21.5 Terms for Data Storage Capacity on Electronic Devices

1 kilobyte (KB)	1024 bytes
1 megabyte (MB)	1024 KB (about 1 million bytes)
1 gigabyte (GB)	1024 MB (about 1 billion bytes)
1 terabyte (TB)	1024 GB (about 1 trillion bytes)

BOX 21.2 How to Prevent Computer Problems

- Hardware should be located on a stable, even surface, away from heat sources.
- Ventilation slots should be clear, allowing air to flow into the device to cool the components.
- Cables and electric cords should be securely plugged in.
- Liquids and food should be kept away from the hardware.

use telephone lines or fiberoptic cables that increase the speed of transmission.

A *router* (ROO tuhr) must be used to allow multiple devices to be on the same network. Most routers used today have wireless connectivity. A router is peripheral hardware that looks like a small box. Many routers have antennas and use **Ethernet** (EE thuhr net). The router allows multiple computers and other devices (e.g., smart devices) to use the same network to send and receive information.

For the **computer network** to have internet access, the ambulatory care facility must do the following:
- Subscribe to an internet services provider (ISP)
- Have its router connected to a **modem** (MOE duhm)

Most routers have a specific port that is designed to connect to the Ethernet port of a cable or digital subscriber line (DSL) modem. DSL is a high-speed internet service. It uses a modem to translate the computer's digital signals into voltage that is then sent over telephone lines.

Maintaining Computer Hardware

The medical assistant must maintain the computer hardware. Typically, the role involves routine cleaning. This helps prevent equipment failure and breakage. Larger facilities usually have their own information technology (IT) department. The IT staff provides technology assistance to the employees and maintains the equipment. If the facility uses an external IT support company, the medical assistant may have additional responsibilities (Boxes 21.2 and 21.3).

VOCABULARY
computer network: A system that links personal computers and peripheral devices to share information and resources.
Ethernet: A communication system for connecting several computers so information can be shared.
modem: Peripheral computer hardware that connects to the router to provide internet access to the network or computer.

CRITICAL THINKING 21.7
Christiana works with an information technology (IT) company that provides hardware, software, and services to the healthcare facility. How might her role with her agency's computer network differ if the healthcare facility had its own IT department?

A disc should be handled with care; grasp its outer edges or center hole. Keep discs clean and dust free. Store them in cases. Use a clean lint-free cloth to clean a disc. Wipe in a straight line from the center of the disc toward the outer edge. Keep discs and flash drives out of sunlight and extreme heat or high-humidity environments. To prevent flash drive data loss, make sure you never unplug the flash drive while it is writing or reading data.

BOX 21.3 Routine Cleaning for Computer Hardware

Before cleaning the computer or peripheral components, turn off and unplug the device. Refer to the operator's manual for cleaning instructions:

- If liquids spill on the keyboard, unplug the keyboard. Tip the keyboard upside down to drain out the liquid. Let the keyboard dry overnight. Sticky liquids are more apt to damage the keyboard.
- Use a damp lint-free cloth to wipe the hardware's casing to remove the grime and dirt.
- Wipe clean all vents and air holes.
- Spray a household glass cleaner on a lint-free cloth, and then wipe the glass monitor screen. Do not spray liquid directly on a component, as the liquid may drip into the device.
- Use a lint-free cloth dampened with water to clean nonglare or antiglare screens.
- Spray a disinfectant on a lint-free cloth or use a disinfectant cloth to disinfect the keyboard.
- Use compressed air dusters (i.e., pressurized air in a can) to blow the dirt out of the keyboard (Fig. 21.9).

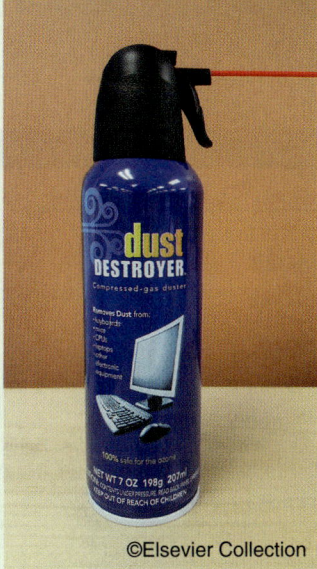

FIG. 21.9 Compressed air dusters provide an efficient means of removing the dust and dirt from keyboards.

Computer Workstation Ergonomics

It is important to arrange the computer workstation correctly to avoid the risk of repetitive stress injuries. Poor posture and straining can cause physical stress and injury to the body. This results in workers' compensation claims for treatment and services. Ergonomics is the field of study that involves reducing strain and injuries by improving the workstation design.

To have an ergonomically friendly workstation, the following are important:

- Torso and neck should be vertical and in line.
- Feet need to be flat on the floor or a footrest (Fig. 21.10A).
- Backrest should help support the upper body in the upright position.
- Backrest lumbar support area should be fitted to the small of the back (Fig. 21.10B).
- Seat should be the appropriate size and height to accommodate the body build so that there is no added pressure on the back of the knees or thighs.
- The armrest should support the forearms with the shoulders in a relaxed position (Fig. 21.10C).
- For standing workstations, legs, torso, head, and neck should be vertical and in line. One foot can be elevated on a step.
- Monitor should be directly in front of the person with the top of the monitor at or just below eye level.
- Use a document holder, so documents are placed at the same distance and height as the monitor (Fig. 21.10D).
- Use an ergonomic split-key or waved keyboard. Place keyboard at a height and an angle that allow the wrists to be in a neutral position.
- The work surface and mouse should be at elbow level for typing. Your wrist should be supported by a foam wrist rest (Fig. 21.10E).
- Headsets should be used for those answering frequent phone calls to prevent muscle strain.

Whether you are standing or sitting at a workstation, it is important to change position every 30 minutes. If you are sitting, adjustments can be made to chairs or backrests. Stretching your fingers, arms, and torso is important. Frequently look away from the computer to a distant object to prevent eyestrain. Stand up and walk around for a few minutes. Preventing repetitive stress injuries is important for all computer users.

Software Used in the Ambulatory Care Center

For hardware to work, the computer must have software. The terms *software* and *program* are mostly synonymous. Programs existed before software. A program is a sequence of instructions. It is written in a language understood by the computer. It directs the computer to perform a specific task. Software contains several programs that together perform a function. Web browsers, email, games, spreadsheets, and word processors are all types of software.

The two main categories of software are system software and application software. System software is a collection of programs that operate and control the computer. The system software loads on the computer. It operates in the background while application software is used. Operating systems and utility software are two types of system software (Table 21.6).

Application software (also called an application, app, or application program) allows the user or other applications to perform specific tasks. Application software may consist of a single program or a collection of programs. A collection can be called a software package or system. In the ambulatory care facility, several types of application software are used, including practice management software and electronic health records (see Table 21.6).

Medical assistants use practice management software. This software can include programs for scheduling, new patient registration, billing, coding, and managing finances. Practice management software features can include appointment reminder email or letter tools, bookkeeping programs, and financial analysis tools. Managers use practice management software for running their business, making processes more efficient.

Many people use the terms **electronic medical record (EMR)** and *electronic health record (EHR)* interchangeably. However, there is a significant difference between these two types of software. When patients'

> **VOCABULARY**
> **electronic medical record (EMR):** An electronic record of health-related information about an individual that can be created, gathered, managed, and accessed by authorized clinicians and staff members within a single healthcare organization. An EMR is an electronic version of a paper record.

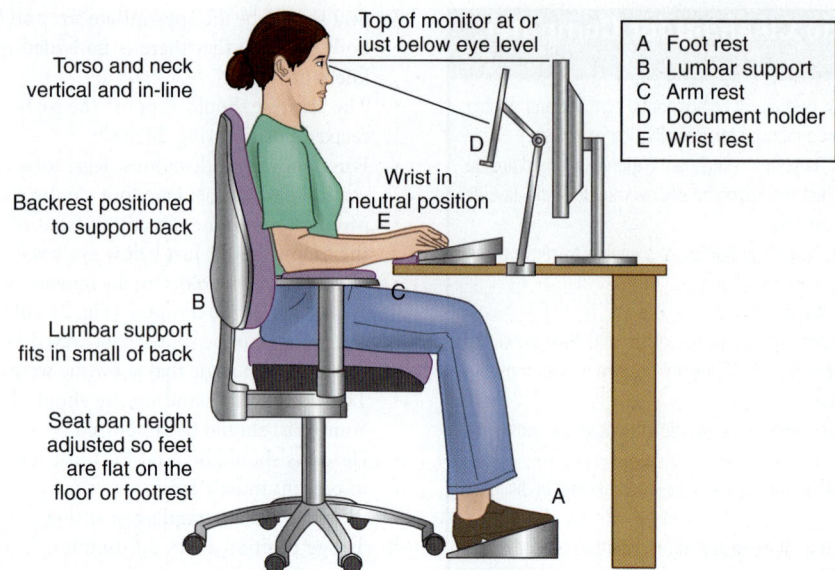

FIG. 21.10 Medical assistants should use an ergonomically correct workstation to prevent repetitive stress injuries. Equipment that helps create this type of workstation includes a footrest (A), lumbar support (B), armrest (C), document holder (D), and wrist rest (E). (From Proctor D, et al: *Kinn's The Medical Assistant*, ed 13, St. Louis, 2017, Elsevier.)

TABLE 21.6	Types of Software	
Main Category	**Types of Software**	**Description**
System software	Operating system	Acts as the computer's software administrator by managing, integrating, and controlling application software and hardware. Windows is an example.
	Utility software	Helps the computer function. Examples include file managers, screensavers, backup software, and clipboard managers.
Application software	Word processing software	Used to compose letters and documents. Microsoft Word is an example.
	Spreadsheet software	Used to manage numbers, data, and expenses. Microsoft Excel is an example.
	Telecommunication software	Used to email patients and vendors.
	Antimalware software	Used to protect computers against viruses (malware), which damage the computer.
	Database software	Allows the user to work with large amounts of data stored in the program. Examples include Microsoft Access, *practice management software* systems, and EHR software.

records became electronic (or computerized), they were called electronic medical records. The EMR software contains limited information, usually related to medical treatment for one healthcare facility. The EMR was a digital version of the paper medical record. The electronic health record has advantages over the EMR. The EHR allows sharing of information with other providers outside the facility, including medical laboratories, nursing homes, hospitals, and specialists. The information from all types of healthcare providers can be stored in the EHR, enhancing functionality and patient care.

It is important for the medical assistant to be aware of the differences between the practice management software and the EHR. You may use both during your day as a medical assistant. The EHR contains a record of patient interactions and health history. The practice management software allows the facility to operate the business side by maintaining schedules and financial information for revenue cycle management for reimbursement.

Computer Network Privacy and Security

We store vast quantities of confidential information in computer files. Electronic security is becoming more important today. Several healthcare facilities have had their network computer systems compromised by hackers and malware. Unsecured patient and employee confidential information can lead to identity theft and other criminal actions.

> **VOCABULARY**
> **practice management software**: A type of software that allows the user to enter demographic information, schedule appointments, maintain lists of insurance payers, perform billing tasks, and generate reports.

BOX 21.4 Making Strong Passwords

Strong passwords have more than eight characters and use a random combination of upper- and lowercase letters, numbers, and symbols. It is important to use different passwords and to change them frequently. Do not share passwords.

The Privacy Rule under the Health Insurance Portability and Accountability Act (HIPAA) and the Health Information Technology for Economic and Clinical Health Act (HITECH) require privacy, security, and confidentiality of patient records. These acts mandate training and procedures to be used in healthcare facilities to keep electronic records safe. Employers must provide privacy and security training to new employees. Periodic refresher courses are important for current staff. Most clinics also need to comply with the **meaningful use requirements**. These requirements include developing a **security risk analysis** process. This process is used to monitor for potential threats to privacy of the EHR and network files. (This process is explained in more detail later in the chapter.) Administrators and employees must work together to keep the computer network safe.

Common network security procedures used by employees include the following:

- *Authentication*: each employee with network access must log in using a unique password.
- Use strong passwords and frequently change passwords (Box 21.4).
- Use **privacy filters** over monitors to prevent others from seeing the information.
- Log out of the network when leaving a workstation.

A logged-in unsupervised workstation allows others to view confidential information. It can also allow individuals to document in an EHR using your electronic signature.

Administrators have additional security responsibilities. To help manage these responsibilities, many healthcare facilities appoint a security officer. This person is usually the IT manager. The security officer has the following responsibilities:

- Oversees the security and privacy of the network
- Helps the facility meet federal regulations related to electronic technology security
- Monitors the network for suspected breaches
- Manages passwords, reminds staff to change passwords, and provides staff with the adequate access levels needed for each job

Many healthcare facilities have banned employees from downloading files. Many times, downloaded files cause malware to be introduced into the network. Table 21.7 describes additional security measures used to keep computer network files secure.

TABLE 21.7 Security Measures Used to Keep Information Confidential

Security Measures	Description
Encryption software	Used to encode or change the information into nonreadable or encrypted data (also called cipher text). Prevents unauthorized users from reading the information. An authorized user must enter a password for **decryption** to occur and make the text readable again.
Firewalls	A program or hardware device that acts as a barrier or filter between the network and the internet. Data coming from the internet must pass through the firewall. Data that do not meet the firewall criteria are not allowed into the network.
Virus protection software	Also called antivirus or antimalware software; used to detect and remove malware (malicious programs). Examples include Norton and AVG Anti-Virus.
Security risk analysis	Potential threats of network breaches are identified, and action plans are instituted to prevent the breaches.
Audit trails	Records of computer activity used to monitor users' actions within software, including additions, deletions, and viewing of electronic records.
Monitoring of log-in activity	Multiple incorrect log-in attempts are flagged, and many times the account is locked. Prevents hackers (unauthorized users who attempt to break into networks) from cracking passwords.
Automatic log-off	Used to safeguard records. After a period of inactivity, the workstation logs off.
Access restrictions	Limit what staff members can see on the computer based on job description. Not all staff members have the same access in software programs, such as EHRs and practice management software.

CRITICAL THINKING 21.8

Like many small healthcare facilities without an IT department, Christiana must assume a leadership role with the EHRs. She has administrator rights, which means she can assign different levels of access for the various staff members. In such a small healthcare facility, what other security measures should she consider using to ensure the privacy of EHRs? What resources might she use to implement the security measures identified?

VOCABULARY

decryption: The computer process of changing encrypted text to readable or plain text after a user enters a secret key or password.

firewall: A program or hardware that acts as a barrier between the network and the internet.

meaningful use requirements: Requirements established by the Centers for Medicare and Medicaid Services (CMS) as part of the Electronic Health Records (EHR) Incentives Program. The program provides financial incentives for healthcare organizations that "meaningfully used" their certified EHR technology. The requirements include implementing security measures to ensure the privacy of patients' EHRs.

privacy filters: Devices attached to the monitor that allow visualization of the screen contents only if the user is directly in front of the screen; also called *monitor filters* or *privacy screens*.

security risk analysis: Identification of potential threats of computer network breaches, for which action plans for corrective actions are instituted.

Performing data backup procedures is also important. Depending on the size of the facility, the network may be backed up once to several times a day. *Backing up* is a process in which the network files are copied, and the copy is stored in a secure offsite location. Many healthcare facilities contract with cloud backup services. These services back up all the data on the network to protect against data loss. Cloud backup services are like cloud storage services in regard to the access of the data anytime and anywhere. Backup companies do not typically provide file sharing services. When computer data are compromised, either by errors, natural causes (e.g., floods, storm damage), or human causes (e.g., fires, hackers, and malware), the data can be restored using the backup copy.

> **CRITICAL THINKING 21.9**
>
> Some healthcare facilities store network backup copies in fireproof safes onsite. Why is it important to store the backup copy offsite? What would be the advantage of using a data backup internet service that has several data storage locations around the country?

Continual Technology Advances in Healthcare

Patients are seeing more technology in healthcare settings today. Receptionists are wearing Bluetooth headsets. These headsets allow them to be more mobile when answering phone calls (Fig. 21.11). Bluetooth is a short-range wireless communication technology. It uses short-wave radio frequencies to interconnect wireless electronic devices like phones and headsets.

To comply with HIPAA, sign-in sheets are being replaced by sign-in kiosks. Some facilities have patients enter health information using the kiosk or a tablet computer. Some clinics use a camera to take the patient's picture for identification. The health information and the photo are then added to the EHR. Receptionists have card readers to use for collecting payments that have been applied to credit and debit cards. The card reader machines can be mounted on the computer monitor or are stand-alone units. Many have a printer feature that allows the receptionist to present the patient with a paper receipt.

Many healthcare facilities provide patients with wristbands that have bar code technology. This practice started in the hospital and is now moving into the ambulatory care setting. The wristband is scanned before diagnostic tests are done or medications are administered. This scanning process creates an automatic entry in the patient's EHR. This process is another step in ensuring patient safety and accuracy in billing.

Ambulatory surgery centers and walk-in clinics use patient tracking systems in both the reception area and the patient care area. Patients sign in or are signed into the system. Their names go into the queue. For confidentiality purposes, patients may be given a unique number. As patients move from one area of the facility to another, their progress shows on monitors in the reception area. This keeps family members informed of their progress. Patients awaiting appointments or laboratory services can see their number moves up in the queue or can observe current wait times. These tracking systems provide cost-effective ways to promote patient satisfaction while improving flow and efficiency.

In the exam room, healthcare workers are using more technology to provide better patient care. Some clinics use wireless mobile workstations called **computer on wheels (COWs)** or workstations on wheels (WOWs). Providers and medical assistants use tablets, smart devices, and wearable computing devices to access EHRs and online resources (Fig. 21.12). **Point-of-care** tools and apps are available for providers to use in the exam room with the patients. This technology gives providers the latest clinical information. Apps are available to provide patients with visuals of surgical procedures, disease processes, and anatomic structures. Wearable computing devices allow healthcare employees to access medical records and information while moving around and providing patient care. Mobile devices and apps help providers to make quicker decisions with a lower rate of error and improved patient care outcomes. With advances in Bluetooth smart technology, more medical equipment can work with apps on smart devices.

> **VOCABULARY**
>
> **computer on wheels (COW):** A wireless mobile workstation; also called a workstation on wheels (WOW).
>
> **point-of-care:** Something designed to be used at or near where the patient is seen; point-of-care tools and apps are resources for the provider to use when working directly with the patient.

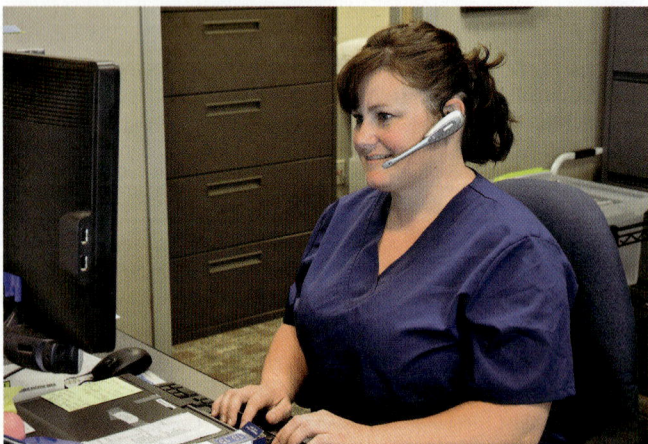

FIG. 21.11 Bluetooth headsets are helpful for receptionists and other healthcare employees who frequently answer or make phone calls. (From Proctor D, et al: *Kinn's The Medical Assistant*, ed 13, St. Louis, 2017, Elsevier.)

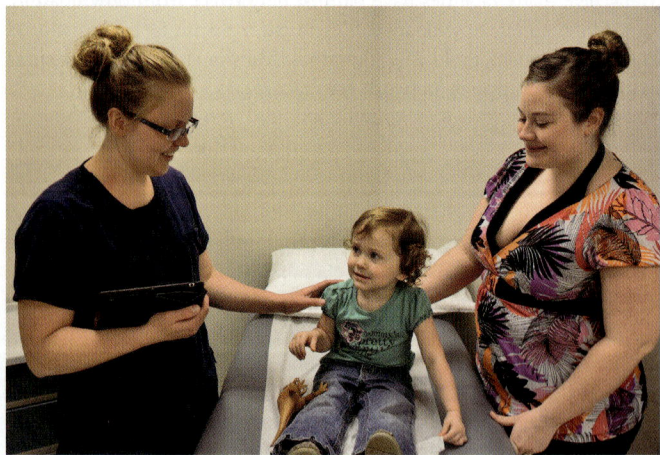

FIG. 21.12 Medical assistants can use tablets to enter information into the electronic health record. (From Proctor D, et al: *Kinn's The Medical Assistant*, ed 13, St. Louis, 2017, Elsevier.)

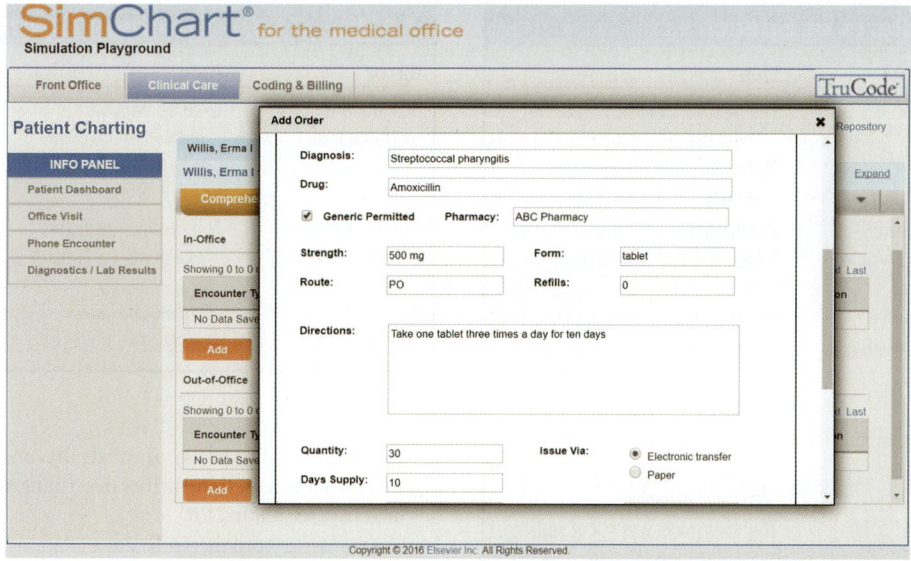

FIG. 21.13 With e-prescribing, providers can enter the prescription information into the EHR and send it to the pharmacy. The pharmacist can easily read the information, which reduces the chance of errors.

Because it uses diagnostic imaging to provide detailed information on internal structures, three-dimensional (3D) printing has become popular in healthcare. Implants, medical devices, and prosthetics can be customized for a patient instead of using a generic model. Surgeons use 3D printing to help with virtual surgical planning. Magnetic resonance imaging (MRI) and computed tomography (CT) create detailed pictures of internal structures. Using 3D printing, an exact replica of the person's internal structures is created. The replica is used as the surgeons rehearse complicated surgical procedures prior to surgery.

With advancements in EHR software and practice management software, new features and programs are being used. **E-prescribing** allows providers to send prescriptions to the pharmacy electronically (Fig. 21.13). With voice-recognition software, providers can dictate notes directly into the patient's EHR. Computerized provider/physician order entry (CPOE) software allows orders for medical laboratory tests, diagnostic tests, and medications to be entered into the computer. In many healthcare facilities, licensed healthcare providers and credentialed medical assistants use CPOE. This improves the efficiency of ordering tests and medications. Some healthcare agencies hire medical scribes. A *medical scribe* enters patient data into the EHR while the provider examines and treats the patient. With all the advances in technology, medical assistants need to remain flexible and willing to adapt to technology changes in the workplace (Box 21.5). Medical assistants must also ensure the privacy and confidentiality of patient records and information.

> **BOX 21.5 Reliable Health Websites**
>
> Often, medical assistants need to research health-related topics. The internet has many sites that offer information. The medical assistant must only use websites that are reliable and respected. The following points should be considered when identifying reliable health websites:
> - Government websites (.gov) and educational institution websites (.edu) can be trusted.
> - Large respected healthcare and educational agencies (e.g., Mayo Clinic, Harvard University, Johns Hopkins) usually have many reliable health-related resources.
> - Wikipedia is not reliable.
>
> If reviewing .com or .org websites, evaluate for bias and accuracy. Research the site by identifying these factors:
> - What is the mission or purpose of the website? Who supports or runs website? Is advertising present on the website pages?
> - Is the information current or less than 3 years old?
> - What is the source of the information? Who is the author of the content? Does a panel of healthcare experts (doctors, nurses, etc.) review the content?
> - Do you need to provide your personal information to view the pages? If so, what will the site do with your personal information?

VOCABULARY

e-prescribing: The use of electronic software to communicate with pharmacies and send prescribing information. It takes the place of writing a prescription by hand and giving it to a patient; most new or refill prescriptions can be submitted electronically, cutting down on fraud and errors.

> **CRITICAL THINKING 21.10**
>
> Christiana had considered applying for a medical scribe position at a local healthcare facility before she was promoted to lead administrative medical assistant. Why would a strong background in EHR be important for a medical scribe position?

TABLE 21.8 Parts of Speech

Part	Example	Use
Noun	computer	The medical assistant used the *computer*.
Verb	greeted	The receptionist *greeted* the patient.
Subject	receptionist	The *receptionist* of the orthopedic and pediatric departments answers the phone.
Dependent clause	because the patient felt sick	The receptionist immediately notified the clinical medical assistant *because the patient felt sick*.
Phrase	warm exam room	A *warm exam room* helps keep the patient comfortable during a physical exam.
Adjective	warm	The *warm* room was full of patients.
Adverb	softly	The patient spoke *softly*.
Preposition	beside	The student sat *beside* the receptionist.

TABLE 21.9 Common Grammatical Errors

Error	Incorrect	Correct
Fragment or incomplete sentence	*Greeted patients before she updated their information.*	*The receptionist always greeted patients before she updated their information.*
Nonagreement of subject and verb	The medical *assistant talk* to the patient. The *patients is* waiting for the doctor.	The medical *assistant talks* to the patient. The *patients are* waiting for the doctor.

FUNDAMENTALS OF WRITTEN COMMUNICATION

Written communication from an ambulatory care facility is a reflection of the provider and the clinic. Medical assistants commonly compose emails and letters to patients and vendors. A poorly worded message or incorrect punctuation in a letter or email gives the reader a negative impression of the sender and thus the clinic. A medical assistant needs to know how to correctly write a letter or message to others. It is important that the sentence structure, grammar, spelling, and tone of the message are professional.

Parts of Speech

A noun is a word or phrase for a person, place, thing, or idea (Table 21.8). A common noun is a general group of people, places, things, and ideas (e.g., *desk, office*). A proper noun names a specific person, place, or thing (e.g., *Zachary, Boston*). A proper noun should start with a capital letter. A pronoun is a word that takes the place of a noun (e.g., *I, he, she, it,* and *they*).

A verb is a word or phrase that shows action or a state of being (e.g., *talks, walks, is,* and *are*) (see Table 21.8). The subject in a sentence is a noun, pronoun, or set of words that performs the verb action (see Table 21.8). A sentence requires at least one main clause, which contains an independent subject and verb and expresses a complete thought. A fragment is a phrase without a main clause and is a major error in writing (Table 21.9). It is important to make sure the subject and verb agree. A singular subject (e.g., *provider, patient*) must be matched with a singular verb (e.g., *is, reads, goes*). A plural subject (e.g., *providers, patients*) must be paired with a plural verb (e.g., *are, read, go*) (see Table 21.9).

Many sentences also contain the following:
- *Dependent clauses*: often begin with words such as *although, since, when, because,* and *if*. A dependent clause needs an independent clause (e.g., subject and verb) to be a complete sentence (see Table 21.8).
- *Phrase*: a group of words without a subject or verb (see Table 21.8).
- *Adjective*: a word or group of words that describes a noun or pronoun; may come before or after the noun or pronoun it describes (see Table 21.8).
- *Adverb*: a word or group of words that answers how, where, when, or to what extent, thus further describing a verb, adjective, or other adverbs (see Table 21.8).
- *Preposition*: a word that indicates a relationship or a location between a noun or pronoun and the rest of the sentence. Examples include *near, besides, about, to, with, by, after,* and *in* (see Table 21.8).

> **CRITICAL THINKING 21.11**
>
> Christiana needs to compose a letter. How can she be sure she does not have any incomplete sentences in her letter? What parts of speech are required for a complete sentence?

Appropriate Use of Words

When composing professional communications, it is important to use language the reader will understand. Refrain from slang, generational terms, and abbreviations used with electronic communication. These can cause miscommunication with the reader. The medical assistant should know the proper use of commonly confused words and misused phrases (Table 21.10). Homonyms (i.e., words that sound alike) can lead to mistakes (Box 21.6). They may not always be identified by word processing software's spell-checker (Table 21.11).

A common mistake when communicating is a mismatch between the noun and pronoun number. When referring to plural nouns, use plural pronouns. Plural pronouns include *we, us, you, they,* and *them*. When referring to singular nouns, use singular pronouns. Singular pronouns include *I, me, you, she, her, he, him,* and *it*. For example, "When the receptionist answers the phone, they need to be polite." The *receptionist* is a singular noun, but *they* is a plural pronoun. The noun and pronouns should agree in number, as in this example: "When receptionists answer the phones, they need to be polite."

To ensure that the message is clear to the reader, make the following adjustments if necessary:
- Refrain from using two negatives in the same sentence.
- Refrain from using vague expressions or overusing the same words within a paragraph.
- Avoid using run-on sentences, which contain several independent clauses together without the required punctuation.

Proper spelling, use of words, and sentence structure are important because they reflect on the writer and the healthcare facility.

Capitalization, Numbers, and Punctuation

Part of composing written communication is using correct capitalization and punctuation. As mentioned earlier, errors can reflect poorly on the writer and the facility. Professional documents should contain correct capitalization, appropriate punctuation, and the right number format.

TABLE 21.10 Commonly Confused Words

Words	Examples
As: used in comparisons	She is *as* fast as he is on the keyboard.
Has: to possess, own, or experience	The medical assistant *has* increased his keyboarding speed by using the computer every day.
Lie: to recline or rest on a surface	I *lie* down to sleep.
Lay: to put or place	I *lay* down the book.
Set: to put or place	She *set* the gown on the table for the patient.
Sit: to be seated	*Sit* on the table when you have changed into a gown.
Who: refers to people; he or she did an action	*Who* placed the order for supplies?
Whom: refers to him or her	Mike saw *whom* yesterday?
That: refers to people, things, and groups of people	The letters *that* are on the printer need to be signed.
Which: refers to things or groups	The letters, *which* are on the printer, need to be signed.
Like: means "similar to"	The child is *like* her mother.
As: means "in the same manner" and requires a verb	He works *as* a phlebotomist.
Farther: refers to a measurable distance	The healthcare facility is *farther* away than I thought.
Further: refers to an abstract length	*Further* research is needed before we purchase a new computer.

BOX 21.6 Commonly Misused Words and Phrases

- Anyway (not *anyways*)
- Supposed to (not *suppose to*)
- Toward (not *towards*)
- Used to (not *use to*)

TABLE 21.11 Meanings of Common Homonyms

Homonyms	Examples
Affect (verb): to influence or transform	The outbreak of influenza will *affect* our patients.
Effect (noun): a result, outcome, consequence, or appearance	The *effect* of influenza was devastating to the city.
Accept (verb): to receive	Will you *accept* this certified letter?
Except (preposition): excluding	She mailed all the envelopes, *except* the certified letter.
Than (conjunction): used to compare	The receptionist was busier *than* the clinical medical assistant.
Then (adverb): tells when	The receptionist finished registering the patient and *then* she scheduled the appointment.
There (adverb): indicates place	*There* were 25 chairs in the reception area.
Their (pronoun): indicates possession	*Their* children remained in the reception area.
They're (contraction): they are	*They're* the only patients in the reception area.
Your (pronoun): indicates possession	*Your* new job is in pediatrics.
You're (contraction): you are	*You're* working in pediatrics today.
To (preposition): indicates direction, action, or condition	She went *to* answer the phone.
Too (adverb): means "also"	The medical assistant's phone was ringing, *too*.
Two (noun): number	Her phone has *two* lines.
Where: to, at, or in what place	*Where* did the patient go?
Were (verb): past tense plural of "be"	*Were* you finished?
Wear (verb): to have something on your body	*Wear* the gown, please.

The first letter of the first word in a sentence or question should be capitalized. The pronoun "I" is always capitalized. The first letter of proper nouns, including names of people, months, institutions, organizations, countries, and national nouns and adjectives (e.g., *French, British*) should be capitalized. Common nouns (e.g., girls, women, boys, men) should not be capitalized unless the word is the first word of a sentence.

A few rules apply to writing numbers. Spell out all numbers at the beginning of a sentence. Hyphenate all compound numbers from 21 to 99 (e.g., twenty-three) and all written-out fractions (e.g., two-thirds). Use commas for figures with four or more digits (e.g., 1,234). It is not advised to include a decimal point or a dollar sign when writing out sums less than a dollar (e.g., 23¢). Use *noon* and *midnight* instead of 12 p.m. and 12 a.m. The format for a.m. and p.m. can vary.

A sentence can end with one of three types of punctuation: a period (.), a question mark (?), or an exclamation point (!). Use a period for a sentence that makes a statement. A period goes inside a closing quotation mark (e.g., "Thank you for coming in today."). Use a question mark after a direct question. Use an exclamation point for sentences that express strong emotion. An exclamation point is rarely used in professional written communication.

Commas are frequently used in written communication (Table 21.12). A semicolon (;) is a common punctuation mark used in professional letters and documentation. The semicolon is used before certain words (*however, therefore, for example*). It is also used when separating phrases in a series (e.g., "The provider is running late; however, our first two patients canceled this morning."). A colon (:) is used to introduce a series of items either in the sentence or bulleted. A colon is also used after the greeting or salutation in a professional letter. Quotation marks (" ") are used to set off direct quotes. They are used frequently when documenting a patient's chief complaint, the main reason for the patient's visit. When using quotation marks, the periods and commas go inside the quotation marks. An apostrophe (') is used to show ownership. To show plural possession, the apostrophe is placed after the "s" (e.g., patients'). These are the most common punctuation marks used in professional correspondence and in charting in a patient's health record.

Using the correct words and punctuation marks is important when composing written correspondence. To reduce the risk of errors, the medical assistant should do the following:

- Perform a spelling and grammar check.
- Proofread the document.
- Double-check the recipient's address.

Many times, the reader develops an impression of the writer, the employer, and the healthcare facility based solely on written correspondence.

TABLE 21.12 Use of Commas

Rule	Examples
Use before a coordinator (*and, but, yet, nor, for, or, so*) that links two main clauses. Do not use a comma before a coordinator that links two names, words, or phrases.	The last patient left, and the receptionist locked the door.
Use to separate items in a list.	The medical assistant escorted the mother, the father, and the child to the exam room.
Use to separate two interchangeable adjectives.	The patient was a strong, healthy child.
Use after certain words at the start of a sentence (i.e., *yes, no, hello*).	Yes, the bill was correct.
Use to set off the name or title or an expression that interrupts the flow of the sentence.	Will you, Michaela, want an appointment in two weeks? I am, by the way, very excited about the job opportunity.
Use after a dependent clause that starts a sentence.	If you have any questions, let me know.
Use to separate the day from the year.	May 24, 20–
Use to separate the city from its state. *(This rule does not apply when addressing envelopes.)*	Madison, Wisconsin
Can be used to separate Sr. or Jr. from the person's name, but this is not mandatory.	Bob Smith, Sr. or Bob Smith Sr. Bob Smith, Sr., has arrived for his appointment.
Use after a degree or title and to enclose the degree or title if it appears in a sentence.	John Williams, M.D. John Williams, M.D., will be the speaker for the event.
Use to set off nonessential words or phrases.	Catherine, the newest secretary, has arrived. My brother, Keith, has an appointment to see Dr. Smith.
Use with direct quotations.	She stated, "I have waited too long." "Why," I asked, "do you want tomorrow off?"

WRITTEN CORRESPONDENCE

Medical assistants are responsible for communicating with vendors or supply companies. They are also required to send written communication to patients and other providers, as directed by their provider-employers. Knowing how to compose a professional letter is an important skill for medical assistants. To compose a letter, you must know the correct content and location for the parts of the letter. Creating an email requires that the writer follow business etiquette guidelines.

Parts of a Professional Letter

A professional letter uses 8.5 × 11-inch paper or letterhead paper. Letterhead paper is 20- to 24-lb. bond paper (e.g., the thicker the paper, the larger the lb. bond number). The letter typically has 1-inch margins on all four sides. The entire letter should be written using single line spacing. Consistency in line spacing is important for a professional appearance. The font should be simple and easy to read, such as Times New Roman or Arial, in a 10- or 12-point size. Limit the use of boldface and italics in the letter.

Sender's Address. The sender's address is usually located in the letterhead (Fig. 21.14). Most facilities use preprinted letterhead paper. Letterhead can also be created at the top of the document using the word processing software's header tool. The letterhead may or may not include the provider's name. It should have the clinic's name, street address or post office box, city, state, and ZIP code. Some letterheads have additional contact information, such as phone numbers, website address, and an email address.

If letterhead is not used for a professional letter, the sender's address is placed at the left margin, 1 inch from the top of the document. Use single spacing and include the facility's address. Do not include the sender's name because that is in the closing section of the letter.

Date. All professional letters must include a date. The date is located either at the left or right margin or starts at the center point of the document (see Fig. 21.14). The location depends on the type of letter format used. When using letterhead, the date line starts on the second line after the letterhead. If letterhead is not used, the date line starts on the second line below the sender's address. In either situation, there should be one blank line between the date and the last line of the letterhead or sender's address.

When keying (typing) the date, write out the name of the month, then the number of the day, followed by a comma and the four-digit year. Make sure to have a blank space between the month and the day and after the comma (e.g., May 14, 20–). Do not use "th" or "st" after the day (e.g., May 14th, 20–).

Inside Address. The inside address starts between the second to the tenth line, below the date line. The placement depends on the length of the letter (see Fig. 21.14). If the body of the letter is long, leave one blank line between the date and the inside address. If the body is short, add up to nine blank lines between the date line and the first line of the inside address. The goal is to have the body of the letter centered vertically on the page.

The inside address is always left justified. It includes the recipient's name and title on the first line. The next lines include the department and healthcare facility name. The last lines include the street address, followed by the city, state, and ZIP code. Always address the letter to a specific person. If the letter relates to a minor, address the letter to the patient's guardian. When writing out the person's name, include the person's personal title (e.g., Miss, Ms., Mrs., Mr., or Dr.). If you are unsure of a woman's title preference, use Ms.

Use the US Postal Service format and abbreviations for the address (Table 21.13). No comma is needed between the city and state. Use the two-letter abbreviations for the states. For all other abbreviations in the address, use only approved abbreviations. For international addresses, key (type) the name of the country in capital letters on the last line.

Reference Line. The reference line may be used occasionally. It starts on the second line below the inside address at the left margin. The salutation then is placed on the second line below the reference line. The purpose of the reference line is to refer to a specific item, such as a file, case number, or product number. It provides easy reference for the reader and sender (e.g., Reference: Invoice #44549).

Salutation. The salutation is the greeting. It starts on the second line below the inside address. It is always left justified (see Fig. 21.14). For business letters, the salutation should be formal. "Dear" is followed

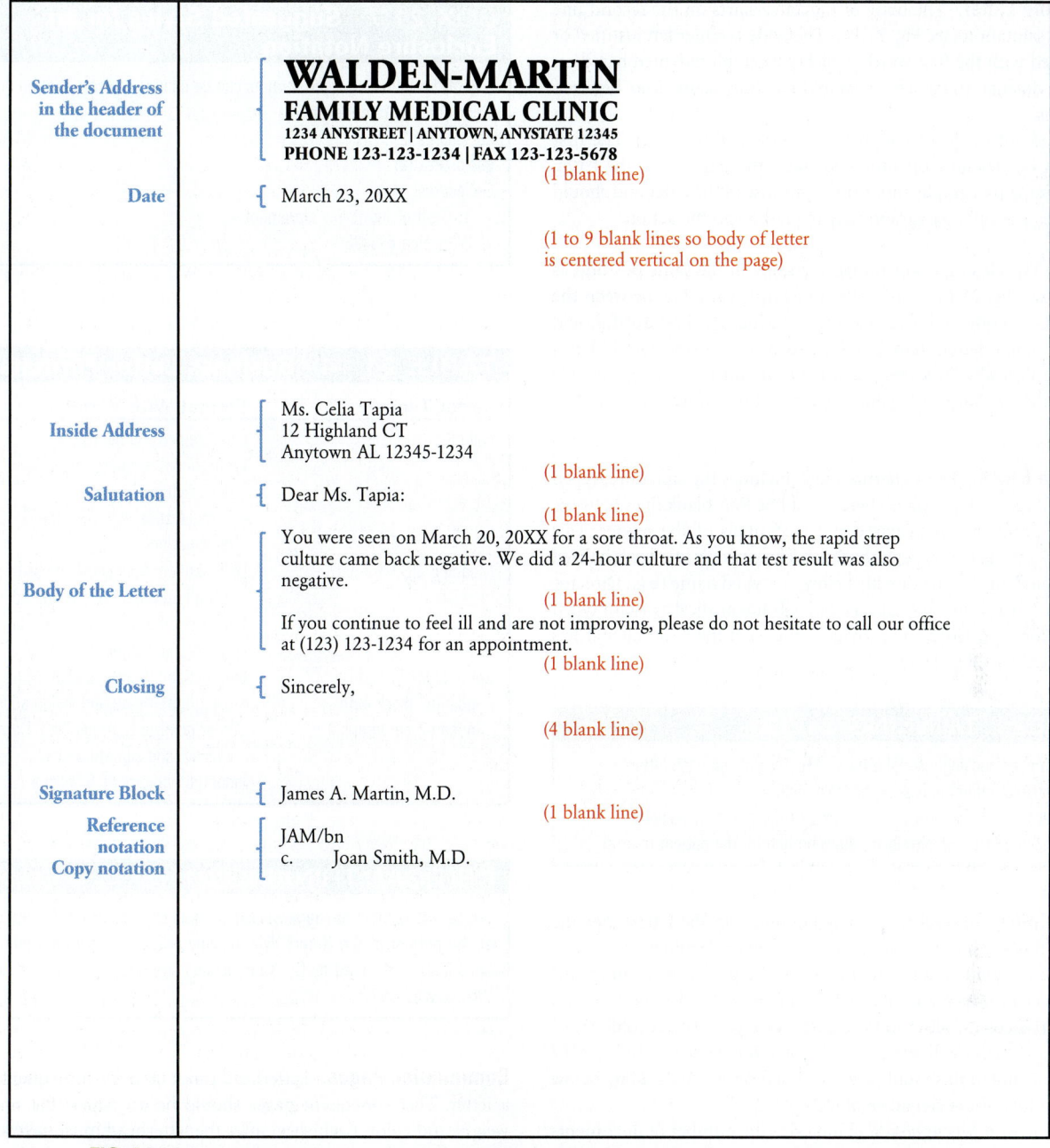

FIG. 21.14 Business letter format. When a medical assistant types a letter for a provider, that provider must sign the letter after it has been printed. (From Proctor D, et al: *Kinn's The Medical Assistant*, ed 13, St. Louis, 2017, Elsevier.)

TABLE 21.13 US Postal Service Standard Street Abbreviations			
Word	**Abbreviation**	**Word**	**Abbreviation**
Alley	ALY	Drive	DR
Avenue	AVE	Estate	EST
Boulevard	BLVD	Highway	HWY
Bridge	BRG	Parkway	PKWY
Bypass	BYP	Road	RD
Center	CTR	Route	RTE
Circle	CIR	Street	ST
Court	CT	Terrace	TER
Crossing	XING	Way	WAY

by the person's title and name and then ends with a colon (e.g., Dear Mr. Smith:). Sometimes the person's first name may be added (e.g., Dear Mr. Ted Smith:). If the person's gender is not known, use the first and last name without the title (e.g., Dear Chris Smith:). The phrase "To Whom It May Concern" can be used if a person's name is not known.

Subject Line. The subject line is not used very often. The purpose of the subject line is to state the main subject of the letter. It is left justified and placed on the second line below the salutation. The body of the letter starts on the second line below the subject line. The subject line should be composed using bold face, underlining, or all capital letters because this would draw the reader's attention (SUBJECT: ORDER NO. 45677-93).

Body of the Letter. The body of the letter starts on the second line below the salutation (see Fig. 21.14). The body is either left justified or left justified with the first word of each paragraph indented based on the letter format used. There should be one blank line between paragraphs.

The body of the letter contains the content of the letter. The first paragraph is a friendly opening and states the purpose of the letter. The remaining paragraphs support the purpose of the letter and should be concise. The final paragraph may request a specific action.

Closing. The closing is positioned vertically in the same position as the date (see Fig. 21.14). There should be one blank line between the last line of the body of the letter and the closing. The first word should include a capital letter. Remaining words in the closing should be in lowercase. Typically, "Sincerely" is used; more formal closings include "Yours truly" or "Very truly yours." The word or phrase is followed by a comma.

Signature Block. The signature block includes the signature, typed name, and title of the sender. There should be four blank lines between the closing and the typed name and credentials of the sender. This space allows the person to sign the letter. The person's title is capitalized and is located on the line directly below the typed name (e.g., Director of Walden-Martin Family Medical Clinic). If the medical assistant typed the letter for a provider, the provider must sign the letter after it has been printed (see Fig. 21.14).

> **CRITICAL THINKING 21.12**
>
> Christiana is composing several letters. Who would sign each letter?
> - A letter to a patient indicating her test results
> - A letter to a vendor asking for specific pricing for a new computer
> - A letter to a referring physician, thanking him for the patient referral

End Notations. Several items may be noted on the letter after the signature block. This may vary among healthcare facilities.
- *Reference notation*: notes the initials of the person who composed the letter in uppercase followed by the initials of the person who keyed (typed) the letter in lowercase (see Fig. 21.14). A colon (:) or a forward slash (/) divides the two sets of initials (e.g., MR:bn, MR/bn). This notation should be left justified on the second line below the last line of the signature block.
- *Enclosure/attachment notation*: indicates the number of documents or attachments that accompany the letter. The enclosure notation is left justified. It starts on the second line below the reference notation. If the reference notation is not present, the enclosure notation is placed on the second line below the last line of the signature block. The enclosure notation can be typed in several ways. It can be indicated with either "Enclosure" or "Enc." If more than one enclosure is sent, the number of enclosures or the names of the enclosures should be indicated (Box 21.7).
- *Copy notation* (c.): used to notify the letter's recipient who else received a copy of the letter. The "c" is left justified and goes on the line immediately following the last notation. It is then followed by a period. Use the tab tool to move a half-inch before typing the person's name (e.g., c. John Smith). Additional names should be aligned vertically on the document.
- *Blind copy* (bc.): used if the sender does not want the recipient to know a copy was sent to another person. The format is the same as it is for "c," but the "bc" is added only to the office copy of the letter. It is not listed on the letter going to the recipient.

> **BOX 21.7 Suggested Styles for an Enclosure Notation**
>
> Any of the following three formats can be used to indicate that an enclosure is included with the letter:
> Enclosures: 2
> Enclosures (2)
> Enclosures:
> 1. Draft of the policy statement
> 2. Invoice #45433

TABLE 21.14 Business Letter Formats

Letter Type	Format With Variations
Full block format	Left justified: All elements
	Professional business letters use "closed" punctuation
	Informal letters can use "open" punctuation
Modified block format	Left justified: Sender's address (if not using letterhead) and inside address
	Center point or right justified: Date, closing, and signature block
Semi–block format (or modified block with indented paragraphs)	Left justified: Sender's address (if not using letterhead) and inside address
	Center point or right justified: Date, closing, and signature block
	Indented paragraphs 5 spaces

> **CRITICAL THINKING 21.13**
>
> For the letters that Christiana will sign, should she include a reference notation at the bottom of the letter? Why or why not? For the letters prepared by Christiana and signed by Dr. Kahn, should she add the reference notation? Why or why not?

Continuation Pages. Letterhead is not used for subsequent pages of a letter. The subsequent pages should be on paper that matches in weight and color. Each sheet after the letterhead must have a heading that includes these elements on separate lines: the recipient's name, the page number, and the date. The name should be on the first line below the top margin, and all three elements should be left justified.

Ms. Celia Tapia
Page 2
March 23, 20–

Business Letter Formats

Three main formats are used to compose a business letter. The formats vary slightly in the position of certain elements of the letter. The line spacing between the elements remains the same (Table 21.14). It is important for a medical assistant to be able to compose a professional letter (Procedure 21.1).

Full Block Letter Format. The full block format is the most common type of business letter (Fig. 21.15). All elements are left justified. This means the elements start at the left margin of the document. Typically, for business letters, "closed" punctuation is used. Closed punctuation

PROCEDURE 21.1 Compose a Professional Business Letter

Task
Compose a professional letter using technology.

Scenario
Create a letter for the following scenario: Nurse practitioner Jean Burke has requested that you compose a letter to the parent (Lisa Parker) of Johnny Parker (date of birth [DOB]: 06/15/2010) to let her know that Johnny's throat culture from last Wednesday was negative. If he is not improving or if she has any questions, she should call the office. Lisa Parker's address is 91 Poplar Street, Anytown, AL 12345-1234. You are working at Walden-Martin Family Medical Clinic. The healthcare facility's address is 1234 Anystreet, Anytown, AL 12345. The phone number is 123-123-1234 and the fax number is 123-123-5678.

Equipment and Supplies
- Patient's health record
- Computer with word processing software and printer
- Paper or letterhead paper
- #10 envelope

Procedural Steps
1. Obtain the intended recipient's contact information and determine the message you want to convey.
   Purpose: This gives you a focus when composing the letter. You will need the recipient's information to create the letter.
2. Using the computer and word processing software, compose the letter using one of the three business letter formats. If using blank paper, create a letterhead in the header of the document. Include the clinic's name, street address or post office box, city, state, and ZIP code.
   Purpose: The information in the letterhead provides the reader contact information for the clinic.
3. Key (type) the date in the correct location using the correct format. Have one blank line between the date line and the last line of the letterhead.
   Purpose: All letters require a date for legal purposes.
4. Key the inside address using the correct spelling, punctuation, and location for the information. Leave one to nine blank lines between the date and the inside address, to center the body of the letter on the page.
   Purpose: The body of the letter must be centered vertically from the top to the bottom of the document. More blank lines can be added to move the body to the correct location.
5. Starting on the second line below the inside address, key the salutation, using the correct format.
   Purpose: A proper greeting sets the tone of the letter.
6. Use your critical thinking skills to compose a concise, accurate message. Type the message in the body of the letter using the proper location and format. There should be a blank line after the salutation and between each paragraph. The message should be clear, concise, and professional. Use proper grammar, punctuation, capitalization, and sentence structure.
   Purpose: Proper grammar helps to convey the message accurately and professionally.
7. Key a proper closing. Leave one blank line between the last line of the body and the closing. Use the correct format and location.
   Purpose: The closing helps end the message with a professional tone.
8. Key the signature block using the correct format and location. If you are preparing the letter for a provider, you must include a reference notation. There should be four blank lines between the closing and the signature block.
   Purpose: The signature block provides the reader with the name of the sender of the letter. The reference notation identifies who typed the letter.
9. Spell-check and proofread the document. Check for the proper tone, grammar, punctuation, capitalization, and sentence structure. Check for proper spacing between the parts of the letter. Make any final corrections. Print the document.
   Purpose: The spell-checker identifies only certain errors; proofreading helps you find incorrect word use, improper tone, and errors in formatting.
10. Address the envelope, using either the computer and word processing software or a pen and following the correct format. After addressing the envelope, fold the letter using the correct technique and place it in the envelope.
    Purpose: Following the post office guidelines on format helps prevent a delay in delivery of the letter. The provider is the sender of the letter and should have the opportunity to review it before it is mailed to the patient.
11. File a copy of the letter in the paper medical record or upload an electronic copy of the letter to the electronic health record (EHR).
    Purpose: A copy of all correspondence should be kept in the patient's health record.

---

means the document is typed using the punctuation marks described earlier in this chapter. Closed punctuation gives the letter a professional appearance.

Informal full block–formatted letters can use open punctuation. *Open punctuation* means that minimal punctuation is used in the letter. The body is the only part of the letter that contains the normal grammatical punctuation. No punctuation appears in the sender's or inside addresses, date, salutation, and closing. This is a current trend with electronic technology and letters produced by word processing. Open punctuation should not be used with professional letters.

Modified Block Letter Format. The body and the inside address are left justified with the modified block format. If letterhead is not used, the sender's address is also left justified. The date, closing, and the signature block start either at the center point of the document or are right justified. If the center point is used, all three elements must start at that point (Fig. 21.16). The text flows toward the right margin. The three elements vertically line up in the document. When you use the right-justified technique, the text for these three elements finish in a vertical line at the right margin (Fig. 21.17).

Semi–Block Letter Format. The semi–block letter format can also be called the modified block with indented paragraphs (see Fig. 21.17). The semi–block format resembles the modified block format with the three elements (i.e., date, closing, and signature block) right justified or starting at the center point of the document. The difference with the semi–block format is the indented paragraph, or paragraphs, in the body of the letter. The paragraphs should be indented five spaces.

Letter Templates

Letter templates are sample letters that can be personalized for each patient. Many practice management or word processing software programs have prebuilt letter templates. These templates can be used, or a medical assistant can design a letter template. For routine communication with patients (e.g., normal laboratory results or appointment reminders), a letter template can be created. You can use the practice

WALDEN-MARTIN
FAMILY MEDICAL CLINIC
1234 ANYSTREET | ANYTOWN, ANYSTATE 12345
PHONE 123-123-1234 | FAX 123-123-5678

March 23, 20XX

Ms. Celia Tapia
12 Highland CT
Anytown AL 12345-1234

Dear Ms. Tapia:

You were seen on March 20, 20XX for a sore throat. As you know, the rapid strep culture came back negative. We did a 24-hour culture and that test result was also negative.

If you continue to feel ill and are not improving, please do not hesitate to call our office at (123) 123-1234 for an appointment.

Sincerely,

James A. Martin, M.D.

JAM/bn
c. Joan Smith, M.D.

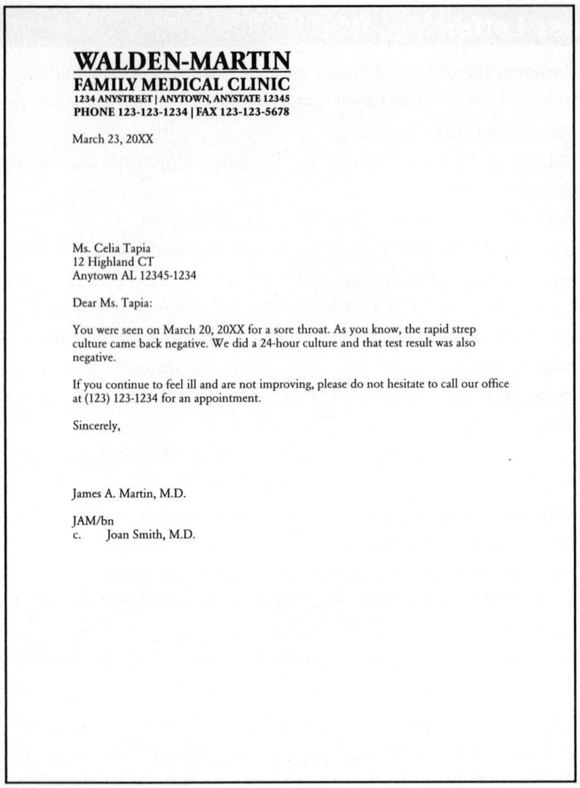

FIG. 21.15 Full block letter format. (From Proctor D, et al: *Kinn's The Medical Assistant*, ed 13, St. Louis, 2017, Elsevier.)

WALDEN-MARTIN
FAMILY MEDICAL CLINIC
1234 ANYSTREET | ANYTOWN, ANYSTATE 12345
PHONE 123-123-1234 | FAX 123-123-5678

March 23, 20XX

Ms. Celia Tapia
12 Highland CT
Anytown AL 12345-1234

Dear Ms. Tapia:

You were seen on March 20, 20XX for a sore throat. As you know, the rapid strep culture came back negative. We did a 24-hour culture and that test result was also negative.

If you continue to feel ill and are not improving, please do not hesitate to call our office at (123) 123-1234 for an appointment.

Sincerely,

James A. Martin, M.D.

JAM/bn
c. Joan Smith, M.D.

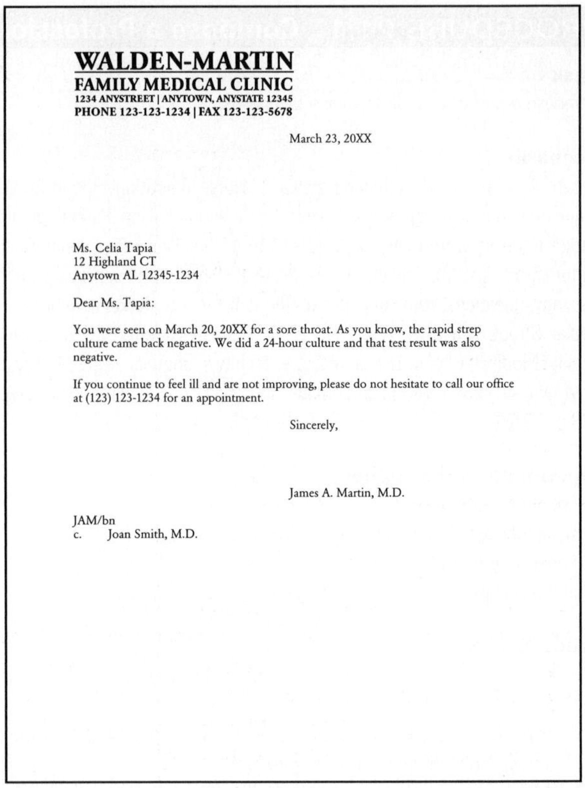

FIG. 21.16 Modified block letter format, showing the date, closing, and signature block starting at the center point of the document. (From Proctor D, et al: *Kinn's The Medical Assistant*, ed 13, St. Louis, 2017, Elsevier.)

management software, EHR, or word processing software to merge the patient's data into the letter template. This creates an individualized letter and is an efficient method of providing a customer-friendly document for a patient.

Preparing the Letter for Delivery

Business letters should be enclosed in standard #10 business-sized envelopes. Standard #10 envelopes measure 4.125 × 9.5 inches. Business envelopes are available with a few variations, including the type of flap, preprinted return address, and presence or absence of a window. The window envelope and the #6 ¾ envelope may be used for billing statements to patients. The envelopes can be white, manila, or made of recycled paper.

When the automated mail processing machine at the post office reads the envelope, it reads the bottom line of the recipient's address (i.e., city, state, and ZIP code) before moving up and reading the next line. To ensure timely delivery, use the following tips when addressing mail:

- Key (type) the envelope using a simple black font of at least 10 points in size. Use all capital letters and no punctuation marks (Fig. 21.18).
- Put one space between the city and state and two spaces between the state and ZIP code.
- If you cannot fit the suite or apartment number on the same line as the delivery address, put it on the line above the delivery address, not below it.
- Use ZIP code + 4 code (e.g., 55555-1111) as often as possible. This allows the piece of mail to be directed to a more precise location than when just using the ZIP code.
- Do not put anything (e.g., logo, slogan, attention line) below the last line of the delivery address. The machine will read it, and your letter may be misrouted or delayed.

WALDEN-MARTIN
FAMILY MEDICAL CLINIC
1234 ANYSTREET | ANYTOWN, ANYSTATE 12345
PHONE 123-123-1234 | FAX 123-123-5678

March 23, 20XX

Ms. Celia Tapia
12 Highland CT
Anytown AL 12345-1234

Dear Ms. Tapia:

You were seen on March 20, 20XX for a sore throat. As you know, the rapid strep culture came back negative. We did a 24-hour culture and that test result was also negative.

If you continue to feel ill and are not improving, please do not hesitate to call our office at (123) 123-1234 for an appointment.

Sincerely,

James A. Martin, M.D.

JAM/bn
c. Joan Smith, M.D.

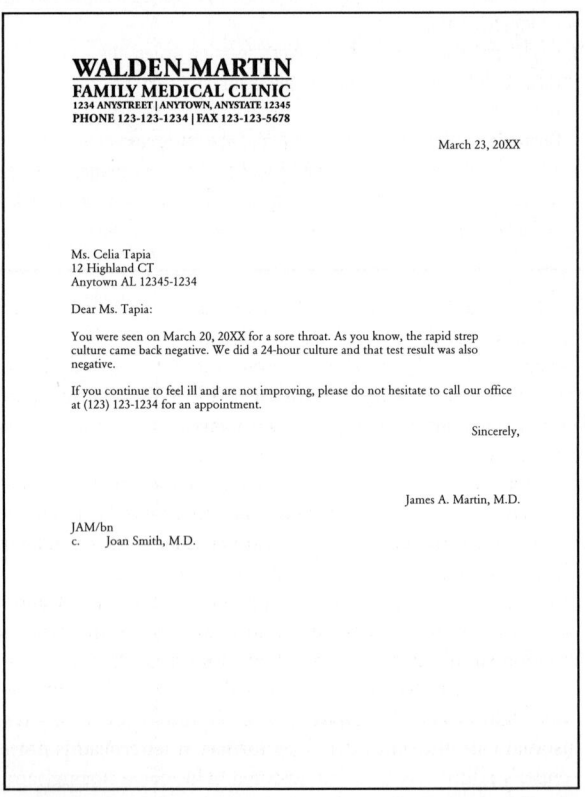

FIG. 21.17 Semi–block letter format (also called modified block with indented paragraph letter format). This letter uses right justification for the date, closing, and signature block. (From Proctor D, et al: *Kinn's The Medical Assistant*, ed 13, St. Louis, 2017, Elsevier.)

TABLE 21.15 US Postal Service Domestic Shipping Sizes

Domestic Shipping	Size
Postcard	Height: 3.5″–4.25″ Length: 5″–6″ Maximum thickness: 0.016″
Letter	Height: 3.5″–6.125″ (6 ⅛″) Length: 5″–11.5″ Maximum thickness: 0.25″
Large envelopes	Height: 6.125″–12″ Length: 11.5″–15″ Maximum thickness: 0.75″
Packages	Maximum length plus **girth**: 108″ (130″ for standard post)

TABLE 21.16 Postage Options

Postage Options	Description
Print postage labels on USPS.com	Can print Priority Mail Express and Priority Mail shipping labels on the facility's printer.
Permit imprints	For bulk mailing (200 or more envelopes); requires a fee and permit. Print postage information on the envelope and pay for postage when mailing is sent.
Precanceled stamps	Complete permit, place precanceled stamps on envelopes and mail. Cannot return unused stamps.
Postage meter printing	Lease a postage meter, pay the fee, and print postage directly on the mail or on a meter tape.

- Use only approved US Postal Service abbreviations.

The medical assistant should fold the letter by pulling up the bottom end until it reaches just below the inside address or two-thirds of the way up the letter. Crease the paper. Then, fold the top of the letter down so that it is flush with the bottom fold and crease the paper. For windowed business envelopes, fold the letter in a Z pattern. With the letter's print side facing up, place the envelope over the top third of the letter. Fold the bottom edge of the paper up to the bottom edge of the envelope and crease the paper. Then, remove the envelope and flip the letter over so the backside of the document is facing up. Fold the top of the letter down to the prior crease line and crease the paper. The letterhead and recipient's addresses should then be visible. Place the letter in the envelope so that the recipient's address shows through the window.

Postage. After addressing the envelope, postage must be added prior to mailing the letter. The postage depends on the following:
- Weight and size of the item (Table 21.15)
- Urgency for arrival
- Delivery **zone**
- Services required

For the ambulatory care facility, there are several postage options for mailings (Table 21.16). The US Postal Service (USPS) website (www.usps.com) provides valuable resources for addressing and shipping mail. It allows you to buy stamps, schedule a pickup, calculate the shipping costs, look up ZIP codes, and track sent mail.

The medical assistant will utilize different types of mail services for the healthcare facility's business. It is crucial to understand the different services. For routine mail, the healthcare facility will use First-Class Mail. Table 21.17 summarizes USPS domestic services available.

The USPS also has a host of optional services that can be added to the standard services for an additional fee. Table 21.18 summarizes additional services available. It is important to note that healthcare facilities use certified mail and return receipt. When using certified mail combined with return receipt, the facility gets a mailing receipt showing the date when the item was mailed. It also gets additional information on when the delivery occurred and the recipient's signature. Many state laws mandate that **termination letters** be sent by certified mail with return receipt. The mailing receipt, the return receipt, and a copy of the letter are uploaded into the EHR or filed in the paper medical record. These items provide proof the law was followed if there is ever a question. For a complete list of services, refer to the USPS website (www.usps.com).

TABLE 21.17 Summary of the US Postal Service's Domestic Services

Type	Description
Priority mail express	Very expensive; 7-days-a-week delivery service with guaranteed overnight scheduled delivery. Insurance is included. For letters and packages up to 70 lb. Cost based on weight and delivery zone. Flat rate boxes available.
Priority mail	Expensive; delivery within 3 days. Insurance is included. For letters and packages up to 70 lb. Cost based on weight and delivery zone. Flat rate boxes available.
First-class mail	Most commonly used service. Provides delivery in 3 days or less. For envelopes and packages weighing up to 13 oz. Cost based on size, shape, and weight. Add-on services are available for an extra fee.
USPS retail ground	Delivery in 2–8 days. Used for oversized packages weighing up to 70 lb. and measuring up to 130 inches in combined girth and length. Cost based on weight, shape, and delivery zone.
Media mail	Use for sending books, electronic media, and educational material, with delivery in 2–8 days. Cost based on weight.

VOCABULARY

authorized agent: A person who has written documentation that he or she can accept a shipment for another individual.

girth: The measurement around something; when referring to mail, it is the measurement around the middle of the package that is being shipped.

termination letters: Documents sent to patients explaining that the provider is ending the physician-patient relationship and the patients need to see other providers.

zone: A region or geographic area used for shipping.

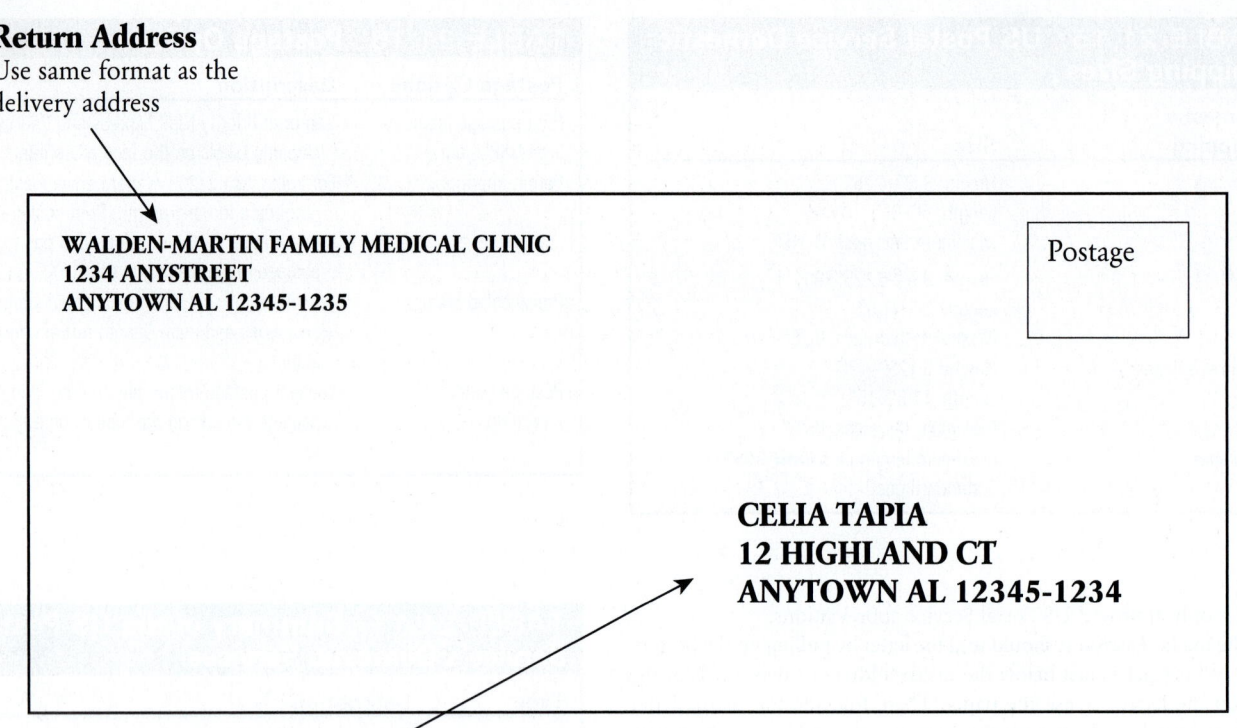

FIG. 21.18 Address format for an envelope. (From Proctor D, et al: *Kinn's The Medical Assistant*, ed 13, St. Louis, 2017, Elsevier.)

Memorandums

Memorandums, or memos, are communication documents shared within a healthcare facility. They address one topic and provide a message to the reader. Use the portrait orientation for the document and 1-inch margins. Memorandums typically have four headings:
- **TO:** Include the name of the recipient or recipients and omit the titles (e.g., Mr., Mrs.). With many recipients, each name can be followed by a comma, or each name can be on its own line.
- **FROM:** Include the name of the sender of the memo. It is optional if the sender initials the memo before it is sent.
- **DATE:** Spell out the month and follow it with the day and year (e.g., May 23, 20–).
- **SUBJECT:** Include the topic of the memo.

The headings are left justified (Fig. 21.20). Boldface and capital letters are used for the headings, and a colon (:) follows the heading. The information should be in regular font, with a mix of capital and lowercase letters. The information should be aligned vertically down the page, using the tab tool in the word processing software. The date should be written out as indicated for professional letters.

The headings may be separated from the body of the memo by a centered black line. The line should extend from 2 inches to the entire width of the page. Whether or not the line is used, there should be two to three blank lines separating the headers from the body of the memo. The body of the memo should be single spaced and left justified. If it consists of multiple paragraphs, skip a single line between paragraphs. The content in the body of the letter should be clear, concise, and informative. The writer does not need to add a closing or signature. Special notations, including reference, copy, and enclosures, can be added to the bottom of the memo. They should be formatted as indicated in the End Notations section.

Professional Emails

The use of electronic communication between the ambulatory care center staff and patients is increasing. Medical assistants need to know how to compose a professional email (Procedure 21.2). Following email etiquette is important for maintaining a customer-friendly environment. Tips on writing customer-friendly emails include the following:
- When sending the email to several people, separate each email address by a semicolon (;).

VOCABULARY

portrait orientation: The most common layout for a printed page; the height of the paper is greater than its width.

CHAPTER 21 Technology and Written Communication

TABLE 21.18 Optional Services Provided by the US Postal Service

Optional Service	Description
Standard insurance	Protects against loss or damage. Cost is based on the item's declared value.
Registered mail	Used to protect expensive items. Mailed item can be insured up to the maximum amount. A mailing receipt is given; upon request, an electronic verification of delivery or delivery attempt can be sent.
Certified mail	Mailing receipt provides evidence the letter was mailed and combined with the return receipt shows delivery information and the recipient's signature (Fig. 21.19).
Signature confirmation	Provides date and time of delivery or when delivery attempt was made, along with the recipient's signature. Copy of delivery record is available upon request.
Return receipt	Provides an automatic electronic or mailed delivery record showing the recipient's signature.
Adult signature restricted delivery	Addressee or authorized agent must verify identity and age (i.e., must be over 21); must sign for delivery.
Restricted delivery	Addressee or authorized agent must verify identity and must sign for delivery.
Certificate of mailing	Provides evidence (i.e., date and time) when an item was mailed. (Limited service because it does not provide evidence of the delivery.)
US Postal Service tracking	Provides updates as an item is being shipped. Will include date and time of delivery or attempted delivery.
Special handling	Used to get preferential handing when shipping very unusual items or items that need extra care.
Collect on delivery (COD)	Recipient pays for merchandise and shipping when the package is received.
Hold for pickup	Option to pick up item from a specified post office within 15 days, depending on service selected.

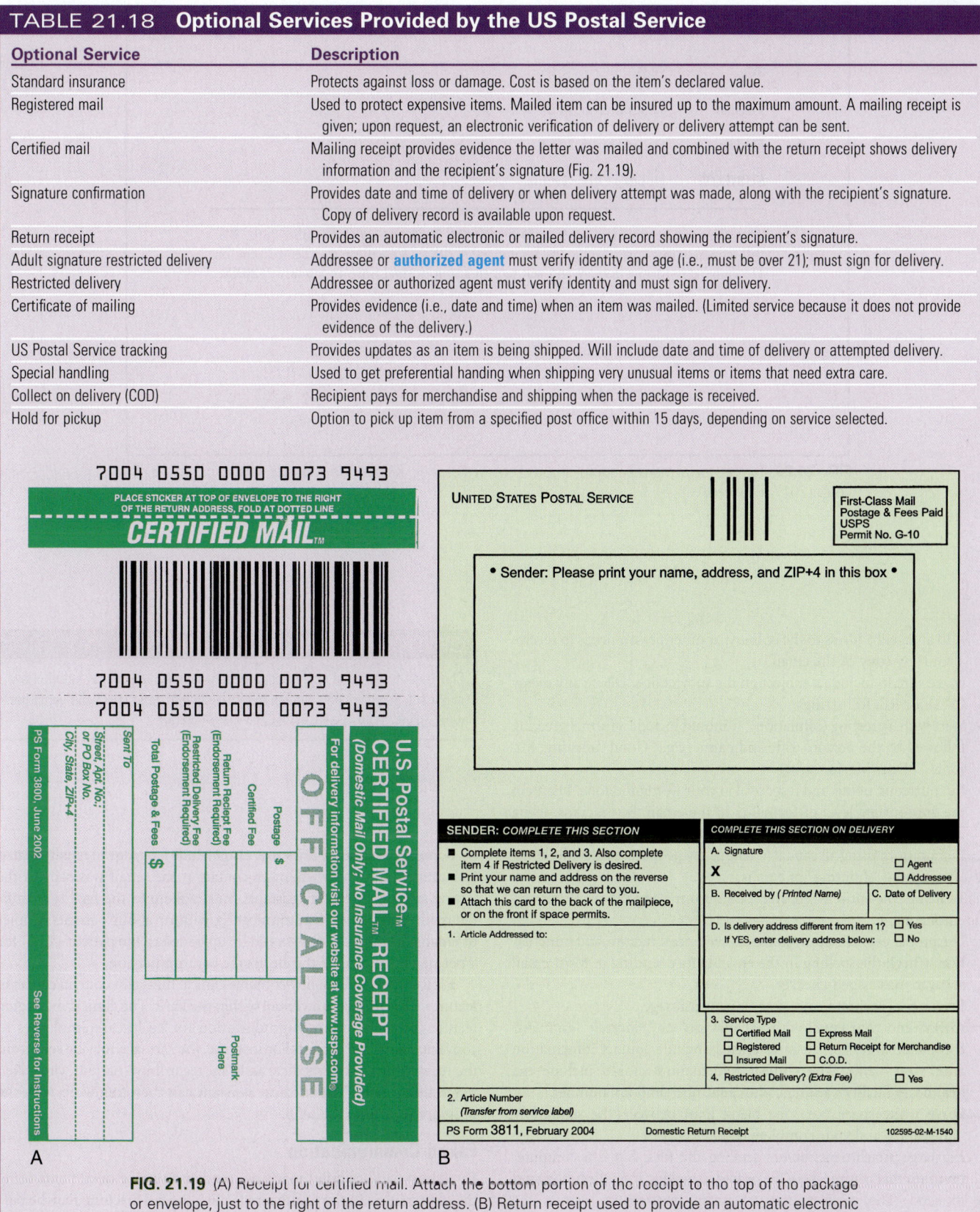

FIG. 21.19 (A) Receipt for certified mail. Attach the bottom portion of the receipt to the top of the package or envelope, just to the right of the return address. (B) Return receipt used to provide an automatic electronic or hardcopy record showing the recipient's signature. (From Proctor D, et al: *Kinn's The Medical Assistant*, ed 13, St. Louis, 2017, Elsevier.)

TO:	Staff
FROM:	James Martin, M.D.
DATE:	December 15, 20XX
SUBJECT:	Holiday Office Hours

The office will be closed at noon on December 24, 20XX through December 26th. We will reopen at our normal time on December 27, 20XX. We will then close at 3 p.m. on December 31st for the holiday and will reopen at our normal time on January 2, 20XX.

FIG. 21.20 Format for a memorandum. (From Proctor D, et al: *Kinn's The Medical Assistant*, ed 13, St. Louis, 2017, Elsevier.)

- Add an email address to the cc line if another person needs to receive a courtesy copy of the email.
- Make sure to include a subject on the subject line. Delete any messy FWD: or RE: RE: strings.
- Start with a greeting (salutation). It should include a formal greeting followed by the person's title and name (e.g., "Good morning, Mr. Jones," "Dear Mr. Jones,").
- Be courteous, polite, and respectful in your words and tone. Maintain the appropriate level of formality in the email. Be gracious, using expressions such as "please" and "thank you."
- Refrain from using all capital letters. Many people consider all capital letters to be "shouting" in emails.
- Write out the entire word, and refrain from using abbreviations and emoticons.
- Use proper capitalization, grammar, sentence structure, and punctuation. Check the spelling in the email before sending it. Most email software has a spell-checker.
- Be concise, accurate, and clear in your message.
- Always end your email with "Thank you" or "Sincerely" and your complete name. For business emails, include contact information after your name. The contact information should include the healthcare facility's address, phone number, and fax number.
- Leave white space (i.e., one blank line) between the salutation, paragraphs, and your complete name.
- Zip large attachments before sending the files. *Zip* is a computer program that compresses a file or folder, making it smaller and easier to send. The receiver uses an unzip program to extract the contents.
- Many email programs have features such as (!) urgent or a response box that sends an email back to the sender when the email is opened by the recipient. Use the urgent feature only for crucial emails.

> **CRITICAL THINKING 21.14**
>
> Christiana receives an email from a patient that is in all capital letters. How might she perceive the situation with the patient? How could she verify her perceptions? How should she handle this situation?

Some healthcare facilities may also include language in emails related to confidentiality and whom to contact if the email was sent to the wrong address. Medical assistants must adhere to the facility's confidentiality rules when communicating with or about patients. Copies of email communications should be uploaded to the patient's EHR for a permanent record of the electronic communication.

EHR software frequently contains clinical messaging or clinical email features. This feature is an email within the EHR. The clinical messaging feature provides secure communication for healthcare employees to converse about the patient. For instance, the message may be sent from the receptionist to the medical assistant regarding a patient who called requesting a refill. The medical assistant can then follow up with the provider regarding the refill.

Faxed Communication

Fax (short for facsimile) machines send and receive documents using the phone lines. In the healthcare facility, the fax machine may be part of a copy machine, or the computers may have software that allows faxes to be sent and received. As communications technology has advanced, the use of fax machines has decreased, but they are still an important piece of equipment in the ambulatory care center.

CHAPTER 21 Technology and Written Communication

PROCEDURE 21.2 Compose a Professional Email

Task
Compose a professional email that conveys the message to the reader clearly, concisely, and accurately.

Scenario
Create an email for the following scenario: Aaron Jackson (DOB: 10/17/2011) has an appointment at 11 a.m. next Thursday. Send his guardian an appointment reminder via email. Aaron will be seeing David Kahn, M.D. The guardian should bring in any medications Aaron is currently taking. You are working at Walden-Martin Family Medical Clinic. The healthcare facility's address is: 1234 Anystreet, Anytown, AL 12345. The phone number is 123-123-1234 and the fax number is 123-123-5678. Your instructor will supply you with the guardian's name and email address.

Equipment and Supplies
- Patient's health record
- Computer with email software

Procedural Steps

1. Obtain the intended recipient's contact information and determine the message you want to convey.
   Purpose: This gives you a focus when composing the email. You will need the recipient's information to create the email.
2. Using the computer and email software, key (type) in the recipient's email address. If the email has two recipients, use a semicolon (;) after the name of the first recipient. Double-check the email addresses for accuracy.
   Purpose: If the email address is incorrect, the email will not get to the recipient.
3. Key in a subject, keeping it simple but focused on the contents of the email.
   Purpose: In many email software packages, the user can search for emails using the subject field. Keeping the subject simple and focused makes it easier for the user to find the message.
4. Key a formal greeting, using correct punctuation.
   Purpose: A proper greeting sets the tone of the letter.
5. Key the message in the body of the email using proper grammar, punctuation, capitalization, and sentence structure. Avoid abbreviations. The message should be clear, concise, and professional.
   Purpose: Using proper grammar and avoiding abbreviations will convey the message accurately and professionally.
6. Finish the email with closing remarks.
   Purpose: In the closing, you can thank the recipient or encourage him or her to follow up with concerns or questions. This gives the email a professional tone.
7. Key a closing, followed by your name and title on the next line. Include the clinic's name and contact information below your name.
   Purpose: The email clearly states who is sending it.
8. Spell-check and proofread the email. Check for proper tone, grammar, punctuation, capitalization, and sentence structure. Check for proper spacing between the parts of the email.
   Purpose: White space or spacing between the elements of an email helps separate the parts of the email, making it easier to read.
9. Make any final revisions, select any features to apply to the email, and then send it.
   Purpose: If the email is urgent (!), that feature should be selected before you send the email. If you require a confirmation email when the email is opened, this feature can also be selected.
10. Print a copy of the email to be filed in the paper medical record or upload an electronic copy of the email to the patient's electronic health record (EHR).
    Purpose: A copy of all correspondence should be kept in the patient's health record.

When sending a fax, the medical assistant must adhere to HIPAA and HITECH rules. Healthcare facilities usually have a required face sheet (the first sheet) that includes confidentiality language, which instructs the recipient, if he or she is not the intended party, to destroy the fax and contact the medical facility. Besides the confidentiality statement, the face sheet should include the contact information for sender and recipient, the date, and the total number of pages.

EXCEPTIONAL CUSTOMER SERVICE

When using computers while interacting with others, it is important to focus on the customer. Often, the customer feels forgotten. The employee's attention seems to be on the computer. Being attentive to our customers is important. Remember that your customers in healthcare can be coworkers, providers, patients and their family members, and vendors. It is critical that you use eye contact and body language that show your customers you are really listening. Body language that indicates listening includes the following:
- Turning your head and upper body toward the speaker
- Leaning forward
- Tilting your head and nodding
- Smiling (if appropriate in the situation)

CLOSING COMMENTS

This chapter discussed technology typically seen in the ambulatory care center. The medical assistant should be familiar with hardware and software commonly used in the facility. The most important consideration in regard to technology is security. The medical assistant has an important role in securing the network and preventing unauthorized users from accessing the network. Simply logging off a workstation before leaving it can keep the network secure.

The medical assistant also has an important role in communicating with internal and external customers. Being able to write a professional email and letter is important. Using proper format, sentence structure, punctuation, and capitalization is critical when composing written communication. Remember, how a medical assistant communicates is a reflection on the provider and the facility.

CHAPTER REVIEW

A personal computer (PC) is a relatively inexpensive piece of hardware that is used by a single person. It can be a desktop, laptop, or tablet computer. The medical assistant should be knowledgeable about input and output hardware used in the healthcare environment. As technology advances, more input devices will be used in ambulatory care facilities.

The computers and output devices in a healthcare facility are all usually connected to the clinic's network. A router is used to allow multiple devices to be used on the same network. The ambulatory care center must subscribe to an internet services provider and be connected to a modem to have internet access.

When sitting at a workstation, your torso and neck should be vertical and in line. The chair should be adjusted so that your feet are flat on the floor or a footrest. Your legs should be comfortably below the workstation. The backrest lumbar support area should be fitted to the small of your back. The backrest should help support the upper body in the upright position. The monitor should be directly in front of you and tilted to avoid glare. The top of the monitor should be at or just below eye level. This prevents you from bending your head or neck. Use a document holder to prevent continual movement of the head.

System software is a collection of programs that operate and control the computer. Operating systems and utility software are two types of system software. The medical assistant should be able to distinguish between the EMR and the practice management system. The EMR is used to document patient-related information. The practice management software is used to run the "business." Scheduling, billing, and coding programs are part of the practice management software typically used in the healthcare facility.

To abide by HIPAA rules and meaningful use requirements, healthcare agencies must ensure that their computer networks are secure. Data backup procedures can help prevent problems if the network files are compromised by a hacker or an environmental situation (e.g., fire, flood).

Medical assistants should be familiar with the components or elements of a professional business letter. They must include the appropriate information and punctuation in each section of the letter to achieve professional results. Proper and consistent spacing in the letter provides the polished, professional appearance that medical assistants should strive for when creating letters.

There are three main business letter formats: full block letter format, modified block letter format, and semi–block letter format. With more patients communicating by email, medical assistants must be able to write professional emails. Emails must send a clear message to the recipient in a professional and respectful manner.

SCENARIO WRAP-UP

Since her promotion, Christiana has learned many helpful administrative and computer procedures. She has also been implementing changes in the administrative area. Her first change was to email, rather than mail, appointment reminders. She uses the appointment reminder feature of the practice management software when emailing the notifications to patients. Not only does this save time, but it also saves postage costs. Christiana has also learned how to create letter and memo templates. She uses templates to notify patients about laboratory and diagnostic test results. She continues to create custom letters for patients, yet she saves time by using predesigned templates.

Christiana has learned a great deal about the healthcare facility's computer network. She is implementing more security measures. She is training staff members to log out of their workstations before leaving the computer. She is also working with a local IT company to increase the network's protection against unauthorized users. She has contracted with an online backup service to protect the network files.

Christiana enjoys her new position and knows that she will need to stay up to date on technology advances and privacy mandates. She plans to do this by reading online articles and attending continuing education events. She understands that learning is an ongoing process that will help her to become the professional she strives to be.

22

Reception and Daily Operations

LEARNING OBJECTIVES

1. Explain tasks for the medical assistant to handle when opening the healthcare facility.
2. Discuss patient processing tasks that should happen upon the patient's arrival to the healthcare facility. Create a brochure and coach patients regarding office policies.
3. Describe how to show consideration for patients' time, escort a patient to the exam room, and handle various challenging situations in the healthcare facility. Explain medical assisting duties related to patient checkout.
4. Explain duties for the medical assistant to handle when closing the healthcare facility, including daily and monthly duties.
5. List the steps involved in completing an inventory, and perform an equipment inventory with documentation.
6. Explain the purpose of routine maintenance of administrative and clinical equipment, and perform routine maintenance of equipment. Discuss service calls, warranties, and purchasing equipment.
7. Do the following related to the many supplies required to run a medical office and treat patients:
   - Discuss inventory management and inventory management control systems.
   - Perform a supply inventory with documentation while using proper body mechanics.
   - Consider prices when ordering supplies.
   - Prepare a purchase order.
8. Discuss how to handle mail in the healthcare facility.
9. Identify the principles of body mechanics, and use proper body mechanics.
10. Evaluate the work environment to identify unsafe working conditions.
11. Identify critical elements of an emergency response plan to use in the event of a natural disaster or other emergency, participate in a mock exposure event, and demonstrate the proper use of a fire extinguisher.
12. Recognize the physical and emotional effects on persons involved in an emergency situation.

CHAPTER OUTLINE

1. Opening Scenario, 494
2. You Will Learn, 494
3. Introduction, 494
4. Opening the Healthcare Facility, 494
   a. Opening Tasks for the Medical Assistant, 494
      i. *The Reception Area, 497*
5. Patient Processing Tasks, 497
   a. Patient's Arrival, 497
      i. *Sign-in Register, 498*
      ii. *Infection Control in the Reception Area, 499*
      iii. *Registration for New Patients, 499*
      iv. *Check-in Procedures for All Patients, 500*
      v. *Patients With Special Needs, 500*
   b. Showing Consideration for Patients' Time, 500
   c. Escorting Patients to the Exam Room, 500
   d. Challenging Situations, 501
      i. *Talkative Patients, 501*
      ii. *Children, 502*
      iii. *Angry Patients in the Reception Area, 502*
   e. Patient Checkout, 502
6. Closing the Healthcare Facility, 502
   a. Daily and Monthly Duties, 503
7. Equipment and Supplies, 503
   a. Equipment, 503
      i. *Equipment Inventory, 503*
      ii. *Equipment Safety and Maintenance, 503*
      iii. *Service Calls and Warranties, 504*
      iv. *Purchasing Equipment, 505*
   b. Supplies, 506
      i. *Inventory Management, 506*
      ii. *Inventory Control Systems, 507*
      iii. *Taking Inventory, 507*
      iv. *Price Consideration When Ordering Supplies, 507*
      v. *Ordering Supplies, 509*
      vi. *Receiving the Order, 509*
8. Handling Mail, 511
   a. Private Delivery Services, 511
   b. Incoming Mail, 511
9. Safety and Security, 512
   a. Body Mechanics, 512
   b. Providing a Safe Environment, 513
      i. *Workplace Violence, 513*
   c. Evaluating the Work Environment, 513
      i. *Preventing Falls and Injuries, 514*
      ii. *Preventing Electrical Issues and Fires, 514*

d. Emergency Response Plan, 514
   i. *Evacuation Procedures, 514*
   ii. *Fire Response, 516*
e. Effects of Stress, 518

10. Closing Comments, 519
11. Chapter Review, 520
12. Scenario Wrap-Up, 520

OPENING SCENARIO

Marie Van Bakel, a certified clinical medical assistant (CMA), is a new medical assistant at Walden-Martin Family Medical (WMFM) Clinic. She was hired to work with the family medicine providers. This is Marie's first job as a new graduate from a medical assistant program. She is excited to work in family medicine. This was the same specialty she worked in during her medical assistant practicum. Because this is a small healthcare facility, Marie's responsibilities are different from what they would be in a larger facility. She and the administrative medical assistant, Catherine, are the only staff members in the office at the start of the day. The providers make hospital rounds at that time. The providers and the rest of the medical assistants come in later.

Marie and Catherine need to open the office and prepare for the patients. Marie is also responsible for the inventory of clinical supplies and administrative and clinical equipment. During Marie's interview, Dr. Walden expressed her concern about the lack of procedures for ordering and maintaining inventory. She would like Marie to develop those procedures. Having little exposure to supplies and ordering during her practicum, Marie realizes she needs to learn about these procedures.

YOU WILL LEARN

1. To perform duties necessary to open and close the healthcare facility.
2. To describe procedures involved with patient processing.
3. To perform inventory on equipment and supplies.
4. To order supplies and to perform the procedures done when supplies are received.
5. To handle incoming mail.
6. To follow safety procedures, including using correct body mechanics, evaluating the work environment, and responding to emergencies.

INTRODUCTION

A first impression is a lasting one. Nowhere is this more important than in the healthcare facility. The facility must appear orderly and clean. The appearance of the reception room and the front desk, as well as a cordial greeting from the medical assistant, will influence patients' perception of the entire facility and of the care that they will receive. We will examine the preparation required before patients arrive, the patient processing procedures, and dealing with special situations.

Additional operational procedures including performing inventory and handling incoming mail are described. The chapter concludes with a discussion on safety, evaluating the environment for risks, and handling emergencies.

OPENING THE HEALTHCARE FACILITY

Employees who are responsible for opening the ambulatory healthcare facility must arrive before the patients in the morning. These employees must prepare for the day. Preparation time will vary based on the size of the practice and the number of patients on the schedule.

In smaller facilities, a few reliable employees are given keys to unlock the doors and deactivate the alarm system. In larger facilities, employees must use the locked employee entrances. Employees can unlock the doors by entering unique codes into a keypad or by using unique keycards (Fig. 22.1A–B). Both systems are developed to monitor who enters the building. Usually security, custodial, or supervisory personnel are responsible for deactivating the alarm system in larger facilities. Staff members then open the main patient doors at a set time.

Opening Tasks for the Medical Assistant

The clinical medical assistant assists the provider with patient treatments and procedures (e.g., injections, wound care, and diagnostic tests). The administrative medical assistant works in the reception area. In larger facilities, both types of medical assistants have opening duties. If the healthcare facility is small, then the medical assistant may be required to perform both administrative and clinical tasks. Often this is called performing "front office" and "back office" activities.

It is important for the clinical medical assistant to prepare the clinical equipment and exam rooms for patient visits. An unprepared area can cause delays in patient care. Facility opening tasks for the clinical medical assistant include the following:

- Prepare the exam rooms by turning on the lights, ensuring supplies are stocked, and making sure the rooms are cleaned appropriately and safe for patients. Prescription pads (if used) need to be stored outside of the exam rooms (Box 22.1).
- Unlock supply cabinets (with the exception of the narcotics cabinet, which remains locked).
- Ensure restrooms have adequate supplies for patients (e.g., urine specimen containers, cleansing towelettes).
- Perform **quality control** tests on laboratory equipment and complete refrigerator and freezer temperature logs.

In addition to these tasks, the clinical medical assistant must follow up on outstanding patient issues from the prior day. The medical assistant also needs to handle new diagnostic test reports (e.g., x-ray reports). For agencies using paper health records, this would require the following:

- Obtaining the patient's paper health record
- Clipping the diagnostic report to the record
- Giving the health record and report to the provider to review

For facilities with electronic health records (EHRs), this process is completed using the electronic messaging system in the software.

Often medical assistants notify patients of normal test results and document the notification in the health record. No test result can be given to the patient unless the provider has authorized it or the facility's procedures allow it. The medical assistant must follow the facility's procedures when notifying the patient of the results.

> **VOCABULARY**
>
> **e-prescribing**: The use of electronic software to communicate with pharmacies and send prescribing information. It takes the place of writing a prescription by hand and giving it to a patient; most new or refill prescriptions can be submitted electronically, cutting down on fraud and errors.
>
> **quality control**: A process to ensure the reliability of test results, often using manufactured samples with known values.

CHAPTER 22 Reception and Daily Operations

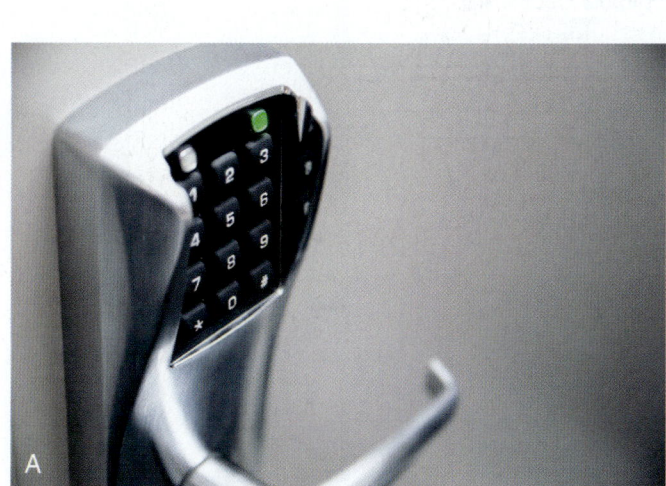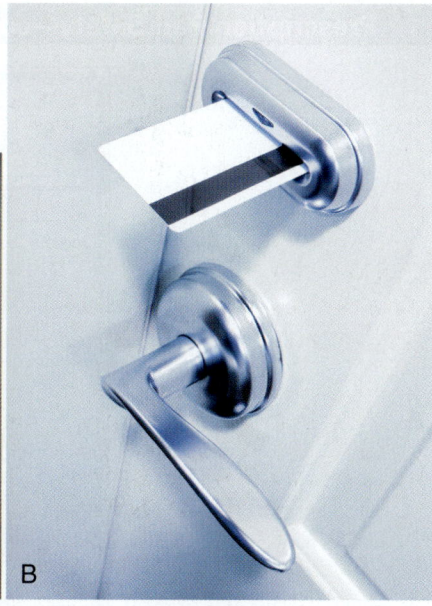

FIG. 22.1 (A) Keyless access locks allow employees to enter unique numbers that open the door and track who has keyed in. Once a person is no longer employed, the number is deleted. (B) Employees can unlock doors using their unique key card. This system can track which keycard was used to open the door. (A from baloon111/istock/Thinkstock. B from nazdravie/iStock/Thinkstock.)

BOX 22.1 Prescription Pad Safety

For ambulatory care facilities that do not use **e-prescribing**, prescription pads should not remain in exam rooms (Figs. 22.2 and 22.3). The providers should keep a pad in their pocket. The extra prescription pads should be stored in a locked cabinet. Prescription pads should never be accessible to patients. Some patients or staff might take the pads and try to forge a prescription, which is illegal.

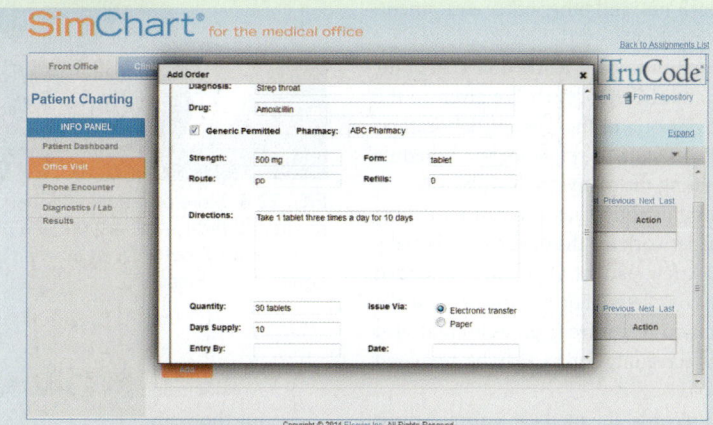

FIG. 22.2 With e-prescribing, providers can enter the prescription information into the electronic health record (EHR) and send it electronically to the pharmacy.

Continued

BOX 22.1 Prescription Pad Safety—cont'd

SECURITY FEATURES LISTED ON BACK – SECURITY FEATURES LISTED ON BACK

THOMAS A. SCOTT, M.D.
General Practice
135 So. Elm St.
Sacramento, CA 94107
DEA # ________ Telephone: (916) 344-5550 LIC. # ________

FOR ________________ DATE ________
ADDRESS ________________
℞

REFILL ________ TIMES ________________
#25-8293V Thomas A. Scott, M.D.

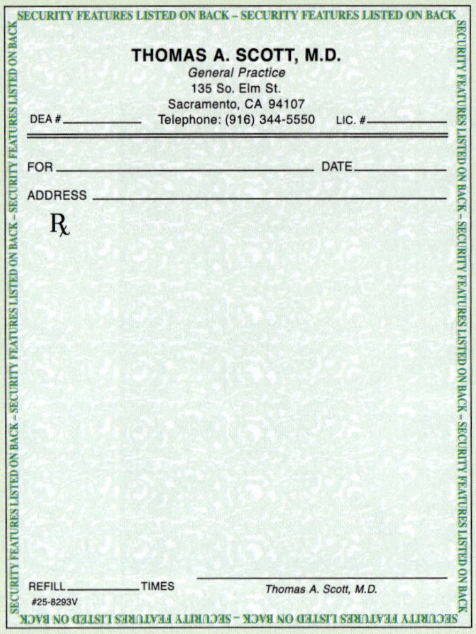

FIG. 22.3 The provider should keep one prescription pad, and extra pads should be locked up. (From Proctor D, et al: *Kinn's The Medical Assistant*, ed 13, St. Louis, 2017, Elsevier.)

Opening tasks for the administrative medical assistant include the following:

- Checking voice mail or **answering service** messages. The answering service may email or fax messages to the facility. All messages need to be addressed and documented in the patient's health record.
- Updating the voice mail message.
- Switching the phone, so patients can reach the facility instead of the answering service.
- Turning on computers, copy machines, and other office equipment.
- Preparing the reception area for patients.
- Printing schedules of the day's appointments. A schedule is kept for the paper health record preparation. Other copies are given to the clinical medical assistants, providers, and the medical laboratory. In some facilities, the EHR allows staff to reference the schedule using the software, thus eliminating the printed schedule.

In addition to these duties, the administrative medical assistant must compile any remaining required paperwork for the day's visits. Usually this is done the prior afternoon. A few patient visits may be added onto the schedule that need to be completed. For healthcare facilities with EHRs, required patient education literature (e.g., well-child visit documents) and preprinted paper screening forms may be prepared (Fig. 22.4).

For facilities with paper health records, the medical assistant must do the following:

- Pull the paper health records, using a copy of the appointment schedule.
- Verify that the correct record was pulled for each patient.
- Check off the patient's name on the copy of the appointment schedule.
- Review each record:
  - Have all recently received documents (e.g., laboratory reports, radiograph readings) been placed correctly and permanently attached to the record?
  - Are documents (e.g., laboratory reports) missing that are needed for the visit?
  - Is there enough space available on the **progress notes** for the provider to write in the record? If not, place additional progress notes pages in the record.

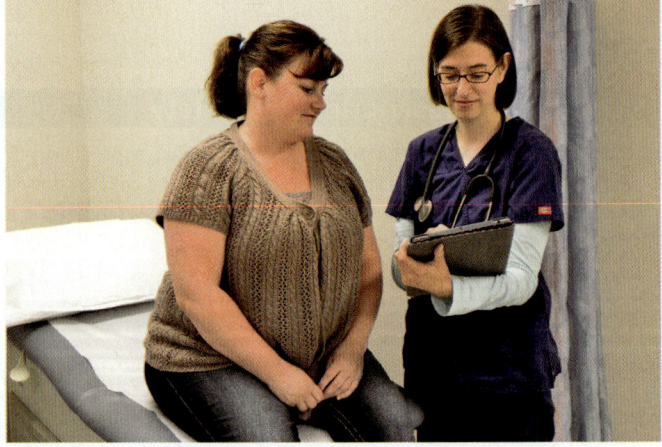

FIG. 22.4 More providers and their staff members use electronic health records to reduce paperwork and provide better, more efficient patient care. (From Proctor D, et al: *Kinn's The Medical Assistant*, ed 13, St. Louis, 2017, Elsevier.)

VOCABULARY

answering service: A commercial service that answers telephone calls for its clients.

progress notes: Documentation in the medical record that can be used to track the patient's condition and progress.

- Arrange the health records in the order in which the patients will be arriving. The record for the first visit of the day should be on top. Larger facilities may alphabetize the health records.

> ### CRITICAL THINKING 22.1
> When opening the family medicine office, what jobs does Marie, the clinical medical assistant, need to do? What jobs does Catherine, the administrative medical assistant, need to do to prepare for the day?

The Reception Area. The reception room is a place to receive patients and visitors. The area should be planned for patients' comfort. It should be as attractive and cheerful as possible. It needs to be kept clean and uncluttered (Fig. 22.5; Box 22.2).

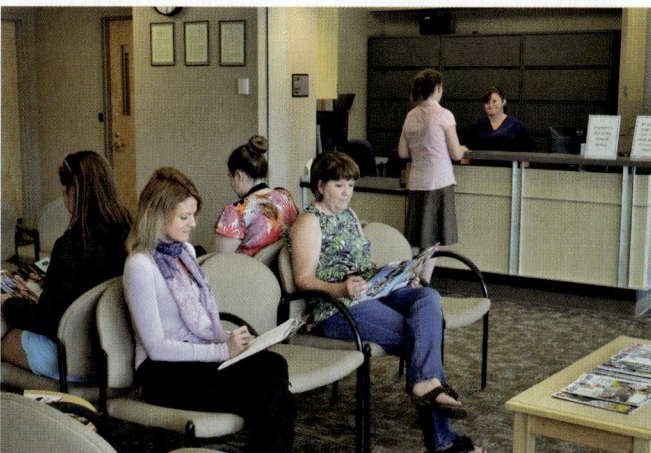

FIG. 22.5 Patients appreciate cleanliness, restful colors, good ventilation, and light to read by when waiting in the reception area. (From Proctor D, et al: *Kinn's The Medical Assistant*, ed 13, St. Louis, 2017, Elsevier.)

> ### BOX 22.2 Maintaining the Reception Area
> Each morning and throughout the day, the medical assistant should ensure the reception area is neat for patients:
> - Magazines should be neatly displayed.
> - Toys should be **disinfected** on a routine basis for infection control.
> - Tissue boxes, hand sanitizers, and face masks should be well stocked and available for sick patients.
> - Beverages (if offered) should be prepared and adequately stocked.
> - The temperature should be comfortable.
> - Lighting should be adequate to allow for reading and safety.

> ### VOCABULARY
> **disinfected**: The state of having destroyed or rendered pathogenic organisms inactive; does not include spores, tuberculosis bacilli, and certain viruses.
> **privacy filters**: Devices attached to the monitor that allow visualization of the screen contents only if the user is directly in front of the screen; also called *monitor filters* or *privacy screens*.
> **triage**: To sort out and classify the injured; used in the military and in emergency settings to determine the priority of a patient to be treated.
> **white noise**: The sound from a television or stereo that muffles or mutes the conversation of others, thus helping to protect the confidentiality of patients.

Most reception areas are well supplied with recent magazines, and some have various books. Any reading material placed in the reception room should be of interest to the public. On donated magazines, mark through the person's name and address so it cannot be read. Providers' professional journals or pharmaceutical company's flyers should not be in the reception area.

Most reception areas have background music that provides **white noise** to help maintain patient confidentiality. A television or DVD player can help the time pass much faster, especially in pediatric practices. A children's corner equipped with small-scale furniture and some safe toys helps occupy children.

> ### CRITICAL THINKING 22.2
> Catherine utilizes low-volume music from a stereo as white noise in the reception area, which is near the reception desk. What are the benefits of the music?

Many healthcare facilities offer a computer for patients to use while waiting to see the provider. Patients often bring in electronic devices to use while waiting. It is important to have Internet access available for patients and visitors. Many facilities have a separate network for guests, thereby safeguarding the confidentiality of patient records. It is important to post or provide the guest log-on information.

The registration desk should be visible when patients enter the facility. The desk should be free of clutter. Patient health and financial records must be protected from the view of others. Keep computer monitors out of patients' view. Use **privacy filters** and screen savers as added protection. This prevents violation of the privacy regulations established by the Health Insurance Portability and Accountability Act (HIPAA). No food, drink, or personal items should be on the registration desk.

PATIENT PROCESSING TASKS

When working at the reception desk, the medical assistant needs to screen the individuals arriving:
- People with emergent conditions: Individuals may be bleeding, having chest pain, or feeling very ill. It is important that the medical assistant immediately contacts the **triage** nurse to see the patient. If the nurse is not available, then the medical assistant should bring the patient back to an exam room and notify the provider right away. Facilities may have procedures in place to indicate when 911 needs to be called immediately.
- Pharmaceutical and equipment representatives: The medical assistant should follow the facility's policies and procedures regarding when these representatives are permitted to see the providers.
- Salespeople and visitors: The medical assistant needs to find out the reason for the visit and then follow the facility's procedures.

The most common visitors to the facility will be patients and family members who have appointments. We will examine the tasks the medical assistant must perform when patients arrive.

Patient's Arrival

When patients arrive, two important things need to occur. First, they need to know where to go and what to do. Second, they need to be greeted as quickly as possible. Signage is helpful to indicate what patients need to do upon arrival.

Every patient has the right to expect courteous treatment in a provider's office. Regardless of the patient's economic or social status, each person who arrives should receive a cordial, friendly greeting (Fig. 22.6). A personal touch, such as greeting the patient by name, is an easy way to develop patient rapport (Box 22.3). Table 22.1 provides appropriate greetings for the medical assistant to use as recommended by HIPAA.

The person sitting at the front reception desk should greet each patient as quickly as possible. Some experts say that a person should be greeted within 30 seconds of arriving. If this is not possible, a simple smile and eye contact will acknowledge the person. Make sure to greet the person verbally as soon as possible. If too much time elapses from the person's entrance to the greeting, the person may feel ignored or unimportant. This can impact a person's perception of the facility and, ultimately, the care provided. If the medical assistant must step away from the reception desk, it is important to check the reception area for new arrivals as soon as she or he returns.

In facilities where the receptionist is behind sliding glass windows, the environment can appear impersonal to patients. Although the closed glass windows increase patient privacy, they can also give the impression that the staff and provider are off limits to the patients. The glass window should be open as much as possible to give the appearance of openness to others. The policy and procedure manual should indicate when the glass window should be closed.

Sign-in Register. Some facilities will have the patient sign a register. A sign-in register that promotes patients' privacy should be used (Fig. 22.7). Remember, other patients can read the prior patients' information. This is not considered a violation of HIPAA policy if the information disclosed is appropriately limited (Table 22.2). This is one type of incidental disclosure under HIPAA.

BOX 22.3 Patients' Names

- Use the patient's last name and title (e.g., Mrs. Crawford) unless the patient insists on the use of his or her first name or prefers a nickname.
- Greet any individual you do not know, and then ask for his or her name.
- Learn how to pronounce each patient's name correctly. Incorrect pronunciations may offend or irritate some people.
- Make a note of the phonetic spelling in the health record for reference. Note if the patient prefers a nickname.
- Avoid calling patients "honey" or "sweetie."

TABLE 22.1 HIPAA Appropriate Communication

HIPAA Violation	HIPAA Appropriate Communication
"How is your leg ulcer today, Mr. Bowden?"	"How are you today, Mr. Bowden?"
"Mr. Biller, Dr. Walden will see you now for your shingles."	"Mr. Biller, the doctor will see you now."

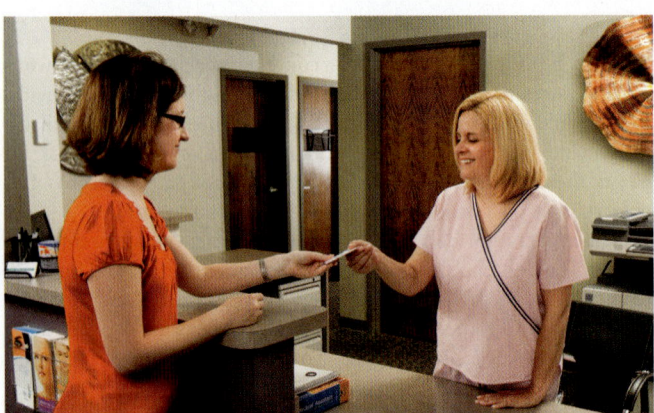

FIG. 22.6 Greet all patients with a warm smile, and assist them with forms they need to complete for the health record. (From Proctor D, et al: *Kinn's The Medical Assistant*, ed 13, St. Louis, 2017, Elsevier.)

Patient Sign-In Date: _____

Please sign-in and notify us if:
- New patient   • Phone/address change   • Insurance change

No.	Patient Name print	Appt. Time	Arrival Time	Appt. with	New patient (✓)	Phone/address change (✓)	Insurance change (✓)
1	PLEASE						
2	2						
3	3						
4	4						
5	5						
6	6						
7	7						
8	8						
9	9						
10	10						

FIG. 22.7 Sign-in sheets contain basic information about the patient and provide information for the medical assistant about changes that need to be made on the patient's record. (From Proctor D, et al: *Kinn's The Medical Assistant*, ed 13, St. Louis, 2017, Elsevier.)

TABLE 22.2 HIPAA Appropriate Sign-in Register

Features Causing a HIPAA Violation	Features of a HIPAA Appropriate Register
Insurance information (e.g., name, number)	Date
Reason for visit	Name
Demographic (dem uh GRAF ik) information (e.g., address, employer, date of birth)	Arrival time
	Appointment time
	Appointment with
	Check boxes to indicate changes (but no information can be given)

BOX 22.4 Facts Listed on Patient Information or Registration Forms

Most patient information or registration forms contain the following:
- Patient's first, middle, and last name
- Date of birth
- Responsible person's name and relationship to the patient
- Address, telephone number (home and cell phone), and email address
- Name, address, and telephone number of a contact person
- Occupation
- Place of employment
- Social Security number
- Driver's license number
- Nearest relative not living with the patient and his or her relationship
- Source of referral, if any

Infection Control in the Reception Area. It is vital for the medical assistant to take steps to protect the other patients in the reception area. The medical assistant may need to ask a few screening questions to identify patients who are ill with specific symptoms or at risk for specific diseases. These questions are set by the healthcare facility and usually recommended by the Centers for Disease Control and Prevention (CDC). Questions may include the following:

- "Have you traveled outside of the United States in the past 21 days?" Travel to specific countries may be included in the question. Patients who answer yes should be taken to an exam room immediately.
- "Are you coughing?" If patients are coughing, they should be encouraged to use masks. This is especially important during flu season or when other respiratory infections are prevalent. Tissues, along with waste containers and hand sanitizer, should be available for patients in the reception area.

Registration for New Patients. When someone visits the provider's office for the first time, the staff must gather information from the new patient, such as demographic and the health history information. The demographic information is usually gathered using the patient information or registration form. The patient's name should appear prominently at the top of the form, followed by other pertinent facts (Box 22.4). The patient's personal history, medical history, and family history may be obtained by using a questionnaire.

There are many ways the healthcare facility can obtain this information. Patients may be mailed the documents a few weeks prior to the appointment or directed to complete the information using the online **patient portal**. In some facilities, patients complete this information as they wait, prior to the appointment. They may complete paper forms or provide the information using an electronic device. In some cases, the medical assistant may take the patient to a private room where he or she can ask the questions and enter the information into the EHR.

The medical assistant must be willing to answer any questions either in person or over the phone (Fig. 22.8). The medical assistant must

CRITICAL THINKING 22.3

Often some time is needed to complete forms when a new patient arrives in the healthcare facility. How might Catherine keep the healthcare facility on schedule when new patients arrive who require health record construction and form completion? What are some ways to trim time from these activities?

VOCABULARY

patient portal: A secure online website that gives patients 24-hour access to personal health information using a username and password.

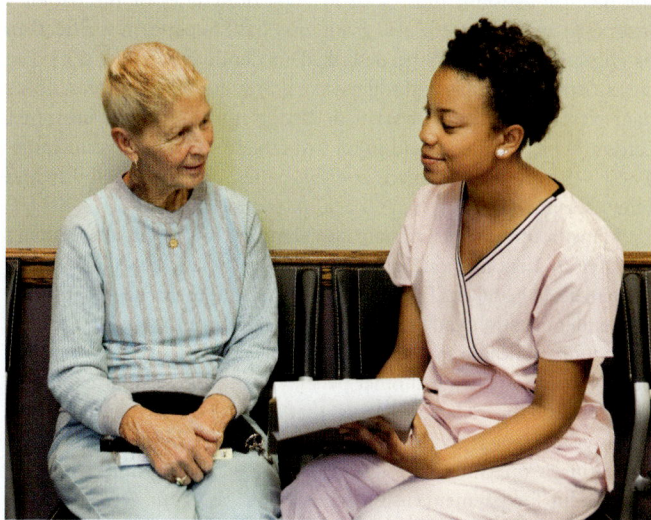

FIG. 22.8 The medical assistant should take time to explain forms the patient does not understand and should always be willing to answer questions. (From Proctor D, et al: *Kinn's The Medical Assistant*, ed 13, St. Louis, 2017, Elsevier.)

then review the completed form and verify that the required information has been provided. The provider also reviews the health history information and can then add information during the patient visit.

In addition to collecting information from the patient, the provider must give the patient the facility's Notice of Privacy Practices (NPP) document. The healthcare provider is legally obligated to give each patient a notice that explains how the health information may be used and shared. HIPAA requires that patients state in writing that they received the NPP document. The healthcare facility may ask the patient to sign a paper or electronic document. This form is then kept in the patient's health record. If the patient refuses to sign, the provider can still use and disclose the health information as permitted by HIPAA. The refusal needs to be documented in the patient's health record.

Many times, new patients are given a brochure on the facility's policies and procedures (Box 22.5). New patient brochures should be designed in a professional manner. The wording should be at a level that patients understand. When coaching a patient regarding the facility's policies, summarize the content of the brochure. Do not read the brochure to the patient. Use active listening skills. Make sure to address any questions the patient may have. Procedure 22.1 describes how to create the brochure and coach the patients regarding the policies.

> **BOX 22.5 New Patient Brochure Content**
>
> The following topics should be addressed in the new patient brochure:
> - Description of the healthcare facility (e.g., type of practice, mission statement)
> - Location or a map of the facility
> - Contact information (i.e., telephone numbers, emails, and website addresses)
> - Providers' names and credentials
> - Services offered
> - Hours of operation
> - How appointments can be scheduled
> - Healthcare facility's policies and procedures (e.g., payment policies, appointment cancellations, medication refills, assistance after hours)
> - Type of medical insurance that is accepted

Check-in Procedures for All Patients. During the check-in process, the medical assistant must scan or copy both sides of the patient's insurance card. The medical assistant may have to perform **verification of eligibility**. (This will be described in depth in Chapter 23.) The patient's phone number and address along with the insurance subscriber's date of birth should also be verified. Patients must show their insurance cards and picture identification for insurance and identity verification. These verifications take place at every patient visit for eligibility and safety reasons.

Many healthcare facilities are also scanning or copying the patient's legal photo identification. Facilities with EHRs may require a photo of the patient to be taken. The photo is uploaded to the EHR. Between the photo identification and the EHR photo, facilities are trying to decrease the amount of healthcare identify fraud. This fraud occurs when a person obtains healthcare using another person's name and insurance.

Some healthcare facilities insist that copays be collected before the office visit. Signage in the reception area often includes a statement indicating "Copayments are due at the time of the appointment." Ask the patient for payment, using phrases such as "Your copay today is $15, Mrs. Crawford. Will you be writing a check or would you like to charge this visit to your Visa?" If the facility is flexible with copayment collection, the medical assistant can give the patient an option. "Mr. Thomas, would you like to pay your copay now?"

Patients With Special Needs. After a patient is checked in, the receptionist may have additional duties if the patient has special needs. Some patients arrive in wheelchairs unattended by family or friends. They may need assistance to get to the reception area. Remember to always ask patients if they need assistance before you try to assist them.

If there is a language barrier, the medical assistant may need to get translation assistance for the visit. Typical options for assistance include having a qualified translator present or using translation technology. There are many online programs that can assist with translation in many different languages. It is important for the administrative medical assistant to communicate special needs of patients to the clinical medical assistant. In all special needs cases, it is important to remain professional and treat everyone with respect.

Showing Consideration for Patients' Time

Patients expect to see the provider at the appointed time. There should be signage in the reception area stating that patients should let the receptionist know if they have been waiting for longer than 15 to 20 minutes. If the provider is delayed, the medical assistant should let the patients know (Fig. 22.9). The medical assistant can also offer to reschedule the appointment. Some facilities will offer patients gift cards (e.g., coffee, gas) if an error occurred in scheduling or if the patient needs to reschedule due to a long wait time. These gestures show the patients that the staff recognizes their inconvenience. It is a great customer service practice.

> **CRITICAL THINKING 22.5**
>
> Catherine offers to reschedule patient appointments if the schedule ever falls more than 15 minutes behind. If a patient becomes belligerent about the delays, how can Catherine handle the situation in a professional manner?

Escorting Patients to the Exam Room

In some facilities, the administrative medical assistant may escort the patient to the exam room. In other facilities the clinical medical assistant comes to the reception area and calls the name of the patient. For confidentiality, it is important to call the patient by the first and last name only. Make sure to clearly pronounce the name. If you are unsure, attempt the pronunciation and then ask the patient. Apologize for pronouncing it incorrectly. Make sure to add the pronunciation to the record for the next visit. Remember, no other information should be given in the public waiting area. When you and the patient are alone or away from the reception area, verify that the patient's date of birth matches your records. If it does not, you have the wrong patient!

Some patients may bring a family member or friend with them to an appointment. On occasion, several people may want to accompany the patient to the exam room. Based on the facility's policy, respectfully explain that the exam room has only two chairs. If the patient still insists, make every attempt to satisfy the patient's needs (Box 22.6). Please be aware that in some cultures, it is expected that multiple people will accompany the patient to see the provider. In those situations, attempt to use a larger room if available.

It is understood that the medical assistant escorts the patient to the exam room. Ask if patients need any assistance, if it appears they might. Do not assume they need assistance—ask first and ask how you can assist them. To show respect for the patient, open doors and walk at the patient's speed.

If a urine specimen is needed, direct the patient to the restroom. Always explain how to collect the specimen and where the specimen should be placed. When you get to the exam room with the patient, instruct the patient based on the provider's wishes. If the patient needs to undress, explain what clothing items need to be removed and how

> **CRITICAL THINKING 22.4**
>
> A patient passes Marie in the hallway as she is leaving for lunch and stops to greet her. The patient's face is familiar, but Marie cannot recall the patient's name. Occasionally, Marie sees a patient outside of the office (e.g., at the store). Everyone forgets someone's name on occasion.
>
> How might Marie and her staff members remember names? What special tips or techniques can help you remember names? What can Marie do the next time she sees a patient and does not remember the person's name?

> **VOCABULARY**
>
> **verification of eligibility:** The process of confirming health insurance coverage for the patient.

PROCEDURE 22.1 Coach Patients Regarding Office Policies

Tasks
Create a new patient brochure, and then role-play ways to coach patients regarding office policies.

Scenario
You work at Walden-Martin Family Medical Clinic. Your supervisor asks you to create a new patient brochure for the clinic. The healthcare facility's information is listed here. After you complete the brochure, you coach the following patients regarding office procedures:
- Mr. Charles Johnson (he has a question regarding the payment policy)
- Ms. Monique Jones (she has a question regarding the medication refill procedure)

Healthcare Facility	Providers
Walden-Martin Family Medical Clinic	Julie Walden, M.D.
1234 Anystreet	James Martin, M.D.
Anytown, Anystate 12345	Angela Perez, M.D.
Phone: 123-123-1234	David Kahn, M.D.
Fax: 123-123-5678	Jean Burke, N.P.

Equipment and Supplies
- Computer with word processing software and printer
- Office procedure manual (optional)

Procedural Steps

1. Using word processing software, design an informational brochure for patients that provides information about the healthcare facility and describes practice procedures. At a minimum, the information should include the following:
   - Description of the healthcare facility (e.g., type of practice, mission statement)
   - Location or a map of the facility
   - Contact information (i.e., telephone numbers, emails, and website addresses)
   - Providers' names and credentials
   - Services offered
   - Hours of operation
   - How appointments can be scheduled
   - Healthcare facility's policies and procedures (e.g., payment policies, appointment cancellations, medication refills, assistance after hours)
   - Insurance plans accepted

   Purpose: Providing patients with a written brochure listing the facility's information, policies, and procedures enables them to use it as a reference.

2. Proofread the brochure. Revise as needed. Print the brochure.
   Purpose: It is important to proofread and revise documents as needed before they are available to patients.

3. Using the scenario for the first patient, give a brief summary of the different parts of the brochure. Use words the patient will understand.
   Purpose: By discussing each part of the brochure with the potential patient, you can explain what is printed. Summarize the information without reading the sections to the patient.

4. Ask if the patient has any questions. Actively listen to the patient's concerns. Address those concerns.
   Purpose: By actively listening, you will be able to identify issues or confusion the patient is experiencing. It is important that the messages during the conversation are clear for both parties.

5. Using the scenario for the second patient, give a brief summary of the different parts of the brochure. Use words that the patient understands.
   Purpose: By reviewing the brochure, you can summarize the policies. If the patient has an immediate question, you can answer it.

6. Ask if the patient has any questions. Actively listen to the patient's concerns. Address those concerns.
   Purpose: By actively listening, you will be able to identify issues or confusion the patient is experiencing. It is important that the messages during the conversation are clear for both parties.

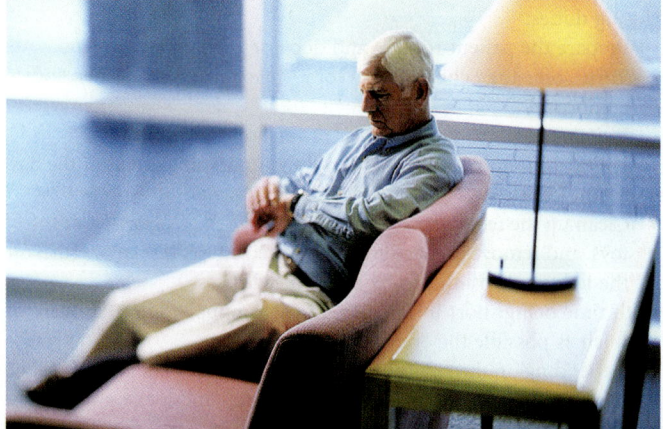

FIG. 22.9 One of the most common patient complaints is the time spent in the reception area. (From Proctor D, et al: *Kinn's The Medical Assistant*, ed 13, St. Louis, 2017, Elsevier.)

BOX 22.6 Interacting With Friends and Relatives of Patients

Patients are sometimes accompanied by a relative or friend. Be cautious if these individuals want to discuss the patient's illness. Avoid a "too casual" attitude, such as "I'm sure there's nothing to worry about." A show of moderate concern and reassurance that "the patient is in good hands" usually takes care of the situation. Remember that health information cannot be released to anyone, including concerned friends and relatives, without the patient's written consent on the release form.

to put on the gown. Make sure to indicate where the patient needs to sit. If the patient has a risk of falling, have the him or her sit on the chair instead of the exam table.

If using the EHR, make sure to log out of the software before leaving the room, and then close the door. If you need to reenter the room, always knock first out of respect for the patient. Pause before opening the door. The pause allows the patients time to prepare and time for them to tell you to enter.

For facilities that use paper health records, often file holders are located on the door or near the door. Place the health record in the holder in such a way that the patient's name is not visible. HIPAA considers names on health records to be incidental disclosures. It is a good practice to protect patient privacy. Many facilities have flags on the door to indicate the status of the patient. Adjust the flagging system so the provider knows the patient is in the room and ready to be seen.

Challenging Situations

Talkative Patients. Any professional office has problem patients. Talkative patients, for example, take up far more of the provider's time than is justified. Many times, the provider and medical assistant will devise a method to help keep everything on schedule. For instance, the medical assistant may have to page the provider after a certain time period. This alerts the provider to the time already spent with the patient. The provider can then complete the visit and move to the next patient.

> **CRITICAL THINKING 22.6**
>
> Catherine has one patient who insists on sitting close to her desk and attempting to chat the entire time she is waiting to see the provider. Even worse, she comes to her appointments at least an hour early. How might Catherine subtly deal with this patient?

Children. Children frequently present special management challenges. The child may be the patient, or he or she may be accompanying the patient. Parents or guardians are responsible for their children's behavior while at the healthcare facility. If children are doing something that could be harmful, quietly speak to the parents and allow them to handle the situation. The medical assistant should not discipline the child (Box 22.7). If the child continues to behave badly, call the parent to the exam room early. They may not be seen early but can wait in the exam room instead of the reception area.

In most cases (other than those that involve teens and suspected abuse situations), parents or guardians accompany the child to the exam room. Sometimes parents of older teens want to be present for the visit. Some providers find teens are more honest with their answers if parents are not present. In these situations, allowing the parent to be in the room for the interview may be helpful, but the parent can then wait in the reception area during the physical exam. This will allow the provider can ask follow-up questions if needed without the parent overhearing the answers. In all cases (unless indicated by state law), parental permission is required for minors to be seen.

Angry Patients in the Reception Area. Every medical assistant eventually is confronted with an angry patient. The anger may simply reflect the patient's pain or fear of what the provider may discover during the exam. If possible, invite the patient into a room out of the reception area. Usually the best course is to let the patient talk out the anger. Present a calm attitude and speak in a low tone of voice. Under no circumstances should the medical assistant return the anger or become argumentative. Medical assistants must use good listening skills with angry people and must be empathetic. Notify the facility's administrator of all difficult patients or ask for help from coworkers.

There should be a policy in place for dealing with potentially dangerous individuals. Policies can include the following:
- Making sure that you can reach the exit if you take the patient to another room
- Having another employee close by
- Knowing under what circumstances you should contact the police or building security for assistance

Patient Checkout

When patients return to the front office for checkout, greet them with a friendly smile and call the individual by name. Form the habit of asking patients if they have any questions. Check the health record to determine when the provider wants the patient to return. Most providers note this information on the encounter form. Make the return appointment. Remember to give the patient choices on the time and day. Give the patient an appointment reminder card.

The medical assistant can convey a sense of caring by terminating the visit cordially. Thank the patient for coming. If the patient will return for another visit, the assistant can say something like, "We'll see you next week." If the patient will not be returning soon, a pleasant "I hope you'll be feeling better soon" is appropriate. In addition, tell patients to call the facility if they have any questions or if they need additional care. Whatever words of goodbye are chosen, all patients should leave the facility feeling that they have received top-quality care and were treated with friendliness, respect, and courtesy.

CLOSING THE HEALTHCARE FACILITY

At the end of the day, the medical assistant needs to help with the closing duties. The clinical medical assistant must ensure that all the patients have left by checking the exam and treatment rooms. The clinical medical assistant will complete the following closing duties:
- **Restock** the rooms and organize any reading materials.
- Disinfect the exam table, writing table, counters, computer keyboards, and chairs (i.e., those made of plastic, metal, or wood).
- Secure (put away) confidential documents.
- Turn off computers and other devices.
- **Sanitize**, disinfect, or **sterilize** equipment and instruments.
- Lock supply and medication cabinets.
- Verify and count the narcotic medication stock, following the facility's procedure.

The administrative medical assistant will complete the following closing duties:
- Prepare the patient records and documents for the next day.
- Turn off the computers, copy machine, and other office equipment.
- Switch phones to voice mail or the answering service.
- Follow office procedures for handling money at the end of the day.
- Secure (put away) any confidential documents.
- Clean up the reception area (neatly arrange the magazines, disinfect toys, and remove garbage and unsolicited advertisements). Turn off the lights, television, stereo, and other devices.

With time being short in the morning, it is important to take care of as much as possible the evening before you leave.

Depending on the facility, the medical assistant may be responsible for turning off the lights, activating the alarms, and locking the doors. In larger facilities, the custodial or security staff handles these responsibilities.

> **BOX 22.7 Strategies to Use With Bad Behavior With Children**
>
> - Move down to his or her level and offer a book or toy.
> - Lead the child away from any objects that could be broken or from other patients.
> - Say to the child, "Let's come over here and play next to your mom!"

> **VOCABULARY**
>
> **restock:** The process of replacing the supplies that were used.
> **sanitize:** The process of cleaning equipment and instruments with detergent and water in order to remove debris and reduce the number of microorganisms.
> **sterilize:** The process of removing all microorganisms.

Daily and Monthly Duties

Medical facilities either employ custodial staff or hire cleaning services to clean. This cleaning takes place after hours each day. Larger facilities that employ custodial staff will have the staff clean high-traffic areas several times a day. These areas include the restrooms and the entrances. During wet weather, it is critical that the floors are kept dry to prevent people from slipping and falling.

> **CRITICAL THINKING 22.7**
>
> The office utilizes a local cleaning service to clean the facility's rooms. The staff members arrive after hours and are gone by the time Catherine and Marie open the office in the morning. Over the past month, Marie has noticed that the rooms do not look as clean as they should. Should she address this concern? If so, with whom should she discuss it?

The medical assistant also is responsible for cleaning and organizing the reception area and exam rooms. During slow times, medical assistants are expected to do extra duties, including restocking medical and office supplies, forms, and patient literature. The cabinets and drawers need to be straightened and reorganized. Medications and supplies that have expiration dates need to be checked monthly. The **crash cart** and other emergency supplies need to be inventoried monthly and after each use (Fig. 22.10). Many facilities use a master list of crash cart supplies with expiration dates. This helps to ensure all supplies are in the crash cart and expiring supplies and medications can be easily identified.

It is important that the healthcare facility be clean and organized. By taking the **initiative** (i NISH eh tiv) to perform those tasks during quiet times, you will be considered a more valuable employee. Supervisors and providers value employees who look for additional activities that can be done during quiet times.

EQUIPMENT AND SUPPLIES

Another medical assistant duty is to manage the equipment and supplies in the medical office. In smaller facilities, this may involve ordering and maintaining an inventory control system. In larger facilities, purchasing department employees are hired for such roles.

Equipment

In a healthcare facility, administrative and clinical equipment are used. The medical assistant needs to know how to operate, maintain, and handle issues with the equipment. For financial and tax purposes, the purchase cost and age of each item needs to be recorded. The process of gathering and creating a list of the equipment in the facility is called managing **inventory**.

Equipment Inventory. For all clinical and administrative equipment, records need to be maintained. These records are used to replace

> **VOCABULARY**
>
> **crash cart**: Emergency medications and equipment (e.g., oxygen, intravenous [IV] and airway supplies) stored in a cart and ready for an emergency.
> **depreciate**: To diminish in value (such as the value of an item) over a period of time; a concept used for tax purposes.
> **initiative**: The ability to start a task and energetically complete it.
> **inventory**: A detailed list of equipment and supplies owned and stored; the process of counting the supplies in stock.

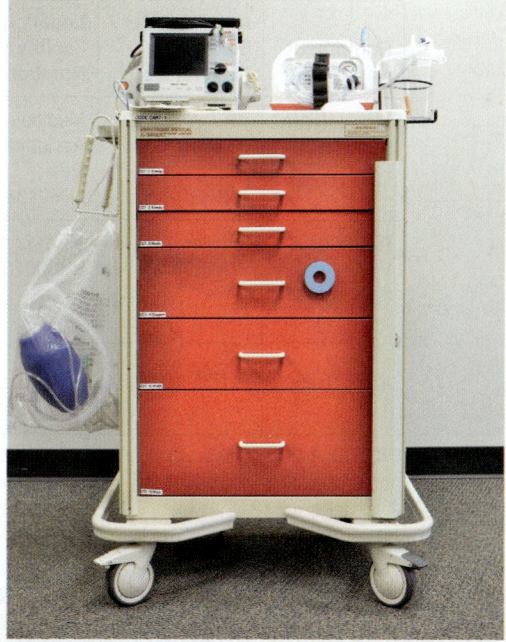

FIG. 22.10 Crash carts must be inventoried monthly or after each use to ensure that medication and supplies have not expired, and all the required supplies are available for an emergency.

equipment lost in a disaster or theft. The healthcare facility's accountant also uses the information when preparing tax paperwork. For instance, records should be maintained for the following items:

- Small equipment (e.g., thermometers, glucose monitors), which is deducted as an expense for the year in which it is purchased.
- Large office equipment (e.g., computer hardware, calculators, and copiers), which **depreciate** (di PREE shee ate) over 5 years.
- Office furniture items (e.g., desks, files, safes, exam tables), which depreciate over 7 years.

Lastly, the equipment inventory is used by supervisors to identify equipment that needs to be replaced. Preplanning equipment purchases is a financial strategy for the practice. It allows the practice to be prepared and plan for future investments.

> **CRITICAL THINKING 22.8**
>
> Marie needs to learn more about managing inventory. She reviews her medical assistant textbook, and reads articles online. She decides to start by creating an inventory list of the equipment in the medical office. What are some advantages of having an updated list of administrative and clinical equipment?

When creating an equipment inventory list, it is helpful to use spreadsheet software (Fig. 22.11). In some situations, you may have inventory forms that you can complete (Procedure 22.2). For all equipment, document the following information:

- Equipment name, manufacturer, and serial number
- Purchase date, cost, and supplier
- Warranty information (e.g., start and end date, warranty coverage)
- Location of the equipment (optional)
- Unique facility number given to that piece of equipment (optional)

Equipment Safety and Maintenance. The owner's or operation manual and warranty information should be kept at a central location

Equipment Name	Manufacturer / Serial Number	Location / Facility Number	Purchase Date / Supplier	Cost	Warranty Information
Laser Printer	HP / HP3598XA	Medical Assistant Desk / LP59483	08/01/20XX / Best Office Supplies	$325	Parts and labor expires 07/31/20XX
AT2 Plus ECG / Spirometry	Schiller / WA4893X	Treatment Room / ES00012	05/02/20XX / Medical Equipment Supplies	$2987	Parts and Labor expires 05/01/20XX

FIG. 22.11 An equipment inventory list can be created in a spreadsheet and provides useful information about the administrative and clinical equipment in the facility. (From Proctor D, et al: *Kinn's The Medical Assistant*, ed 13, St. Louis, 2017, Elsevier.)

PROCEDURE 22.2 Perform an Equipment Inventory With Documentation

Tasks
Perform an equipment inventory. Document the inventory on the equipment inventory form.

Equipment and Supplies
- Pens
- Administrative or clinical equipment
- Purchase information (e.g., date, cost, and supplier) and warranty information (e.g., start and end date, warranty coverage)
- Equipment inventory form

Procedural Steps
1. For the equipment to be inventoried, gather the following information for each piece of equipment:
   - Name of equipment, manufacturer, and serial number
   - Location and facility number (if applicable)
   - Purchase date, cost, supplier, and warranty information

   Purpose: It is important to have the essential information required when creating the spreadsheet.

2. Complete an equipment inventory form by adding the gathered information for each item inventoried (see Fig. 22.11).

   Purpose: Creating an equipment inventory list on the computer will help you organize the information. It will also help you maintain the information easily.

3. Review the document created. Make any necessary revisions.

   Purpose: It is important to proofread your work to ensure it is accurate.

---

and available to users. Many operation manuals are available online. The manuals are used to do the following:
- Problem-solve performance issues.
- Identify service schedules and routine maintenance.
- Identify parts or supplies needed for the operation of the machine.

The medical assistant is responsible for monitoring equipment safety and proper functioning. Routine maintenance helps to ensure the best performance of the equipment. Potential issues should not be overlooked. Actions should be taken to prevent injury to staff or patients and costly damage to the equipment. The medical assistant should do the following:

- Check electrical cords on equipment for damage.
- Address any suspected overheating issues.
- Investigate any unusual noise or change in performance.
- Clean and maintain equipment routinely in accordance with the operation manual.

Routine maintenance varies with the equipment. Copiers and printers may entail changing toner or cartridges. For clinical equipment, maintenance may include changing filters or batteries.

It is important to keep track of routine maintenance. Making a schedule as a reminder for routine maintenance can be helpful. Many facilities utilize logs to track routine maintenance and service calls (Fig. 22.12). Box 22.8 indicates the information that should be on the log. Procedure 22.3 explains the steps involved in creating a maintenance log, performing the maintenance, and then documenting the maintenance.

CRITICAL THINKING 22.9

Marie realized that the facility did not have maintenance logs for the various pieces of equipment. She decided to start making logs, but she realized there were a lot of logs she would have to make. How could she create logs in a time-efficient manner? For a small office, describe options that she could use to organize all the logs so they are easy to locate and use.

Service Calls and Warranties. When equipment is purchased, a warranty is given for a period of time. The warranty is the manufacturer's guarantee. If the piece of equipment needs to be repaired or has a defective part, the manufacturer will pay for the cost of the repair. In some cases, the item may be replaced. Warranty language includes details on what is covered. Some warranties are not honored if someone other than a "recognized" serviceperson attempts to fix the machine. Extended warranties lengthen the protection time and can be purchased for some equipment.

For complex or expensive equipment, the healthcare facility may contract with a service provider for repairs and routine service checks. This assistance is necessary for some equipment. It also helps to extend the lifetime of those machines. For repairs on other equipment, it might be necessary to ship or bring the machine to the repair service. Usually the cost for onsite repairs is more than if the machine is taken or shipped to the service provider for repairs. One of the main concerns when a piece of equipment breaks down is the effect on the healthcare facility. Some service providers will also loan equipment to facilities while the repairs take place. This service greatly lessens the burden on the practice.

CHAPTER 22 Reception and Daily Operations

Maintenance Log

Equipment Name: **Laser Printer** Serial #: **HP3598XA** Location: **Medical Assistant Desk**
Facility #: **LP59483** Manufacturer: **HP** Purchased: **08/01/20XX**
Warranty Information: **Parts and labor expires 07/31/20XX**
Freqency of Inspections: **Every 6 months**
Service Provider: **Best Office Supplies**

Date	Time	Maintenance Activities	Signature
12/15/20XX	0956	Replaced toner cartridge	Marie Van Bakel, CMA (AAMA)
02/11/20XX	1235	Service call: Office Repair Company – to fix stray ink marks on copies	Catherine Black, RMA

Maintenance Log

Equipment Name: **AT2 Plus ECG/Spirometry** Serial #: **WA4893X** Location: **Treatment Room**
Facility #: **ES00012** Manufacturer: **Schiller** Purchased: **05/02/20XX**
Freqency of Inspections: **Every 12 months**
Warranty information: **Parts and Labor expires 05/01/20XX**
Service Provider: **Medical Equipment Suppliers**

Date	Time	Maintenance Activities	Signature
10/23/20XX	1123	Replaced battery	Marie Van Bakel, CMA (AAMA)
05/02/20XX	1445	No tracing, cleaned stylus with alcohol	Marie Van Bakel, CMA (AAMA)

FIG. 22.12 Equipment maintenance logs are utilized by the staff and outside repair agencies to track maintenance activities. (From Proctor D, et al: *Kinn's The Medical Assistant*, ed 13, St. Louis, 2017, Elsevier.)

PROCEDURE 22.3 Perform Routine Maintenance of Equipment

Tasks
Perform routine maintenance of administrative or clinical equipment. Document the maintenance on the log.

Equipment and Supplies
- Maintenance log(s)
- Administrative or clinical equipment (e.g., oral thermometers)
- Supplies for routine maintenance (e.g., battery)
- Operation manual, if needed
- Pens
- Information regarding the equipment (i.e., name, serial number, location, facility number, manufacturer, purchase date, warranty information, frequency of inspections, and service provider)

Procedural Steps
1. Gather information on the piece of equipment identified for routine maintenance, including name, serial number, location, facility number, manufacturer, purchase date, warranty information, frequency of inspections, and service provider.
   Purpose: It is important to have the essential information required when completing the log.
2. Fill in the equipment details on the log (see Fig. 22.12).
   Purpose: Adding the equipment details helps identify the machine. It provides a quick reference to useful information that the service provider might request. The form serves as a log for documenting the maintenance activities performed.
3. To perform the maintenance activities, gather the required supplies. If you are not familiar with the procedure or the required supplies, refer to the operation manual.
   Purpose: You need to be familiar with the supplies and the procedure before you start the maintenance.
4. Perform the maintenance activities as directed in the operation manual. Take any required safety precautions necessary to protect yourself and others.
   Purpose: Following the outlined procedure in the operation manual will help you successfully complete the maintenance without injuring yourself and others or damaging the machine.
5. Clean up the work area.
   Purpose: It is important to clean up after yourself.
6. Using a pen, document the date, time, the maintenance activity performed, and include your signature on the log.
   Purpose: The log, indicating the activities performed, will serve as a communication tool for future reference and services needed on that piece of equipment.

Purchasing Equipment. The process of purchasing equipment can vary depending on the size of the organization. Large agencies have purchasing departments. The staff researches the need and identifies the best equipment to purchase. The medical assistant may be involved with the process in smaller practices.

Many factors are considered when equipment is being replaced:
- Age of the equipment and the availability of parts
- Frequency and cost of repairs
- Utilization of the machine and whether new features will lead to extra **billable services**

> **VOCABULARY**
> **billable service**: Assistance (i.e., service) that is provided by a healthcare provider and can be billed to the insurance company or patient.

> **CRITICAL THINKING 22.10**
>
> Currently, the providers are using an offsite radiology service. They are contemplating creating a small radiology room where they could take x-rays. How could Marie assist the providers with their plans for a potential purchase of x-ray equipment?

Leasing medical equipment is becoming a popular option for smaller facilities. The healthcare facility pays a fee to lease an item (Box 22.9). The fee is less than what it would cost to purchase the item. The lease fees are tax-deductible and allow the healthcare facility to provide extra billable services.

The medical assistant may help identify potential new equipment models to purchase or lease. Using the Internet and contacting the company's salespeople are two ways to get additional information. Some salespeople will meet with the staff and demonstrate the product. In addition to research, the medical assistant may need to explain the usage of the machine and the frequency of repair checks. Usually the supervisor or provider has the final say as to whether the purchase should occur.

Supplies

Many supplies are required to run the medical office and treat patients. Supplies include administrative items (e.g., pens, paper, envelopes, and paperclips) and clinical items (e.g., bandages, vaccines, medications, slings, and splints). The medical assistant must make sure there are enough supplies to treat patients. A lack of supplies can greatly affect the services provided to patients. It can be expensive for the healthcare facility because of last-minute ordering at higher prices. On the other hand, overstocking supplies can be a financial waste to the facility. Many supplies have expiration dates and cannot be used beyond that date. Having adequate amounts of supplies in inventory is crucial.

> **BOX 22.8 Routine Maintenance Log Information**
>
> - Equipment name, serial number, location of machine, and facility's unique equipment number (if applicable)
> - Manufacturer's name
> - Date of purchase
> - Warranty information (e.g., start and end date, warranty coverage)
> - Service provider contact information, such as telephone number
> - Date and time and description of maintenance activities performed
> - Signature of person performing maintenance

Inventory Management. Inventory management involves ordering, tracking inventory, and identifying the quantity of product to purchase. The goal of inventory management is to have adequate supplies on hand. It is important not to have too much stock that will expire or take a long time to use.

The medical assistant in charge of ordering and managing supplies must keep a record on each item in inventory. The record can be a manual entry written in a notebook or on index cards. It can be computerized in a spreadsheet or inventory control system software. For each inventory item, the medical assistant must record the following:

- Item details: item name, size, quantity, item number, supplier's name, and cost (Fig. 22.13).
- *Quantity to reorder*: amount of supplies that need to be ordered. This amount reflects the product used during the **buying cycle**.
  - For instance, the healthcare facility's buying cycle for 2 × 2 nonsterile gauze (100 per pack) is 1 month. The facility typically goes through 25 packs in 1 month. This would be the quantity used during the buying cycle. It would also be the quantity to reorder each time (see Fig. 22.13).
- *Reorder point*: point at which low inventory requires the product to be ordered.
  - For instance, when the inventory of 2 × 2 nonsterile gauze packs gets depleted to 5 packs, the medical assistant must reorder (see Fig. 22.13). Five is the reorder point or the quantity that triggers an order to be placed to replenish the inventory (Box 22.10). The reorder point for medical and administrative supplies can be different for each item because of the usage rate and the time it takes to receive the item after it is ordered.

> **VOCABULARY**
>
> **buying cycle**: Refers to how often an item is purchased and depends on how frequently the item is used and the storage space available for it.

> **BOX 22.9 Examples of Leased Equipment and Furniture**
>
> - Monitoring equipment
> - Diagnostic testing equipment
> - Computer systems
> - Exam tables

Item Name	Size	Quantity	Item Number	Supplier's Name	Reorder Point	Quantity to Reorder	Cost	Stock Available	Order (✓)
Nonsterile gauze sponges, 8 ply	2"x 2"	100/pkg	NG0022	Midwest Medical	5	25	$2.31/pkg		
Sterile gauze sponges, 12 ply, 2/pkg	2"x 2"	25 pkg/box	NG0042	Midwest Medical	4	20	$3.99/box		

FIG. 22.13 A supply inventory list shows details of items in inventory. For efficiency, use two extra columns ("Stock Available" and "Order") as shown. This list can be duplicated and utilized when performing inventory. (From Proctor D, et al: *Kinn's The Medical Assistant*, ed 13, St. Louis, 2017, Elsevier.)

BOX 22.10 How to Calculate the Reorder Point

The reorder point can be calculated based on the number used per day and the number of days it takes to order and receive the product.

For instance, the practice uses 0.5 pack of 2 × 2 nonsterile gauze per day. It takes 4 days to receive the order from the medical supply company. The medical practice may also want 6 extra days' worth of supplies on hand to prevent issues related to running out of the item. Here is how you would figure out the reorder point:

Stock to cover order time: 0.5 pack per day × 4 days to receive order = 2 packs
Extra stock: 6 days × 0.5 pack per day = 3 packs
Reorder point: 2 packs (stock to cover order time) + 3 packs (6-day supply) = 5 packs

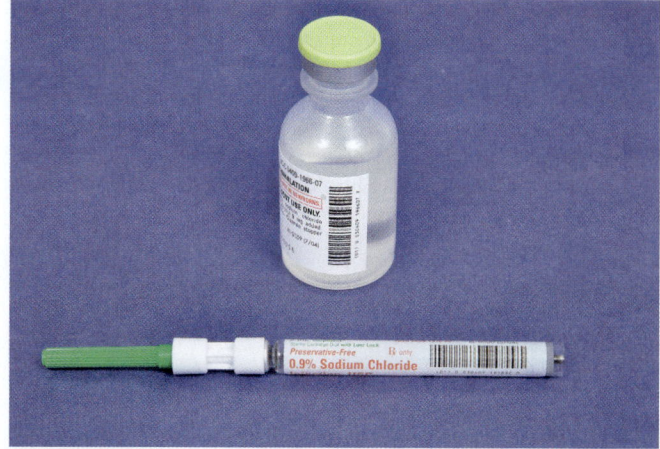

FIG. 22.14 Using bar codes makes inventory control more efficient. (From Proctor D, et al: *Kinn's The Medical Assistant*, ed 13, St. Louis, 2017, Elsevier.)

Inventory Control Systems. An inventory control system helps to make inventory management work well. Large medical facilities utilize computerized inventory control systems. These systems monitor usage and inventory in stock. They also identify items that need to be ordered. Smaller facilities may use simple computerized or manual systems.

To help create an efficient computerized system, many medical facilities utilize bar codes to track inventory and for insurance and patient billing for supplies (Fig. 22.14). With this system, each item has a unique bar code. The bar code is scanned with a bar code reader when items are added or taken from inventory. Software monitors the inventory quantity. For bar codes to work successfully, the staff must be diligent in scanning the bar codes when taking a product from stock. Bar code inventory control systems work successfully in large and small healthcare facilities.

There are several manual systems utilized for identifying what supplies need to be ordered. The following are some of the more common methods utilized in medical facilities:

- When staff identify a product that needs to be ordered, the item is written in a log. This process is like making a list of what you need at the grocery store. The person responsible for ordering supplies then prepares the order based on the information in the log.
- Another system includes using product identification slips, which contain the name of the product. The slips or cards are attached to the product or a box/package of items. When the product is used, the slip is put in a special location like a box or plastic pocket. The medical assistant then uses the slips in the box or pocket to prepare the supply order.
- The two-bin system consists of having a main bin for each item in inventory and then a backup bin for each item. When the main bin is emptied, the backup bin is used, and the product is reordered.
- The medical assistant responsible for ordering performs a hand count of the items in stock to identify what needs to be ordered. This system is explained in the next section.

CRITICAL THINKING 22.11

Marie decided to implement a manual system for inventory. Of the manual systems discussed, which method might work best in the small facility? Discuss your answer.

Taking Inventory. Inventory (counting supplies) must be taken at specific times. Many businesses that utilize automated inventory control systems hand count their inventory at least once a year. Usually this is done around the close of the business year. These companies compare their hand counts to the computer counts and identify discrepancies. The discrepancies are followed up on. The manual inventory procedure provides the company with information on the actual number of items in stock. With this information, the financial value of the inventory can be calculated and used for financial reports and taxes at the close of the business year.

For medical offices that do not implement inventory control systems, performing inventory or counting the items in stock is important before each buying cycle.

One of the most frequent errors when performing inventory is to report a different quantity than what is on the supply inventory list. For instance, a medical assistant counts nonsterile sponges. Each package should be counted as 1 and not as 100 each. Looking at Fig. 22.13, if there were 6 packages of sponges left in the supply cabinet, it should be noted that the stock available was 6 packages. It should not be indicated as 600 sponges or 600 each. Counting each item in a box or package when the product is inventoried by box or package creates conflict and confusion when looking at the reorder point.

The medical assistant should utilize a supply inventory list to be most efficient when counting supplies (Fig. 22.15). The supply inventory list shows all the items in stock. The medical assistant can mark down the inventory counts for each item on the document (Procedure 22.4). If the supply inventory list is not available, then the medical assistant needs to write down the item number, size, quantity (e.g., 100/box), manufacturer, and any other identifying information. This process takes a lot more time. Using abbreviations can be helpful (Box 22.11).

When performing an inventory, work in a systematic manner. Start with one supply cabinet, working from top to bottom, before moving onto another cabinet. All stock areas should be inventoried before preparing the supply order.

Price Consideration When Ordering Supplies. When ordering supplies, price comparison shopping is important. The healthcare facility must balance the time it takes to the money saved. Some medical offices

VOCABULARY

discrepancy: A lack of similarity between what is stated and what is found; for instance, the computer inventory count is different than the physical count.

compare prices only on more expensive items or items that are used in vast quantities. They may compare prices every 6 to 12 months. When comparing prices, consider the following:
- Shipping and handling charges
- Quality and amount (e.g., 10 per box), as these must be the same among products
- Quantity discounts or price breaks when buying a certain amount (Box 22.12)

Some medical facilities join group purchasing organizations (GPOs). These organizations combine orders from many different medical facilities. Combining orders results in volume discounts from specific vendors. GPOs typically purchase both supplies and medications.

> **VOCABULARY**
> **vendors**: Companies that sell supplies, equipment, or services to other companies or individuals.

> **CRITICAL THINKING 22.12**
> Currently the facility orders its clinical supplies from two vendors. Marie would like to do some cost comparisons to get the best deals on supplies. She does not have a lot of time to spend on the research. How might she approach this situation? Where should she start first? What might be a long-term goal for her?

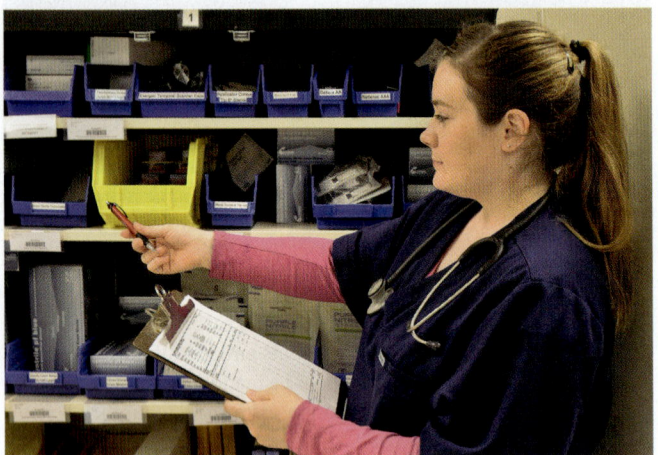

FIG. 22.15 A medical assistant performing an inventory. (From Proctor D, et al: *Kinn's The Medical Assistant*, ed 13, St. Louis, 2017, Elsevier.)

> **BOX 22.11 Common Inventory and Purchase Abbreviations**
>
> BTL: Bottle   PO: Purchase Order
> BX: Box   PPD: Prepaid
> CS: Case   PYMT: Payment
> EA: Each   QTY: Quantity
> PKG: Package

PROCEDURE 22.4 Perform a Supply Inventory With Documentation While Using Proper Body Mechanics

Tasks
Perform a supply inventory using correct body mechanics. Document the inventory on the supply inventory form.

Equipment and Supplies
- Pens
- Administrative or clinical supplies to be inventoried
- Purchase information (e.g., item number, cost, and supplier) for supplies in inventory
- Reorder point and quantity to reorder for each item in inventory
- Supply inventory form

Procedural Steps
1. For the supplies in inventory, gather the following information for each item:
   - Name, size, quantity (e.g., purchased individually, 100 per box)
   - Item number, supplier's name, cost
   - Reorder point and quantity to reorder

   Purpose: This information is required as you create the inventory form.

2. For each supply item, enter information on the inventory form. Make sure the appropriate entry is in the right location (see Fig. 22.13).
   Note: The "Stock Available" column will be empty for now.
   Purpose: Creating a supply inventory list will help you organize the information and maintain the information easily.

3. Review the document. Make any necessary revisions.
   Purpose: Make sure the document is correct so errors do not impact the inventory process.

4. Using the supply inventory list, inventory the supplies in the department. Identify how the supply should be counted (e.g., individually, by the box), and count the number of items in stock.
   Purpose: By identifying the correct quantity that the item is inventoried by, you will increase the accuracy of the inventory. Counting an item by "each" when it comes as a package can cause confusion when identifying what needs to be ordered.

5. Add the number in the appropriate row under the "Stock Available" header.
   Purpose: Making sure you add the number to the correct column and row will keep your inventory form accurate.

6. Compare the reorder point number to the stock available number. If the stock available number is at or below the reorder point, indicate that the item needs to be reordered by checking the appropriate column.
   Purpose: Identify the supplies that need to be ordered.

7. Make sure the supplies are neatly arranged. The older stock should be in front of the newer stock.
   Purpose: It is important to clean up your workspace. The oldest stock must be moved to the front to ensure it is used first.

8. Repeat steps 5 through 7 until all supplies are inventoried.

9. Use proper body mechanics when lifting and moving supplies by maintaining a wide, stable base with your feet. Your feet should be shoulder-width apart, and you should have good footing. Bend at the knees, keeping your back straight. Lift smoothly with the major muscles in your arms and legs. Use the same technique when putting the item down.
   Purpose: Correct body mechanics will decrease your risk for injury when carrying or lifting heavy objects. See Figs. 22.19 and 22.20 for proper body mechanics when lifting boxes.

10. Use proper body mechanics when reaching for an object. Clear away barriers, and use a step stool if needed. Your feet should face the object. Avoid twisting or turning with a heavy load.
    Purpose: Straining when reaching or standing on tiptoes can increase your risk for injury.

CHAPTER 22   Reception and Daily Operations

BOX 22.12   Quantity Discounts

Quantity discounts or price breaks save money when ordering. The more of an item purchased, the cheaper the product becomes, as this example shows:
- Quantity 1 to 5, $1.50 per each item
- Quantity 6 to 15, $1.25 per each item

If the medical assistant purchased a quantity of 6, the price per each would be cheaper than if 4 were purchased. Before ordering extra product, consider the following:
- Storage space
- How quickly the item will be used
- Shelf life (or expiration date) of the item

Buying too much just to get a price break may not be in the best interest of the healthcare facility.

BOX 22.13   Creating an Account for Purchasing

When creating an account for purchasing supplies, consider these points:
- Use the facility's information (address, fax number, and phone number)
- Be prepared to give the provider's license number when ordering medications and needles
- Fax the provider's license number, if required, before ordering
- Provide a copy of the provider's Drug Enforcement Administration (DEA) registration if narcotics are being ordered; narcotics require special tracking documentation and thus a high level of authorization when purchasing them

Physician buying groups (PBGs) offer providers potential cost-saving pricing for vaccines. The drawback is that the provider must exclusively use the vaccines from the contracted manufacturers.

Ordering Supplies. If the facility is not part of a buying group, the medical assistant might need to order supplies. It is important to select just a few vendors if possible. The medical assistant can utilize the following:
- Supplier's printed catalog, though it may only be printed a few times a year and may not provide accurate item availability and pricing.
- Supplier's website store, which would have the most accurate prices, sale prices, and available stock

Many vendors require the creation of an account before ordering (Box 22.13). Some medical facilities utilize **purchase order (PO) numbers**, giving each order a unique reference number. This PO number should be included on the order sheets, added to the online information, or provided during the phone order. Vendors add the PO number to the order's documentation (i.e., **packing slip** and statement). This way both parties can use it as a reference if questions come up. The healthcare facility uses the purchase order number to track the order (Procedure 22.5).

Payment terms may vary among vendors. Payment methods may include credit card, check, money order, or a line of credit. Typically, the line of credit is good for 30 to 60 days. **Invoices** are sent to the facility and should be paid after the purchases have been received. Orders can typically be placed via fax, mail, phone, or online. If the medical assistant is faxing or mailing the order, the vendor usually requires the order to be placed on the vendor's order sheet. The medical assistant should keep a copy of the phone, mailed, or fax order, or a printout of the online order to verify that the order was filled correctly.

Receiving the Order. Orders can arrive via the mail, a national delivery service (e.g., FedEx, United Parcel Service [UPS]), or a local delivery service. The delivery person may require a signature from an employee. This signature is used to track who received the delivery.

VOCABULARY
invoices: Billing statements that list the amount owed for goods or services purchased.
packing slip: A document that accompanies purchased merchandise and shows what is in the box or package.
purchase order number: A unique number assigned by the ordering facility that allows the facility to track or reference the order.

PROCEDURE 22.5   Prepare a Purchase Order

Task
Create an accurate purchase order for supplies.

Equipment and Supplies
- Pens
- Supply inventory list showing item name, size, quantity, item number, supplier's name, reorder point, quantity to reorder, cost, and current stock available
- Computer with internet access
- Printer or order form

Procedural Steps
1. Review the supply inventory list with the current stock counts, and determine what supplies need to be reordered.
   Purpose: By determining what needs to be reordered, you avoid having too much or too little stock of an item.
2. Using the Internet, find the online company used for ordering the needed supplies.
3. Using the search box, type in the item number or description. Verify that the item from the search results is what you need to order.
   Purpose: It is important to verify you have the correct product before you add the product to your basket/cart.
4. Apply critical thinking skills as you identify the quantity to reorder for that item and order this amount. (Either place the item in the cart or complete the information on the order form.)
   Purpose: The "Quantity to Reorder" column will indicate how much to reorder to prevent having too many or too few of the products in inventory.
5. Repeat steps 3 and 4 until all items are ordered.
6. When you have finished, verify the contents in your basket/cart and print a copy of the order. If using an order form, verify the accuracy of the information. Review the supply inventory list to ensure you have ordered everything that needs to be reordered and have ordered the correct quantity of each item.
   Note: For a real order, the payment information would be added, and the order would be submitted at this time
   Purpose: When ordering products, the copy of the order is then compared with the packing slips to ensure you have received the complete order. The copy and the packing slips are then stapled together and verified against the invoice when it is received. For prepaid orders, the packing slips and copy of the order are filed once the entire order has been received.

The medical assistant must check the delivery as soon as possible. Some medications, like vaccines, are shipped in a cold environment and must remain at a cold temperature. These medications need to be placed in the refrigerator or freezer immediately upon arrival (Box 22.14). Storage information for medications can be found in the

BOX 22.14 Vaccine Storage Guidelines

For All Vaccines
- Unpack vaccines immediately.
- Each type of vaccine should be placed in its own tray, which allows for airflow. Place newer vaccines behind older vaccines. Keep vaccine vials in their original boxes to prevent light exposure.

For Refrigerated Vaccines
- The ideal temperature for refrigerated vaccines is 36° F to 46° F.
- Do not store vaccines next to the wall, top shelf, door, or floor of the refrigerator.
- Do not put food or beverages in the vaccine storage refrigerator. Place bottles of water in the crisper bins to maintain the temperature.
- Make sure the door is closed.

For Frozen Vaccines
- Ideal temperature for refrigerated vaccines: −58° F to 5° F.
- Leave 2 to 3 inches between the vaccine and the freezer wall.
- Use water bottles to help maintain the temperature
- Make sure the door is closed.

Temperature Monitoring Equipment
The CDC recommends temperature monitoring equipment (Digital Data Loggers [DDL]) for all vaccines storage units. All vaccine storage units (e.g., refrigerators, freezers, transport containers) must have a temperature monitoring device. Simple thermometers can show the minimum and maximum temperature since the last reset. A DDL records a temperature at least every 30 minutes and provides the most accurate storage temperatures. The CDC recommends keeping the digital data from the DDLs for 3 years. This data may need to be shown to demonstrate compliance when the facility is involved with vaccination programs.

Check Temperature
Use a simple maximum/minimum thermometer to make the following inspections:
- Check and log temperatures twice a day (Fig. 22.16).
- Check the current temperature.
- Check the minimum and maximum temperature. This represents the coldest and warmest temperatures that occurred since you last checked it.
- Reset the thermometer if needed.
- If the temperature is outside the range, contact the vaccine manufacturer and report the total amount of time the temperature was outside the range.

Date	Time	Refrigerator Temperature Range: 36° F to 46° F			Freezer Temperature Range: −58° F to 5° F			Initials	Within Range
		Current	Minimum	Maximum	Current	Minimum	Maximum		
10/11/XXX	0755	40° F	37° F	39° F	3° F	−13° F	−12° F	MVB	Yes
10/11/XXX	1723	38° F	35° F	38° F	−8° F	−28° F	−19° F	BMN	No
10/12/XXX	0752	42° F	36° F	39° F	−13° F	−23° F	18° F	MVB	No
10/13/XXX	0748	47° F	38° F	38° F	−8° F	−27° F	−22° F	MVB	No

FIG. 22.16 Example of a temperature log.

From Resources on Proper Vaccine Storage and Handling, https://www.cdc.gov/vaccines/hcp/admin/storage/index.html. Vaccine Storage & Handling Toolkit, https://www.cdc.gov/vaccines/hcp/admin/storage/toolkit/storage-handling-toolkit.pdf.

---

package insert or on the manufacturer's website. If the medication warms up too much, it may not be good. For instance, vaccines that get too warm can have reduced potency. This means they may not protect patients against the disease.

CRITICAL THINKING 22.13
Using the Vaccine Storage Guidelines (see Box 22.14), answer the following questions:
- Did all the refrigerator temperatures fall within the required range? Explain.
- Did all the freezer temperatures fall within the required range? Explain.
- If a temperature was outside the required range, what should be done?
- Were the temperatures checked twice daily?

When an order arrives, remove the packing slip from the box. Compare the items in the package to the packing slip (Fig. 22.17). Check off all items received. Some vendors may indicate items that are **backordered** and will be arriving later. Note any discrepancies or differences on the packing slip. Any items that are damaged should be noted on the packing slip. The copy of the original order should be compared against the packing slip, and any differences should be noted. Any discrepancies or damaged items should be addressed with the supply company as soon as possible.

The packing slip should be attached to the copy of the order once the supplies have been reviewed. When the complete order has been received, the copy of the order with the packing slips attached should be filed if the order was prepaid. If a line of credit was used, the copy of the order with the attached packing slips is placed in the **accounts payable** folder to wait for the invoice's arrival. The person responsible for paying the healthcare facility's bills will match the invoice with the copy of the order, ensuring everything is in order before paying the bill.

VOCABULARY
accounts payable: Money owed by a company to other companies for services and goods; pertains to paying the facility's bills.
backordered: An order placed for an item that is temporarily out of stock and will be sent later.

The items received should be put away as soon as possible and the boxes should be discarded. When putting supplies away, it is important to rotate stock. This means the new stock should go in the back and the older stock needs to be moved forward so it can be used first. Any items with expiration dates should be placed so that the items expiring first are in front, so they are used first. For stock without expiration dates, consider the saying "First in, first out," which means when new stock comes in, it is placed behind the older stock. The older stock needs to be used first. If removing expired stock, remember to subtract the quantity from the inventory system.

HANDLING MAIL

The medical assistant's responsibility with mail will vary. In large facilities, designated mailroom employees prepare the mail and handle incoming mail. In these facilities, mail is delivered from the mailroom to each department. The administrative medical assistant sorts the department mail. This will be discussed in more detail later in this section. In smaller facilities, the medical assistant may handle both incoming and outgoing mail. Chapter 21 discusses outgoing mail and the United States Postal Service (USPS). In this chapter, we focus on alternative delivery services and incoming mail.

Private Delivery Services

The USPS only handles a portion of the mail delivered in the United States. Private companies have grown by offering competitive rates and additional services compared with USPS. Some companies provide national and international services, but others are more locally based.

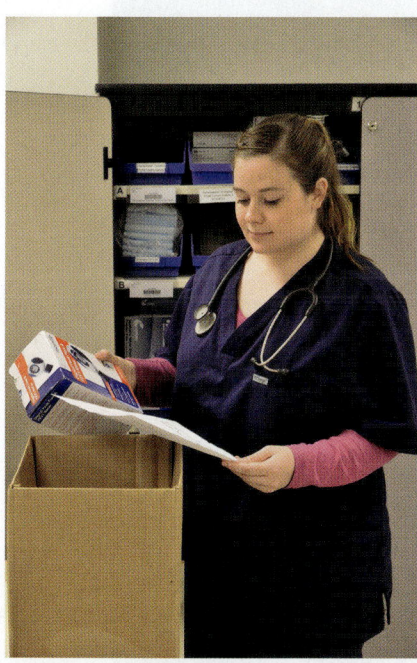

FIG. 22.17 Comparing the packing slip to the contents in the box is an important step in receiving supplies. (From Proctor D, et al: *Kinn's The Medical Assistant*, ed 13, St. Louis, 2017, Elsevier.)

> **VOCABULARY**
> **bonded**: Occurs when an employer obtains a fidelity bond from an insurance company, which will cover losses from employees dishonest acts (e.g., embezzlement, theft).

FedEx, UPS, and DHL are very popular national options for shipping letters and packages. Some offer onsite pickup.

Larger cities have courier services that have become popular options for local deliveries. Some companies have drivers that are **bonded** and trained to handle all aspects of delivery from medical to hazardous deliveries. Some of the services provided include the following:
- Pickup and delivery of medical specimens (e.g., they take patient laboratory samples to a medical laboratory for testing).
- Transportation of health records and documents from one location to another, complying with HIPAA requirements.
- Pickup and delivery of deposits to the bank, with return of cash if requested.

The goal for the healthcare facility is to utilize a mail/courier company that provides the most efficient service at the best price. The medical assistant may have to research the delivery services available in the area to identify the best fit for the facility.

> **CRITICAL THINKING 22.14**
> The providers would like to utilize an offsite laboratory to process specimens. Marie would like to have a local courier service pick up specimens and deliver them to the offsite laboratory. When researching potential delivery couriers for this activity, what factors should Marie consider?

Incoming Mail

Mail can be collected at the post office or be delivered to the healthcare facility. The medical assistant must sort the mail following the facility's procedure for incoming mail. Providers may request the incoming mail be placed on their desks. In larger departments, mailboxes are utilized for each person in the department (Fig. 22.18). The medical assistant can easily sort the mail and place it in the individual mailboxes. The mailboxes need to be safe and secure. They should not be in a patient care area.

If there is a question as to who should get a piece of mail, it is important to ask. If there is a question about opening something, it is better to not open it and ask the provider or office manager. If mail is accidentally opened that should not have been, the medical assistant should tape the envelope shut. A note should be included with the envelope to indicate that it was accidently opened. The note should include the person's name who opened it and the date. The facility will have a procedure for handling the mail while the provider is on vacation.

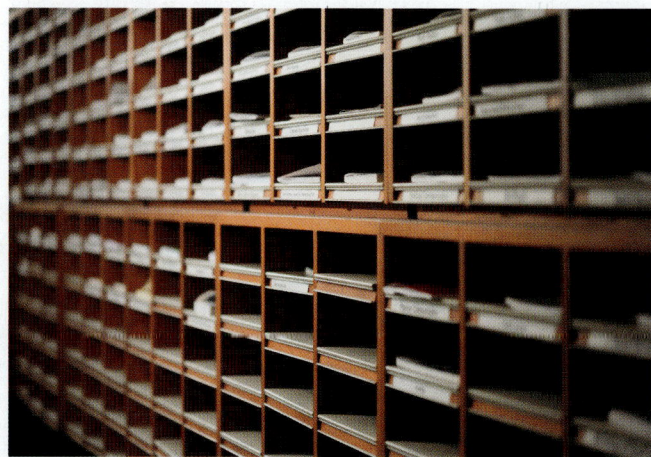

FIG. 22.18 Mailboxes offer an efficient way to sort and store mail for individuals in the department. (Photo copyright calion/iStock/Thinkstock.)

UNIT 3 Administrative Ambulatory Care

> **CRITICAL THINKING 22.15**
>
> Catherine sorts the mail for the healthcare facility. Because the facility is small, the staff does not use the mailbox system. Mail has gotten lost after she placed it on the providers' desks. What other options can Catherine implement to prevent mail from getting lost or misplaced on the providers' desks?

SAFETY AND SECURITY

Body Mechanics

The Occupational Safety and Health Act (OSHA) of 1970 requires that employers provide a workplace that is free from serious recognized hazards. Employers must comply with OSHA standards. In the healthcare environment, most injuries are sprains, strains, and tears. Back injuries are one of the most common injuries. They can result from microtrauma related to repetitive activity over time or from one traumatic experience. Reasons for back injuries include the following:

- Improper lifting or lifting items too heavy for the back to support
- Reaching, twisting, or bending when lifting
- Bad body mechanics when lifting, pushing, pulling, or carrying items
- Poor footing or constrained posture

Proper body mechanics entails using the appropriate muscles and body movements to maintain correct posture and body alignment. Proper body mechanics will increase coordination and endurance. The risk of strain and injury to the body decreases. Medical assistants need to protect themselves from bodily harm while lifting, reaching, and carrying heavy objects (Fig. 22.19A–B and Fig. 22.20A–B). Using proper

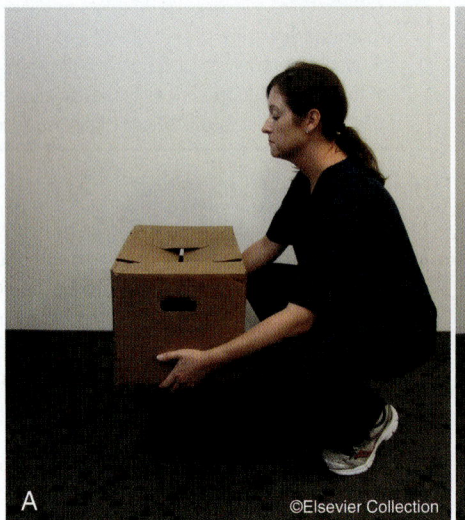 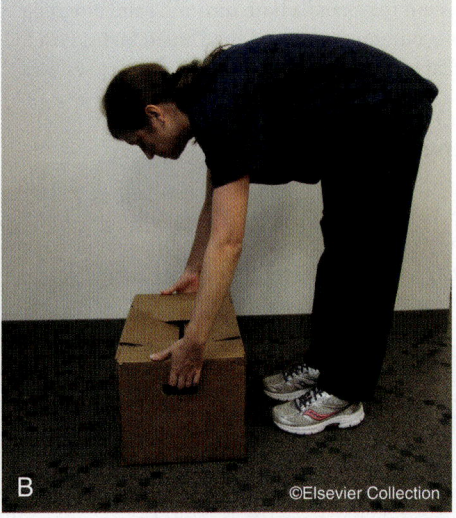

FIG. 22.19 (A) Bend knees for proper lifting technique. (B) Improper lifting technique.

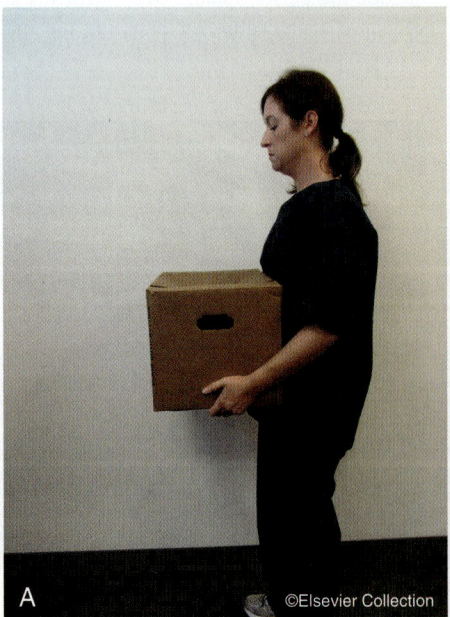 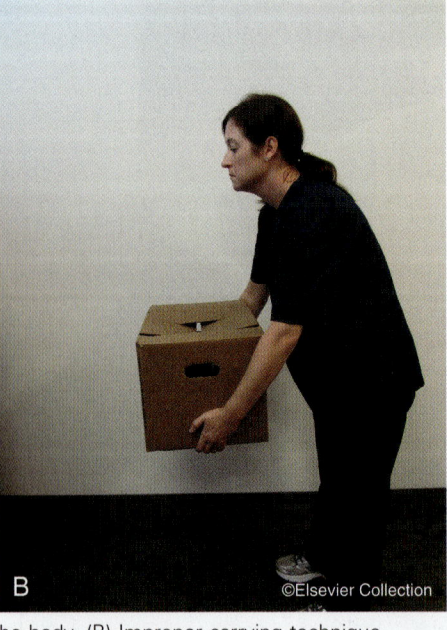

FIG. 22.20 (A) Carrying an item close to the body. (B) Improper carrying technique.

body mechanics is important to prevent injuries (Box 22.15). See Procedure 22.4, which explains how to use correct body mechanics when performing a supply inventory.

Providing a Safe Environment

Security and safety are important to the well-being of the ambulatory care staff, patients, and visitors (Box 22.16). The healthcare facility can draw unwanted attention from those seeking drugs and money. Having plans in place that can be implemented when security is in question is critical for all.

Medical facilities can be a target for those wanting to steal money, narcotic medications, and prescription pads. The staff should implement measures to limit the amount of money available in the building. Cash and checks from patients should be deposited daily to limit the quantities of money in the facility. Cash drawers should be stored out of the sight of patients and visitors. As mentioned earlier, prescription pads should remain out of the view and reach of patients. Narcotic medications, if present in the healthcare facility, should always be in a double-locked cabinet with the keys hidden. Depending on the type of clinic, some will post signs stating there are no narcotic medications on site.

Many facilities have chosen to keep the employee entrance doors locked during business hours. The doors require either a key card or unique code to enter the building. In high-crime areas, low-staffed clinics, or rural clinics, the doors to the patient care areas are also locked. This prevents the unauthorized entry of people to the patient care areas in the back, thereby increasing the security.

> ### CRITICAL THINKING 22.16
> Over the past 6 months, crime and break-ins have increased in the local area around the clinic. Many people believe the healthcare facility has a supply of narcotic medication in stock, which is *not* true. What strategies can the staff implement to increase the security of the healthcare facility?

Workplace Violence. Stories of workplace violence are becoming more common. Healthcare employees face an increased risk of work-related assaults primarily from patients and visitors (Box 22.17). OSHA encourages healthcare employees to take "universal precautions for violence." This means that violence should be expected. Violence can be avoided or lessened by respecting others, protecting the dignity of others, and through teamwork to prevent violence. Medical assistants should report patient incidents or at-risk patient behaviors and situations to the manager.

Healthcare facilities should have violence prevention programs in place. Management and employees should work together to identify hazards and plan preventive strategies (Box 22.18). All employees should be trained to handle workplace violence and facility lockdown procedures (Box 22.19).

Evaluating the Work Environment

It is important to safeguard both the patients and the employees from injuries in the healthcare facility. The medical assistant should continually evaluate the environment for safety. From a flipped-over rug to a burned-out light in the stairway, safety risks can lead to falls and injuries. This section explains how to evaluate the work environment for unsafe working conditions. By fixing or correcting issues, the environment becomes safer for all.

Remember that for all injuries that occur to patients, visitors, and employees, an incident report form must be completed. Incident report forms are discussed in Chapter 17.

> ### BOX 22.15 Principles of Proper Body Mechanics
> - To lift an object, maintain a wide, stable base with your feet. Your feet should be shoulder-width apart, and you should have good footing. Bend at the knees, keeping your back straight. Lift smoothly, using the major muscles in your arms and legs. Use the same technique when putting the item down. Bending over to lift or to set down a heavy object increases your risk of injury.
> - When lifting and carrying heavy items, keep the item directly in front of you to avoid rotating your spine.
> - Keep your movements smooth. Jerky or uncoordinated movements increase the risk for injury.
> - When reaching for an object, your feet should face the object. Twisting or turning with a heavy load can cause injury.
> - Prevent reaching and straining to get an object. Clear away barriers, and utilize a firm and level surface (e.g., a step stool) to get close to the object. Avoid standing on tiptoes.
> - Get help if the item is too heavy to lift by yourself.
> - Store heavy objects at waist level or below.

> ### BOX 22.16 Ways to Keep Safe
> - Stay alert for suspicious people.
> - Listen to your instincts if a situation or person makes you feel strange or on edge.
> - Try to alert another employee if a situation occurs. Many agencies have code words for emergency situations.
> - Use emergency alarms when needed. Many will notify the local police department.
> - Keep yourself at a distance from the person (e.g., try to separate yourself from the person by a desk or another piece of furniture).
> - Position yourself so you are the closest to the door.
> - Discuss the situation with the provider or supervisor if you are uncomfortable rooming a patient.
> - Follow the facility's safety procedures.

> ### BOX 22.17 Increased Risk Factors for Violence in Healthcare
> - Working with patients or family members that
>   - Have a history of violence
>   - Abuse drugs or alcohol
>   - Are gang members
>   - Carry firearms and other weapons
> - Poor workplace design and poorly lit hallways, rooms, parking lots, and other areas (which can limit vision of potential situations and interfere with escape plans)
> - Lack of means of emergency communication (e.g., alarms, healthcare facility's emergency procedures) and training of employees
> - Working in neighborhoods with high crime rates
> - High employee turnover
> - Long waits for patients in overcrowded, uncomfortable reception areas
> - Unrestricted areas, allowing public access to the major areas of the building
> - A perception that violence is tolerated, and police will not be called
>
> From Guidelines for Preventing Workplace Violence for Healthcare and Social Service Workers, https://www.osha.gov/Publications/osha3148.pdf.

> **BOX 22.18 Strategies to Secure the Environment**
>
> - Physical barriers (e.g., locked doors, enclosures, bullet-proof windows, security guards)
> - Bright, effective lighting and accessible exits
> - Closed-circuit video (inside and outside of the building)
> - **De-escalating** (dee es kah LATE ing) areas for patients and visitors
> - Secure work area for those working alone; panic buttons
> - Name badges to identify employees

From Guidelines for Preventing Workplace Violence for Healthcare and Social Service Workers, https://www.osha.gov/Publications/osha3148.pdf.

> **BOX 22.19 Lockdown Procedures**
>
> Lockdown is used when it is safer to stay where you are. This procedure is employed when there is a dangerous person in the building or in the area:
> - Lock or barricade the doors. If the person is in the area, lock windows and pull shades.
> - Keep away from the windows and doors.
> - If the person is in the building,
>   - Silence cell phones.
>   - Contact 911 immediately.
>   - Hide in the locked room.

Preventing Falls and Injuries. Accidents can be expensive for the healthcare facility, as costs can range from losses of employee workdays to lawsuits. Preventing accidents is therefore critical. In the healthcare facility, there are many areas that can be prone to slips, trips, and falls. In the winter months, depending on the geographic location, slips and falls can be common because of the snow and ice. The healthcare facility should have employees that oversee the sidewalks for patients and visitors. Inside the facility, high-risk situations for accidents include the following:

- *Water or trash on floors:* Standing water on floors should be cleaned up. Signage should be used to indicate wet floors. Paper wrappings, covers, and other items should not be tossed on the floor during procedures, due to an increased risk of injury.
- *Dim lighting:* Burned-out light bulbs should be replaced. All stairwells should have adequate lighting.
- *Flooring and rugs:* Rugs and mats need to be smooth and flat. Flooring that is old and pulling up needs to be replaced. Carpeting with holes can catch a shoe heel, causing the person to trip and fall.
- *Cords, cables, and other objects in walkway:* Electrical cords, computer cables, boxes, and other potential tripping hazards should never be in the walkway. Hallways and **fire doors** need to be clear of debris. Unused wheelchairs and walkers should be collapsed if possible and moved out of the way.
- *Heavy objects placed on high shelves:* These items can fall and injure someone. Reaching for a heavy object can also cause injury. Store heavier items on lower shelves so they do not have to be lifted any higher than necessary.
- *Using unsafe objects to stand on:* A chair or box could collapse or move when a person stands on it. Use a stable step stool to reach for things.

Preventing Electrical Issues and Fires. Malfunctioning equipment can also cause accidents. Any equipment that is not functioning or does not sound normal should not be used until it can be serviced and checked out. The medical assistant should follow the facility's procedure in this situation. Usually, the supervisor is notified if equipment is malfunctioning.

The medical assistant can help prevent injuries and fires in many ways:
- Check electrical cords and plugs for cracks, fraying, or other damage.
- Ensure power strips are not overloaded.
- Do not use electricity near water.
- Turn off equipment that appears to be overheating or malfunctioning.
- Store potentially flammable chemicals and supplies according to the manufacturers' guidelines.
- Keep combustibles (e.g., paper, cardboard, cloth, flammable chemicals) away from heat sources.

Many fires are started by smoking materials. It is important to have adequate No Smoking signs at the facility's doors. Deep, nontip ashtrays should be outside the doors, so visitors have an adequate place to dispose of smoking materials.

Cautery equipment and lasers are commonly used in healthcare. Cautery equipment by design gets hot. Inappropriate use can cause fires. Lasers can cause health issues (e.g., burns and blindness) and fires. All staff using or assisting with lasers should take a safety class. Signage should be on the door where the laser is being used. Water should be available if needed. Oxygen, other gases, and combustible chemicals should not be in the room when laser equipment is used.

Procedure 22.6 describes how to evaluate the environment for unsafe working conditions. Remember that when issues are found, it is important to fix them. If you cannot fix the unsafe condition, let your supervisor know immediately. Delays can increase the risk of others getting injured.

Emergency Response Plan

A variety of emergency situations can occur and impact the healthcare facility. Each facility should have a plan to respond to the situations. An emergency response plan addresses possible **workplace emergencies**. This document guides the staff on handling emergencies and may protect the business. The occurrence of natural disasters may vary around the country. The emergency response plan should cover only potential emergencies seen at the facility and in the community (Table 22.3). Table 22.4 provides the critical elements that at the minimum must be in the emergency response plan.

Having a plan is the first step. The employer also needs to train new staff on the procedures. Yearly refresher courses and mock drills help employees remain current on the procedures. The employer should document employee participation at the training sessions.

Evacuation Procedures. Evacuation procedures involve exit routes and procedures for moving employees, patients, and visitors to safe locations. Floor maps with evacuation exit routes and emergency equipment locations should be posted throughout the facility (Fig. 22.21). It is recommended that at least two routes are identified, which provides a backup route in case the primary route is blocked. Exit routes must follow these conventions:

> **VOCABULARY**
>
> **de-escalating**: Reducing the level or intensity; bringing down a person's anger or elevated emotions.
> **fire doors**: Doors made of fire-resistant materials; they close manually or automatically during a fire to prevent it from spreading.
> **workplace emergencies**: Unforeseen situations that threaten the employees and visitors; can disrupt services provided.

CHAPTER 22 Reception and Daily Operations

PROCEDURE 22.6 Evaluate the Work Environment

Tasks
Evaluate the work environment and identify unsafe working conditions.

Equipment and Supplies
- Work environment evaluation form
- Pen

Procedural Steps

1. Observe the environment for slipping, tripping, or fall risks. Document your findings to the following questions:
   - Is the lighting appropriate? Are any lights burned out? Are any areas dim?
   - Is the flooring and carpeting ripped or pulled up? If rugs/mats are present, are they folded?
   - Is water on the floor? Is signage present warning of the water?
   - Are items cluttering the hallway, making walking difficult?
   - Are cords, cables, and other items in the walkway?
   - Is trash on the floor?
   - Are heavy items on high shelves? Is a sturdy step stool available?

   Purpose: When the floor is cluttered, or the flooring is damaged, the risk of falls increases.

2. Observe the environment for safety and security issues. Document your findings to the following questions:
   - Are rooms available that can be locked and used during workplace violence? Is there limited visibility from the hallway into the room?
   - Are there areas in the building with limited visibility?
   - If the building is accessible to the public, are there any safe zones or areas for staff?
   - Are the emergency call lights in the exam rooms and bathrooms functioning?
   - Are the oxygen tanks (if available) checked per the facility's policy?

   Purpose: Having a safe area in a building is important during a workplace violence situation.

3. Observe the environment for fire risks and electrical issues. Document your findings to the following questions:
   - Are electrical cords and plugs free from cracks, fraying, or other damage?
   - Are power strips overloaded?
   - Is electricity being used near a water source?
   - Are flammable chemicals and supplies stored according to manufacturers' guidelines?
   - Are combustibles (e.g., paper, cardboard, cloth, flammable chemicals) away from heat sources?

   Purpose: The risk of fires increases when cords are damaged, or power strips are overloaded. Safe storage of chemicals is important to decrease the fire risk.

4. Observe the environment for fire containment and evacuation strategies. Document your findings to the following questions:
   - Are building diagrams posted on walls? Are exit routes indicated? Are two or more exit routes indicated on the map? Are fire alarms and fire extinguishers indicated?
   - Are exit routes uncluttered?
   - Are exit signs visible and lit?
   - Are fire doors unlocked and able to be closed in an emergency?
   - Are interior rooms available for severe storms?
   - Are smoke detectors located throughout the building? Are fire alarms available?
   - Are fire extinguishers available and checked routinely (per the facility's policy)?
   - Are flammable products (e.g., oxygen tanks, chemicals) stored along the exit routes?

   Purpose: Two or more exit routes should be available. Flammable products should not be stored in the location of the exit routes. Closed fire doors will help contain the fire.

5. Based on your observations, summarize your findings. If risks are present, create a list of issues that need to be addressed. Describe what needs to be done for each risk.

   Purpose: Creating a list of issues that need to be addressed is important in a professional setting.

TABLE 22.3 Potential Emergencies

Event	Type	Examples
Natural	Geological hazards	Tsunami, volcano, landslide, and earthquake.
	Meteorological hazards	Flood, tornado, hurricane, and ice
	Biological hazards	Foodborne illnesses and communicable disease
Human caused	Accidental events	Hazardous spill, fire, and transportation incident (aircraft, vehicle)
	Intentional events	Robbery, lost person, bomb threat, terrorism, and weapons
	Technology caused events	Telecommunication, electrical power, water, and cyber security issues

- Be clearly marked and well lit
- Be wide enough to accommodate several people
- Not pass areas where flammable products (e.g., oxygen tanks, chemicals) are stored
- Be clear of debris and obstructions at all times

Some employees must assist those who need help evacuating. Areas of rescue assistance are available in many multistory buildings (Box 22.20). Evacuation chairs can also be used to move people down the stairs. As people evacuate by priority, it is important that appointed staff remain behind to verify that everyone is out (Table 22.5). All rooms including restrooms need to be checked.

Evacuation procedures vary based on the emergency (Procedure 22.7). There are five types of evacuations:

- *Shelter-in-place evacuation*: A shelter-in-place is an interior room with no windows. In cases of tornados and other severe storms, employees, patients, and visitors should evacuate to shelter-in-place locations. Typically, these locations should be on the lowest level possible. Shelter-in-place locations are also used when a contaminant (e.g., chemical) is released into the environment.
- *Local evacuation*: Involves moving one or more people out of immediate danger (e.g., evacuate a patient out of an exam room where a chemical spill occurred).

TABLE 22.4 Critical Elements That Must Be in an Emergency Response Plan

Critical Elements	Includes
Methods to report a fire and other emergencies	• How to alert employees of the emergency (e.g., alarms, overhead paging system) • How to alert law enforcement and the fire department
Evacuation policy and procedure	• Evacuation conditions • Clear chain of command and designated person to order the evacuation and to account for employees (may be called an evacuation warden) • Patient sign-in sheets or schedules that are used to account for patients. • Evacuation procedures, including routes and meeting locations; maps should be posted
Critical shutdown procedures	• Names of specific employees who must perform certain procedures before leaving • Critical shutdown procedures (describe what needs to be done); examples include turning off the water, gas, electricity, and oxygen (if piped into the exam rooms)
Emergency escape/exit routes and procedures	• Floor plan, workplace map, safe areas, and procedures
Rescue and medical duties	• Names of workers who need to perform rescue and medical duties
Who to contact for additional information	• Names, titles, and contact information of internal and external people who can provide additional information on emergency response plans (internal people would be management and other employees; external people might be community leaders and specialists)

From How to Plan for Workplace Emergencies and Evacuations, https://www.osha.gov/Publications/osha3088.html.

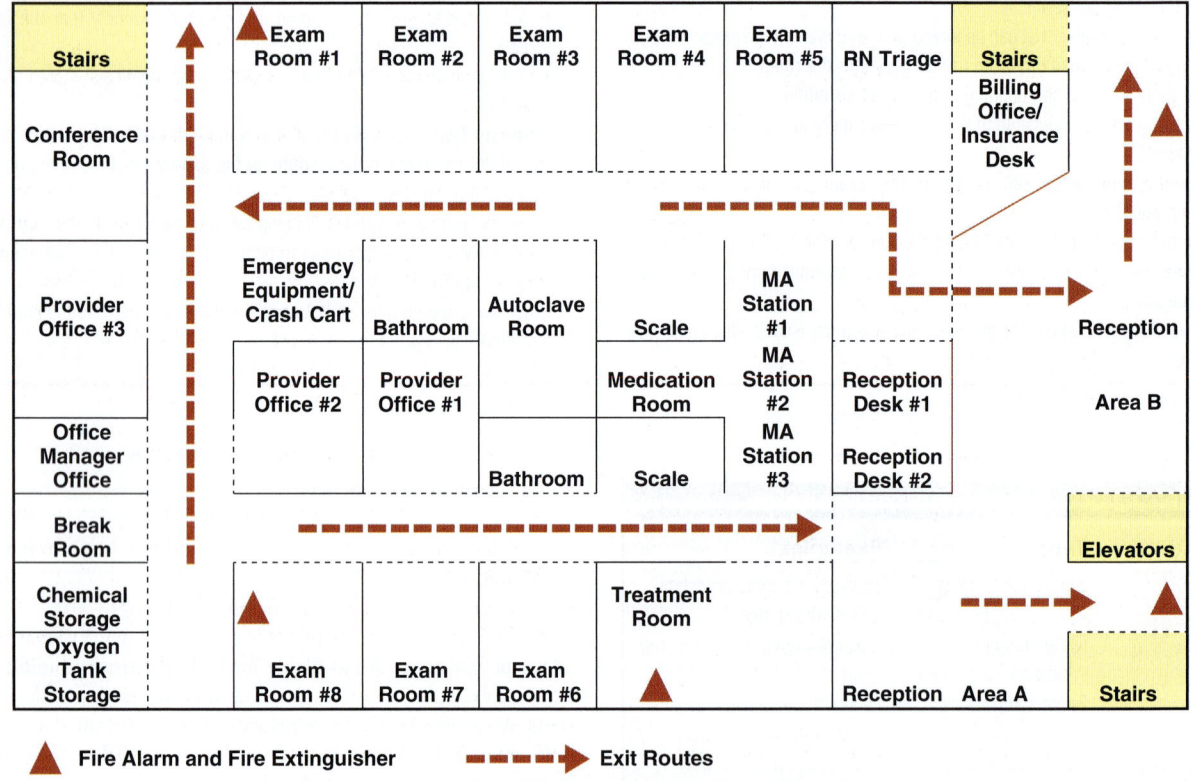

FIG. 22.21 A floor map with exit routes and emergency equipment indicated.

- *Horizontal evacuation*: Involves evacuating people off the same floor as the emergency situation.
- *Vertical evacuation*: Involves evacuating people who are located on the floors above and below the situation.
- *Building evacuation*: Involves evacuating everyone from the building to a safe location outside of the building.

Fire Response. A medical assistant should be aware of the healthcare facility's fire response procedures. It is important to know how to activate

BOX 22.20 Areas of Rescue Assistance

According to the Americans with Disabilities Act (ADA), safety requirements are needed for people in multistory buildings who need access to wheelchairs. Areas of rescue assistance are safe places where people in wheelchairs or those who cannot do stairs can await help in emergency situations. Typically, these areas are stairwells that have alarms that communicate with emergency personnel.

the alarms, evacuate people, and use a fire extinguisher for small fires. Fire response actions include the following:
- A wall-mounted fire extinguisher, manual pull station (alarm), warning alarms, smoke alarms, and automatic sprinkler systems should be located throughout the facility per state code. An employee should be assigned to routinely check this equipment and replace as needed.
- If you smell smoke or suspect a fire, use RACE (Box 22.21). Do not use elevators if a fire is suspected. This will decrease the risk of entrapment.
- If a fire is suspected, immediately disconnect oxygen supplies, or turn off oxygen tanks to prevent an explosion.

TABLE 22.5 Evacuation Priorities

Evacuation Priorities by Location	Evacuation Priorities by People
1. People in immediate danger	1. People nearest the emergency
2. People located on the floor where the emergency is occurring	2. Ambulatory people
	3. Nonambulatory people
3. People on the floor immediately above and below the floor with the situation	
4. People on the rest of the floors	

BOX 22.21 Use RACE for Fires

RESCUE: Rescue individuals threatened by the fire.
ACTIVATE: Activate the alarm if you discover the fire or respond if you hear the alarm.
CONFINE: Confine the fire by closing doors and fire doors to slow the spread of the fire.
EXTINGUISH/ **E**VACUATE: Extinguish only the small fires; otherwise **e**vacuate individuals from the area.

PROCEDURE 22.7 Participate in a Mock Exposure Event

Tasks
Demonstrate self-awareness in an emergency situation. Participate in a mock exposure event, and document specific steps taken. Recognize the physical and emotional effects on individuals involved in an emergency situation.

Scenario
You and Beth are in the autoclave room and two chemicals spill, creating toxic fumes. Beth is having trouble breathing. The staff, patients, and visitors present include:

Rooms
1—Teen and his mother
2—Older woman in a wheelchair
3—Mother with three little children
4—Adult female
5—Empty
6—An older couple
7—Adult male
8—Empty
Procedure room—Empty

Staff and Reception Areas
Reception Area A—Four people waiting
Reception Area B—Five people waiting

Staff
Tim—In MA station 3
Rose—At the insurance desk
Dave and Patty—At the receptionist desk
Julie Walden, MD—In provider office 1
Angela Perez, MD—In room 3
Jean Burke, NP—In room 7

Equipment and Supplies
- Paper
- Pen
- Floor map (see Fig. 22.21)
- Computer with internet access

Procedural Steps
1. Using the scenario, describe how you would handle the emergency exposure situation with Beth.
   - Identify four steps a medical assistant could take to demonstrate self-awareness while responding to this emergency situation.
   - Describe exposure control mechanisms or how you might limit the exposure to other people once you remove Beth for the room.
   Purpose: It is important to be self-aware as to how you would respond in emergency situations. Exposure control mechanisms are ways to limit the exposure to other people. How might you contain the situation? How might you prevent others from being impacted by the exposure?

2. Scenario continues: Dr. Walden informed the staff to evacuate from the building. The outdoor safe meeting location is at the back of the parking lot. Document the steps to handle the exposure event and evacuation from the building.
   - Describe what each staff member and provider should do to help with the evacuation procedure and notify 911.
   - Describe the steps (evacuations) in the order that they should occur.
   - Describe how the staff may ensure all individuals are out of the building.
   Purpose: It is important to know which individuals need to be evacuated first, second, etc. Employees should work with individuals in their area unless they have an appointed duty. Making sure all individuals are out of the building are important before the staff leaves the area.

3. Dr. Walden is in charge during the emergency. Describe what her responsibilities include.
   Purpose: The evacuation warden's name is listed in the emergency response plan. This person is in charge of the evacuation.

4. Dave took the patient registry. Describe why the patient registry is important.
   Purpose: The patient registry lists the patients that have checked in for appointments. It is important to take this document during evacuations.

5. Scenario continues: Two weeks after the event, Beth confides to you that she is not doing well. She recovered from the exposure, but since the event she has had difficulty sleeping. She is anxious when she goes into the autoclave room. She is having trouble concentrating on her job. She mentioned she has had two nightmares of emergencies occurring in the department and she gets injured.
   - Describe what might be occurring with Beth and the symptoms that relate to it.
   - Discuss what you might encourage her to do about the situation.
   Purpose: It is not uncommon after an emergency that individuals involved experience issues related to the emergency.

6. Research the physical and emotional effects of stress on the body. Identify four physical effects and four emotional effects of stress on persons involved in an emergency situation. Cite your resources.

7. Describe how the physical and emotional effects of stress would be different for Beth, you, the providers, and the other employees present.

8. Describe how a medical assistant could limit the physical and emotional effects of stress on each person/group: Beth, the providers, the other employees present in the facility, and yourself.

- For small fires, use the PASS procedure as you operate a fire extinguisher (Box 22.22 and Box 22.23; Procedure 22.8). Make sure you use the correct type of extinguisher for the fire (Table 22.6).

> ### CRITICAL THINKING 22.17
> One morning when the weather was stormy, Marie and Catherine were discussing the facility's emergency policy and procedures. How would you respond to a tornado warning and the need to evacuate to a shelter-in-place? How would you respond if you found a wastebasket on fire in the facility?

Effects of Stress

When a person is involved in an emergency, it can cause physical and emotional symptoms (Box 22.24). For instance, a person who was in a tornado may experience sleeping and anger issues. These may be related to the stress of the situation.

The general adaptation syndrome (GAS) is used to describe the long- and short-term effects of stress on the body. GAS was originally described by Hans Selye. He felt the syndrome impacted the nervous and the endocrine systems. The stages include the following:
- *Stage 1—Alarm reaction*: It is the immediate reaction to the stressor. The "fight or flight" response occurs. The body releases the hormones cortisol, adrenaline, and noradrenaline. This provides energy, preparing the body for physical activities. This stage can impact the immune system, causing the person to be more susceptible to illness.
- *Stage 2—Adaptation stage*: If the stressor continues, the individual's body adapts to the stressor.
- *Stage 3—Exhaustion stage*: The body's resistance had been diminished with the continued stress. The body is more susceptible to disease.

> ### CRITICAL THINKING 22.18
> Ella Rainwater had an appointment to see Dr. Martin. Marie was rooming Ms. Rainwater and had to obtain her medical history. The patient reported that she was going through a divorce and was having issues with sleeping. She said that she cannot concentrate on her job and finds herself crying throughout the day. She cannot think and is not interested in socializing any more. Based on what you learned in this chapter, what might be occurring with Ms. Rainwater?

> ### BOX 22.22 Most Fire Extinguishers Operate Using the PASS Acronym
>
> **P**ULL: Pull the pin.
> **A**IM: Aim the nozzle or hose at the base of the fire.
> **S**QUEEZE: Squeeze the handle to release the extinguishing agent.
> **S**WEEP: Sweep the nozzle or hose from side to side at the base of the fire until the fire is out. *Evacuate if you are not successful or doubt the ability to put out the fire.*

> ### BOX 22.23 New Fire Extinguisher Technology
>
> A new type of fire extinguisher, the Eliminator, changes the way fire extinguishers are used (Fig. 22.22A). This new fire extinguisher has an ergonomically designed handle and spray hose. Most fire extinguishers need to be serviced and maintained to keep them operable. This extinguisher allows facilities to maintain it easier and cheaper than other extinguishers. When using the Eliminator, a person must follow "TPASS" (Fig. 22.22B):
>
> **T**: Twist the lock to break the seal.
> **P**: Push the level down. This will pressure the extinguisher.
> **A**: Aim the valve nozzle at the base of the fire.
> **S**: Squeeze the valve level.
> **S**: Sweep the valve nozzle from side to side to put out the fire.
>
>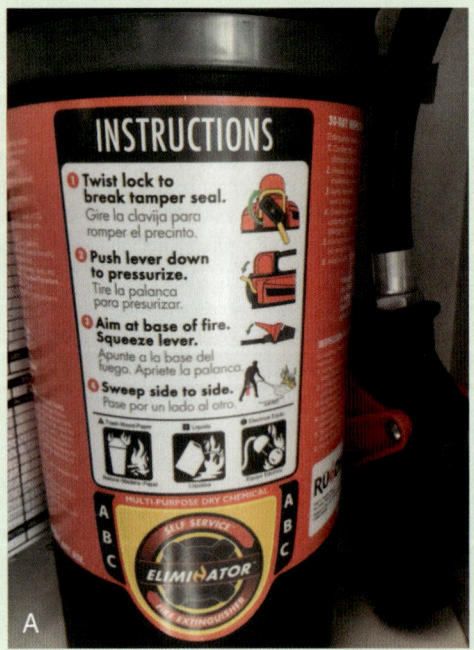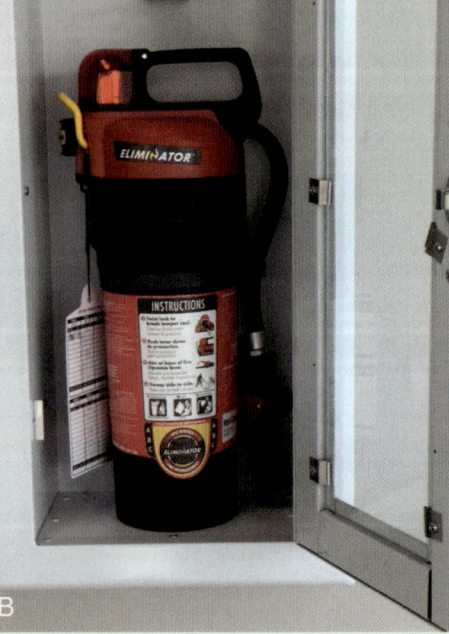
>
> **FIG. 22.22** (A) The Eliminator is a new type of fire extinguisher. (B) Users must follow "TPASS" when using the Eliminator.

CHAPTER 22 Reception and Daily Operations

PROCEDURE 22.8 Use a Fire Extinguisher

Tasks
Select the correct fire extinguisher and demonstrate the correct use.

Scenarios
a. You are working in the medical laboratory and an electrical fire starts.
b. You are working in the clinic and fire starts in a wastebasket.
c. You are working in the medical laboratory and a chemical fire starts (combustible metal fire).

Equipment and Supplies
- Fire extinguisher

Procedural Steps
1. Using the scenario, identify the type of fire extinguisher required to put out the fire.
   Purpose: The correct fire extinguisher must be used to put out the fire. Using the wrong extinguisher can make the fire worse.
2. Hold the extinguisher by the handle with the hose or nozzle pointing away from you. Pull out the pin that is located below the trigger.
   Purpose: Pulling the pin allows the extinguisher to be used.
3. Stand about 10 feet from the fire. Aim the extinguisher hose or nozzle at the base of the fire. Keep the extinguisher in an upright position as you work.
   Purpose: The most efficient method of putting out fires is to work at the base of the fire.
4. Squeeze the trigger slowly and evenly.
   Purpose: Squeezing slowly allows the discharge to come out in a steady flow.
5. Sweep from side to side until the fire is out.
   Purpose: As the fire nearest to you is put out, you can move closer to the rest of the fire.

TABLE 22.6 Uses of Fire Extinguishers

Labeled Class	Used for
A	Water extinguisher: used on *ordinary combustibles* (e.g., paper, wood, rubber, cloth, and many plastics)
B	Carbon dioxide (CO_2) extinguisher: used on flammable liquids; fires in oils and grease
C	Dry chemical extinguisher: used on electrical equipment; fires in wiring, fuse boxes, computers, and other electrical sources
ABC	Multi-purpose dry chemical extinguisher. Used on ordinary combustibles, flammable liquids, or electrical equipment
D	Fires involving combustible metals: may be found in the medical laboratory
K	Fires involving combustible cooking oils and fats: found in the kitchen

BOX 22.24 Symptoms of Stress

- Shock, disbelief
- Irritability, tension
- Fear, anxiety
- Feeling numb and powerless
- Difficulty making decisions
- High blood pressure
- High blood glucose levels
- Back pain
- Loss of interest in normal activities
- Nightmares
- Anger
- Crying, sadness
- Sleep problems
- Trouble concentrating
- Stomach problems

CLOSING COMMENTS

The medical assistant has many important duties to help the healthcare facility operate. From greeting and interacting with individuals arriving at the facility to managing inventory, these duties are important to the success of the facility. Paying attention to detail while performing these duties is important. Patients are not impressed if they are not greeted or if they are called by the wrong name. Keeping the right amount of supplies in stock so providers can treat patients also requires paying attention to details.

The medical assistant also needs to be knowledgeable about the emergency policies and procedures of the healthcare facility. During an emergency is not the time to read the procedure on what to do! It is important for the medical assistant to be calm, cool, and composed during these times. This will help others around you to remain calm.

VOCABULARY
small talk: Polite light conversation about uncontroversial matters.

EXCEPTIONAL CUSTOMER SERVICE

Going to a healthcare facility can be intimidating and uncomfortable for many patients. It is important that the medical assistant try to put everyone at ease. Cultivate the habit of greeting each patient immediately in a friendly, self-assured manner. Establish eye contact and smile while introducing yourself to the patient.

Small talk can help put a patient at ease. Talking about the weather or an uncontroversial topic may make the patient more comfortable.

Asking personalized questions can also help. Providers and staff members sometimes make brief notes in the health record about the current events in the patient's life. On the next visit, the staff or provider can use this information to start a conversation with the patient. For instance, the patient may state she is going to Florida for a vacation. During the next visit, the provider may start the visit off by asking how her Florida trip was. Asking personalized questions will solidify the personal connection with patients. They may feel important, less intimated, and more comfortable. It is a great way to provide excellent customer service.

CHAPTER REVIEW

The medical assistant has many tasks to perform when opening the healthcare facility. Many times, these duties are split between the administrative and the clinical medical assistants. Time must be taken to be prepared. This will make the day run more smoothly.

As patients arrive, the medical assistant must register new patients, update information, and obtain copies of insurance and patient identification cards from patients. The medical assistant must be observant for ill patients that require the triage nurse. The medical assistant must also be watchful of patients waiting for long periods of time. Keeping patients updated on wait times can relieve some of the frustration. If the medical assistant is escorting the patients to the exam room, it is important to be respectful of the patients. Keeping in mind the importance of confidentiality is critical.

Just like with opening the facility, the medical assistant has closing duties. It is important not to put tasks off until the next morning. Completing the facility closing tasks will ease the burden in the morning.

Besides daily duties, the medical assistant also has monthly duties to keep the facility clean and organized.

The medical assistant also has a role in managing equipment and supplies. Managing the inventory and ordering supplies is a large responsibility. When the supplies arrive, it is important for the medical assistant to check them immediately for any items that need to be transferred to the refrigerator or freezer.

There is a lot the medical assistant can do to ensure the safety and security of those in the facility. Using proper body mechanics is an important way for medical assistants to protect themselves from injury. It is also critical for the medical assistant to continually evaluate the work environment for unsafe issues. Items like trash on the floor or flipped-over rugs are real safety hazards that can take just seconds to correct. All healthcare professionals have an obligation to be current on the facility's emergency policies and procedures. This knowledge will pay off when an emergency occurs.

SCENARIO WRAP-UP

Marie has started to implement an inventory management process that is helping her identify when to reorder and how much to reorder. She initially started by hand-counting the inventory, and then she identified how much was utilized each buying cycle. It took a few months for her to identify trends. She found certain times of the year affected the quantity of products used. For instance, providers tend to use more casting products in the winter and summer months, which means Marie will need to increase her stock of those items during these times of the year. Marie knows that the more she learns, the more efficient she can become when managing inventory. She has already helped the facility save money by identifying cheaper vendors for commonly used expensive items. Marie loves her new job and the variety of responsibilities she has. She looks forward to continual learning.

23

Health Insurance Basics

LEARNING OBJECTIVES

1. Discuss the purpose of health insurance and explain the health insurance contract between the patient and the health plan.
2. List the 10 categories of essential health benefits according to the Affordable Care Act (ACA).
3. List and discuss various types of government-sponsored insurance plans.
4. Describe different types of private health insurance plans.
5. Discuss traditional health insurance and differentiate among the different types of managed care models.
6. Explain the health insurance contract between the healthcare provider and the health insurance company.
7. Summarize the medical assistant's role in health insurance. Also, identify information on a health insurance identification (ID) card, and explain the importance of verifying eligibility for services, including documentation.
8. Discuss disability insurance, life insurance, long-term care insurance, and liability insurance.
9. Describe the impact that the ACA has had on health insurance in the United States.

CHAPTER OUTLINE

1. Opening Scenario, 521
2. You Will Learn, 522
3. Introduction, 522
4. Benefits, 522
5. Health Insurance Plans, 522
   a. Government Health Insurance Plans, 523
      i. *Medicare, 523*
      ii. *Medicaid, 524*
      iii. *Government Managed Care Plans, 524*
      iv. *Children's Health Insurance Program, 524*
      v. *TRICARE, 524*
      vi. *Civilian Health and Medical Program of the Veterans Administration, 525*
      vii. *Workers' Compensation, 525*
   b. Private Health Insurance Plans, 525
      i. *Employer Group Plans, 525*
      ii. *Individual Health Insurance Plans, 526*
6. Health Insurance Models, 526
   a. Traditional Health Insurance, 526
   b. Managed Care Organizations, 526
      i. *Models of Managed Care Organizations, 526*
      ii. *Utilization Management/Utilization Review, 527*
7. Participating Provider Contracts, 527
   a. Contracted Fee Schedules, 528
8. The Medical Assistant's Role, 528
   a. Health Insurance Identification Card, 528
   b. Verifying Eligibility, 528
9. Other Types of Insurance, 529
   a. Disability Insurance, 529
   b. Life Insurance, 530
   c. Long-Term Care Insurance, 530
   d. Liability Insurance, 530
10. The Affordable Care Act, 530
11. Closing Comments, 531
12. Chapter Review, 531
13. Scenario Wrap-Up, 531

▶ OPENING SCENARIO

Jon Bimmell, a registered Medical assistant (RMA), has worked for Walden-Martin Family Medical Clinic (WMFM) for 3 years. Jon started with WMFM as a receptionist. Donna Potter, the office manager, recognized that Jon was very detail oriented, so, 2 years ago, she asked him to take charge of the health insurance policies and procedures manual for the practice.

Jon also trains all new medical assistants on how to verify patient health insurance coverage and eligibility. Because Jon has learned quite a bit about health insurance, he can answer most of the patients' questions about their coverage, benefits, and/or the exclusions of their policies. He knows where to direct patients who have more complicated questions and how to follow up – one of the most important duties of a professional medical assistant. He has a great attitude about assisting patients with insurance questions and does not hesitate to call the insurance company on the patient's behalf.

He provides patients with exceptional customer service. When patients call him for assistance, he responds within 24 hours (often within 1 hour) with answers to their questions or a resource to help them. Jon is willing to help any staff member with other duties when necessary and prides himself on being a patient advocate. He is an enthusiastic team player who puts patients first.

YOU WILL LEARN

- To identify the various government health insurance plans.
- To identify private health insurance plans.
- To recognize the different managed care organizations.
- To understand what it means to be a participating provider.

INTRODUCTION

Insurance is something that is purchased to help protect against loss or harm from specified circumstances. Using automobile insurance as an example, the specified circumstances are those related to a car accident. The insurance could pay for damage done to your vehicle or other vehicles. It could also pay for medical expenses for anyone injured in an accident. With health insurance, the specified circumstances are those related to the policyholder's health. This insurance would pay for hospital expenses, provider expenses, and certain supplies and equipment.

A *policy* is purchased with a *premium* or payment. The premium can be paid by:
- An individual
- An employer
- A combination of employer contribution and individual (employee) contribution

The policy is considered a legal contract and will stay in force as long as the premium is being paid. The policy will specify exactly what services are covered. The more services that are covered, the higher the premium cost. The person responsible for the payment of the premium is referred to as a *subscriber*.

Most policies require the patient to pay a portion of the healthcare expenses. This is referred to as *cost-sharing*, which includes the following:
- *Deductible*: A set dollar amount that the policyholder must pay before the insurance company starts to pay for services. It can be as low as $100 and as high as $5,000. The higher the deductible, the lower the premium.
- *Co-insurance*: After the deductible has been met, the policyholder may need to pay a certain percentage of the bill and the insurance company pays the rest. A typical split is 80/20 – the insurance company pays 80%, and the policyholder pays 20%.
- *Copayment*: A set dollar amount that the policyholder must pay for each office visit. It is possible that copayments differ for different types of office visits. For example, there can be one copayment amount for a primary care provider and a different copayment amount (usually higher) to see a specialist or to be seen in the emergency department.

The policy will specify the dollar amounts for the deductible, co-insurance, and copayment. The premium is not usually considered part of cost-sharing.

In order for the insurance carrier to pay for services, a *claim* must be submitted. The claim is reviewed by the insurance company to determine if the services provided are covered under the policy. It is important for a medical assistant to be familiar with the different types of insurance so that claims can be submitted accurately. This will result in faster payment for the healthcare facility.

> **VOCABULARY**
> **claim:** A formal request for payment from an insurance company for services provided.
> **policy:** A written agreement between two parties, in which one party (the insurance company) agrees to pay another party (the patient) if certain specified circumstances occur.

BENEFITS

The Affordable Care Act (ACA) requires all health plans to cover essential health benefits. There are 10 categories of essential health benefits:

- Ambulatory patient services
- Hospitalization
- Mental health and substance use disorder services
- Prescription drugs
- Preventive and wellness services and chronic disease management
- Emergency services
- Maternity and newborn care
- Rehabilitative and habilitative services and devices
- Laboratory services
- Pediatric services, including oral and vision care

In addition to the essential health benefits, an insurance policy may cover other services. For a group policy, an employer can pick and choose the benefits it wants for employees, such as vision or dental coverage. Medical assistants should contact an insurance company to determine if certain services are covered under a patient's policy.

HEALTH INSURANCE PLANS

There are two types of health insurance plans in the United States:
- Government health insurance plans
- Private health insurance plans

Health insurance plans typically cover health services and procedures that are deemed medically necessary. *Medically necessary* services are those that are necessary to improve the patient's current health. Most insurance policies do not cover elective procedures. *Elective procedures* are medical procedures that are not deemed medically necessary, such as a facelift or another cosmetic procedure. The ACA states that health insurance plans must cover preventive care. *Preventive care* includes services provided to help prevent certain illnesses or that lead to an early diagnosis (Box 23.1). Insurance companies must cover preventive care services and cannot impose cost-sharing for those services.

> **BOX 23.1 Preventive Care Services**
>
> The following is a list of services considered to be preventive care services:
> - Alcohol misuse screening
> - Blood pressure screening
> - Cholesterol screening
> - Colorectal cancer screening
> - Depression screening
> - Diabetes (type 2) screening
> - Diet counseling
> - Hepatitis B and C screening
> - Human immunodeficiency virus (HIV) screening
> - Immunization vaccines
> - Lung cancer screening
> - Obesity screening and counseling
> - Tobacco use screening
> - Sexually transmitted infection (STI) prevention counseling

TABLE 23.1 Comparing Medicare Plans

	Covered Services	Monthly Premium	Deductible
Part A	Inpatient hospital care, skilled nursing facilities, home health care, and hospice services	$0	$1,340 deductible for each benefit period (2018); Days 1–60: $0 co-insurance for each benefit period; Days 61–90: $335 co-insurance per day of each benefit period; Day 91 and beyond: $670 co-insurance per each "lifetime reserve day" after day 90 for each benefit period (up to 60 days over a lifetime)
Part B	Outpatient hospital care, durable medical equipment, provider's services, and other medical services	$134	$183 (2018), plus 20% co-insurance for all medical services
Part C	Expanded inpatient hospital and outpatient hospital care benefits	Varies by plan	Varies by plan
Part D	Prescription drugs	Varies by income	Varies by plan

https://www.medicare.gov/your-medicare-costs/costs-at-a-glance/costs-at-glance.html. Accessed February 19, 2018.

Government Health Insurance Plans

Government health insurance plans provide coverage with reduced or no monthly premiums for the **indigent** (IN di juh nt), the elderly, the military, and government employees. There are a number of different plans, but patients need to qualify by:
- Age
- Income
- Government occupation
- Health condition

A patient who is age 65 or older can qualify for *Medicare*. A low-income patient may be eligible for *Medicaid*. Dependents of military personnel are covered by *TRICARE*. Surviving spouses and dependent children of veterans who died in the line of duty are covered by the *Civilian Health and Medical Program of the Veterans Administration* (CHAMPVA). Employees who are injured or become ill due to work related issues are covered under *workers' compensation insurance*.

Medicare. Medicare is a federal health insurance program that provides healthcare coverage for individuals who are age 65 or older; people who are disabled; and patients who have been diagnosed with end-stage renal disease (ESRD). Medicare refers to those covered by Medicare as *beneficiaries*. Medicare currently is the world's largest insurance program. In 2017 there were more than 58 million beneficiaries. The Medicare program is administered by the Centers for Medicare and Medicaid Services (CMS), a division of the Department of Health and Human Services (HHS). Laws enacted by Congress regulate the Medicare program.

The Medicare plan is divided into four parts (Table 23.1):
- Part A covers inpatient hospital charges. It is financed with special contributions deducted from employed individuals' salaries, with matching contributions from their employers. Due to these contributions and regular Social Security contributions, there is no monthly premium for Part A.
- Part B covers ambulatory care, including primary care and specialists. Beneficiaries are required to pay a monthly premium. Beneficiaries can visit any specialist without a referral.
- Part C is an option for Medicare-qualified patients to turn their Part A and Part B benefits into a private plan that can offer some additional benefits. The private plan must cover everything that would be covered under Part A and Part B.
- Part D is a prescription drug program offered to Medicare-qualified individuals that requires an additional monthly premium.

Basic medical coverage for Medicare Part B is 80% of the allowed amount after the deductible. This means that patients are responsible for the remaining 20%. The allowed amount is determined using a **resource-based relative value scale (RBRVS)** (Box 23.2). Some patients choose to purchase a private supplemental health insurance policy to help cover the 20%. These policies can also pay for services not covered by Medicare. These supplemental health insurance plans are known as *Medigap* policies. Federal regulations now require Medicare supplement policies to be uniform to avoid confusion for the purchaser.

BOX 23.2 Resource-Based Relative Value Scale (RBRVS)

The RBRVS is one of the outcomes of the Medicare Physician Payment Reform that was enacted in the Omnibus Budget Reconciliation Act of 1989 (OBRA '89). Originally, Medicare Part B had paid providers using a fee-for-service system based on usual, customary, and reasonable (UCR) charges. However, implementation of the RBRVS in 1992 changed this system to a fee scale consisting of three parts:
- Provider work
- Charge-based professional liability expenses
- Charge-based overhead

The provider work component includes the degree of effort invested by a provider in a particular service or procedure and the time it consumed. The professional liability and overhead components are computed by the Centers for Medicare and Medicaid Services (CMS).

The RBRVS fee schedule is designed to provide nationally uniform payments after adjustment to reflect the differences in practice costs across geographic areas. The fee schedule includes a conversion factor, which is a single national number applied to all services paid under the fee schedule. Conversion factors are changed by Congress, usually annually, at the request of the CMS.

VOCABULARY

indigent: Poor, needy, impoverished.
resource-based relative value system (RBRVS): A system used to determine how much providers should be paid for services rendered. It is used by Medicare and many other health insurance companies.

CRITICAL THINKING BOX 23.1

Jana Green is a Medicare patient who has Part A and Part B coverage. Will Medicare cover her office visit with the cardiologist? What percent of the bill will she be responsible for?

The fee schedule for Medicare Part B is determined using the RBRVS. This system consists of three parts:
- Provider work
- Charge-based professional liability expenses
- Charge-based overhead

The provider work component includes the degree of effort and time needed by a provider to perform a particular service or procedure. The professional liability and overhead components are computed by the CMS.

The RBRVS fee schedule is designed to provide nationally uniform payments to healthcare providers. Payments are adjusted to reflect the differences in practice costs across geographic areas. The fee schedule includes a conversion factor, which is a single national number applied to all services paid under the fee schedule. Conversion factors are set by Congress, and changed annually, at the request of the CMS.

Depending on the contract between the provider and the insurance carrier (especially Medicare, Medicaid, and other government programs), the provider writes off the difference between the RBRVS schedule and his or her fee.

Contracts between the provider of service and the insurance company vary greatly, depending on the insurance. It is important for the medical assistant to know the contract terms for each insurance company. As insurance payments are received, the medical assistant should examine the explanation of benefits (EOB) closely to ensure that all benefits have been reimbursed correctly.

Medicaid. Medicaid is the government program that provides medical care for the indigent. This program is funded by both federal and state governments to provide medical care for people meeting specific eligibility criteria. All states and the District of Columbia have Medicaid programs, but program specifics vary by state. A person eligible for Medicaid in one state may not be eligible in another state, and covered medical services may differ.

The federal government provides funding to each state for Medicaid programs. To receive this funding, each state is required to cover certain services (Box 23.3). The individual states decide what additional services will be covered.

An ambulatory care facility has the right to limit the number of Medicaid patients it accepts into the practice. The medical office cannot pick and choose which Medicaid patients they are willing to see. There can be no discrimination based on age, gender, race, religious preference, or national origin. The Medicaid fee schedule is the lowest of all insurance companies, and it may not be in the medical office's financial interest to accept a large number of Medicaid patients. A provider who accepts Medicaid patients automatically agrees to accept Medicaid's allowed amount as payment in full for covered services. Some patients who are eligible for Medicaid are required to pay a copayment. The provider can collect the copayment from the patient but cannot bill for any amount over the allowed amount.

VOCABULARY

explanation of benefits (EOB): A document sent by the insurance company to the provider and the patient explaining the allowed charge amount, the amount reimbursed for services, and the patient's financial responsibilities.
fee schedule: A list of fixed fees for services.
Qualified Medicare Beneficiaries (QMBs): Low-income Medicare patients who qualify for Medicaid for their secondary insurance.

BOX 23.3 Mandatory Medicaid Benefits

In order to receive federal funds for Medicaid, each state Medicaid plan must cover the following services:

- Inpatient hospital services
- Outpatient hospital services
- Nursing facility services
- Early and periodic screening, diagnostic, and treatment (EPSDT) services
- Home health services
- Physician services
- Rural health clinic service
- Federally qualified health center services
- Laboratory and x-ray services
- Family planning services
- Nurse midwife services
- Certified pediatric and family nurse practitioner services
- Freestanding birth center services
- Transportation to medical care
- Tobacco cessation counseling for pregnant women

https://www.medicaid.gov/medicaid/benefits/list-of-benefits/index.html. Accessed March 27, 2017.

Eligibility for benefits is determined by the respective states, but most Medicaid recipients also are some or all of the following:
- Low-income families
- Qualified pregnant women and children
- Recipients of Temporary Assistance for Needy Families (TANF)
- Individuals who receive Supplemental Security Income (SSI)
- Individuals who receive certain types of federal and state aid
- Individuals who are Qualified Medicare Beneficiaries (QMBs) – Medicaid pays for Medicare Part B premiums, deductibles, and co-insurance for qualified low-income elderly individuals
- Individuals in institutions or receiving long-term care in nursing facilities and intermediate-care facilities

Government Managed Care Plans. In an effort to reduce costs and increase the delivery of efficient care, Medicare and many Medicaid programs offer their members the option to join a managed care plan. These managed care plans must cover all services that would be covered under Medicare or Medicaid. The identification cards will look just like the ones issued to people not on Medicare or Medicaid. The government managed care plan may have a copayment that the patient would be responsible for.

Children's Health Insurance Program. The Children's Health Insurance Program (CHIP) is a state-funded program for children whose family income is above the Medicaid qualifying income limits. Although Medicaid does not typically have a premium, CHIP does. The premiums are typically 5% of the family monthly income. State CHIP programs cover:

- routine checkups
- immunizations
- doctor visits
- prescriptions
- dental care and vision care
- inpatient and outpatient hospital care
- laboratory tests and x-ray services
- emergency services

CHIP programs are similar to managed care plans in that care is covered only through the designated network of providers. There are smaller copayments for medical services for CHIP patients.

TRICARE. TRICARE is the comprehensive healthcare program for uniformed service members and retirees and their families. Members of the National Guard/Reserve and their families can also be covered under TRICARE.

The TRICARE program is managed by the military in partnership with civilian hospitals and clinics. It is designed to:
- expand access to health care
- ensure high-quality care
- promote medical readiness

All military hospitals and clinics are part of the TRICARE program and offer high-quality health care at a low cost. TRICARE offers two types of plans:
- TRICARE Prime
- TRICARE Select

Review Table 23.2 for a comparison of the TRICARE plans.

Civilian Health and Medical Program of the Veterans Administration. CHAMPVA, a health benefits program similar to TRICARE, provides coverage for the families of veterans who were permanently disabled or killed in the line of duty. The Department of Veterans Affairs (VA) shares the cost of certain healthcare services and supplies with eligible beneficiaries.

Workers' Compensation. Workers' compensation is an insurance plan for individuals who are injured on the job or become ill due to job-related circumstances. An example of a job-related illness would be mesothelioma (mez uh thee lee OH muh) caused by inhaling asbestos. The insurance plan covers:
- medical care and rehabilitation benefits
- weekly income replacement benefits
- death benefits to dependents

The provider accepts the workers' compensation reimbursements as payment in full and does not bill the patient. Time limitations are set for the prompt reporting of workers' compensation cases. The employee is obligated to promptly notify the employer. The employer must then notify the insurance company and refer the employee to a healthcare provider.

All 50 states have passed workers' compensation laws to protect workers against the loss of wages and the cost of medical care resulting from an occupational accident or disease, as long as the employee was not proven negligent. State laws differ regarding employees who are included and the benefits provided by workers' compensation insurance. Federal and state legislatures require employers to maintain workers' compensation coverage to meet minimum standards, covering most employees, for work-related illnesses and injuries. The purpose of workers' compensation laws is to provide prompt medical care to an injured or ill worker so that the person may be restored to health and return to full earning capacity in as short a time as possible.

Private Health Insurance Plans

Health insurance plans that are available from commercial insurance companies are considered private plans. The majority of people are part of an employer group plan. Those that are not eligible for an employer plan can purchase insurance on their own. This is referred to as an *individual health insurance plan*. Most private plans use managed care to reduce the costs of delivering quality health care.

Employer Group Plans. Many businesses offer a *group policy*, a private health insurance plan purchased by an employer for a group of employees. These plans can cover the employee, their spouse (i.e., domestic partner), and their children. Typically, an employer pays a certain percentage of the premium for full-time employees. This makes the cost of the insurance plan more affordable for the employee. Part-time employees can be part of the group policy, but most employers do not pay a part of the premium for part-time employees. Employers also determine the health insurance benefits under the group policy. Health insurance monthly premiums and benefits can vary from employer to employer. For example, the health insurance plan for Employer A covers chiropractic care, but the health insurance plan for Employer B does not. The premium for a group policy is usually lower than that for an individual plan because

TABLE 23.2 Comparing TRICARE Plans

Active Duty Family Members

	TRICARE Prime	TRICARE Select
Annual deductible	None	$150/individual or $300/family for E-5 and above; $50/$100 for E-4 and below
Annual enrollment fee	None	None currently; 1/1/2020 $150/individual or $300/family
Civilian outpatient visit	No cost	Primary Care -$21 Specialty - $31
Civilian inpatient admission	No cost	$18.60 a day ($25 minimum)
Civilian inpatient mental health	No cost	$18.60 a day ($25 minimum)
Civilian inpatient skilled nursing facility care	$0 per diem charge per admission; no separate copayment/cost-share for separately billed professional charges	$18.60 a day ($25 minimum)

Retirees (Under 65), Their Family Members, and Others

	TRICARE Prime	TRICARE Select
Annual deductible	None	$150/individual or $300/family
Annual enrollment fee	$289.08/individual or $578.16/family	None
Civilian copays	None	20% of negotiated fee
Outpatient emergency care mental health visit	$12 per visit	$20 Primary $30 Specialty
Civilian inpatient cost-share	$11 a day ($25 minimum) charge per admission	Lesser of $250 a day or 25% of negotiated charges plus 20% of negotiated professional fees
Civilian inpatient skilled nursing facility care	$11 a day ($25 minimum) charge per admission	$250 per diem copayment or 20% cost-share of total charges for institutional care, whichever is less, plus 20% cost-share of separately billed professional charges

https://tricare.mil/Costs/HealthPlanCosts. Accessed February 19, 2018.

> **BOX 23.4 Self-Funded Group Health Plans**
>
> Many large companies or organizations have enough employees that they can fund their own insurance program. This is called a *self-funded plan*. Technically, a self-funded plan does not fit the true definition of insurance. The employer pays employee healthcare costs from the funds collected from employee monthly premiums. Usually, the costs of benefits and premiums for self-funded plans are similar to those for group plans. Self-funded plans tend to work best for companies that are large enough to offer good benefit coverage and reasonable premium rates and are able to pay large claims for expensive medical services. Often a **third-party administrator (TPA)** handles paperwork and claim payments for a self-insured group.
>
> Self-funded health care is an arrangement in which an employer provides health or disability benefits to employees with its own funds. This is different from fully insured plans, in which the employer contracts with an insurance company to cover the employees and dependents. In self-funded health care, the employer assumes the direct risk for payment of the claims for benefits. The terms of eligibility and coverage are stated in the insurance plan document, which includes provisions similar to those found in a typical group health insurance policy.

of the large pool of employees. The insurance company will receive premiums from a larger number of people, and just a few of them will need a lot of services. The employees' share of the premium is often paid through payroll deductions (Box 23.4).

Individual Health Insurance Plans. An individual health insurance plan is one that is not offered by an employer or another group. An individual policy can cover just one person or a family. These policies can be purchased through a **health insurance exchange** or directly from an insurance company. Premiums for an individual plan are generally higher than for a group plan.

HEALTH INSURANCE MODELS

There are basically two different models of health insurance today:
- Traditional health insurance
- Managed care organizations

You can find these options in both employer group plans and individual plans.

> **VOCABULARY**
>
> **gatekeeper:** The primary care provider, who is in charge of a patient's treatment. Additional treatment, such as referrals to a specialist, must be approved by the gatekeeper.
> **health insurance exchange:** An online marketplace where you can compare and buy individual health insurance plans. State health insurance exchanges were established as part of the Affordable Care Act.
> **preauthorization:** A process required by some insurance carriers in which the provider obtains permission to perform certain procedures or services.
> **provider network:** An approved list of physicians, hospitals, and other providers.
> **referral:** An order from a primary care provider for the patient to see a specialist or to get certain medical services.
> **third-party administrator (TPA):** An organization that processes claims and provides administrative services for another organization. Often used by self-funded plans.

Traditional Health Insurance

Traditional health insurance plans pay for all or a share of the cost of covered services, regardless of which provider, hospital, or other licensed healthcare provider is used. Because providers are paid for each office visit, test, procedure, or other service they deliver, traditional insurance plans are often called *fee-for-service plans*. This was the first type of health insurance. Tradition health insurance plans provide the most flexibility for the patient, but are also the costliest option.

Policyholders of fee-for-service plans and their dependents choose when and where to get healthcare services. When the policy is purchased, the subscriber is often given a fee schedule, which explains the benefit payment amounts. Benefits are usually paid to the insured, unless that person has authorized payment to be made directly to the provider. This is referred to as *assignment of benefits*.

The fee schedule amounts can be determined by a process called *usual, customary, and reasonable* (UCR). UCR is the amount paid for a medical service in a geographic area based on what providers in the area usually charge for the same or similar service.

Managed Care Organizations

Managed care organizations (MCOs) are health insurance companies whose goal is to provide quality, cost-effective care to its members. MCOs negotiate reduced rates with contracted providers and hospitals. In return, the managed care plan increases the provider's patient load. Many MCOs require the patient to choose a *primary care provider (PCP)*, who coordinates the patient's care. Managed care plans can also require **referrals** for their patients to be treated by a specialist, thus limiting patient access to more expensive care. The **preauthorization** process can further control patient care costs. Medical care, testing, or medication therapy is provided only when it is justified to the health insurance plan. It is important that medical assistants be familiar with the various models of managed care to fully understand their effects on healthcare costs.

Models of Managed Care Organizations. Patient care is coordinated through a network of providers and hospitals. There are different types of managed care plans, such as health maintenance organizations (HMOs), preferred provider organizations (PPOs), and exclusive provider organizations (EPOs). They provide health care in return for scheduled payments and coordinate health care through a defined network of PCPs, hospitals, and other providers.

Health maintenance organization. HMOs are health plans that are regulated by HMO laws, which require them to include preventive care as part of their benefits package. The goal of the HMO health insurance plan is to reduce the cost of health care while still providing quality health care. HMO plans typically have the lowest monthly premiums among other health insurance plans. The patient's out-of-pocket expenses are also very low. Patient are not required to pay a deductible or co-insurance.

Patients are required to select a PCP, who acts as the **gatekeeper** to more specialized care. The insurance plan will not pay for services that are not included in its **provider network**; patients are 100% financially responsible for medical expenses incurred outside the HMO network of providers. For example, patients wanting to visit the dermatologist for eczema must visit their PCP first; they would be fully responsible financially if they made an appointment with a dermatologist directly. The PCP can either treat the patient or refer him or her to the specialist.

TABLE 23.3 Health Maintenance Organization (HMO) Models

Model	Structure	Payment Structure
IPA (Independent Practice Association)	General or family practice provider or provider group that practices independently and may contract with several HMOs. Can see patients outside of the HMO.	Capitation or fee-for-service
Staff	One or more providers hired by an HMO. Providers see only HMO patients.	Salaried
Group	Multispecialty group with or without a primary care provider (PCP; i.e., gatekeeper); may contract with several HMOs.	Capitation or fee-for-service
Network	HMOs contract with multiple provider groups. Those providers can see patients outside of the HMO. Provides wider geographic coverage for members.	Capitation or fee-for-service

PCPs receive financial incentives when they reduce the cost of patient care. In the earlier example, prescribing medicine to the patient is more cost-effective than referring the patient to the specialist. HMOs always require:
- referrals from the PCP to specialists
- precertification and preauthorization for hospital admissions, outpatient procedures, and treatments.

HMOs can be set up using several different models. The payment structure can be different for each of those models (Table 23.3).

CRITICAL THINKING BOX 23.2

Noemi Rodriguez is a patient who called to make an appointment with the endocrinologist because she is having trouble managing her diabetes. She told Jon over the phone when she was making the appointment that she has Aetna HMO. Will Jon be able to schedule Ms. Rodriguez's appointment with the endocrinologist? Why or why not? What would she need to make an appointment?

VOCABULARY

capitation: A payment arrangement for healthcare providers. The provider is paid a set amount for each enrolled person assigned to him or her, per period of time, whether or not that person has received services.

utilization management: A decision-making process used by managed care organizations to manage healthcare costs. It involves case-by-case assessments of the appropriateness of care.

Preferred provider organization. A PPO is a managed care network that contracts with a group of providers. The providers agree on a predetermined list of charges for all services, including those for both normal and complex procedures. The PPO model of managed health care uses the fee-for-service concept that many providers prefer. Typically, the patient's financial responsibilities represent, on average, 20% to 25% of the allowed charge, but this depends on the patient's health insurance policy. A provider who joins a PPO does not need to change the manner of providing care and continues to treat and bill patients on a fee-for-service basis. When a patient covered under a PPO plan comes for treatment, the provider treats the patient and bills the PPO. Patients do not need to visit their PCP to obtain a referral to a specialist for more specialized care. And, they typically have more control over healthcare choices.

PPOs provide their subscribers with a list of participating providers and healthcare facilities from which they can access in-network health care at PPO reduced rates. Rates are quite often lower than those charged to non-PPO patients. This gives the patient more choices for providers. If the patient chooses to see a provider that is not in the PPO network the deductible, co-insurance, and copayments will higher.

Although patients have the option to visit a specialist when they feel the need, they are still required to obtain preauthorization for more expensive services, such as diagnostic imaging.

CRITICAL THINKING BOX 23.3

Diego Lupez called Jon; he was upset because he had received a patient statement with a balance owing. He told Jon that he has full-coverage insurance through his employer and did not know why he had a balance. What information can Jon share with Mr. Lupez to explain his financial responsibility?

Exclusive provider organization. An EPO combines features of an HMO (e.g., an enrolled group or population, PCPs, and an authorization system) and a PPO (e.g., flexible benefit design and fee-for-service payments). Patients with EPO coverage will not be covered for services outside the designated network of providers (unless there is an emergency), but they may not need to obtain a referral for specialized care. Unlike HMO members, EPO plan members are not required to choose a PCP.

Table 23.4 compares the different types of managed care plans.

Utilization Management/Utilization Review. Utilization management is a form of patient care review by healthcare professionals who do not provide the care but are employed by health insurance companies. It is a necessary component of managed care to control costs. A *utilization review committee* reviews individual cases to ensure that medical care services are medically necessary. For this committee to function properly, having the correct diagnosis code is critical. This committee also reviews all provider referrals and cases of emergency department visits and urgent care. For referrals, the committee reviews the referral and either approves or denies it, so it is important to submit accurate documentation. The medical assistant should contact the utilization review department directly; it should never be left to the patient to contact this department.

PARTICIPATING PROVIDER CONTRACTS

With all government health plans and most private health plans, healthcare providers must become *participating providers* (PARs): These

TABLE 23.4 Managed Care Plans

Plan	Providers	Access to Specialized Care	Deductible, Co-Insurance, Copayment
Health maintenance organization (HMO)	Must see only HMO providers and choose a primary care provider (PCP).	Referral required for specialized care.	Usually no deductible or coinsurance. Copayments required for office visits and prescriptions.
Preferred provider organization (PPO)	No PCP required. There is a network of providers, but out-of-network providers can be seen.	No referral required. Preauthorization needed for expensive services.	Lower deductible and co-insurance if an in-network provider is used. Copayments required for office visits and prescriptions.
Exclusive provider organization (EPO)	Must see network providers. No PCP required.	No referral needed.	Usually no deductible or co-insurance. Copayments required for office visits and prescriptions.

providers are contracted with the insurance plan and have agreed to accept the contracted fee schedule as payment in full. Healthcare providers can apply to become PARs through a process called *credentialing*. Credentialing is the process of confirming the healthcare provider's qualifications, including the healthcare provider's license to practice medicine, affiliated organizations, and his or her education and professional background.

Once the healthcare provider is credentialed, the health insurance plan issues a contract to become an in-network PAR. The contract includes a fee schedule that the health insurance company will use to reimburse the provider for health services rendered. By signing the contract, the provider agrees to accept the health insurance plan's fee schedule, even if it is lower than the provider's fee schedule.

Contracted Fee Schedules

Payment for services is typically made after the health services are provided. Once the service has been provided to the patient, the healthcare provider must submit a health insurance claim, which includes the diagnosis and procedure codes, in addition to the total charges. Although the healthcare provider establishes his or her own fee schedule, health insurance plans maintain their own rates at which they reimburse.

When setting up a fee schedule a healthcare provider considers three things:
- Time
- Expertise
- Services

In every case, healthcare providers must place an estimate on the value of these services. Fees for medical procedures and services differ from office to office based on the type of practice. An office visit with a family practice provider may cost less than an office visit with a specialist. In the past, most providers worked on a fee-for-service basis; that is, patients were charged for the provider's service based on each individual service performed.

In recent years, health insurance plans, particularly government plans and managed healthcare organizations, have greatly influenced what healthcare providers can be reimbursed by establishing the allowable charge. The *allowable charge* is the maximum that the insurance plan will pay for a procedure or service. The patient cannot be charged for the amount above the allowable charge if the provider and/or the healthcare facility are a PAR provider.

THE MEDICAL ASSISTANT'S ROLE

A medical assistant can be involved in many different tasks related to health insurance. Being familiar with the technology and forms that are used will make you more efficient at your job.

Health Insurance Identification Card

When a patient is enrolled in a health insurance plan, he or she will be issued a health insurance ID card that supplies the following information:

- Health insurance company
- Health plan type
- Subscriber identification number
- Copay amounts
- Health plan name
- Subscriber's name and covered dependents
- Policy group number
- Health plan contact phone numbers

Review Fig. 23.1 for a sampling of different insurance ID cards for common insurance companies.

Verifying Eligibility

Verification of eligibility is the process of confirming health insurance coverage for the patient. When scheduling an appointment, health insurance information should be collected (unless it is an emergency situation). If the healthcare facility is not part of the patient's network of providers, the individual should be informed of this. The patient can then decide if he or she still wants to schedule an appointment. The medical assistant should also verify the *effective date*, or date the insurance coverage began, and confirm that the patient will be covered on the date the medical services are provided. The medical assistant should make it a practice to review each insurer's **online insurance web portal**, which can verify insurance eligibility, benefits, and exclusions, prior to the patient's appointment. If the online insurance web portal is not available, the medical assistant should contact the provider services desk; the phone number should be listed on the patient's health insurance ID card.

> **VOCABULARY**
> **online insurance web portal:** An online service provided by various insurance companies for providers to look up a patient's insurance benefits, eligibility, claims status, and explanation of benefits.

> **CRITICAL THINKING BOX 23.4**
> Robert Caudill, an elderly patient, called to make an appointment, but was unsure what his benefits were. How can Jon find out what benefits he qualifies for? Is it appropriate for Jon to educate Mr. Caudill on his health insurance benefits? Why or why not?

In the recent past, the medical assistant would have to call the health insurance company to verify eligibility for each and every patient. Each call to the health insurance company automated system would take at

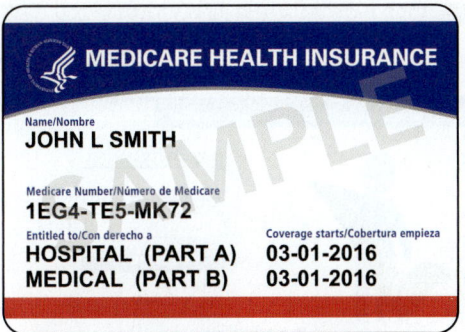
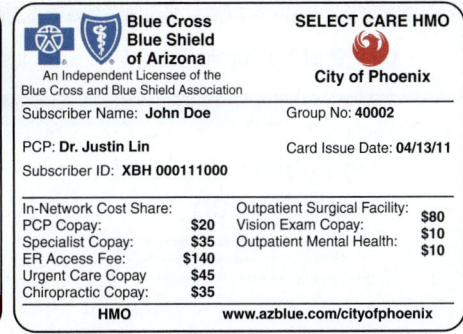
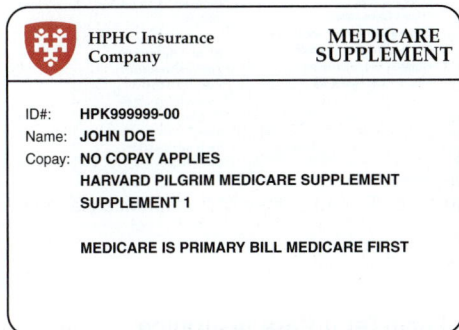
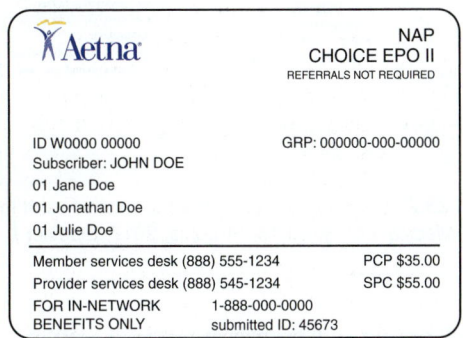
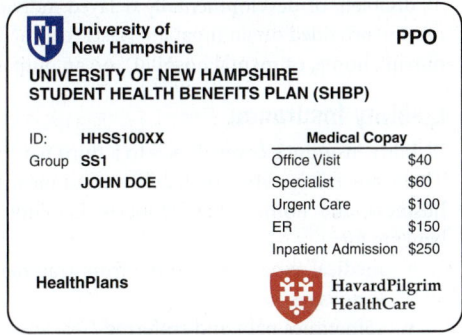

FIG. 23.1 A variety of different health insurance identification cards. (From Proctor D, Niedzwiecki B: *Kinn's The Medical Assistant*, ed 13, St Louis, 2017, Elsevier.)

least 5 minutes, and the medical assistant would not have access to all of the patient's benefit information unless he or she spoke to a member services agent, which would take even more time. Today, most privately sponsored health insurance plans have offered online insurance provider portals, which allow for quick and easy verification of eligibility (Fig. 23.2). The healthcare facility will have to apply for access to the online web portal. Once it has been approved, patient benefits can be looked up in their entirety in seconds instead of minutes. Information on a patient's benefit plan can be uploaded to the electronic health record (EHR) very quickly; this process reduces the use of paper in the healthcare facility.

OTHER TYPES OF INSURANCE

When you work in a healthcare facility, the most common type of insurance you will see is health insurance. However, there are other types of insurance that can require the involvement of a healthcare provider. These other types of insurance will be discussed below.

Disability Insurance

Disability insurance is a form of insurance that provides income replacement if the patient has a disability that is not work related. The disability means that the employee is unable to perform his or her work functions or duties. It could involve either short-term disability or long-term disability benefits. Both provide 40% to 70% of the individual's predisability income. Many employers offer a disability policy to their employees. Generally, the employee pays the monthly premium. These policies can also be purchased by an individual.

Short-term disability means that a person is unable to work for 9 to 52 weeks. Long-term disability policies pick up when short-term benefits are exhausted. Long-term disability coverage will pay out until the patient returns to work or for the number of years specified in the

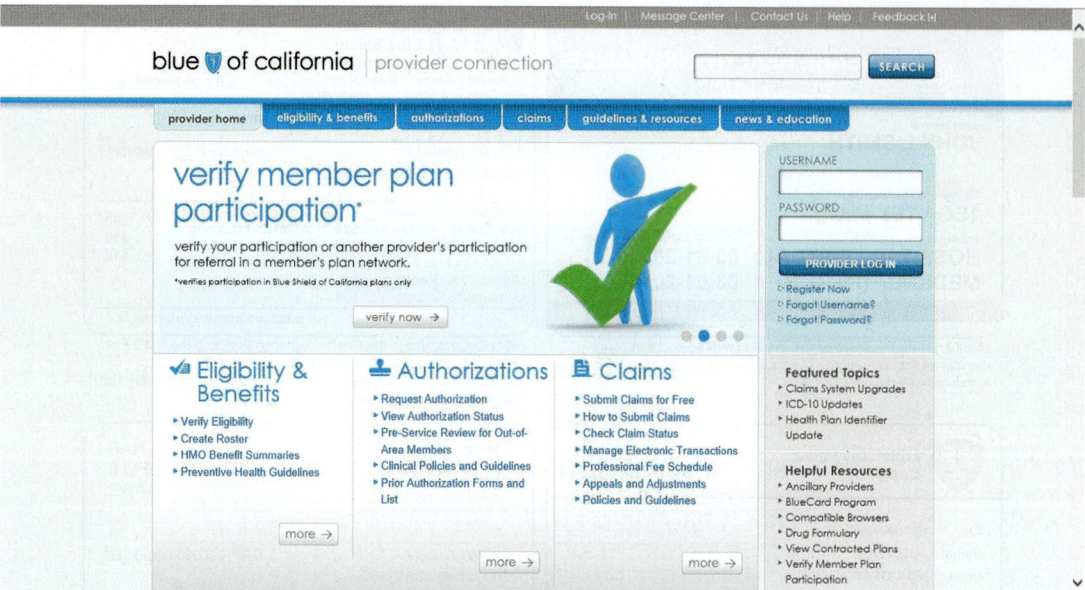

FIG. 23.2 A provider's web portal for online health insurance. (From Fordney MT: *Insurance Handbook for The Medical Office,* ed 14, St Louis, 2017, Elsevier.)

policy. Some policies will pay out until the patient reaches the age of 65 and then is eligible for Social Security benefits. There may be a *waiting period* before benefits can be paid. Sick time can be used for the waiting period days.

Weekly or monthly cash benefits are provided to employed policyholders who become unable to work as a result of an accident or illness. The accident or illness must not be related to work, because that would be covered under workers' compensation. Payments are made directly to the insured and are intended to replace lost income resulting from an illness or other disability. Disability payments are not intended for payment of specific medical bills, and a disability insurance policy should not be confused with a regular health insurance plan.

The medical office may be involved in the examination of the patient to determine the level of disability and when the disability ends. There are forms that must be completed by a healthcare provider and then submitted to the insurance carrier.

Life Insurance

Life insurance provides payment of a specified amount, upon the insured's death, either to his or her estate or to a designated *beneficiary*. Annuity life insurance policies provide monthly cash benefits if the policyholder becomes permanently and totally disabled. Sometimes the proceeds from life insurance are used to meet the expenses of the insured person's last illness.

The healthcare facility may be required to complete physical examination forms when a patient is applying for life insurance. If there is an annuity policy, the healthcare provider may have to determine if there is a permanent disability and submit documentation.

Long-Term Care Insurance

Long-term care insurance is a relatively new type of insurance that covers a broad range of maintenance and health services for chronically ill, disabled, or developmentally delayed individuals. Medical services may be provided on an inpatient basis (e.g., at a rehabilitation facility, nursing home, or mental hospital), on an outpatient basis, or at home.

Liability Insurance

Liability insurance covers losses to a third party caused by the insured. There are many types of liability insurance, including automobile, business, and homeowners' policies. Liability policies often include benefits for:

- medical expenses resulting from traumatic injuries
- lost wages
- sometimes pain and suffering

All liability insurance policies are payable to victims injured by the insured person's home or car, without regard to the insured person's actual legal liability for the accident.

THE AFFORDABLE CARE ACT

In the early 2000s it became clear that a large number of Americans lacked basic health insurance. *Preexisting conditions* made it difficult for Americans who did not work full time or were self-employed to obtain health insurance. In addition, the health insurance market was discriminating against young adults 18 years or older, who may not have been qualified to receive health benefits because they could not find full-time employment.

In 2010 the Patient Protection and Affordable Care Act, also known as the *Affordable Care Act* (also Obamacare), was enacted. It increased the quality, availability, and affordability of private and public health insurance for more than 44 million uninsured Americans. The legislation includes new qualifying regulations, taxes, mandates, and subsidies. The federal mandate not only opens opportunities for more Americans to obtain affordable health insurance, but also works to reduce overall healthcare spending in the long run. Other patient protections and provisions under the Affordable Care Act include:

VOCABULARY

beneficiary: A designated person who receives funds from an insurance policy.
waiting period: The length of time a patient waits for disability insurance to pay after the date of injury.

- Insurance companies are prohibited from dropping patient health coverage if the individual gets sick or makes an unintentional mistake on the health insurance application.
- It eliminates preexisting conditions and gender discrimination, so patients cannot be charged more based on their health status or gender.
- Young adults can remain on their parent's or guardian's insurance policy until age 26.
- It creates *health insurance marketplaces,* where low- to middle-income Americans can compare plans and lower their costs on healthcare coverage.
- States will expand Medicaid coverage to 15.9 million Americans to include those who qualify for cost assistance through the marketplace.
- Individuals seeking health insurance can apply only during the open enrollment period, which is established by each state.

With more Americans having health insurance, the number of office visits to providers across the country is expected to increase. Thus, efficient health insurance management policies should be instituted to meet the new demand for services.

> **EXCEPTIONAL CUSTOMER SERVICE**
>
> It is important for patients to understand how their insurance plan works. Many people, especially the elderly, believe that if they have health insurance, all charges for their health care will be paid for. To provide excellent customer service, a medical assistant should have a basic understanding of the insurance policies seen most often in the healthcare facility. That way, you can answer questions from patients about their benefits and exclusions. Often healthcare facilities provide their patients with a brochure that explains how health insurance and reimbursement work. The brochures often also provide patients with definitions of some of the more common terms used in the insurance claims process. If patients are well advised and comfortable with insurance facts before treatment begins, the medical experience will go more smoothly, and the collection of the amount owed will be easier. The medical assistant must practice good communication skills, patience, and tact when discussing reimbursement and financial responsibilities with patients.

CLOSING COMMENTS

Health insurance and benefits coverage can be confusing to the patient. Medical assistants should educate themselves on the specific details of all plans accepted at the healthcare facility. Managed care has often been criticized in the media for its cost-saving practices. Extra efforts made by medical assistants to overcome these challenges and educate their patients on how to use their health insurance plans will improve the quality of care delivered to their patients. Providers and healthcare facilities need to evaluate their ability to accept the fee schedule of insurance plans they are contracted with, especially since Medicaid's fee schedule is the lowest in the industry.

CHAPTER REVIEW

Most patients who visit a provider are covered by some type of insurance plan. The insurance coverage could be from a government plan such as:

- Medicare
- Medicaid
- CHIP
- TRICARE
- CHAMPVA
- Workers' compensation

It could also be from a private health insurance plan from either an employer group plan or a privately purchased plan. Wherever the coverage is from, it is important for a medical assistant to be familiar with the plans commonly seen in the healthcare facility.

There are basically two different health insurance models, traditional and managed care. Within managed care there are several types, including:

- HMOs
- PPOs
- EPOs

Managed care organizations use utilization management/utilization review to help contain the cost of providing healthcare coverage.

Providers who have a contract with a health insurance plan are considered PAR providers and must honor the contracted fee schedule. This means that they will write off the difference between their billed amount and the contracted allowed amount. This reduces the out-of-pocket expenses for the patient.

Medical assistants are responsible for verifying whether or not patients are eligible for insurance coverage. This can be done by using online resources, such as a provider's web portal, or by calling the insurance carrier. Medical assistants should also be able to interpret the information found on a patient's insurance identification card.

SCENARIO WRAP-UP

Although he was initially nervous about explaining fees to patients and asking for payment, Jon has become more comfortable in doing this aspect of his job, because he now understands the business aspect of the practice. Patients understand that providers must charge for their services and have become accustomed to copayments and co-insurance amounts. Many times these fees are collected in advance, before the patient sees the provider. This practice saves time on checkout, and most patients believe that the copay is a small cost compared with the entire fee that providers charge to manage their care in one office visit.

Jon has noticed that the usual, customary, and reasonable fees that Dr. Crawford, a member of the practice, charges his patients directly affect the reimbursements that are paid by various insurance and managed care companies. Jon has attended several health insurance billing seminars sponsored by Medicare and Blue Cross/Blue Shield, and he believes that this extra training has resulted in a drop in health insurance claim rejections at WMFM.

24

Diagnostic Coding Basics

LEARNING OBJECTIVES

1. Discuss diagnostic coding, explain where diagnostic statements are found, and define medical necessity as it applies to diagnostic coding.
2. Identify the structure and format of the ICD-10-CM.
3. Describe how to use the Alphabetic Index to select main terms, essential modifiers, nonessential modifiers, and the appropriate code (or codes) and code ranges.
4. Do the following related to the Tabular List:
   - Explain how to use the Tabular List to select main terms, essential modifiers, nonessential modifiers, and the appropriate code (or codes) and code ranges.
   - List and discuss the conventions used in the Tabular List.
   - Summarize coding conventions as defined in the ICD-10-CM coding manual.
5. Explain how to abstract diagnostic statements from the patient's health record.
6. List the eight basic steps required for accurate ICD-10-CM coding, and perform coding using the current ICD-10-CM manual or an encoder.
7. Explain the importance of coding guidelines for accuracy, and discuss special rules and considerations that apply to the code selection process.
8. Discuss the importance of maximizing third-party reimbursement, and use tactful communication skills with medical providers to ensure accurate code selection.

CHAPTER OUTLINE

1. Opening Scenario, 532
2. You Will Learn, 533
3. Introduction, 533
4. What Is Diagnostic Coding?, 533
5. Getting to Know the ICD-10-CM, 533
   a. Structure and Format of the ICD-10-CM, 533
   b. The Alphabetic Index, 534
      i. *Supplementary Sections of the Alphabetic Index*, 535
   c. The Tabular List, 536
      i. *Conventions Used in the Tabular List*, 536
6. Preparing for Diagnostic Coding, 538
   a. Abstracting Diagnostic Statements, 538
      i. *Encounter Form*, 538
      ii. *History and Physical Exam*, 538
      iii. *Progress Notes*, 538
      iv. *Discharge Summary*, 538
      v. *Operative Report*, 539
      vi. *Radiology, Laboratory, and Pathology Reports*, 539
7. Steps in ICD-10-CM Coding, 539
   a. Using the Alphabetic Index, 539
   b. Using the Tabular List, 542
   c. Encoder Software, 542
8. Understanding Coding Guidelines, 543
   a. Coding of Signs and Symptoms, 543
   b. Coding the Etiology and Manifestation, 543
   c. Coding Organism-Caused Diseases, 543
   d. Coding Human Immunodeficiency Virus (HIV) Infection and Acquired Immunodeficiency Syndrome (AIDS), 543
   e. Coding Neoplasms, 544
      i. *Six Steps for Coding Neoplasms*, 545
   f. Coding for Diabetes Mellitus, 545
   g. Coding for Complications of Pregnancy, Childbirth, and the Puerperium, 545
   h. Coding for Burns and Corrosions, 545
   i. Coding for External Causes of Morbidity, 546
   j. Place of Occurrence Guideline, 546
   k. Activity Codes, 546
   l. Coding for Health Status and Contact with Health Services, 546
9. Maximizing Third-Party Reimbursement, 546
10. Providers and Accurate Coding, 546
11. Closing Comments, 547
12. Chapter Review, 547
13. Scenario Wrap-Up, 547

 OPENING SCENARIO

Mike Simeone, a recent medical assistant graduate, excelled in his diagnostic coding course. Recently, he found an entry-level coding position at the Walden-Martin Family Medicine Clinic (WMFM).

Mike is a little nervous but also excited about starting ICD-10-CM coding. Mike has used encoder software in some of his classes, which helped him determine the most specific and accurate code. Mike noticed that the new software update in the medical office has the most recent ICD-10-CM codes.

CHAPTER 24 Diagnostic Coding Basics

Mike has had some previous experience working in health records, which gives him a strong understanding of the importance of accurate, quality documentation. He knows where to look to find diagnostic statements in providers' orders, treatment plans, progress notes, surgical reports, and other medical reports.

YOU WILL LEARN

- How the format, layout, and conventions of the ICD-10-CM manual help the medical assistant locate the most accurate and specific diagnostic code.
- To identify the diagnostic statement from various sources.
- To apply coding guidelines to coding situations that are seen in the healthcare facility.

INTRODUCTION

A *diagnosis* (dahy uh g NOH sis) has many purposes in health care. Patient treatment plans are based on the diagnosis. *Reimbursement* (ree im BURS ment) from insurance companies is based, in part, on the diagnosis. Researchers use diagnoses for their studies. Diagnostic coding has been used to standardize diagnoses. It was initially developed to study causes of *mortality*. Over time, diagnostic coding has been expanded to include all diseases and conditions. The World Health Organization (WHO) has established the International Classification of Diseases. This classification system is in its tenth revision and is known as the International Classification of Diseases, Tenth Revision, Clinical Modification (ICD-10-CM). These codes are used for:

- mortality data
- *epidemiological* (ep i dee mee o LOJ i kuh l) data
- billing purposes

The ICD-10-CM allows providers to be much more specific in diagnostic coding than was possible with previous revisions. This will, in turn, result in more accurate data collection and billing practices. Every year the Centers for Medicare and Medicaid Services (CMS) reviews the ICD-10-CM coding manual. The update is published on October 1. Additions, revisions, and deletions are made to many of the diagnostic codes, code descriptions, and guidelines. *You must always use the current year's coding manual to ensure accurate coding and to comply with regulatory guidelines.*

The Health Insurance Portability and Accountability Act (HIPAA) has mandated that specific code sets be used to help standardize the process of claims submission. The ICD-10-CM is the mandated diagnostic code set.

In this chapter we will look at the structure of the ICD-10-CM codes and how to accurately determine the correct code.

WHAT IS DIAGNOSTIC CODING?

Diagnostic coding changes written descriptions of diseases, illnesses, or injuries into alphanumeric codes. The ICD-10-CM code set uses up to seven characters to identify the disease or injury. Using the ICD-10-CM can help ensure both accurate health record documentation and efficient claims processing.

The ICD-10-CM code set is available through online resources, within the electronic health record (EHR) as an *encoder*, or as a print manual. The print manual is produced by several publishers and may use different layouts, symbols, color coding, and some other features. For the coding manual, however, the format, conventions, tables, appendices, content, and basic structure are the same.

When you use the ICD-10-CM, you will be choosing a standardized alphanumeric code for the *diagnostic statement* assigned by the provider. Diagnostic statements are found in:

- operative reports
- discharge summaries
- history and physical exam (H&P) reports
- reports on *ancillary diagnostic services* (e.g., radiology, pathology, and laboratory reports)

All of these should provide the patient's diagnosis or diagnoses. These reports are used by healthcare providers to code and report clinical information. Diagnostic coding is required for participation in Medicare and Medicaid programs and by most insurance companies. The diagnostic codes are used on insurance claims. The ICD-10-CM codes tell the insurance company why the procedures were done. These codes are linked to the procedures that are performed. This linking can determine if a procedure or service is paid for. The diagnostic code can show that a procedure or service was *medically necessary*. If it was not medically necessary, the insurance company will not pay for it. The ICD-10-CM is also used to keep track of various healthcare statistics related to disease and injury. Practice management software, clearinghouses, and insurance companies recognize these codes, which simplifies the coding process and speeds reimbursement to healthcare providers.

GETTING TO KNOW THE ICD-10-CM

Structure and Format of the ICD-10-CM

The ICD-10-CM has two sections:
- Alphabetic Index (the ICD-10-CM Index to Diseases and Injuries)
- Tabular List (officially, the ICD-10-CM Tabular List of Diseases and Injuries)

Determining an ICD-10-CM code starts in the Alphabetic Index and is confirmed in the Tabular List. These codes have three to seven characters (Fig. 24.1). Every ICD-10-CM code begins with an alphabetic letter that indicates the chapter in the Tabular List from which the code originates (Table 24.1). All the letters of the English alphabet are used except U, which WHO has reserved to assign to new diseases of uncertain *etiology* (ee tee OL uh jee). Some conditions use more than one alphabetic letter

---

VOCABULARY

diagnosis: Determining the cause of a condition, illness, disease, injury, or congenital defect.

diagnostic statement: Information about a patient's diagnosis or diagnoses that has been taken from the medical documentation.

encoder: Software that will apply diagnostic or procedure codes to medical conditions or procedures.

epidemiological: The branch of medicine dealing with the incidence, distribution, and control of disease in a population. It also involves the prevalence of disease in large populations, in addition to detection of the source and cause of epidemics of infectious disease.

etiology: The study of the causes or origin of diseases.

medically necessary: Accepted healthcare services that are appropriate for the evaluation and treatment of a disease, condition, illness, or injury, and are consistent with the applicable standard of care.

mortality: The relative frequency of deaths in a specific population.

reimbursement: To make repayment for an expense or a loss incurred.

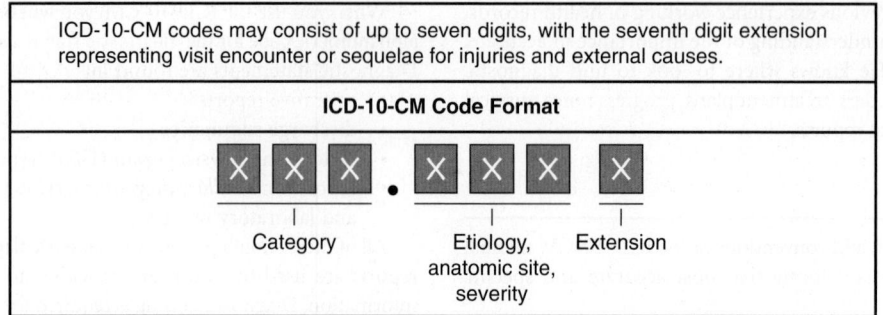

FIG. 24.1 Code structure and format of ICD-10-CM codes. (From Proctor D, Niedzwiecki B: *Kinn's The Medical Assistant*, ed 13, St Louis, 2017, Elsevier.)

TABLE 24.1 ICD-10-CM Tabular List of Diseases and Injuries

Chapter	Title	Code Range	Possible Diagnosis[a]	ICD-10-CM Code
1	Certain Infectious and Parasitic Diseases	A00–B99	Measles	B05.9
2	Neoplasms	C00–D49	Colon cancer	C18.9
3	Diseases of the Blood and Blood-Forming Organs, and Certain Disorders Involving the Immune Mechanism	D50–D89	Iron-deficiency anemia	D50.9
4	Endocrine, Nutritional, and Metabolic Diseases	E00–E89	Type I diabetes	E10
5	Mental, Behavioral, and Neurodevelopmental Disorders	F01–F99	Dementia	F03
6	Diseases of the Nervous System	G00–G99	Parkinson's disease	G20
7	Diseases of the Eye and Adnexa	H00–H59	Glaucoma	H40.9
8	Diseases of the Ear and Mastoid Process	H60–H95	Otitis media, left ear	H60.92
9	Diseases of the Circulatory System	I00–I99	Hypertensive heart disease	I11.9
10	Diseases of the Respiratory System	J00–J99	Acute sinusitis	J01.91
11	Diseases of the Digestive System	K00–K95	Inguinal hernia	K40
12	Diseases of the Skin and Subcutaneous Tissue	L00–L99	Pressure ulcer of right heel	L89.619
13	Diseases of the Musculoskeletal System and Connective Tissue	M00–M99	Rheumatoid arthritis	M05
14	Diseases of the Genitourinary System	N00–N99	Endometriosis	N80.9
15	Pregnancy, Childbirth, and the Puerperium	O00–O94	Ectopic pregnancy	O00.9
16	Certain Conditions Originating in the Perinatal Period	P00–P96	Neonatal jaundice	P59.9
17	Congenital Malformations, Deformations, and Chromosomal Abnormalities	Q00–Q99	Cleft lip	Q37.9
18	Symptoms, Signs, and Abnormal Clinical and Laboratory Findings, Not Elsewhere Classified	R00–R99	Abdominal pain	R10.9
19	Injury, Poisoning, and Certain Other Consequences of External Causes	S00–T88	Left ankle fracture	S82.92xA
20	External Causes of Morbidity	V00–Y99	Snowboard accident	V00.318A
			Fall from cliff	W15
			Exposure to excessive natural cold	X31
21	Factors Influencing Health Status and Contact With Health Services	Z00–Z99	Pregnancy state	Z33.1

[a]All diagnoses presented are not otherwise specified (NOS).

in their code ranges. For example, the codes in Chapter 1, Certain Infectious and Parasitic Diseases (A00–B99), begin with the letter A or B. The second character is always numeric. The remaining characters can be a combination of letters and numbers. A decimal is required after the third character. There are only certain codes that require the 7th character. Box 24.1 describes the 7th character requirements in more detail.

The CMS prepares the Official Guidelines for Coding and Reporting to be used with the ICD-10-CM codes, in addition to instructions on how to report the codes on insurance claim forms. The guidelines are a set of rules that have been developed to accompany and complement the official conventions and instructions provided in the ICD-10-CM proper.

The Alphabetic Index

The Alphabetic Index consists of an alphabetic list of diagnostic terms and related codes. This index includes main terms, nonessential modifiers, essential modifiers, and subterms:

- *Main terms:* These terms appear in bold type.
- *Nonessential modifiers:* These terms follow the main term and are enclosed in parentheses. They are supplementary words or explanatory information. They do not need to be in the actual diagnostic statement.
- *Essential modifiers:* These terms are indented under the main term. They can modify the main term by describing different sites or etiology. They must be included in the diagnostic statement.

Fig. 24.2 shows an example of an entry in the Alphabetic Index:
- the main term
- nonessential modifiers
- essential modifiers

Let's use the example of chronic ischemic (ih SKEE mick) colitis (koh LYE tis). You would start with the main term: Colitis. You can see that the main term is followed by the nonessential modifiers (acute, catarrhal, chronic, noninfective, hemorrhagic) that do not affect the code assignment. Follow the list to the modifying term: Ischemic. Indented under ischemic, you will find "chronic" with the code K55.1. You will look up K55.1 in the Tabular List.

> **MEDICAL TERMINOLOGY**
> **isch/o:** to hold back
> **-emic:** pertaining to blood condition
> **col/o:** colon
> **-itis:** inflammation

> **BOX 24.1   ICD-10-CM 7th Character Requirements**
>
> Seventh characters are used for many ICD-10-CM codes. The following list shows the chapters that require a 7th character, and also what the character identifies.
> - Chapter 13: Diseases of the Musculoskeletal System – Encounter
> - Chapter 15: Pregnancy, Childbirth and the Puerperium – Fetus identification
> - Chapter 18: Symptoms, Signs, and Abnormal Clinical and Laboratory Findings, Not Elsewhere Classified – Coma Scale
> - Chapter 19: Injury, Poisoning, and Certain Other Consequences of External Causes – Encounter
> - Chapter 20: External Causes of Morbidity – Encounter
> - Chapter 21: Factors Influencing Health Status and Contact with Health Services – Encounter
>
> As you can see, this character most often indicates the encounter type. The most letters used for an encounter type are A, D, and S:
> - A: Initial encounter
> - D: Subsequent encounter
> - S: *Sequela,* complications or conditions that occur as a direct result of a condition

> **CRITICAL THINKING BOX 24.1**
>
> Mike is working with the ICD-10-CM manual and is trying to refresh his memory about nonessential and essential modifiers. In your own words, define an essential modifier and a nonessential modifier. Compare your definitions with those of a classmate.

> **VOCABULARY**
> **chronic:** Developing slowly and lasting for a long time, generally 3 or more months.

Supplementary Sections of the Alphabetic Index. The Alphabetic Index section includes two important tables.
- *Table of Neoplasms:* This table lists neoplasms by anatomical location. For coding purposes, neoplasms are further classified into six categories:
  - Malignant Primary
  - Malignant Secondary
  - Ca (cancer) in situ

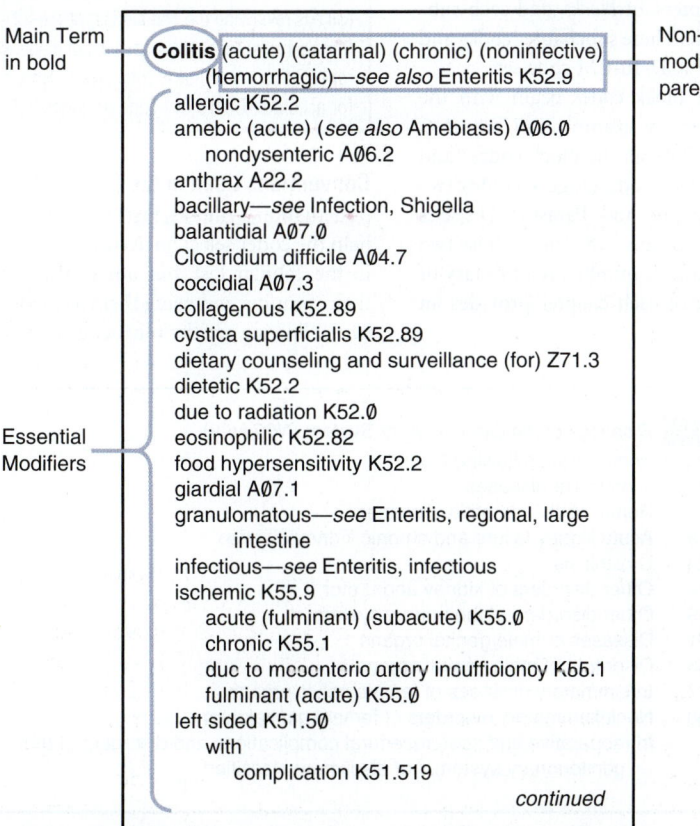

FIG. 24.2 ICD-10-CM Alphabetic Index with main term, nonessential modifiers, and essential modifiers.

- Benign
- Uncertain Behavior
- Unspecified Behavior
- *Table of Drugs and Chemicals:* This table presents a classification of drugs and other chemical substances; it is used to identify poisonings and external causes of adverse effects. The six coding classifications are:
  - Poisoning, Accidental (Unintentional)
  - Poisoning, Intentional Self-Harm
  - Poisoning, Assault
  - Poisoning, Undetermined
  - Adverse Effect
  - Underdosing

The Tabular List

The Tabular List is divided into 21 chapters. Most chapter titles specify a particular group of diseases and injuries, and all titles are followed by a code range in parentheses; for example, Chapter 1, Certain Infectious and Parasitic Diseases (A00–B99) (see Table 24.1). Some chapters use a body part or an organ system to group the codes; for example:
- Chapter 7, Diseases of the Eye and Adnexa (H00–H59)
- Chapter 9, Diseases of the Circulatory System (I00–I99)

Other chapters group conditions by etiology or the nature of the disease process; for example:
- Chapter 2, Neoplasms (C00–D49)
- Chapter 15, Pregnancy, Childbirth, and the Puerperium (O00–O94) – groups codes related to the prenatal and postnatal periods
- Chapter 20, External Causes of Morbidity (V00–Y99) – also groups codes related to external causes of injury and poisoning
- Chapter 21, Factors Influencing Health Status and Contact With Health Services (Z00–Z99).

Each chapter is divided into subchapters, or *blocks*, and each subchapter has a designated 3-character code. These subchapter codes and code ranges form the foundation of the ICD-10-CM code set.

In each chapter, all the 3-character block codes begin with the alphabetic letter assigned to that chapter. For example, in Chapter 6, Diseases of the Nervous System (G00–G99), all the block codes (and their versions) begin with G. If a chapter's code range includes two letters [e.g., Chapter 1, Certain Infectious and Parasitic Diseases (A00–B99)], each 3-character block code begins with one of those two letters. The letter is followed by a 2-character number. A summary of the blocks (Fig. 24.3) at the beginning of each chapter provides an overview of the chapter.

As mentioned, the ICD-10-CM manual is produced by a variety of publishers, but many of the optional features are similar (remember, the important elements are always the same, regardless of the publisher). For instance, to enable the coder to better maneuver through the Alphabetic Index, each page has *guide words*, which are the first and last words on that page (this is the same arrangement used for the pages of a dictionary). Each chapter of the Tabular List has a different-colored border strip; in some manuals, this strip shows the chapter title and the range of codes found on that specific page. In the chapters in the Tabular List, the codes for each category/block are arranged alphabetically (by the initial alpha character) and then numerically. Familiarizing yourself with these tools can help you improve your proficiency as you work through the manual to find the most accurate code.

It is important to note that some codes do not need to be extended beyond the 3-character code, and these are considered valid codes as is; for example, code **I10** {**Essential (primary) hypertension**}. If a code has only three characters, do not add a decimal after the 3rd character. If a code has more than three characters, add a decimal point after the 3rd character; for example, **K11.7** {**Disturbances of salivary secretion**}. Most ICD-10-CM codes have 4 to 7 characters (Box 24.2).

> **MEDICAL TERMINOLOGY**
> **sinus/o:** sinus
> **-itis:** inflammation

> **VOCABULARY**
> **specificity:** The quality or state of being specific.

> **CRITICAL THINKING BOX 24.2**
>
> Mike is reviewing the Tabular List of the ICD-10-CM coding manual. He notices that each chapter begins with a list of diagnostic categories with a corresponding range of codes. What is this called? How can this feature be used as a tool for accurate ICD-10-CM code assignment?

Conventions Used in the Tabular List. *Conventions* are abbreviations, punctuation, symbols, instructional notations, and related entities that help the coder select an accurate, specific code. Conventions are found in the Tabular List, but not in the Alphabetic Index. Understanding their meaning and using them as guides are crucial to accurate coding. The following are the most common conventions.

Chapter 14	*Diseases of the Genitourinary System (N00-N99)*
	This chapter contains the following blocks:
N00-N08	Glomerular diseases
N10-N16	Renal tubulo-interstitial diseases
N17-N19	Acute kidney failure and chronic kidney disease
N20-N23	Urolithiasis
N25-N29	Other disorders of kidney and ureter
N30-N39	Other disorders of the urinary system
N40-N51	Diseases of male genital organs
N60-N65	Disorders of male genital organs
N70-N77	Inflammatory diseases of female pelvic organs
N80-N98	Noninflammatory disorders of female genital tract
N99	Intraoperative and postprocedural complications and disorders of the genitourinary system, not elsewhere classified

FIG. 24.3 Chapter blocks in the Tabular List. (From Proctor D, Niedzwiecki B: *Kinn's The Medical Assistant*, ed 13, St Louis, 2017, Elsevier.)

CHAPTER 24   Diagnostic Coding Basics

BOX 24.2   Reporting NEC and NOS Codes

In some cases, because of limited documentation in the patient's health record, the medical assistant coder can find it difficult to assign an ICD-10-CM code with a higher **specificity** (spes uh FIS i tee). The ICD-10-CM code set accommodates these coding circumstances by establishing "not elsewhere classified" (NEC) and "not otherwise specified" (NOS) guidelines.

- *NEC* means that the diagnostic statement contains specific wording, but no specific classification exists to match the wording. For example, an NEC code would be assigned if a patient seeks medical attention for chronic postoperative pain. The ICD-10-CM code would be **G89.28 {Other chronic postprocedural pain}**. For all NEC codes, the last character is always 8.

- *NOS* means that the diagnostic statement does not contain any more specific wording. For example, **sinusitis** (sye nuh SYE tis) with no documentation of the specific sinus site is assigned the NOS code **J32.9 {Chronic sinusitis, unspecified}**. The coder should keep in mind that the lack of documentation does not mean that all the patient's sinuses are inflamed. There must be no documentation of the exact site of the sinusitis for a non-NOS code to be assigned. As providers recognize that ICD-10-CM codes are more specific than ICD-9-CM codes, their documentation also is becoming more specific. For all NOS codes, the last character is always 9.

Convention	Explanation	Example
Placeholder Character	ICD-10-CM uses the dummy placeholder X in two different ways. The dummy placeholder can be used as the 5th character in certain six-character codes; this allows for future expansion of the code set without interruption of the six-character structure.	T43.4X1A Poisoning by butyrophenone and thiothixene neuroleptics, accidental, initial encounter (unintentional)
	Specific categories have a 7th character, but may not use the 4th, 5th, or 6th characters. In these cases, the dummy placeholder X is used to fill the empty character spaces. Note that a dummy placeholder would not be needed for codes with less than 7 characters.	S50.01XA Contusion of right elbow
Punctuation	Four basic forms of punctuation are used in the Tabular List: brackets, parentheses, colons, and braces. Each form serves a different purpose to help you read and understand the code descriptions.	[ ] Brackets enclose synonyms, alternative wording, or explanatory phrases ( ) Parentheses are used to enclose supplementary words, which may be present or absent in the statement of a disease or procedure : Colons are used in the Tabular Index after an incomplete term that needs one or more of the modifiers or adjectives that follow to make it assignable { } Braces enclose a series of terms, each of which is modified by the statement appearing to the right of the brace
Instructional Notations	Instructional notations, which are found in both the Alphabetic Index and the Tabular List, are critical to correct coding practices. They are located directly under the main term.	**Includes**: further defines or gives examples of the content of the category **Excludes**: The ICD-10-CM uses two types of exclusion notes: Excludes1: This is a clear "NOT CODED HERE!" message. It means that the excluded code should never be used with the code above the Excludes1 note. For example, code **G14 {Postpolio syndrome}**, has this Excludes1 note: **sequelae** (si KWEL uh) of poliomyelitis (B91). Excludes2: This means "not included here." The excluded condition is not part of the condition represented by the code; however, a patient may have both conditions. When an Excludes2 note is present, the coder may code both conditions if the patient presents with both. For example, code F02 {**Dementia** (dih MEN shah) in other diseases classified elsewhere} has the following Excludes2 note: **vascular** (VAS kyoo lur) **dementia** (F01.5). This means that vascular dementia is not part of the condition coded as F02; therefore, you can code both dementia (F02) and vascular dementia (F01.5) if the patient has both. **Code first/Use additional code**: *Code first* notes appear under *manifestation* codes. Manifestation codes specify the way in which an underlying condition appears, or manifests, as a result of an underlying etiology; the main terms of most manifestation codes include the words "in diseases classified elsewhere." A *Code first* note indicates that the underlying condition must be coded first. For example, Code F02 {Dementia in other diseases classified elsewhere} states, Code first the underlying physiological condition, such as: Alzheimer's (G30.-)

Continued

Convention	Explanation	Example
Relational Terms	These terms are used in both the Alphabetic Index and the Tabular List to clarify the context of the disease or injury.	• *And:* In the Tabular List code titles, *and* should be interpreted as meaning "and/or." • *With:* The term *with* should be interpreted as meaning "associated with" or "due to" when it appears in the Alphabetic Index, or in an instructional note or code title in the Tabular List. In the Alphabetic Index, the word *with* follows immediately after the main term, not in alphabetical order. • *Due to:* In both the Tabular List and the Alphabetic Index, the term *due to* signifies relationship between two conditions. This assumption can be made when both conditions are present or when the diagnostic statement indicates this relationship.

CRITICAL THINKING BOX 24.3

Mike is looking for the ICD-10-CM code for morbid obesity. From the Alphabetic Index, Mike finds the code E66. When he goes to verify the code in the Tabular List, he finds that the main term, Overweight and obesity, has a symbol indicating that a 4th character is needed. What is Mike's next step to assign the most accurate code? Can Mike just use E66? Why or why not? Share your answer with the class.

PREPARING FOR DIAGNOSTIC CODING

Now that you have a basic understanding of the ICD-10-CM system, let's take a look at how you find the information you need to determine diagnostic codes.

Abstracting Diagnostic Statements

To prepare for diagnostic coding, you must analyze the patient's health record and **abstract** the diagnostic statement documented in the various reports. Sources of diagnostic statements include the encounter form, treatment notes, discharge summary, operative report, and radiology, pathology, and laboratory reports. Let's take a look at those documents.

Encounter Form. The **encounter form** (also known as a *superbill*) can be viewed in the EHR or as a paper document. The most commonly used diagnostic and procedure codes are listed. The provider then indicates what services and/or procedures were done and the diagnosis code for the visit. It is important to update the encounter form with the new diagnostic and procedure codes. If outdated codes are used, it can delay or reduce the amount paid by the insurance company.

History and Physical Exam. The history and physical exam are the starting point of the patient's medical evaluation. The H&P begins with a statement in the patient's own words that describes the reason for the visit. This statement, called the *chief complaint (CC)*, is often abbreviated in the history documentation in the health record. After the chief complaint, the provider documents any other pertinent history:
- Medical, current illness and past medical history
  - History of present illness (HPI)
  - Previous illnesses
  - Previous hospitalizations
  - Previous surgeries
- Family history
  - Family members
    - Current ages
    - If deceased, age at death
    - Any medical conditions
- Social history
  - Tobacco use
  - Alcohol use
  - Drug use

After recording the patient's history, the provider performs a physical examination. This includes both objective and subjective assessments of the patient's physical status. The final sections of an H&P include an assessment and a plan. The assessment is the provider's evaluation of the findings from the H&P, and it includes a diagnostic statement. The plan is the treatment plan for the conditions noted in the assessment; it may include x-ray studies, laboratory tests, surgery, administration of medications, or other treatments.

Progress Notes. Progress notes are the second most common medical document from which diagnostic statements can be extracted. The format healthcare providers most commonly use for their notes is *SOAP notes*, a system of charting in which information is divided into subjective findings, objective findings, assessment, and plan for treatment. Just as in the H&P, the diagnostic statement can most often be found in the assessment section of the SOAP notes.

Discharge Summary. The discharge summary is used primarily for abstracting diagnostic information for patients who were hospitalized,

VOCABULARY

abstract: Collecting important information from the health record.
dementia: A mental disorder in which the individual experiences a progressive loss of memory, personality alterations, confusion, loss of touch with reality, and stupor (seeming unawareness of, and disconnection with, one's surroundings).
encounter form: A document used to capture the services/procedures and diagnoses for a patient visit. The fees for the services/procedures are usually included on the encounter form.
sequela (singular), **sequelae** (plural)**:** An abnormal condition resulting from a previous disease.

MEDICAL TERMINOLOGY

vascul/o: vessel
-ar: pertaining to

rather than those seen in a provider's office. The main elements of a discharge summary are:
- admission date
- date of discharge
- H&P findings
- clinical course during hospitalization
- health condition on discharge
- discharge diagnosis
- aftercare plan.

Diagnostic statements are abstracted from the discharge diagnosis section. This diagnosis would be used to bill for the provider's visits to the patient while the person was in the hospital. The medical office can use a discharge summary as an overview of the patient's condition, especially if the discharge was recent.

Operative Report. For patients who have surgery as an outpatient or inpatient, the operative report also is used to abstract diagnostic statements. An operative report includes:
- preliminary diagnosis
- final diagnosis
- detailed description of the operative procedure from start to finish

The medical assistant uses the final diagnosis when searching for and selecting a diagnostic code.

Radiology, Laboratory, and Pathology Reports. Radiology, laboratory, and pathology reports are used to support and/or establish the diagnostic statement. Any findings from these reports must be documented in the progress notes in the health record so that they can be used for diagnostic coding, charge entry, or insurance billing purposes.

CRITICAL THINKING BOX 24.4

While reviewing an encounter form, Mike notices that the diagnostic statement indicated that the patient needed to be treated for a left inguinal (IN gwin null) **hernia** (HER nee ah). However, Mike also notes that the surgical report indicates that the left inguinal hernia was obstructed. What should Mike use as the final diagnostic statement? Should he ask the provider which diagnostic statement to use?

MEDICAL TERMINOLOGY

inguin/o: groin
-al: pertaining to

VOCABULARY

hernia: protrusion of a loop of intestine through a weakness in the abdominal wall.

STEPS IN ICD-10-CM CODING

Accurate ICD-10-CM coding requires eight basic steps (Table 24.2). The first step involves abstracting the diagnostic statement from the health record and figuring out the main and modifying terms. Use the Alphabetic Index to search for the code or code ranges that best fit the diagnostic statement. The remaining steps are performed using the Tabular List to verify and confirm that the code or codes located in the Alphabetic Index fully match the diagnostic statement and that they are the most specific and accurate diagnostic codes. Procedure 24.1

TABLE 24.2 Diagnostic Coding Step-by-Step: Parkinson's Disease

Step 1	• Determine the correct diagnosis from the diagnostic statement. Parkinson's Disease
Step 2	• Use the main term to look up the diagnosis in the Alphabetic Index. **Parkinson's disease, syndrome or tremor**—see Parkinsonism
Step 3	• Look up the "see" term in the Alphabetic Index. **Parkinsonism** (idiopathic) (primary) G20

Step 4	• Review the essential modifiers under the main term.
	Parkinsonism (idiopathic) (primary) G20
	  with neurogenic orthostatic hypotension (symptomatic) G90.3
	  arteriosclerotic G21.4
	  dementia G31.83 [F02.80]
	    with behavioral disturbance G31.83 [F02.81]
	  due to
	    drugs NEC G21.19
	      neuroleptic G21.11
	  neuroleptic induced G21.11
	  postencephalitic G21.3
	  secondary G21.9
	    due to
	      arteriosclerosis G21.4
	      drugs NEC G21.19
	        neuroleptic G21.11
	      encephalitis G21.3
	      external agents NEC G21.2
	      syphilis A52.19
	  specified NEC G21.8
	  syphilitic A52.19
	  treatment-induced NEC G21.19
	  vascular G21.4

Step 5	• Choose the correct essential modifier based on the diagnostic statement. Because the diagnostic statement only indicates Parkinson's Disease, code G20 should be chosen.
Step 6	• Look up code G20 in the Tabular List. **G20 Parkinson's disease**

Step 7	• Check for any coding guidelines, conventions, inclusion or exclusion notes, or an additional character symbol.
	Includes Hemiparkinson's
	Excludes 1 Idiopathic Parkinsonism or Parkinson's disease
	              Paralysis agitans
	              Parkinsonism or Parkinson's disease NOS
	              Primary Parkinsonism or Parkinson's disease dementia with Parkinsonism (G31.83)

Step 8	• Assign the final ICD-10-CM code. **G20 Parkinson's disease**

---

details the basic coding steps using the ICD-10-CM manual and also encoder software (i.e., TruCode).

Using the Alphabetic Index

After the diagnostic statement has been abstracted from the health record, identify the main term and start searching for the best code, or code range, in the Alphabetic Index. It is important to note that the

PROCEDURE 24.1 Perform Coding Using the Current ICD-10-CM Manual or Encoder

Task:
To perform accurate diagnosis coding using the ICD-10-CM manual or an encoder.

Equipment and Supplies
- ICD-10-CM manual (current year), or
- Encoder software, such as TruCode

Scenario
The encounter form and progress notes both show that the diagnosis for this patient encounter is acute colitis. Locate the most accurate ICD-10-CM code for this diagnostic statement.

Procedural Steps

Alphabetic Index

1. Determine and locate the main terms from the diagnostic statement in the Alphabetic Index.
   Purpose: To provide a starting point for searching the Alphabetic Index.
2. Locate the essential modifiers listed under the main term in the Alphabetic Index.
   Purpose: To ensure further specificity of the codes found in the Alphabetic Index.
3. Review the conventions, punctuation, and notes in the Alphabetic Index.
   Purpose: To ensure that no additional searches, exclusions, or similar terms are needed to complete the search in the Alphabetic Index.
4. Choose a tentative code, codes, or code range from the Alphabetic Index that matches the diagnostic statement as closely as possible.
   Purpose: To prevent backtracking and repeated searches in the Alphabetic Index.

Tabular List

1. Look up the codes chosen from the Alphabetic Index in the Tabular List.
   Purpose: To begin the process of determining whether the codes selected from the Alphabetic Index are appropriate and accurate.
2. Review notes, conventions, and the Official Coding Guidelines associated with the code and code description in the Tabular List.
   a. Review conventions and punctuation.
   b. Review instructional notations:
      - *Includes* and *excludes* notes
      - *Code first, code also,* and *code additional* notes
      - *and, or,* and *with* statements
   Purpose: To ensure that the code or codes selected are appropriate for use and to determine whether they require additional codes or further specificity, or are excluded from use.
3. Verify the accuracy of the tentative code in the Tabular List.
   a. Make sure all elements of the diagnostic statement are included in the codes selected.
   b. Make sure the code description does not include anything not documented in the diagnostic statement.
   Purpose: To ensure that the most accurate and specific code is selected and that no contraindication exists to use of the code or codes selected.
4. Extend the codes to their highest level of specificity (up to the 7th character, if required). If a 7th character is required and no codes are present for the 4th, 5th, or 6th characters, it is appropriate to use the dummy placeholder X for these positions.
5. Assign the code (or codes) selected from the Tabular List as the appropriate code for the patient's condition by documenting it in the patient's health record.
   Purpose: To ensure that the health record and/or electronic encounter form contain documentation of the code or codes assigned.

Using the TruCode Encoder Software

1. Type in the main term from the diagnostic statement in the search box, as shown in the following figure.

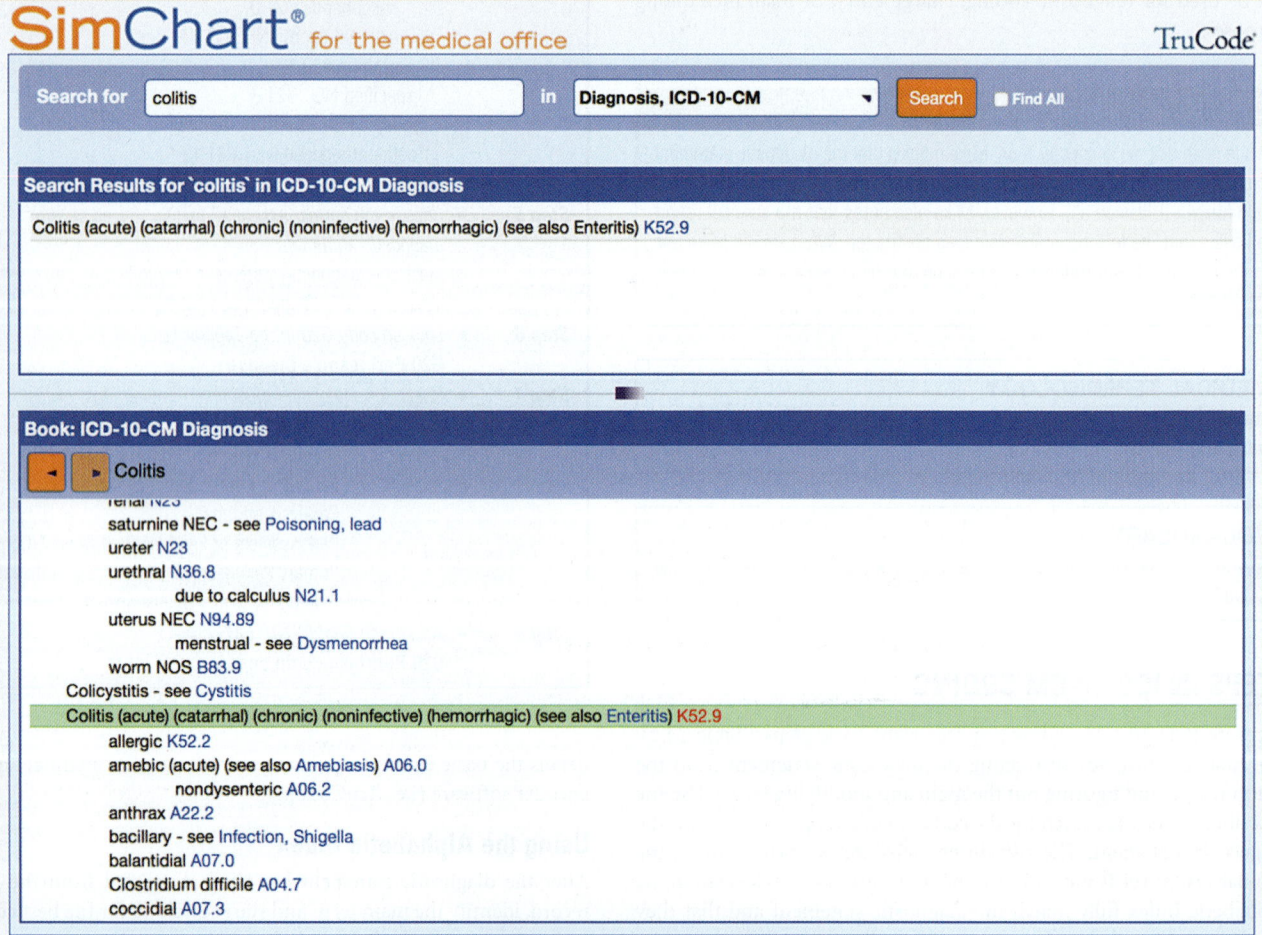

CHAPTER 24 Diagnostic Coding Basics

PROCEDURE 24.1 Perform Coding Using the Current ICD-10-CM Manual or Encoder—cont'd

2. The software will provide a list of main terms that could be related to the diagnosis typed in the search box. The coder chooses the main term that best represents the diagnostic statement.
3. Based on the main term chosen, a list of essential modifiers is presented (see the following figure). The coder must review the diagnostic statement to ensure that all documented modifying terms are identified. If the provider does not document a modifying term, the coder should not assume that a modifying term was implied.

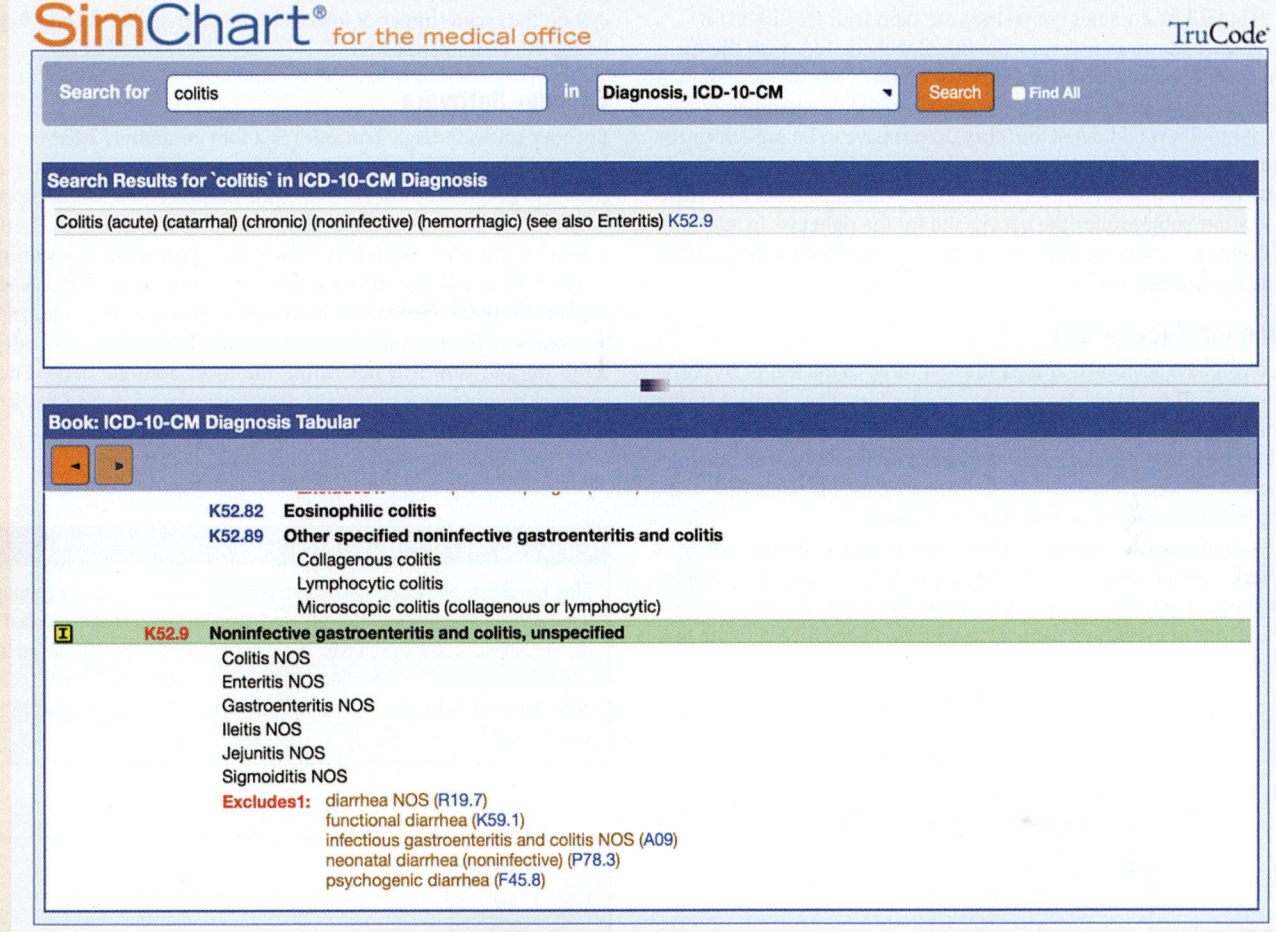

4. In the preceding figure, note the yellow on the left of the chosen diagnosis. In the TruCode program, click on the yellow area, and an instructional notes textbox, which includes coding guidelines, will appear, as shown in the following figure. To determine the most accurate code, follow these coding guidelines.

> **Noninfective enteritis and colitis (K50-K52)**
>
> K50—K52
>   Includes: noninfective inflammatory bowel disease
> K50—K52
>   Excludes1: irritable bowel syndrome (K58.-) megacolon (K59. 3)
>
> **Chapter 11: Disease of the digestive system (K00-K95)**
>
> K00—K95
>   Excludes2: certain conditions originating in the perinatal period (P04-P96)
>   certain infectious and parasitic diseases (A00-B99)

5. Once all the menus of essential modifiers have been presented, choose the most accurate and specific code based on the diagnostic statement.

Alphabetic Index should be used only as a tool to locate the appropriate code or code range. The Tabular List, with its conventions, punctuation, notes, and guidelines, must always be used to confirm that the code or codes selected are accurate and specific and that there are no contraindications to the use of the code found in the Alphabetic Index. For this reason, never assign a code directly from the Alphabetic Index. Even if only one code is found in the Alphabetic Index, it may be used only if a thorough review of the conventions and instructional notations in the Tabular List does not contraindicate (kon truh IN di keyt) it.

Fig. 24.4 shows an excerpt from the Alphabetic Index for the main term Cyst. The first essential modifier is "eyelid." Note the nonessential modifier – sebaceous – in parentheses after eyelid. (Remember, nonessential modifiers add detail, but they do not have to be present in the diagnostic statement for the code to be acceptable for use.) Directly below the essential modifier eyelid are the subterms. Note that there are separate subterms for the left eye and for the right eye. In addition, the diagnostic codes for each eye are further modified by the location of the cyst (upper or lower).

Using the Tabular List

Once you have identified at least the first three characters of the code in the Alphabetic Index, turn to the Tabular List. The chapters in the Tabular List are arranged alphabetically according to the initial letter of the 3-character code or codes assigned to each chapter. For example, Chapter 1 has code range A00–B99; Chapter 2 has code range C00–D49; Chapter 3 has code range D50–D89, and so on.

From the above example, you've determined that the code you probably need is in the H02 code range. Turn to the chapter that includes that range (Chapter 7). Fig. 24.5, an excerpt from the Tabular List, shows **Cysts of eyelid** as a main term, with the code H02.82. (Note that the nonessential modifier, sebaceous, is not shown in parentheses; rather, it appears under the main term in the nonbold phrase "Sebaceous cyst of eyelid.")

In the coding manual you would see the "additional character" symbol, which indicates that code H02.82 requires one more character. All possible diagnoses with 6-character codes are indented below the main term. A closer look at the disorders and their codes shows that the 6th character specifies the right or left eye and the location of the cyst on the eyelid (upper or lower). For the not-specified code, 9 would be the 6th character position.

Encoder Software

Encoder software (e.g., TruCode) is a tool commonly used by coders to assist in medical coding. This software performs computer-aided coding to assign the most accurate code possible. (TruCode is especially helpful to students because it allows them to search the ICD-10-CM manual using a few key terms.) The coder types a few key words into a search box, and the software finds the most likely matches in the Alphabetic Index. The coder then clicks on a specific code, and the software searches the Tabular List. From the Tabular List, the coder can scroll up and down to determine the most accurate code. Encoder software can increase the speed and efficiency of coding for a wide variety of medical cases.

CRITICAL THINKING BOX 24.5

Mike has determined a diagnostic statement to be "Perforation of the **tympanic** (tim PAN ick) membrane in the left ear." What keyword should be used for the TruCode software search box? What main term will the encoder go to in the Alphabetic Index? What should Mike click to get to the Tabular List? At what point can Mike be sure that he has assigned the most accurate and specific code?

VOCABULARY

cyst: A small, capsule-like sac that is filled with a semisolid material, such as a keratinous or sebaceous cyst.
contraindicate: Suggest that it should not be used.

MEDICAL TERMINOLOGY

tympan/o: eardrum
-ic: pertaining to

```
Cyst—continued
    eyelid (sebaceous) H02.829
        infected—see Hordeolum
        left H02.826
            lower H02.825
            upper H02.824
        right H02.823
            lower H02.822
            upper H02.821
```

FIG. 24.4 Excerpt from the Alphabetic Index: **Cyst** (main term), eyelid (essential modifier), sebaceous (nonessential modifier). (From Proctor D, Niedzwiecki B: *Kinn's The Medical Assistant*, ed 13, St Louis, 2017, Elsevier.)

H02.82	Cysts of eyelid
	Sebaceous cyst of eyelid
H02.821	Cysts of right upper eyelid
H02.822	Cysts of right lower eyelid
H02.823	Cysts of right eye, unspecified eyelid
H02.824	Cysts of left upper eyelid
H02.825	Cysts of left lower eyelid
H02.826	Cysts of left eye, unspecified eyelid
H02.829	Cysts of unspecified eye, unspecified eyelid

FIG. 24.5 Excerpt from the Tabular List: Cysts of the Eyelid. (From Proctor D, Niedzwiecki B: *Kinn's The Medical Assistant*, ed 13, St Louis, 2017, Elsevier.)

UNDERSTANDING CODING GUIDELINES

All ICD-10-CM coding manuals, regardless of the publisher, have comprehensive instructional notations and conventions to help the coder select the most accurate diagnostic code or codes. When there is a difference between reference sources (including this text), the current year's ICD-10-CM coding manual is the final authority – this fact cannot be emphasized enough. When coding, you must always refer to and thoroughly review the conventions, instructional notations, code definitions, and other guidelines in the Alphabetic Index and Tabular List in the current year's version of the ICD-10-CM.

The following instructions are designed to provide some additional guidance in selecting diagnostic codes from various chapters in the ICD-10-CM. But they are not to be considered a replacement for the ICD-10-CM manual, nor do they provide all the coding information, definitions, or explanations found in the manual. The steps for diagnostic coding (see Procedure 24.1) are the same for all chapters of the ICD-10-CM; however, special rules and considerations apply to some chapters that affect the code selection process.

Coding of Signs and Symptoms

Signs and symptoms are coded only if the provider has not yet determined the final diagnosis. For example, if the provider's notes state:
- "rule out"
- "suspected"
- "probable"
- "suspected"

the coder should use the patient's documented signs and symptoms, including subjective and objective findings. Subjective findings include the patient's chief complaint or statements about why the patient is seeking medical care. Objective findings are any measurable indicators found during the physical examination. If a patient comes in to see the provider because he or she has had a sore throat and fever for the past 3 days and the provider states "suspected strep throat" as the diagnosis, you would code sore throat and fever.

In the Tabular List, ill-defined conditions, signs, and symptoms are found in Chapter 18, Symptoms, Signs, and Abnormal Clinical and Laboratory Findings, Not Elsewhere Classified (R00–R99).

Conditions, signs, and symptoms included in Chapter 18 include the following:
- Not elsewhere classified (NEC) cases, even after all the facts of the medical case have been examined
- Signs or symptoms that existed on the first encounter but were temporary and for which causes could not be determined
- Conditional diagnosis for a patient who failed to return for further care and the cause of whose condition had not yet been determined
- Medical cases referred elsewhere for treatment before a diagnosis could be made
- Not otherwise specified (NOS) cases in which a more precise diagnosis was not available for any reason
- Certain symptoms, for which supplementary information is provided, that represent important problems in the medical care provided

Coding the Etiology and Manifestation

Etiology refers to the underlying cause or origin of a disease. *Manifestation* describes the signs and symptoms of the disease. In the Alphabetic Index, the etiology and manifestation codes are listed together. The etiology code is always listed first, and the manifestation code is listed beside it in italics and enclosed within brackets. If the diagnosis in the health record indicated cataract (KAT ur ackt) due to myxedema (mick suh DEE mah), you would find the following listed in the Alphabetic Index:
- cataract (cortical) (immature) (incipient) H26.9
- the essential modifier would be myxedema E03.9 *[H28]*

E03.9 takes you to the Other hypothyroidism section, which is the etiology for this cataract. H28 takes you to the cataract, which is the manifestation. You would need to verify both codes in the Tabular List and list both codes in the documentation.

Coding Organism-Caused Diseases

The two-step process of coding organism-caused diseases begins with the affected anatomical site. In the case of a throat infection caused by enterovirus, you should first assign the diagnostic code for throat infection, or pharyngitis (fair in JYE tis). In the Tabular List, code J02.8 {Acute pharyngitis due to other specified organism} is accompanied by the following *Use additional code* note: "Use additional code (B95–B97) to identify infectious agent" (Fig. 24.6). In the Tabular List, the B95–B97 category/block (found in Chapter 1) is titled Bacterial and Viral Infectious Agents. Starting with code B95, search for the code that specifies enterovirus; this happens to be code B97.1 {Enterovirus as the cause of diseases classified elsewhere}. Note that code B97.1 requires a 5th character; however, no other information is provided by the medical record. Therefore, you can assign code B97.19 {Other enterovirus as the cause of diseases classified elsewhere} as the final organism code.

> **VOCABULARY**
> **cataract:** Progressive loss of transparency of the lens of the eye.
> **myxedema:** Advanced hypothyroidism in adulthood.

> **MEDICAL TERMINOLOGY**
> **pharyng/o:** throat (pharynx)
> **-itis:** inflammation

Coding Human Immunodeficiency Virus (HIV) Infection and Acquired Immunodeficiency Syndrome (AIDS)

To correctly code HIV infection and AIDS, it is essential to first understand the descriptions of the codes available. The key is whether the patient has symptoms.

- J02.8 Acute pharyngitis due to other specified organisms

    Use additional code (B95-B97) it identify infectious agent
    Excludes1   pharyngitis due to coxsackie virus (B08.5)
                   pharyngitis due to gonococcus (A54.5)
                   acute pharyngitis due to herpes [simplex] virus (B00.2)
                   acute pharyngitis due to infectious mononucleosis (B27.-)
                   enteroviral vesicular pharyngitis (B08.5)

FIG. 24.6 Excerpt from the Tabular List: Acute pharyngitis due to other specified organism.

	Malignant Primary	Malignant Secondary	Ca in situ	Benign	Uncertain Behavior	Unspecified Nature		Malignant Primary
bladder (urinary)	C67.9	C79.11	D09.0	D30.3	D41.4	D49.4	marrow NEC	C96.9
dome	C67.1	C79.11	D09.0	D30.3	D41.4	D49.4	unspecified side	C40.10
neck	C67.5	C79.11	D09.0	D30.3	D41.4	D49.4	marrow NEC	C96.9
orifice	C67.9	C79.11	D09.0	D30.3	D41.4	D49.4	cartilage NEC	C41.9
ureteric	C67.6	C79.11	D09.0	D30.3	D41.4	D49.4	clavicle	C41.3
urethral	C67.5	C79.11	D09.0	D30.3	D41.4	D49.4	marrow NEC	C96.9
overlapping lesion	C67.8	—	—	—	—	—	clivus	C41.0
sphincter	C67.8	C79.11	D09.0	D30.3	D41.4	D49.4	marrow NEC	C96.9
trigone	C67.0	C79.11	D09.0	D30.3	D41.4	D49.4	coccygeal vertebra	C41.4
urachus	C67.7	—	D09.0	D30.3	D41.4	D49.4	marrow NEC	C96.9
wall	C67.9	C79.11	D09.0	D30.3	D41.4	D49.4	coccyx	C41.4
anterior	C67.3	C79.11	D09.0	D30.3	D41.4	D49.4	marrow NEC	C96.9
lateral	C67.2	C79.11	D09.0	D30.3	D41.4	D49.4	costal cartilage	C41.3
posterior	C67.4	C79.11	D09.0	D30.3	D41.4	D49.4	costovertebral joint	C41.3
blood vessel—*see* Neoplasm, connective tissue							marrow NEC	C96.9
							cranial	C41.0

FIG. 24.7 Excerpt from the Table of Neoplasms. (From Proctor D, Niedzwiecki B: *Kinn's The Medical Assistant*, ed 13, St Louis, 2017, Elsevier.)

- HIV: This indicates only that the virus is present.
- AIDS: AIDS is a syndrome; a syndrome is defined as a "group of symptoms occurring together." AIDS is the manifestation of signs and/or symptoms that can occur as a result of HIV infection.

Never code a patient as having HIV infection unless it is clearly documented as confirmed. Probable and suspected cases are never coded; instead, the signs and symptoms present should be coded. If a patient is seen for an HIV-related condition, the principal diagnosis should be B20 {Human immunodeficiency virus [HIV] disease}, followed by additional diagnostic codes for all reported HIV-related conditions.

Remember that strict restrictions are placed on the disclosure of medical information about patients with HIV infection and/or AIDS. Make sure the patient has signed the appropriate release of medical information form before any disclosures are made to third parties.

Coding Neoplasms

A **neoplasm** (NEE uh plaz uh m), or new growth, is coded by the site or location of the neoplasm and its behavior. The Table of Neoplasms (Fig. 24.7) is located just after the Alphabetic Index in the coding manual. This table lists the ICD-10-CM codes for neoplasms by anatomical site in alphabetic order. Six possible code numbers exist for each anatomical site, depending on whether the neoplasm:
- is malignant or benign
- exhibits uncertain behavior
- is of an unspecified nature

VOCABULARY
histologic: The study of body tissues.

MEDICAL TERMINOLOGY
hist/o: tissue
log/o: study of
neo-: new
-ic: pertaining to
-plasm: formation

In the Table of Neoplasms, malignant neoplasms are categorized into three separate subclassifications (Box 24.3):
- Malignant Primary
- Malignant Secondary
- Ca in situ (carcinoma in situ)

Definitions of benign, uncertain behavior, and unspecified nature can be found in Box 24.4.

BOX 24.3 Terms Defining Malignant Neoplasm Sites

- *Primary:* Identifies the originating anatomical site of the neoplasm. A primary malignancy is defined as the original site or sites of the cancer.
- *Secondary:* Identifies sites to which the primary neoplasm has metastasized (muh TAS tuh sahyzd) (spread). A secondary malignancy is defined as a second location to which the cancer has spread from the primary location.
- *Ca in situ:* Carcinoma in situ (kahr suh NOH muh in SAHY too) is defined as situated in the original place or position. Tumor cells are undergoing malignant changes but are still confined to the point of origin, without invasion of surrounding normal tissue. The *Ca in situ* column is used only if the provider documents that precise terminology.

BOX 24.4 Definitions of Benign, Uncertain Behavior, and Unspecified Nature Neoplasms

- *Benign:* The growth is noncancerous, nonmalignant, and has not invaded adjacent structures or spread to distant sites.
- *Uncertain Behavior:* The pathologist is unable to determine whether the neoplasm is benign or malignant.
- *Unspecified Nature:* Neither the behavior nor the histologic (hi STOL ah jic) type of neoplasm is specified in the diagnostic statement

Most coding decisions on malignant neoplasms are between the primary and secondary classifications. Other terms are used in the following cases:
- *In situ* is used only when the diagnostic statement contains that exact phrase.
- *Unspecified* is used only when no pathologic study has been done, and the neoplasm is still described with a term such as "tumor" or "growth."
- *Uncertain* is used by the provider when it has not been determined whether the neoplasm is malignant or benign.

Six Steps for Coding Neoplasms. The following steps can help determine the most specific and accurate diagnostic code for a neoplasm. These steps can be used in addition to the basic diagnostic steps:
1. In the Table of Neoplasms, find the site (anatomical location) of the neoplasm.
2. Determine, from the documentation, whether the neoplasm is malignant or benign.
3. If the neoplasm is benign, select the correct column in the table by reviewing the diagnostic statement.
4. If the neoplasm is malignant, select the column in the table that best fits its behavior: Malignant Primary, Malignant Secondary, or Ca in situ.
5. Link the appropriate column to the appropriate row.
6. Check the code shown in the table with the code in the Tabular List, to make sure the former complies with the guidelines, conventions, and instructional notations of the latter.

The ICD-10-CM manual always provides additional information, definitions, and guidelines for coding neoplasms in the Tabular List, just as it does for all other diseases, illnesses, and injuries.

Coding for Diabetes Mellitus

Diabetes mellitus (DM) (dahy uh BEE tis MEL ih tus) is classified as type 1 or type 2. Patients with DM type 1 develop the disease because the pancreas is unable to produce insulin. In individuals with DM type 2, the pancreas has become unable to maintain the level of insulin the body needs to function, or the person has developed target cell resistance to insulin.

The diabetes mellitus codes are combination codes. This means that they include the type of diabetes mellitus, the body system affected, and the complications affecting that body system. Use as many codes within a particular category/block as necessary to describe all the complications of the disease. These codes should be sequenced according to the reason for a particular encounter. Assign as many codes from category/block E08 to E13 (Diabetes Mellitus) as needed to identify all the patient's associated conditions.

Coding for Complications of Pregnancy, Childbirth, and the Puerperium

Coding for the obstetric patient is like using a specialty codebook within the ICD-10-CM coding manual. This is challenging for coders who do not code obstetrics often. Some important clinical terms regarding pregnancy are:

> **MEDICAL TERMINOLOGY**
> **ante-:** before, forward
> **post-:** after, behind
> **peri-:** around, surrounding
> **-partum:** delivery

- *antepartum* (AN tee PAHR tuh m): Pregnancy (applies as soon as a pregnancy test result is positive)
- *childbirth:* Delivery
- *postpartum:* The *puerperium* (pyoo ur Per ee um), or first 6 weeks after delivery
- *peripartum:* The period from the last month of pregnancy to 5 months' postpartum

Obstetrics cases use codes from Chapter 15, Pregnancy, Childbirth, and the Puerperium (O00–O9A). Additional codes from other chapters may be used in conjunction with Chapter 15 codes to further specify conditions. If the provider documents that the pregnancy is incidental to the encounter, **Z33.1 {Pregnant state, incidental}** should be used instead of any Chapter 15 codes. This would be the case if the patient were being seen for a sprained ankle. The sprained ankle is not related to the pregnancy, but is an incidental diagnosis. It is the provider's responsibility to state that the condition being treated is not affecting the pregnancy. Codes from Chapter 15 are documented only in the maternal health record; they are never used in the health record of the newborn.

Most of the codes in Chapter 15 have a 6th character, which indicates the trimester of pregnancy. Assignment of the final character for trimester should be based on the provider's documentation of the trimester (or number of weeks) for the encounter. This applies to the assignment of trimester for preexisting conditions, in addition to those that develop during or are due to the pregnancy. The provider's documentation of the number of weeks may be used to assign the appropriate code identifying the trimester. The seventh character in this chapter is used to identify the fetus when there is more than one. (Box 24.5).

Coding for Burns and Corrosions

The same principles for multiple coding apply to burns. Code each burn separately unless specific combination codes are given in the Tabular List. There are many combination codes. Most burn codes are found in Chapter 19 (Injury, Poisoning, and Certain Other Consequences of External Origin); the applicable codes are T20–T32. Because burns are coded by site and degree and by the extent of body surface involvement, all burn cases should have at least two codes, and a third if the wound is infected. Other types of wounds, lacerations, punctures, and so on use a different 5th character to show that they are infected and, therefore, complicated. However, burn codes use the 5th character for other information. Therefore, these diagnoses require an additional code to indicate infection.

The ICD-10-CM makes a distinction between burns and corrosions. The burn codes are used for the following: thermal burns (except sunburns) caused by a heat source, such as a fire or hot appliance; burns resulting from electricity; and burns resulting from radiation. Corrosions, on the other hand, are burns caused by chemicals. The guidelines are the same for burns and corrosions.

> **BOX 24.5 7th Character for Fetus Identification**
>
> Some codes in Chapter 15, Pregnancy, Childbirth, and the Puerperium (O00–O9A), require a 7th character. In this chapter the 7th character is used when there are multiple fetuses to indicate which fetus is affected. The 7th character options are:
> 0 not applicable or unspecified
> 1 fetus 1
> 2 fetus 2
> 3 fetus 3
> 4 fetus 4
> 5 fetus 5
> 9 other fetus

Current burns (T20–T25) are classified by depth, extent, and burn agent (X code). Depth is categorized as first degree (redness), second degree (blistering), and third degree (full-thickness involvement). Burns of the eye and internal organs (T26–T28) are classified by site but not by degree.

Coding for External Causes of Morbidity

External cause codes are intended to provide data for research on injuries and for evaluation of injury prevention strategies. These codes capture:
- how the injury or health condition happened (cause)
- the intent (unintentional or accidental; or intentional, such as suicide or assault)
- the place where the event occurred
- the activity of the patient at the time of the event, and the person's status (e.g., civilian, military).

These codes are often used for workers' compensation claims.

Place of Occurrence Guideline

Codes from category Y92 {Place of occurrence of the external cause} are secondary codes. They are used after other external cause codes to identify the location of the patient at the time of the injury or other condition.

A place of occurrence code is used only once, at the initial encounter for treatment. No 7th character is used in Y92 codes. Only one code from category Y92 should be recorded on the patient's health record. Do not use place of occurrence code Y92.9 {Unspecified place or not applicable} if the place is not stated or if it is not applicable.

Activity Codes

Category Y93 codes {Activity codes} are used to define the activity the patient was involved in at the time of injury or when the health condition developed. Only one code from category Y93 should be recorded in the patient's health record. An activity code should be used in conjunction with a place of occurrence code (Y92). The activity codes are not applicable to poisonings, adverse effects, misadventures, or sequelae.

Do not assign code Y93.9 {Unspecified activity} if the activity is not stated.

A code from category Y93 can be used with external cause (Y99) and occurrence (Y92) codes if identifying the activity provides additional information about the event.

For example, you are coding a closed ankle fracture that occurred while the patient was playing soccer in a public park. First, you must identify what should be coded first. In this case, the ankle fracture is coded first: S92.111A {Displaced fracture of neck of right talus} (Remember, "A" indicates initial encounter). The second code is the activity code; the patient was playing soccer, so the code for this activity is Y93.66 {Activity, soccer}. Remember, if the report did not state an activity, do not add Y93.9 {Unspecified activity}. Finally, when an activity code is used, a place of occurrence code should also be used. In this scenario, the patient was playing in a public park; therefore, the place of occurrence code is Y92.830 {Public park}.

Coding for Health Status and Contact With Health Services

In the ICD-10-CM, Chapter 21, Factors Influencing Health Status and Contact with Health Services (Z00–Z99) are used to describe circumstances or encounters with a healthcare provider when no current illness or injury exists, such as:
- inoculations (ih nok yuh LEY shuh n) and vaccinations
- health status
- personal and/or family history of particular diseases
- screening
- observation
- follow-up
- donor counseling
- encounters for obstetric and reproductive services
- supervision of newborns and infants
- routine and administrative examinations
- other health encounters that do not fall into any one of the mentioned categories

MAXIMIZING THIRD-PARTY REIMBURSEMENT

The most important thing to remember in using the ICD-10-CM is to code the diagnosis to the highest level of specificity. Obtaining the correct reimbursement is important to the practice's cash flow, and it depends on proper coding and billing techniques. Some other crucial points to remember when submitting diagnostic codes for claims include:
- Use the current year ICD-10-CM manual and stay informed of all changes, revisions, and additions published for that year to both the codes and the official coding guidelines.
- Code accurately from documented information, making sure the appropriate code or codes are assigned for all parts of the diagnostic statement, with no additions or omissions.
- Be sure the diagnosis corresponds to the symptoms and treatment. Many codes are specific to age and gender.
- Review data entry to make sure no digits have been transposed.
- Know the insurance carrier's rules and requirements for completion and submission of claims.
- Incomplete or inaccurate codes may result in delay or denial of reimbursement. An inaccurate diagnosis may have a lifelong negative effect on the patient.

PROVIDERS AND ACCURATE CODING

Detailed documentation in the patient's health record can help coders to code to the highest specificity. Therefore, providers should be trained in how to document patient health records appropriately. Respectfully discuss with providers that diagnostic codes cannot be assigned unless clear documentation is found in the patient's health record. Some providers may feel that because they care for the same type of cases, specialized diagnostic statements should be implied. However, the medical assistant should stress to providers the importance of detailed documentation and how developing this practice not only improves ICD-10-CM code assignment, but may also result in higher health insurance reimbursements.

Staff meetings to review third-party requirements should be held regularly by the medical billing supervisor. Medical assistants should be respectful to the healthcare provider when discussing third-party requirements for more detailed documentation. An understanding and patient attitude toward the healthcare provider goes a long way in building a trusting relationship.

> ### EXCEPTIONAL CUSTOMER SERVICE
>
> Most patients know very little about medical coding, so they may not understand how the codes on their encounter forms relate to their diagnosis. If the patient has questions, explain that the codes represent his or her diagnosis to the most specific and accurate level. Because the coding system is much like a foreign language to patients, be patient when explaining this process and answering questions. This will help the patient to understand the insurance billing process.

CLOSING COMMENTS

Diagnostic coding using the ICD-10-CM, with its almost 70,000 codes, can seem overwhelming. Successful medical coders follow specific steps to assign the most accurate ICD-10-CM code. Encoder software (e.g., TruCode) can search ICD-10-CM electronically to aid in faster coding. Detailed documentation in the patient's health record and accurate coding work hand-in-hand to maximize reimbursement for services provided. When working with providers on issues related to coding and documentation, show respect and patience. Medical assistants are expected to follow ethical standards by assigning and reporting only codes that are clearly supported by the documentation in the patient's record. When in doubt, a medical assistant should consult the provider for clarification. A coding professional is responsible for maintaining and continually enhancing his or her coding skills and for staying current with the changes in the codes, guidelines, and regulations.

CHAPTER REVIEW

When assigning diagnostic codes, the medical assistant needs to be familiar with the format of the ICD-10-CM manual and the various documents in which the diagnostic statement can be found. The ICD-10-CM manual is made up of two sections: the Alphabetic Index and the Tabular List. Coding begins in the Alphabetic Index, and the actual diagnostic code is determined in the Tabular List. You should always review the instructional notes to ensure that you have the most specific code.

Diagnostic statements can be found in a number of different documents. In a clinic setting, the diagnosis is most commonly found on the encounter form or in the progress notes. When billing for services provided in the hospital, you may need to review the discharge summary or operative report.

Once the diagnostic statement has been identified, you must follow the coding guidelines. If the diagnostic statement includes words such as "rule out" or "possible," then you must code the signs and symptoms. When indicated, you should be sure to include both the etiology and manifestation codes.

Diagnostic coding can affect reimbursement from the insurance carrier. The diagnostic codes tell the insurance carrier why the services were provided. If the diagnostic code does not match the service provided, the insurance company will not pay for the service. An example would be if the diagnostic code was for pharyngitis, yet the service it was linked to was for a blood glucose test. In this scenario, the insurance company would say that a blood glucose test is not medically necessary for pharyngitis.

Being proficient at diagnostic coding makes you a valuable member of the healthcare team.

SCENARIO WRAP-UP

Mike's experience using the ICD-10-CM coding manual and encoder software on actual medical office cases has made him even more enthusiastic about his new responsibilities, and he enjoys the coding process more. He knows that as he gains experience in ICD-10-CM coding, he will be able to set a positive example for the staff. As Mike progresses with diagnostic coding, he will also be able to help the providers and medical assistant staff be attentive to details when documenting in a health record.

Although the electronic encounter form for entering billing codes is an easy tool, Mike has learned that knowing how to use the ICD-10-CM Alphabetic Index and Tabular List is a necessary skill to ensure accurate coding. He also knows that it is important when coding a diagnosis to make sure the medical documentation matches the encounter form and that all elements of the diagnostic statement are included. Furthermore, he must ensure that the diagnosis listed on the encounter form is fully documented in the patient's health record. Mike is feeling more comfortable about referring to coding guidelines to ensure the most accurate code and to make certain that every character for the ICD-10-CM code is present. Every feature of the manual provides guidance in choosing and confirming a diagnostic code that matches the diagnostic statement on the encounter form and in the health record. Searching for codes in the encoder also has helped Mike develop his coding skills more quickly.

25

Procedural Coding Basics

LEARNING OBJECTIVES

1. Describe the organization of the *Current Procedural Terminology* (CPT) manual.
2. Distinguish between the Alphabetic Index and the Tabular List in the CPT code set.
3. Discuss coding guidelines, and explain the importance of modifiers in assigning CPT codes.
4. Review various conventions in the CPT code set.
5. Identify the required medical documentation for accurate procedural coding.
6. Discuss how to use the Alphabetic Index.
7. Discuss how to use the Tabular list. Also, perform procedural coding of a surgery.
8. Identify common CPT coding guidelines for evaluation and management (E/M) procedures and perform procedural coding of an office visit and an immunization.
9. Identify common CPT coding guidelines for surgical procedures. Also, discuss coding factors for the integumentary system and the muscular system, and for maternity care and delivery.
10. Identify common CPT coding guidelines for the Common CPT Coding Guidelines: Pathology and Laboratory section.
11. Do the following related to the HCPCS code set and manual:
    - Identify procedures and services that require HCPCS codes.
    - Describe how to use the most current HCPCS level II coding system.
12. Summarize common HCPCS coding guidelines and use tactful communication skills when working with providers to ensure accurate code selection.

CHAPTER OUTLINE

1. Opening Scenario, 549
2. You Will Learn, 549
3. Introduction to Procedural Coding, 549
4. Introduction to the CPT Manual, 549
5. Code Categories in the CPT Manual, 549
   a. Category I Codes, 549
   b. Category II Codes, 550
   c. Category III Codes, 550
6. Organization of the CPT Manual, 550
   a. The Alphabetic Index, 550
   b. The Tabular List, 550
7. Unlisted Procedure or Service Code, 550
8. CPT Coding Guidelines, 551
   a. Modifiers, 551
9. CPT Conventions, 552
10. Documentation for CPT Coding, 552
11. Using the Alphabetic Index, 552
    a. Searching the Alphabetic Index, 554
    b. Using See and See Also in the Alphabetic Index, 554
    c. Single Codes and Code Ranges, 554
12. Using the Tabular List, 554
    a. Use of the Semicolon, 555
13. Common CPT Coding Guidelines: Evaluation and Management, 555
    a. Identifying the Place of Service, 555
    b. Identifying the Patient Status, 555
    c. Determining the Level of Service Provided, 555
        i. *Key Components and Contributing Factors, 555*
        ii. *History, 559*
        iii. *Examination, 560*
        iv. *Medical Decision Making, 560*
    d. Factors that Contribute to E/M Complexity, 560
        i. *Counseling, 560*
        ii. *Nature of the Presenting Problem, 560*
        iii. *Coordination of Care, 560*
        iv. *Time, 560*
14. Common CPT Coding Guidelines: Surgical Section, 561
    a. Surgical Package Definition, 561
    b. Integumentary System – Excision of Lesions—Benign or Malignant, 561
        i. *Levels of Closure, 561*
        ii. *Listing Services for Wound Repair, 561*
    c. Musculoskeletal System, 561
        i. *Fractures, 561*
    d. Maternity Care and Delivery, 562
15. Common CPT Coding Guidelines: Pathology and Laboratory Section, 562
16. HCPCS Code Set and Manual, 562
17. Common HCPCS Coding Guidelines, 563
    a. Medical and Surgical Supplies, 563
    b. Durable Medical Equipment, 563
18. Closing Comments, 564
19. Chapter Review, 564
20. Scenario Wrap-Up, 564

CHAPTER 25 Procedural Coding Basics

TABLE 25.1 Comparison of Procedural Code Sets

Code Set	Used For	Code Features	Example	Description	Developer	Updated
ICD-10-PCS	Inpatient hospital procedures	7-digit alphanumeric code	0TTJ0ZZ	Appendectomy	National Center for Health Statistics	Annually, October 1
CPT	Outpatient procedures; professional and technical services	5-digit numeric code; a 2-digit modifier can be added	44970	Laparoscopic appendectomy	American Medical Association (AMA)	Annually, January 1
HCPCS	Auxiliary medical treatment, including vaccines, medical transport, drugs, durable medical equipment	5-digit alphanumeric code; a 2-digit modifier can be added	A0428	Ambulance service, basic life support, nonemergency transport	Centers for Medicare and Medicaid Services (CMS)	Annually, October 1

▶ OPENING SCENARIO

Sherald Vogt, a medical assisting student, works at Walden-Martin Family Medical Clinic (WMFM). Sherald really enjoyed learning about diagnostic coding in the *International Classification of Diseases, Tenth Revision, Clinical Modification* (ICD-10-CM), and now she looks forward to learning about procedural coding. Sherald recognizes that a strong understanding of anatomy and physiology are vital to correct diagnostic coding. She also believes the knowledge she has gained will help her in procedural coding. Sherald will be using the *Current Procedural Terminology* (CPT) coding system for most procedures and services provided in the medical office. In addition, she will use the *Healthcare Common Procedure Coding System* (HCPCS; pronounced "hic-pix") for medical products and services not found in the CPT.

As she did with the ICD-10-CM, Sherald is learning that accurate coding begins with the proper analysis of documentation found in the health record. With that information, she will abstract the correct data to assign an accurate procedure code. As does the ICD-10-CM, the CPT has coding guidelines, symbols, and formal steps specific to procedural coding. However, unlike in ICD-10-CM diagnostic coding, in CPT and HCPCS coding Sherald must determine how and when to use modifiers. The office manager wants to give Sherald some experience, so he allows her to review some healthcare records so she can practice coding.

YOU WILL LEARN

- How the format, layout, and conventions of the CPT and HCPCS manuals help the medical assistant locate the most accurate and specific procedural code.
- To identify the documents in which the procedures and services can be found.
- To apply coding guidelines necessary for procedural coding.
- When to use a modifier for procedure codes.
- To define upcoding and downcoding and the reasons they should not be done.

INTRODUCTION TO PROCEDURAL CODING

Procedural coding changes the written descriptions of procedures and services delivered in a healthcare facility into numeric or alphanumeric codes. These codes are used for a variety of different purposes. They can be used to track the services that are being provided to patients and on claims sent for payment from insurance companies. There are three procedure code sets used for these purposes:

- International Classification of Diseases, Tenth Revision, Procedural Coding System (ICD-10-PCS)

BOX 25.1 Format of the CPT Coding Manual

- Comprehensive instructions for using the manual, including the steps for coding
- Tabular List, which includes the following six sections:
  - Evaluation and Management
  - Anesthesia
  - Surgery
  - Radiology
  - Pathology and Laboratory
  - Medicine
- Coding Guidelines, Conventions, and Notes
- Appendices (16; A–P)
- The Alphabetic Index

- Current Procedural Terminology (CPT)
- Healthcare Common Procedure Coding System (HCPCS)

Table 25.1 compares the three different code sets. Medical assistants most often work in an outpatient setting. This chapter will focus on the CPT and HCPCS code sets. The medical biller is responsible for maintaining accurate medical records and for processing insurance claims. This can be done efficiently by using the CPT and HCPCS codes. These codes identify procedures and services commonly used in an outpatient healthcare facility.

INTRODUCTION TO THE CPT MANUAL

The Current Procedural Terminology (CPT) system was developed and is maintained by the American Medical Association (AMA). It is updated each year and released on January 1. The CPT coding manual consists of descriptive terms and identifying codes for reporting professional and technical services. CPT codes convert written descriptions of procedures and services into numeric codes. They establish a standard system that accurately describes medical and surgical services.

CODE CATEGORIES IN THE CPT MANUAL

There are three different categories of codes in the CPT. Category I codes are used most frequently and are required for insurance claim submission. Category II and Category III codes are used for data collection.

Category I Codes

Category I codes are located in the Tabular List of the CPT manual and arranged by sections (Box 25.1). For example, codes beginning

> **BOX 25.2 Use of Category II Codes**
>
> If a patient was seen by the provider for asthma, a Category I code of 99213 could be used for the visit. In addition, a Category II code of 2015F Asthma impairment assessed (Asthma) could be used.

with 7 (e.g., 70100—radiologic examination of the mandible, partial, with less than four views) are located in the Radiology section of the manual. Each code has a description of the service or procedure performed. These codes are 5-digit numeric codes.

Category II Codes

Category II codes are a set of supplemental tracking codes that healthcare facilities use for *performance measurement*. Category II codes are optional. They cannot be used as a substitute for Category I codes, and they are not used as part of the insurance billing process. When these codes are used, it can reduce the need for abstracting information from the health record. These codes describe clinical components that may be typically included in Evaluation and Management services, or clinical services. In a Category II code, the 5th digit is the letter F (Box 25.2).

Category II codes are described and listed in their own section, which is located after the Medicine section and before the appendices. Category II codes are reviewed by the Performance Measures Advisory Group. This group is composed of members from various medical organizations and government agencies.

Category III Codes

Category III codes are temporary codes used for emerging and new technology, services, and procedures that have not been officially added to the Tabular List. The 5th digit in a Category III code is the letter T. Category III codes may be used in billing and reporting if:
- no code in the Tabular List correctly describes the technology, service, or procedure performed.
- no Category I code matches the documentation.

In most publishers' editions of the CPT manual, Category III codes are also listed in their own section, after the Medicine section and before the appendices.

ORGANIZATION OF THE CPT MANUAL

The CPT coding manual is separated into the Alphabetic Index and the Tabular List.

The Alphabetic Index

CPT coding starts with the Alphabetic Index. It is found in the back of the CPT manual and is an alphabetic listing of main terms. These terms represent the type of surgery, the anatomical site, or *eponym* (EP uh num) (Fig. 25.1). Much like the Alphabetic Index in the ICD-10-CM manual, the Alphabetic Index in the CPT gives a code, codes, or a code range that must be verified in the Tabular List of the CPT manual.

> **CRITICAL THINKING 25.1**
>
> To practice her coding skills, Sherald is reviewing a surgical report for a gallbladder removal. Will she be able to find the main term "gallbladder" in the Alphabetic Index? Why or why not? What other main term could she be looking for? Once she finds the range of codes in the Alphabetic Index, what is her next step?

The Tabular List

The Tabular List is divided into six sections, with codes listed in numeric order in each section. As in the ICD-10-CM, the codes in the Tabular List include definitions, guidelines, and notes. These enable the coder to select the most specific code based on the procedural statement and service descriptions documented in the health record. The six sections of the Tabular List and their CPT code ranges are:
- Evaluation and Management (99201-99499)
- Anesthesia (00100-01999, 99100-99157)
- Surgery (10021-69990)
- Radiology, including nuclear medicine and diagnostic ultrasound (70010-79999)
- Pathology and Laboratory (80047-89398)
- Medicine (90281-99199, 99500-99607)

Sections are subdivided into *subsections*; *subsections* are subdivided into *subheadings*; and *subheadings* can be subdivided into *categories*. Each level of a section provides more *specificity* (spes hu FIS i tee) about the procedure or service performed and the anatomical site or organ system involved (Fig. 25.2). Each section and subsection provides coding guidelines and, if needed, a reference to the *CPT Assistant*. In most instances, all four levels are found, although this is not a hard-and-fast rule.

In the CPT manual, the subsection is listed below the section and indented. The subsection usually describes an anatomical site or an organ system, as in the following examples:
- Anatomical site: heart, femur, or skull
- Organ system: digestive, integumentary, or cardiovascular

A subheading is listed below the subsection. It generally refers to a specific procedure or service, but it can also indicate a more specific anatomical site:
- Procedures: esophagoscopy, incision and drainage, or cardiac catheterization
- Specific anatomical site: mitral valve, distal femur, or occipital bone

Category is the lowest level of code description. The subcategory is listed below the subheading. It provides even more specificity about an anatomical site or the procedure or service performed.

UNLISTED PROCEDURE OR SERVICE CODE

Occasionally, even with the most detailed documentation, an accurate code to match the procedure or service performed cannot be found in the CPT manual. For this reason, in each section, nonspecific codes have been provided. These codes are known as Unlisted Procedures and Services. For example, code 29999 is found in the Surgery section, Musculoskeletal subsection. It describes an "unlisted procedure,

> **VOCABULARY**
>
> ***CPT Assistant***: An online CPT coding journal, supported by the AMA, which addresses subjects such as appealing insurance denials, validating coding to auditors, training staff members, and answering day-to-day coding questions.
>
> **eponym:** In medical terms, a medical diagnosis or procedure named for the person who discovered it.
>
> **performance measurement:** The regular collection of data to assess whether the correct processes are being performed and desired results are being achieved.
>
> **specificity:** The quality or state of being specific.

CHAPTER 25 Procedural Coding Basics

Fracture
Acetabulum
  Closed Treatment 27220-27222
  Open Treatment 27226-27228
    with Manipulation 27222
    without Manipulation 27220
Alveolar Ridge
  Closed Treatment 21440
  Open Treatment 21445
Ankle
  Bimalleolar 27808, 27810, 27814
  Lateral 27786, 27788, 27792, 27808, 27810, 27814
  Medial 27760, 27762, 27766, 27808, 27810, 27814
  Posterior 27767-27769, 27808, 27810, 27814
  Trimalleolar 27816, 27818, 27822-27823
Ankle Bone
  Medial 27760-27762
Bennett's
  See Thumb, Fracture
Blow-Out Fracture
  Orbital Floor 21385-21387, 21390, 21395
Bronchi
  Reduction 31630
Calcaneus
  Closed Treatment 28400-28405
  Open Treatment 28415-28420
  Percutaneous Fixation 28406
  with Manipulation 28405-28406
  without Manipulation 28400

FIG. 25.1 Alphabetic Index: Fractures. (From Proctor D, Niedzwiecki B: *Kinn's The Medical Assistant*, ed 13, St Louis, 2017, Elsevier.)

Section: Surgery (10021-69990)

Subsection: Integumentary System

Subheading: Skin Subcutaneous and Accessory Structures

Category: Débridement

FIG. 25.2 Format of Tabular List.

---

arthroscopy." Unlisted codes can be used only when no other Category I or Category III code exactly matches the documentation. When an unlisted code is used, a **special report** must be sent with the insurance claim that describes the procedure or service in detail.

> **VOCABULARY**
> **special report:** Additional medical documentation required to confirm the need for the use of unlisted, unusual, or newly adopted medical procedures code.

CPT CODING GUIDELINES

At the beginning of each section and some subsections are coding guidelines. These guidelines add definitions and descriptions needed to interpret and report the procedures and services in that section or subsection. Coding guidelines enhance the coder's understanding of when and under what circumstances specific codes may be used. It is important to thoroughly read and apply the coding guidelines provided. Because coding guidelines are updated every year on October 1, it is also important to reread the guidelines after every new edition is released. Selecting a code without reading the guidelines usually leads to selection of the wrong code. Not only will this result in possibly delayed or denied reimbursement, but also, continued inappropriate code selection can be considered fraud or abuse, and can result in serious civil or criminal penalties.

Modifiers

Category I code *modifiers* are two-digit, numeric codes that report or indicate:
- specific criteria
- specific condition
- special circumstance

Category II code modifiers are alphanumeric. In either situation, they are used with CPT codes to indicate that a service or procedure performed was altered by specific circumstances (Table 25.2). Modifiers are included with the 5-digit CPT code to supply additional information or to describe extenuating circumstances that affected the procedure or service. For instance, modifier –50 adds the detail that a procedure was performed **bilaterally** (bye LAT er uhl ee), or on both sides of the body. When an assistant surgeon is needed for a surgical procedure, modifier –80 is used. This allows the assistant surgeon to submit charges for his or her time. Modifiers can also show which side of the body a medical procedure was performed on. For example, the code 19100-RT indicates that the right breast was

TABLE 25.2 Commonly Used CPT Code Modifiers

Modifier	Description
–50	Bilateral procedure. If the procedure was performed on both sides of the body (e.g., both knees, both eyes) and the code description does not indicate that the procedure or service was performed bilaterally, modifier –50 is used.
–62	Two surgeons. When two surgeons work together as primary surgeons performing distinct parts of a procedure, each surgeon should report the procedure he or she performed to the insurance carrier using modifier –62. This prevents the insurance carrier from possibly rejecting a surgical charge as a duplicate.
–26	Professional component. This modifier is used when a technician performs the service to provide his or her professional opinion.
–RT, –LT	Indicates the side of the body on which the procedure took place. (e.g., 19100–LT – Breast biopsy, left side)

Symbols

- ▲ Revised code
- ● New code
- ▶◀ New or revised text
- ⟿ Reference to *CPT Assistant*, *Clinical Examples in Radiology*, and *CPT Changes*
- ✚ Add-on code
- ⊘ Exemptions to modifier 51
- ⊙ Moderate sedation
- ⁄ Product pending FDA approval
- ○ Reinstated or recycled code
- # Out-of-numerical sequence code

FIG. 25.3 CPT conventions. (From Proctor D, Niedzwiecki B: *Kinn's The Medical Assistant*, ed 13, St Louis, 2017, Elsevier.)

biopsied. A list of modifiers can be found in the CPT coding manual in Appendix A.

MEDICAL TERMINOLOGY
bi–: two
later/o: side
–al: pertaining to

CPT CONVENTIONS

Conventions, or special symbols (Fig. 25.3), are used to provide additional information about specific codes. Let's look at a skin graft procedure for a wound that is 50 sq cm:
- Code 15271, Application of skin substitute graft to trunk, arms, legs, total wound surface area up to 100 sq cm; first 25 sq cm or less wound surface area
- Code +15272, each additional 25 sq cm wound surface area, or part thereof

To accurately code for this skin graft, two codes would be used: 15271 and 15272.

In the Tabular List in most CPT manuals, the legend explaining the meanings of the convention symbols is found at the bottom of each page.

CRITICAL THINKING 25.2

Sherald is trying to look up the CPT code for a left arm cyst biopsy. She has found the code, but how can she show that the procedure took place on the left side?

Sherald also came across CPT code 32440 (removal of lung, pneumonectomy), but she needs to also code for the repair of a portion of the bronchus. The code has a (+) in front of it; what does this mean?

DOCUMENTATION FOR CPT CODING

Medical records used for procedural coding can include any or all of the following:
- Encounter form (Fig. 25.4)
- History and physical report (H&P)
- Progress notes
- Discharge summary
- Operative report
- Pathology report
- Anesthesia record
- Radiology report

When comparing the documentation to the codes, make sure all the elements of the description match substantially, with nothing added or missing. For example, review CPT codes 21315 and 21320. Both codes describe the closed treatment of a nasal bone fracture. However, 21315 indicates that there is no stabilization, and 21320 indicates that there is stabilization. The coder reviews the procedures and then assigns the CPT codes with the description that most closely resembles the documentation.

Some providers have CPT and ICD-10-CM codes printed on their encounter forms; however, these codes should be treated only as a reference. Medical coders must also review the health record carefully, abstracting all the procedures and services rendered during an encounter. For example, a provider may circle the procedure for a preventive health visit for a 4-year-old on the encounter form but forget to record the injections provided during the encounter. When the medical assistant reviews the patient's electronic health record (EHR), he or she discovers that the provider's notes state routine injections were administered. If the medical assistant had not reviewed the EHR, the clinic would have lost reimbursement because the claim would not have included all the CPT codes for the visit. Encounter forms should be updated annually to ensure that code additions, changes, and revisions are current.

USING THE ALPHABETIC INDEX

Procedural coding starts with identifying the main term and then locating it in the Alphabetic Index. Although the Alphabetic Index is a comprehensive, alphabetical listing of all main terms, there are no code descriptions. It is not effective to assign a CPT code simply by finding it through the Alphabetic Index. The Alphabetic Index is not a substitute for the Tabular List. Even if an individual is only looking for one code, the Tabular List must be used to ensure the code is accurate.

The Alphabetic Index is used as a guide to search for one or more codes or code ranges. The index is similar to that found in the back of any textbook; it is an alphabetic list of main and modifying terms found in the Tabular List of the coding manual. In a typical index, the term or concept listed in the index is followed by the page numbers on which detailed information is presented in the body of the book. The Alphabetic Index in the CPT coding manual is used in the same way, except that it provides codes or code ranges rather than page numbers. As discussed

CHAPTER 25 Procedural Coding Basics

YOUR NAME CLINIC
Walden-Martin Family Medical Clinic,
1234 Anystreet, Anytown AK 12345
Phone: 123-123-1234   Fax: 123-123-5678

Julie Walden, M.D.   David Kahn, M.D.
James Marin, M.D.   Jean Burke, N.P.
Angela Perez, M.D.

TELEPHONE:
FAX:

PATIENT'S NAME   CHART #   DATE

☐ MEDI-MEDI   ☐ MEDICAL
☐ MEDICARE   ☐ PRIVATE
☐ SELF PAY   ☐ HMO

✓	CPT/Md	DESCRIPTION	FEE	✓	CPT/Md	DESCRIPTION	FEE	✓	CPT/Md	DESCRIPTION	FEE	✓	CPT/Md	DESCRIPTION	FEE
	OFFICE VISIT—NEW PATIENT				**LAB STUDIES**				**PROCEDURES (continued)**				**INJECTIONS**		
	99202	Focused Ex.			36415	Venipucture			93235	Holter, 24 Hour			90724	Influenza	
	99203	Detailed Ex.			81000	Urinalysis			10061	I & D Abscess Comp.			90732	Pneumococcal	
	99204	Comprehensive Ex.			81003	–w/o Micro			10060	I & D Abscess Simple			J0295	Ampicillin, 1 gr	
	99205	Complex Ex.			84703	HCG (Urine, Pregnancy)			94761	Oximetry w/Exercise			J0696	Rocephine	
	OFFICE VISIT—ESTABLISHED PATIENT				82948	Glucose			93720	Plethysmography			J1030	Depomedrol 40 mg	
	99212	Focused Ex.			82270	Hemoccult			94760	Pulse Oximetry			J2000	Lidocaine 50 cc	
	99213	Expanded Ex.			85023	CBC-diff.			10003	Rem. Sebaceous Cyst			J2175	Demerol	
	99214	Detailed Ex.			85024	CBC w/part diff			11100	Skin Bx			J3360	Valium 5 mg	
	99215	Complex Ex.			85018	Hemoglobin			94010	Spirometry			J1885	Toradol 30 mg IV	
	PREVENTATIVE MEDICINE—NEW PATIENT				88155	Pap Smear			92801	Visual Acuity			J1885	Toradol 60 mg IM	
	99381	< 1 year old			87210	KOH/Saline Wet Mount			17100	Wart Removal			90720	DTP–HIB	
	99382	1–4 year old			87430	Strep Antigen			17101	Wart Removal, 2nd			90746	HEP B—HIB	
	99383	5–11 year old			87060	Throat Culture			17102	Wart Removal, 3–15			90707	MMR	
	99384	12–17 year old			80009	Chem profile			11042	Wound Debrid.			86580	PPD	
	99385	18–39 year old			80061	Lipid profile				**X-RAY**			86580	PPD w/control	
	99386	40–64 year old			82465	Cholesterol			70210	Sinuses			90732	Pneumovax	
	99387	65+ year old			99000	Handling fee			70360	Neck Soft Tissue			90716	Varicella	
	PREVENTATIVE MEDICINE—ESTABLISHED PATIENT				**PROCEDURES**				71010	CXR (PA only)			82607	Vitamin B12 Inj.	
	99391	< 1 year old			92551	Audiometry			71020	Chest 2V			90712	Polio	
	99392	1–4 year old			29705	Cast Removal			72040	C-Spine 2V			90788	TD Adult	
	99393	5–11 year old			2900_	Casting (by location)			72100	Lumbrosacral			95115	Allergy inj., single	
	99394	12–17 year old			92567	Ear Check			73030	Shoulder 2V			95117	Allergry inj., multiple	
	99395	18–39 year old			69210	Ear Wax Rem. 1 2			73070	Elbow 2V					
	99396	40–64 year old			93000	EKG			73120	Hand 2V					
	99397	65+ year old			93005	EKG tracing only			73560	Knee 2V					
					93010	EKG. Int. and Rep			73620	Foot 2V					
					11750	Excision Nail			74000	KUB					
					94375	Flow Volume									

DESCRIPTION   ICD-10-CM

- Abdominal pain/unspec...... R10.9
- Abscess...... L02._
- Allergic reaction...... T78.40_
- Alzheimer's disease...... G30
- Anemia/unspec...... D64.9
- Angina/unspec...... I20.9
- Anorexia...... R63.0
- Anxiety/unspec...... F41.9
- Apnea, sleep...... G47.30
- Arrhythmia, cardiac...... I49.9
- Arthritis, rheumatoid...... M06.9
- Asthma/unspec...... J45.909
- Atrial fibrillation...... I48.0
- B-12 deficiency...... E53.8
- Back pain, low...... M54.5
- BPH...... N40
- Bradycardia/unspec...... R00.1
- Broncitis, acute...... J20._
- Bronchitis, chronic...... J42
- Bursitis/unspec...... M71.9
- CA, breast...... C50._
- CA, lung...... C34._
- CA, prostate...... C61
- Cellulitis...... L03._
- Chest pain/unspec...... R07.9
- Cirrhosis, liver/unspec...... K74.60
- Cold, common...... J00
- Colitis/unspec...... K51.90
- Confusion...... R41.0
- CHF...... I50.9
- Constipation...... K59.00
- COPD...... J44.9
- Cough...... R05
- Crohn's disease/unspec...... K50.90
- CVA...... I63.9
- Decubitus ulcer...... L89._
- Dehydration...... E86.0
- Dementia/unspec...... F03
- Depression, major/unsp...... F32.9
- Diab I, no complications...... E10.0
- Diab II, no complications...... E11.9
  - w/kidney complic...... E11.2_
  - w/ophthalmic compl...... E11.3_
  - w/neurolog compl...... E11.4_
  - w/circulartory compl...... E11.5_
- Insulin use...... Z79.4
- Diarrhea/unspec...... R19.7
- Diverticulitis...... K57.92
- Diverticulosis...... K57.90
- Dizziness...... R42
- Dysuria...... R30.0
- Edema/unspec...... R60.9
- Endocarditis...... I38
- Esophageal reflux...... K21.0
- Fatigue (lethargy)...... R53.83
- FUO...... R50.9
- Gastritis...... K29.70
- Gastroenteritis (colitis)...... K52.9
- G.I. bleed...... K92.2
- Gout/unspec...... M10.9
- Headache...... R51
- Health exam...... 200._
- Hematuria/unspec...... R31.9
- Herpes simplex...... B00.9
- Herpes zoster...... B02.9
- Hiatal hernia...... K44.9
- HTN (HBP)...... I10
- Hyperlipidemia/unspec...... E78.5
- Hypothyroidism/unspec...... E03.9
- Impotence...... N52._
- Influenza, respiratory...... J10.1
- Insomnia...... G47.0
- IBS, diarrhea...... K58._
- Lupus, systemic erythim...... M32.9
- MI, acute...... I21._
- MI, old...... I25.2
- Migraine...... G43.9
- Myalgia...... M79.1
- Neck pain...... M54.2
- Neuropathy...... G62.9
- Nausea...... R11.1
- Nausea/vomitting...... R11.0
- Obesity/unspec...... E66.9
- Osteoarthritis (site)...... M19._
- Otitis media...... H66.9_
- Parkinson's disease...... G20
- Pharyngitis, acute...... J02.9
- Pleurisy...... R09.1
- Pneumonia...... J18.9
- Pneumonia, viral...... J12.9
- Prostatitis/unspec...... N41.9
- PVD...... I73.9
- Radiculopathyp...... M54.1_
- Rectal bleeding...... K62.5
- Renal failure...... N19
- Sciatica...... M54.3_
- Shortness of breath...... R03.02
- Sinusitis, chr./unspec...... J32.9
- Syncope...... R55
- Tachycardia/unspec...... R00.0
- Tachy., supraventric...... I47.1
- Tedinitix/unspec...... M77.9
- TIA...... G45.9
- Ulcer, duodenal/unspec...... K26.9
- Ulcer, gastric/unspec...... K25.9
- Ulcer, peptic/unspec...... K27.9
- URI/unspec...... J06.9
- UTI...... N39.0
- Vertigo...... R42
- Weight gain...... R63.5
- Weight loss...... R63.4

DIAGNOSIS: (IF NOT CHECKED ABOVE)

PROCEDURES: (IF NOT CHECKED ABOVE)

RETURN APPOINTMENT INFORMATION:

( ) DAYS ( ) WKS. ( ) MOS. ( ) PRN

REC'D BY:
☐ CASH
☐ CR. CARD
☐ CHECK
#

TODAY'S FEE

AMT. REC'D.

BALANCE

FIG. 25.4 Encounter form. (From Proctor D, Niedzwiecki B: *Kinn's The Medical Assistant*, ed 13, St Louis, 2017, Elsevier.)

earlier, the Tabular List is divided into sections, and the procedures and services are listed in numeric order by the Category I code.

The Alphabetic Index is organized by main terms, and modifying terms that are indented below the main term. Modifying terms further describe and add information needed to narrow the search for an appropriate procedure or service code. A main term can be a procedure, such as an excision. Each modifying term could provide further information such as:
- anatomical location
- organ excised
- type of instrument used
- special technique
- other procedures performed at the same time (e.g., obtaining biopsy tissue for examination)

Modifying terms affect the selection of appropriate codes; therefore, it is important to review the list of modifying terms when selecting a code or code range.

Searching the Alphabetic Index

Begin the search of the Alphabetic Index by using one of the four primary classifications (or types) of main and modifying terms:
- Procedure or service (e.g., examination, excision, scope, revision, repair, drainage)
- Organ or anatomical site (e.g., clavicle, mandible, humerus, liver, colon, uterus)
- Condition, illness, or injury (e.g., *cholelithiasis* [koh lee lih THY is sis[, ulcer, fracture, pregnancy, fever)
- Eponym, synonym, abbreviation, or acronym (e.g., Naffziger operation, MRI [magnetic resonance imaging], TURP [transurethral resection of the prostate])

> **MEDICAL TERMINOLOGY**
> **chol/e:** gall, bile
> **lith/o:** stones
> **–iasis:** presence of

> **VOCABULARY**
> **cholelithiasis:** Presence of stones in the gall bladder.

When searching the Alphabetic Index, use:
- the name of the performed procedure or service (anastomosis, splint, repair, stress test, therapy, vaccination)
- the organ or other anatomical site of the procedure (tibia, colon, salivary gland, aorta)
- the condition, illness, or injury (abscess, fracture, cholelithiasis, strabismus)
- synonyms, eponyms, or abbreviations (ECG [electrocardiography], Stookey-Scarff procedure, Mohs' micrographic surgery)

Sometimes searching for a main term may not yield any results. When a main term cannot be found, search by another primary classification in the Alphabetic Index. Let's search the following procedural statement: Removal of Skin Tags on Neck. Begin by identifying the Main terms that closely match the four primary classifications in the Alphabetic Index:
1. Procedure of Service: Removal
2. Organ or Anatomic Site: Neck Skin
3. Condition, Illness, or Injury: Skin Tag
4. Eponym: None in this case

Once all possible main terms have been abstracted, the coder can quickly search through the Alphabetic Index for the code or code range that matches the procedural statement.

Using *See* and *See Also* in the Alphabetic Index

The *see* statement in the Alphabetic Index points to another location in the Alphabetic Index to find the code or code range. The *see also* statement points to additional codes or code ranges in the Alphabetic Index that may be useful to the code found in the original search.

Single Codes and Code Ranges

In the Alphabetic Index, a procedure or service may list a single code or a range of possible codes that may match the documentation. Remember that the Alphabetic Index is an index; it is designed as a guide to the most suitable codes that match the documentation. At this point, the search is only for the closest match or matches to the procedural statement.

Some medical procedures and diagnostic tests can be quite complex. There may be a single code or a code range that may include one main term but has several modifying terms for the main term. For example, the code for Acromioplasty has a range of codes: 23415–23420. The same main term, Acromioplasty, with a modifying term, partial, has a single code: 23130. The code range is shown with a hyphen to indicate that all codes within that range could be appropriate.

In some cases, a single code and a range of codes are listed for the same service or procedure. For example, Craterization, femur, lists both the single code 27360 and the code range 27070–27071. Once a single code or code range has been found in the Alphabetic Index, the next step is to look up each of those in the Tabular List. Select the code or codes that most closely match the documentation (Box 25.3).

> **CRITICAL THINKING 25.3**
>
> Sherald is having trouble finding a procedural code for removal of a cataract in the Alphabetic Index. What are some options and/or alternative ways she can perform an Alphabetic Index search?

USING THE TABULAR LIST

Once the code or code ranges have been selected from the Alphabetic Index, the next stop is the Tabular List. This is where the procedural coding decision takes place. In the Tabular List, the conventions, symbols, guidelines, notes, and even the punctuation all play a part in choosing the most accurate code possible.

In the Tabular List, look up each code or code range found numerically in the Alphabetic Index. Read the description of each code thoroughly to ensure that the main terms abstracted from the procedural statement in the medical documentation are all included in the code description, with nothing substantial omitted or added. Read the section guidelines

> **BOX 25.3 Steps for Using the CPT Alphabetic Index**
>
> 1. Abstract the procedural statement from the medical documentation and determine the main and/or modifying terms.
> 2. Select the most appropriate main term to begin searching in the Alphabetic Index.
> 3. Once the main term has been located, select one or more modifying terms, if needed, to narrow the search.
> 4. If no main or modifying term produces an appropriate code or code range, repeat steps 2 and 3 using a different main term.
> 5. Find the code or code ranges that include all or most of the description of the procedure or service found in the medical record.

> **BOX 25.4 Steps for Using the CPT Tabular List**
>
> Except for the special considerations required for coding from the Evaluation and Management (E/M) and Anesthesia sections, the following steps apply to all sections of the CPT manual.
> 1. Look up the code or code range from the Alphabetic Index Search in the Tabular List numerically.
> 2. Compare the description of the code with the procedural statement from the documentation. Verify that all or most of the health record documentation matches the code description and that there is no additional element or information in the code description that is not found in the documentation.
> 3. Read the guidelines and notes for the section, subsection, and code to ensure that there are no contraindications to the use of the code.
> 4. Evaluate the conventions, especially add-on codes (+) and exemption from modifier −51.
> 5. Determine whether any special circumstances require the use of a modifier or whether a Special Report is required.
> 6. Record the CPT code selected in the health record documentation next to the procedure or service performed and in the appropriate block of the insurance claim form.

and notes to determine whether additional codes should be used, add-on codes or modifiers are required, or use of the code is contraindicated.

Use of the Semicolon

A semicolon (;) at the end of a main description indicates that modifying terms and descriptions follow. Every indented description below a stand-alone code is related to that stand-alone code. To get the full description for an indented code, you use the description of the stand-alone code up to the semicolon and then include the description of the indented code. Let's look at excision of the spleen as an example. In the CPT manual you will see the following entry:

Hemic and Lymphatic Systems
Spleen
Excision
38100 Splenectomy; total (separate procedure)
38101 partial (separate procedure)
38102 total, en bloc for extensive disease, in conjunction with other procedure (List in additional to code for primary procedure)

The description for code 38100 is a splenectomy, total. The description for code 38101 is splenectomy, partial. The description for code 38102 is splenectomy, total, en bloc for extensive disease, in conjunction with other procedure. If you were to use 38102, you would also have to have the code for the other procedure. You could not use just 38102 (Box 25.4).

For practice on CPT surgery coding, refer to Procedure 25.1.

COMMON CPT CODING GUIDELINES: EVALUATION AND MANAGEMENT SECTION

Evaluation and Management codes are commonly referred to as E/M codes. These codes are used to reflect what the provider does during the time spent with the patient. To properly code for that, the medical assistant must apply different techniques from the basic steps outlined earlier. Assigning the correct E/M code includes:
- identifying the following for the procedure or service:
  - section
  - subsection
  - category
  - subcategory
- reviewing the reporting instructions and guidelines for the code chosen
- reviewing the level of E/M service
  - determining the extent of the history obtained and the examination performed
  - determining the complexity of medical decision making

The E/M section is divided into broad subsections, such as office visit, emergency room visit, hospital visit, and consultation. These subsections are further divided into subcategories, which include the place where the services were rendered, such as:
- provider's office
- hospital emergency department
- skilled nursing facility
- patient's home
- patient status
  - new
  - established

Procedure 25.2, Part A, explains how to perform CPT coding for an office visit.

The first two steps in choosing an E/M code are:
1. Identify the place of service (POS)
2. Identify the patient status (new or established)

Identifying the Place of Service

The place of service (POS) is the healthcare facility where the provider delivered care to the patient. The two most common places of service are "office" and "hospital." Table 25.3 presents a list of common POS locations and their 2-digit identifying numbers, or POS codes.

Identifying the Patient Status

The patient status choices are "new" or "established" patient. A new patient (NP) is one who has not received any professional services from the provider, or from another provider of the exact same specialty and subspecialty who belongs to the same group practice, within the past 3 years.

An established patient (EP) is one who has received professional services from the provider, or from another provider of the exact same specialty and subspecialty who belongs to the same group practice, within the past 3 years.

Once the POS and patient status have been established, the next step in selection of an E/M code is to determine the level of service provided.

Determining the Level of Service Provided

Key Components and Contributing Factors. The three key components for determining the level of service for E/M coding are:
- History
- Examination
- Medical decision making

The four contributing factors are:
- Counseling
- Nature of the presenting problem
- Coordination of care
- Time

The history, examination, and medical decision-making components are considered the three most important components for deciding the level of service. Counseling, the nature of the presenting problem, coordination of care, and time are secondary considerations. Fig. 25.5 presents criteria for choosing the appropriate E/M code.

PROCEDURE 25.1   Perform Procedural Coding: Surgery

Task
To use the steps for CPT procedural coding to find the most accurate and specific CPT surgery code.

Equipment and Supplies
- CPT coding manual (current year) or
- TruCode encoder software
- Operative report (see the following figure)

Operative Report

PATIENT NAME: Sonia Sample
ROOM NUMBER: 222 West
MR NUMBER: 12-34-56

DATE OF PROCEDURE: 04/22/00
PREOPERATIVE DIAGNOSIS: Acute cholecystitis
POSTOPERATIVE DIAGNOSIS: Acute cholecystitis
NAME OF PROCEDURE: 1. Laparoscopic cholecystectomy
   2. Intraoperative cystic duct cholangiogram
SURGEON: Claude St. John, M.D.
ASSISTANT: Mark Weiss, D.O.
ANESTHESIOLOGIST: Angela Adams, M.D.
ANESTHESIA: General

DESCRIPTION OF THE OPERATION:
   The patient was placed in the supine position under general anesthesia. The oral gastric tube was placed. The Foley catheter was placed. The patient received appropriate antibiotics. The abdomen was prepped with iodine and draped in the usual fashion. Using a midline subumbilical incision, we entered the subcutaneous fat to find the aponeurosis of the rectus abdominis. Two stay sutures were placed 0.5 cm from the midline bilaterally and we left on these sutures, creating an opening in the linea alba.
   Under direct vision, the catheter was placed. The Hasson cannula was placed in the abdominal cavity and all was normal except an acute necrotizing and probably gangrenous gallbladder. There were multiple omental adhesions. Three other trocars were placed in the right subcostal plane in the midline, midclavicular line, and midaxillary line using a #10, #5, and #5 mm trocar, respectively. The gallbladder was punctured and emptied of clear white bile indicating a hydrops of the gallbladder. It was grasped at its fundus and at Hartmann's pouch retracted cephalad and to the right, respectively. We found the cystic duct and the cystic artery after circumferential dissection and isolated the cystic duct completely.
   When we were sure that this structure was a deep cystic duct, the clip was placed at the most distal aspect to make an opening immediately proximally and we placed a Reddick cholangiocatheter into it via #14 gauge percutaneous catheter. The cholangiogram showed normal arborization of the liver radicals. Normal bifurcation of the common hepatic duct. Normal common hepatic duct. Long large cystic duct. The common bile duct had numerous stones within it. They could not be emptied from the common bile duct. There was good flow into the duodenum.
   The impression was choledocholithiasis. This was corroborated by the radiologist. The decision was made to prepare the patient most probably for endoscopic retrograde cholangiopancreatography postoperatively, and no further intervention of the common bile duct was done in this setting.
   The cholangiocatheter was removed. An attempt was made to milk the bile out, but no stones came out. Three clips were placed on the proximal aspect of the cystic duct and the duct was then cut distally. The artery was isolated and double clipped proximally and single clipped distally and cut in the intervening section. We then peeled the gallbladder off the gallbladder bed with some difficulty because of the intense edema and inflammation. It was then removed from the liver bed completely. Cautery, suctioning and irrigation were used copiously to create a bloodless field. A last check was made and there was no bleeding and no bile leaking. A #15 Jackson-Pratt type drain was placed into Morrison's pouch and brought out through the lateral most port. We then removed, with great difficulty, the gallbladder from the umbilicus. Because of its enormous size and a 3 cm stone within it that was very difficult to macerate, the opening of the umbilicus had to be enlarged.
   As this was done, we removed the gallbladder completely and sent it for pathologic section. Two separate figure-of-eight 0 PDS were used to close the abdominal fascia. The Jackson-Pratt drain was then sutured in place with 2.0 nylon. The skin was closed throughout with subcuticular 3-0 PDS after copious irrigation of the subcutaneous plane. Mastisol and Steri-Strips were placed on the wound. The patient remained stable although she did have bigeminy during surgery and was on a Lidocaine drip. She will be going to the intensive care unit but as she left, she was extubated in the recovery room and was fully alert. She is moving all limbs.
   I will discuss with the gastroenterologist postoperative endoscopic retrograde cholangiopancreatography.
   SPECIMEN: Gallbladder.

Claude St. John, M.D.
CSJ/ld:
D: 04/22/00
T: 04/22/00 9:21 am
CC: Maria Acosta, M.D.

PROCEDURE 25.1   Perform Procedural Coding: Surgery—cont'd

Procedural Steps
Using the CPT Coding Manual
1. Abstract the procedures and/or services from the procedural statement in the surgical report.
2. Select the most appropriate main term to begin the search in the Alphabetic Index.
3. Once the main term has been located in the Alphabetic Index, review and select the modifying term or terms if required.
   Purpose: For additional specificity and to narrow the search for the most accurate CPT code or code range in the Alphabetic Index.
4. If the main term cannot be found in the Alphabetic Index, repeat steps 2 and 3 using a different main term possibly based on the procedural statement.
5. Once the CPT code or code range is identified in the Alphabetic Index, disregard any code or code range containing additional descriptions or modifying terms not found in the health record.
6. Record the code or code ranges that best match the procedural statements in the surgical report.
   Purpose: To prevent repeated reference to the Alphabetic Index by recording all possible matches to the code or code range sought. This saves time and prevents redundant effort.
7. Turn to the Tabular List and find the first code or code range from your search of the Alphabetic Index.
   Purpose: To begin the process of finding the most specific and accurate code.
8. Compare the description of the code with the procedural statement in the surgical report. Verify that all or most of the health record documentation matches the code description and that there is no additional information in the code description that is not found in the documentation.
9. Review the coding guidelines and notes for the section, subsection, and code to ensure that there are no contraindications to use of the code. Review the coding conventions and add-on codes, if any.
   Purpose: To ensure there are no instructions that would prevent the use of the code selected.
10. Determine whether a modifier is needed.
    Purpose: To select any appropriate modifiers that provide additional information for the chosen code to explain certain circumstances or provide additional detail.
11. Determine whether a Special Report is required.
    Purpose: To clarify and add additional detail when an unusual or extenuating circumstance exists or if a Category III or unlisted procedure Category I code is used.
12. Record the CPT code selected in the health record documentation next to the procedure or service performed and in the appropriate block of the insurance claim form.
    Purpose: To complete the documentation and recording requirements.

Using the TruCode Software
1. Abstract the procedures and/or services from the procedural statement in the surgical report.
2. Type the main term into the encoder Search box and select the CPT. Then click on Show All Results.
3. If the main term cannot be found through the search, repeat steps 2 and 3 using a different main term based on the procedural statement.
4. Choose the procedure description that is closest to the procedural statement in the surgical report (see the following figure).
   Purpose: To prevent upcoding or downcoding errors or other possible fraud and/or abuse circumstances.

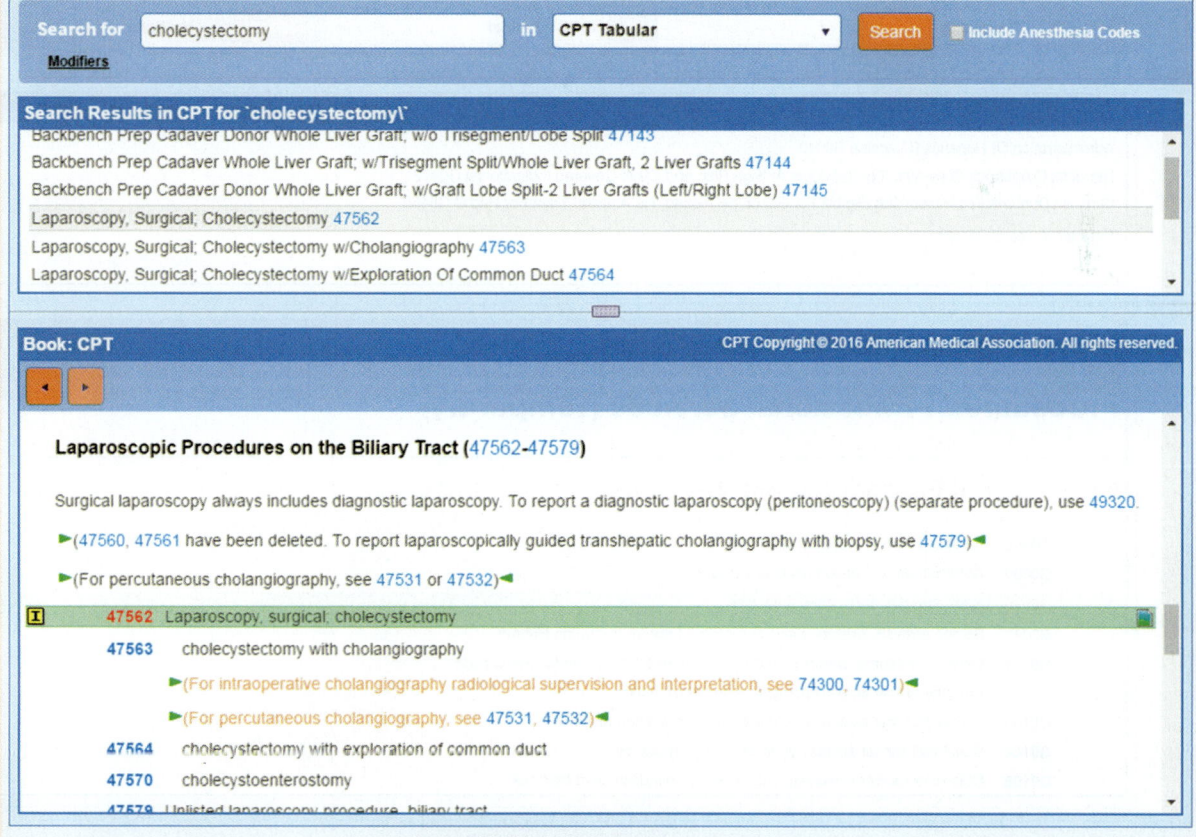

5. Record the CPT code that best matches the procedural statements in the surgical report in the patient's health record.
   Purpose: To prevent repeated reference to the Alphabetic Index by recording all possible matches to the code or code range being sought. This saves time and prevents redundant effort.

PROCEDURE 25.2   Perform Procedural Coding: Office Visit and Immunizations

Task
To use the steps for CPT Evaluation and Management coding and HCPCS coding to find the most accurate and specific CPT E/M and HCPCS codes using the coding manuals or the TruCode encoder.

Equipment and Supplies
- CPT coding manual (current year)
- HCPCS coding manual (current year) or
- TruCode encoder software
- Progress note

Progress Note for Daniel Miller (DOB 03/12/2012)
04/08/20XX Daniel was seen today for a follow-up visit for his recent case of otitis media in the left ear. The ear infection has completely cleared, and he is now able to receive his hepatitis B vaccine. The office visit involved a problem-focused history, problem-focused examination, and medical decision making of low complexity.

Procedural Steps
Part A: CPT E/M Coding
1. Determine the place of service from the encounter form.
   Purpose: To determine the most accurate CPT E/M code, the place of service needs to be identified.
2. Determine the patient's status.
   Purpose: To determine the most accurate CPT E/M code, the patient should be identified as new or established.
3. Identify the subsection, category, or subcategory of service in the E/M section.
   Purpose: To ensure that the correct place of service and patient status are used and the appropriate level of service is selected.
4. Determine the level of service:
   - Determine the extent of the history obtained.
   - Determine the extent of the examination performed.
   - Determine the complexity of medical decision making.
   Purpose: To ensure that the correct level is chosen for the history, examination, and medical decision making.
5. If necessary, compare the medical documentation against examples in Appendix C, Clinical Examples, of the CPT manual.
   Purpose: To help the coder select the appropriate level of service.
6. Select the appropriate level of E/M service code, and document it in the patient's health record.
   Purpose: To complete the documentation and reporting requirements.

Part B: HCPCS Coding With TruCode Encoder Software
1. Review the provider documentation.
   Purpose: To ensure that all procedures and/or services are listed on the encounter form; that all procedures and services on the encounter form match the health record; and that nothing documented in the health record is missing from the encounter form.
2. Type the main term into the Search box of the encoder and choose the HCPCS Tabular code set for accurate coding (see the following figure).

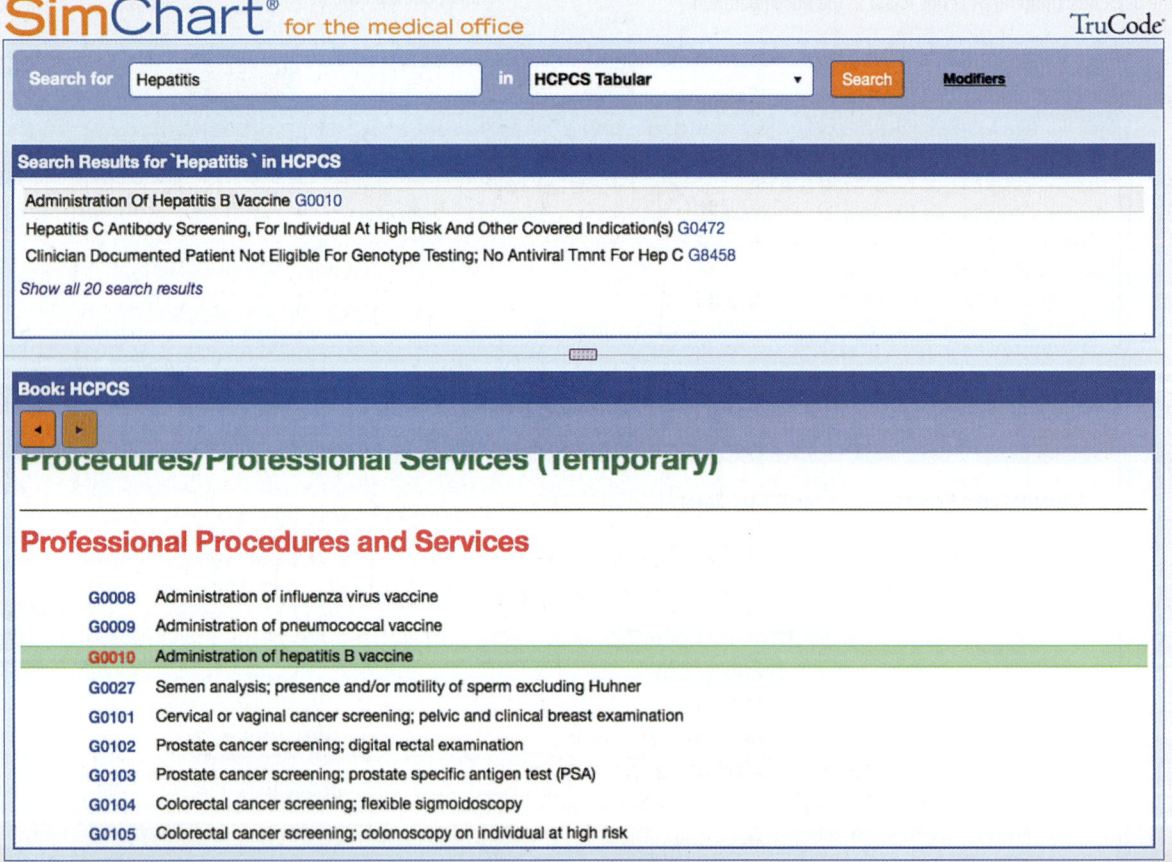

1

3. If no modifying term produces an appropriate code or code range, repeat steps 2 and 3 using a different main term.
   Purpose: To help find the most appropriate code or code range by using alternative methods of searching the Alphabetic Index.
4. Compare the description of the code with the medical documentation.
   Purpose: To avoid upcoding and downcoding errors and to ensure there are no contraindications to use of the code selected.
5. Select the appropriate HCPCS immunization code, and document it in the patient's health record.
   Purpose: To complete the documentation and reporting requirements.

TABLE 25.3 Commonly Used Place of Service (POS) Codes

Code	Name
01	Pharmacy
11	Office
12	Home
13	Assisted Living Facility
14	Group Home
15	Mobile Unit
17	Walk-In Retail Health Clinic
20	Urgent Care Facility
21	Inpatient Hospital
22	Outpatient Hospital
23	Emergency Room–Hospital
24	Ambulatory Surgery Center
31	Skilled Nursing Facility
34	Hospice
51	Inpatient Psychiatric Facility
60	Mass Immunization Center
65	End-Stage Renal Disease Treatment Facility
71	Public Health Clinic
72	Rural Health Clinic
81	Independent Laboratory

History. To understand the history levels, it is important to know the definition and components of the patient's history. The history relates to the patient's clinical picture and depends on the patient for answers to specific questions.

Levels of history. The following are the four levels of history taking.

- *Problem-focused history:* A problem-focused history concentrates on the chief complaint; it looks at the symptoms, severity, and duration of the problem. It usually does not include a **review of systems (ROS)** or the family and social histories.
- *Expanded problem-focused history:* The expanded problem-focused history includes:
  - symptoms, severity, and duration of the chief complaint
  - review of systems that relate to the chief complaint.

Usually the past, family, and social histories are not included.

- *Detailed history:* The detailed history includes:
  - chief complaint
  - extended history of present illness

> **VOCABULARY**
>
> **review of systems:** A list of questions related to each organ system, designed to uncover potential disease processes.

Select the Appropriate Level of E/M Services Based on the Following

1. For the following categories/subcategories, **all of the key components**, ie, history, examination, and medical decision making, must meet or exceed the stated requirements to qualify for a particular level of E/M service: office, new patient; hospital observation services; initial hospital care; office consultations; initial inpatient consultations; emergency department services; initial nursing facility care; domiciliary care, new patient; and home, new patient.

2. For the following categories/subcategories, **two of the three key components** (ie, history, examination, and medical decision making) must meet or exceed the stated requirements to qualify for a particular level of E/M services: office, established patient; subsequent hospital care; subsequent nursing facility care; domiciliary care, established patient; and home, established patient.

3. When counseling and/or coordination of care dominates (more than 50%) the encounter with the patient and/or family (face-to-face time in the office or other outpatient setting or floor/unit time in the hospital or nursing facility), then **time** shall be considered the key or controlling factor to qualify for a particular level of E/M services. This includes time spent with parties who have assumed responsibility for the care of the patient or decision making whether or not they are family members (eg, foster parents, person acting in loco parentis, legal guardian). The extent of counseling and/or coordination of care must be documented in the medical record.

FIG. 25.5 Appropriate assignment of E/M codes. (From Proctor D, Niedzwiecki B: *Kinn's The Medical Assistant*, ed 13, St Louis, 2017, Elsevier.)

- problem-pertinent system review, including a review of a limited number of additional systems
- pertinent past, family, and/or social histories directly related to the patient's problems.
- *Comprehensive history:* A comprehensive history includes:
  - chief complaint
  - extended history of present illness
  - ROS that is directly related to the problem or problems identified in the history of the present illness
  - review of all additional body systems, in addition to complete past, family, and social histories

Examination. The examination is the objective part of the patient's visit. The provider examines the patient, obtains measurable findings, and makes notes referring to body areas and/or organ systems as follows:
- *Body areas:* Head, including face and neck; chest, including breasts and axillae; abdomen; genitalia, groin, and buttocks; and back, including spine and extremities
- *Organs and organ systems:* General (e.g., vital signs, general appearance); eyes; ears, nose, throat, and mouth; cardiovascular; respiratory; gastrointestinal (GI); genitourinary; musculoskeletal; skin; neurologic; psychiatric; and hematologic, lymphatic, and immunologic

Levels of examination. The examination is divided into the following levels:
- *Problem-focused examination:* The examination is limited to the affected body area or single system mentioned in the chief complaint.
- *Expanded problem-focused examination:* In addition to the limited body area or system, related body areas or organ systems are examined.
- *Detailed examination:* An extended examination is performed on the affected body area and related body areas or organ systems.
- *Comprehensive examination:* A complete multisystem examination is performed or a complete examination of a single organ system.

Medical Decision Making. When a provider makes medical decisions, the decisions are based on many years of education and experience. Three elements comprise the medical decision-making process:
1. The number of diagnoses and/or management options
2. The amount and/or complexity of data obtained, reviewed, and analyzed
3. The risk of significant complications and/or morbidity and/or mortality

Number of diagnoses and management options. The provider's notes during the history and examination should help identify whether the patient's problem is minor, acute, stable, or worsening. The documentation should also identify whether a new problem exists or whether the provider plans to order any diagnostic tests to further investigate the patient's illness or injury.

Amount and complexity of data reviewed. The documentation should also identify what laboratory tests, x-ray diagnostic procedures, and other tests have been ordered or reviewed.

Risk of complications and morbidity or mortality. Risk is often involved in medical care, either from the treatment given to the patient or from the lack of treatment and professional care. *Morbidity,* the

TABLE 25.4 Complexity of Medical Decision Making

Number of Diagnoses or Management Options	Amount and/or Complexity of Data to Be Reviewed	Risk of Complications and/or Morbidity or Mortality	Type of Medical Decision Making
Minimal	Minimal or none	Minimal	Straightforward
Limited	Limited	Low	Low complexity
Multiple	Moderate	Moderate	Moderate complexity
Extensive	Extensive	High	High complexity

relative incidence of disease, and *mortality,* which relates to the number of deaths from a given disease, are integral parts of the provider's assessment of risks.

Complexity levels in medical decision making. The complexity of medical decision making is categorized into four levels:
- straightforward
- low complexity
- moderate complexity
- high complexity

Table 25.4 presents descriptions of the different levels of complexity of medical decision making.

Factors That Contribute to E/M Complexity

Counseling. Counseling is a discussion with a patient and/or family members about:
- diagnostic results
- impressions
- recommended diagnostic studies
- prognosis
- risks and benefits of management or treatment options
- instructions for management, treatment, and/or follow-up.

Almost all E/M services involve a degree of counseling with the patient and/or family. This is factored into the E/M code. As long as the counseling does not exceed 50% of the time spent with the patient, it is included in the E/M code. It can be considered a contributing factor when the counseling exceeds 50% of the encounter.

Nature of the Presenting Problem. The presenting problem is usually explained in the chief complaint. It can range from something as simple as a cold in an otherwise healthy patient to a life-threatening problem. Unless dealing with the nature of the presenting problem exceeds half of the patient encounter, it is included in the E/M code description and is not a factor in selecting the level of service.

Coordination of Care. Some patients need help in arranging for care beyond the visit or hospitalization. Some will need care in a skilled nursing facility or home health care. Others will need hospice care. The primary provider usually coordinates this care. Coordination of care is also factored into the E/M code and is a consideration for determining the level of service only when it exceeds 50% of the patient encounter.

Time. Time is included in the E/M code descriptions only to assist providers in selecting the most appropriate level of E/M service. The times stated in the code descriptions are averages. Time is not a

---

VOCABULARY

chief complaint: A statement in the patient's own words that describes the reason for the visit.

determining factor in code selection unless counseling exceeds more than 50% of the encounter. Only then can time be used as a determining component to code level selection.

At first, E/M coding can be difficult to understand and put into practice. The E/M coding process provided here can serve as a guide to help medical assistants in determining:
- place of service
- patient status
- level of care provided

You can then select the most accurate E/M code. Using the clinical examples in Appendix C of the CPT manual and comparing them to the medical documentation also can help medical assistants acquire a better understanding of E/M coding.

COMMON CPT CODING GUIDELINES: SURGICAL SECTION

Specific guidelines and notes related to surgery coding must be considered when assigning a CPT code. Always review the current year's guidelines for the Surgery section for the most up-to-date information. The following sections discuss a few of the more common guidelines. When coding procedures and services, be sure to read the guidelines and notes thoroughly for accurate coding assignment.

Surgical Package Definition

The CPT code set is designed to include patient prep, surgical care, and postsurgical care in a single code. These are considered **global services** because they are already built into the surgical package cost of the assigned CPT code. Medical coders that include any of these global services as a separate CPT code are committing fraud. The CPT code descriptions of global surgical services typically include the following:
- Local infiltration, digital block, and/or topical anesthesia
- After the decision for surgery, one related E/M encounter on the day of, or the day before, the date of the procedure
- Immediate postoperative care, including documentation in the patient's health record and talking with family and/or other physicians
- Writing orders for postsurgical care
- Evaluating the patient in the post anesthesia recovery area
- Typical postoperative follow-up care (includes care for approximately 6 to 8 weeks after surgery and is usually done at the provider's office)

Integumentary System – Excision of Lesions— Benign or Malignant

Excision of benign lesions includes a simple closure and anesthesia. If a wound (incision, excision, or traumatic lesion) requires intermediate or complex closure, the repair by intermediate or complex closure is coded and reported separately from the incision or excision. For example, if the provider excised a benign lesion measuring 1 cm from the patient's arm that required intermediate repair (closure), two codes would be used:
- 11401 – Excision, benign lesion including margins; excised diameter 0.6 to 1 cm
- 12031 Repair, intermediate, wounds of scalp, axillae, trunk and/or extremities (excluding hands and feet); 2.5 cm or less

Levels of Closure (Repair).
- *Simple repair:* Performed when the wound is superficial (epidermis, dermis, or subcutaneous) without significant involvement of deeper structures. This includes local anesthesia and chemical or electrocauterization of wounds not closed.
- *Intermediate repair:* Includes simple repair with a need for a layered closure of one or more of the deeper layers of subcutaneous tissue and superficial fascia in addition to the skin closure. Single-layer closure of heavily contaminated wounds that required extensive cleaning or removal of particulate matter also constitutes an intermediate repair.
- *Complex repair:* Includes wounds that require more than layered closure (e.g., scar revision, extensive undermining, or stents or retention sutures). Necessary preparation includes creation of a limited defect for repairs or **débridement** of complicated lacerations. Complex repair does not include excision of benign or malignant lesions, excisional preparation of a wound bed, or débridement, or the removal of damaged tissue or foreign objects from a wound, an open fracture, or an open dislocation.

Listing Services for Wound Repair.
- The repaired wound or wounds should be measured and recorded in centimeters; it also should be indicated whether the wound was curved, angular, or in a star-like pattern.
- When multiple wounds are repaired, add together the lengths of those in the same classification (simple, intermediate, or complex) and from all anatomical sites that are grouped together into the same code descriptor.
- When wounds of more than one classification are repaired, list the more complicated repair as the primary procedure and the less complicated repair as the secondary procedure, using modifier –59.
- Débridement is considered a separate procedure only when gross contamination requires prolonged cleansing; when a large amount of dead or contaminated tissue must be removed; or when débridement is carried out separately without immediate primary closure.
- Wound repair that involves nerves, blood vessels, and/or tendons should be reported under the appropriate system for repair of those structures. The repair of these associated wounds is included in the primary procedure unless it qualifies as a complex repair, in which case modifier –59 applies.

Musculoskeletal System
Fractures.
- *Closed fracture:* The fractured bone does not protrude through the dermis or epidermis.
- *Open fracture:* The fractured bone cuts through the skin layers and can be directly visualized.
- *Closed treatment:* The fracture site is not surgically opened. The three methods of closed treatment of fractures are:
  - without manipulation
  - with manipulation
  - with or without traction
- *Manipulation:* Attempted reduction or restoration of a fracture or dislocated joint into its normal anatomical alignment by manually applied forces.
- *Open treatment:* Used when (1) the fractured bone is surgically opened or (2) an opening is made remote from the fracture site to insert an intramedullary nail across the fracture site.

> **VOCABULARY**
> **débridement:** The surgical removal of dead, damaged, or infected tissue to improve the function of healthy tissue.
> **global services:** For purposes of CPT coding, medical services and procedures performed for the patient before, during, and after a surgical procedure, that are included with the assigned CPT code.

- *Percutaneous skeletal fixation:* Fracture treatment that is neither open nor closed. The fracture fragments are not visualized, but a fixation device (e.g., pins) is placed across the fracture site, usually under x-ray imaging.

Maternity Care and Delivery

The services normally provided in uncomplicated maternity cases include antepartum care, delivery, and postpartum care.

- *Antepartum* care includes:
  - initial and subsequent history
  - physical examinations
  - recording of weight, blood pressure, and fetal heart tones
  - routine chemical urinalysis
  - monthly visits up to 28 weeks' gestation
  - biweekly visits to 36 weeks' gestation
  - weekly visits until delivery.

Any other visits or services provided within this period should be coded separately, including any routine tests (e.g., sonography, routine laboratory tests).

- *Delivery* includes:
  - admission to the hospital, the admission history, and the physical examination
  - management of uncomplicated labor
  - vaginal delivery (with or without forceps or episiotomy), or cesarean delivery.

Medical problems complicating labor and delivery should be identified by using the codes in the Medicine and E/M sections in addition to codes for maternity care.

- *Postpartum* care includes:
  - hospital and office visits after vaginal or cesarean section delivery

COMMON CPT CODING GUIDELINES: PATHOLOGY AND LABORATORY SECTION

Assigning CPT codes for the Pathology section is the same procedure as for the Surgery section. For purposes of coding from the Laboratory section, organ or disease panels are groupings of numerous tests performed to diagnose the health or disease status of specific organ systems. A panel code can be used only if all the tests listed under the code selected were performed. These are considered *bundled codes* and must be billed under the single CPT code (Box 25.5). If they are not all present, the individual tests should be billed using a separate code for each. There are two types of drug testing, qualitative and quantitative. The codes for drug testing are *qualitative*; that is, they are based on the type of drug found. *Quantitative* assays, on the other hand, are performed to determine the amount of drug present.

CRITICAL THINKING 25.4

Sherald reviewed a coded medical record for a Basic Metabolic Panel with total Calcium that had listed specific CPT codes for each panel test. Is this the correct way to code for the organ panel? According to Box 25.5, how should this organ panel be coded?

HCPCS CODE SET AND MANUAL

Healthcare Common Procedure Coding System (HCPCS) codes have 5 alphanumeric characters, beginning with one letter followed by 4 numbers. HCPCS uses coding conventions for special instructions relating to specific codes (Fig. 25.6). The modifiers for HCPCS are codes composed of 2 alphanumeric characters. The HCPCS modifiers do not change the description of the code, but rather provide additional information or describe extenuating circumstances. Like the CPT manual, the HCPCS manual is divided into an Alphabetic Index and a Tabular List. As with the CPT, procedures and services are looked up in the Alphabetic Index, and the code (or codes) is then confirmed as the most accurate and appropriate using the Tabular List. The HCPCS manual has no subsections, categories, or subcategories; it has only sections. An appendix contains all the HCPCS modifiers and their descriptions.

The coding steps for HCPCS are almost identical to those for CPT codes. Clinical documentation is the starting point for HCPCS coding. The final code selected should add nothing to or omit anything from the description in the medical documentation. The final step is determining whether the code selected can stand alone or requires a modifier to further define or add needed information.

Sometimes HCPCS codes are used along with CPT codes, especially in the medical office setting (Fig. 25.7 and Box 25.7). For example, a well-baby visit would include the E/M code for the patient visit and also HCPCS codes for the administration of immunizations. Procedure 25.2, Part B, explains how to code an office visit involving immunizations.

BOX 25.5 CPT Tabular List Basic Metabolic Panel

80047 Basic Metabolic Panel (Calcium, Ionized)
This panel must include the following:
  Calcium, ionized (82330)
  Carbon dioxide (bicarbonate) (82374)
  Chloride (82435)
  Creatinine (82565)
  Glucose (82947)
  Potassium (84132)

The codes in parentheses after the individual tests are CPT codes. Those CPT codes would be used if not all of these tests were ordered at the same time.

Other Basic Metabolic Panel Components
Sodium (84295)
Urea Nitrogen (BUN) (84520)

BOX 25.6 Upcoding and Downcoding

Upcoding is the use of a higher level procedure code than is supported in the documentation or medical necessity. An example would be using E/M code 99213 (detailed history, detailed examination, and low complexity medical decision making) when the documentation supports 99202 (Expanded problem focused history and examination, and straightforward medical decision making). This would be considered fraud.

Downcoding is the use of a lower level procedure code than is justified. This also can be damaging to the healthcare facility, because it would result in lower reimbursement.

In procedural coding, the coder must always choose the code that most accurately describes the services provided.

- ● New. Additions to the previous edition.
- ▲ Revised. Revisions with the line or code from the previous edition.
- ▢ Reinstated. A code that was previously deleted and has now been reactivated.
- ✪ Special coverage instructions. Indicates that there are instructions provided regarding circumstances in which the code might be included for reimbursement.
- ⊘ Not covered by or valid by Medicare. These codes might result in reimbursement by private health insurance payers but not by Medicare.
- ✱ Carrier discretion. The individual third-party payer must be contacted to find out if coverage is available.

FIG. 25.6 HCPCS coding conventions. (From Proctor D, Niedzwiecki B: *Kinn's The Medical Assistant*, ed 13, St Louis, 2017, Elsevier.)

BOX 25.7 Healthcare Common Procedure Coding System (HCPCS)

HCPCS is a collection of codes and descriptions for procedures, supplies, products, and services not covered by or included in the CPT coding system (see Fig. 25.7). As are CPT codes, HCPCS codes are updated annually by the Centers for Medicare and Medicaid Services (CMS). These codes are designed to promote standardized reporting and collection of statistical data on medical supplies, products, services, and procedures.

Humidifiers/Compressors/Nebulizers for Use with Oxygen IPPB Equipment

Code	Description
E0550	Humidifier, durable for extensive supplemental humidification during IPPB treatments or oxygen delivery
E0555	Humidifier, durable, glass or autoclavable plastic bottle type, for use with regulator or flowmeter
E0560	Humidifier, durable for supplemental humidification during IPPB treatment or oxygen delivery
E0561	Humidifier, nonheated, used with positive airway pressure device
E0562	Humidifier, heated, used with positive airway pressure device
E0565	Compressor, air power source for equipment which is not self-contained or cylinder driven
E0570	Nebulizer, with compressor
E0571	Aerosol compressor, battery powered, for use with small volume nebulizer
E0572	Aerosol compressor, adjustable pressure, light duty for intermittent use
E0574	Ultrasonic/electronic aerosol generator with small volume nebulizer
E0575	Nebulizer, ultrasonic, large volume
E0580	Nebulizer, durable, glass or autoclavable plastic, bottle type, for use with regulator or flowmeter
E0585	Nebulizer, with compressor and heater

FIG. 25.7 Healthcare Common Procedure Coding System (HCPCS) Tabular List. (From Proctor D, Niedzwiecki B: *Kinn's The Medical Assistant*, ed 13, St Louis, 2017, Elsevier.)

COMMON HCPCS CODING GUIDELINES

Medical and Surgical Supplies

HCPCS codes for medical and surgical supplies range from A4000 to A6513. The HCPCS manual provides some figures that offer guidance as to what the medical and surgical supplies look like, so that they can be billed properly. Medical assistants can code only for surgical supplies purchased by the medical office. For example, pharmaceutical and medical equipment representatives can provide the medical office with some supplies that can be used for patient care. However, it is unethical to bill the patient's insurance company for supplies that were given to the provider for free. All medical and surgical supplies used during patient care should be documented on the encounter form in the patient's health record.

Durable Medical Equipment

HCPCS codes for durable medical equipment range from E0100 to E1841. Examples of durable medical equipment include crutches, wheelchairs, walkers, and other products that assist patients with mobility. Some equipment is kept in the medical office inventory. If the practice purchases the medical equipment wholesale, it is allowed to bill patients and/or their insurance company for the retail value of the equipment. Just as with medical and surgical supplies, it is important for the provider to document the dispensing of durable medical equipment on the encounter form or health record (Procedure 25.3).

EXCEPTIONAL CUSTOMER SERVICE

It is important for anyone who does coding to be able to explain to patients what those codes mean. When statements are sent to patients, many call the healthcare facility and ask for an explanation of the charges. A common question is, "Why is the charge for my office visit so high?" By looking at the CPT E/M code, you can see the level of history taking, physical examination, and medical decision making for that visit. You can help patients understand that it is not just the face-to-face time that determines the level of an office visit. If there is an extensive history and examination that is done and a lot of tests to review, the E/M code will be at a higher level. That higher level warrants a higher charge. Most patients understand once all the criteria have been explained to them. Doing this with a pleasant attitude also will help with patient satisfaction.

PROCEDURE 25.3 Working With Providers to Ensure Accurate Code Selection

Using tactful communication skills means using good manners as you provide truthful, sensitive information to another person, while considering the person's feelings. Tactful communication skills include verbal and nonverbal communication that shows respect, discretion, compassion, honesty, diplomacy, and courtesy. When you use tactful behaviors, you demonstrate professionalism and you preserve relationships, by avoiding conflicts and finding common ground.

Many times the medical coder is the expert on the accurate CPT and ICD code selections. The highest level of specificity must be used when coding so that appropriate reimbursement can occur. It is not uncommon for the medical coder to interact with providers and assist them in understanding the coding process. During these interactions, it is crucial that the medical coder provide the information in a professional, organized, and logical manner. Using tactful communication skills is critical to maintaining a healthy working relationship with the providers.

Using the following case study, role-play with two peers how you would use tactful communication skills with medical providers to ensure accurate code selection.

You are a new medical coder for the medical practice. You have been on the job for 6 weeks and have been seeing a trend that charges are being downcoded. The required documentation is present in the health records, but the providers have been selecting less specific codes for the appointments types. Your goal today is to explain to the providers accurate code selection for the appointment types.

CLOSING COMMENTS

The CPT and HCPCS coding manuals are updated and published every year. The updated manuals should be ordered in the early fall so that they arrive in time for the medical assistant to review them. Always use the current year's manuals so that the codes are accurate. The Introduction in each manual discusses and highlights changes and/or new coding guidelines. Annual updates should be uploaded to reflect any coding changes in the encoder to ensure that all codes are up-to-date for the current year.

CHAPTER REVIEW

In this chapter, you have learned how to determine CPT and HCPCS codes. For both types of codes, the coding process starts with the Alphabetic Index. CPT Category I codes are made up of five numerals. Category II and Category III codes have a letter at the end of the code. You must first determine the main term for the procedure or service and then locate it in the Alphabetic Index. From there you will see a single code, multiple codes, or a code range. All codes must be verified in the Tabular List. Once in the Tabular List, you must look at all of the coding conventions to make sure you have the most accurate code.

The Evaluation and Management codes in the CPT require some extra steps because you will need to determine the place of service and the patient status. Once those have been determined, you then need to look at all of the codes available in that section, referring to the documentation in the health record if needed. The key components for determining the correct E/M code are history, examination, and level of medical decision making.

HCPCS codes are used for services and supplies that are not found in the CPT. These codes always start with a letter and are followed by 4 numerals. In a medical office, HCPCS codes are most often used for medical and surgical supplies and durable medical equipment.

Modifiers are used with both CPT and HCPCS codes to further explain the services provided, such as right or left side. These modifiers can be numeric or alphabetic.

SCENARIO WRAP-UP

Sherald has learned that procedural coding using the CPT is similar in many ways to ICD-10-CM diagnostic coding. The two coding manuals have unique but also similar steps, conventions, and guidelines. She has learned that proper abstraction of procedural data from the health record is equally important for ICD-10-CM and CPT coding. Sherald also has learned that HCPCS codes are used to describe procedures and services not found in the CPT, such as vaccinations, ambulance services, and durable medical equipment.

Sherald uses documentation by the provider in the encounter form to identify the procedures performed. However, she realizes that she also must know how to use the CPT manual because some procedures or services must be coded from the documentation. As with diagnostic coding, Sherald reviews the patient's health record documentation if any questions come up about a claim. She knows that coding to the highest level of specificity helps to ensure accuracy and also enables the practice to obtain the maximum reimbursement allowed. She realizes the importance of keeping up-to-date with the CPT and HCPCS codes, so she plans to order the updated manuals every year. As Sherald continues to learn procedural coding, she envisions herself becoming well rounded in her knowledge of the practice's administrative operations.

26

Billing and Reimbursement

LEARNING OBJECTIVES

1. Identify the types of information contained in the patient's billing record.
2. Apply managed care policies and procedures; also, describe processes for precertification, and obtain precertification, including documentation.
3. Identify steps for filing a third-party claim.
4. Explain how to submit health insurance claims, including electronic claims, to various third-party payers.
5. Review the guidelines for completing the CMS-1500 Health Insurance Claim Form, and complete an insurance claim form.
6. Differentiate between fraud and abuse.
7. Discuss methods of preventing the rejection of claims, and display tactful behavior when speaking with medical providers about third-party requirements.
8. Describe ways of checking a claim's status.
9. Review and read an Explanation of Benefits.
10. Discuss reasons for denied claims.
11. Define "medically necessary" as it applies to diagnostic and procedural coding, and follow medical necessity guidelines.
12. Explain a patient's financial obligations for services rendered; also, inform a patient of these obligations, and show sensitivity when speaking with patients about third-party requirements.

CHAPTER OUTLINE

1. Opening Scenario, 566
2. You Will Learn, 566
3. Introduction, 566
4. Medical Billing Process, 566
5. Types of Information Found in the Patient's Billing Record, 567
6. Managed Care Policies and Procedures, 569
   a. Precertification/Preauthorization, 569
7. Submitting Claims to Third-Party Payers, 571
8. Generating Electronic Claims, 571
   a. Electronic Claims Submission, 571
      i. *Direct Billing, 571*
      ii. *Clearinghouse Submissions, 571*
9. Completing the CMS-1500 Health Insurance Claim Form, 572
   a. Section 1: Carrier – Block 1, 572
   b. Section 2: Patient and Insured Information – Blocks 1a through 13, 572
      i. *Blocks 1a, 4, 7, and 11 a-d, 572*
      ii. *Blocks 2, 3, 5, 6, and 10 a-c, 572*
      iii. *Block 9, 572*
      iv. *Blocks 12 and 13, 572*
   c. Section 3a: Physician or Supplier Information – Blocks 14 through 23, 573
      i. *Block 14, 573*
      ii. *Block 15, 573*
      iii. *Block 16, 574*
      iv. *Block 17 and 17b, 574*
      v. *Block 18, 574*
      vi. *Block 19, 574*
      vii. *Block 20, 574*
      viii. *Block 21, 574*
      ix. *Block 22, 574*
      x. *Block 23, 574*
   d. Section 3b: Physician or Supplier Information – Blocks 24 through 33, 575
      i. *Block 24, 575*
      ii. *Block 25, 576*
      iii. *Block 26, 576*
      iv. *Block 27, 576*
      v. *Block 28, 576*
      vi. *Block 29, 576*
      vii. *Block 30, 576*
      viii. *Block 31, 576*
      ix. *Block 32, 576*
      x. *Block 33, 576*
      xi. *Block 33a, 576*
10. Accurate Coding to Prevent Fraud and Abuse, 577
11. Preventing Rejection of a Claim, 580
    a. Communication with Providers About Third-Party Requirements, 580
12. Checking the Status of a Claim, 581
13. Explanation of Benefits, 581
    a. Reading an Explanation of Benefits, 581
    b. Rejected Claims, 581
14. Denied Claims, 581
    a. Medical Necessity, 582
15. The Patient's Financial Responsibility, 582
    a. Calculating the Co-insurance and Deductible, 582
    b. Allowed Amount, 583
    c. Discussing the Patient's Financial Responsibility, 583
    d. Showing Sensitivity When Discussing the Patient's Finances, 584
16. Closing Comments, 586
17. Chapter Review, 586

OPENING SCENARIO

Ann Snyder, a recent medical assisting graduate, has been hired to work in the billing office for Walden-Martin Family Medical Clinic (WMFM). During her medical assistant program, her instructor, Grant Wilson, helped her realize that working with health insurance can be quite rewarding. Mr. Wilson worked with Ann and her classmates, answering their questions and helping them to see that medical insurance is not as complicated as it may seem.

Ann is detailed oriented, and she enjoys billing and coding activities. She understands that performing these duties in the provider's office is crucial because tasks related to billing have a significant effect on the healthcare facility. She also understands that income generated is used to pay the clinic's expenses, including payroll, so the facility's staff indirectly counts on accurate and timely billing. Medical assistants who continually develop their coding skills are assets to the practice and can look forward to a long and rewarding career.

Ann gained an understanding of the insurance process while in school. Mr. Wilson showed the students several different Explanation of Benefits (EOBs) forms from a variety of insurance companies so that the students could learn how the reimbursement process works for a variety of health insurance plans. Ann also learned about the importance of verifying patient billing information, in addition to the steps for obtaining precertification for medical procedures. She also learned how to discuss the patient's billing record professionally. Ann is looking forward to using all of the skills she gained in school.

YOU WILL LEARN

- The importance of collecting accurate billing information
- How to obtain precertification/preauthorization for services
- How to complete a CMS-1500 claim form
- How to use the information found on explanation of benefits

VOCABULARY

claims clearinghouse: An organization that accepts the claim data from the provider, reformats the data to meet the specifications outlined by the insurance plan, and submits the claim.

CMS-1500 Health Insurance Claim Form (CMS-1500): The standard insurance claim form used for all government and most commercial insurance companies.

co-insurance: After the deductible has been met, the policyholder may need to pay a certain percentage of the bill and the insurance company pays the rest. A typical split is 80/20; the insurance company pays 80%, and the policy holder pays 20%.

copayment: A set dollar amount that the patient must pay for each office visit. There can be one copayment amount for a primary care provider, a different copayment amount (usually higher) to see a specialist or to be seen in the emergency department.

deductible: A set dollar amount that the policyholder must pay before the insurance company starts to pay for services.

eligibility: Meeting the stipulated requirements to participate in the healthcare plan.

explanation of benefits (EOB): A document sent by the insurance company to the provider and the patient explaining the allowed charge amount, the amount reimbursed for services, and the patient's financial responsibilities.

precertification The process of determining if a procedure or service is covered by the insurance plan and what the reimbursement is for that procedure or service.

INTRODUCTION

Medical billing and reimbursement represent the financial lifeline of the healthcare facility. Collecting accurate patient health insurance information is essential to submitting accurate health insurance claims. Each health insurance company has its own claims submission policies and procedures for timely reimbursement. A successful medical assistant in insurance billing learns the insurance company requirements and submits accurate claims. Many health insurance companies have online provider web portals. This has made the process of checking the status of a claim quick and easy. The medical assistant also needs to be able look at a patient's insurance card and interpret the information found there, including **copayment** amounts. An **explanation of benefits (EOB)** from the insurance carrier will indicate the patient's **deductible** and/or **co-insurance**. Clear communication with the patient about his or her financial responsibilities takes patience and sensitivity.

MEDICAL BILLING PROCESS

The medical billing process starts when a patient makes an appointment and is complete when payment has been received. The following steps are typically taken for medical billing.

- Collect patient information when the patient calls to schedule an appointment. This includes information about the insured, his or her employer, demographic information, and health insurance data.
- When the patient arrives for the appointment, you should:
    - make a copy or scan both sides of the patient's insurance card and government-issued ID card.
    - inform the patient of his or her copayment responsibility and collect it before services are provided (Procedure 26.1).
- Verify the patient's **eligibility** (EL i juh bill i tee), confirming that the patient's contract with the insurance company is valid for the date of service. Patient eligibility can be confirmed by:
    - calling the provider services phone number on the back of the health insurance ID card
    - using the provider web portal sponsored by the patient's health insurance company
- Review patient benefits and exclusions for certain medical procedures and services.
    - If **precertification** is needed, contact the health insurance company to request it.
- After services have been provided to the patient, code the diagnosis and procedures, and review the encounter form/superbill for completeness. The charges for the procedure or procedures should be provided automatically by the medical billing software.
- Complete the **CMS-1500 Health Insurance Claim Form (CMS-1500)** or an electronic claim form. Submit the form to the insurance company. Electronic claim information may be submitted to a **claims clearinghouse**.
- Review the electronic claims submission report to ensure that the claim was submitted accurately. Correct any discrepancies through the claims clearinghouse and resubmit denied claims.
- Meet the timely filing requirements of each of the different health insurance carriers. Health insurance companies do not pay claims submitted after the established filing period, and this balance cannot be billed to the patient.
- Post payments in the patient's account using the EOB to identify the line items that were paid, reduced, or denied. Patient account statements for the person's financial responsibility should be mailed out. Health insurance claims for patient accounts with secondary insurance should be submitted to the secondary carrier.

PROCEDURE 26.1   Interpret Information on an Insurance Card

Task:
To identify essential information on the health insurance identification (ID) card, so as to confirm copayment obligations and obtain accurate health insurance information for claims submission.

Equipment and Supplies
- Patient's health insurance ID card, both sides (see following figure)

Front

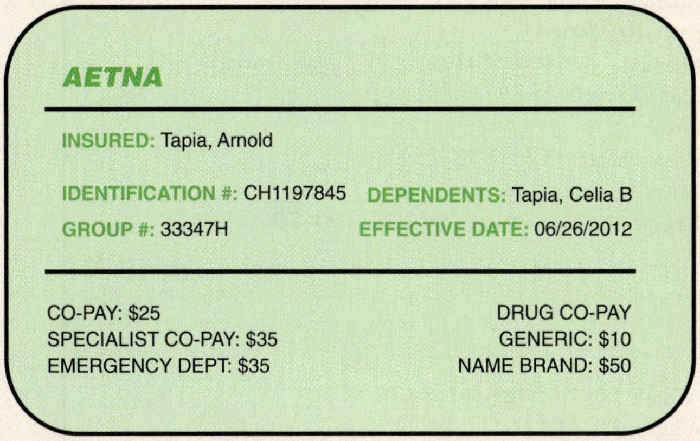

AETNA

INSURED: Tapia, Arnold
IDENTIFICATION #: CH1197845   DEPENDENTS: Tapia, Celia B
GROUP #: 33347H   EFFECTIVE DATE: 06/26/2012

CO-PAY: $25
SPECIALIST CO-PAY: $35
EMERGENCY DEPT: $35

DRUG CO-PAY
GENERIC: $10
NAME BRAND: $50

Back

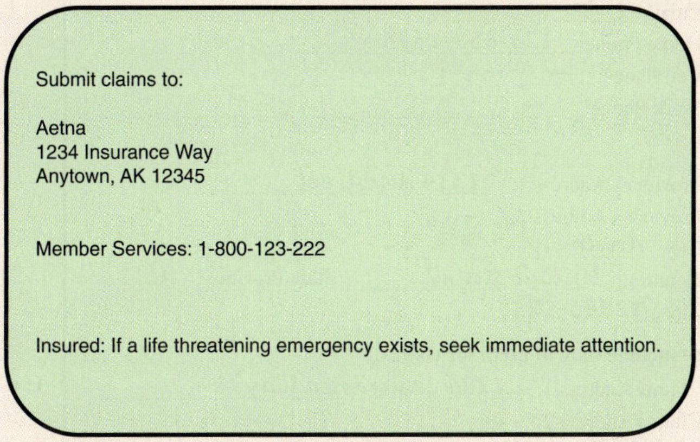

Submit claims to:

Aetna
1234 Insurance Way
Anytown, AK 12345

Member Services: 1-800-123-222

Insured: If a life threatening emergency exists, seek immediate attention.

Procedural Steps
1. Review the patient's health insurance ID card and identify the insured on the health insurance ID card. If the patient is someone other than the insured, obtain the relationship with the insured and the insured's date of birth and gender.
   Purpose: To submit an accurate health insurance claim, the insured's date of birth and gender are required.
2. Identify the insurance plan.
   Purpose: To confirm that the provider is a participating provider for the insurance plan or the HMO network. If the provider is out of network, the patient should be informed that they would either have to pay more out of pocket or the medical services rendered will not be covered by the insurance plan.
3. Identify the insured's identification number and group number.
   Purpose: To accurately submit the health insurance claim under the correct insurance policy number and group number.
4. Identify the patient's copayment, which is due before the appointment. Collect the correct amount. (For example, if the provider is a specialist, collect the copayment listed for specialist.)
   Purpose: To ensure that the proper copayment is paid by the patient.
5. On the back of the health insurance ID card, make sure that a customer service phone number and medical claims address are present.
   Purpose: To ensure that the provider can contact customer service and has the correct mailing address.

CRITICAL THINKING BOX 26.1

The medical billing manager informs Ann that she has noticed an increase in the number of insurance claim rejections that state the patient cannot be identified. Which step of the medical billing process might be addressed to resolve this problem?

TYPES OF INFORMATION FOUND IN THE PATIENT'S BILLING RECORD

The claim submission process begins after the patient receives services from the provider. When a patient makes a first appointment, it is routine to ask the patient for insurance billing information. Much of this information is collected on the patient information form (Fig. 26.1). This form can be sent to the patient ahead of time or completed when the patient comes to the medical office for the first visit. This form should always be completed for every new patient. For established patients, demographic and insurance information should be verified.

Accurate patient information for submitting a health insurance claim is important, but a medical **release of information** form, signed by the patient, should also be kept in the person's health record. The release form allows the release of medical information to the insurance company. Even though the patient expects the insurance claim to be submitted for payment, this cannot be done without a signature in the patient's health record granting permission.

VOCABULARY

release of information: A form completed by the patient that authorizes the medical office to release medical records to the insurance company for health insurance reimbursement.

WALDEN-MARTIN
FAMILY MEDICAL CLINIC
1234 ANYSTREET | ANYTOWN, ANYSTATE 12345
PHONE 123-123-1234 | FAX 123-123-5678

Patient Information

Patient Information (Please use full legal name.)
Last Name: Tapia
First Name: Celia
Middle Initial: B
Medical Record Number: 11012373
Date of Birth: 05/18/1970
Age: 42
Sex: Female
SSN: 857-62-1594
Emergency Contact Name: Arnold Tapia

Address 1: 12 Highland Court
Address 2: Apt 101
City: Anytown
Country: United States   State/Province: AL
Zip: 12345-1234
Email: —
Home Phone: 123-858-1545
Driver's License: —
Emergency Contact Phone: 123-200-5006

Guarantor Information (Please use full legal name.)
Relationship of Guarantor to Patient: Spouse
Guarantor/Account #: Tapia, Arnold / 12088787
Account Number: 12088787
Last Name: Tapia
First Name: Arnold
Middle Initial: —
Date of Birth: 05/18/1970
Age: 42
Sex: Male
SSN: 812-93-1341
Employer Name: Anytown String Shop
School Name: —

Address 1: 12 Highland Court
Address 2: Apt 101
City: Anytown
Country: United States   State/Province: AL
Zip: 12345-1234
Email: —
Home Phone: 123-858-1545
Cell Phone: —
Work Phone: —

Provider Information
Primary Provider: James A. Martin, MD
Referring Provider: —
Date of Last Visit: August 28, 2013
Phone: 123-123-1234

Provider's Address 1: 1234 Anystreet
Provider's Address 2: —
City: Anytown
Country: United States   State/Province: AL
Zip: 12345-1234

Insurance Information (If the patient is not the Insured party, please include date of birth for claims.)
Insurance: Aetna
Name of Policy Holder: Arnold Tapia
SSN: 812-93-1341
Policy/ID Number: CT5487854
Group Number: 41554T

Claims Address 1: 1234 Insurance Way
Claims Address 2: —
City: Anytown
Country: United States   State/Province: AL
Zip: 12345-1234
Claims Phone: 180-012-3222

Secondary Insurance
Insurance: —
Name of Policy Holder: —
SSN: —
Policy/ID Number: —
Group Number: —

Claims Address 1: —
Claims Address 2: —
City: —
Country: —   State/Province: —
Zip: —
Claims Phone: —

"I hereby authorize direct payment of all insurance benfits otherwise payable to me for services rendered. I understand that I am financially responsible for all charges not covered by insurance for services rendered on my behalf to my dependents. I authorize the above prociders to release any information required to secure payment of benefits. I authorize the use of this signature on all insurace submissions."

Signature: Celia Japia
Date: 05/06/20XX

FIG. 26.1 Completed patient information form.

PROCEDURE 26.2 Show Sensitivity When Communicating With Patients Regarding Third-Party Requirements

Task:
To demonstrate sensitivity through verbal and nonverbal communication when discussing third-party requirements with patients.

Scenario
Ken Thomas saw Jean Burke, N.P., for his asthma today. He was prescribed a fluticasone inhaler, 220 mcg, and a refill on his Albuterol inhaler. When Ken stops at the check-out desk to make a follow-up appointment, he looks concerned. You inquire how you can help him, and he states that he is wondering if his new insurance will pick up the fluticasone inhaler. He further explains that he has used one in the past, with great results, but he recently switched insurance plans, and he is finding it doesn't have the same coverage as his old plan.

Role-play 1: You call the insurance company and discuss the coverage with the insurance carrier's representative. The representative tells you that the fluticasone inhaler is not covered. The representative gives you names of two other inhalers that would be covered.

Role-play 2: You must explain to Ken, who is upset over his insurance coverage, that he would have to cover the $250 cost of the fluticasone inhaler.

Equipment and Supplies
- Copy of patient's health insurance ID card
- Prescription for new medication

Procedural Steps
1. Obtain a copy of the patient's health insurance ID card and the prescription for the new medication.
   Purpose: Having the required documents will help you to be more efficient as you perform the task.
2. Review the insurance card for coverage information and the phone number for providers.
   Purpose: You will need the phone number from the ID card to call the insurance company. You will also need to provide the insurance representative with the patient's information.
3. Using role-play 1, call the insurance company and clearly state the patient's information, the patient's question, and the name of the new medication.
   Purpose: The insurance representative will need the patient's information and the question to assist you. Speaking clearly as you provide the information will help the listener understand what you are asking.
4. Demonstrate professionalism in verbal communication skills by stating a respectful, clear, and organized message, pronouncing medical terminology and medication names correctly.
5. Using role-play 2, explain the insurance representative's message to the patient using language the person can understand.
   Purpose: For the patient to understand your message, you need to use language that he or she can understand.
6. Demonstrate sensitivity to the patient by paying attention and responding appropriately to his or her body language and verbal message.
   Purpose: Demonstrating sensitivity can be done through verbal messages and body language. Paying attention to the patient and responding appropriately to his or her message and nonverbal communication are important.
7. Demonstrate sensitivity to the patient by showing empathy and clarifying that you understand what the patient is stating. Give the patient your full attention during the conversation and reserve judgment.
8. Demonstrate sensitivity to the patient by using a pleasant, courteous tone of voice. Use body language to communicate respect (e.g., eye contact if culturally appropriate, keeping arms uncrossed and relaxed).
   Purpose: As the patient's frustration and anger increase, it is important to use a pleasant, courteous, and normal tone of voice. Keeping your body appearance relaxed (e.g., arms uncrossed, hands relaxed) will help to show the patient you are calm.
9. Provide the patient with options if appropriate.
   Purpose: Providing the patient with choices also shows the patient that you care.

BOX 26.1 Health Plan–Sponsored Training in Medical Billing

Some major health plans offer annual training for newly implemented medical billing policies and procedures. These sessions can range from 1 day to a week of informative seminars. Although these training sessions can be expensive, the knowledge gained ensures that the most accurate claims are being submitted. The experts conducting the seminars also can answer specific questions about medical billing situations. This can prove valuable for future claims submissions. Medical billers should visit the insurance company's website to see whether any training sessions are scheduled. Ideally, an office representative would attend a workshop at least once a year for most of the insurance companies that the practice submits claims to.

MANAGED CARE POLICIES AND PROCEDURES

Medical billers should be familiar with procedures commonly used by managed care organizations (MCOs), such as precertification. If the procedures are not followed, the MCO might not pay for the services. For example, pain management services typically require a preauthorization. If a pain management facility were to provide these services to the patient without preauthorization, the MCO could deny all insurance claims. To submit accurate health insurance claims, medical assistants should follow office procedures for applying MCO policies and procedures (Procedure 26.2). Box 26.1 presents more about training offered by MCOs for medical billing purposes.

Precertification/Preauthorization

In an effort to control costs, many MCOs require precertification for certain procedures and services. Precertification is the process of proving to the insurance company that the service is medically necessary. The insurance company, in turn, will determine if it is a covered service and what the reimbursement will be. Precertification must be done before the procedure or service is performed.

To obtain precertification, the medical assistant:
- calls the provider services phone number on the back of the patient's health insurance ID card.
- provides the insurance company with procedures and/or services requested and the diagnoses.
- documents the outcome of the call in the patient's health record, including the precertification number.

Precertification does not guarantee payment of services. The process ensures that both the healthcare provider and the patient are informed both of the amount that the insurance company will pay and also the amount that the patient will have to pay.

Each insurance company has its own precertification requirements. Almost every MCO requires precertification, but medical assistants must confirm this by contacting the insurance company. Successful medical billers are diligent in obtaining precertification.

The precertification and preauthorization processes (see Procedure 26.3) are very similar. The insurance company is contacted after the primary care provider (PCP) recommends the procedure or service. In fact, many health insurance companies use the terms precertification and preauthorization interchangeably. However, precertification specifically determines whether the procedure is medically necessary, and preauthorization gives the provider approval to render the medical service. Precertification and preauthorization can be requested through an insurance company's online web portal (Box 26.2 and Procedure 26.3).

MEDICAL TERMINOLOGY
esophagi/o: esophagus
-eal: pertaining to

VOCABULARY
endoscopy: Nonsurgical procedure that uses an endoscope to view inside the body.

BOX 26.2 Preauthorization/Precertification Examples

1. Dr. David Khan is the primary care provider (PCP) for Janine Butler, who has heartburn that has not improved with medication.
2. Because Ms. Butler's condition is not improving, Dr. Khan requests preauthorization for her to see Dr. Eduard Hamilton, a gastrointestinal (GI) specialist. Ms. Butler is insured by a managed care organization (MCO).
3. The MCO authorizes Ms. Butler to see Dr. Hamilton; this authorization is sent to Ms. Butler, Dr. Khan, and Dr. Hamilton. When Ms. Butler receives the authorization, she schedules an appointment with Dr. Hamilton.
4. After evaluating Ms. Butler, Dr. Hamilton orders an **esophageal** (eh soff uh JEE ul) **endoscopy**. However, Ms. Butler is concerned about her financial responsibility. Therefore, Dr. Hamilton's office requests precertification for the endoscopy on Ms. Butler's behalf.
5. The MCO notifies Dr. Hamilton that the plan would reimburse a total of $1,500, and Ms. Butler would be financially responsible for $400. The precertification is sent both to Dr. Hamilton and Ms. Butler, who agree to its financial terms and schedule the procedure.

PROCEDURE 26.3 Perform Precertification With Documentation

Task:
To obtain precertification from a patient's insurance carrier for requested services or procedures.

Equipment and Supplies
- *Paper method:* Patient's health record, prior authorization (precertification) request form, copy of patient's health insurance ID card, pen
- *Electronic method:* Electronic health record system, such as SimChart for the Medical Office (SCMO)

Scenario
You are working with Dr. Julie Walden at Walden-Martin Family Medical Clinic. Erma Willis (DOB 12/09/19XX) is seen for excessive snoring, and Dr. Walden orders a sleep study. You need to complete a prior authorization/certification form for the sleep study, which will be conducted by Dr. Jim Sandman. You checked, and there is a signed release of information form.

Insurance Information
Aetna
1234 Insurance Way
Anytown, AL 112345-1234
Member ID Number: EW8884910
Group Number: 66574W

Clinic and Provider Information
Walden-Martin Family Medicine Clinic
1234 Anystreet
Anytown, AL 12345
Provider: Julie Walden, MD
Fax: 123-123-5678
Phone: 123-123-1234
Provider Contact Name: (your name)

Service Information
Place: Walden-Martin Family Medicine Clinic
Service Requested: Sleep study
Starting Service Date: 1 week from today
Ending Service Date: 1 week from today
Service Frequency: once
ICD-10-CM code: R06.83
CPT code: 95807
Not related to an injury or workers' compensation

Procedural Steps
1. For the paper method, gather the health record, precertification/prior authorization request form, copy of the health insurance ID card, and a pen. For the electronic method, access the Simulation Playground in SCMO.
2. Using the health record, determine the service or procedure that requires precertification/preauthorization.
3. For the paper method, complete the precertification/prior authorization request form. For the electronic method, click on the Form Repository icon in SCMO. Select Prior Authorization Request from the left INFO PANEL. Use the Patient Search button at the bottom to find the patient. Complete the remaining fields of the form.
   Purpose: This provides information on the ordered procedure or service to the insurance company, which will notify the provider's representative if the procedure or service will be covered under the plan.
4. Proofread the completed form and make any revisions needed.
   Purpose: To ensure the accuracy of the information.
5. With the paper method, file the document in the health record after it has been faxed to the insurance carrier. With the electronic method, print and fax or electronically send the form to the insurance company and save the form to the patient's record.
   Purpose: Copies of all forms completed for the patient need to be maintained in the health record.

Referrals

Patients seeking specialized care must first visit their assigned PCP to obtain a referral to a specialist or for more specialized therapy or care. Patients with HMO plans can only obtain a referral to the specialist by visiting their assigned PCP. HMOs will measure how many patients are referred to specialists by individual PCPs. Approval or denial of a referral can take anywhere from a few minutes to a few days. The three types of referrals are as follows:
- A *regular referral* usually takes 3 to 10 working days for review and approval. This type of referral is used when the provider believes that the patient must see a specialist to continue treatment.
- An *urgent referral* usually takes about 24 hours for approval. This type of referral is used when an urgent but not life-threatening situation occurs.
- A *STAT referral* can be approved online when it is submitted to the utilization review department through the provider's Web portal. A STAT referral is used in an emergency situation as indicated by the provider.

A *regular referral* is the most common type and can be inconvenient for the patient. With most managed care plans, preauthorization needs to be obtained for a referral. Remember this cardinal rule: never tell the patient the referral has been approved unless you have a hard copy of the authorization. A referral is authorized after the approval has been received. When a referral is approved the PCP's office and the patient should receive a copy of the authorization. Always review the authorization thoroughly and confirm details such as approved diagnosis and procedure codes and the exact period of time the authorization lasts. The patient will receive a letter with an authorization number and details regarding the approved services. The patient must bring the authorization to the specialist's office on the date of the appointment.

SUBMITTING CLAIMS TO THIRD-PARTY PAYERS

All health insurance companies accept:
- CMS-1500 as the standard claim form
- ICD-10-CM for diagnostic codes
- CPT and HCPCS procedural codes

However, each health insurance company has its own policies and procedures for the submission of claims.

Guidelines for Medicare and Medicaid claims can be found on the administrator websites for each state. MCO plans associated with capitation agreements have specific guidelines on the types of medical services that are billable. Private health insurance plans have their own policies and procedures for submitting claims. The medical assistant should research the health plans commonly seen in the healthcare facility.

The medical assistant can successfully manage the requirements of the different insurance plans by keeping a medical billing manual. The manual should contain the billing policies and procedures for the most common third-party payers. The person in charge of the manual should make sure that every medical biller has a copy and that the policies and procedures are up-to-date. For example, Medicare's billing procedures and policies are updated on October 1. Whenever an update is released, the medical billing manual also should be updated.

GENERATING ELECTRONIC CLAIMS

Since 2006 Medicare has required that claims be sent electronically. Most health insurance plans have followed suit. If the majority of claims are submitted electronically, why is it important to learn the different fields of the CMS-1500 paper form? The data used to submit electronic claims is the same data used on the CMS-1500. A medical assistant who is familiar with a paper CMS-1500 will have no problem collecting the proper data for an electronic claim.

Electronic claims are insurance claims that are transmitted over the internet from the provider to the health insurance company through *electronic data interchange*. Electronic data interchange is the electronic transfer of data between two or more entities. When submitting electronic claims, a healthcare facility transmits the data for the claim, and the health insurance company accepts it. Most medical billing software is designed to generate electronic claims.

As with paper claims, when electronic claims are submitted, accurate data are essential. When the medical assistant reviews the claim for accuracy, the claim is prepared for submission.

Electronic Claims Submission

Electronic claims are submitted in the 5010 format established by the Health Insurance Portability and Accountability Act (HIPAA) and can be directly transmitted to the insurance carrier or to a claims clearinghouse.

Direct Billing. Direct billing is the process by which an insurance company allows a provider to electronically submit claims directly to the company. Most major insurance companies, including Medicare and Medicaid, provide software packages that are used to enter the following:
- Patient's information
- Insured's information
- Charges
- Provider details

Many carrier-direct systems are supplied free of charge to the provider, but the direct system can transmit only to specific carriers. If the majority of claims for the healthcare facility are submitted to just one insurance company, direct billing would be a good way to submit claims.

Clearinghouse Submissions. A claims clearinghouse is an organization that acts as a go-between for the healthcare facility and the insurance company. The clearinghouse:
- accepts electronically submitted claims information from healthcare agencies.
- audits the claims for completeness.
- reformats claims to meet the insurance companies' specifications.

The claims are sorted by insurance plans and sent in batches electronically to the appropriate companies. The insurance companies then send a report through the data clearinghouse to:
- confirm the receipt of claims.
- report the status of previously submitted claims.
- serve as claim payment notification.

A clearinghouse charges the healthcare facility a small fee for:
- sending and receiving claims transmissions.
- checking and preparing the claims for processing.
- consolidating claims so that one transmission can be sent to each carrier.
- submitting claims in correct data format to the appropriate insurance payer.

VOCABULARY

audit: A process completed before claims submission in which claims are examined for accuracy and completeness.

capitation: A payment arrangement for healthcare providers. The provider is paid a set amount for each enrolled person assigned to him or her, per period of time, whether or not that person has received services.

A typical fee is 25¢ per submitted claim. Other services that clearinghouses typically provide include:
- Reporting the number of claims submitted, and the number of errors and their specifics
- Forwarding claims to insurance carriers that accept electronic claims (e.g., Medicare, Medicaid, Blue Cross/Blue Shield, and others) or to another clearinghouse that may hold the contracts with specific payers
- Keeping provider offices updated as new carriers are added to the database
- Generating informative statistical reports

COMPLETING THE CMS-1500 HEALTH INSURANCE CLAIM FORM

The CMS-1500 Health Insurance Claim Form is the form required by HIPAA for paper claim submission. The form has 33 blocks. These blocks are divided into three sections:
- *Section 1: Carrier.* The first section indicates the type of insurance plan to which the claim is being submitted; this section includes only Block 1.
- *Section 2: Patient and Insured Information.* The second section contains information about the patient and the insured; it includes Blocks 1a through 13.
- *Section 3: Physician or Supplier Information.* The third section contains information about the provider or supplier; it includes Blocks 14 through 33.

Table 26.2 presents a summary of the information needed to complete the CMS-1500 accurately.

Section 1: Carrier – Block 1 (Fig. 26.2)

Block 1 shows the type of insurance the patient has. Indicate the type of health insurance coverage for this claim by putting an X in the appropriate box, marking only one box. This information directs the claim to the correct payer.

Section 2: Patient and Insured Information – Blocks 1a Through 13 (Fig. 26.3)

The CMS-1500 distinguishes between the patient and the insured. The insured is the individual who is directly contracted with the insurance company. For example, if an insurance claim for Sabrina Rudman is submitted and Blue Cross covers her through her employer, she is both the patient and the insured. However, if the insurance claim is for Chris Rudman, her son, Sabrina Rudman is the insured, and Chris Rudman, her dependent, is the patient. Every CMS-1500 requires the name, gender, and birth date of both the insured and the patient, even if they are different individuals. The blocks in Fig. 26.3 highlighted in yellow are for the patient's information, and the blocks highlighted in blue are for the insured's information.

Blocks 1a, 4, 7, and 11 a-d. Information required for the insured includes:
- person's health plan ID number
- name
- address
- policy and group numbers
- birth date (MM/DD/YYYY) and gender
- employer's name (if applicable)
- name of the insurance plan
- whether the insured has another health benefit plan

Blocks 2, 3, 5, 6, and 10 a-c. Required information for the patient includes:
- person's name
- birth date (MM/DD/YYYY) and gender
- address
- relationship to the insured
- patient's status
- whether the patient's condition is related to his or her job, an automobile accident, or some other accident

> ### CRITICAL THINKING BOX 26.2
>
> Ann is preparing an insurance claim to bill to Blue Cross. She notes that the patient is the dependent of the insured, so she reviews the patient registration intake form and finds that the date of birth for the insured is not present. Can Ann accurately complete the CMS-1500?

Block 9. Block 9 is for recording information about any secondary insurance plan that may be applicable. (Box 26.3) The data required includes:
- the other insured person's name
- policy or group number
- name of the other insurance plan.

Blocks 12 and 13. Block 12 requires the signature of the *patient* or an authorized person, and Block 13 requires the signature of the *insured* or an authorized person. In Block 12, the signature authorizes the release

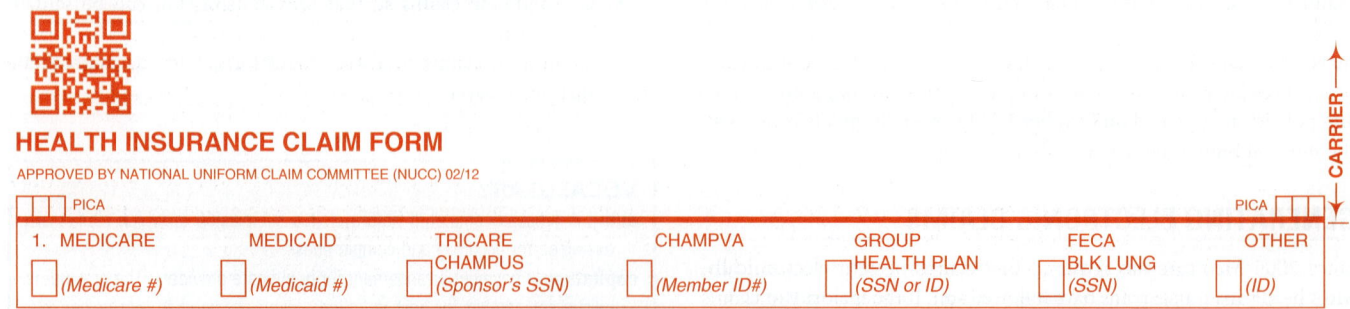

FIG. 26.2 Section 1 Carrier (Block 1). (From Proctor D, Niedzwiecki B: *Kinn's The Medical Assistant*, ed 13, St Louis, 2017, Elsevier.)

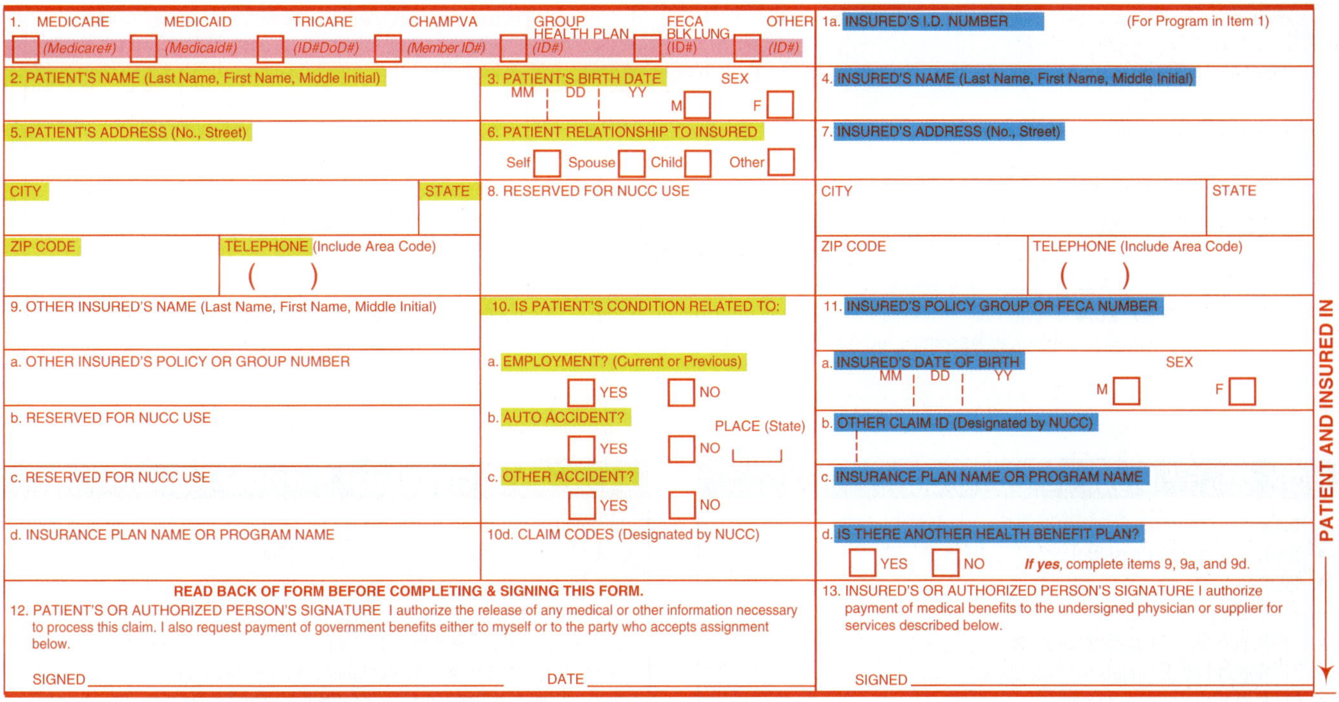

1. MEDICARE (Medicare#) | MEDICAID (Medicaid#) | TRICARE (ID#DoD#) | CHAMPVA (Member ID#) | GROUP HEALTH PLAN (ID#) | FECA BLK LUNG (ID#) | OTHER (ID#)

1a. INSURED'S I.D. NUMBER (For Program in Item 1)

2. PATIENT'S NAME (Last Name, First Name, Middle Initial)

3. PATIENT'S BIRTH DATE MM | DD | YY SEX M F

4. INSURED'S NAME (Last Name, First Name, Middle Initial)

5. PATIENT'S ADDRESS (No., Street)

6. PATIENT RELATIONSHIP TO INSURED Self Spouse Child Other

7. INSURED'S ADDRESS (No., Street)

CITY STATE

8. RESERVED FOR NUCC USE

CITY STATE

ZIP CODE TELEPHONE (Include Area Code) ( )

ZIP CODE TELEPHONE (Include Area Code) ( )

9. OTHER INSURED'S NAME (Last Name, First Name, Middle Initial)

10. IS PATIENT'S CONDITION RELATED TO:

11. INSURED'S POLICY GROUP OR FECA NUMBER

a. OTHER INSURED'S POLICY OR GROUP NUMBER

a. EMPLOYMENT? (Current or Previous) YES NO

a. INSURED'S DATE OF BIRTH MM | DD | YY SEX M F

b. RESERVED FOR NUCC USE

b. AUTO ACCIDENT? YES NO PLACE (State)

b. OTHER CLAIM ID (Designated by NUCC)

c. RESERVED FOR NUCC USE

c. OTHER ACCIDENT? YES NO

c. INSURANCE PLAN NAME OR PROGRAM NAME

d. INSURANCE PLAN NAME OR PROGRAM NAME

10d. CLAIM CODES (Designated by NUCC)

d. IS THERE ANOTHER HEALTH BENEFIT PLAN? YES NO *If yes*, complete items 9, 9a, and 9d.

READ BACK OF FORM BEFORE COMPLETING & SIGNING THIS FORM.

12. PATIENT'S OR AUTHORIZED PERSON'S SIGNATURE I authorize the release of any medical or other information necessary to process this claim. I also request payment of government benefits either to myself or to the party who accepts assignment below.

SIGNED ______ DATE ______

13. INSURED'S OR AUTHORIZED PERSON'S SIGNATURE I authorize payment of medical benefits to the undersigned physician or supplier for services described below.

SIGNED ______

PATIENT AND INSURED INFORMATION

FIG. 26.3 Section 2: Patient and Insured Information (Blocks 1a to 13). (From Proctor D, Niedzwiecki B: *Kinn's The Medical Assistant*, ed 13, St Louis, 2017, Elsevier.)

BOX 26.3 Primary and Secondary Insurance Determination

When a patient is covered by more than one insurance policy, it is important to determine which policy is considered primary. The primary insurance pays the claim first, and if there is anything left over, it is submitted to the secondary insurance company. One of the most common situations is a patient with coverage under two policies, such as a dependent whose parents each have family coverage through employer group insurance.

In the case of a child whose mother and father both carry the child as a dependent on their employer health insurance plans, primary and secondary insurance status is determined by the *birthday rule*. Whichever parent's birth date falls first in a calendar year is considered to have the primary insurance. The year of the parent's birth is not used. If the mother's birth date is February 20 and the father's birth date is May 1, the mother's insurance is the primary insurance and the father's insurance is the secondary insurance. This means the claim will be submitted to the mother's insurance first, and if there is any balance left, it will be submitted to the father's insurance.

Medicare is usually the primary insurance, and there is a secondary policy to cover the patient's responsibility. In some cases, however, Medicare can be the patient's secondary insurance. This typically happens when a Medicare patient is still covered under an employer-sponsored group policy because the patient works full time.

Medicaid is always the payer of last resort. That means if there is any other type of insurance coverage for the patient, that insurance is responsible for the claim. If there is any balance left over, it will be submitted to Medicaid.

of any medical or other information necessary to process or **adjudicate** (uh JOO di keyt) the claim. In Block 13, the signature affirms that the insured has a signature on file authorizing payment of medical benefits directly to the provider (whose name appears in Block 31). The phrase "Signature on File" or "SOF" may be entered in these fields (Box 26.4).

BOX 26.4 Assignment of Benefits

In the health insurance contract between the third-party payer and the patient, the patient receives the payment when a claim is submitted. For the healthcare facility to receive the reimbursement directly from the insurance company, the patient must sign an *assignment of benefits*. The assignment of benefits transfers the patient's legal right to collect benefits for medical expenses to the provider of those services, authorizing the payment to be sent directly to the provider. In other words, the assignment of benefits authorizes the provider to not only submit the insurance claim on behalf of the patient, but also to be reimbursed directly by the third-party payer. There is usually a statement about the assignment of benefits on the Patient Information form. When the patient has signed the assignment of benefits, the medical assistant completes Blocks 12 and 13 on the CMS-1500 form with the statement "Signature on File" or "SOF" and the claim filing date.

Section 3a: Physician or Supplier Information – Blocks 14 Through 23 (Fig. 26.4)

Block 14

Date of current illness, injury, or pregnancy (LMP). Block 14 requires the date of the current illness, injury, or pregnancy (LMP). The date should be the date on which the current illness or condition began; the date an injury occurred; or, in the case of pregnancy, the date of the last menstrual period (LMP), all in MM/DD/YYYY format.

Block 15

Other date. This block is used for another date related to the patient's condition or treatment. Enter the applicable qualifier (Box 26.5) to identify which date is being reported.

VOCABULARY

adjudicate: To settle or determine judicially.

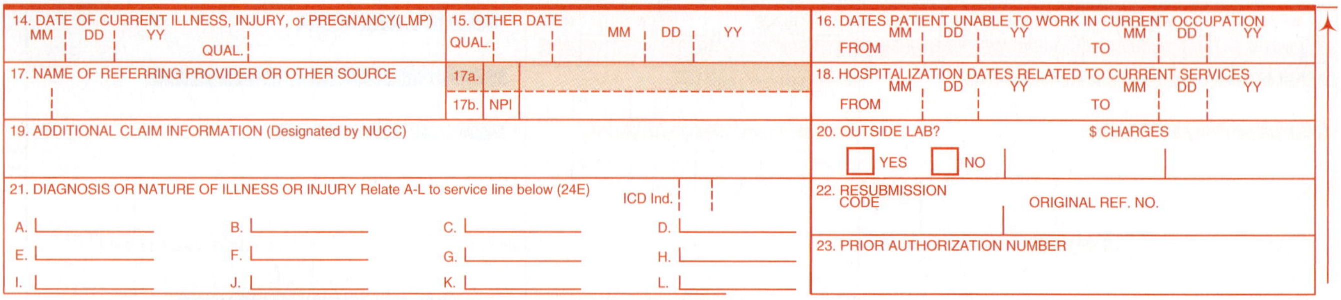
14. DATE OF CURRENT ILLNESS, INJURY, or PREGNANCY(LMP) MM DD YY QUAL.
15. OTHER DATE QUAL. MM DD YY
16. DATES PATIENT UNABLE TO WORK IN CURRENT OCCUPATION MM DD YY FROM TO MM DD YY
17. NAME OF REFERRING PROVIDER OR OTHER SOURCE
17a.
17b. NPI
18. HOSPITALIZATION DATES RELATED TO CURRENT SERVICES MM DD YY FROM TO MM DD YY
19. ADDITIONAL CLAIM INFORMATION (Designated by NUCC)
20. OUTSIDE LAB? YES NO $ CHARGES
21. DIAGNOSIS OR NATURE OF ILLNESS OR INJURY Relate A-L to service line below (24E) ICD Ind.
A. B. C. D.
E. F. G. H.
I. J. K. L.
22. RESUBMISSION CODE ORIGINAL REF. NO.
23. PRIOR AUTHORIZATION NUMBER

FIG. 26.4 Section 3a: Physician or Supplier Information (Blocks 14 to 23) (From Proctor D, Niedzwiecki B: *Kinn's The Medical Assistant*, ed 13, St Louis, 2017, Elsevier.)

BOX 26.5 Block 15 Qualifiers

- 454 Initial Treatment
- 304 Latest Visit or Consultation
- 455 Last X-ray
- 471 Prescription
- 090 Report Start (Assumed Care Date)
- 091 Report End (Relinquished Care Date)
- 444 First Visit or Consultation
- 439 Accident
- 453 Acute Manifestation of a Chronic Condition

BOX 26.6 National Provider Identifier (NPI)

Government insurance claims require that National Provider Identifiers (NPIs) be used for the referring providers (Block 17b) and rendering providers (Block 24J). Every healthcare entity is required to have an NPI. The NPI is an identifier assigned by the CMS that classifies the healthcare provider by license and medical specialty. The Administrative Simplification provisions of the Health Insurance Portability and Accountability Act (HIPAA) required the adoption of standard unique identifiers for healthcare providers and health plans. The purpose is to improve the efficiency of electronic transmission of health information.

Some private insurance companies may require claims to be submitted with the NPI. However, each privately sponsored insurance plan in each state has its own policies and procedures. Medical assistants will find that some third-party payers require NPIs and others do not.

Block 16

Dates patient unable to work in current occupation. These dates are used to help determine an employee's long- or short-term disability payments.

Block 17 and 17b

Name of referring provider or other source. Block 17 is for the name of the provider who referred or ordered the services or supplies. The following qualifier can be added:

- DN Referring Provider
- DK Ordering Provider
- DQ Supervising Provider

The providers' National Provider Identifier (NPI) (Box 26.6) is entered in Block 17b.

VOCABULARY

National Provider Identifier (NPI): An identifier assigned by the Centers for Medicare and Medicaid Services (CMS) that classifies the healthcare provider by license and medical specialties.

Block 18

Hospitalization dates related to current services. If inpatient services are provided, the admission and discharge dates are entered here.

Block 19

Additional claim information (designated by the National Uniform Claim Committee [NUCC]). Some insurance plans ask for specific identifiers in Block 19. The medical assistant should check the instructions from the applicable third-party payer.

Block 20

Outside lab charges. Applies to diagnostic laboratory services purchased from an independent or a separate provider (who is listed in Block 32). Put an X in the YES box to indicate that the diagnostic test was performed by an entity other than the provider billing for the service (i.e., the provider listed in Block 33), and that the provider in Block 33 paid the laboratory directly. Include the amount the provider was charged by the diagnostic laboratory.

Block 21

Diagnosis or nature of illness or injury. The ICD-10-CM diagnosis code or codes are entered. Up to 12 diagnostic codes can be entered here. The primary diagnosis should be recorded in the first field. Do not include the decimal point in the diagnosis code. Relate lines A to L to lines of service in Block 24E by the letter of the line. This will link the diagnosis to the service provided.

Block 22

Resubmission code and/or original reference number. Both the resubmission code and the original reference number assigned by the insurance payer must be entered in this block. Resubmission codes:

- 7 Replacement of prior claim
- 8 Void/cancel of prior claim

Block 23

Prior authorization number. The preauthorization/precertification number obtained from the insurance company is entered.

CHAPTER 26 Billing and Reimbursement

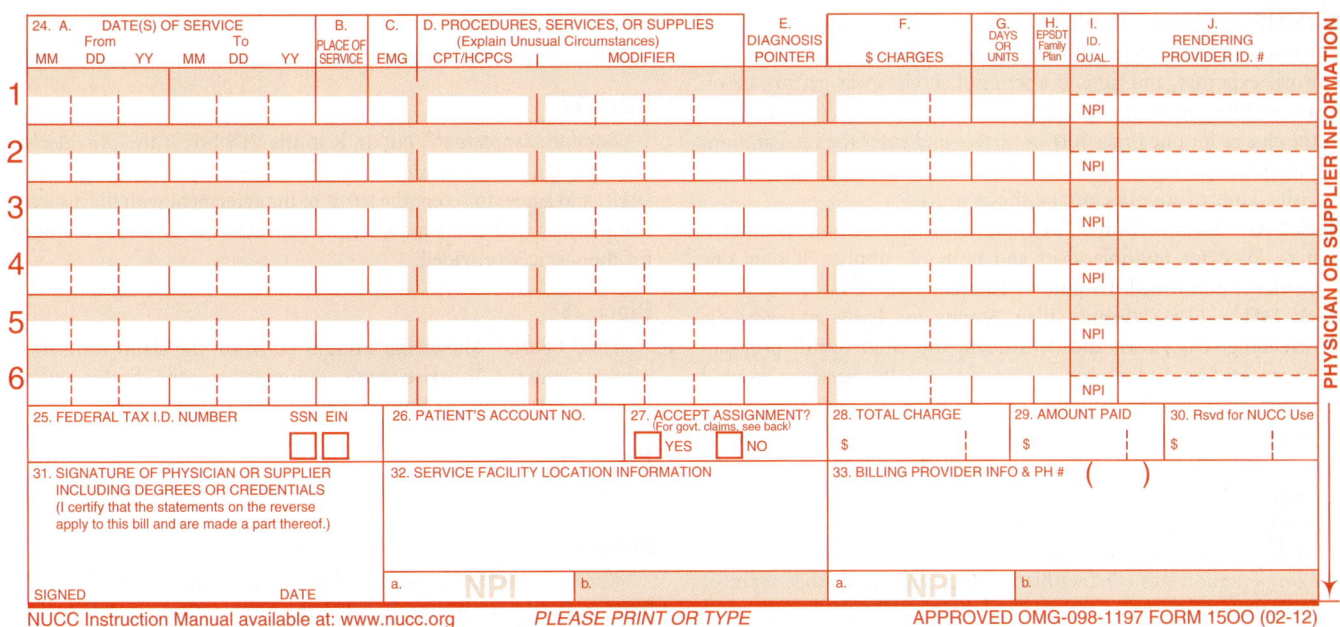

FIG. 26.5 Section 3b: Physician or Supplier Information (Blocks 24 to 33) (From Proctor D, Niedzwiecki B: *Kinn's The Medical Assistant*, ed 13, St Louis, 2017, Elsevier.)

Section 3b: Physician or Supplier Information – Blocks 24 Through 33 (Fig. 26.5)

Procedure codes, such as the Current Procedural Terminology (CPT) codes and/or the Healthcare Common Procedure Coding System (HCPCS) codes, are listed in Block 24. Each procedure code is considered a line item; the line numbers are found to the left of Block 24. All data in one line belongs to the coordinated CPT/HCPCS code. For claims that require more than six line-items, a second CMS-1500 form should be generated. Check with the insurance company to confirm how to indicate that the claim has multiple pages; some insurance companies require the statement "Continued" or "Page 1 of 2" in Block 28, Total Charges.

Block 24

Procedures and charges

Block 24A – Date(s) of Service. Note that there is space for both "From" and "To" dates. If the service was provided on just one day, you would only enter a From date, in a MM/DD/YY format. If the service was provided on multiple days, such as an inpatient hospital stay, the first day the service was provided would in the From field and the last day the service was provided would be entered in the To field. The number of times that that service was provided would be indicated in Block 24G.

Block 24B – Place of Service. The Place of Service (POS) codes indicate where the services were provided. As shown in Table 26.1, 11 would indicate that the procedure took place in a doctor's office.

Block 24C – EMG (emergency). A Y in this field indicates that the service was an emergency.

Block 24D – Procedures, Service or Supplies. There are two sections in this block, CPT/HCPCS and Modifier. There is space for a single 5-digit code and up to four separate 2-digit modifiers. No space is provided for a written description of the code; only the code is required.

Block 24E – Diagnosis Pointer. This block indicates which diagnosis is used for each line item. The letter from diagnosis listed in Block 21 should be used here to link the diagnosis to the service. Do not enter the ICD-10-CM codes in this block.

TABLE 26.1 Common Place of Service Codes

Code	Description
11	Doctor's office
12	Patient's home
21	Inpatient hospital
22	Outpatient hospital
23	Emergency department—hospital
24	Ambulatory surgical center
25	Birthing center
26	Military treatment facility/uniformed service treatment facility
31	Skilled nursing facility (swing bed visits)
32	Nursing facility (intermediate/long-term care facilities)
33	Custodial care facility (domiciliary or rest home services)
34	Hospice (domiciliary or rest home services)
35	Adult living care facilities (residential care facility)
41	Ambulance—land
42	Ambulance—air or water
50	Federally qualified health center
51	Inpatient psychiatry facility
52	Psychiatric facility—partial hospitalization
53	Community mental health care (outpatient, 24-hour/day services, admission screening, consultation, and educational services)
54	Intermediate care facility/mentally retarded
55	Residential substance abuse treatment facility
56	Psychiatric residential treatment center
60	Mass immunization center
61	Comprehensive inpatient rehabilitation facility
62	Comprehensive outpatient rehabilitation facility
65	End-stage renal disease treatment facility
71	State or local public health clinic
72	Rural health clinic
81	Independent laboratory
99	Other unlisted facility

Block 24F – $ Charges. The dollar amount of the provider's fee for the service is entered here. This fee is calculated in the office based on work, expertise, and time. If a series of services was performed on any one line, multiply the number of days or units (Block 24G) by the charge for one procedure or service and enter the total amount for all days or units. This field is most commonly used for multiple visits, units of supplies, or anesthesia units.

Block 24G – Days or Units. The number of days or units is entered here. Used for multiple visits and units of supplies. If only one service is performed, 1 would be entered.

Block 24H – EPSDT/Family Plan. Stands for Early and Periodic Screening, Diagnosis, and Treatment, the child health program under Medicaid. This block identifies specific services covered under state health insurance plans. Refer to the appropriate insurance payer's guidelines (typically Medicaid or the Medicaid intermediary) for instructions on completing this block. Leave the block blank for Medicare, TRICARE, and the Civilian Health and Medical Program of the Department of Veterans Affairs (CHAMPVA) (military insurance plans), group health plans, Federal Employees Compensation Act (FECA)/Black Lung, and most other types of insurance.

Block 24I – ID Qual. Used if the number in Block 24J is not an NPI. The following are the qualifiers:
- 0B State License Number
- 1G Provider UPIN Number
- G2 Provider Commercial Number
- LU Location Number
- ZZ Provider Taxonomy

Block 24J – Rendering Provider ID #. Enter the NPI of the provider who rendered the service, as identification.

Block 25
Facility information. The Federal Tax ID Number of the provider filing the claim can be listed as a Social Security number (SSN) or an Employer Identification Number (EIN); mark the appropriate box with an X.

Block 26
Patient's account no. Enter the account number or medical record number assigned to the patient by the provider of the service. This information will be included on the EOB from the insurance company to help with posting the payment.

Block 27
Accept assignment? Put an X in the YES box if the provider will accept assignment; this means that he or she is a *participating provider (PAR)* and agrees to accept the terms of the agreement with the insurance company, as well as accept what the plan states as an allowed amount for the services provided.

Block 28
Total Charge. Shows the amount billed on the claim form for all services rendered. To arrive at this amount, add up the charges reported in Block 24F for all the lines of service on the claim form.

Block 29
Amount Paid. The amount received from the patient or other payers.

Block 30
Reserved for NUCC Use. Some secondary insurance claims use this box for the claim amount due after the primary insurance has paid.

Block 31
Signature of Physician or Supplier. The signature of the authorized or accountable person for the services on the claim, verifying that he or she provided the services listed, and they have been checked for accuracy.

Block 32
Service Facility Location Information. Enter the name, address, city, state, and ZIP code for the site where the services listed in the claim were provided. Enter the facility's NPI in Block 32a only if it is different from the Billing Provider NPI (Block 24J).

Block 33
Billing Provider Info & PH #. Enter the address and phone number of the provider asking to be paid on this claim.

Block 33a
Enter the same NPI number listed in Block 24J.

TABLE 26.2 Information Required for Completion of the CMS-1500 Health Insurance Claim Form

Block	Information Needed	Block	Information Needed
	Completed patient registration/intake form	5	Patient's address and telephone number
	Photocopy of insurance card or cards (front and back)		• Permanent address (including apartment number if appropriate)
	Encounter form		• City, state, ZIP code
	Preauthorization or precertification number (when applicable)		• Telephone number
Section 1: Carrier		6	Patient's relationship to insured
1	Type of insurance	7	Insured's address and telephone number
Section 2: Patient and Insured Information			• Permanent address (including apartment number if appropriate)
1a	Insured's identification (ID) number (primary insurance)		• City, state, ZIP code
2	Patient's full name		• Telephone number
3	Patient's date of birth and gender	9	Other insured's name (secondary insurance)[a]
4	Insured's name (primary insurance)	9a	Policy or group number (secondary insurance)[a]

TABLE 26.2 Information Required for Completion of the CMS-1500 Health Insurance Claim Form—cont'd

Block	Information Needed	Block	Information Needed
9b	Secondary insured's date of birth and gender[a]	23	If prior authorization and/or referral is required, provide authorization (approval) number from insurance payer (preauthorization or precertification number)
9c	Secondary insured's employer or school name[a]		
9d	Secondary insured's insurance plan or program name[a]		
10a-c	If patient's condition or illness is related to employment, auto accident, or some other type of accident, make sure information is obtained as outlined in Block 1	24A	From–To dates of service for current encounter
		24B	Place of service (POS) code
		24C	If an emergency, put a Y in this box
10d	Claim codes as designated by NUCC	24D	CPT and/or HCPCS code
11	Insured's policy, group, or FECA number (primary insurance)		CPT and/or HCPCS modifier(s) (maximum of four per charge line)
11a	Primary insured's date of birth and gender	24E	Block 21 field or reference number (1, 2, 3 and/or 4)
11b	Other claim ID designated by NUCC	24F	Total charge for CPT- or HCPCS-coded services listed in Block 24D
11c	Primary insured's insurance plan or program name		• If more than 1 day or unit is indicated in Block 24G, multiply the charge for the service(s) coded in Block 24D by the number of days/units in Block 24G; enter the result in Block 24F
11d	Determine whether the patient also is covered by a secondary health insurance plan		
12	Confirm that the patient's release of information form has been signed dated and is in the patient's record		
		24G	Total number of days or units
13	Confirm that the insured's authorization of benefits form has been signed dated and is in the patient's record	24H	EPSDT or Family Plan code (Medicaid or AFDC)
		24I	Qualifier ID code (if no NPI available)
		24J	Rendering (treating) provider's NPI – unshaded field
Section 3: Physician or Supplier Information			PIN (if no NPI is available) – shaded field
14	Date current illness, injury, or pregnancy began	25	Rendering provider's federal tax ID number (EIN or SSN)
15	Determine whether patient has had the same or similar symptoms	26	Patient's account number with rendering provider
16	From–To dates if patient was unable to work at current occupation	27	Determine whether contract or agreement between provider and insurance carrier allows provider to accept assignment
17	Name of ordering or referring provider		
17a	Not required	28	Total charges from Block 24F, lines 1–6
17b	Ordering or referring provider's NPI	29	Amount paid by patient, insured, or other insurance
18	From–To dates if patient encounter included an inpatient hospital stay	30	Balance due (if any amount paid is shown in Block 29)
		31	Signature of provider performing service or procedure
19	Determine whether insurance carrier in Carrier block and Block 1 requires any information to be entered in this field	32	Address of facility where services were rendered
		32a	NPI number of service facility listed in Block 32
20	Determine whether an outside laboratory was used; if so, enter charges billed to provider for outside lab services	32b	Qualifier ID number and PIN of facility listed in Block 32 (if no NPI available)
21	ICD-10-CM code or codes for patient's condition, illness, or injury (maximum of four per claim)	33	Name, address, and phone number of performing (rendering) provider
22	Is Medicaid claim being resubmitted? If yes, provide reference number from original Medicaid claim submitted	33a	NPI of provider listed in Block 33
		33b	Qualifier ID number and PIN of provider listed in Block 33 (if no NPI available)

[a]Only required if a secondary insurance exists and is to be submitted to the insurance carrier.
AFDC, Aid to Families with Dependent Children; *CPT*, Current Procedural Terminology coding system; *EIN*, Employer Identification Number; *EPSDT*, Early and Periodic Screening, Diagnosis, and Treatment; *FECA*, Federal Employees Compensation Act; *HCPCS*, Health Care Common Procedural Coding System coding method; *ICD-10-CM*, International Classification of Diseases, Tenth Revision, Clinical Modification coding method; *NPI*, National Provider Identifier; *NUCC*, National Uniform Claim Committee; *PIN*, personal identification number; *POS*, place of service; *SSN*, Social Security number.

Procedure 26.4 shows how to complete a health insurance claim form using the information from an insurance card and an encounter form (Fig. 26.6).

CRITICAL THINKING BOX 26.3

Ann is reviewing an encounter form that has one CPT code and two HCPCS codes with one diagnosis code for the same office visit. How many lines in Box 24 of the CMS-1500 will she need to use? Will all three CPT/HCPCS codes point to the same diagnosis? Why or why not?

ACCURATE CODING TO PREVENT FRAUD AND ABUSE

In any healthcare environment, accurate coding is essential to prevent fraud and abuse in reimbursement. According to HIPAA:

Fraud is defined as knowingly and willfully executing or attempting to execute a scheme to defraud any healthcare benefit program or to obtain by means of false or fraudulent pretenses, representations, or promises any of the money or property owned by any healthcare benefit program.

Abuse in medical billing would be actions that are contrary to ethical standards in the medical office. *Abuse* is an unintended action that directly or indirectly results in an overpayment to the healthcare provider. Abuse is similar to fraud, except that it is unclear if the unethical practice

BOX 26.7 Patient-Centered Medical Home (PCMH)

Patient-centered medical home (PCMH) is model of patient care. In this model, patient care is looked at from a holistic approach. The healthcare team wants to be able to assist the patient with any issues that come up about his or her care. This means having multiple team members available. The provider and the medical assistant would provide the primary care. There would also be a nurse who coordinates all of the care for the patient, including issues about home healthcare, financial issues, transportation issues, and so on. Many models include a clinical pharmacist who is available to discuss medication questions and concerns with the patient.

The goal of PCMH is to improve patient outcomes and reduce costs. There are accreditation processes that must be completed for a healthcare facility to be recognized as a PCMH.

Billing for the services provided can be a challenge for the medical biller. When do you bill for the pharmacist visit or phone contact? It is important to have billing policies and procedures in place when your healthcare facility is a PCMH so that services are billed consistently and accurately.

was committed on purpose. The term *intentional* is important when determining whether fraudulent medical billing practices were done on purpose or were an accident.

Violations of the laws governing reimbursement may result in:
- nonpayment of claims
- civil monetary penalties (CMPs)
- exclusion from the payer program
- criminal and civil liability
- in extreme cases, jail time

These laws may be changed or updated. The person who is responsible for coding must pay close attention to detail and act as a sort of "medical detective" to prevent a case against a provider or clinic. The ICD-10-CM and CPT/HCPCS manuals are updated annually. New coding manuals have a few pages dedicated to the updates for that particular year. Accurate use of ICD-10-CM and CPT/HCPCS manuals is essential for correct translation of the claim information in the health record into the correct codes (Box 26.8).

PROCEDURE 26.4 Complete an Insurance Claim Form

Task:
To accurately complete a CMS-1500 Health Insurance Claim Form (see Fig. 26.6).

Equipment and Supplies
- Patient's health record
- Copy of patient's insurance ID card or cards
- Patient registration/intake form
- Encounter form
- Insurance claims processing guidelines
- Blank CMS-1500 Health Insurance Claim Form

Procedural Steps
Almost all medical billing is done electronically through a practice management billing software. The paper CMS-1500 Health Insurance Claim Form is provided only to help students practice and develop their medical billing skills.

Complete each block (as appropriate) of the CMS-1500 (see Table 26.2 for block descriptions).

1. Gather the documents required to complete the claim form.
2. Complete the claim form using a pen. Use capital letters. Do not use punctuation (commas or dollar signs) unless indicated in the insurance manual or guidelines. Use a hyphen to hyphenate last names.
3. Using the patient's health insurance ID card, determine the type of insurance, and the insurance ID number. Enter this information into Blocks 1 and 1a.
    Purpose: After selecting the appropriate type of health insurance, the medical assistant can refer to the claims processing guidelines for that plan.
4. Using the ID card, the encounter form, and the registration/intake form, determine the patient's information and the insured individual's information. Accurately complete Blocks 2, 3, 5, 6, 9, and 10 a-c by entering the patient's information. Complete Blocks 4, 7, and 11 a-d with the insured's information.
    Purpose: By distinguishing between the patient and the insured, the medical biller can determine whether the insurer requires additional information for submission of an accurate claim.
5. Complete Blocks 12 and 13 by entering "signature on file" and the date.
    Note: The Assignment of Benefit form should have been signed by the patient and/or the insured at registration. Enter the dates in either the six (6)-digit format (MM/DD/YY) or the eight (8)-digit format (MM/DD/YYYY).
    Purpose: To submit an insurance claim, the medical practice must be authorized to release the service information on behalf of the patient or the insured.
6. Accurately enter the physician or supplier information by completing Blocks 14 through 23. Use the eight (8)-digit format (MM/DD/YYYY) when needed.
7. Using the encounter form, complete Block 24 and the appropriate blocks from 24A through 24H. Note the following:
    - *Block 24A:* Enter the dates of service, both From and To. For ambulatory services, enter the same date in the FROM and TO fields. Enter a date for each procedure or service in eight (8)-digit format (MM/DD/YYYY).
    - *Block 24F:* Enter the charge for the listed service or procedure. *Do not use commas when reporting dollar amounts.* The cents column is the small column to the right.
    - *Block 24G:* Enter the number of days or units. This block is usually used for multiple visits, units of supplies, anesthesia units or minutes, or oxygen volume. If only one service was performed, enter 1.
8. Complete Blocks 24I through 27 by entering information on the provider, or on the healthcare facility where the service was provided, and the patient's account number. Check the correct box to indicate acceptance of assignment of benefits.
9. Complete Blocks 28 and 29 by entering the total charges, total amount paid, and the total amount due. Complete Blocks 31 through 33a by entering the provider's and facility's information.
10. Review the claim for accuracy and completeness before submitting. Correct any errors and provide any missing information.
    Note: Before sending the claim, make a copy of the form and file the copy in the patient's insurance claim file.
    Purpose: It is important to double-check the form for accuracy and for required information that has not been provided.

FIG. 26.6 Completed CMS-1500 Health Insurance Claim Form. (From Proctor D, Niedzwiecki B: *Kinn's The Medical Assistant*, ed 13, St Louis, 2017, Elsevier.)

BOX 26.8 Guidelines for Reviewing Claims Before Submission

The following guidelines can help ensure that clean insurance claims are submitted.

- Proofread the form carefully for accuracy and completeness.
- Make certain any necessary attachments are included with the completed form.
- Follow office policies and guidelines for claim review and signatures.
- Forward the original claim to the proper insurance carrier either by mail or electronically.
- Make sure the patient's and/or insured's name, address, and ID, group, and/or policy number are identical to the information printed on the insurance card.
- Make sure the patient's birth date and gender are the same as in the medical record.
- Section 2, Patient and Insured Information **(Blocks 1–13)**: Complete these blocks accurately, according to the insurance carrier's guidelines.
- **Block 11:** Enter the word NONE if Medicare is the primary payer.
- **Block 12:** Make sure the patient has authorized the release of information, and that Block 12 has a handwritten signature, the words "Signature on File," or the acronym SOF.
- **Blocks 17** and **17b:** If applicable, enter the referring, provider's name and NPI number.
- Make sure the diagnosis is not missing or incomplete.
- Check that the diagnosis has been coded accurately, according to the ICD-10-CM coding manual, and is linked to the treatment.
- **Blocks 14–24J** (required fields for diagnosis and procedure): Make sure these blocks are completed accurately, according to the guidelines of the third-party payer or insurance company.
- List the fees for each charge individually; or, if more than 1 day or unit is entered in **Block 24G**, the fees must be computed correctly.
- **Block 25:** Double-check the provider's federal Social Security number (SSN) or Employer Identification Number (EIN) to ensure accuracy.
- **Block 27** (Accept Assignment?): Put an X in the YES box if the provider is a PAR provider or has an agreement with the insurance company to accept assignment.
- **Block 31:** Check for the provider's signature, which must be on the form.
- **Block 24J** and **Blocks 33a, 33b:** Make sure the provider's NPI, corresponding to the insurance carrier being billed, has been entered in Block 24J and again in Block 33a.

PREVENTING REJECTION OF A CLAIM

It is important for the medical assistant to understand and comply with the specific guidelines for completing a CMS-1500 established by each insurance company. This prevents delays in reimbursement and denial of payment. The guidelines for Medicare, Medicaid, TRICARE, and workers' compensation can be found online at the websites for these healthcare insurers. Most practice management billing systems have built-in claim scrubbers that help in the process. If claims are sent electronically through a clearinghouse, claims auditing is done before the clearinghouse transmits the claim to the insurance company. Claims without errors of any type are called *clean claims*. Claims with incorrect, missing, or insufficient data are called *dirty claims*.

> **VOCABULARY**
> **claim scrubbers:** Software that finds common billing errors before the claim is sent to the insurance company.

Communicating With Providers About Third-Party Requirements

It can be challenging for a provider to keep up with the annual changes made by the government plans, private health insurance companies, and the coding updates. This is why healthcare providers trust their medical office staff to stay up-to-date on the various changes in the health insurance industry.

Some providers may be so focused on patient care that they feel uncomfortable with change. This may be the case with the encounter form/superbill used in patient care. A provider may feel comfortable using the same form, but over time, some codes may have changed or become obsolete, or new medical services offered may not be listed on the form.

A medical coder should tactfully discuss with the provider the benefits of using an updated encounter form. If the provider is still reluctant to change the form, even though it is outdated, the medical coder may suggest that the form will not be changed, just the codes on it. Adjust the encounter form to include an open text box for the provider to add medical procedures that he performs occasionally.

When communicating with the provider about coding issues, you must always have a respectful attitude. The many changes occurring in medical coding and billing can be overwhelming and confusing for some providers. The approach of coding professionals should be to guide them patiently through these changes.

CRITICAL THINKING BOX 26.4

Being tactful means using good manners as you provide truthful, sensitive information or honest, critical feedback to another person. Tactful behaviors include showing respect, discretion, compassion, honesty, diplomacy, and courtesy while you deliver a message. Tactful behaviors encompass both nonverbal and verbal communication, including what you say, how you say it, and your body language during the communication. A critical element of being tactful is considering the other person's feelings and reactions as you deliver the information. When you use tactful behaviors, you demonstrate professionalism and you preserve relationships by avoiding conflicts and finding common ground.

Many times the medical biller is the expert on the third-party requirements, and providers rely on the biller to help them understand the requirements. Being tactful with providers as you communicate third-party requirements is critical to your working relationship with the provider and also important in the overall financial scope of the agency. It is crucial to assist the provider in a tactful manner, understanding his or her role in meeting third-party requirements.

Using the following case study, role-play with two peers how you would display tactful behaviors when communicating with medical providers about third-party requirements.

You are the medical biller for your clinic. The two providers have not been communicating with you about procedures that need prior authorization from the insurance companies. As a result, multiple claims are being denied, and the clinic has had to write off much of the cost. Today you are talking with the providers, explaining common procedures that require prior authorizations and the process of getting preauthorizations.

CHECKING THE STATUS OF A CLAIM

The medical biller should keep track of every submitted claim to ensure timely reimbursement. Clearinghouses send a confirmation report after submission of a claim. The medical biller should always confirm that the claims submitted to the clearinghouse match the claims listed on the confirmation report. If direct billing is used, the medical biller must set up a system to track the claims that were submitted. Medical assistants should maintain this practice to ensure that every claim is submitted correctly.

The claim submission confirmation report also indicates claims that were rejected because they were incomplete. These claims should be corrected and resubmitted electronically immediately. Often these claims are rejected for data entry errors. The medical biller should compare the patient's information in the practice management software to the information on the patient's registration form and scanned insurance card, to ensure accuracy.

It typically takes 10 to 14 business days for insurance companies to process insurance claims electronically. If no response has been received from the insurance company after 30 days, the medical biller should inquire about the status of the claim. This can be done through the company's provider web portal or by a call to the provider services number on the back of the patient's insurance ID card. To verify the claim status, you must provide:

- insured subscriber's member number and birth date
- patient's name and birth date
- date of service

With this information, the insurance company should be able to tell if the claim has been paid, is still in process, was denied, or was never received. The medical biller will use this information for the proper follow-up. This could be:

- investigating the records at the clinic to see if the payment came in but was applied to the incorrect patient account
- researching the denial and resubmitting the claim
- determining why the claim was not received and resubmitting it.

The state insurance commission has standards that insurance companies must abide by, including claim processing times and payment guidelines. Medical assistants should keep the commission's contact information in the office medical billing manual as a reference, in case a claim should be reported.

EXPLANATION OF BENEFITS

An explanation of benefits is sent by the insurance company to the provider who submitted the insurance claim and to the patient. It comes with a check or a document indicating that funds were electronically transferred. Medicare sends a remittance advice (RA) with confirmation of electronic funds transfer. Although it has a different name, the document is the same as the EOB.

The healthcare facility cannot just deposit the check and disregard the EOB, which provides detailed accounting for the submitted insurance claim. The EOB breaks down each line item charge from Block 24 on the CMS-1500 into the charged amount, the amount allowable, and the amount paid. Most EOBs will also indicate how much was applied to the deductible, what the patient's co-insurance amount is, and if any services were denied.

Reading an Explanation of Benefits

The EOB contains essential information about the submitted health insurance claim. To properly apply payments to a patient's account, it is vital that the medical assistant understand all the elements of an EOB. When interpreting the EOB, review the following steps:

1. Verify that the EOB applies to the correct patient by comparing the account number and date of service on the EOB with the submitted claim.
2. Confirm that the EOB shows the same charged amount as the submitted claim. In other words, the line items and charges should match. Sometimes the EOB summarizes the entire claim in one charged amount. In this case, confirm that the total charged is the same as in the submitted claim.
3. Post the payment and adjusted amount per line item. In the practice management billing software, these are posted on the same line. The patient's responsibility, as determined by the primary insurance EOB, is calculated using the following equation:

   Charged amount – Payment amount – Adjustment amount
   = Patient s responsibility

4. Once the patient's responsibility has been determined, check for a secondary insurance. If one is listed, submit a health insurance claim with the balance due determined by the primary insurance EOB. If no secondary insurance is listed, the patient is billed for the balance due.
5. Review the *remark codes* on the EOB for any additional messages or information about the claim. The remark codes area is where the insurance company indicates the conditions under which the claim was paid. For example, code 01 states that the claim amount allowed was established by the contract between the health insurance plan and the provider. Other remarks codes give the reasons a claim was denied or rejected. Some remarks codes indicate that the claim is pending, awaiting specific information.
6. All remarks codes on pending or denied claims should be followed up immediately upon receipt of the EOB, to prevent further delay in payment for other claims.

Rejected Claims

The EOB provides detailed information on rejected claims. All rejected claims have a code, with a legend toward the bottom of the page. Some of the reasons claims are rejected are:

- The time period for filing the claim had expired (check the insurance plan's billing policies manual for details).
- Incorrect ICD-10-CM, CPT, and/or HCPCS codes or combinations of codes were entered.
- The insurer claims that the ICD-10-CM code and the CPT/HCPCS codes do not match; that is, the claim lacks **medical necessity**.
- More than one CPT/HCPCS code was filed on the same date of service, and they are mutually exclusive when billed together.
- The claim was submitted to the wrong insurance company.

Rejected claims should be resubmitted as soon as possible to prevent further delay in reimbursement.

> **VOCABULARY**
> **medical necessity:** Services or supplies (CPT and HCPCS codes) that are used to treat the patient's diagnosis (ICD codes) meet the accepted standard of medical practice.

DENIED CLAIMS

The two main reasons for denial of payment are technical errors and insurance policy coverage issues. Technical errors include incorrect,

incomplete information, data entry and/or mathematical errors. Common reasons for denial include:
- The patient was not covered by the insurance plan on the date of service.
- A listed procedure was not an insurance benefit.
- Preauthorization for the service was not obtained.
- Medical necessity

Medical Necessity

Insurance companies determine medical necessity based on the diagnostic and procedural codes submitted on the claim. The diagnostic code is the reason that the procedure was necessary. For example, if a claim submitted to the insurance company indicated that a bunionectomy was performed for tonsillitis, the insurer will deny the claim based on medical necessity. Procedure codes are linked to diagnostic codes in the claim. The health record must support the reason for each service provided.

If an insurance claim is denied for medical necessity, the medical assistant should review the claim information and the health record. If there is an error on the claim, such as the wrong diagnostic coded on the encounter form, then a new claim should be submitted.

If an insurance claim is denied for medical necessity and the medical assistant believes that it was coded correctly, an appeal letter should be sent to the insurance company. The appeal letter should identify the denied claim, and include a statement from the provider detailing the medical reasoning for performing the procedure. Additional medical reports (e.g., laboratory reports, operative reports, and history and physical examination findings [H&P]) should be sent if they support the provider's treatment decision (Procedure 26.5).

THE PATIENT'S FINANCIAL RESPONSIBILITY

Most MCO health insurance contracts require patients to pay a copayment, which is collected at the time of service (Table 26.3). Copayments can range from $10 to $75 for office visits. They vary, depending on whether the patient is seen by a PCP or a specialist, in urgent care, or in the emergency department. Office visit and prescription copayments do not count toward the yearly deductible. The medical assistant must make sure that the proper copayments are received and credited to patients' accounts.

A *deductible* is a set dollar amount that the policyholder is responsible for each year before the insurance company begins to reimburse the healthcare provider. The deductible amount is stated in the insurance policy.

Co-insurance means that the insured and the insurance company share the cost of covered medical services after the deductible has been met. The insurance company and the patient split the cost of the services. An 80/20 split is very common, especially for traditional insurance. This means that after the yearly deductible has been met, the insurance company pays 80% of the fee and the insured pays 20%. The patient's deductible or co-insurance responsibility is shown on the EOB.

To help patients understand their health insurance benefits, the medical assistant must be confident in defining the terms *copayment*, *co-insurance*, and *deductible*.

The medical office can contact the insurance company on the patient's behalf to determine the amount of the deductible the patient has already paid in the calendar year. The process of precertification enables the healthcare provider to inform patients of how much the procedure will cost them.

Calculating the Co-insurance and Deductible

Consider this example: Mrs. Anita Jones' health insurance plan has a $500 annual deductible, after which the insurance company pays 95% of all charges. Mrs. Jones, therefore, has a 5% co-insurance expense, in addition to the deductible. Mrs. Jones has incurred a $10,000 charge for cardiac surgery performed by her provider.

In Fig. 26.7, Column A shows that Mrs. Jones paid the $500 deductible, and 5% of $10,000 (i.e., an additional $475). The insurance company then paid the remaining balance of $9,025.

Also in Fig. 26.7, Column B shows that Mrs. Jones' cardiac surgery cost $20,000. Mrs. Jones' total out-of-pocket expense is now $975, and the insurance company is responsible for payment of the balance of $18,525.

PROCEDURE 26.5 Use Medical Necessity Guidelines: Respond to a "Medical Necessity Denied" Claim

Task:
To resolve the insurance company's denial of a claim for medical necessity by completing an accurate claim.

Scenario
You are working at the Walden-Martin Family Medicine Clinic, 1234 Anystreet, Anytown, AL 12345 (phone: 123-123-1234).

You receive a letter indicating that Medicare has denied the following claim for not being medically necessary.

Patient: Norma B. Washington
DOB: 08/07/1944
Policy/ID Number: 847744144A
Date of Service: 06/13/20XX
ICD: G43.101 (Migraine)
CPT: J3420 (B-12 injection)
Provider: Julie Walden MD

You do some research and find that the information above was the only information sent to Medicare for that encounter. The following information was the correct information for the encounter.

Patient: Norma B. Washington
DOB: 08/01/1944
Date of Service: 06/15/20XX
ICD: G43.101 (Migraine)
CPT: J1885 (Toradol 15 mg—$15.50) and 90772 (Injection, Ther/Proph/Diag—$25.00)
ICD: D51.0 (Vitamin B_{12} deficiency anemia)
CPT: J3420 (B-12 injection—$24.00) and 90772 (Injection, Ther/Proph/Diag—$25.00)
To be billed to: Medicare, 1234 Insurance Road, Anytown, AL 12345-1234

Equipment and Supplies
- *Paper method:* Patient's health record, copy of patient's insurance ID card or cards, patient registration form, encounter form, blank CMS-1500 Health Insurance Claim Form, pen
- *Electronic method:* SimChart for the Medical Office
- Insurance denial letter or scenario (see above)

PROCEDURE 26.5 Use Medical Necessity Guidelines: Respond to a "Medical Necessity Denied" Claim—cont'd

Procedural Steps

1. Review the insurance denial letter (scenario) carefully. Compare the patient's information from the denial letter to the health record, claim, and encounter form. Look for errors in the patient's name and date of birth.
   Purpose: Errors in patient information can be a reason for denial.
2. Compare the insurance denial letter (scenario) to the health record, claim, and encounter form. Look for errors in the date of service, the diagnosis, and the procedure codes. The procedure must be medically necessary for the diagnosis indicated.
   Purpose: Errors related to the encounter must be corrected for the claim to be accepted. The procedure codes must indicate an acceptable standard of treatment for the diagnosis listed. In some cases, the encounter form may contain a diagnosis that did not make it into the original claim form. Review the patient's health record to determine whether the procedure was medically necessary.
3. Complete a claim (either CMS-1500 or an electronic claim using SimChart) by entering the information about the carrier, patient, and insured.
4. Enter the information about the physician, procedures, and diagnosis. Make sure to include all the information from the encounter.
5. Proofread the claim form for accuracy before submitting the claim.

TABLE 26.3 Comparing Patient Financial Responsibilities

Patient Financial Responsibility	When Patient Pays	Amount Patient Pays
Copayment	At the time of medical service	Fixed amount, $10 to $75 per visit
Deductible	Before the insurance company will pay	Variable amount, $250 to $5,000
Co-insurance	After the provider has been paid	Variable amount, up to 30%

	Column A	Column B
Total Charge	$10,000	$20,000
Deductible (paid by Mrs. Jones)	$500	$500
Coinsurance (5% paid by Mrs. Jones)	5% of $9500 (Total charge minus the deductible) = $475	5% of 19,500 (Total charge minus the deductible) = $975
Total amount paid by Mrs. Jones	$975	$1475
Total amount paid by insurance	95% of $9500 (Total charge minus the deductible) - $9025	95% of $19,500 (Total charge minus the deductible) - $18,525

FIG. 26.7 Deductible and Co-insurance.

	PAR	NonPAR
Total Charge	$10,000	$10,000
Allowed amount	$8,500	$8,500
$1500 difference between charged amount and allowed amount	Written off as an adjustment	Billed to the patient
Deductible (paid by Mrs. Jones)	$500	$500
Coinsurance (paid by Mrs. Jones)	$8500 – $500 (deductible) X 5% = $400	$8500 – $500 (deductible) X 5% = $400
Total amount paid by Mrs. Jones	$900	$2400
Total amount paid by insurance	$7,600	$7,600

FIG. 26.8 PAR vs. NonPAR.

CRITICAL THINKING BOX 26.5

The providers in the practice where Ann works are not in-network for a preferred provider organization (PPO) that is often used in their geographic area. Many patients are confused when they have to pay a larger out-of-pocket fee for their medical services. How can Ann explain the reason for these higher fees to patients?

Allowed Amount

Another factor to be considered when determining the patient's financial responsibility is whether the provider is a PAR provider or not. To become a participating provider in an insurance network, the provider must agree to accept the insurance plan's fee schedule as payment in full for services rendered. This means that if the provider's fee is higher than the plan's allowed amount, the difference should be adjusted. For example, a provider may charge $80 for a Level I office visit; however, the insurance plan's allowable amount may be only $60. If the provider is a participating provider, he or she is obligated to adjust the difference between these two amounts – $20. The patient is not responsible for that $20. However, if the provider is not a participating provider, he or she can bill the patient for the $20 balance. Because contracts between insurance companies and providers vary greatly, it is important for the medical assistant to closely examine the EOB to ensure that the proper adjustments are done.

Let's look at how this would affect the example in Fig. 26.7. If the allowable amount for Mrs. Jones' $10,000 cardiac surgery is $8,500, the $1,500 difference between the provider's charge and the allowed amount would be either written off or passed on to the patient. Fig. 26.8 demonstrates the differences in the patient's responsibility and provider reimbursement.

Discussing the Patient's Financial Responsibility

The *guarantor* is the person legally responsible for the entire bill. It is important the that patient and the guarantor understand what the financial responsibilities are for services provided. Some patients expect insurance to pay all costs simply because they are paying a premium. Often patients do not even read their insurance policies and have no idea what is and is not covered.

The medical assistant may need to educate patients about their policies and help patients work with their insurance company to get answers to questions and make sure they are receiving all the benefits to which they are entitled. If problems come up with the insurance company, it is in the practice's best interest to actively assist the patient. The medical billing staff is usually more knowledgeable than the patient about health insurance. Helping patients with issues can help ensure that provider is compensated for his or her services.

Medical assistants gain knowledge about the insurance industry when they actively assist patients with their concerns. The more experience a medical assistant has in working with insurance, the more helpful he or she can be to patients. As mentioned previously, medical assistants should keep a manual of medical billing policies and procedures for most of the insurance plans they handle; this can serve as an excellent source of guidance and suggestions for working with a particular payer.

PROCEDURE 26.6 Inform a Patient of Financial Obligations for Services Rendered

Task:
To inform the patient of his or her financial obligation and to demonstrate professionalism and sensitivity when discussing the patient's billing record.

Scenario
During this role play, Christi Brown is meeting with you regarding the bill she received in the mail. When she called to make the appointment, she voiced her confusion about the bill, stating she thought her insurance covered everything. You check her record and see that she met her deductible and now needs to pay 20% of the billed amount. She owes $170.

Equipment and Supplies
- Patient's account record
- Copy of patient's insurance card.

Procedural Steps
1. Determine the patient's financial responsibility under the insurance plan by reviewing the copy of the patient's insurance card.

    Purpose: Having an understanding of the patient's financial responsibility from the insurance plan will help you to explain the terms to the patient.
2. Determine the amount the patient owes by reviewing the patient's account record.

    Purpose: It is important that when working with a patient, you are familiar with the facts of the situation.
3. Discuss the situation with the patient. (Role-play the above scenario.)
4. Demonstrate professionalism when discussing the situation with the patient. Verbal and nonverbal communication should demonstrate patience, understanding, and sensitivity. The medical assistant should refrain from inappropriate and unprofessional behavior, including eye rolling, harsh words, disrespectful comments, and similar behaviors.
5. Demonstrate professionalism by respectfully providing the patient with payment options based on the clinic's policies and what the patient can pay on a monthly basis.

    Purpose: The medical assist should not force or harass the patient in to paying. The medical assistant will be more successful if the communication with the patient is respectful.

Always be sure to obtain the guarantor's signature on an agreement to pay for services. Most patient information sheets have a section referring to the guarantor. A statement may be included that serves as an agreement to pay the costs of medical care. States have statutes that deal with guarantors, so be sure the office's policies comply with those laws. It is especially important to secure a written agreement to pay for services when the care will be long term or involves costly treatment or surgical procedures. Procedure 26.6 explains how to inform patients of their financial obligations for services rendered (Box 26.9 and Fig. 26.9).

Showing Sensitivity When Discussing the Patient's Finances

Most patients use health insurance, but they do not always recognize that they will have financial obligations after the insurance plan pays its share. This is common among Medicare patients, who often feel that they should have all their medical expenses paid because they have government insurance. It usually falls to the medical assistant to inform patients of their financial responsibilities.

Patients seeking medical care are not usually feeling like themselves because they may be suffering through pain and discomfort. As a result, their behavior may not be typical when the medical assistant suggests discussing their financial responsibilities.

Medical assistants should show patience and sensitivity when discussing a patient's financial obligations (Fig. 26.10). Patients should never be harassed to make a payment or forced into payment arrangements. Medical assistants should always be courteous when discussing payments with patients. In addition, the medical practice should offer a variety of payment options to meet patients' needs, including credit card and online payment options.

BOX 26.9 Advance Beneficiary Notice (ABN)

Medicare does not cover some healthcare services. The Advanced Beneficiary Notice (ABN) is presented to patients in these circumstances. The ABN provides an option for patients to pay the provider's fee in full so as to receive services that Medicare does not cover. The patient decides whether he or she still wants to receive the services from the provider and completes the information on the form (see Fig. 26.9).

EXCEPTIONAL CUSTOMER SERVICE

Most patients are unaware of their benefits and coverage through their insurance policies. The medical assistant should encourage patients to read the entire policy to become familiar with its limitations and exclusions. Inform patients that when they call the insurance company with questions, they should always write down the date, the time, and the name of the person with whom they spoke. Using email is helpful because a record of the correspondence can easily be saved or printed. Making sure that patients have a general understanding of their health insurance coverage is well worth the effort.

Often patients do not dispute the decision or question the insurance company when a claim is rejected or not paid in the expected amount. Encourage them to call the company and question rejections if they do not understand why the claim was denied.

CHAPTER 26 Billing and Reimbursement   585

A. Notifier: John Doe, MD, College Clinic, 4567 Broad Avenue, Woodland Hills, XY 12345 555-486-9002
B. Patient Name: Mary Judd   **C. Identification Number:** 0920XX7291

Advance Beneficiary Notice of Noncoverage (ABN)

NOTE: If Medicare doesn't pay for D. _B12 injections_ below, you may have to pay.
Medicare does not pay for everything, even some care that you or your health care provider have good reason to think you need. We expect Medicare may not pay for the D. _B12 injections_ below.

D.	E. Reason Medicare May Not Pay:	F. Estimated Cost
B12 injections	Medicare does not usually pay for this injection or this many injections	$35.00

WHAT YOU NEED TO DO NOW:
- Read this notice, so you can make an informed decision about your care.
- Ask us any questions that you may have after you finish reading.
- Choose an option below about whether to receive the D. _B12 injections_ listed above.
  Note: If you choose Option 1 or 2, we may help you to use any other insurance that you might have, but Medicare cannot require us to do this.

G. OPTIONS: Check only one box. We cannot choose a box for you.

☑ **OPTION 1.** I want the D. _B12 injections_ listed above. You may ask to be paid now, but I also want Medicare billed for an official decision on payment, which is sent to me on a Medicare Summary Notice (MSN). I understand that if Medicare doesn't pay, I am responsible for payment, but **I can appeal to Medicare** by following the directions on the MSN. If Medicare does pay, you will refund any payments I made to you, less co-pays or deductibles.

☐ **OPTION 2.** I want the D. _____ listed above, but do not bill Medicare. You may ask to be paid now as I am responsible for payment. **I cannot appeal if Medicare is not billed.**

☐ **OPTION 3.** I don't want the D. _____ listed above. I understand with this choice I am **not** responsible for payment, and **I cannot appeal to see if Medicare would pay.**

H. Additional Information:

This notice gives our opinion, not an official Medicare decision. If you have other questions on this notice or Medicare billing, call **1-800-MEDICARE** (1-800-633-4227/**TTY:** 1-877-486-2048).
Signing below means that you have received and understand this notice. You also receive a copy.

I. Signature: *Mary Judd*	J. Date: *March 20, 20XX*

According to the Paperwork Reduction Act of 1995, no persons are required to respond to a collection of information unless it displays a valid OMB control number. The valid OMB control number for this information collection is 0938-0566. The time required to complete this information collection is estimated to average 7 minutes per response, including the time to review instructions, search existing data resources, gather the data needed, and complete and review the information collection. If you have comments concerning the accuracy of the time estimate or suggestions for improving this form, please write to: CMS, 7500 Security Boulevard, Attn: PRA Reports Clearance Officer, Baltimore, Maryland 21244-1850.

Form CMS-R-131 (03/11)   Form Approved OMB No. 0938-0566

FIG. 26.9 Advance Beneficiary Notice for Medicare Patients. (From Fordney MT: *Insurance Handbook For The Medical Office,* ed 14, St Louis, 2017, Elsevier.)

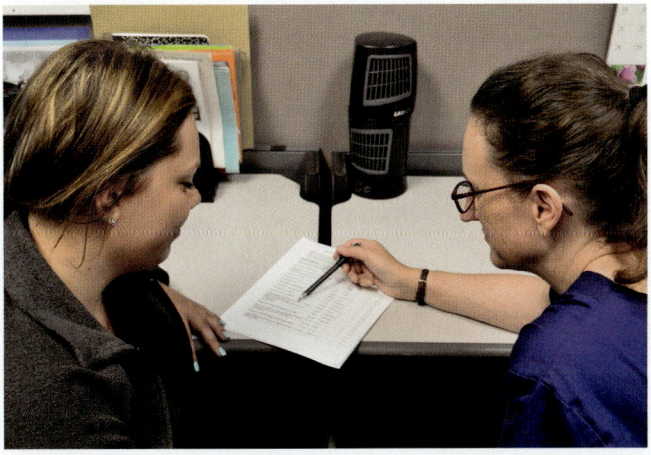

FIG. 26.10 Medical assistants must show respect and sensitivity when discussing financial issues with patients (From Proctor D, Niedzwiecki B: *Kinn's The Medical Assistant,* ed 13, St Louis, 2017, Elsevier.)

CLOSING COMMENTS

Accurate insurance billing practices are essential for the financial success of every healthcare facility. Medical assistants are strong assets to the healthcare facility when they can submit claims electronically, manage denied and rejected claims, and discuss financial responsibilities with patients professionally. Medical assistants should always maintain a positive attitude toward patients and keep in mind that those who are ill or facing challenges are not always at their best and may not respond in a positive way when discussing their financial responsibilities.

CHAPTER REVIEW

It is important for medical assistants to be familiar with the information needed to submit insurance claims. Not all insurance cards are in the same format. A medical assistant should be able to look at any patient's insurance card and determine the copay amount, identification and group numbers, where claims should be submitted, and where to call to get preauthorization for services.

Most MCOs require precertification/preauthorization. The medical billing specialist should be familiar with how to accomplish this. It can be done with a paper form, or it can be done electronically. If precertification is not done, the services may not be paid for by the insurance company.

Submitting claims can be done either with a paper claim form or electronically. All of the information needed to complete a paper form is also required for an electronic form. If a medical assistant understands the information needed for the paper form, he or she will know what information needs to be in the computer system for an electronic claim.

Whenever medical assistants work with billing, they need to be sure that they are completing the tasks in a legal and ethical manner. Fraud and abuse should be avoided at all costs. By keeping up-to-date on all regulations for health insurance billing, the medical assistant can avoid fraud and abuse.

After submitting a claim, the medical biller must continue to track the progress of that claim to ensure that payment is received. Once payment has been received, the medical biller must ensure that the payment was correct. Looking for rejections and denials is part of the reimbursement process. Those rejections and denials must be researched and then claims should be resubmitted.

Helping patients understand their financial obligations is one of the responsibilities of a medical assistant. Many patients do not understand what deductibles, copayments, or co-insurance are. Using a sensitive manner in helping them to understand is one way of providing excellent customer service.

SCENARIO WRAP-UP

Ann realizes that the best way to keep track of all the carriers is to keep an up-to-date manual that contains the addresses, phone numbers, and medical billing policies and procedures for each insurance plan that the healthcare facility accepts. This manual can help prevent the rejection and denial of many claims because the claims will be submitted accurately the first time.

The medical assistant's understanding of how to calculate deductibles, co-insurance, and allowed amounts for procedures and services benefits both the provider and the patient. The provider's productivity, income, and losses can be easily tracked, and the patient can be educated as to the exact amounts he or she is responsible for paying.

Ann also has learned the importance of being courteous to patients when discussing their financial obligations. She has learned how to use the Assignment of Financial Responsibility form to communicate what the patient owes in a clear, straightforward manner.

27

Accounts, Collections, and Banking

LEARNING OBJECTIVES

1. Define bookkeeping and bookkeeping terms, and discuss all the different transactions recorded in patient accounts.
2. Discuss the patient ledger.
3. Perform accounts receivable procedures for patient accounts, including posting charges, payments, and adjustments.
4. Discuss payment at the time of service. Also, give an example of displaying sensitivity when requesting payment for services rendered.
5. Describe the impact of the Truth in Lending Act on collections policies for patient accounts.
6. Discuss monthly patient account statements, and list the necessary data elements on each monthly statement. Also, review policies and procedures for collecting outstanding balances on patient accounts.
7. Do the following related to collection procedures:
   - Describe successful collection techniques for patient accounts.
   - Discuss strategies for collecting outstanding balances through personal finance interviews.
   - Describe types of adjustments made to patient accounts, including a nonsufficient funds (NSF) check and collection agency transactions.
8. Do the following related to banking in today's business world:
   - Explain the purpose of the Federal Reserve Bank and the types of banks it manages.
   - Identify common types of bank accounts.
   - Discuss the importance of signature cards.
   - Explain how online banking has made standard banking processes more efficient.
9. Do the following related to checks:
   - Compare different types of negotiable instruments.
   - Identify precautions in accepting checks from patients.
   - Explain how checks are processed from one account to another.
   - Review the procedure followed when the healthcare facility receives an NSF check.
10. Identify precautions in accepting cash. Also, discuss the use of debit and credit cards, including advantages and precautions.
11. Do the following related to banking procedures in the ambulatory care setting:
    - Describe banking procedures as related to the ambulatory care setting.
    - Explain the importance of depositing checks daily.
    - Prepare a bank deposit.
    - Compare types of check endorsements.
    - Review check-writing procedures used to pay the operational expenses of a healthcare facility.
12. Understand the purpose of bank account reconciliation for auditing purposes, and how to pay bills in order to maximize cash flow.
13. Discuss the process of employee payroll.

CHAPTER OUTLINE

1. **Opening Scenario,** 588
2. **You Will Learn,** 588
3. **Introduction,** 588
4. **Managing Funds in the Healthcare Facility,** 588
5. **Bookkeeping in the Healthcare Facility,** 589
6. **Accounts Receivable (A/R),** 589
   a. Patient Ledger, 589
      i. *Entering and Posting Transactions in the Patient Ledger, 589*
      ii. *Posting Charges, 591*
      iii. *Posting Payments, 592*
      iv. *Posting Adjustments, 593*
      v. *Payment at the Time of Service, 596*
      vi. *Payment Agreements, 596*
   b. Monthly Patient Account Statements, 597
      i. *Billing Minors, 597*
      ii. *Medical Care for Those Who Cannot Pay, 597*
      iii. *Fees in Hardship Cases, 598*
   c. Collection Procedures, 598
      i. *When to Start Collection Procedures, 598*
      ii. *Preparing Patient Accounts for Collections Activity, 598*
      iii. *Collection Telephone Calls, 598*
      iv. *General Rules for Telephone Collections, 599*
      v. *Collection Letters, 600*
      vi. *Personal Finance Interviews, 600*
      vii. *Special Collection Situations, 601*
      viii. *Using a Collection Agency, 601*
      ix. *Small Claims Court, 603*
7. **Accounts Payable (A/P),** 604
   a. Banking in Today's Business World, 604
      i. *Common Types of Bank Accounts, 605*
      ii. *Signature Cards, 605*
      iii. *Online Banking, 605*

b. Checks, 605
      i. *Routing and Account Numbers,* 606
      ii. *Types of Negotiable Instruments,* 606
      iii. *How Checks Are Processed from One Bank to Another,* 606
   c. Patient Payment Management, 606
      i. *Cash Payments,* 606
      ii. *Checks,* 608
      iii. *Debit Cards,* 608
      iv. *Credit Cards,* 608
      v. *Precautions for Accepting Credit and Debit Cards,* 609
   d. Banking Procedures in the Ambulatory Care Setting, 609
      i. *Making Bank Deposits,* 609
      ii. *Preparing the Deposit,* 609
      iii. *Check Endorsements,* 609
      iv. *Overdraft,* 611
      v. *Stop-Payments,* 611
   e. Bank Statements and Reconciliation, 611
      i. *What to do When the Balances Do Not Match,* 611
   f. Paying Bills to Maximize Cash Flow, 613
      i. *Invoices and Statements,* 614
      ii. *Online Bill Pay,* 614
      iii. *Direct Deposit,* 614
8. **Employee Payroll,** 614
9. **Closing Comments,** 615
10. **Chapter Review,** 615

▶ OPENING SCENARIO

Laura Casper has been working in the back office at Walden-Martin Family Medical Clinic (WMFM) for the past 3 years. Her primary job has been working with patient accounts. She has recently been asked to also take on some of the accounts payable responsibilities. This will involve banking procedures and bill paying.

While working with patient accounts, Laura has become familiar with the billing cycle and collection procedures, and she is training new employees. It can be a complicated process, but Laura finds it challenging and enjoyable.

After the addition of the banking responsibilities to her work duties, Laura met with a bank representative. They discussed some time-efficient ways to bank with mobile depositing and online banking. Laura realizes that she still has much to learn about the daily financial duties in a healthcare facility, including working with the patient account management software, making daily deposits, reconciling bank statements, and many other banking responsibilities.

Laura wants to increase the value of the healthcare facility's bank accounts by looking for bank accounts that pay a higher interest rate and by reducing the office's operational expenses. Laura also wants to encourage patients at the healthcare facility to use debit or credit cards, instead of checks, to pay for services, because she knows that returned patient checks have created problems in the past.

YOU WILL LEARN

- To define the bookkeeping transactions that occur in a healthcare facility.
- How to perform accounts receivable procedures, including posting charges, payments, and adjustments.
- To describe special bookkeeping procedures, including credit balances, NSF checks, and bankruptcy.
- To understand the need for sensitivity when discussing payment options with patients.
- How the Truth in Lending Act affects collection policies.
- To describe successful collection techniques for patient accounts.
- To explain the purpose of the Federal Reserve Bank.
- To identify common types of bank accounts.
- To explain how online banking has made banking processes more efficient.
- To describe the different methods for patient payments and the precautions needed with each.
- To describe payroll procedures in a healthcare facility.
- To differentiate between hourly and salaried employees.

INTRODUCTION

Managing the finances in a healthcare facility is an important task. Every patient encounter creates a financial transaction for the facility. Transactions generated by the patient encounter include a variety of charges, payments, and adjustments that need to be accounted for on a daily basis. Financial management is essential if the healthcare facility is to pay the business operating expenses. This includes maintaining patient accounts and performing collection activities and banking duties. If the expenses of operating the healthcare facility exceed the fees collected for services rendered, the business will be forced to close.

A medical assistant who works in the back office is responsible for posting charges, accepting and posting a variety of payments and adjustments, endorsing and depositing checks, writing checks for office expenses, and regularly reconciling bank and credit card statements. Mobile deposit allows healthcare facilities to deposit checks on the date payments are received, because it is conveniently done in the office. The medical assistant will have to master basic math skills (e.g., addition and subtraction) for all banking functions.

MANAGING FUNDS IN THE HEALTHCARE FACILITY

The purpose of financial management is to ensure that the healthcare facility earns enough money to cover its operating expenses. The financial records of the healthcare facility should show the following:
- how much money was earned in a given period
- how much money was collected
- how much money is owed
- the distribution of all operational expenses

An accountant can prepare monthly and annual financial records from daily **bookkeeping** records. Periodic analyses of these reports result in:
- improved business practices
- improved time management
- elimination of unprofitable services
- more efficient expense budgeting

In order to be able to properly manage finances, it is crucial that the medical assistant understand the difference between accounts receivable and accounts payable.

CHAPTER 27 Accounts, Collections, and Banking

BOX 27.1 Credit vs. Debit

There are two terms used in bookkeeping that can be confusing – credit and debit.

Credit: A bookkeeping entry that increases accounts receivable, or what is owed to the provider. Example: posting charges to a patient's account.

Debit: A bookkeeping entry that increases accounts payable, or what is owed by the provider. Example: posting a patient payment and insurance payment to a patient's account that results in an overpayment.

- *Accounts receivable (A/R)* is money that is expected but has not yet been received. The amount charged on the encounter form is an example of accounts receivable for the healthcare facility. When a payment is made on the patient account, the received payment becomes **cash on hand**.
- *Accounts payable (A/P)* is the management of debt **incurred** and not yet paid. All invoices, statements, and operating expenses are included in accounts payable. When expenses have been paid, they are no longer categorized as accounts payable.

BOOKKEEPING IN THE HEALTHCARE FACILITY

Most healthcare facilities use practice management software for daily bookkeeping transactions. A/R transactions come from the encounter form. The charges documented on the encounter form are used to complete the health insurance claim form. *Payments* to the healthcare facility come as reimbursement from the insurance company, or from a patient payment. *Adjustments* are made to a patient's account when it is necessary to add or subtract an amount, which is not a payment, from the balance; for example, the difference between the provider's charged amount and the contracted insurance payment amount. Box 27.1 presents an explanation of the bookkeeping terms *credit* and *debit*.

A/P transactions also require bookkeeping entries. Writing checks and maintaining the checking account register are examples of A/P bookkeeping entries. Expenses are tracked by category (e.g., rent, clinical supplies, and administrative supplies).

ACCOUNTS RECEIVABLE (A/R)

The majority of the money owed to the healthcare facility comes from patient accounts. It is important for a medical assistant to have an understanding of how the patient account system works.

Patient Ledger

A **patient account** is created when the healthcare provider renders services. Charges are applied to the patient account when an *encounter form* (Fig. 27.1) is completed during the office visit. The ledger is where all the procedures and charges for services rendered are listed.

> **VOCABULARY**
> **bookkeeping:** The process of recording financial transactions.
> **cash on hand:** The amount of money the healthcare facility has in the bank that can be withdrawn as cash.
> **incurred:** To come into or acquire.
> **patient account:** A running balance of all financial transactions for a specific patient.

BOX 27.2 Manual Bookkeeping

Although we live in a technology-savvy world, some providers still use a manual pegboard system. In many cases, providers who have been in practice for many years do not want to invest in a practice management software system because of the cost associated with moving to practice management software. Also, if the office computers go down, employees will have to use a manual system until the system is back up.

The medical assistant must be familiar with both manual and electronic patient account management systems. The pegboard system is the most popular manual system for this purpose. It is simple to operate and contains the same components as a computer system. Once a medical assistant learns the pegboard system, computer systems are much easier to understand.

The pegboard system gets its name from a board that is used. This board has a row of pegs along the side or top that holds the forms in place. The patient account ledger cards are perforated for alignment on the pegs (see Fig. 27.3). All the forms used in any system must be compatible so that they can be aligned perfectly on the board.

The pegboard system generates all the necessary financial records for each transaction (by writing once with carbonless forms) as follows:

- Encounter form
- Receipt
- Patient account ledger card
- Bookkeeping transaction entry

The system also may include a statement and bank deposit slip. It provides current accounts receivable totals and a daily record of bank deposits and cash on hand, in addition to the record of income and expenses. The need for separate posting to patient accounts is eliminated, and the chance for error is reduced.

The pegboard system allows the medical assistant to keep control over cash, collections, and receivables, and ensures that every cent is accounted for and properly entered. It provides a record of every patient, every charge, and every payment, plus a daily recap of earnings – a running record of receivables and an audited summary of cash – and requires little time.

All transactions for professional services are posted to the patient's ledger daily. In this way, the ledger becomes the source for answering questions from patients about their financial obligations. The patient ledger should include all information related to collecting the balance due, such as:

- Name and address of the guarantor
- Insurance identification information
- Home, work, and cell phone numbers
- Any special instructions for billing
- Emergency or alternative contact information

The patient ledger (Fig. 27.2) provides a running balance, the result of all of the different financial transactions performed in the account, including charges, payments, and adjustments. This same information can be found in practice management software in an electronic format.

Entering and Posting Transactions in the Patient Ledger. When a **pegboard system** is used (Fig. 27.3 and Box 27.2), transactions are initiated before the patient goes to the exam room. The patient account ledger card is inserted under the first or next available receipt, and the first available writing line of the card is aligned with the carbonized strip on the receipt. Enter the receipt number and the date; enter the account balance in the space labeled *previous balance*; and then enter the patient's name. A copy of the receipt is detached and clipped to the patient's chart to be routed to the provider.

UNIT 3 Administrative Ambulatory Care

Walden-Martin Family Medical Clinic
1234 Anystreet, Anytown, AK 12345-1234
Phone: 555-486-9002

STATE LIC.# C1503X
SOC. SEC. # 000-11-0000
PIN #

☐ Private ☒ Bluecross ☐ Ind. ☐ Medicare ☐ Medi-cal ☐ Hmo ☐ Ppo

Patient's last name	First	Account #:	Birthdate	Sex ☒ Male	Today's date
Thomas	Ken	11594111	10 / 25 / 1961	☐ Female	09 / 17 / 20XX
Insurance company	Subscriber		Plan #	Sub. #	Group
Blue Cross Blue Shield	Ken Thomas			KT4496785	55124T

ASSIGNMENT: I hereby assign my insurance benefits to be paid directly to the undersigned physician, I am financially responsible for non-covered services.
SIGNED: Patient, or parent, if minor *Ken Thomas*   Today's date 09 / 17 / 20XX

RELEASE: I hereby authorize the physician to release to my insurance carriers any information require to process this claim.
SIGNED: Patient, or parent, if minor *Ken Thomas*   Today's date 09 / 17 / 20XX

✓	DESCRIPTION	CODE		FEE	✓	DESCRIPTION	CODE	FEE	✓	DESCRIPTION	CODE	FEE
	OFFICE VISITS	NEW	EST.			Venipuncture	36415			OFFICE PROCEDURES		
	Blood pressure check		99211			TB skin test	86580			Anoscopy	46600	
	Level II	99202	99212			Hematocrit	85013			Ear lavage	69210	
	Level III	99203	99213			Glucose finger stick	82948			Spirometry	94010	
X	Level IV	(99204)	99214	$175		IMMUNIZATIONS				Nebulizer Rx	94664	
	Level V	99205	99215			Allergy inj. X1	95115			EKG	93000	
	PREVENTIVE EXAMS	NEW	EST.			Allergy inj. X2	95117			SURGERY		
	Age 65 and older	99387	99397			Trigger pt. inj.	20552			Mole removal (1st)	17110	
	Age 40 - 64	99386	99396			Therapeutic inj.	96372			(2nd to 14th)	17003	
	Age 18 - 39	99385	99395			VACCINATION PRODUCTS				Flat warts (1st - 14th)	07110	
	Age 12 - 17	99384	99394			DPT	90701			15 or more	17111	
	Age 5 - 11	99383	99393			DT	90702			Biopsy, 1 lesion	11100	
	Age 1 - 4	99382	99392			Tetanus	90703			Addt'l. lesions	11101	
	Infant	99381	99391			MMR	90707			Endometrial Bx	58100	
	Newborn ofc		99432			OPV	90712			Skin tags to 15	11200	
	OB/NEWBORN CARE					Polio inj.	90713			Each addt'l. 10	11201	
	OB package		59400			Flu	90662			I & D abscess	10060	
	Post-partum visit N/C					Hemophilus B	90645			SUPPLIES/MISCELLANEOUS		
	LAB PROCEDURES					Hepatitis B vac.	90746			Surgical tray	99070	
	Urine dip		81000			Pneumovax	90670			Handling charge	99000	
	UA qualitative		81005			VACCINE ADMINISTRATION				Special report	99080	
X	Pregnancy urine		81025			Age: Through 18 yrs. (1st inj.)	90460			DOCTOR'S NOTES:		
	Wet mount		87210			Age: Through 18 yrs. (ea. addt'l. inj.)	90461					
	kOH prip		87220			Adult (1st inj.)	90471					
	Occult blood		82270			Adult (ea. addt'l. inj.)	90472					

DIAGNOSES ICD-10-CM

- Abdominal pain/unspec. . . R10.9
- Absess . . . . L02._
- Allergic reaction . . . . T78.40_
- Alzheimer's disease G30
- Anemia/unspec. D64.9
- Angina/unspec. I20.9
- Anorexia R63.0
- Anxiety/unspec. F41.9
- Apnea, sleep G47.30
- Arrhythmia, cardiac I49.9
- Arthritis, rheumatoid M06.9
- Asthma/unspec. J45.909
- Atrial fibrillation I48.0
- B-12 deficiency E53.8
- Back pain, low M54.5
- BPH N40
- Bradycardia/unspec. R00.1
- Broncitis, acute . . . . J20._
- Bronchitis, chronic J42
- Bursitis/unspec. M71.9
- CA, breast . . . . C50._
- CA, lung . . . . C34._
- CA, prostate C61
- Cellulitis . . . . L03._
- Chest pain/unspec. R07.9
- Cirrhosis, liver/unspec. . . K74.60
- Cold, common J00
- Colitis/unspec K51.90
- Confusion R41.0
- CHF I50.9
- Constipation K59.00
- COPD J44.9
- Cough R05
- Crohn's disease/unspec . K50.90
- CVA I63.9
- Decubitus ulcer . . . . L89._
- Dehydration E86.0
- Dementia/unspec. F03
- Depression, major/unsp. . F32.9
- Diab I, no complications . E10.0
- Diab II, no complications . E11.9
-   w/kidney complic. . . . . E11.2_
-   w/ophthalmic compl. . E11.3_
-   w/neurolog.compl. . . . E11.4_
-   w/circulatory cmpl. . . . E11.5_
- Insulin use Z79.4
- Diarrhea/unspec. R19.7
- Diverticulitis K57.92
- Diverticulosis K57.90
- Dizziness R42
- Dysuria R30.0
- Edema/unspec. R60.9
- Endocarditis I38
- Esophageal reflux K21.0
- Fatigue (lethargy) R53.83
- FUO R50.9
- Gastritis K29.70
- Gastroenteritis (colitis) . . K52.9
- G.I. bleed K92.2
- Gout/unspec. M10.9
- Headache R51
- Health exam . . . . 200._
- Hematuria/unspec. R31.9
- Herpes simplex B00.9
- Herpes zoster B02.9
- Hiatal hernia K44.9
- HTN (HBP) I10
- Hyperlipidemia/unspec. . E78.5
- Hypothyroidism/unspec. . E03.9
- Impotentce . . . . N52._
- Influenza, respiratory . . . J10.1
- Insomnia G47.0
- IBS, diarrhea . . . . K58.
- Lupus, systemic erythem. M32.9
- MI, acute . . . . I21._
- MI, old I25.2
- Migraine G43.9
- Myalgia M79.1
- Neck pain M54.2
- Neuropathy G62.9
- Nausea R11.1
- X Nausea/vomiting R11.0
- Obesity/unspec. E66.9
- Osteoarthritis (site) . . . . . M19._
- Otitis media . . . . H66.9_
- Parkinson's disease G20
- Pharyngitis, acute J02.9
- Pleurisy R09.1
- Pneumonia J18.9
- Pneumonia, viral J12.9
- Prostatitis/unspec. N41.9
- PVD I73.9
- Radiculopathy . . . . M54.1_
- Rectal bleeding K62.5
- Renal failure N19
- Sciatica . . . . M54.3_
- Shortness of breath R03.02
- Sinusitis, chr./unspec. . . . J32.9
- Syncope R55
- Tachycardia/unspec. R00.0
- Tachy., supraventric I47.1
- Tendinitis/unspec. M77.9
- TIA G45.9
- Ulcer, duodenal/unspec. . K26.9
- Ulcer, gastric/unspec. . . . K25.9
- Ulcer, peptic/unspec. . . . K27.9
- URI/unspec. J06.9
- UTI N39.0
- Vertigo R42
- Weight gain R63.5
- Weight loss R63.4

Diagnosis/additional description:
Headache

Doctor's signature/date
Dr. Martin   09-17-20XX

Return appointment information:	-with whom	(Self) other	Rec'd. by:	Total today's fee	$175
Days Wks. (Mos.) 1 month			☐ Cash ☐ Check ☐ Credit # _____	Co-payment	$50
				Amount rec'd. today	

PLEASE RMEMBER THAT PAYMENT IS YOUR OBLIGATION, REGARDLESS OF INSURANCE OR OTHER THIRD PARTY INVOLVEMENT.

INSUR-A-BILL ® BIBBERO SYSTEMS, INC. • PETALUMA, CA • © 7/90 (BM1092)   (REV. 7/11)

FIG. 27.1 Encounter form with charges. (Courtesy Bibbero Systems, an InHealth Company, Petaluma, CA (800) 242-2376 • www.bibbero.com)

CHAPTER 27 Accounts, Collections, and Banking

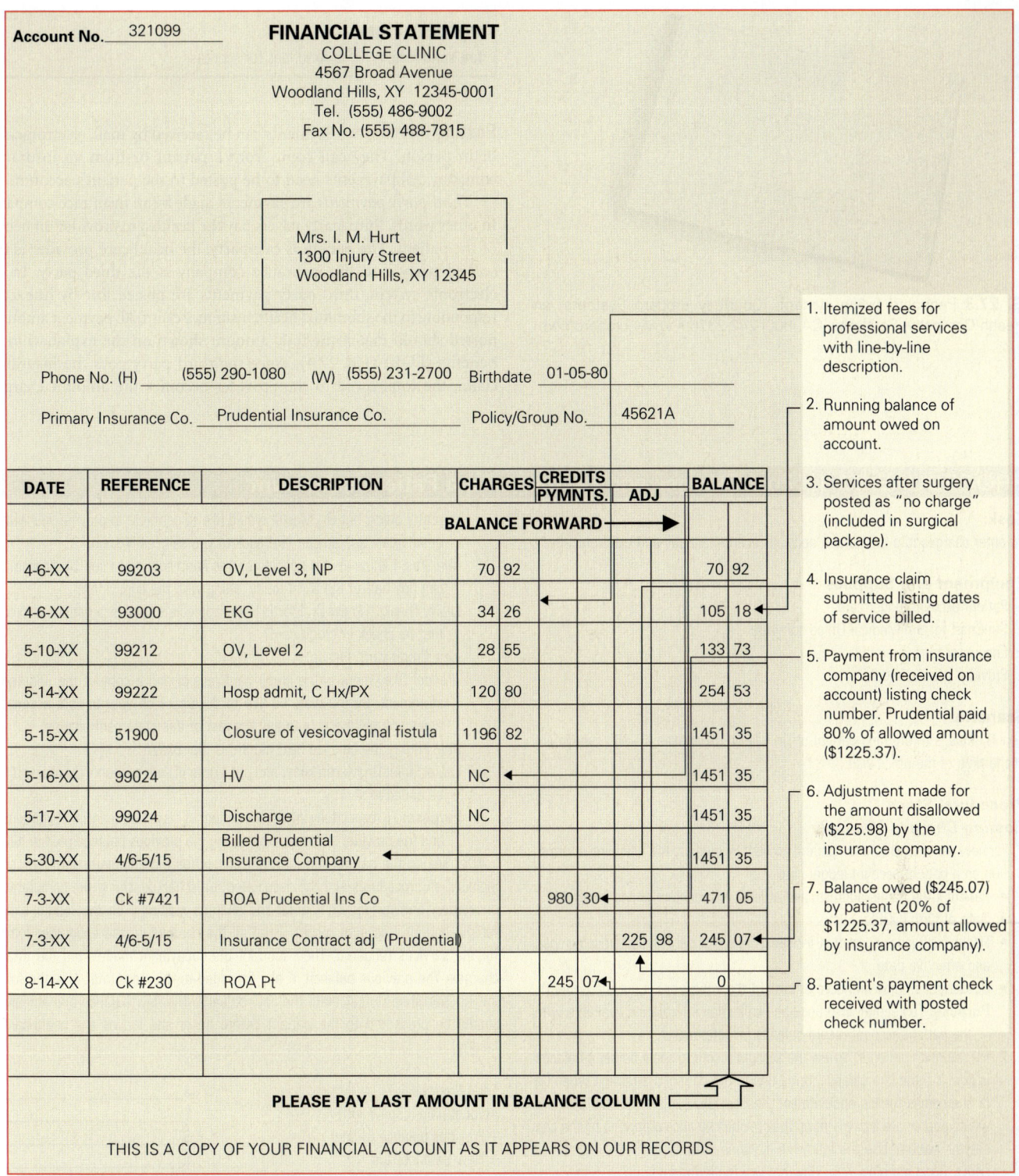

FIG. 27.2 Patient ledger. (From Fordney WT: *Insurance Handbook For The Medical Office*, ed 14, St. Louis, 2017, Elsevier.)

VOCABULARY

pegboard system: A manual bookkeeping system that uses a day sheet to record all financial transactions for the date of service and maintains patient account balances by using physical ledger cards.

Posting Charges. When a practice management software system is used, charges are entered into the ledger automatically from the encounter form after the office visit (Procedure 27.1). The fees for services rendered come from the **fee schedule**. Most practice management systems will automatically determine the fee based on the CPT/HCPCS code and insurance company.

UNIT 3 Administrative Ambulatory Care

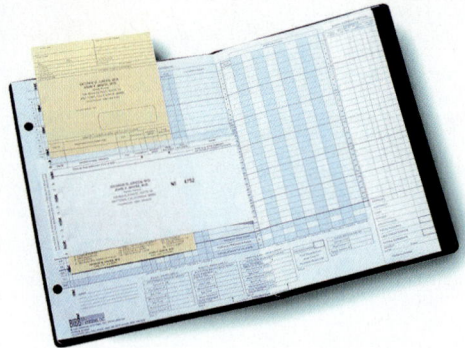

FIG. 27.3 Pegboard billing system. (Courtesy Bibbero Systems, an InHealth Company, Petaluma, CA (800) 242-2376 • www.bibbero.com)

> **VOCABULARY**
> **fee schedule:** A list of fixed fees for services.

Posting Payments. Payments can be received by mail, electronically, or in person. They can come from a patient or from an insurance company. All payments need to be posted to the patient's account.

Third-party payments are payments made by an insurance company. In other words, third-party payers pay the healthcare provider on behalf of the patient. The patient is one party, the healthcare provider is the second party, and the insurance company is the third party. In an electronic system, third-party payments are posted line by line, corresponding to the submitted health insurance claim. All payment amounts posted should match the total amount shown on the *explanation of benefits (EOB)* (Fig. 27.4). Once the third party pays the insurance claim, the total owed to the provider becomes the amount charged

---

PROCEDURE 27.1 Post Charges and Payments to a Patient's Account

Task:
To enter charges into the patient account record manually and electronically.

Equipment and Supplies
- Patient account ledger card
- SimChart for the Medical Office software
- Encounter form/superbill
- Provider's fee schedule

Scenario
Ken Thomas is a returning patient of Dr. Martin. He makes his $50 copayment at the time of the office visit.

Procedural Steps
Posting Charges Manually
1. For new patients, create the patient account by entering the following information on a patient account ledger card:
   - Patient's full name, address, and at least two contact phone numbers
   - Date of birth (DOB)
   - Health insurance information, including the subscriber number, group number, and effective date
   - Subscriber's name and date of birth (if the subscriber is not the patient)
     Purpose: To keep all insurance and collection information available with the patient account record balance for reference.
2. For returning patients, review the account record to see whether a balance is due. If there is a balance, bring this to the patient's attention when he or she comes for the appointment. Respectfully explain that the provider would appreciate a payment on the previous balance before he or she can see the patient. Use the following dialogue:
   Laura: Good morning, Ken. How are you feeling today?
   Ken: Not so good, I really need to see Dr. Martin again because my headaches have been getting worse.
   Laura: I'm sorry to hear that. Let's get you in to see the doctor right away. I can collect the $50 copayment for today's visit, and here is a statement for your previous balance of $214. How would you like to take care of that today?
   Ken: Oh, I didn't know about the previous balance. Can I just pay the copayment today?
   Laura: Dr. Martin would like at least half of this previous balance paid before seeing you today, please. I know that medical bills can pile up

   pretty quick, but Dr. Martin would like to continue to provide you with quality care so you can feel back to yourself really soon.
   Ken: Yes, I know you're right. I need to keep coming to see Dr. Martin. I can pay half of the $214 today, along with the copayment.
   Laura: Thanks, I know Dr. Martin really appreciates you as a patient. Would that be check or credit card?
   Ken: Credit card, please.
   Brenda: Okay, here is the credit card receipt and a copy of the updated statement. By the way, I'd like to document on your patient account when you will be able to pay the rest of this statement amount.
   Ken: I'll pay the balance next month; is that okay?
   Laura: I'll let Dr. Martin know and put a note in your account. Thanks; you'll be called in shortly.
   Purpose: To respectfully inform the patient of his or her financial obligations and the provider's intention of having the previous balance paid in full.

   After seeing the patient, the provider completes the encounter form, which includes all procedures and the associated fee schedule. Using the completed encounter form in Fig. 27.1, enter the charges manually on the ledger card for the patient's account record. Total all the charges on the encounter form for the services rendered. Then subtract the copayment made from the total charges. The previous balance, if any, is added to this new total. Use the following worksheet to calculate the new balance. The new balance-due amount should be presented to the patient before he or she leaves the healthcare facility.

Total Charges	$_____
Amount paid (copayment)	$_____
+ Previous balance (if any)	$_____
= New Balance Due	$_____

Posting Charges in Simchart for the Medical Office
1. After logging into SimChart, locate the established patient by clicking on Find Patient; enter the patient's name, verify the DOB, and click on the radio button. This will bring you to the Clinical Care tab. If there is no encounter shown, create an encounter by clicking on Office Visit under Info Panel on the left, select a visit type, and click on Save. Once an encounter has been created, return to the Patient Dashboard and click on the Superbill link on the right (or click on the Coding and Billing tab as seen in the following figure.

PROCEDURE 27.1 Post Charges and Payments to a Patient's Account—cont'd

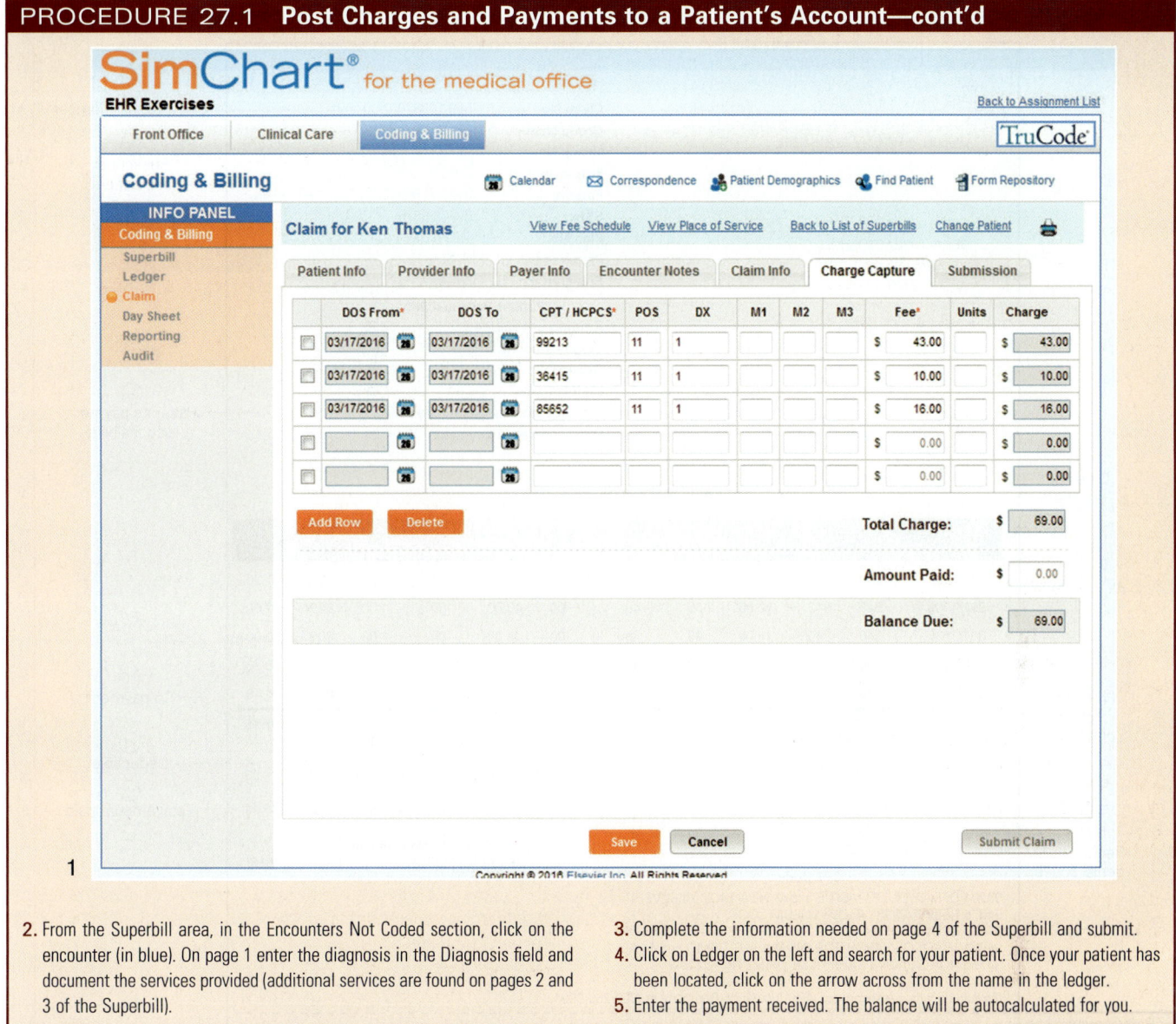

1.

2. From the Superbill area, in the Encounters Not Coded section, click on the encounter (in blue). On page 1 enter the diagnosis in the Diagnosis field and document the services provided (additional services are found on pages 2 and 3 of the Superbill).

3. Complete the information needed on page 4 of the Superbill and submit.

4. Click on Ledger on the left and search for your patient. Once your patient has been located, click on the arrow across from the name in the ledger.

5. Enter the payment received. The balance will be autocalculated for you.

---

minus the payment amount and the amount adjusted by the third party. The remaining balance is still owed to the provider by the patient:

Insurance payment amount + Adjustment amount + Patient responsibility = Total charged

> **VOCABULARY**
> **explanation of benefits (EOB):** A document sent by the insurance company to the provider and the patient explaining the allowed charge amount, the amount reimbursed for services, and the patient's financial responsibilities.

Posting Adjustments. Adjustments are used to either credit or debit a patient's account. Credit adjustments are posted to the patient ledger when an amount needs to be subtracted from a patient's balance. An example would be when the provider's fee exceeds the amount allowed stated on the EOB. The difference between the billed amount and the allowed amount would need to be adjusted (written off). Credit adjustments should always be posted to the patient account record at the same time as the payment. The patient ledger should have a column for the adjustments. *Remember: payments and credit adjustments are both credits*; however, payments are money that is received in the healthcare facility, and credit adjustments simply reduce the balance that the patient owes on the account. When the payments and credit adjustments are subtracted from the charged amount, the balance is either the patient responsibility or the amount billed to the secondary insurance.

Before continuing to post to the next EOB line item, confirm that the payment amount, the adjusted amount, and the patient responsibility/secondary insurance balance exactly match the amounts calculated on the EOB.

Debit adjustments are posted to the patient ledger when an amount needs to be added to the patient's balance but is not a charge for services. An example would be if a check the patient had written to the healthcare facility was returned for nonsufficient funds. The amount had initially been credited to the account, but the healthcare facility never actually got the funds. A debit adjustment must be made to add the amount of the check back to the patient's balance (Box 27.3 and Fig. 27.5).

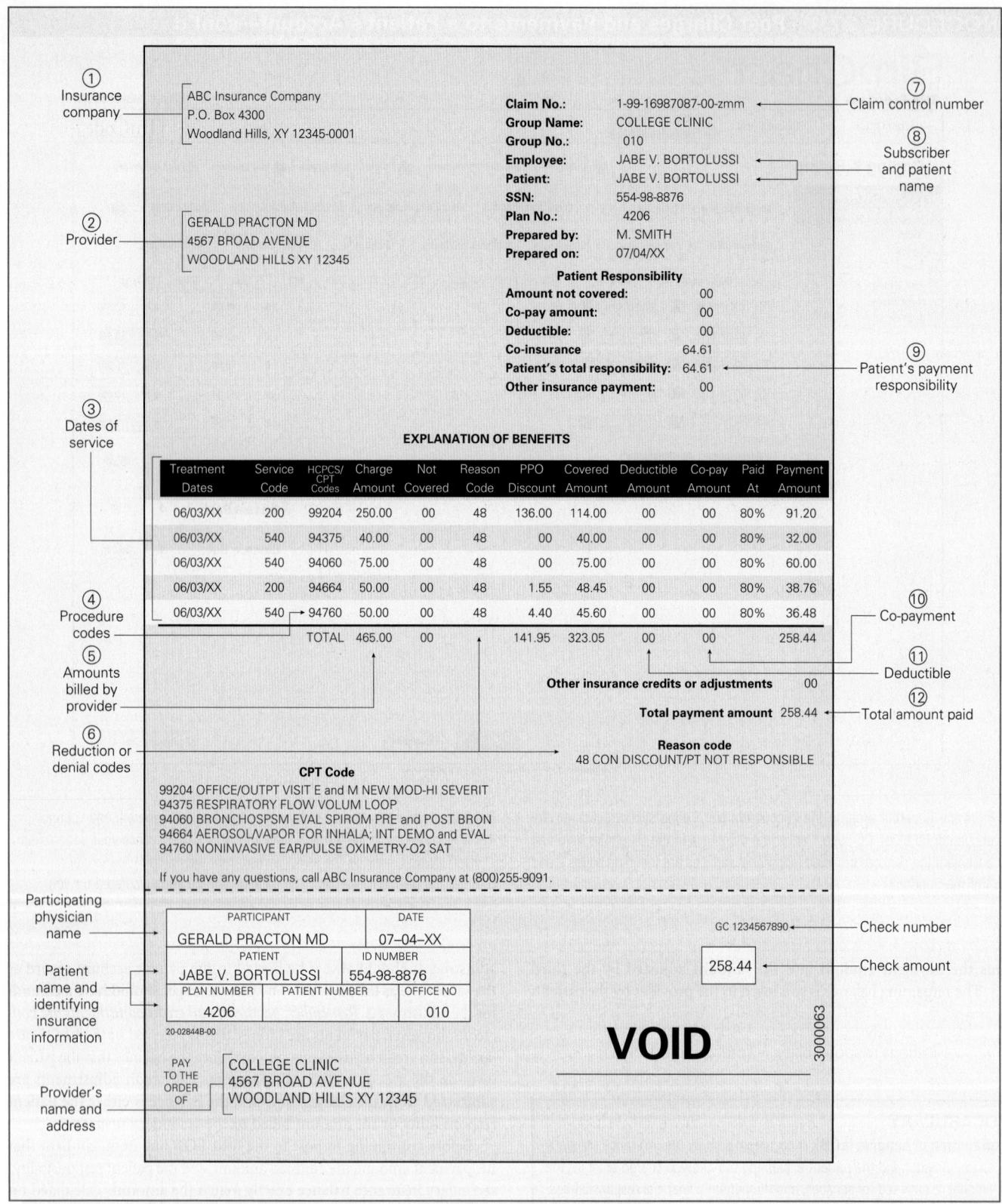

FIG. 27.4 Explanation of Benefits (EOB). (From Fordney MT: *Insurance Handbook For The Medical Office*, ed 14, St Louis, 2017, Elsevier.)

BOX 27.3 Nonsufficient Funds (NSF) Checks

Nonsufficient funds (NSF) checks occur when a patient pays with a check without having sufficient funds in the bank to cover the payment. The bank will return the check to the healthcare practice marked NSF and will charge the practice's bank account a returned check fee. The payment posted to the patient account must be reversed. It is important to note that the original payment is not deleted; instead, a charge line item is added to the patient account record with the amount of the NSF check (see Fig. 27.5). Many medical offices add additional line items for NSF fee charges, but this is up to the discretion of the provider.

If the healthcare facility receives an NSF check, call the signer of the check immediately and ask him or her to stop by the office to pay the amount needed to cover the check and the additional fee. Most offices require that such payment be made by another form of payment, preferably credit card. Legal remedies are available for the provider if the check remains unpaid.

Many NSF problems can be cleared up quickly and easily with courtesy and tact, assuming the situation was simply a mistake or an oversight. Bad checks may be reported to several organizations, and once the writer is in their databases, the person will have difficulty writing a check to any business. Turn the account over to a qualified collection agency if you are unable to collect on the account within a short time.

CRITICAL THINKING BOX 27.1

The bank calls Laura to inform her that three of the patient checks deposited last week were NSF. What steps should Laura take to collect the NSF check amounts from the patients? Are there additional charges she can add to the patients' balances to cover the inconvenience?

Credit balances. A *credit balance* occurs when a patient has paid in advance, or an overpayment or duplicate payment is made. For example, an overpayment occurs if the patient makes a partial payment, and later the insurance payment is more than the remaining balance. When this happens, the patient account will show a credit balance, or an amount that the provider owes. The medical assistant should investigate to whom the credit balance is owed (i.e., the patient or the insurance company). The first place to look is the EOB from the insurance company; this document shows the exact amount of the patient's financial responsibility. The medical assistant should confirm that all the line items match the corresponding amounts on the EOB because many credit balances are created when an error is made in payment posting. If the patient's payment exceeded the amount indicated on the EOB, the provider must send a check for the balance to the patient. A credit balance creates a *debit* in the patient account, or an amount that is due by the provider to the patient or the insurance company, depending on which party made the overpayment. A debit adjustment is done showing that the patient or insurance company was refunded. This debit adjustment should bring the account balance to zero.

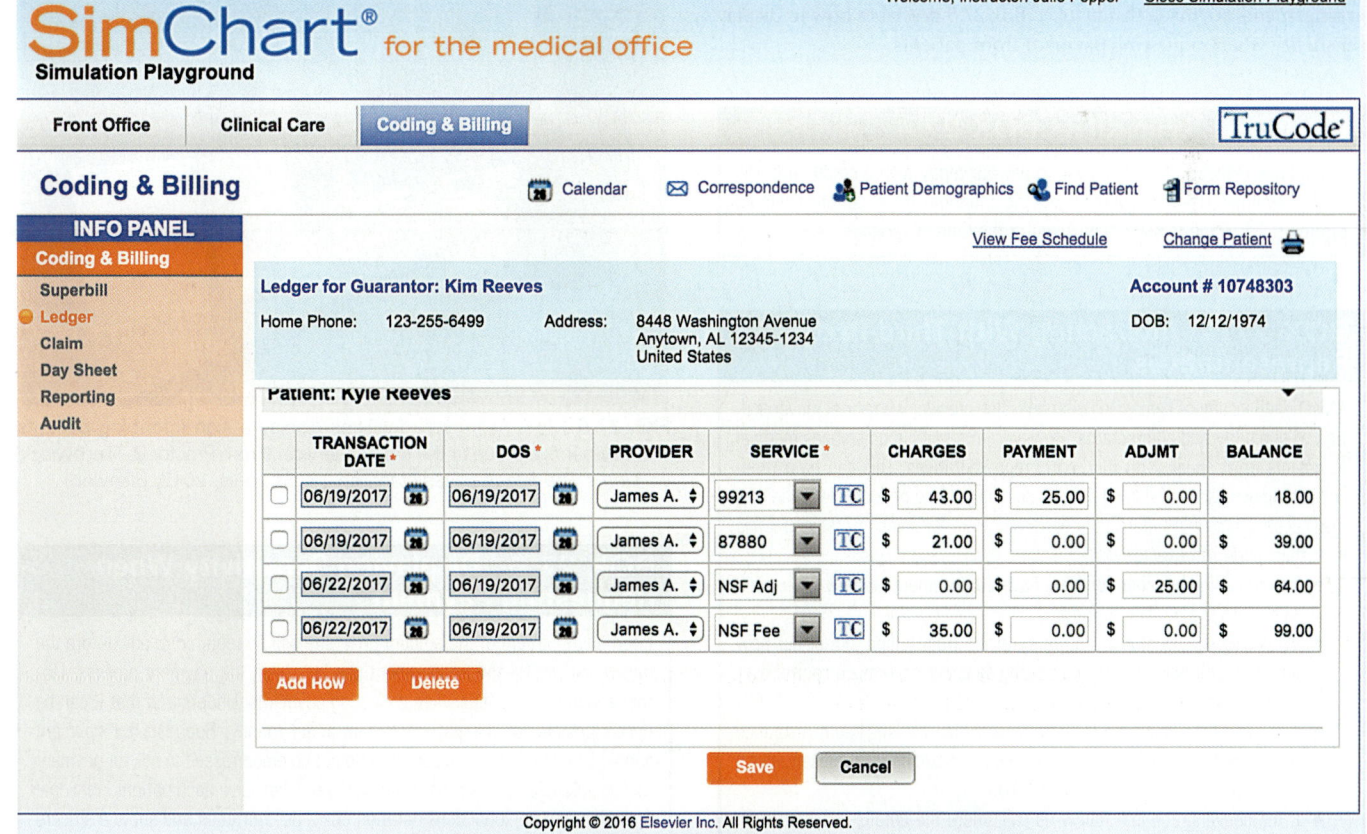

FIG. 27.5 NSF Adjustments in Simchart for the Medical Office.

Most patient account management software can enter charges, payments, and adjustments. As discussed previously, charges increase what is owed to the provider, whereas payments reduce what is owed to the provider, and adjustments can do both. Box 27.4 and Procedure 27.1 present tips for interacting with third-party representatives,

> ### CRITICAL THINKING BOX 27.2
>
> The healthcare facility receives two checks for a patient, Kelly Washington, from Blue Cross for the same date of service. One check is for $438, and the other is for $534. Can Laura post the larger payment and just refund the smaller payment to Blue Cross? What must Laura do before she posts either payment?

> ### CRITICAL THINKING BOX 27.3
>
> Laura received a claim denial for a patient, Clara Martin, for date of service 1/11/20XX. The denial stated that Ms. Martin was not covered on this date of service. Laura reviewed her notes in the patient's account and found the verification of eligibility that was done on 1/11/20XX for Clara Martin. What should Laura do to prepare to call the insurance company?

Payment at the Time of Service. For the most part, patients are expected to pay their copayment at the time of service unless previous arrangements have been made (Fig. 27.6). Patients without health insurance should pay after the visit has been completed. When an appointment is made, patients should be informed that payment is expected at the time of service. That way they are not surprised when asked for payment at the healthcare facility. The medical assistant may say, "Your charge for today is $25. Will that be cash, check, credit, or debit card?" If a patient asks to be billed, the medical assistant may say, "Our normal procedure is to pay at the time of service unless other arrangements are made in advance." Box 27.5 describes how to display sensitivity when requesting payment from patients.

> ### CRITICAL THINKING BOX 27.4
>
> Adam Page comes to the front desk to pay his copay with a credit card. His card is declined. How can Laura handle the situation? What options could be offered to Mr. Page to make a payment at the time of service?

> ### BOX 27.4 Interacting With Third-Party Representatives
>
> Most health insurance companies offer an online provider web portal for verification of eligibility and claim status. However, in some circumstances medical assistants must speak with third-party representatives. This can be a time-consuming process involving waiting on hold on for long periods. Nevertheless, medical assistants must interact professionally. Here are some tips for interacting with third-party representatives:
> - Before calling provider services, have all documents readily accessible to discuss the patient account.
> - When the representative answers, refrain from telling him or her how long the wait was; the person usually does not have much control over wait times.
> - Document the details of the phone conversation with the health insurance representative in the patient account record, including the representative's name and the date and time of the call.
> - If the conversation is a follow-up call, share the details collected from the previous call from notes documented in the patient account record.

Payment Agreements. With the increase in high-deductible insurance plans, there has been an increase in the need for payment agreements. If the patient is having an elective procedure, payment can be made before or at the time of service. If the procedure or therapy is expensive, the patient may need to spread the payments out over time. Therefore, the medical assistant must explain to the patient the fees and the office credit policies. In most healthcare practices, the appropriate staff member sits down with the patient for a financial consultation before a payment arrangement contract is offered. The payment arrangement contract states the monthly payment; how many months it must be paid; the payment due date; whether interest will be charged; and the penalties of nonpayment. If the patient is going to be making more than four payments, the Truth in Lending Act comes into play.

Truth in Lending Act. It is considered an offer of credit when the healthcare facility allows the patient to make more than four payments on his or her balance. When offering credit options for patients, the healthcare facility should be in compliance with Regulation Z of the Truth in Lending Act (TILA). TILA is enforced by the Federal Trade Commission (FTC) and is part of the Consumer Credit Protection Act. TILA requires that individuals be provided certain information when credit is extended, including:
- the annual percentage rate (APR)
- the monthly interest rate
- the total costs to the borrower
- when payments are due
- the amount of any late payment charges and when they will be applied

If the healthcare facility and patient agree that payment will be made in more than four installments, the practice must provide a Federal

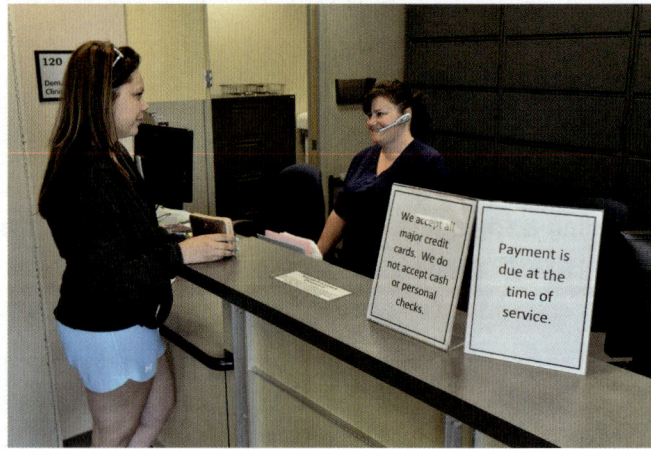

FIG. 27.6 Most healthcare facilities display a sign informing patients that payments are due at the time of service. (From Proctor D, Niedzwiecki B: *Kinn's The Medical Assistant*, ed 13, St Louis, 2017, Elsevier.)

> ### BOX 27.5 Displaying Sensitivity When Requesting Payment
>
> Informing a patient of the amount he or she will be required to pay before the person arrives for the appointment can help with the payment process. Use tact and good judgment when collecting payments. Understand that it can be uncomfortable for the patient to talk about money. Requests for payment should be made in a private setting. Do not be embarrassed to ask for payment for the valuable services that have been provided. Give each patient individual attention and personal consideration; also, be courteous and show a sincere desire to help the patient with financial problems.

Truth in Lending Statement (Fig. 27.7). This should be in place even if no finance fees are charged. The statement is signed by the practice's representative and the patient.

Monthly Patient Account Statements

Healthcare facilities should send monthly statements for all patient accounts that have a balance due (Box 27.6). Statements should be printed on clean, good-quality paper. Payment options, such as check, e-check, online payments, and/or credit card, should be presented clearly. The statement should provide itemized details on the following:
- Date(s) of service
- Services provided
- Insurance payments and adjustments
- Patient payments, including copayments

Envelopes should be printed with "Address Service Requested" in the appropriate place to maintain up-to-date mailing lists. A self-addressed return envelope included with the statement is convenient for the patient and encourages prompt payment. The statement should also indicate how old the balance is, such as 30, 60, 90, 120, or >120 days. For accounts that are more than 60 days past due, some offices apply neon-colored stickers to emphasize the need to pay the balance as soon as possible, thus avoiding further collection activity.

Billing Minors. According to federal regulations, a minor cannot be held financially responsible for his or her account balance unless the individual is an *emancipated minor*. Bills for minors are usually addressed to the *guarantor*. If a bill is addressed to a minor, parents could take the attitude that they are not responsible because they never received a statement.

If the parents are separated or divorced, the parent who brings the child in for treatment is responsible for payment. Whatever financial agreement exists between the parents is strictly their personal business and should not concern the healthcare practice. The responsible parent should be so informed from the first appointment.

If a minor appears in the office and requests treatment, you should determine if the person is legally emancipated. If he or she is, the minor will be financially responsible. Minors can be treated for certain conditions, such as sexually transmitted diseases (STDs), pregnancy, and birth control, without parental consent. Each state has differences in the laws in these cases. Medical assistants must be familiar with their state laws and office polices to determine where the statement should be sent.

Medical Care for Those Who Cannot Pay. The medical profession traditionally has accepted the responsibility of providing medical care occasionally for individuals who are unable to pay for these services. There are government programs to help care for the medically *indigent* (IN di juh nt), but there are still patients who are not covered. In many instances, medical care for the indigent is available through social service agencies. Medical assistants should learn about local organizations and agencies that can aid patients in obtaining the necessary assistance. The provider can provide only medical services. Other agencies can:
- help pay for hospitalization
- arrange for and help pay for special therapy, rehabilitation, or medications

Unfortunately, another segment of the population consists of uninsured or underinsured employees who are not eligible for public assistance, are not covered under a group policy, and cannot afford the high premiums for private medical insurance. Give special attention to helping these people arrange payment of their medical bills. If a provider knows in advance that a patient cannot pay for services and decides to still provide care, complete records must still be kept on the patient. The only difference in procedure is that an adjustment would be made to the account so that balance would be zero.

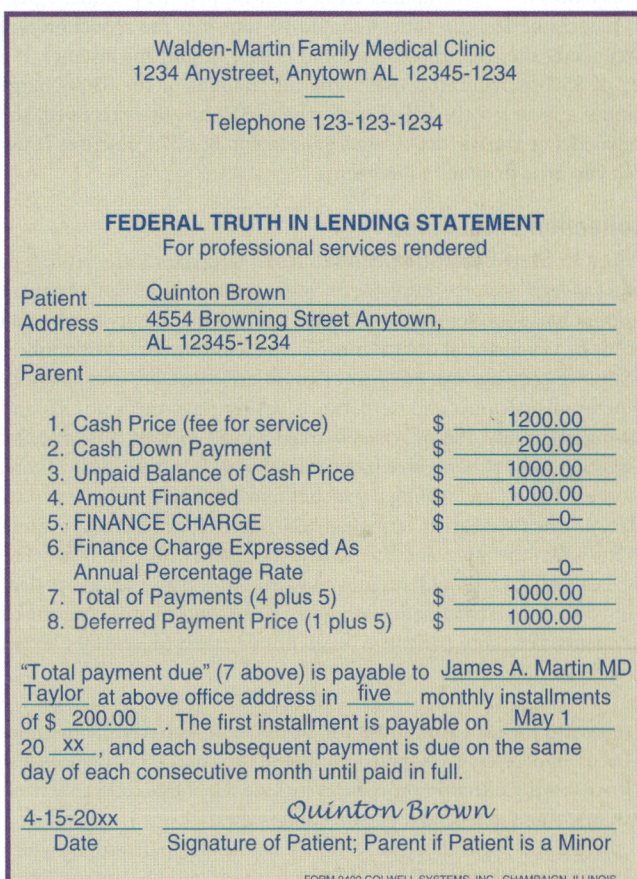

FIG. 27.7 Truth in Lending Statement. (From Courtesy Colwell Systems, Champaign, IL.)

VOCABULARY

emancipated minor: A minor who has been granted emancipation by the court; the minor can assume the rights and responsibilities of adulthood.
guarantor: The person legally responsible for the entire bill. This is usually the patient, but in the case of a minor it would be a parent or legal guardian.
indigent: Poor, needy, impoverished.

BOX 27.6 Billing Cycle

The healthcare facility should establish a set schedule for sending statements to patients. Sending them monthly is most common, but they can be sent every 2 weeks or even quarterly. When a monthly system is used, patient accounts are divided into equal segments, usually alphabetically. One segment is sent out each week of the month. This keeps an even flow of money into the healthcare facility. It can also spread out patients' calls about their statements.

Fees in Hardship Cases. Sometimes a healthcare practice is faced with the problem of deciding whether to reduce or cancel a fee in a hardship case. Before adjusting or canceling a fee, the provider or medical assistant should have a frank discussion with the patient about his or her financial situation. Find out whether the patient is entitled to or qualifies for medical assistance. If the patient's injuries are the result of a car accident, there may be medical insurance through the automobile policy. The patient may qualify for local or state public assistance, such as crime victim assistance. Maintain information about such agencies in the area and direct the patient to the appropriate one.

If the provider is aware of the hardship before services are provided, the fee can be discussed and payment arrangements made. The healthcare facility may suggest that a medically indigent patient seek care at a clinic that provides public assistance. A provider should be free to choose his or her form of charity and should not feel obligated to substantially reduce or cancel a fee when the circumstances are known in advance.

The provider and the patient may agree on a fee, but special circumstances may come up that create a hardship. If the provider agrees to reduce the fee, the patient should be told that the reduction will occur only after the adjusted amount is paid in full. For instance, if a fee of $500 is reduced to $350, the full amount of the $500 charge should appear on the ledger, and when $350 has been received, the remainder can be written off as an adjustment. Box 27.7 describes issues that can arise from fee adjustments.

Collection Procedures

When to Start Collection Procedures. *Collection* is the process of using all legal resources available to collect payment for past due patient account balances. Sometimes a patient may have difficulty meeting all of his or her financial obligations. The patient may have lost a job or insurance coverage. An emergency could arise that depletes finances. When patients must choose between paying their medical bills and having electricity, the provider is often forced to wait for payment. Although a few patients absolutely refuse to pay for their medical care, most are honest and willing to pay but may need help with a payment plan. As discussed earlier, terms can be arranged for collecting payment in full when the office and the patient cooperate with each other. The medical assistant should attempt to work out a plan that the patient can abide by, and the patient should be expected to make promised payments. For those patients who do not pay their bill, further action is necessary.

Preparing Patient Accounts for Collection Activity. Sometimes it becomes necessary to aggressively attempt to collect the balances that patients owe. Collection procedures include telephone calls, collection reminders and letters, and personal interviews.

Before you begin collection action, it is essential to determine which accounts have a balance due and how old the account balance is. Some accounts are grouped together, or "aged," according to the dates of the last payment activity, whereas others are grouped according to the original date of service (Fig. 27.8). Common account aging categories are:
- Current
- 31–60 days
- 61–90 days
- 91–120 days
- >120 days

Most bills with balances less than 30 days old are probably waiting for the health insurance to pay, so no collection action is needed. Patient account balances more than 90 or 120 days old require a final demand letter before the account is turned over to a collection agency. Always allow the provider to review and approve the list of patient accounts being sent to a collection agency.

The medical assistant can use a variety of techniques to collect patient accounts, such as collection phone calls, collection letters, and skip tracing. Often more than one technique must be used to obtain payment. Always be courteous and kind when using all collection techniques.

Collection Telephone Calls. Whenever attempts are made to collect a debt, the Fair Debt Collection Practices Act must be kept in mind (Box 27.8). A telephone call at the right time, with the right presentation, is more successful than notes, patient account statements, or collection letters. The personal contact call often prompts patients to mail in their payment or to make payments over the phone with a credit card. If the staff does not have enough time to make calls, the collection letter is the next best approach. If collections are a serious problem, it may be worth an extra salary to hire a person to make the phone calls.

Always treat patients with the utmost respect on the telephone. Keep their financial record nearby in case they have questions about their bill; also, have their insurance company's phone number handy. Remember that some patients may not understand anything about insurance or third-party payers. Helping them to understand, and acting as their advocate in getting as much reimbursement as possible, can reduce the patient's share. Never simply insist that the insurance plan has paid and the patient's balance is due. This puts the patient in a negative mindset. Try using phrases such as the following:
- "Mrs. Diggs, it looks as if your insurance company paid late last month. You have co-insurance for your surgery that amounts to $450. Let me review some payment options to help make that as easy as possible for you to pay."
- "Mr. Hildebrand, we're showing that you have a balance due from your surgery. Your insurance has paid, and it looks as if you owe $700. We would be happy to help you by splitting that into two or three payments. When can I schedule that first payment for you?"
- "Mrs. Crumley, it seems that you have a balance due of $450 from your surgery, and I called to see whether I could help you budget that. For example, you could pay $50 this week

---

> **BOX 27.7 Pitfalls of Fee Adjustments**
>
> Problems can come up when a provider begins to reduce his or her fees. Patients may begin to expect fees to be reduced in all circumstances. Patients may even doubt the competency of a provider who habitually reduces fees. Make fee reductions the exception rather than the norm.
>
> Take great care in reducing the fee for care of a patient who dies. This could be misinterpreted and result in a suit for malpractice. The family may suspect that the fee was reduced because the provider knew he or she made an error.

> **BOX 27.8 Fair Debt Collection Practice Act**
>
> In March, 1978, the Fair Debt Collection Act went into effect. It was designed to eliminate abusive, deceptive, and unfair debt collection practices. The act states that collection calls cannot be made:
> - at any time or place that is unusual or known to be inconvenient to the patient; before 8 a.m. or after 9 p.m.
> - when the creditor is aware that the debtor is represented by an attorney with respect to the debt.
> - to the patient's place of work if the patient's employer prohibits such contacts.

Patient Account Aging Report: Walden-Martin Family Medical Clinic

Starting Date: 9/1/2017   Ending Date: 9/30/2017   Report Date 9/30/2017

Jacob Abraham (3406) — Last Payment: 7/12/2017 — 15.00
Guarantor: Self — Home: 954-233-9033 — Work: NA

Date	Code	Billed	Current	31–60	61–90	91–120	>120	Total
7/12/2017	99201	45.00			45.00			45.00
7/12/2017	Cash	(15.00)			(15.00)			(15.00)
Patient Total		30.00	0.00	0.00	30.00	0.00	0.00	30.00

Frank Bullock (3412) — Last Payment: 8/20/2017 — 45.00
Guarantor: Wife — Home 954-388-0196 — Work: 954-233-5803

Date	Code	Billed	Current	31–60	61–90	91–120	>120	Total
8/20/2017	99205	195.00		195.00				195.00
8/20/2017	Check	(45.00)		(45.00)				(45.00)
Patient Total		150.00	0.00	150.00	0.00	0.00	0.00	150.00

Cynthia Dearing (3433) — Last Payment: 7/25/2017 — 10.00
Guarantor: Self — Home: 953-518-2100 — Work: 954-333-9003

Date	Code	Billed	Current	31–60	61–90	91–120	>120	Total
6/12/2017	99386	185.00				185.00		185.00
7/15/2017	BCBS	(160.00)				(160.00)		(160.00)
7/25/2017	Check	(10.00)				(10.00)		(10.00)
Patient Total		15.00	0.00	0.00	0.00	15.00	0.00	15.00

Kirsha Macken (3462) — Last Payment: 7/10/2017 — 50.00
Guarantor: Parent — Home: 954-736-7227 — Work: FT Student

Date	Code	Billed	Current	31–60	61–90	91–120	>120	Total
4/23/2017	58900	230.00					230.00	230.00
4/23/2017	Cash	(50.00)					(50.00)	(50.00)
7/10/2017	99214	90.00			90.00			90.00
7/10/2017	90658	30.00			30.00			30.00
7/10/2017	Cash	(50.00)			(50.00)			(50.00)
Patient Total		250.00	0.00	0.00	70.00	0.00	180.00	250.00

Larry Nerod (3501) — Last Payment: 6/22/2017 — 15.00
Guarantor: Self — Home: 953-736-7227 — Work: 954-332-001

Date	Code	Billed	Current	31–60	61–90	91–120	>120	Total
6/22/2017	99204	140.00				140.00		140.00
6/22/2017	CCard	(15.00)				(15.00)		(15.00)
Patient Total		125.00	0.00	0.00	0.00	125.00	0.00	125.00

Emanuel Perez (3513) — Last Payment: 7/12/2017 — 46.00
Guarantor: Self — Home: 956-303-2070 — Work: 953-322-5500

Date	Code	Billed	Current	31–60	61–90	91–120	>120	Total
7/12/2017	68500	403.00			403.00			403.00
7/12/2017	Check	(46.00)			(46.00)			(46.00)
Patient Total		357.00	0.00	0.00	357.00	0.00	0.00	357.00

| **Report Totals** | | | 0.00 | 150.00 | 457.00 | 140.00 | 180.00 | 927.00 |
| **Percent of Total** | | | 0.00% | 16.18% | 49.3% | 15.10% | 19.41% | 100.00% |

FIG. 27.8 Sample Aging Report.

---

and split the remaining $400 into two payments over the next 2 months."

Always abide by office policy when making payment arrangements in collection situations. Never be **belligerent** (buh LIG er uh nt) with a patient. If the person becomes angry, simply state that he or she can call back when ready to discuss a solution for paying the account, say good-bye, and gently hang up the phone. Never listen to **expletives** (EK spli tiv) or allow verbal abuse. Respectfully end the phone call by saying thank you and good-bye; do not slam down the phone.

Before a final demand for payment is made, a letter must be sent indicating that legal or collection proceedings will be started.

General Rules for Telephone Collections
What to do:
- Call the patient when it can be done privately.
- Call only between 8 a.m. and 9 p.m.
- Determine the identity of the person with whom you are speaking. If you ask, "Is this Mrs. Noble?" and she answers, "Yes," it could be the patient's mother-in-law or daughter-in-law, who may also be "Mrs. Noble." Use the person's full name. Include suffixes, such as "Thomas Melborn, III." This may sound too formal, but it helps to ensure that the correct person is on the phone.
- Be respectful. One can be friendly and professional at the same time.
- Ask the patient whether it is a convenient time to talk. Unless you have the attention of the patient, there is little to be gained by continuing. If you are told that it is an inopportune time, ask for a specific time to call back or get a promise that the patient will call the office at a specified time.

VOCABULARY
belligerent: Hostile and aggressive.
expletive: An oath or swear word.

- After a brief greeting, state the purpose of the call. Make no apology for calling, but state the reason in a friendly, businesslike way. The provider expects payment, and the medical assistant is interested in helping the patient meet the financial obligation. Open the call with a phrase such as, "This is Alice, Dr. Walden's medical assistant. I'm calling about your account." A well-placed pause at this point in the call sometimes gets an immediate response from the debtor with regard to the nonpayment.
- Assume a positive attitude. For example, convey the impression that the patient intended to pay, and it is only a matter of working out some suitable arrangements.
- Keep the conversation brief and to the point; do not make threats of any kind.
- Try to get a definite commitment – payment of a certain amount by a certain date.
- Follow up on promises made by the patient. This is best accomplished by using a tickler file or a note on the calendar. If the payment does not arrive by the promised date, remind the patient with another call. If the medical assistant fails to do this, the whole effort has been wasted.
- Document the call in the patient's record.

What *not* to do:
- Do not call between 9 p.m. and 8 a.m. To do so may be considered harassment.
- Do not make repeated telephone calls on the same day.
- Do not call the patient's place of work if the employer prohibits personal calls.
- If a call is placed to the patient at work and the person cannot take the call, leave a message asking the patient to "call Ms. Black at 951-727-9238" without revealing the nature of the call; that is, do not state that the call is from "Dr. Walden's office" or "Dr. Walden's medical assistant."
- Refrain from showing any kind of hostility. An angry patient is a poorly paying patient. Insulted patients often do not pay at all.

> **VOCABULARY**
> **tickler file:** A chronologic file used as a reminder that something must be dealt with on a certain date.

Collection Letters. Some experts believe that a printed collection letter or reminder enclosed with a statement is more effective than a personal letter. The idea is that a patient may be embarrassed by a personal letter and feel that he or she has been singled out for attention. An impersonal printed message will probably encourage the patient to send a payment.

Letters that are friendly requests for an explanation of why payment has not been made are effective in most cases. These letters should indicate that the provider is sincerely interested in the patient's health and well-being and wants to help resolve the financial obligation. Invite the patient to the office to explain the reasons for nonpayment so that payment arrangements can be made. To lessen the patient's embarrassment, these letters can suggest that previous statements may have been overlooked.

When receiving these letters, most patients make some effort to explain their failure to make payment. If a patient really is having financial difficulties, he or she may be able to get some type of assistance. If it is a temporary financial problem, the provider and the patient may work together to come up with a satisfactory installment plan for payment.

The medical assistant is often given a free hand in designing collection patterns and composing collection letters. Many medical assistants compose a series of collection letters using example letters they have found effective. Such a series usually includes at least five letters in varying degrees of forcefulness.

Sometimes even a person with poor paying habits will pay, as long as he or she is treated with respect and consideration. The medical assistant should never go beyond the authority granted by the provider in pursuing collections. If questions come up about special collection problems, always check with the provider or office manager before proceeding. The provider and the medical assistant should agree on general collection policies, as outlined earlier in this chapter, and the policies should be followed. In all cases when an account is to be assigned to a collection agency, make sure the provider is aware and approves.

In most healthcare facilities, the medical assistant signs collection letters using his or her title, such as "Medical Assistant" below the typewritten signature. Do not list "Collections" below the name, because the patient may assume that the account has been placed with a collection agency. Some providers want to sign these communications personally, but generally the medical assistant who handles the patient accounts also signs the collection letters.

Personal Finance Interviews. Personal finance interviews with patients can sometimes be more effective than a whole series of collection letters. Often times speaking with a patient face-to-face can result in a better understanding of the problem, and an agreement about future payment plans can be reached (Fig. 27.9).

Occasionally a patient may undergo a long course of treatment and yet make no attempt to pay anything on the account. The patient may be waiting for the provider or the medical assistant to suggest that a payment be made. When it is known in advance that the patient requires extensive treatment, the matter of payment should be discussed early in the course of treatment. The credit policy should be explained, and some agreement should be reached on a payment plan.

Because medical services are far more intangible than any commercial service, collection efforts must not be delayed too long. Most responsible, sincere patients will call the provider's office after receiving a second statement and explain the delay in payment or ask for a payment plan. This is best accomplished in a private, personal interview.

If the account ultimately must be referred to a collection agency, find a good agency with a high recovery rate. All collection activity is costly. Know when to stop and call on the services of a professional agency.

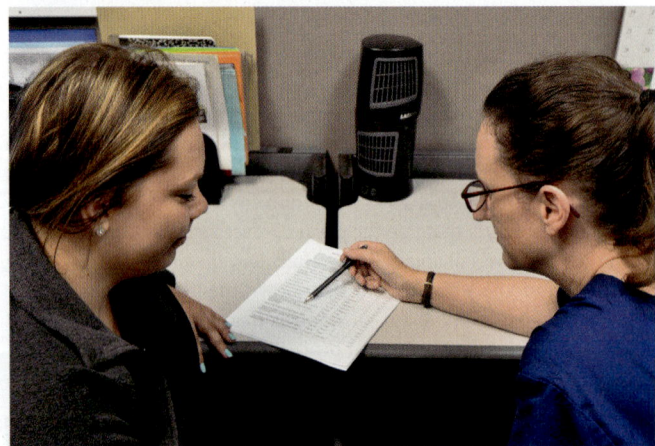

FIG. 27.9 A face-to-face personal finance interview may motivate patients to take steps to settle their account balances. (From Proctor D, Niedzwiecki B: *Kinn's The Medical Assistant,* ed 13, St Louis, 2017, Elsevier.)

BOX 27.9 Suggestions for Tracing Skips

- Review the patient's original office registration card.
- Call the telephone number listed in the patient account record. Occasionally a patient may move without leaving a forwarding address but will transfer the old telephone number.
- If you are unable to contact the individual by telephone, make a few discreet calls to the references listed on the registration card to get leads.
- Check the internet to find the names and telephone numbers of neighbors or the landlord and contact these people to obtain information about the debtor's whereabouts.
- Do not inform a third party that the patient owes money. Simply state that you are trying to locate or verify the location of the individual.
- Check the guarantor's place of employment for information. If the person is a specialist in his or her field of work, the local union or similar organizations may be contacted. Although they may not give you the person's current address, they will relay the message that you are seeking to contact the person. Often people are prompted to pay if they think their employer may learn of their failure to pay.

Special Collection Situations

Tracing "skips." When a patient account statement is returned marked "Moved—no forwarding address," you may consider this account a skip. This could be an innocent error on the part of the patient, who may have forgotten to provide a forwarding address to the post office. The patient could also be attempting to avoid liability for debts. Whichever is the case, immediate action should be taken. Do not wait until the next billing cycle to attempt to trace the debtor.

The internet can be a valuable tool in tracing skips. You can use the online white pages to search for the patient's name. Patients might even be found on social networking sites, such as Facebook, and that information may provide clues about the person's whereabouts. Investigate the search results carefully so that collection efforts are directed at the right person. If all attempts fail, turn the account over to a collection agency without delay. Do not keep a skip account too long because as time passes, the trail may become so cold that even collection experts won't be able to follow it. Box 27.9 presents tips for tracing skips.

Claims against estates. The patient account for a deceased patient may be handled a little differently from regular accounts. Courtesy dictates that a bill not be sent immediately, but do not delay longer than 30 days. The executor will expect to receive the statements from all healthcare providers. Use the following format to address the statement:

- Estate of (name of patient)
- c/o (spouse, next of kin, or executor if known)
- Patient's last known address

A will generally is filed within 30 days of a death. The name of the executor usually can be obtained by sending a request to the Probate Department of the Superior Court, County Recorder's Office, in the county where the person lived. The time limits for filing an estate claim are determined by the state where the person resided.

An itemized statement should be sent to the executor of the estate by certified mail, return receipt requested. If no response is received in 10 days, contact the executor or the county clerk where the estate is being settled and obtain forms for filing a claim against the estate. This claim against the estate must be made within a certain time. This time frame varies from 2 to 36 months, depending on the state where it is filed.

The executor of the estate either accepts or rejects the claim. If it is accepted, the executor will send an acknowledgment of the debt. Payment can be delayed because of the legal complications involved in settling an estate. If the claim has been accepted, the provider eventually receives the payment. If the executor rejects the claim, file a claim against the executor according to state laws. The time limit in such cases starts with the date on the letter of rejection.

States have different time limits and statutes with regard to these issues. The medical assistant should contact the provider's attorney or the local court for the exact procedure to follow. Or, the provider may prefer to turn such matters over to his or her legal counsel immediately.

Bankruptcy. Bankruptcy laws were passed to ensure equal distribution of the assets of an individual among the individual's creditors. These are federal laws that apply in all the states. When notified that a patient has declared bankruptcy, do not send statements or make any attempt to collect on the account from the patient.

Chapter 7 bankruptcy is usually a "no asset" situation. Because the provider's charges are considered an unsecured debt, there is little purpose in pursuing collection. Chapter 13 is known as *wage-earner bankruptcy*, which means that the patient-debtor pays to a trustee a fixed amount agreed upon by the court. This money is passed on to the creditors. During this period, none of the creditors can attach the debtor's wages or otherwise attempt to collect the debt. However, the debts are paid in order, secured debts first. Consequently, the provider may never receive payment from a debtor who has filed bankruptcy.

Using a Collection Agency.
The medical assistant should try every means possible to collect on accounts before they become delinquent. An account should be sent to a collection agency as soon all collection activities have been exhausted. If the patient has failed to respond to the final letter or has twice failed to send a promised payment, the account should be considered uncollectable. Skips should be sent immediately.

Even though the collection agency will keep 40% to 60% of the amount owed, waiting only reduces the chances of recovery by the professional collector. If the agency finds that the case deserves special consideration, it will ask the provider's advice before proceeding further.

The collection agency represents the healthcare facility. Therefore, the healthcare facility should ensure that its patients are treated with as much respect and dignity as possible throughout the collection process. There are many different collection agencies. If one doesn't work out, prepare to switch to another that can better represent the healthcare practice.

VOCABULARY

assets: All property available for the payment of debts.
executor: An individual assigned to make financial decisions about the estate of a deceased patient.
intangible: Something of value that cannot be touched physically.
unsecured debt: Debt that is not guaranteed by something of value; credit card debt is the most common type of unsecured debt.
trustee: The coordinator of financial resources assigned by the court during a bankruptcy case.

A collection agency needs certain data to begin collection procedures on overdue accounts:
- Guarantor's full name
- Spouse's full name
- Last known address
- Full amount of the debt
- Date of the last entry (charge, payment, or adjustment) on account
- Occupation of the debtor
- Employer's address and phone number

After an account has been sent to a collection agency, the healthcare facility can make no further collection attempts. Once the agency has begun its work, a number of guidelines and procedures should be followed:
- Send no more patient statements.
- The patient account should be closed for activity because the account was forwarded to a collection agency. The balance should be written off.
- Refer the patient to the collection agency if he or she contacts the office about the account.
- Promptly report any payments made directly to your office to the collection agency and pay the collection agency's fee.
- Call the agency if any information is obtained that will be of value in tracing or collecting the account.

Posting collection agency transactions. Collection agencies charge the healthcare practice different percentages of the amount owed to collect delinquent accounts; the agency with the cheapest fee is rarely the most effective. Agencies pay the *net back*, which is the amount of money paid to the practice after the agency has been paid its fee. The net back is the figure that should be considered when a collection agency is used, not simply the fee percentage. If a patient sends a payment after the account has been turned over to a collection agency, the payment must be recorded in the patient account record. Because the agency charges a fee for its collection efforts, the amount sent to the healthcare facility might be less than the actual payment amount. For instance, if the agency charges 25%, a $100 payment results in a $75 payment to the healthcare facility and the agency keeps $25. When the payment is posted, the patient account must credit the full amount paid to the collection agency. This would be done by posting a $75 payment and $25 adjustment (Fig. 27.10 and Procedure 27.2).

CRITICAL THINKING BOX 27.5

Laura has had several complaints about the collection agency used by the office. Patients have called to report that the collectors are threatening and unprofessional. The collection agency's supervisor has been disrespectful to patients and has said that because they owe the money, the collection agency's job is to collect the account in whatever way necessary. How should the healthcare facility approach the collection agency about these complaints?

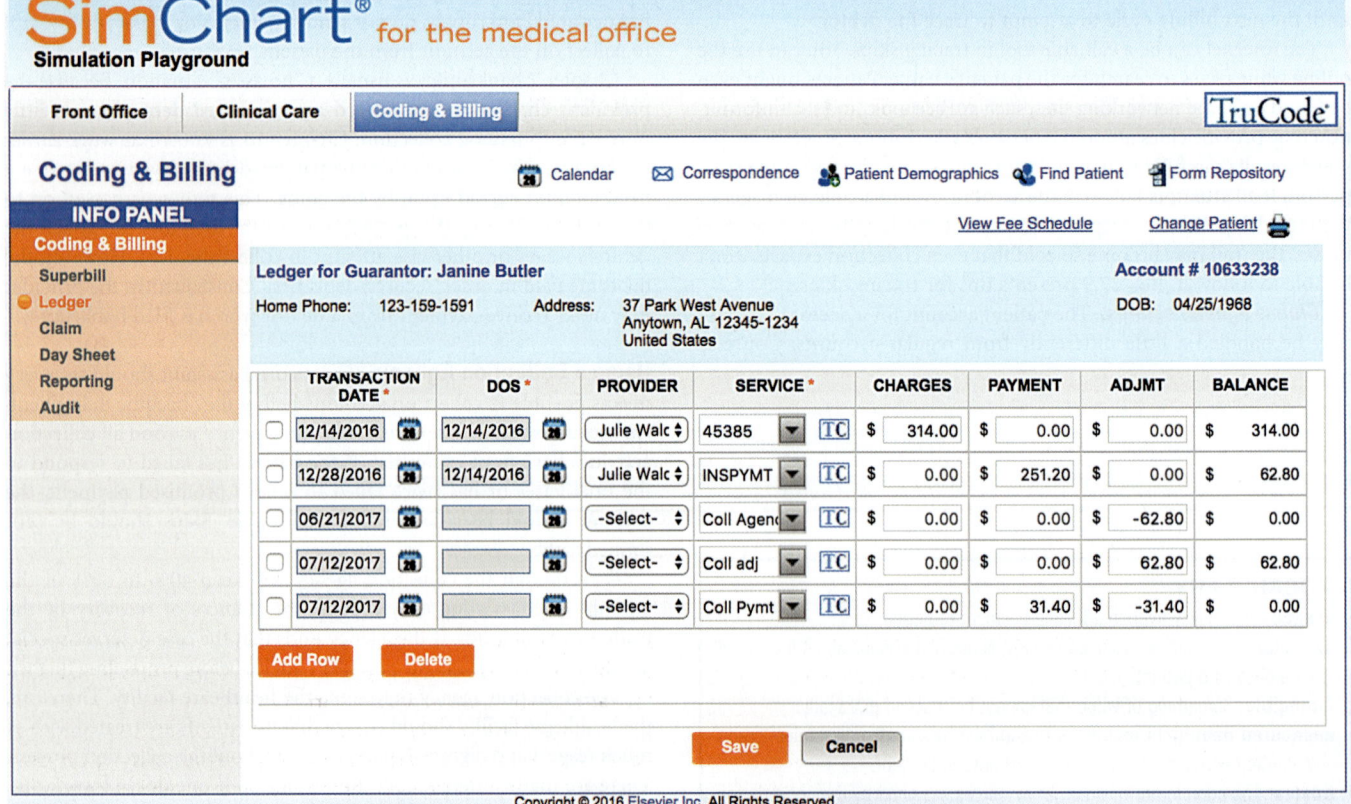

FIG. 27.10 Posting a collection agency payment in SimChart for the Medical Office.

CHAPTER 27 Accounts, Collections, and Banking

PROCEDURE 27.2 Post Payments and Adjustments to a Patient's Account

Task:
To post payments and adjustments to patient accounts accurately.

Scenario
Monique Jones (06/23/1985) was seen 6 months ago for a wellness visit and lab work. Her insurance had lapsed, and she is completely responsible for the bill. She did not make any payments and resisted all attempts at collection of the balance of $172.00. Her account was turned over to a collection agency, which was able to collect the balance in full. The collection agency retains 50% of what it collects as payment. Post the collection agency payment and adjustment to Ms. Jones' account.

Equipment and Supplies
- Patient account ledger card, or SimChart for the Medical Office software

Procedural Steps
1. Look up the ledger card for the patient account (or the patient ledger in SimChart). Confirm that you have the correct patient account.
   Purpose: All transactions need to be posted to the correct account.
2. Post an adjustment to reverse the adjustment done when the account was turned over to the collection agency.
   Purpose: The account should show a zero balance. If the reverse adjustment is not done, the account will have a credit balance.
3. Post the payment and adjustment that reflects the actual dollar amount received from the collection agency and the amount that was retained as payment as seen in the following figure.
   Purpose: Both the payment amount and adjustment must be posted, to give the patient credit for the full payment that was sent to the collection agency.

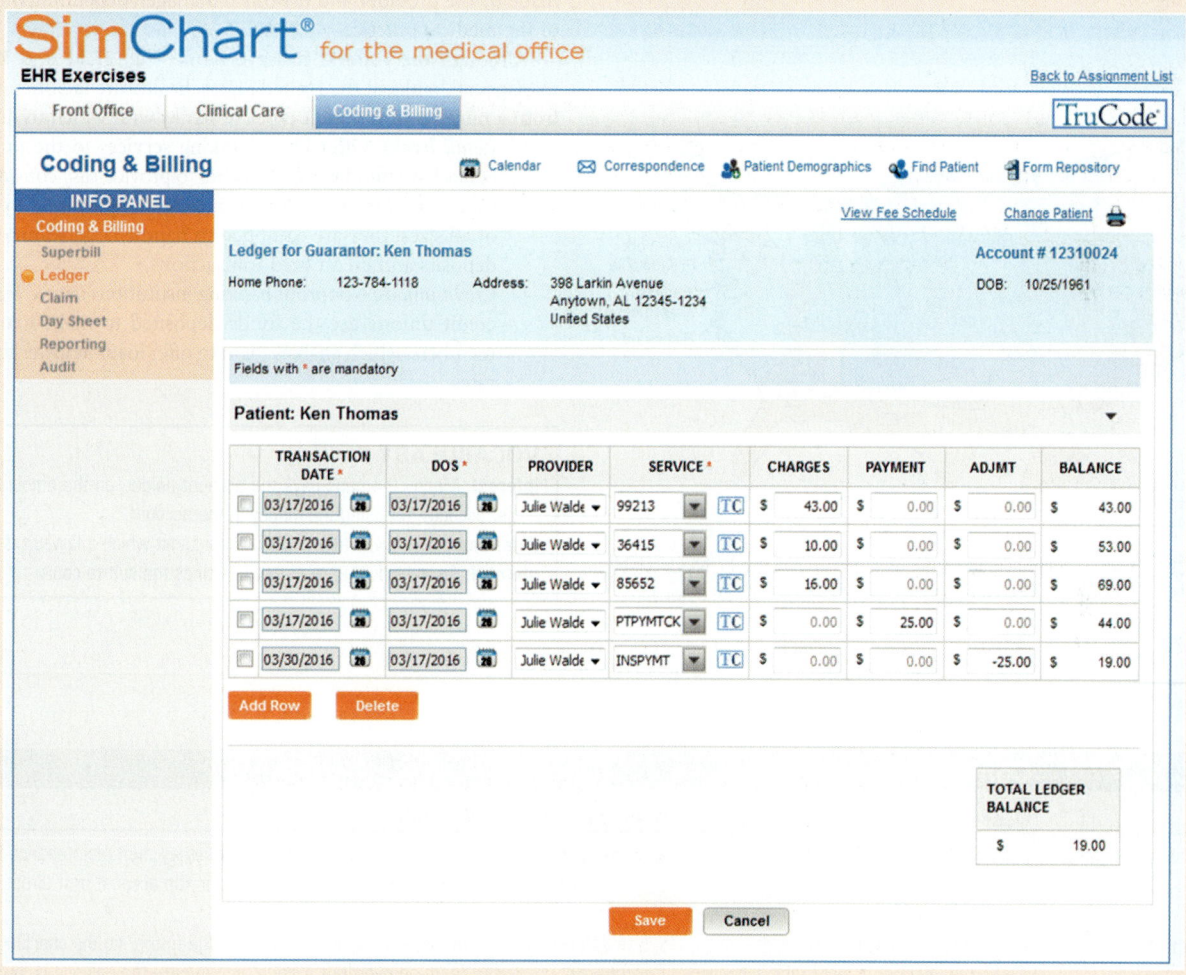
1

Small Claims Court. Many healthcare practices find small claims court a satisfactory, inexpensive means of collecting delinquent accounts. State law places a limit on the amount of debt for which relief may be sought in small claims court. This limit should be determined before the small claims court process is started.

Parties to small claims actions are not represented by an attorney at the hearing but may send another person to court on their behalf to produce records supporting the claim. Providers often send their medical assistant with records of unpaid accounts to show the judge.

> **VOCABULARY**
> **small claims court:** A special court established to handle small claims or debts without the services of lawyers.

If the court awards a judgment for the amount owed, the **plaintiff** in small claims court may also recover the costs of the suit. For a very small investment in time and money, the provider who uses this method saves the time of a civil court action and eliminates attorneys' fees.

After being awarded a judgment, the healthcare practice must still collect the money. The only person in a small claims action who has the right of appeal is the **defendant**. An appeal by the defendant may have the judgment set aside. The plaintiff cannot file an appeal in a small claims action; the decision of the court is final.

The necessary papers for filing action and full instructions on the course to follow may be obtained from the clerk of the local small claims court. It would be wise for a medical assistant who has never appeared in court to attend once as a spectator to preview the procedure; this should allow him or her to feel more at ease when appearing for the provider.

ACCOUNTS PAYABLE (A/P)

Managing accounts payable may be the responsibility of the medical assistant. There are many aspects of accounts payable, which will be discussed in the next section.

Banking in Today's Business World

Banks can be used to centralize all financial transactions for a healthcare facility. The bank account tracks all deposits, withdrawals, and transfers. Monthly bank account balances can help healthcare facilities establish and maintain a monthly operational budget. Banks also provide opportunities to earn **interest** and to invest for future financial gain. Overall, banks organize funds for the financial management of the healthcare facility.

Fees for banking services depend on the bank and products used (Table 27.1). The type of bank the medical practice will use is a decision made by the provider and the office manager, depending on the needs of the medical practice.

Although the **Federal Reserve Bank** (Fig. 27.11 and Box 27.10) manages all banks in the United States, healthcare facilities can choose from a number of different types of banks with which to do business.

- *Retail banks:* Offer basic banking services to the public; these banks have hundreds of branches to provide easy consumer access.
- *Commercial banks:* Offer business banking services to businesses of all sizes; they are equipped to handle large volumes of check deposits and credit card transactions.
- *Credit unions:* Nonprofit banking institutions owned by members; credit unions use the funds deposited to make loans to their members, which enables them to offer loans at lower than market rates.

> **VOCABULARY**
> **interest:** Money the bank pays the account holder, on the amount in his or her account, for using the money in the account.
> **defendant:** An individual or a business against which a lawsuit is filed.
> **plaintiff:** An individual or a party who brings the suit to court.

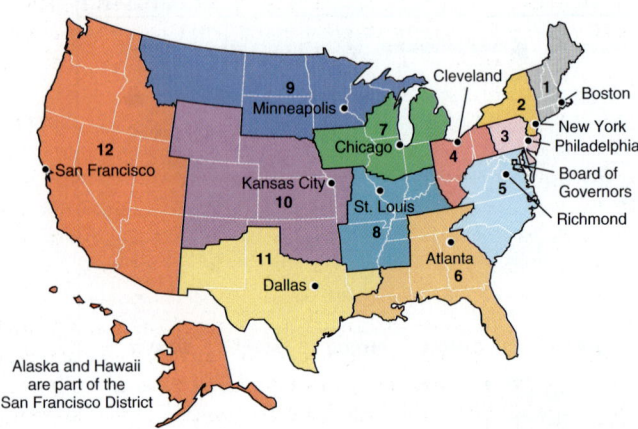

FIG. 27.11 The 12 Federal Reserve districts. (From Proctor D, Niedzwiecki B: *Kinn's The Medical Assistant*, ed 13, St Louis, 2017, Elsevier.)

TABLE 27.1 Common Banking Fees

Fee	Description	Average Fee	Waivable?
Account maintenance fee	Fee for using the bank account	$5 to $25 per month	Some bank accounts waive monthly account maintenance fees if a specific balance is maintained in the account or if direct deposit is used.
Overdraft fee	Fee for the bank paying a check or debit when the balance is not in the account	$25 to $40 per occurrence	Not usually. To avoid the fee in the future, tie the checking account with an overdraft account just in case the balance is low.
Returned deposit fee	Fee charged when a deposited check is returned from the drawer's account	$5 to $10 per occurrence	Not usually. However, the practice can require the check drawer to cover this expense because the check did not clear his or her account.
Hard copy statement fee	Fee for the bank to send paper copies of bank statements	$5 to $10 per statement	This fee can be avoided by downloading all electronic bank statements when they are released.
Nonsufficient funds (NSF) fee	Fee charged when a check is written against an account with not enough funds and the check is returned unpaid	$25 to $40 per occurrence	Not usually. To avoid the fee in the future, tie the checking account with an overdraft account just in case the balance is low.
Transaction fee	Fee charged when too many transactions are made on a bank account	$.50 to $1.00 per transaction	Online banking is usually free, but nowadays banks are charging fees to visit bank branches and to complete transactions with customer service over the phone.

CHAPTER 27   Accounts, Collections, and Banking

> **BOX 27.10 The Federal Reserve**
>
> In 1913 Congress created the Federal Reserve Banking System. This was to provide the nation with a safer, more flexible, and stable monetary and financial system. The system consists of:
> - a seven-member Board of Governors with headquarters in Washington, D.C.
> - 12 Federal Reserve banks in major cities throughout the country (see Fig. 27.11)
>
> The Federal Reserve Bank monitors the movement of money, in the form of checks, from one bank account to another. Each check has:
> - a routing number
> - an account number
>
> These numbers identify which Federal Reserve Bank jurisdiction, bank location, and specific bank accounts are used in each transaction.
>
> For additional information on the Federal Reserve System and its regional banks, visit the system's website: https://www.federalreserve.gov.

- *Online banks:* Offer basic banking services at competitive rates because all banking transactions are done online; there are no branch locations to visit.

The medical assistant will most likely manage only the bank accounts set up for the income and operational expenses of the healthcare facility.

Because of their large volume of bookkeeping transactions, many healthcare facilities use accounting management software. Most online banking systems allow for the download of bank account data. These software systems can be complicated to use, so the medical assistant should be in regular contact with the accountant chosen by the provider, who can answer questions when needed.

Common Types of Bank Accounts

Checking accounts. By placing an amount of money in a bank, a depositor can set up a checking account. Simply stated, a checking account is a bank account against which checks can be written, or debit cards used, and funds can be transferred to the payable party. Banks typically charge a monthly account maintenance fee. In addition, there may be fees associated with banking services, such as transferring funds to other banks or using the checking overdraft (see Table 27.1).

Savings accounts. Money that is not needed for current expenses can be deposited into a savings account. In most cases, savings accounts earn a higher interest rate than checking accounts. Interest rates fluctuate with the financial market.

A standard savings account earns interest at the lowest prevailing rate and has no minimum balance requirement and no check-writing privileges. However, penalties apply for withdrawing funds from a savings account more than four times per month. The provider may deposit a certain percentage of **discretionary income** into a savings account each month to earn interest. The money in a savings account can be transferred to a checking account when needed.

Money market savings account. An insured money market savings account combines features of a checking and savings account. A minimum balance is required (anywhere from $500 to $5,000). It earns interest at money market rates (usually a higher percentage rate than for a regular savings account), and it allows only a specified number of checks (frequently three) to be written per month. Such checks are usually written to transfer funds to a checking account. Some businesses transfer excess funds from the business checking account to a money market account over the weekend, or over an extended holiday period to earn higher interest on the funds.

Signature Cards. When an account is opened at a bank branch, the account signer is required to provide his or her handwritten signature on a physical or electronic card, which is kept on file with the bank. If a check comes through and some suspicion arises that the depositor's signature has been forged, bank personnel compare the signature on the check with the original on the signature card.

The task of paying bills is often delegated to a responsible medical assistant. In this case, any staff member who has been authorized to sign the medical facility's checks must go to the bank and add his or her handwritten signature to the signature card. Only those whose names appear on the signature card are authorized to sign checks, and the bank is responsible for verifying any questionable signatures.

Online Banking. Internet banking has changed the way financial institutions manage money. People once had to fight traffic and wait in line at crowded banks; now, they can bank from their offices any time of day. A healthcare facility's banking transactions, such as paying bills and transferring funds between accounts, can be done online. In addition, staff members have access to supply companies online and can easily review costs from the office instead of driving to numerous companies to compare prices.

Online banking is a means of performing banking services electronically via the internet. All banks and credit unions have this capability, and most of them offer both basic and advanced services. With basic services, a customer usually can do the following:
- Check account balances
- Transfer funds between accounts in the same bank
- Pay bills electronically and create checks
- Determine whether a check has cleared the bank
- Download account information
- View images of transactions

More advanced services include being able to deposit checks online.

A major concern with online banking is fraud. Concern that unauthorized users may gain access to the healthcare facility's account balances are valid. Some experts believe that online banking involves a slightly greater risk of fraud than does conventional banking. Despite the disadvantages, studies show that internet banking is now mainstream.

Checks

A *check* is a bank draft, or an order to pay a certain sum of money, on demand, to a specified person or entity. When a check is presented for payment, the *drawee* (the bank on which the check is drawn or written) pays the specified sum of money written on the face of the check to the *holder* (the person presenting the check for payment).

> **VOCABULARY**
>
> **discretionary income:** Money in a bank account that is not assigned to pay for any office expenses.
>
> **Federal Reserve Bank:** The central bank of the United States. The Federal Reserve system consists of a seven-member Board of Governors with headquarters in Washington, D.C., and 12 Federal Reserve banks in major cities throughout the country.

A check is considered a **negotiable** (ni GOH shee uh buh l) **instrument**. For a check to be negotiable, it must:
- Be written and signed by the *drawer* (the person who writes the check)
- Contain a promise or order to pay a sum of money
- Be payable on demand or at a fixed future date

To ensure that the amount is taken from the correct account number, the routing and account numbers are printed with magnetic ink on the bottom of the check. The check should have the amount written as a number and as text to confirm the amount. Finally, the check must be signed and dated by the drawer of the account.

Routing and Account Numbers. A *routing transit number* (RTN) is a nine-digit code printed on the bottom left side of checks. A RTN is assigned to every banking institution under the Federal Reserve Banking System. It identifies the bank upon which the check was drawn. RTNs are also used for direct deposits and the transfer of funds between banks. The first two digits indicate the Federal Reserve district where the bank is located. The third digit indicates the specific district office. And the rest of the digits represent the individual accounts that belong to the bank.

Bank account numbers are assigned to each individual account. No two account numbers in the same financial institution can be the same. *Wire transfers* and *automated clearinghouse (ACH) transfers* use the routing and account numbers to transfer funds between exact accounts. Wire transfers are between two separate banking institutions in which both accounts are verified, so funds are available quickly. ACH transfers also involve two different banking institutions, but because both accounts are not verified, a few extra days are needed for funds to be available.

Types of Negotiable Instruments. The following are different types of negotiable instruments:
- Personal check
- Cashier's check
- Money order
- Business check
- Voucher check

Personal check. A personal check is drawn by a bank against funds deposited to a personal account in another bank. Patients typically write these checks for copayments and other financial responsibilities.

Cashier's check. A cashier's check is a bank's own check, drawn on itself and signed by the bank cashier or other authorized official. A cashier's check is obtained by paying the bank the amount of the check, in cash. Many banks charge a fee for this service. Cashier's checks often are issued for a savings account customer who does not have a checking account.

Money order. Money orders can be purchased at banks, some retail stores, and the U.S. Postal Service. Money orders are often used to pay bills by mail when a person does not have a checking account. The maximum face value varies, depending on the source. Cashier checks are preferable to money orders when larger amounts need to be paid.

Business checks. The checkbook most widely used in the professional office is a ledger-type book with three checks per page and a perforated stub at the left side of the check. The stubs serve as the checking account register, where the balance of the account is tracked. The checks and matching stubs are numbered in sequence and preprinted with the depositor's name and account number, along with any additional information, such as address and telephone number. Business checks can also be printed through accounting management software programs when vendors submit invoices. Today, most business checks can be prepared through online banking.

Voucher check. A voucher check has a detachable voucher form or could be attached to an EOB. The voucher portion is used to itemize or specify the purpose for which the check was drawn. The voucher portion of the check is removed before the check is presented for deposit. The voucher is then used to post the payment in the patient account ledger (Fig. 27.12).

How Checks Are Processed From One Bank to Another. Checks received by the drawee's bank are turned over daily to a regional banking clearinghouse, which clears each one. The identifying code numbers, printed on the face of the check with magnetic ink, enable this "clearing" process to be accomplished quickly and efficiently. Checks due from and to all banks outside a specific region are settled by electronic entries. The bank keeps the canceled checks, and an electronic copy of the check is returned to the *drawer,* or the writer of the check. When the drawer needs proof of payment, a copy of the check can be requested from the bank, or the drawer can review monthly bank statements for printed copies of cleared checks. Check copies can also be obtained online through the banking portal.

Electronic checks. In an effort to prevent check fraud, many healthcare facilities accept only electronic checks. When the patient presents a personal check to the healthcare facility, the bottom of the check, which includes the routing and account numbers, is scanned. The funds are then automatically transferred from the patient's checking account and into the healthcare facility's account. Once the transaction has been approved, the paper check is returned to the patient with "VOID" printed across it to show that it has already been used. Electronic checks reduce the time involved in transferring funds from one account to another.

Patient Payment Management

Cash Payments. Some patients may prefer to pay in cash instead of by check or debit or credit card. Cash transactions can occur with little or no paperwork; therefore, an audit trail is harder to establish.

To prevent the mismanagement of cash, many healthcare facilities do not allow patients to pay cash for services. Healthcare facilities that have a no-cash payment policy should post a sign in the lobby to inform patients of this in advance. If a patient does not have a bank account, the medical staff can kindly refer the patient to a local money order dealer. Patients may see this as an inconvenience, but the medical assistant should explain that the policy is intended to protect the patient's account.

If the healthcare facility chooses to accept cash payments, keep in mind the following precautions:
- Make sure the cash is not **counterfeit** (KOUN ter fit); use a marker or tool designed for this purpose to confirm its authenticity. If you suspect that the cash may be counterfeit, do not accept the payment and contact the local law enforcement office.
- Establish a checks-and-balance system in which the employee accepting cash must document cash payments on a register and in the patient's account to establish an audit trail.
- Inform patients that change cannot be made for larger bills.

VOCABULARY

counterfeit: An imitation intended to be passed off fraudulently or deceptively as genuine; forgery.

negotiable instrument: A document guaranteeing payment of a specific amount of money to the payer named on the document.

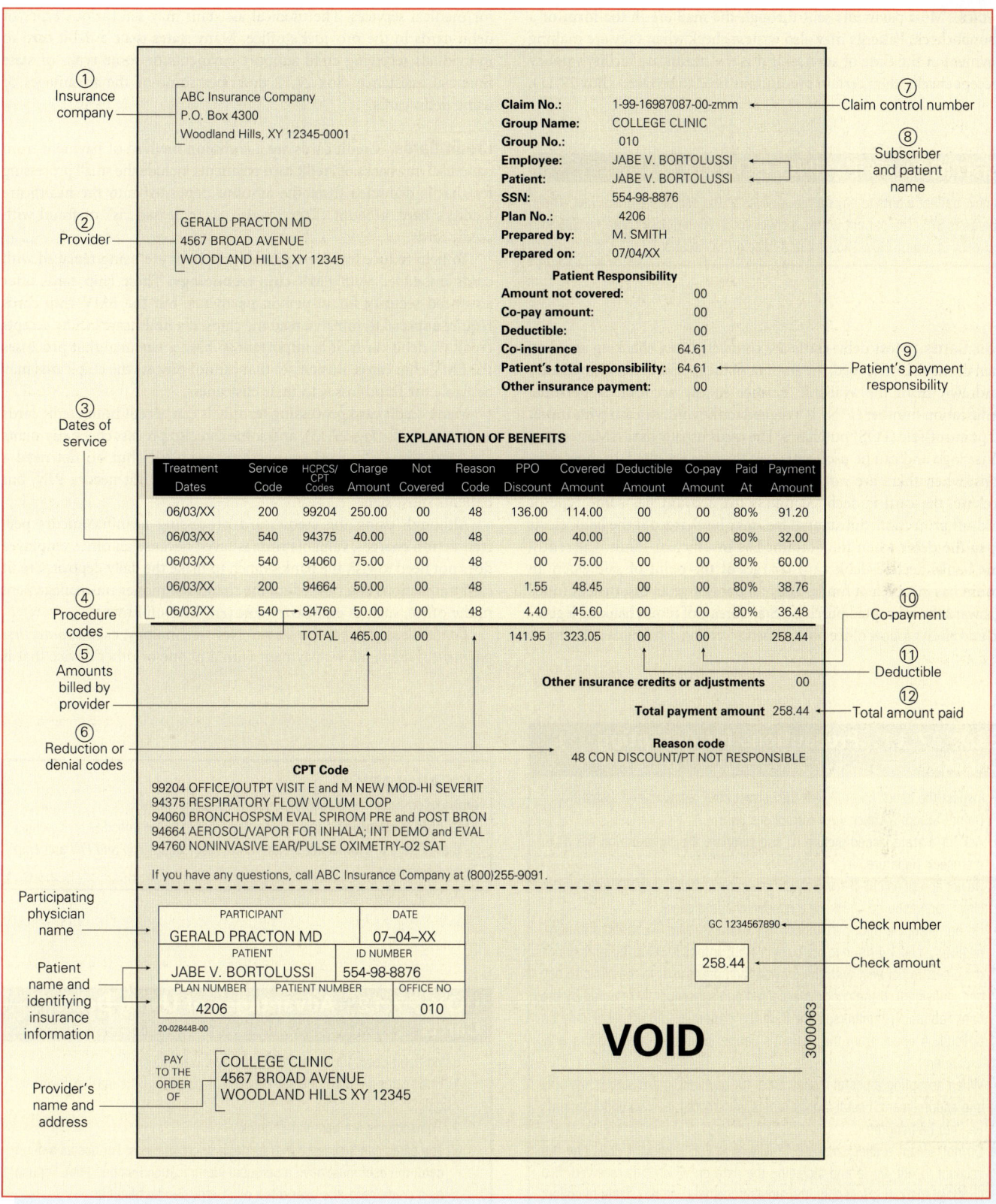

FIG. 27.12 Sample voucher check. (From Fordney MT: *Insurance Handbook For The Medical Office*, ed 14, St Louis, 2017, Elsevier.)

Checks. Most payments sent through the mail are in the form of a personal check. Patients may also write a check when they are making a payment at the time of service. If it is the healthcare facility's policy to accept checks, then certain precautions need to be taken (Box 27.11).

> ### CRITICAL THINKING BOX 27.6
> A new patient wants to pay for his services at the end of the office visit. The charge is $75. The patient writes a check for $100 and asks Laura for $25 in currency in return. How should Laura handle the situation?

Debit Cards. Most debit cards are connected to a checking account. When the debit card is used, the amount of the transaction is immediately withdrawn from the available balance in the account. A personal identification number (PIN) is assigned to the card for cash withdrawal and point-of-sale (POS) purchases. The cards usually have a MasterCard or Visa logo and can be used wherever they are accepted. In most situations, when there are not enough funds in the account to make a purchase, the card is declined unless the account has some type of overdraft protection. Substantial fees may be charged if the bank elects to pay the debit when the account has insufficient funds. Currently, some banks decline debit card charges at the point of sale when an account has insufficient funds. They do not charge an insufficient funds fee toward the attempted purchase. Stay abreast of recent banking legislation and always follow office policy when accepting debit cards as payment for medical services. The medical assistant may see various types of debit cards in the provider's office. Many states issue a debit card to individuals receiving child support payments or some types of state financial assistance. Box 27.12 describes some of the advantages of using debit cards.

Credit Cards. Credit cards are a common method of payment from patients. Drawbacks of credit card payments include the small processing fee that is deducted from the amount deposited into the healthcare facility's bank account. There is also an increased risk of fraud with credit cards.

To help reduce fraud, magnetic strip cards are being replaced with cards imbedded with **EMV chip technology**. These chip cards offer advanced security for in-person payments, but the EMV chip cards require a special terminal to read the chips. If a healthcare facility accepts credit or debit cards, it is important to have a terminal that processes the EMV chip cards. Businesses that cannot process the chip cards may be liable for fraud losses to their customers.

Many credit card processing terminals can accept both credit cards and debit cards (Fig. 27.13), and some can also process check payments electronically. Debit card transactions use a PIN but do not need a patient's signature. Credit card transactions do not need a PIN, but patients must sign.

Although using the credit card processing terminal incurs per-transaction charges, valuable time is saved because an office employee does not need to visit the bank branch to make the daily deposit. Credit card transactions also can reduce the chances of money mismanagement in the office, such as **embezzlement** (em BEZ uh l ment).

Contactless payment systems. New technology, called *contactless payment systems,* allows payment with a phone or other device that is

> ### BOX 27.11 Precautions for Accepting Checks
> - Inspect the check carefully for the correct date, amount, and signature.
> - Do not accept a check with corrections on it.
> - Ask for a state-issued picture ID and compare the signature on the ID to the check signature.
> - Do not accept an out-of-town check, government check, payroll check, starter check, unnumbered check, or a nonpersonalized check.
> - Do not accept a third-party check. For example, Mrs. Richards, a patient, receives a check written to her by her neighbor for $30. Mrs. Richards brings the check to her visit with the provider and presents it to the clinic to pay her copayment. If the check is accepted and subsequently returned by the bank, obtaining reimbursement from the patient or the neighbor may be difficult. A check from the patient's health insurance carrier is the only exception.
> - When accepting a postal money order for payment, make sure it has only one endorsement. Postal money orders with more than two endorsements will not be honored.
> - Do not accept a check marked "Payment in Full" unless it does pay the account in full, up to and including the date on which it is received. If a check so marked is less than the amount due, you will be unable to collect the balance on the account once you have accepted and deposited such a check. It is illegal to cross out the words "Payment in Full."
> - Do not accept a check written for more than the amount due; returning cash for the difference between the amount of the check and the amount owed is poor policy. If the check is not honored by the bank, your office suffers the loss not only of the amount of the check, but also of the amount returned in cash.

> ### VOCABULARY
> **embezzlement:** The misuse of funds for personal gain.
> **EMV chip technology:** Global technology that includes imbedded microchips that store and protect cardholder data; also called *chip and PIN* and *chip and signature*.

> ### BOX 27.12 Advantages of Using Debit Cards
> Using debit cards for payment has many advantages:
> 1. Debit cards are both safe and convenient, particularly for making payments online.
> 2. Transactions are completed quickly.
> 3. The cards can be used either as debit or credit cards. For use as a debit card, the user must have a personal identification number (PIN). For use as a credit card, the user often must provide identification.
> 4. If stolen or lost, the debit card can be cancelled quickly with minimum liability.
> 5. Receipts and statements provide a permanent, reliable record of disbursements for tax purposes.
> 6. The debit card statement provides a summary of receipts.
> 7. The cards usually can be used anywhere that accepts MasterCard or Visa.

CHAPTER 27 Accounts, Collections, and Banking

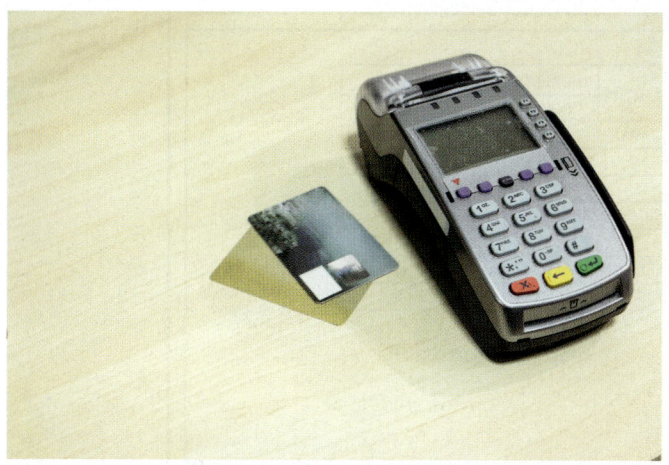

FIG. 27.13 Card reader terminal, both EMV chip and magnetic strip readers. (From mumemories/iStock/Thinkstock.)

> **BOX 27.13 Accounting Management Software**
>
> Accounting management software can simplify the banking transactions of healthcare facilities. This type of software is compatible with many online banking portals. That means that daily transactions can be downloaded directly into the accounting program. Attentive medical assistants who download daily can manage all account balances on a regular basis. Office expenses and invoices can be entered into the accounting management software as accounts payable, and payments can be scheduled for entered invoices. Checks to vendors can be printed at any time from the accounting software, documenting the transaction — and documented transactions make bank reconciliation a snap!

linked to a credit or debit card. If office policy allows this type of payment to be made, special equipment will be purchased to accommodate it.

Online payment options. Many offices choose to accept payment online. Patients can use their patient portal to make payments by debit or credit card, electronic check, or direct transfer. If your office uses this for payments, it should be noted in patients' bills, so they know they have this option for payments.

Precautions for Accepting Credit and Debit Cards. Just as the medical assistant must take precautions when accepting checks, care must be taken when accepting a credit or debit card as payment for medical services. Make sure that the person presenting the card is the person to whom it was issued. Always ask for a state-issued ID. Compare the name and signature to the one on the credit card. Follow the healthcare facility's policy on verifying identity if the name on the state-issued ID does not match the name on the credit card. Some patients may use a prepaid credit card, which is purchased with cash and does not have the patient's name printed on it, to make payments on their accounts. These cards, if allowed by office policy, pay just like a normal credit card. If a patient becomes belligerent when his or her credit card is denied, refer him or her to the office manager.

Banking Procedures in the Ambulatory Care Setting

Healthcare facilities use bank accounts to deposit funds (as cash, checks, debit card, or credit card transactions) and to pay their operational expenses by check or credit card (Box 27.13).

Making Bank Deposits. The medical assistant should make daily bank deposits, which minimizes the risks of keeping large sums of money on hand and also makes the money available for paying expenses. Depositing checks daily is important for these reasons:
- Checks may have a restricted time payment or may be lost, misplaced, or stolen over time.
- A stop-payment order may be placed on a check, or it may be returned for insufficient funds.
- Prompt processing is a courtesy to the payer.

Prompt check processing ensures that the money is available for the healthcare facility to use, or to be used to build interest.

Preparing the Deposit. The medical assistant must prepare a deposit slip (ticket) that accompanies the funds being deposited. The deposit slip, which can be paper or electronic, itemizes the cash or checks being deposited. It provides the information for the bank account into which the funds need to be deposited (Fig. 27.14). All details of the daily deposit should be recorded in the accounting software program; each check should be entered separately. The check number, payer, and check amount should also be recorded in the accounting software program so that the deposit amount from the software matches the bank deposit record. Many banks will not credit deposits made after 3 p.m. until the following business day (Procedure 27.3).

Another option for depositing checks is using a credit card terminal that electronically processes checks at the time of payment. Also, small healthcare facilities can snap a picture of the check and use the bank's app to do a mobile deposit. Facilities receiving a high volume of checks can use a mobile check scanner (Fig. 27.15). Checks are scanned individually and documented as a bank transaction on the monthly statement. Mobile deposits can save staff time and do not require a deposit slip because the software (app) is linked to the bank account being used. When mobile deposits are used, the daily deposit amount must match the exact daily deposit amount in the accounting management software.

Check Endorsements. An endorsement is a signature plus any other writing on the back of a check by which the endorser transfers all rights in the check to another party. Endorsements are made with either a pen or rubber ink stamp. The medical assistant needs to endorse the back of the check in the box indicated. Regardless of how checks are deposited, they all need to be endorsed.

Types of endorsements. Four principal kinds of endorsements can be used: blank, restrictive, special, and qualified (Table 27.2). Blank and restrictive endorsements (Fig. 27.16) are most commonly used.

Methods of endorsement. Any endorsement should exactly match the name on the Pay To line of the check. If the name of the payee is misspelled, the payee usually must endorse the check the way the name is spelled on the face, followed by the correctly spelled signature.

A stamp can be used to endorse checks from patients and other sources. As they arrive, these checks should be recorded in the ledger and immediately stamped with the restrictive endorsement "For Deposit

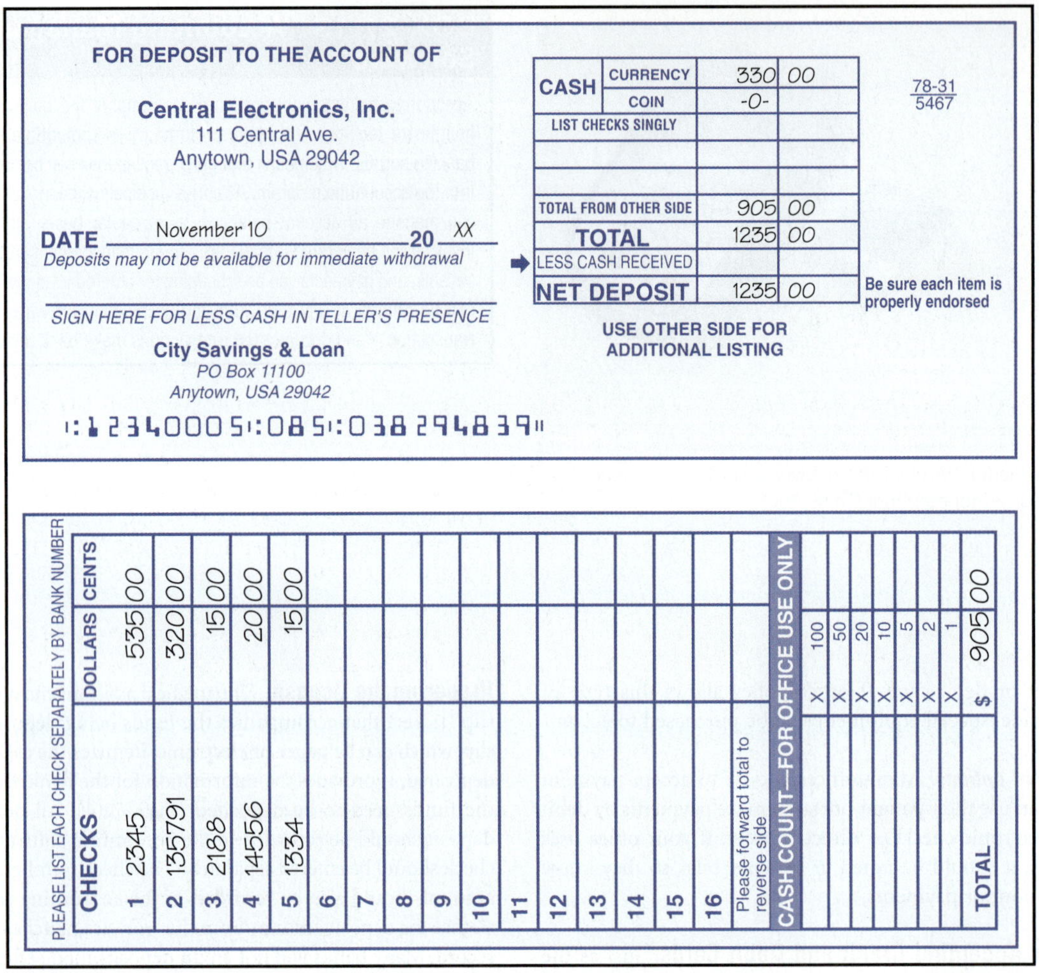

FOR DEPOSIT TO THE ACCOUNT OF

Central Electronics, Inc.
111 Central Ave.
Anytown, USA 29042

DATE November 10 20 XX
Deposits may not be available for immediate withdrawal

SIGN HERE FOR LESS CASH IN TELLER'S PRESENCE

City Savings & Loan
PO Box 11100
Anytown, USA 29042

⑆1234000 5⑆085⑆038 2948 39⑈

CASH	CURRENCY	330	00
	COIN	-0-	
LIST CHECKS SINGLY			
TOTAL FROM OTHER SIDE		905	00
TOTAL		1235	00
LESS CASH RECEIVED			
NET DEPOSIT		1235	00

78-31
5467

Be sure each item is properly endorsed

USE OTHER SIDE FOR ADDITIONAL LISTING

PLEASE LIST EACH CHECK SEPARATELY BY BANK NUMBER

	CHECKS	DOLLARS	CENTS
1	2345	535	00
2	135791	320	00
3	2188	15	00
4	14556	20	00
5	1334	15	00
6			
7			
8			
9			
10			
11			
12			
13			
14			
15			
16			
Please forward total to reverse side			
TOTAL	$	905	00

CASH COUNT—FOR OFFICE USE ONLY

X	100
X	50
X	20
X	10
X	5
X	2
X	1

FIG. 27.14 Front and back of a deposit slip. (From Proctor D, Niedzwiecki B: *Kinn's The Medical Assistant,* ed 13, St Louis, 2017, Elsevier.)

PROCEDURE 27.3 Prepare a Bank Deposit

Task:

To prepare a bank deposit for currency and checks.

Scenario

The following checks need to be deposited: #3456 for $89; #6954 for $136; #9854-10 for $1366.65; #8546 for $653.36; and #9865 for $890.22. The following currency and coins need to be deposited: (19) $20 bills; (10) $10 bills; (46) $5; (73) $1. The healthcare facility's name is Walden-Martin Family Medicine Clinic, account number 123-456-78910, and the bank is Clear Water Bank, Anytown, Anystate.

Equipment and Supplies

- Checks and currency for deposit (see Scenario)
- Check for endorsement
- Calculator
- Paper method: bank deposit slip
- Electronic method: SimChart for the Medical Office (SCMO)

Procedural Steps

1. Gather the documents to be used. For the electronic method, enter the Simulation Playground in SCMO. Click on the Form Repository icon. On the INFO PANEL, click on Office Forms and then select Bank Deposit Slip.
2. Enter the date on the deposit slip.
3. Using the calculator, calculate the amount of currency to be deposited. Enter the amount in the CURRENCY line, completing the dollar and cent boxes.
4. Enter the total amount in the TOTAL CASH line.
5. For each check to be deposited, enter the check number, the dollars, and cents. List each check on a separate line.
   Purpose: The bank requires that each check be listed separately; this also helps when verifying the checks before the deposit.
6. Calculate the total to be deposited and enter the number in the TOTAL FROM ATTACHED LIST box.
7. Enter the number of items deposited in the TOTAL ITEMS box.
8. Before completing the deposit slip, verify the check amounts listed and recalculate the totals. For the electronic method, click on SAVE.
   Purpose: It is crucial to verify the accuracy of check amounts and totals.
9. Place a restrictive endorsement on the check(s).
   Purpose: To prevent cashing of checks in case of loss or theft.

CHAPTER 27 Accounts, Collections, and Banking

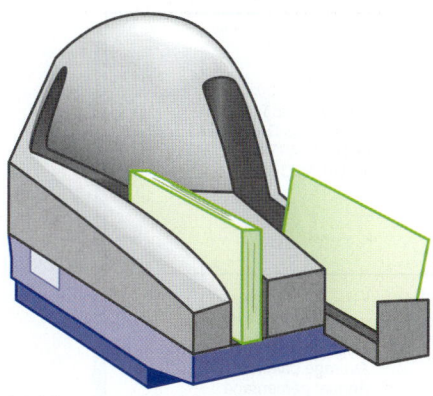

FIG. 27.15 Mobile check scanner. (From Proctor D, Niedzwiecki B: *Kinn's The Medical Assistant*, ed 13, St Louis, 2017, Elsevier.)

```
Pay to the Order of
Midwest National Bank
     Main Branch
   For Deposit Only
  ROBERT SPALDING
      301-012697
```

FIG. 27.16 Example of a restrictive endorsement. (From Proctor D, Niedzwiecki B: *Kinn's The Medical Assistant*, ed 13, St Louis, 2017, Elsevier.)

TABLE 27.2	Types of Endorsements
Type	**Description**
Blank endorsement	The payee signs only his or her name. This makes the check payable to the bearer. It is the simplest and most common type of endorsement on personal checks but should be used only when the check is to be cashed or deposited immediately.
Restrictive endorsement	Specifies the purpose of the endorsement (see Fig. 27.16). It is used in preparing checks for deposit to the provider's checking account.

Special endorsement	Includes words specifying the person to whom the endorser makes the check payable. For instance, a check written to Helen Barker as the payee may be endorsed to the provider by writing on the back of the check as follows:
	   Pay to the order of
	   Theodore F. Wilson, M.D.
	   Helen Barker
	The check is still negotiable but requires Dr. Wilson's signature or endorsement.

Qualified endorsement	The effect of the endorsement is qualified by disclaiming or destroying any future liability of the endorser. Usually the words "without recourse" are written above by an attorney who accepts a check on behalf of a client but who has no personal claim in the transaction.

Only." This is a safeguard that prevents the cashing of lost or stolen checks. Most banks accept routine stamp endorsements that are restricted to For Deposit Only if the customer is well known and maintains an established account.

A signature can also be used as an endorsement. Some insurance checks or drafts require a personal signature endorsement; a stamped endorsement is not acceptable. This is stated on the back of the check. In such cases ask the payee to endorse the check, then stamp immediately below the signature the restrictive endorsement For Deposit Only.

Overdraft. When a depositor writes a check for more than the amount available in the account, the account is overdrawn. Issuing a check for more than the amount on deposit in the bank is illegal. Such a check is said to "bounce." Should this happen through error or oversight and a check is written by an established depositor, the bank may honor the check and notify the depositor that the account is overdrawn. If the bank pays or covers the check, it issues an overdraft on the depositor's account. Considerable fees ($10 to $35) normally are charged for an overdraft. If the bank does not cover the amount of the check, it will be returned as NSF.

Stop-Payments. A depositor or check writer who wants to take back the check has the right to request that the bank stop payment on it. Stop-payment orders should be used only when absolutely necessary; as with overdrafts, most banks charge a fee for this service. Reasons for stop-payment requests include:
- Loss of a check
- Disagreement about a purchase
- Disagreement about a payment

Bank Statements and Reconciliation

The bank creates a statement at the end of each month. The medical assistant can download the bank statement directly into the accounting management software, which has a *reconciliation* (rek uh n sill ee EY shuh n) feature. The purpose of reconciliation is to start with the beginning balance, add all deposits, and subtract all checks and other debit transactions. This will then leave the ending statement balance. The ending balance should match the ending balance on the bank statement. If it does, the account has been reconciled. Bank statement reconciliation is used as an audit, or to ensure that the bank is managing the funds in the account accurately. It can also help to locate any errors made in the checking account register. Any errors on the bank statement should be immediately reported to the bank. Bank statements typically contain the following elements (Figs. 27.17 and 27.18):
- Beginning balance
- Deposits made
- Checks paid (including images of all cleared checks)
- Transfer transactions
- Online payment transactions
- Bank charges
- Ending balance

> **VOCABULARY**
> **reconciliation:** To bring into agreement.

What to Do When the Balances Do Not Match. When there are a large number of transactions from check deposits and bill payment activities, it can be challenging to match the closing balance of the bank statement with the closing balance indicated in the accounting management software. Keeping accurate records of deposits and bill payment

```
0621-402054
                                    #821
        ||I||ɪɪ|ɪI|ɪ|ɪ|ɪɪ|ɪ||ɪɪɪ||ɪɪ||I||ɪ|ɪɪ|ɪɪɪɪ|ɪɪI|ɪɪI    N    Call (888) 555-2932
                                                            2    24 HOURS/DAY, 7 DAYS/WEEK
                                                                 FOR ASSISTANCE WITH
                                                                 YOUR ACCOUNT.

Page 1 of 2      This statement covers: 6/22/02 through 7/22/02
```

Interest Checking 0621-402054	Summary			
	Previous balance	252.10	Minimum balance	142.55
	Deposits	68.74 +	Average balance	220.00
	Interest earned	.18 +	Annual percentage	
	Withdrawals	109.55 −	yield earned	.95%
	Customer service calls	.00 −		
	Interlink/purchase fee	.00 −	Interest earned	2.23
	Monthly checking fee and other charges	.00 −		
	▶ New balance	211.47		

Use your express card to make unlimited purchases at retailers displaying the interlink symbol (a $1 monthly fee may apply.)
Try it today at Arco…Mobil…Lucky…Ralphs…Safeway and more!

Checks and withdrawals	Check	Date paid	Amount	Check	Date paid	Amount
	202	7/05	15.05	203	7/15	94.50

Deposits		Date posted	Balance
	Customer deposit	7/22	68.74
	interest payment this period	7/22	.18

Balance information	Date	Balance	Date	Balance	Date	Balance
	6/22	252.10	7/05	237.05	7/15	142.55
					7/22	211.47

24 Hour Customer Service	Each account comes with 3 complimentary calls per statement period. Calls to 24 hour customer service this statement period: 0

Interest information	From 6/22	Through 7/22	Interest rate 1.00%	Annual percentage yield (APY) 1.01%

Interest rate/APY as of 7/22/02 if your balance is

$0–4,999…………………………1.00%   1.01%
$5,000–$9,999……………………1.00%   1.01%
$10,000 and over…………………1.00%   1.01%

Call 1-800-555-2932 in California anytime for current rates.

Member FDIC

STATEMENT

FIG. 27.17 Example of a regular checking account statement. (From Proctor D, Niedzwiecki B: *Kinn's The Medical Assistant*, ed 13, St Louis, 2017, Elsevier.)

activities makes the bank reconciliation much smoother. All deposit copies should be maintained with a copy of the calculator tape totaling the day's deposit. Every online bill pay transaction should be recorded accurately in the accounting management system.

If you have carefully recorded every transaction and the balances still do not match, ask yourself the following questions:
- Is your math correct? Could a deposit, check, or online bill pay amount be transposed?
- Did you forget to include one of the outstanding checks?
- Did you fail to record a deposit or did you record one twice?

Most banks ask to be notified within a reasonable time (e.g., 10 days) of any error found in the statement. The bank statement should be reconciled as soon as it is received. Most banks provide a form for reconciliation (bank statement reconciliation formula) on the last page of the bank statement:

Bank statement balance	$ _____
Minus outstanding checks	$ _____
Plus deposits not shown	$ _____
Corrected bank statement balance	$ _____
Checkbook balance	$ _____
Minus any bank charges	$ _____
Corrected checkbook balance	$ _____

If the two corrected balances agree, stop there. If they do not agree, subtract the lesser figure from the greater figure; the difference usually provides a clue to the error. For instance, if the shortage is $35, examine all the transactions for $35 on the statement and checkbook register and determine whether one of them has a posting error. Check the math and make sure all figures were added and subtracted correctly. Look at each figure and make sure none has been transposed. These

CHAPTER 27 Accounts, Collections, and Banking

FIG. 27.18 Reverse side of a bank statement, which is used for reconciling a checking account. (From Proctor D, Niedzwiecki B: *Kinn's The Medical Assistant*, ed 13, St Louis, 2017, Elsevier.)

tips usually catch the mistake. Box 27.14 provides suggestions for preventing check fraud in the healthcare facility.

Another medical assistant function is maintaining the petty cash fund in the healthcare facility. This process is described in Box 27.15.

Paying Bills to Maximize Cash Flow

It is important to establish a systematic plan for paying bills. Some offices use an online bill paying system and pay bills as soon as they are received. Some pay bills monthly. In establishing the procedure for accounts payable, a medical assistant should keep in mind that most vendors allow 30 days to pay. When each invoice is received, check the "terms," which are usually located at the top of the document. Sometimes a bill will be discounted if it is paid within a specified time, such as 10 days. Such discounts usually are indicated at the bottom of invoices or

BOX 27.14 Preventing Check Fraud in the Healthcare Facility

The National Check Fraud Center suggests the following steps to minimize the chance of check fraud in the healthcare facility:

- Check bank statements immediately after receiving them. If check fraud is not reported within 30 days of receipt of a monthly statement, the bank usually does not have to reimburse the loss.
- Make sure all extra checks, deposit slips, bank statements, and records are stored securely (e.g., locked in a file cabinet or a secure electronic folder).
- Bank statements and records should be maintained for up to 7 years and then shredded before disposal.

For more information on how to prevent check fraud or what to do if fraud occurs, consult the National Check Fraud Center's website: http://ckfraud.org.

BOX 27.15 Petty Cash

Petty cash is a small amount of money kept on hand for small, miscellaneous expenses, such as:
- parking money for a conference
- postage due
- lunch for the provider
- deliveries
- minor office supplies

Although it is a small amount of money, records still need to be kept and expenses tracked. If an employee is being reimbursed for expenses, a receipt should be written out and the disbursement tracked in the petty cash log. Periodically the petty cash fund should be balanced, much like the checking account reconciliation.

If funds are running low in the petty cash fund, a check should be written and the addition of the new funds noted on the petty cash register.

---

billing statements. If the terms say, "Net 30," this means the total amount of the bill is due within 30 days.

Remember to allow a certain number of days for mailing (2 to 5, depending on where the payment is sent). If the business checking account is an interest-bearing one, do not pay bills before their due date. In this way, the funds in the account continue to earn interest until the check is cashed. Also, if the practice has a weekly service (e.g., a laundry or cleaning service) that bills several times a month, accumulate the invoices and issue only one check per month.

Invoices and Statements. The vendor usually includes an *invoice* for payment with delivery of the merchandise. An invoice describes the products delivered and shows the amount due. Always verify that the items listed on the packing slip and invoice are included in the delivery.

Invoices should be placed in a designated accounts payable folder until paid. The healthcare facility may make more than one purchase from the same vendor during the month and send only a single payment at the end of the month for all deliveries.

CRITICAL THINKING BOX 27.7

Laura does not recall ordering a certain item from the office supply company. However, it was included in her last shipment and was shown on the packing list. How can she determine whether the item was ordered?

Online Bill Pay. Online banking is a common practice for personal and business accounts. The healthcare facility can set up the account so that bills are paid automatically. This results in debiting the customer's account and crediting the merchant's account. This works well for those bills that occur every month or on a regular cycle, such as insurance premiums, rent payments, and utility bills. All banking transactions can be downloaded into an accounting management program for efficient money management. Online banking also is an excellent way to research the checks that have cleared the bank and to compute accurate bank balances.

Direct Deposit. *Direct deposit,* also known as *electronic funds transfers* (EFT), is the electronic payment of payroll, money owed to vendors or business establishments, and payments from government agencies. Direct deposit payments are safe, secure, efficient, and less expensive than paper checks. Their greatest advantage is the cost savings: the U.S. government pays $1.03 to issue each check payment, but only $0.105 to issue a direct deposit. Electronic processing becomes more common each day, and business transactions are processed faster and more efficiently through electronic means.

EMPLOYEE PAYROLL

A medical assistant is often times responsible for processing employee payroll for the healthcare facility. Employees can be paid either on an hourly basis or with a salary. If the employee is salaried, his or her net paycheck will always be the same dollar amount. If the employee is paid hourly, the net paycheck will depend on how many hours the person worked during the pay period. The hourly rate is multiplied by the number of hours worked to determine these individuals' gross pay. In either situation, the gross amount earned is used to determine how much is withheld for taxes.

VOCABULARY
gross: The amount earned before any tax deductions or adjustments.
net: The amount someone is paid after taxes and other deductions have been subtracted.
salary: A fixed compensation periodically paid to a person for regular work.

Each employee must complete a W-4 form, Employee's Withholding Allowance Certification. This form indicates the person's tax status and how many allowances he or she is claiming. This information is used to determine how much money is withheld for income taxes.

Other deductions from an employee's paycheck could be for insurance premiums, retirement savings, health savings accounts, or flexible spending accounts.

All employers are required to provide their employees with a W-2 form on a yearly basis. This must be sent to employees by January 30. This form lists the amounts that were withheld for income tax purposes. The employee needs this information to compute his or her taxes for the year.

It is important for the healthcare facility to keep exact records regarding payroll, withholding, and deductions. The employer is responsible for submitting the withheld tax amounts to the federal and state governments in a timely fashion. These are usually submitted on a quarterly basis (i.e., every 3 months).

EXCEPTIONAL CUSTOMER SERVICE

It should be emphasized that patients are financially responsible for balances on their accounts. Patients should be informed of the healthcare facility's payment policy at the very first appointment. If a patient submits an NSF check, the medical assistant should call the patient and explain the problem, requesting that he or she correct the matter as soon as possible. It is important to remember that most overdrafts are simply the result of mathematical errors or a delay in deposited funds being available for withdrawal. Therefore, the medical assistant should be patient and courteous when discussing NSF issues with patients. However, patients need to know that overdrafts are costly not only to them but also to the medical facility.

CLOSING COMMENTS

Patient accounts management and collections are critical responsibilities in the healthcare facility, and a responsible medical assistant is a great asset in this important area. Always maintain a positive attitude with patients when discussing financial matters. Remember that people who are ill or facing challenges are not always cordial, so they may not respond positively to discussion of their patient account balances. Make every attempt to work with each patient to develop a financial plan for settling the account balance. The healthcare facility works hard to collect every dollar, so effective financial management is essential for practice success.

An equally important financial aspect for the healthcare facility is accounts payable. This must also be handled in an efficient manner. Being aware of the different banking options can help with depositing funds and paying bills. Making sure that there are policies in place for patient payment methods is crucial. Patients should also be made aware of those policies.

CHAPTER REVIEW

The first step in understanding the financial side of a healthcare facility is learning about patient accounts. Whether the healthcare facility uses a manual bookkeeping method or a computerized system, the process is similar. A patient ledger is used to track all of the charges, payments, and adjustments made to a patient's account. The ledger is used to answer questions and concerns that may come up regarding patient financial issues. The information found there is used to make decisions about payment agreements and collection activities.

A billing cycle needs to be established so that patient statements are sent on a regular basis. Determining policies regarding the billing of minors, providing care for those who cannot pay, and hardship cases can ensure that those unusual circumstances are handled fairly.

When patients do not make regular payments on their account, collection procedures need to be followed. This could mean telephone calls, collection letters, or even turning an account over to a collection agency. When doing in-house collection activities, it is important to keep in mind the Fair Debt Collection Practices guidelines.

Banking procedures are used for depositing funds and also for paying bills. The increased use of online banking has made both of those processes more efficient. Patients will make payments using cash, checks, credit and debit cards, and/or other electronic payment options. The medical assistant should understand the precautions needed for each of those payment types.

Employee payroll is another financial aspect for the healthcare facility. Making sure that all of the deductions are done correctly is essential for the employer as well as the employee. A salaried employee is one who receives a set dollar amount that is paid regardless of how many hours are worked. An hourly employee is paid a set dollar amount for each hour the person works. Meticulous records must be kept for all withholdings and deductions.

SCENARIO WRAP-UP

Laura has learned a lot about the different types of bookkeeping transactions performed daily in the healthcare facility. As she has gained more experience, she has come to appreciate the important role of patient accounts collection in the practice's cash flow and ability to cover its operating expenses.

After the visit with the bank representative, Laura implemented a few changes in bank account management, which have increased productivity in the office. For one, Laura requested that the bank send a mobile deposit machine so this could be done in-house, which has saved Laura a lot of time.

Laura has also set up an online bill pay system and manages all invoice payments through the banking portal online. She sits down once a month and sets up all payments for the month. In this way, she can budget the office expenses for the month and can transfer unused funds to a money market account that pays a higher interest rate.

Laura is working closely with the providers at WMFM to make some financial policy changes in the office to streamline banking processes. As of January 1 of the new year, the sign at the healthcare facility's lobby window will explain that cash will no longer be accepted for services and that a $35 fee will be charged for NSF checks.

28

Infection Control

LEARNING OBJECTIVES

1. Describe the characteristics of pathogenic microorganisms.
2. Do the following related to the chain of infection:
   - Apply the chain of infection process to the healthcare practice.
   - Compare viral and bacterial cell invasion.
   - Differentiate between humoral and cell-mediated immunity.
3. Summarize the impact of the inflammatory response on the body's ability to defend itself against infection.
4. Analyze the differences among acute, chronic, latent, and opportunistic infections.
5. Do the following related to the Occupational Safety and Health Administration (OSHA) standards for the healthcare setting:
   - Specify potentially infectious body fluids.
   - Integrate OSHA's requirement for a site-based exposure control plan into facility management procedures.
   - Explain the major areas included in the OSHA Compliance Guidelines.
- Discuss protocols for disposal of biologic chemical materials.
- Remove contaminated gloves while following the principles of Standard Precautions.
- Summarize the management of postexposure evaluation and follow-up, and participate in bloodborne pathogen training and a mock exposure event.
6. Apply the concepts of medical and surgical asepsis to the healthcare setting.
7. Discuss proper hand washing, and demonstrate the proper hand-washing technique for medical asepsis.
8. Differentiate among sanitization, disinfection, and sterilization procedures, and select barrier/personal protective equipment while demonstrating the correct procedure for sanitizing contaminated instruments.
9. Discuss the role of the medical assistant in asepsis.

CHAPTER OUTLINE

1. Opening Scenario, 616
2. You Will Learn, 616
3. Introduction, 617
4. Disease, 617
5. Chain of Infection, 617
6. Inflammatory Response, 620
7. Types of Infection, 621
   a. Acute Infection, 621
   b. Chronic Infection, 621
   c. Latent Infection, 621
   d. Opportunistic Infections, 622
8. Occupational Safety and Health Administration Standards for the Healthcare Setting, 622
   a. Bloodborne Pathogens Standard, 622
   b. Compliance Guidelines, 625

   i. *Barrier Protection,* 625
   ii. *Environmental Protection,* 625
   iii. *Housekeeping Controls,* 627
   iv. *Hepatitis B Vaccination,* 629
   v. *Postexposure Follow-Up,* 629
9. Aseptic Techniques: Preventing Disease Transmission, 630
   a. Hand Hygiene, 632
   b. Sanitization, 632
      i. *Ultrasonic Sanitization,* 632
   c. Disinfection, 634
   d. Sterilization, 634
10. Role of the Medical Assistant in Asepsis, 634
11. Closing Comments, 635
12. Chapter Review, 635
13. Scenario Wrap-Up, 635

▶ OPENING SCENARIO

Rosa Lucia is a certified medical assistant working for Walden-Martin Family Medical (WMFM) Clinic. She is quite concerned about contracting an infectious disease while caring for her patients. Rosa learned about Standard Precautions while enrolled in her medical assisting program and now must implement that knowledge in the workplace. Two important factors in preventing the spread of infection are (1) understanding how to break the chain of infection and (2) recognizing the importance of correct and frequent hand washing.

YOU WILL LEARN

1. To identify the various infectious agents.
2. To recognize the components of the chain of infection.

CHAPTER 28 Infection Control

3. To describe how the Bloodborne Pathogens Standard impacts healthcare.
4. To differentiate among sanitization, disinfection, and sterilization.

INTRODUCTION

To gain an understanding of the importance of infection control, you must comprehend the concepts of disease transmission and the body's response to infection. One of the easiest ways to prevent the spread of disease is to wash your hands or use alcohol-based hand sanitizers. Every procedure must begin and end with hand hygiene practices. Making sure that **sterile** (STER il) technique is used is another huge component of infection control. The fundamental concepts of this chapter should be used whenever you are faced with an infection control issue. The guidelines established by the Occupational Safety and Health Administration (OSHA) have stated this as well. The guidelines in this chapter are basic to all clinical skills, and following them can reduce the transmission of disease organisms and lessen the severity of disease. They also may save a patient's or coworker's life, or even your own.

DISEASE

Disease is defined as a specific illness with a recognizable group of signs and symptoms and a clear cause (e.g., infection, environment). We recognize and categorize many types of diseases: **hereditary** (huh RED i ter ee) (genetic), drug-induced, **autoimmune**, degenerative (degenerative), *communicable* (kuh MYOO ni kuh buh l), and infectious, to name only a few. Sometimes a specific disease may fit two or more categories.

Any disease caused by the growth of pathogenic microorganisms in the body falls into the category of **infectious diseases**. The entrance of a living microbe into the body is not a disease until the infected cell or individual shows harmful changes in structure, physiology, or biochemistry. In fact, a pathogen may be **ingested**, injected, or inhaled and never cause disease. However, an unaffected person can still transmit the infection to another person. In this case we call the unaffected person a *carrier*.

Microorganisms are almost everywhere. We carry them on our skin, in our bodies, and on our clothing. They can be in ice, boiling water, the soil, and the air. The only places free of microorganisms are certain internal body organs and tissues, and sterilized medical equipment and supplies. In the normal state, organs and tissues that do not connect with the outside by means of mucus-lined membranes are free of all living microorganisms.

CHAIN OF INFECTION

Certain factors are required for an infectious disease to spread. These factors, or links, make up the chain of infection. Break the chain and you break the infection process (Fig. 28.1).

The chain of infection starts with the infectious agent. There are five types of potentially pathogenic agents or microorganisms: viruses, bacteria, *fungi* (FUHN jahy), *protozoa* (proh tuh ZOH uh), and *helminths* (HEL minths). Infection cannot occur without the presence of an infectious microorganism. The best way for healthcare workers to prevent the spread of disease is to use infection control procedures, such as the following:

- Consistent hand washing
- Proper use of **antiseptics** (an tuh SEP tiks)
- Effective disinfection and sterilization methods

Viruses, the smallest of all pathogens, lead the list of important disease-causing agents. Viral particles insert their own deoxyribonucleic acid (DNA) or ribonucleic acid (RNA) into a host cell and then use the host cell to help reproduce more viral particles. Viral invasion may not cause immediate symptoms because host cells infected with viruses can produce a substance called **interferon** (in ter FEER on). This protects nearby cells. Interferon leaves the infected cell and acts somewhat like Paul Revere, warning neighboring cells that "a virus is coming!" The neighboring cells then produce antiviral proteins, which prevent the virus from replicating inside the cells, slowing or halting the infection.

Antibiotics are unable to destroy viral invaders. The only way to destroy a viral invader is to destroy the host cell. Therefore the treatment for viral infections typically focuses on relieving symptoms, or *palliative* (PAL ee ey tiv) treatment, and antiviral medications that slow the rate of viral replication. Interferon and the antiviral agents (Box 28.1) may be prescribed, depending on the specific viral agent. Viral diseases include the following:

- Common cold
- Influenza
- Herpes
- Infectious hepatitis (e.g., hepatitis B and C)
- Acquired immunodeficiency syndrome (AIDS), which is caused by the human immunodeficiency virus (HIV)

VOCABULARY

antiseptics: Substances that inhibit the growth of microorganisms on living tissue (e.g., alcohol and povidone-iodine solution [Betadine]); they are used to cleanse the skin, wounds, and so on.
autoimmune: A disease in which the body produces antibodies that attack its own tissues, leading to the deterioration of tissue.
hereditary: Passed from parents to offspring through the genes.
ingested: Taken, as food, into the body.
interferon: A protein formed when a cell is exposed to a virus; the protein blocks viral action on the cell and protects against viral invasion.
sterile: Free of all microorganisms, pathogenic and nonpathogenic.

MEDICAL TERMINOLOGY

-genic: pertaining to, produced by
path/o: disease

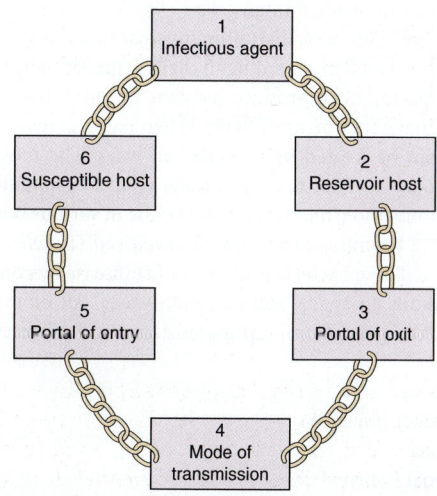

FIG. 28.1 The chain of infection. (From Proctor D, et al: *Kinn's The Medical Assistant*, ed 13, St. Louis, 2017, Elsevier.)

BOX 28.1 Antiviral Agents

- Acyclovir (Zovirax)
- Adefovir dipivoxil (Hepsera)
- Famciclovir (Famvir)
- Oseltamivir (Tamiflu)
- Penciclovir (Denavir)
- Valacyclovir hydrochloride (Valtrex)

BOX 28.2 Bacteria Morphology

Spherical
- Coccus (singular), cocci (plural)

Rod Shaped
- Bacillus (singular), bacilli (plural)

Spiral Shaped
- Spirilla (singular), spirillum (plural)
- Spirochete (singular), spirochetes (plural)
- Vibrio (singular), vibrios (plural)

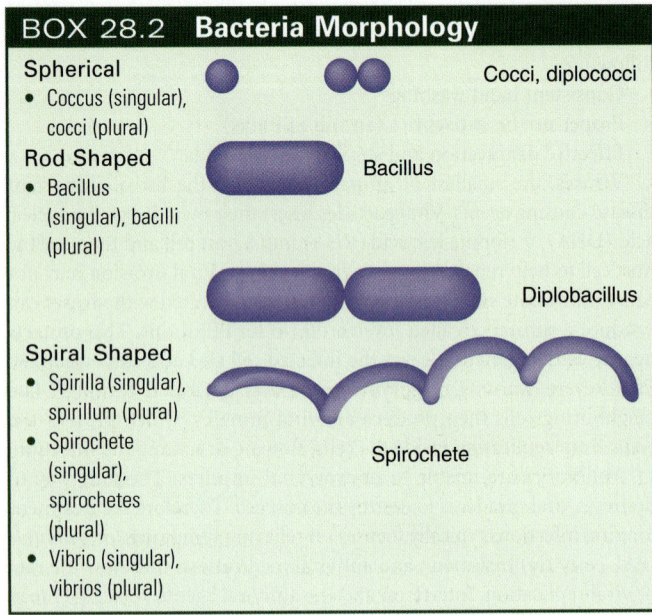

Figures from Proctor D, et al: *Kinn's The Medical Assistant*, ed 13, St. Louis, 2017, Elsevier.

BOX 28.3 Antibiotic Resistance

Antibiotic resistance is one of the world's most significant public health problems. Infectious microorganisms that once were easily treated with antibiotics are growing increasingly resistant to the actions of these drugs. The Centers for Disease Control and Prevention (CDC) reported that at least 2 million people in the United States become infected with antibiotic-resistant bacteria, and at least 23,000 people die each year as a direct result of these infections. Resistance occurs when an antibiotic is used inappropriately to treat an infection. This allows the pathologic organism to change or mutate in some way, which reduces or eliminates the effectiveness of the drug. The mutation can occur in the following situations:
- An antibiotic is prescribed when it is not needed (e.g., for a viral infection).
- The antibiotic is prescribed inaccurately (e.g., lower dosage, fewer days than recommended).
- The antibiotic is not taken as prescribed.

Although mutations are rare, overuse of antibiotics provides more opportunity for them to occur. Antibiotics should be used to treat bacterial infections; however, they are not effective against viral infections, such as the common cold, most sore throats, and the flu. Cautious use of antibiotics is the key to preventing the spread of resistance. The CDC makes the following recommendations for providers:
- Prescribe antibiotic therapy only when it will benefit the patient.
- Treat the patient with an antibiotic that is specific to the infecting pathogen.
- Prescribe the recommended dose and treatment duration of the medication.

VOCABULARY

spore: A thick-walled, dormant form of bacteria that is very resistant to disinfection measures.

CRITICAL THINKING 28.1

Susie Chen, a 3-year-old patient, is being seen today. She has been complaining of a cough and nasal congestion. Susie's father does not understand why the pediatrician did not order an antibiotic for his daughter's viral infection. Rosa needs to reinforce the doctor's decision. How can she help the father understand the proper use of antibiotics?

Bacteria are tiny, simple cells that produce disease in a variety of ways. Pathogenic bacteria can secrete toxic substances that do the following:
- Damage human tissues
- Act as parasites inside human cells
- Grow on body surfaces, disrupting normal functions

Bacteria are classified according to their shape, or *morphology* (Box 28.2). Some bacteria can produce resistant internal structures, called spores, that make treatment difficult. When bacteria invade the body, the patient can be treated in a number of ways. The most common approach is to use antibiotics to destroy the invader or inhibit its growth. We all have nonpathogenic bacteria that reside in various body systems. For example, a harmless form of *Escherichia coli (E. coli)* lives in the large intestine. These bacteria protect against disease by competing for nutrients, taking up space, and excreting waste. All of these actions discourage pathogens. Common diseases caused by bacteria include the following:
- Tuberculosis
- Urinary tract infections
- Pneumonia
- Strep throat

Bacteria can mutate and become resistant to antibiotic treatments. To learn more about antibiotic resistance, see Box 28.3.

Fungi may be unicellular or multicellular; they include such organisms as mushrooms, molds, and yeasts. Many forms are pathogenic and can cause disease, such as candidiasis (kan di DAHY us sis) and tinea (TIN ee uh) infections. Fungi grow best in warm, moist environments. Treatment with antifungal agents includes the application of topical preparations (e.g., clotrimazole [Lotrimin]) for tinea infections; vaginal suppositories (e.g., miconazole [Monistat]) for candidiasis; and oral medications, such as fluconazole (Diflucan), ketoconazole (Nizoral), and terbinafine (Lamisil). Fungal infections also are called *mycotic* infections.

CHAPTER 28   Infection Control   619

> **BOX 28.4 Reservoirs**
> - People
> - Water
> - Insects
> - Food
> - Animals
> - Contaminated instruments and equipment

> **BOX 28.5 Means of Exit and Entry**
> Means of exit and entry include the following:
> - Mouth
> - Nose
> - Eyes
> - Ears
> - Intestines
> - Urinary tract
> - Reproductive tract
> - Open wounds

Protozoa are unicellular parasites that can replicate and multiply rapidly once inside the host. Examples of diseases caused by protozoa include giardiasis, which is typically caused by the ingestion of water contaminated by feces, and malaria, in which *Plasmodium* organisms invade the blood system. Protozoal infections frequently are seen in tropical climates, which have large insect populations. These insects serve as vectors for many protozoal diseases. For example, the mosquito transmits the organisms that cause malaria. Protozoa and helminths (worms) are usually grouped together as parasites.

Helminths are multicellular and include tapeworms, roundworms, and flatworms (flukes [flooks]). Tapeworms live in the intestines of some animals and can be transferred to humans who eat undercooked meat from infected animals. Most parasitic roundworm eggs are found in the soil and enter the human body when a person picks them up on the hands and then transfers them to the mouth. Roundworms eventually end up or live in human intestines and cause infection and disease. Flatworms with an external sucker are referred to as flukes. Flukes are found in raw or improperly cooked fish.

The second link in the chain of infection is the reservoir (Box 28.4). Most pathogens must gain entrance into a host or else they die. The reservoir host supplies all of the conditions needed for microbial growth, allowing it to multiply. The pathogen either causes infection in the host or, in the case of vector-borne diseases, exits the host in great enough numbers to cause disease in another host.

The chain of infection continues with the means, or *portal*, of exit—that is, how the pathogen escapes the reservoir host (Box 28.5). The use of Standard Precautions (e.g., gloves, masks, proper wound care, correct disposal of contaminated products, and hand washing) helps control the ability of infectious material to spread from one host to another.

After exiting the reservoir host, the organism needs a *mode of transmission*. Transmission is either direct or indirect. *Direct transmission* occurs from contact with an infected person, with discharges from an infected person (such as feces or urine), or with infected soil. Direct transmission includes droplet transmission. This refers to the droplets that come from sneezing, coughing, or even talking. Those droplets land on the next potential host. *Indirect transmission* refers to the transfer of microorganisms by suspended particles in the air, inanimate objects, or animals and insects. When microorganisms are suspended particles, this is considered airborne transmission. Transmission occurs through inhalation (in huh LEY shuh n) of the microorganisms. *Vectors* are animals or insects that harbor pathogens and can transmit them. Transmission can also occur through contaminated food or drink or through contact with contaminated objects (called *fomites* [FOH mahyt]). Proper sanitation of water and food; the use of sanitization, disinfection, and sterilization procedures; and the use of germicides (JUR muh sahyds) (e.g., Wavicide and Cidex) all help control the transmission of pathogens.

The next link in the chain of infection is the means, or portal, of entry. This is how the transmitted pathogen gains entry into a new host (see Box 28.5). The first line of defense against pathogenic invasion is made up of the body's physical and chemical barriers. An intact *integumentary system*, or skin, serves as a physical barrier to infection. Other anatomic defense mechanisms include the following:

- Tears
- Cilia
- Mucous membranes
- pH of body fluids
- Defecation (DEF i kay shun) and vomiting

The body's second line of defense is nonspecific chemical and cellular responses. *Phagocytic* cells engulf and destroy the microbes. Inflammation occurs, bringing white blood cells to the area. The inflammatory response produces swelling, redness, heat, and pain.

The third line of defense involves specific immunity. The immune system responds by producing antibodies specifically designed to combat the presence of a foreign substance, or *antigen*. This process is called *humoral immunity* (Box 28.6) and is the responsibility of the body's B cells. Another immune system response involves T cells. This is called *cell-mediated immunity* and causes the destruction of pathogenic cells at the site of invasion. More information on the immune system can be found in Chapter 9.

> **VOCABULARY**
> **antibodies**: Protein substances produced in the blood or tissues in response to a specific antigen, which destroy or weaken the antigen; part of the immune system.
> **candidiasis**: An infection caused by a yeast, Candida albicans, that typically affects the vaginal mucosa and skin.
> **defecation**: The act of voiding waste from the bowels through the anus; the act of having a bowel movement.
> **germicides**: Agents that destroy pathogenic organisms.
> **inanimate**: Not animate; lifeless.
> **inhalation**: The act of breathing in.
> **tinea**: Any fungal skin disease that results in scaling, itching, and inflammation; examples include ringworm and athlete's foot.
> **transmission**: The passage or spread disease.
> **vectors**: Animals or insects (e.g., ticks) that transmit a pathogen.

BOX 28.6 How Humoral Immunity Is Acquired

There are two ways that antibodies can be acquired: actively or passively. These groups can be further categorized as artificial or natural.

With actively acquired immunity, the body actively makes antibodies after exposure to the disease-causing organism. This could result from having the actual disease or from a vaccination.

With passively acquired immunity, the body is given the antibodies without having to work for them. This could be the result of placental transfer, breastfeeding, or an injection of immunoglobulins.

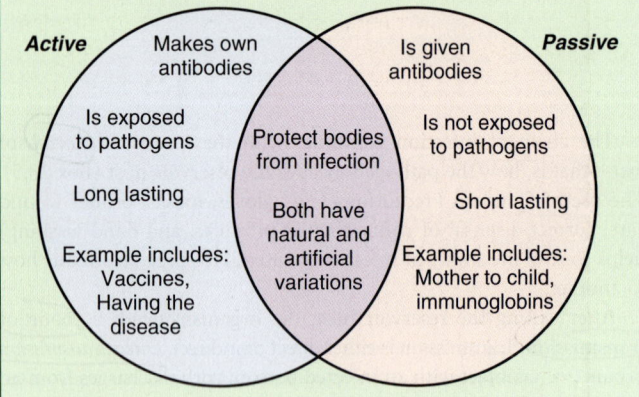

BOX 28.7 The Body's Natural Protective Mechanisms

The body has many levels of protection against the invasion of pathogenic microorganisms:
- Intact skin serves as a natural barrier to disease.
- Mucous membranes lining the openings of the body help protect underlying tissues and trap foreign substances.
- Tiny, hairlike projections, called *cilia*, line the respiratory tract and move in a coordinated upward motion to expel trapped foreign substances.
- Trapped substances can be expelled with sneezing and coughing before the organisms invade underlying tissue.
- Some body secretions, such as tears, have antimicrobial properties that help destroy invading pathogens.
- The natural pH of many of the body's organs discourages the growth of microbes. The acidic pH of urine, the vaginal mucosa, and the stomach helps prevent pathogenic invasion. The body's resident microbes create and maintain this environment.

The final link in the chain of infection is exposure of the pathogen to a susceptible host. If the host is *susceptible* (suh SEP tuh buh l) (i.e., capable of supporting the growth of the infecting organism), the organism multiplies. Various factors contribute to a host's susceptibility:
- Genetic factors
- Quantity of organisms
- State of the individual's health
  - Stress
  - Poor health
  - Poor nutrition
  - Poor hygiene

If conditions are right, the organism reaches infectious levels, and the susceptible host can start the chain of infection all over again.

CRITICAL THINKING 28.2

Tommy Anderson, a 5-year-old patient, is in the office because of an outbreak of impetigo. Rosa must apply the concepts of the chain of infection and infection control methods to teach Tommy and his mother how to prevent the spread of the infection to other members of the family. What procedures should she follow after Tommy's visit to prevent the spread of the infection to other patients, other staff members, and herself?

Immunizations trigger the development of antibodies. These antibodies mean that an individual is not susceptible to that disease even if she or he is exposed to the pathogen. However, some people do not develop immunity to diseases even after following immunization guidelines. The Centers for Disease Control and Prevention (CDC) estimated that, depending on the vaccine, individuals do not develop immunity 1% to 5% of the time. The provider can check for immunity by ordering an antibody titer. A *titer* is a laboratory test that measures the level of antibodies in a blood sample. If a vaccine stimulated a person's immune system to create antibodies to a disease, the antibodies will be present in adequate amounts in the titer. If not, the provider decides whether another dose of the vaccine should be given to try to boost the person's immune response. To learn more about how the human body protects itself, see Box 28.7.

INFLAMMATORY RESPONSE

The *inflammatory response* (Fig. 28.2) starts when the body experiences trauma or is exposed to pathogens. To defend itself, the body starts certain responses to destroy and remove pathogenic organisms and their by-products. If this is not possible, it will limit the damage caused by the invading pathogen. This process results in the four classic symptoms of inflammation:

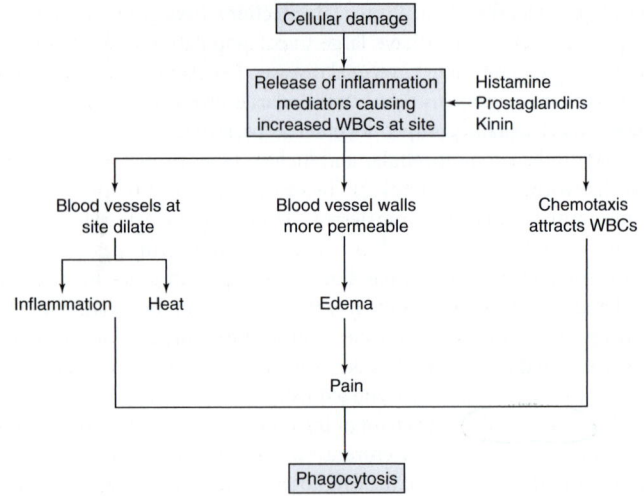

FIG. 28.2 The inflammatory response. (From Proctor D, et al: *Kinn's The Medical Assistant*, ed 13, St. Louis, 2017, Elsevier.)

MEDICAL TERMINOLOGY

cyt/o: cell
-ic: pertaining to
phag/o: eat, swallow

- *Erythema* (redness)
- *Edema* (swelling)
- Pain
- Heat

When the body is exposed to an infectious agent or a foreign substance, cellular damage occurs at the site. Inflammation mediators (i.e., *histamine* [HIS tuh meen], *prostaglandins* [pros tuh GLAN din], and *kinins* [KAHY nin]) are released, causing three different responses at the cellular level. All three actions are designed to increase the number of white blood cells (WBCs) at the injury site.

First, blood vessels at the site dilate, causing an increase in local blood flow, which results in redness (inflammation) and heat. Blood vessel walls become more *permeable*, which allows for the movement of WBCs through the vessel wall to the site. The WBCs begin to form a fibrous capsule around the site to protect surrounding cells from damage or infection. Blood plasma also filters out of the more permeable vessel walls, resulting in edema (swelling), which puts pressure on the nerves and causes pain. Finally, *chemotaxis* (kee moh TAK sis), or the release of chemical agents, occurs, attracting even more WBCs to the site. The increased number of WBCs at the site results in phagocytosis. Destroyed pathogens, cells, and WBCs collect in the area and form a thick, white substance called *pus*. If the pathogenic invasion is too great for localized control, the infection may collect in the body's lymph nodes, where more WBCs are present to help fight the battle. This causes swollen glands, or *lymphadenopathy* (lim fad uh NOP puh thee). If the body is too weak or the number of pathogens is too great, the infection may spread to the bloodstream. A systemic infection, called *septicemia* or *blood poisoning*, may occur, which ultimately could affect the entire body. Another term for septicemia is **pyemia** (pahy EE mee uh). Without appropriate medical intervention, death can occur from a systemic infection.

> **BOX 28.8 Stages of an Infection**
>
> An acute infection will go through the following stages:
> Incubation: The period of time between exposure to the pathogen and the appearance of the first symptoms. It can be from a few days to a few months. The incubation period for mononucleosis is 4 to 6 weeks.
> Prodromal: The short period of time when the first symptoms appear. With mononucleosis the patient may have 1 to 2 weeks of **fatigue** (fuh TEEG), **malaise** (ma LEYZ), *myalgia* (mye AL jah), and a low-grade fever.
> Acute: The disease is at its peak and symptoms are fully developed. With mononucleosis, *pharyngitis* (fair in JYE tis), *tonsillitis* (ton suh LAHY tis), and *lymphadenopathy* (lim fad n OP uh thee) are common symptoms.
> Declining: The symptoms of the disease start to subside. If patients have been prescribed antibiotics, this when they may decide to stop taking them. It is important to stress to patients that they must take all of the medication. With mononucleosis, the declining stage can take several weeks or even months.
> Convalescent: In this stage, patients will regain their strength and return to a state of good health.

TYPES OF INFECTION

Acute Infection

An *acute infection* has a rapid onset of symptoms but lasts a relatively short time. The *prodromal stage* (Box 28.8) of an acute infection is that time when the patient first shows vague, nonspecific symptoms of disease. For example, the person is not vomiting, nor does he or she have a fever, but the individual just does not feel well. In an acute viral infection, the host cell typically dies within hours or days. In most acute infections, such as the common cold, the body's defense mechanisms eliminate the virus within 2 to 3 weeks.

Chronic Infection

A *chronic infection* is one that persists for a long period of time, sometimes for life. In the case of chronic hepatitis B infection, patients are *asymptomatic*, or without symptoms. The virus is still detectable with blood tests and remains transmissible throughout the person's life. Hepatitis B infection is transmitted by blood or blood products and by all body fluids. It is a serious health hazard to those who work in healthcare. All individuals employed in a healthcare setting should be immunized against hepatitis B. OSHA requires all employers to offer hepatitis B vaccination to their employees.

Latent Infection

A *latent infection* is a persistent infection in which the symptoms cycle through periods of **relapse** and **remission**. Cold sores and genital herpes are latent viral infections caused by the herpes simplex virus (HSV) types 1 and 2, respectively. The virus enters the body and causes the original lesion. It then lies dormant, in nerve cells away from the surface, until a certain trigger (illness with fever, sunburn, or stress) causes it to leave the nerve cell and seek the surface again. Once the virus reaches the superficial tissues, it becomes detectable for a short time and causes a new outbreak at the site. Another herpes virus, varicella-zoster virus, causes chickenpox (varicella). This virus may lie dormant along a nerve pathway for years and later erupt as the painful disease shingles (herpes zoster).

> **CRITICAL THINKING 28.3**
>
> Rosa's next patient appears to have a localized inflammatory response to a splinter. What signs and symptoms should she expect the patient to show?
>
> Rosa answers a telephone call from a patient who had surgery 3 days ago. The patient is concerned that the incision site is red, swollen, and hot. Is this a normal postoperative response? How might Rosa know whether the response is abnormal?

MEDICAL TERMINOLOGY
-algia: pain
-itis: inflammation
lymphaden/o: lymph gland
my/o: muscle
-pathy: disease
-pathy: disease process
pharyng/o: throat
tonsil/o: tonsil

VOCABULARY
fatigue: Extreme tiredness.
malaise: A condition of general bodily weakness or discomfort.
pyemia: The presence of pus-forming organisms in the blood.
relapse: The recurrence of the symptoms of a disease after apparent recovery.
remission: The partial or complete disappearance of the clinical and subjective characteristics of a chronic or malignant disease.

BOX 28.9 Other Potentially Infectious Materials

Items contaminated with any of the following potentially infectious materials require special handling:
- Body fluids:
  - Semen
  - Vaginal secretions
  - Cerebrospinal fluid (CSF)
  - Synovial fluid
  - Pleural fluid
  - Pericardial fluid
  - Peritoneal fluid
  - Amniotic fluid
- Any unfixed tissue
- Any pathogenic microorganism
  - Saliva in dental procedures
  - Any body fluid that is visibly contaminated with blood
- All body fluids in situations where it is difficult or impossible to differentiate between body fluids

Opportunistic Infections

Opportunistic (AH per too NIS tik) *infections* are caused by organisms that are not typically pathogenic but cause disease under certain circumstances. A host with an impaired immune system response, such as an individual infected with HIV, is susceptible to opportunistic infections. Over time, the person's immune system becomes weakened, and diseases result that are not typically seen in patients with a healthy immune system, such as *Pneumocystis carinii* (noo muh SIS tis KAHR in ee i) pneumonia and oral candidiasis. People without a compromised immune system can have an opportunistic infection.

OCCUPATIONAL SAFETY AND HEALTH ADMINISTRATION STANDARDS FOR THE HEALTHCARE SETTING

In 1987, in response to concern about the increasing prevalence of HIV and hepatitis B virus (HBV), the CDC recommended a new approach to potentially infectious materials called *Universal Precautions*. The underlying concept of Universal Precautions is that because healthcare workers do not know whether a patient has an infectious organism, all blood and certain body fluids must be treated as if they contain infectious bloodborne pathogens. Therefore precautions must be implemented for all patients, regardless of the information available about the person's individual health history. In turn, Universal Precautions protect patients from any bloodborne infection the healthcare worker may carry.

In 2001 OSHA developed the Bloodborne Pathogens Standard (Standard Precautions) that includes Universal Precautions. The goal of the Bloodborne Pathogens Standard is to safeguard all healthcare employees and their patients who are at risk of exposure from blood and other potentially infectious materials (OPIM) (Box 28.9).

Bloodborne Pathogens Standard

In 2000 Congress passed the Needlestick Safety and Prevention Act. This was in response to the CDC's concern about employee risk when working with sharps. Employers are required to keep a sharps injury log that describes the device involved in the incident and the details of how and where the incident occurred. Employers must also make available to employees effective sharps management devices, such as these:
- Syringes with self-sheathing needles

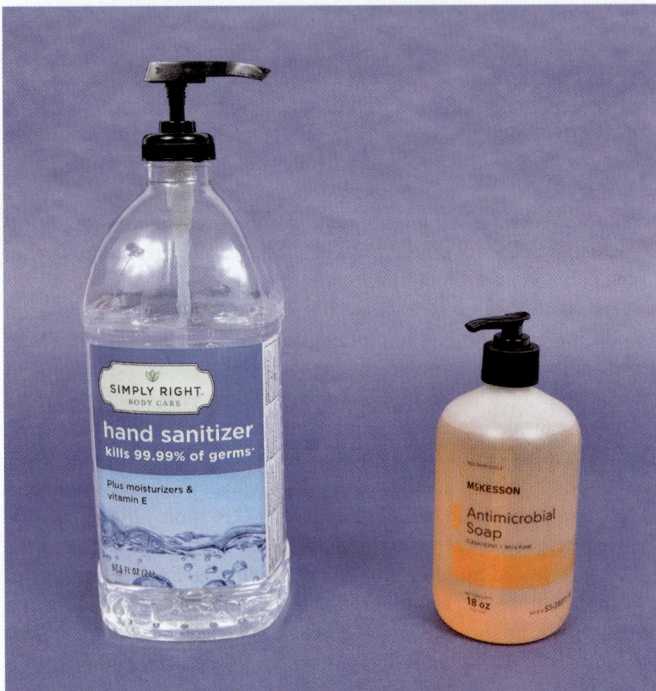

FIG. 28.3 Alcohol-based hand sanitizer and soap. (From Proctor D, et al: *Kinn's The Medical Assistant*, ed 13, St. Louis, 2017, Elsevier.)

- Needles that retract after use
- Needleless intravenous (IV) systems

Parenteral (pa REN ter uh l) exposure includes accidental needlesticks, occupation-related human bites, and exposure of nonintact skin (e.g., cuts and abrasions on the employee's hands) to OPIM. An employer who fails to comply with OSHA's Bloodborne Pathogens Standard could face a maximum penalty of $7000 for the first violation and up to $70,000 for repeated violations.

The Bloodborne Pathogens Standard also clarifies the use of washing or flushing of any exposed body area or mucous membrane immediately, or as soon as possible, after exposure to OPIM. This includes hand washing after the removal of gloves or other personal protective equipment.

Hands should be washed with soap and warm, running water when available. When running water is not available, alcohol-based hand sanitizers can be used. Studies have shown that correct use of alcohol-based hand sanitizers significantly reduces the number of microorganisms on the skin. It also takes less time than traditional hand washing and causes less irritation to the skin (Fig. 28.3).

The CDC's recommendations for adequate hand hygiene are as follows:
- Visibly soiled hands should be washed for a minimum of 15 seconds with soap and warm, running water (see Procedure 28.1).
- Alcohol-based hand sanitizers should be used before and after contact with each patient, and also after removing gloves, to prevent cross-contamination among patients and healthcare workers (see Procedure 28.1, presented later in the chapter).

VOCABULARY
parenteral: Taken into the body by any route other than the digestive tract (e.g., subcutaneous, intravenous, or intramuscular administration).
Standard Precautions: A set of infection control practices used to prevent the transmission of diseases that can be acquired by contact with blood, body fluids, nonintact skin, and mucous membranes.

PROCEDURE 28.1 Perform Hand Hygiene

Task
Minimize the number of pathogens on the hands, thus reducing the risk of transmission of pathogens.

Equipment and Supplies
- Sink with warm running water
- Liquid soap in a dispenser (bar soap is not acceptable)
- Disposable nailbrush or orange stick
- Paper towels in a dispenser
- Water-based lotion
- Covered waste container with foot pedal
- Alcohol-based hand sanitizer

Procedural Steps for Medical Aseptic Hand Washing

1. Remove all jewelry except your wristwatch, if it can be pulled up above your wrist, and a plain wedding ring.
   Purpose: Jewelry can harbor microorganisms.
2. Turn on the faucet and regulate the water temperature to lukewarm.
   Purpose: Water that is too hot can cause skin to become dry and chapped.
3. Wet your hands, apply soap, and lather using a circular motion with friction while holding your fingertips downward (Fig. 1). Rub well between your fingers. If this is the first hand wash of the day, use a nailbrush or an orange stick and clean under every fingernail. Inspect your nails thoroughly.
   Purpose: Friction removes soil and contaminants from the hands and wrists.

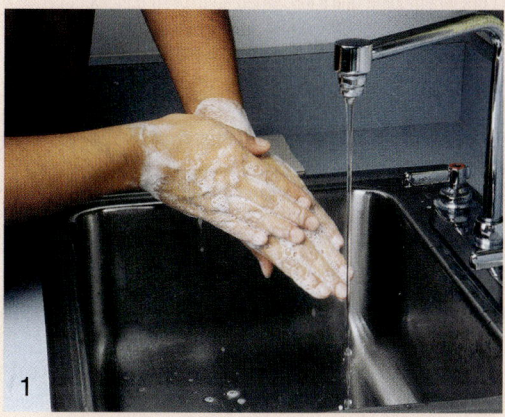

4. Rinse well, holding your hands so that the water flows from your wrists downward to your fingertips (Fig. 2).
   Purpose: Soil and contaminants will wash off the skin and down the drain.

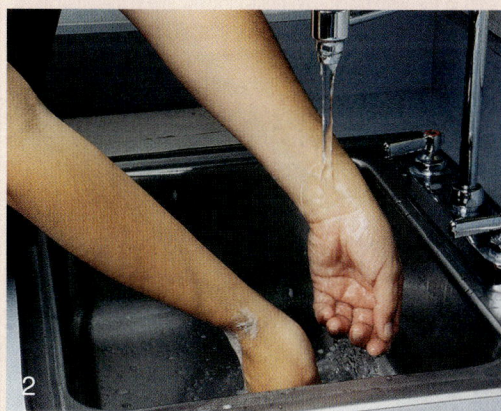

5. If this is the first hand wash of the day or if your hands are obviously contaminated, wet your hands again and repeat the scrubbing procedure using a vigorous, circular motion over the wrists and hands for at least 1 to 2 minutes.
   Purpose: Time is required for friction and motion to eliminate all possible soil and contaminants.
6. Rinse your hands a second time, keeping the fingers lower than your wrists.
   Purpose: To ensure removal of all transient flora.
7. Dry your hands with paper towels. Do not touch the paper towel dispenser as you are obtaining towels (Fig. 3).
   Purpose: Touching the dispenser contaminates your hands, and you will need to start over.

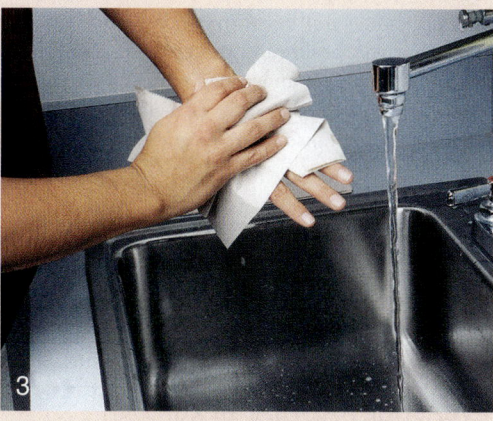

8. If the faucets are not foot operated, turn them off with a dry paper towel (Fig. 4).
   Purpose: The faucet is dirty and will contaminate your clean hands.

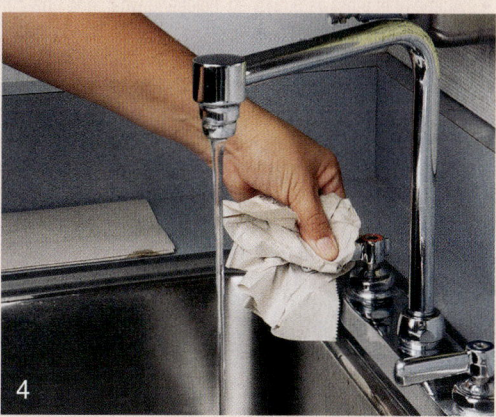

9. After you finish drying your hands and turning off the faucets, place used towels into a covered waste container.
   Purpose: Always discard contaminated waste in a covered waste container immediately to eliminate the source of infection.
10. If needed, apply a water-based antibacterial hand lotion to prevent chapped or dry skin.
    Purpose: Chapped skin eliminates the first line of defense against infectious organisms.
11. Repeat the procedure as indicated throughout the day.
    Purpose: To eliminate contaminants and prevent the transmission of pathogens to yourself and others.

Procedural Steps for Applying an Alcohol-Based Hand Sanitizer

1. Inspect hands to ensure they are not visibly soiled.
   Purpose: If hands are visibly soiled, then the medical aseptic hand wash should be performed.
2. Remove watch or push up on arms, and remove rings.
   Purpose: Watches and rings can harbor microorganisms.
3. Apply alcohol-based hand sanitizer to the palm of one hand; gel or lotion should be dime sized, and foam should be walnut sized.
   Purpose: Using too much alcohol-based hand sanitizer can be drying to the skin. Dry skin cracks and chaps, creating portals of entry for microorganisms.
4. Thoroughly spread sanitizer over all surfaces of both hands including around and under fingernails.
   Purpose: All surfaces need to be exposed to the alcohol-based hand sanitizer to effectively kill all microorganisms.
5. Rub hands until dry (20–30 seconds).

- Use an alcohol-based hand sanitizer properly, applying the label-recommended amount to the palm of one hand and rubbing the hands together, covering all surfaces until the hands are dry.
- Artificial nails should not be worn; studies show that even after careful hand hygiene, healthcare workers with artificial nails have more pathogenic microbes under their nails and on their fingertips than workers with natural nails. Artificial nails also cause nail changes that contribute to the transmission of microbes.
- Natural nail tips should be no longer than one-fourth of an inch to prevent microbial growth under the nail.

The best way to reduce the risk of infection is to follow the Bloodborne Pathogens Standard. Healthcare workers must take adequate and consistent precautions to protect themselves and their patients. Fig. 28.4 summarizes the Bloodborne Pathogens Standard. Healthcare facilities must establish specific policies and procedures for the management of an exposure incident (e.g., accidental needlestick) and the exposed employee.

Requirements of Employers: OSHA Bloodborne Pathogens Standard

EXPOSURE CONTROL PLAN
Each medical office must develop a written exposure control plan (ECP). The purpose of an ECP is to identify tasks where there is the potential for exposure to blood and other potentially infectious materials.
- A timetable must be published indicating when and how communication of potential hazards will occur.
- The employer must offer employees the hepatitis B vaccine within 10 working days of employment (at no cost to the employee). If employees sign a form to refuse the vaccine, they can change their mind at no cost to the employee.
- The employer must document the steps that should be taken in case of an exposure incident, including a postexposure evaluation and follow-up, strict record keeping, implementation of engineering controls, provision for personal protective equipment, and general housekeeping standards. This plan must be posted in the medical office.
- There must also be written procedures for evaluating the circumstances of an exposure incident.
- Training records must be kept for 3 years.

ENGINEERING CONTROLS AND WORK PRACTICES
The employer must provide engineering controls, or equipment and facilities that minimize the possibility of exposure. Examples of engineering controls include the following:
- Providing puncture-resistant containers for used sharps.
- Providing handwashing facilities that are readily accessible.
- Equipment for sanitizing, decontaminating, and sterilizing.

The employer must also enforce work practice controls. Work practice controls also minimize the possibility of exposure by making sure employees are using the proper techniques while working. Examples include the following:
- Enforcing proper handwashing or sanitizing procedures.
- Enforcing proper technique for using and handling needles to prevent needle sticks.
- Enforcing proper techniques to minimize the splashing of blood.

PERSONAL PROTECTIVE EQUIPMENT
Employers must provide, and employees must use, personal protective equipment (PPE) when the possibility exists of exposure to blood or contaminated body fluids. This equipment must not allow blood or potentially infectious material to pass through to the employee's clothes, skin, eyes, or mouth. Examples of PPE include the following:
- Gowns
- Face shields
- Goggles
- Gloves

If an employee has an allergy to powder or latex, the employer must provide hypoallergenic or powderless gloves. The employee cannot be charged for PPEs.

EXPOSURE INCIDENT MANAGEMENT
An exposure incident is contact with blood or biohazard infectious material that occurs when doing one's job. When an exposure incident is reported, the employer must arrange for an immediate and confidential medical evaluation. The information and actions required are as follows:
- Documenting how the exposure occurred.
- Identifying and testing the "source" individual, if possible.
- Testing the employee's blood, if consent is granted.
- Providing counseling.
- Evaluating, treating, and following up on any reported illness.

Medical records must be kept for each employee with occupational exposure for the duration of employment plus 30 years.

COMMUNICATION OF POTENTIAL HAZARDS TO EMPLOYEES
A medical assistant will be exposed to hazardous chemicals on the job. Most chemicals handled by assistants are not any more dangerous than those used in the home. In the workplace, however, exposure is likely to be greater, concentrations higher, and exposure time longer.

The "right to-know" law, OSHA's hazard communication standard, states that each employee has a right to know what chemicals he or she is working with in the workplace. The right-to-know law is intended to make the workplace safer by making certain that all information regarding chemical hazards is known to the employee. This information is supplied in the material safety data sheet (MSDS), a fact sheet about a chemical that includes the following information:
- Identification of the chemical
- Listing of the physical and health hazards
- Precautions for handling
- Identification of the chemical as a carcinogen
- First-aid procedures
- Name, address, and telephone number of manufacturer

Many SDS information sheets can be obtained in repositories on the internet. An SDS should be updated at least every 3 years. Employers must ensure that all products have an up-to-date SDS when they enter the workplace.

Potential hazards are also communicated with labels and color. Any containers with biohazard waste must be orange (or reddish orange) and must display the biohazard symbol. These labels and colors alert employees to the risk of possible exposure.

FIG. 28.4 Requirements of Employers: OSHA Bloodborne Pathogens Standard. (From the Occupational Safety and Health Administration, www.osha.gov.)

BOX 28.10 Types of Personal Protective Equipment Used in Healthcare Settings

- Gloves
- Gowns/aprons, shoe covers
- Laboratory coats
- Masks and respirators
- Protective eyewear
- Face shields

- Touching a patient's blood, body fluids, mucous membranes, or skin that is not intact.
- Handling items and surfaces contaminated with blood and body fluids.
- Performing venipuncture, finger sticks, injections, and other vascular procedures.
- Assisting with any surgical procedure. If a glove is torn during the procedure, the glove should be removed, the hands washed carefully, and new gloves put on as soon as possible.
- Handling, processing, and disposing of all blood and body fluid specimens.
- Cleaning and decontaminating spills of blood or other body fluids.

The same pair of gloves cannot be worn for the care of more than one patient; new disposable gloves must be used for each individual patient.

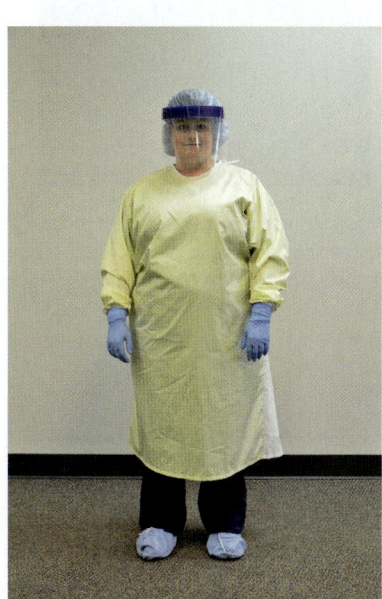

FIG. 28.5 Personal protective equipment. (From Proctor D, et al: *Kinn's The Medical Assistant*, ed 13, St. Louis, 2017, Elsevier.)

SAFETY ALERT

Protective equipment contaminated with body fluids of any kind must be removed and placed in a designated area or biohazard waste container. The hands or any other exposed areas must be washed or flushed as soon as possible. Face shields that cover the mouth, nose, and eyes must be worn whenever splashes, sprays, or droplets are possible. Utility gloves may be reused if they are intact (i.e., have no cracks, tears, or punctures). All PPE must be removed before the medical assistant leaves the medical facility (Fig. 28.6).

CRITICAL THINKING 28.4

Rosa is caring for an injured 3-year-old child with an open wound on his right knee. She puts on disposable gloves to clean the wound, and the mother demands to know why. How can she explain her actions?

Compliance Guidelines

The Bloodborne Pathogens Standard is for anyone working in the healthcare field. Only some of the regulations apply to the ambulatory care setting. Safety and infection control go beyond hand washing and knowledge of the disease cycle. The information presented here applies to the medical assisting profession.

Barrier Protection. Barrier protection, or *personal protective equipment (PPE)*, should be used when contact with blood or OPIM is expected. PPE includes specialized clothing or equipment that prevents the healthcare worker from coming in contact with blood or other potentially infectious material. This prevents or minimizes the entry of infectious material into the body (Box 28.10, Fig. 28.5).

Gloves are the most commonly used PPE in a healthcare facility. Gloves must be worn if the medical assistant is at all likely to be involved in any of the following activities (Procedure 28.2):

Environmental Protection. Environmental protection refers to minimizing the risk of injury by isolating or removing any physical or mechanical health hazard in the workplace. Every medical assistant must adhere to these safety rules:

- Read warning labels on biohazard waste containers and equipment.
- Minimize splashing or spraying of OPIM. Blood that splatters onto exposed areas of the skin or mucous membranes is a proven mode of HBV transmission.
- Bandage any breaks or lesions on your hands before gloving.
- If any body surface is exposed to potentially infectious material, scrub the area with soap and warm, running water as soon as possible after the exposure.

PROCEDURE 28.2 Remove Contaminated Gloves and Discard Biohazardous Material

Task
Minimize exposure to pathogens by aseptically removing and discarding contaminated gloves.

Equipment and Supplies
- Disposable gloves
- Biohazard waste container with labeled red biohazard bag

Procedural Steps

1. With the dominant hand, grasp the glove of the opposite hand near the palm and begin removing the first glove (Fig. 1). The arms should be held away from the body with the hands pointed down.
   Purpose: Holding the hands down and away from the body helps prevent possible contamination.

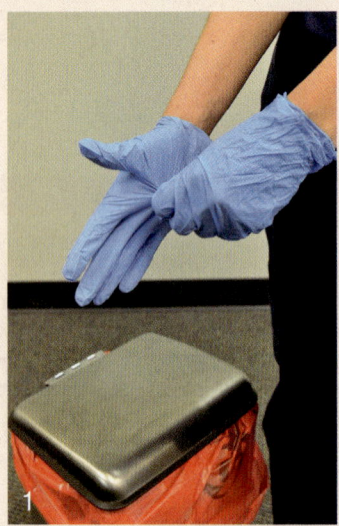

2. Pull the glove inside out (Fig. 2). After removal, ball it into the palm of the remaining gloved hand.
   Purpose: Taking off the glove inside out prevents transmission of pathogens to another surface.

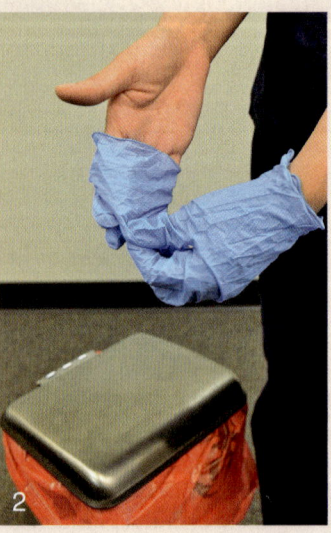

3. Insert two fingers of the ungloved hand between the edge of the cuff of the other contaminated glove and the hand (Fig. 3).

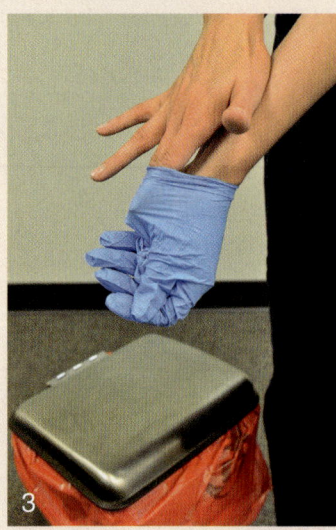

4. Push the glove down the hand, inside out, over the contaminated glove being held, leaving the contaminated side of both gloves on the inside.
   Purpose: This technique protects the wearer from the contaminated surfaces of both gloves.

5. Properly dispose of the inside-out, contaminated gloves in a biohazard waste container (Fig. 4).
   Purpose: To prevent the spread of infection.

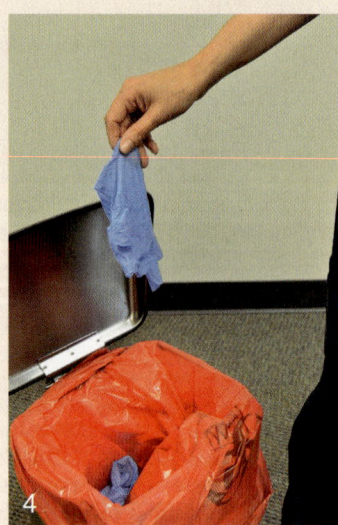

6. Perform a medical aseptic hand wash as described in Procedure 28.1, or sanitize the hands with an alcohol-based sanitizer.
   Purpose: To minimize the number of pathogens on the hands, thereby reducing the number of transient flora and the risk of transmission of pathogens.

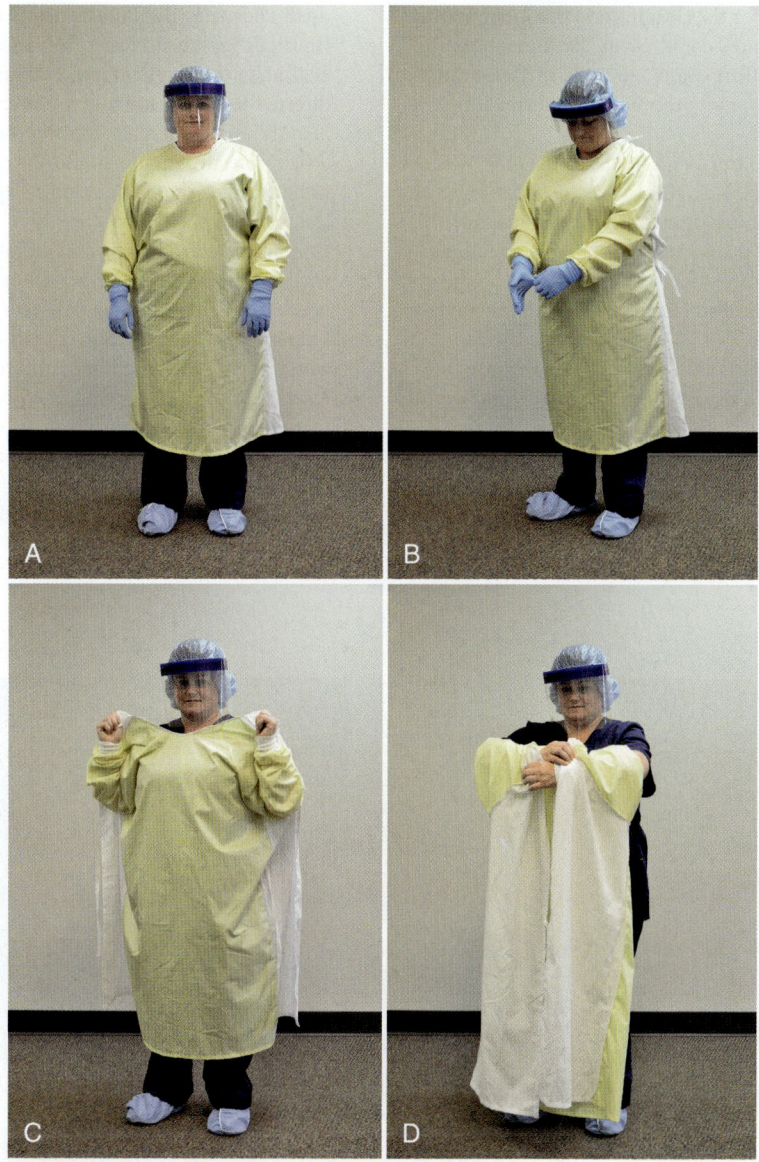

FIG. 28.6 Removing a contaminated gown. (From Proctor D, et al: *Kinn's The Medical Assistant*, ed 13, St. Louis, 2017, Elsevier.)

- If your eyes come in contact with body fluids, continuously flush them with water as soon as possible for a minimum of 15 minutes using an eye wash unit. A stationary unit connected to warm, running water is the best method for properly flushing potentially infectious material out of the eyes (Procedure 28.1).
- Contaminated needles and other sharps should never be recapped, bent, broken, or resheathed; needle units must have protective safety devices to cover the contaminated needle after injection.
- Contaminated sharp instruments, such as operating scissors, should not be processed in a way that requires employees to reach into containers to grasp them.
- Immediately after use, dispose of syringes and needles, scalpel blades, and other disposable sharp items in a labeled, leakproof, puncture-resistant biohazard container. The container must be located as close as possible to the area where the item is used.
- All specimens must be placed in a container that prevents leakage during collection, handling, processing, storage, transport, and shipping. Avoid contaminating the outside of the container or the label with the specimen substance. The container must have a biohazard label to alert others that it holds potentially infectious material. Gloves should be worn throughout this procedure.
- Equipment requiring repair that has been contaminated with blood or body fluids should be decontaminated before being repaired in the office or transported for repair. There is no documented evidence of HIV transmission from contaminated environmental surfaces, but surface contamination is a proven mode of transmission of HBV.
- Smoking, eating, drinking, applying cosmetics or lip balm, and handling contact lenses are prohibited in work areas where there is a reasonable likelihood of contamination by pathogens.
- Food and beverages cannot be kept in refrigerators, freezers, or cabinets or on countertops where infectious materials could be present.

Housekeeping Controls. The Bloodborne Pathogens Standard requires certain housekeeping measures to ensure a sanitary work area. A schedule must be posted for the cleaning and decontaminating of each work area where exposures could occur. Documentation of these procedures must include information about the surface cleaned, the type of waste encountered, and procedures performed in the designated area.

- After accidental spills of blood or body fluids, at the end of each procedure, and at the end of each shift, work surfaces must be immediately cleaned and then disinfected with a **disinfectant** (dis in FEK tuh nt) registered with the Environmental Protection Agency (EPA).
- All reusable containers must be disinfected and decontaminated on a routine basis.
- Sharps containers must be kept as close as possible to the work area. Never attempt to reach inside a sharps container, and do not overfill them. Replace containers on a routine basis, and be certain that the lid is closed securely before preparing them for biohazard waste disposal.
- Never pick up spilled material or broken glassware with the hands. Brooms, brushes, dustpans, and pickup tongs or forceps should be used. The material should be placed immediately into an **impervious** (im PUR vee uh s) biohazard waste container at the spill site (Fig. 28.7). Use an absorbent, professional biohazard spill preparation as directed to decontaminate the site.
- Handle soiled linen as little as possible and always wear gloves or other protective equipment during disposal. Linens soiled with blood or body fluids should be double-bagged and transported in labeled, leakproof biohazard bags.
- Contaminated materials and/or infectious waste must be handled with extreme caution to prevent exposure. Biohazard waste must be collected in impermeable, red polyethylene or polypropylene biohazard-labeled bags or containers and sealed (Fig. 28.8). This waste must be disposed of in accordance with all federal, state, and local regulations. Disposal methods include treatment by heat, incineration, steam sterilization, chemical treatment, or other equivalent methods that will render the waste inactive before it is placed in a landfill.

For additional information about the disposal of biologic chemical materials, see Box 28.11.

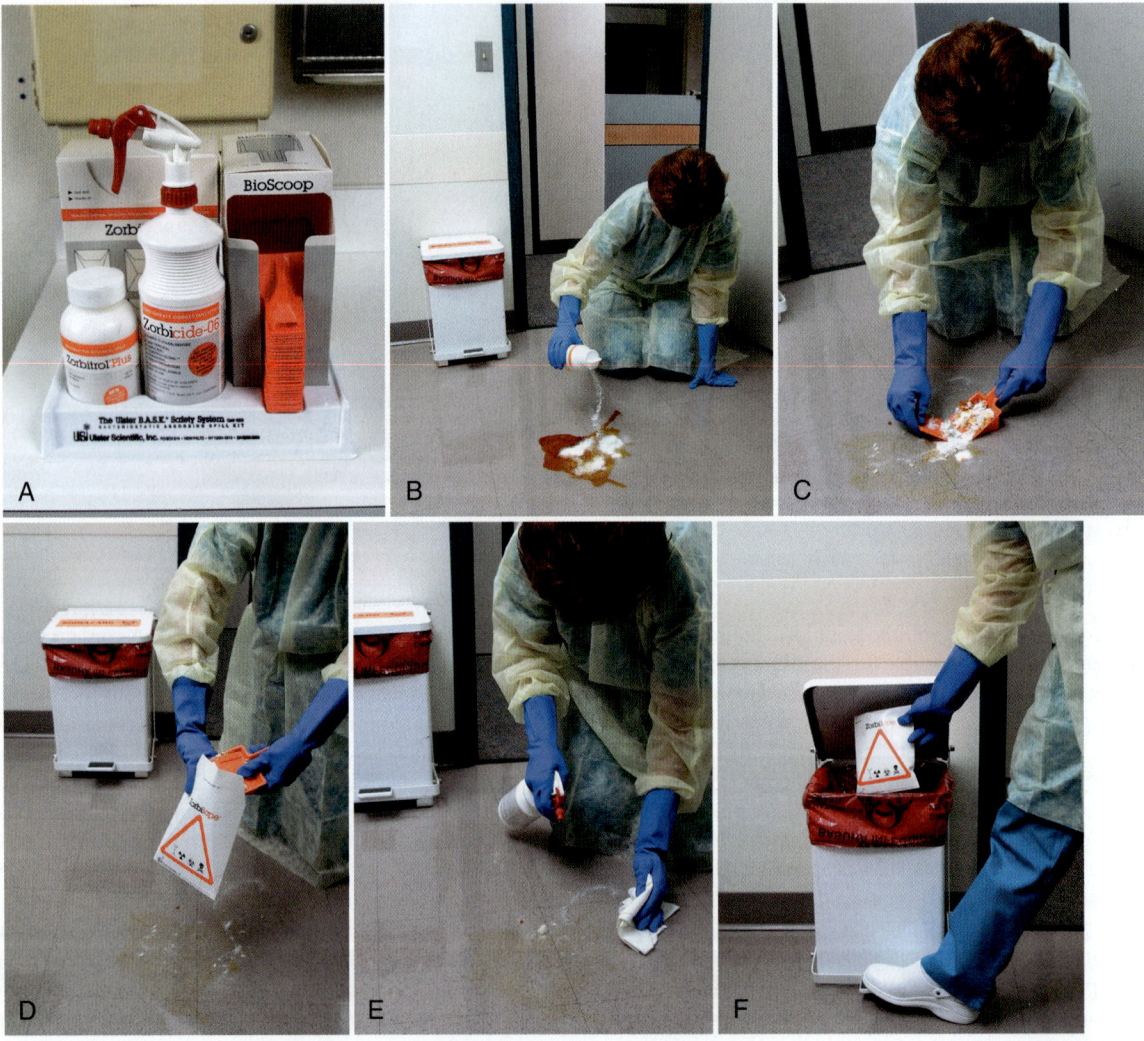

FIG. 28.7 Cleaning up spilled material. (A) Cleanup kit with printed instructions. (B) Sprinkle congealing powder over the spill. (C) Scoop up the spill. (D) Place the contents in a biohazard bag. (E) Wipe the area thoroughly with a germicide. (F) Place all contaminated material in a biohazard bag or container. (From Proctor D, et al: *Kinn's The Medical Assistant,* ed 13, St. Louis, 2017, Elsevier.)

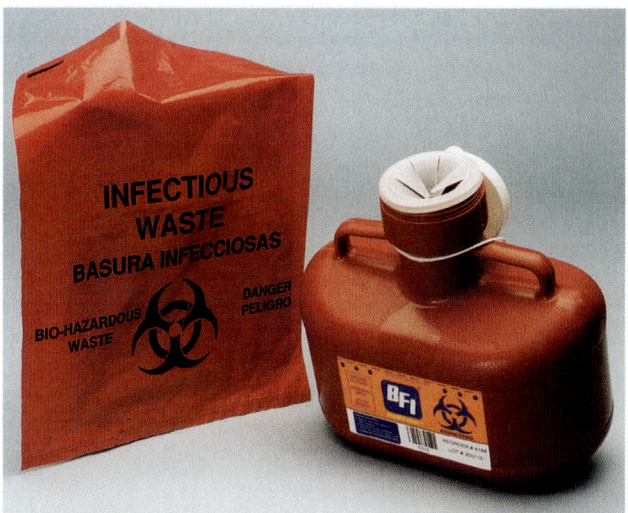

FIG. 28.8 Biohazard bag and biohazard sharps container. (From Proctor D, et al: *Kinn's The Medical Assistant*, ed 13, St. Louis, 2017, Elsevier.)

> **CRITICAL THINKING 28.5**
>
> Your office manager asks you to prepare a fact sheet for your coworkers that summarizes the details of OSHA's Bloodborne Pathogens Standard. What should you include?

Hepatitis B Vaccination. HBV vaccination must be available free of charge to all employees at risk for occupational exposure to bloodborne pathogens, within 10 days of starting employment. The vaccine is given by intramuscular injection in three doses. The second injection is given 4 weeks after the first, and the third injection 6 months after the first. Boosters for the hepatitis B immunization are not currently recommended. However, if they are recommended in the future, boosters must be made available to eligible employees without cost.

After three doses of hepatitis B vaccine, more than 90% of healthy adults and more than 95% of infants, children, and adolescents develop adequate antibody responses. Despite this, healthcare workers with a high risk of exposure should have a titer drawn after completing the series to determine whether they have antibodies against the disease. Antibody testing should be done 1 to 2 months after completion of the vaccine series. If the employee did not respond to the first series, or if the series was not completed, revaccination with a second three-dose series is recommended. If antibodies still do not develop, no further vaccination is given.

Employees have the right to decline hepatitis B immunization, but they are required to sign a declination form (Fig. 28.9) that is kept on file as a record of their refusal. The statement can be signed only after the employee has received training about the following:
- Hepatitis B and the hepatitis B vaccination
- Safety, route of administration, and benefits of vaccination

In addition, the employee must be informed that the vaccine will be administered free of charge. Employees who change their mind may receive the vaccine at a future date free of charge.

Postexposure Follow-Up. If an employee is exposed through an accidental needlestick, a human bite, exposure to broken skin, or from a splash or splatter onto mucous membranes, such as the eyes, certain procedures must be followed. The following specific steps should be taken after exposure to contaminated waste:
- Immediately, or as soon as possible after exposure, the worker should wash or flush the exposed area.
- The exposure incident must be immediately reported to the supervisor.
- The employee must immediately receive a confidential medical evaluation. The provider caring for the exposed employee must receive written details of the exposure incident, including the route and circumstances surrounding the incident. All documentation related to the exposure must do the following:
  - Remain confidential.
  - Not be disclosed to any individual without the employee's express written permission.
  - Be kept for at least the duration of the worker's employment plus 30 years.
- An incident report must be filed that documents the details surrounding the exposure incident, the route or type of exposure, and the identity, if known, of the source individual. The source individual is the person, living or dead, whose blood or potentially infectious material was the source of the occupational exposure.
- The source individual is screened for HBV, hepatitis C virus (HCV), and HIV. Depending on state regulations, consent may or may not be required from the source individual to perform the screening. If

---

BOX 28.11 Protocols for Disposal of Biologic Chemical Materials

The Medical Waste Tracking Act set the standards for governmental regulation of medical waste; however, that law expired in 1991. The states were then given responsibility for regulating the disposal of medical waste. Each state varies in its degree of regulation, ranging from no regulation to strict rules. The following are some examples of regulations covering the disposal of hazardous materials:

- Biomedical waste should be collected in containers that are leakproof and strong enough to prevent breakage during handling; the containers must be labeled with the biohazard symbol.
- Workers who handle biomedical waste should observe Standard Precautions.
- Biologic waste containers and boxes should not be held in the healthcare facility for longer than 30 days.
- Sharps are instruments intended to cut or penetrate the skin; they include lancets, scalpel blades, needles, and syringe/needle combinations. Sharps must be placed in red, hard plastic sharps boxes after use; sharps boxes should be closed when three-fourths full.
- Boxes for disposal of chemicals should be labeled with the chemicals' names and any other pertinent data; they must be adequately sealed to prevent breakage or leakage.
- Each healthcare facility must hire a biomedical waste disposal service whose employees are trained to collect and haul away biomedical waste in special containers (usually cardboard boxes or reusable plastic bins) for treatment at a facility designed to handle biomedical waste.

The cost to the healthcare facility for biomedical waste disposal is typically based on the weight of the contaminated items collected (i.e., the weight of filled sharps containers, biohazard boxes, and bags).

VOCABULARY

disinfectant: Any chemical agent used on nonliving objects to destroy or inhibit the growth of harmful organisms; not effective against bacterial spores.

impervious: Not permitting penetration.

Hepatitis B Vaccine Declination

I understand that due to my occupational exposure to blood or other potentially infectious materials I may be at risk of acquiring hepatitis B virus (HBV) infection. I have been given the opportunity to be vaccinated with hepatitis B vaccine, at no charge to myself. However, I decline hepatitis B vaccination at this time. I understand that by declining this vaccine, I continue to be at risk of acquiring hepatitis B, a serious disease. If in the future I continue to have occupational exposure to blood or other potentially infectious materials and I want to be vaccinated with hepatitis B vaccine, I can receive the vaccination series at no charge to me.

Name: _____ Date: _____

FIG. 28.9 Sample hepatitis B declination form. (From the Occupational Safety and Health Administration, https://www.osha.gov/SLTC/etools/hospital/hazards/bbp/declination.html.)

BOX 28.12 Postexposure Management

- *Hepatitis B virus (HBV):* Hepatitis B vaccine series started in any unvaccinated person; postexposure prophylaxis (PEP) with hepatitis B immune globulin or hepatitis B vaccine series if the postvaccination antibody test is negative.
- *Hepatitis C virus (HCV):* Immune globulin and antiviral agents (e.g., interferon with or without ribavirin) are not recommended for PEP of hepatitis C; determine the HCV status of the source and the exposed person; provide follow-up HCV testing for the employee if the source is HCV positive.
- *Human immunodeficiency virus (HIV):* Four-week PEP regimen of two drugs (zidovudine [ZDV] and lamivudine [3TC], 3TC and stavudine [d4T], or didanosine [ddI] and d4T) for most HIV exposures, and a third drug for HIV exposures that pose an increased risk for transmission; employees should receive follow-up counseling, postexposure testing, and medical evaluation, regardless of whether they receive PEP. After baseline testing at the time of exposure, follow-up testing could be performed at 6 weeks, 12 weeks, and 6 months after exposure.

consent is required but not given, the employer must document that consent was not received from the source individual. If screening is done, OSHA requires that the employee be informed of the results of the source individual's tests.

- The exposed employee is tested for HBV, HCV, and HIV if consent is given to determine whether the employee already has one of these infectious diseases. If the employee refuses the tests but blood is drawn, the sample must be stored 90 days for the worker to decide whether screening is wanted.
- If the employee has not been vaccinated against HBV, vaccination is offered.
- The injured employee must receive a copy of the healthcare provider's written opinion within 15 days of completion of the evaluation.
- The exposed employee must receive health counseling about the risk of illness or other adverse outcomes of exposure and the potential for and consequences of transmission of the disease to family, patients, and others.

Healthcare students are at risk for bloodborne pathogen exposure and should follow all OSHA guidelines designed to protect individuals from exposure. A complete, unabridged copy of OSHA's Bloodborne Pathogens Standard may be obtained at the OSHA website (www.osha.gov). For additional information on postexposure management, see Box 28.12.

The CDC has developed a checklist that ambulatory care facilities can use to systematically assess employee adherence to infection prevention and to ensure that the facility has policies and procedures in place and has adequate supplies available to prevent infections at the site. If the answer to any of the questions is no, the facility must do all it can to correct the problems with either staff or supplies (Table 28.1).

For information about the risk of infection after an occupational exposure, see Box 28.13.

BOX 28.13 Risk of Infection After an Occupational Exposure

Hepatitis B Virus (HBV)
Healthcare workers who have received hepatitis B vaccine and have developed immunity to the virus are at virtually no risk for infection. For an unvaccinated person, the risk from a single needlestick or a cut exposure to HBV-infected blood ranges from 6% to 30%.

Hepatitis C Virus (HCV)
The estimated risk for infection after a needlestick or cut exposure to HCV-infected blood is approximately 1.8%. The risk after a blood splash is unknown but is believed to be very small.

Human Immunodeficiency Virus (HIV)
The average risk for HIV infection after a needlestick or cut exposure to HIV-infected blood is about 0.23%; the risk after exposure of the eye, nose, or mouth is near zero; the risk after exposure of the skin to HIV-infected blood is estimated to be less than 0.1%.

From the Occupational Safety and Health Administration, https://www.cdc.gov/hiv/workplace/healthcareworkers.html.

ASEPTIC TECHNIQUES: PREVENTING DISEASE TRANSMISSION

Asepsis (ey SEP sis) means free from infection or infectious material. *Medical asepsis* is defined as the destruction of disease-causing organisms. By using principles of medical asepsis, we can prevent the spread of disease. The goal is to eliminate or minimize pathogens by following OSHA's Bloodborne Pathogens Standard and disinfecting objects as soon as possible after contamination. This creates a healthcare environment as free of pathogens as possible.

Surgical asepsis is the destruction of all organisms. This technique is used for any procedure that enters the body's skin or tissues, such as surgery or injections. Anytime the skin or a mucous membrane is

CRITICAL THINKING 28.6

Rosa's office has been especially busy today. While administering an injection to a frightened 6-year-old child, a coworker accidentally sticks herself with the needle. She tells Rosa about the incident, but she does not know what to do next. What steps should be taken to manage the situation?

TABLE 28.1 Modified CDC Infection Prevention Checklist[a]

Facility Policies	Practice Performed		If Answer Is No, Document Plan for Remediation
1. Administrative Policies and Facility Practices			
a. Written infection prevention policies and procedures are available, current, and based on evidence-based guideline, regulations, or standards.	Yes	No	
b. Infection prevention policies and procedures are reassessed at least annually or according to state or federal requirements, and updated if appropriate.	Yes	No	
c. At least one individual trained in infection prevention is employed by or regularly available to the facility.	Yes	No	
d. Supplies necessary for adherence to Standard Precautions are readily available.	Yes	No	
e. Healthcare personnel for whom contact with blood or other potentially infectious material is anticipated are trained on the OSHA bloodborne pathogens standard upon hire and at least annually.	Yes	No	
f. The facility maintains a log of needlesticks, sharps injuries, and other employee exposure events.	Yes	No	
g. Following an exposure event, postexposure evaluation and follow-up, including prophylaxis as appropriate, are available at no cost to employee.	Yes	No	
h. Hepatitis B vaccination is available at no cost to all employees at risk of occupational exposure.	Yes	No	
i. Postvaccination screening for hepatitis B surface antibodies is conducted.	Yes	No	
j. All personnel are offered annual influenza vaccination at no cost.	Yes	No	
k. All personnel with potential exposure to tuberculosis (TB) are screened for TB upon hire and annually (if negative).	Yes	No	
2. Surveillance and Disease Reporting			
a. Updated list of reportable diseases is readily available to all personnel.	Yes	No	
3. Hand Hygiene			
a. Facility provides training and supplies necessary for adherence to hand hygiene.	Yes	No	
4. Personal Protective Equipment (PPE)			
a. Facility provides training and supplies for appropriate PPE.	Yes	No	
b. Impermeable gowns are worn during procedures where contact with blood or body fluids is anticipated.	Yes	No	
c. PPE is removed and discarded prior to leaving the exam room.	Yes	No	
d. Hand hygiene is performed immediately after removal of PPE.	Yes	No	
5. Environmental Cleaning			
a. Policies and procedures exist for routine cleaning and disinfection of environmental surfaces.	Yes	No	
b. Cleaning procedures are periodically monitored and assessed to ensure that they are consistently and correctly performed.	Yes	No	
c. The facility has a policy/procedure for decontamination of spills of blood or other body fluids.	Yes	No	

[a]The complete checklist is available at the CDC website for Infection Prevention in Outpatient Settings: Modified from the Occupational Safety and Health Administration, www.cdc.gov/HAI/settings/outpatient/checklist/outpatient-care-checklist.html.

punctured, pierced, or incised, surgical aseptic techniques are practiced. Everything that comes in contact with the patient should be sterile:
- Gowns
- Drapes
- Instruments
- Gloves

Minor surgery, urinary catheterization, injections, and some specimen collections, such as blood collection and biopsies, are performed using surgical aseptic technique.

Because skin cannot be sterilized, the goal of hand hygiene is to reduce the amount of microorganisms. Hand washing uses mechanical friction, soap, and warm, running water. Alcohol-based hand sanitizers are also effective in reducing the number of microorganisms. The alcohol kills the microorganisms. If the hands are visibly soiled, hand washing should be done.

Normally, two types of microorganisms are found on the skin: normal *resident flora* (REZ i duh nt FLOHR uh) and *transient flora* (TRAN see ent FLOHR uh). Normal resident flora lives harmlessly on the skin.

Transient flora includes bacteria, viruses, and other organisms picked up on the hands. Resident flora is firmly attached to the skin, whereas transient flora is not. This means that transient flora is easily removed by thorough hand hygiene, preventing the transfer to patients.

The most effective barrier against infection is intact skin. If the skin and mucous membranes are intact, medical asepsis can be used for most **noninvasive procedures**, such as pelvic and proctologic examinations. Instruments and objects used in medical aseptic procedures must be sanitized and disinfected or sterilized before being used on another patient. Medical aseptic procedures may include the use of gowns and masks, but these are not sterile and are worn to protect the healthcare worker more than the patient.

Another practical application of medical aseptic technique is to set up work areas in the medical office's laboratory. One side of the laboratory is the "clean" side, where only noninfectious procedures are performed. The other side is the "dirty" side, where potentially infectious materials are processed or cleaned.

Hand Hygiene

Hand hygiene (HAHY jeen) can be accomplished in two different ways. If the hands are visibly soiled, they must be washed using a medical aseptic technique. If the hands are not visibly soiled, alcohol-based hand sanitizer can be used. Hand hygiene, using the correct technique, must be done before and after each patient is examined or treated, and also when stipulated by the Bloodborne Pathogens Standard.

When washing hands for the first time in the morning, at least 1 minute should be spent on the scrub. For subsequent hand washing, the CDC recommends 15 seconds. Each office sink should be equipped with a liquid soap dispenser. A water-soluble lotion may be rubbed into the hands after they have been washed and dried. Dry, cracked, chapped skin is no longer intact and can provide a means of entry for microorganisms.

Proper hand washing depends on two factors: running water and friction. The water should be warm. Water that is too hot or too cold causes the skin to become chapped. Friction is the firm rubbing of all surfaces of the hands and wrists. Remember that your fingers have four sides, and fingernails have two sides. For medical aseptic hand washing, all jewelry except a plain wedding band is removed. A wristwatch may be left on if it can be moved up on the forearm away from the wrist area. The hands are washed under running water with the fingertips pointing downward. Soap and friction are applied to the hands and wrists. The water is allowed to wash debris away from the wrists and down toward the fingertips (see Procedure 28.2).

When using an alcohol-based hand sanitizer, it should take 20 to 30 seconds to rub all it into the skin. Be sure to cover all surfaces and continue rubbing it in until your hands are dry (Procedure 28.2). Evidence suggests that hand hygiene with an alcohol-based hand sanitizer is more effective at reducing **nosocomial** (nos uh KOH mee uh l) **infections** than plain hand washing. Antimicrobial-impregnated wipes (e.g., towelettes) are not a substitute for an alcohol-based hand sanitizer or soap.

Remember, the goal of hand hygiene is to protect you from infection and prevent cross-contamination from one patient to another (Box 28.14).

According to the CDC, proper hand hygiene must be performed in the following instances even if disposable gloves are worn:
- Before and after contact with the patient or his or her immediate care environment
- Before performing an aseptic task (e.g., giving an injection, drawing blood)
- After contact with blood, body fluids, or contaminated surfaces
- When hands move from a contaminated body site to a clean body site during patient care

Sanitization

Instruments and other items used in the healthcare facility must be carefully cleaned before proceeding with disinfection or sterilization. *Sanitization* (SAN i tah zaa shun) is the cleaning process that reduces the number of microorganisms to a safe level. This cleansing process removes debris such as blood and other body fluids from instruments or equipment. This debris can protect the microorganisms from disinfection or sterilization (Procedure 28.3).

The medical assistant should always wear gloves while performing sanitization. Thick utility gloves will help protect your hands when working with instruments that have sharp or pointed edges. Gloves prevent possible personal contamination with OPIM that may be present on the articles being cleaned. The procedure should be completed immediately after use of the instruments. A separate workroom or on the "dirty" side of the utility room is used to prevent cross-contamination of clean instruments and equipment. If sanitization cannot be done immediately, rinse the used items under cold water immediately after the procedure and place them in a detergent solution. Never allow blood or other substances to dry on an instrument.

When you are ready to sanitize instruments, rinse each instrument in cold running water. Sharp instruments should be kept separate from the other instruments. Metal instruments may damage the cutting edges, and sharp instruments may damage other instruments or injure you. Clean all sharp instruments at the same time, when you can concentrate on preventing injury. Open all hinges, and scrub serrations and ratchets with a small scrub brush or toothbrush. Rinse the instruments in hot water, and then check carefully that they are in proper working order before they are disinfected or sterilized. The items should be hand dried with a towel to prevent spotting and allowed to air dry before further processing.

Sanitization is a very important step, and it cannot be overlooked or done carelessly. The use of disposable instruments minimizes the need for sanitization, disinfection, and sterilization.

Ultrasonic Sanitization. Sound waves can be used to sanitize instruments. The instruments are placed in an ultrasonic bath of cleaner and

---

BOX 28.14   When to Use Hand Hygiene

Medical aseptic hand washing or alcohol-based hand sanitizer should be used in the following situations:
- After you finish with one patient and before you attend to another patient
- After you finish handling one specimen and before you handle another specimen
- After you use toilet facilities
- Whenever you touch something that causes your hands to become contaminated
- When you arrive at work and before you leave the facility
- Before and after eating

VOCABULARY

noninvasive procedures: Procedures that do not penetrate human tissue.
nosocomial infections: Infections acquired in a healthcare setting.

PROCEDURE 28.3 Sanitizing Soiled Instruments

Task
Remove all contaminated matter from instruments in preparation for disinfection or sterilization while following Standard Precautions and wearing appropriate personal protective equipment (PPE).

Equipment and Supplies
- Sink with cold and hot running water
- Sanitizing agent or low-sudsing soap with enzymatic action
- Decontminated utility gloves that show no signs of deterioration
- Chin-length face shield or goggles and face mask if contamination with bloodborne pathogens is possible
- Impermeable gown
- Disposable brush
- Disposable paper towels
- Utility gloves
- Disinfectant cleaner prepared according to the manufacturer's directions
- Covered waste container with foot pedal
- Biohazard waste container with labeled red biohazard bag

Procedural Steps
1. Put on an impermeable gown and face shield or goggles and mask if potential for splashing of infectious material exists (Fig. 1).
   Purpose: To provide personal protection against potentially infectious matter.

   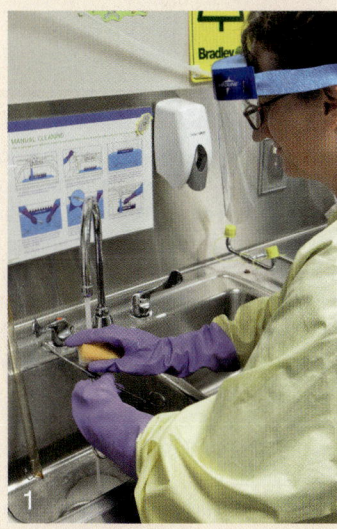

2. Put on utility gloves.
   Purpose: To provide personal protection against potentially infectious matter and sharp instruments.
3. Separate the sharp instruments from other instruments to be sanitized.
   Purpose: To prevent possible self-injury and exposure to infectious matter.
4. Rinse the instruments under cold running water.
   Purpose: To help remove debris and body fluids.
5. Open hinged instruments and scrub all grooves, crevices, and serrations with a disposable brush (Fig. 2).
   Purpose: Microorganisms can hide under contaminants and may not be destroyed by the disinfection process.

   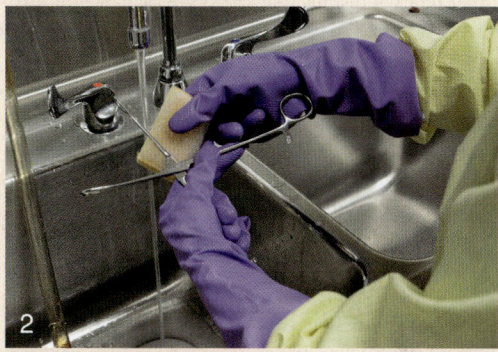

6. Rinse well with hot water.
   Purpose: Hot water removes all soap and contaminant residue.
7. Towel-dry all instruments thoroughly, and dispose of contaminated towels and disposable brush in a biohazard waste container. Do not touch the paper towel dispenser as you are obtaining towels.
   Purpose: All contaminated material must be discarded in a labeled biohazard container or a labeled red biohazard bag. Touching the dispenser with the utility gloves contaminates the dispenser. Wet instruments can rust or become dull.
8. Remove the utility gloves, and wash your hands according to Procedure 28.1.
   Purpose: To remove any possible contaminants.
9. Towel-dry your hands and put on gloves. Decontaminate the utility gloves and work surfaces using disinfectant.
   Purpose: To prevent personal exposure to contaminants. All equipment and working surfaces should be cleaned and decontaminated with a disinfectant to prevent transmission of infectious organisms.
10. Dispose of the contaminated towels in a covered waste container.
    Purpose: All contaminated material must be disposed of in a labeled biohazard container or a labeled red biohazard bag.
11. Place sanitized instruments in a designated area for disinfection or sterilization.
    Purpose: Sanitized instruments must be removed from the cleaning area to prevent possible cross-contamination.
12. Remove the gloves according to Procedure 28.2. Dispose of the gloves in a biohazard waste container. Sanitize the hands.
    Purpose: To prevent the spread of infectious organisms and to remove any possible contaminants.

water. Sound waves cause the solution to vibrate, which loosens the materials attached to the instruments. Ultrasonic cleaners are beneficial because they do not damage even the most delicate instruments, and workers do not run the risk of an accidental sharps injury.

Disinfection

Disinfection is the process of killing pathogenic organisms or of rendering them inactive. It is not always effective against spores, tuberculosis bacilli, and certain viruses. Some disinfectant chemicals can kill microbes within a short time, but they are usually hard on instruments. Some chemicals, such as Cidex, are effective enough to kill all organisms, but the usual immersion time for these sterilants is 10 hours or longer. For exam tables and countertop surfaces, there are two common disinfectants: hydrogen peroxide and bleach. Both are low cost and are effective.

Many other types of disinfecting agents are available for instruments and equipment (Box 28.15). It is important to follow the manufacturer's guidelines on the following factors:
- How to use each product properly
- Advantages and disadvantages
- Possible sources of error

Here are common errors that can cause chemicals to lose their effectiveness:
- Instruments are not thoroughly sanitized. Attached organic matter inhibits or prevents the action of the disinfectant. No chemical can kill unless it reaches all instrument surfaces; therefore complete sanitization is absolutely necessary.
- The disinfectant solution is left in an open container, and evaporation changes its concentration.
- Solutions are not changed after the recommended period for use has expired.
- Solutions are not prepared properly or are not mixed properly before use.
- The manufacturer's recommended temperature for use and storage is not maintained.

Chemical disinfectants cannot be used on skin or tissues because they can damage them. Therefore antiseptics, such as alcohol, are used on the skin to reduce the number of pathogens. Alcohol is the most widely used antiseptic, but studies indicate that it is not as effective as other products in inhibiting the growth and reproduction of microorganisms on the skin's surface. Other antiseptic chemicals, such as povidone-iodine solution (Betadine), are effective antimicrobial agents that are safe to use on a patient's skin.

> **MEDICAL TERMINOLOGY**
> **-scope:** instrument to view
> **sigmoid/o:** sigmoid colon

Sterilization

Sterilization is essential for surgical asepsis. Sterilization can be achieved with moist heat, dry heat, ultraviolet, ionizing radiation, gas, or chemicals. Medical facilities typically use the autoclave method, which uses moist heat. Steam under pressure in the autoclave offers an excellent method of sterilization because it kills all pathogens and spores. You will learn more about surgical asepsis and the sterilization process in Chapter 34.

> **CRITICAL THINKING 28.7**
> Rosa is responsible for the orientation of the new medical assistant in the office's sanitization and disinfection procedures. Outline the important concepts and methods of each one.

> **BOX 28.15 Levels of Disinfectants**
> The CDC defines three levels of disinfectants:
> - Low-level disinfectants can kill most vegetative bacteria, some fungi, and some viruses. Used for exam tables and countertops. Example: hydrogen peroxide.
> - Intermediate-level disinfectants can kill mycobacteria, vegetative bacteria, most viruses, and most fungi, but they do not kill spores. Used for noncritical items such as stethoscopes and percussion hammers. Example: isopropyl alcohol.
> - High-level disinfectants will kill all microorganisms except large numbers of bacterial spores. Used for semicritical items such as a flexible fiberoptic *sigmoidoscope*. Example: Cidex OPA.

ROLE OF THE MEDICAL ASSISTANT IN ASEPSIS

Asepsis is one of the few procedures that will directly affect the health of the patient, the provider, and the staff. The spread of pathogens in the ambulatory care setting can be controlled only through the effective, consistent application of the Bloodborne Pathogens Standard and by proper sanitization, disinfection, and sterilization of supplies, equipment, and work surfaces.

The medical assistant must develop the skills needed for performing aseptic procedures properly. It is important that these techniques be done on such a routine basis that they become an unbreakable habit. The use of disposable items is highly recommended for infection control purposes. However, when disposable equipment is used, the assistant must follow recommended disposal guidelines to ensure infection control.

> **EXCEPTIONAL CUSTOMER SERVICE**
> The medical assistant should take every opportunity to educate patients about the infection process and ways to prevent the transmission of disease. The best time to instruct a patient in aseptic techniques that can be used at home is while performing the aseptic procedure. Consider these examples:
> - While washing your hands, explain to the patient that this routine is particularly important for patients who are very young or old or who seem to get sick frequently. Instruct the patient that the hands should be washed before and after meals; after sneezing, coughing, or blowing the nose; after using the restroom; before and after changing a dressing; and after changing an infant's diaper.
> - Advise the patient to carry an alcohol-based hand sanitizer and to use it as indicated throughout the day.
> - Explain to the patient that coughing or sneezing into a bent elbow is an effective method for preventing the spread of disease.
> - Instruct the patient in the differences between sterile and clean dressings and bandages. Demonstrate each step in changing a dressing properly, and explain how to dispose of contaminated items.
>
> A medical assistant can help patients live healthier lives in many ways. For example, here are a few more suggestions for teaching the patient about asepsis and infection control:
> - Set up an information table in the waiting room with take-home pamphlets and literature.
> - Mail, email, or post on the healthcare facility's website a periodic newsletter to patients about infection control, especially during flu season.
> - Demonstrate and explain aseptic procedures to patients and family members, inviting them to participate.

CLOSING COMMENTS

One of the medical assistant's main responsibilities is to perform sanitization, disinfection, and sterilization procedures with precision and total effectiveness. There is no room for compromise. These procedures have a huge impact on infection control. Patients should have absolute confidence that they are being treated in an aseptic atmosphere and under aseptic conditions. This assurance is just as important for the protection of the provider and staff as it is for the patient. Allowing the provider to assume that the correct aseptic techniques were used when preparing a procedure and allowing him or her to use contaminated equipment on a patient may result in a malpractice lawsuit. Honesty on the part of the medical assistant builds self-respect and contributes to professional achievement.

CHAPTER REVIEW

To understand infection control, you must first know what can cause disease. The different pathogenic microorganisms include viruses, bacteria, fungi, protozoa, and helminths. The chain of infection starts with those infectious agents. In order for it to grow, the pathogen must have a reservoir host that provides all of the proper conditions. The next link in the chain is the means or portal of exit, mode of transmission, and means or portal of entry. It ends with a susceptible host. Breaking any one of those links will stop the spread of infection.

If someone does become infected with a pathogen, the inflammatory response and the immune response will try to take care of the pathogen. Cell-mediated and humoral immune responses do battle with the pathogen.

OSHA standards have been developed to reduce the risk of infection for both patients and healthcare professionals. Following the Bloodborne Pathogens Standard is crucial for infection control.

Sanitization is washing with soap and water to remove blood and other debris so that disinfection and sterilization can occur. Disinfection removes most pathogens but is not effective against spores. Sterilization is destruction of all microbial life.

SCENARIO WRAP-UP

Implementing Standard Precautions throughout daily practice is crucial to the welfare and protection of both the patient and the healthcare worker. Rosa must be sure to wash her hands routinely or to use an alcohol-based hand sanitizer. She also must familiarize herself with the office's exposure control plan, follow OSHA's Bloodborne Pathogens Standard, use PPE when needed, follow environmental protection guidelines, use appropriate procedures for cleaning up contaminated spills and other housekeeping controls, and understand postexposure follow-up if an accidental exposure occurs. In addition, Rosa must follow guidelines for sanitization, disinfection, and sterilization of appropriate instruments and equipment.

29

Vital Signs

LEARNING OBJECTIVES

1. Do the following related to temperature:
   - Cite the average body temperature for various age groups.
   - Describe emotional and physical factors that can cause body temperature to rise and fall.
   - Convert temperature readings between the Fahrenheit and Celsius scales.
   - Obtain and record an accurate patient temperature using three different types of thermometers.
2. Do the following related to pulse:
   - Cite the average pulse rate for various age groups.
   - Describe pulse rate, volume, and rhythm.
   - Locate and record pulse at multiple sites.
3. Do the following related to respiration:
   - Cite the average respiratory rate for various age groups.
   - Demonstrate the best way to obtain an accurate respiratory count.
4. Do the following related to blood pressure:
   - Cite the approximate blood pressure range for various age groups.
   - Specify physiologic factors that affect blood pressure.
   - Differentiate between essential and secondary hypertension.
   - Interpret current hypertension guidelines and treatment.
   - Describe how to determine the correct cuff size for individual patients.
   - Identify the different Korotkoff phases.
   - Accurately measure and document blood pressure.
5. Discuss and perform pulse oximetry.
6. Accurately measure and document height and weight, use the body mass index scale, and convert kilograms to pounds and pounds to kilograms.

CHAPTER OUTLINE

1. **Opening Scenario,** 637
2. **You Will Learn,** 637
3. **Introduction,** 637
4. **Factors That May Influence Vital Signs,** 637
5. **Temperature,** 637
   a. Fever, 638
6. **Sites,** 638
   a. Types of Thermometers and Their Uses, 639
      i. *Digital Thermometer,* 639
      ii. *Tympanic Thermometer,* 640
      iii. *Temporal Artery Thermometer,* 640
7. **Pulse,** 641
   a. Pulse Sites, 643
   b. Characteristics of a Pulse, 646
      i. *Rate,* 646
      ii. *Rhythm,* 646
      iii. *Volume,* 646
   c. Determining the Pulse Rate, 648
      i. *Radial and Apical Pulse Rates,* 648
      ii. *Femoral, Popliteal, and Pedal Pulses,* 649
8. **Respiration,** 649
   a. Characteristics of Respirations, 649
   b. Counting Respirations, 650
9. **Blood Pressure,** 651
   a. Factors Affecting Blood Pressure, 651
   b. Evaluating the Blood Pressure, 651
   c. Measuring Blood Pressure, 653
      i. *Effects of Body Position on Blood Pressure Measurement,* 654
   d. Korotkoff Sounds, 656
      i. *Phase I,* 656
      ii. *Phase II,* 656
      iii. *Phase III,* 656
      iv. *Phase IV,* 656
      v. *Phase V,* 657
   e. Palpatory Method, 657
10. **Pulse Oximetry,** 658
11. **Anthropometric Measurements,** 658
    a. Measuring Weight and Height, 658
       i. *Weight,* 660
       ii. *Height,* 661
12. **Closing Comments,** 661
13. **Chapter Review,** 661
14. **Scenario Wrap-Up,** 661

CHAPTER 29 Vital Signs

OPENING SCENARIO

Carlos Ricci, CMA (AAMA), is a certified medical assistant that works at Walden-Martin Family Medical (WMFM) Clinic. Carlos graduated from a medical assistant program 3 years ago and enjoys the variety of patients and the patient contact involved in working on the clinical side of WMFM Clinic. One of Carlos' primary responsibilities is to accurately measure and record each patient's vital signs before the patient is seen. Over the past 3 years, he has come to understand the importance of taking accurate vital sign measurements, and accurately documenting those results.

YOU WILL LEARN

1. To recognize why vital signs are an important part of the patient examination.
2. To identify the factors that can affect vital signs and how to minimize them.
3. To list the three most common types of thermometers and describe how they should be used.
4. To locate the pulse sites.
5. To identify the characteristics of a pulse and describe what must be assessed.
6. To identify the characteristics of respirations and describe what must be assessed.
7. To evaluate blood pressure.
8. To define Korotkoff sounds.
9. To define pulse oximetry.
10. To accurately determine a patient's height and weight.

INTRODUCTION

Almost every patient who visits the healthcare facility will have some vital signs measured. These signs are the body's indicators of internal **homeostasis** (hoh mee oh STAY sis) and the patient's general state of health. Medical assistants are often responsible for obtaining these measurements. It is crucial that they have confidence in the theory and practical applications of vital sign measurements. A medical assistant who understands the principles of and the reasons for these measurements is a valuable asset to any healthcare facility.

> **VOCABULARY**
> **homeostasis**: The internal environment of the body that is compatible with life. A steady state that is created by all the body systems working together to provide a consistent and unvarying internal environment.

Accuracy is essential. A change in one or more of the patient's vital signs may indicate a change in general health. Variations may suggest the presence or disappearance of a disease process. This may lead to changes in the treatment plan. Taking vital signs is a task that requires consistent attention to accuracy and detail. These findings are necessary to come up with a correct diagnosis. Vital signs should never be measured in an indifferent or casual manner. In addition to performing accurate measurement, care must be taken when documenting the findings in the patient's health record.

The *vital signs* are the patient's temperature, pulse, respiration, and blood pressure. These four signs are abbreviated *TPR* and *BP* and may be referred to as *cardinal signs*. Many organizations consider pulse oximetry, SpO$_2$, a vital sign also. The medical assistant must understand the significance of the vital signs and must measure and record them accurately. *Anthropometric* (an thruh POH me trik) *measurements* are not considered vital signs but are usually obtained at the same time as vital signs. These measurements include height, weight, body mass index (BMI), and other body measurements, such as fat composition.

FACTORS THAT MAY INFLUENCE VITAL SIGNS

Vital signs are influenced by many factors, both physical and emotional. A patient may have had a hot or cold beverage just before the examination or may be anxious or fearful about what the provider may find. For example, consider that a patient has been asked to return for a repeat Papanicolaou (Pap) test because the first one showed the presence of suspicious cells. The medical assistant measures the patient's blood pressure and finds it significantly elevated compared with previous readings. The patient may be anxious and concerned about the test results. The elevated blood pressure readings likely reflect her anxiety.

What impact would it have on a temperature reading if a patient could not find a parking place and had to walk four blocks to the office, knowing he would be late for his appointment? If you said it would be elevated, you are right. Certainly, this patient's metabolism would increase because of the physical exercise. As a result, his temperature would be elevated, along with his pulse, respirations, and blood pressure. The medical assistant should give the patient some time to recover from his sprint to the office before taking any vital sign measurements.

Vital signs are often altered if the patient is in pain. Pay attention to nonverbal signs that might indicate discomfort or pain, especially if the patient's blood pressure, pulse, and respirations are elevated. In addition, many patients are uneasy about being seen by the provider. This may alter vital signs. The medical assistant must help the patient relax before taking any readings. Measurements sometimes must be obtained a second time, after the patient is more calm or comfortable. For a better picture of the patient's vital signs, the medical assistant may be asked to take the vital signs twice: at the beginning of the visit and just before the patient leaves the examination room.

TEMPERATURE

Body temperature is defined as the balance between heat lost and heat produced by the body. It is measured in degrees Fahrenheit (F) or degrees Celsius (C). The process of chemical and physical change in the body that produces heat is called *metabolism*. Body temperature is a result of this process. The core body temperature is maintained within a normal range by the *hypothalamus* (hye puh THAL uh mus). The average body temperature varies from person to person and is different in each person at different times throughout the day. In a healthy adult, this **diurnal** (dahy UR nl) **variation** ranges from 97.7° to 99.5°F (36.5° to 37.5° C); the average daily temperature is 98.6°F (37°C). Body temperature is lowest in the morning and highest in the late afternoon. Factors that may affect body temperature include the following:

- *Age:* The body temperature of infants and young children **fluctuates** (FLUHK choo eyts) more rapidly in response to external environmental temperatures. Aging adults lose the insulation of subcutaneous fat and thermoregulatory control.
- *Stress and physical activity:* Both exercise and emotional stress can increase the metabolic rate, causing an elevation in temperature.
- *Gender:* Hormone secretions result in fluctuations of the core body temperature in women throughout the menstrual cycle.
- *External factors:* Smoking, drinking hot fluids, and chewing gum can temporarily elevate an oral temperature. Environmental factors can change body temperature as well. Cold weather tends to decrease body temperature and hot weather tends to increase it.

In illness, an individual's metabolic activity increases. This causes an increase in internal heat production, which in turn raises the body temperature. The increase in body temperature is thought to be the body's defensive reaction, because heat inhibits the growth of some bacteria and viruses.

When a fever is present, superficial blood vessels (those near the surface of the skin) constrict. The small papillary muscles at the base of hair follicles also constrict, creating goose bumps. Chills and shivering may follow, producing internal heat. As this process repeats itself, more heat is produced, and the body temperature rises above the normal range. When more heat is lost than is produced, the opposite effect occurs, and body temperature drops below the normal range.

Fever

Infection, either bacterial or viral, is the most common cause of fever in both children and adults.

Infants do not usually develop **febrile** (FEB ruh l) illnesses during the first 3 months of life; if one is present, it usually is very serious. However, fever, or **pyrexia** (pahy REK see uh), is very common in young children and accounts for an estimated 30% of office visits. Fevers are classified according to the 24-hour pattern they follow. The three most common patterns are as follows (Fig. 29.1):

- *Continuous fever*, which rises and falls only slightly during a 24-hour period. The temperature consistently remains above the patient's average normal temperature range and fluctuates less than 3 degrees.
- *Intermittent fever*, which comes and goes, alternating between elevated and normal levels.
- *Remittent fever*, which fluctuates considerably (i.e., by more than 3 degrees) and never returns to the normal range.

Variation from the patient's average body temperature range may be the first warning of an illness or a change in the patient's current condition. Patients with fever usually have the following indicators:
- Loss of appetite (*anorexia* [an uh REK see uh])
- Headache
- Thirst
- Flushed face
- Hot skin
- General **malaise**

Some patients experience an acute onset of chills and shivering, followed by an increase in body temperature. A serious possible complication in young children with high fevers is a febrile seizure. Medication to reduce the fever, or *antipyretic* drugs (e.g., acetaminophen or ibuprofen), should be taken as instructed to prevent dangerous spikes in temperature. Box 29.1 describes when a temperature is considered a fever.

SITES

Several types of thermometers and various sites can be used to take temperature readings. A digital thermometer is placed under the tongue, in the armpit, or in the rectum; a tympanic thermometer is inserted into the ear; and a temporal artery thermometer is moved across the forehead. Temperatures can be read in either Fahrenheit or Celsius (Box 29.2). Most thermometers will convert from one scale to the other. Average temperature values for adults are shown in Table 29.1.

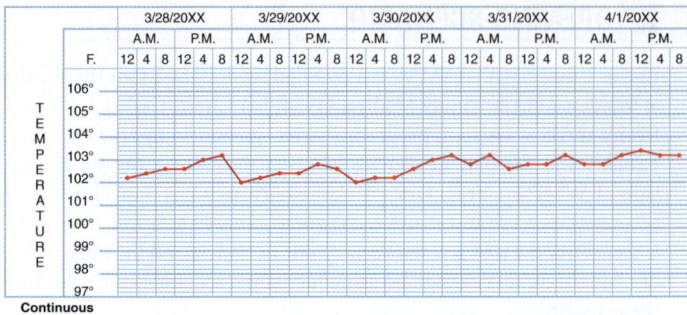
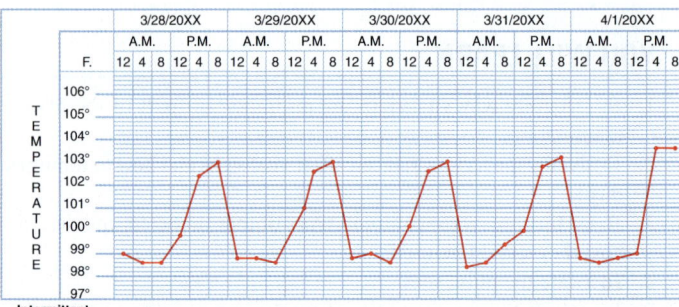
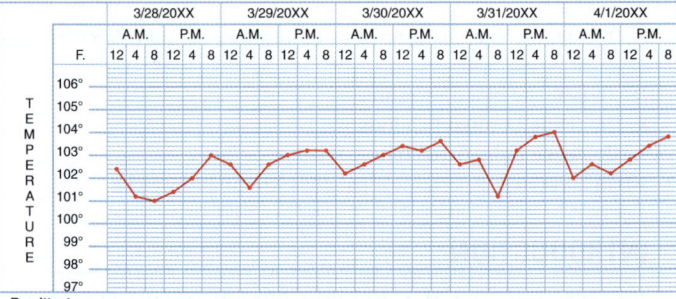

FIG. 29.1 Fever patterns.

BOX 29.1 Temperatures Considered Febrile

- Rectal, temporal, or *aural* (AWR uh l) (ear) temperature over 100.4°F (38°C)
- Oral temperature over 100°F (37.8°C)
- Axillary temperature over 99°F (37.2°C)

VOCABULARY
diurnal variation: Fluctuations that occur during each day.
febrile: Pertaining to an elevated body temperature.
fluctuate: To shift back and forth.
malaise: A condition of general bodily weakness or discomfort, often marking the onset of a disease.
pyrexia: A febrile condition or fever.

CRITICAL THINKING 29.1

Using the correct formula, convert the following temperatures from one system to the other (see Box 29.2):
1. 99°F = _____ °C
2. 102°F = _____ °C
3. 38°C = _____ °F
4. 39.5°C = _____ °F

BOX 29.2 Converting Temperatures

There are many options for converting temperatures between the Fahrenheit and Celsius scales. Most EHRs will do the conversion when the temperature is entered. There are online options as well. If you need to do the conversion manually, the following formulas will help you out.

Fahrenheit to Celsius
°C = (°F − 32)/1.8
Example: 101°F
°C = (101−32)/1.8
°C = 69/1.8
°C = 38.3

Celsius to Fahrenheit
°F = (°C × 1.8) + 32
Example: 39°C
°F = (39 × 1.8) + 32
°F = 70.2 + 32
°F = 102.2

TABLE 29.1 Average Adult Temperatures

Site	Fahrenheit	Celsius
Axillary	97.6°	36.4°
Oral	98.6°	37°
Tympanic	99.6°	37.6°
Rectal	99.6°	37.6°
Temporal artery	99.6°	37.6°

There are a number of factors to consider when determining which site should be used.

Factor	
Age	Birth–3 months: rectal or temporal artery
	3 months–4 years: rectal, axillary, temporal artery; after the age of 6 months a tympanic thermometer may be used
	4 years and older: oral, axillary, tympanic, temporal artery, rectal
Condition	Mouth breathing; oral is not an option
	Ear infection or occlusion; tympanic is not an option
	Diarrhea; rectal not an option
	Open wound or rash on forehead; temporal artery not an option
State of consciousness	If unconscious; oral not an option
Thermometers available in the facility	May only have one or two types of thermometers available
Healthcare facility procedures	Based on patient's condition or provider's preference

When an oral temperature is obtained, you do not have to indicate the site when documenting the reading in the patient's health record. If you use an alternate site, you should document the following identifiers after recording the temperature:
- (T) for tympanic
- (A) for axillary
- (R) for rectal
- (TA) for temporal artery

For example, T: 99.4°F (T) clarifies that an alternate site was used.

Axillary temperatures (A) are approximately 1°F (0.6°C) lower than oral readings because axillary readings are not taken in an enclosed body cavity. Tympanic, rectal, and temporal artery temperatures are approximately 1°F (0.6°C) higher than oral readings. The actual reading from the thermometer should be documented with the correct abbreviation for the site.

The oral site is not typically used with young children. This site requires the patient to hold the thermometer under the tongue and keep the mouth closed, a task that can be difficult for children under the age of 3. A rectal temperature is most often used for infants. It is important to use the proper technique to avoid damaging the rectal tissue (see Procedure 29.3, presented later). However, most pediatricians prefer that infants' temperatures be taken with a temporal artery thermometer (see Procedure 29.5, presented later) because it is more comfortable for the baby, less invasive, and eliminates the possible complication of a perforated rectum.

When taken correctly, the tympanic (ear/aural) temperature (T) is an accurate measure because it records the temperature of the blood closest to the hypothalamus. However, research on the temporal artery (TA) thermometer indicates that this method is more accurate than tympanic measurement for identifying elevated temperatures in infants. Pediatricians therefore may prefer TA temperatures in infants suspected of having a fever. The TA thermometer also records accurate temperature readings in all age groups. The tympanic method still is considered a fast, accurate, and noninvasive way of recording temperatures for older children and adults.

For patients younger than 3 years and for those unable to hold a thermometer properly in their mouth during the procedure, a tympanic or temporal artery thermometer can be used; if not, a less accurate axillary temperature can be obtained.

CRITICAL THINKING 29.2

The mother of a 3-year-old calls the office to report that her child had an axillary temperature of 101°F at 9 o'clock this morning. The schedule is full today, so Carlos has to decide whether the child should be seen today or first thing tomorrow. When should Carlos schedule the appointment? What is the significance of the axillary temperature reading?

Types of Thermometers and Their Uses

Digital Thermometer. Digital thermometers are battery operated. Disposable covers fit snugly over the probes and are easily and quickly removed by pushing in the colored end of the probe. The instrument sounds a beep when the process is complete (in 10 to 60 seconds), and the reading appears on a screen on the face of the instrument. Because the only part of the instrument that comes in contact with the patient is the probe, which is covered, the risk of cross-infection is greatly reduced (Fig. 29.2).

When using a digital thermometer to take an oral temperature (Procedure 29.1), it is important to ask if the patient has recently had anything to eat, drink, or smoke. These factors may artificially alter the patient's temperature. Wait 10 to 15 minutes before taking an oral temperature if those factors have occurred. In addition, the patient must be able to hold the thermometer under the tongue with the lips tightly sealed around the probe if an accurate oral reading is to be obtained. Be sure to use the blue probe for an oral temperature.

A digital thermometer with a blue probe can also be used for an axillary temperature (Procedure 29.2). It is important make sure that there is a tight seal around the probe. This can be done by having the patient hold his or her arm snugly across the chest. Remember, this site is considered the least accurate.

A digital thermometer with a red probe is used for rectal temperatures (Procedure 29.3). This site is used most often for infants. To take an infant's temperature rectally, lubricate the probe tip (most facilities use

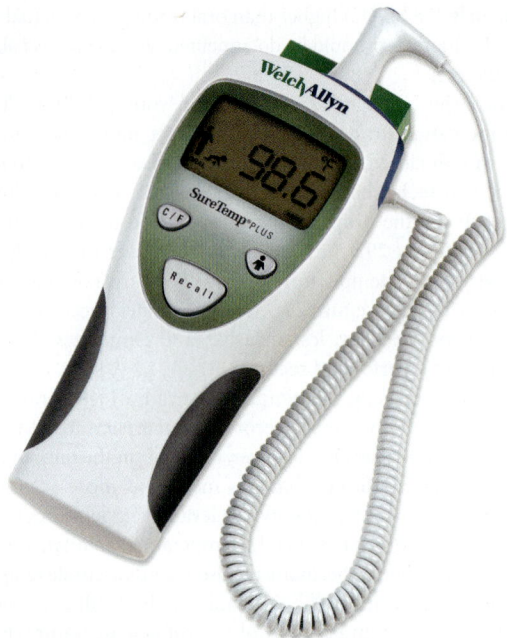

FIG. 29.2 Digital thermometer. (Courtesy Welch Allyn.)

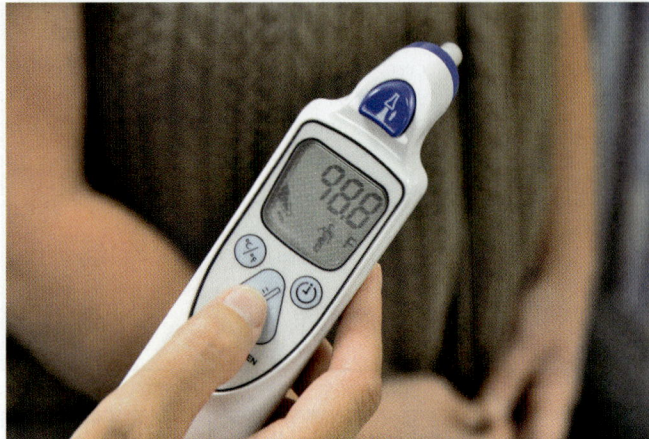

FIG. 29.3 Tympanic thermometer. (From Proctor D, et al: *Kinn's The Medical Assistant*, ed 13, St. Louis, 2017, Elsevier.)

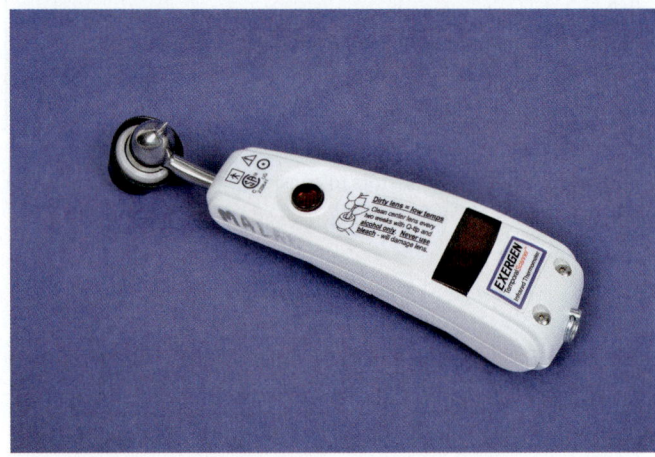

FIG. 29.4 Temporal artery thermometer. (From Proctor D, et al: *Kinn's The Medical Assistant*, ed 13, St. Louis, 2017, Elsevier.)

a lubricating product such as K-Y Jelly), hold the baby securely with the legs elevated, and insert the probe approximately 1 inch; hold the probe carefully and continue to secure the infant's legs throughout the procedure to prevent rectal damage.

The digital unit or individual digital thermometers should be routinely cleaned with disinfectant. When ejecting the probe cover, be careful not to contaminate the probe or the processing unit. The probe cover should be deposited directly into a biohazard waste container. If a chance exists that a patient's body fluids touched the unit, wipe it with disinfectant before returning it to the storage area.

Tympanic Thermometer. The tympanic membrane of the ear can be used for quick, accurate, and safe assessment of a patient's temperature. It shares the blood supply with the hypothalamus, which is the brain's temperature regulator. The ear canal is a protected cavity. This means factors such as an open mouth, hot or cold drinks, or even a stuffy nose do not affect aural temperature.

The tympanic thermometer system consists of a handheld unit equipped with a tympanic probe, which is covered with a disposable probe cover (Fig. 29.3). When the probe is placed into the ear canal, it gently seals the external opening of the canal, and the sensor detects the infrared energy produced by the tympanic membrane. This signal is digitized by the thermometer and shown on the display screen. Accurate readings are obtained in less than 2 seconds (Procedure 29.4). The tympanic thermometer is popular due to the speed of obtaining the temperature and the comfort it affords the patient. This site should not be used if the patient is complaining of pain in both ears when the ear is touched. He or she may have bilateral **otitis externa**, making the procedure uncomfortable for the patient. In addition, if the patient has a history of or has impacted **cerumen** (si ROO muh n) in both ears, do not use a tympanic thermometer because the reading may be inaccurate.

> **VOCABULARY**
> **cerumen:** A waxy secretion in the ear canal; commonly called *ear wax*.
> **otitis externa:** Inflammation or infection of the external auditory canal; commonly called *swimmer's ear*.

Insert the probe into the ear canal far enough to seal the opening without applying pressure. To expose the tympanic membrane in children younger than age 3, gently pull the earlobe down and back; for patients older than age 3, gently pull the pinna (top of the ear) up and back.

Temporal Artery Thermometer. The temporal artery thermometer uses an infrared beam to assess the temperature of the blood flowing through the temporal artery of the forehead, where the artery lies about 1 mm below the skin (Fig. 29.4). Because the artery is so close to the skin, it provides good surface heat conduction, allowing the thermometer to obtain a fast, accurate, and noninvasive measurement of body temperature. To perform the procedure, place the probe in the center of the forehead, halfway between the eyebrows and the hairline. Bangs should be pushed back off the forehead (this method cannot be used if bandages cover the area). Depress the button on the scanner and gently stroke the probe across the forehead toward the hairline (at the temples), keeping the probe flat on the patient's skin. As the scanner moves across the forehead, repeated temperature measurements are taken and the highest measurement is recorded; keeping the button depressed, lift the scanner from the temporal area and lightly place the probe behind the earlobe. Release the button and remove the probe. Recording an accurate temperature takes about 3 seconds (Procedure 29.5). Depending on the facility's infection control procedures, disposable covers can be used on the scanner, or it can be cleaned between patients with an alcohol wipe.

CHAPTER 29 Vital Signs

PROCEDURE 29.1 Obtain an Oral Temperature Using a Digital Thermometer

Task
Accurately determine and record a patient's oral temperature using a digital thermometer.

Equipment and Supplies
- Patient's record
- Digital thermometer and probe covers
- Biohazard waste container

Procedural Steps
1. Wash hands or use hand sanitizer.
   Purpose: To ensure infection control.
2. Assemble the needed equipment and supplies.
3. Greet the patient. Identify yourself. Verify the patient's identity with full name and date of birth. Explain the procedure to be performed in a manner that the patient understands. Answer any questions the patient may have about the procedure. Make sure the patient has not eaten, consumed any hot or cold fluids, smoked, or exercised during the 15 minutes before the temperature is measured.
   Purpose: Identification of the patient prevents errors, and explanations are a means of gaining implied consent and patient cooperation. The temperature will be inaccurate if hot or cold food or fluids have been consumed or if the patient has exercised within 15 minutes.
4. Prepare the probe for use as described in the directions (Fig. 1). Make sure probe covers are always used.
   Purpose: To ensure infection control.

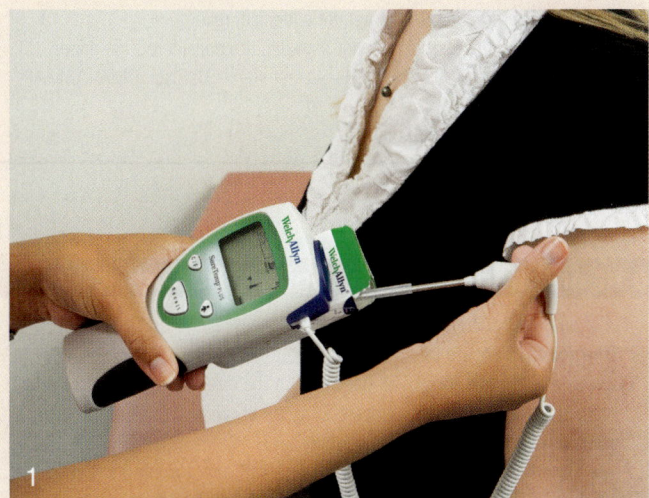

5. Place the probe under the patient's tongue (Fig. 2) and instruct the patient to close the mouth tightly without biting down on the thermometer. Help the patient by holding the probe end, or the patient can hold the probe end if that is more comfortable.
   Purpose: Air seeping into the mouth interferes with an accurate body temperature reading.

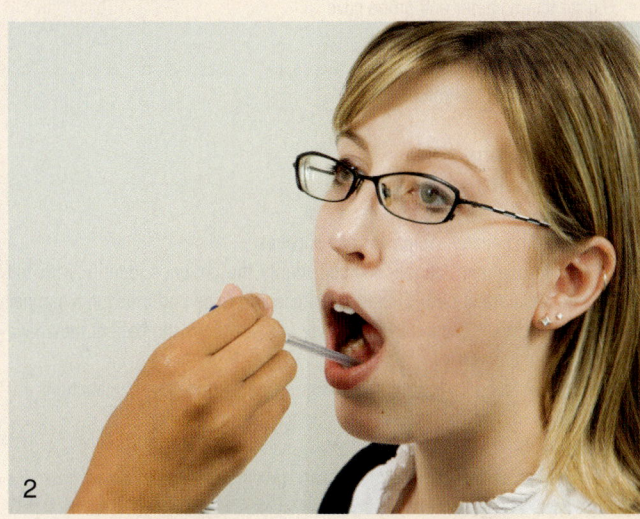

6. When a beep is heard, remove the probe from the patient's mouth and immediately eject the probe cover into an appropriate biohazard waste container.
   Purpose: The probe cover is contaminated and must be discarded in a biohazard waste container.
7. Note the reading on the display screen of the thermometer.
8. Document the reading in the patient's medical record (e.g., T: 97.7°F).
   Purpose: Procedures that are not documented are considered not done.
9. Wash hands or use hand sanitizer, and disinfect the equipment as indicated.
   Purpose: To observe infection control measures and Standard Precautions.

6/29/20XX 10:05 a.m. T: 97.7 ———————————— C. Ricci, CMA (AAMA)

CRITICAL THINKING 29.3
How should the medical assistant adapt temperature-taking techniques in the following scenarios?
- Patient who talks continuously with the thermometer in his mouth
- 7-year-old patient with bilateral otitis externa
- 3-month-old patient when a temporal artery thermometer is available
- 46-year-old patient with a severe asthma attack
- 72-year-old patient with bilateral impacted cerumen
- 28-year-old patient who has just smoked a cigarette

PULSE

A patient's pulse rate reflects the palpable beat of the arteries throughout the body as they expand in response to contraction of the heart. With every beat, the heart pumps an amount of blood, known as the *stroke volume*, into the aorta. Arteries branch off the aorta as it travels down through the center of the abdomen, transferring the pulse beat throughout the body. To measure the pulse, an artery is used that is close to the body surface and can be pushed against a bone. Palpating a **peripheral** (puh RIF er uh l) pulse gives the rate, rhythm, and volume of the heartbeat and local information about the condition of the artery used.

PROCEDURE 29.2 Obtain an Axillary Temperature Using a Digital Thermometer

Task
Accurately determine and record a patient's axillary temperature using a digital thermometer.

Equipment and Supplies
- Patient's record
- Digital thermometer and probe cover
- Supply of tissues
- Patient gown as needed
- Biohazard waste container

Procedural Steps
1. Wash hands or use hand sanitizer.
   Purpose: To ensure infection control.
2. Gather the needed equipment and supplies.
3. Greet the patient. Identify yourself. Verify the patient's identity with full name and date of birth. Explain the procedure to be performed in a manner that the patient understands. Answer any questions the patient may have about the procedure.
   Purpose: Identification of the patient prevents errors, and explanations are a means of gaining implied consent and patient cooperation.
4. Prepare the thermometer in the same manner as for oral use.
5. Expose the axillary region. If necessary, provide the patient with a gown for privacy.
6. Pat the patient's axillary area dry with tissues if needed.
   Purpose: To ensure an accurate reading. Do not rub the area because this may cause an elevated reading.
7. Place the probe tip into the center of the armpit, making sure the thermometer is touching only skin, not clothing.
   Purpose: To obtain the most accurate axillary reading; contact with clothing alters the reading.
8. Instruct the patient to hold the arm snugly across the chest or abdomen until the thermometer beeps (Fig. 1).
   Purpose: To prevent air from leaking in and interfering with the temperature reading.

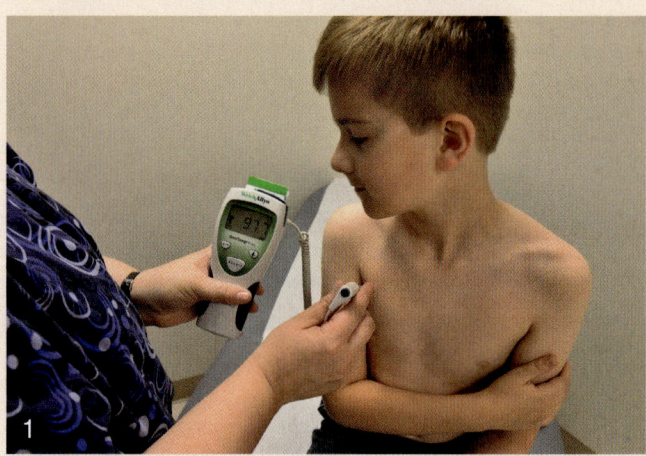

9. Remove the thermometer, note the digital reading, and dispose of the cover in the biohazard waste container.
10. Disinfect the thermometer if indicated.
    Purpose: To ensure infection control.
11. Wash hands or use hand sanitizer.
12. Document the reading in the patient's medical record.
    Purpose: Procedures that are not recorded are considered not done.

6/29/20XX 10:05 a.m. T: 98.2°F (A) ——————— C. Ricci, CMA (AAMA)

PROCEDURE 29.3 Obtain a Rectal Temperature of an Infant Using a Digital Thermometer

Task
Accurately determine and record a patient's rectal temperature using a digital thermometer.

Equipment and Supplies
- Patient's record
- Digital thermometer and probe covers
- Disposable gloves
- Biohazard waste container
- Water soluble lubricant (KY jelly)

Procedural Steps
1. Wash hands or use hand sanitizer.
   Purpose: To ensure infection control.
2. Assemble the needed equipment and supplies. Make sure that the red probe is used.
3. Greet the patient's parent or caregiver. Identify yourself. Verify the patient's identity with full name and date of birth. Explain the procedure to be performed in a manner that the patient's parent or caregiver understands. Answer any questions about the procedure.
   Purpose: Identification of the patient prevents errors, and explanations are a means of gaining implied consent and cooperation.
4. Have the parent or caregiver undress the infant.
5. Put on disposable gloves.
   Purpose: To ensure infection control.
6. Prepare the probe for use as described in the directions. Make sure probe covers are always used. Lubricate 2 inches of probe.
   Purpose: To ensure infection control.
7. Gently insert the thermometer probe one-half inch for infants (this would change to five-eighths inch for children and 1 inch for adults). Remain with the patient at all times, and hold the thermometer in place until a beep is heard.
8. Remove the probe, and immediately eject the probe cover into an appropriate biohazard waste container.
   Purpose: The probe cover is contaminated and must be discarded in a biohazard waste container.
9. Note the reading on the display screen of the thermometer.
10. Remove soiled gloves, and discard them into an appropriate biohazard waste container.
11. Wash hands or use hand sanitizer, and disinfect the equipment as indicated.
    Purpose: To observe infection control measures and Standard Precautions.
12. Document the reading in the patient's medical record.
    Purpose: Procedures that are not documented are considered not done.

6/29/20XX 2:10 p.m. T: 100.7°F (R) ——————— C. Ricci, CMA (AAMA)

PROCEDURE 29.4 Obtain a Temperature Using a Tympanic Thermometer

Task
Accurately determine and record a patient's temperature using a tympanic thermometer.

Equipment and Supplies
- Patient's record
- Tympanic thermometer
- Disposable probe covers
- Alcohol wipes
- Biohazard waste container

Procedural Steps
1. Wash hands or use hand sanitizer.
   Purpose: To ensure infection control.
2. Gather the necessary equipment and supplies.
3. Greet the patient. Identify yourself. Verify the patient's identity with full name and date of birth. Explain the procedure to be performed in a manner that the patient understands. Answer any questions the patient may have about the procedure.
   Purpose: Identification of the patient prevents errors, and explanations are a means of gaining implied consent and patient cooperation.
4. Clean the probe with an alcohol wipe if indicated. Place a disposable cover on the probe (Fig. 1).
   Purpose: To ensure a clean surface and prevent cross-contamination.

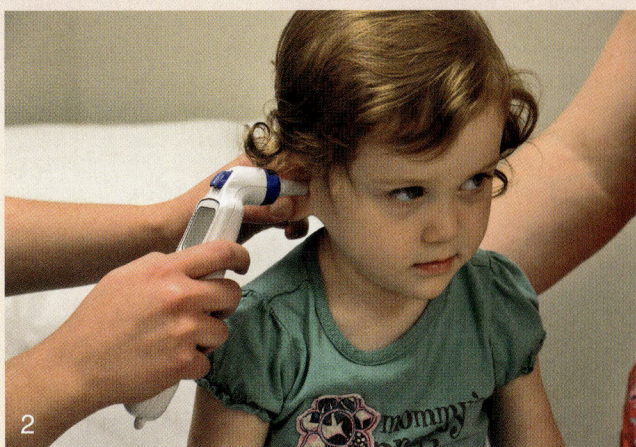

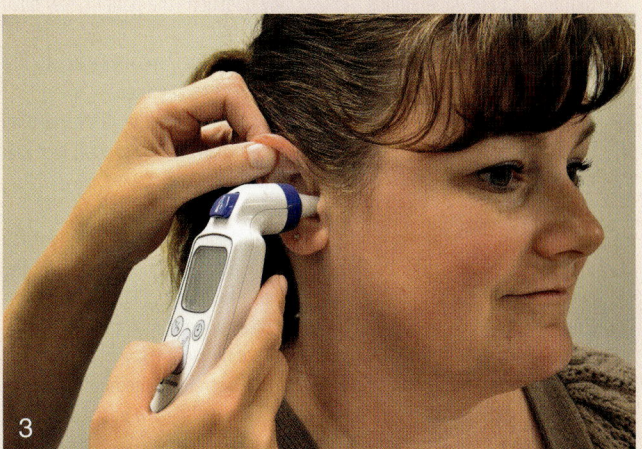

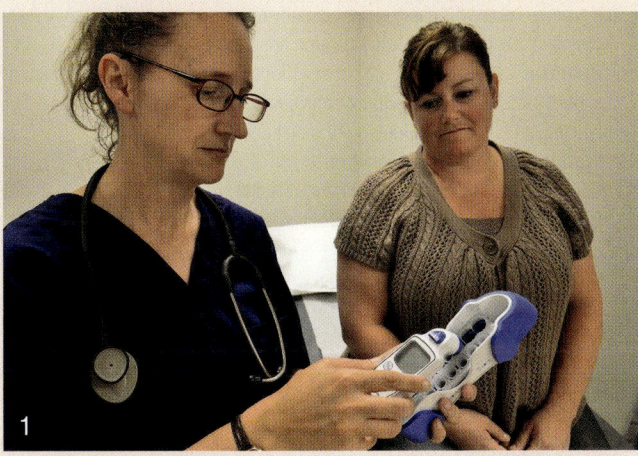

5. Insert the probe into the ear canal far enough to seal the opening. Do not apply pressure. For children younger than age 3, gently pull the earlobe down and back (Fig. 2); for patients older than age 3, gently pull the top of the ear (pinna) up and back (Fig. 3).
   Purpose: The external ear must be pulled gently to open the external auditory canal and expose the tympanic membrane for an accurate reading.
6. Press the button on the probe as directed. The temperature will appear on the display screen in 1 to 2 seconds.
7. Remove the probe, note the reading, and discard the probe cover into a biohazard waste container without touching it.
   Purpose: The probe cover is contaminated and must be discarded in a biohazard waste container.
8. Wash hands or use hand sanitizer, and disinfect the equipment if indicated. See the manufacturer's manual for cleaning the probe tip. Many recommend cleaning the probe lens with alcohol wipes.
   Purpose: To ensure infection control.
9. Document the reading in the patient's medical record
   Purpose: Procedures that are not recorded are considered not done.
   7/11/20xx 2:20 p.m. T: 101.2°F (T) ——————— C. Ricci, CMA (AAMA)

VOCABULARY
peripheral: Refers to an area outside of or away from an organ or structure.

Pulse Sites

A pulse rate may be counted anyplace an artery is near the surface of the body and the vessel can be pressed against a bone. The most common pulse sites are the temporal, carotid, brachial, radial, femoral, popliteal, and dorsalis pedis arteries (Fig. 29.5). The apical pulse is taken by listening with a stethoscope.

The *temporal* (TEM per uh l) pulse is located in the temple area of the skull, parallel and lateral to the eyes (Fig. 29.6). It is seldom used as a pulse site but may be used as a pressure point to help control bleeding from a head injury.

The *carotid* (kuh ROT id) artery is located between the larynx and the *sternocleidomastoid* muscle in the front and to the side of

PROCEDURE 29.5 Obtain a Temperature Using a Temporal Artery Thermometer

Task
Accurately determine and record a patient's temperature using a temporal artery thermometer.

Equipment and Supplies
- Patient's record
- Professional temporal artery thermometer with probe covers
- Alcohol wipes
- Biohazard waste container

Procedural Steps
1. Wash hands or use hand sanitizer.
   Purpose: To ensure infection control.
2. Gather the necessary equipment and supplies.
3. Greet the patient. Identify yourself. Verify the patient's identity with full name and date of birth. Explain the procedure to be performed in a manner that the patient understands. Answer any questions the patient may have about the procedure.
   Purpose: Identification of the patient prevents errors, and explanations are a means of gaining implied consent and patient cooperation.
4. Remove the protective cap on the probe. Depending on the facility's infection control procedures, disposable covers can be used on the scanner, or it can be cleaned by lightly wiping the surface with an alcohol wipe.
   Purpose: To ensure infection control.
5. Push the patient's hair up off the forehead to expose the site. Gently place the probe on the patient's forehead, halfway between the edge of the eyebrows and the hairline, at the center of the face (just above the nose).
   Purpose: This places the probe directly over the temporal artery.
6. Depress and hold the SCAN button, and lightly glide the probe sideways across the patient's forehead to the hairline just above the ear (Fig. 1). As you move the sensor across the forehead, you will hear a beep, and a red light will flash.
   Purpose: This verifies that the scanner is recording temperatures as it moves across the surface of the temporal artery.

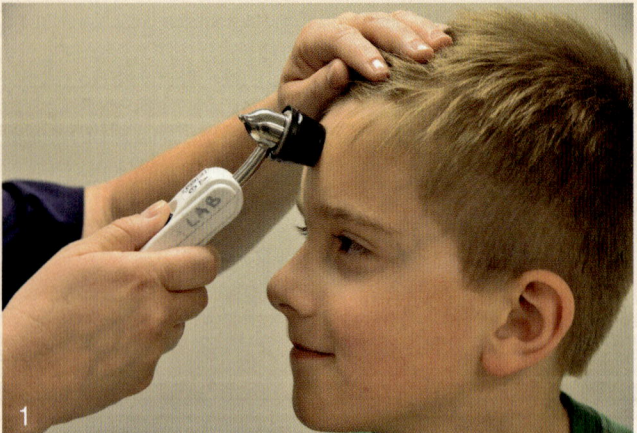

7. Keeping the button depressed, lift the thermometer, and place the probe behind the ear lobe (Fig. 2). The thermometer may continue to beep, indicating that the temperature is rising.
   Purpose: To continue scanning of the temporal artery until the highest temperature is recorded on the thermometer.

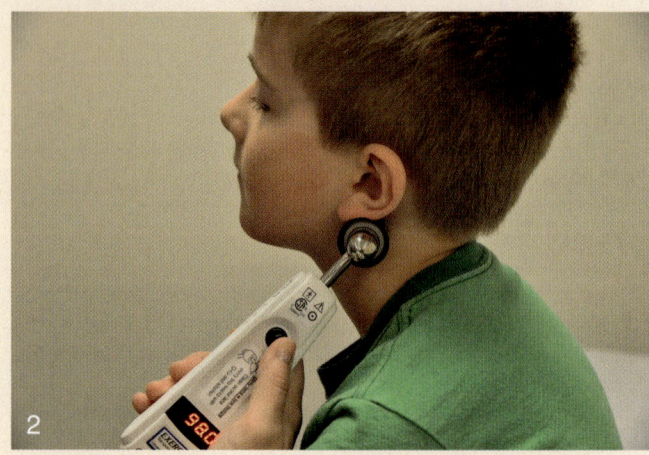

8. When scanning is complete, release the button and lift the probe. Note the temperature recorded on the digital display. The scanner automatically turns off 15 to 30 seconds after release of the button.
9. If a probe cover was used, eject it directly into a biohazard waste container. Disinfect the thermometer if indicated and replace the protective cap.
   Purpose: To ensure infection control. Depending on the facility's infection control procedures, disposable covers can be used on the scanner, or it can be cleaned between patients with a disinfectant wipe.
10. Wash hands or use hand sanitizer.
11. Document the reading in the patient's medical record.
    Purpose: Procedures that are not recorded are considered not done.
    8/1/20XX 11:20 a.m. T: 101.6°F (TA) ———————— C. Ricci, CMA (AAMA)

---

the neck (Fig. 29.7). It most frequently is used in emergencies and to check the pulse during cardiopulmonary resuscitation (CPR). It can be felt by pushing the muscle to the side and pressing against the larynx.

VOCABULARY
larynx: The voice box.

MEDICAL TERMINOLOGY
cleid/o: clavicle (collarbone)
mast/o: mastoid process
stern/o: sternum

The *brachial* (BREY kee uh l) pulse is felt at the inner (*antecubital* [an tuh KYOO bit uhl]) aspect of the elbow. This is the artery that is felt and listened to when blood pressure is measured (Fig. 29.8). It also

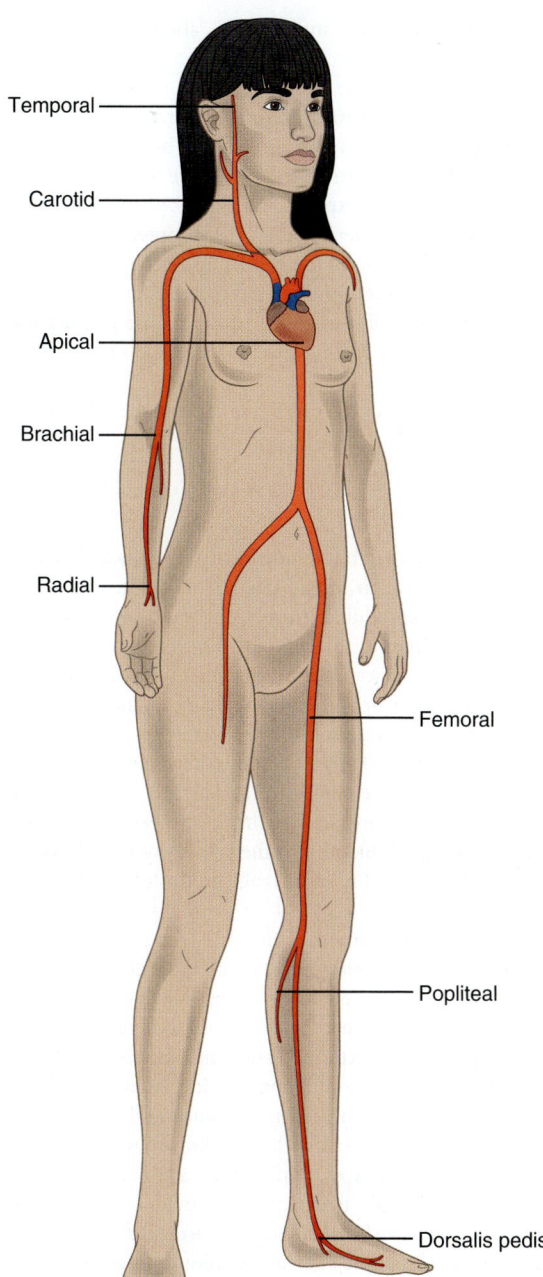

FIG. 29.5 Pulse sites. (From Proctor D, et al: *Kinn's The Medical Assistant*, ed 13, St. Louis, 2017, Elsevier.)

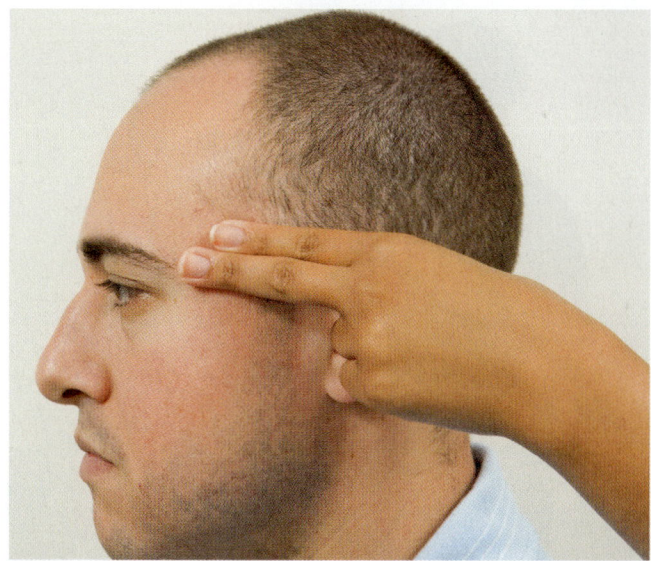

FIG. 29.6 Temporal pulse. (From Proctor D, et al: *Kinn's The Medical Assistant*, ed 13, St. Louis, 2017, Elsevier.)

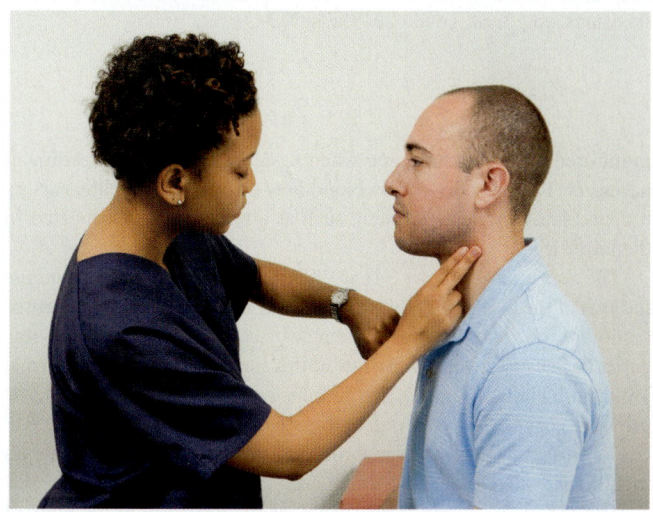

FIG. 29.7 Carotid pulse. (From Proctor D, et al: *Kinn's The Medical Assistant*, ed 13, St. Louis, 2017, Elsevier.)

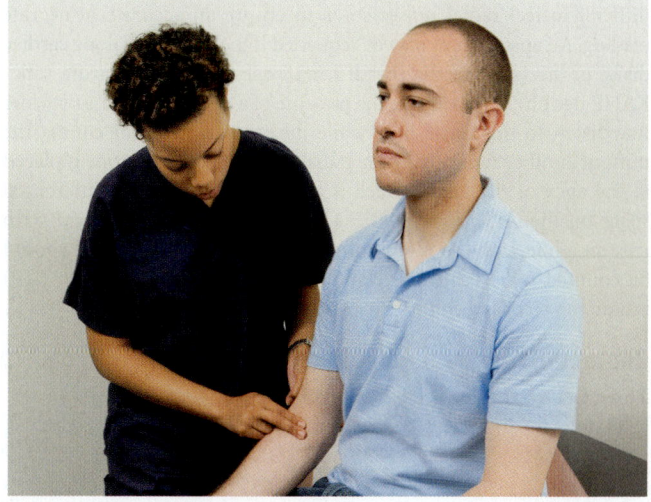

FIG. 29.8 Brachial pulse. (From Proctor D, et al: *Kinn's The Medical Assistant*, ed 13, St. Louis, 2017, Elsevier.)

can be felt in the groove between the biceps and triceps muscles on the inner surface of the middle upper arm. This is the pulse that is checked on infants and young children receiving CPR.

The *radial* (REY dee uh l) artery is the most commonly used site for counting the pulse rate. It is found on the thumb side of the wrist, 1 inch below the base of the thumb (Fig. 29.9).

The *femoral* (FEM er uh l) pulse is located at the site where the femoral artery passes through the groin (see Fig. 29.5). The examiner must press deeply below the *inguinal* (ING gwuh nl) ligament to palpate this pulse.

The *popliteal* (pop LIT ee uh l) pulse is found at the back of the leg behind the knee (see Fig. 29.5). Palpation of this pulse requires the patient to be in a recumbent position with the knee slightly flexed. The popliteal artery is deep and difficult to feel. It is palpated and also

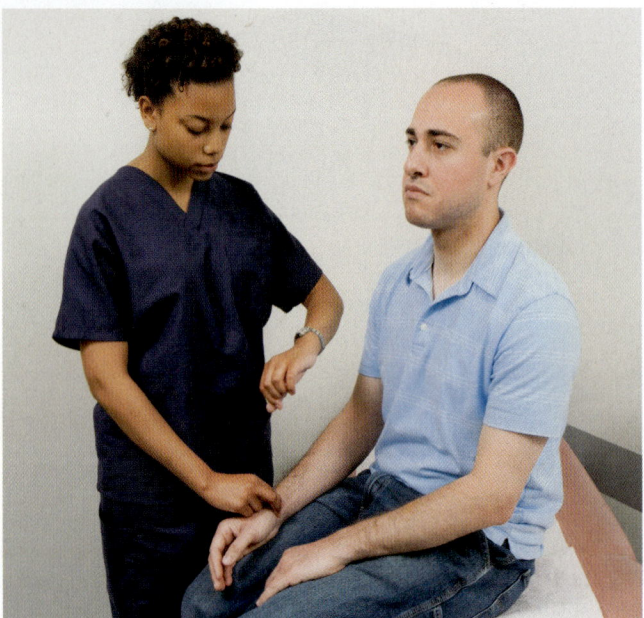

FIG. 29.9 Radial pulse. (From Proctor D, et al: *Kinn's The Medical Assistant*, ed 13, St. Louis, 2017, Elsevier.)

monitored with a stethoscope when a leg blood pressure reading is necessary. The provider checks blood flow through the popliteal artery if a circulatory system problem, such as a blood clot, is suspected in the lower leg.

The *dorsalis pedis* (dawr SAL is PEE diss) (pedal) artery is felt across the arch of the foot, just slightly lateral to the midline, beside the extensor tendon of the great toe. This pulse may be congenitally absent in some patients. Because a good pulse rate at this site is an indicator of normal lower limb circulation and arterial *sufficiency* (suh FISH uh n see), the provider checks the pedal pulses in patients with *peripheral* (phy RIF er uh l) *vascular* (VAS kyuh ler) problems, such as patients with diabetes mellitus.

The *apical* (EY pi kih l) heart rate, or the heartbeat at the apex of the heart, is heard with a stethoscope. It is used for infants and young children because the radial pulse is difficult to palpate in young patients. Apical rates are also recorded on adult patients who have irregular or difficult-to-feel radial pulses so as to ensure an accurate heart rate reading. An apical count may be requested if the patient is taking cardiac drugs or has **bradycardia** (bradi KAHR dee uh) or **tachycardia** (tak i KAHR dee uh). To determine the presence of a **pulse deficit**, the provider may listen to the apical beat while the medical assistant counts the pulse at another site (usually the radial pulse). The stethoscope is placed at the apex of the heart, which is located in the left fifth intercostal space on the midclavicular line—that is, between the fifth and sixth ribs on a line with the midpoint of the left clavicle. The pulse should be counted for 1 full minute and should be documented with (AP) beside the recorded count (Procedure 29.6).

Characteristics of a Pulse

Three factors are assessed when taking a pulse:
- Rate
- Rhythm
- Volume

These characteristics vary with the size and elasticity of the artery and the strength and regularity of the heart's contractions. A patient's pulse can reveal valuable information about the cardiovascular system.

Rate. The pulse rate is a measure of the number of beats felt from the movement of blood through an artery. When the heart contracts, blood is pumped into the arteries. The pressure throughout the arteries increases, and the arteries expand. When the heart relaxes, little blood is moving through the arteries, and arterial pressure decreases. Each contraction and relaxation of the heart muscle is a beat. The resulting expansion and relaxation of the arteries creates a pulsation. This is the pulse rate. Normally, the beat (rate) and the pulse rate are the same. The rate of the pulse is the number of beats (pulsations) that occur in 1 minute.

Factors that can affect the pulse rate include the following:
- Age
- Body size
- Gender
- Health status

The rate is also affected by an individual's activities and psychological state as well as by certain medications. Children tend to have more rapid pulse rates than adults. It usually is faster in women (70 to 80 beats per minute) than in men (60 to 70 beats per minute). The rate is more rapid when a person is sitting than when he or she is lying down, and it increases when an individual stands, walks, or runs. During sleep or rest, the pulse rate may drop to as low as 45 to 50 beats per minute. Well-conditioned athletes tend to have pulse rates of 50 to 60 beats per minute because consistent aerobic exercise strengthens the heart muscle (the myocardium) so that each heart contraction ejects an increased volume of blood into the arterial system. Table 29.2 lists the normal pulse ranges for various age groups of patients.

Rhythm. The pulse rhythm is the time between pulse beats. A normal rhythm pattern has an even tempo, which indicates that the intervals between the beats are of equal duration. An abnormal rhythm, or *arrhythmia*, is described according to the rhythm pattern detected. An **intermittent pulse** may occur in healthy individuals during exercise or after drinking a beverage containing caffeine. A common irregularity found in children and young adults is a **sinus arrhythmia**. The heart rate varies with the respiratory cycle, speeding up with inspiration and slowing to normal with expiration. If beats are frequently skipped or if the beats are markedly irregular, the provider should be advised, because this may indicate heart disease. If an irregular rhythm is detected, the pulse should be counted for a full minute to ensure accuracy. A note also should be made that the patient's pulse was irregular—for example, "P: 86 irregular."

Volume. The volume (*pulse amplitude* [AM pli tood]) reflects the strength of the heart when it contracts. Volume can be assessed by feeling the strength of the pulse as blood flows through the vessel. The

---

VOCABULARY

bradycardia: A slow heartbeat; a pulse below 60 beats per minute.
intermittent pulse: A pulse in which beats occasionally are skipped.
pulse deficit: A condition in which the radial pulse is less than the apical pulse; it may indicate a peripheral vascular abnormality.
sinus arrhythmia: An irregular heartbeat that originates in the sinoatrial node (pacemaker).
tachycardia: A rapid but regular heart rate; one that exceeds 100 beats per minute.

CHAPTER 29 Vital Signs

PROCEDURE 29.6 Obtain an Apical Pulse

Task
Accurately determine and record the patient's apical heart rate.

Equipment and Supplies
- Patient's record
- Watch with a second hand
- Patient gown as needed
- Stethoscope
- Alcohol wipes

Procedural Steps

1. Wash hands or use hand sanitizer, and clean the stethoscope earpieces and diaphragm with alcohol wipes.
   Purpose: To ensure infection control and to follow Standard Precautions.
2. Greet the patient. Identify yourself. Verify the patient's identity with full name and date of birth. Explain the procedure to be performed in a manner that the patient understands. Answer any questions the patient may have about the procedure.
   Purpose: Identification of the patient prevents errors, and explanations are a means of gaining implied consent and patient cooperation.
3. If necessary, assist the patient in disrobing from the waist up and provide the patient with a gown that opens in the front.
   Purpose: To expose the chest and provide privacy and warmth.
4. Assist the patient into the sitting or supine position.
   Purpose: To allow easier access to the apical site at the apex of the heart.
5. Hold the stethoscope's diaphragm against the palm of your hand for a few seconds.
   Purpose: To warm the diaphragm, promoting patient comfort.
6. Place the stethoscope at the left midclavicular line at the fifth intercostal space over the apex of the heart (Figs. 1 and 2). Do not touch the bell end of the stethoscope.
   Purpose: This is the point of maximum contractile strength, where the heartbeat can be heard best. Touching the bell end of the stethoscope may interfere with the sound.
7. Listen carefully for the heartbeat. Count the pulse for 1 full minute. Note any irregularities in rhythm and volume.
   Purpose: The apical pulse is always measured for 1 full minute to obtain the most accurate reading.
8. Help the patient to sit up and dress.
9. Disinfect the stethoscope with an alcohol wipe.
   Purpose: To ensure infection control.
10. Wash hands or use hand sanitizer.
11. Document the reading in the patient's medical record.
    3/3/20XX 4:10 p.m. AP: 93 irregular ——————— C. Ricci, CMA (AAMA)

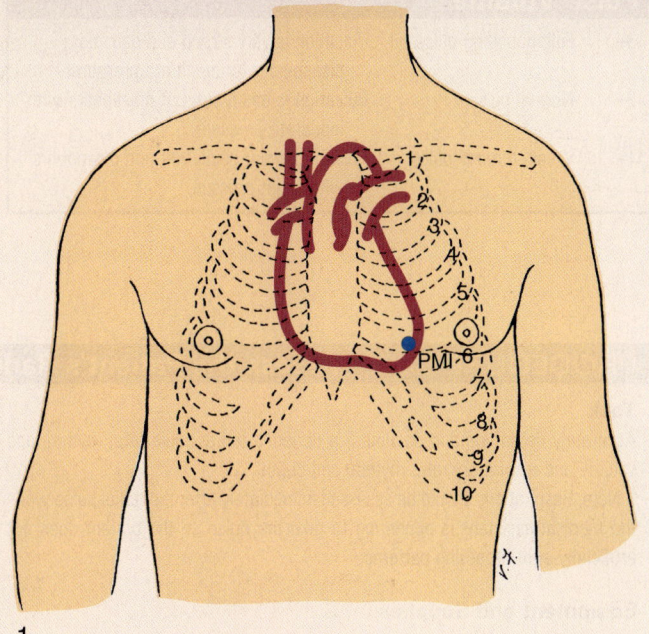

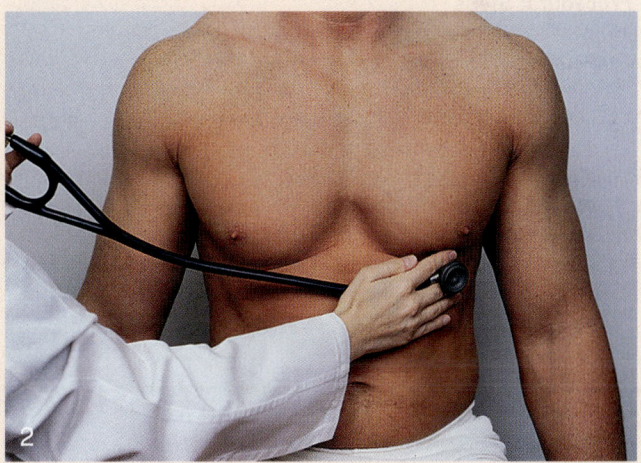

TABLE 29.2 Approximate Age-Related Pulse Rates		
Age	Range (beats/min)	Average
Newborn	120–160	140
1–2 years	80–140	120
3–6 years	75–120	100
7–11 years	75–110	95
Adolescence to adulthood	60–100	80

force of each pulse beat is described as **bounding**, or full; strong, or normal; or **thready**, or weak. The force of the heartbeat and the condition of the arterial wall (whether hard or soft) influence the volume of the pulse beat. The pulse may vary only in intensity and otherwise may be perfectly regular. This condition also can indicate heart disease. The pulse volume is recorded using a three-point scale (Box 29.3).

> **VOCABULARY**
> **bounding:** Describes a pulse that feels full because of the increased power of cardiac contraction or as a result of increased blood volume.
> **thready:** Describes a pulse that is thin and feeble.

BOX 29.3 Three-Point Scale for Measuring Pulse Volume

3+	Full, bounding pulse	Pulsation is very strong and does not disappear with moderate pressure.
2+	Normal pulse	Pulsation is easily felt but disappears with moderate pressure.
1+	Weak, thready pulse	Pulsation is not easily felt and disappears with slight pressure.

Determining the Pulse Rate

Radial and Apical Pulse Rates. To record an accurate radial pulse, you must have the patient in a comfortable position with the artery to be used at the same level as or lower than the heart (Procedure 29.7). The limb should be well supported and relaxed. The patient may be lying down or sitting. As with all palpated pulse readings, the pads of the first two or three fingers are placed over the artery. Never use your thumb to determine the pulse rate. The thumb has its own pulse, and you may confuse your pulse rate with the patient's rate. Push the radial

PROCEDURE 29.7 Assess the Patient's Radial Pulse and Respiratory Rate

Task
Accurately determine and document a patient's radial pulse rate, rhythm, and volume and respiratory rate, rhythm, and depth.

Note: Respirations should be assessed immediately after the radial pulse while the medical assistant is appearing to take the pulse so the patient does not artificially alter breathing patterns.

Equipment and Supplies
- Patient's record
- Watch with a second hand

Procedural Steps
1. Wash hands or use hand sanitizer.
   Purpose: To ensure infection control.
2. Greet the patient. Identify yourself. Verify the patient's identity with full name and date of birth. Explain the procedure to be performed in a manner that the patient understands. Answer any questions the patient may have about the procedure.
   Purpose: Identification of the patient prevents errors, and explanations are a means of gaining implied consent and patient cooperation.
3. Place the patient's arm in a relaxed position, palm at or below the level of the heart.
   Purpose: The patient's radial artery is more easily palpated when the patient is relaxed and in this position.
4. Gently grasp the palm side of the patient's wrist with your first two or three fingertips approximately 1 inch below the base of the thumb (Fig. 1).
   Purpose: This position puts your fingertips directly over the radial artery. Press firmly (but do not press too hard, or you will occlude the artery and feel nothing).
5. Count the beats for 1 full minute using a watch with a second hand.
   Purpose: Counting for 1 full minute allows you to obtain an accurate count, including any irregularities in rhythm and volume. Once you become more adept at taking a pulse, you can reduce this to 30 seconds and multiply that number by 2 to record the patient's heart rate.
6. While counting the beats, also assess the rhythm and volume of the patient's pulse.
7. While continuing to hold the patient's arm in the same position used to count the radial pulse, observe the rise and fall of the patient's chest (see Fig. 29.12). If you have difficulty noticing the patient's breathing, place the arm across the chest to detect movement.
   Purpose: The respiratory count may be altered if the patient is aware that you are counting his or her breaths; placing the arm across the chest allows you to feel or see the rise and fall of the chest wall.
8. Inhalation and exhalation make up one complete breathing cycle or respiration. Count the respirations for 30 seconds and multiply by 2.
   Purpose: Counting for 30 seconds allows you to obtain an accurate count and determine any irregularities in rhythm or depth or unusual breathing patterns. If respirations are abnormal in any way, count for 1 full minute.
9. While counting, also assess the rhythm and depth of the patient's respirations.
10. Release the patient's wrist.
11. Wash hands or use hand sanitizer.
    Purpose: To ensure infection control.
12. Document the reading in the patient's medical record.
    Purpose: Procedures that are not recorded are considered not done.

5/6/20XX 8:35 a.m. P: 72 regular, 1+ R: 18, regular, normal —————
                                                    C. Ricci, CMA (AAMA)

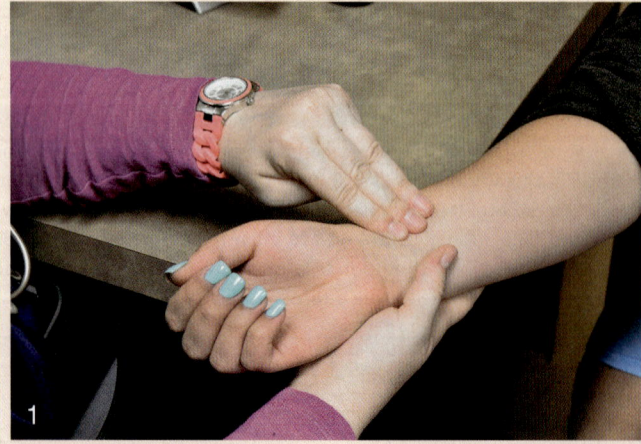

1

artery against the bone until the strongest pulsation is felt. Both you and the patient should be in a relaxed position. Too much pressure occludes the artery, and too little pressure prevents detection of irregularities or of all the beats. The pulse should be counted for 1 full minute A 30-second interval may be used once you become proficient at performing the skill. In either case you should document the number of beats in 1 minute. A 30-second interval may be used once you become proficient at performing the skill.

While counting the rate, you must also be aware of the rhythm and volume. Variations from normal should be noted, such as an arrhythmia or a pulse that is thready or bounding. Some pulses are more difficult to feel than others, and finding the correct pressure to be used for each patient and site requires repeated practice and experience.

For an apical pulse, the patient can be sitting or lying down. Place the stethoscope at the junction of the fifth intercostal space and the midclavicular line on left side of the patient's chest. You will hear a lubb-dubb sound. Each lubb-dubb sound is one heartbeat. The apical pulse should always be auscultated (AW skuh l teyt ed) for a full minute to detect any irregularities in rate and rhythm. Remember, one reason you would decide to take an apical pulse on an adult patient is that you noted irregularities in the heart rate when palpating the radial pulse. Therefore you should listen to an apical pulse for a full minute to make sure you are accurately counting the number of beats per minute. If the pulse rate is counted at any site other than the radial artery, the rate should be documented along with a notation of the site used.

Femoral, Popliteal, and Pedal Pulses. Pulses in the lower extremities may be difficult to find and equally difficult to hear. A Doppler unit, an ultrasound unit that magnifies the pulsation, may be used to locate and count these pulses accurately (Fig. 29.10). A Doppler unit is battery operated and can be attached to a stethoscope so that only the provider can hear the beat, or it can be set so that both the provider and the patient can hear the pulsations.

RESPIRATION

Respiration allows for the exchange of oxygen and carbon dioxide with the atmosphere, the blood, and the body cells. Oxygen is taken into the body to be used for life-sustaining body processes, and carbon dioxide is released as a waste product.

One complete *inhalation* (in hull LAY shun) and *exhalation* (ex hull LAY shun) is called a *respiration*. During the inhalation phase, the diaphragm contracts and drops down. The *intercostal* muscles pull the ribs up and outward; this causes the lungs to expand and fill with air. During the exhalation phase, the diaphragm returns to its normal elevated position and the intercostal muscles relax; this causes the lungs to expel the waste air out of the body.

> **VOCABULARY**
> **auscultated:** Listened to with a stethoscope.
> **occlude:** To close, shut, or stop up.

> **MEDICAL TERMINOLOGY**
> **-al:** pertaining to
> **-ation:** process of
> **cost/o:** rib
> **ex-:** out
> **hal/o:** to breathe
> **in-:** in
> **inter-:** between

> **CRITICAL THINKING 29.4**
> Mrs. Arnez has a documented thready pulse. What site should Carlos use to measure the pulse? Why should he take the pulse for a full minute?

Both internal and external respirations occur. *External respiration* is the exchange of oxygen and carbon dioxide in the lungs. *Internal respiration* occurs at the cellular level. Oxygen in the bloodstream is transferred into the cells for energy. Carbon dioxide is released as a waste product and transported back to the lungs for exhalation.

The respiratory center in the *medulla oblongata* (muh DOO lah ob lon GAH tah) is sensitive to changes in blood oxygen and carbon dioxide levels. When carbon dioxide levels rise, the respiratory control center sends a message that triggers breathing. Respiration is controlled by the involuntary nervous system. This means that we breathe automatically. Because respiration can be controlled to a certain extent, it also is a voluntary function. However, breathing ultimately is under the control of the medulla oblongata. This is why we can hold our breath only for a short period of time. Once cells become oxygen starved, a stimulus is sent to the respiratory muscles (the diaphragm and intercostal muscles) and breathing begins involuntarily.

Characteristics of Respirations

Normally, a person's breathing is relaxed, automatic, and silent. However, respiratory disease or chronic conditions can influence the

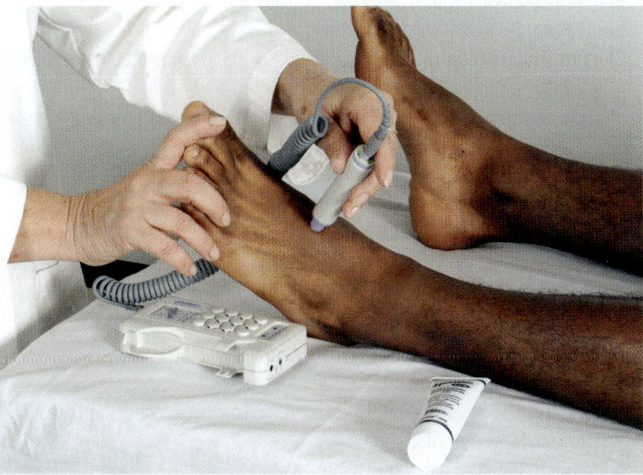

FIG. 29.10 Doppler ultrasound unit measuring the pedal pulse. (From Jarvis C: *Physical Examination and Health Assessment,* ed 7, St. Louis, 2016, Saunders.)

characteristics of an individual's respirations. **Dyspnea** (DISP nee uh) occurs in patients with pneumonia, asthma, or **chronic obstructive pulmonary disease (COPD)**. It also occurs after physical exertion or at very high altitudes. Other alterations in breathing are **bradypnea** (brad IP nee ah), **apnea** (AP nee ah), **tachypnea** (tack ip NEE ah), and **hyperpnea** (hye PURP nee ah). Hyperpnea usually is accompanied by **hyperventilation** (hye pur ven tih LAY shun) and often occurs when the patient is extremely anxious or in pain. **Orthopnea** (or THOP nee ah) frequently occurs in patients with congestive heart failure (CHF) and COPD. **Wheezing** (WHEE zeeng) signals difficulty breathing in patients with asthma.

When assessing a patient's respirations, you must note three important characteristics: rate, rhythm, and depth:

- *Rate:* The rate of respiration is the number of respirations per minute. Fig. 29.11 shows sample rate patterns recorded with a **spirometer**. A ratio of four pulse beats to one respiration is typical. As a rule, both the pulse and respiratory rates respond to exercise or emotional upset. Table 29.3 lists normal respiratory ranges for patients in various age groups.
- *Rhythm:* Rhythm refers to the breathing pattern, the space between each breath. A regular breathing pattern is normal in adults; however, the breathing pattern for infants varies. Automatic interruptions, such as sighing, are also considered normal. The terms *regular* or *irregular* are used to document rhythm.
- *Depth:* The *depth* of respiration is the amount of air inhaled and exhaled. When a patient is at rest, normal respirations have a consistent depth, which can be noted as you watch the rise and fall of the chest. Rapid, shallow breathing at rest occurs with some diseases, such as asthma and emphysema. An alteration in the depth and sometimes the rate of breathing is also seen in **Cheyne-Stokes respirations**. The terms *normal, deep, shallow,* and *gasping* should be used to document depth.

Normally, no noticeable breath sounds occur during the breathing process, except during snoring. Noticeable breath sounds are a sign of certain diseases, such as pneumonia, asthma, and pulmonary edema. After listening to breath sounds with a stethoscope, the provider can describe the characteristics of breath sounds by using specific terminology (e.g., **rales** [rayls], **rhonchi** (RON kye), or **stertorous** (STUR ter uh s) breathing).

When an individual cannot breathe in enough oxygen to supply all body cells with oxygenated blood, normal skin coloring, particularly around the mouth and the nail beds, changes to a bluish, dusky color. This coloration, which indicates an increased level of carbon dioxide in the blood, is called *cyanosis.* The patient also may have other signs and symptoms, such as **vertigo** (VUR tih goh), chest pain *(angina),* and numbness in the fingers and toes.

Counting Respirations

Because most people can control their breathing to a certain extent, do not mention that you will be counting the person's respirations (see Procedure 29.7). Patients may self-consciously alter their breathing rate when they know they are being watched. Count the respirations while appearing to count the radial pulse. Keep your eyes alternately on the patient's chest and your watch while you count the pulse rate; then, without removing your fingers from the pulse site, determine the respiratory rate (Fig. 29.12). If the patient is lying down, the arm on which you are taking the radial pulse may be crossed over the chest so that respirations can be felt with the rise and fall of the chest. Another way of observing respirations is to watch the movement of the patient's

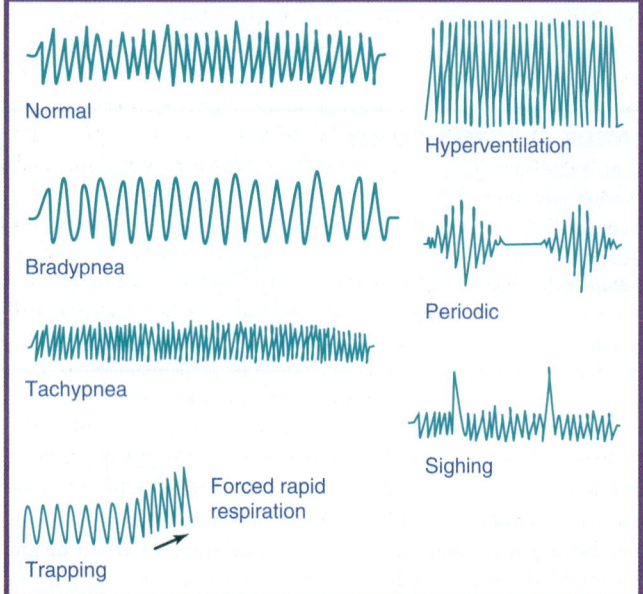

FIG. 29.11 Respiratory rate patterns, called spirograms, are recorded using a spirometer. (From Proctor D, et al: *Kinn's The Medical Assistant*, ed 13, St. Louis, 2017, Elsevier.)

TABLE 29.3 Approximate Age-Related Respiration Ranges

Age	Range (breaths/min)	Average
Newborn	30–50	40
1–3 years	20–30	25
4–6 years	18–26	22
7–11 years	16–22	19
Adolescence to adulthood	12–20	16

VOCABULARY

apnea: Abnormal, periodic cessation of breathing.
bradypnea: Abnormally slow breathing.
Cheyne-Stokes respiration: Deep, rapid breathing followed by a period of apnea.
chronic obstructive pulmonary disease (COPD): A progressive, irreversible lung condition that results in diminished lung capacity.
dyspnea: Difficult or painful breathing.
hyperpnea: Excessively deep breathing.
hyperventilation: Abnormally increased breathing.
orthopnea: Condition of difficult breathing unless in an upright position.
rales: An abnormal lung sound heard on auscultation, characterized by discontinuous bubbling noises.
rhonchi: An abnormal rumbling sound heard on auscultation, caused by airways blocked by secretions or muscle contractions.
spirometer: An instrument that measures the volume of air inhaled and exhaled.
stertorous: Heavy, as related to snoring.
tachypnea: Rapid, shallow breathing.
vertigo: Dizziness; an abnormal sensation of movement when there is none.
wheezing: Whistling sound made during breathing.

CHAPTER 29 Vital Signs 651

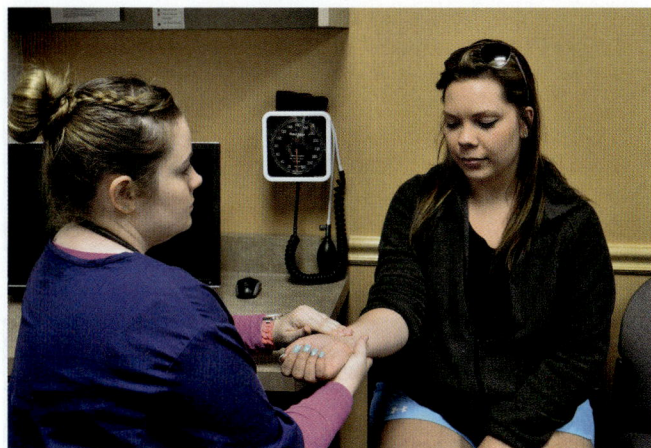

FIG. 29.12 Hand position when counting respirations. The hands should be left in place as if still counting the patient's pulse. (From Proctor D, et al: *Kinn's The Medical Assistant*, ed 13, St. Louis, 2017, Elsevier.)

TABLE 29.4 Approximate Age-Related Blood Pressure Ranges

Age	RANGE	
	Systolic	Diastolic
Newborn	60–96	30–62
1–3 years	78–112	48–78
4–6 years	78–112	50–79
7–11 years	85–114	52–79
Adolescent	94–119	58–79
Adult	100–119	60–79

shoulders with each inspiration. Count the respirations for 30 seconds and multiply the number by 2. Do not use the 15-second interval because this count can vary by a factor of ±4, which is significant when dealing with such a small number. Note any variation or irregularity in the rhythm or depth. Record the respirations in the health record.

> **CRITICAL THINKING 29.5**
>
> Tina Anderson, a 36-year-old patient who is obese, is wearing a heavy knit sweater, and Carlos needs to obtain a respiratory count. What could he do to obtain an accurate measurement of Tina's respiratory rate?

BLOOD PRESSURE

A blood pressure (BP) reading reflects the pressure of the blood against the walls of the arteries. Each time the ventricles contract, blood is pushed out of the heart and into the aorta, exerting pressure on the walls of the arteries. There are actually two BP readings:

- The *systolic* (SIS tol ic) pressure is the highest pressure level that occurs when the heart is contracting and is the first sound heard.
- The *diastolic* (dye AS tol ic) pressure is the lowest pressure level when the heart is relaxed and is the last sound heard.

Systole (heart contraction) and diastole (heart relaxation) together make up the cardiac cycle. The difference between systolic and diastolic pressures is the pulse pressure.

Blood pressure is read in millimeters of mercury, abbreviated *mm Hg*. However, you need not include the abbreviation when documenting the reading in the patient's health record. BP is recorded as a fraction, with the systolic reading serving as the numerator (top) and the diastolic reading serving as the denominator (bottom) (e.g., 130/80). Table 29.4 lists normal BP ranges for patients of various age groups.

Factors Affecting Blood Pressure

Factors that determine blood pressure include the following:
- Blood volume
- Peripheral resistance created by blood *viscosity* (vi SKOS it tee) (the thickness of the blood)
- Vessel elasticity
- Condition of the heart muscle and arterial walls

Volume is the amount of blood in the arteries. An increased blood volume raises BP, and a decreased blood volume lowers BP. With extensive bleeding or hemorrhage, the blood volume drops, and so does the BP.

The *peripheral resistance* of blood vessels refers to the lumen (the diameter of the vessel) and the amount of blood flowing through it. The smaller the lumen, the greater the resistance to blood flow. BP is higher with a small or reduced-size lumen and lower with a large lumen. Vessels affected by fatty cholesterol deposits (*atherosclerotic plaque* [ath uh roh skluh ROH tic plak]) become narrower over time. This results in smaller vessel lumens and therefore higher blood pressure.

Vessel elasticity is the ability of an artery to expand and contract to supply the body with a steady flow of blood. With advancing age, certain lifestyle factors, or the presence of arteriosclerosis (ar teer ee oh sklah ROH sis), vessel elasticity may decrease. This causes the arterial walls to become firm and resistant, increasing the BP.

The condition of the myocardium (mye oh KAR dee um) is a primary determinant of the volume of blood flowing through the body. A strong, forceful contraction empties the heart and tends to keep the BP within normal limits. If the myocardium becomes weak, pressure in the vessels begins to increase in an attempt to maintain an adequate level of circulating blood to meet the oxygen and nutrient needs of the body.

Evaluating the Blood Pressure

The American Heart Association (AHA) guidelines for the diagnosis and management of hypertension include four categories for diagnostic and treatment purposes (Table 29.5). The goal of the AHA recommendations is to reduce the number of people who die each year from hypertension-related illnesses, such as these:

> **VOCABULARY**
>
> **arteriosclerosis:** Thickening, decreased elasticity, and calcification of arterial walls.
> **pulse pressure:** The difference between the systolic and diastolic blood pressures (30 to 50 mm Hg is considered normal).
> **myocardium:** Middle layer and the thickest layer of the heart; composed of cardiac muscles.

TABLE 29.5 Stages and Treatment of Hypertension

Blood Pressure	Treatment
Prehypertension 120–139 systolic OR 80–89 diastolic	Lifestyle modification (reduced sodium, low saturated and trans fat diet; regular aerobic activity; moderate alcohol intake; smoking cessation; weight loss; stress reduction) Drug therapy for patients with diabetes mellitus or chronic kidney disease
Stage 1 hypertension 140–159 systolic OR 90–99 diastolic	Consider coexisting conditions Thiazide-type diuretics (e.g., furosemide [Lasix] or hydrochlorothiazide plus triamterene [Dyazide]) for most patients
Stage 2 hypertension ≥160 systolic OR ≥100 diastolic	Consider coexisting conditions Two-drug combination for most patients
Hypertensive Crisis >180 systolic >110 diastolic	Requires emergency medical attention

Modified from the Seventh Report of the Joint National Committee on Prevention, Detection, Evaluation, and Treatment of High Blood Pressure at http://www.nhlbi.nih.gov/health-pro/guidelines/current/hypertension-jnc-7/.

BOX 29.4 Signs and Symptoms of Hypertension

- Blurred vision
- Vertigo
- Fatigue
- Flushing
- Angina
- Dyspnea
- Headache
- Nosebleeds (*epistaxis* [ep uh STAK sis])

BOX 29.5 Races Associated With Greater Risk of Developing Hypertension

- African Americans
- Native Americans
- Some Asian Americans
- Mexican Americans
- Native Hawaiians

BOX 29.6 Metabolic Syndrome

Metabolic syndrome occurs when a patient has at least three of the five following conditions:
- Abdominal obesity
- Elevated blood pressure
- Elevated fasting plasma glucose
- High serum triglycerides
- Low high-density lipoprotein (HDL) levels

Metabolic syndrome is associated with an increased risk of developing cardiovascular disease and type 2 diabetes. It is estimated that one-quarter of adults in the United States have metabolic syndrome.

- Coronary artery disease
- Heart attack
- Heart failure
- Kidney disease
- Stroke

Hypertension can occur in children or adults, but individuals of African American descent, middle-aged and older adults, patients with diabetes mellitus, and those with kidney disease are at greatest risk. Hypertension has been called *the silent killer* because it frequently has no symptoms. Individuals may go for long periods without knowing they have a problem (Box 29.4). Hypertension often is discovered during treatment for another problem. Table 29.5 summarizes the stages and recommended treatment for the different levels of elevated blood pressure.

Essential hypertension (stage 1 primary hypertension) (see Table 29.5) is the most common type of hypertension. It is **idiopathic** (id ee uh PATH ik) but is associated with obesity, a high blood level of sodium, elevated cholesterol levels, family history, and race (Box 29.5).

VOCABULARY
essential hypertension: Elevated blood pressure of unknown cause that develops for no apparent reason; sometimes called *primary hypertension*.
idiopathic: Of unknown cause.

When there is a concern about a patient's BP, the individual is often asked to track it. These readings should be taken at about the same time of day and by the same person using the same-size cuff and the same arm. *Secondary hypertension* is caused by another underlying pathologic condition, such as the following:
- Renal disease
- Complications of pregnancy
- Endocrine imbalance
- Brain injury

Temporary hypertension may occur with stress, pain, exercise, and exhaustion. Many patients experience "white coat syndrome." This is when their BP becomes elevated in the medical environment, but it is normal when they are away from the healthcare facility.

If a patient's BP is persistently in the prehypertension range at two or more office visits over time, essential hypertension is diagnosed. If the patient's BP is elevated initially, it should be checked again after the patient has been allowed to sit comfortably for at least 2 minutes. Check the BP in both arms with a cuff that is the proper size. If the readings are different, the provider uses the higher value for diagnostic purposes. All of the readings must be documented in the patient's record.

Hypertension is also linked to metabolic syndrome. For more information on metabolic syndrome see Box 29.6.

Treatment guidelines for hypertension have four basic aspects:
1. Individuals with prehypertension should be diagnosed and encouraged to make lifestyle changes before they require treatment or move into the hypertensive category. The AHA recommends limiting one's intake of salt and eating a diet rich in potassium, calcium, magnesium, and protein while reducing total fat intake, especially saturated fat. Individuals with prehypertension also should restrict their alcohol intake, engage in regular physical activity, and lose weight if necessary to maintain a healthy BMI range (see Box 29.8, presented later in the chapter). Many times, just losing 10% of a person's weight lowers the blood pressure.
2. In people older than 50 years of age, the systolic reading is more important than the diastolic reading. Individuals over 50 should be treated if they have a systolic pressure of 140 mm Hg or higher, regardless of their diastolic blood pressure. Medical treatment at

this age can reduce the development of cardiac and kidney disease later in life.
3. Most patients with hypertension require two or more medications to achieve desired blood pressure levels. The goal of treatment is to maintain blood pressure below 140/90 mm Hg, or below 130/80 mm Hg in patients with diabetes or kidney disease. Patients should be treated with both a diuretic, to help the body excrete excess amounts of fluid and sodium, and an antihypertensive medication.
4. A patient-centered treatment approach should be implemented to motivate patients and to maintain compliance with hypertension management. The medical assistant can play an active role in establishing a therapeutic relationship with the patient by providing ongoing education and support to ensure compliance with provider-recommended treatment. Using community resources, such as local dietitian referrals, may also help patients comply with treatment.

Hypotension is an abnormally low blood pressure, which may be caused by emotional or traumatic shock, hemorrhage, central nervous system (CNS) disorders, and chronic wasting diseases. Persistent readings of 90/60 mm Hg or lower usually are considered hypotensive. Orthostatic (postural) hypotension can cause patients to experience vertigo or syncope (SING kuh pee). Some medications can cause orthostatic hypotension.

> ### CRITICAL THINKING 29.6
> Mr. Samuel Long, a 43-year-old patient, recently was diagnosed with essential hypertension. What should Carlos discuss with Mr. Long to emphasize the dangers of his disease and to teach him about possible lifestyle modifications that he must make to improve his health? Are any community resources available that might help Mr. Long and his family effectively manage his disease?

> ### VOCABULARY
> **hypotension:** Blood pressure that is below normal (systolic pressure below 90 mm Hg and diastolic pressure below 50 mm Hg).
> **orthostatic (postural) hypotension:** A temporary fall in blood pressure when a person rapidly changes from a recumbent position to a standing position.
> **syncope:** Fainting; a brief lapse in consciousness.

Measuring Blood Pressure

The instrument used to measure blood pressure is called a *sphygmomanometer* (sfig moh man NAW meh ter) or blood pressure cuff. It consists of an inflatable cuff, an inflation bulb with a control valve, and a pressure gauge. The blood pressure mechanism consists of an aneroid dial attached to an inflatable cuff (Fig. 29.13A); the device may be handheld, wall mounted, or a floor model (Fig. 29.13B). Some systems have a trigger-style air release valve; these can be pumped up and then the air slowly released simply by pushing the trigger (Fig. 29.14). With the more traditional sphygmomanometers, the valve must be unscrewed.

> ### MEDICAL TERMINOLOGY
> **man/o:** scanty pressure
> **-meter:** instrument to measure
> **sphygm/o:** pulse

Sphygmomanometers are delicately calibrated (KAL uh breyt d) instruments that must be handled carefully. They should be recalibrated regularly and checked for accuracy by you or by a medical supply dealer. The needle on the aneroid dial sphygmomanometer should rest within the small square or circle at the bottom of the dial. If the sphygmomanometer is not correctly calibrated, the patient's blood pressure reading will be inaccurate.

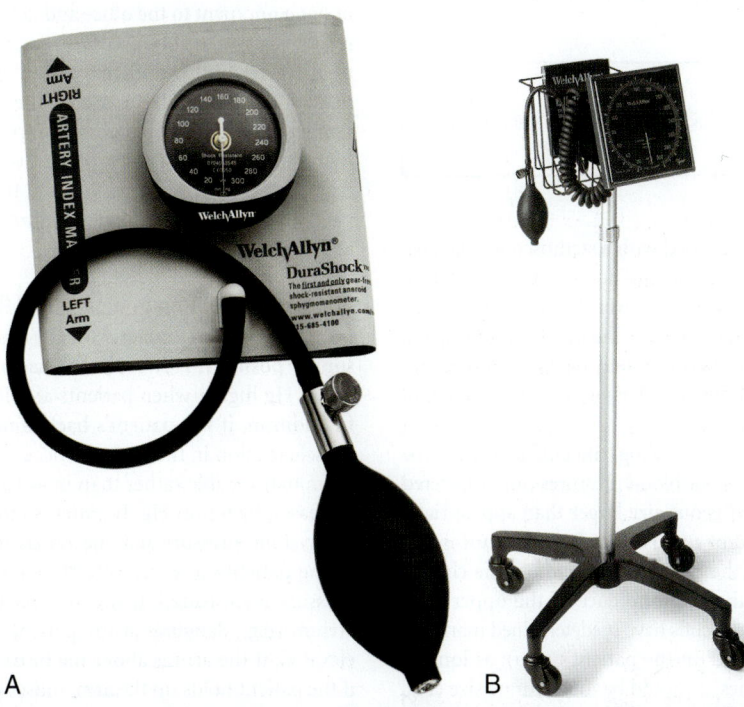

FIG. 29.13 (A) Aneroid dial system with an inflatable cuff. (B) Aneroid floor model with a large slanted face. (From Proctor D, et al: *Kinn's The Medical Assistant*, ed 13, St. Louis, 2017, Elsevier.)

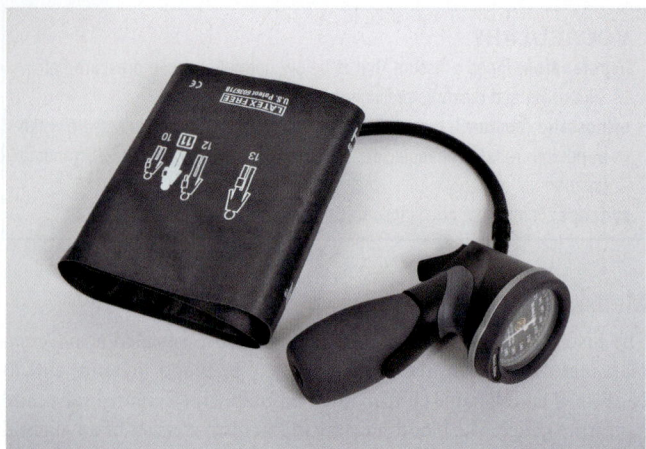

FIG. 29.14 Trigger-release aneroid blood pressure valve. (From Proctor D, et al: *Kinn's The Medical Assistant*, ed 13, St. Louis, 2017, Elsevier.)

TABLE 29.6	Blood Pressure Cuff Sizes	
	ARM CIRCUMFERENCE	
Cuff	**Centimeters**	**Inches**
Small adult	22–26	9
Adult	27–34	Up to 13
Large adult	35–44	14–17
Adult thigh	45–52	18–20

Data from Pickering TG, Hall JE, Appel LJ, et al: Recommendations for blood pressure measurement in humans and experimental animals: Part 1. Blood pressure measurement in humans: a statement for professionals from the Subcommittee of Professional and Public Education of the American Heart Association Council on High Blood Pressure Research, *Hypertension* 45:142–161, 2005.

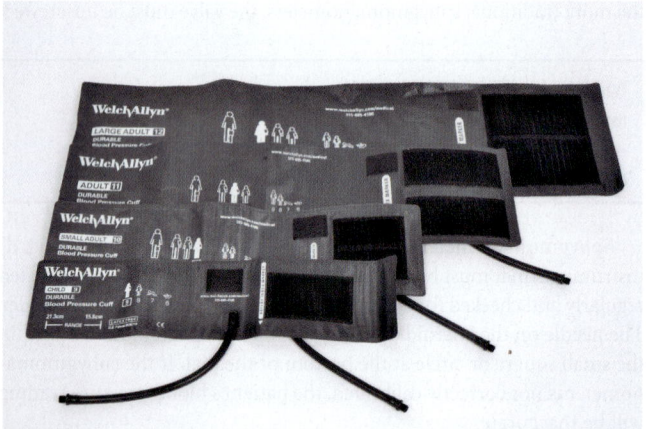

FIG. 29.15 Variety of blood pressure cuff sizes. (From Proctor D, et al: *Kinn's The Medical Assistant*, ed 13, St. Louis, 2017, Elsevier.)

> **VOCABULARY**
>
> **calibrated:** Determined by or checked against those of a standard (as in readings).

The sphygmomanometer must be used with a stethoscope. The goal of the procedure is to use the inflatable cuff to stop the circulation through an artery. The stethoscope is placed over the artery just below the cuff. As the cuff is slowly deflated to allow the blood to flow again, cardiac cycle sounds are heard through the stethoscope, and readings are taken when the first (systolic) and last (diastolic) sounds are heard (Procedure 29.8).

To obtain a correct blood pressure reading, the cuff used must be the proper size. The systolic and diastolic blood pressures can be lowered by as much as 5 mm Hg if the cuff is one size larger than appropriate; the blood pressure can be elevated by up to 6 mm Hg if the cuff is one size smaller. The inflatable part (the bladder) of a cuff of the correct size should cover about 80% of the circumference of the upper arm. To help with this, most blood pressure cuffs have predetermined markings on the internal side (the side placed on the patient's arm); as long as the cuff is secured within these lines, it should be the accurate size (Fig. 29.15). Table 29.6 presents the various sizes of blood pressure cuffs available.

When placed on the patient's arm, the cuff should cover two-thirds of the distance from the elbow to the shoulder. The lower edge of the cuff should be 2 to 3 cm (about 2 finger widths, or 1 inch) above the elbow or antecubital space to allow plenty of room to place the stethoscope without touching the cuff. If the stethoscope touches the cuff during the blood pressure reading, the sound of the deflating cuff may interfere with your ability to hear the correct reading. The patient's sleeve must be above the antecubital space; if the sleeve is tight, ask the patient to remove the arm from the sleeve. This is done for two reasons: tight clothing can restrict normal blood flow in the brachial artery, altering the blood pressure, and placing the stethoscope over clothing makes it difficult to hear blood pressure sounds. Provide a patient gown if needed to maintain the patient's privacy.

Blood pressure cuffs and stethoscopes are available in drug and retail stores for patients to use to measure their own blood pressure at home. These units can be aneroid, electronic, or computerized sphygmomanometers (Fig. 29.16). If you have patients who are monitoring their pressure at home, be sure they understand the mechanics of obtaining an accurate reading. It is best to have the patient bring his or her equipment to the office and demonstrate its use. While the patient is showing you the home equipment, you will have an ideal opportunity to check technique and calibration and to answer any questions the patient may have about use of the equipment. This is also a good opportunity to reinforce treatment plans, such as medication, diet, and exercise. It is helpful for a patient who is monitoring blood pressure readings at home to keep a log and review it with the provider during visits to help detect blood pressure variations during normal daily activities.

Effects of Body Position on Blood Pressure Measurement. Blood pressure is usually taken with the patient in either the sitting or the supine position. However, the diastolic pressure can be as much as 5 mm Hg higher when patients are sitting than when they are supine. In addition, if the patient's back is not supported and there is some muscle tension in the body (as occurs when the patient is seated on an examination table rather than in a chair), the diastolic pressure may be increased by 6 mm Hg. If patients cross their legs during the reading, the systolic pressure may be raised by 2 to 8 mm Hg. The position of the patient's arm can also have a major influence when the blood pressure is measured. If the upper arm is below the level of the right atrium (e.g., dangling at the patient's side), the reading is artificially elevated; if the arm is above the heart level, the reading is lowered. Or if the patient holds up the arm, muscular tension will raise the pressure. The arm should be placed at the level of the heart on a table next to an exam room chair or resting on the arm of the chair to avoid these

PROCEDURE 29.8   Determine a Patient's Blood Pressure

Task
Perform a blood pressure measurement that is correct in technique, accurate, and comfortable for the patient.

Equipment and Supplies
- Patient's record
- Sphygmomanometer
- Stethoscope
- Antiseptic wipes/alcohol wipes

Procedural Steps
1. Wash hands or use hand sanitizer.
   Purpose: To ensure infection control.
2. Assemble the equipment and supplies needed. Clean the earpieces and diaphragm of the stethoscope with alcohol wipes.
   Purpose: For infection control and to follow Standard Precautions.
3. Greet the patient. Identify yourself. Verify the patient's identity with full name and date of birth. Explain the procedure to be performed in a manner that the patient understands. Answer any questions the patient may have about the procedure.
   Purpose: Identification of the patient prevents errors, and explanations are a means of gaining implied consent and patient cooperation.
4. Select the appropriate arm for application of the cuff (no mastectomy on that side, no injury or disease). If the patient has had a bilateral mastectomy, the blood pressure should be taken using a large thigh cuff with the stethoscope over the popliteal artery.
   Purpose: The pressure of the cuff temporarily interferes with circulation to the limb.
   Caution: If a female patient has had a mastectomy, the blood pressure should never be taken on the affected side. Compressing the arm may cause complications. If she has had a bilateral mastectomy, another site such as the popliteal artery must be used, which requires use of a thigh cuff.
5. Seat the patient in a comfortable position with the legs uncrossed and the arm resting, palm up, at heart level on the arm of a chair or a table next to where the patient is seated.
   Purpose: To expose the brachial artery; also, to promote patient relaxation and ensure a true reading. Crossed legs may increase the blood pressure, and positioning of the arm above heart level may cause an inaccurate reading.
6. Roll the sleeve to about 5 inches above the elbow, or have the patient remove the arm from the sleeve.
   Purpose: Tight clothing prevents an accurate reading.
7. Select the correct cuff size.
   Purpose: An incorrect cuff size prevents accurate measurement of blood pressure. The cuff should fit comfortably around the patient's arm, and the bladder should be located over the brachial artery between the lines designated on the cuff. Pediatric, normal adult, and large adult cuff sizes should be available. Thigh cuffs may be needed for obese patients.
8. Palpate the brachial artery at the antecubital space in both arms. If one arm has a stronger pulse, use that arm. If the pulses are equal, select the right arm.
   Purpose: A stronger pulse is easier to measure; the right arm is the universal arm of choice.
9. Center the cuff bladder over the brachial artery with the connecting tube away from the patient's body and the tube to the bulb close to the body (Fig. 1).
   Purpose: Pressure must be applied directly over the artery for an accurate reading. The cuff and its tubing should not touch the stethoscope. Noise from the tubing can interfere with a correct reading.
10. Place the lower edge of the cuff about 1 inch above the palpable brachial pulse, normally located in the natural crease of the inner elbow, and wrap it snugly and smoothly.

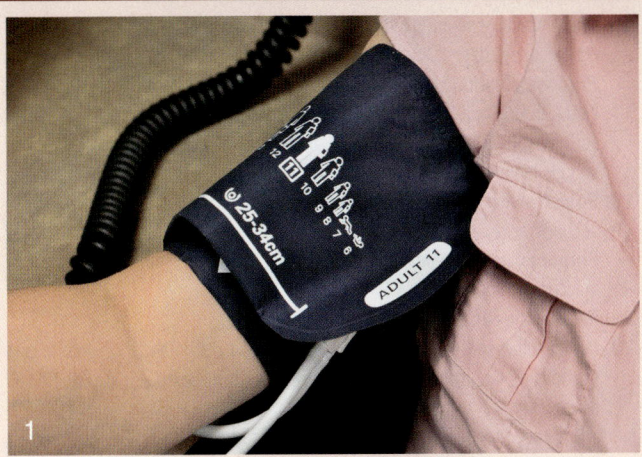

   Purpose: To help ensure an accurate reading. The cuff should be high enough on the arm that the stethoscope does not touch it and so that cuff sounds do not interfere with listening to the blood pressure sounds. A loose cuff results in an inaccurate reading.
11. Position the gauge of the sphygmomanometer so that it is easily seen.
    Purpose: An aneroid gauge should show the needle within the zero mark.
12. Palpate the radial pulse, tighten the screw valve on the air pump, and inflate the cuff until the pulse can no longer be felt. Make a note at the point on the gauge where the pulse could no longer be felt. Mentally add 30 mm Hg to the reading. Deflate the cuff, and wait 15 seconds.
    Purpose: The point where the radial pulse is no longer felt provides an estimate of the systolic pressure. Pumping the cuff above that level ensures that phase I of the Korotkoff sounds will be heard.
13. Insert the earpieces of the stethoscope turned forward into the ear canals.
    Purpose: With the earpieces in this position, the openings follow the anatomic line of the ear canal and the blood pressure will be accurately heard.
14. Place the stethoscope's diaphragm over the palpated brachial artery for an adult patient or the bell for a pediatric patient. Press firmly enough to obtain a seal but not so tightly that the artery is constricted. Only touch the edges of the stethoscope head.
    Purpose: Forming a seal around the head of the stethoscope aids listening for blood pressure sounds. Placing your fingers directly over the stethoscope head will cause interference with the sound.
15. Close the valve and squeeze the bulb to inflate the cuff, rapidly but smoothly, to 30 mm above the palpated systolic level, which was previously determined (Fig. 2).

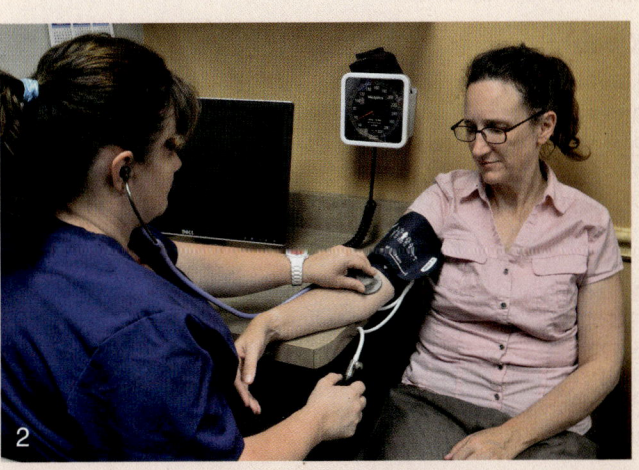

Continued

PROCEDURE 29.8 Determine a Patient's Blood Pressure—cont'd

16. Open the valve slightly and deflate the cuff at a constant rate of 2 to 3 mm Hg per heartbeat.
    Purpose: Careful, slow release allows you to listen to all sounds.
17. Listen throughout the entire deflation; note the point on the gauge at which you hear the first sound (systolic), the last sound (diastolic), and until the sounds have stopped for at least 10 mm Hg.
18. Do not reinflate the cuff once the air has been released. Wait 30 to 60 seconds to repeat the procedure if needed.
    Purpose: Not allowing the blood to refill in the brachial artery results in inaccurate readings.
19. Remove the cuff from the patient's arm.
20. Remove the stethoscope from your ears, and document the systolic and diastolic readings and the arm used as BP systolic/diastolic (e.g., BP: 120/80 R arm).
    Note: It is recommended that the blood pressure be checked and documented in each arm during the initial assessment of the patient and then bilaterally periodically after that for patients with hypertension.
21. Clean the earpieces and the head of the stethoscope with an alcohol wipe and return both the cuff and the stethoscope to storage.
22. Wash hands or use hand sanitizer.
    Purpose: To ensure infection control.
23. Document the reading in the patient's medical record.
    Purpose: Procedures that are not recorded are considered not done.
    Addendum: The provider may direct the medical assistant to record the blood pressure with the patient in three different positions to determine whether orthostatic hypotension is a factor. Complete the following steps to perform this skill:

1. Measure and record the patient's blood pressure (as detailed earlier) while the patient is supine.
2. Leave the cuff in place.
3. Have the patient sit, and immediately measure the blood pressure again.
4. Leave the cuff in place.
5. Have the patient stand, and immediately measure the blood pressure again.
6. Record the second blood pressure and any patient symptoms, such as complaints of (c/o) vertigo or lightheadedness.

5/19/20XX 11:00 a.m. BP: 120/80 arm, supine, 124/82 arm sitting, 130/90 arm standing. ————————————————— C. Ricci, CMA (AAMA)

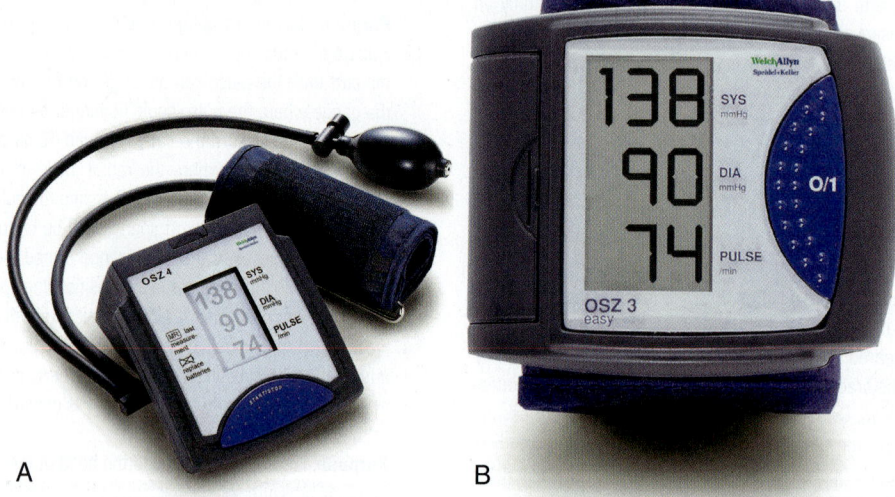

FIG. 29.16 Personal blood pressure systems. (A) Digital arm cuff. (B) Digital wrist cuff. (From Proctor D, et al: *Kinn's The Medical Assistant*, ed 13, St. Louis, 2017, Elsevier.)

issues (Fig. 29.17). Box 29.7 discusses the common causes of errors in blood pressure readings.

Korotkoff Sounds

Korotkoff sounds are the sounds heard during auscultation of blood pressure. Vibrations of the arterial wall produce these sounds when the blood surges back into the vessel after it has been compressed by the blood pressure cuff. The sounds were first discovered and classified into five distinct phases by Russian neurologist Nikolai Korotkoff.

Phase I. Phase I is the first sound heard as the cuff deflates. The blood is resurging into the patient's artery and can be heard clearly as a sharp, tapping sound. Note the gauge reading when this first sound is heard. Record this as the systolic blood pressure.

Phase II. As the cuff deflates, even more blood flows through the artery. The movement of the blood makes a swishing sound. If you did not follow proper procedure in inflating the cuff, you may not hear these sounds because of their soft quality. Occasionally blood pressure sounds completely disappear during this phase. Loss of the sounds, followed by their reappearance later, is called the *auscultatory* (AW skuh l tah tohr ee) *gap*. The silence may continue as the needle falls another 30 mm Hg. Auscultatory gaps occur particularly in hypertension and certain types of heart disease, so if you notice such a gap, make sure to report it to the provider.

Phase III. In phase III, a great deal of blood is moving down into the artery. The distinct, sharp tapping sounds return and continue rhythmically. If you do not inflate the cuff enough, you will miss the first two phases completely and you will incorrectly interpret the beginning of phase III as the systolic blood pressure (phase I).

Phase IV. At this point, the blood is flowing easily. The sound changes to a soft tapping, which becomes muffled and begins to grow fainter.

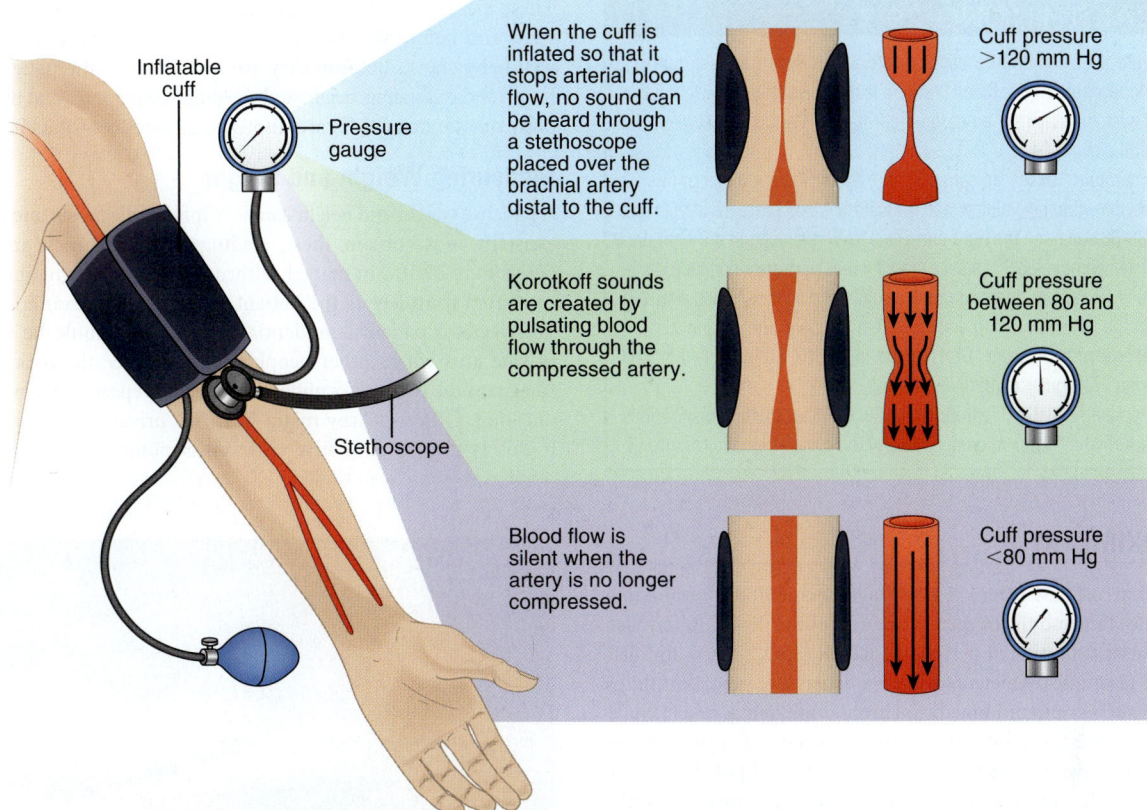

FIG. 29.17 The science of taking a patient's blood pressure. (From Proctor D, et al: *Kinn's The Medical Assistant*, ed 13, St. Louis, 2017, Elsevier.)

BOX 29.7 Common Causes of Errors in Blood Pressure Readings

- The limb used for measurement is above the level of the heart.
- The bladder in the cuff is not completely deflated before a reading is started or retaken.
- The pressure in the cuff is released too rapidly.
- The patient is nervous, uncomfortable, or anxious (may cause a reading to be higher than the patient's actual blood pressure).
- The patient drank coffee or smoked cigarettes within 30 minutes of the blood pressure measurement.
- The cuff was applied improperly.
- The cuff is too large, too small, too loose, or too tight.
- The cuff was not placed around the arm smoothly.
- The bladder is not centered over the artery, or the bladder bulges out from the cover.
- There was a failure to wait 1 to 2 minutes between measurements.
- Instruments are defective:
  - Air leaks in the valve
  - Air leaks in the bladder
  - Aneroid needle not calibrated to zero

Occasionally these sounds continue to zero. This may occur in children, in patients of any age after exercise or with a fever, or in a pregnant patient with anemia. The AHA recommends that the beginning of phase IV be recorded as the diastolic reading for a child. Some providers call the change at phase IV the *fading sound* and want it recorded between systolic and diastolic recordings (e.g., 120/84/70, with 84 representing the gauge reading when the sounds of phase III have ended and those of phase IV are beginning). Other providers consider phase IV the true diastolic pressure.

Phase V. All sounds disappear in this phase. Note the gauge reading when the last sound is heard. Record this as the diastolic pressure.

Palpatory Method

The systolic pressure may be checked by feeling the radial pulse rather than hearing it with the stethoscope. Place the cuff in the usual position and palpate the radial pulse, noting rate and rhythm. Inflate the cuff until the pulse disappears, then add 30 mm Hg more of inflation to get above the systolic pressure. Do not remove your fingers from the pulse or change the pressure of your fingers. Carefully watch the gauge while slowly releasing the pressure in the cuff, and wait until you feel the first pulse beat. Note the reading on the gauge, and document the first pulse felt as the systolic pressure. For example, if you first felt the radial pulse return at 102 mm Hg, the palpated blood pressure is recorded as 102/P, with P indicating that the systolic reading was palpated. The diastolic and Korotkoff phases cannot be determined by this method. This method can be very useful in times of a medical emergency, such as shock, when the patient's blood pressure cannot be auscultated. The palpatory method can be used to determine how far you need to pump the cuff to hear that first beat. This is useful for a new patient.

CRITICAL THINKING 29.7

Vital signs are documented in a paper record in this order: temperature (T), pulse (P), and respirations (R). Blood pressure is recorded after TPR. Depending on the EHR system, they may be ordered differently. Correctly document the following vital signs:

1. Oral temperature 101.2°; apical pulse 90 regular rhythm; respirations 22 regular rhythm, shallow volume; and orthostatic blood pressure in the right arm is 138/88 supine in the right arm and 110/70 standing in the right arm
2. Tympanic temperature 36.8°; radial pulse 66, irregular rhythm, normal volume; respirations 18, regular rhythm, normal volume; and bilateral blood pressure 128/76 in the left arm, sitting and 132/80 in the right arm, sitting
3. Temporal artery temperature 102.4°; apical pulse 102, irregular rhythm; and respirations 27, regular rhythm, normal volume
4. Axillary temperature 97.7°; carotid pulse 58, irregular rhythm; respirations 24, regular rhythm, deep volume; and palpated systolic blood pressure 62

PULSE OXIMETRY

Pulse oximetry (ok SIM i tree) is a noninvasive method of evaluating both the pulse rate and the oxygen saturation of the blood. It may also be referred to as saturation of peripheral oxygen (SpO_2). Many ambulatory settings use pulse oximeters to assess a patient's oxygenation status in disorders such as pneumonia, bronchitis, emphysema, or asthma.

To perform the procedure, the medical assistant clips a probe on the patient's earlobe or finger (Fig. 29.18). Fingernail polish must be removed before the clip is applied. If the patient has artificial nails, the earlobe should be used. A beam of infrared light passes through the tissue, and the amount of light absorbed by oxygenated hemoglobin is measured. This is displayed on the digital screen as a percentage. At the same time, the light measures the patient's pulse rate, which also is shown on the screen. A normal pulse oximetry reading is 95% or higher. Treatment, such as oxygen or bronchodilator therapies, usually is started when readings are 90% to 92% or lower (Procedure 29.9).

ANTHROPOMETRIC MEASUREMENTS

Anthropometry (an thruh POM i tree) is the science that deals with measurement of the size, weight, and proportions of the human body. These measurements often are included in the initial recording of vital signs and before the provider performs a physical examination or a well-baby check. Because they are indicators of the patient's state of health and well-being, height and weight measurements and the associated body mass index (BMI) are discussed as aspects of the vital signs.

Measuring Weight and Height

A patient's weight and height can be helpful in diagnosis, and the medical assistant must obtain these readings with accuracy and empathy (Procedure 29.10). In many healthcare facilities, weight and height are measured routinely as the patient is taken to the examination room. To safeguard patient confidentiality, the scale should be located in a private area where other people are cannot see the patient's weight. Safeguard the patient's confidentiality by not repeating the measurement out loud. Others nearby might hear this private patient information. If this is the patient's first visit, anthropometric measurements are

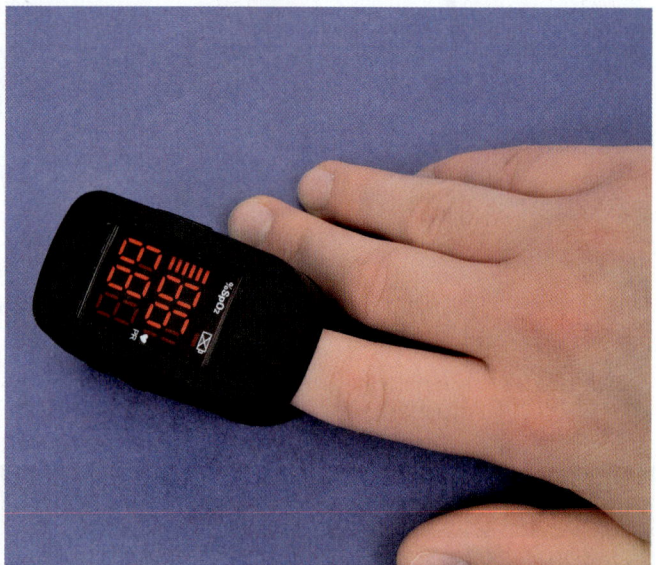

FIG. 29.18 Pulse oximeter. (From Proctor D, et al: *Kinn's The Medical Assistant*, ed 13, St. Louis, 2017, Elsevier.)

PROCEDURE 29.9 Perform Pulse Oximetry

Task
Assess the adequacy of oxygen levels (or oxygen saturation) in the blood using a pulse oximeter.

Equipment and Supplies
- Patient's health record
- Pulse oximeter and probe of the appropriate size

Procedural Steps
1. Assemble the equipment.
2. Greet the patient. Identify yourself. Verify the patient's identity with full name and date of birth. Explain the procedure to be performed in a manner that the patient understands. Answer any questions the patient may have about the procedure.
   Purpose: An informed patient is more cooperative.
3. Wash hands or use hand sanitizer.
   Purpose: Standard Precautions must be followed to prevent the spread of disease.
4. Turn on the monitor, and attach the probe to the finger (preferred) or ear lobe so it is flush with the skin.
5. The light-emitting diode (LED) should be placed on top of the nail. If the patient is wearing nail polish or has artificial nails, these may have to be removed to get a strong pulse signal.
   Purpose: To measure the pulse and oxygen saturation level.
6. Sanitize the patient probe and the external portion of the monitor with an aseptic cleaner.
   Purpose: To follow Standard Precautions.
7. Wash hands or use hand sanitizer.
   Purpose: To ensure infection control.
8. Document the oxygen saturation percentage and pulse in the patient's health record. Include date, time, and if the patient is receiving supplemental oxygen record the amount in liters.
   Purpose: Procedures that are not documented are considered not done.

PROCEDURE 29.10 Measuring a Patient's Weight and Height

Task
Accurately weigh and measure a patient as part of the physical assessment procedure.
Note: Make sure the scale is located in an area away from traffic to maintain the patient's privacy.

Equipment and Supplies
- Balance beam scale with a measuring bar
- Paper towel
- Patient record

Procedural Steps
1. Wash hands or use hand sanitizer.
   Purpose: To ensure infection control.
2. Greet the patient. Identify yourself. Verify the patient's identity with full name and date of birth. Explain the procedure to be performed in a manner that the patient understands. Answer any questions the patient may have about the procedure.
   Purpose: Identification of the patient prevents errors, and explanations are a means of gaining implied consent and patient cooperation.
3. Have the patient remove his or her shoes. Place a paper towel on the scale platform. Check to see that the balance bar pointer floats in the middle of the balance frame when all weights are at zero.
   Purpose: A floating pointer indicates that the scale is properly adjusted and in balance.
4. Help the patient onto the scale. Make sure the patient has removed any heavy objects from pockets and is not holding anything such as a jacket or purse.
5. Move the large weight into the groove closest to the patient's estimated weight. The grooves are calibrated in 50-lb increments. If you choose a groove that is more than the patient's weight, the pointer will immediately tilt to the bottom of the balance frame. You then must move it back one groove (Fig. 1).

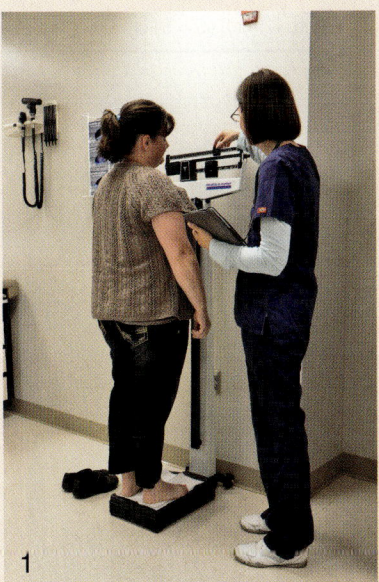

6. While the patient is standing still, slide the small upper weight to the right along the pound markers until the pointer balances in the middle of the balance frame.
   Purpose: The pointer floats between the bottom and the top of the frame when both lower and upper weights together balance the scale with the patient's weight.
7. Leave the weights in place.
8. Ask the patient to step off the scale, and move the height bar to a point above the patient's height. Extend the bar, and ask the patient step back on the scale. On some scales, the patient may need to turn with his or her back to the scale.
9. Adjust the height bar so that it just touches the top of the patient's head (Fig. 2).

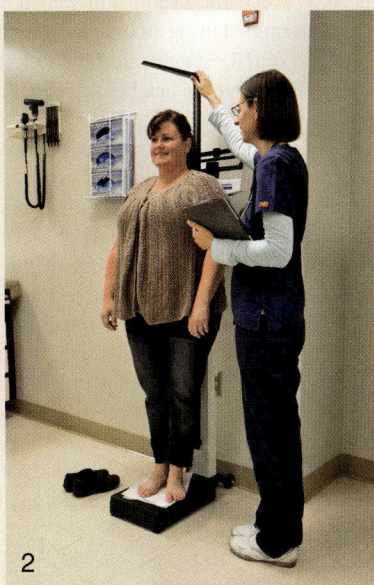

10. Leave the elevation bar set.
    Purpose: To maintain the height recording while protecting the patient from possible injury.
11. Assist the patient off the scale. Make sure all items that were removed for weighing are given back to the patient.
12. Read the weight scale. Add the numbers at the markers of the large and small weights, and document the total to the nearest quarter of a pound in the patient's health record (e.g., Wt: 136½ lb).
13. Read the height. Read the marker at the movable point of the ruler, and document the measurement to the nearest quarter of an inch on the patient's medical record (e.g., Ht: 5" 6½") (Fig. 3).

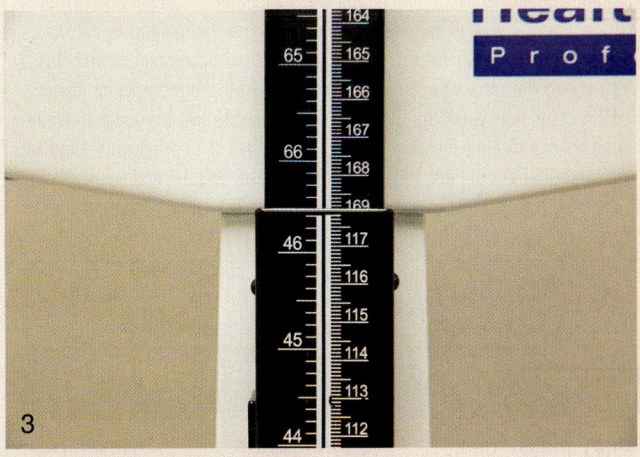

14. Use the patient's weight and height to determine the BMI if the EHR program does not do it automatically.
15. Return the weights and the measuring bar to zero.
16. Remove the paper towel and dispose of in the waste container. Wash hands or use hand sanitizer.
17. Document the results in the patient's health record.

5/26/20XX 11:07 a.m. Wt: 136½ lb, Ht: 5'6½" ——————— C. Ricci, CMA (AAMA)

recorded in the history database and are used as reference information during future visits as needed.

Many providers use the BMI (Box 29.8) to determine the risk for certain diseases, so the medical assistant may have to use the accurately measured height and weight to determine and record the patient's BMI. This is typically done using a BMI chart that converts the patient's height and weight ratio into a BMI number, or with a wheeled device that calibrates the BMI when the height and weight intersect. BMI numbers also can be determined using an online conversion calculator. Electronic health record (EHR) systems automatically calculate and document the patient's BMI after the height and weight measurements are entered.

Certain medical specialties and specific medical problems may require continuous monitoring of weight. Hormone disorders (e.g., diabetes), growth patterns (seen in children), and eating disorders (e.g., obesity, bulimia) require accurate weight checks as part of every medical visit. In addition, pregnant patients must have their weight monitored to make sure they are gaining weight, but also as a precaution against too much weight gain, which may indicate fluid retention. Patients with cardiovascular disorders who tend to retain fluid should have their weight checked each time they are seen in the office. Many healthcare facilities document weight in kilograms, but most Americans understand the pound measurements better. When weight must be converted from one to the other, use the formulas shown in Box 29.9 or an online conversion calculator. EHR systems do the conversion automatically.

Accurate height or length measurements are particularly important for children (see Chapter 32). The provider also may request routine height screening for patients diagnosed with osteoporosis because these patients may lose height over time.

CRITICAL THINKING 29.8

- A patient weighs 87 kg. How many pounds does he weigh?
- A patient weighs 148 lb. How many kilograms does she weigh?

Weight. Weight can be a sensitive issue for many patients. Maintain a professional attitude when obtaining a patient's weight. Make sure heavy items are removed from pockets and that the patient is not holding a purse. Shoes should also be removed. If patients have difficulty with balance or stability, assist them onto the scale and help them balance themselves. A scale with built-in handrails is ideal for patients who are unable to maintain their balance. If the facility does not have this type of scale, a walker can be placed over the scale for the patient to use as hand support when getting on or off, or to maintain balance while on the scale (Fig. 29.19).

BOX 29.9 Weight Conversion Formulas

To Convert Kilograms to Pounds
1 kg = 2.2 lb
  Multiply the number of kilograms by 2.2.

Example
A patient weighs 68 kg: 68 × 2.2 = 149.6 lb.

To Convert Pounds to Kilograms
1 lb = 0.45 kg
  Multiply the number of pounds by 0.45, or divide the number of pounds by 2.2 kg.

Example
A patient weighs 120 lb: 120 × 0.45 = 54 kg, or 120 ÷ 2.2 = 54.5 kg.

BOX 29.8 Body Mass Index (BMI)

To determine how healthy an adult patient's weight level is, the provider may ask the medical assistant to calculate the patient's BMI. The BMI is the relationship of weight to height that mathematically correlates the patient's measurements with health risks. It is a more accurate predictor of weight-related diseases than traditional height-weight charts because it provides a good estimate of the degree of body fat.

A patient's BMI can be calculated by dividing the weight in kilograms by the square of the height in meters: BMI = Weight (kg) ÷ Height (m^2). However, to determine the BMI, clinics can use a wheel device that compares the patient's height to weight, an online BMI calculator, or a BMI chart. This is not necessary with EHR systems because the program automatically calculates the BMI after the patient's height and weight have been documented. Table 29.7 shows the correlation between a patient's BMI and the risks for disease.

Individuals with a BMI of 19 to 22 are thought to live the longest. Death rates are significantly higher for people with a BMI of 25 or above. If the BMI indicates that the patient is overweight or obese, dietary modifications may be needed. The provider makes this decision after evaluating all of the patient's data.

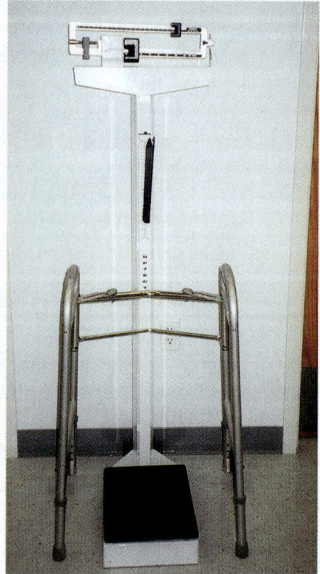

FIG. 29.19 A walker is placed over the scale to aid the patient's balance. (From Proctor D, et al: *Kinn's The Medical Assistant*, ed 13, St. Louis, 2017, Elsevier.)

TABLE 29.7 Body Mass Index and Disease Risk

Body Mass Index	Classification	Disease Risk
≤18.5	Underweight	Low
18.5–24.9	Normal weight	Low
25–29.9	Overweight	Increased
30–34.9	Obese	High
35–39.9	Obese	Very high
≥40	Extremely obese	Extremely high

If the provider prescribes weight measurement at home, make sure the patient understands the importance of getting weighed at the same time each day in clothing of similar weight. Body weight may vary considerably from early morning to late afternoon, so it is usually best if the patient is weighed in the morning. If it is important that the patient be weighed each day, make sure you remind the patient to document each weight and notify the clinic as directed if there are major shifts.

Height. Height can be measured in inches or centimeters. Measurement is easily accomplished by moving the parallel bar attached to a wall ruler or on the scale. Height is usually measured annually for adult patients and documented in feet and inches. If an adult patient has certain medical conditions, such as osteoporosis, height may be measured at each visit. Length measurements used in pediatrics and pediatric BMIs are discussed in Chapter 32.

> ### CRITICAL THINKING 29.9
> Mrs. Johnson is being seen at WMFM Clinic for the first time. In what order should Carlos take her vital signs and her anthropometric measurements? Should blood pressure be measured in both arms, with the patient both sitting and standing? If so, what is the rationale?

> ### EXCEPTIONAL CUSTOMER SERVICE
> Measuring and documenting vital signs are a crucial part of the medical assistant's responsibilities. We must keep in mind that the results can cause the patient anxiety and concern. For example, if you have a patient who is struggling to maintain a healthy blood pressure, it is important that you are sensitive to his or her concerns. If you have a patient who is having difficulty maintaining or losing weight, he or she can be quite apprehensive, embarrassed, or even depressed about weight results. Being aware of the patient's concerns about vital signs and showing sensitivity to his or her needs are part of being a medical assistant.

CLOSING COMMENTS

Taking accurate vital signs and anthropometric measurements is an important aspect of a medical assistant's responsibilities. These measurements give the provider a strong indication of the patient's overall health. Being confident in the process of obtaining these measurements is crucial. Taking vital signs will become second nature over time, but a medical assistant must always take care to be as accurate as possible. It is also important to remember that our patients may be concerned about those measurements. Practicing empathy and good listening skills are also part of being a good medical assistant.

CHAPTER REVIEW

We started this chapter with a discussion of TPR and then moved on to BP and SpO_2. We ended with a discussion of weight and height.

A medical assistant should be familiar with the different sites for taking a temperature and the different thermometers used. Using the correct site and thermometer will ensure that a proper temperature is obtained.

Pulse and respiration are often measured at the same time. This way patients are unaware that you are watching them breathe. Until you are proficient at taking a radial pulse, it should be counted for a full minute. An apical pulse is done using a stethoscope. You will hear two sounds, lubb-dubb. Each lubb-dubb is one beat.

When taking a blood pressure, it is important to use the correct size cuff and have it positioned correctly over the brachial artery. By taking a palpated systolic blood pressure first, you can be certain that you do not miss the first Korotkoff sounds.

Pulse oximetry is often done when there is question about a patient's ability to transport enough oxygen. A finger or earlobe can be used for this procedure. If a finger is used, it should be free of fingernail polish.

Weight and height are anthropometric measurements that are typically taken at a healthcare facility. Weight is usually taken at every visit. Height is usually measured annually for adults, unless the patient has a specific medical condition. These measurements should be taken in a private location for the comfort of the patient. Accurate weight and height measurements are crucial for an accurate BMI calculation. Many providers use BMI to counsel patients about lifestyle changes.

SCENARIO WRAP-UP

Carlos recognizes the significance of measuring and documenting each patient's vital signs and anthropometric measurements. The providers at WMFM rely on Carlos to provide this information accurately. Carlos has never let these procedures become routine. He is always focused on the task, because vital signs are an important reflection of a person's health status.

Carlos knows that a number of factors can alter a patient's vital signs, including the external environment, smoking, drinking hot beverages, exercise, anxiety, and pain. Carlos evaluates patient factors such as age, gender, level of compliance, and the presence of disease to determine the best method of accurately measuring vital signs. In addition, Carlos is sensitive to the need for safeguarding the patient's privacy. When he was first hired by WMFM, he was concerned about privacy and confidentiality when he discovered that the patient scale was in the hall next to the waiting room. After he discussed this with the office manager, the scale was moved to an examination room so that patients could be weighed in privacy.

Carlos attended a workshop last year on the AHA guidelines for the diagnosis and treatment of hypertension, and he is prepared to explain those recommendations to patients. He recognizes his role in motivating patients diagnosed with prehypertension to stick with recommended lifestyle changes and follow the provider's treatment protocol.

30

Physical Examination

LEARNING OBJECTIVES

1. Describe the components of the patient's medical history and how to collect the history information.
2. Do the following related to understanding and communicating with patients:
   - Discuss how to successfully understand and communicate with patients, and display sensitivity to diverse populations.
   - Demonstrate therapeutic communication feedback techniques to obtain information when gathering a patient history.
   - Obtain and document patient information.
   - Respond to nonverbal communication when interacting with patients.
   - Compare open-ended and close-ended questions.
3. Do the following related to the patient interview:
   - Discuss the patient interview.
   - Identify barriers to communication and their impact on the patient assessment.
   - Detect a patient's use of defense mechanisms and the resultant barriers to therapeutic communication.
   - Demonstrate professional patient interviewing techniques.
4. Discuss the use of therapeutic communication techniques with patients across the life span.
5. Compare and contrast signs and symptoms.
6. Document patient care accurately in the medical record.
7. Do the following related to the physical examination:
   - Outline the medical assistant's role in preparing for the physical examination.
   - Summarize the instruments and equipment the provider typically uses during a physical examination.
8. Identify the principles of body mechanics, and demonstrate proper body mechanics.
9. Outline the basic principles of gowning, positioning, and draping a patient for examination. Also, position and drape a patient in different examining positions while remaining mindful of the patient's privacy and comfort.
10. Describe the methods of examination, and give an example of each one.
11. Outline the sequence of a routine physical examination. Also, prepare for and assist in the physical examination of a patient, correctly completing each step of the procedure in the proper sequence.
12. Differentiate among the major types of refractive errors, and discuss the treatment of refractive errors.
13. Do the following related to diagnostic procedures for the eye:
    - Define the various diagnostic procedures for the eye.
    - Perform a visual acuity test using the Snellen chart.
    - Assess color acuity using the Ishihara test.
14. Describe the conditions that can lead to hearing loss, including conductive and sensorineural impairments.
15. Do the following related to diagnostic procedures for the ear:
    - Explain diagnostic procedures for the ear.
    - Use an audiometer to measure a patient's hearing acuity accurately.

CHAPTER OUTLINE

1. Opening Scenario, 663
2. You Will Learn, 663
3. Introduction, 663
4. Medical History, 664
   a. Collecting the History Information, 664
   b. Components of the Medical History, 664
5. Understanding and Communicating With Patients, 665
   a. Sensitivity to Diverse Patient Groups, 666
   b. Therapeutic Techniques, 668
      i. *Active Listening Techniques,* 668
      ii. *Nonverbal Communication,* 669
      iii. *Open-Ended Questions or Statements,* 669
      iv. *Closed Questions,* 670
6. Interviewing the Patient, 670
   a. Interview Barriers, 671
      i. *Providing Unwarranted Assurance,* 671
      ii. *Giving Advice,* 672
      iii. *Using Medical Terminology,* 672
      iv. *Leading Questions,* 672
      v. *Talking Too Much,* 672
      vi. *Defense Mechanisms,* 672
   b. Communication Across the Life Span, 672
7. Assessing the Patient, 674
   a. Signs and Symptoms, 674
8. Documentation, 675
   a. Documentation Guidelines, 675
9. Physical Examination, 675
   a. Preparing the Examination Room, 675
   b. Assisting the Patient, 676
   c. Assisting the Provider, 677
   d. Supplies and Instruments Needed for the Physical Examination, 677
10. Principles of Body Mechanics, 679
    a. Transferring a Patient, 679

11. Assisting With the Physical Examination, 680
    a. Positioning and Draping the Patient for the Physical Examination, 680
        i. *Fowler Position*, 682
        ii. *Semi-Fowler Position*, 682
        iii. *Supine (Horizontal Recumbent) Position*, 683
        iv. *Dorsal Recumbent Position*, 683
        v. *Lithotomy Position*, 684
        vi. *Sims Position*, 684
        vii. *Prone Position*, 684
        viii. *Knee-Chest Position*, 685
        ix. *Trendelenburg Position*, 685
    b. Methods of Examination, 685
        i. *Inspection*, 686
        ii. *Palpation*, 686
        iii. *Percussion*, 686
        iv. *Auscultation*, 687
        v. *Mensuration*, 687
        vi. *Manipulation*, 688
    c. Examination Sequence, 688
        i. *General Appearance*, 689
        ii. *Speech*, 689
        iii. *Skin*, 689
        iv. *Head*, 689
        v. *Eyes*, 689
        vi. *Ears*, 689
        vii. *Nose and Sinuses*, 690
        viii. *Mouth and Throat*, 690
        ix. *Neck*, 690
        x. *Chest*, 690
        xi. *Abdomen*, 690
        xii. *Reflexes*, 690
        xiii. *Breast and Testicles*, 690
        xiv. *Rectum*, 691
12. Vision and Hearing Screenings, 691
    a. Disorders of the Eye, 691
        i. *Refractive Errors*, 691
        ii. *Treatment of Refractive Errors*, 693
    b. Diagnostic Procedures, 693
        i. *Distance Visual Acuity (DVA)*, 694
        ii. *Near Visual Acuity (NVA)*, 696
        iii. *Ishihara Color Vision Test*, 696
    c. Disorders of the Ear, 698
        i. *Hearing Loss*, 698
    d. Diagnostic Procedures, 699
        i. *Tuning Fork Testing*, 699
        ii. *Audiometric Testing*, 699
13. Closing Comments, 702
14. Chapter Review, 702
15. Scenario Wrap-Up, 702

OPENING SCENARIO

Chris Isaacson, CMA (AAMA), works for Walden-Martin Family Medical (WMFM) Clinic. He is responsible for initial patient interviews, taking medical histories, and documentation. Chris struggles with gathering the information needed from some patients. They do not always respond openly and honestly. Chris is also responsible for assisting with physical examinations. His duties include preparing and maintaining the examination room and equipment; getting the patient ready for specific physical examinations; and gowning, draping, and positioning the patient as needed. Because Chris assists with examinations, he must be familiar with the physical examination procedure and order in which the provider needs various pieces of medical equipment. Throughout the physical examination process, Chris needs to be aware of proper body mechanics.

YOU WILL LEARN

1. To develop helping relationships so that the patient's medical history is as comprehensive as possible.
2. To recognize nonverbal communication.
3. To prepare the equipment for a physical examination.
4. To position patients properly for all aspects of the physical examination.
5. To use proper body mechanics when working in a healthcare facility.
6. To perform vision and hearing screening tests.

INTRODUCTION

Medical assistants are directly involved in gathering information from patients about their health. It is important to remember that a healthy state is more than the absence of disease. The assessment process should be a reflection of the entire patient, not just a report about signs and symptoms. Individual lifestyles and environmental factors can be the cause of disease and should be considered when information is gathered about the patient's **chief complaint**. For example, if a patient smokes or works in a stressful occupation, he or she may be more prone to hypertension. Health professionals should consider all patient factors when gathering information about the patient's health status. The method of analyzing all factors that may contribute to the development of disease is based on a **holistic** (hoh LIS tik) perspective. Holistic patient care recognizes that illness is the result of many factors, not just physical ones.

> **VOCABULARY**
> **chief complaint:** A statement in the patient's own words that describes the reason for the visit.
> **holistic:** Considering the patient as a whole; includes the physical, emotional, social, economic, and spiritual needs of the person.

As the first step in treating a disease process, the provider must determine the patient's medical diagnosis. A *differential diagnosis* considers which one of several diseases may be producing the patient's symptoms. The possible causes for a set of symptoms are considered in order to arrive at a diagnosis. For example, if a patient presents with moderate to severe knee pain, the provider might consider causes like an injury or arthritis. A differential diagnosis is based on information gathered from the patient about symptoms; contributing family, personal, and social histories; and a complete physical examination. Multiple causes are not ruled out in a differential diagnosis because it is possible for patients to be sick with more than one thing at once. Once the provider has considered all the possible factors, he or she comes up with a working diagnosis and begins treatment. A working diagnosis is also called a *clinical diagnosis.* The clinical diagnosis is arrived at after taking a detailed history and doing a comprehensive physical examination, but before any laboratory tests or x-rays, diagnostic testing is done. For the patient with knee pain, after gathering detailed patient information and conducting a comprehensive physical examination, the provider decides that the clinical diagnosis is arthritic changes in the joint. The provider orders x-rays and a magnetic resonance image (MRI) of the knee to confirm the clinical diagnosis. The final diagnosis is determined after all diagnostic studies are completed.

However, patient care does not start with the physical examination; it begins when the patient first makes contact with the office. Even before the examination, the medical assistant has the opportunity to interact with the patient to ensure that he or she feels comfortable during the process and that all of the necessary information is obtained.

Interviewing patients, assisting with examinations, and preparing documentation are important responsibilities for a medical assistant. You must know the components of a medical history and the techniques for interviewing patients, because these will help the provider diagnose and treat the patient. The more complete the medical history, the better able the provider will be to treat the patient.

A medical assistant must also know how to best assist the provider during the physical examination. Having an understanding of what supplies and instruments are needed will make the visit go more smoothly for both the patient and the provider. During a complete physical exam, the patient is placed in various positions to facilitate examination. It is often the medical assistant's responsibility to assist the patient into the correct position and drape him or her for modesty.

MEDICAL HISTORY

Collecting the History Information

A new patient is asked to complete a health history form. This form is useful for diagnosing and treating the patient. This self-history also allows the patient to be more involved in the process. The form may be mailed to the patient's home before the appointment or may be completed in the office during the first visit. Some healthcare facilities use electronic forms. These can be emailed to the patient before the first appointment and incorporated into the patient's electronic health record (EHR) when the completed form is emailed back. The patient may also be able to complete the form online through a **patient portal**. If a paper form is used, it can be scanned into the patient's EHR after it is completed.

If you are responsible for taking a portion of the medical history, conduct the interview in a private area, free of distractions and where others cannot hear anything. Patients will not talk freely where they may be overheard or interrupted. Legally and ethically, the patient has the right to privacy, and access to the patient's health record is permitted only for healthcare workers directly involved in the patient's care or individuals the patient has specified on his or her Health Insurance Portability and Accountability Act (HIPAA) release form.

Listen to the patient. Do not express surprise or displeasure at any of the patient's statements. Remember, you are not there to pass judgment but to collect medical data. The medical assistant should document the information in an organized manner, exactly as given by the patient, without opinion or interpretation. The documentation should include the following:

- Purpose of the patient's visit, written as the chief complaint (CC)
- Patient's vital signs (VS)
- Height and weight
- Pain; documented using a scale of 1 to 10, with 1 being the least amount of pain and 10 being the greatest amount

In some facilities, the provider takes the medical history during the patient's initial visit. The provider **correlates** (KAWR uh leyts) the physical findings in the examination with the information in the history. The complete medical history and the physical examination are the starting point and foundation of all patient-physician contacts. EHR systems incorporate the patient's history and physical examination data directly into the health record (Fig. 30.1).

Components of the Medical History

Medical history forms vary, depending on the provider's preference, the practice specialty, and the EHR system used in the facility. The most commonly used medical history forms include these components:

- *Database:* The record of the patient's **demographic** (dem uh GRAF ik) information along with history, physical examination, and initial laboratory findings. As new information is added, it becomes part of this database.
- *Chief complaint (CC):* The purpose of the patient's visit. Generally, this is documented in the patient's own words.
- **History of present illness (HPI):** The medical assistant should gather as much information about the health problem as possible and document it concisely in **chronologic** (kroon l OJ ick) order.
- *Past history (PH)* or *past medical history (PMH):* A summary of the patient's previous health. It includes dates and details about the patient:
  - Usual childhood diseases (UCD or UCHD)
  - Major illnesses
  - Surgeries
  - Allergies (Box 30.1)
  - Accidents
  - Immunization record

Included in the patient's medication history should be a record of frequently used over-the-counter (OTC) medications, including supplements and currently prescribed drugs.

- *Family history (FH):* Details about the patient's parents and siblings and their health; if they are deceased, the age and cause of death. This information is important because certain diseases and disorders have **familial** (fuh MIL yuh l) or hereditary tendencies.
- *Social history (SH):* This section includes information about the patient's lifestyle:
  - Whether he or she feels safe at home
  - Use of tobacco, alcohol, or recreational drugs
  - Sleeping and exercise habits
  - Typical diet
  - Education and occupation
  - Dental care history
  - For female patients, their last menstrual period (LMP), pregnancy history, and method of birth control if sexually active

---

VOCABULARY

chronologic: Arranged in the order of time.
correlate: To establish an orderly relationship or connection.
demographics: Statistical data of a population. In healthcare this includes the patient's name, address, date of birth, employment, and other details.
history of present illness (HPI): Describes the signs and symptoms from the time of onset.
patient portal: A secure online website that gives patients 24-hour access to personal health information using a username and password.

CHAPTER 30   Physical Examination   665

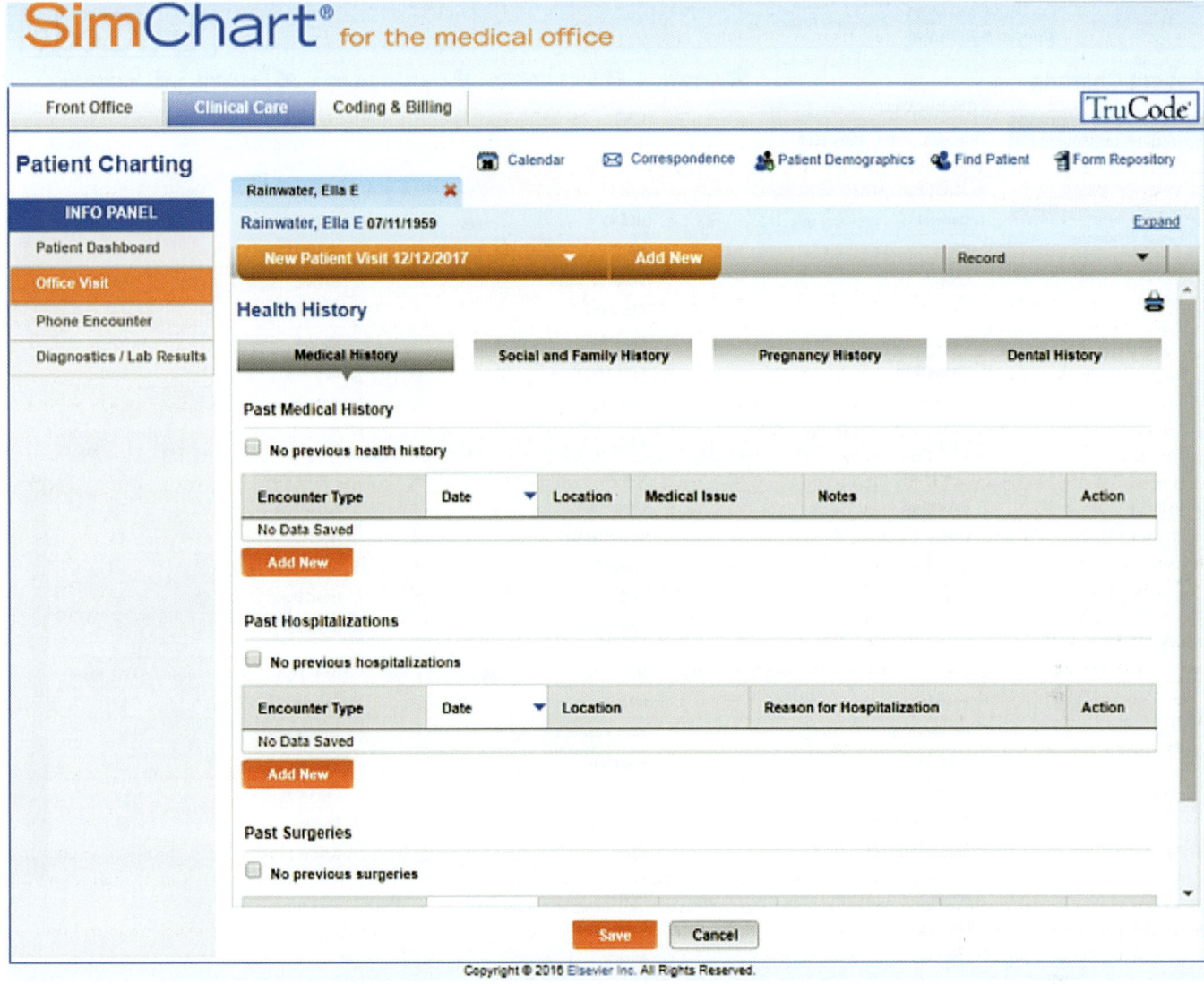

FIG. 30.1 Example of an electronic health record (EHR) system.

BOX 30.1   Allergy Documentation

Each medical practice has a policy on how to document a patient's allergies. In a paper record, they typically are written in red ink or identified by a colored sticker so that all healthcare workers can easily see it. EHR systems have methods for including allergy information on all pertinent screens in the patient's record.

about the state of health of body systems, beginning with the head and proceeding downward (Fig. 30.2). The provider typically completes this section of the medical history while conducting the physical examination.

It may be important to note the patient's cultural and religious background, because these factors could influence certain lifestyle and dietary choices. This information helps the physician to plan treatment for the patient or to determine causative factors for disease. It also provides a holistic picture of the patient's health.
- *Systems review (SR)* or *review of systems (ROS):* These questions provide a guide to the patient's general health and help detect conditions other than those covered under the present illness. Often a patient may think certain health problems are irrelevant and may fail to mention them. However, these problems may help the provider determine the cause of the disorder currently being explored. A systems review is obtained through a logical sequence of questions

VOCABULARY
familial: Occurring in or affecting members of a family more than would be expected by chance.

UNDERSTANDING AND COMMUNICATING WITH PATIENTS

To provide high-quality patient care, we must communicate effectively with the patient and provide a warm, caring environment. Positive reactions and interactions with the patient are vital. A medical assistant

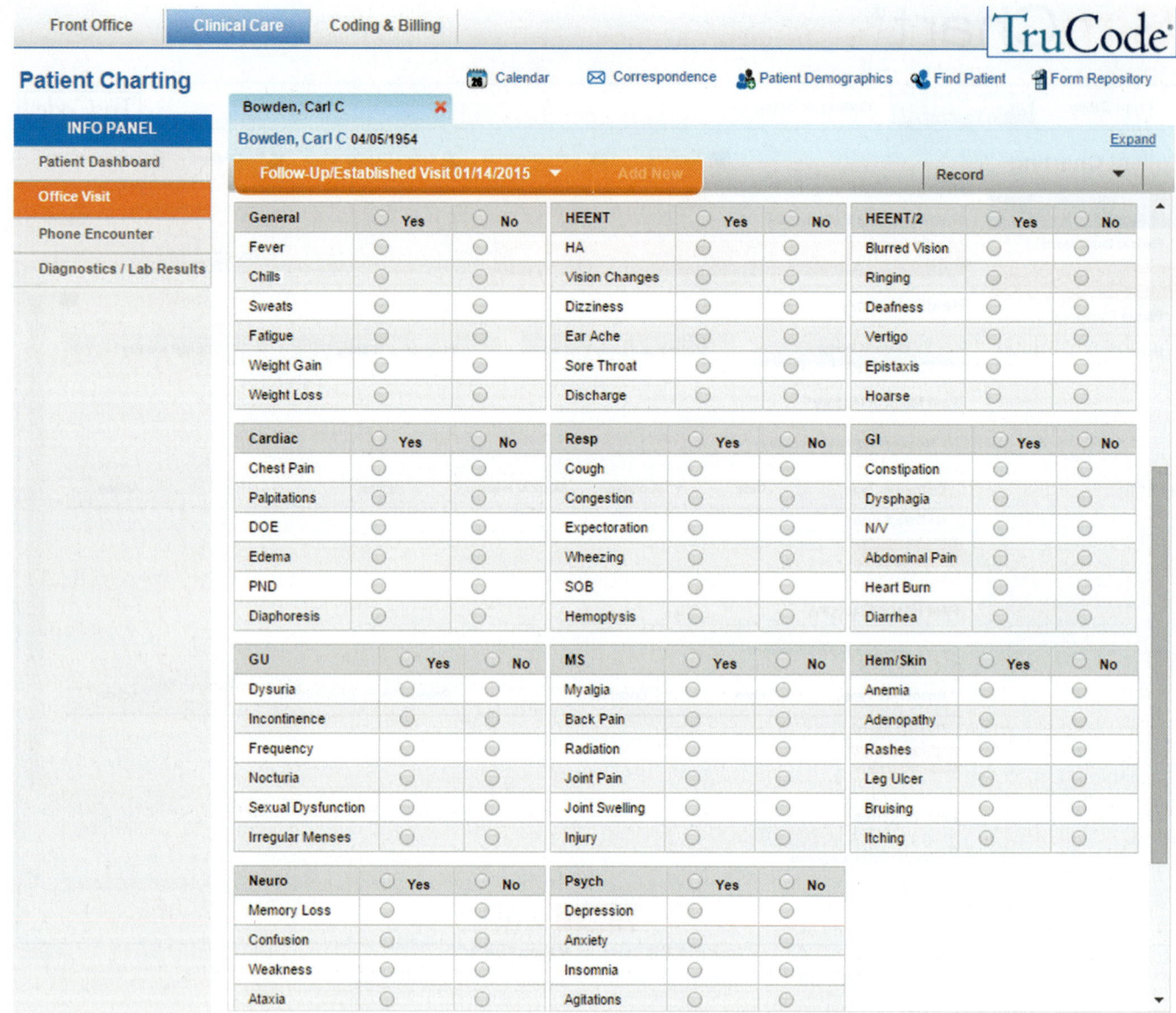

FIG. 30.2 Example of review of systems (ROS) questions in an EHR.

must always remember that each patient is an individual with certain anxieties. These anxieties often cause people to act and react in different ways; therefore effective verbal and nonverbal communication with each patient is essential.

Healthcare professionals accept the responsibility of developing helping relationships with their patients. The interpersonal nature of the patient–medical assistant relationship means that the focus should be on the patient's needs. A medical assistant can bring out either a positive or a negative response simply by the way he or she treats and interacts with patients. You are usually the first person with whom the patient communicates; therefore you play a vital role in therapeutic patient interactions (Procedure 30.1).

Another important aspect of communicating with patients is an awareness of self-boundaries. See Box 30.2 for information about self-boundaries.

Sensitivity to Diverse Patient Groups

Most healthcare facilities have a diverse patient population. The diversity could be based on race, age, culture, religion, or physical qualities such as being deaf/hard of hearing. Whatever the origin of the diversity,

> **BOX 30.2 Self-Boundaries**
>
> When working in healthcare, it is important to develop a solid professional relationship with our patients. By establishing realistic self-boundaries, that relationship can be protected. It is important to keep the focus on the patient. When working with patients who are seen frequently, it is easy to start to think of them as friends. With a friend you are likely to share personal information that is not appropriate with a patient. Patients may feel that they cannot share important health-related information because you are their friend and it would be embarrassing to share that information with a friend.
>
> Self-boundaries can also be thought of as professional boundaries. You need to treat patients with respect and keep the relationship professional. Be friendly to patients and always keep the focus on the patient.

practicing respectful patient care is extremely important. *Empathy* is the key to creating a caring, therapeutic environment. Empathy is different from sympathy. A medical assistant who is empathetic respects the individuality of the patient and attempts to see the person's health problem through his or her eyes. He or she also recognizes the effect

PROCEDURE 30.1   Obtain and Document Patient Information

Task
Use restatement, reflection, and clarification to obtain patient information and document patient care accurately.

Equipment and Supplies
- History form or EHR system with the patient history window opened
- If using a paper form, a red pen for recording the patient's allergies and a black pen to meet legal documentation guidelines
- Quiet, private area

Directions
Complete this procedure with another student playing the role of the patient. To make the experience more realistic, choose a student about whom you know very little. To maintain the student's privacy, he or she does not have to share any confidential information.

Procedural Steps

1. Greet the patient. Identify yourself. Verify the patient's identity with full name and date of birth. Explain your role.
   Purpose: To make the patient feel comfortable and at ease.
2. Take the patient to a quiet, private area for the interview, and explain why the information is needed.
   Purpose: A quiet, private area is necessary to protect confidentiality and prevent interruptions. An informed patient is more cooperative and therefore more likely to provide useful information.
3. Complete the history form by using therapeutic communication techniques, including restatement, reflection, and clarification. Make sure all medical terminology is adequately explained. A self-history may have been mailed to the patient before the visit. If so, review the self-history for completeness.
   Purpose: Therapeutic communication techniques help the medical assistant gather complete information; the self-history is designed to save time and to involve the patient in the process.
4. Speak in a pleasant, distinct manner, remembering to maintain eye contact with your patient.
   Purpose: Positive nonverbal behaviors create a friendly, caring atmosphere.
5. Remain sensitive to the diverse needs of your patient throughout the interview process.
   Purpose: Incorporate awareness of your personal biases into treating all patients with respect despite their diverse backgrounds.
6. Record the following statistical information:
   Patient's full name, including middle initial
   Address, including apartment number and ZIP code
   Marital status
   Sex (gender)
   Age and date of birth
   Telephone numbers for home, cell, and work
   Insurance information if not already available
   Employer's name, address, and telephone number
7. Record the following medical history:
   - Chief complaint
   - Present illness
   - Past history
   - Family history
   - Social history

   Purpose: The provider needs this information to make an accurate assessment and diagnosis. The provider usually completes the review of systems (ROS) during the preexamination interview.
8. Ask about allergies to drugs and any other substances, and record any allergies in red ink on every page of the history form, on the front of the patient record, and on each progress note page; in the EHR, enter allergy information where designated.
   Purpose: The presence of an allergy may alter medication and treatment procedures.
9. If using a paper form, record all information legibly and neatly, and spell words correctly. Print rather than writing in cursive. Do not erase, scribble, or use whiteout. Do not leave any blank spaces or skip lines between documentation entries. If you make an error, draw a single line through the error, write "error" above it, add the correction, and initial and date the entry. If recording the information in the patient's EHR, accurately locate each box; errors in the EHR should be corrected and are automatically tracked within the system.
   Purpose: To maintain a medical record that is understandable and defensible in a court of law.
10. Thank the patient for cooperating, and direct him or her back to the reception area.
11. Review the record for errors before you pass it to the provider or exit the EHR health history area.
12. Protect the integrity of the health record and the confidentiality of patient information. Safeguards mandated by the Health Insurance Portability and Accountability Act (HIPAA) include the following:
    - Passwords to secure access to all EHRs
    - Computer monitor shields to protect patient information if data are left on the screen
    - Turning monitors away from patient traffic areas to prevent accidental release of information
    - Securing all medical records

    Purpose: Patient information may be legally and ethically shared only with a member of the healthcare team who is directly providing care to the patient.

---

of all holistic factors on the patient's well-being. Empathetic sensitivity to diversity requires you to examine your own values, beliefs, and actions; you cannot treat all patients with care and respect until you first recognize and evaluate personal biases. We think and act a certain way for many reasons. The first step in understanding the process is to evaluate your individual value system. Why do you have certain attitudes or beliefs about the worth of individuals or things?

Many factors influence the development of a value system. Value systems begin as learned beliefs and behaviors. Families and cultural influences shape the way we respond to a diverse society. Other factors that influence reactions include socioeconomic and educational backgrounds. To develop therapeutic relationships, you must recognize your own value system to determine whether it could affect how you interact with patients. Preconceived ideas about people because of their race, religion, income level, ethnic origin, sexual orientation, or gender can act as barriers to the development of a therapeutic relationship. You cannot treat your patients empathetically unless you can connect with them in some way. Personal biases or prejudices are huge barriers to the development of therapeutic relationships (Fig. 30.3).

For strategies for working with diverse patient populations, see Box 30.3.

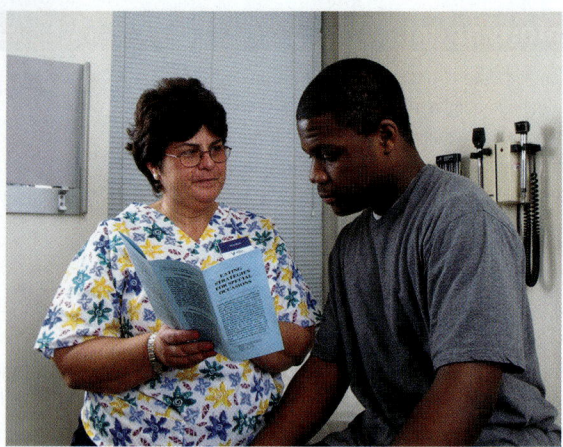

FIG. 30.3 Respectful patient care. (From Proctor D, et al: *Kinn's The Medical Assistant*, ed 13, St. Louis, 2017, Elsevier.)

> ### CRITICAL THINKING 30.1
>
> Honestly evaluate your personal biases. What do you find unacceptable in people? Do you prejudge an individual based on his or her affiliation with a particular group or because of a certain lifestyle decision? Do these biases create barriers to the development of therapeutic relationships? If so, how can you get beyond these barriers?
>
> Consider the following scenarios, and discuss them with your classmates:
> - While you are conducting a patient interview, the patient informs you that he has tested positive for the human immunodeficiency virus (HIV). Do you think this will affect your therapeutic relationship?
> - You are responsible for recording an in-depth interview on a homeless person with very poor hygiene. Will this cause a problem with your professional manner?
> - Your office manager tells you that an inmate of the county prison is being brought in this afternoon for an examination. Do you think his status will affect your interaction with the patient?
> - You are attempting to interview a 20-year-old patient who brought her two young children with her to the office today She is a single mother who is pregnant with her third child and receives public assistance. What do you think? Will you have difficulty being empathetic?

Therapeutic Techniques

Communication is an interactive process involving the sender of the message, the receiver, and feedback. Feedback is a crucial component to confirm that the message was received. The message can be sent by a number of methods:
- Face-to-face communication
- Telephone
- Email
- Letter

Feedback lets us know that the receiver got the message and how they interpreted it. This completes the communication cycle by providing a means for us to know exactly what message the patient received and whether it requires **clarification** (KLAR uh fa kay shuh n).

> **VOCABULARY**
>
> **clarification**: Allows the listener to get additional information.

> ### BOX 30.3 Sensitivity to Diverse Patient Populations
>
> Regardless of the type of healthcare facility you work in, you will care for a wide variety of patients. The medical assistant should take the initiative to learn about the cultures represented in the healthcare practice. Some points to consider about diverse groups include the following:
> - Patients of Asian backgrounds may have been raised in a culture that considers it extremely rude to establish eye contact. Americans view an unwillingness to establish eye contact as a sign of distrust or embarrassment; however, for people from Japan or China, lack of eye contact may be a way of demonstrating respect.
> - Personal space may be an issue for patients from diverse backgrounds. If a patient appears very uncomfortable with touch or lack of personal space, attempt to accommodate him or her as much as possible during the office visit.
> - Research has shown that older people face unique communications problems in the healthcare environment. The healthcare facility should have tools available to help patients with hearing or vision issues. When caring for an aging individual, it is important to focus patient teaching and information on the patient, rather than the family member who may be present.
> - Patients may use their religious beliefs and values to understand and cope with their health problems. However, using religion to guide healthcare decisions may result in a conflict with the provider's recommendations. Healthcare workers may need to find a balance between respect for a patient's beliefs and the delivery of high-quality healthcare.

For example, as a medical assistant, one of your responsibilities will be to provide patient education on how to prepare for diagnostic studies. Let's say you have to explain to an older adult patient how to prepare for a **colonoscopy** (kohl uh NOS kuh pee). You provided a detailed explanation of the preparation procedure and a handout explaining the step-by-step process. How do you really know whether the patient understands? You ask the patient to provide feedback by explaining the process back to you. As a member of the healthcare team, you must become an effective communicator. You will play a vital role in collecting and documenting patient information. If your methods of communication are faulty, the quality of patient care may be seriously impaired.

> **VOCABULARY**
>
> **colonoscopy:** A procedure in which a fiber-optic scope is used to examine the large intestine.

> **MEDICAL TERMINOLOGY**
>
> **col/o:** colon (large intestine)
> **-scopy:** process of viewing

Active Listening Techniques. Hearing is a physical act. Someone speaks, and we hear what the person has said. Listening is something we consciously choose to do. Active listeners go beyond hearing the patient's message to concentrating, understanding, and listening to the main points. Active listening techniques encourage patients to expand on and clarify the content and meaning of their messages. These techniques are very useful communication tools when a patient is agitated or upset. They help the medical assistant clarify the important details of the patient's chief complaint.

Three processes are involved in active listening: restatement, reflection, and clarification. Restatement is simply paraphrasing or repeating the patient's statements with phrases such as, "My understanding of what you are saying is …" or "You are telling me the problem is …"

Reflection involves repeating the main idea of the conversation while also identifying the sender's *feelings*. For example, if the mother of a young patient is expressing frustration about her child's behavior, a reflective statement identifies that feeling with the response, "It sounds like you are frustrated about …" Or if a patient who has been newly diagnosed with insulin-dependent diabetes shows anxiety about administering injections, an appropriate reflective statement recognizes the patient's feelings: "You appear anxious about …" Reflective statements clearly demonstrate to patients that you are not only listening to their words; you also are concerned and are attending to their feelings.

Clarification seeks to summarize or simplify the sender's thoughts and feelings and to resolve any confusion in the message. Questions or statements that begin with "Give me an example of …" or "Explain to me about …" or "So what you're saying is …" help patients focus on the chief complaint and give you the opportunity to clear up any misconceptions before documenting patient information.

Listening is not a passive role in the communication process; it is active and demanding. You cannot be preoccupied with your own needs, or you will miss something important. For the duration of the patient interview, no one is more important than this particular patient. Listen to the way things are said, the tone of the patient's voice, and even to what the patient may not be saying out loud but is saying very clearly with body language (see Procedure 30.1).

Nonverbal Communication. Experts say that more than 90% of communication is nonverbal. Much of what we communicate to our patients is conveyed through the use of body language. Our nonverbal actions, such as gestures, facial expressions, and mannerisms, are learned behaviors that are greatly influenced by our family and cultural backgrounds. The body naturally expresses our true feelings.

Most of the negative messages communicated through body language are unintentional. It is important to remember while conducting patient interviews that nonverbal communication can seriously affect the therapeutic process.

The purpose of observing nonverbal communication is to become aware of the message conveyed by these behaviors rather than the words. This enables you to adapt your behavior to these feelings. You can deliberately select your response, either verbal or nonverbal, to have a favorable effect on others. The favorable effect may consist of the following:
- Providing emotional support
- Conveying that you care
- Defusing the patient's fear or anger
- Providing an invitation to release pent-up feelings by talking about the situation that aroused the feelings

Table 30.1 lists some nonverbal behaviors by patients that may indicate anxiety, frustration, or fear. Box 30.4 provides some helpful listening guidelines.

Your tone of voice can put a patient at ease. Your facial expression and the ease and confidence of your movements demonstrate a sincere interest to the patient. Therapeutic use of space and touch are also important ways of sending nonverbal messages to your patients. You should establish eye contact, sit in a relaxed but attentive position, and avoid using furniture as a barrier between you and the patient. Give the patient your undivided attention, and let your body language inform each patient that you are interested in his or her medical problems (Fig. 30.4 and Procedure 30.2).

The key to successful patient interaction is **congruence** (kuh n GROO uh ns) between verbal and nonverbal messages. Although choosing the correct words is very important, less than 10% of the message received is verbal; therefore to be seen as honest and sensitive to the needs of your patients, you must be aware of your nonverbal behavior patterns. The nonverbal message the patient receives from the medical assistant's listening behavior should be "You are a person of worth, and I am interested in you as a unique individual." Box 30.5 has some suggestions for nonverbal language behaviors that can help with communicating with patients.

TABLE 30.1 Observations of Nonverbal Communication in Patients

Area	Observation	Indication
Breathing patterns	Rapid respirations, sighing, shallow thoracic breathing	Anxiety, boredom, pain
Eye patterns	No eye contact, side-to-side movement, looking down at the hands	Anxiety, distrust, embarrassment
Hands	Tapping fingers, cracking knuckles, continuous movement, sweaty palms	Anxiety, worry, fear
Arm placement	Folded across chest, wrapped around abdomen	Anxiety, worry, fear, pain
Leg placement	Tension, crossed or tucked under, tapping foot, continuous movement	Frustration, anger

From Proctor D, et al: *Kinn's The Medical Assistant*, ed 13, St. Louis, 2017, Elsevier.

BOX 30.4 Helpful Listening Guidelines

- Listen to the main points in the discussion.
- Respond to both verbal and nonverbal messages.
- Be patient and nonjudgmental.
- Do not interrupt.
- Never intimidate your patient.
- Use active listening techniques: restatement, reflection, and clarification.

VOCABULARY

congruence: Agreement; the state that occurs when the verbal expression of the message matches the sender's nonverbal body language.

Open-Ended Questions or Statements. An open-ended question or statement asks for general information or states the topic to be discussed, but only in general terms. This communication tool is used in various ways:
- To begin the interview
- To introduce a new section of questions
- Whenever the person introduces a new topic

It is an effective method of gathering more details from the patient about the chief complaint or health history. Consider these examples:

"What brings you to the doctor?"
"How have you been getting along?"
"You mentioned having dizzy spells. Tell me more about that."

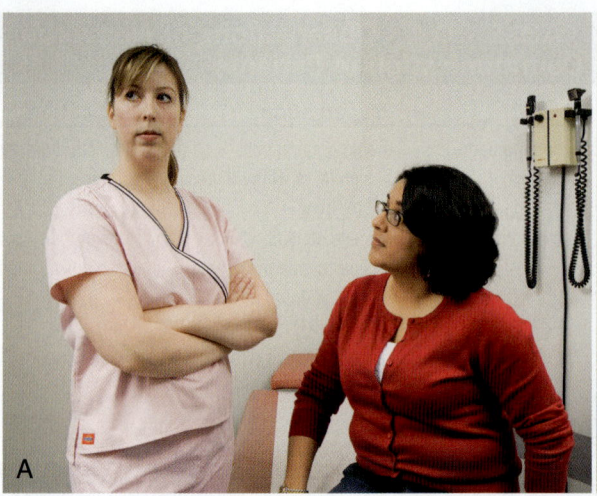 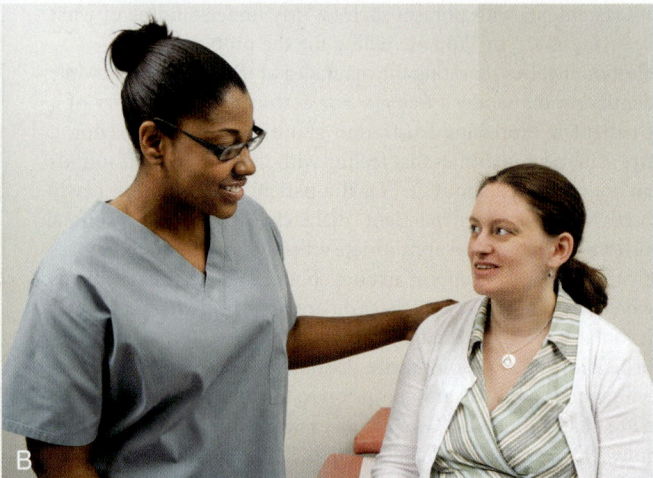

FIG. 30.4 (A) Ineffective nonverbal language. (B) Therapeutic nonverbal language. (From Proctor D, et al: *Kinn's The Medical Assistant*, ed 13, St. Louis, 2017, Elsevier.)

PROCEDURE 30.2 Respond to Nonverbal Communication

Task
Observe the patient and respond appropriately to nonverbal communication.

Equipment and Supplies
- Patient's record

Directions
Complete this procedure with another student playing the role of the patient. To make the experience more realistic, choose a student about whom you know very little. To maintain the student's privacy, he or she does not have to share any confidential information.

Scenario
Monique Jones is a new patient with the CC of intermittent abdominal pain with alternating diarrhea and constipation. Ms. Jones has experienced this discomfort for several months and appears frustrated. She is sitting on the end of the exam table with her arms wrapped around her abdomen. She sighs frequently and refuses to maintain eye contact. What is her nonverbal behavior telling you, and how can you establish therapeutic communication with this patient?

Procedural Steps
1. Greet the patient. Identify yourself. Verify the patient's identity with full name and date of birth. Explain your role.
   Purpose: To make the patient feel comfortable and at ease.
2. Ask the patient the purpose of her visit and the onset, duration, and frequency of her symptoms. Pay close attention to her body language to determine whether what she is telling you is congruent with her body language.
   Purpose: Nonverbal language naturally expresses the patient's true feelings. Closely observing body language will help you reach more accurate conclusions about the patient's information.
3. Use restatement, reflection, and clarification to gather as much information as possible about the patient's CC. Make sure all medical terminology is adequately explained.
   Purpose: Therapeutic communication techniques help the medical assistant gather complete information; using feedback techniques and making sure the patient understands medical terms can help to relieve anxiety.
4. Speak in a pleasant, distinct manner, remembering to maintain eye contact with your patient.
   Purpose: Positive nonverbal behaviors create a friendly, caring atmosphere. Remain sensitive to the diverse needs of your patient throughout the interview process.
5. Continue to observe nonverbal patient behaviors, and select the appropriate verbal response to demonstrate your sensitivity to her discomfort, frustration, and anxiety.
   Purpose: Displaying sensitivity to and awareness of the patient's nonverbal body language demonstrates your concern for the patient and can help defuse the patient's concerns.

This type of question or statement encourages patients to respond in a manner they find comfortable. It allows patients to express themselves fully and provide comprehensive information about their chief complaint.

Closed Questions. Direct, or closed, questions ask for specific information. This form of questioning limits the answer to one or two words—in many cases, yes or no. Use this form of question when you need confirmation of specific facts, such as when asking about past health problems. Here are some examples:

"Do you have a headache?"
"What is your birth date?"
"Have you ever broken a bone?"

INTERVIEWING THE PATIENT

The interview, or gathering the patient's medical history, is the first and most important part of data collection. The medical history identifies the patient's health strengths and problems and is a bridge to the next step in data collection, the physical examination performed by the provider. At this point, the patient knows everything about his or her own health status and you know nothing. Your interview skills help glean the necessary information and build **rapport** (ra POHR) for a successful working relationship.

Consider the interview a type of contract between you and your patient. The contract consists of spoken and unspoken language and addresses what the patient needs and expects from the healthcare visit.

BOX 30.5 Nonverbal Language Behaviors

Nonverbal behavior—your body language—can have either a positive or a negative effect on patient interactions. Positive nonverbal behaviors enhance the patient's experience in the healthcare setting. Communication experts recommend the following:
- When gathering a health history, lean toward the patient to show interest.
- Face the patient squarely and at eye level to make the process more comfortable and to demonstrate sensitivity and empathy.
- Eye contact is essential for therapeutic communication unless the patient is from a culture that discourages this.
- A closed posture (crossed arms or legs) may indicate disinterest.
- Be sensitive to the patient's personal space when possible. Maintain a comfortable distance from the patient, at least an arm's length, when conducting the interview.
- Be careful with body gestures, such as hand and arm movements. Gestures, such as nodding your head when the patient talks, can display interest, but too much body movement can be distracting.
- Your tone of voice should reflect your interest in the patient. Speaking too quietly or too loudly can detract from therapeutic communication.
- Continually observe the patient's body language during the interview; watch for signs of confusion, boredom, worry, and so on so that you can respond appropriately.
- Documenting in an EHR can be distracting to both the medical assistant and the patient. Remind yourself to look at the patient frequently and use encouraging body language to maintain a personal interaction.

BOX 30.6 Preparing the Appropriate Environment

- *Ensure privacy:* Make sure the room you use is unoccupied for the entire time allowed for the interview. The patient needs to feel sure that no one can overhear the conversation or interrupt.
- *Prevent interruptions:* Inform your coworkers of the interview, and ask them not to interrupt you during this time. You need to concentrate on the patient and establish rapport. An interruption can destroy in seconds what you have spent many minutes building up.
- *Prepare comfortable surroundings:* Conducting the interview in comfortable surroundings reduces the patient's anxiety. Keep the distance between you and the patient at arm's length. Arrange chairs so that you and the patient are comfortably seated at eye level and the desk or table does not act as a barrier between you.
- *Take judicious notes:* Note taking should be kept to a minimum while you try to focus your attention on the person. Note taking during the interview has disadvantages, such as breaking eye contact and shifting your attention away from the patient, which diminishes the patient's sense of importance. However, it is important to write down pertinent details as you are interviewing, because you may forget important facts if you do not note them at the time of the discussion. With experience, you will develop a personal type of shorthand that you can use during the interview process. If using an EHR medical history template, efficiently open boxes and choose the appropriate data, maintaining eye contact and using active listening techniques periodically throughout the interview.

The patient interview consists of three stages: the initiation or introduction, the body, and the closing. Box 30.6 provides steps to take to prepare the environment for the interview process.

> **VOCABULARY**
> **judicious:** Using good judgment; being discreet, sensible.
> **rapport:** A relationship of harmony and accord between the patient and the healthcare professional.

The initiation of the interview is the time to introduce yourself, to identify the patient, and to determine the purpose of the interview (Fig. 30.5). If you are nervous about how to begin, remember to keep it short. The patient probably is nervous, too, and is anxious to get started. Address the patient by his or her last name and give the reason for the interview—for example, "Mr. Coleman, my name is Stacey, and I am a certified medical assistant who works with Dr. Perez. I have some questions to ask you about your health history."

After the brief introduction, move on to the body of the interview. This is when you use various therapeutic communication techniques to determine the following:
- The reason the patient is seeking healthcare
- The patient's perception of the problem
- The characteristics of the problem
- The patient's expectations of care

During this time, use active listening skills, meaningful silence, congruent verbal and nonverbal communication, and a combination of open-ended and closed statements and questions to gather the details of the patient's history and current health problem (Table 30.2).

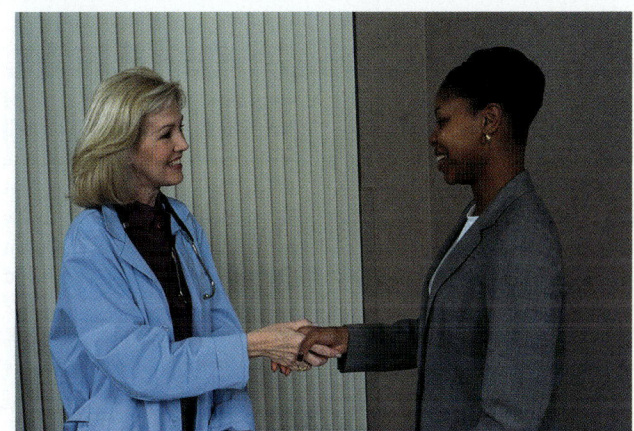

FIG. 30.5 Greeting the patient. (From Proctor D, et al: *Kinn's The Medical Assistant*, ed 13, St. Louis, 2017, Elsevier.)

Conclude the interview by summarizing the results of your interaction. The closing of the interview should clarify the patient's chief complaint, the purpose of the visit, and the patient's expectations of care. This is the patient's opportunity to add any additional details or to explain further the characteristics of the health problem.

Interview Barriers

Providing Unwarranted Assurance. Mrs. Miller says to you, "I know this lump is going to turn out to be cancer." The typical reply is almost automatic: "Don't worry, I'm sure everything will be fine." This type of answer indicates that her anxiety is insignificant and denies her the opportunity to further discuss her fears. A reflective response, such as "You sound really worried about …" acknowledges her feelings and demonstrates empathy and a willingness to listen to her concerns.

TABLE 30.2 Therapeutic Communication Techniques

Technique	Value
Open-ended questions and statements	Encourage the patient to respond in more detail
Direct or closed questions	Ask for specific information; usual reply is yes or no
Active listening	Nonverbally communicates your interest in the patient
Silence	Nonverbally communicates your acceptance of the patient and willingness to wait until the patient is ready to answer
Establishing guidelines	Informs the patient of what to expect during the interview
Acknowledgment	Shows the importance of the patient's role and respect for autonomy
Restating	Checks your interpretation of the patient's message for validation
Reflecting	Shows the patient your acknowledgment of his or her feelings
Summarizing	Helps the patient separate relevant from irrelevant material; provides clarity to the interview

From Proctor D, et al: *Kinn's The Medical Assistant*, ed 13, St. Louis, 2017, Elsevier.

Giving Advice. Mrs. Thompson has just finished talking to the doctor. She looks at you and says, "Dr. Rowe says I need surgery to get rid of these gallstones. I just don't know. What would you do?" If you tell her how you would handle the situation, you may have shifted the accountability for decision making from her to you, and she has not worked out her own solution. Does this woman really want to know what you would do? Probably not. You could respond to her question by saying, "Based on what the doctor told you, what do you think you should do?" or "Do you need further information to make your decision?" If the patient continues to question the provider's recommendations, the medical assistant should encourage further discussion with the provider.

Using Medical Terminology. You must adjust your vocabulary to fit the patient. The more the patient understands about what is happening and how to manage the problem, the better the outcome. Misinterpreted communication is the most common error in patient care. One of the biggest problems for the patient is understanding medical terminology. Closely observe the patient's body language while he or she receives instructions or patient education. If the patient shows signs of not understanding the procedure, ask the patient to repeat back to you the information or instructions. This demonstration–return demonstration form of providing feedback ensures that the patient completely understands what is happening. It also gives the medical assistant the opportunity to clarify any misconceptions.

Leading Questions. During the interview, you ask the patient, "You don't smoke, do you?" By asking questions in this manner, you indicate the preferred answer. Telling you that he or she does smoke would surely meet with your disapproval. Keep your questions positive. A better way of asking would be, "Have you ever smoked?" or "Do you use tobacco?"

Talking Too Much. Some medical assistants associate helpfulness with verbal overload. The patient may let the interviewer talk at the expense of his or her own need to explain what is wrong. Always remember that when interviewing a patient, you should listen more than you talk. Pay close attention to the patient's body language to make sure you are giving the patient ample opportunity to discuss the health problem.

Defense Mechanisms. Many individuals respond to anxiety-provoking situations by automatically relying on defense mechanisms. Defense mechanisms are used consciously or unconsciously to block an emotionally painful experience. It is understandable that patients facing a traumatic diagnosis or a difficult treatment feel the need to protect themselves from the reality of the situation. Ensuring compliance with treatment becomes an issue if the patient is in denial, projecting feelings onto the healthcare worker, or repressing the need for treatment or diagnostic follow-up. The medical assistant must be sensitive to patients' use of defense mechanisms. Consistently applying therapeutic communication techniques to interactions with patients will help to overcome the defense mechanisms. For more information about defense mechanisms, see Box 30.7.

> **CRITICAL THINKING 30.2**
>
> Mr. Gonzales, a 48-year-old patient recently diagnosed with hypertension, did not show up today for his follow-up appointment. Chris calls to find out why he failed to keep the appointment, and the patient tells Chris he forgot to come, even though an appointment reminder call was made yesterday. He also tells Chris he has not been taking his medicine and does not understand why it is so important for him and his wife to meet with the dietitian. Is this patient using defense mechanisms? How should Chris respond? What communications skills might promote a therapeutic relationship?

Communication Across the Life Span

The key to effectively communicating with patients is using an age-specific approach. Given the age and developmental level of your patient, how can you best interact with the person and with significant family members?

For example, Tasha, a 2-year-old patient, is scheduled for a physical examination. How can you best interact with her and her father to ensure that the history phase of the visit is complete and accurate? Therapeutic use of nonverbal language is essential to interacting with children of all ages. Getting down on the child's level, establishing eye contact, and using a gentle but firm voice are ways of gaining the child's confidence and cooperation. Children fear the unknown, so explaining all procedures with language that the child understands is important. At the same time, the medical assistant must communicate with the child's caregiver so that he or she can contribute to the intake process (Fig. 30.6). The following are some important guidelines for obtaining the health history of a child:

- Make sure the environment is safe and attractive.
- Do not keep children and their caregivers waiting any longer than necessary because children become anxious and distracted quickly.
- Do not offer a choice unless the child can truly make one. If part of the treatment requires an injection, asking the child whether she would like her shot now is most likely to get an automatic "No!" However, giving her a choice of stickers after the injection is appropriate.
- Praising the child during the examination helps reduce anxiety and boosts self-esteem. When possible, direct questions to the child so that he or she feels like part of the process.

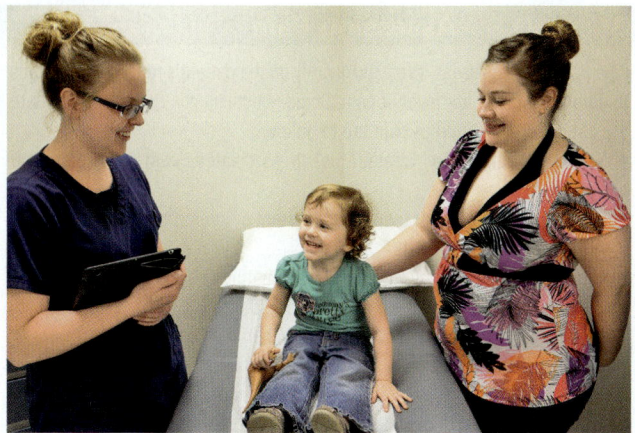

FIG. 30.6 Interacting with a parent and child. (From Proctor D, et al: *Kinn's The Medical Assistant*, ed 13, St. Louis, 2017, Elsevier.)

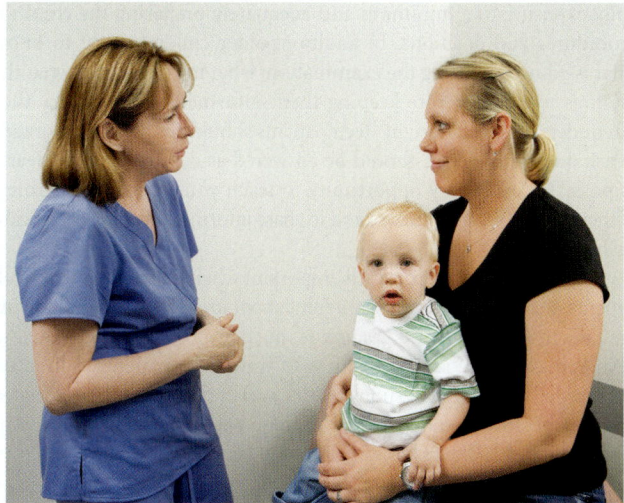

FIG. 30.7 Responding to parental concerns. (From Proctor D, et al: *Kinn's The Medical Assistant*, ed 13, St. Louis, 2017, Elsevier.)

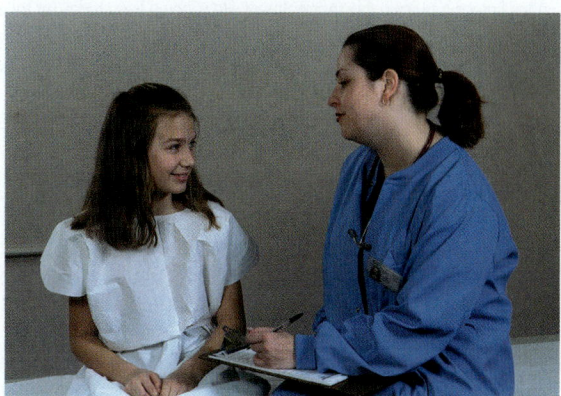

FIG. 30.8 Interacting with a school-aged child. (From Proctor D, et al: *Kinn's The Medical Assistant*, ed 13, St. Louis, 2017, Elsevier.)

BOX 30.7 Defense Mechanisms

Patients may use defense mechanisms to protect themselves from a situation they cannot manage psychologically. Defense mechanisms may hide any of a variety of thoughts or feelings: anger, fear, sadness, despair, or helplessness. A patient who uses defense mechanisms can be difficult to deal with. If the medical assistant is aware of the patient's need for psychological protection, he or she may be able to find a way to provide care for the patient while maintaining a therapeutic relationship. For example, Mrs. Alicia Simone, a 48-year-old patient, has just been told she has breast cancer. The following are defense mechanisms she might display to protect herself from the psychological reality of her disease.

- *Denial:* The patient completely rejects the information. Example: "I couldn't possibly have breast cancer. You must be mistaken."
- *Suppression:* The patient is consciously aware of the information or feeling but refuses to admit it. Example: "I don't think the test is accurate. My mammograms are always normal."
- *Reaction formation:* The patient expresses her feelings as the opposite of what she really feels. Example: If she is angry at the medical assistant for insisting that a biopsy be scheduled, she may express the opposite emotion: "I appreciate your trying to help me, but I just can't come to the hospital that day."
- *Projection:* The patient accuses someone else of having the feelings that she has. Example: If the patient is angry about the diagnosis, she may say to the medical assistant, "You don't have to lose your temper about this," even though the medical assistant's demeanor is completely professional.
- *Rationalization:* The patient comes up with various explanations to justify her response. Example: "I think the results are wrong. I didn't follow the directions for the tests like I should have, and besides, there's no history of breast cancer in my family."
- *Undoing:* The patient tries to reverse a negative feeling by doing something that indicates the opposite feeling. Example: If the patient feels angry and violated about the diagnosis but she finds those feelings unacceptable, she may say, "Don't worry, dear, I'm not upset with you for telling me about this."
- *Regression:* The patient reverts to an old, usually immature behavior to vent her feelings. Example: Perhaps instead of discussing the diagnosis and the need for treatment, she just storms out of the office. Or she may say, "I can't possibly schedule a procedure without discussing this with my mother."
- *Sublimation:* The patient redirects her negative feelings into a socially productive activity. Example: Mrs. Simone eventually becomes an active member of a local support group for women recovering from breast cancer.

- Involving the child in the examination by permitting him or her to manipulate the equipment may help relieve anxiety. If possible, use your imagination and make a game of the assessment or the procedure.
- A typical defense mechanism seen in sick or anxious children is regression. The child may refuse to leave the mother's lap or may want to hold a favorite toy during the procedure as a comfort measure. Look for signs of anxiety, such as thumb sucking or rocking during the assessment, and encourage caregivers to be involved in the process to help make the child feel as safe as possible.
- Listen to parents' concerns and respond truthfully to questions (Fig. 30.7).

Older children may also have difficulty during the health visit (Fig. 30.8). To help school-aged children gain a sense of control, give them the opportunity to make certain decisions about treatment. For example, Heather, a 13-year-old patient with diabetes, could be given the choice of having her father present during the visit. Or if she requires an insulin injection, she could choose the site of the injection or perhaps administer the medication herself. This gives the medical assistant an opportunity to observe her technique and allows Heather to exert her independence.

Privacy is an important issue to consider with older children, especially adolescents. During the physical examination, respect privacy by keeping body exposure to a minimum and adequately preparing the child for procedures and positions. In addition, older children want to know what is going on during the examination, what to expect, and what the findings mean; therefore keeping them informed in a language they can understand is important. Teen patients should always be encouraged to ask questions, which should be answered as completely and clearly as possible. Take every opportunity to teach your patients, regardless of their age, about their disease and to share information about significant wellness factors.

Patient education is extremely important when interacting with adult patients. Using language that the adult patient understands and involving the patient in treatment decisions as much as possible are essential to developing a helping relationship with your older patients. Adults are bombarded by multiple responsibilities, which means that stress-related health problems are not unusual in these patients. Get to know your adult patients, and emphasize preventive healthcare when possible.

CRITICAL THINKING 30.3

Toby Anderson, a 52-year-old, was recently diagnosed with hypertension and prescribed Lotensin twice a day for treatment. He is being seen today for follow-up measurement of his blood pressure. Mr. Anderson is 45 pounds overweight and was given information about a reduced-calorie, low-sodium diet 1 month ago, but he has not lost any weight. He tells Chris that he has been having side effects from the medication. He is sitting with his arms across his chest, tapping his foot, and occasionally cracking his knuckles.

Communication factors Chris should consider include the following:
- What nonverbal language is Mr. Anderson using, and how should Chris interpret it?
- Mr. Anderson tells Chris he is not following that crazy diet and never will. What therapeutic communication skills can Chris use to get more information out of Mr. Anderson and to reinforce the provider's recommendations?
- During the discussion, Mr. Anderson tells Chris he stopped taking the Lotensin because of the side effects. What communication techniques and therapeutic body language can Chris use to emphasize the need for Mr. Anderson to take his medicine as prescribed?

ASSESSING THE PATIENT

After the interview is complete, the patient is escorted to an examination room and prepared for the physical examination. During the examination, the healthcare provider methodically checks all the body's systems. For each system, the provider mentally compares the system with established norms. Normal and abnormal findings are documented in the patient's health record. The physical examination typically starts with the head and progresses downward to the feet. However, the order may vary, depending on the provider's specialty.

Signs and Symptoms

All the signs and symptoms are documented in the health record. To better understand the examination procedure, the medical assistant must know the difference between a sign and a symptom.

Subjective findings, or **symptoms**, are perceptible only to the patient; they are what the patient feels and can be interpreted only by the patient. For example, only the patient experiences and can describe his or her discomfort, pain, nausea, or dizziness. Symptoms of the greatest significance in identifying a disease are called *cardinal symptoms*. For example, crushing chest pain and difficulty breathing are cardinal symptoms of a possible heart attack. Box 30.8 provides more information regarding assessing pain.

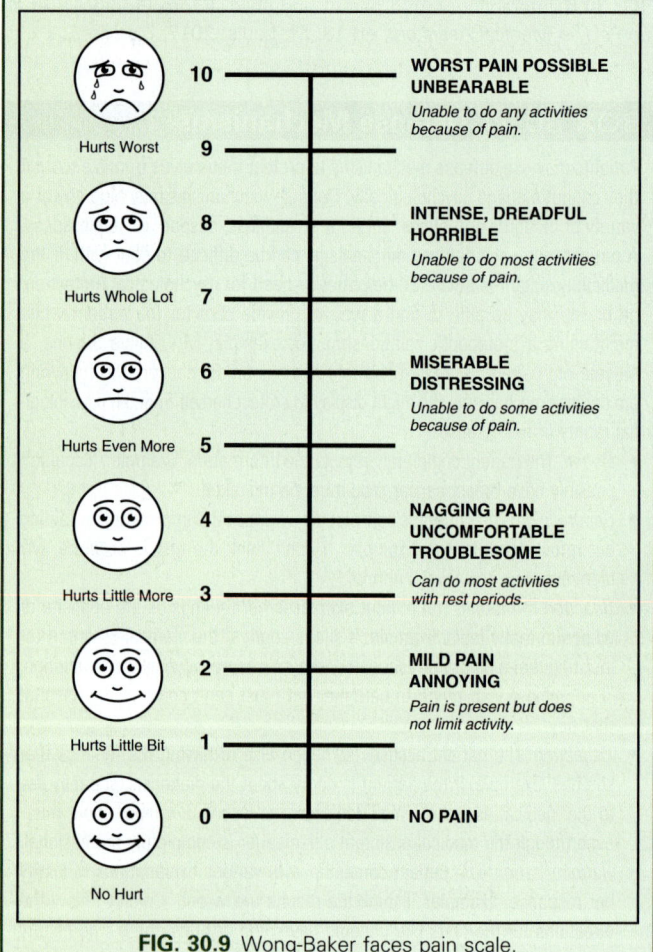

FIG. 30.9 Wong-Baker faces pain scale.

VOCABULARY
symptoms: Subjective complaints reported by the patient, such as pain or nausea.

Objective findings, or **signs**, can be observed or measured by the provider or medical assistant. They are the indicators of health or disease that a provider detects when examining a patient. The provider feels, sees, hears, or measures the signs that often are associated with a certain disease or abnormal condition. For example, a mass that a provider palpates, or feels, in the patient's abdomen is an objective finding and a sign of an abnormal condition. In addition, objective data can be measured and recorded, and repeat measurements can be taken to confirm the presence of or changes in the sign. The patient's temperature, pulse, respirations, and blood pressure are objective signs the medical assistant measures and regularly records.

> **VOCABULARY**
> **signs:** Objective findings determined by a clinician, such as a fever, hypertension, or rash.

DOCUMENTATION

Various methods can be used for documentation, depending on the healthcare provider's preference or the facility's EHR system. However, certain documentation procedures have been standardized to meet the legal requirements for maintaining medical records accurately and concisely. Complete, accurate documentation is one of the primary responsibilities of a medical assistant.

Documentation Guidelines

- Check the name on the record and make sure the information being documented is recorded on the correct form in the correct patient's health record or, with an EHR system, that the correct information is recorded using the correct system prompts. Confirm the patient's identity by checking his or her birth date.
- The month, day, and year must precede the entry; many facilities also require the time of the documentation.
- All unusual complaints, symptoms, or reactions must be noted in detail. Include complete information about the onset (when the problem started), duration (how long episodes last), and frequency (how often episodes occur) of each reported sign and symptom.
  Example: Pt reports night cough, which started 2 days ago, lasts approximately 10 minutes, and occurs 3–4 times per night.
- Describe objective data, such as the presence of a wound, using correct anatomic medical terminology.
  Example: Observed wound on left distal anterior leg approximately 2 cm long and 1 cm wide.
- If the patient reports pain, record the quality and intensity of the pain using a pain scale of 1 to 10.
  Example: Pt c/o dull pain at wound site, a 4 on a scale of 1–10.
- If the patient's comments are entered in the patient's own words, enclose them in quotation marks.
  Example: Pt states, "I fell against a stone foundation while cutting the grass and slashed my leg."
- Document the complete medication history, including both prescription and OTC medications taken on a regular basis, the last dose taken of the medication, its effectiveness, and any other pertinent details.
  Example: Pt reports taking 2 ibuprofen tablets for pain with moderate relief; last dose taken 45 minutes ago.
- Record details about the previous history of the current CC.
  Example: Pt reports having a similar cough 3 weeks ago.
- When entering information in the medical record, sign the entry, including the appropriate initials after your name (e.g., CMA).
- Learn to be observant and to note anything that seems pertinent.
- Use accurate abbreviations, symbols, and terminology (Table 30.3).
- Review your documentation immediately after completion so that you can detect errors while the information is fresh in your mind.
- The electronic record system will automatically track any corrections made to the original documentation entry.
- If documenting in a paper record:
  - Do all charting in black ink except for noting allergies in red ink; never use pencil.
  - Write in a clear, legible manner.
  - Do not leave any blank spaces on the paper record, and do not skip lines between documentation entries.
  - Never scribble, erase, or use whiteout on an error. For legal purposes, it is crucial that the corrected error be readable.
  - Correct the error by drawing one line through it. Write "error" above the corrected word or words and date and initial the correction. Then write in the correction.
- If details are omitted, add information by documenting after the last entry. Record "late entry," include date and time of note, and document the omitted information.

PHYSICAL EXAMINATION

The purpose of a physical examination is to determine the patient's overall state of well-being. All major organs and body systems are checked during a physical examination. As the provider examines the entire body, he or she interprets the findings. By the time the examination has been completed, the provider has formed an initial diagnosis of the patient's condition. Often laboratory and other diagnostic tests are ordered to supplement the provider's clinical diagnosis. The results of these tests are used to do the following:
- Refine the patient's diagnosis
- Help the provider plan or revise treatment for the patient
- Evaluate and maintain current drug therapy
- Determine the patient's progress

Before the examination, the medical assistant has the opportunity to make sure the patient feels comfortable during the examination process and that all the necessary medical information has been obtained. The medical assistant's duties include preparing and maintaining the examination room and equipment, preparing the patient, and assisting the provider during the physical examination.

Preparing the Examination Room

The medical assistant is responsible for making sure the examination room is ready for any procedure that might be performed during the physical examination. The area should be as comfortable as possible for the patient and free of any potential dangers, such as contaminated equipment or unlocked drug cabinets. You should prepare the examination room as follows:
- Check the area at the beginning of each day and between patients to make sure it is completely stocked with equipment and supplies and that all equipment is functioning properly. You must understand how to take care of and operate all equipment and instruments, and you should refer to operation manuals supplied by manufacturers as needed.
- Regularly check expiration dates on all packages and supplies; discard expired materials.
- Make sure the room is private, well lit, and at a comfortable temperature for the patient during the physical examination.
- Clean and disinfect the area daily and between patients to prevent the spread of infection and to ensure patients' comfort. When the patient leaves the room, discard the used exam table paper. Using disinfectant wipes, clean the table and any other potentially contaminated surface. When the table dries, replace the exam table paper.
- Arrange drapes, gowns, and all other patient supplies before the patient enters the room so that they are ready for use.
- To save time, prepare the instruments and equipment needed for the examination, arranging them for easy access, before the provider enters the room.

TABLE 30.3 Medical Abbreviations

Abbreviation	Definition	Abbreviation	Definition
abd	abdomen	FUO	fever of unknown origin
ABG	arterial blood gases	fx	fracture
ac	before eating	GC	gonorrhea
ACLS	advanced cardiac life support	GI	gastrointestinal
ad lib	as desired	GTT	glucose tolerance test
AFP	alpha-fetoprotein	GU	genitourinary
AKA	above the knee amputation	HCT	hematocrit
ASAP	as soon as possible	Hgb	hemoglobin
ASHD	atherosclerotic heart disease	HIV	human immunodeficiency virus
BE	barium enema	h/o	history of
bid	twice a day	HPI	history of present illness
BM	bowel movement	hs	at bedtime or hour of sleep
BMR	basal metabolic rate	HTN	hypertension
BOM	bilateral otitis media	Hx	history
BP	blood pressure	I&D	incision and drainage
BUN	blood urea nitrogen	I&O	intake and output
bx	biopsy	IG	immunoglobulin
$\bar{c}$	with	lytes	electrolytes
C&S	culture and sensitivity	MI	myocardial infarction
CA	cancer	NG	nasogastric
CABG	coronary artery bypass graft	NKA	no known allergies
CAD	coronary artery disease	NPO	nothing by mouth
CBC	complete blood count	N/V	nausea and vomiting
CC	chief complaint	p	after
CHF	congestive heart failure	PE	pulmonary embolism
CHO	carbohydrate	prn	as needed
CNS	central nervous system	pt	patient
c/o	complains of	PE	physical examination
COPD	chronic obstructive pulmonary disease	PT	physical therapy
CPK	creatinine phosphokinase	q	every
CPR	cardiopulmonary resuscitation	RBC	red blood cells
CSF	cerebrospinal fluid	R/O	rule out
CT	computed tomography	ROM	range of motion
CVA	cerebrovascular accident	R/T	related to
CXR	chest x-ray	Rx	treatment
DAT	diet as tolerated	$\bar{s}$	without
dc	discontinue	SOB	shortness of breath
D&C	dilation and curettage	s/s	signs and symptoms
DDx	differential diagnosis	STD	sexually transmitted disease
DM	diabetes mellitus	STAT	immediately
DNR	do not resuscitate	Sx	symptoms
DVT	deep vein thrombosis	Tx	treatment
Dx	diagnosis	UA	urinalysis
ECG	electrocardiogram	URI	upper respiratory infection
EENT	eyes, ears, nose, throat	UTI	urinary tract infection
FBS	fasting blood sugar	VS	vital signs
f/u	follow up	WNL	within normal limits

Modified from Proctor D, et al: *Kinn's The Medical Assistant*, ed 13, St. Louis, 2017, Elsevier.

- Make sure the examination room has all materials required for observing Standard Precautions, including gloves, a sink with soap, paper towels, biohazard waste containers, sharps containers, and impervious gowns and face guards. Sharps containers are replaced when they are two-thirds full, as indicated by Standard Precautions.

Assisting the Patient

Getting the patient ready for the examination includes taking care of paperwork before the patient enters the examination room and performing related clinical skills.

CHAPTER 30 Physical Examination

- Make sure the health record is complete and that any needed consent forms have been signed; document current medications and allergies; identify any medications that need refills. The medical assistant is not responsible for obtaining informed consent, but he or she should review the paperwork to make sure that informed consent forms were reviewed by the provider and that the patient signed the forms.
- Introduce yourself, verify the patient's identity, and address the patient by his or her preferred name, making sure to show respect at all times. Pay close attention to the patient's nonverbal language to make sure he or she understands what to expect.
- Obtain specimens (e.g., urine, blood) if the provider has preordered them or if this practice is part of the office policy.
- Measure and record the patient's height, weight, body mass index (BMI), and vital signs.
- Conduct the initial investigation into the reason for the visit, and explain the examination procedure to the patient. Be prepared to answer the patient's questions and ease any fears. If needed, refer the patient's questions to the provider.
- Ask whether the patient needs to empty his or her bladder before the examination, because a full bladder may interfere with the examination and may be uncomfortable for the patient.
- Help the patient physically prepare for the examination. Explain to the patient what clothing should be removed and in what direction to put on the gown (open to the front or to the back, depending on the type of examination); provide a drape to ensure the patient's privacy, and offer assistance as needed.
- Assist the patient into and out of various examination positions as needed.
- Throughout this sequence of events, explain what is happening, and consistently maintain the patient's privacy and confidentiality.
- Help the patient with dressing as needed after the examination.

Assisting the Provider

The medical assistant should be prepared to help the provider complete the physical examination as comprehensively and efficiently as possible. During the examination, the provider may expect the medical assistant to do the following:

- Hand him or her instruments and equipment as requested, and provide supplies as needed.
- Alter the position of the light source to better illuminate the area being examined, and turn lights on and off during specific phases of the examination.
- Position and drape the patient during different phases of the examination.
- Assist in collecting and properly labeling specimens such as urine, Pap test specimens, and throat cultures.
- Conduct any diagnostic tests preordered by the provider, including hearing and visual screenings.
- Conduct follow-up diagnostic procedures as ordered, including an electrocardiogram (ECG), urinalysis, and phlebotomy.
- Document patient data in the health record, completing all forms required.
- Schedule postexamination diagnostic procedures, such as mammography, x-ray examination, or colonoscopy.

> **VOCABULARY**
> **electrocardiogram (ECG, EKG):** A record or recording of electrical impulses of the heart produced by an electrocardiograph.

Supplies and Instruments Needed for the Physical Examination

The instruments typically used during the physical examination are shown in Fig. 30.10. They enable the provider to see, feel, inspect, and

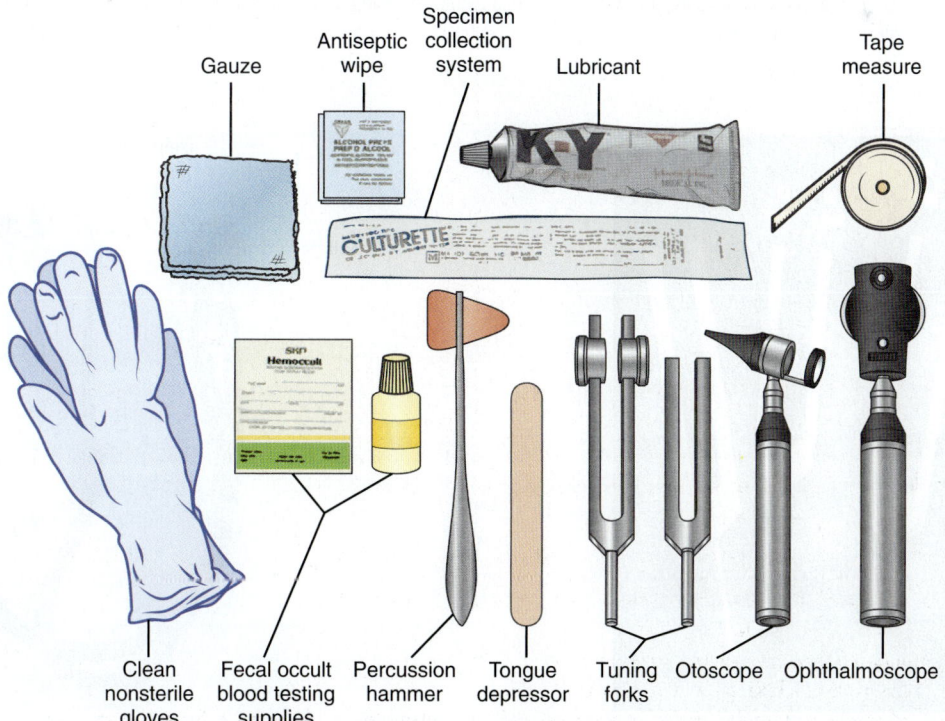

FIG. 30.10 Instruments for the physical examination. (From Proctor D, et al: *Kinn's The Medical Assistant*, ed 13, St. Louis, 2017, Elsevier.)

listen to parts of the body. All equipment must be in good working order, properly disinfected, and readily available for the provider's use during the examination. The instruments most frequently used for a physical examination are described in Table 30.4. Physical examinations typically are performed from the head to the feet; the instruments are listed in the order in which the provider typically would request them.

> **VOCABULARY**
> **auscultate:** To listen with a stethoscope.
> **peripheral neuropathy:** A problem with the function of the nerves outside the spinal cord; symptoms include weakness, burning pain, and loss of reflexes; a frequent complication of diabetes mellitus.

TABLE 30.4 Instruments Needed for the Physical Examination

Instrument	Use
Ophthalmoscope	To inspect the inner structures of the eye. It consists of a stainless-steel handle containing batteries and an attached head, which has a light, magnifying lenses, and an opening through which the eye is viewed.
Tongue depressor	A flat, wooden blade used to hold down the tongue when the throat is examined.
Otoscope	To examine the external auditory canal and tympanic membrane. It has a stainless-steel handle containing batteries or is part of a wall-mounted electrical unit. The head of the otoscope has a light that is focused through a magnifying lens; it should be covered with a disposable ear speculum. The light also may be used to illuminate the nasal passages and throat.
Tuning fork	An aluminum, fork-shaped instrument that consists of a handle and two prongs (Fig. 30.11). The prongs produce a humming sound when the provider strikes them against his or her hand. Tuning forks are available in different sizes, and each size produces a different pitch level. A tuning fork is used to check the patient's auditory acuity and to test bone vibration. A tuning fork can also be used to test for diabetic **peripheral neuropathy**.
Tape measure	A flexible ribbon ruler that is usually printed with inches and feet on one side and centimeters and meters on the reverse side. Measurements may be used to assess length and head circumference in infants, wound size, and so on.
Stethoscope	A listening device used when certain areas of the body are **auscultated** (AW skuh l teyt d), particularly the heart and lungs. This instrument is available in many shapes and sizes. All have two earpieces that are connected to flexible rubber or vinyl tubing (Fig. 30.12). At the distal end of the tubing is a diaphragm or bell (many have both); when it is placed securely on the patient's skin, it enables the provider to hear internal body sounds.
Reflex hammer	Sometimes called a percussion hammer. This stainless-steel instrument has a hard rubber head that is used to strike the tendons of the knee and elbow to test the neurologic reflexes.
Gloves	Gloves protect the healthcare worker and the patient from microorganisms. According to Standard Precautions, gloves must be worn whenever the potential exists for contact with any body fluid, broken skin or wounds, or contaminated items.
Additional supplies	Gauze, cotton balls, cotton-tipped applicators, disposable tissues, specimen containers, fecal occult blood test cards, Pap test supplies for female patients, lubricating jelly for vaginal and rectal examinations, and laboratory request forms should be easily accessible during the examination.

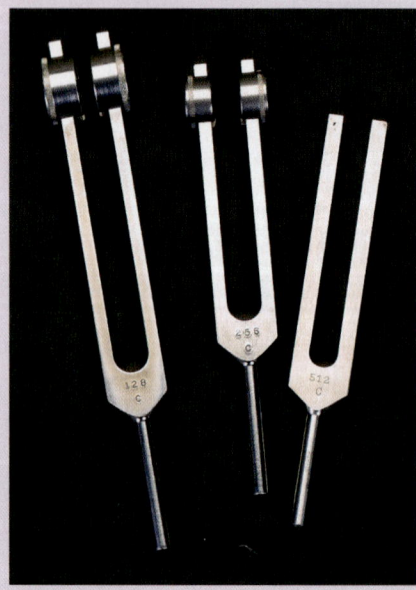

FIG. 30.11 Tuning forks. (From Proctor D, et al: *Kinn's The Medical Assistant*, ed 13, St. Louis, 2017, Elsevier.)

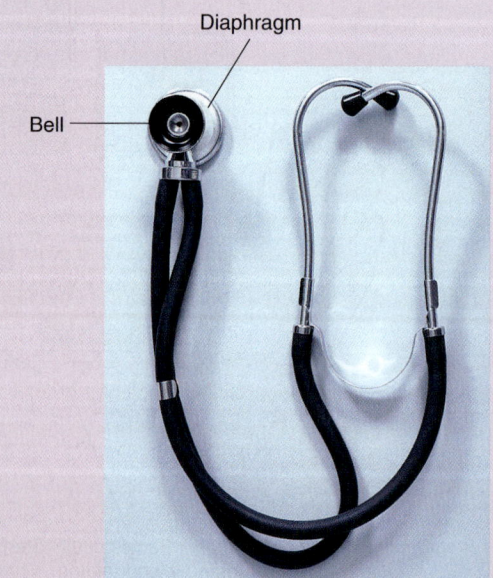

FIG. 30.12 Stethoscope. (Modified from Ball JW, et al: *Seidel's Guide to Physical Examination*, ed 8, St. Louis 2015, Mosby.)

PRINCIPLES OF BODY MECHANICS

Medical assistants should use proper body mechanics consistently throughout the work environment when sitting or standing, lifting or carrying objects, pushing or pulling, or transferring patients. Without consistent application of correct anatomic alignment, injuries, especially lower back injuries, easily occur.

Proper body alignment begins with good posture. Maintaining posture requires a combination of muscle efforts. Good posture keeps the spine balanced and aligned while a person is sitting or standing. A person in good body alignment can maintain balance without undue strain on the musculoskeletal system.

When reaching for an object, avoid twisting or turning; instead, move the feet to face the object needed; this prevents undue strain on the lumbar region. Do not cross the legs while sitting because this interferes with circulation to the legs and feet. When sitting, keep the popliteal area (behind the knees) free of the edge of the chair. Pressure in this area interferes with circulation and may damage nerves behind the knees. Do a mental check of your posture regularly. Hold the head erect, the face forward and the chin slightly up, the abdominal muscles contracted up and in, the shoulders relaxed and back, the feet pointed forward and slightly apart, and the weight evenly distributed to both legs, with the knees slightly bent. Always be on the alert for poor body mechanics that may cause injury (Figs. 30.13 and 30.14). See Box 30.9 for tips on lifting items safely.

Transferring a Patient

Patients may need assistance in moving from a chair to the examination table or back again. Patients can be transferred in multiple ways, but all should focus on correct body mechanics. If the patient is in a wheelchair, move the chair at a 45-degree angle toward the footrest that extends from the bottom of the exam table (Fig. 30.15), lock the wheels, and lift the footrests of the wheelchair out of the way. Explain the procedure to the patient, and ask for his or her assistance.

If one side of the patient is stronger than the other, always provide support on the strong side. Support the patient close to your body on the strong side, with one hand under the axillary region and the other either grasping the patient's hand or holding the forearm. When bending, always bend at the knees and maintain the back's three natural curves, allowing the leg muscles to help in lifting. Give the patient a signal and lift as the patient assists. Help the patient step up onto the footrest with the strong leg first, then pivot. Ease the patient down onto the table, bending your knees while keeping your back aligned. Make sure the patient is comfortable and safely positioned on the table.

Use a gait belt as needed to help transfer patients, prevent injury to yourself, and safeguard patients from falling. A gait belt is a safety device that is used to help transfer a patient from a wheelchair to the exam table or to help a patient walk. The gait belt helps you support the patient while keeping your body in proper alignment to prevent back injuries. A gait belt should be used if the patient is weak and at risk of falling. Follow these steps to use a gait belt:

- Place the belt around the individual's waist over clothing with the buckle in front.
- Insert the belt through the teeth of the buckle, and pull it tight to lock it.
- The belt should be tight, with just enough room to place your fingers under it.
- Grip the belt tightly, bend your knees, and keep your back straight.
- Ask the patient to assist you; then lift, using your arm and leg muscles.
- Avoid twisting or turning as you help the patient stand.
- Keep your body close to the patient with your knees in front of his or hers at all times to stabilize the patient and prevent falls.
- Complete the transfer without bending or twisting your body; encourage the patient to bear as much weight as possible and to gently sit down on the table.
- After transferring the patient, remove the gait belt for the provider's examination, and replace it to help transfer the patient back to the wheelchair after the provider is finished.
- If the patient should start to fall during a transfer, do not try to stop the fall because you may be injured; use the gait belt to help guide the patient to the floor as gently as possible.

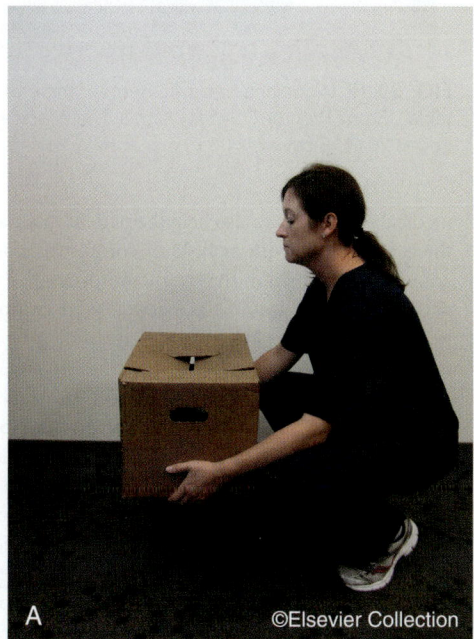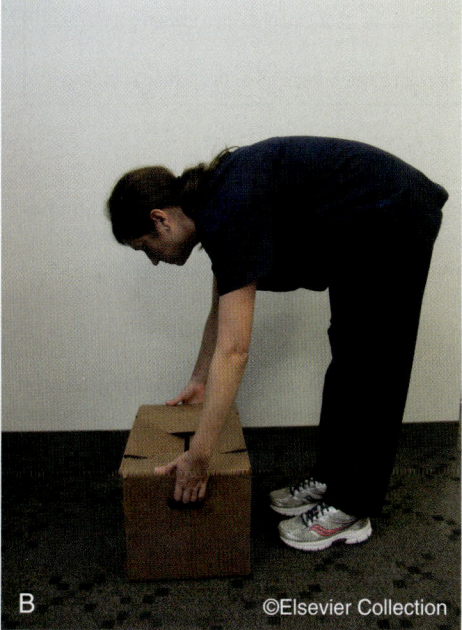

FIG. 30.13 (A) Proper lifting technique. (B) Improper lifting technique. (From Proctor D, et al: *Kinn's The Medical Assistant*, ed 13, St. Louis, 2017, Elsevier.)

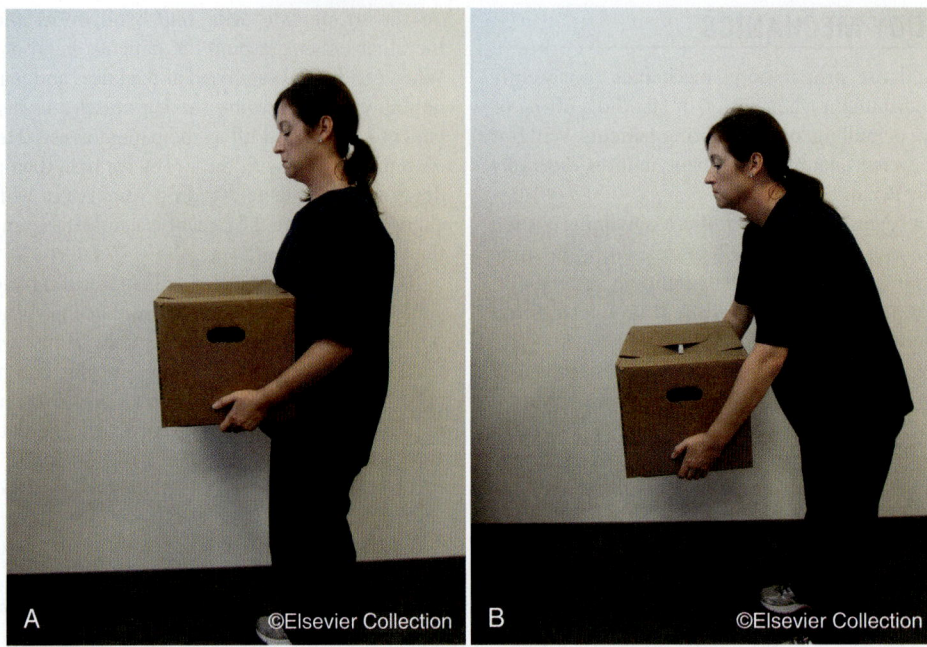

FIG. 30.14 (A) Carrying an item close to the body. (B) Improper carrying technique. (From Proctor D, et al: *Kinn's The Medical Assistant*, ed 13, St. Louis, 2017, Elsevier.)

> **BOX 30.9 Safe Lifting Techniques**
>
> - Always get help if the load is too heavy.
> - Maintain correct body alignment, with the legs spread apart for a broad base of support.
> - Do not reach for items; clear barriers out of the way and get as close as possible to what needs to be lifted.
> - Bend at the knees with the feet shoulder width apart, and keep the back straight. Use the major muscle groups of the arms and legs rather than the weaker ones of the back to help lift a heavy item (see Fig. 30.13).
> - When carrying a heavy item, keep the weight as close to the body as possible (see Fig. 30.14).
> - Move the feet in the direction of the lift. Do not twist or turn on fixed feet.
> - Bend the knees while keeping the back straight when lowering an item at the completion of a lift.
> - If possible, slide, roll, or push a heavy item rather than lifting or pulling it.

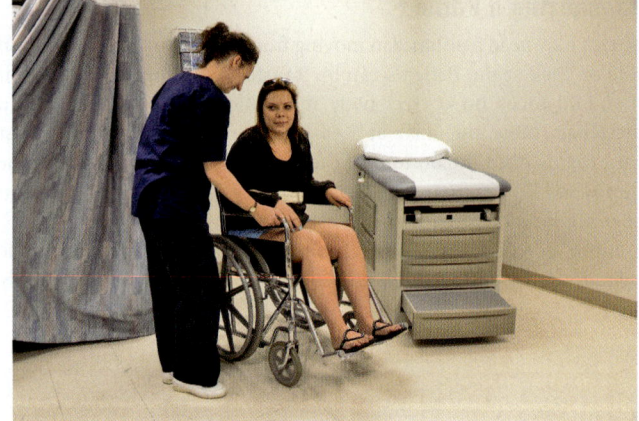

FIG. 30.15 Wheelchair at a 45-degree angle at the end of the exam table. (From Proctor D, et al: *Kinn's The Medical Assistant*, ed 13, St. Louis, 2017, Elsevier.)

You may need to remain with the patient until the examination has been completed to ensure his or her safety. If the provider prefers that the patient be in a supine position, place one arm across the patient's shoulders and the other under the knees, and smoothly lower the patient's upper body to the table while raising the legs. Use the same pivoting techniques with proper body mechanics to help transfer the patient from the examination table back to the locked wheelchair. If the patient must hold onto you, have the person hold your waist or shoulders, not your neck (Procedure 30.3).

ASSISTING WITH THE PHYSICAL EXAMINATION

Positioning and Draping the Patient for the Physical Examination

Various patient positions are used to facilitate a physical examination. The medical assistant instructs the patient and assists the patient into these positions, ensuring as much ease and modesty as possible. The medical assistant may also help the patient maintain the position during the examination with as little discomfort as possible. Do not place a patient into a position that is uncomfortable or that compromises the patient's privacy until it is necessary to complete that part of the examination. Never leave the patient's side if he or she is in a position that could result in a fall.

Draping the patient with a sheet protects the individual from embarrassment and keeps the patient warm. However, the sheet must be positioned so that it allows complete visibility for the examiner and does not interfere with the examination. During the general examination, each part of the body is exposed one portion at a time. For gynecologic and rectal examinations, the sheet is positioned on the diagonal across the patient, or in a diamond shape, to provide maximum comfort for the patient while allowing the provider to perform the examination.

The following sections describe a number of the positions used during medical examinations.

PROCEDURE 30.3 Use Proper Body Mechanics

Task
Safely transfer a patient from a wheelchair to an examination table using proper body mechanics.

Equipment and Supplies
- Patient's record
- Wheelchair
- Examination table with pull-out footrest
- Gait belt

Procedural Steps
1. Wash hands or use hand sanitizer.
   Purpose: Hand sanitization is an important step for infection control.
2. Greet the patient. Identify yourself. Verify the patient's identity with full name and date of birth. Explain the procedure to be performed in a manner that the patient understands. Determine how much assistance the patient will need to transfer from the wheelchair to the examination table. Do not proceed if you think you will need additional help.
   Purpose: To promote the patient's cooperation during the transfer and prevent personal injury.
3. Place the wheelchair at a 45-degree angle toward the footrest at the base of the examination table (Fig. 30.15).
4. Lock the brakes on the wheelchair, and move the footrests of the wheelchair out of the way (Fig. 1).
   Purpose: Never transfer a patient into or out of a wheelchair until the brakes are locked on both sides of the chair.

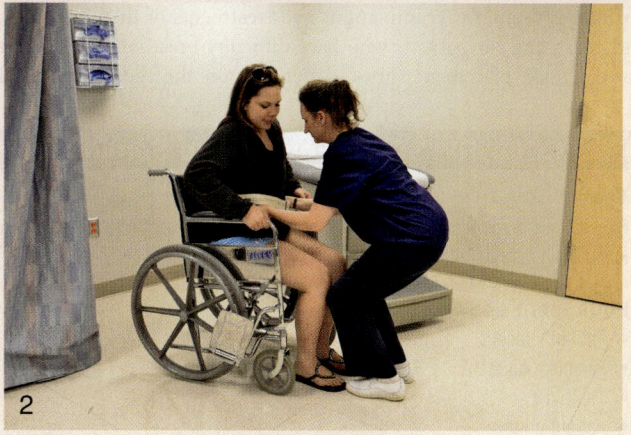

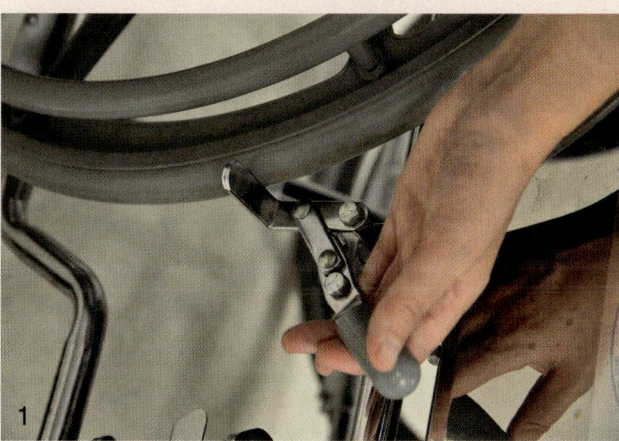

5. Place the gait belt around the patient's waist over clothing with the buckle in front. Insert the belt through the teeth of the buckle, and pull it tight to lock it. The belt should be tight with just enough room to place your fingers under it.
6. Request that the patient place both feet flat on the floor with the hands on the armrests.
   Purpose: This position helps you grasp the gait belt; the patient can use the wheelchair armrests to help push her or him into an upright position, and feet flat on the floor help with patient stability.
7. Stand directly in front of the patient with your feet apart, back straight, and knees bent (Fig. 2).
   Purpose: This position helps you maintain good body mechanics during the transfer.
8. Slide your fingers under the gait belt on opposite sides of the patient's waist.
9. Instruct the patient at the count of 3 to push off from the armrests while you at the same time grasp the gait belt and, using your leg muscles, straighten your knees so that the patient is in a standing position.
   Purpose: This position allows the patient to assist as much as possible while you are using the large muscles of your legs to help lift the patient.
10. Ask the patient to step up onto the footrest at the bottom of the exam table, and assist the person in pivoting and sitting down on the examination table. Remove the gait belt until the provider has completed the examination (Fig. 3).

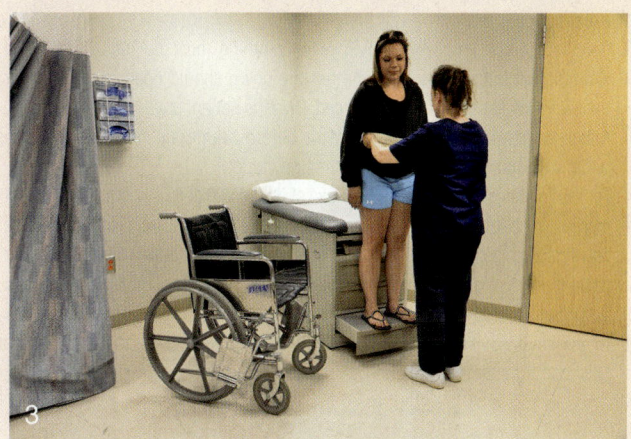

11. After the examination is complete, place the wheelchair at an angle next to the exam table and lock the wheels. Replace the gait belt. Make sure the patient is positioned at the edge of the table.
    Purpose: To prepare for transfer back to the wheelchair.
12. Place yourself directly in front of the patient with your back straight and your knees bent. Slide your fingers under the gait belt on opposite sides of the patient's waist.
13. Grasp the gait belt on both sides at the waist. Instruct the patient at the count of 3 to push off from the examination table and, using your leg muscles, straighten your knees so that the patient is in a standing position on the footrest.
14. Maintaining your hold on the gait belt, ask the patient to step down. Pivot the person so that she or he can slowly sit in the wheelchair; at the same time, bend your knees but keep your back straight.
15. Remove the gait belt. Replace the wheelchair footrests, and unlock the brakes on the wheelchair.

Fowler Position. In the Fowler position, the patient sits on the examination table with the head of the table elevated 90 degrees. This position is useful for examinations and treatments of the head, neck, and chest, and for patients who have difficulty breathing while lying down. Drape placement varies, depending on the type of physical examination done and the need to maintain the patient's modestly (Procedure 30.4).

Semi-Fowler Position. The semi-Fowler position is a modification of the Fowler position. The head of the table is positioned at a 45-degree

---

PROCEDURE 30.4 Fowler and Semi-Fowler Positions

Task
Position and drape the patient for examinations of the head, neck, and chest, or position and drape patients who have difficulty breathing when lying flat.

Equipment and Supplies
- Patient's record
- Examination table
- Table paper
- Patient gown
- Drape
- Disinfectant wipes
- Gloves

Procedural Steps

1. Wash hands or use hand sanitizer.
   Purpose: Hand sanitization is an important step for infection control.
2. Greet the patient. Identify yourself. Verify the patient's identity with full name and date of birth. Explain the procedure to be performed in a manner that the patient understands. Answer any questions the patient may have about the procedure.
   Purpose: To promote the patient's understanding and cooperation during the examination.
3. Give the patient a gown. Explain what clothing must be removed for the examination being done and whether the gown should open in the front or the back. Provide assistance as needed. Give the patient privacy while changing. Knock on the examination room door before reentering to make sure the patient has completed undressing and gowning.
4. For the Fowler position, elevate the head of the bed 90 degrees. Patients who feel more comfortable can sit at the end of the table (Fig. 1). Extend the footrest as needed for patient comfort. The patient may be more comfortable in the semi-Fowler position. In this modification of the Fowler position, the head of the table is elevated 45 degrees. The semi-Fowler position may be used for postoperative follow-up or for patients with a fever, head injury, or pain. It also is a comfortable, supportive position for patients with breathing disorders (Fig. 2).

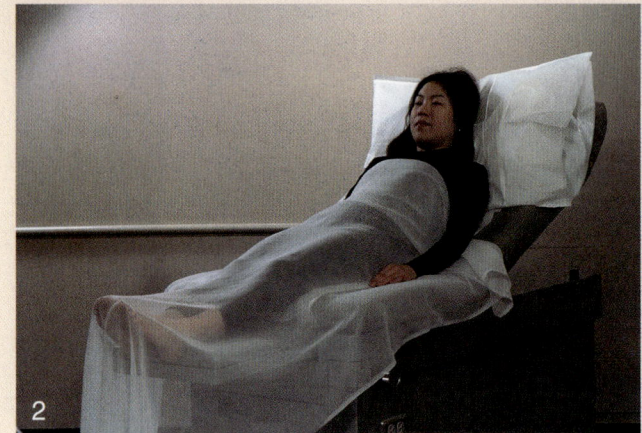

5. Drape the patient according to the type of examination and the required patient exposure.
   Purpose: Draping the patient provides warmth and privacy while giving the provider access to the examination site.
6. After the examination has been completed, assist the patient as needed to get off the table and get dressed.
7. Put on gloves, and use disinfectant wipes to clean the exam table and all potentially contaminated surfaces. Dispose of used gloves and examination table paper according to facility policies. Pull clean paper over the table.
   Purpose: To ensure infection control and to prevent the transmission of pathogens from one patient to another.
8. Wash hands or use hand sanitizer.
9. Follow up with the provider's orders regarding scheduling of diagnostic studies, collection of specimens, or scheduling of future appointments.

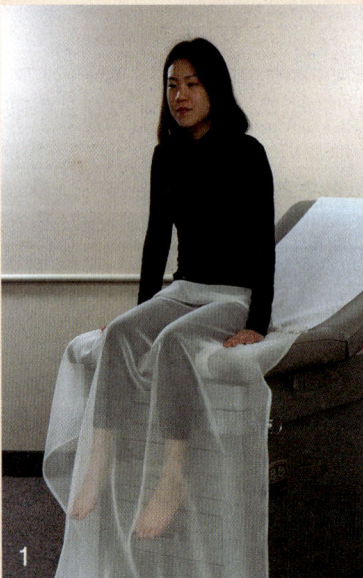

angle instead of at a full 90-degree angle. This position is useful for postoperative examination, for patients with breathing disorders, and for patients suffering from head trauma or pain (see Procedure 30.4). The drape or gown should cover the entire patient from the nipple line down.

> **VOCABULARY**
> **trauma:** A physical injury or wound caused by external force or violence.

Supine (Horizontal Recumbent) Position. In the supine position, the patient lies flat with the face upward and the lower legs supported by the table extension (Procedure 30.5). This position is used for examination of the front of the body, including the heart, breasts, and abdominal organs. The patient's gown should open down the front, and the drape should be placed over any exposed area that is not being examined.

Dorsal Recumbent Position. In the dorsal recumbent position, the patient lies face upward, with the weight distributed primarily to the surface of the back. This is accomplished by flexing the knees so that the feet are flat on the table. This position relieves muscle tension in the abdomen and may be used for examination or inspection of the rectal, vaginal, and perineal (pair ih NEE uhl) areas. It may also be used if the patient experiences back discomfort when lying supine. This position can be used for digital examination of the vagina and rectum, but it is not used if an instrument such as a speculum is needed. To ensure the patient's privacy, it is important to keep the patient completely draped, with the drape in a diamond shape, until the provider is present (see Procedure 30.5).

PROCEDURE 30.5 Supine (Horizontal Recumbent) and Dorsal Recumbent Positions

Task
Position and drape the patient for examinations of the abdomen, heart, and breasts in the horizontal recumbent (supine) position and exams of the rectal, vaginal, and perineal areas in the dorsal recumbent position.

Equipment and Supplies
- Patient's record
- Examination table
- Table paper
- Patient gown
- Drape
- Disinfectant wipes
- Gloves

Procedural Steps
1. Wash hands or use hand sanitizer.
   Purpose: Hand sanitization is an important step for infection control.
2. Greet the patient. Identify yourself. Verify the patient's identity with full name and date of birth. Explain the procedure to be performed in a manner that the patient understands. Answer any questions the patient may have about the procedure.
   Purpose: To promote the patient's understanding and cooperation during the examination.
3. Give the patient a gown. Explain the clothing that must be removed for the examination being done and whether the gown should open in the front or in the back. Provide assistance as needed. For the horizontal recumbent position, the gown should be open in the front. Give the patient privacy while changing. Knock on the examination room door before reentering to make sure the patient has completed undressing and gowning.
4. Do not place the patient in the necessary positions until the provider is ready for that part of the examination.
   Purpose: To ensure the patient's privacy, comfort, and modesty.
5. Pull out the table extension that supports the patient's legs. For the horizontal recumbent (supine) position, help the patient lie flat on the table with the face upward (Fig. 1). For the dorsal recumbent position, have the patient lie flat on the back and flex the knees so the feet are flat on the table (Fig. 2). If needed, help the patient move down toward the foot of the table for the examination.

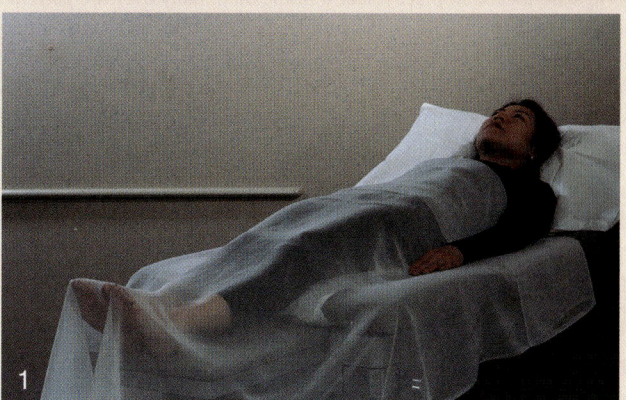

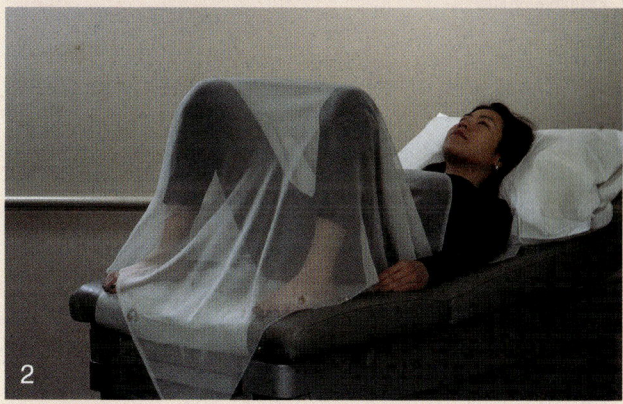

6. Drape the patient from nipple line to feet in the supine position, and diagonally with the point of the drape between the feet for the dorsal recumbent position.
   Purpose: Draping the patient provides warmth and privacy while giving the provider access to the examination site.
7. After the examination has been completed, assist the patient as needed to get off the table and get dressed.
8. Put on gloves, and use disinfectant wipes to clean the exam table and all potentially contaminated surfaces. Dispose of used gloves and examination table paper according to facility policies. Pull clean paper over the table.
   Purpose: To ensure infection control and to prevent the transmission of pathogens from one patient to another.
9. Wash hands or use hand sanitizer.
10. Follow up with the provider's orders regarding scheduling of diagnostic studies, collection of specimens, or scheduling of future appointments.

> **VOCABULARY**
> **perineal:** Pertaining to the area between the vaginal opening and the rectum (perineum).

Lithotomy Position. The patient should not be placed in the *lithotomy* (li THOT uh mee) position until the provider is in the examination room and is ready for this part of the examination. Place the patient on his or her back with the knees sharply flexed and the arms at the sides or folded over the chest; have the patient slide the buttocks down to the bottom edge of the table. Support the feet in stirrups placed wide apart and somewhat away from the table, with the stirrup arms extended to match the length of the patient's legs. If the heels are too close to the buttocks, the possibility of leg cramps increases, and it is more difficult for the patient to relax the abdominal muscles. Make sure the stirrups are locked in place. Place a drape diagonally over the patient's abdomen and knees. The drape must be long enough to cover the knees and touch the ankles and wide enough to prevent the sides of the thighs from being exposed. The provider lifts the drape away from the pubic area when the examination begins (Procedure 30.6). The lithotomy position is used primarily for vaginal examinations that require the use of a speculum and for Pap tests.

Sims Position. The Sims position is sometimes called the *left lateral position*. The patient is placed on the left side; the left arm and shoulder are drawn back behind the body so that the body's weight is predominantly on the chest. The right arm is flexed upward for support. The left leg is slightly flexed, and the buttocks are pulled to the edge of the table. The right leg is sharply flexed upward. The drape extends diagonally from under the arms to below the knees. The provider can raise a small portion of the sheet from the back of the patient to expose the rectum sufficiently. The remaining portion of the sheet covers the patient's chest area and thighs. This position is used for rectal examinations, for instillation of rectal medication, and for some perineal and pelvic examinations (Procedure 30.7).

Prone Position. In the prone position, the patient lies face down on the table on the ventral surface of the body. This is the opposite of the supine position and is another of the recumbent positions. The drape should cover from the middle of the back to below the knees, with the gown opening in the back (Procedure 30.8). This position is used for examination of the back and for certain surgical procedures.

PROCEDURE 30.6 Lithotomy Position

Task
Position and drape the patient primarily for vaginal and pelvic examinations and Pap tests.

Equipment and Supplies
- Patient's record
- Examination table
- Table paper
- Patient gown
- Drape
- Disinfectant wipes
- Gloves

Procedural Steps
1. Wash hands or use hand sanitizer.
   Purpose: Hand sanitization is an important step for infection control.
2. Greet the patient. Identify yourself. Verify the patient's identity with full name and date of birth. Explain the procedure to be performed in a manner that the patient understands. Answer any questions the patient may have about the procedure.
   Purpose: To promote the patient's understanding and cooperation during the examination.
3. Give the patient a gown. Instruct the patient to undress from the waist down with the gown open in the back. If the provider also will be doing a breast examination, the patient should undress completely and put on the gown so that it opens in the front. Provide assistance as needed. Give the patient privacy while changing. Knock on the examination room door before reentering to make sure the patient has completed undressing and gowning.
4. Do not place the patient in the lithotomy position until the provider is ready for that part of the examination.
   Purpose: To promote the patient's privacy, comfort, and safety.
5. Pull out the table extension that supports the patient's legs, and help the patient lie face upward on the table. Pull out the stirrups, adjust their extension length for the patient's comfort, and lock them in place.
6. Reinsert the table extension, and have the patient move toward the foot of the table with her buttocks on the bottom table edge. Gently place the patient's legs in the stirrups, checking for comfort. Some offices may stock cloth or paper stirrup covers to protect the patient and make the position more comfortable. The patient's arms can be placed alongside the body or across the chest (Fig. 1).

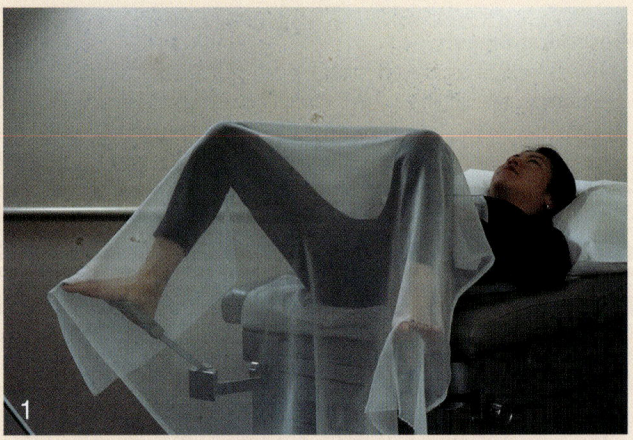

7. Drape the patient diagonally, with the point of the drape between the feet. The drape should be large enough to cover the patient from the nipple line to the ankles and wide enough so the patient's thighs are not exposed.
   Purpose: To provide warmth and privacy for the patient while giving the provider access to the examination site.
8. After the examination has been completed, assist the patient as needed to get off the table and get dressed.
9. Put on gloves, and use disinfectant wipes to clean the exam table and all potentially contaminated surfaces. Dispose of used gloves and examination table paper according to facility policies. Pull clean paper over the table.
   Purpose: To ensure infection control and to prevent the transmission of pathogens from one patient to another.
10. Wash hands or use hand sanitizer.
11. Follow up with the provider's orders regarding scheduling of diagnostic studies, collection of specimens, or scheduling of future appointments.

PROCEDURE 30.7 Sims Position

Task
Position and drape the patient for examination of the rectum, instillation of rectal medication, perineal examination, and some pelvic examinations.

Equipment and Supplies
- Patient's record
- Examination table
- Patient gown
- Table paper
- Drape
- Disinfectant wipes
- Gloves

Procedural Steps

1. Wash hands or use hand sanitizer.
   Purpose: Hand sanitization is an important step for infection control.
2. Greet the patient. Identify yourself. Verify the patient's identity with full name and date of birth. Explain the procedure to be performed in a manner that the patient understands. Answer any questions the patient may have about the procedure.
   Purpose: To promote the patient's understanding and cooperation during the examination.
3. Give the patient a gown, and explain what clothing must be removed for the examination being done. Tell the patient that the gown should open in the back. Provide assistance as needed. Give the patient privacy while changing. Knock on the examination room door before reentering to make sure the patient has completed undressing and gowning.
4. Do not place the patient in the Sims position until the provider is ready for that part of the examination.
   Purpose: To promote the patient's privacy, comfort, and safety.
5. Help the patient turn onto the left side; the left arm and shoulder should be drawn back behind the body so that the patient is tilted onto the chest. Flex the right arm upward for support, slightly flex the left leg, and sharply flex the right leg upward. Help the patient move the buttocks to the side edge of the table (Fig. 1).

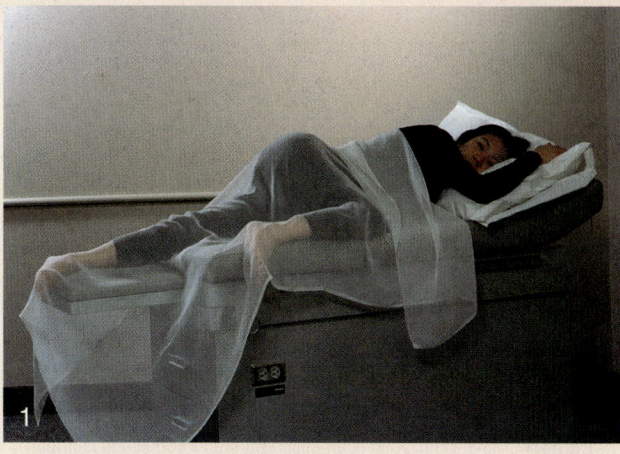

6. Drape the patient diagonally in a diamond shape, with the point of the diamond dropping below the buttocks. Make sure the drape is large enough to prevent exposure of the patient.
   Purpose: Draping the patient provides warmth and privacy while giving the provider access to the examination site.
7. After the examination has been completed, assist the patient as needed to get off the table and get dressed.
8. Put on gloves, and use disinfectant wipes to clean the exam table and all potentially contaminated surfaces. Dispose of used gloves and examination table paper according to facility policies. Pull clean paper over the table.
   Purpose: To ensure infection control and prevent the transmission of pathogens from one patient to another.
9. Wash hands or use hand sanitizer.
10. Follow up with the provider's orders regarding scheduling of diagnostic studies, collection of specimens, or scheduling of future appointments.

Knee-Chest Position. For the knee-chest position, the patient rests on the knees and the chest with the head turned to one side. The arms can be placed under the head for support and comfort, or they can be bent and placed at the sides of the table near the head. The thighs are perpendicular to the table and slightly separated. The buttocks extend up into the air, and the back should be straight. The patient will need assistance to assume the knee-chest position correctly. Most patients have difficulty maintaining this position, so they should not be placed into it until it is required. The medical assistant must remain next to the patient for assistance and support the entire time the knee-chest position is needed. If the correct knee-chest position cannot be obtained, the patient may have to be placed in a knee-elbow position. This position puts less strain on the patient and is easier to maintain. These positions are used for *proctologic* (prok TOL loj ick) examination and for *sigmoid* (SIG moid), rectal, and occasionally vaginal examinations. The patient's gown should open in the back, and a fenestrated (opening) drape or a single sheet should be draped diagonally over the patient's back at the sacral area (Procedure 30.9).

Trendelenburg Position. The Trendelenburg position is rarely used in the ambulatory care setting, but it may be needed if a patient has severe hypotension. This position can be achieved only if the examination table separates so that the legs can be elevated higher than the head (Fig. 30.16).

> **CRITICAL THINKING 30.4**
>
> Determine the correct patient position and method of gowning and draping for the following examinations:
> - Insertion of a rectal suppository
> - Annual Papanicolaou (pap) test
> - Examination of the back
> - Patient with dyspnea
> - Breast examination

Methods of Examination

Examinations are performed as both a routine confirmation of wellness and a means of diagnosing disease. Healthcare providers use six methods to examine the human body:

- Inspection
- Palpation (PAL pey taa shuh n)
- Percussion (per KUHSH uh n)
- Auscultation

PROCEDURE 30.8   Prone Position

Task
Position and drape the patient for examination of the back and certain surgical procedures.

Equipment and Supplies
- Patient's record
- Examination table
- Patient gown
- Table paper
- Drape
- Disinfectant wipes
- Gloves

Procedural Steps
1. Wash hands or use hand sanitizer.
   Purpose: Hand sanitization is an important step for infection control.
2. Greet the patient. Identify yourself. Verify the patient's identity with full name and date of birth. Explain the procedure to be performed in a manner that the patient understands. Answer any questions the patient may have about the procedure.
   Purpose: To promote the patient's understanding and cooperation during the examination.
3. Give the patient a gown, and explain what clothing must be removed for the examination being done. Tell the patient that the gown should open in the back. Provide assistance as needed. Give the patient privacy while changing. Knock on the examination room door before reentering to make sure the patient has completed undressing and gowning.
4. Do not place the patient in the prone position until the provider is ready for that part of the examination.
   Purpose: To promote the patient's privacy, comfort, and safety.
5. Pull out the table extension, and help the patient lie down on his or her stomach (Fig. 1).

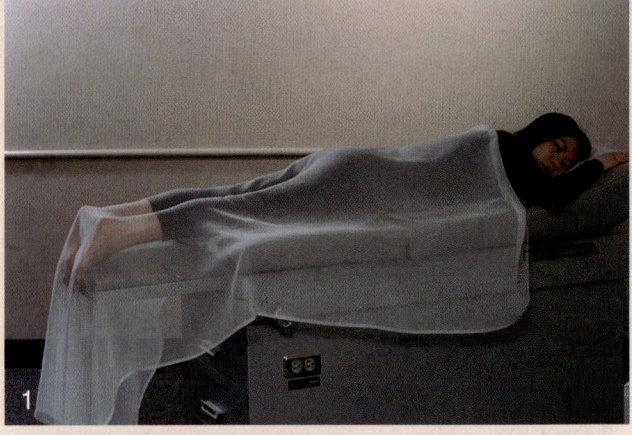

6. Drape the patient over any exposed area that is not included in the examination. For female patients, the drape should be large enough to cover from the breasts to the feet so that the patient is not exposed accidentally if she is asked to roll over.
   Purpose: Draping the patient provides warmth and privacy while giving the provider access to the examination site.
7. After the examination has been completed, assist the patient as needed to get off the table and get dressed.
8. Put on gloves, and use disinfectant wipes to clean the exam table and all potentially contaminated surfaces. Dispose of used gloves and examination table paper according to facility policies. Pull clean paper over the table.
   Purpose: To ensure infection control and to prevent the transmission of pathogens from one patient to another.
9. Wash hands or use hand sanitizer.
10. Follow up with the provider's orders regarding scheduling of diagnostic studies, collection of specimens, or scheduling of future appointments.

- Mensuration (men shuh REY shuh n)
- Manipulation (muh nip yuh LEY shuh n)

All six are part of a complete physical examination.

Inspection. During the inspection, the examiner uses observation to detect significant physical features or objective data. This method of examination ranges from focusing on the patient's general appearance (general state of health, including posture, mannerisms, and grooming) to more detailed observations, including body contour, **gait**, symmetry, visible injuries and deformities, tremors, rashes, and color changes. Inspection will be done before palpation or percussion so that there will be no changes made to the appearance of the skin.

> **VOCABULARY**
> **gait:** The manner or style of walking.

Palpation. In **palpation**, the examiner uses the sense of touch (Fig. 30.17A). A part of the body is felt with the hand to determine its condition or the condition of an underlying organ. Palpation may involve touching the skin or performing a firmer exploration of the abdomen for underlying masses. With this technique, the provider is assessing the following:
- Temperature
- Vibration
- Consistency
- Form
- Size
- Rigidity
- Elasticity
- Moisture
- Texture
- Position
- Contour

Palpation is performed with one hand, both hands (bimanual), one finger (digital), the fingertips, or the palmar aspect of the hand. A pelvic examination is done bimanually, whereas an anal examination is performed digitally. Do not confuse palpation with *palpitation*, which is a throbbing pulsation felt in the chest.

> **VOCABULARY**
> **palpation:** The use of touch during the physical examination to assess the size, consistency, and location of certain body parts.

Percussion. *Percussion* (per KUHsh uh n) involves tapping or striking the body, usually with the fingers or a small hammer. This will cause sounds, vibratory sensations, or involuntary reactions. Percussion can help to determine the position, size, and density of an underlying organ or cavity. The examiner both hears and feels the effect of percussion. It is helpful in determining the amount of air or solid matter in an underlying organ or cavity. The two basic methods of percussion are

PROCEDURE 30.9 Knee-Chest Position

Task
Position and drape the patient for examinations of the back and rectum and for certain surgical procedures.

Equipment and Supplies
- Examination table
- Table paper
- Patient gown
- Drape
- Disinfectant wipes
- Gloves

Procedural Steps
1. Wash hands or use hand sanitizer.
   Purpose: Hand sanitization is an important step for infection control.
2. Greet the patient. Identify yourself. Verify the patient's identity with full name and date of birth. Explain the procedure to be performed in a manner that the patient understands. Answer any questions the patient may have about the procedure.
   Purpose: To promote the patient's understanding and cooperation during the examination.
3. Give the patient a gown, and explain what clothing must be removed for the examination being done. Tell the patient that the gown should open in the back. Provide assistance as needed. Give the patient privacy while changing. Knock on the examination room door before reentering to make sure the patient has completed undressing and gowning.
4. Do not place the patient in the knee-chest position until the provider is ready for that part of the examination.
   Purpose: To promote the patient's privacy, comfort, and safety.
5. Pull out the table extension if necessary. Help the patient lie down on his or her back and then turn over into the prone position. Ask the patient to move up onto the knees, spread the knees apart, and lean forward onto the head so that the buttocks are raised. Tell the patient to keep the back straight and turn the face to either side. The patient should rest his or her weight on the chest and shoulders (Fig. 1).

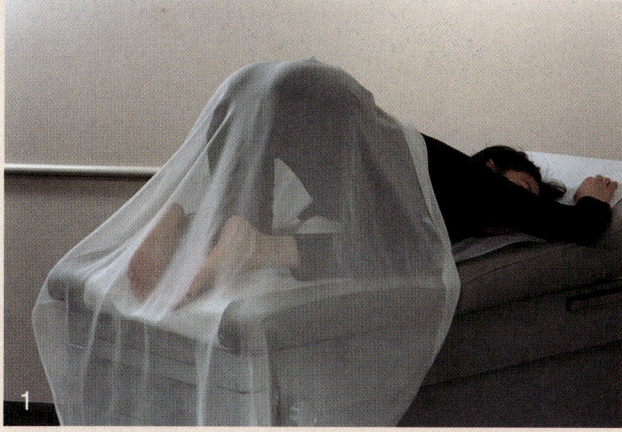

6. If the patient has difficulty maintaining this position, an alternative is to place weight on bent elbows with the head off the table.
7. Drape the patient diagonally so that the point of the drape is on the table between the legs.
   Purpose: Draping the patient provides warmth and privacy while giving the provider access to the examination site.
8. After the examination has been completed, assist the patient as needed to get off the table and get dressed.
9. Put on gloves, and use disinfectant wipes to clean the exam table and all potentially contaminated surfaces. Dispose of used gloves and examination table paper according to facility policies. Pull clean paper over the table.
   Purpose: To ensure infection control and to prevent the transmission of pathogens from one patient to another.
10. Wash hands or use hand sanitizer.
11. Follow up with the provider's orders regarding scheduling of diagnostic studies, collection of specimens, or scheduling of future appointments.

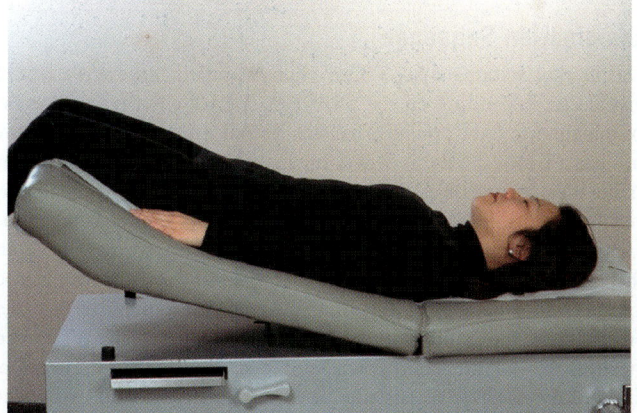

FIG. 30.16 Trendelenburg position. (From Proctor D, et al: *Kinn's The Medical Assistant*, ed 13, St. Louis, 2017, Elsevier.)

direct percussion and indirect percussion. Direct percussion is performed by striking the body with a finger or a reflex hammer. With indirect percussion, which is used more frequently, the provider places his or her hand on the area and then strikes the placed hand with a finger of the other hand (see Fig. 30.17B). Both a sound and a sense of vibration are evident. The examiner assesses the sound in terms of pitch, quality, duration, and resonance.

Auscultation. For *auscultation* (aw skuh l TEY shuh n), the provider uses a stethoscope to listen to sounds from the body. Auscultation is a complex method of examination because the provider must distinguish between a normal sound and an abnormal sound (see Fig. 30.17C). It is particularly useful for evaluating sounds originating in the lungs, heart, and abdomen, such as a **murmur**, a **bruit** (broot), and bowel sounds.

> ### VOCABULARY
> **bruit:** An abnormal sound or murmur heard on auscultation of an organ, vessel (e.g., carotid artery), or gland.
> **murmur:** An abnormal sound heard during auscultation of the heart that may or may not have a pathologic origin; it is associated with valve disease or a congenital heart defect.

Mensuration. Mensuration is the process of measuring. Measurements that are recorded include the following:
- Height and weight
- Size and depth of a wound

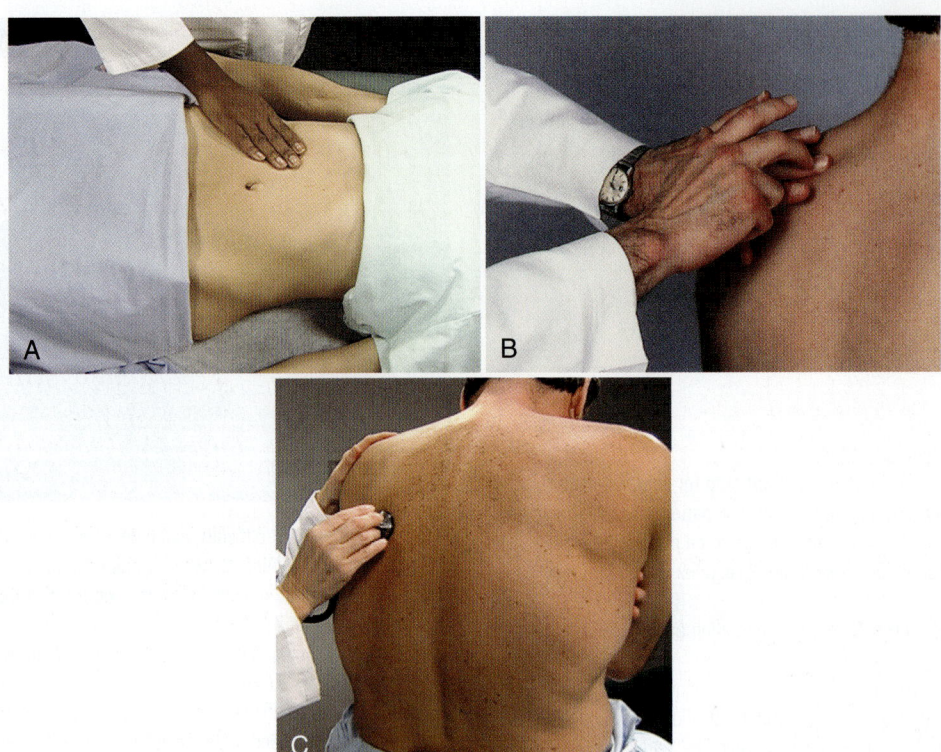

FIG. 30.17 (A) Demonstration of palpation. (B) Demonstration of percussion. (C) Demonstration of auscultation. (From Ball JW, et al: *Seidel's Guide to Physical Examination,* ed 8, St. Louis, 2015, Mosby.)

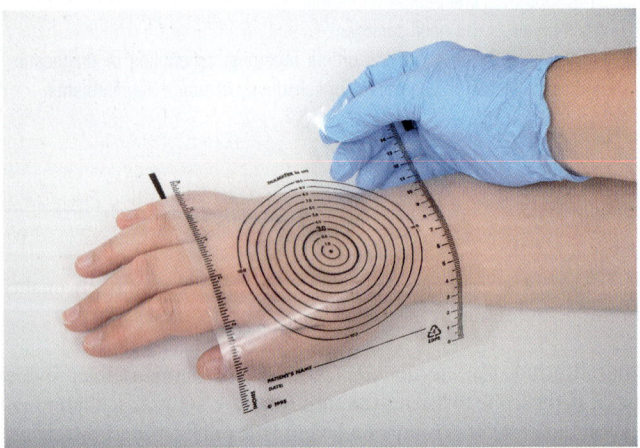

FIG. 30.18 Circular wound measurement device.

- Size of the uterus during pregnancy
- Pressure of a grip
- Length and diameter of an extremity

Measurements are taken with a flexible tape measure, a circular wound measurement device (Fig. 30.18), or a specialized piece of equipment (e.g., a goniometer, which is used to measure joint angles) and usually are recorded in centimeters.

Manipulation. Manipulation is the passive movement of a joint to determine the range of extension or flexion of a part of the body. Insurance and industrial reports often request this information in detail. For example, a patient involved in a work-related accident that caused joint damage may have to perform assisted range-of-motion (ROM) exercises to the joint, with subsequent measurements of joint flexion and extension to demonstrate improvement or lack thereof.

> **VOCABULARY**
> **extension:** The process of stretching out; increasing the angle of a joint.
> **flexion:** The process of decreasing the angle of a joint.
> **manipulation:** Movement or exercise of a body part by means of an externally applied force.

Examination Sequence

The physical examination sequence is fairly standard; however, variations may occur, depending on the provider's specialty, the reason for the examination, and the provider's preference. Patients are more cooperative and less anxious if they understand what is expected of them. Start by giving the patient a brief explanation of the examination process. Many healthcare facilities provide the option for patients to have a chaperone present during physical examinations. For more information about chaperones, see Box 30.10. Assemble all supplies and instruments needed for the examination before the provider enters the room. As the provider proceeds with the examination, make sure the patient remains unexposed by adjusting the drape and gown as needed. During the examination, the medical assistant assists the provider by handing him or her the correct instruments and needed supplies. When the provider begins the examination, the medical assistant should keep conversation to a minimum and remain inconspicuous (in kuh n SPIK yoo uh s). The examination usually starts with the patient seated at the end of the exam table, or in the Fowler position, if the patient needs support. If the provider uses reflected light, the light source should be behind the patient's right shoulder. If illuminated instruments are used, standard overhead lights are sufficient. Take care not to shine a light directly into the patient's eyes; this can be done by turning on lights while they are

> **BOX 30.10 Chaperones During Physical Examinations**
>
> It is becoming common for chaperones to be present during physical examinations. Having a third person in the exam room provides protection for both the patient and the provider. A medical assistant may be asked to be a chaperone.
>
> A chaperone can reassure the patient about the professional character of the healthcare facility. The patient has the right to refuse having a chaperone present in the room, but most are accepting. When the chaperone is another health professional, such as a medical assistant, she or he can serve two purposes: as a chaperone and as an assistant to the provider.
>
> If a healthcare facility is going to have chaperones present, there should be a written policy that describes the role of the chaperone. This policy should allow for a private conversation between the patient and the provider.

directed away from the patient and carefully moving the light toward the area.

General Appearance. The provider starts the physical examination by observing the patient's appearance, using an inspection technique. The general appearance explains whether the patient appears well and in good health (e.g., note whether the patient appears disoriented or in distress, well nourished or undernourished, and answers questions with ease or confusion).

The patient's gait often provides important information. The patient may limp, walk with the feet wide apart, have a shuffle step, or have difficulty maintaining his or her balance. Posture also is checked for indications of pain, stiffness, or difficulty with limb movement. The provider notes body build and proportions. Any *gross* (immediately obvious) deformities are recorded. Sometimes abnormalities in height or body proportion may be caused by hormonal imbalances. If the medical assistant notices any of these or the patient reports any complaints, these should be documented in the patient's health record, along with the vital signs, before the provider begins the examination.

Speech. Speech may reveal a pathologic condition. Some basic speech defects include *aphonia* (ey FOH nee uh), the inability to speak because of loss of the voice, which is commonly seen with severe *laryngitis* (lar uh n JAHY tis) or overuse of the voice; *aphasia* (uh FEY zhuh), the loss of expression by speech or writing because of an injury or disease of the brain; and *dysphasia* (dis FEY zhuh), lack of coordination and failure to arrange words in proper order, usually caused by a brain lesion. With *motor aphasia,* the patient knows what he or she wants to say but cannot use muscles properly to speak; for example, this may be noted as slurred or incoherent speech that might occur after a cerebrovascular accident (CVA). In *sensory aphasia,* the patient pronounces words easily but uses them inaccurately, as in jumbled speech. Speech is also assessed in well-child checkups. A delay in speech development can indicate an issue (e.g., a neurologic deficit or possible autism spectrum disorder) and the need for a referral.

Skin. The condition of the skin can be a reflection of the patient's nutritional status and hydration level. If dehydration is suspected, skin turgor (TUR ger) is checked by pinching the skin on the posterior surface of the hands. The tissue is observed to see how quickly it returns to the normal location. A delay indicates a decrease in tissue fluid, confirming the diagnosis of dehydration. Extreme dryness, scaling, extended time for wound healing, or frequent breaks in the skin may indicate systemic disease.

Fingernails and toenails often give some indication of a person's health. Brittle, grooved, or lined nails may indicate local infection or systemic disease. Clubbing of the fingertips is associated with some congenital heart or lung diseases. Spooning of the nail is seen in some patients with severe iron-deficiency anemia. *Beau lines,* deep grooved horizontal lines, appear after an acute illness but grow out and disappear. The provider may refer a patient with skin disorders to a dermatologist for diagnosis and treatment.

Head. Once the provider makes the overall observations of the patient's general condition, the physical examination typically begins with the head and face and moves downward to the feet. The face reflects the patient's state and tells the provider a great deal about how the patient handles stress and illness. The skull, scalp, and face are palpated for size, shape, and symmetry. The distribution or lack of hair and hair texture may indicate hormonal changes. Excessive hair, especially facial hair in females, indicates a hormonal imbalance. As the head is palpated, the provider assesses possible nodules, masses, or signs of trauma.

Eyes. The pupils are checked for reaction by shining a light into one eye at a time. If the pupils constrict equally and smoothly to a light stimulus, the provider documents "PERRLA" (which means the pupils are equal, round, react to light, and accommodation). The sclera (SKLEER uh) is checked for color, which ranges from white to pale yellow. If the eye is inflamed, it will be evident in the sclera. A sclera with a yellow tone indicates liver disease. Movements of the eyes are tested by having the patient follow the provider's finger. If eye movement is within average range, "extraocular movement (EOM) intact" is documented. The *ophthalmoscope* (op THAL muh skohp) is used to examine the interior of the eye, including the retina and intraocular vessels. Some diseases, such as diabetes mellitus or hypertension, damage the blood vessels of the retina.

Ears. The ears are examined with an otoscope covered with a disposable speculum. The external ear is checked first for inflammation of the external auditory canal or for earwax (cerumen). The tympanic membrane (eardrum) is examined and should appear pearly gray. Scars on the eardrum are frequently the result of earlier, chronic ear infections

> **MEDICAL TERMINOLOGY**
>
> **a-:** without
> **dys-:** bad, difficult, painful, abnormal
> **-ia:** condition, state of
> **-itis:** inflammation
> **laryng/o:** larynx (voice box), throat
> **phas/o:** speech
> **phon/o:** sound, voice

> **VOCABULARY**
>
> **clubbing:** Abnormal enlargement of the distal phalanges (fingers and toes) associated with cyanotic heart disease or advanced chronic pulmonary disease.
> **inconspicuous:** Not noticeable or prominent.
> **nodules:** Small lumps, lesions, or swellings that are felt when the skin is palpated.
> **turgor:** Referring to normal skin tension; the resistance of the skin to being grasped between the fingers and released. Turgor decreases with dehydration and increases with edema.
> **sclera:** The white part of the eye that forms the orbit.

or perforations. The color of the eardrum is important to the diagnosis because it may indicate fluids such as blood or pus behind the eardrum in the middle ear. The patient may be asked to swallow several times to allow observation of movement of the tympanic membrane, which occurs because of pressure changes in the eustachian (yoo STA shun) tube. The eustachian tube equalizes air pressure between the middle ear and the throat. The ability of the tympanic membrane to move is crucial to the hearing process.

Nose and Sinuses. The mucosa of the nasal cavity is examined for color and texture. The sinuses cannot be seen, but the frontal and maxillary (MAK suh ler ee) sinuses may be examined by firm palpation over the area and by transillumination (trans i LOO muh ney shun). When disorders of the eyes, ears, nose, and throat are observed and the provider believes that the condition warrants the attention of a specialist, the patient is referred to an *ophthalmologist* (op thuh l MOL uh jist) or an *otorhinolaryngologist* (oh toh rahy noh lar ing GOL uh jist) (ear, nose, and throat specialist).

Mouth and Throat. The mouth, or oral cavity, is usually thought of in terms of oral hygiene and dental care. Dental hygiene includes the condition of the teeth, how the patient cares for the teeth and gums, and whether the teeth of the upper and lower jaws meet properly (occlude) for chewing. Healthy gums are pale pink, glossy, and smooth and do not bleed when pressure from a tongue depressor is applied. The palatine tonsils are usually visible. The provider may use a tongue depressor and a piece of gauze to grasp the tongue to examine it carefully. The floor of the mouth is examined by both inspection and palpation for enlarged lymph nodes, salivary gland function, and ulcerations. The insides of the cheeks and the gum line are also examined for any abnormal marks or color. The provider may use the otoscope light to help with the examination.

Neck. The neck is examined for ROM by having the patient move the head in various directions. The thyroid gland is given special attention for symmetry, size, and texture. The provider manually palpates the thyroid area while the patient swallows several times because this action elevates the thyroid lobes. The carotid artery is palpated and auscultated for possible bruits. The lymph nodes are palpated. *Lymphadenopathy* (lim fad uh NOP puh thee) (enlargement of the lymph nodes) can occur if the patient has an infection of the face, head, or neck.

Chest. While the patient is still in the sitting position, the chest, heart, and lungs are examined. The chest is examined for symmetric expansion. A tape measure may be used, especially if variation exists between the upper and lower chest expansion. A patient with a history of emphysema (em fuh ZEE muh) may have a barrel-shaped chest. The provider may use percussion to determine the density of lung tissues.

Placing a stethoscope on the patient's back, the examiner auscultates lung sounds. The patient is asked to take deep, regular breaths. This may produce slight dizziness, but the patient should be assured that it is only the result of the deep respirations and will rapidly pass. The provider notes the types of respirations and the presence of lung sounds in all lobes.

Because considerable concentration is required to interpret heart sounds, the provider must have complete silence when listening to the patient's heart. In patients with heart disease, the provider may spend an extended time listening to heart sounds. If lung or heart abnormalities are found, the provider typically orders further diagnostic tests, including blood analysis, x-ray evaluation, and an ECG. Once the results of these studies have been analyzed, the provider may refer the patient to a *cardiologist* (kahr dee OL uh jist) for treatment of a heart condition, or a *pulmonologist* (PUHL muh nal uh jist) or a respiratory care specialist for treatment of a breathing disorder.

Abdomen. For the abdominal part of the examination, the patient is lowered to the dorsal recumbent or supine position, and the drape is lowered to the pubic hairline. The gown is raised to just under the breasts. The patient's arms may be placed at the side, or the hands may be crossed over the chest or under the head. Relaxation of the abdominal muscles is needed for the abdominal examination. To assist in this goal and to promote patient comfort, a small pillow can be placed under the head and knees. The provider auscultates the abdomen in all quadrants to confirm the presence of complete bowel sounds and palpates the abdomen for any abnormalities. The provider also may use percussion to determine the density, position, and size of underlying abdominal organs.

Reflexes. The patient's reflexes are checked with the patient sitting, in the Fowler position, or supine. While the patient is sitting, the biceps are checked with the patient's arm flexed and supported by the examiner. The knee jerk (patellar reflex) and the ankle jerk (Achilles reflex) are checked using *tapotement* (tuh POHT ment) (a tapping or percussing movement) with either the fingers or the reflex hammer. The plantar reflexes (Babinski reflex and Chaddock reflex) are tested with the patient in an upright or a supine position.

Breast and Testicles. Careful breast examination is part of the physical examination for every female, even if she is asymptomatic. The breasts are examined both by inspection and by palpation with the patient in the supine position. The arm on the side that is being examined is bent and tucked under the head. Breast cancer is the most common malignancy in women, and early detection is the key to successful treatment. This is a good opportunity to discuss and reinforce the consistent use of

---

VOCABULARY

emphysema: Thinning and eventual destruction of the alveoli; usually accompanies chronic bronchitis.
symmetry: Similarity in size, form, and arrangement of parts on opposite sides of the body.
transillumination: Inspection of a cavity or organ by passing light through its walls.

MEDICAL TERMINOLOGY

cardi/o: heart
-logist: one who specializes in the study of
lymphaden/o: lymph gland (lymph node)
ophthalm/o: eye
ot/o: ear
-pathy: disease process
pulmon/o: lung
rhin/o: nose

monthly breast self-examination (BSE). For male patients who have reached puberty or are 14 years of age or older, the provider performs a testicular examination. The testicular self-examination (TSE) is an important self-examination for all males to perform each month because testicular carcinoma is a major health risk that has a high cure rate if discovered early.

> **CRITICAL THINKING 30.5**
>
> Alice Greenbaum, a 68-year-old patient of Dr. Walden, is scheduled for an annual physical examination, including a breast check and Pap test. Mrs. Greenbaum appears anxious and asks Chris whether the gynecologic examination is necessary. How should Chris answer this patient? What might help to ease the patient's fears and prepare her for the examination?

Rectum. The rectal examination usually follows the abdominal examination or may be part of the examination of the genitalia. Preserving the patient's comfort and dignity is vital. For this part of the examination, the provider needs gloves and water-soluble lubricating jelly (e.g., K-Y Jelly). The examination light should be directed at the perineal area during the examination.

Fecal occult blood test specimens are often collected at the time of the digital rectal examination. If this is a procedure the provider performs, be sure to include the necessary collection folder with the examination equipment. Patients diagnosed with gastrointestinal (GI) disorders may be referred to a *gastroenterologist* (gas troh en tuh ROL uh jist). Procedure 30.10 presents the steps for assisting with the physical examination.

VISION AND HEARING SCREENINGS

There are basic screening procedures that medical assistants perform during a physical examination. Eye procedures would include distance visual **acuity** (ah KYOO ih tee), near visual acuity, and color vision screening. Ear procedures would include hearing screening using tuning forks or audiometers. Before we discuss those procedures, you should have some understanding of the disorders that are being screened for.

Disorders of the Eye

Vision requires light and depends on the proper functioning of all parts of the eye (Chapter 13). A visual impulse begins with the passage of light through the cornea, where the light is **refracted**; it then passes through the aqueous humor and the pupil into the lens. The ciliary muscle adjusts the curvature of the lens to again refract the light rays so that they pass into the retina, triggering the photoreceptor cells of the rods and cones. At this point, the light energy is converted into an electrical impulse, which is sent through the optic nerve to the visual cortex of the *occipital* (ok SIP i tl) lobe of the brain; there, the light impulse is interpreted and a picture is created. There can be issues with vision when the light is not correctly refracted. There can be other issues with the shape of the eyeball and the muscles that control the eyeball. These issues are discussed in the following section.

Refractive Errors. Four major types of refractive errors result when the eye is unable to focus light effectively on the retina. Refraction is the ability of the lens of the eye to bend parallel light rays coming into the eye so that the rays are focused simultaneously on the retina. An *error of refraction* means that the light rays are not refracted or bent properly and consequently do not focus correctly on the retina. Defects in the shape of the eyeball can cause a refractive error. Most refractive errors can be corrected with corrective lenses, contacts, or surgery (Fig. 30.19). Signs and symptoms of refractive errors are described in Box 30.11.

Hyperopia (farsightedness). When light enters the eye and focuses behind the retina, a person has *hyperopia* (hahy per OH pee uh) (Fig. 30.19B). This disorder occurs when the eyeball is too short from the anterior to the posterior wall. An individual with hyperopia has difficulty seeing objects that are close, at reading or working level. A convex corrective lens helps the eye's internal lens place objects directly on the retina and creates a sharp, detailed image. Refractive surgery may also be done to correct the shape of the lens.

Myopia (nearsightedness). Myopia (mahy OH pee uh) occurs when light rays entering the eye focus in front of the retina (Fig. 30.19A). This causes objects at a distance to appear blurry and dull. Objects viewed at reading or working level are seen clearly. In this disorder, the eyeball is elongated from the anterior to the posterior wall. The internal lens of the eye cannot sharpen the image. A concave corrective lens is used to focus the light rays on the retina. Surgery can also be done to change the shape of the cornea. However, the surgery is performed only on adults who have had a stable eye prescription for at least 1 year.

Presbyopia. As people age, the lens of the eye becomes less flexible, and the ciliary muscles weaken. This means changing the point of focus from distance to near becomes difficult. This is called *presbyopia* (prez bee OH pee uh). The condition results in difficulty seeing at reading level. A combination corrective lens, known as a *bifocal lens* or a *progressive lens correction,* is used to focus both near and far objects directly on the retina. Presbyopia actually starts at approximately age 10, but most people do not report a change in vision until their early 40s. Corrective lens such as bifocals, trifocals, or progressive can correct presbyopia. Conductive *keratoplasty* (KAIR uh toh plas tee) is a laser surgical procedure used to treat presbyopia.

Astigmatism. Astigmatism (uh STIG muh tiz uh m) occurs when light rays entering the eye are focused irregularly. This usually occurs because the cornea or the lens is not a smooth sphere but rather has an irregular shape. Ophthalmologists describe the lens as being shaped like a football rather than a sphere, such as a basketball. This causes light rays to be unevenly or diffusely focused on the retina, resulting

> **VOCABULARY**
> **acuity:** Test of the clearness or sharpness of vision.
> **refracted:** The bending of light rays.

> **MEDICAL TERMINOLOGY**
> **enter/o:** small intestine
> **gastr/o:** stomach
> **hyper-:** excessive
> **kerat/o:** cornea
> **-opia:** vision condition
> **-plasty:** surgical repair
> **presby-:** old age

PROCEDURE 30.10 Assist Provider With a Patient Exam

Task
Aid the provider in the examination of a patient by preparing the patient and the necessary equipment and ensuring the patient's safety and comfort during the examination.

Equipment and Supplies
- Patient's record
- Stethoscope
- Gauze
- Ophthalmoscope
- Pen light
- Scale with height measurement bar
- Tuning fork
- Tongue depressor
- Biohazard waste container
- Cotton balls
- Examination light
- Laboratory request forms
- Percussion hammer
- Specimen bottles and laboratory requisitions
- Lubricating gel
- Gloves
- Patient gown
- Sphygmomanometer
- Drapes
- Otoscope with disposable speculum
- Thermometer
- Cotton-tipped applicators
- Tape measure
- Fecal occult blood test supplies
- Disinfectant wipes
- Table paper

Procedural Steps

1. Check the examination room at the beginning of each day and between patients to make sure it is completely stocked with equipment and supplies and that the equipment functions properly.
   Purpose: The room must be ready for patient services.
2. Check expiration dates on all packages and supplies regularly, and discard expired materials.
   Purpose: To ensure the patient's safety.
3. Prepare the examination room before and between patients according to acceptable medical rules of asepsis.
   Purpose: The room must be aseptically clean to prevent the spread of infection.
4. Wash hands or use hand sanitizer.
   Purpose: Hand sanitization is an important step for infection control.
5. Locate the instruments for the procedure. Set them out in order of use within reach of the provider, and cover them until the provider enters the examination room.
   Purpose: To promote time management and ensure that all needed equipment and supplies are ready.
6. Greet and identify the patient, introduce yourself, and determine whether the patient understands the procedure. If the patient does not, explain what to expect. Refer any unanswered questions to the provider.
   Purpose: To promote the patient's understanding and cooperation during the examination.
7. Review the medical history with the patient, and investigate the purpose of the visit. Review current medications, and document any changes or prescription refills needed. Document the interview results.
   Purpose: To verify that all information is current and complete.
8. Measure and record the patient's vital signs, height, weight, and body mass index (BMI). Instruct the patient on how to collect a urine specimen, if ordered, and hand the patient a properly labeled specimen container. Obtain blood samples for any tests ordered.
   Purpose: To gather data needed before the examination begins.
9. Hand the patient a gown and drape. Explain what clothes should be removed for the examination and whether the gown should open in the front or the back. Help the patient with undressing as needed (most patients prefer to undress in privacy). Knock on the door before reentering the room to protect the patient's privacy.
   Purpose: To assist the patient in preparing for the examination and to safeguard the patient's privacy, comfort, and safety.
10. Assist the patient as needed in sitting at the foot of the examination table; place the drape over the patient's lap and legs. If the patient is an older adult, confused, or feeling faint or dizzy, do not leave him or her alone.
    Purpose: To provide for the patient's warmth and privacy and to prevent a fall or injury.
11. Place the patient's paper health record in the designated area, or make sure the computer is ready for the provider to log in and access the patient's electronic health record (EHR). Be careful to safeguard patient confidentiality during this step of the procedure.
12. Assist during the examination by handing the provider instruments as needed and by positioning and draping the patient.
13. When the provider has completed the examination, allow the patient to rest for a moment, then help the patient from the table. Assist with dressing, if necessary. Use proper body mechanics if assistance in transfer is needed.
    Purpose: To ensure the patient's stability and safety and to protect yourself from injury.
14. Return to the patient, and ask whether he or she has any questions. Give the patient any final instructions, and schedule tests as ordered by the provider or the next appointment.
    Purpose: To clarify instructions, eliminate any misunderstandings, and allow the patient to discuss any concerns. If the patient's misunderstandings or concerns are beyond your scope of experience or skill, arrange for the provider to speak with the patient again.
15. Put on gloves, and dispose of used supplies and linens in designated biohazard waste containers. Dispose of exam table paper. Use disinfectant wipes to clean the examination table and any other potentially contaminated surface. Disinfect all equipment.
    Purpose: To prevent cross-contamination with any potential infectious materials.
16. Remove the gloves, discard them in the biohazard waste container, and wash hands or use hand sanitizer.
    Purpose: To ensure infection control.
17. Cover the exam table with fresh paper, replace used supplies, and prepare the room for the next patient.

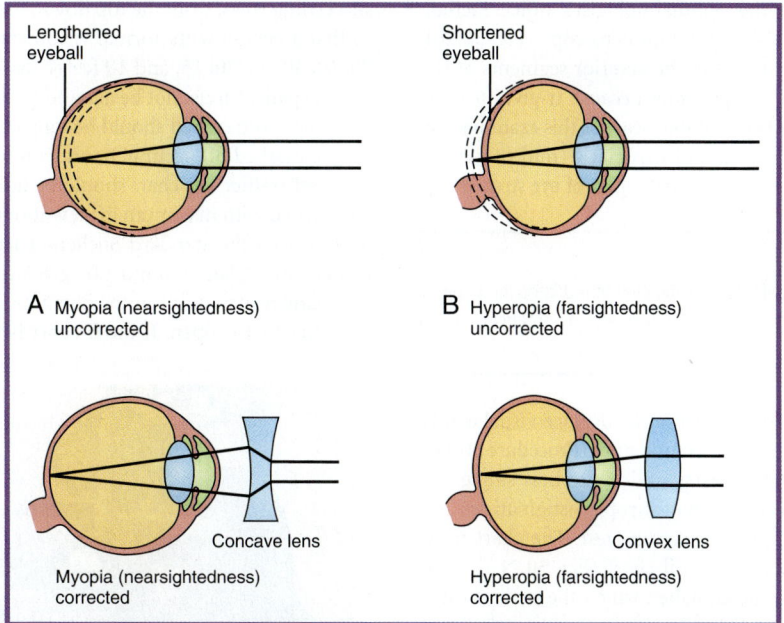

FIG. 30.19 Errors of refraction. (A) Myopia. (B) Hyperopia. (From Proctor D, et al: *Kinn's The Medical Assistant*, ed 13, St. Louis, 2017, Elsevier.)

BOX 30.11 Signs and Symptoms of Refractive Errors
Refractive errors in vision can lead to squinting, frequent rubbing of the eyes, and headaches. The individual notices blurred vision, fading of words at reading level, or both. Some refractive errors are familial in nature.

BOX 30.12 PERRLA
P Pupils
E Equal
R Round
R Reactive to
L Light [and]
A Accommodation

in blurred vision. It is like attempting to focus on objects seen through a wavy piece of window glass. Astigmatism can be corrected with glasses, contacts, or surgery. Surgical correction attempts to reshape the cornea into a more spherical or uniformly curved surface.

Treatment of Refractive Errors. Eyeglasses and contact lenses are the traditional treatments for visual acuity problems caused by refractive errors. However, problems with the shape of the lens can be surgically corrected. Surgery is performed on an outpatient basis and requires only a short stay in the facility. Medical assistants employed in an outpatient eye surgery facility must be trained to fulfill this specialized role.

CRITICAL THINKING 30.6
Chris is performing visual acuity examinations. Dr. Martin asks him whether he understands the causes of refractive errors. Chris has difficulty explaining why refractive errors occur, so he tells Dr. Martin he will research the topic and get back to him. What have you learned about the different refractive disorders and why they occur?

Diagnostic Procedures

A complete examination of the eye is technical and requires expensive equipment and the expertise of an ophthalmologist or optometrist. However, a primary care provider performs some basic examinations and treatments of the eye. The ophthalmoscope is used to examine the interior of the eye. It projects a bright, narrow beam of light through the lens and illuminates the interior parts of the eye and retina. It is helpful for detecting disorders of the eyes and certain systemic disorders, such as capillary changes that occur with diabetes mellitus.

The eyelids are examined for edema, which may be the result of nephrosis, heart failure, allergy, or thyroid deficiency. *Blepharoptosis* (bleff ah rop TOH sis), also called *ptosis*, is drooping of the upper eyelid that can be caused by a disorder of the third cranial nerve, muscular weakness as seen in muscular dystrophy, or *myasthenia gravis* (my as THEE nee ah GRAV is).

MEDICAL TERMINOLOGY
blephar/o: eyelid
-ptosis: drooping

The pupils of the eyes are normally round and equal. Normal pupils constrict rapidly in response to light. This is demonstrated by shining a bright, pinpoint light into one eye from the side of the patient's head. The pupil of an illuminated eye constricts, and the pupil of the other eye constricts equally. This test is called *light and accommodation* (L&A). An older patient's eyes do not accommodate as well as those of a younger person. Each eye is checked this way. The patient then is asked to look at the provider's finger as it is moved directly toward the patient's nose to check for eye coordination. If the pupils are equal and round, respond normally to light, and adjust and focus on objects at different distances in a reasonable length of time, the provider charts the acronym PERRLA (Box 30.12).

Special techniques used in the ophthalmologist's office include examinations performed with a slit lamp biomicroscope (Fig. 30.20). This device is used to view fine details in the anterior segments of the eye. It may be used to view a foreign body because it gives a well-illuminated and highly magnified view of the area. For this examination, the provider first orders administration of **mydriatic** (mid ree AT ik) eyedrops to dilate the pupil and enhance visualization of eye structures.

> **VOCABULARY**
>
> **mydriatic:** Describes a topical ophthalmic medication that dilates the pupil; it is used in diagnostic procedures of the eye and as treatment for glaucoma.

Distance Visual Acuity (DVA). Determining distance visual acuity frequently is part of a complete physical examination (Procedure 30.11). It is widely used in schools and industry and is the best single test available for vision screening. Many cases of myopia, astigmatism, and hyperopia have been detected with this routine test. The chart most commonly used is the Snellen alphabetical chart (Fig. 30.21A). This chart displays various letters of the alphabet, which the patient must identify in ever smaller font sizes. Patients with limited knowledge of the English alphabet can be tested with the E chart (Fig. 30.21B). In addition, a chart that uses pictures as symbols is available. This chart is used for young children or individuals who do not know the alphabet (Fig. 30.21C). To avoid patient confusion over the E chart or the symbol chart, the medical assistant should review the charts with patients first to make sure they know how to demonstrate the E visualized or the meaning of each picture or symbol. People with normal vision can read the symbol on the top line of the chart at 200 feet. In each of the succeeding rows, from the top down, the size of the symbols is reduced so that a person with normal vision can see them at distances of 100, 70, 50, 40, 30, 20, 15, and 10 feet, consecutively.

The patient must not be allowed to study the chart before taking the test. The room or hall should be long enough that the 20-foot distance can be marked off accurately, and without interruptions from patient and staff traffic. The chart should be hung at the patient's eye level and illuminated with maximum light, without glare on the chart. Most adults do not need the standard Snellen chart explained, but if the E chart is used, an explanation must be given as to how the E's are to be read. The patient may point up or down or right or left toward the part of the letter that is open. If the E chart is to be used for a child, practice

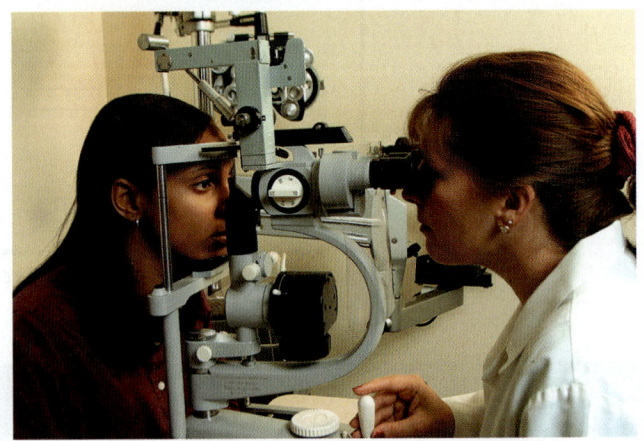

FIG. 30.20 Slit lamp. (From Proctor D, et al: *Kinn's The Medical Assistant*, ed 13, St. Louis, 2017, Elsevier.)

PROCEDURE 30.11 Measuring Distance Visual Acuity

Task
Determine the patient's degree of visual clarity at a measured distance of 20 feet using the Snellen chart and established protocols.

Equipment and Supplies
- Patient's health record
- Provider's order
- Snellen eye chart
- Disposable eye occluder or an alcohol wipe to clean the occluder before use
- Pen or pencil and paper

Procedural Steps
1. Wash hands or use hand sanitizer.
   Purpose: Hand sanitization is an important step for infection control.
2. Prepare the area. Make sure the room is well lit and that a distance marker is 20 feet from the chart.
3. Greet the patient. Identify yourself. Verify the patient's identity with full name and date of birth. Explain the procedure to be performed in a manner that the patient understands. Answer any questions the patient may have about the procedure. Instruct the patient not to squint during the test because squinting temporarily improves vision. The patient should not have an opportunity to study the chart before the test is given. If the patient wears corrective lenses, they should be worn during the test.
   Purpose: Explanations help gain the patient's cooperation and alleviate apprehension.
4. Position the patient in a standing or sitting position at the 20-foot marker.
   Purpose: Twenty feet is the standard testing distance.
5. Check that the Snellen chart is positioned at the patient's eye level.
6. If the occluder is not disposable, disinfect it before the procedure starts. Then, instruct the patient to cover the left eye with the occluder and to keep both eyes open throughout the test to prevent squinting (Fig. 1).
   Purpose: Traditionally, the right eye is tested first.

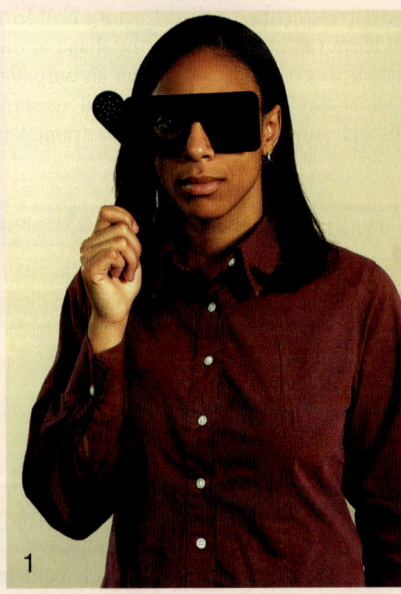

PROCEDURE 30.11 Measuring Distance Visual Acuity—cont'd

7. Stand beside the chart, and point to each row as the patient reads it aloud, starting with the 20/70 row (Fig. 2).
   Purpose: Starting with larger letters gives the patient confidence and allows for accommodation of vision.

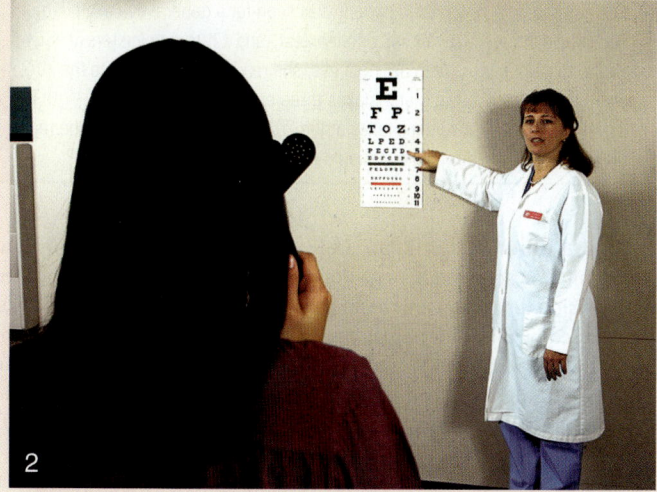

8. Proceed down the rows of the chart until the smallest row the patient can read with a maximum of two errors is reached. If one or two letters are missed, the outcome is recorded with a minus sign and the number of errors (e.g., 20/40–2). If more than two errors are made, the previous line should be documented.

9. Record any of the patient's reactions while reading the chart.
   Purpose: Reactions such as squinting, leaning, tearing, or blinking may indicate that the patient is having difficulty with the test.

10. Repeat the procedure with the left eye, covering the right eye.
11. Repeat the procedure with both eyes uncovered.
12. Disinfect the occluder, if it is not disposable, and wash hands or use hand sanitizer.
    Purpose: To follow infection control procedures.
13. Document the procedure in the patient's record, including the date and time, visual acuity results, and any reactions by the patient. Also record whether corrective lenses were worn.
    Purpose: Procedures that are not recorded are considered not done.

Documentation Exercise
The medical assistant conducted a Snellen exam on Carlene Anderson, who wears contacts. The results were as follows: right eye 20/60; left eye 20/30, but she missed one letter at the 20/30 line; both eyes 20/40. Carlene did not squint or strain during the exam.

Correct Documentation
8/01/20XX 2:20 p.m.: DVA completed Snellen chart. Right eye 20/60, left eye 20/30–1, both eyes 20/40 corrective lenses. No squinting noted. ————————
Kim Tau, CMA (AAMA)

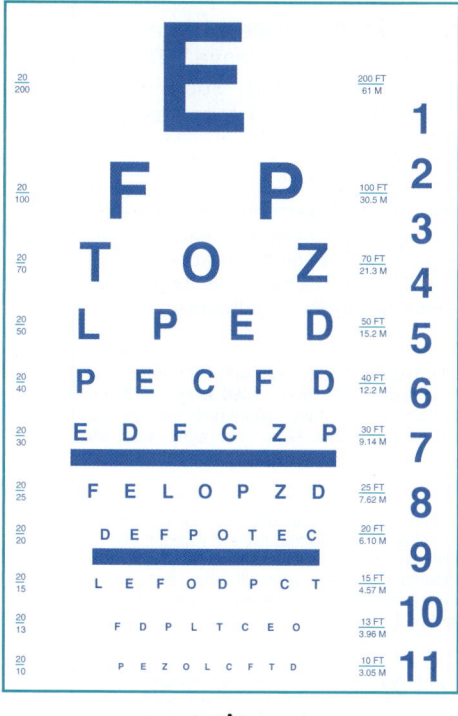
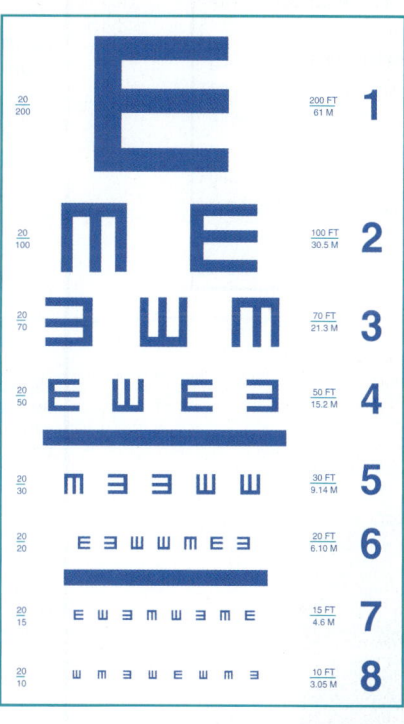
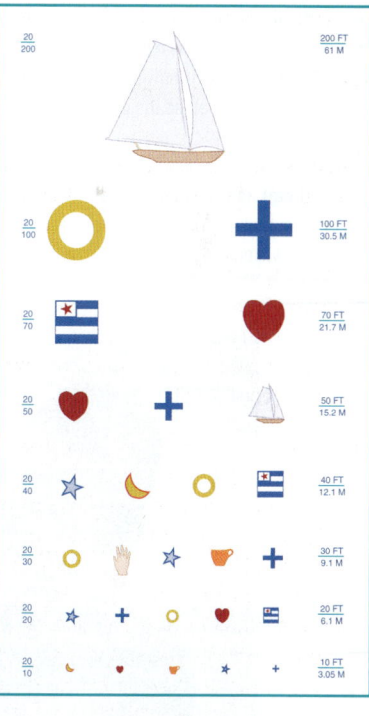

A   B   C

FIG. 30.21 Different types of Snellen charts. (From Proctor D, et al: *Kinn's The Medical Assistant*, ed 13, St. Louis, 2017, Elsevier.)

with an index card that has a large E drawn on it before the child is tested. Turn the card in different directions to simulate the position of the "fingers" of the E on the chart, and give the child the opportunity to demonstrate the direction of the E fingers by pointing his or her own fingers in the same direction (Fig. 30.22).

Because this is a gross screening of distance visual acuity, the eyes are typically tested with corrective lenses; therefore the patient should not remove glasses or contact lenses unless the provider requests it. Indicate in the patient's health record whether the assessment was done with or without corrective lenses. Record the results of each eye separately and as fractions. The numerator (top number) is the distance of the patient from the chart (always 20 feet), and the denominator (bottom number) is the lowest line read satisfactorily by the patient. For example, if the patient reads the 20 line at 20 feet, the fraction 20/20 is recorded for that eye. *The last line the patient can read without squinting or straining and with no more than two mistakes is the line recorded in the patient's record for that eye.* The medical assistant should document the outcomes of the test, specifying the results for each eye and for both eyes. The Joint Commission no longer recommends the use of medical abbreviations for the eyes and ears because they are frequently confused or misinterpreted; therefore the medical assistant must now document right eye, left eye, and both eyes. Box 30.13 provides more information about interpreting Snellen results.

Near Visual Acuity (NVA). Near visual acuity can be tested with the near vision acuity chart (Fig. 30.23). This test is given to screen for presbyopia or hyperopia. If the patient wears corrective lenses, they should be worn during the test. The size of the type on the card varies. The test should be given in a well-lit room, with the patient holding the card approximately 14 to 16 inches away. As with the Snellen examination, the near visual acuity test is given for each eye, starting with the right eye. The eye not being tested should be covered with an occluder but remain open. The patient should be monitored for indications of difficulty, such as squinting or tearing. The patient reads the card, starting at the top, until reaching the smallest print that can be read. The medical assistant should document the number at which the patient had no more than two errors for each eye and also the two eyes together, whether corrective lenses were worn, and any signs of eyestrain.

BOX 30.13 Interpreting Snellen Results

- The patient always stands 20 feet from the chart.
- Each result is a record of how well the patient can see compared with normal vision.
- Example: A patient with a 20/40 reading can see that line correctly standing at 20 feet, but an individual with normal vision can see the same line correctly at 40 feet, so the patient's vision is not as acute as someone with normal vision.
- Example: A patient with a 20/15 reading can see that line accurately standing at 20 feet, but a person with normal vision must stand at 15 feet to have the same vision, meaning the patient's vision is better than someone with normal vision.

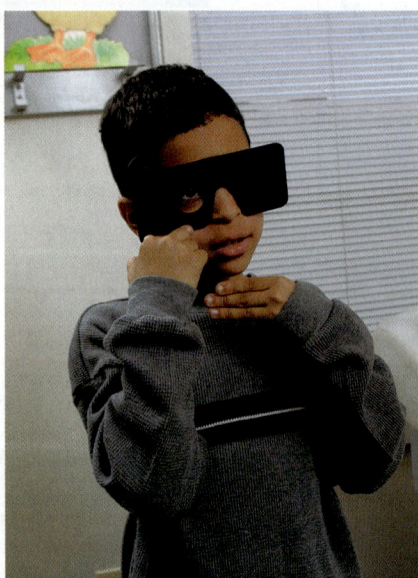

FIG. 30.22 Visual acuity test with the E chart. (From Proctor D, et al: *Kinn's The Medical Assistant*, ed 13, St. Louis, 2017, Elsevier.)

CRITICAL THINKING 30.7

Susie Anthony, a 19-year-old patient was seen for a general eye examination. The provider orders a routine Snellen test, and Chris administers it. Susie wears contact lenses. With her right eye, she reads without errors to the 20-25 line; however, she squints and makes three errors at the 20/20 line. With her left eye, Susie makes two mistakes at the 20/20 line; with both eyes she reads the 20/25 without errors. How should Chris document this procedure?

Ishihara Color Vision Test. Defects in color vision are classified as congenital or acquired. Congenital defects are caused by an inherited color vision defect and are found most often in males. Acquired defects are caused by eye injury or disease. The Ishihara test is a simple, convenient, and accurate procedure. It detects total color blindness, in addition to the red-green blindness prevalent in congenital blindness (Procedure 30.12). The test assesses the perception of primary colors and shades of colors.

The test booklet contains plates made up of colored dots in numeric patterns. The numbers are one color, and the background dots are a different color. Patients with average visual acuity can read the number

60

Nothing can take the place of "the only pair of eyes you will ever have." That is why you are exercising such good judgment in taking care of them as you are now doing.

50

For this reason, you will welcome the suggestion about lenses which are designed and made to give you "greater comfort and better appearance." In man's earliest days he had little use for glasses. He used his eyes chiefly for long distance.

40

He worked by daylight and at tasks with little detail. But now, you use your eyes for much close work—reading, writing, sewing and many other uses which the eyes of primitive man did not know. Now your eyes meet all sorts of lighting conditions, artificial and natural.

30

Many of these conditions produce "overbrightness" or glare. Sometimes it is the direct or reflected glare of sunlight; often it is direct or reflected from artificial light. And very often this glare is uncomfortable—impairs your efficiency. But special lenses, developed by America's leading optical scientists, combat this glare.

25

These lenses give you more comfortable vision and blend harmoniously with your complexion. These lenses are less conspicuous. We are glad to recommend them because they will give you greater comfort and better appearance. Thousands of satisfied wearers testify to their real benefits.

20

You are wise in taking good care of "the only pair of eyes you will ever have." You know how valuable they are, that you can never have another pair. For this reason, you will welcome the suggestion about lenses which are designed and made to give you "greater comfort and better appearance." In man's earliest days he had little use for glasses.

The above letters subtend the visual angle of 5' at the designated distance in inches.

FIG. 30.23 Near vision acuity chart.

CHAPTER 30 Physical Examination

PROCEDURE 30.12 Assess Color Acuity Using the Ishihara Test

Task
Assess a patient's color acuity correctly, using established protocols and record the results.

Equipment and Supplies
- Patient's health record
- Provider's order
- Room with natural light, if possible
- Ishihara color plate book
- Pen, pencil, and paper
- Watch with a second hand

Procedural Steps
1. Assemble the equipment, and prepare the room for testing. The room should be quiet and illuminated with natural light.
   Purpose: Natural light is needed to test colors correctly.
2. Greet the patient. Identify yourself. Verify the patient's identity with full name and date of birth. Explain the procedure to be performed in a manner that the patient understands. Answer any questions the patient may have about the procedure. Use a practice card during the explanation and make sure the patient understands that he or she has 3 seconds to identify each plate.
   Purpose: To make sure you have the right patient. Also, an informed patient is a cooperative patient. The first plate is a practice plate and is designed to be read correctly.
3. Hold up the first plate at a right angle to the patient's line of vision and 30 inches from the patient. Be sure both of the patient's eyes are kept open during the test (Fig. 1).
4. Ask the patient to tell you the number on the plate. Record the plate number and the patient's answer (Fig. 2).

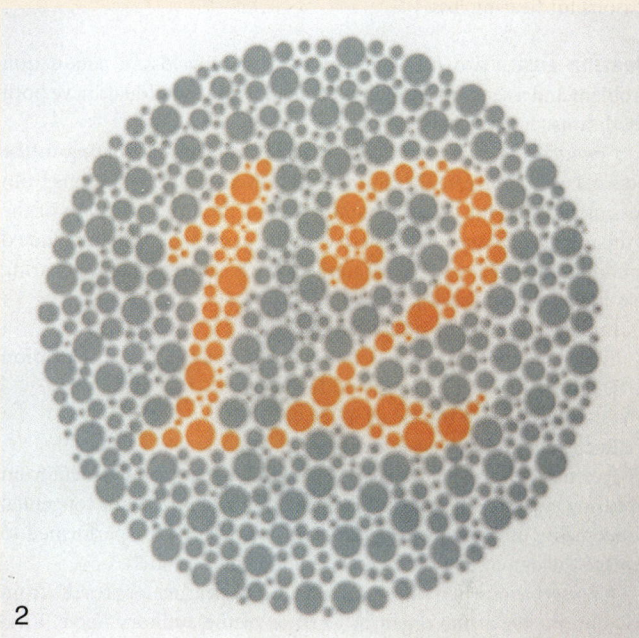

2

5. Continue this sequence until all 11 plates have been read. If the patient cannot identify the number on the plate, place an X in the record for that plate number. Your record should look like this:
   Plate 1 = pass, Plate 2 = pass, Plate 3 = X, Plate 4 = pass, and so on
6. Include any unusual symptoms in your record, such as eye rubbing, squinting, or excessive blinking.
7. Place the book back into its cardboard sleeve, and return it to its storage space.
   Purpose: The Ishihara color plates must be stored in a closed position away from external light to protect the colors.
8. Document the procedure in the patient's health record, including the date and time, the testing results, and any patient symptoms shown during the test.
   Purpose: Procedures that are not recorded are considered not done.

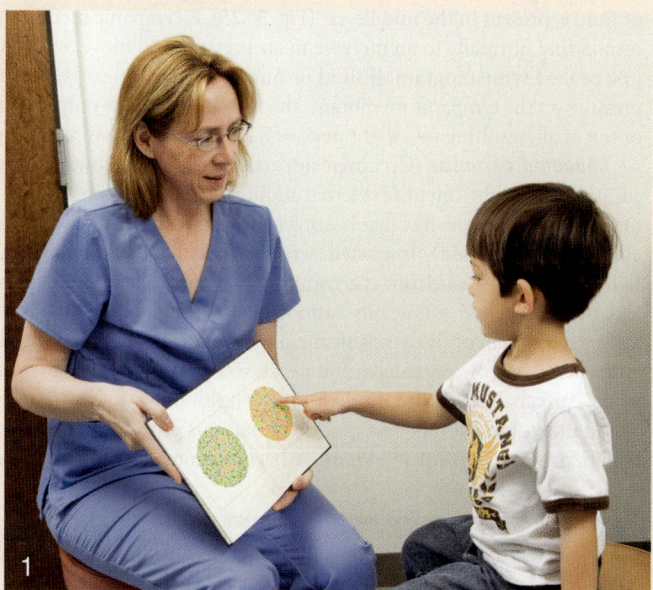

1

within the dot matrix without difficulty. Patients with color vision defects are unable to read the number, or they see a totally different number. A section of plates is included that contains colored line trails through a background of dots. These plates are designed to be used with children and adults who are unable to read numbers. In this situation, the patient uses a finger to follow the dotted trail through the picture.

The test should be administered in a quiet room that is well illuminated by sunlight, not by artificial lighting. If this is not doable, create the best situation possible by adjusting lights to resemble the effect of natural daylight. The test uses 14 color plates. The basic test consists of plates 1 through 11. Plates 12 through 14 are used if the patient appears to be having difficulty with red-green differentiations. The medical assistant records the number of plates read correctly. If the score is 10 or higher, the patient is within the average range. If the score is 7 or lower, the patient is suspected of having a color deficiency, and the ophthalmologist performs additional assessment tests using more precise color vision testing equipment.

Disorders of the Ear

The most common screening tests done in a healthcare facility involving the ear are for hearing. These tests can involve tuning forks or an audiometer. The following section discusses the two most common reasons for hearing loss.

Hearing Loss. Two problems result in hearing loss: a conduction problem and a sensorineural impairment. Some individuals have both conditions.

Conductive hearing loss is caused by a problem originating in the external or middle ear. These problems prevent sound vibrations from passing through the external auditory canal, limit the vibration of the tympanic membrane, or interfere with the passage of bone-conducted sound in the middle ear. Common factors causing conductive hearing loss include the following:
- Impacted cerumen (si ROO muh n)
- Trauma to the tympanic membrane, especially with scar formation
- Hemorrhage or fluid in the middle ear
- Otosclerosis (oh toh sklair ROH sis)
- Recurrent chronic ear infections

Patients with conductive hearing loss receive the greatest benefit from a hearing aid. If the hearing loss is caused by a malfunction or congenital abnormality of the ossicles, a surgical procedure can be performed to replace the damaged ossicles with manufactured models.

A *sensorineural* (sen suh ree NYOO R uhl) hearing loss results from an abnormality of the organ of Corti or of the auditory nerve. Viral infection (e.g., rubella, influenza, herpes) can result in hearing loss, as can head trauma or certain ototoxic (oh tuh TOK sik) medications. The first sign of ototoxic drug complications usually is *tinnitus* (TIN i tuh s), a ringing in the ears. This sometimes occurs with high doses of aspirin, certain antibiotics (erythromycin and vancomycin), and chemotherapeutic agents. A sensorineural hearing loss also can occur because of prolonged exposure to loud noise, such as repetitive noise in the workplace or loud music, which damages the delicate cilia lining the organ of Corti.

Presbycusis (prez bee KOO sis), the hearing loss that affects aging people, is caused by a reduction in the number of receptor cells in the organ of Corti and also is classified as a sensorineural loss. Children can be born with a congenital hearing deficit or deafness because of an intrauterine infection, such as measles (rubella).

Mixed hearing loss is a combination of conductive and sensory deafness. This type of loss can result from tumors, toxic levels of certain medications, hereditary factors, and stroke.

Otitis. Two common types of otitis are seen in patients in an otology or family practice. The first affects the external ear canal and is called *otitis externa*, or swimmer's ear. Otitis externa may be caused by dermatologic conditions, such as seborrhea (seb uh REE uh) or psoriasis (suh RAHY us sis), trauma to the canal, or continuous use of earplugs or earphones. Swimmers frequently have otitis externa because water collects in the ears and mixes with cerumen to form an ideal culture medium for bacteria and fungus. Patients with otitis externa complain of severe pain and have inflammation and swelling of the external auditory canal, hearing loss, and possibly *purulent* (PYOO R uh luh nt) (containing pus) or serous (SEER uh s) drainage. The inflammation is treated with antibiotic or steroid eardrops, and the canal must be kept clean and dry or the condition can become chronic.

Otitis media is an inflammation of the normally air-filled middle ear that results in a collection of fluid behind the tympanic membrane. Otitis media can be serous or suppurative (SUHP yuh rey tiv). Serous otitis media occurs because of a buildup of clear fluid in the middle ear; patients complain of a full feeling and some hearing loss. In suppurative otitis media, purulent fluid is present in the middle ear, and the patient has fever, pain, and hearing loss. Otitis media often is associated with an upper respiratory tract infection caused by a virus or an allergic reaction that results in swelling and inflammation of the sinuses and eustachian tubes. A child's eustachian tube is shorter, narrower, and more horizontal than that of an adult. The small size and decreased angle for drainage increases the chance that inflammation will block the tube and cause fluid to collect in the middle ear, which not only is uncomfortable but also interferes with the conduction hearing process.

An otoscopic examination reveals that the normally pearly gray tympanic membrane is inflamed (bright pink or red) and bulging (Fig. 30.24). Areas of fluid or pus may be visible through the membrane. A *tympanogram* may be done to determine the air pressure of the middle ear and the mobility of the tympanic membrane. During a tympanogram test, a small earphone is placed into the ear canal and the air pressure is gently changed. This test is helpful for showing whether an ear infection or fluid is present in the middle ear (Fig. 30.25). A tympanic membrane responding normally to an increase in air pressure will move, resulting in a peaked tympanogram. If fluid or pus in the middle ear is putting pressure on the tympanic membrane, the membrane moves only slightly or not at all, resulting in a slight peak or a flat tympanogram recording.

Impacted cerumen. Cerumen normally is a soft, yellowish, waxy substance that lubricates the external auditory canal. Excessive secretion of cerumen can gradually cause hearing loss, tinnitus, a feeling of fullness, and *otalgia* (ear pain). Impacted cerumen that has been pushed up tightly against the eardrum is a common cause of conductive hearing loss because sound vibrations cannot pass through the cerumen to initiate movement of the tympanic membrane. Individuals with psoriasis, abnormally narrow ear canals, or an excessive amount of hair growing in the ear canals are more prone to this condition.

An otoscopic examination quickly reveals this problem. If impacted cerumen is found, it must be removed. This can be done by softening

> **VOCABULARY**
> **otosclerosis:** The formation of spongy bone in the labyrinth of the ear, which often causes the auditory ossicles to become fixed and unable to vibrate when sound enters the ears.
> **ototoxic:** Describes medications that have a harmful effect on the eighth cranial nerve or the organs of hearing and balance.
> **psoriasis:** A usually chronic, recurrent skin disease marked by bright red patches covered with silvery scales.
> **seborrhea:** An excessive discharge of sebum from the sebaceous glands, forming greasy scales or crusty areas on the body.
> **serous:** A thin, watery serum-like drainage.
> **suppurative:** Characterized by the formation or discharge of pus.

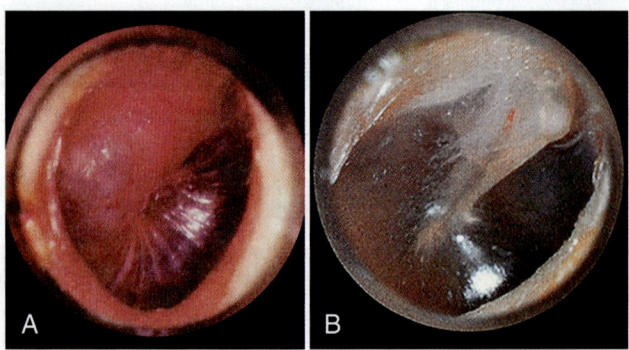

FIG. 30.24 (A) Tympanic membrane with otitis media. (B) Normal tympanic membrane. (From LaFleur Brooks M: *Exploring Medical Language*, ed 9, St. Louis, 2014, Mosby.)

> BOX 30.14 Useful Questions for Gathering a History of Ear Problems
>
> - Are you experiencing nausea, vomiting, dizziness, ear pain, fever, headache, upper respiratory infection, ringing of the ears, drainage, loss of balance, or hearing loss?
> - What are the onset, duration, and frequency of symptoms?
> - Have you taken any medication for the symptoms? If so, what medication? Has it been helpful?
> - Do you have the problem in both ears?
> - Are you experiencing pain? On a scale of 1 to 10, with 10 being the worst pain, how would you rate the pain? Is it localized or radiating, in one ear or both?
> - Has anything you have tried relieved the symptoms?

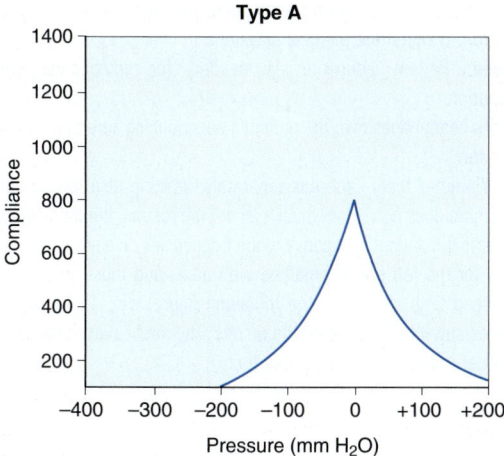

FIG. 30.25 A normal tympanogram shows a peak at normal pressure (0). An ear with fluid produces a flat tympanogram. (From Proctor D, et al: *Kinn's The Medical Assistant*, ed 13, St. Louis, 2017, Elsevier.)

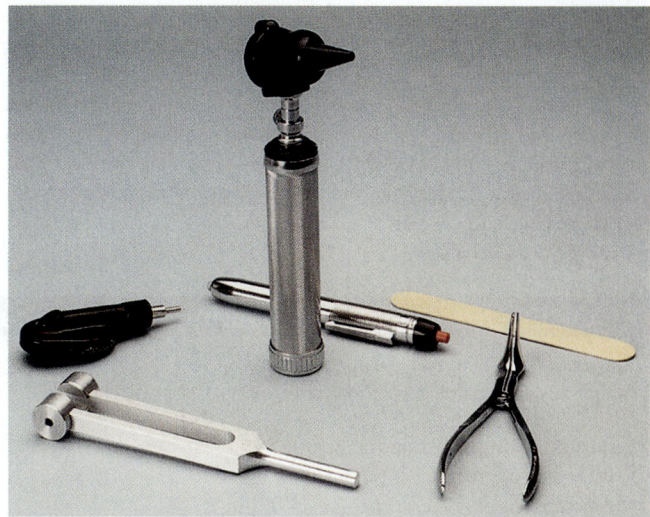

FIG. 30.26 Instruments used in an otoscopic examination. (From Proctor D, et al: *Kinn's The Medical Assistant*, ed 13, St. Louis, 2017, Elsevier.)

that it vibrates 512 cycles per second, the level of normal speech patterns. To activate the fork, the provider holds it by the stem and strikes the tines softly on the palm of the hand. Striking the tines too forcefully creates a tone that is too loud for diagnostic use. The two tests used to evaluate hearing are the Weber and Rinne tests. Both of these procedures are commonly used to evaluate conductive and sensory losses.

> **VOCABULARY**
>
> **hertz**: The unit of measurement used in hearing examinations; a wave frequency equal to 1 cycle per second.

The Weber test is used if the patient reports that hearing is better in one ear than in the other. The vibrating fork is placed in the center of the top of the head, and the patient is asked in which ear the tone is louder or if the tone is the same in both ears. Because the patient is hearing the tone by bone conduction through the head, a normal result is hearing the sound equally in both ears.

The Rinne test is designed to compare air conduction sound with bone conduction sound. In this test, the stem of the vibrating fork is placed on the patient's mastoid process, and the patient is instructed to raise a hand when the sound disappears. The fork is quickly inverted so that the vibrating tines are approximately 1 inch in front of the external ear canal. If hearing is normal, the patient should still hear a sound. In normal hearing, the sound is heard twice as long by air conduction as by bone conduction.

Audiometric Testing. An audiometric test may be done in an otology or a family practice and is performed by medical assistants who have received additional training. Audiometry measures the lowest intensity of sound an individual can hear (Fig. 30.27). The patient, frequently a child, is assisted in placing headphones over the ears.

Newer machines give the operator the choice of performing a traditional manual hearing test or an automated one. In the automatic mode, the patient is prompted through the ear phones to press a hand button as soon as he hears a tone. The advantages of automated machines are that voice prompts are available in multiple languages and the test requires less time to complete. The medical assistant can watch the progress of the test on the audiometer's screen. Whether the test is delivered manually

the wax with oily drops, such as carbamide peroxide (Debrox), and then irrigating the ear with warm water until the plug is removed. Because this condition can recur, the patient may need to schedule periodic examinations. If the patient is experiencing hearing loss because of the impaction, it is immediately remedied with removal of the cerumen.

Box 30.14 provides questions that are helpful with taking a history of a patient with ear problems.

Diagnostic Procedures

An ear examination involves viewing the external auditory canal with an otoscope covered by an ear speculum (Fig. 30.26). Disposable plastic speculum covers should be used each time to prevent disease transmission. A normal otoscopic examination reveals an external auditory canal with a small amount of cerumen and a pearly gray and concave tympanic membrane. In addition to performing the otoscopic examination, the provider palpates the area around the pinna for abnormalities or sensations. A number of tests are used to assess hearing acuity, ranging from simple tuning fork tests to quantitative and qualitative audiometric testing. If a hearing loss is suspected, the next test usually is performed with a tuning fork.

Tuning Fork Testing. Tuning fork tests measure hearing by air conduction and bone conduction. Remember that in bone conduction, the sound vibrates through the cranial bones to the inner ear. Tuning forks are available in different sizes, each with a different frequency. The most commonly used tuning fork is the 512 **hertz** (hurts) (Hz), which means

or with an automated model, each ear is tested by delivering a single frequency at a specific intensity, starting with low-frequency tones and going up to very high frequencies. The patient is asked to signal when he or she hears the sound. The results are printed on a graph, called an *audiogram*, or the medical assistant charts the results on a graph sheet (Procedure 30.13). An adult with normal hearing can hear tone frequencies below 25 decibels, and children with normal hearing can hear those below 15 decibels.

If initial screening indicates a hearing deficit, the provider may recommend an appointment with an **audiologist** (aw dee OL uh jist) for audiometric evaluation.

> **VOCABULARY**
> **audiologist**: An allied healthcare professional who specializes in the evaluation of hearing function, detection of hearing impairment, and determination of the anatomic site of impairment.

PROCEDURE 30.13 Measuring Hearing Acuity With an Audiometer

Task
Perform audiometric testing of hearing acuity, using established protocols.

Equipment and Supplies
- Patient's health record
- Provider's order
- Audiometer with adjustable headphones and graph paper
- Quiet area

Procedural Steps
1. Wash hands or use hand sanitizer, assemble the equipment, and bring the patient into a quiet area.
   Purpose: The testing room should be free of distractions and noise so the patient can concentrate completely on the hearing evaluation.
2. Greet the patient. Identify yourself. Verify the patient's identity with full name and date of birth. Explain the procedure to be performed in a manner that the patient understands. Answer any questions the patient may have about the procedure.
   Purpose: To make sure you have the right patient. Also, explanations help gain the patient's cooperation and ease apprehension.
3. Explain that the audiometer measures whether the patient can hear various sound wave frequencies through the headphones. Each ear is tested separately. When the patient hears a frequency, he or she should raise a hand or push the button to signal the medical assistant.
   Purpose: Patient education is needed for compliance with the examination.
4. Place the headphones over the patient's ears, making sure they are adjusted for comfort.
5. The audiometer tests each ear separately, starting at a low frequency. If the machine does not automatically record the results, the medical assistant documents the patient's response to the frequencies on a graph or audiogram. Results for the left ear are marked with an X, and those for the right ear are marked with an O (see the following figure) (Fig. 1). More advanced machines automatically record the results. The medical assistant must have specialized training to conduct this test.

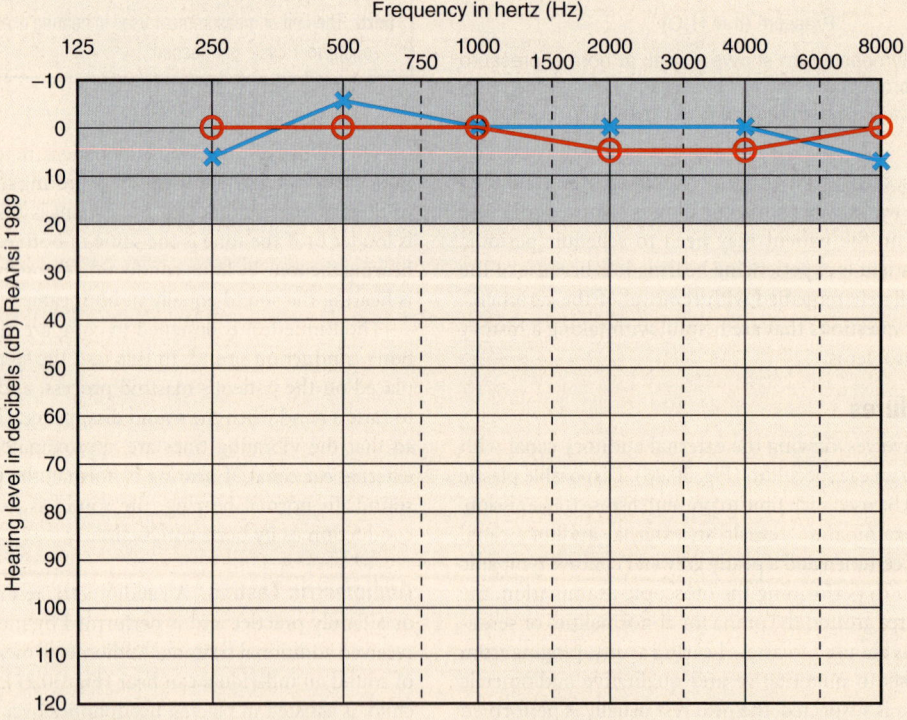

6. Frequencies are increased gradually to test the patient's ability to hear. Each response by the patient is documented.
7. After one ear has been tested, the other ear is then tested, and the results are documented.
8. The results are given to the provider for interpretation or downloaded into the patient's electronic health record for the provider to review.
9. The equipment is sanitized and disinfected according to the manufacturer's guidelines.
10. Wash hands or use hand sanitizer.

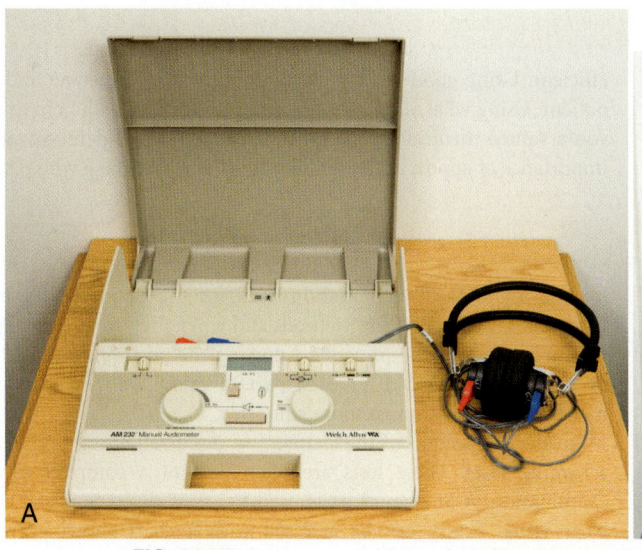 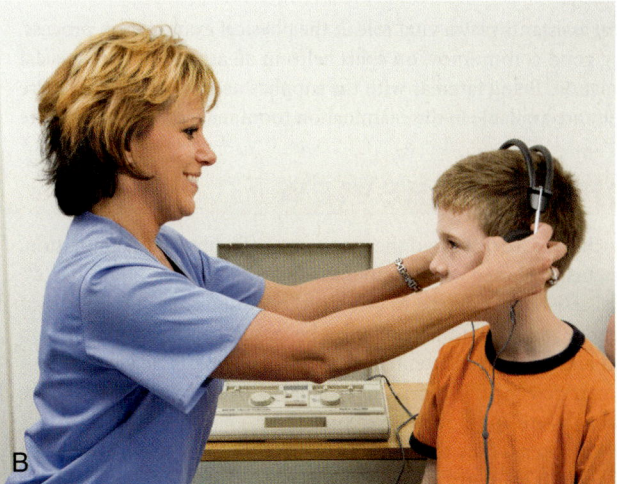

FIG. 30.27 Audiometer with headset. (From Proctor D, et al: *Kinn's The Medical Assistant*, ed 13, St. Louis, 2017, Elsevier.)

PROCEDURE 30.14 Demonstrate Appropriate Self-Boundaries

Task
Use respectful and tactful communication while demonstrating the principles of self-boundaries.

Background
For the medical assistant to have a professional therapeutic relationship with a patient, the medical assistant must guard against crossing self-boundaries, which is also called professional boundaries. The relationship between the medical assistant and the patient needs to be professional. It cannot be a dual relationship, where the medical assistant also becomes a friend to the patient. This means the medical assistant cannot share personal intimate information, contact the patient outside of the work environment, befriend the patient on social media, or engage in a flirty or romantic relationship with the patient.

Scenario #1
You are rooming Morgan, who frequently sees the provider you work for. You have gotten to know Morgan over the time you have worked for the provider. Today, Morgan asks you for your personal phone number and social media information.

Scenario #2
You are rooming Sam, who you have gotten to know well over the time you have worked for your provider. Sam is outgoing, enjoys talking, and has many of the same interests as you do. You have just split up with your significant other and have been feeling a bit down. Sam asks you if you would be available for coffee sometime.

Directions
Role-play the scenarios with a peer. Your peer will play the patient in the scenario and you are the medical assistant.

EXCEPTIONAL CUSTOMER SERVICE

The ability to communicate effectively is crucial to the role of the professional medical assistant and allows for excellent customer service. Effective communication includes the use of all of the therapeutic tools discussed in this chapter. The professional medical assistant should do the following:

- Watch for nonverbal behaviors to verify congruence between what the patient states verbally and demonstrates via body language.
- Modify communication methods as needed to meet the needs of a diverse patient population.
- Use restatement, reflection, and clarification to gather pertinent and comprehensive patient information.
- Utilize electronic communication appropriately and effectively.

CLOSING COMMENTS

Medical assistants play a vital role in the physical examination process. Having good communication skills helps in all aspects of the physical examination. Being familiar with the supplies needed and making sure that they are available in the examination room makes the process more efficient. Using good body mechanics helps to protect you and your patient. Using what you have learned in this chapter will help to make you a valued medical assistant. Procedure 30.14 will demonstrate the importance of appropriate self-boundaries when working with patients.

CHAPTER REVIEW

In this chapter we discussed the many parts of a physical examination. The discussion started with communication techniques. To be an effective medical assistant, you need to be able to communicate well. To obtain an accurate medical history, you must be familiar with the information needed and use therapeutic techniques to obtain it. The barriers to a good interview include defense mechanisms. We discussed what those mechanisms are and how to overcome them.

How to prepare for the physical examination was also discussed in this chapter. It is important to have the room well supplied so that the exam can proceed efficiently. Knowing the instruments needed for the exam will help you to assist the provider. Knowing the positions needed will help you to assist the patient. Using good body mechanics will help to keep you and your patient safe.

The methods of examination used for the exam are presented. Understanding each of the methods and when they are used will allow you to better help the provider. Knowing the positions and methods of examination needed for each part of examination sequence will make the examination go more smoothly.

In the last section of the chapter, we discussed vision and hearing screening tests. These tests are often part of a complete physical examination. A Snellen chart is used to assess distance visual acuity. Near visual acuity can be assessed with a chart showing type in different sizes. Ishihara plates are used to assess color vision. For hearing screening, a set of tuning forks can be used as well as an audiometer.

SCENARIO WRAP-UP

Chris has met with the office supervisor and reviewed essential techniques for gathering patient information. Therapeutic communication includes demonstrating respectful patient care, using active listening skills, observing nonverbal behaviors, and using a combination of both open-ended and closed questions to gather the best possible detail about the patient's chief complaint. The supervisor gave Chris a variety of information on meeting the needs of a diverse patient population and also gave him suggestions on how to develop empathetic, helping relationships with patients.

Chris has also taken responsibility for making sure that exam rooms are fully supplied and equipment is in working order. He is able to place patients in all of the appropriate positions during the examination and run the vision and screening tests ordered by the providers. He is also aware of using correct body mechanics when working at the healthcare facility.

31

Assisting With Obstetrics and Gynecology

LEARNING OBJECTIVES

1. Outline the medical assistant's role in a gynecologic examination (including breast, abdominal, and pelvic examinations) and demonstrate how to assist with a gynecologic examination.
2. Prepare for and assist with the collection of specimens, including those for a Pap test, a maturation index, and tests for various types of vaginal infections.
3. Compare and contrast current contraceptive methods.
4. Discuss post-examination duties.
5. Describe three of the most common gynecologic procedures performed in the medical office:
    - Cryotherapy
    - Colposcopy with or without a biopsy
    - Loop electrosurgical excision procedure (LEEP).
6. Specify the signs, symptoms, and treatments for conditions related to menopause.
7. Summarize the process of pregnancy and postpartum care, including the prenatal record, the first prenatal examination, return prenatal visits, and the postpartum visit.
8. Describe the common specialized tests and procedures for obstetric patients.
9. Describe the possible signs of domestic abuse and know how to report it.

CHAPTER OUTLINE

1. **Opening Scenario, 704**
2. **You Will Learn, 704**
3. **Introduction, 704**
4. **Gynecology, 704**
    a. Setting Up for a Gynecologic Examination, 704
    b. Preparation for the Gynecologic Examination, 704
    c. Assisting with an Examination, 704
    d. Breast Examination, 705
    e. Abdominal Examination, 706
    f. Pelvic Examination, 706
    g. Specimen Collection, 706
        i. *Pap Test, 706*
        ii. *Maturation Index, 707*
        iii. *Vaginal Infections, 707*
    h. Contraception, 707
        i. *Barrier Methods, 708*
        ii. *Hormonal Contraceptives, 708*
        iii. *Intrauterine Devices, 710*
        iv. *Permanent Methods, 710*710
    i. Post-Examination Duties, 710
    j. Special Procedures, 710
        i. *Cryotherapy, 710*
        ii. *Colposcopy With or Without a Biopsy, 710*
        iii. *Loop Electrosurgical Excision Procedure, 711*
    k. Menopause, 711
5. **Obstetrics, 713**
    a. Prenatal Record, 713
        i. *Demographic Information, 713*
        ii. *Menstrual History, 713*
        iii. *Obstetric History, 713*
        iv. *Medical and Surgical History, 714*
        v. *Family and Social History, 715*
    b. First Prenatal Examination, 716
    c. Return Prenatal Visits, 716
        i. *Fetal Heart Tones, 717*
        ii. *Fundal Height Measurement, 717*
    d. Postpartum Visit, 717
    e. Special Tests and Procedures, 717
        i. *Ultrasound, 718*
        ii. *Laboratory Testing, 718*
        iii. *Amniocentesis, 718*
        iv. *Chorionic Villi Sampling (CVS), 719*
6. **Recognizing Domestic Abuse, 719**
7. **Closing Comments, 720**
8. **Chapter Review, 720**

UNIT 4 Basic Clinical Procedures

 OPENING SCENARIO

Peggy St. John has been working in the obstetrics and gynecology (OB/GYN) department for about 5 years. She loves what she does and feels grateful that she can be there for her patients as they go through the pregnancy process. She also gets a lot of satisfaction from working with patients who come in with gynecologic issues. She especially likes the patient education that she can do with all of her patients. Her supervisor recognizes that Peggy enjoys teaching and has asked her to mentor a medical assistant student, Jill Snow, who is just starting her practicum. Peggy is excited to share how she works with patients in the OB/GYN department.

YOU WILL LEARN

- The components of a gynecologic examination.
- The components of prenatal and postpartum examinations.
- To assist providers with specialty examinations.
- How and why fundal height measurements are done.
- About special testing done during pregnancy.

INTRODUCTION

The branch of medicine that deals with pregnancy, labor, and the postpartum period is known as *obstetrics* (awb STE triks), and the branch of medicine that deals with diseases of the reproductive system in women is called *gynecology* (gy neh KAW loh jee). Frequently, a provider practices both specialties and is known as an *OB/GYN provider*. Assessment of the female reproductive system is an important part of health care. Patients are often hesitant and uncomfortable talking about sexual matters, so they wait until the symptoms are uncomfortable or until the disease is advanced before they seek medical care. The medical assistant needs to be familiar with signs and symptoms of the diseases and conditions related to this specialty, as discussed in Chapter 7, Reproductive System. In addition, the medical assistant must be aware of the patient's emotional state and must give support when needed.

In this chapter, we will be discussing the medical assistant's role in gynecologic and obstetric procedures. A medical assistant has two roles in these situations:

- To assist the provider in any way needed
- To be there for the patient; helping her to be as comfortable as possible during her time in the healthcare facility

When we make the patient feel comfortable, we help to establish a trusting relationship with her. This enables her to share the information the provider needs so as to give her the best possible care.

GYNECOLOGY

The need for an annual pelvic examination is being debated in the medical community. Currently the American College of Obstetricians and Gynecologists (ACOG) recommends annual pelvic examinations for patients 21 years or older. This examination is done to evaluate the reproductive organs and to diagnose and treat any abnormalities of those organs.

A breast examination is considered part of the gynecologic examination. A clinical breast examination should be done annually. The provider examines the breast, underarm area, and just below the clavicle.

Setting Up for a Gynecologic Examination

A medical assistant is responsible for setting up the examination room and making sure that all of the supplies are available for a gynecologic examination. The following is a list of supplies needed for a routine gynecologic examination:

- Patient's health record
- Laboratory requisition slips
- Patient gown and drape
- Lubricant
- Examination light
- Cervical spatula and/or cytobrush
- Microscope slides (direct smear method)
- Fixative (direct smear method)
- Plastic-fronded broom (liquid-based method)
- Liquid preparation container (liquid-based method)
- Vaginal speculum
- Sterile swabs
- Fecal occult blood test cards with developer
- Biohazard waste container

All items should be placed within easy reach for the provider and organized in a logical manner.

Preparation for the Gynecologic Examination

At the time the appointment was made, the patient should have been advised not to douche or have sexual intercourse for 24 hours before the examination. This allows the vaginal discharge to be properly evaluated and ensures accurate results of cytologic studies. Before the provider begins the pelvic examination, the medical assistant should obtain a complete gynecologic history. After documenting the patient's history and chief complaint, the medical assistant should prepare the room and the patient for the examination (Procedure 31.1).

The following should be included in the gynecologic history:

- Age at **menarche**
- Details about the regularity of the menstrual (MEN stroo al) cycle; the amount and duration of menstrual flow; and a history of menstrual disturbances and their treatment
- Any current indicators of infection, including vaginal discharge, pelvic pain, and urinary difficulties
- Description of any breast abnormalities and the date of the patient's last mammogram
- Date of the last Pap test
- Sexual history; sexually transmitted infection (STI) history
- Number of times pregnant and the number of pregnancies carried to more than 20 weeks
- Date of last menstrual period (LMP)
- Lifestyle factors, including diet, exercise, smoking, and alcohol use

> **VOCABULARY**
> **menarche:** The first menstrual period.

Assisting With an Examination

The pelvic and breast examination can an embarrassing and emotionally difficult medical experience. In our society, reproduction is not openly talked about. Aside from the embarrassment, many women fear the provider's findings. By behaving in a professional manner, explaining what is going to happen, and showing a genuine interest in the patient's concerns, the medical assistant can help lay to rest most of the patient's anxieties and fears.

The medical assistant is responsible for supporting the patient and assisting the provider during the procedure. To prevent unnecessary embarrassment and discomfort, the procedure should be fully explained to the patient. During the explanation, the medical assistant has the opportunity to provide patient education. This should be done using

CHAPTER 31 Assisting With Obstetrics and Gynecology

PROCEDURE 31.1 Set Up for and Assist the Provider With a Gynecology Examination

Task:
Prepare equipment for a gynecologic examination and assist the provider by placing the patient in the appropriate positions.

Equipment and Supplies
- Disposable examination gloves
- Fecal occult blood test kit
- Water soluble lubricant
- Vaginal speculum
- Slide and fixative or liquid preparation container
- Cervical spatula or plastic-fronded broom
- Laboratory requisition form
- Cotton-tipped applicator
- Patient gown
- Patient drape sheet
- Tray or Mayo stand

Procedural Steps

1. Sanitize hands.
   Purpose: Hand sanitization is an important step for infection control.
2. Assemble equipment needed for the gynecologic examination. Place on a tray or Mayo stand in a logical order.
   Purpose: Having the equipment in a logical order allows you to assist the clinician in an efficient manner.
3. Change the table paper if needed.
   Purpose: Clean table paper prevents the transmission of microorganisms from one patient to another.
4. Greet the patient. Identify yourself. Verify the patient's identity with full name and date of birth. Explain the procedure to be performed in a manner that is understood by the patient. Answer any questions the patient may have about the procedure.
   Purpose: It is important to identify the patient in two different ways to ensure that you have the correct patient. Explaining the procedure can make the patient feel more comfortable and helps to reduce anxiety.
5. Ask if the patient needs to empty her bladder, and collect a urine specimen if needed.
   Purpose: An empty bladder will make the pelvic examination more comfortable for the patient.
6. Instruct the patient to undress and put on the gown.
   Purpose: The patient will need to be completely undressed for the examination.
7. Assist the patient onto the examination table; she should remain in the sitting position. Place the drape across her lap.
   Purpose: The first position used for the gynecologic examination is the sitting position. In this position the provider will visually inspect the breasts.
8. Assist the patient into the supine position, providing a pillow for under her head for comfort. Pull out the leg extension on the examination table.
   Purpose: For the rest of the breast examination and the abdominal examination, the patient will need to be in the supine position.
9. With the stirrups in place on the examination table, assist the patient into the lithotomy position. The leg extension should be pushed in.
   Purpose: The lithotomy position is used for the pelvic examination.
10. When the examination is complete, assist the patient into the sitting position. Instruct the patient that she can get dressed.
    Purpose: At the end of the examination the patient can get dressed.
11. After the patient has dressed and left the exam room, clean the room and prepare specimens for transport to the laboratory.
    Purpose: By cleaning the examination room it will be prepared for the next patient. It is the medical assistant's responsibility to properly prepare specimens for transport to the laboratory.

---

terms that are easy for the patient to understand. The medical assistant should remain in the examination room to provide reassurance to the patient and legal protection for the provider.

The patient should be instructed to empty her bladder, completely disrobe, and put on an examination gown. Some providers prefer the patient put the gown on with the opening in the front, whereas others prefer the opening in the back. As the medical assistant, you should be aware of your provider's preference and instruct the patient accordingly (Box 31.1).

Breast Examination

The first part of the gynecologic examination is the breast examination. The exam begins with the patient in the sitting position for a visual check of the breasts. The gown should be adjusted so that the breast tissue can be easily exposed. After the visual inspection, the patient will be placed in the supine position. The medical assistant should be prepared to help the patient to lie down on the examination table. The foot rest should be extended, and a small pillow may be placed under the patient's head for comfort. If needed, the gown and drape should be adjusted to protect the patient's modesty. Palpation will be used to determine if there is thickening or lumps in the breast and collar bone area. The provider will instruct the patient to place her arms above her head to allow assessment of the underarm area using palpation. When the examination is complete, the gown is readjusted to cover the breasts. The provider may choose to discuss breast self-examination with the patient at this time or may inform the patient that the medical assistant will be explaining the technique at the end of the examination. Breast

BOX 31.1 Pap Test and Other Guidelines for Women

- Women ages 21 to 29 should have a Pap test alone every 3 years. HPV testing is not recommended.
- Women ages 30 to 65 should have a Pap test and an HPV test (co-testing) every 5 years (preferred). It also is acceptable to have a Pap test alone every 3 years.

If you have had a hysterectomy, you still may need screening. The decision is based on whether your cervix was removed, why the hysterectomy was needed, and whether you have a history of moderate or severe cervical cell changes or cervical cancer. Even if your cervix is removed at the time of hysterectomy, cervical cells can still be present at the top of the vagina. If you have a history of cervical cancer or cervical cell changes, you should continue to have screening for 20 years after the time of your surgery.

You should stop having cervical cancer screening after age 65 years if:

You do not have a history of moderate or severe abnormal cervical cells or cervical cancer, and

You have had either three negative Pap test results in a row or two negative co-test results in a row within the past 10 years, with the most recent test performed within the past 5 years.

Cervical cancer screening. Patient Education FAQ085. Washington, DC: ACOG: 2017. Available at https://www.acog.org/Patients/FAQs/Cervical-Cancer-Screening. Retrieved January 19, 2018.

self-examination will be discussed in more detail in Chapter 35, Patient Coaching with Health Promotion.

Abdominal Examination

While the patient is in the supine position, the provider will palpate the abdomen. This is done to confirm normal **symmetry** (SIM i tree) of the pelvic organs and to detect any masses. The provider also watches for any signs of discomfort or pain that could indicate a problem.

Pelvic Examination

For the pelvic examination, the patient is placed in the lithotomy (li THOT uh mee) position. This can be an awkward position for the patient to assume without assistance, and it may be embarrassing to the patient. If needed, the medical assistant should be available to help the patient into this position. Never place the patient in the lithotomy position until the provider is ready to begin the examination. When you assist the patient into the lithotomy position, always keep her totally covered.

The medical assistant should stand at the patient's side to observe the patient, yet still be able to move quickly (if needed by the provider). First, the provider inspects the external genitalia (jen ih TAY lee ah) and palpates the **perineal** (pair ih NEE al) area. The patient may be asked to bear down to show any muscular weaknesses that may be the result of lacerations of the perineal body during childbirth. A third-degree laceration may have involved the rectal sphincter and may cause rectal incontinence.

Next, the vaginal speculum (SPEK yuh luh m) is inserted for examination of the cervix and the vaginal canal and to obtain the Pap specimen. The speculum should be prewarmed with warm water. Have the patient take some deep breaths to help relax the abdominal muscles. The normal cervix points posteriorly and has smooth, pink, squamous epithelium. Abnormalities most frequently seen are ulcerations (erosions), **Bartholin** (BAR thoh lin) **cysts**, and cervical polyps. Because erosions cannot be palpated, inspection is the only method of detecting them. Healed lacerations from childbirth are common in a patient who has had multiple deliveries. Pregnancy increases the size of the cervix, and hormone deficiency causes it to atrophy. The vaginal wall is reddish pink and has a corrugated appearance from the overlapping tissue (rugae [ROO jee]) lining. Vaginal infections change the appearance of the vaginal mucosa.

After the inspection of the vaginal wall, the provider may collect a specimen for a Pap test. When the specimen has been obtained, the medical assistant may be responsible for labeling the specimen and preparing it for transport to the cytology laboratory. Be sure to follow laboratory instructions during the preparation to avoid having to repeat the examination.

After removal of the vaginal speculum, the provider does a bimanual examination. For a bimanual examination, two gloved fingers are lubricated with a water-soluble jelly (lubricant) and inserted into the vaginal canal, and the other hand palpates the abdomen over the pelvic organs and the mons pubis (Fig. 31.1). The uterus is examined for shape, size, and consistency, and its position is noted. A normal uterus is freely movable with limited discomfort. A laterally displaced uterus is usually the result of pelvic adhesions or displacement caused by a pelvic tumor. The fallopian tubes and ovaries are evaluated. Normal tubes and ovaries are difficult to palpate, which is why the provider may have to press firmly in the pelvic area, causing minor discomfort for the patient. A digital rectal exam may be done at this time. This involves the insertion of a gloved finger into the rectum. A small amount of stool is left on the glove and can be used for a fecal occult blood test.

Specimen Collection

During a pelvic examination, there are several types of specimens that may be collected. If the pelvic exam is part of a wellness examination, a specimen for a Pap test may be collected. If the provider wants to evaluate the endocrine function, a maturation index may be ordered. If the pelvic examination is for a possible vaginal infection, a specimen may be collected for culture or observation under a microscope.

Pap Test. The two methods of specimen collection for a Pap test are the direct smear method and the liquid-based method.

Direct smear method
1. The specimen is collected with a cervical spatula.
2. The cells are placed (smeared) directly on a microscope slide.
3. A fixative must be applied immediately to the slide before it is sent to the laboratory.

Liquid-based method
1. The specimen is collected with a plastic-fronded broom.
2. Cells are suspended in a bottle of preservative by rinsing the broom in the specimen vial

---

MEDICAL TERMINOLOGY
-al: pertaining to
perine/o: perineum

VOCABULARY
Bartholin cyst: A fluid-filled cyst in one of the vestibular glands located on either side of the vaginal orifice.
perineal: Pertaining to the area between the vaginal opening and the rectum (perineum).
symmetry: Similarity in size, form, and arrangement of parts on opposite sides of the body.

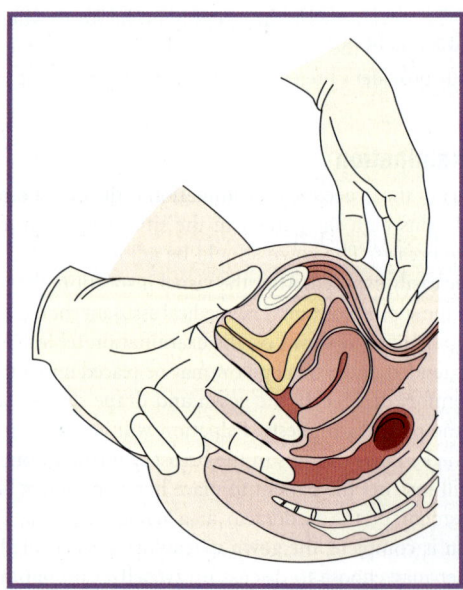

FIG. 31.1 Bimanual examination. (From Proctor D, Niedzwiecki B: *Kinn's The Medical Assistant*, ed 13, St Louis, 2017, Elsevier.)

3. The results of the Pap test are often reported using the Bethesda System (see Box 31.2).

Maturation Index. A *maturation index* is an endocrine evaluation that can assist in the diagnosis and treatment of infertility issues, amenorrhea (ah men uh REE ah), menopause, or postmenopausal bleeding. Cells are collected from the vaginal wall and treated much like a Pap test specimen. If the provider orders a maturation index, it much be indicated on the cytology request form.

> **VOCABULARY**
> **amenorrhea:** Lack of menstrual flow.
> **microcephaly:** Abnormally small head associated with incomplete brain development.

Vaginal Infections. In Chapter 7, Reproductive System, common vaginal infections were discussed. To collect a specimen to determine what type of vaginal infection is occurring, a pelvic exam needs to be done (Box 31.3). For many vaginal infections, a sterile swab is used to collect a sample of the discharge. The secretion is then swabbed on the microscope slide, and the provider looks at it under the microscope. Common infections, the infectious agents, and the type of specimen and test used to identify each include:

- Candidiasis (yeast infection): The provider tests for the presence of *Candida albicans*. A small amount of discharge is placed on a slide, and a drop of 10% solution of potassium hydroxide (KOH) is added. The KOH dissolves other cellular debris so that the provider can see the yeast buds.
- Trichomoniasis: A small amount of discharge is placed on a slide, and a drop of saline is added. The provider is looking for *Trichomonas vaginalis*, which appears as a pear-shaped organism with a flagellum (tail) that moves it around.
- Chlamydia: A sterile swab is used to collect a specimen from the endocervical canal. The swab is then placed in a tube containing a transport medium and sent to the lab for testing. The causative organism frequently is *Chlamydia trachomatis*.

> **MEDICAL TERMINOLOGY**
> **a-:** without
> **cephal/o:** head
> **men/o:** menses
> **micro-:** small
> **-rrhea:** discharge
> **-y:** condition; process of

Contraception

At the time of a gynecologic examination, a provider may discuss contraception (con trah SEP shun) with the patient. A woman's choice of a contraceptive method is based on many factors. To make an informed choice, a patient should know the risks, benefits, side effects, costs, failure rates, and convenience of each available method. In addition, although condoms are only moderately successful at preventing pregnancy, they should be used consistently to prevent transmission of STIs. The medical assistant may help provide patient education on

---

> **BOX 31.2 Pap Test Results**
>
> The Bethesda System is often used to report the results of a Pap test. This system looks at the squamous cells and the glandular cells separately.
>
> **Squamous Cells**
> - Negative for intraepithelial lesion of malignancy: normal epithelial cells, no precancerous findings
> - Atypical squamous cells (ASC)
>   - Atypical squamous cells of undetermined significance (ASC-US): Squamous cells do not appear completely normal but do not clearly suggest precancerous cells. Most often means there is an infection.
>   - Atypical squamous cells, cannot exclude a high-grade squamous intraepithelial lesion (ASC-H): Minor changes with unknown causes that are at risk of progressing to high-grade lesion (HSIL).
> - Low-grade squamous intraepithelial lesions (LSILs): Mild cell changes that may be classified as mild dysplasia. These abnormalities are often caused by human papilloma virus (HPV) infection.
> - High-grade squamous intraepithelial lesions (HSILs): Severe abnormalities that have a higher likelihood of progressing to cancer if left untreated. Maybe classified as moderate or severe dysplasia.
> - Squamous cell carcinoma: Cervical cancer
>
> **Glandular Cells**
> - Atypical glandular cells (ACG): Glandular cells do not appear normal, but it is not clear what is causing the changes.
> - Endocervical adenocarcinoma in situ (AIS): Severely abnormal cells are found, but they have not spread beyond the glandular tissue of the cervix.
> - Adenocarcinoma: Cancer of the endocervical canal and possibly endometrial, extrauterine, and other cancers.

> **BOX 31.3 Patient Education: Gynecology**
>
> Zika virus is frequently transmitted by mosquito bites, but it can also be sexually transmitted and transmitted from a pregnant woman to her fetus.
>
> According to the Centers for Disease Control and Prevention (CDC), Zika virus is found in semen and vaginal fluids and can be passed to sex partners. At this time, there is no medicine or vaccine for the Zika virus. Treating the symptoms are the best we can do at this point. Symptoms include fever, rash, joint pain, red eyes, headache, and muscle pain. In order to prevent the sexual transmission of the Zika virus, the CDC recommends the following:
> - abstaining from sex
> - using condoms
>
> Zika virus infection during pregnancy can have serious consequences for the fetus. Congenital Zika syndrome is a group of birth defects found in babies who were infected with the Zika virus during pregnancy. Congenital Zika syndrome has the following features:
> - Severe microcephaly (my kroh seh FAL lee)
> - Decreased brain tissue with a specific pattern of brain damage
> - Damage to the back of the eye
> - Joints with limited range of motion
> - Too much muscle tone, restricting body movement
>
> Not all babies will have all of these problems.
>
> To prevent the mosquito bites that may contain the Zika virus:
> - Use insect repellant
> - Wear long-sleeved shirts and long pants
> - Use screens on windows and doors and repair holes in screens

contraceptive methods. Table 31.1 summarizes the characteristics of various contraceptive methods.

Barrier Methods. Barrier methods of contraception either kill sperm (through the use of a chemical spermicide) or prevent them from entering the cervical os. These methods, which are relatively inexpensive, include the condom, diaphragm (DY ah fram), and cervical cap or sponge. Each method must be used every time the person has intercourse, which means the patient must be motivated to follow through on using it. Patient education on the use of a diaphragm includes the following instructions:

- Examine the diaphragm before each use by holding it up to a bright light to check for holes or cracks.
- Place 1 to 2 tablespoons of spermicidal jelly or cream into the diaphragm dome before insertion.
- Leave the diaphragm in place for 6 hours after intercourse; do not douche until after you have removed it.
- Before repeated intercourse, add spermicide to the outside of the diaphragm with an applicator. Do not remove the diaphragm until 6 hours after the last intercourse.
- After removal, wash the diaphragm with soap and water, allow it to air dry, and inspect it for breaks or holes before storing.
- Have the diaphragm refitted if:
  - You gain or lose more than 10 to 15 pounds.
  - You have a miscarriage, give birth, or undergo any type of pelvic surgery.
  - You have difficulty voiding or moving your bowels with the diaphragm in place.

The cervical cap is a thimble-sized, domed barrier device that fits over the end of the cervix. It also is used with spermicidal jelly (Fig. 31.2).

If used properly, the cervical cap is 92% to 96% effective. An advantage of this barrier method is that the cap can be inserted up to 12 hours before intercourse and can stay in place up to 72 hours without a decrease in effectiveness or safety. The cervical sponge contains spermicide and can also be inserted hours before intercourse and is effective for 24 hours. If always used as directed, the sponge is 80% to 91% effective.

Hormonal Contraceptives. Hormonal contraceptives are a highly effective and reversible form of contraception. They work by preventing ovulation, changing the cervical mucosa, affecting sperm mobility, and

TABLE 31.1 Commonly Used Contraceptive Methods

	Failure Rate	Characteristics	Contraindications	Side Effects
Male or female condom (barrier method)	2%–10%	No prescription or examination needed; easily available; inexpensive	Latex allergy in either partner	Possible allergic response to latex or spermicide
Diaphragm, cervical cap, cervical sponge (barrier method)	2%–19%	Must be fitted by clinician; requires instruction on how to insert and remove; spermicide must be used each time; diaphragm and sponge must be left in place for 6 hours after intercourse	Latex, rubber, or spermicide allergy; uterine prolapse; severe cystocele or rectocele	Increased risk for UTI (diaphragm); increased risk of abnormal Pap test result (cap)
Intrauterine device (IUD)	2%–6%	Copper type releases copper, which slows sperm in the cervix; hormonal type release progestin, which reduces sperm mobility and prevents thickening of the endometrial wall	Cervicitis, vaginitis, endometriosis, pelvic infection, history of STI or ectopic pregnancy	Copper type may temporarily increase vaginal bleeding and menstrual pain; hormonal IUDs decrease menstrual flow and cramping
Birth control implants	1%	Flexible plastic implant inserted under skin of upper arm; releases progestin to prevent ovulation, thickens cervical secretions to block semen, thins endometrial wall; effective for up to 3 years	Certain antibiotics, HIV drugs, seizure medications may make it less effective; history of blood clots, liver disease, or breast cancer	Irregular bleeding in first 6–12 months; nausea, headache, sore breasts, scarring at implantation site
Depo-Provera (DMPA)	0.5%	Requires 150-mg IM injection every 3 months	Intention of becoming pregnant within 1 year; breast cancer; liver disease	Return of fertility may be delayed 10–18 months; should not be used more than 2 years in a row because it can cause a temporary loss of bone density; headache, weight gain, possibly depression
Oral contraceptives (OCPs) Hormonal patch Vaginal ring	1%	Suppress ovulation; atrophy of the endometrium	Thrombolytic, liver, or coronary artery disease; breast, liver, reproductive tract cancer; smoker over age 35; diabetes; sickle cell disease	Nausea, breakthrough bleeding, breast tenderness, fluid retention; hypertension, elevated lipid levels, blood clots, strokes

HIV, Human immunodeficiency virus; *IM*, intramuscular; *PID*, pelvic inflammatory disease; *STI*, sexually transmitted infection; *UTI*, urinary tract infection.

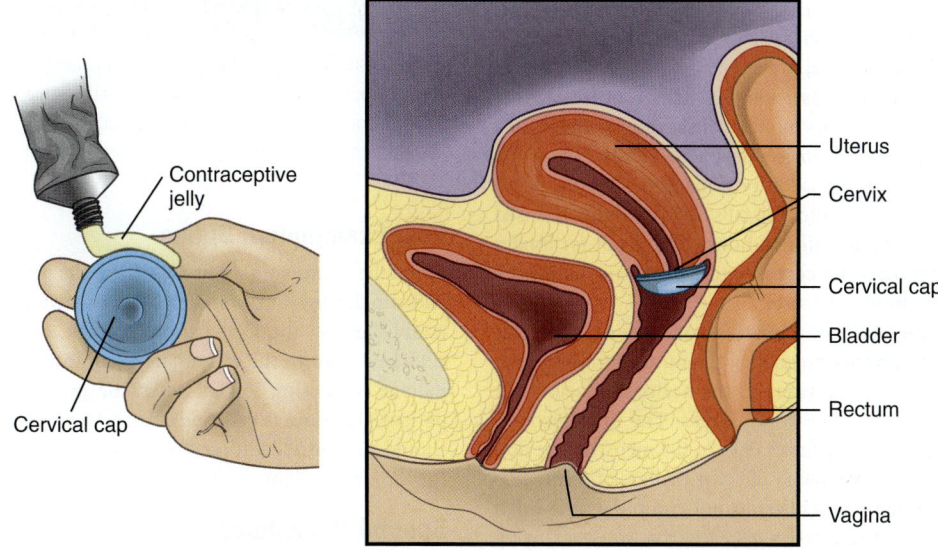

FIG. 31.2 Cervical cap with spermicide. (From Proctor D, Niedzwiecki B: *Kinn's The Medical Assistant*, ed 13, St Louis, 2017, Elsevier.)

preventing thickening of the endometrial wall. Hormonal contraceptives include:
- Birth control pills or patch
- Vaginal ring
- Depo-Provera injections
- Hormonal implants

Besides being a highly effective method of birth control, oral contraceptives can be used to treat a wide range of gynecologic conditions, including menstrual irregularities, premenstrual syndrome (PMS) symptoms, and **anovulation**. They also can be used to prevent ovarian cysts and may be prescribed to increase bone density. However, to be effective, the pills must be taken daily, at the same time each day. Failure rates are associated with noncompliance and can range from less than 1% (in highly compliant women) to greater than 15% (in those who do not take the pills as prescribed). Oral contraceptive pills (OCPs) can have serious side effects. Patients should be informed of conditions that require immediate medical attention. These can be remembered with the mnemonic ACHES: *a*bdominal pain (new and severe), *c*hest pain (new and severe), *h*eadaches (new or more frequent), *e*ye problems (blurred vision or vision loss), and *s*evere leg pain. These symptoms may indicate the formation of a blood clot in the abdomen, chest, or leg. They may also be signs of a stroke. Blood clot formation and stroke are the most serious complications of OCPs.

A type of oral contraception, the extended cycle pill, limits the number of menstrual periods to four a year. Patients are more likely to have spotting and breakthrough bleeding with this hormone therapy than with the traditional 28-day birth control pill. The extended cycle pill is designed to be taken once a day for 84 days, and then an inactive dose is taken for a week, during which the woman would menstruate. A combination birth control pill that contains both estrogen (ES truh juh n) and progestin (proh JES tin) may be prescribed for women suffering from a severe form of **premenstrual syndrome (PMS)** called **premenstrual dysphoric** (dis FOR ik) **disorder (PMDD)**; it also is useful for treating acne in female patients at least 14 years of age who have started menstruating.

As mentioned, hormonal contraception also can be delivered via a transdermal patch. The patch is a 1¾-inch square that slowly releases estrogen and progestin through the skin into the bloodstream. It is considered as effective as oral contraceptives in women who weigh less than 198 pounds; however, the patch is still a very effective method for women who weigh more than this. Current research shows that the risk of blood clots with the contraceptive patch is similar to the risks observed with oral contraceptives. However, cigarette smoking increases the risk of serious cardiovascular side effects, especially if the patient is over age 35. Patients should be told not to apply any creams or oils at the application site, to change the patch weekly for 3 consecutive weeks, and to go patch free the fourth week, allowing menstruation to occur. The patch can be applied to the buttocks, lower abdomen, and upper body, but not to the breasts. The woman can bathe, shower, and swim while wearing the patch, but if it comes off, it should be replaced immediately.

The vaginal ring contraceptive device is made of flexible plastic and is inserted into the vagina. The ring slowly releases estrogen and progestin

---

MEDICAL TERMINOLOGY

an-: no, not, without
ovul/o: ovum
-ation: process of

VOCABULARY

anovulation: Failure of the ovaries to release an ovum at the time of ovulation.
premenstrual dysphoric disorder (PMDD): A mood disorder that includes depression, irritability, fatigue, changes in appetite or sleep, and difficulty in concentrating; it occurs 1 to 2 weeks before the onset of the menstrual flow.
premenstrual syndrome (PMS): A poorly understood group of symptoms that occur in some women on a cyclical basis; breast pain, irritability, fluid retention, headache, and a lack of coordination are some of the symptoms.

in order to prevent pregnancy and provide effective contraceptive action for 1 month after insertion. The device is 2 inches in diameter and can be inserted anywhere in the vagina; however, the deeper it is placed, the less likely it is to be felt after insertion. Side effects of the vaginal ring are similar to those of other hormonal contraceptives, and it may increase the risk of heart attack, stroke, and blood clots. When the patient first starts using the ring, an additional method of birth control must be used for the first week. If the ring falls out, it should be rinsed with warm water and reinserted within 3 hours. If it is out for longer than 3 hours, contraception is not certain and the patient should use another birth control method for 1 week.

Depo-Provera is an injectable contraceptive that contains high doses of progestin. Each dose prevents pregnancy for up to 3 months, but women must be compliant in returning to the healthcare facility for follow-up and repeat doses every 9 to 13 weeks. The first injection should be administered within the first 5 days of the menstrual period for birth control coverage. This is a highly effective method of contraception and is ideal for women who either do not comply with a birth control regimen or do not want to take a pill every day. However, using Depo-Provera for 2 years or longer may increase the risk of bone loss and the eventual development of osteoporosis. Almost all patients using the injections experience some menstrual irregularities, but these usually subside after two doses. Women using this form of hormonal contraception are not at risk for the side effects of estrogen exposure, such as increased risk of blood clots and cardiovascular disease.

A birth control implant is a single, flexible rod, about the size of a match, that is inserted under the skin of the upper arm. The birth control implant releases a low, steady dose of progestin. This suppresses ovulation, thickens cervical mucus to block the passage of sperm, and thins the endometrial wall to prevent implantation. It prevents pregnancy for up to 3 years after insertion. Hormonal implants have risks and contraindications similar to those of other hormonal types of contraception.

Intrauterine Devices. The intrauterine device (IUD) (Fig. 31.3) is a T-shaped plastic frame with threads attached that is inserted by the provider into the uterus to prevent pregnancy. Two general types of IUDs are available: the copper type and the hormonal type. Both products inhibit fertilization by blocking the sperm's journey to the fallopian tubes, and, if fertilization does occur, they prevent the embryo from implanting in the uterine wall. In addition, the copper type of IUD releases copper, which acts to slow sperm in the cervix. The hormonal types of IUD release progestin, which reduces sperm mobility and prevents the thickening of the endometrial wall during the menstrual cycle. Both types of IUDs are extremely effective at preventing pregnancy (over 99%); the copper type can remain in place as long as 12 years, whereas the hormonal types must be replaced every 3 to 5 years. The copper IUD may temporarily increase vaginal bleeding and menstrual pain. The hormonal IUD results in both decreased menstrual flow and cramping. To remove an IUD, the provider gently withdraws it by pulling on the IUD string. In rare instances, it must be removed surgically.

Permanent Methods. Both male and female patients can undergo surgical procedures that are considered permanent contraceptive methods. Vasectomies in the male were addressed in Chapter 7, Reproductive System. For the female, a bilateral tubal ligation can be performed in which a portion of both fallopian tubes is excised or ligated. The cost and rate of complications are higher for tubal ligations than for vasectomies. In addition, tubal ligations must be done on an outpatient basis with general anesthesia, so the woman has that additional risk. Both procedures can be reversed, but not always successfully.

> **CRITICAL THINKING BOX 31.1**
>
> When directed by the provider, Peggy provides patient education regarding contraceptives. She has asked Jill to create a reference sheet that covers all birth control options, their characteristics and side effects, and any patient education details that might be appropriate. What should Jill include?

Post-Examination Duties

When the examination is finished, help the patient into a sitting position and into the dressing room if needed. Following the Standard Precautions established by the Occupational Safety and Health Administration (OSHA), remove the examination equipment and supplies while the patient is dressing so that when the provider returns to talk to the patient, the room is neat and clean. Once the patient has left, the room should be sanitized, disinfected, and restocked as necessary so it is ready for the next patient.

Special Procedures

There are a number of gynecology-related special procedures that a patient may undergo related to an abnormal Pap test result. Let's look at the three most commonly performed procedures:

- cryotherapy
- colposcopy with or without a biopsy
- loop electrosurgical excision procedure (LEEP)

Cryotherapy. Depending on the condition of the cervix, *cryotherapy*, or the application of freezing temperatures, may be used to treat chronic cervicitis and cervical erosion. Freezing causes cellular necrosis, and in approximately 1 month, the dead cells are replaced with healthy cells. The procedure involves placing a probe against the problem area on the cervix and applying liquid nitrogen to the area for approximately 3 to 4 minutes or until the site is frozen. The patient may experience some pain for 30 minutes or so after the procedure, and a slight watery discharge for up to a week. If any signs of infection, foul discharge, or pain develop, the patient should call the provider's office. Advise the patient not to engage in sexual intercourse for 1 month and to expect a heavier than usual menstrual flow for the first cycle after the procedure.

Colposcopy With or Without a Biopsy. *Colposcopy* is the visual examination of the vagina and cervical surfaces with a colposcope (Fig. 31.4). The *colposcope* is a microscope with a light source and a magnifying lens that can be used during a vaginal examination to:

- locate and evaluate abnormal cells.
- detect cancer of the cervix in the early stages.
- examine tissue from which an abnormal Pap test result has been obtained.
- monitor areas of the cervix where malignant lesions have been removed.

In combination with a colposcopy, a cervical biopsy may be performed (Box 31.4). A major advantage of obtaining a biopsy during colposcopy

> **MEDICAL TERMINOLOGY**
>
> **colp/o:** vagina
> **cry/o:** extreme cold
> **necr/o:** death, dead
> **-osis:** abnormal condition
> **-scopy:** process of viewing
> **-therapy:** treatment

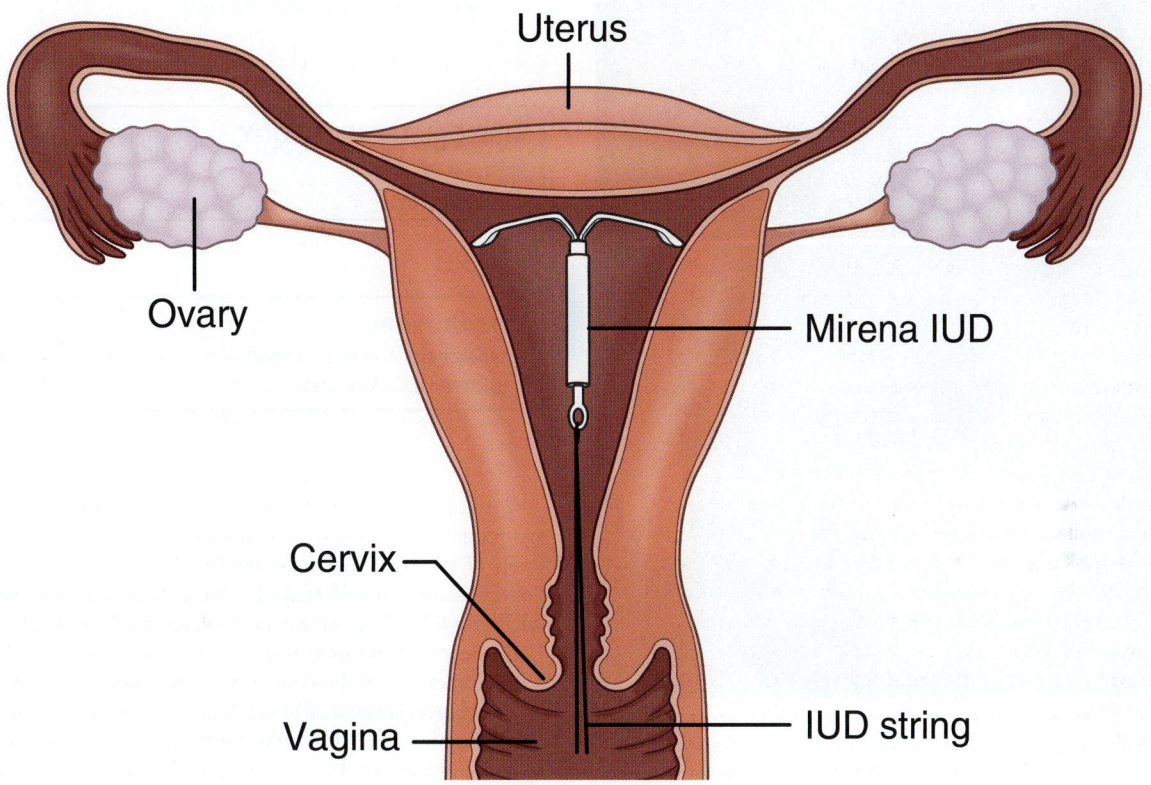

FIG. 31.3 Intrauterine device. (From Proctor D, Niedzwiecki B: *Kinn's The Medical Assistant*, ed 13, St Louis, 2017, Elsevier.)

BOX 31.4 Assisting With a Cervical Biopsy

When a cervical biopsy is being performed, there may be multiple biopsies taken. The provider is looking for abnormalities on the cervix and will take a biopsy specimen when one is seen. You may be receiving the sample from the provider. It is very important to accurately label each specimen container with the location of the biopsy. The provider uses the face of a clock for determining the location of the biopsy. The specimen container label should indicate that location (e.g., 2:00).

is that the instrument permits visualization of the suspicious area so that the biopsy can be taken from the most atypical site.

Colposcopy is a relatively safe, painless procedure performed in the provider's office. Discomfort may occur when the speculum is inserted into the vagina to improve visualization of the tissue. Discomfort and bleeding can occur when tissue is taken in a biopsy.

Loop Electrosurgical Excision Procedure. Depending on the results of the cervical biopsy, the patient may need a more extensive procedure, *conization*, in which a cone-shaped wedge of cervical tissue is removed for treatment or further analysis. More often a less-invasive LEEP is performed. With this technique, a local anesthetic is injected into the cervix, and a wire loop is inserted into the vagina. A high-frequency electrical current running through the wire is used to remove abnormal tissue from both the cervix and the endocervical canal. Like conization, LEEP can be used as a diagnostic tool to collect biopsy samples and as a treatment to remove abnormal tissue (Fig. 31.5).

Menopause

Conditions and disorders related to the menstrual cycle are a big part of a gynecologic specialty. *Menopause* is the permanent ending of menstruation as a result of the end of ovarian function. It usually occurs between 45 and 55 years of age but can occur as early as the 30s and as late as the 60s. Menses may stop suddenly, flow may decrease over time, or the time between menses may lengthen until menstruation

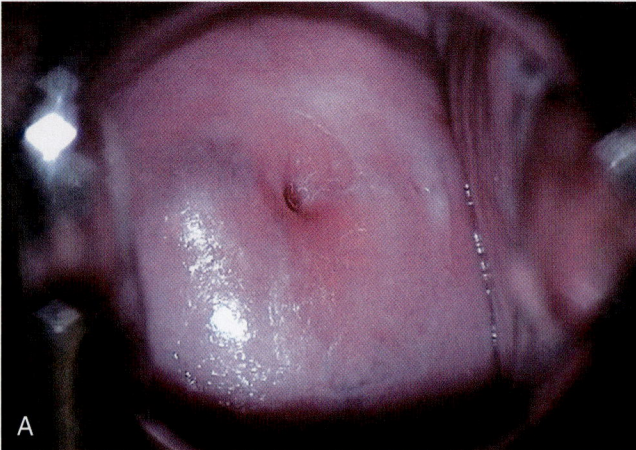

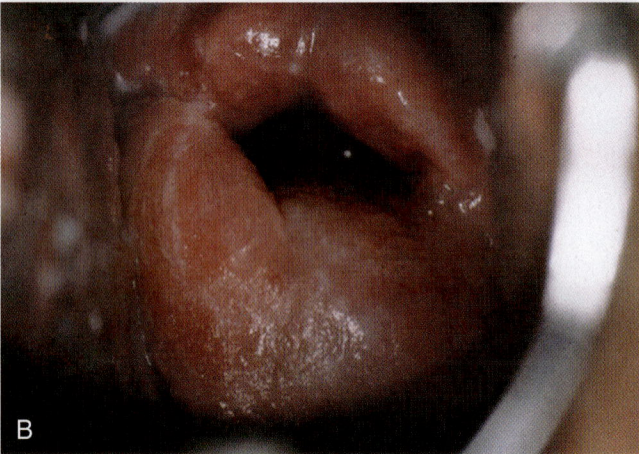

FIG. 31.4 Colposcopic appearance of a normal cervix (A) and an abnormal cervix (B). (**A** from Swartz MH: *Textbook Of Physical Diagnosis,* ed 7, Philadelphia, 2014, Saunders; **B** from Pfenninger JL, Fowler GC: *Pfenninger and Fowler's Procedures For Primary Care,* ed 3, Philadelphia, 2011, Saunders.)

completely stops. Menopause can be diagnosed only retrospectively. Only after 12 months of amenorrhea is a woman said to be in menopause, and the years after this are called *postmenopause.*

Perimenopause begins when hormone-related changes start to appear, and it lasts until the final menses; this can be as long as 10 years before menopause. During this time, women are still ovulating, but the uneven rise and fall of estrogen and progesterone may cause symptoms. Some women experience few or no symptoms, whereas others may have:
- hot flashes
- concentration problems
- mood swings
- irritability
- migraines
- vaginal dryness
- urinary incontinence
- dry skin
- sleep disorders

Treatment focuses on relieving these signs and symptoms. The provider may prescribe very-low-dose oral contraceptives to balance estrogen and progesterone levels or short-term hormone replacement therapy (HRT) to treat symptoms. The provider also may recommend that the patient consume soy products or take soy supplements for a plant source of estrogen. Vitamin E may help ease hot flashes, and vitamin B_6 helps create natural serotonin, a neurotransmitter that affects mood. Other methods that help with symptoms include:
- avoiding caffeine and spicy foods (to reduce hot flashes)
- using relaxation techniques (to aid with sleep disorders)
- consuming a low-fat diet high in calcium and vitamin D
- performing regular weight-bearing exercise (to help prevent osteoporosis and heart disease)

> **MEDICAL TERMINOLOGY**
> **oste/o:** bone
> **por/o:** passage

> **VOCABULARY**
> **osteoporosis:** Abnormal thinning of the bone structure, causing bones to become brittle and weak.

Medical treatment of menopause focuses on managing uncomfortable symptoms and preventing conditions associated with a drop in blood levels of estrogen, such as osteoporosis and coronary artery disease. Providers traditionally treated perimenopause and menopause with long-term HRT for most women; however, studies indicate that although HRT does protect the menopausal woman from osteoporosis, hip fracture, and colon cancer, at the same time, it increases the risk of heart attack, stroke, breast cancer, and blood clotting. It is now recommended that providers prescribe HRT to meet individual patient needs over a short term (i.e., no longer than 5 years) rather than as routine treatment for all menopausal women. Studies show that the risk for heart disease and other complications increases after 5 years of HRT. The medical assistant must be aware of the provider's recommendations regarding HRT.

Other medications that may be prescribed include antidepressants to prevent hot flashes. Gabapentin and clonidine also may be prescribed to reduce the frequency of hot flashes. Because the development of osteoporosis is a concern in perimenopausal and postmenopausal women, the provider may prescribe alendronate, risedronate, or ibandronate to reduce bone loss and the risk of fracture. Another drug that may be used to improve postmenopausal bone density is raloxifene; however, hot flashes are a common side effect of this medication. Vaginal dryness can be treated with estrogen administered locally by vaginal tablet, ring, or cream, or the patient can use K-Y Jelly or some other vaginal moisturizer as a lubricant.

> **CRITICAL THINKING BOX 31.2**
>
> Peggy and Jill room Rose Conrad, a 53-year-old patient. Mrs. Conrad is here to see Dr. Walden regarding her hormone replacement therapy, which she has been on for 3 years. Mrs. Conrad is willing to have Jill in the room during her discussion with Dr. Walden so that Jill can observe and learn. Mrs. Conrad recently read that her therapy may be dangerous. Dr. Walden agrees that if she is concerned, she can stop taking the medication; however, Dr. Walden recommends that Mrs. Conrad try some alternative therapies. What suggestions might Dr. Walden make for nonpharmaceutical treatment of perimenopausal symptoms?

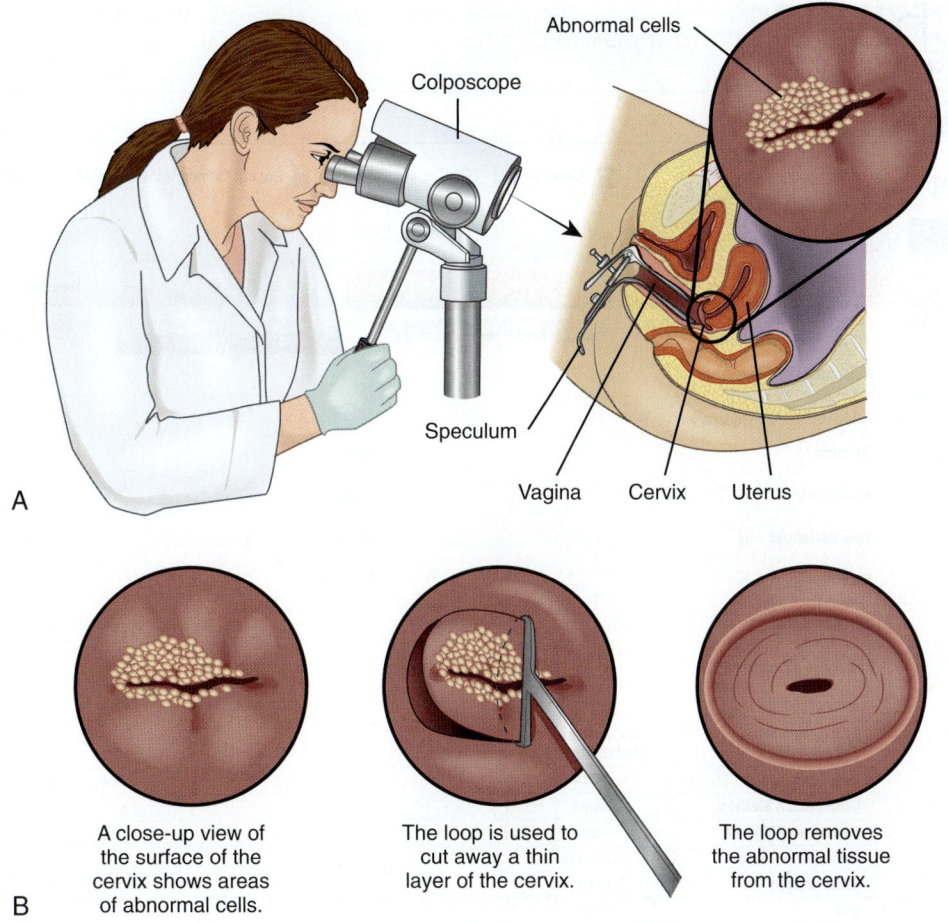

FIG. 31.5 Colposcopic view of the cervix (A) and LEEP biopsy of abnormal cells (B). (From Proctor D, Niedzwiecki B: *Kinn's The Medical Assistant*, ed 13, St Louis, 2017, Elsevier.)

OBSTETRICS

Pregnancy can be the most exciting and most terrifying experience for a patient, especially the first time around. As a medical assistant working in obstetrics, it is important to be able to reassure the patient while remaining professional. The next section will discuss the examinations and procedures related to prenatal and postpartum care.

Prenatal Record

At the first prenatal examination, an extensive health history will be taken. This history can help to identify any risk factors for the patient. Frequently, the first prenatal visit is the first comprehensive physical examination that the patient has had in a long time. The health history can point out pregnancy-related risk factors and overall health-related risk factors that can also be addressed. The following information should be collected when creating the prenatal record for a patient:
- Demographic information
- Menstrual history
- Obstetric history
- Medical and surgical history
- Family and social history

Demographic Information. The healthcare facility must have accurate and up-to-date demographic information, including the following:
- Address and phone numbers (land line and cellular)
- Employment
- Insurance
- Emergency contact
- Language
- Self-identified ethnicity
- Religious preference

This information is necessary for billing purposes and for preauthorization of services. It also can help to ensure that we are providing all of the services needed for the patient by making sure that we have an interpreter available (if needed, based on language) and having any special dietary needs met for the patient at the hospital.

Menstrual History. The prenatal record should include the first day of the last menstrual period. This is used to determine the estimated date of delivery (EDD). It is also important to know the normal cycle length for the patient and if this last menstrual period was "normal." The medical assistant should also ask if the patient was using contraception when she became pregnant. If she was, the method being used should be documented.

Obstetric History. The provider will need to have a complete history of previous pregnancies. This will help to determine any risk factors for the current pregnancy. The following information should be included in the obstetric history (Fig. 31.6):
- Dates of deliveries
- Types of deliveries (vaginal or cesarean)
  - If cesarean, the type of incision should be noted
- Birth weight and gestational age of previous infants
- Complications of previous pregnancies

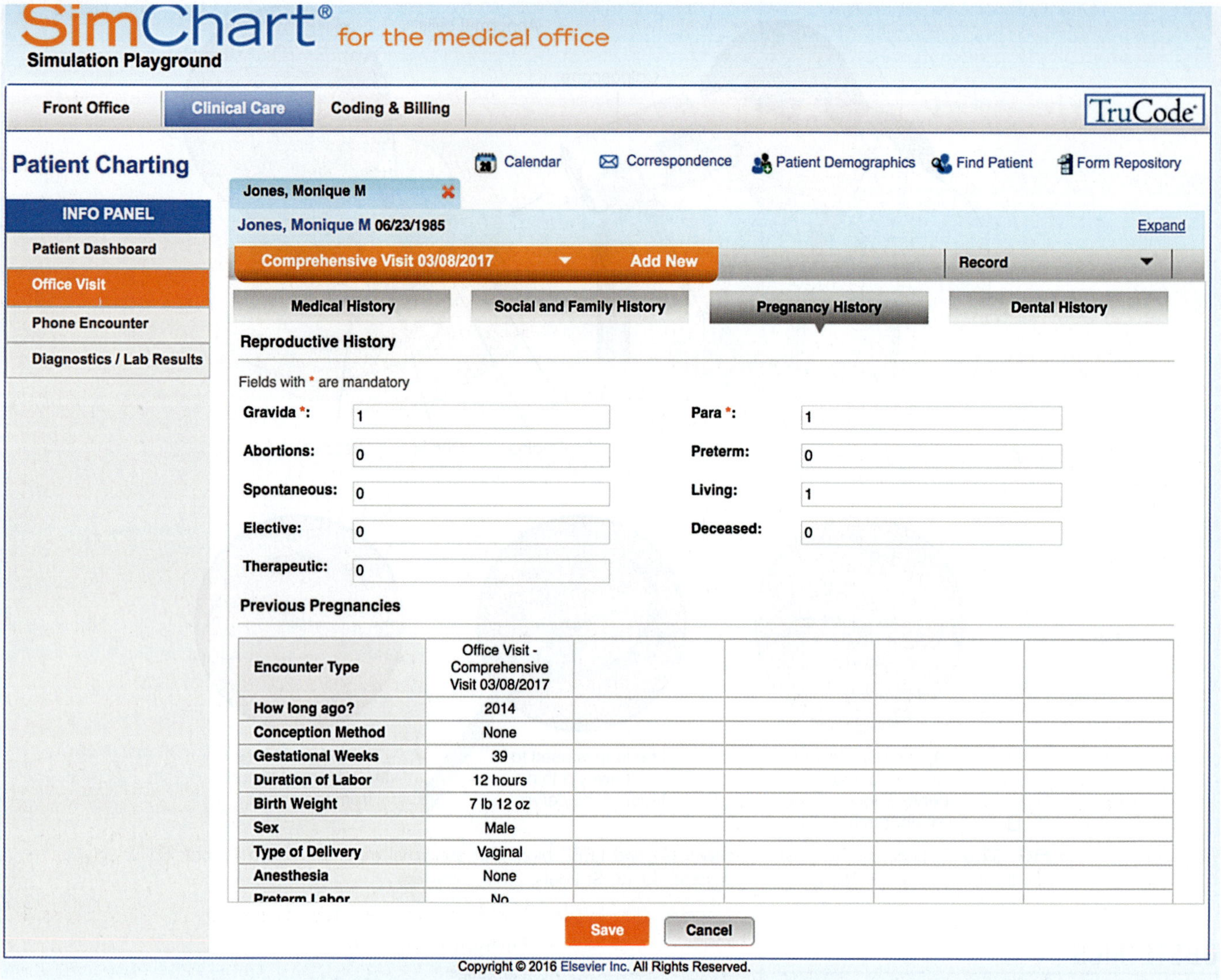

FIG. 31.6 Pregnancy history form from SimChart for the Medical Office.

There are some specific terms related to an obstetric history that you should be familiar with. Table 31.2 provides you with those terms and their definitions.

A prenatal record includes documenting the gravida, para, and abortion information. As a medical assistant, you should be able to determine those numbers after obtaining the obstetric history from a patient. It is important to remember that gravida and para refer to the number of pregnancies and not the number of babies. A twin pregnancy is considered just one pregnancy. If this was the first pregnancy for the patient and the pregnancy went to term (38 to 40 weeks), she would be gravida: 1 and para: 1.

> **MEDICAL TERMINOLOGY**
> -gravida: pregnancy
> par/o: giving birth
> primi-: first
> multi-: many
> nulli-: none

> **VOCABULARY**
> viability: Ability to live.

Medical and Surgical History. There are medical and surgical conditions that could affect a patient's current pregnancy. Common chronic conditions, such as diabetes, hypertension, asthma, and mitral valve prolapse, should be included in the prenatal record. The management of those conditions could change with pregnancy. Less common conditions, such as thyroid disorders, systemic lupus erythematosus, and bleeding disorders, can also affect the patient and the fetus. In order to help both, the provider needs to be aware of those conditions and the treatment that is being followed for each.

> **CRITICAL THINKING BOX 31.3**
> Jill is interviewing a new OB patient. The patient tells Jill that this is her fourth pregnancy, and she has two children. She had two early miscarriages. What would her gravida number be? What would her para number be? What would her abortion number be?

CHAPTER 31 Assisting With Obstetrics and Gynecology

TABLE 31.2 Obstetric History Terms

Term	Definition
gravida (GRAV i duh)	Number of pregnancies
primigravida (pree ma GRAV i duh)	A woman who is pregnant for the first time
multigravida (muhl ti GRAV i duh)	A woman who has been pregnant two or more times
nulligravida (nuh li GRAV i duh)	A woman who has never been pregnant
para (PEAR uh)	Number of pregnancies that have gone to the age of fetal viability (vahy uh BIL i tee) (20 weeks' gestation)
primipara (pree ma PEAR uh)	A woman who has carried one pregnancy to the age of fetal viability
multipara (muhl ti PEAR uh)	A woman who has carried two or more pregnancies to the age of fetal viability
nullipara (nuh li PEAR uh)	A woman who has not carried a pregnancy to the age of fetal viability
abortion (ah BOR shun)	Termination of a pregnancy before the fetal age of viability Miscarriage, spontaneous, elective
spontaneous abortion	Natural death of an embryo or fetus before the fetal age of viability. Also called a *miscarriage*
therapeutic or elective abortion	A procedure for the planned termination of a pregnancy
stillbirth	Fetal death after 20 weeks' gestation. Also called *intrauterine fetal death (IUFD)*

Certain infections can affect a pregnancy. A history of certain STIs can put the patient at risk for complications. Pelvic inflammatory disease (PID) can cause scarring of the fallopian tubes, which increases the risk of an ectopic (eck TAH pick) pregnancy. Genital herpes and other infections can be transmitted to the newborn during delivery. If the provider is aware of those conditions, plans can be made to protect both the mother and the baby.

If the patient has had any type of abdominal surgical procedure, it could affect the pregnancy and/or delivery. If there is a history of prior ectopic pregnancy, this would be a risk factor for another one. If there is a history of a uterine puncture or any uterine incision, the patient and provider will need to talk about a possible cesarean section.

Family and Social History. There are many conditions that have a genetic component to them. Obtaining an accurate family history can help to determine if the patient and/or the infant is at risk. With this knowledge, the patient and the provider can be prepared. Additional testing may be included during the prenatal period for a patient with certain factors in the family history. Conditions that could be of concern include:
- Diabetes
- Hypertension
- Heart disease
- Autoimmune disorders (e.g., lupus, rheumatoid arthritis)
- Kidney disease
- Seizures
- Depression
- Thyroid disease
- Preeclampsia (pree eh KLAMP see ah)

A family history of genetic disorders should also be documented in the patient's family history. These disorders could include the following:
- Down syndrome
- Neural (NYOOR al) tube defects (spina bifida [SPY nah BIF id dah], meningocele [meh NING goh seel], anencephaly [an en SEF uh lee])
- Hemophilia (hee moh FEE lee ah)
- Sickle cell anemia
- Cystic fibrosis (CF)
- Phenylketonuria (PKU)

> **MEDICAL TERMINOLOGY**
> - **-cele:** herniation, protrusion
> - **spin/o:** spine
> - **bi-:** two
> - **-fida:** split
> - **mening/o, meningi/o:** meninges
> - **encephala/o:** brain
> - **-y:** process of; condition
> - **hem/o:** blood
> - **-philia:** increase; condition of attraction

> **VOCABULARY**
> **anencephaly:** Congenital absence of part or all of the brain.
> **cystic fibrosis (CF):** A disorder that affects all the exocrine cells, but affects the respiratory system the most. Mucus is abnormally thick and blocks the alveoli, causing dyspnea.
> **Down syndrome:** A genetic disorder in which abnormal cell division results in an extra chromosome 21.
> **ectopic pregnancy:** Implantation of the embryo in any location other than the uterus.
> **hemophilia:** A group of inherited blood disorders characterized by a deficiency of one of the factors necessary for the coagulation of blood.
> **meningocele:** The protrusion of the meninges through an opening in the spinal column or skull.
> **phenylketonuria (PKU):** A deficiency in the enzyme phenylalanine hydroxylase, which is responsible for converting phenylalanine into tyrosine.
> **preeclampsia:** An abnormal condition of pregnancy of unknown cause, marked by hypertension, edema, and proteinuria.
> **sickle cell anemia:** An inherited anemia characterized by crescent-shaped red blood cells (RBCs). This causes RBCs to block capillaries, reducing the oxygen supply to the cells.
> **spina bifida:** A condition in which the spinal column has an abnormal opening that allows protrusion of the meninges and/or the spinal column.

Other family history information that should be noted would include a history of twins in the family, food allergies, and a family history of recurrent miscarriages or stillbirths.

The social history includes tobacco, alcohol, and recreational drug use. This information can be used for patient education as it relates to pregnancy. Nutrition and exercise are an important part of pregnancy. Finding out if the pregnant patient follows a particular diet, such as vegan or vegetarian, will provide the opportunity for patient education regarding the nutritional needs during pregnancy. Employment is also part of a social history. This can point out any occupational duties that could be affected by pregnancy, such as working with certain chemicals, or physical activities that should not be done when pregnant.

Collecting all of the components discussed previously is a great start to the patient's prenatal record, in addition to supplying the provider with the information needed to provide excellent care during the patient's pregnancy.

The prenatal record will continue to be updated throughout the pregnancy. There will be clinical data added at each prenatal visit. You will also be checking with the patient to see if there have been any changes or additions to the initial demographic and history information.

First Prenatal Examination

The physical examination during a first prenatal visit includes an overall assessment of the woman's health status. This would include vital signs, weight, and urinalysis. The medical assistant must prepare the patient. The patient should be asked if she needs to empty her bladder. If she does, she should collect a urine specimen for a routine urinalysis and a possible pregnancy test. The medical assistant should also prepare the exam room, ensuring that the supplies and equipment necessary to obtain pelvic measurements, perform serologic tests, and prepare for laboratory tests are available. The provider will assess the heart, lung, and thyroid. A physical examination will be done to rule out any other abnormalities. Next, the provider performs an obstetric examination that includes measurement of the height of the uterus and an internal or pelvic examination. A Pap test may be performed if one has not been done in the past year.

The estimated date of delivery or due date will be determined at this visit. There are a number of different ways to determine the due date. One method is using a gestational wheel (Fig. 31.7). With this method the arrow is lined up with the first date of the LMP, and the EDD is shown at the 40-week mark. The EDD may also be calculated by the electronic health record (EHR) or determined by ultrasound.

- Hematocrit and hemoglobin levels, to check for anemia.
- Blood type and Rh with antibody screening for possible Rh incompatibility.

A series of blood tests also is performed during the initial prenatal visit (Fig. 31.8 and Box 31.5). Prenatal blood and laboratory tests include the following:
- Rubella titer to determine whether the mother is immune to German measles; rubella infection during pregnancy can cause multiple birth defects, including deafness, vision disorders, and mental retardation.
- Syphilis screening; if the result is positive, antibiotic treatment is initiated to protect the fetus from congenital syphilis.
- Hepatitis B screening, because this virus can be passed to the fetus in utero.
- Human immunodeficiency virus (HIV) screening is suggested; if the result is positive, treatment of the mother greatly reduces the risk of transmission to the fetus.
- Gonorrhea and chlamydia cultures to prevent infection of the baby at birth.
- Urinalysis to detect protein, white blood cells, or glucose.

Any concerns that the patient has should be noted and reported to the provider. The medical assistant should be prepared to suggest community resources that can provide assistance to new parents, such as:
- Childbirth and parenting classes
- Infant cardiopulmonary resuscitation (CPR) courses
- Nutritional counseling, if needed
- Contact information for the Special Supplemental Nutrition Program for Women, Infants, and Children (WIC), which helps lower income expectant mothers get nutritious food

Return Prenatal Visits

The return prenatal visits follow a regular schedule:
- Every 4 weeks through 28 weeks' gestation
- Every 2 weeks through 35 weeks' gestation
- Every 1 week until delivery

In follow-up prenatal visits, the medical assistant should collect a urine specimen for urinalysis, weigh the patient, measure her blood pressure, and answer questions about diet and health habits. The mother should gain approximately 10 to 12 pounds in the first half of pregnancy and another 15 to 17 pounds during the second half. Experts believe that a healthy weight gain is somewhere between 25 and 35 pounds.

> ### BOX 31.5 Hemolytic Disease of the Newborn (HDN)
>
> To determine if someone's blood type is Rh positive or Rh negative, the blood is tested for the presence of D antigens. Rh-positive blood has D antigens present. Rh-negative blood does not. If the blood type with Rh factor shows that the mother has Rh-negative blood, there is a concern that hemolytic disease of the newborn (HDN) could develop if the fetus is Rh positive. HDN is also known as *erythroblastosis fetalis*. If the mother is Rh negative and her fetus is Rh positive, the mother will form antibodies to the Rh-positive factor. Future Rh-positive pregnancies will be in jeopardy because the mother's anti-Rh antibodies will cross the placenta and destroy fetal blood cells.
>
> HDN can be prevented by giving the mother Rh immune globulin products. RhoGAM, or anti-D immune globulin, is given at 28 to 30 weeks of gestation to Rh-negative mothers, regardless of the father's Rh type. After delivery, the cord blood is tested, and a dose of RhoGam is given within 72 hours of delivery only if the baby is Rh positive. RhoGam is also given for miscarriages or abortions. The immune globulin prevents the infant's Rh positive cells from stimulating the mothers immune system, thus preventing HDN.

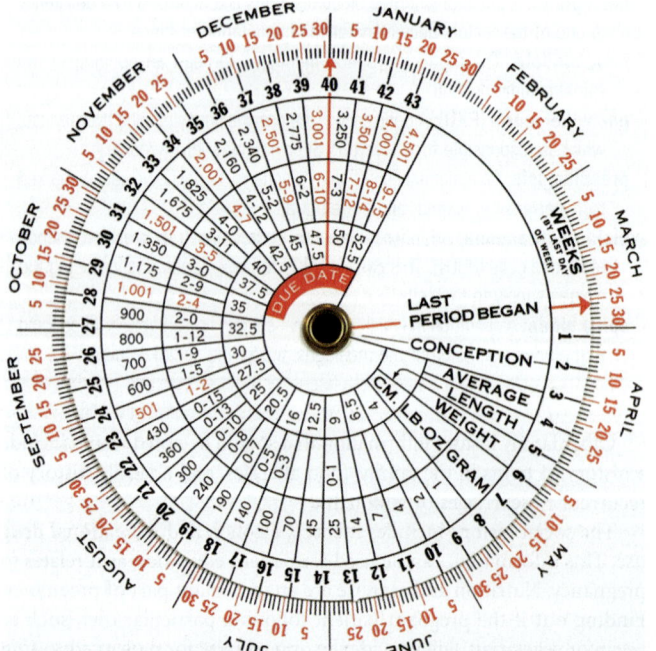

FIG. 31.7 Gestational wheel. (From Jarvis C: *Physical Examination And Health Assessment,* ed 6, St Louis, 2012, Saunders.)

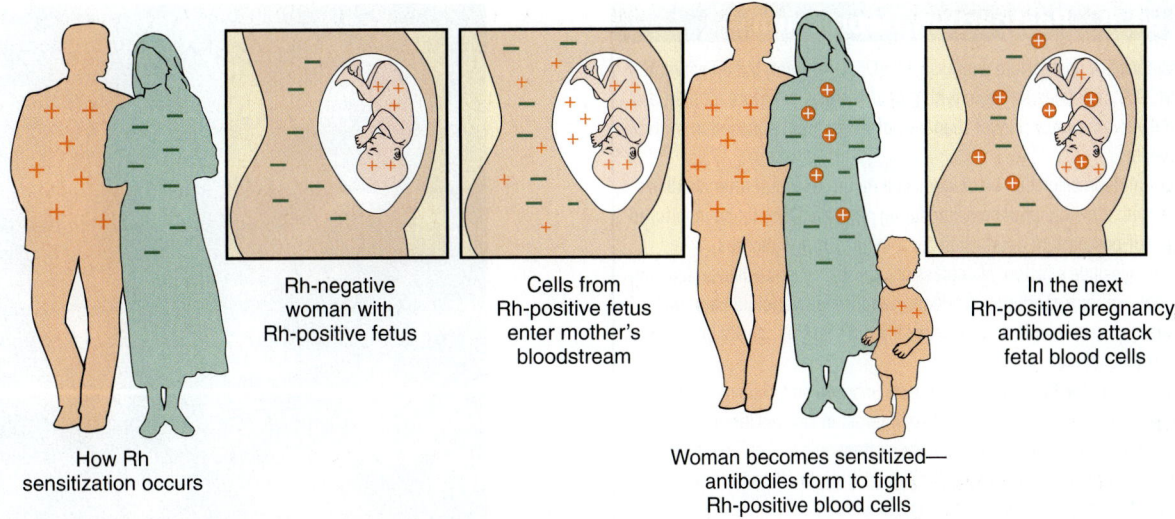

FIG. 31.8 Hemolytic disease of the newborn. (From Hagen-Ansert SL: *Textbook Of Diagnostic Sonography*, ed 7, St Louis, 2012, Mosby.)

Fetal Heart Tones. A Doppler monitor may be used to hear the baby's heart tones somewhere between 9 and 12 weeks' gestation. Once recorded, the fetal heart rate is assessed at each subsequent visit. It is important to remember that a fetal heart rate would be between 120 and 160 beats per minute. If you get a reading between 60 and 100 beats per minute, you may be assessing the patient's heart rate and not the fetal heart rate.

Fundal Height Measurement. Fundal height measurement is routinely done during the return prenatal visit. As the uterus grows during pregnancy, it will rise into the abdominal cavity. Between week 8 and week 13 the fundus (the top of the uterus) can be palpated above the symphysis pubis. The fundal height measurement is taken with a flexible tape measure, measuring from the symphysis pubis to the fundus of the uterus. The height is measured in centimeters (cm) and most often matches the number of weeks the patient has been pregnant. For example, if the patient is 25 weeks pregnant, the provider would expect to see a fundal height measurement of 25 cm (Fig. 31.9). This is only considered accurate for the first and second trimesters. If the fundal height measurement does not match the number of weeks pregnant, this could signal an issue with the pregnancy. Fundal height measurements that either are larger or smaller than expected could indicate:
- Slow fetal growth (intrauterine growth restriction)
- A significantly larger than average baby (*fetal macrosomia*)
- Too little amniotic fluid (*oligohydramnios* [oh lih goh hy DRAM nee ohs])
- Too much amniotic fluid (*polyhydramios* [paw lee hy DRAM nee ohs])

If the provider suspects an issue, an ultrasound would likely be ordered to determine what was causing the unusual measurements.

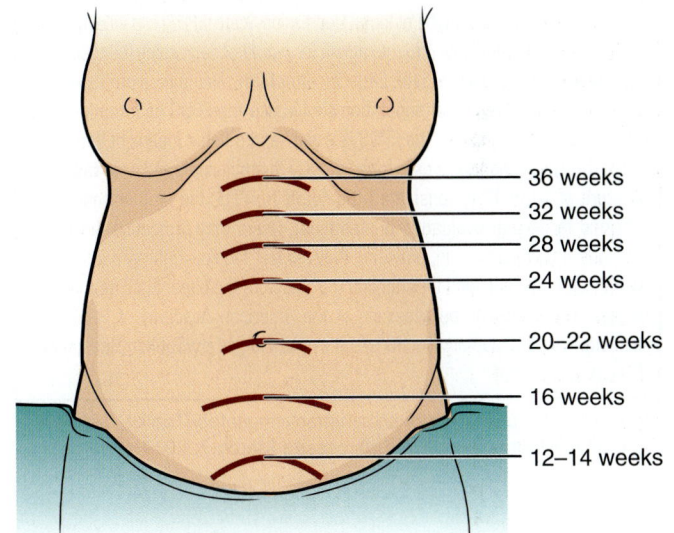

FIG. 31.9 Fundal height measurement.

Postpartum Visit

The patient should return about 6 weeks after delivery for a **postpartum** visit. At this visit, the provider will do a pelvic examination to make sure that everything is healing. If a cesarean section was done, the incision site also will be checked for healing. If the patient is interested in using contraceptives, the provider will talk about contraceptive choices. If a diaphragm had been used previously, the fit will need to be checked. There may also be discussion about how breast-feeding is going. Any of the patient's questions about care for the baby should be answered at this visit.

The postpartum visit is also an opportunity to see how the patient is doing emotionally. The provider will ask questions related to the patient's moods and check for signs of postpartum depression (Box 31.6).

The medical assistant should set up for this visit just as you would set up for a pelvic examination. You should also be aware of the patient's mood and body language. These can alert you to potential issues with postpartum depression. You should also have a list of provider-approved resources for the patient regarding postpartum depression and/or breast-feeding issues.

Special Tests and Procedures

Throughout the pregnancy, there are special tests and procedures that may done to assess the status of the pregnancy. In the next section we will explore some of the more common tests and procedures.

MEDICAL TERMINOLOGY
olig/o: scanty, few
hydr/o: water
-amnios: amnion, inner fetal sac
poly-: many, much, excessive, frequent

BOX 31.6 Postpartum Depression

- The incidence of postpartum depression (PPD) is not clear, but an estimated 10% to 20% of women struggle with major depression before, during, and after delivery of a baby. Fewer than half of these are diagnosed in routine office visits.
- Postpartum depression can be diagnosed a month to a year after childbirth. Women with a history of depression during pregnancy should be monitored for signs of postpartum depression for a minimum of 4 months.
- Risk factors include a history of depression, abuse, or mental illness; smoking or alcohol use; anxiety during pregnancy and fears over child care; lack of financial resources and secure relationships; a fussy or colicky infant; and lack of social support.
- Symptoms of postpartum depression include anorexia and insomnia; irritability and anger; overwhelming fatigue; loss of interest in sex and lack of a feeling of joy in life; feelings of shame, guilt, or inadequacy; severe mood swings; difficulty bonding with the baby; withdrawal from family and friends; and thoughts of harming herself or the baby.
- Postpartum depression must be detected as soon as possible so that treatment can begin; untreated postpartum depression may last for a year or longer. Treatment includes both counseling and antidepressant medication.

The 10-question Edinburgh Postnatal Depression Scale (EPDS) is a valuable and efficient way of identifying patients at risk for *perinatal* depression (between the 28th week of pregnancy and the 28th day after birth). Healthcare professionals working with the perinatal population should use the EPDS as a routine part of postnatal care, because the EPDS is a valid and reliable means of detecting PPD. This screening tool is user friendly, easy to administer, and easy to score. A score of 10 to 12 is considered the cutoff for PPD; the mother should be referred for further evaluation or treatment. Users may reproduce the scale without further permission, providing they respect the copyright by quoting the names of the authors and the title and the source of the paper in all reproduced copies. The EPDS can be accessed at the American Academy of Pediatrics website: www2.aap.org/sections/scan/practicingsafety/Toolkit_Resources/Module2/EPDS.pdf

From www2.aap.org/sections/scan/practicingsafety/Toolkit_Resources/Module2/EPDS.pdf. Accessed March 7, 2017.

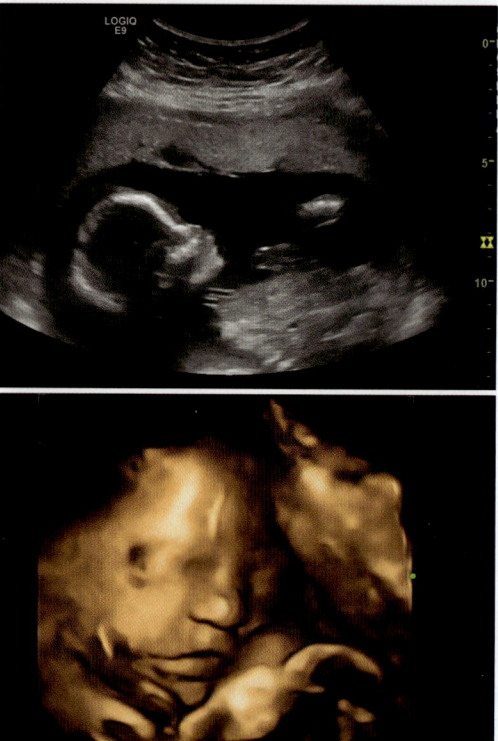

FIG. 31.10 Ultrasound of a fetus. (Courtesy Megan Pepper.)

Ultrasound. Ultrasound exams are typically done once during the first trimester and then again between weeks 18 and 20, in order to assess fetal development to confirm the age of the fetus and proper growth (Fig. 31.10). The gender of the baby can also be determined at that time. It is best if the patient has a full bladder for the ultrasound. The full bladder provides a great "window" for the sound waves to travel through, allowing for the best possible images. The patient should be instructed to drink two or three 8-ounce glasses of water 1 hour before the scheduled ultrasound.

Laboratory Testing. Between weeks 15 and 18 of pregnancy, the provider may suggest that the patient have a maternal blood screen, in order to detect any risk of fetal and chromosomal disorders. This could be a Triple Screen Test (also known as AFP Plus and Multiple Marker Screening) or a Quad Screen Test. Both tests screen for:
- alpha-fetoprotein (AFP)
- human chorionic gonadotropin (hCG)
- estriol

The Quad Screen also tests for inhibin-A. These tests are used to evaluate if there is an increased chance of certain chromosomal conditions, such as Down syndrome. The alpha-fetoprotein evaluates the chances of neural tube defects, such as spina bifida.

If the patient is at risk for gestational diabetes, the provider will likely order a glucose challenge test. Risk factors for gestational diabetes include:
- A body mass index (BMI) before pregnancy of 30 or higher
- Mother, father, sibling, or child with diabetes

For a glucose challenge test, the patient must drink a glucose solution. One hour later, a blood test will be done to measure the glucose level. A blood glucose level of 130 to 140 milligrams per deciliter (mg/dL) is considered normal. If the result is higher than that, a glucose tolerance test may be ordered. The glucose tolerance test involves having the patient fast overnight before coming in for a blood glucose reading. The patient will then drink another glucose solution and have her blood glucose level checked every hour for the next 3 hours. If two out of the three readings are higher than normal, the patient would be diagnosed with gestational diabetes.

Group B streptococcus is a common bacterium found in the intestines. It is usually harmless in adults, but in newborns it can cause group B strep disease. This is a serious illness for newborns. A group B streptococcus culture of the lower vagina can be performed between weeks 32 and 36. If the result is positive, the mother is treated with intravenous (IV) antibiotics to prevent fetal exposure during vaginal birth.

Amniocentesis. Amniocentesis involves needle aspiration of approximately 2 tablespoons of amniotic fluid after week 14 of pregnancy, in order to detect genetic and chromosomal abnormalities or inherited metabolic disorders (Fig. 31.11). Potential complications include:
- Miscarriage
- Fetal injury

MEDICAL TERMINOLOGY
post-: after, behind
-partum: parturition (delivery)

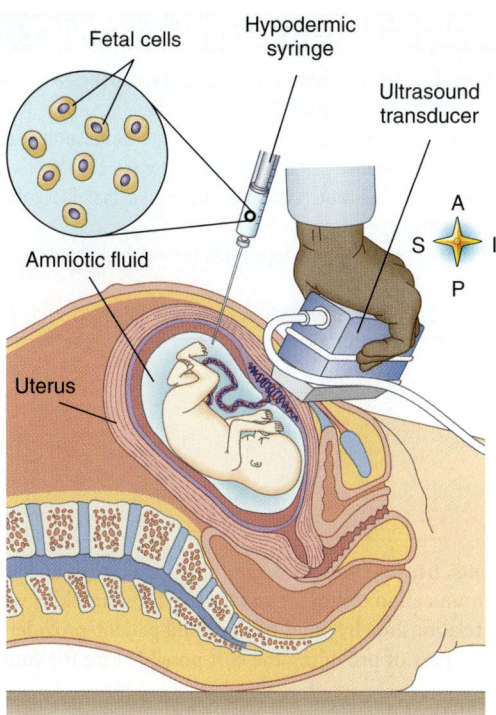

FIG. 31.11 Amniocentesis. (From Shiland B: *Mastering Healthcare Terminology*, St Louis, 2016, Elsevier.)

- Infection
- Premature labor
- Maternal hemorrhage

Results take up to 2 weeks.

Chorionic Villus Sampling (CVS). *Chorionic villi* are tiny placental projections, the cells of which have the same genetic material found in fetal cells. CVS involves the removal of a small piece of the chorionic villi, either transvaginally or through a small incision in the abdomen (Fig. 31.12). Cellular screening at 8 to 12 weeks' gestation provides early detection of genetic or chromosomal disorders. Potential complications include:

- Accidental abortion
- Infection, bleeding
- Fetal limb deformities

Results are available within several days.

Patient education is vital for a woman who is planning to become pregnant or has just discovered that she is pregnant. Box 31.7 presents important tips the medical assistant can provide to these women.

RECOGNIZING DOMESTIC ABUSE

There are federal laws in place that require that many insurance plans provide coverage for certain preventive health services without any cost-sharing for the patient. Included in the preventive health services is screening and counseling for interpersonal and domestic violence. Working in healthcare gives us an opportunity to provide support and resources for someone who is dealing with domestic violence. As a medical assistant, you should be looking for possible signs of abuse, such as:

- Unusual or frequent bruises or fractures
- Attempts to hide the bruises with makeup or clothing
- Low self-esteem
- Being extremely apologetic and meek
- References to the partner's temper

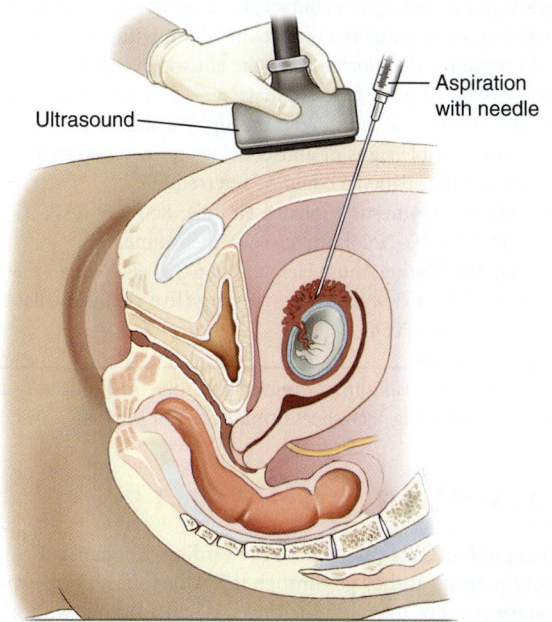

FIG. 31.12 Chorionic villus sampling (CVS). (From Shiland B: *Medical Terminology And Anatomy For ICD-10 Coding*, St Louis, 2012, Mosby.)

BOX 31.7 Patient Education: Obstetrics

A woman who is planning a pregnancy or who has just found out that she is pregnant may benefit from some simple guidelines for healthy living.

- *Nutrition:* Before pregnancy, emphasize the need for folic acid to prevent neural tube defects. The woman can take a supplement or can eat dark green, leafy vegetables. Many women have iron-deficiency anemia, and eating foods high in iron (red meat, spinach, or enriched cereal) is helpful. A pregnant woman must meet the calcium needs of both herself and her fetus; therefore, she needs about 1,000 mg of calcium a day. Most pregnant women should consume about 1,800 calories per day during the first trimester, 2,200 per day during the second trimester, and 2,400 calories per day during the third trimester. Women of average weight should gain 25 to 35 pounds, but underweight women should gain 35 to 45 pounds for a healthy infant.
- *Alcohol:* Alcohol passes through the placenta to the fetus and can cause serious problems. No one knows how much is safe, so it is a good idea for pregnant women to avoid alcohol completely.
- *Smoking:* Smoking can cause premature birth and low-birth-weight full-term infants. Smoking is linked to an increased risk of otitis media, heart problems, and upper respiratory infection in infants, and also to sudden infant death syndrome (SIDS). Pregnant women should not smoke and should not be exposed to secondhand smoke.
- *Medicine:* All chemicals pass through the placenta; therefore, a pregnant woman should never take any medicine (even over-the-counter drugs) without the knowledge and approval of her obstetrician. If the medical assistant is managing telephone screening, having a list of provider-approved medications next to the phone helps in answering patients' questions.
- *STI screening:* STI screening should be done before a woman becomes pregnant. Many STIs are asymptomatic in women but treatable. Infants are at risk for serious health problems if exposed to certain STIs in utero or during the birth process.

If you notice any of these signs, you should make the provider aware of them. Even a patient who shows no signs of abuse should be asked if he or she feels safe in the home.

The healthcare facility should put together a list of resources for patients who may be victims of domestic abuse. Having a list of shelters, advocacy groups, emergency contact phone numbers, and transportation services to give to patients may provide them with the resources they need to make the decision to leave the abusive situation.

Abuse does not just happen in marriages or committed relationships; it can also occur in a dating relationship. We should be observing all patients for possible signs of abuse. Below are two national help lines with websites that patients could be referred to[a]:

- National Domestic Violence Hotline: 800-799-SAFE (7233) or TTY 800-787-3224; https://www.thehotline.org
- National Dating Abuse Helpline: 866-331-9474 or TTY 866-331-8453; https://www.loveisrespect.org (live chat is available); text "loveis" to 77054

[a]https://www.womenshealth.gov/publications/our-publications/fact-sheet/screening-counseling-fact-sheet.html. Accessed March 7, 2017.

> **EXCEPTIONAL CUSTOMER SERVICE**
>
> To provide excellent customer service while working in obstetrics and gynecology, a medical assistant should do the following:
> - Behave in a professional manner at all times, because this can be an uncomfortable and embarrassing situation for the patient.
> - During patient education sessions, make sure that the patient truly understands the content.
> - Stay current with the new topics and technology related to obstetrics and gynecology.
> - Treat all patients as you would want to be treated.

CLOSING COMMENTS

Working in OB/GYN can be a very rewarding experience. Being there for your patients as they go through this sometimes trying experience can make it more tolerable for them. When working with obstetric patients, you have an opportunity to develop a strong relationship with your patients, because you are seeing them on a regular basis. Using good communication techniques and active listening skills will help to build that relationship. By building that solid patient-provider relationship, you are part of providing the best possible care for your patient.

CHAPTER REVIEW

Obstetrics and gynecology are very closely linked. Gynecology is the study of the female reproductive system. Obstetrics deals with pregnancy, labor, and the postpartum period. In order to sustain a pregnancy, the reproductive system needs to be healthy. The gynecologic examination, which includes a breast and pelvic examination, is done to determine if there are any abnormalities in the female reproductive system. The medical assistant is involved in the following ways:

- Setting up for the examination
- Preparing the patient for the examination
- Assisting the provider and patient during the examination
- Providing patient education as directed by the provider
- Processing specimens obtained during the examination
- Cleaning and restocking the examination room

During obstetric visits, the medical assistant has those same duties, with the addition of obtaining vital signs and other measurements.

Whether the patient is being seen for a gynecologic examination or an obstetric examination, the medical assistant has a duty to look for signs of abuse. If the medical assistant sees those signs, they must be reported to the provider.

As always, medical assistants have a duty to provide excellent customer service to all patients. This can be done by behaving in a professional manner, having resources available for all patients, and treating everyone (patients and coworkers) as you would want to be treated.

Medical Terminology in This Chapter

Word Part	Definition	Word Part	Definition
a-	without	necr/o	death, dead
-al	pertaining to	nulli-	none
-amnios	amnion, inner fetal sac	olig/o	scanty, few
an-	no, not, without	-osis	abnormal condition
-ation	process of	oste/o	bone
bi-	two	ovul/o	ovum
-cele	herniation, protrusion	par/o	giving birth
cephal/o	head	-partum	parturition (delivery)
colp/o	vagina	perine/o	perineum
cry/o	extreme cold	-philia	increase; condition of attraction
encephal/o	brain	poly-	many, much, excessive, frequent
-fida	split	por/o	passage
-gravida	pregnancy	post-	after, behind
hem/o	blood	primi-	first
hydr/o	water	-rrhea	discharge
men/o	menses	-scopy	process of viewing
mening/o, meningi/o	meninges	spin/o	spine
micro-	small	-therapy	treatment
multi-	many	-y	condition; process of

SCENARIO WRAP-UP

Jill Snow has enjoyed her time in the OB/GYN department and has learned a lot from Peggy. She was able to observe several procedures and saw how Peggy prepped the patient and the exam room for those procedures. Peggy has been an amazing mentor for Jill. She has taken the time to explain the reasons for how each procedure is done. Peggy's knowledge and expertise in OB/GYN along with her willingness to teach others has made Jill decide to pursue a position in this field after she graduates. Peggy's supervisor recognizes her talents in this area and has asked her to take over the practicum program for their department.

32

Assisting in Pediatrics

LEARNING OBJECTIVES

1. Describe childhood growth patterns.
2. Discuss developmental patterns and therapeutic approaches for infants, toddlers, preschoolers, school-aged children, and adolescents.
3. Describe various developmental theories.
4. List and describe common pediatric diseases and disorders.
5. Discuss the current immunization schedule for children from newborn to 18 years old. Also, detail guidelines for childhood immunization, and document immunizations.
6. Do the following related to the pediatric patient:
   - Describe how the Apgar scoring system works.
   - List the recommendations of the American Academy of Pediatrics when it comes to the frequency of well-child visits.
- Discuss sick-child visits, as well as important questions for telephone screening of an older child who can communicate symptoms.
7. Describe the medical assistant's role in pediatric procedures, including measuring the circumference of an infant's head. Citing reference ranges for pediatric vital signs should be the last thing listed here as measuring an infant's length and weigh should be after measuring the circumference of an infant's head.
8. Discuss the unique challenges and needs of the adolescent patient.
9. Specify child safety guidelines for injury prevention and management of suspected child abuse.

CHAPTER OUTLINE

1. **Opening Scenario, 722**
2. **You Will Learn, 722**
3. **Introduction, 722**
4. **Normal Growth and Development, 723**
    a. Growth Patterns, 723
    b. Developmental Patterns, 723
    c. Developmental Theories, 725
5. **Pediatric Diseases and Disorders, 725**
    a. Colic, 725
    b. Diarrhea, 725
    c. Failure to Thrive, 726
    d. Obesity, 726
    e. Otitis Media, 726
6. **Immunizations, 727**
7. **The Pediatric Patient, 729**
    a. Well-Child Visits, 729
    b. Sick-Child Visits, 733
8. **The Medical Assistant's Role in Pediatric Procedures, 733**
    a. Measurements, 734
    b. Assisting with the Examination, 734
    c. Obtaining a Urine Sample, 739
9. **The Adolescent Patient, 739**
10. **Injury Prevention, 739**
11. **Child Abuse, 740**
12. **Closing Comments, 741**
13. **Chapter Review, 741**

▶ OPENING SCENARIO

Allison Kwong, CMA (AAMA), who has 2 years of experience, has accepted a new position with the pediatric department of the Walden-Martin Family Medical Clinic (WMFM). Allison's primary responsibility will be to assist in the clinical area, but she also will have to rotate through the message screening center in the office. Office policy states that telephone screening employees should manage problems as much as possible. However, if patient callbacks are needed, they are to be referred to the provider on call that day by noon for morning calls and no later than 5 p.m. for afternoon calls. Although Allison has worked in the healthcare field for 2 years, she does not have much experience with pediatrics. She is glad that she has been assigned a mentor for the first few weeks.

YOU WILL LEARN

- To recognize expected growth and developmental patterns.
- What conditions should be seen right away.
- To understand the Centers for Disease Control and Prevention (CDC) schedule of immunizations.
- The importance of Vaccine Information Statements (VISs).
- What needs to be documented when immunizations are given.
- How to assist the provider during a pediatric examination.

INTRODUCTION

Pediatrics (pee dee A triks) is the medical specialty that deals with the development and care of children and with the treatment of childhood diseases. Pediatric patients range in age from newborn to puberty. Some practices continue to see the child until he or she graduates from high school. Subspecialties within pediatrics include surgery, cardiology, and psychiatry.

Approximately 50% of the patients in a pediatric office are there for well-baby or well-child visits. The roles of the provider and the medical office staff are to supervise and help maintain the health of these patients. The medical assistant can help by encouraging therapeutic communication among the patient, parents, caregivers, and medical staff. The trust that a child develops in these relationships and the consideration the family receives in the provider's office form the basis of good medical care.

Pediatric care actually starts before the child is born, with good prenatal care. The confidence and enthusiasm of the parents can have a significant impact on an infant's physical and emotional well-being.

NORMAL GROWTH AND DEVELOPMENT

The terms *growth* and *development* are often used together. They refer to the combination of changes a child goes through as he or she matures. *Growth* refers to measurable changes, such as height and weight. The first determinant of these physical characteristics is the genetics inherited from the parents; however, a child's growth can be influenced by many factors, including nutritional status, environmental factors, and the presence of disease. *Development* refers to the stages of physical, cognitive, and social growth. A provider looks at how the child is progressing in motor, mental, social, and language skills. A child's development is determined by a combination of prenatal, environmental, and caregiver factors. Each child has his or her own pattern of growth and development. Pediatric assessments are individualized for each child according to age, developmental level, health condition, family characteristics, and past experiences with healthcare professionals. National standards are used to help pinpoint irregularities in growth and development. The child's physical, intellectual, and social levels are compared with the published national standards. This comparison indicates whether the child is at the appropriate stage of growth and development for his or her chronologic age.

Growth Patterns

Physical growth is one of the most visible changes in childhood. The average birth weight is 7 to 7½ pounds, and in 6 months, the baby's birth weight doubles. Growth then slows slightly over the next 6 months and even more over the next couple of years (Table 32.1). Between ages 2 and 3 most children slim down, so that by the time the third birthday arrives, the potbellied toddler has become the characteristic preschooler.

By age 4, the child usually has doubled the birth length. During this time, the legs are the fastest growing part; fatty connective tissue continues to increase slowly until approximately age 7. This same growth rate continues through the school-aged period (6 to 12 years), and as this period of development ends, the child usually is into a growth spurt that indicates impending puberty.

The growth spurt continues for approximately 2 years, and the child then reaches *adolescence* (ages 12 to 18 years). During this period, the adolescent gains almost half of his or her adult weight, and the skeleton and organs double in size. Weight increases in girls by 20 to 25 pounds and in boys by 15 to 20 pounds. Girls grow 5 to 6 inches, and boys grow 4 to 5 inches. As the growth spurt is completed, the teenager reaches sexual maturity. In girls, sexual maturity is signaled by the onset of the menstrual cycle; in boys, it is determined by the presence of sperm in the semen. The timing of sexual maturity in both genders varies greatly.

Skeletal growth is complete in girls between 15 and 16 years of age and in boys between ages 17 and 18. Skeletal growth is considered complete when the growth plates (epiphyseal [eh PIFF ih see uhl] plates) of the long bones of the extremities have completely fused.

> **VOCABULARY**
> **epiphyseal plate:** A thin layer of cartilage located at the ends of a long bone where new bone forms.

Growth charts are used to compare the child's individual growth pattern with national standards. The CDC has developed growth charts that can track growth continuously through the age of 20. The growth charts are gender specific. Length, weight, and head circumference are tracked on the birth-to-36-months growth chart. Stature and weight are tracked on the 2-to-20-years growth chart. There are also CDC growth charts for body mass index (BMI) for infants and young adults 2 to 20 years of age, giving providers another weapon in the fight against childhood obesity. BMI for adults was discussed in Chapter 30, Physical Examination. BMI is a means of assessing the relationship between height and weight. BMI conversion charts typically are available, or they are calculated automatically in electronic health record (EHR) programs. The actual formula to calculate is:

$$BMI = \frac{Weight\ (kg)}{Height\ (m)^2}$$

For adults, the BMI itself is used as the screening tool. In pediatrics, the BMI needs to be plotted on the gender-specific growth chart, and the growth chart percentile is the screening tool. The CDC has developed four weight status categories (Box 32.1).

Developmental Patterns

General patterns of child development occur rapidly during the first year of life (Box 32.2) as the infant progresses from reflex activities (e.g., grasping fingers and sucking) to learning to manipulate simple

TABLE 32.1	Early Childhood Growth Patterns
6 months	birth weight doubles
1 year	birth weight triples, length increased by 50%
2 years	gains 6 pounds in 1 year
3 years	gains 3–5 pounds in 1 year and grows 2–2½ inches
3–6 years	gains 3–5 pounds per year, grows 1½–2½ inches per year

BOX 32.1 CDC Weight Status Categories	
Weight Status Category	**Percentile Range**
Underweight	Less than the 5th percentile
Normal or Healthy Weight	5th percentile to less than the 85th percentile
Overweight	85th percentile to less than the 95th percentile
Obese	Equal to or greater than the 95th percentile

Source: https://www.cdc.gov/healthyweight/assessing/bmi/childrens_bmi/about_childrens_bmi.html. Accessed July 13, 2017.

> **BOX 32.2 Therapeutic Approaches for Infants (Newborn to 12 Months)**
>
> - Crying is normal; use distraction, but do not overstimulate.
> - It is important to keep the infant close to the caregiver; either have the parent hold the infant, or keep the parent in the child's line of vision.
> - Involve the parent as much as possible, depending on the task and the parent's level of comfort.
> - Place a familiar object near the infant, and keep frightening ones out of view.
> - An infant's negative response to strangers usually develops at approximately 8 months; do not take the rejection personally.
> - Do not restrain the infant any more than necessary, but be ready to use restraint at times (e.g., when giving an injection) to keep the infant safe.
> - Encourage the caregiver to cuddle and hug the child after the procedure is complete.
> - Unpleasant procedures are associated with other objects, so do not use play areas for treatment, and do not use a favorite toy or object during the procedure; offer it afterward for comfort.

> **BOX 32.3 Therapeutic Approaches for Toddlers and Preschoolers (2 to 6 Years)**
>
> - Toddlers and preschoolers often fear visits to the doctor; ignore temper tantrums and negative behavior.
> - Praise the child as much as possible.
> - Perform unpleasant procedures as quickly as possible; the fear of the procedure is worse than the actual discomfort.
> - Allow the child to keep on as much clothing as possible for security and comfort.
> - Use words familiar to the child, and do not use words the child could misinterpret. For example, "The test uses dye" (the child may think you mean "die"); "The doctor will put you to sleep so it doesn't hurt" (the family dog may have been put to sleep).
> - Explain a procedure as the child would sense it; that is, what it will look like, how it will smell, how it will feel, and so on.
> - Allow the child to handle equipment when possible.
> - Do not use the child's favorite doll or stuffed animal to demonstrate; the child may believe the toy feels pain.
> - Explain procedures to the parents away from the child when possible; the child may misinterpret the information.

> **BOX 32.4 Therapeutic Approaches for School-Aged Children (7 to 11 Years)**
>
> - Allow choices when possible, such as which arm to use for an injection.
> - A parent or caregiver should always be present during examinations.
> - Remove only as much clothing as needed for the examination or procedure.
> - Explain procedures in concrete terms; use pictures and diagrams when possible.
> - Give the child time to ask questions.
> - School-aged children often are curious, and they can be cooperative if they know what is expected of them.
> - Address the conversation to the child; involve the child in decision making as much as possible.
> - Provide privacy.

Verbal communication has increased to full simple and even complex sentences but remains quite literal. For example, if you tell a preschool child that you are going to fly to visit Aunt Sue, the child thinks you are going to flap your arms and fly. Nonverbal communication skills are also being mastered. The vocabulary now includes more than 2,000 words. During this period, children need to develop social skills, such as sharing and taking part in peer group activities.

> **CRITICAL THINKING BOX 32.1**
>
> Allison receives a call from the mother of a 6-month-old child. The woman is concerned that her child may not be reaching his developmental milestones. What type of information about the child's growth and development should Allison gather? If Allison is unable to answer the mother's questions, what should she do?
>
> Based on what you have learned about therapeutic approaches for the pediatric patient, what would be the best way to deal with the following patient situations?
>
> 1. A crying 3-month-old being seen for a well-child visit
> 2. A 10-month-old with otitis media
> 3. A 2-year-old who needs the dressing changed on an infected wound
> 4. A 5-year-old scheduled for vision and hearing screening
> 5. An 8-year-old who needs a throat culture to rule out a strep infection
> 6. A 12-year-old who needs a penicillin injection in the dorsogluteal site
> 7. A 15-year-old girl who complains of abdominal pain and is accompanied by her mother

objects (e.g., pulling open drawers or throwing toys out of the crib). In addition to these motor skills, the child learns verbal patterns, progressing from cooing and crying for attention to speaking his or her first words.

By age 3, the child is showing increased autonomy (aw TON uh mee). Now the child can walk, is toilet trained, sits at the table and eats with the family, can make simple sentences, understands the word "No," and even imitates the parent by using verbal gestures that he or she has seen used. The child's vocabulary consists of up to 900 words.

> **VOCABULARY**
> **autonomy:** The ability to function independently.

During the preschool stage, the child becomes increasingly independent and initiates activities (Box 32.3). Preschoolers have mastered many gross motor skills and are perfecting their fine motor development.

School-aged children have perfected fine motor skills and can paint, draw, and play an instrument (Box 32.4). They enjoy team activities and are expanding their reading and writing skills. Their intellectual skills are developing, and social skills are going through refinement as a sense of self-achievement and self-worth is developed. During this time, the child learns and tests the rules for socializing outside the immediate family as an independent individual.

Adolescence, or the transition stage, is the time when the individual attempts to establish an adult identity. The teenager proceeds by trial and error, experimenting with adult roles and behavior patterns (Box 32.5). Traditional values learned in childhood may be questioned, and peer relationships take on new importance. During this time teenagers must develop the emotional maturity and motivation to make reasonable decisions. They look to family members for encouragement and guidance in making decisions that will help them develop self-confidence and to become patient, in addition to less impulsive and self-centered.

> **BOX 32.5 Therapeutic Approaches for Adolescents (12 to 18 Years)**
>
> - Adolescents are self-conscious and strongly influenced by peers.
> - Privacy is very important to them.
> - Address how a procedure might affect the adolescent's appearance.
> - Do not be judgmental; listen without condemning.
> - Encourage the adolescent to verbalize his or her concerns and fears.
> - The adolescent may regress to more childish behaviors when sick.
> - Teenagers want to be treated as adults; they want to know what is being done and why.
> - To promote honest discussion about lifestyle issues, encourage the teenager to see the provider without the parent present.

Developmental Theories

Psychologists have been researching and developing theories about human behavior since the beginning of the 20th century. Erik Erikson, a developmental psychologist, expanded on Sigmund Freud's work. Erikson's theory recognizes the cultural and social influences on individual development. His theory is based on stages of development that the individual must pass through and master. Each stage focuses on a developmental crisis, starting in infancy and ending in old age. According to Erikson, the following are the stages that children must master:

- *Trust versus mistrust:* Infants learn to rely on caregivers; mistrust occurs if needs are not met.
- *Autonomy versus shame and doubt:* Toddlers learn language skills and gain independence; they may feel shame and doubt if they cannot meet parental expectations or are overprotected.
- *Initiative versus guilt:* Preschoolers actively seek out new experiences; children become hesitant if restrictions or reprimands make them feel guilty or afraid to try more challenging skills.
- *Industry versus inferiority:* School-aged children enjoy finishing projects and receiving recognition; they develop feelings of inferiority if not accepted by peers or if they cannot please their parents.
- *Identity versus role confusion:* Adolescents face many physical and hormonal changes in this stage. Teenagers work at figuring out who they are and where they fit; they are looking for a direction for their lives. If they are unable to establish an identity and sense of direction, they become role confused.

When working in pediatrics, it can be helpful to understand Erikson's stages and how you can help someone master those stages.

PEDIATRIC DISEASES AND DISORDERS

The disease process in pediatric patients poses special problems, because children are constantly changing both physically and functionally. As a child grows and develops, the immune system matures, and with the aid of routine prophylactic immunizations, the child acquires long-term protection against certain infectious diseases.

Colic

Colic usually is seen in the newborn period or in early infancy. The problem is intermittent. The classic situation is an infant between 2 weeks and 4 months of age who has crying episodes that occur at least three times a week for longer than 3 hours a day and lasting 3 weeks. During an attack, the infant draws up the legs, clenches the fists, and cries inconsolably. The abdominal distress of colic usually occurs in the late afternoon and evening. Many theories have been suggested for why infants have colic, but none has been proven correct. If the baby is fed infant formula, physicians recommend switching formulas to a non–cow's milk type, because this may help relieve the infant's discomfort. Treatment consists of determining the cause; however, the child frequently outgrows the condition before the causative agent can be identified. Drugs have not been found to be helpful. Parents need reassurance that they are not responsible for the child's discomfort, and they may find counseling and assistance in developing coping techniques helpful.

Diarrhea

Diarrhea can be caused by a variety of microorganisms, including bacteria, viruses, and parasites. However, children sometimes can have diarrhea without having an infection. It could be caused by food allergies or by certain medications, such as antibiotics. Diarrhea is diagnosed when the child has two or more watery or apparently abnormal stools within 24 hours. The child may not show other signs of illness or may have nausea, vomiting, stomach ache, headache, or fever. If the diarrhea continues for longer than 2 days, medical intervention is needed. Prolonged diarrhea can cause dehydration and electrolyte imbalance because of excessive fluid loss. In addition, diarrhea can cause diaper rash and excoriation (ik skawr ee EY shun n), which can be very painful.

> **CRITICAL THINKING BOX 32.2**
>
> Allison receives a call from the grandmother of a 3-year-old child who has had diarrhea since last night. What are some questions Allison should ask to determine the seriousness of the problem? Should the child be seen today, even though appointments are already overbooked?

Pediatric diarrhea needs to be followed closely. In the case of bloody stools, laboratory analysis should be ordered to determine the cause. If the patient is an infant or small child, a follow-up telephone call should be made after 12 hours and then daily until the diarrhea has stopped. Parents should know the indications of dehydration:

- lack of tears when crying
- lethargy (LETH er jee)
- fewer wet diapers or decreased urination
- dry mouth and lips
- weight loss

The provider may recommend the use of oral rehydration therapy, such as Pedialyte or Infalyte; small amounts (approximately 2 tablespoons) are offered at a time (i.e., every 15 minutes) to prevent vomiting. Soft drinks, juices, sports drinks, and tea should be avoided because they lack electrolytes and may lead to even more diarrhea. Parents should be informed that the child's diarrhea may not stop when the child is given oral rehydration therapy, but the fluids prevent the child from becoming dehydrated. It is important to continue to feed the child because lack of food can damage the villi in the small intestine. If breast-fed, the baby should continue to nurse because breast milk is shown to protect the gastrointestinal lining.

> **VOCABULARY**
>
> **excoriation:** Inflammation and irritation of the skin.
> **lethargy:** The state of being drowsy and dull, listless and unenergetic.

The banana, rice, applesauce, and toast (BRAT) diet has been the traditional approach for children with diarrhea, but it is no longer recommended because there is no evidence that it is useful. In fact, the poor protein content of the BRAT diet may contribute to continued diarrhea and poor nutrition. Providers now recommend that children resume their prediarrhea diet as soon as possible so that they continue to eat something they prefer while the intestine heals. Probiotics found in certain yogurt products can also be helpful in stabilizing the child while the intestinal tract gets back to normal. The child should not be given over-the-counter (OTC) antidiarrheal medications, such as Pepto-Bismol, Kaopectate, Imodium, or Lomotil, because these can cause serious side effects, including decreased motility of the bowel, respiratory depression, and drowsiness. The provider may prescribe antibiotics if stool cultures test positive for pathogens. Children with severe dehydration require hospitalization and intravenous (IV) hydration to replace electrolytes and fluids.

Failure to Thrive

Failure to thrive refers to children whose current weight or rate of weight gain is much lower than that of other children of similar age and gender. It is a symptom more than a disease. An infant or a young child whose weight is consistently below the 3rd percentile on standardized growth charts, or who is 20% below the ideal body weight for length, may be diagnosed with failure to thrive. Physical, mental, and social skills also are delayed in these children. This could include failure to roll over, smile, coo, stand, or walk at age-appropriate developmental levels. Failure to thrive can be caused by a physiologic factor (e.g., malabsorption disease or cleft palate), or it may be related to a problem with the parent-child relationship. The provider needs an accurately recorded history of the child's birth weight and subsequent length, weight, and head circumference measurements. A comprehensive family history is important to rule out genetic growth abnormalities or a history of malabsorption problems, such as cystic fibrosis or celiac disease.

Children with failure to thrive need more calories than usual – approximately 150% of their normal calorie load – to catch up to their target weight. Both medical and social factors are evaluated in the treatment of children with this problem. Experts believe that infants may suffer from this problem if they are being neglected; however, low weight gains also are possible with extremely attentive and cautious parents. The family must be considered as a whole to treat nonorganic (nahn or GAN ik) causes effectively. Treatment may include the use of support groups and parental counseling.

Obesity

Just as with adult weight patterns, children are assessed according to their BMI. A child's level of body fat varies as the child grows; for example, children normally slim down as they reach school age, and very often their weight increases as they mature from adolescence to adulthood. In addition, body fat levels vary between boys and girls as they reach puberty. Providers use growth charts that plot the child's BMI-for-age to determine whether the child's weight, in comparison with height, is within healthy limits (see Box 32.1). Obesity now affects nearly 20% of all children and adolescents in the United States. Children who are overweight or obese as preschoolers are five times as likely as normal-weight children to be overweight or obese as adults. Studies have shown that a child who is obese between the ages of 10 and 13 has an 80% chance of becoming an obese adult.

The reasons for childhood obesity vary; they include a family history of obesity, inactivity, high-calorie diets, and stress. In rare cases, childhood obesity may be caused by metabolic or endocrine disorders. Overweight and obese children are at greater risk of developing serious health conditions, including asthma, diabetes mellitus type 2, sleep apnea, and hypercholesterolemia, which increases the risk of cardiovascular disease and hypertension. The psychosocial impact of obesity can be overwhelming for many children because isolation, loneliness, and lack of self-esteem are common. The provider can provide assistance by recommending a comprehensive diet and exercise program that emphasizes healthy living. The medical assistant can help by providing educational materials, encouragement for the child and parents, and referral to community education and support programs.

Otitis Media

Infection or inflammation of the middle ear usually is a side effect of a cold or other upper respiratory tract disorder, but it also can be caused by allergies. Otitis media (OM) usually occurs in children younger than

> ### CRITICAL THINKING BOX 32.3
> Juanita Johnston is a 12-year-old patient who was recently diagnosed as being obese. You are asked to help Juanita and her mother access online information about healthy nutrition options. What websites would be most appropriate for Juanita and her family? What other community resources can you recommend to support the family in making healthier nutrition decisions?

3 years of age. Signs include inflammation of the middle ear, with fluid building up behind the tympanic membrane. The child may cry persistently, tug at the ear, have a fever, be irritable, and have diminished hearing in the affected ear. These symptoms sometimes may be accompanied by diarrhea, nausea, and vomiting.

Otitis media is classified as either serous (SEER uh s) (Fig. 32.1) or suppurative (SUHP yuh rey tiv) (Fig. 32.2), depending on the fluid in the middle ear. In Fig. 32.2, pus is in the middle ear and shows up as white in the image. Because otitis media may be caused by bacteria or a virus, determining the most appropriate treatment can be difficult.

> **VOCABULARY**
> **nonorganic:** Not having an organic or physiologic cause; a disorder that does not have a cause that can be found in the body.
> **serous:** A thin, watery serum-like drainage.
> **suppurative:** Characterized by the formation and/or discharge of pus.

In 2013 the American Academy of Pediatrics (AAP) and the American Academy of Family Physicians (AAFP) released an updated clinical practice guideline for the diagnosis and management of otitis media

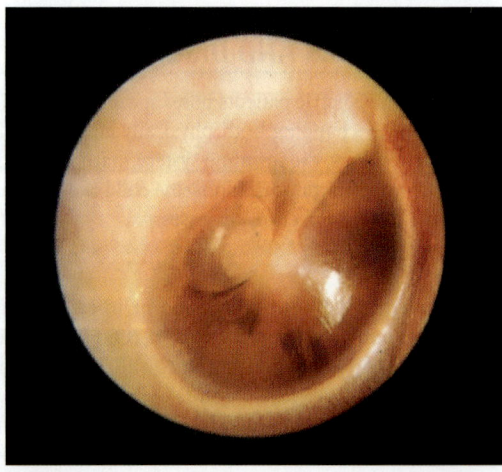

FIG. 32.1 Serous otitis media. (From Swartz MH: *Textbook of Physical Diagnosis*, ed 5, Philadelphia, 2006, Saunders.)

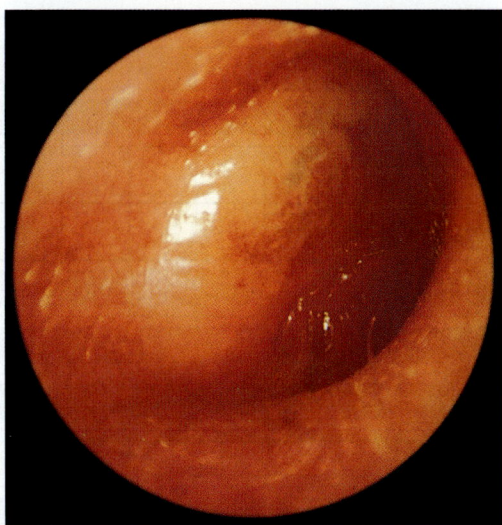

FIG. 32.2 Suppurative otitis media. (Courtesy of Dr. Michael Hawke, MD. From Zitelli BJ, Davis HW: *Atlas of Pediatric Physical Diagnosis*, ed 5, St Louis, 2007, Mosby.)

> **BOX 32.6 Common Childhood Diseases**
>
> - Conjunctivitis – also called *pinkeye*, is a common infection in children and is highly contagious, especially in day care centers and schools. It can be caused by a bacterial or viral infection that produces white or yellowish pus, which may cause the eyelids to stick shut in the morning.
> - Fifths disease – also called *erythema infectiosum, parvovirus infection,* or *slapped cheek disease,* is an infection caused by parvovirus B19. Outbreaks are most common in the winter and spring. Symptoms begin with a mild fever and general malaise. After a few days, the cheeks take on a flushed appearance, making the face look as if it has been slapped. A lacy rash also may be seen on the trunk, arms, and legs, but not all those infected develop the rash.
> - Hand-foot-and-mouth disease – caused by the coxsackievirus, which is transmitted by direct contact with nose and throat drainage, saliva, or the stool of an infected individual. The disease is seen most often in day care settings, where children can easily come in contact with infected bodily secretions. Symptoms include a combination of fever; sore throat; painful red blisters on the tongue, mouth, palms, and soles; headache; anorexia; and irritability (Fig. 32.3).
> - Reye's syndrome – the cause of Reye's syndrome is unknown, but the disorder has been linked to the use of aspirin during a viral illness. Reye's syndrome is an acute and sometimes fatal illness characterized by fatty invasion of the inner organs, especially the liver, and swelling of the brain. It most often is seen in children from infancy through puberty (age 16). Prevention is the best treatment, which means children up to age 14 should never be given aspirin unless prescribed by a provider for a chronic condition such as juvenile rheumatoid arthritis.

in children age 6 months to 12 years. Antibiotics (typically amoxicillin or azithromycin [Zithromax]) should be prescribed for children 6 months or older who have severe signs and symptoms. Antibiotics can also be prescribed for patients under 24 months of age who are experiencing nonsevere bilateral infections. However, in children over 6 months with nonsevere symptoms, observation and a follow-up within 48 to 72 hours before initiating antibiotics may be offered to assess patient improvement. If no improvement is noticed or symptoms have worsened, antibiotic therapy should be started. In all cases, if the child has not improved in 48 to 72 hours, the current antibiotic should be switched. Because antibiotics do not provide immediate relief from symptoms, children can be given oral acetaminophen and/or ibuprofen for pain relief.

If fluid in the middle ear persists for longer than 3 months and/or if the child experiences hearing loss, the provider may recommend a *myringotomy*; in this operation, a small incision is made in the tympanic membrane and a tube is inserted to drain the fluid and balance the pressure between the outer and middle ear. The tube typically stays in the eardrum for 6 to 12 months and falls out as the child grows.

Other common childhood diseases are discussed in Box 32.6. Autism spectrum disorder is discussed in Box 32.7.

IMMUNIZATIONS

Over the years, immunizations have helped dramatically reduce potentially lethal childhood infections. Fig. 32.4 shows the 2017 immunization schedule from the CDC for children 0 through 18 years of age. All of the immunization schedules can be found at the CDC's website: http://www.cdc.gov/vaccines/schedules/downloads/child/0-18yrs-child-combined-schedule.pdf.

The schedules are updated periodically as new vaccines become available and/or research indicates a better method for giving the vaccine. The CDC recommends immunization against infectious diseases for all children, except those for whom a particular vaccination would pose a risk. However, each state develops its own immunization program and methods of enforcement. Parents/guardians do have the right to refuse immunizations.

The vaccines consist of a suspension of attenuated (uh TEN yoo eyt d) organisms or their toxins, which is administered to stimulate an active immune response in the body. This results in the production

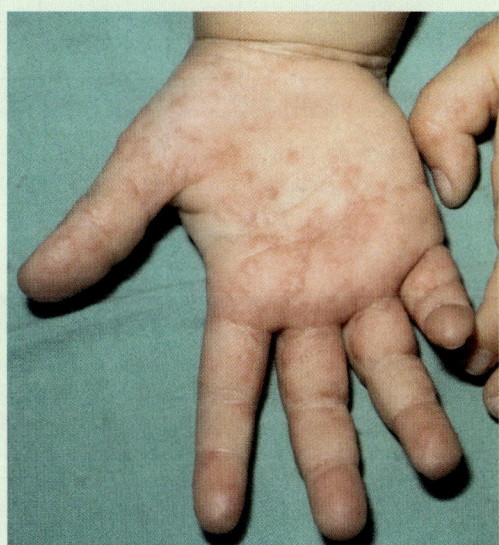

FIG. 32.3 Vesicular palm lesion in hand-foot-and-mouth disease. (From Fitzpatrick JE, Morelli JG: *Dermatology Secrets Plus*, ed. 4, St. Louis, 2011, Mosby.)

of antibodies against the specific pathogens. Booster doses are usually equivalent to a single dose of the initial immunization. For some immunizations (e.g., tetanus) boosters are prescribed at designated intervals to ensure maintenance of immune levels.

> **VOCABULARY**
> **attenuated**: Weakened or changed.

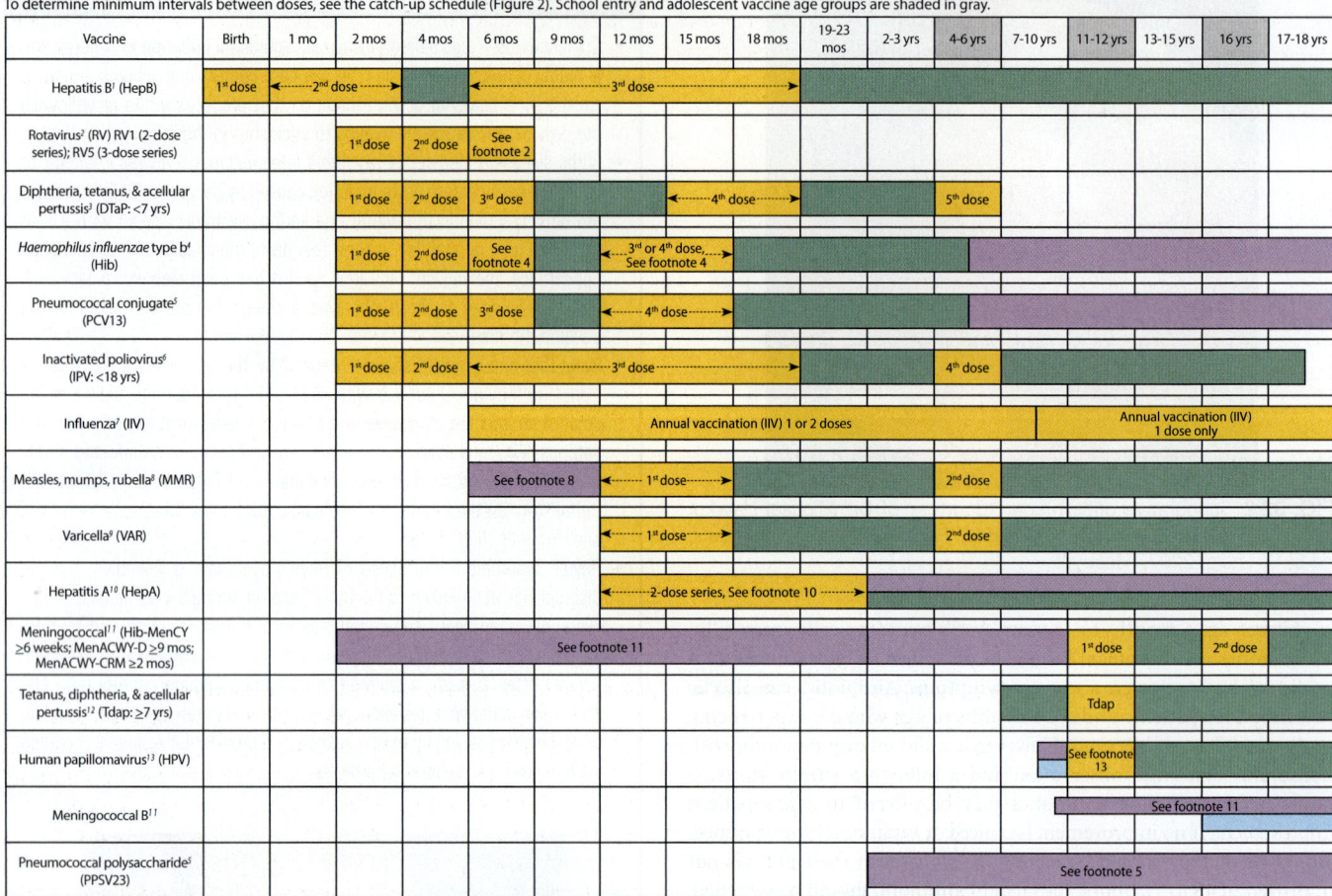

FIG. 32.4 Recommended immunization schedule for children ages birth to 18 years. (From http://www.cdc.gov/vaccines/schedules/downloads/child/0-18yrs-child-combined-schedule.pdf. Accessed July 14, 2017.)

BOX 32.7 Autism Spectrum Disorder

- Children diagnosed with autism spectrum disorder (ASD) show a wide range of neurologic and developmental behaviors. The most severe form is autism, or classical ASD; a milder form may present as Asperger syndrome; and sometimes a child cannot be categorized into a specific diagnosis and so is labeled with a pervasive developmental disorder (PDD).
- ASD occurs in all ethnic and socioeconomic groups and affects every age group.
- The Centers for Disease Control and Prevention (CDC) estimates the prevalence of ASD to be 1 in 68; it is almost five times more common among boys (1 in 42) than among girls (1 in 189).
- Children with autism have impaired social interaction, do not respond to their name, avoid eye contact, and show limited interest in their surroundings. They rarely communicate with others and display repetitive movements or mannerisms, such as rocking or twirling. They may also have self-abusive behaviors, such as biting and head banging. Many children with autism have a very high pain tolerance but are extremely sensitive to noise, touch, or other sensory stimulation.
- The cause of this developmental disorder is unknown, but researchers believe it is due to a combination of genetic errors and environmental factors, perhaps a problem with fetal brain development. Although many parents are concerned about a connection with vaccines, extensive studies have failed to show a link between the two.
- The American Academy of Pediatrics (AAP) recommends a general developmental screening at every well-child visit and a developmental screening using a standardized tool at 9, 18, and 30 months, or whenever a caregiver expresses concern. In addition, autism-specific screening is recommended for all children at the 18- and 24-month visits.
- Treatment involves coordinated educational and behavioral interventions to help the child develop social and language skills. Medications may be prescribed to treat depression, anxiety, and obsessive-compulsive behaviors.

From https://www.aap.org/en-us/about-the-aap/Committees-Councils-Sections/Council-on-Children-with-Disabilities/Pages/Autism.aspx. Accessed July 13, 2017.

Vaccine manufacturers have trade names for each product and have established protocols to ensure potency and stability. All vaccines are tested for safety and effectiveness. Every vaccine package has an insert that fully describes:
- the vaccine and its use
- the route of administration
- adverse reactions
- signs and symptoms the parent might observe after immunization that would indicate a potential problem.

Unfavorable responses include high fever, swelling at the site of the injection, urticaria (ur ti KAIR ee uh), breathing difficulties, severe headache, and convulsions. Any of these should be immediately reported to the provider. Vaccine storage should follow the manufacturer's guidelines (e.g., some vaccines must be refrigerated; others must not be exposed to sunlight).

> **VOCABULARY**
> **urticaria:** Hives.

Some vaccines are grown in birds' eggs or in a medium made of animal organs, or are weakened with chemicals. Therefore, a child who is allergic to eggs cannot receive some of the vaccines, such as influenza. The medical assistant must know the potential allergic problems, common symptoms, and adverse reactions to immunizations and must make sure the parent is informed. Table 32.2 details guidelines for childhood immunizations.

Before a child or adult receives a vaccine, the healthcare provider is required by the National Childhood Vaccine Injury Act (NCVIA) to provide a copy of a VIS to either the adult patient or the child's parent or legal guardian. A VIS provides information about the risks and benefits of each vaccine. If providing the parent or guardian with the VIS is the medical assistant's responsibility, he or she should do the following (Procedure 32.1):
- Before administering the vaccine, give the parent the most current VIS available for that particular vaccine. Give the parent enough time to review the information and then answer any questions or refer the parent's concerns to the provider before administering the vaccine. VIS forms are available online in a number of different languages to meet the needs of a diverse patient population.
- Document in the child's health record the date the VIS was given and the publication date of the VIS (which appears on the bottom of the form).
- To make sure the office has the most current VIS forms, either call the state health department or refer to the CDC's website: www.cdc.gov/vaccines/hcp/vis/current-vis.html. Forms can be printed directly from the site.
- If an informed consent form is required in your state, it must be signed and attached to the child's health record or electronically signed in the child's EHR before immunizations are given. Documentation of immunization administration must include the date the vaccine was administered, the manufacturer of the vaccine, the manufacturer's lot number, the type of vaccine, the exact site of administration if an injection was given, any reported or observed side effects, the name and title of the person who administered the vaccine, and the address of the medical office where the vaccine was administered.
- An immunization record should be given to the parent. If it is in a paper form (e.g. a booklet), it should be updated as needed to reflect the child's current immunization status. Most EHRs allow for the immunization record to be printed after each immunization. The medical assistant should not only document the required details in the patient's health record, but also complete the parent's immunization record each time the child receives another vaccination or booster. These parent records help schools and day care centers determine the child's immunization status. Some states are developing computerized immunization record systems.
- It is very important that vaccine vials be handled and stored properly to maintain the compound's ability to fight disease (Box 32.8). The CDC's recommendations for vaccine management practices can be found at its website: http://www.cdc.gov/vaccines/recs/storage/.

> **CRITICAL THINKING BOX 32.4**
>
> Allison will be administering pediatric immunizations during the well-baby visits scheduled for today. To prepare for this responsibility, she looked up the primary vaccinations, their routes of administration, contraindications, and possible side effects. The first child arrives for her 4-month checkup. She has been receiving all her previous immunization on schedule. What immunizations should the child receive, and how should they be administered? The baby's father asks whether she will get sick from the vaccines. What should Allison tell him? What does Allison need to do to meet the requirements of the National Childhood Vaccine Injury Act?

THE PEDIATRIC PATIENT

An infant's first physical assessment comes at the time of delivery, when the provider assesses the newborn's ability to thrive outside the uterus. The Apgar score is a system for evaluating the infant's physical condition at 1 and 5 minutes after birth (Table 32.3). Developed by pediatrician Virginia Apgar, the scoring system evaluates the following: *a*ppearance (color); *p*ulse (heart rate); *g*rimace (reflex; response to stimuli); *a*ctivity (muscle tone); and *r*espiration (breathing). These parameters are each rated 0, 1, or 2. The maximum total score is 10. Infants with low scores require immediate medical attention.

Well-Child Visits

The frequency of well-child visits varies with the provider and the community. The American Academy of Pediatrics recommends the following pattern:

- 2 to 5 days
- 1 month
- 2 months
- 4 months
- 6 months
- 9 months
- 12 months
- 15 months
- 18 months
- 2 years
- Annually

These visits focus on maintaining the child's health through basic system examinations, immunizations, and updating of the child's medical history record.

The decision on whether the child is to be seen alone or with the parent depends on the provider and the child's age. Often the child looks to the parent for approval before answering or performing a skill; for this reason, the provider may want to assess the child alone. If this is the case, explain to the parent that the provider wants to evaluate the child's independent abilities and that as soon as testing is complete, the provider will explain the results of the tests.

The medical history is an essential guide to the pediatric examination. With an infant, the provider depends on the caregiver for the history, but as the child gets older, some history may be obtained from the child and clarified or amplified by the parent. Close observation also gives the provider considerable information. Box 32.9 discusses lead paint exposure.

TABLE 32.2 Guidelines for Childhood Immunizations

Vaccine	Trade Name	Route of Administration	Contraindications[a]	Side Effects
DTaP Diphtheria, tetanus, pertussis (whooping cough)	Daptacel, Infanrix	IM; Td (tetanus and diphtheria) boosters at 11–12 yr if at least 5 yr since last dose; subsequent booster every 10 yr	Moderate or severe acute illness; neurologic problem; complication after previous dose (e.g., fever, convulsions)	Mild fever, anorexia, irritability, drowsiness
HAV Hepatitis A (can use either Havrix or Vaqta)	Havrix, Vaqta	IM; all children 1 yr; 2 doses 6 mo apart	Hypersensitivity to product, acute infection or fever	Localized injection site reaction, fever, headache
HBV Hepatitis B	Engerix-B, Recombivax HB	IM; may give with all other vaccines but at a separate site; requires 3 injections	Moderate or severe acute illness; yeast allergy; severe cardiovascular disease	Fever, pain at site, headache, malaise, vomiting
Hib *Haemophilus influenzae* serotype B meningitis	COMVAX, PedvaxHIB, ActHIB, Hiberix	IM; may give with all other vaccines but at a separate site. Three doses of ActHIB, MenHibrix, or Pentacel at 2, 4, and 6 months or 2 doses PedvaxHib or COMVAX at 2 and 4 months of age; booster dose at 12 through 15 months	Not routinely given to children older than 5; moderate or severe acute illness	Minimal
HPV Human papillomavirus	HPV2 (Cervarix) females only; HPV4 (Gardasil), HPV9 (Gardasil 9) males and females	IM; routine vaccination at age 11 or 12 years; second dose 1 to 2 months after first dose; third dose 16 weeks after second dose	Hypersensitivity to ingredients; pregnancy	Relatively few; mild headache and GI upset
Influenza Trivalent inactivated vaccine for 6 months; at 2 years, use live, attenuated vaccine	Afluria, Fluad, Flublok, Flucelvax, FluLaval, Fluarix, Fluvirin, Fluzone, FluMist (nasal spray)	IM; annually each fall	Allergy to eggs; recent fever	Uncommon; fever, local irritation at injection site, general malaise
IPV Inactive poliovirus for polio	Ipol	SC or IM; 4 doses; may give with all other vaccines but at a separate site	Moderate or severe acute illness; egg allergy	Uncommon
Meningococcal vaccine for meningitis (MCV4)	Menactra, Menomune, MenHibrix, Bexsero, or Trumenba	IM; single dose of Menactra or Menveo vaccine at age 11 through 12 years, with a booster dose at age 16 years; aged 16 through 23 years vaccinated with a 2-dose series of Bexsero or a 3-dose series of Trumenba vaccine to provide short-term protection	Moderate or severe acute illness; history of allergic reaction to MCV4	Uncommon
MMR Measles, mumps, rubella	M-M-R II	SC; may give with all other vaccines but at a separate site	Moderate or severe acute illness; immunocompromised patients (may be given if HIV positive); pregnancy or possible pregnancy in 3 mo; egg allergy	Fever
Pneumococcal (PCV) Pneumococcal pneumonia	Pneumovax 23, Prevnar 13	IM or SC; all children 2–23 mo; administer every 6 yr for high-risk patients	Moderate or severe acute illness; hypersensitivity	Drowsiness, local irritation at site, mild fever
Rotavirus (Rota) RotaTeq for prevention of rotavirus gastroenteritis	Rotarix	PO; 3 doses at 6–12 wk; subsequent doses at 4–10 wk intervals	Hypersensitivity	GI upset and blood disorders
Varicella (chickenpox)	Varivax	SC; may give with all other vaccines but at a separate site; 2-dose series at ages 12 through 15 mo and 4 through 6 yr	Confirmed history of chickenpox; pregnancy or possible pregnancy in 1 mo; moderate or severe acute illness; immunocompromised patients; egg allergy	No salicylates for 6 wk afterward to prevent risk of Reye's syndrome
May give combination vaccine: measles, mumps, rubella, varicella (MMRV)	ProQuad	SC; may give with all other vaccines but at a separate site; all susceptible children 12 mo or older	Confirmed history of chickenpox; pregnancy or possible pregnancy in 1 mo; moderate or severe acute illness; immunocompromised patients; egg allergy	No salicylates for 6 wk afterward to prevent risk of Reye's syndrome

[a]Mild illness is not a contraindication.
GI, Gastrointestinal; *HIV*, human immunodeficiency virus; *IM*, intramuscular; *PO*, oral; *SC*, subcutaneous.

CHAPTER 32 Assisting in Pediatrics

BOX 32.8 Safe Handling and Storage of Vaccines

The Centers for Disease Control and Prevention (CDC) have devised a list of important rules and steps to ensure safekeeping of a practice's vaccine supply. This list can be used as a checklist in the office.

_____ 1. One person should be in charge of the handling and storage of vaccines at the facility, with a backup person to ensure proper management.

_____ 2. A vaccine inventory log should be maintained that includes the following:
  _____ (1) Vaccine name
  _____ (2) Number of doses
  _____ (3) Date vaccine was received
  _____ (4) Condition of vaccine on arrival
  _____ (5) Manufacturer
  _____ (6) Lot number
  _____ (7) Expiration date

_____ 3. Vaccines should be stored in separate, self-contained units that refrigerate or freeze only. A household-style combination unit can be used to store only refrigerated vaccines; frozen vaccines must be kept in a separate, stand-alone freezer.

_____ 4. The vaccine refrigerator and freezer should not be used for food or drinks.

_____ 5. Vaccines should be stored in the middle of the refrigerator or freezer, not in the door.

_____ 6. New supplies should be placed behind the vials with the closest expiration date; the vials with the nearest expiration date should be used first.

_____ 7. A sign should be posted on the refrigerator door identifying which vaccines should be stored in either the refrigerator or the freezer.

_____ 8. One thermometer should be kept in the refrigerator and one in the freezer; the refrigerator temperature should be maintained at 35° to 46° F (2° to 8° C) and the freezer temperature at −58° to 5° F (−50° to 15° C) or colder.

_____ 9. Containers of water should be kept in the refrigerator and ice packs in the freezer to help maintain cold temperatures.

_____ 10. A temperature log should be kept on the refrigerator door; the refrigerator and freezer temperatures should be recorded twice a day: first thing in the morning and at the end of the day.

_____ 11. A "Do Not Unplug" sign should be posted next to the refrigerator's electrical outlet.

_____ 12. If the refrigerator or freezer stops working, the following steps should be taken:
- Immediately place the vaccines in another refrigerator or freezer, and mark them so that they can be separated from vaccines that were not affected.
- Record the temperature of the refrigerator or freezer, and contact the vaccine manufacturer or state health department. Follow their instructions on the use, alteration of expiration dates, or disposal of the vaccines.

_____ 13. The facility should have a copy of the health department's general and emergency vaccine management policies.

PROCEDURE 32.1 Document Immunizations

Task:
To document accurately the administration of a pediatric immunization.

Equipment and Supplies
- Patient's record
- Vaccine administration record (VAR)
- Parent's immunization record (if used in the medical practice)
- Vaccine Information Statement (VIS) for hepatitis B (a link to the current VIS forms can be accessed at this website: http://www.cdc.gov/vaccines/hcp/vis/current-vis.html)

Scenario
Samantha Anderson, a 5-week-old infant, has just received her second dose of the hepatitis B (HBV) vaccine. Document the administration of the vaccine.

Procedural Steps
1. Gather the necessary forms.
2. Make sure the provider obtained informed consent from the parent (if required by your state), that the hepatitis B VIS form was given, and that all the parent's questions were answered before the vaccine is dispensed and administered.
   Purpose: To follow risk management practices.
3. Administer the vaccine intramuscularly (see Chapter 38, Administering Medication).
4. Complete the information required on the VAR, including the name of the vaccine, the date given, the route of administration and site, the vaccine lot number and manufacturer, the date on the VIS form, the date it was given to the parent, and your signature or initials.
   Purpose: To meet the legal requirements of the National Childhood Vaccine Injury Act.
5. In the parent's copy of the immunization record, record the date of administration, the name and address of the provider's practice, and the type of vaccine administered.
   Purpose: To maintain an accurate and comprehensive parental record of childhood immunizations for school and/or day care purposes.
6. After administering the HBV vaccine, record the following details in the child's health record:
   - Date the vaccine was administered
   - Vaccine's manufacturer, batch and lot numbers, and expiration date
   - Type of vaccine administered and dose
   - Route of administration and exact site if an injection was given
   - Any reported or observed side effects
   - Publication date of the VIS form given to the parent (on the bottom of the form)
   - Parent education about possible side effects of the vaccine
   - Name and title of the person who administered the vaccine

Documentation Example
4/2/20XX 3:25 pm: Mother given VIS form for Hep B. Had no questions. Administered second dose of Hep B IM to Φ vastus lateralis per Dr. Walden's order. No problems noted after injection. _____
           _____ A. Kwong, CMA (AAMA)

Continued

PROCEDURE 32.1 Document Immunizations—cont'd

Vaccine Administration Record for Children and Teens

(Page 1 of 2)

Patient name: _____
Birthdate: _____ Patient ID number: _____
Clinic name and address

Before administering any vaccines, give copies of all pertinent Vaccine Information Statements (VISs) to the child's parent or legal representative and make sure he/she understands the risks and benefits of the vaccine(s). Always provide or update the patient's personal record card.

Vaccine	Type of Vaccine[1]	Date given (mo/day/yr)	Funding Source (F,S,P)[2]	Route & Site[3]	Vaccine Lot #	Mfr.	Vaccine Information Statement (VIS) Date on VIS[4]	Date given[4]	Vaccinator[5] (signature or initials & title)
Hepatitis B[6] (e.g., HepB, Hib-HepB, DTaP-HepB-IPV) Give IM.[3]									
Diphtheria, Tetanus, Pertussis[6] (e.g., DTaP, DTaP/Hib, DTaP-HepB-IPV, DT, DTaP-IPV/Hib, Tdap, DTaP-IPV, Td) Give IM.[3]									
Haemophilus influenzae **type b**[6] (e.g., Hib, Hib-HepB, DTaP-IPV/Hib, DTaP/Hib, Hib-MenCY) Give IM.[3]									
Polio[6] (e.g., IPV, DTaP-HepB-DTaP-IPV/Hib, DTaP-IPV) Give IPV SC or IM.[3] Give all others IM.[3]									
Pneumococcal (e.g., PCV7, PCV13, conjugate; PPSV23, polysaccharide) Give PCV IM.[3] Give PPSV SC or IM.[3]									
Rotavirus (RV1, RV5) Give orally (po).[3]									

See page 2 to record measles-mumps-rubella, varicella, hepatitis A, meningococcal, HPV, influenza, and other vaccines (e.g., travel vaccines).

How to Complete This Record

1. Record the generic abbreviation (e.g., Tdap) or the trade name for each vaccine (see table at right).
2. Record the funding source of the vaccine given as either F (federal), S (state), or P (private).
3. Record the route by which the vaccine was given as either intramuscular (IM), subcutaneous (SC), intradermal (ID), intranasal (IN), or oral (PO) and also the site where it was administered as either RA (right arm), LA (left arm), RT (right thigh), or LT (left thigh).
4. Record the publication date of each VIS as well as the date the VIS is given to the patient.
5. To meet the space constraints of this form and federal requirements for documentation, a healthcare setting may want to keep a reference list of vaccinators that includes their initials and titles.
6. For combination vaccines, fill in a row for each antigen in the combination.

Abbreviation	Trade Name and Manufacturer
DTaP	Daptacel (sanofi); Infanrix (GlaxoSmithKline [GSK]); Tripedia (sanofi pasteur)
DT (pediatric)	Generic DT (sanofi pasteur)
DTaP-HepB-IPV	Pediarix (GSK)
DTaP/Hib	TriHIBit (sanofi pasteur)
DTaP-IPV/Hib	Pentacel (sanofi pasteur)
DTaP-IPV	Kinrix (GSK)
HepB	Engerix-B (GSK); Recombivax HB (Merck)
HepA-HepB	Twinrix (GSK), can be given to teens age 18 and older
Hib	ActHIB (sanofi pasteur); Hiberix (GSK); PedvaxHIB (Merck)
Hib-HepB	Comvax (Merck)
Hib-MenCY	MenHibrix (GSK)
IPV	Ipol (sanofi pasteur)
PCV13	Prevnar 13 (Pfizer)
PPSV23	Pneumovax 23 (Merck)
RV1	Rotarix (GSK)
RV5	RotaTeq (Merck)
Tdap	Adacel (sanofi pasteur); Boostrix (GSK)
Td	Decavac (sanofi pasteur); Generic Td (MA Biological Labs)

Technical content reviewed by the Centers for Disease Control and Prevention

For additional copies, visit www.immunize.org/catg.d/p2022.pdf • Item #P2022 (4/14)

This form was created by the Immunization Action Coalition • www.immunize.org • www.vaccineinformation.org

BOX 32.9 Lead Paint Exposure

Children are especially vulnerable to lead levels in their environment. High blood lead levels can result in serious brain injury, including seizures, coma, and death. Lower levels can cause learning problems, stunted growth, and behavior disorders. The most common causes of lead exposure are lead-based paint in homes and on imported toys, and chronic exposure to lead-contaminated dust and water. The Centers for Disease Control and Prevention (CDC) recommend a screening blood test for lead levels in all children between 1 and 2 years of age. For children who show elevated levels, follow-up should include home and school environmental testing to determine the cause of lead exposure.

TABLE 32.3 Apgar Scoring System[a]

Clinical Sign	0	1	2
Heart rate	Absent	<100 beats per minute	>100 beats per minute
Respiratory effort	Absent	Slow and irregular	Good and crying
Muscle tone	Limp	Some flexion of the arms and legs	Active movement
Reflex irritability	No response	Grimace	Coughing, sneezing, or vigorous cry
Color	Blue and pale	Body pink and extremities blue	Pink all over

[a]Readings are taken by the provider at 1 minute and 5 minutes after birth. At *1 minute:* If the score is 7 or lower, some nervous system problems are suspected. If the score is below 4, resuscitation usually is necessary. At *5 minutes:* If the score is at least 8, the child probably is reacting normally.

TABLE 32.4 Important Questions for Telephone Screening of Pediatric Problems

Complaint	Screening Questions
Pain	• What are the onset, frequency, and duration of the pain? • On a scale of 1 to 10, how severe is the pain? • Where is the exact location? • Was any accident involved (include details)? • Has the pain gotten worse over time? • Has the pain interfered with sleep? • Is there associated fever, vomiting, diarrhea, or rash?
• Gastrointestinal	• What are the onset, duration, and frequency of the symptoms? Has the child been vomiting longer than 24 hours without improvement? • Is the child drinking and/or eating? • Is the child dehydrated (e.g., dry mouth, no urination in 8–10 hours, listless)? • If the child has diarrhea, have there been more than five or six watery stools in 12 hours? • Does the child have other symptoms (e.g., vomiting, fever of 101° F [38.3° C], rapid breathing)?
• Respiratory	• What are the onset, duration, and frequency of the symptoms? • How would you describe the child's breathing? • Has the child been diagnosed with a breathing disorder? • Is a prescribed treatment being used? • Are any other signs or symptoms present (e.g., severe headache, stiff neck, fever, cough)? • If the child is coughing, what does it sound like? • Are there signs of a sore throat or earache?

Sick-Child Visits

Sick-child visits occur whenever needed, usually on short notice. For this reason, most pediatric offices keep open appointments in the schedule to accommodate calls for sick-child visits. The length and frequency of this type of visit depends entirely on the child and the illness. The medical assistant is frequently the first point of contact for a sick child and the child's caregiver.

Determining whether the child should be seen immediately or the problem can wait for an opening in the schedule is crucial to pediatric care. The medical assistant should follow established office policies, but when in doubt about the seriousness of the problem, he or she should ask the office manager or provider for advice. Usually the provider prefers to see the child rather than delay seeing a patient with a potentially serious condition. The child should be seen right away, if the child is young (under 2 years old) and the parent reports:

- Frequent cycles of crying, lethargy, vomiting that lasts longer than 24 hours
- Diarrhea (more than six stools in the past 12 hours)
- Fever of 101° F (38.3° C) or higher
- He or she cannot verbalize associated pain or problems

Table 32.4 summarizes some important questions for telephone screening of an older child who can communicate symptoms. It is important to focus on the *onset* (when symptoms first started), *frequency* (are symptoms constant, or do they cycle through recurrences), and *duration* (how long the episodes last) of the problem, in addition to attempted treatments and their effectiveness. As with any other patient, all telephone communication should be documented to record the reason for the call; the information gathered; the action taken, including whether the provider was consulted; any orders given; and whether and when an appointment was scheduled.

THE MEDICAL ASSISTANT'S ROLE IN PEDIATRIC PROCEDURES

The medical assistant is responsible for:
- assisting the provider with examinations
- updating patient histories
- performing ordered screening tests (e.g., vision, hearing, urinalysis, and hemoglobin checks)
- administering immunizations
- measuring and weighing children as needed
- providing patient and caregiver support

A medical assistant must develop a relationship with the pediatric patient that encourages cooperation and compliance with tests and treatment plans.

Interacting with children requires special techniques, depending on the child's age. A calm, unhurried manner is essential to gaining cooperation. The tone of voice should be gentle but confident. Using a firm, direct approach about expected behavior is important in gaining the cooperation of older children. Offer reasonable choices when possible, such as, "Would you like your shot in your left leg or your right leg?" not, "Are you ready for your shot now?" Offering sincere praise for the child during the examination or procedures helps ease anxiety and builds self-esteem. If the child is having an unusually difficult time, try to discover the reason. If he or she has had a bad medical experience in the past, the child may be afraid of what might happen. Each step should be explained in a language the child (and parent) can understand. Children younger than age 2 feel better when the parent holds them or remains very close (Fig. 32.5). Preschool children enjoy playing, so making a game out of the situation is helpful (Fig. 32.6).

Whatever the child's age, the medical assistant should be sensitive to his or her individual needs and should adapt the examination and procedures as much as possible to meet those needs.

The sequence of the provider's examination varies and frequently is based on the child's cooperation. The provider will probably leave procedures and tests that are likely to cause the most objections until the end of the appointment. The provider is constantly evaluating the child's growth and development. A child's alertness and responses tell the provider a considerable amount. With infants and young children of preschool age, the parent is closely questioned about the child's eating, sleeping, and elimination habits. A school-aged child is usually a little more cooperative during an examination and can answer most questions without parental assistance. Adolescent patients should be given the option of not having parents present during an examination. This may permit teenagers to respond more honestly about lifestyle factors, and also protects their privacy.

Measurements

Examination of the child during routine well-child care includes measurement of the circumference of the infant's head to determine normal growth and development (Procedure 32.2). The size of the child's head reflects the growth of the brain. Brain growth is 50% complete by 1 year of age, 75% by age 3, and 90% by age 6. Routine head measurement is recommended in children until 36 months of age and in older children whose head size is not within norms. If the circumference of the head deviates greatly from normal measurements, **hydrocephaly** (hye droh SEFF ul lee) or **microcephaly** (may kroh suh FAL lee) may be suspected. It is important to discover any congenital problem as early as possible so that appropriate treatment can be started.

> **VOCABULARY**
> **hydrocephaly**: Enlargement of the cranium caused by abnormal accumulation of cerebrospinal fluid in the cerebral system.
> **microcephaly**: Abnormally small head associated with incomplete brain development.

Along with the head circumference, the medical assistant should record the child's length (or height) and weight (Procedure 32.3) on growth charts so that the provider can compare the child's measurement statistics with national standards. Growth charts consist of a series of percentile curves that illustrate the distribution of selected body measurements.

The CDC has gender-specific growth charts for:
- Birth to 36 months (Figs. 32.7 and 32.8)
  - Length for age
  - Weight for age
  - Head circumference for age
  - Weight for length
- 2 to 20 years
  - Stature for age
  - Weight for age
  - BMI for age

There are 20 CDC charts (10 for boys and 10 for girls). As mentioned previously, the BMI is the recommended method of determining whether children or adults are overweight or obese. The BMI growth charts can be used beginning at 2 years of age, when height can be measured accurately.

EHRs may automatically plot the measurements on the appropriate growth chart and calculate the percentile.

Assisting with the Examination

The provider will have a designated set of procedures that the medical assistant completes before the provider sees the child. Vital signs are measured first (Table 32.5). Depending on the child's age and level of cooperation, the temperature may be obtained by the axillary, oral, rectal, tympanic, or temporal artery method. The rectal and temporal artery methods are considered most accurate in infants; however, the temporal artery method is easiest, quickest, and less invasive. It is important to remember that the younger the child, the more immature the ability to regulate body heat. Therefore, the temperature of an infant may fluctuate easily and rapidly. The child's pulse rate is affected similarly to that of an adult; it can increase as a result of activity, anxiety, illness, and environmental temperature. If the child is younger than age 2, the pulse is measured apically by placing the stethoscope on the left side

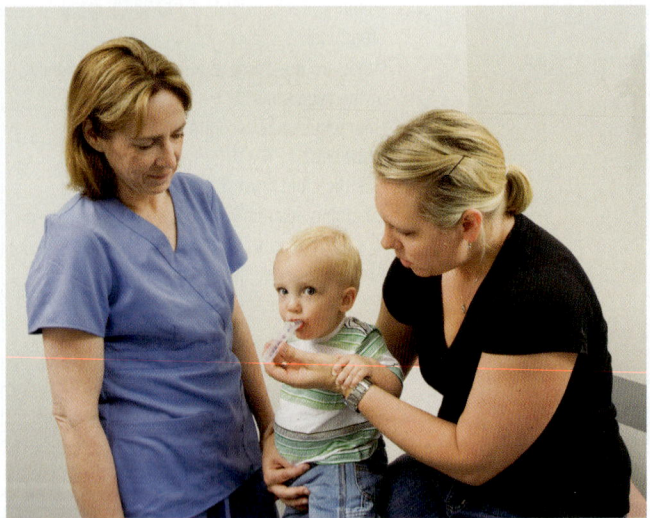

FIG. 32.5 Sometimes a pediatric patient is more comfortable when held by a parent. (From Proctor D, et al: *Kinn's The Medical Assistant*, ed 13, St. Louis, 2017, Elsevier.)

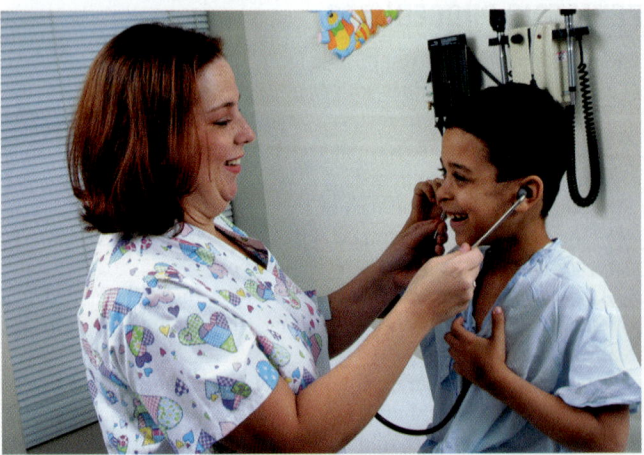

FIG. 32.6 Making a game out of a procedure. (From Proctor D, et al: *Kinn's The Medical Assistant*, ed 13, St. Louis, 2017, Elsevier.)

CHAPTER 32 Assisting in Pediatrics 735

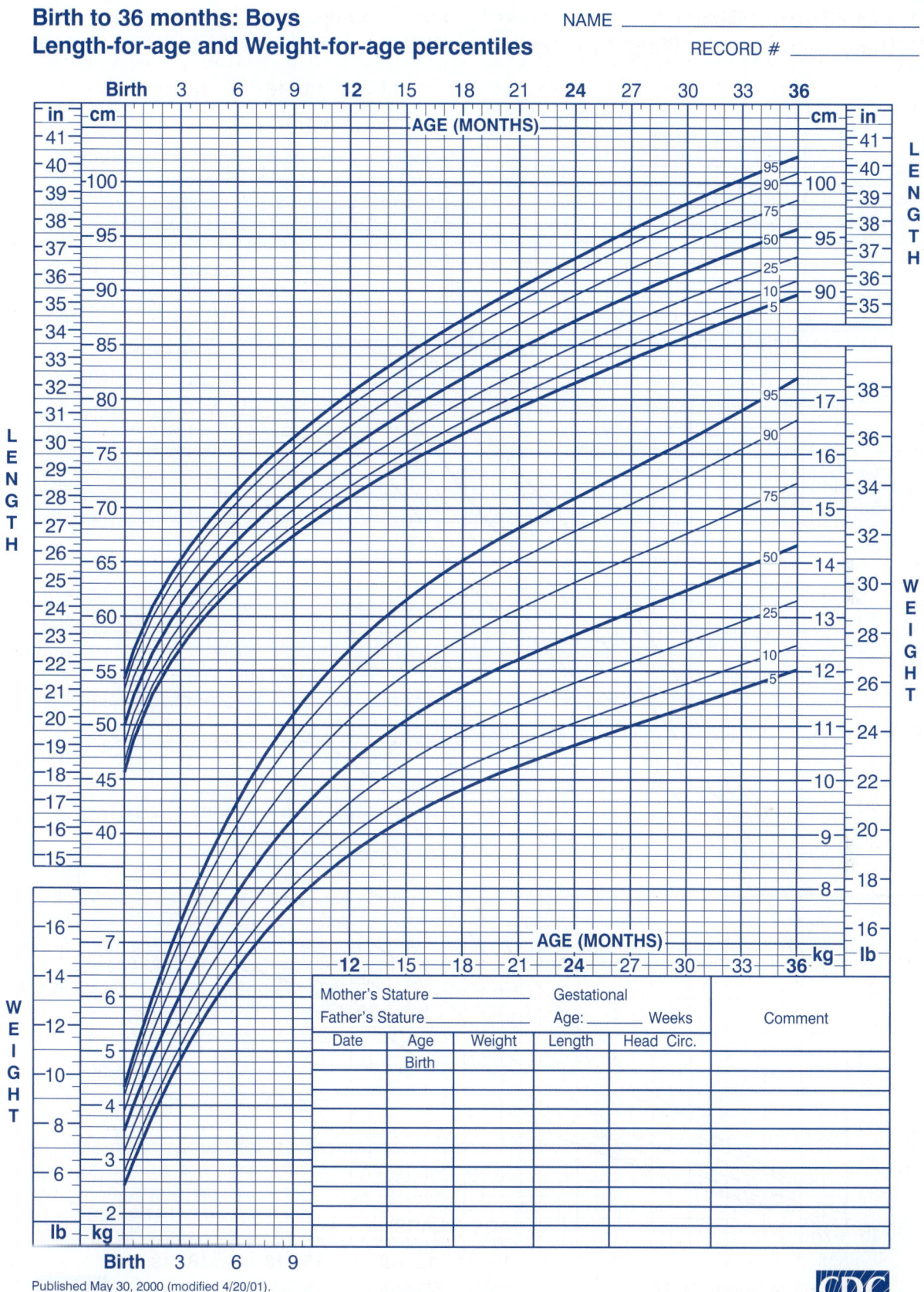

FIG. 32.7 Growth chart: boys (birth to 36 months).

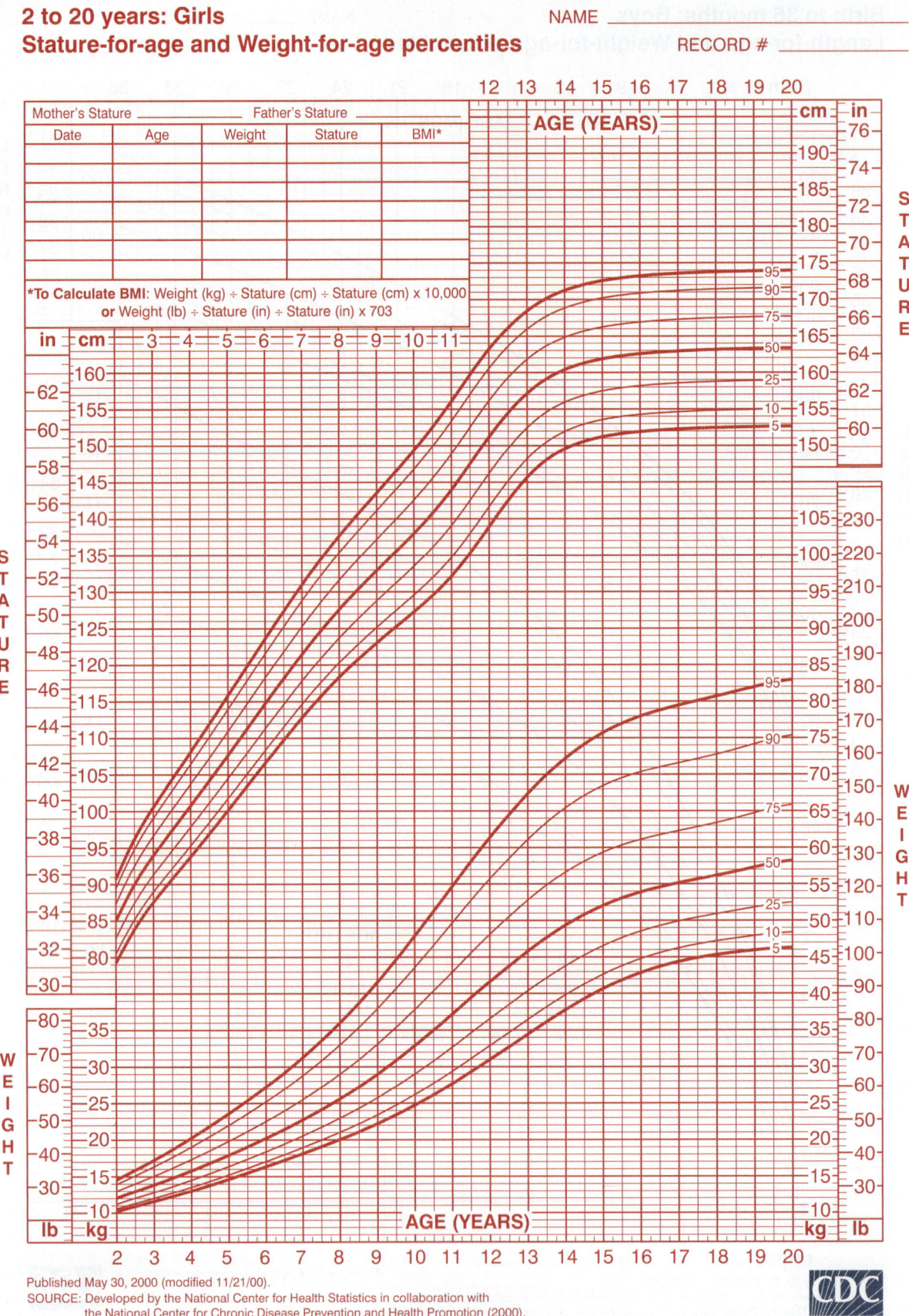

FIG. 32.8 Growth chart: girls (birth to 36 months).

CHAPTER 32 Assisting in Pediatrics

PROCEDURE 32.2   Measure the Head Circumference of an Infant

Task:
To obtain an accurate measurement of the circumference of an infant's head and plot the result on the patient's growth chart.

Equipment and Supplies
- Patient's record
- Flexible disposable tape measure
- Age- and gender-specific growth chart
- Pen

Procedural Steps
1. Wash hands or use hand sanitizer.
   Purpose: To ensure infection control.
2. Greet the patient and the parents or caregivers. Identify yourself. Verify the patient's identity with full name and date of birth. Explain the procedure to be performed in a manner that is understood by the patient (if old enough) or the parent or caregiver. Answer any questions about the procedure. If the child is old enough, gain his or her cooperation through conversation.
   Purpose: To alleviate anxiety and gain the child's trust.
3. Place an infant in the supine position, or the infant may be held by the parent. An older infant may sit on the examination table.
4. Hold the tape measure with the zero mark against the infant's forehead, slightly above the eyebrows and the top of the ears. Ask the parent for assistance if necessary.
5. Bring the tape measure around the head, just above the ears, until it meets (see the following figure).
6. Read to the nearest 0.5 cm or ¼ inch.
7. Record the measurement on the growth chart and in the patient's health record.
   Purpose: A procedure is not done until it is recorded.
8. Dispose of the tape measure.
9. Wash hands or use hand sanitizer.
   Purpose: To ensure infection control.

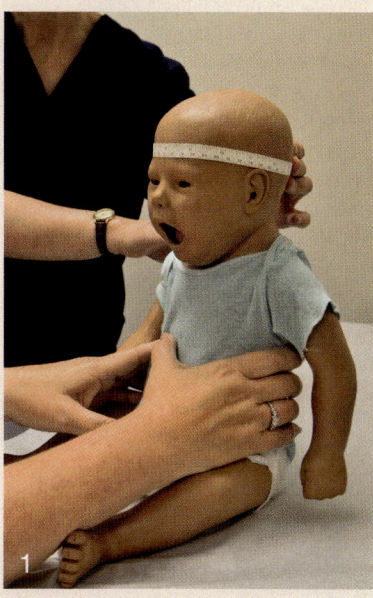

PROCEDURE 32.3   Measure an Infant's Length and Weight

Task:
To measure an infant's length and weight accurately so that growth patterns can be monitored and recorded.

Equipment and Supplies
- Patient's record
- Infant scale with paper cover
- Flexible measuring tape
- Examination table paper
- Pen
- Pediatric length board, if available
- Gender-specific infant growth chart
- Waste container

Procedural Steps
Measuring an Infant's Length
1. Wash hands or use hand sanitizer; assemble the necessary equipment.
2. Greet the patient and parents or caregivers. Identify yourself. Verify the patient's identity with full name and date of birth. Explain the procedure to be performed in a manner that is understood by the patient (if old enough) and the parent or caregiver. Answer any questions about the procedure.
3. Undress the infant. The diaper may be left on.
4. Cover the examination table with smooth, flat paper. Ask the caregiver to place the infant on his or her back on the examination table. If the table is a pediatric table with a headboard, ask the caregiver to hold the infant's head gently against the headboard while you straighten the infant's leg and note the location of the heel on the measurement area. If there is no headboard, ask the caregiver to gently hold the infant's head still while you draw a line on the paper at the top of the baby's head and at the heel after extending the leg (see the following figure).

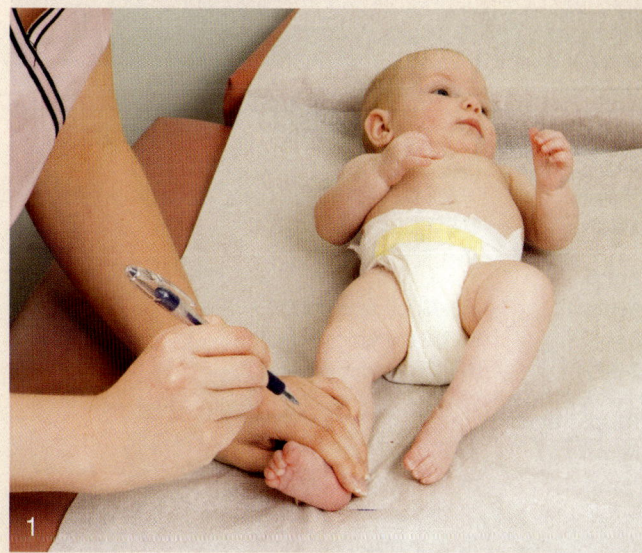

Measure the infant's length with the tape measure and record it. Document the results in either inches or centimeters, depending on office policy, on the infant's growth chart, in the progress notes, and in the caregiver's record if requested.

Continued

PROCEDURE 32.3   Measure an Infant's Length and Weight—cont'd

Weighing an Infant

1. Wash hands or use hand sanitizer, assemble the necessary equipment, and explain the procedure to the infant's caregiver.
2. Greet the patient and parents or caregivers. Identify yourself. Verify the patient's identity with full name and date of birth. Explain the procedure to be performed in a manner that is understood by the patient. Answer any questions the parents or caregivers may have on the procedure.
3. If the scale is not a digital model, prepare the scale by sliding weights to the left; line the scale with disposable paper to reduce the risk of pathogen transmission.
4. Completely undress the infant. If the diaper is clean and dry it can remain on.
   Purpose: It is important to get the most accurate weight possible, and a wet diaper will add to the total weight.
5. Place the infant gently on the center of the scale, keeping your hand directly above the infant's trunk for safety (see the following figure).

Purpose: To protect the infant from possible injury.

6. If the scale is not a digital model, slide the weights across the scale until balance is achieved. Read the infant's weight while he or she is still.
7. If the scale is not a digital model, return the weights to the far left of the scale and remove the baby. Discard the paper lining the scale. If the scale became contaminated during the procedure, follow Occupational Safety and Health Administration (OSHA) guidelines for use of gloves and disposal of contaminated waste. Disinfect the equipment according to the manufacturer's guidelines.
   Purpose: Infection control.
8. Wash hands or use hand sanitizer.
9. Document the results in either pounds or kilograms, depending on office policy, on the infant's growth chart, in the progress notes, and in the caregiver's record if requested.

Documentation Example
8/24/20XX 10:20 am: Wt 17 lb 4 oz. Length 27 in. _____ A. Kwong, CMA (AAMA)

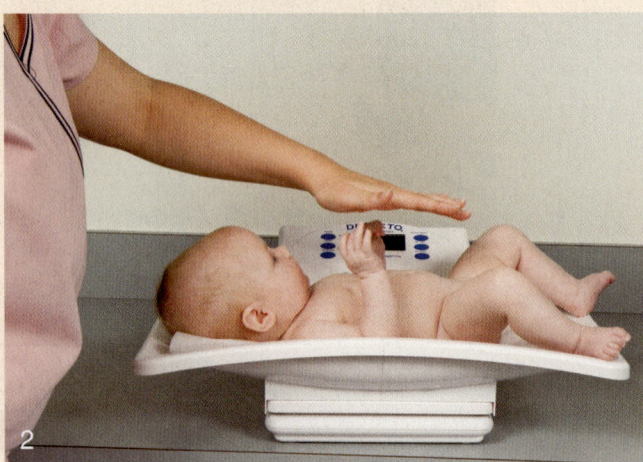

TABLE 32.5   Reference Ranges for Pediatric Vital Signs

Vital Sign	Reference Range
Temperature	
Oral	98.6° F (37° C)
Tympanic	99.6° F (37.6° C)
Axillary	97.6° F (36.4° C)
Pulse	
Newborn	100–180 beats per minute
3 mo–2 yr	80–150 beats per minute
2–10 yr	65–130 beats per minute
Respirations	
Newborn	30–50 breaths per minute
1–3 yr	25–30 breaths per minute
4–6 yr	23–25 breaths per minute
7+ yr	16–20 breaths per minute
Blood Pressure	
Newborn	Systolic 90 mm Hg; diastolic 70 mm Hg
1–5 yr	Systolic 100 mm Hg; diastolic 70 mm Hg
6–12 yr	Systolic 120 mm Hg; diastolic 84 mm Hg
13+ yr	Systolic, 100 mm Hg + age; diastolic, 30–40 mm Hg less

of the chest medial to the nipple. Always count the beats for 1 full minute for accuracy.

An alternative method of obtaining the pulse of a very young child is to use the brachial artery in the upper arm. After age 2, the child's pulse may be taken at the radial pulse site. Anticipate a pulse rate higher than that of an adult; the younger the child, the faster the pulse. The respiratory rate is easily obtained in a child because the chest can be readily observed. Expect the rate to be increased according to the child's age (the younger the child, the faster the normal respiratory rate) and health. The ratio of 4 pulse beats to 1 respiration should remain constant in a healthy child.

It is recommended that blood pressure be checked for children aged 3 years or older. The cuff must be the appropriate width to obtain an accurate reading, and the bell of the stethoscope must be small enough to seal over the site. It is best to use a pediatric stethoscope with a pediatric bell when obtaining an infant's pressure. Blood pressure readings in a young child are lower than those in an adult (see Table 32.5).

To prevent a small child or infant from rolling the head from side to side during the provider's examination, stand at the head of the table and support the child's head between your hands, taking care not to press on the ears or on the anterior or posterior fontanelles (font n EL s). An infant need not be draped, but privacy is important to an older child. Sincere respect and friendly conversation at the child's level accomplishes a great deal. Always be patient with children. Make sure they understand what is expected. Always involve the parents or caregivers as much as possible.

> **VOCABULARY**
> **fontanelle**: A space covered by thick membranes between the sutures of an infant's skull; called the baby's "soft spots"; there are both anterior and posterior fontanelles.

Accurately judging the level of pain a young patient is experiencing can be difficult. If the child is able to communicate, the Wong-Baker FACES Pain Scale could be used, which shows simple drawings of faces that express varying levels of pain on a 0 to 10 scale (Fig. 32.9).

Obtaining a Urine Sample

The easiest way to obtain a urine sample from a child who is toilet trained is to give the parent the container and instructions ahead of time. Then, when the child arrives at the office for the examination, the sample is available to be tested. If the sample is needed while the child is at the office, consult with the parent for the best method to use. If the child is not toilet trained, a pediatric urine collection device can be put on him or her to collect the sample (Fig. 32.10). This device is placed as soon as the child is checked in to increase the chance of obtaining the needed sample before the child leaves. Once the device is in place, the child can be diapered to help hold it properly. Make sure the adhesive sticks tightly so that the specimen collects in the device when the child urinates.

In some cases, the child may need to be catheterized to obtain the specimen. Pediatric catheterization kits contain all the supplies needed for this procedure. When preparing the kit, always remember that this is a sterile procedure. The provider usually asks the parent to help with the infant while the medical assistant labels and prepares the specimen for the laboratory. In some practices, a registered nurse (RN) or a specially trained medical assistant may perform a catheterization procedure to collect a pediatric urine sample.

THE ADOLESCENT PATIENT

The adolescent patient may present the greatest challenge to health education and disease management. Adolescence begins with the onset of puberty, a time when the child's reproductive system matures. This is a period marked by rapid changes in the endocrine and musculoskeletal systems. The adolescent undergoes rapid growth spurts and the development of secondary sexual characteristics.

Health examinations for patients in this age group should include:
- screening for height and weight
- gathering details about diet and exercise routines
- screening for sexually transmitted infections (STIs)
- Pap test (for sexually active female adolescents), especially to screen for infection with the human papillomavirus [HPV])
- reviewing the vaccination history and administering boosters as indicated
- assessing for high-risk behaviors, such as substance abuse, smoking, and sexual behavior

Health problems most frequently seen in adolescent patients include eating disorders (anorexia nervosa and bulimia nervosa), obesity, and injury-related problems. Accidents are the leading cause of death and injury in adolescence, and suicide is the third leading cause of death. All healthcare personnel should be on the alert for indicators of suicide, including:
- Signs of depression, such as headaches, abdominal discomfort, anorexia, fatigue, aggressiveness, drug or alcohol abuse, and sexual promiscuity
- Verbal statements that hint at the adolescent's intention to commit suicide; talking about dying
- Actions such as giving away prized objects, withdrawing from social groups, suddenly changing normal behavior patterns, or writing a suicide note

INJURY PREVENTION

Unintentional injuries are the leading cause of death and disability in children in the United States. Injuries cause more childhood deaths

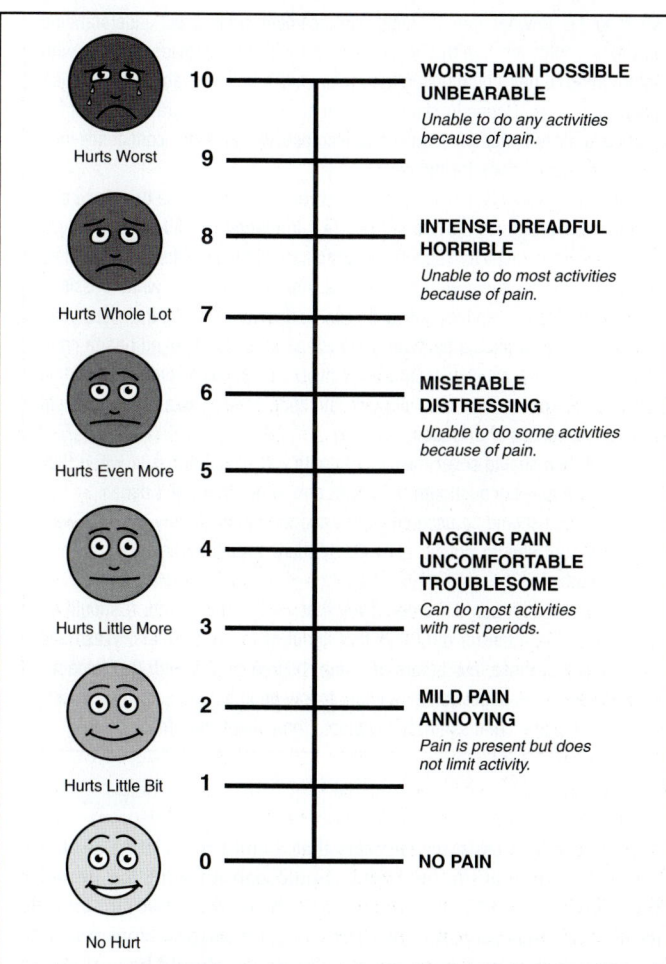

FIG. 32.9 Wong-Baker FACES Pain Scale.

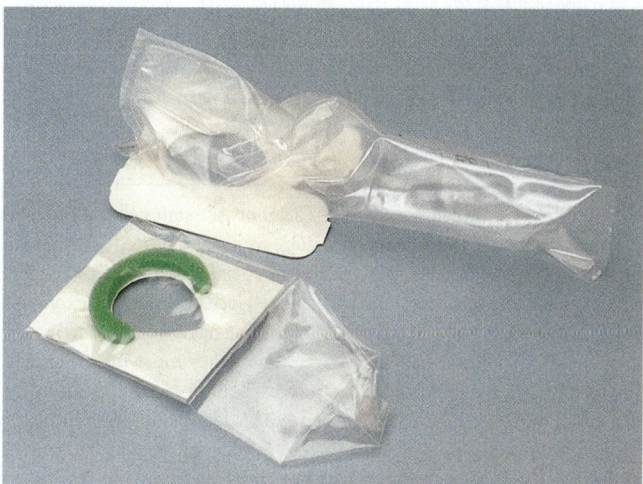

FIG. 32.10 Urine collection devices. (From Proctor D, et al: *Kinn's The Medical Assistant*, ed 13, St. Louis, 2017, Elsevier.)

> **BOX 32.10 Signs of Child Abuse**
>
> **Obvious Signs**
> - Previously filed reports of physical or sexual abuse of the child
> - Documented abuse of other family members
> - Different stories from the parents and the child on how an accident happened
> - Stories of incidents and injuries that are suspicious
> - Injuries blamed on other family members
> - Repeated visits to the emergency department for injuries
>
> **Examination Findings**
> - Trauma to the nervous system
> - Internal abdominal pain
> - Discolorations/bruising on the buttocks, back, and abdomen
> - Elbow, wrist, and shoulder dislocations
>
> **Changes in Child's Behavior**
> - Too eager to please the parent
> - Overly passive and too compliant
> - Aggressive and demanding
> - Parenting the parent (role reversal)
> - Delays in the normal growth and development patterns
> - Erratic school attendance
>
> **Physical Indicators**
> - Poor hygiene
> - Malnutrition
> - Obvious dental neglect
> - Neglected well-baby procedures (e.g., immunizations)

than all diseases combined. The primary causes of childhood injuries are:
- motor vehicle accidents
- drowning
- burns
- falls
- poisoning
- aspiration with airway obstruction
- firearm accidents

Childhood injuries are linked to the child's growth and development level and usually are preventable. Young children are totally dependent on caregivers to keep them safe, so constant supervision and a childproof environment are essential for this age group. Older children need to be aware of health hazards and should be encouraged to protect themselves from injury (e.g., use bike helmets, protective padding when skateboarding, seat belts, and so on). The highest incidence of accidental injuries is seen in children under age 9, but as children grow older, the percentage of deaths from injuries increases. In the United States, more than 9,000 children die each year – about 25 deaths a day – from injuries. Healthcare workers play a major role in injury prevention. The medical assistant is responsible for making sure the ambulatory care office is safe and parents are educated about potential hazards.

CHILD ABUSE

The Child Abuse Prevention and Treatment Act states that all threats to a child's physical and/or mental welfare must be reported. This means that every teacher, healthcare worker, and social worker – in fact, every citizen – who suspects that a child is being neglected, abused, or exploited, must report this to the proper authority. The agency must record the report, and after three similar reports, the agency must investigate.

When suspected abuse, neglect, or exploitation are reported, the individual must provide his or her name. This is considered confidential information and is not given to the child's parent or guardian, nor is it given to the investigating officer. The individual making the report is also protected under the law from any liability for reporting suspicions of child abuse.

> **EXCEPTIONAL CUSTOMER SERVICE**
>
> In a pediatric practice, the child usually is joined by one or both parents during visits to the provider. Parents need reinforcement, praise, and understanding in dealing with the health and welfare of their child. Provide parents with information to help them understand their child's behavior and improve their parenting skills. Understanding the normal behavioral characteristics of a particular developmental stage may increase the parents' confidence and reinforce expectations for the child.
>
> The waiting room is an ideal place for parent education. Use the space and resources available to provide up-to-date information on child health issues and on local resources for support and assistance. If the provider has pamphlets available, discuss them with the parents. Answer questions when possible, or alert the provider so that questions can be answered during the office visit. Every opportunity should be taken to teach parents about sound health care. Because so many ambulatory care visits involve infectious disorders, educating children and parents on the following infection control measures may help reduce the spread of disease:
> - Children should cover their mouth with a disposable tissue when they cough and/or cough into their bent arm rather than their hands.
> - A tissue should be used only once and then immediately thrown away.
> - Children should not be allowed to share toys they have put in their mouth.
> - After a child has discarded a toy that was in the mouth, it should be placed in a bin for dirty toys that is out of reach of others. Wash and disinfect these toys before allowing children to play with them again.
> - Make sure all children and adults follow good hand-washing practices. Have pump hand sanitizers available throughout the office.

If the medical assistant suspects that a child is a victim of abuse, neglect, or exploitation, he or she should consult with the provider immediately (Box 32.10). In most states, the medical assistant and the provider can make separate reports to the authorities. However, state laws vary, so state and local reporting protocols should be outlined in the office procedures manual.

CLOSING COMMENTS

Working in pediatrics can be one of the most challenging and rewarding jobs a medical assistant can have. The patient population is diverse. You are dealing with all ages. You must also establish a solid relationship with the patient's parents and/or caregivers. Having solid communication skills will help to develop those relationships.

CHAPTER REVIEW

In this chapter, we have discussed the growth patterns that children go through. Having an understanding of those patterns can help you deal with all of the patients seen in pediatrics. In addition, it will help you recognize when there is a potential problem that the provider should be aware of. Erik Erikson's development theories can also provide insight on how to work with patients of all ages.

There are certain diseases and disorders that are more common in children than adults. Colic, diarrhea, and failure to thrive are conditions that can be very upsetting for parents and caregivers. As a medical assistant, your role is to reinforce the instructions and information given by the provider regarding these conditions.

Immunizations are a big part of well-child visits. Following the CDC's schedule of immunizations can help ensure that the vaccines protect the child. VISs are part of the immunization procedure. A VIS must be given to an adult patient or to the parents or caregivers of a child before the immunization is given, and all their questions must be answered. Documentation is the key for immunizations. Be sure to document all needed information.

For well-child visits, the medical assistant will obtain certain vital signs, based on age. It is important to remember the normal range for most vital signs changes that correspond to the age of the patient.

Working with a child can be challenging, but if you can establish a positive relationship with the child. things will go more smoothly. Adolescent patients pose their own set of challenges, some of them legal. You should be aware of the laws in your state regarding the treatment and release of information regarding adolescents.

SCENARIO WRAP-UP

After working with the telephone screening staff, Allison has come to realize the importance of becoming familiar with childhood diseases and disorders, and the management policy of her provider-employers. Many times Allison has had to refer to the office procedure manual to make sure she is asking the right questions and gathering all the information needed for the provider who will make the daily response calls. From working in the clinical area, Allison has also realized that a pediatric practice actually has two groups of patients: the child and the caregivers. She must be sensitive to the needs of both groups and develop communication skills that build trust with the child and his or her parents.

Allison is working on developing a comprehensive education site in the office for interested parents and is creating a community resource guide for interested caregivers. She recognizes the need to stay up-to-date on the CDC's recommendations for childhood immunizations, and she routinely refers to the CDC's website to make sure the office has the most recently published VIS forms. Allison regularly attends her local American Association of Medical Assistants (AAMA) chapter meetings to maintain her certification and to continue to learn about the pediatric practice specialty.

33

Assisting in Geriatrics

LEARNING OBJECTIVES

1. Do the following related to the cardiovascular, endocrine, gastrointestinal, integumentary, and musculoskeletal body systems:
   - Explain the changes in the anatomy and physiology caused by aging.
   - Summarize the major related diseases and disorders faced by older patients.
2. Do the following related to the nervous system, pulmonary system, sensory organs, urinary system, and reproductive systems:
   - Explain the changes in the anatomy and physiology caused by aging.
   - Summarize the major related diseases and disorders faced by older patients.
   - Describe various screening tools for dementia, depression, and malnutrition in aging adults.
3. Explain the effect of aging on sleep.
4. Differentiate among independent, assisted, and skilled nursing facilities.
5. Summarize the role of the medical assistant in caring for aging patients; also, list and describe the principles of effective communication with older adults.

CHAPTER OUTLINE

1. Opening Scenario, 742
2. You Will Learn, 742
3. Introduction, 742
4. Changes in Anatomy and Physiology, 744
   a. Cardiovascular System, 744
   b. Endocrine System, 745
   c. Gastrointestinal System, 746
   d. Integumentary System, 746
   e. Musculoskeletal System, 747
      i. *Osteoporosis*, 748
      ii. *Falls*, 748
   f. Nervous System, 749
      i. *Alzheimer's Disease*, 749
   g. Pulmonary System, 750
   h. Sensory Organs, 750
      i. *Vision*, 750
      ii. *Hearing*, 751
      iii. *Taste and Smell*, 752
   i. Urinary System, 753
   j. Reproductive System, 754
   k. Sleep Disorders, 754
   l. Living Arrangements, 754
5. The Medical Assistant's Role in Caring for the Older Patient, 755
6. Closing Comments, 756
7. Chapter Review, 756

OPENING SCENARIO

Bill Novelli, CMA (AAMA), works at Walden-Martin Family Medical Clinic (WMFM). Although patients of all ages are seen in the practice, many patients are age 65 or older. Through his work with Dr. Stephanie Kennedy, Bill has learned to recognize the unique communication needs of aging individuals and the importance of using family and community resources to maintain optimum health in this special population.

YOU WILL LEARN

- How the aging population will impact the delivery of healthcare.
- To describe the changes in anatomy and physiology in body systems in geriatric patients.
- To adjust your communication style when working with geriatric patients.

INTRODUCTION

According to the National Institutes of Health, the aging population in the United States (those age 65 or older) is expected to nearly double over the next 30 years. By 2050, it is projected that there will be 88 million people age 65 or over.

The average life expectancy of an individual who reaches age 65 is an additional 19.3 years (20.6 years for females and 18 years for males). A child born in 2014 can expect to live 78.9 years, about 30 years longer than a child born in 1900. Older women outnumber older men; 25.1 million women are over age 65, as are 19.6 million men. About 30% of older people who live outside of institutions live alone; half of women over age 75 live alone. More than half a million grandparents over the age of 65 are the primary caregivers for their grandchildren, who live with them. Most older people have at least one chronic medical condition, and many have multiple conditions. Hypertension, arthritis, heart disease, cancer, and diabetes are the health problems most commonly seen in the elderly, and a significant number also suffer from strokes, asthma, emphysema, and chronic bronchitis.

What does all this mean to those who have chosen careers in health care? As the aging population expands, it will affect all aspects of society. One area in particular will be these individuals' increased use of health services. To provide quality care to aging patients, medical assistants must understand the aging process, including the physical and sensory changes that occur with aging (Procedure 33.1). This knowledge enables medical assistants to recognize the special needs of the aged and to develop therapeutic management and communication skills that can help them effectively care for the older patient. Ongoing research and education about the aging process have dispelled many of the old stereotypes.

Aging is a complex physiological, psychological, and social process. Old age is not an illness, but rather a normal life process that people experience in different ways. Lack of exercise, poor nutrition, substance abuse, continual stress, and air pollutants are all factors that cause a person to show the effects of aging decades earlier than someone who has practiced healthy living habits.

As people age, changes occur in their physical appearance and abilities, along with sensory changes in vision, hearing, taste, and smell. These changes do not occur at the same time in everyone; however, sensorimotor changes can have a profound effect on the individual's ability to interact with his or her environment. Box 33.1 describes some of the common stereotypes and myths about aging.

> **BOX 33.1 Stereotypes and Myths About Aging**
>
> - *Most aging people will develop dementia.* Dementia is not part of the normal aging process. However, the older the person, the greater the risk of dementia. About 6% of those over age 65 and almost 50% of those over age 85 are diagnosed with significant memory and disorientation issues.
> - *Disease is a normal and an unavoidable part of the aging process.* Recent research verifies that individuals who have established healthy lifestyles as they age remain healthy well into their older years. Aging people are more likely to have health issues, but these are not inevitable for all persons over age 65.
> - *Older workers are less productive than younger ones.* Individuals with a strong work ethic continue to perform in this way. It may take aging people longer to learn new material, but they continue to be capable of learning and applying new knowledge.
> - *Most older people end up in long-term care facilities.* At any given time, approximately 5% of the aging population lives in long-term care facilities; 80% of aging individuals live independently, with or without a partner.
> - *Most aging people have no interest in or capacity for sexual relations.* Sexual interest does not change significantly with age; a decrease in sexual activity is usually related to the loss of a partner.
> - *Damage to health because of lifestyle factors is irreversible.* It is never too late to benefit from healthy lifestyle choices.

PROCEDURE 33.1 Understand the Sensorimotor Changes of Aging

Task:
To role-play an older adult so as to better understand the needs of aging people.

Equipment and Supplies
- Yellow-tinted glasses, ski goggles, or laboratory goggles
- Pink, white, yellow "pills" (e.g., various colors of Tic Tacs)
- Petroleum jelly (e.g., Vaseline)
- Cotton balls
- Eye patches
- Tape
- Utility gloves
- Tongue depressors
- Elastic bandages
- Medical forms in small print
- Pennies
- Button shirts
- Walker

Procedural Steps
1. Role-play vision and hearing loss.
   - Put two cotton balls in each ear and an eye patch over one eye. Follow your partner's instructions.
   - *Partner:* Stand out of the line of vision (to prevent lip-reading). Without using gestures or changing your voice volume, tell your partner to cross the room and pick up a book.
2. Role-play yellowing of the lens of the eye.
   - Line up "pills" of different pastel colors.
   - *Partner:* Pick out the different colors while wearing the yellow-tinted glasses.
3. Role-play difficulty with focusing.
   - Put on goggles smeared with petroleum jelly and follow your partner's directions.
   - *Partner:* Stand at least 3 feet in front of your partner and motion for him or her to come to you (your partner is deaf, so talking will not help).
4. Role-play loss of peripheral vision.
   - Put on goggles with black paper taped to the sides.
   - *Partner:* Stand to the side, out of the field of vision, and motion for your partner to follow you.
5. Role-play aphasia and partial paralysis.
   - You are unable to use your right arm or leg. Place tape over your mouth. Let your partner know you need to go to the bathroom.
   - *Partner:* Stand at least 3 feet away with your back to your partner and wait for instructions.
6. Role-play problems with dexterity.
   - Put thick gloves on your hands and try to sign your name, button a shirt, tie your shoes, and pick up pennies.
7. Role-play problems with mobility.
   - Use the walker to cross the room.
   - *Partner:* After your partner starts to use the walker, hand him or her a book to carry.
8. Role-play changes in sensation.
   - Put a rubber utility glove on; turn on very warm water; test the difference in temperature between the gloved hand and the ungloved hand.
9. Summarize and share with the group your impressions of the effect of age-related sensorimotor changes.

> **CRITICAL THINKING BOX 33.1**
>
> When Bill first started working with aging patients, he believed many of the stereotypes about people over age 65. Through his work with Dr. Kennedy, he has come to realize that many of these myths have no foundation in actual practice. Based on the myths mentioned in the text, what do you think about these beliefs on aging? Share your thoughts with your classmates.

CHANGES IN ANATOMY AND PHYSIOLOGY

The aging process brings about changes in all of the body's systems. Table 33.1 summarizes these changes and what can be done to promote healthy aging.

Cardiovascular System

Cardiovascular disease is the most frequent cause of illness and disability in the aging population, and congestive heart failure (CHF) (see Chapter 10, Cardiovascular System) is the most common reason for hospitalization. Age-related changes can occur in the cardiovascular system. Disease and lifestyle habits such as lack of exercise, poor diet, and stress can greatly contribute to these changes. Heart disease is ranked as the leading cause of death among men and women. Proper management of cardiovascular disease can help maintain the health of an aging population and reduce *mortality* (mawr TAL i tee) rates.

> **VOCABULARY**
> **mortality:** The relative frequency of deaths in a specific population.

The aging process causes structural changes in the heart. Myocardial cells enlarge, and deposits of fat and connective tissue increase. These combine to make the myocardial wall stiffer and to increase the time needed for the relaxation phase of the cardiac cycle. As a result, cardiac output declines, making aging people more susceptible to CHF. The reduction in cardiac output leads to pooling of blood in the legs, cold extremities, and edema (Table 33.2). In addition, the heart cannot respond as quickly or as forcefully to an increased workload. Exercise, sudden movements, and changes in position can result in dizziness and loss of balance. Aging typically brings with it an increase in blood pressure, requiring the heart to work harder to pump blood into the systemic circulation. Hypertension increases the workload of the left ventricle, and this may result in **hypertrophy** (hahy PUR troh fee) of the chamber and weakening of the myocardial (mahy uh KAHR dee all) wall. The valves of the heart tend to thicken and become more rigid, making it more difficult for blood to circulate through the cardiopulmonary vessels. With these cardiovascular problems, arrhythmias (ey RITH mee uh) become more common.

> **MEDICAL TERMINOLOGY**
> **hyper-:** excessive, above
> **-trophy:** process of nourishment, development

TABLE 33.1 System Changes With Aging and Measures to Promote Health

System	Age-Related Changes	Health Promotion
Cardiovascular system	Arteriosclerosis and atherosclerotic plaque buildup reduces blood flow to major organs; 50% of the aging population have hypertension; CVD is the number one killer of women and men in their 60s.	Regular exercise; weight control; diet rich in fruits, vegetables, and whole grains; cholesterol, blood glucose monitoring
Central nervous system	Brain shrinks by 10% between ages 30 and 90; takes longer to learn new material; attention span and language remain the same; signs and symptoms may be caused by depression, vascular disease, and drug reactions.	Aerobic exercise to increase blood flow to CNS; maintaining mental activities (e.g., reading, interacting with others)
Endocrine system	After age 50, women have a sharp decline in estrogen; men have a more gradual decline in testosterone.	Possible hormone replacement therapy or natural soy supplements
Gastrointestinal system	Decline in gastric juices and enzymes by age 60; decreased peristalsis with increased constipation; some nutrients are not absorbed as well.	High-fiber diet and adequate fluid intake; regular exercise to prevent constipation
Musculoskeletal system	Muscle mass decreases; tendency to gain weight; gradual loss of bone density; deterioration of joint cartilage.	Strength training to increase muscle mass; stretching to remain limber; exercise; vitamin D and calcium supplements
Pulmonary system	At age 55 the lungs become less elastic and the chest wall gradually stiffens, making oxygenation more difficult.	Quit smoking; regular aerobic exercise
Sensory organs	Hearing is intact through the mid-50s but declines by 25% by age 80; oral problems are common; skin thins and loses elasticity; presbyopia after age 40; cataracts common after age 60.	Avoid exposure to loud noise, use hearing aids; good dental hygiene; prevention of sun damage to the skin; annual eye examinations; diet rich in dark green, leafy vegetables to prevent cataracts and macular degeneration
Urinary system	Kidneys become less efficient; bladder muscles weaken; one third of seniors experience incontinence; prostate enlargement is common.	Pelvic exercises, drugs, or surgery for incontinence; annual PSA with digital rectal exam monitoring for men
Sexuality	*Men:* Impotence is not a symptom of normal aging; men over age 50 may have some altered function. *Women:* Menopause causes vaginal narrowing and dryness, resulting in painful intercourse.	*Men:* Maintenance of cardiovascular health with exercise, weight control, no smoking, diabetes management *Women:* Use of vaginal lubricants or estrogen cream

From Proctor D, et al: *Kinn's The Medical Assistant*, ed 13, St. Louis, 2017, Elsevier.
CNS, Central nervous system; *CVD*, cardiovascular disease; *PSA*, prostate-specific antigen.

TABLE 33.2 Normal Changes in Cardiac Output With Age

Age	Blood Pumped by Resting Heart (quarts/min)	Maximum Heartbeat During Exercise (beats/min)
30	3.6	200
40	3.4	182
50	3.2	171
60	2.9	159
70	2.6	150

Data from American Heart Association. www.americanheart.org. Accessed July 20, 2012.

Aging causes the walls of the veins to weaken and stretch. This damages the valves, especially in the veins of the legs, where the walls are subject to greater pressure as blood struggles to return to the heart against the force of gravity. As a result, edema and varicose veins of the lower extremities are common in the elderly, increasing the risk of phlebitis and the formation of thrombi in the deep veins, or *deep vein thrombosis* (DVT).

Arteriosclerosis (ar teer ee oh sklah ROH sis) is considered part of the aging process. The vessel walls thicken and become less elastic as a result of the calcification and buildup of connective tissue. In addition, the arteries' ability to dilate and contract diminishes. To maintain an adequate blood supply throughout the body, the heart must work harder to overcome the resistance caused by stiffened vessels. Older adults have a higher incidence of orthostatic hypotension. The clinical criterion for alterations in blood pressure from sitting to standing is:

- a drop of 20 mm Hg or more in the systolic pressure, or
- 10 mm Hg or more in the diastolic pressure

When a person with orthostatic hypotension stands, gravity causes blood to pool in the legs, resulting in a drop in the amount of blood returning to the heart for circulation. This decrease in circulating blood volume causes a sudden drop in blood pressure. The provider may have the medical assistant take orthostatic blood pressures as part of the routine intake protocol for aging patients. To perform this procedure, apply a blood pressure cuff and take the individual's blood pressure and pulse while the patient is lying down. Leave the cuff in place, have the patient sit up, and take the blood pressure and pulse after 1 minute. Leave the cuff in place, have the patient stand, take the blood pressure and pulse immediately, and then again after 3 minutes. Record the blood pressure immediately, including the position for each of the readings.

Endocrine System

Hormonal changes that occur with aging are related to a general decrease in hormone production combined with changes in tissue receptor binding. The most common endocrine system disorder seen in aging patients is *diabetes mellitus (DM) type 2*. As a person ages, insulin production by the beta cells in the pancreas decreases and insulin resistance at the tissue level increases. According to the National Institutes of Health, more than half of the 16 million Americans diagnosed with diabetes type 2 are over age 65. Elderly patients with diabetes are at increased risk of developing vascular disease, including:

- renal disorders
- retinopathy (ret in OP ah thee)
- neuropathy (noo ROP ah thee)
- myocardial ischemia (mye oh KAR dee ul ih SKEE mee uh)
- angina (an JYE nuh)
- myocardial infarction (mye oh KAR dee ul in FARCK shun)
- cerebrovascular accidents
- peripheral vascular disease, such as lower extremity ulcers

Older patients do not always experience the classic symptoms of diabetes, which are **polyuria** (pah lee YOO ree ah), **polydipsia** (pah lee DIP see ah), and **polyphagia** (pah lee FAY jee ah). They may show a variety of problems, including:

- unexplained weight loss
- slow wound healing
- recurrent bacterial or fungal infections
- changes in mental state
- cataracts
- macular disease
- muscle weakness and pain
- angina
- foot ulcers
- **uremia** (yoo REE mee uh)

The range of symptoms is due to the insidious (in DID ee uh s) onset of diabetes in older people, who may have gradually developing **hyperglycemia** (HI per gly SEE mee uh) for years before diagnosis.

The treatment protocol for aging patients with diabetes is the same as for other age groups; however, special consideration must be given to the patient's ability to understand and comply with the therapeutic plan. In addition, the person may have other health problems that are being treated with medications. Therefore, an aging patient newly diagnosed with diabetes may face a complicated treatment plan that requires explicit (ik SPLIS it) instruction and continual follow-up in the ambulatory care setting.

The medical assistant must be aware of any sensory abnormalities, such as diminished vision or problems with fine motor skills, that may interfere with the patient's ability to follow treatment guidelines. Teaching

---

VOCABULARY

insidious: Stealthily treacherous.
orthostatic hypotension: A temporary fall in blood pressure when a person rapidly changes from a recumbent position to a standing position.

MEDICAL TERMINOLOGY

-al: pertaining to
-ar: pertaining to
arteri/o: artery
cardi/o: heart
cerebr/o: cerebrum
-dipsia: condition of thirst
-emia: blood condition
glyc/o: sugar, glucose
hyper-: excessive, above
-ia: condition
my/o: muscle
neur/o: nerve
-pathy: disease process
phag/o: to eat, swallow
poly-: excessive
retin/o: retina
-sclerosis: abnormal condition of hardening
ur/o: urine
vascul/o: vessel

> **BOX 33.2 Factors That Can Affect Diabetes Management in Older People**
>
> - Modifying lifestyle risk factors may be more difficult because of poor nutrition, inability to exercise, and long-standing habits, such as smoking and a diet high in saturated fats and calories.
> - Previously diagnosed health conditions, such as hypertension and heart disease, in addition to an age-related decline in kidney and liver function, increase the challenge of treating diabetes.
> - Older people are more likely to be prescribed multiple medications, which increases the risk of adverse drug interactions.
> - Elderly patients with diabetes are more prone to hypoglycemia and may not recognize and respond quickly to the signs of low blood glucose levels.
> - Diabetic complications can develop quickly because of a long history of prediabetes before diagnosis.
> - Older people may have decreased physical and/or mental abilities that make it difficult for them to understand and adhere to a complicated treatment regimen.
> - Older patients may not be able to afford the medications and supplies needed to maintain health.

> **CRITICAL THINKING BOX 33.2**
>
> Quite a few of the elderly patients at WMFM have diabetes type 2. Based on what you have learned about the difficulty of managing diabetes in aging people, what factors do you need to consider when conducting patient education for an elderly person with diabetes? Are there any community resources that might be useful for patients and their families?

and treatment plans must be adapted to meet the individual needs of each patient. For example, if the patient has vision difficulties, an injector pen, with audible clicks, can be used to deliver a preset amount of insulin. Box 33.2 presents more information about factors that can affect diabetes management in older people.

Gastrointestinal System

Age-related changes in the gastrointestinal system begin in the mouth with dental problems:
- a decrease in the number of taste buds
- a decrease in the production of saliva
- a diminishing sense of smell

Older people generally find eating less pleasurable, have a reduced appetite, and are unable to chew and lubricate their food as well as younger people. This makes *dysphagia* (dis FAY jee ah) (difficulty swallowing) a common age-related problem. Aging also brings a decrease in the production of hydrochloric acid, which affects the digestion of calcium and iron. Secretion of intrinsic factor, a protein that is needed for the absorption of vitamin B_{12}, also declines. This affects the function of the nervous system. It also affects the formation of red blood cells, resulting in excessive fatigue. It is not unusual for aging patients to be on regular vitamin B_{12} replacement therapy, either by oral dosage or by injection.

Food passes more quickly through the small intestine, resulting in poorer absorption of vitamins and minerals. **Peristalsis** (per uh STAHL suhs) in the colon decreases, making aging patients more susceptible to constipation and diverticular (dahy ver TICK yoo luhr) disease. Poor eating habits, a reduced fluid intake, and some medications (e.g., antidepressants, diuretics, antacids containing aluminum or calcium, and medications for Parkinson's disease) also contribute to constipation. The liver decreases in size and weight after age 70. It is still able to

> **VOCABULARY**
>
> **explicit:** Fully and clearly expressed or demonstrated; leaving nothing merely implied.
> **peristalsis:** Rhythmic contraction of involuntary muscles lining the gastrointestinal tract.

perform vital functions, but more time is required to metabolize drugs and alcohol. All of these factors combine to increase the potential for adverse drug reactions in older adults.

Aging individuals have a higher incidence of several gastrointestinal system diseases, such as:
- **gastroesophageal** (gass troh eh say fah JEE ul) reflux disease (GERD)
- peptic ulcers
- **diverticulosis** (dye vur tick yoo LOH sis) (related to lack of dietary fiber and constipation)
- **cholelithiasis** (koh lee lih THY ih sis)
- colorectal cancer

Dietary counseling and annual screenings should be part of the routine care of aging patients.

> **MEDICAL TERMINOLOGY**
>
> **gastr/o:** stomach   **-itis:** inflammation
> **esophag/o:** esophagus   **chol/e:** gall, bile
> **-eal:** pertaining to   **lith/o:** stone
> **diverticul/o:** diverticulum **-iasis:** presence of

Integumentary System

The skin is the body's first line of protection against infection, and it also is responsible for preventing the loss of body fluids and regulating body temperature. Changes in the appearance and function of the integumentary system are usually caused by a combination of ordinary age-related changes and environmental factors, especially the amount of sun exposure over time. Exposure to ultraviolet light from the sun frequently is the cause of:
- wrinkles
- age spots
- blotches
- leathery, dry, loose skin

All of which are associated with aging. Changes caused by the ultraviolet light from the sun or by the normal aging process can affect all three layers of the skin: the epidermis, dermis, and subcutaneous tissue.

The cells in the epidermis reproduce more slowly as people age, and this slower regeneration causes the skin to appear thinner. The skin becomes more prone to tearing and blistering. The risk of infections increases, the healing process takes longer, and older people are more susceptible to bruising. Because the skin can be easily torn, it is important to be very careful when performing phlebotomy or covering a wound on an older patient. The use of tape should be avoided. Vitamin D synthesis, a major function of the epidermis, significantly declines in aged skin, and a decrease in the number of melanocytes increases photosensitivity.

The dermis loses 20% of its mass during the aging process, resulting in the paper-thin or transparent skin seen in older adults. The number of **collagen** (KAW lah jen) cells in the dermis also declines with age, causing the skin to sag and wrinkle. Because both sweat and sebaceous (se BEY shuh s) glands decrease in number, aging people have difficulty tolerating higher temperatures because they perspire less. At the same time, the blood supply to the dermis decreases; this makes it difficult to regulate the body temperature and leads to an increased susceptibility to both hypothermia and heat stroke in aging individuals. Any situation in which an older adult would be exposed to extremes of cold or heat should be avoided. Make sure a blanket is available in the examining room if the air conditioning is on. Ask the person if he or she is too

> **VOCABULARY**
>
> **collagen:** The most abundant structural protein found in skin and other connective tissues. It provides strength and cushioning to many parts of the body.

cold or too hot and take the necessary steps to make the patient feel more comfortable.

Atrophy of the subcutaneous layer increases the skin's susceptibility to trauma, so patients bruise much more easily. The skin is denied natural lubrication, and dry skin is one of the most common complaints among older people. In addition, fat deposits increase in the abdomen in men and in the abdomen and thighs in women as they age.

Suggestions that might help older people prevent and treat dry skin include:
- Use a room humidifier to moisten the air
- Bathe less frequently and use warm rather than hot water
- Use a mild soap or cleansing cream (e.g., Aveeno, Basis, or Dove)
- Wear protective clothing in cold weather
- Moisturize dry skin

Pain receptors are distributed throughout the skin. Because of age-related changes in the receptors, older people have a higher pain threshold. They may not notice a cut or burn as quickly as a younger person would, so a more serious burn may occur before it is noticed. In addition, wound healing becomes a problem because of decreased blood flow to dermal tissues.

Other changes occur in the skin's appendages. Hair changes in color, growth, and distribution. Hair grays because of the decreased rate of melanin production and the replacement of pigmented hair with nonpigmented hair. Women lose hair on the trunk and have increased facial hair. Although *alopecia* (al oh PEE shee uh) (loss of hair) is caused by an inherited trait, aging also causes hair loss. Hair on the eyebrows, nose, and ears becomes coarser and longer in men. The nails of older people take longer to grow and are more brittle. Nails, particularly toenails, thicken as a result of trauma or nutritional deficiencies. It is not unusual for nails to split, making them more susceptible to fungal infections.

> **MEDICAL TERMINOLOGY**
>
> **a-:** no, not, without
> **dermatome:** Skin surface areas supplied by a single afferent spinal nerve.
> **kerat/o:** hard, horny
> **postherpetic neuralgia:** Nerve pain that occurs after a shingles outbreak and may become chronic.
> **-rrheic:** pertaining to discharge
> **seb/o:** oil
> **troph/o:** development
> **-y:** process of

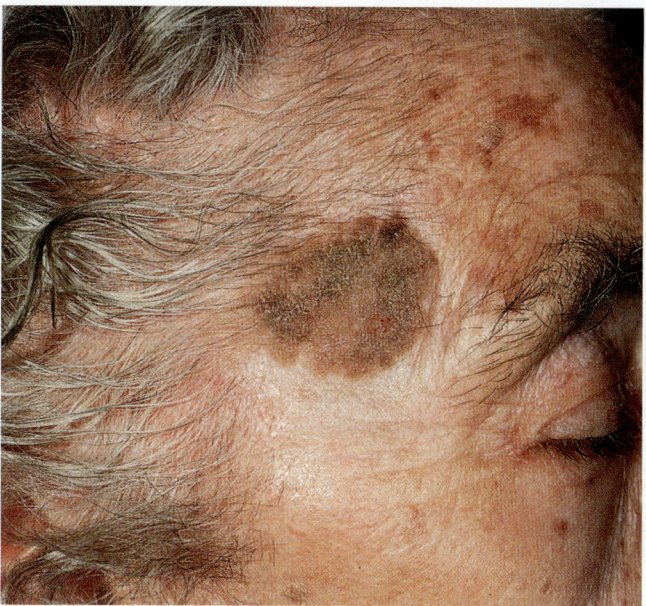

FIG. 33.1 Seborrheic keratosis. (From Habif TP: *Clinical Dermatology: A Color Guide To Diagnosis And Therapy*, ed 6, St Louis, 2016, Mosby.)

Seborrheic keratoses (seb oh REE ick kair ah TOE sus), usually referred to as "age spots," are one of the most common benign skin disorders found in the aging population. They appear as waxy, scaly papules that vary from tan to dark brown (Fig. 33.1) and typically are found in areas of sun exposure, such as the trunk, back, face, neck, extremities, and scalp. They are not dangerous but may be removed for cosmetic purposes.

Shingles is another condition that shows up on the skin. It is caused by the same virus that causes chickenpox. A person who has had chickenpox in the past is at risk for developing shingles. Box 33.3 describes two ways to reduce the risk for developing shingles.

> **CRITICAL THINKING BOX 33.3**
>
> Rose Deluca, a 71-year-old patient of Dr. Martin, is unhappy about the changes in her skin that have occurred in the past several years. Based on what Bill knows about the normal changes that occur in the skin as people age, how can he explain these changes to Mrs. Deluca, and what can he suggest to help with dryness and other typical aging changes?

Musculoskeletal System

As the body ages, changes occur in the muscles, bones, and joints that affect the individual's appearance, strength, and mobility (Box 33.4). The extent of change depends on the person's diet, exercise pattern, and heredity. Cartilage loss and degeneration, which produce **osteoarthritis** (os TEE oh arth RYE tis), commonly occur in the weight-bearing joints of older people. Joint range of motion is affected, and the intervertebral disc spaces are decreased, causing loss of height as a person ages. A breakdown in joint structures may lead to inflammation, pain, stiffness, and deformity.

Aging brings a decrease in the strength and speed of muscle contractions in the extremities but only a slight decline in overall muscle endurance. Muscular changes in the aging patient are directly related to the individual's activity level. Research shows that musculoskeletal

BOX 33.3 Shingles Risk Reduction

The varicella-zoster virus causes both shingles and chickenpox. After an active chickenpox infection, the virus lies dormant in a nerve **dermatome** (DUR mah tome). As people age, their risk increases that the virus will reactivate, causing the formation of blisters and varying degrees of pain along the affected nerve pathway. It is estimated that one in three adults will develop shingles in their lifetime. There are currently two shingles vaccines approved in the United States.

The older vaccine, Zostavax, was developed to reduce the risk of shingles in people age 60 and older. Zostavax is a live virus vaccine that boosts immunity against the varicella-zoster virus. The vaccine is administered as a single subcutaneous injection. Studies have shown that the vaccine reduces the risk of shingles by about half (51%) and the risk of **postherpetic neuralgia** by 67%; it is most effective in people ages 60 to 69 years.

The newer vaccine, Shingrix, also reduces the risk of shingles. Shingrix is a recombinant vaccine that also boosts immunity against the varicella-zoster virus. This vaccine is administered as an intramuscular injection. It is recommended that the two doses should be given 6 months apart. This vaccine is recommended for healthy adults 50 years and older. The two doses are 90% effective at preventing shingles and postherpetic neuralgia.

For individuals who develop shingles even though they were immunized, the duration of symptoms is shorter. The vaccine is recommended even if an individual has had shingles in the past, to help prevent future occurrences of the disease.

A shingles vaccination can be quite expensive ($200 to $300). Therefore, it is important that the patient or the medical assistant first check with the individual's insurance carrier to see whether the injection is covered.

BOX 33.4 Suggestions for Helping the Older Adult With Mobility, Dexterity, and Balance

- Encourage the person to use assistive devices, such as adaptive silverware, a tub seat or shower chair, electric razor, and reaching devices.
- Assist the person with gripping devices as needed (wait for the patient to place his or her hand around a cup or help him or her with it before letting go).
- Provide older adults with enough time to complete tasks independently.
- For a post-stroke patient who is ambulatory but has one weak side, use a gait belt when transferring the patient from a chair to an examination table.
- The provider may recommend physical therapy for range-of-motion exercises.
- Encourage activity approved by the provider; lack of activity results in a decline in the ability to function.

disease is not an inevitable result of the aging process; however, 40% to 50% of women over age 50 have a serious problem with bone demineralization. Men also experience bone loss, but at a later age, and at a much slower rate than women.

Osteoporosis. Osteoporosis (os tee oh puh ROH sis) is the primary cause of hip fractures, which can lead to a loss of independence and also to complications that ultimately can end in death. The spinal vertebrae also can collapse, producing the stooped posture associated with "dowager's hump." Sometimes bones break because of the sheer weight of the body on them. Often people say they fell and broke a bone, when in reality the bone fractured, causing them to fall. Multiple factors contribute to the development of osteoporosis, but it is most common in postmenopausal women. Risk factors for osteoporosis include:

- Female gender (women have a five times greater risk than men)
- Thin; small-boned frame
- Family history of osteoporosis
- Estrogen deficiency before age 45, either from early menopause or oophorectomy (oo for ECK tuh mee)
- Estrogen deficiency resulting from an abnormal absence of menses (eating disorders, excessive aerobic exercise, fibrocystic ovaries)
- Racial background (Caucasian and Asian women have the highest risk)
- Aging
- Extended use of anticonvulsant drugs, prednisone, and excessive thyroid hormone medications

VOCABULARY
osteoporosis: Abnormal thinning of the bone structure causing bones to become brittle and weak.
oophorectomy: Surgical removal of the ovaries.

- Sedentary lifestyle, smoking, excessive alcohol intake, and lack of calcium and vitamin D when growing up

Weight-bearing exercises and calcium and vitamin D supplements are recommended to prevent demineralization of the bones. Medications used to prevent and/or treat osteoporosis include:

- alendronate (Fosamax) and risedronate (Actonel), which reduce the rate of demineralization
- raloxifene (Evista) and ibandronate (Boniva), which slow bone thinning and cause some increase in bone thickness
- denosumab (Prolia), an injectable medication, which helps increase bone mass
- calcitonin (Calcimar, Miacalcin), which is either injected or inhaled as a nasal spray and results in a decrease in the rate of bone thinning and relieves the pain associated with spinal compression

Another option is an intravenous (IV) medication, zoledronic acid (Reclast), for the once yearly treatment of postmenopausal women with osteoporosis. Reclast helps increase bone density in the spine and hip, thus reducing the risk of fractures.

Falls. The risk of injuries from falls increases with age; falls cause the greatest number of injuries in people over age 70. Aging individuals are at greater risk of falling because of sensorimotor changes in vision and mobility, osteoporosis, and cerebrovascular accidents (CVAs). Falls in older patients usually result in fractures because a large percentage of these individuals have osteoporosis. Serious fractures, such as those of the hip, require the patient to be immobile for extended periods, and this opens the door to a wide range of debilitating complications, such as:

- decubitus (deh KYOO bih tus) ulcers
- pneumonia
- placement in long-term care facilities
- death

MEDICAL TERMINOLOGY
arthr/o: joint	**-osis:** abnormal condition
-ectomy: removal	**osteo:** bone
-itis: inflammation	**oste/o:** bone
oophor/o: ovary	**por/o:** passage

Falls are largely preventable. The medical assistant can play an active role in helping family members and patients become aware of risk factors and safety measures. Suggestions that can help patients prevent falls are:

- Have regular vision tests.
- Understand the side effects of medications, especially those that cause vertigo.
- If you experience orthostatic hypotension, rise slowly and stand still for a moment with support before moving.
- Limit the use of alcohol.
- If needed, consistently use assistive devices, such as a cane or walker, for support.
- Wear low-heeled, rubber-soled shoes with good support.
- Avoid going outside in icy weather.
- Engage in regular weight-bearing exercise for muscle and bone strength.
- Keep hallways, stairs, and bathrooms well lit.
- Assess the home for possible danger areas; remove throw rugs; use handrails on steps and grab bars in bathrooms; keep emergency numbers handy.

VOCABULARY

decubitus ulcers: Sores or ulcers that develop over a bony prominence as the result of ischemia from prolonged pressure; also called *bed sores* or *pressure sores*.

CRITICAL THINKING BOX 33.4

The family of Rita Schaeffer, a 73-year-old patient, is concerned about the risk of falls. Mrs. Schaeffer recently was diagnosed with osteoporosis, and she lives alone. What information should Bill give the family to help them prevent accidents in their mother's home? Also, Mrs. Schaeffer's 45-year-old daughter is concerned about developing osteoporosis. What steps should the daughter take to prevent the disease?

Nervous System

Cognitive ability (i.e., the ability of a person to think) is influenced by many factors, including a person's general state of health, educational background, and genetic code. The normal process of aging may contribute to a change in the thinking process. The brain begins to get smaller at approximately age 50 and continues to get smaller as we age because of a loss of fluid within the neurons and shrinkage of dendrites. Thinning of the dendrites makes transmitting messages from one neuron to the next more difficult. As a result of all these factors, the aging brain is smaller, weighs less, and has started to pull away from the sheath or cortical mantle. Older neurons process information more slowly, so retrieving old information and learning new information takes longer. Reaction time also slows, and aging individuals are distracted more easily; however, recent research shows that the loss of brain cells is minimal and that the older brain is still capable of generating new neurons. Researchers believe that continued, moderate physical and mental activity can maintain the cognitive abilities of aging individuals.

Dementia (dih MEN shuh), the severe loss of intellectual ability, is not an inevitable part of aging but rather the result of an organic disorder. Most men and women remain mentally competent until the end of their lives. Sudden loss of memory, disorientation, and trouble performing the daily tasks of life indicate a problem that should be investigated. Many conditions can cause signs and symptoms of dementia, including:

- depression
- reactions to prescription and over-the-counter (OTC) drugs
- alcoholism
- malnutrition
- thyroid, liver, heart, and vascular disorders
- Parkinson's disease

Multiple factors can interfere with mental judgment and motor skills, giving the impression of decreased mental status.

The best way to ensure mental functioning in later life is to remain mentally and physically stimulated. Exercise improves memory and thinking because of its positive effect on vascular health, increasing the amount of oxygen delivered to the aging brain. Other ways to maintain mental function are to keep socially active; practice stress-reduction activities; quit smoking; drink alcohol in moderation; use hearing aids and glasses if needed to stay in touch with the world; and receive treatment for depression, diabetes, hypertension, and high cholesterol levels. Risk factors for cognitive decline include:

- Hypertension, diabetes, and heart disease (these reduce blood flow to the brain)
- Environmental exposure to lead
- High stress levels
- Sedentary lifestyle and lack of social interaction
- Low education level
- Smoking and substance abuse

Alzheimer's Disease. Alzheimer's (AWLZ hy mers) disease (AD) is a progressive deterioration of the brain caused by the destruction of central nervous system (CNS) neurons, leading to problems with memory, language, thinking, and behavior. Three major changes occur in the brain:

- Amyloid plaques (AM uh loid plaks) form.
- Neurofibrillary (nyoo r fahy bral air ee) tangles clump together, affecting neuron function (neurons eventually die).
- The connections between neurons that are responsible for memory and learning are lost, resulting in neuron destruction; as neurons die throughout the brain, the affected regions begin to atrophy, or shrink. By the final stage of AD, damage is widespread and brain tissue has shrunk significantly.

Patients who show signs and symptoms of dementia are first evaluated for organic causes, such as systemic disease or depression. AD has no definitive diagnostic test because it can be confirmed only through examination of the brain at autopsy. If the patient shows a gradual onset of progressive difficulty with memory, functional abilities, and behavior, and has no evidence of other causes of these disturbances, the physician makes the diagnosis of AD. Imaging studies, including computed tomography (CT), magnetic resonance imaging (MRI), and positron emission tomography (PET), may help show the structural and functional changes in the brain associated with Alzheimer's disease.

Researchers estimate that about 5 million Americans suffer from AD. The disease typically begins after age 60, and the risk of developing the disorder increases with age, although younger people as early as age 30 have been diagnosed with AD. Research shows that 1 in 10 Americans over age 65 have Alzheimer's disease; almost 50% of people age 85 or older are diagnosed with the disease. Despite these statistics, AD is not considered a normal part of the aging process. Alzheimer's disease is the sixth leading cause of death (across all ages) in the United States and the fifth leading cause of death for those age 65 to 85.

AD is a slowly progressive disease that begins with mild memory problems and ends with severe brain damage. The course the disease takes and how fast changes occur varies among individuals, but on average, patients live for 8 to 10 years after they have been diagnosed. Currently no treatment can stop the progression of the disease. However, a great deal of research on the diagnosis and treatment of AD is under way.

TABLE 33.3 Medications Approved for the Treatment of Alzheimer's Disease

Drug	Stage of Treatment	Common Adverse Effects
Cholinesterase Inhibitors		
donepezil (Aricept)	All stages	• Appetite loss
galantamine (Razadyne)	Mild to moderate	• Dizziness
rivastigmine (Exelon) – tablet, liquid, or topical patch	All stages	• Fatigue
		• Increased frequency of bowel movements and diarrhea
		• Insomnia
		• Muscle cramps
		• Nausea, vomiting
		• Weight loss
Receptor Antagonist		
memantine (Namenda) – prescribed alone or in combination with donepezil	Moderate to severe	• Confusion
		• Constipation
		• Diarrhea
		• Dizziness
		• Headache

From http://www.alz.org/alzheimers_disease_standard_prescriptions.asp?gclid=EAIaIQobChMI2O2e_7WT1QIVTZF-Ch1jGAGwEAAYAiAAEgKyq_D_BwE. Accessed July 18, 2017.

The goal of treatment is to maintain normal activities as long as possible. Currently no medicines can slow the progression of AD, but the U.S. Food and Drug Administration (FDA) has approved four medications for the treatment of AD symptoms (Table 33.3). These drugs help individuals carry out the activities of daily living by maintaining thinking, memory, or speaking skills. They can also help with some of the behavioral and personality changes associated with AD. However, they will not stop or reverse AD, and they appear to help individuals for only a few months to a few years. Cholinesterase inhibitors improve the production of neurotransmitters in the brain, which helps prevent memory loss from becoming worse for a limited time. These drugs do not help everyone; as many as 50% of patients show no improvement in mental function. Memantine (Namenda) was the first drug to be approved for the treatment of moderate to severe AD, although it also has limited effects. Individuals with AD frequently experience changes in behavior, so medications may be prescribed to help control sleeplessness, agitation, wandering, anxiety, and depression. Treating these problems helps make the patient more comfortable while easing the burden on caregivers.

Supportive care for family members is absolutely essential because they are faced with caring for a loved one who is suffering progressive memory loss. The medical assistant can be especially helpful in recommending educational workshops, support groups, and stress management skills for caregivers. Multiple resources are available, including online information and support groups, which family members may find helpful.

Pulmonary System

Maximum lung function decreases with age. The rate of airflow through the bronchi slowly declines after age 30, and the maximum force one is able to achieve on inspiration and expiration declines. The lungs lose their elasticity because of changes in **elastin** (ih LAS tin) and collagen. They become smaller and flabbier. The alveoli enlarge, their walls become thinner, and the number of capillaries is reduced. As a result, the area for gas exchange in the lungs is reduced. The chest wall may stiffen from osteoporosis of the ribs and vertebrae and calcification of the **costal** (KOS tl) cartilage. The respiratory muscles become weaker, making it harder to move air into and out of the lungs. To compensate, older adults rely more on accessory muscles, such as the diaphragm. Weakening of the respiratory muscles and stiffening of the chest wall make it harder to cough deeply enough to clear mucus from the lungs. Pulmonary function tests reveal a decrease in vital capacity and an increase in residual volume. The incidence of sleep apnea and sleep disorders increases, causing a potential problem with nocturnal hypoxemia. All these factors combine to put the older adult at greater risk for pneumonia and aspiration and for reactivation of tuberculosis.

The larynx also changes with aging, causing a change in the pitch and quality of the voice. The voice sounds quieter and slightly hoarse. The individual's voice may sound weaker, but it should not interfere with the ability to effectively communicate.

> **VOCABULARY**
> **elastin:** A highly elastic protein in connective tissue that allows tissues to resume their shape after stretching or contracting; found abundantly in the dermis of the skin.

> **MEDICAL TERMINOLOGY**
> **cost/o:** ribs
> **-al:** pertaining to

Sensory Organs

Vision. By the time a person reaches age 50, structural and functional changes in the eye become noticeable (Table 33.4). The eyebrows and eyelashes start to gray. The skin around the eyelids wrinkles, and the loss of orbital fat allows the eye to sink deeper into the orbit. The cornea increases in thickness and has reduced refractive power. A yellow-gray ring (arcus senilis [AHR kuhs suh NAHY lis]) may develop on the periphery of the cornea. The iris loses pigmentation, and as a result older people appear to have gray eyes.

The lens of the eye continues to grow. As new lens fibers grow, old lens fibers are compressed and pushed to the center, causing the lens to become denser. The lens becomes flatter, thicker, less elastic, and more opaque, progressively yellowing with age. By age 70, the lens has tripled in mass. Clouding of the lens causes light rays to scatter, creating glare.

TABLE 33.4 Age-Related Changes in the Anatomic Structures of the Eye

Structure	Age-Related Change	Effects
Lens	Thickens, becomes more opaque	Decreased refraction, causing blurred vision; decreased color acuity; cataracts
Anterior chamber	Decrease in size and volume	May develop increased intraocular pressure and glaucoma
Ciliary muscles	Affects pupil constriction and dilation	Limits light accommodation; night blindness
Cornea	Thickens, curve decreases	Problems with refraction
Retina	Decrease in number of rods and nerves	Decreased clarity; requires increase in minimum amount of light needed to see clearly

From Proctor D, et al: *Kinn's The Medical Assistant*, ed 13, St Louis, 2017, Elsevier.

The pupil is designed to adjust to control the amount of light entering the eye. The ciliary muscle that causes the pupil to dilate weakens during the aging process. As a result, a reduction in the size of the pupil occurs, limiting the amount of light available to reach the retina. Tear production normally decreases. Tear glands do not make enough tears, or the tears are of poor quality and do not keep the eyes wet enough. Eye irritation and excessive tearing are a result of decreased **lacrimation** (lack rih MAY shun).

> **VOCABULARY**
> **lacrimation**: The secretion or discharge of tears.

By the early to mid-40s, presbyopia (prez bee OH pee uh) develops, which makes it difficult to focus in detail on objects close at hand. This requires the use of corrective lenses to accommodate age-related farsightedness. The ability to refocus quickly from far to near or near to far decreases. Also, the ability to follow a moving object is decreased. The yellowing of the lens causes it to act like a filter, making it difficult to distinguish certain color intensities. Blues, greens, and violets are hard to differentiate, whereas yellows, reds, and oranges are easier to identify. The loss in the ability to discriminate closely related colors can affect the older person's ability to judge distances or his or her depth perception. This increases an aging person's susceptibility to falls and accidents. Stairs become a potential hazard because the edges of the steps cannot be seen clearly.

Older people need as much as six times more light to read; however, increasing the level of light does not completely compensate for visual decline because the elderly also experience an increased sensitivity to glare. Glare is probably one of the most painful experiences for the aging eye. Exposed light bulbs, such as those used in chandeliers, and light from highly reflective surfaces, such as glass tables and floors, can produce excessive glare. The eye has a decreased ability to respond to abrupt changes from light to dark or dark to light. Going from a well-lit waiting room into a dim hallway or negotiating the way down dimly lit aisles in a movie theater could be treacherous for an older person.

Cataracts, glaucoma, and macular degeneration. Eye diseases and disorders that occur frequently in older individuals are:
- cataracts
- glaucoma
- macular degeneration

Cataracts (KAT uh rakts) are cloudy or opaque areas in the lens that cause blurring of vision; rings or halos around lights and objects; and a blue or yellow tint to the visual field. Surgical lens extraction and implantation with an artificial lens improves vision in 95% of cases. The procedure, which is performed in an outpatient facility, involves a small incision to remove the lens, laser therapy, or phacoemulsification (fak oh i muhl suh fi KEY shun) (ultrasonic vibrations), which breaks up the lens and removes it without the need for an incision. After the procedure, patients must avoid bending or lifting heavy objects for 3 to 4 weeks; wearing an eye shield at night and glasses during the day helps protect the eye until it heals. Recovery takes about 2 weeks.

Glaucoma (glaw KOH muh) is a result of blockage of the outflow of aqueous humor, which causes an increase in intraocular pressure and damage to the optic nerve. If not treated, glaucoma can cause progressive loss of peripheral vision and ultimately lead to blindness; however, it can be treated with medication.

The *macula* (MAK yuh luh) is the part of the eye responsible for sharp vision and color. Damage to or breakdown of the macula is called *macular degeneration*, which causes progressive loss of the central field of vision. Macular degeneration is the leading cause of blindness in aging people. (All three of these eye disorders are discussed in more detail in Chapter 13, Sensory System.)

Box 33.5 presents suggestions on how to assist a visually impaired older adult.

> **BOX 33.5 Suggestions for Helping the Visually Impaired Older Adult**
>
> - When escorting an older person, regardless of whether he or she is visually impaired, allow the patient to place his or her hand above your elbow. It is easier for the person to follow your movements. This method also provides a source of support and security.
> - Use high levels of evenly distributed, glare-free light.
> - Ask the pharmacist to use large lettering when labeling medicine bottles.
> - Use paper that has a non-glare finish and large print for forms and educational materials.
> - Make distinct differences (e.g., size of containers or color coding with bright primary colors) for pills that are similar in size and color.
> - Place all objects within the visual field and prevent clutter.

Hearing. Hearing loss can have a profound psychological effect on aging people, causing depression, social withdrawal, and feelings of isolation. Hearing loss occurs gradually over a long period and may go undetected by the older person and healthcare providers. Lack of attention when addressed, inappropriate responses, asking to have statements repeated, and speaking too loudly or too softly often are signs of hearing loss. Changes in hearing begin around age 30. By age 65, one out of three people has a hearing loss, and the number increases to 65% of those over age 80. Age-related hearing loss usually is caused by a dysfunction or loss of cochlear cilia, resulting in an inability to hear high-frequency sounds and difficulty understanding speech. Hearing impairment is compounded by impacted cerumen, otitis media, **otosclerosis** (oh toh sklair ROH sis), **Ménière's** (meyn YAIRZ) **disease**, long-term exposure to intense noise, and certain **ototoxic** drugs, such as aspirin.

MEDICAL TERMINOLOGY	
-cusis: hearing	presby-: old age
-ic: pertaining to	-sclerosis: condition of hardening
ot/o: ear	tox/o: poison

VOCABULARY

Ménière's disease: Chronic disease of the inner ear causing recurrent episodes of vertigo, progressive sensorineural hearing loss, and tinnitus.

ototoxic: A medicine or substance capable of damaging cranial nerve VIII or the organs of hearing and balance.

BOX 33.6 Suggestions for Helping the Hearing-Impaired Older Adult

- Stand in the patient's direct line of vision and gently touch the person to get his or her attention.
- Use gestures, pictures, and large, bold print to communicate.
- Talk in short sentences into the ear with better hearing.
- Do not increase the volume of your speech; this also raises the frequency of the voice, which is the hearing most impaired in aging people. Use expanded speech; lower the tone of your voice and talk in distinct syllables.
- Avoid background noise. Give instructions in a quiet room with the door closed. If the patient has a hearing aid, make sure it is on.

Presbycusis (prez by cue sees) is associated with normal aging and causes a decreased ability to hear high frequencies and to discriminate sounds. Parts of a conversation may be missed because the sound of the word goes above the 2,000-cycle frequency. Often words that sound similar are difficult to differentiate. Consonants such as *g, f, s, sh, t,* and *z* produce high-pitched sounds that are more difficult to hear and differentiate. Low-frequency pitched sounds, such as the vowels *a, e, i, o,* and *u,* may be more easily heard by people with presbycusis. Inability to hear different frequencies combined with low background noise from groups of people talking, noise from appliances, or busy public places compromises an older person's ability to hear clearly. Hearing aids, which can be used to amplify speech, may increase background noises, resulting in sensory overload.

Another hearing disorder common among older people is *tinnitus* (tin EYE tis), a ringing or buzzing in the ear. It can be caused by:

- impacted cerumen
- ear infection
- use of antibiotics
- reaction to a medication
- nerve disorder

Tinnitus can cause difficulty understanding conversational speech and can make sleeping difficult because of the continuous sensation of ringing in the ears.

Hearing loss, with its resultant isolation, is directly related to the development of depression in older adults. Treatable depression often is overlooked in elderly people because of coexisting physical illnesses that mask the symptoms of depression. The medical assistant may be able to contribute to information about depression in elderly patients through conversations with the individual and family members. The provider may use or may train the medical assistant to use the Geriatric Depression Scale Short Form, which includes questions for the patient about daily activities, interests, and feelings to help diagnose depression in the ambulatory setting (Fig. 33.2). Box 33.6 lists suggestions on how to assist a hearing-impaired older adult.

Taste and Smell. During the aging process the abilities to taste and smell decline subtly. Deterioration and atrophy of the taste buds are part of the aging process. The ability to taste salt and sweet flavors is reduced, whereas the ability to detect bitter and sour flavors remains relatively the same. As a result, food frequently tastes bland and unappetizing. Patients on salt-restricted diets and patients with diabetes must be cautioned about the use of excessive amounts of salt and sugar. A decrease in the sense of smell accompanies the decrease in taste. Not only does this affect the individual's enjoyment of food, it also puts him or her at risk of environmental dangers, such as gas leaks, smoke, and other dangerous odors that may go undetected. Checking for gas leaks around stoves and heaters and using smoke alarms reduce some of the danger. Also, dating food when it is put in the refrigerator is a good idea.

Nutritional status. Because of the many environmental, social, economic, and physical changes of aging, older people are at greater risk for poor nutrition, which can adversely affect their health and energy level. It is estimated that 25% of the aging population suffers from malnutrition. Nutrition screening should be part of routine primary care, to identify nutritional deficiencies and correct them before a disease process develops or to assist in the treatment of chronic disease. Patients with chronic conditions, such as cardiovascular disease, hypertension, and diabetes, can benefit from nutrition assessments and interventions. Malnourished older patients get more infections; their injuries take longer to heal; surgery is riskier for them; and their hospital stays are longer and more expensive.

The most effective method of assessing a patient's nutritional status is through a comprehensive patient interview that considers all potential stumbling blocks to adequate nutrition. The medical assistant can help determine the nutritional status of older patients by considering the following factors when conducting patient interviews:

- *Oral health:* Does the patient wear dentures, and if so, do they fit properly? Does the patient have mouth pain? Can he or she swallow without difficulty?
- *Gastrointestinal complaints:* Does the patient have anorexia, nausea, vomiting, diarrhea, or constipation? Is the patient lactose intolerant (the incidence increases with age)?
- *Sensorimotor changes:* Does the patient have loss of vision or hearing or changes in taste and smell? Can the patient feed herself or himself? Does the patient need adaptive utensils?
- *Diet influences:* Can the patient afford, shop for, and prepare food? Are ethnic or religious influences a factor? Does the patient have any disease-related diet restrictions? What is the patient's alcohol consumption?
- *Social and mental influences:* Is the patient depressed, lonely, or isolated? Are support systems available?

See Box 33.4 for more information regarding the sensorimotor changes that occur as people age.

CRITICAL THINKING BOX 33.5

Multiple sensory changes occur as people age. Dr. Kennedy asks Bill to develop a handout for patients and family members to help them understand these normal, age-related sensorimotor changes and also adaptations that can improve communication. What information should Bill include?

GERIATRIC DEPRESSION SCALE (SHORT FORM)

Choose the best answer for how you have felt over the past week:
1. Are you basically satisfied with your life? YES / **NO**
2. Have you dropped many of your activities and interests? **YES** / NO
3. Do you feel that your life is empty? **YES** / NO
4. Do you often get bored? **YES** / NO
5. Are you in good spirits most of the time? YES / **NO**
6. Are you afraid that something bad is going to happen to you? **YES** / NO
7. Do you feel happy most of the time? YES / **NO**
8. Do you often feel helpless? **YES** / NO
9. Do you prefer to stay at home, rather than going out and doing new things? **YES** / NO
10. Do you feel you have more problems with memory than most? **YES** / NO
11. Do you think it is wonderful to be alive now? YES / **NO**
12. Do you feel pretty worthless the way you are now? **YES** / NO
13. Do you feel full of energy? YES / **NO**
14. Do you feel that your situation is hopeless? **YES** / NO
15. Do you think that most people are better off than you are? **YES** / NO

Answers in **bold** indicate depression. Although differing sensitivities and specificities have been obtained across studies, for clinical purposes a score >5 points is suggestive of depression and should warrant a follow-up interview. Scores >10 are almost always depression.

FIG. 33.2 Geriatric Depression Scale. (From Proctor D, et al: *Kinn's The Medical Assistant*, ed 13, St Louis, 2017, Elsevier.)

Urinary System

As the body ages, structural changes in the kidneys cause the urinary system to become less efficient. Between the ages of 40 and 80, the kidney loses about 20% of its mass. The number of functional nephron units decreases. Blood flow to the kidneys is reduced because of a decrease in cardiovascular efficiency. Because of the reduction of blood flow to the kidneys and the decreased number of nephrons, the kidneys become less efficient at filtering waste from the blood. This results in a more diluted, less concentrated urine. The kidneys require more water to excrete the same amount of waste. Medication takes longer to be removed from the body. Older adults are at increased risk for toxic levels of medication in the bloodstream because of this reduced filtration rate.

Fibrous connective tissue replaces the smooth muscle and elastic tissue in the bladder. This thickening of the bladder wall reduces the bladder's ability to expand. The bladder's capacity to store fluid comfortably is reduced from 400 to 250 mL. These structural changes lead to increased frequency of urination and urinary retention. Older adults are at increased risk of urinary tract infections because of residual urine. Sleep is interrupted by the need to void during the night. The sensation of bladder fullness is not recognized as quickly by the older brain. Reduced time between awareness of the need to void and involuntary urination can cause anxiety. Often, older adults reduce their fluid intake to prevent possible embarrassment. Unfortunately, this causes dehydration and an increased risk of urinary tract infections. Another change is loss of muscle tone in the urethra. In addition, the pelvic floor muscles in an aging woman relax as a result of decreased estrogen levels or previous pregnancy and childbirth.

Despite these changes, the kidneys have great reserve capacity and are able to continue functioning normally. *Urinary incontinence* (in KON tn uh nens), the involuntary loss of urine, is a significant problem for aging patients but is not a normal part of the aging process. Changes in the urinary system make older people more vulnerable to incontinence, but factors such as infection, confusion, difficulty with mobility, and side effects of medications contribute to the development of the problem. Incontinence is both an emotional and a physical problem. To avoid the risk of an embarrassing accident, people with this problem may avoid social occasions or activities they enjoy. Often people are too embarrassed to admit they have this condition, or they believe it is just part of aging. Once the condition has been diagnosed by a urologist, pelvic floor muscle exercises, medication, or surgery may be recommended.

Reproductive System

Aging brings a decrease in circulating levels of the female hormones estrogen and progesterone, whereas androgen levels increase. The results of this decrease are changes in the genital tract. The vagina diminishes in width and length and becomes less elastic. The cervix, uterus, and ovaries decrease in size. Vaginal secretions decline; therefore, lubrication diminishes, resulting in vaginal dryness. Bacterial or yeast infections may occur because vaginal secretions are less acidic. Estrogen cream applied to vaginal tissue may be prescribed by the provider for help with dryness and thinning of the vaginal tissue. The patient should discuss the benefits and risks of estrogen replacement therapy with the provider to determine whether it should be used.

Even though sperm production may decline in men over age 50, men remain virile well into old age. However, they experience a change in hormonal levels of testosterone, and these changes can affect the prostate gland. The prostate enlarges over time and presses down on the urethra, causing difficulty with urination. Surgery may be required to remove excess portions of the gland. Unfortunately, the operation may cause impotence, which can be treated medically with erectile dysfunction medications.

Men experience some changes in sexual functioning as they age. It takes longer for the penis to become erect, longer for an orgasm to occur, and longer to recover. Direct stimulation may be required before an erection occurs, and when it does, it may be less firm than in younger years.

Some drugs and illnesses can interfere with sexual function. Drugs used to control high blood pressure, antihistamines, antidepressants, and some stomach acid blockers, in addition to the diseases diabetes, arthritis, and arteriosclerosis, can have an adverse effect on sexual function. Often people who have had heart surgery or a heart attack are concerned about sexual activity. Patients need to feel comfortable and should not be embarrassed to discuss their concerns openly with their provider. It is important for healthcare practitioners to dismiss the myth that older patients have lost the desire for and interest in sexual intercourse.

Sleep Disorders

Complaints of sleeping difficulties increase with age. The amount of time spent sleeping may be slightly longer than in a younger person, but the quality of sleep declines. Older people are often light sleepers and have periods of wakefulness in bed. Rapid eye movement (REM) sleep is the stage of sleep in which people experience dreaming. Non-REM sleep is the period of deepest sleep. The amount of time spent in the deepest stages of sleep decreases with age. Sleep that is disturbed or that leaves the person feeling tired is not part of the aging process and may indicate some underlying emotional or physical problem. Lack of sleep can result in restlessness, disorientation, "thick" speech, and mispronounced words. Often, these symptoms are mistaken for signs of dementia. Other factors that might influence sleep patterns are medications, caffeine, alcohol, depression, and environmental or physical changes.

Common sleep problems in older adults include **dyssomnias** (dih SAHM nee ah), such as periodic limb movement disorder (PLMD), in which periodic jerking of the legs occurs during sleep, and sleep apnea. This is common among overweight individuals and can occur frequently during the night, interrupting sleep. Numerous medical conditions can interfere with sleep, including:

- joint and bone pain
- Parkinson's disease (because of difficulty changing positions)
- congestive heart failure
- chronic obstructive pulmonary disease (COPD)
- diabetes mellitus, which increases nocturia (nok TOO R ee uh)
- depression
- certain medications (e.g., beta blockers can cause nightmares, antidepressants increase PLMD, and barbiturates may result in nightmares or hallucinations)

It is important to be aware of the effect of sleep problems because often these can be confused with dementia. Patients who are experiencing

> **MEDICAL TERMINOLOGY**
> **dys-:** difficult
> **somn/o:** sleep
> **-ia:** condition

> **VOCABULARY**
> **nocturia:** Frequent urination at night.

difficulty with sleeping should be encouraged to document their sleeping patterns, napping patterns, medications, diet, exercise routines, and any events that have resulted in a change of lifestyle. They should discuss this problem with their provider. Simple modification of behavioral patterns may resolve the problem. Taking fewer naps, completing exercise several hours before bedtime, changing eating times, reducing the amount of alcohol and caffeine ingested, drinking a glass of milk before bedtime, or changing medications or the time they are taken all are suggestions that might alter the factors responsible for sleep disturbances.

If behavioral approaches are not effective, medications may be considered for short-term use only, because they have a high incidence of physical and psychological dependence. Elderly people are especially susceptible to side effects from these drugs, such as next-day drowsiness and temporary memory loss. Sedatives or hypnotics that may be prescribed include zolpidem (Ambien), eszopiclone (Lunesta), zaleplon (Sonata), and ramelteon (Rozerem).

Living Arrangements

At any given time, only 5% of the elderly population lives in long-term care facilities. According to information published by the National Institute on Aging, older people live close to their children and are in frequent contact with them. People prefer to age in place; that is, they want to live in their own home environment as long as possible. Individuals are admitted to nursing homes because they are no longer able to perform activities of daily living, such as bathing, dressing, eating, walking, and maintaining bladder and bowel continence. They also have difficulty with grocery shopping, housekeeping, and money management. Chronic health conditions and accidents interfere with the older person's ability to perform these tasks.

Many resources are available to help seniors maintain their independence. Outreach programs, such as Meals on Wheels, deliver nutritious meals to the homes of older adults. Senior centers serve as a focal point for many activities and as a source of information. Transportation services provide rides to doctors' appointments, day care centers, shopping centers, and community events. Home health agencies provide several types of services, including personal care, shopping, transportation, and meal preparation. Some home health agencies provide a range of activities, from patient education to IV therapy; medical-social services; physical, speech, and occupational therapies; and nutrition and dietary counseling. Advanced technology allows people to receive services at home that formerly were provided only in a hospital or a physician's office.

Adult day care centers provide socialization, recreation, meals, and, in some centers, physical therapy, occupational therapy, and transportation. These centers offer supervision for older adults who may be taken care of by family members in the evening but need care during the day. They also serve as respite for a caregiver.

Assisted-living facilities can be retirement homes or board-and-care homes. These facilities are appropriate for older adults who need assistance with some activities of daily living, such as bathing, dressing, and walking. Skilled nursing facilities provide 24-hour medical care and supervision. In addition to medical care, residents receive care that may include physical, occupational, and speech therapies. The objective of treatment is to improve or maintain the person's abilities.

THE MEDICAL ASSISTANT'S ROLE IN CARING FOR THE OLDER PATIENT

Elderly patients in the ambulatory care setting present a specific set of needs that require a certain amount of accommodation by the staff. For example, aging patients typically require more time to perform tasks and have questions answered. The office staff may want to hurry them so that the day's schedule can be maintained. In the best interests of the patient, however, he or she should be treated with respect and given whatever time is needed to prepare for examinations, ask questions and receive answers, and have procedures explained. A system that is sensitive to the needs of older patients:

- schedules longer periods for appointments
- has adequate lighting in the waiting room
- provides forms in large print
- has an examination room equipped with furniture, magazines, and treatment folders especially designed for older adults
- invites a professional in the management of older patients for in-service training

The primary issue in elder care is effective communication. How you communicate with people is often influenced by what you know or do not know about them. Older people are subject to many changes that affect how they are able to interact with their environment. It is important to recognize these changes and to investigate one's personal perception of older people to break down the barriers that prohibit effective communication.

As people age, they frequently experience a loss of control over their lives because of physical disabilities, economic constraints, and institutional living. Part of the medical assistant's job is to help aging people maintain their dignity and independence while in the ambulatory care setting. Remember, each patient, regardless of his or her education, socioeconomic status, or age, deserves to be treated with compassion and respect. Ask the patient directly what is wrong rather than discussing the patient with family members. It also is important to listen carefully and to be specific and sincere when responding. When a patient is talking, take time to allow him or her to complete the sentence; do not finish it for the person. Give the patient your full attention rather than continuing with other tasks while he or she is speaking. Older people may take a little longer to process information, but they are capable of understanding. Do not hurry through explanations or questions; rather, take time to review a form or give instructions as needed.

Box 33.7 provides suggestions for effective communication with aging patients.

BOX 33.7 Suggestions for Effective Communication With Aging Patients

- Address the patient as Mr., Mrs., or Ms. unless the patient has given you permission to use his or her first name.
- Introduce yourself and explain the purpose of a procedure before performing the procedure.
- Face the aging person and softly touch the individual to get his or her attention before beginning to speak.
- Use expanded speech, gestures, demonstrations, or written instructions in block print.
- If the message must be repeated, paraphrase or find other words to say the same thing.
- Observe the patient's nonverbal behavior for cues indicating whether he or she understands.
- Provide adequate lighting without glare.
- Allow patients time to process information and take care of themselves unless they ask for assistance.
- Conduct communication in a quiet room without distractions.
- Involve family members as needed for continuity of care.
- When leaving a telephone message, remember to speak slowly and clearly and repeat the message in the same manner. It is difficult to interpret a message, and even more difficult to write it down, if the message was delivered in a hurried manner.
- Use referrals and community resources for support, such as the following:
  - Alzheimer's Association: http://www.alz.org/ (1-800-272-3900).
- American Council of the Blind: http://acb.org/ (1-800-424-8666): Provides referrals to state and other organizations that provide services and equipment for the blind.
- American Speech-Language-Hearing Association: http://www.asha.org/ (1-800-638-8255): Offers information on hearing aids, hearing loss, and communication problems in older people and provides a list of certified audiologists and speech pathologists.
- Arthritis Foundation Information Line: http://www.arthritis.org (404-872-7100): Makes referrals to local chapters and provides information on various types of arthritis.
- American Diabetes Association: http://www.diabetes.org/ (1-800-342-2383): Provides information and support for those with diabetes.
- Eldercare Locator: http://www.eldercare.gov/Eldercare.NET/Public/Index.aspx (1-800-677-1116): Run by the National Association of Area Agencies on Aging; help line provides information on contacting local chapters that oversee services to older adults.
- National Institute on Aging Information Center: http://www.nia.nih.gov/ (1-800-222-2225): Provides information on aging health issues for patients, families, and healthcare professionals.
- National Meals-on-Wheels Foundation: http://www.mowaa.org/ (1-888-998-6325).
- National Hospice and Palliative Care Organization: http://www.nhpco.org/ (703-837-1500): A nonprofit organization committed to improving end of life care and expanding access to hospice care.

CRITICAL THINKING BOX 33.6

New staff members in the practice are complaining of having to repeat information to older patients, who, they say, do not pay attention when procedures are explained. Dr. Kennedy has decided to invite a gerontologist from the local university to present an in-service workshop on healthy aging. She asks Bill to coordinate the in-service workshop and prepare materials requested by the guest speaker. What information about caring for the ambulatory aging patient should be included in the workshop?

EXCEPTIONAL CUSTOMER SERVICE

The medical assistant must keep in mind the sensorimotor changes that accompany aging, and also respectful patient communication, when conducting patient education with older patients. Remember, the aging process does not affect a person's ability to learn; it just may take longer to process the information, and the material may need to be repeated for understanding. Showing sensitivity to the needs of aging learners ensures successful patient education and improves compliance with prescribed treatment plans. The current aging population generally is respectful toward authority; therefore, if the medical assistant cannot gain the patient's cooperation, the provider may be able to provide authoritative reinforcement of material. General guidelines for effective patient education with older adults include the following:

- The patient may have short-term memory loss, so you may need to repeat the information using different words.
- The patient may be distracted more easily, so learning in a group may be difficult.
- The patient may take longer to process information, so teach at a pace that matches the patient's needs.
- Provide the patient with handouts that have large print and block letters for reviewing information at home.
- Involve family members as needed for continuity of care; supply provider-approved websites for reference.

CLOSING COMMENTS

Your future employers will expect you to use problem-solving techniques, including recognizing and defining a problem, analyzing the issue, and developing a plan of action. Elderly patients typically have multiple health problems that are frequently complicated by physical, psychological, and environmental factors. To provide quality care for these individuals, you must look at their health issues in a holistic way, taking into consideration all the factors that affect their eventual ability to follow treatment plans and improve their health status. Part of the process involves identifying resources that might help the aging person be better equipped to take care of himself or herself. Consistently using community and online resources may mean the difference between an aging person being able to stay in the home or having to go to long-term care. The professional medical assistant can play a crucial role in providing assistance to aging clients.

CHAPTER REVIEW

In this chapter, we discussed the impact of a growing aging population on society and what that means to the healthcare system. Most older people have at least one chronic medical condition and may have multiple conditions. As healthcare professionals, we need to be aware of the stereotypes and myths associated with aging. We need to understand that stereotypes cannot be applied to all people. To provide respectful care medical assistants should be educated about the realities of aging and elderly population.

The changes in the anatomy and physiology caused by aging were discussed. All body systems are affected by the aging process. There are normal changes that occur, but these changes can be intensified by poor health habits. It is important to stress the importance of regular exercise, a healthy diet, and annual physical examination with health screenings.

Cognitive ability is influenced by many factors, including the aging process. This must be taken into account when working with elderly patients. Using all of the appropriate communication tools is very important when working with elderly patients.

Taste and smell declines as patients age. These factors can affect their nutritional status and their safety. With decreased taste, food doesn't taste as good, so there is less incentive to eat. In order to increase the flavor, the patient may use more salt, which can affect other health issues. Smell also affects taste, but it can be a safety concern. The patient may not be able to smell smoke or gas.

Because aging affects the patient's ability to live on his or her own, the healthcare facility may need to provide living options for its patients. Having an understanding of assisted living and skilled nursing facilities in your area can help you help your patients and their families.

SCENARIO WRAP-UP

Bill has learned to understand the special needs of aging patients. He used to think that most older people were chronically sick and would ultimately end up in long-term care facilities. Now he understands that most aging people lead healthy, active lives and that the disorders that occur in later life usually are the result of lifestyle factors, such as diet and lack of exercise. Bill also has learned how to communicate effectively with older patients and to conduct patient interviews so as to evaluate the patient's physical, mental, emotional, and nutritional health.

34

Assisting With Minor Surgery

LEARNING OBJECTIVES

1. Describe typical solutions and medications used in minor surgical procedures.
2. Summarize methods for identifying surgical instruments used in minor office surgery, and then identify some surgical instruments.
3. Outline the general classifications of surgical instruments.
4. Discuss miscellaneous instruments, and identify drapes and different types of sutures and surgical needles.
5. Differentiate between asepsis and surgical asepsis, and describe the care and handling of surgical instruments.
6. Differentiate between sanitization and disinfection, summarize tips for improving autoclave techniques, and demonstrate how to prepare items for autoclave sterilization.
7. Explain how to wrap materials, discuss the types and uses of sterilization indicators, and describe the need for quality assurance records for office sterilization.
8. Summarize the correct methods of loading, operating, and unloading an autoclave.
9. Summarize common minor surgical procedures.
10. Detail the medical assistant's role in minor office surgery when it comes to preparation of the patient and the room. Also, explain how to perform skin prep for surgery.
11. Outline the rules for setting up and maintaining a sterile field; explain how to perform the following procedures related to sterile techniques:
    - Perform a surgical hand scrub
    - Open a sterile pack and create a sterile field
    - Transfer sterile instruments and pour solutions into a sterile field
    - Perform a two-person sterile tray set-up
    - Apply sterile gloves without contaminating them
12. Discuss how to assist the provider during surgery and demonstrate how to assist with a minor surgical procedure and suturing.
13. Summarize postoperative instructions and explain how to remove sutures and surgical staples.
14. Explain the process of wound healing.
15. Explain how to properly apply dressings and bandages to surgical sites.

CHAPTER OUTLINE

1. **Opening Scenario, 758**
2. **You Will Learn, 758**
3. **Introduction, 758**
4. **Minor Surgery Room, 758**
5. **Surgical Solutions and Medications, 758**
6. **Surgical Instruments, 759**
7. **Classifications of Surgical Instruments, 761**
    a. Cutting and Dissecting Instruments, 761
        i. *Disposable Scalpels, 761*
    b. Grasping and Clamping Instruments, 761
    c. Retractors, 761
        i. *Senn Retractor, 765*
    d. Probes and Dilators, 765
8. **Miscellaneous Instruments, 766**
9. **Drapes, Sutures, and Needles, 767**
    a. Sutures, 767
        i. *Absorbable Sutures, 767*
        ii. *Nonabsorbable Sutures, 767*
        iii. *Suture Sizing and Packaging, 767*
    b. Other Closure Materials, 768
10. **Surgical Asepsis and Assisting With Surgical Procedures, 769**
11. **Care and Handling of Instruments, 769**
    a. Sterilization, 770
        i. *Autoclave, 770*
        ii. *Chemical Sterilization, 775*
    b. Surgical Procedures, 775
        i. *Electrosurgery, 776*
        ii. *Laser Surgery, 776*
        iii. *Microsurgery, 777*
        iv. *Endoscopic Procedures, 777*
        v. *Cryosurgery, 777*
    c. Assisting With Surgical Procedures, 777
        i. *Preparation of the Patient, 777*
        ii. *Preparation of the Room, 778*
        iii. *Sterile Technique, 778*
        iv. *Assisting the Provider During Surgery, 786*
    d. Wound Care, 793
        i. *Wound Healing, 793*
        ii. *Dressings, 796*
12. **Closing Comments, 797**
13. **Chapter Review, 797**

757

▶ OPENING SCENARIO

Callie Casper, CMA (AAMA), works for the Walden-Martin Family Medical Clinic. Callie was hired to work as an administrative medical assistant at the front desk, but one of the clinical medical assistants unexpectedly quit, and the office manager has offered Callie the position. Callie is excited about this opportunity, especially the chance to work with Dr. Juanita Perez, but she is also concerned about her skill level in sterile procedures. At least she is familiar with a number of the patients, most of the staff, and the types of outpatient surgeries performed in the facility. Surgical asepsis and assisting with surgery were her favorite topics when she was in her medical assisting program. However, before she can assist with surgeries, Callie must demonstrate her knowledge of surgical instruments and her ability to set up a sterile field without contaminating the site. She also must show that she can perform wound care skills, including applying sterile dressings and changing bandages.

YOU WILL LEARN:

- To identify common surgical instruments.
- What is required for various minor surgery tray setups.
- How to properly sanitize instruments.
- How to properly prepare instruments for the autoclave.
- The proper handling of autoclaved packages.
- To describe the various types of surgical procedures performed in an ambulatory care setting.
- How prepare a patient for a minor surgical procedure.
- How to assist the provider with a minor surgical procedure.
- To describe the different phases of wound healing.
- How to properly apply a dressing and bandage to a wound.

INTRODUCTION

Office surgery is restricted to the management of minor problems and injuries. The medical assistant is expected to:
- prepare the patient and the sterile field
- assist the provider as needed
- take care of the patient after the procedure
- properly disinfect the area
- document appropriately

Some medical assistants are employed in outpatient surgical facilities and are expected to assist with procedures that were once performed in hospitals. In addition, medical assistants often assist with minor surgical procedures in an office setting. This chapter will focus on preparing for and assisting with minor surgery only. This will include a discussion of surgical supplies and instruments, the care and handling of instruments, and the different types of surgical sutures and needles, sterilization, preparation of the sterile field, specific minor surgical procedures, and care of the patient.

Conscientious (kon shee EN shuh s) attention must be given to all sterile techniques and procedures. Frequently checking and rechecking

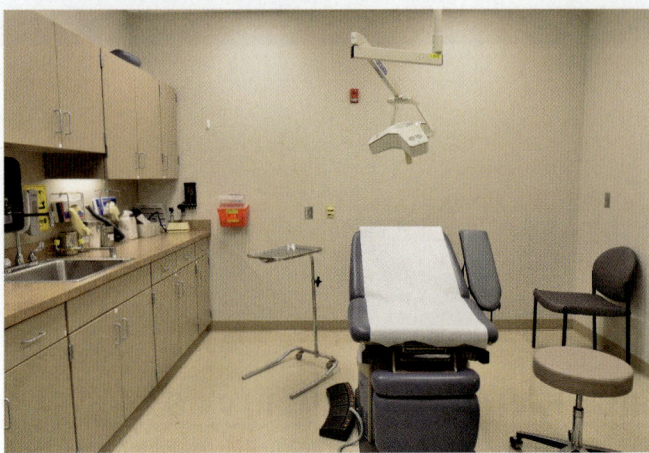

FIG. 34.1 Typical surgical procedure room in an ambulatory care setting. (From Proctor D, et al: *Kinn's The Medical Assistant*, ed 13, St Louis, 2017, Elsevier.)

procedures helps ensure that they are effective and are used without any "breaks" in technique. Single-use, disposable items offer the best method of infection control and are used frequently in healthcare facilities. However, when disposable equipment is used, the assistant must know the specific disposal guidelines for contaminated instruments and supplies.

MINOR SURGERY ROOM

When minor surgery is routinely performed, a minor surgery room that is separate from the other examining rooms may be used. Recovery rooms and family waiting areas may also be available and are common in the larger surgery centers. The minor surgery room in a provider's office, often called the *procedure room,* should be near a workroom with a sink and an autoclave. In some facilities, the sink and autoclave will be located in the procedure room. Cabinets with countertops serve as a side or back table during surgical procedures. Regardless of the setup, it should be easy to disinfect the area, and it should remain uncluttered to allow for easy access to the patient and necessary supplies.

Surgical supplies, wound care equipment, medications, and biopsy containers are stored in the cabinets. The exam table should be easy to adjust. In addition, the room should have bright lighting, a Mayo stand for instruments, vital signs equipment, and possibly an electrocardiograph (ECG) machine as part of the standard equipment for a procedure room (Fig. 34.1).

SURGICAL SOLUTIONS AND MEDICATIONS

Procedure room supplies include the standard solutions and medications used in minor surgery and dressing changes. Although the solutions and medications listed here are basic, every healthcare facility has preferred items and methods of applying them. The medical assistant is responsible for their care and for maintaining up-to-date supplies.

Sterile water is kept in two forms. Multiple-dose or single-use vials are used as a **diluent** for medications. Larger containers of sterile water are for irrigating wounds or rinsing instruments that have been in a chemical disinfectant solution.

VOCABULARY

conscientious: Meticulous, careful.
diluent: A liquid substance that dilutes or lessens the strength of a solution or mixture; it is added to vials of powdered medications to create a solution of the drug for injection.

Sterile normal saline solution is also stocked in two sizes. The small vial is used for injection (e.g., 0.9% Sodium Chloride Injection USP single-dose vials, Bacteriostatic 0.9% Sodium Chloride Injection USP multiple-dose vials). A larger plastic container of sterile saline (e.g., 0.9% Sodium Chloride Irrigation USP) is used for cleaning, rinsing, and irrigating wounds. These commercially prepared products are ordered from a medical supply company.

Before surgery, the surgical site on the patient must be disinfected with an antiseptic skin cleansing preparation. This will reduce the number of **pathogens**. Although it is not possible to remove all microorganisms from the skin, using an antiseptic cleanser will remove most of the **transient** (tran zee uh nt) and pathogenic microorganisms. Resident flora will also be reduced. Research indicates that chlorhexidine gluconate products (Hibiclens), and povidone-iodine (Betadine) are safe and effective antiseptics.

The provider's hands and those of the medical assistant should be scrubbed to reduce the chances of wound contamination, even though the hands will be covered by sterile gloves. Surgical scrub preparations should:

- be effective against bacterial spores
- work to reduce transient bacteria
- show evidence of persistent activity on the skin
- work despite the presence of organic matter, such as blood or wound drainage

Research has shown that the use of a hand sanitizer can be as effective as an extensive surgical scrub.

Even minor surgical procedures require the use of **anesthetics** (an uh s THET iks), which either are injected locally at the site of the procedure or may be applied topically to the skin. For patients who find injections of a local anesthetic painful or traumatic, the provider may first apply a topical anesthetic. Topical anesthetics come in many forms, including sprays, gels, lotions, swabs, and foams. Immediately after applying the topical anesthetic, the provider injects the local anesthetic around the surgical area.

Another topical anesthetic is an ethyl chloride spray, a vapocoolant that controls pain associated with minor surgical procedures (e.g., lancing boils, incision and drainage of small **abscesses**), by causing freezing of the affected area. Because ethyl chloride is highly flammable, it should never be used in the presence of electrical cauterizing equipment. In addition, petroleum jelly must be applied to the surrounding areas to protect them from the cooling action of the spray. Ethyl chloride spray has a short duration of action, so all equipment must be prepared and the provider must be ready to perform the procedure before the spray is applied.

Local anesthetics are injected into the subcutaneous tissue. These produce a temporary numbing at the site of injection by blocking the generation and conduction of nerve impulses. Many different types of local anesthetics are available, but all share the same suffix, *-caine* (Box 34.1). Local anesthetics are purchased in multiple-dose vials of 30 to 50 mL and in various strengths, such as 0.5%, 1%, and 2%. They begin

> **BOX 34.1 Common Local Anesthetics**
>
> - lidocaine (Xylocaine)
> - procaine (Novocain)
> - chloroprocaine (Nesacaine)
> - bupivacaine (Sensorcaine).

acting relatively quickly, within 5 to 15 minutes; the duration of action depends on the type of anesthetic, but they usually last 1 to 3 hours. When highly vascular areas are involved, local anesthetics containing epinephrine (ep uh NEF rin) may be used. Epinephrine causes **vasoconstriction** (vey zoh kuh n STRIK shuh n) at the site, which keeps the anesthetic in the tissues longer, prolonging its effect. It also minimizes bleeding. However, epinephrine is not used in areas where decreased circulation may cause problems with healing, such as fingertips or toes.

All tissues removed or biopsied are sent to the pathology laboratory for analysis. A 10% formalin solution typically is used to preserve excised tissue for specimens. Specimen bottles are purchased with preservatives included and should be part of the supplies prepared for a surgical procedure, if a biopsy is to be done. The provider places the specimen in the container. The medical assistant is responsible for accurately labeling the container with:

- patient's name and date of birth
- medical history number
- date of collection
- type of specimen

Sometimes the provider may want to use topical silver nitrate ($AgNO_3$) solution or coated applicator sticks to stop localized bleeding, such as with *epistaxis* (ip uh STAK sis) (nosebleed) or capillary bleeding at the site of a wound. The applicators must be kept in lightproof containers. The applicator sticks are convenient for use in the mouth or nose. Box 34.2 presents a list of additional surgical supplies.

> **CRITICAL THINKING 34.1**
>
> Callie is ready to do an inventory of supplies in the minor surgery room. What solutions, medications, and miscellaneous supplies should she make sure are on hand for the busy surgical schedule planned for next week?

SURGICAL INSTRUMENTS

The medical assistant must know which instruments are used for each procedure and should be able to identify and understand the function of the surgical instruments preferred by the provider. Instruments have clearly identifiable parts and can be visually differentiated from one another. The basic components are the handle, the closing mechanism, and the part that comes in contact with the patient, commonly called the *jaws*. Many instruments can have either straight or curved tips, depending on the operator's preference and the task to be performed.

Instruments have either ring handles (finger rings) (Fig. 34.3A–B) or spring handles (Fig. 34.3C); these sometimes are called *thumb-handled* or *thumb grasp* instruments. Scissors are an example of a ring-handled instrument; forceps (tweezers) have spring handles. Some instruments have a hinge-type mechanism called a *box lock* (Fig. 34.5C).

VOCABULARY

abscesses: Localized collections of pus, which may be under the skin or deep in the body, that cause tissue destruction.
anesthetic: An agent that causes partial or complete loss of sensation.
pathogen: A disease causing-organism.
transient: Not lasting, enduring or permanent; transitory.
vasoconstriction: Contraction of the muscles causing the narrowing of the inside tube of the vessel.

UNIT 4 Basic Clinical Procedures

> **BOX 34.2 Additional Surgical Supplies**
>
> - Sterilized gauze squares or strips saturated with petroleum jelly or petrolatum – used to pack wounds
> - Sterilized iodoform gauze strips, ¼ inch to 2 inches wide and impregnated with iodoform iodine (see Fig. 34.2) – used to pack abscesses to act as a wick to draw out the infection; also used as a local antibacterial agent
> - Surgical sponges – used to absorb blood and protect tissues during surgery
> - Syringes and needles – used to inject local anesthetics and irrigate wounds
> - Sterile dressing and bandaging materials

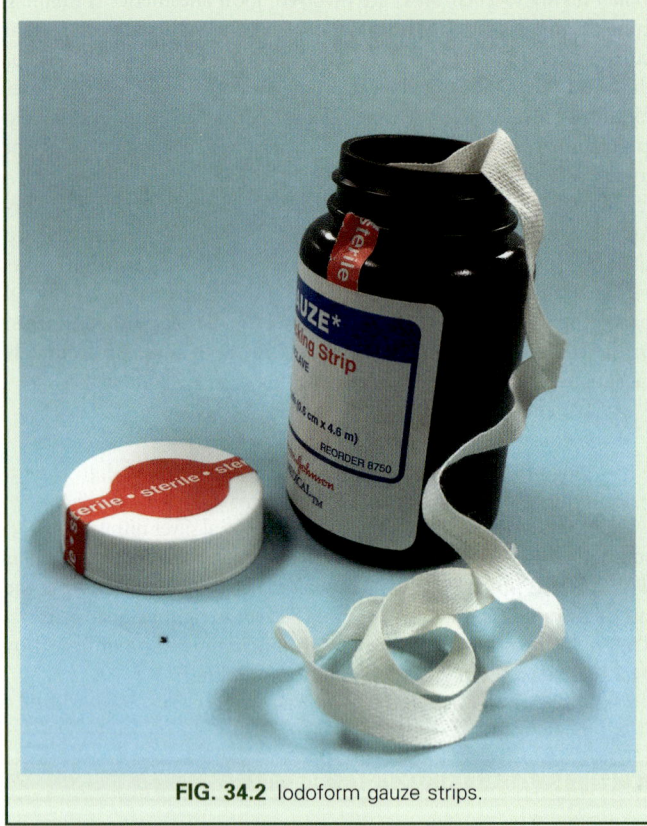

FIG. 34.2 Iodoform gauze strips.

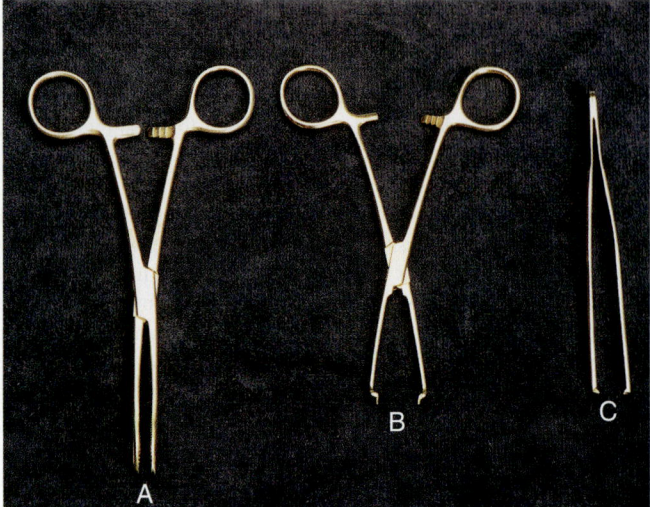

FIG. 34.3 (A) and (B) Ring-handle forceps. (C) Spring-handle thumb forceps. (From Proctor D, et al: *Kinn's The Medical Assistant*, ed 13, St Louis, 2017, Elsevier.)

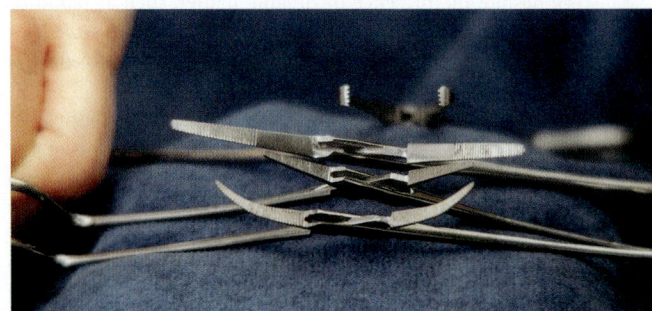

FIG. 34.4 Instruments with serrations. (From Proctor D, et al: *Kinn's The Medical Assistant*, ed 13, St Louis, 2017, Elsevier.)

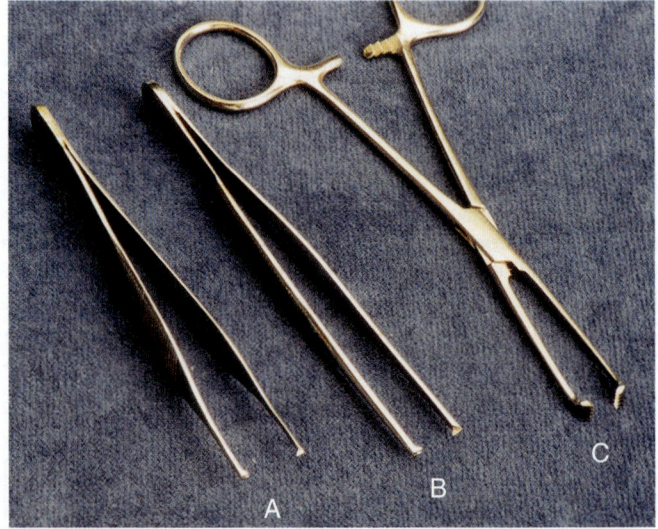

FIG. 34.5 (A) and (B) Toothed jaws. (C) Teeth of Allis tissue forceps. (From Proctor D, et al: *Kinn's The Medical Assistant*, ed 13, St Louis, 2017, Elsevier.)

Ratchets resemble gears and are located just below or next to the ring handle (see Fig. 34.3A–B). They are used to lock an instrument into position. Most ratchets can be closed at three or more positions, depending on the thickness of the tissue or materials being grasped.

The inner surfaces of the jaws on some instruments have ridged teeth, called *serrations* (se REY shuh n); both ring-handled and thumb-type instruments may have them. These serrations may be crisscross, horizontal, or lengthwise (Fig. 34.4). Serrations prevent small blood vessels and tissue from slipping out of the jaws of the instrument.

Instrument tips or jaws may be plain tipped or toothed (Fig. 34.5A–B). Tissue forceps usually are toothed instruments and are identified by the number of intermeshing teeth (e.g., 1×2, 2×3, 3×4). Allis forceps (Fig. 34.5C) are used to grasp delicate, soft tissues, so the teeth are finer, shallower, and more rounded. Other forceps have teeth that are sharper and deeper. Still others have sharp, hook-like, single or double teeth, such as a tenaculum (tuh NAK yuh luh m) (see Fig. 34.14C). Toothed instruments commonly have ratchets for locking into towels or human tissues. Instrument tips may also be either straight or curved, depending on their use.

An instrument can be named for its use (e.g., splinter forceps, for removing splinters) or after the person or people who developed it (e.g., Mayo-Hegar needle holder). Many general instruments are identified by the part of the body on which they are used (e.g., rectal speculum and nasal speculum).

Thousands of surgical instruments have multiple names. The same instrument may have two or three different names, depending on the provider identifying it or the part of the country in which the practice is located. For example, a provider may ask for a clamp or forceps when he or she wants a Kelly hemostat. It is important to learn the provider's preference in terminology. Learn to recognize the distinctive parts of instruments and the reasons for each part, and you will quickly build a working knowledge of hundreds of instruments.

CLASSIFICATIONS OF SURGICAL INSTRUMENTS

Surgical instruments are generally classified according to their use, and most belong to one of four groups:
- Cutting
- Grasping
- Retracting
- Probing and dilating

Cutting and Dissecting Instruments

Cutting and dissecting instruments, which are used for cutting, incising, scraping, punching, and puncturing, include scissors (Table 34.1), scalpels, chisels, elevators, curettes, punches, drills, and needles. Instruments with a sharp blade or surface can cut, scrape, or *dissect*.

> **VOCABULARY**
> **dissect:** To cut or separate tissue with a cutting instrument or scissors.

Disposable Scalpels. Most scalpels used in minor procedures are disposable (Fig. 34.9), with different handle sizes and types of blades already attached to the handles. However, stainless steel, reusable scalpel handles can be used. A variety of blades can be used, which must be attached to the handle using forceps and sterile technique. After the procedure, the handles are sterilized and the blades are discarded in a sharps container. Once used, disposable scalpel/blade units are discarded in a sharps container.
- *Handles:* No. 3 is the standard handle; No. 3L and No. 7 are used in deeper cavities.
- *Blades:* No. 15 is commonly used; Nos. 10, 11, and 12 are used for specialty incisions.

Grasping and Clamping Instruments

Clamping instruments are used for many different tasks. Many have a sharp tooth or teeth and are used to retract, hold, and manipulate fascia (fash EE uh). The most common clamping instruments are hemostats, which originally were designed to stop bleeding or to clamp severed blood vessels. Some clamping instruments are used to grasp other instruments or sterilized materials. Sometimes hemostats and other clamping instruments are used interchangeably. Table 34.2 lists the most common grasping and clamping instruments.

Retractors

Retracting instruments hold tissue away from the surgical wound (incision). Depending on the provider's preference, handheld skin hooks

TABLE 34.1 Scissors

Instrument	Description
Lister bandage scissors (Fig. 34.6A)	• Blunt probe tip • Easily inserted under bandages with relative safety • Used to remove bandages and dressings
Operating scissors (Fig. 34.6B)	• 5 to 6 inches long • Curved or straight blade tips • Used to cut and dissect tissue
Suture scissors (Fig. 34.7)	• Blade has beak or hook to slide under sutures • Used to remove sutures

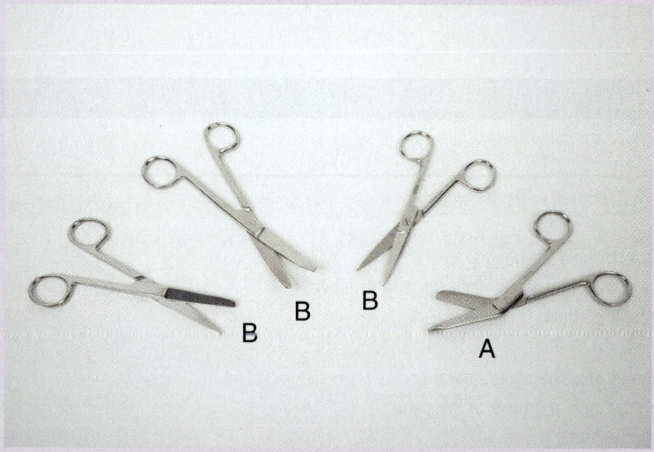

FIG. 34.6 Scissors. (A) Lister bandage scissors. (B) Operating scissors.

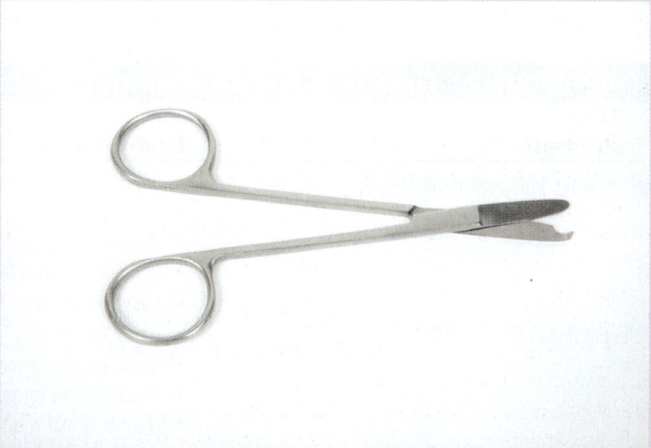

FIG. 34.7 Suture scissors.

Continued

TABLE 34.1 Scissors—cont'd

Instrument	Description
Uterine curette (Fig. 34.8)	• Available in several sizes • Hollow and spoon shaped; used for scraping • Used to remove polyps, secretions, and bits of placental tissue

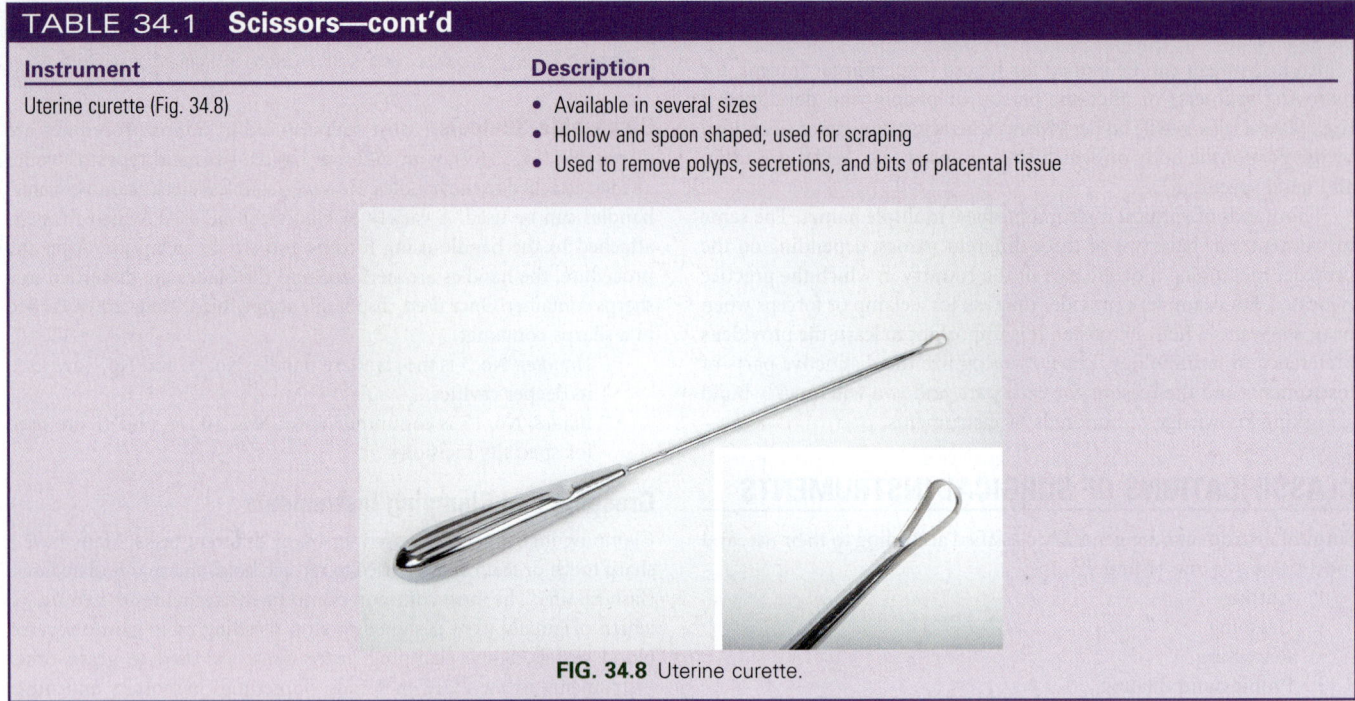

FIG. 34.8 Uterine curette.

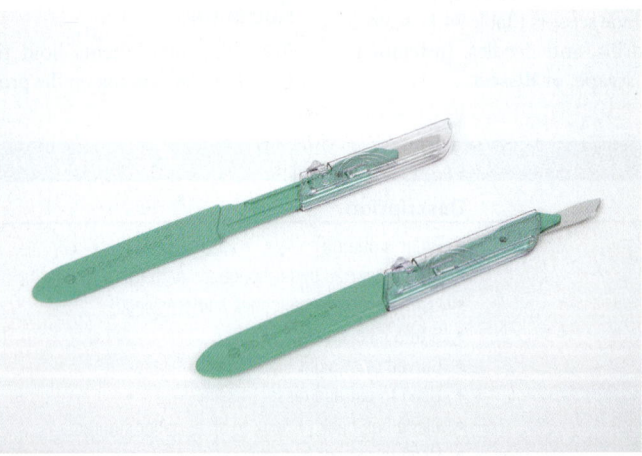

FIG. 34.9 Disposable scalpels.

TABLE 34.2 Grasping and Clamping Instruments

Instrument	Description
Hemostatic forceps (Fig. 34.10A–B)	• Jaws may be fully or partly serrated, without teeth • May be curved or straight • Used to clamp small vessels or hold tissue • Mosquito forceps (4 inches) are smaller and used for very small vessels • Kelly forceps (6 to 7 inches) are larger
Needle holder (Fig. 34.10C)	• 4 to 7 inches long • Jaws are shorter and stronger than hemostat jaws • Jaws may be serrated or may have a groove in the center • Used to grasp a suture needle firmly

CHAPTER 34 Assisting With Minor Surgery

TABLE 34.2 Grasping and Clamping Instruments—cont'd

Instrument	Description

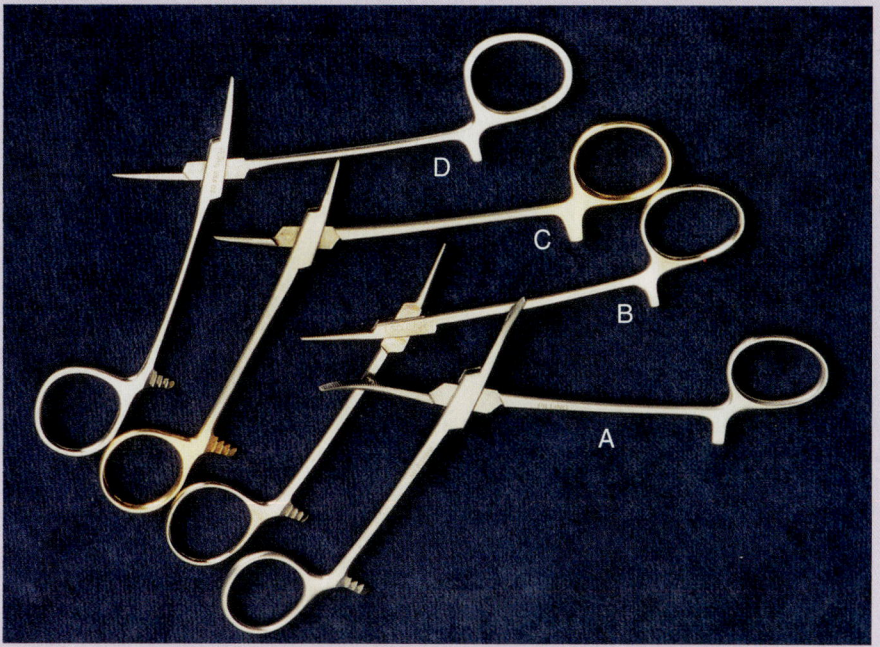

FIG. 34.10 (A) Kelly hemostatic forceps. (B) Mosquito hemostatic forceps. (C) Needle holder. (D) Smooth-tip needle holder. (From Proctor D, et al: *Kinn's The Medical Assistant*, ed 13, St Louis, 2017, Elsevier.)

Instrument	Description
Splinter forceps (Fig. 34.11B)	• Design and construction vary • Fine tip for foreign object retrieval
Plain thumb (dressing) forceps (Fig. 34.11A)	• Manufactured in lengths from 4 to 12 inches • Varying types of serrated jaws but no teeth • Used to insert packing into or remove objects from deep cavities

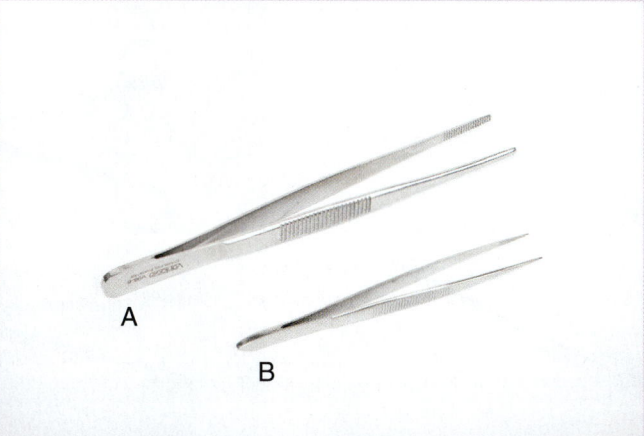

FIG. 34.11 (A) Plain-thumb (dressing) forceps. (B) Splinter forceps.

Instrument	Description
Towel forceps (Fig. 34.12)	• Various lengths from 3 to 8½ inches • May have sharp or atraumatic (dull-edged) tips • Used to hold drapes in place during surgery
Allis tissue forceps (Fig. 34.13A)	• Available in different lengths and jaw widths • Used to grasp tissue, muscle, or skin surrounding a wound

Continued

TABLE 34.2 Grasping and Clamping Instruments—cont'd

Instrument	Description

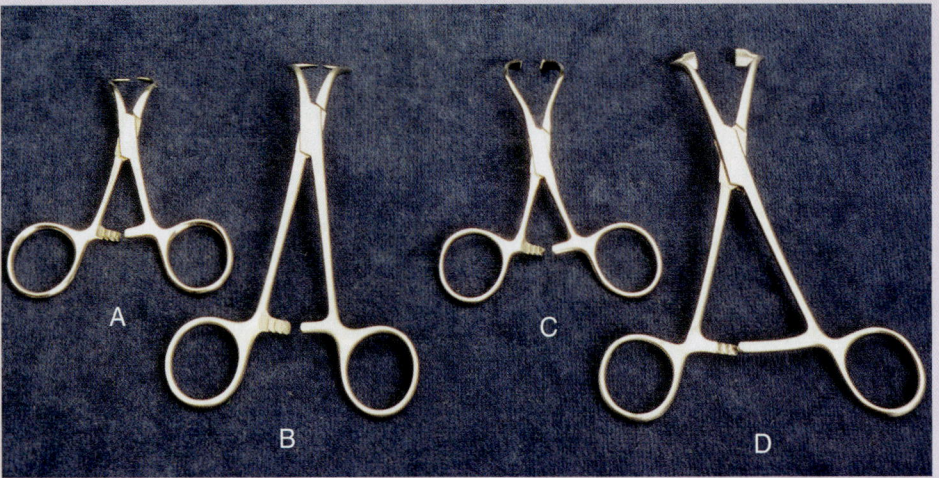

FIG. 34.12 (A) Small sharp towel forceps. (B) Large sharp towel forceps. (C) Small atraumatic towel forceps. (D) Large atraumatic towel forceps. (From Proctor D, et al: *Kinn's The Medical Assistant*, ed 13, St Louis, 2017, Elsevier.)

Instrument	Description
Toothed tissue forceps (Fig. 34.13B)	• Manufactured in 4- to 18-inch lengths • Pincher grip • Used to grasp tissue, muscle, or skin surrounding a wound
Foerster sponge forceps (Fig. 34.14A)	• Used to hold gauze squares to sponge the surgical site • Used as transfer forceps to arrange items on a sterile tray • Straight or curved, with or without serrations
Bozeman sponge forceps (Fig. 34.14B)	• Designed to hold sponges or dressings • Capable of reaching the cervix through the vagina • Used to swab the area or apply medication
Tenaculum forceps (Fig. 34.14C)	• Very sharp, pointed tips • Used to hold tissue (e.g., the cervix) while a tissue specimen is obtained or to lift the cervix so that the fornix can be seen

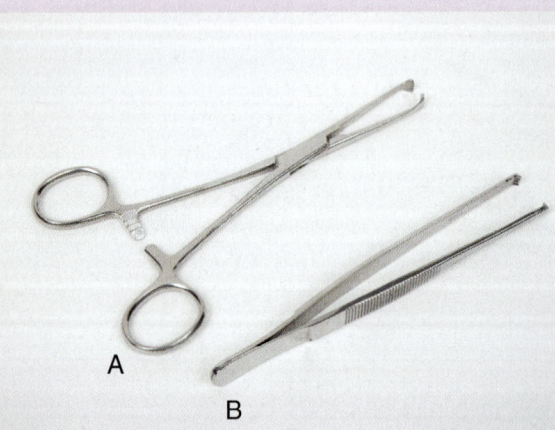

FIG. 34.13 (A) Allis tissue forceps. (B) Toothed tissue forceps.

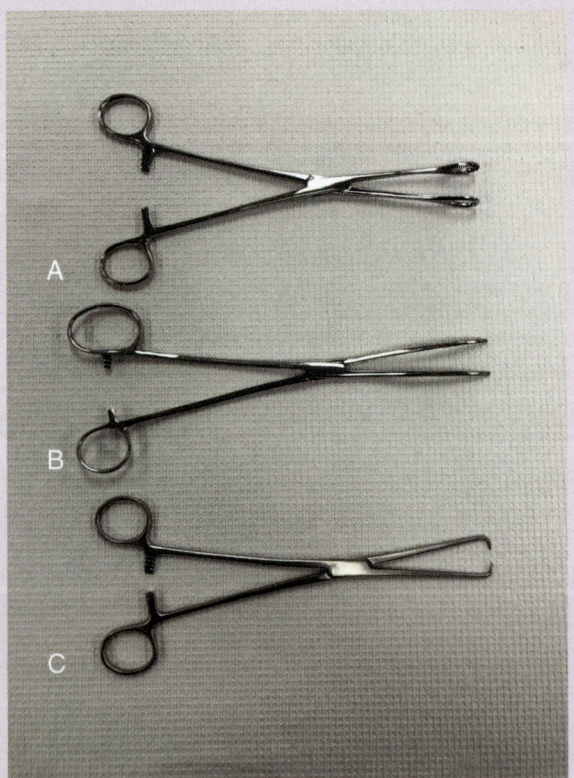

FIG. 34.14 (A) Foerster sponge forceps. (B) Bozeman sponge forceps. (C) Tenaculum forceps.

and Senn retractors are used to retract during most minor surgical procedures.

Senn Retractor (Fig. 34.15)
- Flat end is a blunt retractor.
- Three-prong end may be sharp or dull.

- Used to retract small incisions or to secure a skin edge for suturing.

Probes and Dilators

Probes and dilators are used both for surgery and for examinations. Probes can be used to search for a foreign body in a wound or to enter a fistula. Dilators are used to stretch a cavity or opening for examination or before inserting another instrument to obtain a tissue specimen. Table 34.3 lists the most common probes and dilators.

> **VOCABULARY**
>
> **cannula** (KAN yuh la): A rigid tube that surrounds a blunt trocar or a sharp, pointed trocar, which is inserted into the body; when the trocar is withdrawn, fluid may escape from the body through the cannula, depending on the insertion site.
>
> **obturator** (O(B) tuh reyt oar): A metal rod with a smooth, rounded tip that is placed in hollow instruments to reduce injury to body tissues during insertion.
>
> **stylus** (STAHY luh s): A metal probe that is inserted into or passed through a catheter, needle, or tube used for clearing purposes or to facilitate passage into a body orifice.

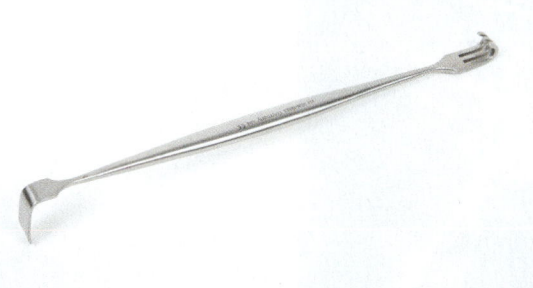

FIG. 34.15 Senn retractor.

TABLE 34.3 Probes and Dilators

Instrument	Description
Probes (Fig. 34.16A–C)	• Lengths range from 4 to 12 inches; available with or without bulbous tip • May be smooth or may have a grooved director • Used to find foreign bodies embedded in dermal tissue or muscle or to trace a wound tract
Trocars and obturators (Fig. 34.16D–G)	• Available in various sizes • Consist of a sharply pointed **stylus** (STAHY luh s) (**obturator** [O(B) tuh reyt or]) contained in a **cannula** (KAN yuh luh) • Used to withdraw fluids from cavities or for draining and irrigating with a catheter

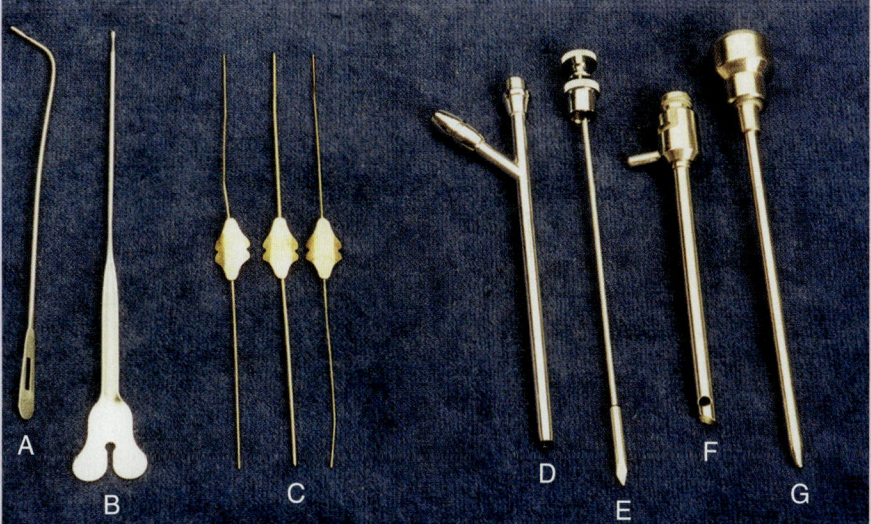

FIG. 34.16 (A) Probe. (B) Grooved dilator. (C) Lacrimal duct probes. (D) Double-ended cannula. (E) Sharp trocar. (F) Canula. (G) Blunt-tip obturator. (From Proctor D, et al: *Kinn's The Medical Assistant*, ed 13, St Louis, 2017, Elsevier.)

Continued

TABLE 34.3 Probes and Dilators—cont'd

Instrument	Description
Specula (Fig. 34.17)	• Most common dilators used • Valves are spread apart, dilating the opening • Used to open or distend a body orifice or cavity • The most common of these is the vaginal speculum used during gynecologic examinations (see Fig. 34.17C). Vaginal specula can be stainless steel (reusable) or plastic (disposable) and can also have a light source for illumination.

FIG. 34.17 (A) Long nasal speculum. (B) Short nasal speculum. (C) Graves vaginal speculum. (D) Anal speculum, self-retaining. (From Proctor D, et al: *Kinn's The Medical Assistant*, ed 13, St Louis, 2017, Elsevier.)

MISCELLANEOUS INSTRUMENTS (Table 34.4)

TABLE 34.4 Miscellaneous Instruments

Instrument	Description
Biopsy forceps (Fig. 34.18A)	• Available in different lengths and styles • Inserted with the jaws closed
Wilde ear forceps (Fig. 34.18B)	• Angled, with serrated tips • Provides easier access to the ear canal and nasal cavities. • Used for packing after ear or nasal procedures • Can be used to remove foreign bodies
Ear curette (Fig. 34.18C)	• Manufactured in various sizes • Available as disposable curettes in many different sizes • Can have a loop or spoon at the end • Made with sharp or blunt scraper ends • Used to remove foreign matter from the ear canals

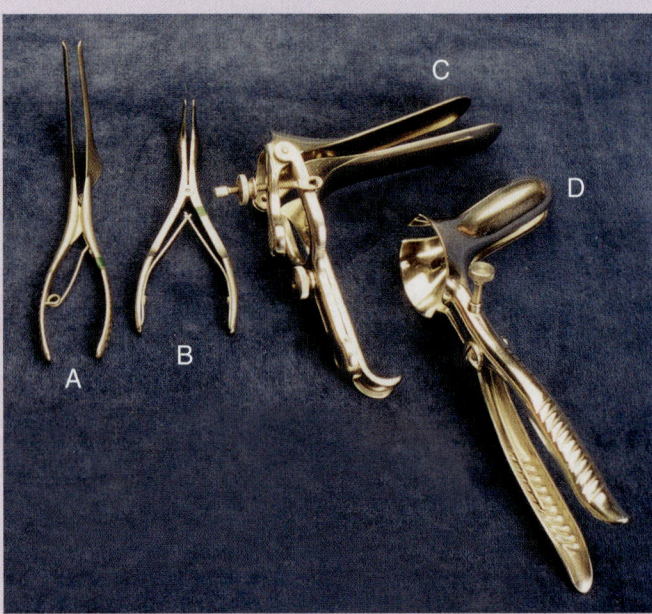

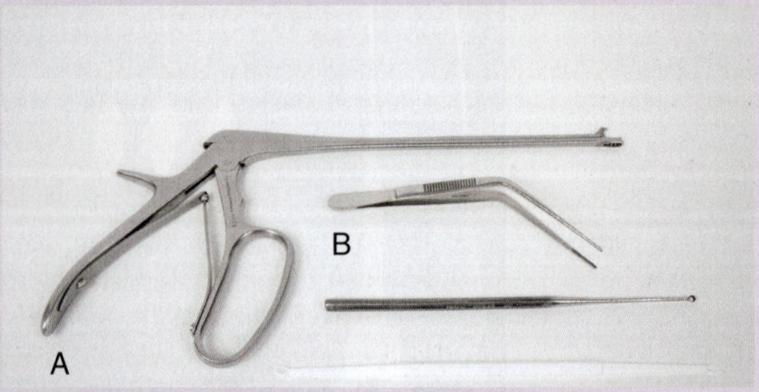

FIG. 34.18 (A), Biopsy forceps. (B) Wilde ear forceps. (C) Ear curettes.

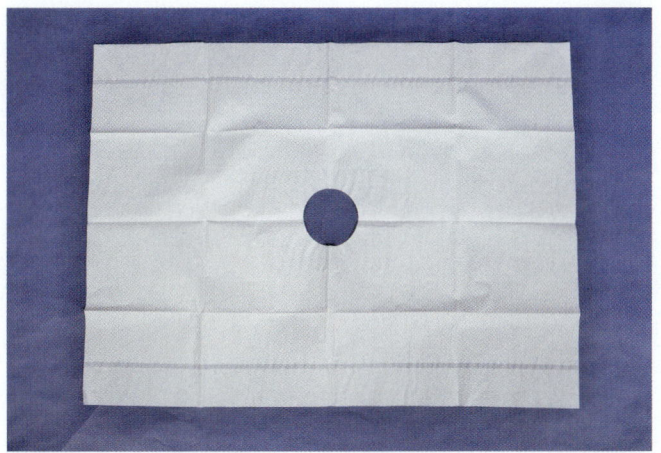

FIG. 34.19 Fenestrated drape. (From Proctor D, et al: *Kinn's The Medical Assistant*, ed 13, St Louis, 2017, Elsevier.)

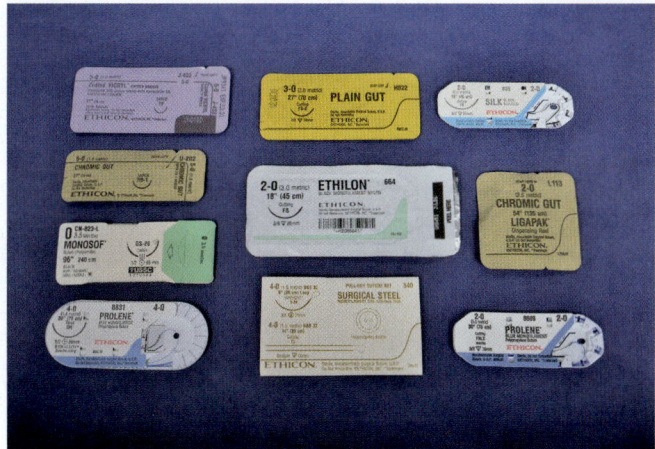

FIG. 34.20 Suture packets labeled according to size, type, length, and type of needle point and shape. (From Proctor D, et al: *Kinn's The Medical Assistant*, ed 13, St Louis, 2017, Elsevier.)

BOX 34.3 Properties of Suture

- Desirable rate of absorption
- Size of the suture
- Type of needle

BOX 34.4 Suture Sizes[a]

Suture Size	Diameter
6-0	0.07 mm
5-0	0.10 mm
4-0	0.15 mm
3-0	0.20 mm
2-0	0.30 mm
0	0.35 mm
1	0.40 mm
2	0.50 mm

[a]Sutures are sized according to the U.S. Pharmacopoeia (USP) scale.

DRAPES, SUTURES, AND NEEDLES

Disposable surgical drapes are available in several different materials and sizes. These typically have an opening (fenestrated [FEN uh strey tid]) for the operative site (Fig. 34.19). The drape is placed over the operative area, using sterile technique, after the patient's skin preparation has been completed. If a fenestrated drape is not available, multiple nonfenestrated drapes can be used to create a sterile field around the surgical site.

Sutures

The word *suture* is used as both a noun and a verb. As a noun, it refers to a surgical stitch or to the material used to close a wound. As a verb, it refers to the act of stitching. The primary purpose of a suture is to hold the edges of a wound together until natural healing occurs.

A suture may also be used as a *ligature* (LIG u cher). This is a strand of suture material used to tie off a blood vessel or to strangulate tissue. If a ligature is used to tie off an internal tubular structure, it must last permanently or long enough for the structure itself to disintegrate. The ideal suture material has certain characteristics:
- Easy to handle and makes a secure knot
- Does not cause a localized tissue reaction and is nonallergenic
- Has adequate strength without cutting through tissue
- Can be sterilized

The provider will request a certain type of suture based on the specific properties of the suture material (Box 34.3). Both natural and synthetic suture materials are available. Sutures may be classified as either absorbable or nonabsorbable. Many different suture materials are available, each having its advantages and disadvantages. Suture materials commonly used in minor surgical procedures are described in the following paragraphs (Fig. 34.20).

Absorbable Sutures. Absorbable sutures are dissolved by the body's enzymes during the healing process. They are used when deep incisions or lacerations require inner layers of sutures to close the wound. Absorbable suture material is also used in areas where suture removal is difficult (e.g., oral surgery). Catgut (sheep, cattle, or pig intestine) was once the absorbable suture material of choice, but it has largely been replaced in recent years by synthetic absorbable suture material (e.g., Vicryl). Other synthetic absorbable suture materials include Dexon, PDS, and Maxon. These materials remain stable longer than natural catgut (up to 11 weeks), allowing the wound to heal completely before absorption occurs.

Nonabsorbable Sutures. Nonabsorbable suture material is left in place until healing is complete. It frequently is used in minor surgical procedures performed in the medical office because most of the suturing required is superficial. It can be used in areas where sutures can be easily removed after healing has taken place. Silk is a common nonabsorbable suture material because it is strong and easy to tie. It is treated with a coating to prevent tissue drag and flaking. Polyester fiber sutures (e.g., Dacron and Prolene) are among the strongest nonabsorbable sutures, along with surgical steel. These fine filaments are braided and have great strength. Nylon suture is strong and has a high degree of elasticity. It is used primarily for skin closure. Due to its elasticity and stiffness, many knots must be used because the knots tend to untie if placed incorrectly.

Suture Sizing and Packaging. Suture material is available in a variety of diameters and lengths (Box 34.4). The diameter of the suture strand determines its size; the smaller gauges are numbered below 0 (pronounced *aught*), and the larger gauges are identified with numbers above 0. For instance, 2-0 suture is thinner than size 0, which is thinner than size 2.

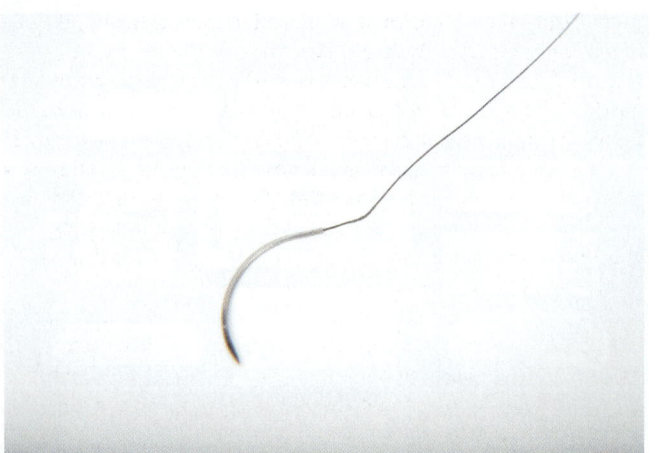

FIG. 34.21 Swaged suture needle.

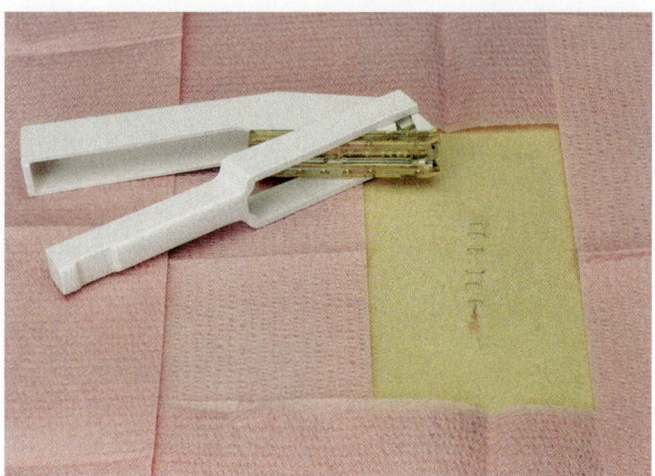

FIG. 34.22 Disposable skin stapler. (From Proctor D, et al: *Kinn's The Medical Assistant*, ed 13, St Louis, 2017, Elsevier.)

The sizes from 6-0 to 2-0 are used most frequently in the medical office. The length of the suture material may vary, with strands precut in 18-, 24-, 54-, and 60-inch lengths.

Needles. Surgical needles are chosen according to the area in which they are to be used and the depth and width of the desired suture. They are classified according to shape, which may be straight or curved. Most sutures are applied with curved needles because they allow the provider to penetrate the surface and then come back up on the other side. The sharper the curve of the needle, the deeper the provider can pass it into the tissue. The point of a needle can be a taper or a cutting edge. A taper is used on delicate tissues. The cutting-edge needle is used on the skin. It lacerates the skin as the needle is passed through. This is advantageous on tougher tissues, such as connective tissue.

Needles are manufactured with the suture material attached, or *swaged*, to the needle. These atraumatic needles do not have an eyelet and cause the least amount of trauma as they are passed through the tissue. Manufacturers package suture strands with the suture needle attached in peel-apart sterile, disposable packages. These may be obtained as single, individually packed, or multipack sutures in a variety of needle types and sizes with a wide range of suture materials and lengths. The most common needle type for minor skin repair is the curved, cutting-edge, swaged needle (Fig. 34.21).

Other Closure Materials

Surgical staples can also be used for skin closure. They are made of stainless steel or titanium and are available in different sizes. Surgical staples are applied (Fig. 34.22) and removed (Fig. 34.23) with specific staple instruments.

Another technique for wound closure is the use of Steri-Strips, which are self-adhesive tapes that are placed over the wound, pulling the wound edges together. Using a tincture of benzoin prior to the application of Steri-Strip can help them remain in place longer. Tincture of benzoin is applied parallel to the edges of the wound. Care should be taken so that it does not go into the wound because it can cause a burning pain. The compound becomes tacky, and the Steri-Strips stay on longer. Steri-Strips can be used to support a wound if there is potential tension at the site, or for superficial wounds (Fig. 34.24). Frequently, small, clean lacerations may be closed with Steri-Strips (see Fig. 34.24). These strips reduce the chance of infection and do not leave suture scars. Steri-Strips are used on areas of the body that are protected from movement and stress. They often are used on the face. A medical assistant can place Steri-Strips as ordered by the provider. They are placed on the wound in the same sequence and at the same intervals as interrupted sutures and are left in place until they fall off or the wound heals.

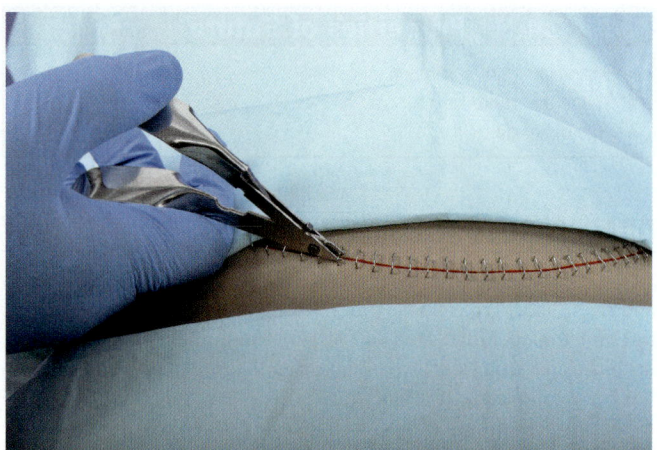

FIG. 34.23 Surgical staple remover. (From Proctor D, et al: *Kinn's The Medical Assistant*, ed 13, St Louis, 2017, Elsevier.)

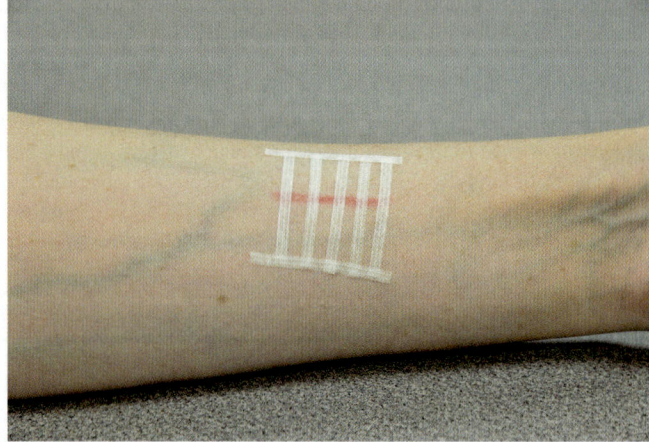

FIG. 34.24 Wound closed with Steri-Strips. (From Proctor D, et al: *Kinn's The Medical Assistant*, ed 13, St Louis, 2017, Elsevier.)

Tissue adhesives, similar to glue, can also be used for superficial wounds (Box 34.5). Examples of tissue adhesives are Histoacryl, Dermabond, and SurgiSeal. Tissue adhesives form a strong bond across wound edges, allowing normal healing to occur below. Skin adhesives are also an alternative to sutures. They are frequently used for closure

BOX 34.5 Advantages of Tissue Adhesive

- Saves time during wound repair
- Creates a flexible, water-resistant protective coating for the wound
- Eliminates the need for suture removal
- Results in better cosmetic outcomes because there is no scarring from suture entry
- May also be used on larger wounds for which subcutaneous sutures are needed
- Especially helpful in pediatric patients or individuals afraid of needles

of facial lacerations, especially in pediatric patients, because they are effective for wound closure without requiring the use of needles and sutures.

SURGICAL ASEPSIS AND ASSISTING WITH SURGICAL PROCEDURES

Asepsis (ey SEP sis) is the condition of being free of **infection** or infectious material. *Medical asepsis* is the reduction of microorganisms and the prevention of the transfer of microorganisms. This creates an environment that is clean but not *sterile* (i.e., free of microorganisms). The principles of medical asepsis are implemented to prevent reinfection of a patient and cross-infection of another patient or ourselves. To prevent cross-contamination, potential microorganisms and pathogens must be isolated by following standard blood and body fluid precautions and by sanitizing, disinfecting, and/or sterilizing objects as soon as possible after they become contaminated.

> **VOCABULARY**
> **infection:** Invasion of body tissues by microorganisms, which then multiply and damage tissues.

Surgical asepsis is the complete destruction of microorganisms. This technique is mandatory for any procedure that invades the body's skin or tissues, such as surgery. In surgical asepsis, everything that comes in contact with the surgical site must be sterile, including surgical gowns, drapes, instruments, and the gloved hands of the surgeon and surgical assistants. Anytime the skin or a mucous membrane is punctured or pierced, as in venipunctures or injections, surgical aseptic techniques must be practiced. Urinary catheterizations, biopsies, and dressing changes on open wounds are performed using sterile technique.

CARE AND HANDLING OF INSTRUMENTS

Because instruments are expensive and the success of the procedure depends on their quality, the medical assistant must properly care for each instrument to maximize its life and ensure that every part is in safe working order.

Instruments that are not disposable are made of fine-grade stainless steel. The term *stainless* usually is taken too literally. Although stainless steel does resist rust and keeps a fine edge and tip longer, even the best stainless steel may develop water spots and stains. Proper hardness and flexibility are important. Inexpensive instruments that are chrome plated may be too brittle or too soft. In addition, mistreatment of chrome-plated instruments can cause minute breaks in the finish, which may become a source of contamination or may tear the provider's gloves.

All instruments should be carefully examined when they are purchased. Scissors should be tested to see whether they shear the full length of the blades completely to the tip. If the scissors cut a piece of cloth cleanly and do not chew at any point, even at the tip, they are functioning correctly. Teeth and serrations should be checked to see whether they intermesh completely and whether the jaws are even on the sides and tip. Each instrument should be felt over its entire surface for any rough areas that may tear or snag the provider's gloves or act as a future source of contamination. Box locks and hinges must work freely but should not be too loose. Thumb- and spring-handled instruments must have the correct tension and meet evenly at the tips. After inspection, instruments should be sanitized and checked again for possible faulty workmanship before sterilization.

Under no circumstances should instruments be bundled together or allowed to become entangled. Do not mix stainless steel instruments with others made of different metals, including chrome-plated instruments, because this may cause electrolysis and result in etching. If an instrument is accidentally dropped, it may be permanently damaged. If scissors are dropped with the blades partly open, there may be a nick at the point where the blades cross. Any damaged or malfunctioning instrument must be disposed of to prevent complications during a surgical procedure.

After a surgical procedure, contaminated instruments should be placed in a basin of disinfectant solution. Heavier instruments should be on the bottom of the basin and lighter, more delicate instruments on top. Always unlock each instrument before immersing it in the chemical decontaminant to permit sanitization of the entire surface area. Never allow blood or other substances to dry on an instrument because they will be difficult to remove. If immediate sanitization and disinfection are not possible, the instruments should be rinsed well and placed in a cold-water solution with a blood solvent and mild detergent. It is best to use a detergent that has neutral pH and low suds and can be rinsed off easily. The manufacturer's recommendations for the correct dilution and time of immersion of the various sanitizing agents, disinfectants, and blood solvents must be strictly followed for the chemicals to be effective.

When the surgical procedure is completed, the receiving basin for instruments should be transferred from the surgical area to the disinfection and sterilization room. It is important to remove used instruments from the patient's view as soon as possible. After sanitization is complete, instruments should be rinsed thoroughly and either washed by hand or washed mechanically using an ultrasonic device. Some delicate instruments, such as microsurgical and lensed instruments, should be washed by hand with a mild, low-sudsing, neutral-pH detergent solution, and a soft brush.

All instruments should be cleaned while submerged to prevent the airborne spread of microorganisms. Throughout the sanitization process, the medical assistant should wear heavy utility gloves to prevent possible exposure to contaminants. Some clinical policies require the medical assistant to wear disposable gloves under utility gloves for added protection from contaminants. Instruments then should be rinsed, dried with a lint-free cloth, and inspected for proper functioning before they are packed for sterilization.

Mechanical washing, such as with an ultrasonic device, can be used for most instruments and is an especially good method for sanitizing sharp instruments to prevent injuries (Fig. 34.25). In an ultrasonic cleaning unit, the instruments are immersed in a cleaning solution and the device produces sound waves that clean contaminants from the instruments' surfaces. Some units then rinse and dry the instruments, leaving them ready for the sterilization process. However, manufacturers' guidelines should be followed for rubber and plastic materials.

After sanitization and inspection, the instruments are ready for the sterilization process. Commercially prepared, disposable packs are available for most minor surgical procedures. They save time and eliminate the need for sanitization, disinfection, and sterilization of

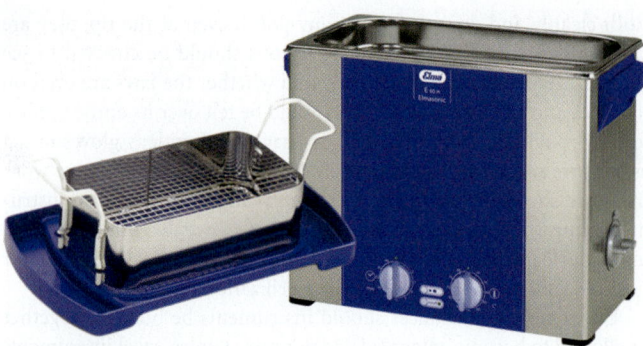

FIG. 34.25 Elmasonic E ultrasonic cleaner unit. (Courtesy Tovatech Elma Ultrasonic, South Orange, NJ.)

BOX 34.6 Utility Room

To ensure proper sterilization for surgical aseptic procedures, an area should be set aside for just this purpose. The area should be divided into two sections, one dirty and one clean. The dirty section is used for receiving contaminated instruments and other materials at the end of surgical procedures. This area should have a sink, receiving basins, proper sanitizing and disinfecting agents, brushes, utility gloves, autoclave wrapping paper or cloth, autoclave envelopes and tape, sterilizer indicators, and gloves. Designated biohazard waste containers are needed for gloves worn when handling contaminated items. Personal protective equipment (PPE) for sanitization, disinfection, and autoclave procedures includes:

- Fluid-resistant gloves to prevent contact with contaminants
- A laboratory coat or impervious gown, if needed, to protect against splashes
- A face shield and/or goggles if a splash hazard exists
- Heat-resistant autoclave gloves for unloading

The clean section of the utility room should be reserved for receiving the sterile items after they have been removed from the autoclave. Clear, clean plastic bags in which to store sterile packs may be kept in the clean area. Both areas should be spotlessly clean and well organized.

reusable stainless steel instruments, but they may also be too costly for individual practices.

CRITICAL THINKING 34.2

Callie is preparing instrument and supply packs for specific procedures performed by Dr. Martin. One of the packs she is preparing for the autoclave is for removal of a nasal polyp. Based on your understanding of typical and specialty instruments and supplies, what items should Callie include in the instrument pack?

Sterilization

Before an instrument or piece of equipment can be used in a surgical procedure, it must first be sanitized, then disinfected, and finally sterilized to remove all forms of microorganisms. It is essential that you understand the concepts of sanitization and disinfection before learning sterilization methods. Written sanitization, disinfection, and sterilization procedures should be in place for each workplace. Box 34.6 presents details regarding the use of a utility room.

Instruments and other items used in ambulatory surgery, examination, or treatment must be carefully cleaned before proceeding with the steps of disinfection or sterilization. *Sanitization* (SAN i tah zay shun) is the cleansing process that removes organic material and reduces the number of microorganisms to a safe level. This cleansing process removes debris, such as blood and other body fluids, from instruments or equipment. Sanitization should be completed immediately after instruments are used. This should occur in a separate workroom or area or on the "dirty" side of the utility room to prevent cross-contamination of clean instruments and equipment. If it is not possible to sanitize instruments immediately after a procedure, rinse them under cold water immediately after the procedure and place them in a low-sudsing, rust-inhibiting, enzyme-containing detergent solution. Blood and debris must be removed so that later disinfection with chemicals and/or sterilization can penetrate to all the instruments' surfaces. Never allow blood or other substances that can coagulate to dry on an instrument.

The medical assistant should always wear utility gloves while performing sanitization to prevent possible personal contamination with potentially infectious body fluids that may be present. When you are ready to sanitize instruments, drain the soaking solution and rinse each instrument in cold, running water.

Clean all sharp instruments at one time, when you can concentrate on preventing injury to yourself. Open all hinges and scrub serrations and ratchets with a small scrub brush or toothbrush. Rinse the instruments in hot water and then check carefully that they are in proper working order before they are disinfected or sterilized. Generally, these instruments are then left out to air dry, but they may be hand dried with a microfiber towel to prevent spotting. Follow facility policy as to how instruments should be dried.

Disinfection is the process of killing pathogenic organisms or rendering them inactive. Many types of disinfecting agents are available, and they have varying degrees of effectiveness. It is important to follow the manufacturer's guidelines on how to use each product properly and to understand its advantages and disadvantages and possible sources of error. Disinfectants are used on equipment that cannot be sterilized (e.g., blood pressure cuffs and stethoscopes); on countertops and other physical surfaces in the healthcare facility; and for soaking instruments and equipment before sterilization. It is important to wear proper protective equipment when using disinfectants because they are generally strong enough to damage human tissue and will often leave burns if allowed prolonged contact with the skin.

CRITICAL THINKING 34.3

The office manager tells Callie she needs to review the office policy and procedures manual on sanitization, disinfection, and sterilization methods. Why is this important to accomplish before Callie starts performing sterilization procedures? What information in this manual would be most important to Callie as she starts this new position? Why?

Autoclave. Sterilization can be achieved by moist heat, dry heat, ultraviolet or ionizing radiation, gas, with chemicals. Medical facilities typically use the autoclave method, which uses moist heat and pressure to achieve sterilization. Steam under pressure in the autoclave (Fig. 34.26) is an excellent method of sterilization because it kills all pathogens and spores.

VOCABULARY

spore: A thick-walled, dormant form of bacteria that is very resistant to disinfection measures.

Pressurized steam is fast, convenient, and dependable. The pressure allows for heat higher than the boiling point (Box 34.7), and when combined with moisture, these two factors create a very effective

CHAPTER 34 Assisting With Minor Surgery

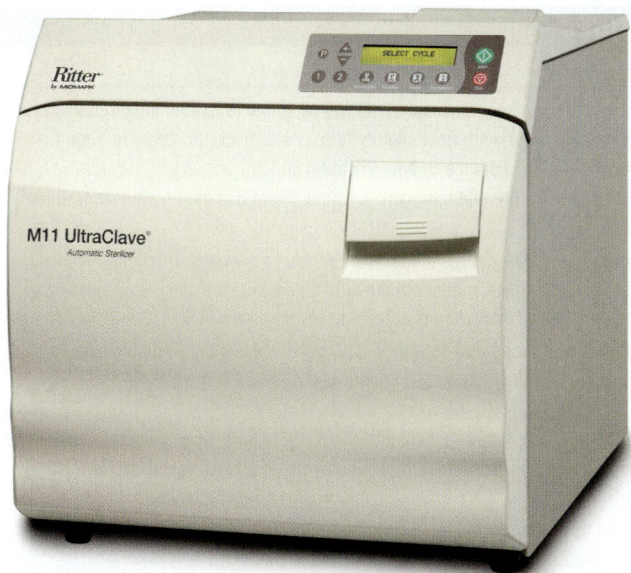

FIG. 34.26 Steam autoclave. (Courtesy Midmark Corp., Dayton, OH.)

BOX 34.7 Steam Temperature

Steam from a pot of boiling water on a stove is about 100° C (212° F). We know that spores can survive temperatures of up to 115° C (240° F) for 4 hours. In an autoclave, the steam is contained within a chamber and is under 15 pounds per square inch (psi) of pressure. This pressure allows the steam to reach 121° C (250° F). No organism can last at that temperature for more than 15 minutes.

TABLE 34.5 Common Factors Influencing the Effectiveness of Sterilization

Causes	Potential Problem
Improper sanitization of instruments	Protein and salt debris may prevent direct contact with pressurized steam and heat in the autoclave.
Improper packaging	Prevents penetration of the sterilizing agent; packing material may melt.
Wrong packaging material for the method of sterilization Excessive packaging material	Reduces penetration of the steam and heat.
Improper loading of the sterilizer Overloading	Increases heat-up time and decreases penetration of pressurized steam and heat to the center of the sterilizer load.
No separation between packages, even without overloading	May prevent or reduce thorough contact of the sterilizing agent with all the items in the chamber.
Improper timing and temperature Incorrect operation of the sterilizer	Insufficient time at proper temperature to kill organisms.

Adapted from CDC: Infection Control. https://www.cdc.gov/infectioncontrol/guidelines/disinfection/sterilization/sterilizing-practices.html. Accessed June 28, 2017.

mechanism for killing all microorganisms. When steam enters the autoclave chamber, it simultaneously heats and wets the object, coagulating the proteins present in all living organisms. When the cycle is complete and the chamber has cooled, the steam condenses and explodes the cells of microorganisms, thus destroying them. To be effective, the steam moisture must come in contact with all surfaces being sterilized. Steam under pressure is capable of much faster penetration of fabrics and textiles than dry heat, but its use has definite limitations if the proper techniques are not followed.

The recommended temperature for sterilization in an autoclave is 121° to 123° C (250° to 255° F). Follow the guidelines that come with the autoclave; in general, unwrapped items are sterilized for 20 minutes, small wrapped items for 30 minutes, and large or tightly wrapped items for 40 minutes. Processing time starts *after* the autoclave reaches normal operating conditions of 121° C (250° F) and 15 pounds per square inch (psi) pressure. There are different autoclave cycles for different materials; ambulatory care facilities do not autoclave liquids or dressing material, so the most used cycle will be the gravity cycle, which is used to sterilize stainless steel instruments. In the *gravity ("fast exhaust") cycle*, the autoclave fills with steam and is held at a set temperature for a set period. When the cycle is complete, a valve opens and the chamber rapidly returns to atmospheric pressure. Drying time may be added to the end of the cycle.

Incorrect operation of an autoclave may result in superheated steam. If steam is brought to too high a temperature, it is literally dried out, and the advantage of a higher heat is diminished. Wet steam is another cause of incomplete sterilization. Wet steam results from failing to preheat the chamber, which causes excessive condensation in the interior of the chamber. Condensation is necessary, but too much prevents the sterilization process from being completed properly. It can be compared with taking a hot shower in a cold bathroom, which results in heavily steamed mirrors, walls, and towels. If packs become too saturated to dry during the drying cycle, the packs pick up and absorb bacteria from the air or any surface on which they are placed after removal from the autoclave. Placing cold instruments in a hot chamber also increases condensation. Other causes of wet steam include opening the door too wide at the end of the cycle or allowing a rush of cold air into the chamber. Overfilling the water reservoir may produce this same effect (Table 34.5).

The main cause of incomplete sterilization in the autoclave is the presence of residual air. Without the complete elimination of air, an adequately high temperature cannot be reached. Air and steam do not mix. Because air is heavier than steam, it pools wherever possible. One tenth of 1% (0.1%) residual air trapped around an instrument prevents complete sterilization. This is especially dangerous in older autoclaves that do not have a chamber thermometer separate from the pressure gauge. Adequate chamber pressure does not guarantee a proper chamber temperature. Table 34.6 provides tips for improving autoclave techniques.

Wrapping materials. Maintaining the sterility of the autoclaved package depends completely on the wrapper and method of wrapping (Procedure 34.1). The wrapping material must be **permeable** (PUR mee uh buh l) to steam but **impervious** (im PUR vee uh s) to contaminants. Acceptable wrapping materials for autoclaving should allow the steam to penetrate and also prevent pathogens from entering during storage and handling. A wrapper should not be used if it is torn or has a hole in it.

The types of wrapping material used for instruments that are to be autoclaved are disposable double-ply autoclave paper and peel-apart polypropylene bags (Fig. 34.27). Multiple layers of autoclave paper are recommended to maintain the integrity of sterilization during handling and storage of autoclaved instrument packs. Double-layered autoclave paper provides these multiple layers of protection for surgical instruments from contamination and saves time because wrapping is done only once.

TABLE 34.6 Tips for Improving Autoclave Techniques

Problem	Causes	Correction
Damp autoclave paper	Clogged chamber drain; items removed from chamber too soon after cycle; improper loading	Remove strainer; free openings of lint. Allow items to remain in sterilizer an additional 15 min with door slightly open. Place packs on edge; arrange for least possible resistance to flow of steam and air.
Stained autoclave paper	Dirty chamber	Clean chamber with mild detergent solution; never use strong abrasives, such as steel wool; rinse thoroughly after cleaning.
Corroded instruments	Poor sanitization; residual soil; exposure to hard chemicals (e.g., iodine, salt, and acids); inferior instruments	Improve sanitization process; do not allow soil to dry on instruments — sanitize first. Do not expose instruments to hard chemicals; if exposure occurs, rinse immediately. Use only top-quality instruments.
Spotted or stained instruments	Mineral deposits on instruments; residual detergents from cleaning; mineral deposits from tap water	Wash with soft soap and detergent with good wetting properties. Rinse instruments thoroughly with distilled water.
Instruments with soft hinges or joints	Corrosion or soil in joint; instrument parts out of alignment	Clean with warm, weak acid solutions (e.g., 10% nitric acid solution); rinse thoroughly. Have instrument realigned by qualified instrument repair professional.
Steam leakage	Worn gasket; door closed improperly	Replace gasket; reopen door and shut carefully; have serviced if unable to close door properly.
Chamber door does not open	Vacuum in chamber (check chamber pressure gauge)	Turn on controls to start steam pressure; wait until equalized, then vent and open door.

From Proctor D, et al: *Kinn's The Medical Assistant*, ed 13, St Louis, 2017, Elsevier.

PROCEDURE 34.1 Wrap Instruments and Supplies for Sterilization in an Autoclave

Task:
To place dry, inspected, and sanitized supplies and instruments inside appropriate wrapping materials for sterilization and storage without contamination.

Equipment and Supplies
- Dry, inspected, and sanitized instruments
- Double-ply autoclave paper
- Autoclave tape
- Sterilization strip
- Waterproof, felt-tipped pen
- Gloves (if part of office policy)

Procedural Steps
1. Wash or sanitize your hands. Collect and assemble already inspected, sanitized instruments to be wrapped. Gloves may be worn.
2. Place the double-ply autoclave paper on a clean, flat surface.
3. Place the instruments diagonally at the approximate center of the double-ply autoclave paper. Make sure the size of the square is large enough for the items (see the following figure).
   Purpose: Each of the four corners must fold over and completely cover the instruments, with a few extra inches of overlap for folding.
4. Open any hinged instruments. If the instrument is sharp, its teeth or tip should be shielded with cotton or gauze.
   Purpose: To prevent puncture of the package or injury to the operator.
5. Place a sterilization strip in the center of the pack to check for sterilization standards.
   Purpose: To ensure that the autoclave is reaching effective levels of heat and pressure to destroy all microorganisms.
6. Bring up the bottom corner of the wrap and fold back a portion of it.
   Purpose: This folded-back flap is the only part of each wrapper corner that can be touched when a sterile package is opened (see the following figure).

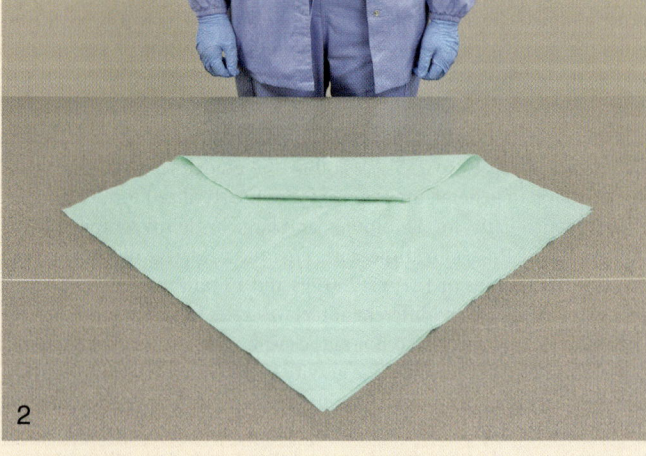

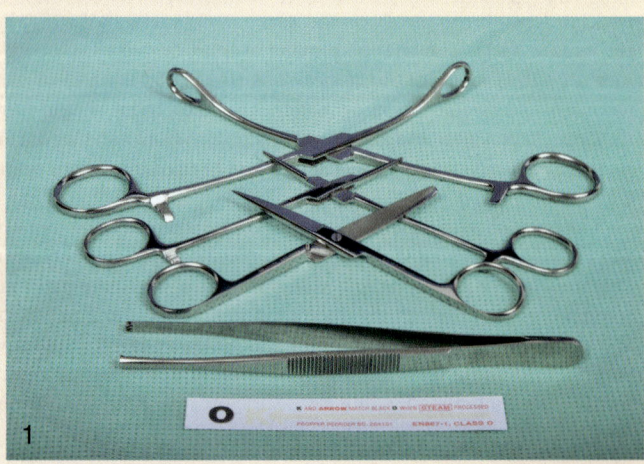

CHAPTER 34 Assisting With Minor Surgery

PROCEDURE 34.1 Wrap Instruments and Supplies for Sterilization in an Autoclav—cont'd

7. Repeat the previous step with each corner, making sure to turn back a portion each time (see the following figures).

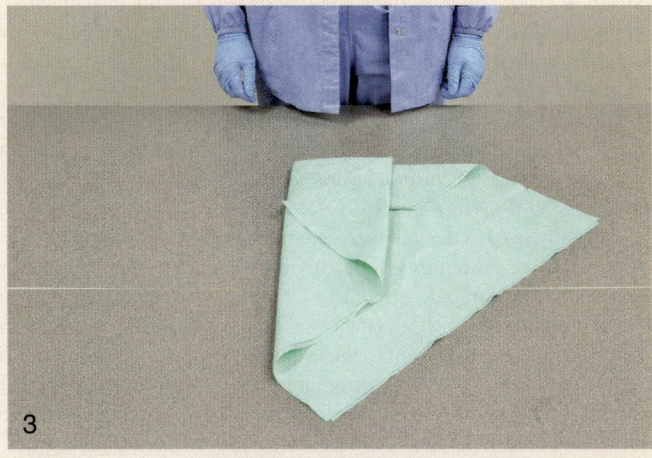

3

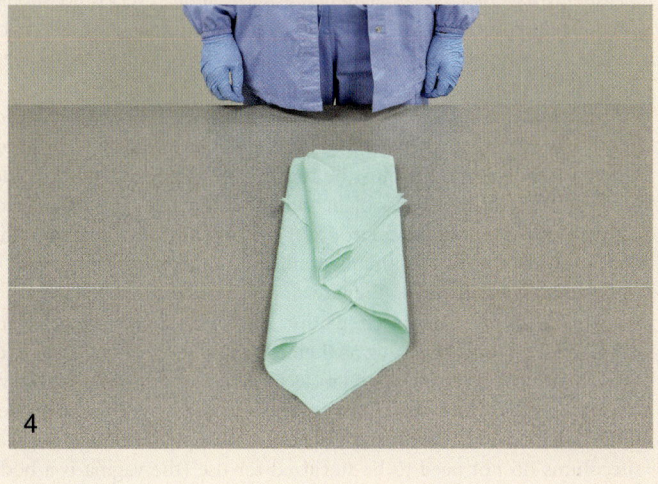

4

8. Fold the last flap over (see the following figure).

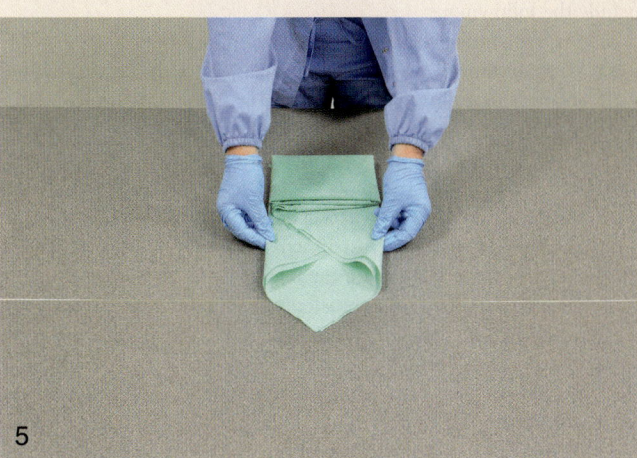

5

9. Secure with autoclave tape (see the following figure) and label the package with the date, including the year, contents, and your initials.
   Purpose: So that staff members will know what is in the pack, when it was autoclaved, and who performed the task.

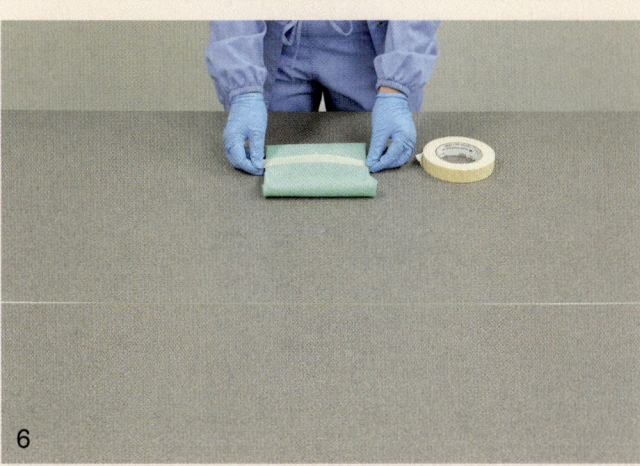

6

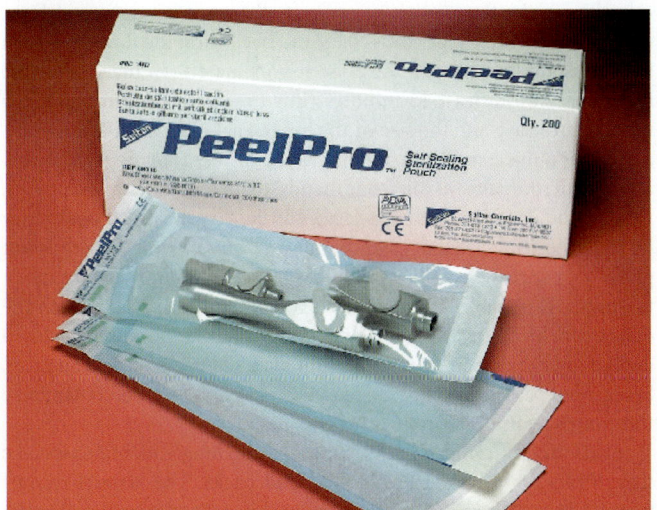

FIG. 34.27 Sterilization pouches with sterilization indicators on the outside and inside of the envelope. The puncture-resistant, tinted plastic front is safety sealed to an autoclave paper backing. (Courtesy Practicon, Inc., Greenville, NC.)

CRITICAL THINKING 34.4

Callie is processing instruments and trays when she notices that one of her co-workers never places gauze squares around the tips of sharp instruments before wrapping a pack. She also notices that not all of the packs are labeled properly. What is the significance of Callie's observation? How should she handle this situation? Why?

VOCABULARY

permeable: Allowing for penetration.
impervious: Not permitting penetration.

Wrapping instruments. The method used to wrap instruments for autoclave sterilization must allow the pack to be opened without becoming contaminated. The rules for protecting package contents include the following:
- Discard autoclave paper that is torn or has holes.
- Wrap all hinged instruments in the open position to allow full steam penetration of the joint.
- Place a gauze square around the tips of sharp instruments to prevent them from piercing the wrapping material.
- If a number of instruments are to be placed on a stainless steel tray for wrapping, first place a double-folded towel on the tray, and then position the instruments. This helps to protect them.
- Polypropylene is a plastic capable of withstanding autoclaving but is resistant to heat transfer. Therefore, materials in a polypropylene pan take longer to autoclave than the same materials in a stainless steel pan.
- When using sterilizing bags, insert the handles of the instruments into the end of the bag that will be opened first to ensure that the grasping end of the instrument can be reached easily when the bag is opened.
- When using two-ply autoclave paper, use specialized autoclave tape to seal the package.
- Label each pack according to the instrument contents and sterilization date, and write your initials. Use a permanent marker; never use a ballpoint pen.

Whether you are wrapping one item or many items together on a tray as a surgical pack, the procedure is the same; be sure the wrapper is large enough to cover the items to be sterilized.

Sterilization indicators. Sterilization is achieved only when steam reaches the optimum temperature for a designated length of time and has penetrated to the center of the articles. Sterilization indicators must be used routinely to determine whether all microorganisms have been destroyed. The two basic types of sterilization indicators are chemical indicators (e.g., autoclave tape) and biologic indicators.

Chemical sterilization indicators. Autoclave tape, a commonly used sterilization indicator, contains a chemical dye that changes color when exposed to steam (Fig. 34.28). The tape is not an absolute indication that the proper sterilization time, temperature, and steam have been maintained. It merely indicates that a high temperature was reached while the article was in the autoclave. The tape strip must completely change color (colors vary by manufacturer) or reveal the word "autoclaved" to show effective operation. The main function of autoclave tape, besides holding the wrapping material together, is to verify at a glance that the package was autoclaved. Other chemical indicators are placed inside the instrument packages to verify steam and heat penetration of the wrapping. Some instruments are autoclaved unwrapped, such as stainless steel vaginal specula. A chemical indicator should be placed in the autoclave with unwrapped instruments in an area most difficult for steam to access, such as under the tray or between the instruments.

Biologic sterilization indicators. The healthcare facility should have a policy for how frequently the autoclave is tested using biologic sterilization indicators. The Centers for Disease Control and Prevention (CDC) recommends that this procedure should be performed weekly. Spore strip indicators have been replaced by rapid-readout biologic indicators that use ampules of *Bacillus stearothermophilus,* which is destroyed at 121° C (250° F). The ampule is placed in the center of the largest pack that is autoclaved in the facility to determine the accuracy of the autoclave and autoclave procedures in destroying all microbes. On completion of the cycle, the ampule is sent to a laboratory for analysis of any type of microbial growth. If tests show that microbes are present in the sample, then a report is sent to the facility notifying it that the autoclave, or possibly its sterilization procedures, are not effective in achieving sterilization. Results from the biologic indicator testing must be documented. Failed tests must be investigated and the causes resolved.

Quality-assurance records for office sterilization. Every office should have specific protocols to follow for quality-assurance evaluations of the autoclave, including regular maintenance. This is done at specified intervals, depending on the volume and frequency of autoclave use. A log must be kept of the type of control test done, when it was performed, and the testing results. If the testing results indicate that sterilization was inadequate, a report must be made and filed. The report should identify the nature of the problem and how and when it was corrected. The report also should contain proof of correction by indicating the date and time of a first, subsequent and successful sterilization run.

Loading the autoclave. Prepare all packs and arrange the load in a way that allows maximum circulation of steam and heat (Procedure 34.2). Articles should be resting on their edges and should not be crowded. Placing the packs in stainless steel racks prevents packing of the autoclave too tightly. Instruments may be autoclaved unwrapped if they do not need to be sterile when used later. For example, although vaginal speculums do not need to be sterilized for use (the vagina is a body cavity that is naturally open to the external environment), they must be sanitized and sterilized to prevent cross-contamination among patients. They can be placed, unwrapped, on a perforated stainless steel tray in the autoclave and then stored in a clean area for future use.

Unloading guidelines. When the autoclave's sterilization cycle is complete, release the pressure according to the manufacturer's guidelines. Once the pressure gauge reads "0," stand back from the door and, with heat-resistant gloves, open the door approximately $\frac{1}{4}$ inch. Allow the load to dry for at least 15 minutes (this time varies according to the type of autoclave and the size of the load). Packs can act like a sponge, attracting outside moisture and microorganisms. Touching a wet pack allows microorganisms on your hands to penetrate the wrappings, making the contents of the pack nonsterile. Dry, wrapped packs may be removed with clean, dry hands, but it is safer to wear heat-resistant gloves to reduce the possibility of burns from the hot instruments inside the packs. If possible, allow all packs to cool in the autoclave with the door open. Place the packs on a dry, dust-free surface inside an enclosed cupboard or drawer for storage. Do not place the packs on cold surfaces, because hot packs may cause condensation, and moisture will contaminate the contents (Box 34.8).

Shelf life of sterilized packs. The CDC no longer identifies specific time limits for the shelf life of sterilized packs. The general recommendation is that as long as the sterilized items are stored so that the packaging material remains intact and undamaged, then the pack is considered sterile. All sterile packs should be stored on dry, dust-free,

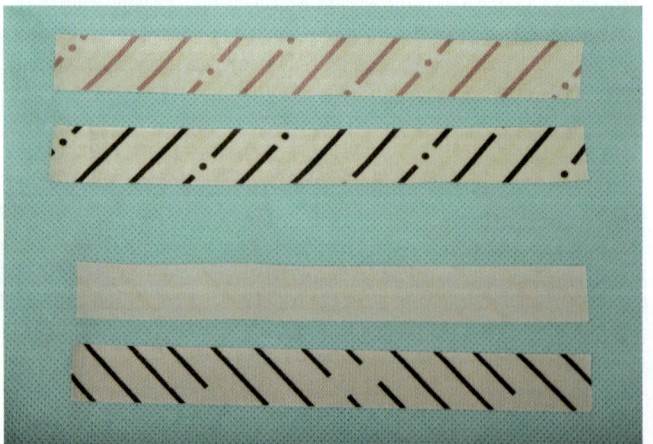

FIG. 34.28 Autoclave tape.

CHAPTER 34 Assisting With Minor Surgery

PROCEDURE 34.2 Operate the Autoclave

Task:
To sterilize properly prepared supplies and instruments using the autoclave.

Equipment and Supplies
- Autoclave
- Wrapped items ready to be sterilized
- Heat-resistant gloves

Procedural Steps
NOTE: The specific instructions for operating an autoclave may vary based on the model number and manufacturer. Refer to the instructions that accompany the autoclave to be sure the appropriate steps are followed.

1. Check the water level in the reservoir and add distilled water as necessary.
   Purpose: Too much or too little water may alter the effectiveness of the equipment. Tap water leaves lime deposits in the chamber.
2. Turn the control to "Fill" to allow water to flow into the chamber. The water flows until you turn the control to its next position. Do not let the water overflow.
3. Load the chamber with wrapped items, spacing them for maximum circulation and penetration.
   Purpose: To ensure sterilization of all items.
4. Close and seal the door.
   Purpose: The door must be closed, or the heated water in the chamber evaporates.
5. Turn the control setting to "On" or "Autoclave" to start the cycle.
6. Watch the gauges until the temperature gauge reaches at least 121° C (250° F) and the pressure gauge reaches 15 pounds of pressure.
   Purpose: The proper temperature and pressure must be reached before sterilization can begin.
7. Set the timer for the desired time.
8. At the end of the timed cycle, turn the control setting to "Vent."
   Purpose: This releases the steam and pressure. The water at the bottom of the chamber drains back into the reservoir. Newer autoclaves automatically perform this step.
9. Wait for the pressure gauge to reach zero.
10. Standing behind the autoclave door, carefully open the chamber door ¼".
    Purpose: To allow steam to escape faster. Be careful to prevent accidental burns.
11. Leave the autoclave control at "Vent" to continue releasing heat.
    Purpose: To dry the items faster.
12. Allow complete drying of all articles.
13. Using heat-resistant gloves, remove the items from the chamber and place the sterilized packages on dry, covered shelves or open the autoclave door and allow the items to cool completely before removal and storage.
14. Turn the control knob to "Off" and keep the door slightly ajar.
    Purpose: To allow the inside of the autoclave to dry completely.

BOX 34.8 Guidelines for Unloading an Autoclave

- Stand behind the door when opening it to prevent accidental steam burns.
- Slowly open the door only a crack, allowing the items to cool for 15 to 20 minutes before removing them.
- If for any reason the integrity of the sterilization process is in question, the load should be considered contaminated and autoclaved again. Reasons for concern include:
  - Any load that fails to convert a sterilization indicator strip (autoclave tape)
  - Any loads processed after a biologic test indicates that the autoclave is not working properly

covered shelves or in drawers. Some facilities continue to date every sterilized package and use shelf-life practices such as first in, first out; other facilities have switched to event-related practices. With event-related practices, items remain sterile until some event causes contamination (e.g., a pack becomes wet or packing material is torn). The quality of the packaging material, storage conditions, and how much the packs are handled all affect the possibility of contamination. Therefore, sterile packs should be inspected before they are used to verify the integrity of wrapping material. Any package that is wet, torn, dropped on the floor, or damaged in any way should be sanitized, disinfected, wrapped in new autoclave paper or placed in new autoclave pouches, and autoclaved again.

CRITICAL THINKING 34.5

Callie discovers a number of packages of paper-wrapped sterile instruments that appear to have water marks on them. The indicator tape shows that they have been autoclaved. What should she do with these packs? Why?

Chemical Sterilization. In the medical office, chemical sterilization is used for instruments that cannot be exposed to the high temperatures of steam sterilization. The sterilizing chemical solution must be mixed exactly according to the instructions on the bottle. The solution must be marked with the date of preparation and expiration. Materials to be sterilized must be submerged in this chemical bath with a closed lid for 8 hours or longer. Items are removed with sterile forceps and must be rinsed with water to remove all traces of the chemical before the items are used on a patient. You must avoid skin contact with the sterilizing solution because it is very **caustic** (KAW stik).

> **VOCABULARY**
> **caustic:** Capable of burning, corroding, or destroying living tissue.

The use of chemicals for sterilization is not very practical in the ambulatory facility. The instruments or equipment cannot be wrapped during processing in the liquid chemical. Once they are removed from the liquid, they are no longer considered sterile. In addition, because of the caustic nature of the chemicals, instruments must be rinsed with water after removal from the chemical fluid. This water is typically not sterile. However, high-level chemical disinfectants do have a place in healthcare. They can be used on instruments (e.g., endoscopes) that would be damaged by autoclaving. Because of the limitations of using liquid chemicals for sterilization, their use should be restricted to reprocessing critical devices that are heat sensitive and incompatible with other sterilization methods.

Surgical Procedures

Common surgical procedures that are routinely performed in the primary care facility include suturing, cyst removal, incision and drainage (I&D)

of abscesses, and collection of biopsy specimens. The medical assistant should be proficient in:
- explaining each of these procedures to the patient
- preparing the patient and the room
- assisting the provider with the surgery
- applying a sterile dressing and bandage after the procedure is finished

Each surgical procedure requires appropriate skin preparation and draping with a *fenestrated* drape. This is a surgical drape with an opening in the center. The size of the opening depends on the size of the surgical field. The opening is placed directly over the surgical site after the site has been prepared (or "prepped," as it is called in healthcare practice). A minor surgery tray is opened, and a sterile field is created on a Mayo stand. Sutures, scalpels, and any other instruments needed are added to the field, according to the provider's preference. An injectable and/or a spray local anesthetic should also be ready for the provider's use with the needed injection supplies.

After achieving suitable local anesthesia, the provider opens the skin with an incision. If a cyst is being removed, the provider dissects around it and usually tries to "deliver" it from the wound intact. If the procedure is an I&D, foul matter will start oozing from the wound immediately after the skin is incised. The wound is drained completely and flushed with copious amounts of sterile saline solution. If the procedure is a biopsy, a small amount of tissue is removed and placed in a specimen container with preservative. The specimen container must be carefully labeled with the appropriate patient information, the date, and specifics about the specimen type and location. It then is sent to the laboratory, where it is examined microscopically for changes or abnormalities.

Electrosurgery. Electrosurgery is also known as *electrocautery*. An electrosurgical unit (ESU) uses high-frequency current to cut through tissue and coagulate blood vessels. A small probe with an electric current running through it is used to *cauterize* (i.e., burn or destroy) the tissue. This process seals blood vessels, minimizing cellular oozing and bleeding. Electrosurgery may be used to destroy granulations and small polyps or to take a tissue sample for pathology examination. The loop electrosurgical excision procedure (LEEP) uses a wire loop heated by electric current to remove cells and tissue as part of the diagnosis and treatment of abnormal or cancerous conditions of the uterine cervix.

Necessary components are the ESU's power source, the grounding cable and pad, and the active electrode (i.e., a pencil-like instrument with a tip and cord). The grounding pad (Box 34.9) is a gel-covered adhesive electrode that provides a safe return path for the electrosurgical current. Electrode tips are disposable and are used according to the type of procedure performed. The two most commonly used tips are the needle and flat designs.

> **BOX 34.9 Important Tips About the Grounding Pad**
>
> - Carefully inspect the pad, cable, and skin before the procedure.
> - Place the pad close to the operative site.
> - The pad must be tight against the patient's skin.
> - Apply the pad to a fleshy area, such as the thigh.
> - Do not place the pad over a bony area.
> - Do not place the pad over body hair.
> - Do not place the pad over metal implants or a pacemaker.
> - Carefully inspect the pad site on the skin after the procedure for signs of burns.

Holding the pencil-like instrument, the provider touches the tissue with the tip and activates the electric current with a switch on the instrument. The electric current is delivered to the tissues, and tissue is vaporized at the site of contact, or a specimen can be removed for pathology (Fig. 34.29).

Laser Surgery. *Laser* is an acronym for *l*ight *a*mplification by *s*timulated *e*mission of *r*adiation. Because a laser beam is so small and precise, it can be used to safely treat specific tissue with minimal damage to surrounding tissues and limited scar formation. Lasers were first used in medicine to treat diseases of the retina, and they now are used for many procedures, including:
- excision of lesions
- cauterization of blood vessels
- removal of warts or moles
- cosmetic surgical procedures

Several types of lasers are used, including the carbon dioxide, yttrium-aluminum-garnet (YAG), and pulsed dye lasers. Each laser has a specific use. The color of the laser light beam is directly related to the type of surgery performed.

A medical assistant must be specially trained to operate a laser before assisting with laser surgery. Laser equipment requires very careful handling, care, and maintenance. Laser light destroys tissue and can harm the patient, the provider, and you if handled improperly. The medical assistant should complete a full laser safety program before assisting in laser procedures. Once trained, the medical assistant's role during laser surgery includes:
- Protecting the patient's eyes from the potential damaging light of the laser
- Observing the surgical field through safety goggles for possible contamination
- Keeping wet sponges ready
- Removing any flammable items from the laser's path
- Assisting with suctioning of the **plume** to maintain a clear visual field
- Providing a basin of sterile normal saline solution and a filled irrigating syringe
- Watching each application of the laser beam and anticipating the need for protective supplies, special equipment, or instruments

> **VOCABULARY**
> **plume:** Vapor, smoke, and particle debris produced by laser procedures.

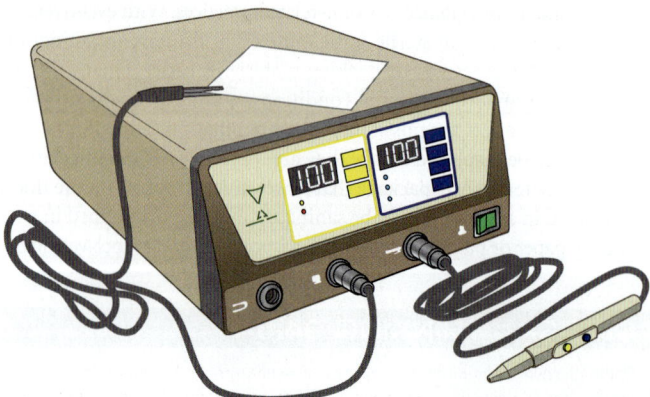

FIG. 34.29 Electrosurgical unit. (From Proctor D, et al: *Kinn's The Medical Assistant*, ed 13, St Louis, 2017, Elsevier.)

Microsurgery. Microsurgery involves the use of an operating microscope to perform delicate surgical procedures. One of its major uses is in **ophthalmologic** (op thuh MOL oj ick) surgery. It also is used in **otologic** (OH toe loj ick), **rhinologic** (RYE no loj ick) and sinus, **laryngologic** (luh RIN jee oh loj ick), neurosurgical, microvascular, **gynecologic** (gahy ni KOL oj ick), and **genitourinary** (jen ih toh YOOR ih nair ee) procedures. A medical assistant must acquire a basic knowledge of the operation and care of a microscope before becoming qualified to assist in these types of procedures.

The basic components of an operating microscope are the light source, eyepieces (also called the *oculars*), lenses, and cord. Accessory pieces include assistant and observer lenses, cameras, video recorders, television monitors, and printers. These are all valuable for documentation and teaching purposes. Disposable sterile drapes and handle covers are used on the microscope during surgical procedures.

Surgical microscopes are expensive, delicate instruments that require extreme care in handling and cleaning. All lenses and cords should be carefully inspected before and after each use.

Endoscopic Procedures. An endoscope is a medical device consisting of a miniature camera mounted on a flexible tube with an optical system and a light source that is used to examine the area inside an organ or a cavity. Many types of endoscopes are used, and they are named according to the organs or areas they are used to explore, such as the urinary bladder, bronchus, larynx, colon (Fig. 34.30), stomach, uterus, abdomen, and various joints. Small instruments can be used to take samples of suspicious tissues through the endoscope.

Direct visualization with an endoscope is used for diagnostic purposes or to perform surgical procedures. Endoscopes may be rigid (e.g., **laparoscope** [LAP ar oh skohp] or **hysteroscope** [HIS ter oh skohp]), semirigid, or flexible (e.g., **colonoscopes** [kohl on AW skohp], **bronchoscopes** [BRONG koh skohp], **gastroscopes** [gas TRAW skohp]). All are delicate and expensive and require extreme care in handling to protect them from damage.

Accessory equipment used with endoscopes includes fiberoptic light cables and light source; irrigators for solution instillation and suction; and a camera, monitor, printer, and video recorder. The fiberoptic light cable consists of hundreds of glass fibers. It is important to protect it from being bent, dropped, kinked, squashed, or smashed. The light source can become very hot and must be kept out of contact with the patient, the provider, the staff, and any flammable material, such as surgical draping. All equipment must be checked before and after use. Always follow the manufacturer's recommendations for use, care, and maintenance of equipment. Endoscopic instruments would be damaged by the high temperature and steam under pressure in autoclaves. Special care must be taken in sanitizing and using high-level disinfectants after each procedure to destroy pathogenic organisms and prevent cross-contamination to subsequent patients.

Cryosurgery. Cryosurgery (KRY oh sur juh ree) involves the use of a very-low-temperature probe to destroy tissue by freezing it on contact. The probe's temperature is usually below −20° C (4° F). This cold temperature is achieved by circulating liquid nitrogen through the tip of the probe. A local anesthetic is usually administered before cryosurgery. Cryosurgery is used to treat warts and cancers of the skin. In many situations, cryosurgery is less invasive than traditional surgery and therefore generally has fewer associated complications. Cryosurgery often is performed in an ambulatory setting or in an outpatient surgery center.

Assisting With Surgical Procedures

Surgery performed in a medical office is restricted to the management of minor problems and injuries. The medical assistant is expected to assist with preparing the patient and setting up the sterile field. The following procedures must be used without exception when assisting with minor surgery. Individual facilities may have specific guidelines for some of these procedures; however, the theory behind sterile technique is universal, regardless of where you work.

Preparation of the Patient. Whether minor surgery is performed because of an unforeseen accident or is a planned, elective procedure, the patient needs both psychological and physical support. A patient facing a surgical procedure may be concerned about pain, disfigurement, and the possible diagnosis. An injured patient may feel anxious about medical bills or possible loss of employment. Because surgery is a frightening experience, the medical assistant must take the time, both preoperatively and at the time of surgery, to help the patient deal with fears and anxieties. The best way to help is to make sure that the patient

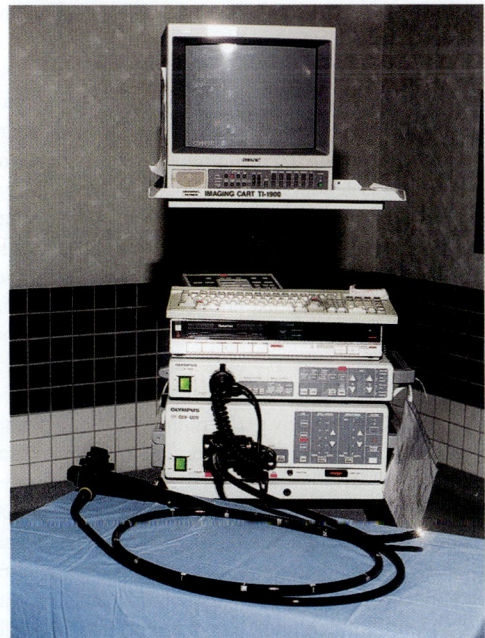

FIG. 34.30 Flexible colonoscope with monitor and video recorder. (From Proctor D, et al: *Kinn's The Medical Assistant*, ed 13, St Louis, 2017, Elsevier.)

MEDICAL TERMINOLOGY
-ary: pertaining to
bronch/o: bronchus
colon/o: large intestine
cry/o: extreme cold
gastr/o: stomach
genit/o: genitalia
gynec/o: female, woman
hyster/o: uterus
lapar/o: abdomen
laryng/o: larynx (voice box)
ophthalm/o: eye
ot/o: ear
rhin/o: nose
-scope: instrument to view
urin/o: urine, urinary system

> **BOX 34.10 Preoperative Instructions**
>
> When office surgery is planned, certain procedures are followed before the appointment. These include:
> - Having the necessary consent forms ready to sign
> - Giving the patient the necessary preoperative instructions, such as medications to be used and special skin-cleansing instructions
> - Telling the patient to bring a relative or friend to drive him or her home after the surgery
> - Instructing the patient to leave jewelry and other valuables at home
> - Calling the patient the day before the scheduled surgery to confirm any special instructions

> **CRITICAL THINKING 34.6**
>
> Callie is preparing a patient for a biopsy of a suspected cancer of the skin. The consent form has been signed and is in the health record. While Callie is chatting with the patient during completion of the final setup for the procedure, it becomes clear the patient thinks she is having a "skin tag" removed from her back. What action should Callie take, if any? What is the significance of what the patient said in this situation?

understands the details of the procedure, that all questions are answered by the provider, and that the patient has the opportunity to talk about the procedure and voice any concerns.

Questions should be answered directly, but you should answer only the questions that are within your scope of knowledge and the policies of the office. If you cannot answer a question, assure the patient that you will relay it to the provider before the procedure and then be sure to do so. What may seem to be a minor or unimportant question to you may be a very frightening concern to the patient. The minor surgery room can be intimidating, so unless the patient is sedated, try to make conversation with him or her while you prepare for the provider's arrival.

Preoperative preparation may include:
- blood and urine tests
- completion of a consent form
- gathering of the current history concerning any recent illnesses
- medications, and allergies

Patient preparations before surgery may include a shave prep, cleansing enemas, food intake restrictions, special bathing, and administration of a sedative medication (Box 34.10). On the day of surgery, the patient is instructed to empty the bladder, and undress and gown as requested. The vital signs are recorded in preparation for the procedure.

Informed consent. The provider must have the patient's written informed consent before beginning any surgical procedure. To sign an informed consent form permitting the provider to legally perform the surgery, the patient must understand:
- what procedure will be performed
- why it should be done
- the potential risks and benefits of the surgery
- alternative treatments (including no treatment)
- possible risks of any alternative treatment

This legal requirement is not met simply by having the patient sign a consent form; a discussion must occur, during which the provider gives the patient or the patient's legal representative enough information to enable the person to decide whether to proceed with the proposed surgical treatment. After this discussion, the patient either consents to or refuses the surgery. The patient then signs or refuses to sign the consent form. The discussion must be fully documented in the patient's health record. A copy of the signed form must also be included in the patient's record. Sometimes the patient will sign the form directly on the electronic record. Treatment may not exceed the scope of the consent form.

The patient must not be under the influence of any sedative medication at the time he or she signs the consent form. An interpreter must be used if the patient does not understand English. This condition must *never* be violated.

Positioning. Have the patient disrobe sufficiently to expose the surgical site completely so that accidental contamination does not occur during the procedure. Clothing may also act as a tourniquet or may make applying a proper dressing or bandage difficult. In addition, the patient's clothing may be stained by the skin prep solution or may interfere with adequate site preparation.

The patient needs to be positioned as comfortably as possible for the procedure. An uncomfortable position can be held for only a limited time, and the patient may have to move, perhaps in the middle of a procedure, if you have not ensured his or her comfort from the beginning. When deciding on the correct position, consider where you and the provider will stand or sit, where the instruments will be placed, and where other needed equipment will be located. If the patient has an open wound, wear gloves to assist the patient into position. If there is active and profuse bleeding, wear an impermeable gown and gloves. If there is danger of blood and body fluid contamination to your face or eyes, wear a face shield.

Skin preparation. The human skin is a reservoir of bacteria, but it cannot be sterilized without the risk of damaging cells and tissues. The goal of adequate skin preparation for a surgical procedure is to reduce the number of transient flora so that transfer of harmful organisms at the incision site is limited. Cleansing the patient's skin before surgery with surgical soap and an antiseptic and shaving the area if needed is called a *skin prep* (Procedure 34.3). Sometimes the patient may be instructed to repeatedly cleanse the surgical area with bacteriostatic or antiseptic soap several days before the surgery. Disposable skin prep trays and electric razors should be available in the ambulatory facility.

Preparation of the Room. If you are to assist in a minor surgical procedure, study the provider's care preferences, review the procedure, and note the materials needed. Next, prepare the room and gather the supplies to be used. Sterile supplies are opened just before the procedure. Opened materials that have been exposed longer than 1 hour, usually because of a delay, are considered nonsterile. Supplies should not be placed where they can be knocked over or dropped. Wrapped sterile supplies that fall to the floor must not be used. Make sure the patient and family members understand that they should not approach or touch the sterile field.

Sterile Technique. Accurately performing surgical aseptic technique requires a great deal of concentration and planning of all movements and procedural steps. The procedures covered in this chapter are for minor surgery, but they are the same techniques used during major surgery. To develop a sound knowledge of sterility and sterile technique, use the following memory aid: *Everything sterile is white and everything that is not sterile is black. There is no gray!* Sterile surfaces must *never* come in contact with nonsterile surfaces. If this occurs, the sterile surface immediately is considered contaminated or nonsterile. Constant **vigilance** (VIJ uh luh ns) and absolute honesty are essential for maintaining sterile techniques. When a sterile surface comes in contact with a

CHAPTER 34 Assisting With Minor Surgery

PROCEDURE 34.3   Perform Skin Prep for Surgery

Task:
To prepare the patient's skin and remove hair from the surgical site to reduce the risk of wound contamination.

Equipment and Supplies
Disposable skin prep kit, or collect the following:
- Gauze
- Cotton-tipped applicators
- Soap
- Gloves
- Electric clippers
- Two small bowls
- Antiseptic or antiseptic swabs (e.g., Betadine swabs)
- Sterile normal saline solution
- Optional: cotton balls, nail pick, scrub brush
- Sterile drape
- Biohazardous waste/sharps containers
- Patient's record

Procedural Steps

1. Wash hands or use hand sanitizer.
   Purpose: To follow Standard Precautions.
2. Greet the patient. Identify yourself. Verify the patient's identity with full name and date of birth. Explain the procedure to be performed in a manner that is understood by the patient. Answer any questions the patient may have on the procedure.
   Purpose: To ensure cooperation and demonstrate awareness of possible patient concerns.
3. Ask the patient to remove any clothing that might interfere with exposure of the site and provide a gown if needed.
4. Assist the patient into the proper position for site exposure. Provide a drape if necessary to protect the patient's privacy.
5. Expose the site. Use a light if necessary.
6. If hair is present, the area may need to be shaved. Put on gloves and shave the required area with electric clippers.
   Purpose: Hair should be removed before any invasive procedure to limit the potential for infection; follow Standard Precautions regarding sharps.
7. While wearing gloves, open the skin prep pack and add the soap to the two bowls.
8. Start at the incision site and begin washing with the soap on a gauze sponge in a circular motion, moving from the center to the edges of the area to be scrubbed (see the following figure).
   Purpose: A circular motion from inside to outside drags contaminants away from the incision site.

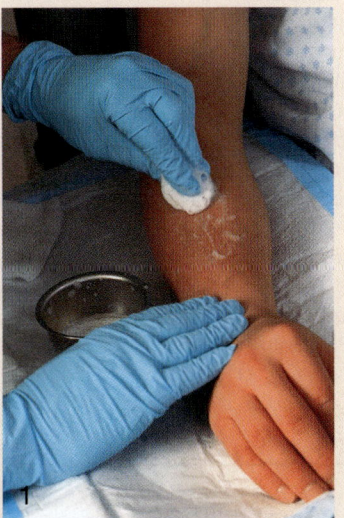

9. After one complete wipe, discard the sponge and begin again with a new sponge soaked in the antiseptic solution.
   Purpose: After one circular sweep, the sponge is contaminated with skin bacteria and debris.
10. Repeat the process, using sufficient friction for 5 minutes (or follow office policy for the length of time required for a particular prep).
11. Rinse the area with sterile normal saline solution (see the following figure).

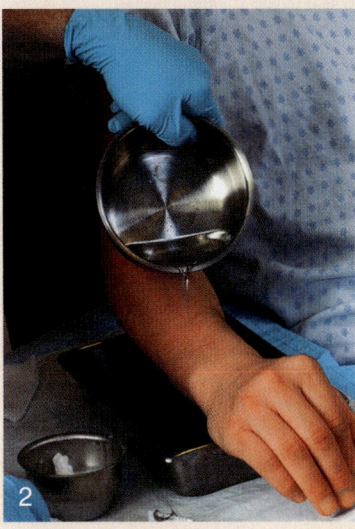

12. Dry the area, using the same circular technique with dry sponges. The area may be dried by blotting with a sterile towel.
13. Paint on the antiseptic with the cotton-tipped applicators or gauze sponges, using the same circular technique and never returning to an area that has already been painted.
14. Place a sterile drape and/or towel over the area.
15. Answer all the patient's questions to relieve anxiety about the upcoming surgical procedure.
16. Document completion of the skin prep in the patient's health record.

nonsterile item, this is called a "break" in sterility or a "break" in the sterile field. During any procedure, everything must stop at this point and the "break" must be corrected immediately. This usually means the assistant must start over again at the very beginning of the procedure. Any break could lead to serious wound contamination, postoperative infection, and even death.

> **VOCABULARY**
> **vigilance:** Keen watchfulness to detect danger.

Before assisting with minor surgery, the medical assistant must perform a series of procedures to ensure surgical asepsis (Procedure 34.4 to 34.7). These skills must be learned, practiced, and followed precisely to establish and maintain the sterile environment required during a surgical procedure. Surgical asepsis directly affects the health and well-being of the patient, the provider, and the office staff, and must be practiced without fail.

> **CRITICAL THINKING 34.7**
> After completing a surgical scrub before assisting with a minor surgical procedure, Callie remembers that she forgot to lay out the practitioner's sterile glove package. She opens up the storage cabinet and quickly adds this to the collection of sterile supplies. Can she go ahead with putting on her sterile gloves? Why or why not?

Text continued on p. 786

PROCEDURE 34.4 Perform a Surgical Hand Scrub

Task:
To scrub the hands with surgical soap, using friction, running water, and a disposable sterile brush to sanitize the skin before assisting with any procedure that requires surgical asepsis.

Equipment and Supplies
- Sink with foot, knee, or arm control for running water
- Surgical soap in a dispenser
- Towels (sterile towels if indicated by office policy)
- Nail file or orange stick
- Sterile disposable brush

Procedural Steps
1. Remove all jewelry.
   Purpose: Jewelry harbors bacteria and is not permitted in surgical asepsis.
2. Roll long sleeves above the elbows.
3. Inspect your fingernails for length and your hands for skin breaks.
4. Turn on the faucet and regulate the water to a comfortable temperature, being careful to stand away from the sink to prevent contamination of clothing from contact with the sink or counter top.
5. Keep your hands upright and held at or above waist level (see the following figure).
   Purpose: Water running from the unscrubbed area above the elbow down to the hands can carry bacteria back onto the hands. All areas below the waist are considered contaminated during all surgical procedures.

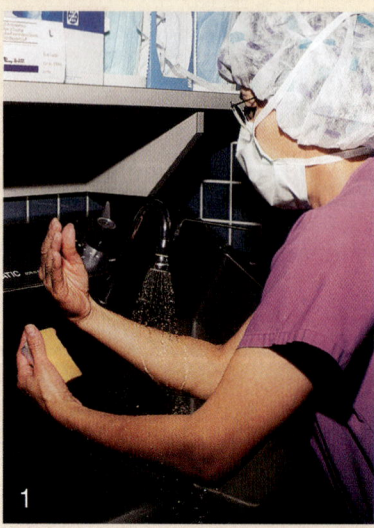

6. Clean your fingernails with a file, discard it (in most situations you will drop the file into the sink and discard it later to prevent contamination by lowering your hands and/or touching a waste receptacle), and rinse your hands under the faucet without touching the faucet or the inside of the sink basin (see the following figure).

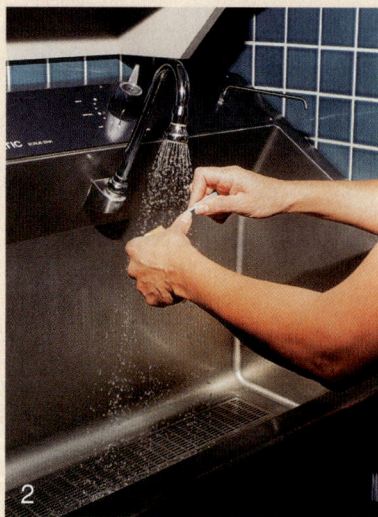

7. Allow the water to run over your hands from the fingertips to the elbows without moving the arm back and forth under the water.
   Purpose: Water running from the elbow down to the hands can carry bacteria back onto the hands.
8. Apply surgical soap from the dispenser to the sterile brush (or use a prepared disposable brush) and start the scrub by scrubbing the palm of the hand in a circular fashion.
9. Continue from the palm to the base of the thumb, then move on to the other fingers, scrubbing from the base, along each side, and across the nail, holding the fingertips upward and remembering to rub between the fingers (see the following figure). After the fingers have been completely scrubbed, clean the posterior surface of the hand in a circular fashion and then proceed to the wrist. The scrub process should take at least 5 minutes for each hand and arm.
   Purpose: The surfaces of the fingers have four sides that all need to be thoroughly cleaned.

CHAPTER 34 Assisting With Minor Surgery

PROCEDURE 34.4 Perform a Surgical Hand Scrub—cont'd

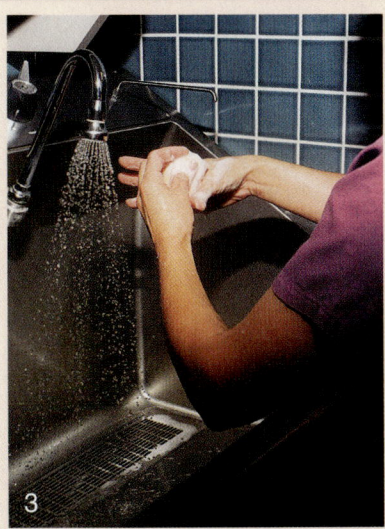

10. Do not return to a clean area after you have moved to the next part of the hand.
    Purpose: Once an area has been scrubbed, it is considered surgically clean, and rubbing that area again contaminates it.
11. Wash the wrists and forearms in a circular fashion around the arm while holding your hands above waist level (see the following figure).

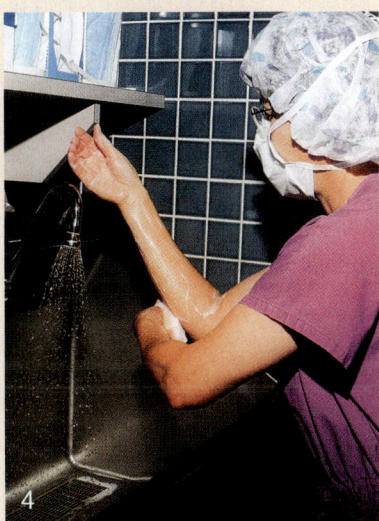

12. Rinse the arms and forearms from the fingertips upward, holding the fingers up, without touching the faucet or the inside of the sink basin (see the following figure).
    Purpose: Keep the fingers higher than the rest of the arm to prevent contamination from water running downward from the elbow. Touching the dirty faucet and/or basin causes contamination.

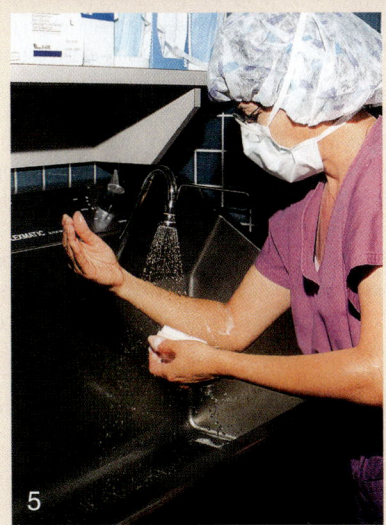

13. Apply more solution without touching any dirty surface and repeat the scrub on the other side, remembering to wash and use friction between each finger with a firm, circular motion.
14. Scrub all surfaces, being careful not to abrade your skin. The second hand and arm should take at least 5 minutes.
15. Rinse thoroughly, keeping your hands up and above waist level. Discard the scrub brush without lowering the arms below the waist (see the following figures).

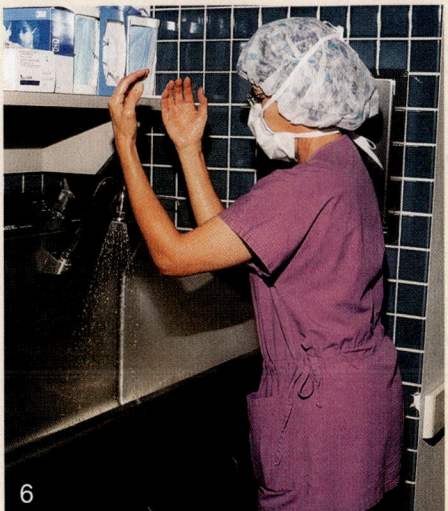

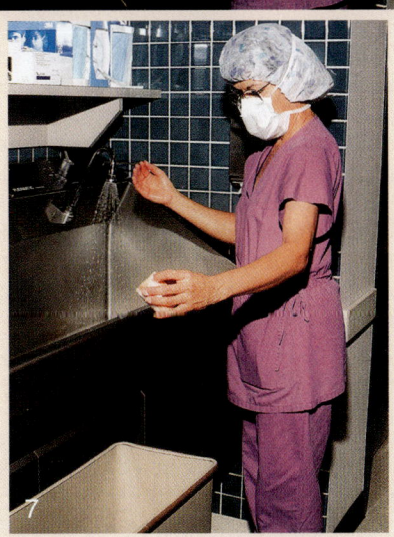

Continued

PROCEDURE 34.4 Perform a Surgical Hand Scrub—cont'd

16. Turn off the faucet with the foot, knee, or forearm lever, if available.
    Purpose: To prevent clean hands from touching the contaminated faucet handles.
17. Dry your hands with a sterile towel, being careful to keep the fingers pointing upward and your hands above the waist. Do not rub back and forth, dragging contaminants from the dirtier area of the upper arm down toward the hands (see Procedure 34.3, Step 11, and Procedure 34.4, Step 5). Use the opposite end of the towel for the other hand.
    Purpose: To keep your clean hands from touching the part of the towel that comes in contact with your forearms, which are not as clean as your hands. If you are to gown and glove for a procedure, you must use a sterile towel.
18. Using a patting motion, continue to dry the forearms. Discard the towel and keep your hands up and above waist level (see the following figure).

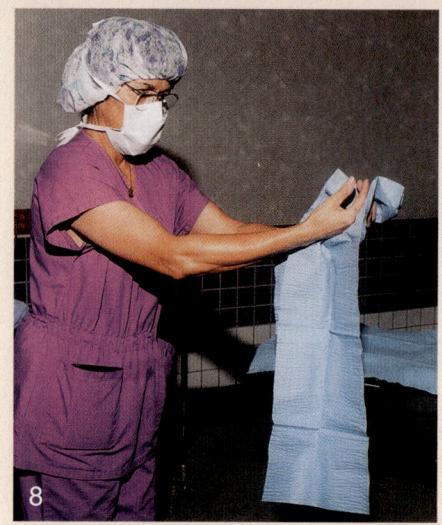

PROCEDURE 34.5 Prepare a Sterile Field, Use Transfer Forceps, and Pour a Sterile Solution Into a Sterile Field

Task:
To open a sterile instrument pack using correct aseptic technique and to create a sterile field; move sterile items on a sterile field or transfer sterile items to a gloved team member; pour a sterile solution into a sterile stainless steel bowl or container sitting at the edge of a sterile field.

Equipment and Supplies
- A sterile instrument pack wrapped with autoclave paper that, when opened, will serve as a sterile table drape or field
- Mayo stand or countertop
- Disinfectant and gauze sponges or disinfectant wipes
- Sterile item to move or transfer
- Sterile wrapped transfer forceps
- Bottle of sterile solution
- Sterile bowl or container
- Sink or waste receptacle

Procedural Steps
1. Check that the Mayo stand or countertop is dust free and clean. If it is not, disinfect and allow to air dry.
   Purpose: Although some areas cannot be sterile, steps must be taken to keep contamination to a minimum; moisture on a tray contaminates the pack.
2. Wash or sanitize your hands and make sure they are completely dry. If you will be assisting with a surgical procedure immediately after opening the sterile pack, perform the surgical hand scrub as explained in Procedure 34.4.
   Purpose: To reduce the number of transient flora on your hands and forearms; moisture on your hands contaminates the pack.
3. Gather supplies. Check the label of the ordered solution. Check the solution name and the expiration date.
4. If using an autoclaved pack, check the indicator tape for a color change.
   Purpose: Autoclave indicator tape changes color after the sterile processing cycle.
5. Open the outside cover (see the following figure). Position the package so that the outer envelope flap is at the top and with the tab facing you.

Purpose: This positions the pack for correct opening so that you do not have to cross over the sterile pack to open it.

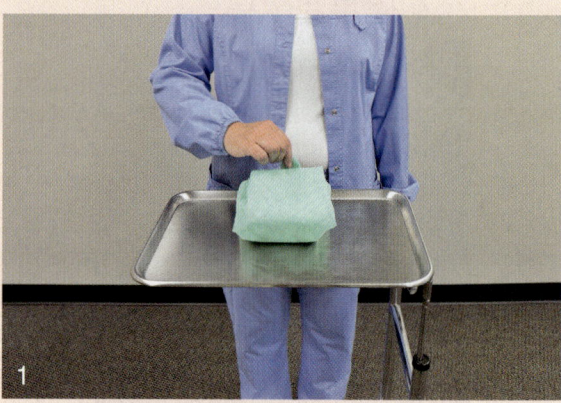

6. Open the outermost flap (see the following figure). Next, open the first flap away from you. You can cross over the uncovered portion of the Mayo stand because it is not sterile. Do not cross over the pack.

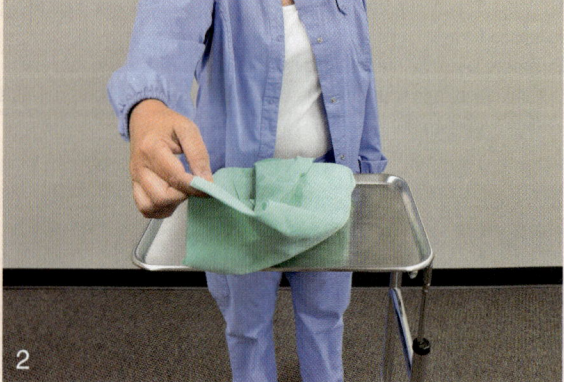

CHAPTER 34 Assisting With Minor Surgery

PROCEDURE 34.5 Prepare a Sterile Field, Use Transfer Forceps, and Pour a Sterile Solution Into a Sterile Field—cont'd

7. Open the second corner, pulling to side (see the following figure).
   Purpose: To prevent contamination of the sterile field.

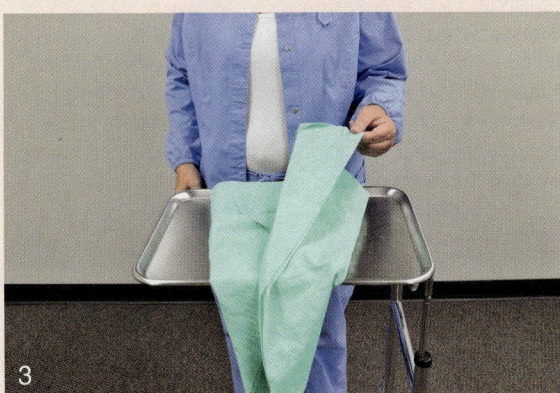

8. Be careful to lift the flaps by touching only the small, folded-back tab and without touching or crossing over the inner surface of the pack or its contents. Open the remaining two corners of the pack (see the following figure).

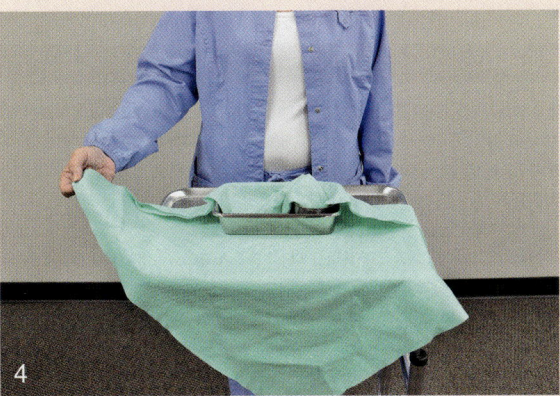

9. You now have a sterile drape as a sterile field from which to work and for the distribution of additional sterile supplies and instruments (see the following figure).

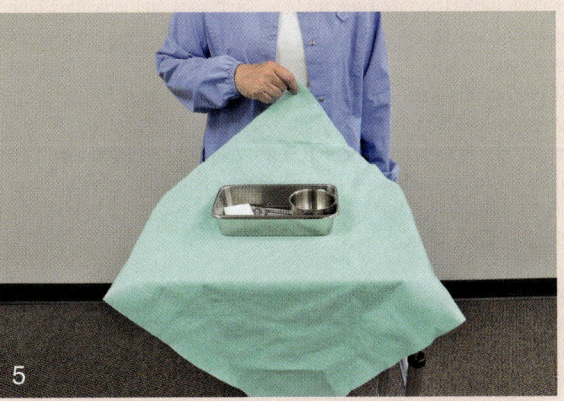

10. Open a package containing sterile transfer forceps (see the following figure). Using sterile technique, handle the sterile forceps by the ring handle only. Always point the forceps tips down.
    Purpose: If the tips are turned upward, any solution encountered will run onto the nonsterile area, and then back down over the sterile end when the tips are turned down again, thus contaminating the forceps.

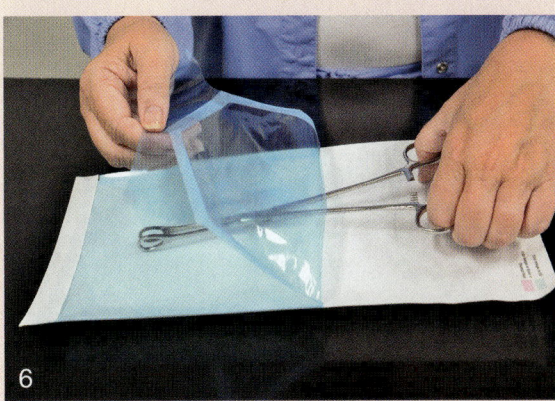

11. Grasp an item on the sterile field with the sterile forceps, points down, and move it to its proper position for the procedure, making sure not to cross the sterile field with the hand or contaminated end of the forceps (see the following figure).

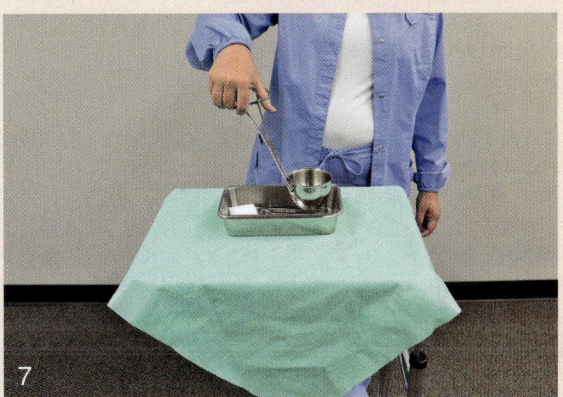

12. Set the forceps aside after one-time use.
    NOTE: The sterile bowl should be placed, using sterile transfer forceps, near one edge of the field and the perimeter of the 1-inch barrier.
13. Check the label of the ordered solution when first obtaining the solution.
    Purpose: Always perform the three label checks before administering any solution or medication.
14. Check the label of the solution for the second time. Place your hand over the label and lift the bottle.
    NOTE: If the container has a double cap, set the outer cap on the counter inside up and then proceed.
15. Lift the lid of the bottle straight up and then slightly to one side; hold the lid in your nondominant hand facing downward.
    Purpose: Air currents carry contaminants that could settle on the inside of the lid.

Continued

PROCEDURE 34.5 Prepare a Sterile Field, Use Transfer Forceps, and Pour a Sterile Solution Into a Sterile Field—cont'd

16. Pour away from the label without allowing any part of the bottle to touch the bowl and without crossing over the sterile field (see the following figure).
    Purpose: Spills down the side of the bottle can stain the label or make it unreadable. The bottle exterior is not sterile, so it cannot pass over the sterile field.

17. If the container does not have a double cap, before pouring the solution into the sterile container, pour off a small amount of the solution into a waste receptacle.
    Purpose: To rinse any contaminants off the bottle lip.

18. Tilt the bottle up to stop the pouring while it is still over the bowl.
    Purpose: Solutions spilled on the sterile field may contaminate the field.

19. Check the label of the solution for the third time. Replace the cap (or caps) off to the side, away from the sterile field, being careful not to touch and therefore contaminate the internal surface of the lid.

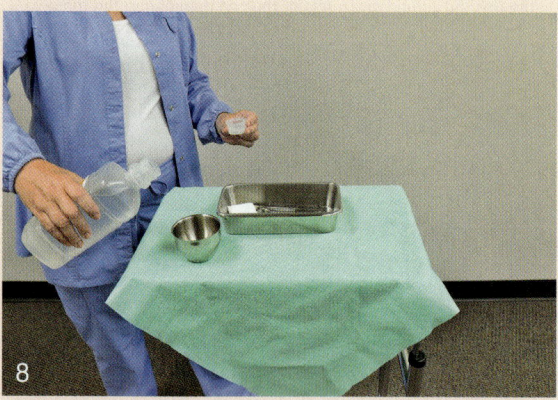

PROCEDURE 34.6 Two-Person Sterile Tray Setup

Task:
Perform a sterile tray setup for a cyst removal.

Equipment and Supplies
- Sterile drape
- Sterile gloves
- In a sealed autoclave pouch: needle holder, operating scissor, tissue forceps, hemostatic forceps
- Suture material with needle
- Sterile 4×4s
- Disposable scalpel

Note: This procedure involves two people. One person will act as the nonsterile person, and the other will have on sterile gloves and will place the items on the sterile tray.

Procedural Steps
Nonsterile Person
1. Check that the Mayo stand or countertop is dust free and clean. If it is not, disinfect and allow to air dry.
   Purpose: Although some areas cannot be sterile, steps must be taken to keep contamination to a minimum; moisture on a tray contaminates the pack.
2. Wash or sanitize your hands and make sure they are completely dry. If you will be assisting with a surgical procedure immediately after opening the sterile pack, perform the surgical hand scrub as explained in Procedure 34.4.
   Purpose: To reduce the number of transient flora on your hands and forearms; moisture on your hands contaminates the pack.
3. Place the package containing the sterile drape on a flat surface near the Mayo stand/tray. Check the integrity of the outer package. Open the package without touching the barrier field.
4. Pick up the barrier field, by the corner, as you move away from table and allow it to unfold without touching anything else. Drape over the Mayo stand.
   Purpose: This maintains the sterility of the barrier field creating the sterile field on the Mayo stand.
5. Inspect the sterile drape for holes and tears, discard if seen and start over. Maintain control of the item inside the package by opening only far enough for a sterile person to grab the item. Allow the sterile person to take the 4×4s. Inspect the package for holes and tears and indicators before the sterile person places the item on the sterile field. Inspect and discard the wrapper.
   Purpose: By inspecting the package after the item has been removed, you can ensure that it is truly sterile.
6. Slowly pull the sides of the peel pack of suture away from each other. Maintain control of the item inside the package by opening only far enough for the sterile person to grab the item. Allow the sterile person to take the suture package. Inspect the package for holes and tears and indicators before the sterile person places the item on the sterile field. Inspect and discard the wrapper.
7. Slowly pull the sides of the peel pack of a scalpel away from each other. Maintain control of the item inside the package by opening only far enough for the sterile person to grab the item. Allow the sterile person to take the scalpel. Inspect the package for holes and tears and indicators before the sterile person places the item on the sterile field. Inspect and discard the wrapper.
8. Slowly pull the sides of the peel pack of instruments away from each other. Maintain control of the items inside the package by opening only far enough for the sterile person to grab the items. Allow the sterile person to take all of the instruments. Inspect the package for holes and tears and indicators before the sterile person places the items on the sterile field. Inspect and discard the wrapper.

Sterile Person
1. Wash or sanitize your hands and make sure they are completely dry. If you will be assisting with a surgical procedure immediately after opening the sterile pack, perform the surgical hand scrub as explained in Procedure 34.4.
   Purpose: To reduce the number of transient flora on your hands and forearms; moisture on your hands contaminates the pack.
2. Remove an item from a peel pack and maintain sterile technique.
3. After the nonsterile person has indicated that the peel pack has not been compromised, place the item on the sterile tray. Repeat for all items. Arrange items on the sterile tray.
4. Maintain sterility of sterile field and sterile supplies.

PROCEDURE 34.7 Put on Sterile Gloves

Task:
To put on sterile gloves correctly before performing sterile procedures.

Equipment and Supplies
- Pair of packaged sterile gloves in your size

Procedural Steps
1. Perform the surgical hand scrub as explained in Procedure 34.4 before putting on sterile gloves.
2. Open the glove pack, being careful not to cross over the open area in the middle of the pack. Remember, a 1-inch area around the perimeter of the glove wrapper is considered not sterile.
   Purpose: The open glove pack is a sterile field.
3. Glove your dominant hand first.
   Purpose: This sets up your dominant hand to do the more difficult step, which is to put on the second glove.
4. With your nondominant hand, pick up the glove for your dominant hand with your thumb and forefinger, grabbing the edge of the folded cuff closest to you, which is the inside of the glove, being careful not to cross over the other sterile glove (see the following figure).
   Purpose: The inside of the glove will be next to your skin and is considered not sterile.

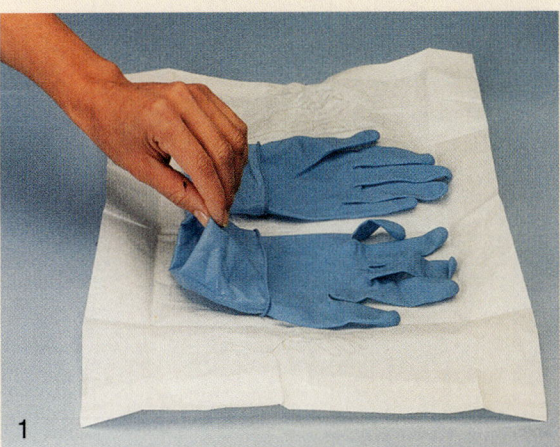

5. Lift the glove up and away from the sterile package.
   Purpose: To prevent accidental contamination from touching the glove on the 1-inch area around the perimeter of the glove wrapper.
6. Hold your hands up and away from your body and slide the dominant hand into the glove (see the following figure).

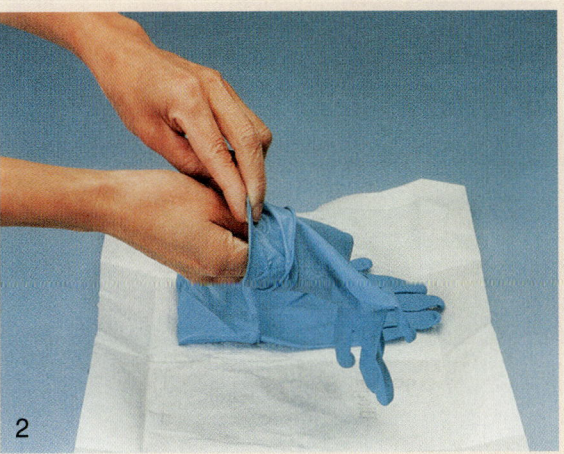

7. Leave the cuff folded (see the following figure).
   Purpose: You will unfold the cuff later.

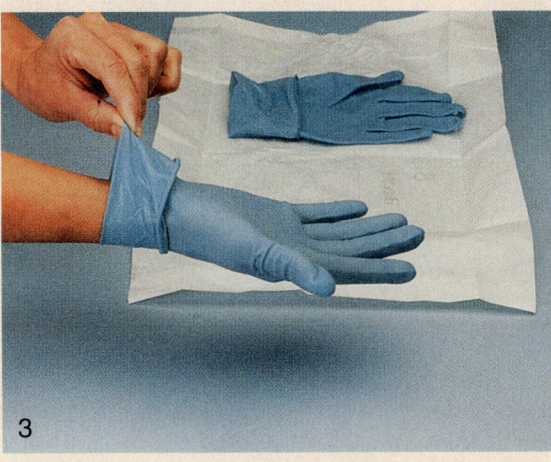

8. With your gloved dominant hand, pick up the second glove by slipping your gloved fingers under the cuff, extending the thumb up and away from the glove (thumbs up position), so that your gloved fingers touch only the outside of the second glove (see the following figure).
   Purpose: Sterile surfaces must always touch sterile surfaces.

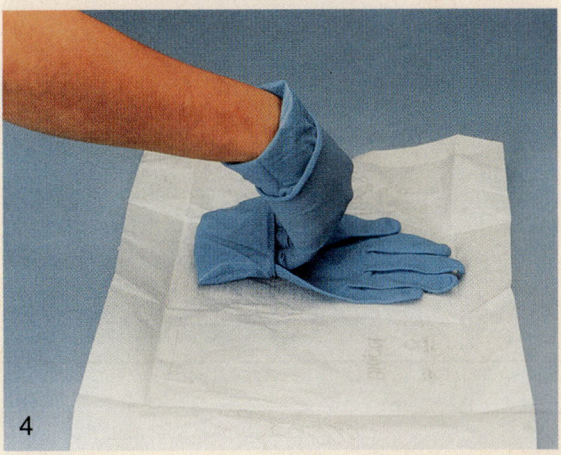

9. Slide your nondominant hand into the glove without touching the exterior of the glove or any part of the gloved hand (see the following two figures).

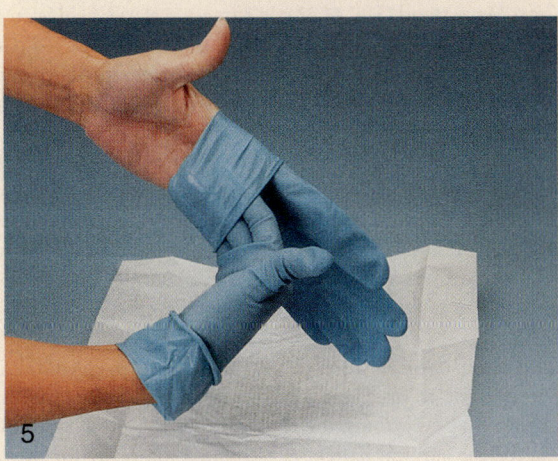

Continued

PROCEDURE 34.7 Put on Sterile Gloves—cont'd

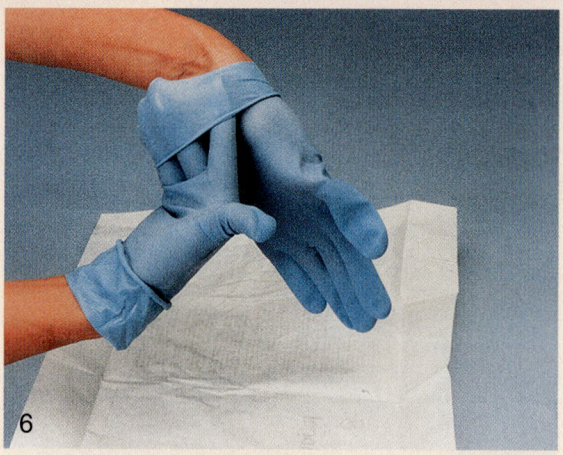

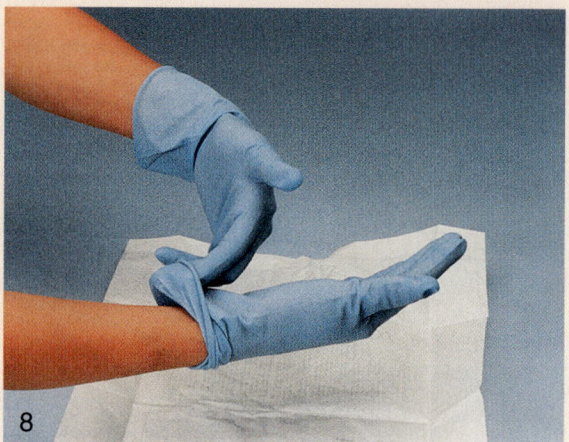

11. Now, slip your gloved fingers up under the first cuff and unroll it, using the same technique (see the following figure).

10. Still holding your hands away from you, unroll the cuff by slipping the fingers into the cuff and gently pulling up and out. Do not touch your bare arm or the internal surface of the glove with any part of the sterile glove (see the following figure).

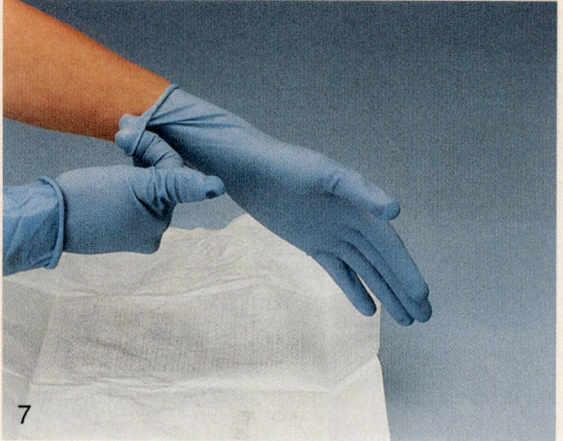

Sterile field. A sterile field is any sterile surface on which sterile items are placed. In the ambulatory facility, a sterile field most often is set up on a Mayo stand (Fig. 34.31). In surgery, a sterile field is created by draping sterile towels (either disposable or from autoclaved packs) over a Mayo stand or table. The surgical site on the patient's skin is prepared and then draped with sterile towels or drapes so that it, also, becomes a sterile field.

Hands and hair are two of the greatest sources of contamination when a sterile field is set up. With practice, you will learn to know what may be touched with your hands and what must be touched only with sterile gloved hands. Hair that falls freely over the shoulders and forward gives off a cloud of bacteria with every movement. It must always be secured back and up, not touching the shoulders (Box 34.11).

Assisting the Provider During Surgery. The provider ultimately is responsible for the patient. The medical assistant is responsible for ensuring that everything the assistant and the provider will use in caring for the surgical patient is accounted for, ready for use, and prepared in a safe and sterile manner (Procedure 34.8). Every team has preferences about the sequence it follows during routine minor surgery.

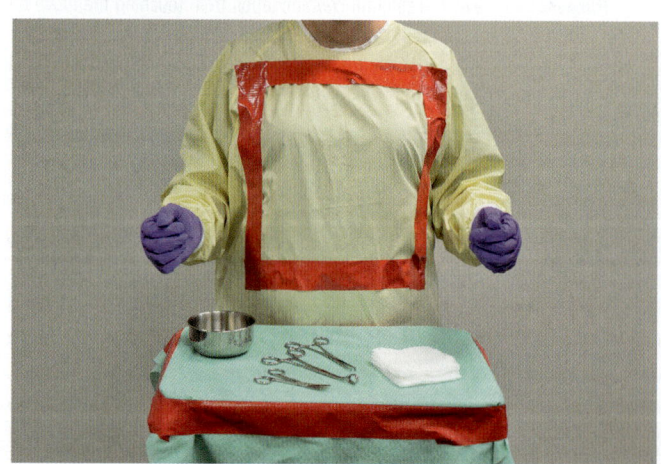

FIG. 34.31 Sterile field *(red outline).*

BOX 34.11 Rules for Maintaining a Sterile Field

- Talking should be kept to a minimum because air currents carry bacteria.
- Sterile team members should always face one another.
- Always keep the sterile field in your view. If you turn your back on a sterile field or lose sight of it, it is considered contaminated.
- Nonsterile body parts (e.g., hands or elbows) and items should never cross over the sterile field.
- Tables and trays are sterile only at table level; anything that falls below the edge of the Mayo tray is considered contaminated. A 1-inch border around the edge of the tray is considered contaminated, so anything placed on the tray within that 1-inch border is contaminated.
- Consider a sterile barrier contaminated if it has been wet, cut, or torn.
- Packages placed on a clean surface are contaminated on the outside, but the inside of the sterilized package may be used as a sterile field.
- Keep sterile gloved hands above waist level at all times; do not let hands drop below the waist.
- Never remove and then replace any item in the field (e.g., using sterile forceps to cleanse a wound), or the field is contaminated.
- The inside of a sterile package remains so if the package is peeled open properly; it should be opened the entire way, and the contents then tossed onto the field without crossing over the sterile area; a two-person transfer can be used, in which one person opens the sterile supplies and another, wearing sterile gloves, removes the contents from the package and places them on the sterile tray.
- If a sterile package falls to the floor, it must be discarded.
- *If you are in doubt about the sterility of anything, consider it contaminated.*

Once a routine has been established, it should be followed in every case. Sample setups for various types of minor surgery are provided in Table 34.7.

The medical assistant sorts and places the scalpels, hemostats, scissors, tissue forceps, and retractors on the sterile field according to their sequence and frequency of use. Scalpels and sharp instruments should be conspicuously placed so that they do not accidentally injure a team member. The provider enters the room after scrubbing and then puts on gloves. The provider drapes the patient with towels or a fenestrated drape as the medical assistant hands him or her the drapes, one at a time. Once the site has been draped, the Mayo stand with the sterile field is positioned below the site, and the medical assistant stands opposite the provider over the patient, ready to help as needed.

Passing instruments. During a procedure, the medical assistant must protect the sterile field from contamination. Notify the provider if a break in sterile technique occurs, dispose of soiled sponges in the biohazardous waste container, and anticipate the provider's need for instruments. The provider may request instruments or may use hand signals. As the team works together over time, the provider may not need to give any signals, because the assistant will be able to anticipate the instrument needed next during the procedure.

Instrumentation is logical; if the practitioner requests a suture, scissors will be needed next to cut the suture strand. In the case of sudden hemorrhage from a bleeding vessel, the provider will need an appropriately sized hemostat. While gaining experience, the assistant watches, listens, and learns to judge what will be needed or performed next. Pass instruments with a firm, purposeful motion so that the provider does not have to look up. Wait until you feel the provider grasp the instrument so that it does not drop onto the patient or the floor, and be careful that you and the provider are protected from injury. Pass the scalpel

PROCEDURE 34.8 Assist With Minor Surgery

Task:
To maintain the sterile field and to pass instruments in a prescribed sequence during a surgical procedure that involves the making of a surgical incision and the removal of a growth.

Equipment and Supplies
- Open patient drape pack on the side counter
- Mayo stand covered with a sterile drape
- Packaged sterile gloves (two pairs)
- Needle and syringe for local anesthetic medication
- Vial of local anesthetic medication
- Sterile drape
- Disposable scalpel with No. 15 blade
- Tissue forceps
- Skin retractor
- Three hemostats
- Needle holder
- Supply of sterile gauze sponges
- Biohazardous waste container
- Sharps container
- Needle with suture material
- Specimen cup
- Laboratory requisitions
- Patient's record

Procedural Steps
1. Prep the patient's skin with surgical soap and antiseptic solution as explained in Procedure 34.3. Explain the prep procedure to the patient.
   Purpose: To ensure infection control and to demonstrate awareness of possible patient concerns.
2. Perform the surgical hand scrub as explained in Procedure 34.4.
3. Instruct and prepare the patient for the procedure. Explain the following: what will occur, what the patient should do during the procedure, how long the procedure will take, and what the patient will sense (e.g., feel, smell, etc.)

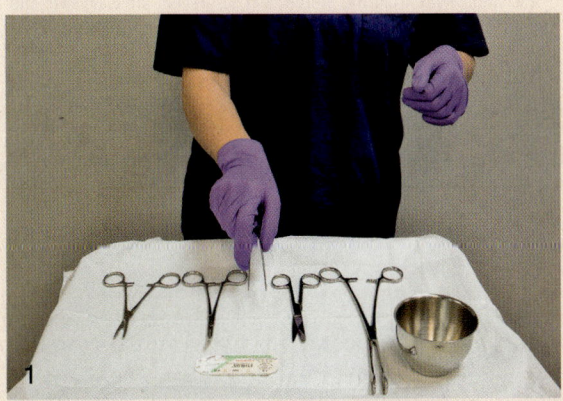

Continued

PROCEDURE 34.8 Assist With Minor Surgery—cont'd

4. Position the Mayo stand near the patient and the operative site, making sure the patient understands not to touch the sterile field (see the following figure).
   Purpose: To prevent contamination of supplies and provide easy access for the provider.

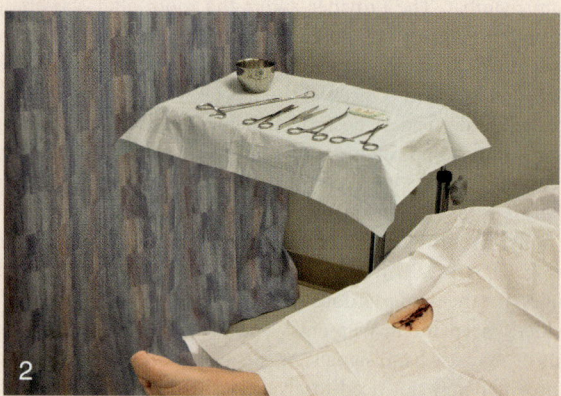

5. Put on sterile gloves using surgical technique.
6. Grasp the patient drape by holding one edge or corner in each hand (see the following figure).

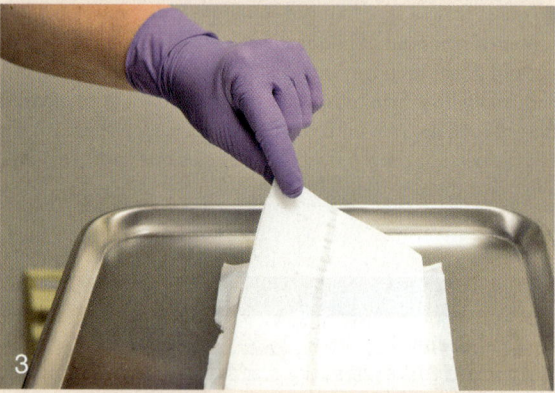

7. Drape the surgical site without touching any part of the patient or the operating area with your gloved hands.
8. If the provider requests medication, such as a local anesthetic, a second circulating assistant holds the vial of local anesthetic so that the provider can read the label. The provider withdraws the desired amount using sterile technique (see the following figure).
   Purpose: The vial of local anesthetic medication must be held by the second assistant away from the sterile field to prevent crossing over the field with a nonsterile item. The medication label must be checked before a medication is dispensed or administered.

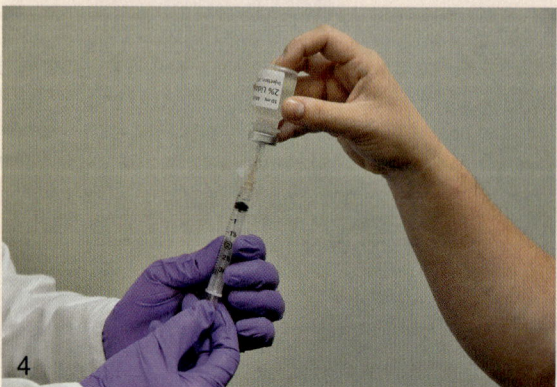

9. The provider injects the local anesthetic and waits a few minutes for it to take effect.
10. Position yourself across from the practitioner. Arrange the sterile field. Check the placement location on the Mayo stand (see the following figure).

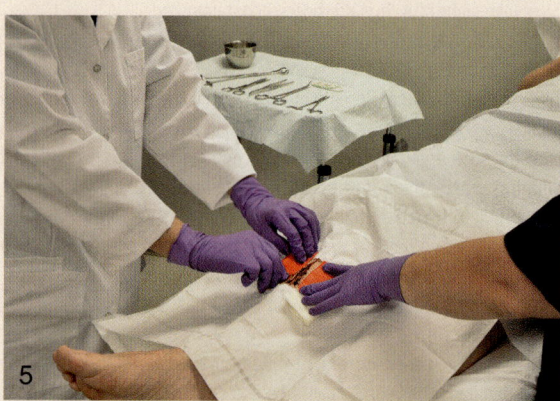

11. Keep all sharp equipment conspicuously placed on the sterile field.
    Purpose: Sharp instruments that are not clearly visible may injure a team member.
12. Pass the scalpel, blade down and handle first, to the provider, or the provider will reach for it. The provider will take the scalpel with the thumb and forefinger in the position ready for use (see the following figure).
    Purpose: To protect the practitioner and yourself from injury.

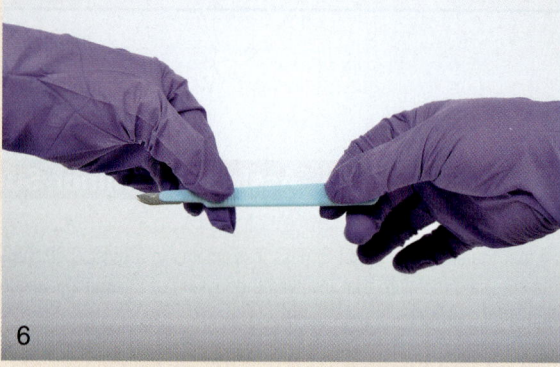

13. Pick up a tissue forceps by the tips and pass it to the provider to grasp a piece of the tissue to be excised (see the following figure).

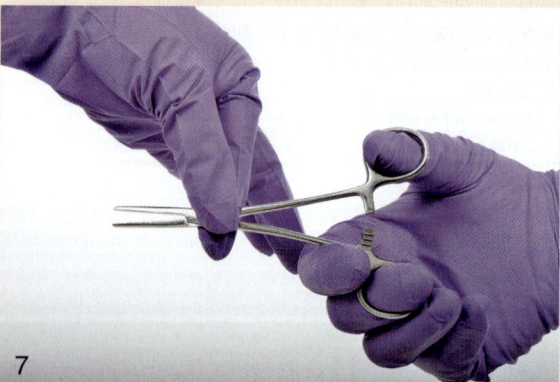

14. Dispose of soiled sponges in the biohazardous waste container, being careful to keep your hands above your waist and to avoid touching any nonsterile items.
15. Hold clean sponges in your hand to pat or sponge the wound as needed.

PROCEDURE 34.8 Assist With Minor Surgery—cont'd

16. Safely position the specimen (if any) where it will not be disturbed in a sterile container on the sterile field.
17. If there is a bleeding vessel or if a hemostat is requested, pass the hemostat in the manner described in Step 13.
18. Continue to sponge blood from the wound site.
19. Retract the wound edge, as needed, with a skin retractor.
20. Continue to monitor the sterile field and assist the provider as needed.
21. Pass the needle and suture material to close the wound and apply a sterile dressing as requested (see the following figure).
22. Monitor the patient and provide assistance as needed.
23. When the provider is finished, clean the surgical site using sterile technique.
24. Collect the specimen using Standard Precautions, place it in a labeled specimen cup, and send it to the laboratory with the proper requisitions.
25. Wash hands or use hand sanitizer. Document the procedure, wound condition, and patient education on wound care.

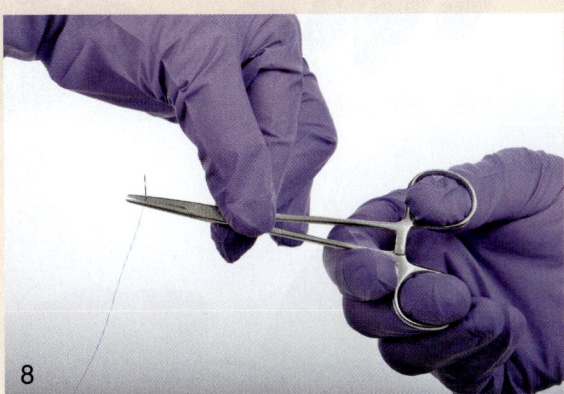

8

TABLE 34.7 Setups for Minor Surgeries

Procedure	Side Counter	Sterile Field	Comments	Postoperative Care
Suture repair	Local anesthetic, dressings and bandages, splints or guards, tape, drape, gloves, sterile normal saline solution	Syringe and needle, hemostats (three), scissors, sponges, suture material and needle, tissue forceps or skin hook, needle holder	If a patient arrives with a pressure dressing over a laceration, follow Standard Precautions. Do not remove the pressure dressing until the provider is ready to suture. If the patient's pressure cloth must be removed, have ample sterile dressings ready to apply immediately. Ask the patient the approximate length, depth, and exact location of the laceration. Follow the provider's directions regarding cleansing of the wound.	Clean lacerations in a moderately protected area; may not require a dressing. The patient is instructed to keep the area clean and dry. Some lacerations may be closed with Steri-Strips or a topical skin adhesive.
Needle biopsy	Specimen container with prepackaged fixative or preserving solution, laboratory form and label, local anesthetic, gloves	Biopsy needle, syringe and needle, sponges	A biopsy is the examination of tissue removed from the living body. Biopsies usually are done to determine whether a growth is malignant or benign; however, a biopsy may be done as a diagnostic aid in other diseases or infections. A needle biopsy may be done by aspiration with a needle and syringe or with a special biopsy needle. The specimen then is sent to a pathologist for either a cytologic or a histologic examination.	Usually no special dressing is required after a needle biopsy. An adhesive bandage strip (e.g., Band-Aid) often is sufficient.
Cyst removal	Local anesthetic, disinfectant (skin prep), laboratory form, dressing (size depends on site), gloves, drape, specimen container with prepackaged fixative or preserving solution	Kelly hemostats (two straight and two curved), dressing forceps (two), suture and needle, scissors, dissector (provider's choice), skin hook, syringe and needle, disposable scalpel with No. 11 or No. 15 blade, tissue forceps (two), Allis forceps, needle holder, sponges	A sebaceous cyst is a benign retention cyst of a sebaceous gland containing fatty substance from the gland. The cyst is attached to the skin and moves freely over the underlying tissue. For cosmetic reasons the provider makes the incision on the natural skin crease lines if possible.	See suture repair, earlier, or apply a small sterile dressing, depending on the size of the incision.

From Proctor D, et al: *Kinn's The Medical Assistant*, ed 13, St Louis, 2017, Elsevier.

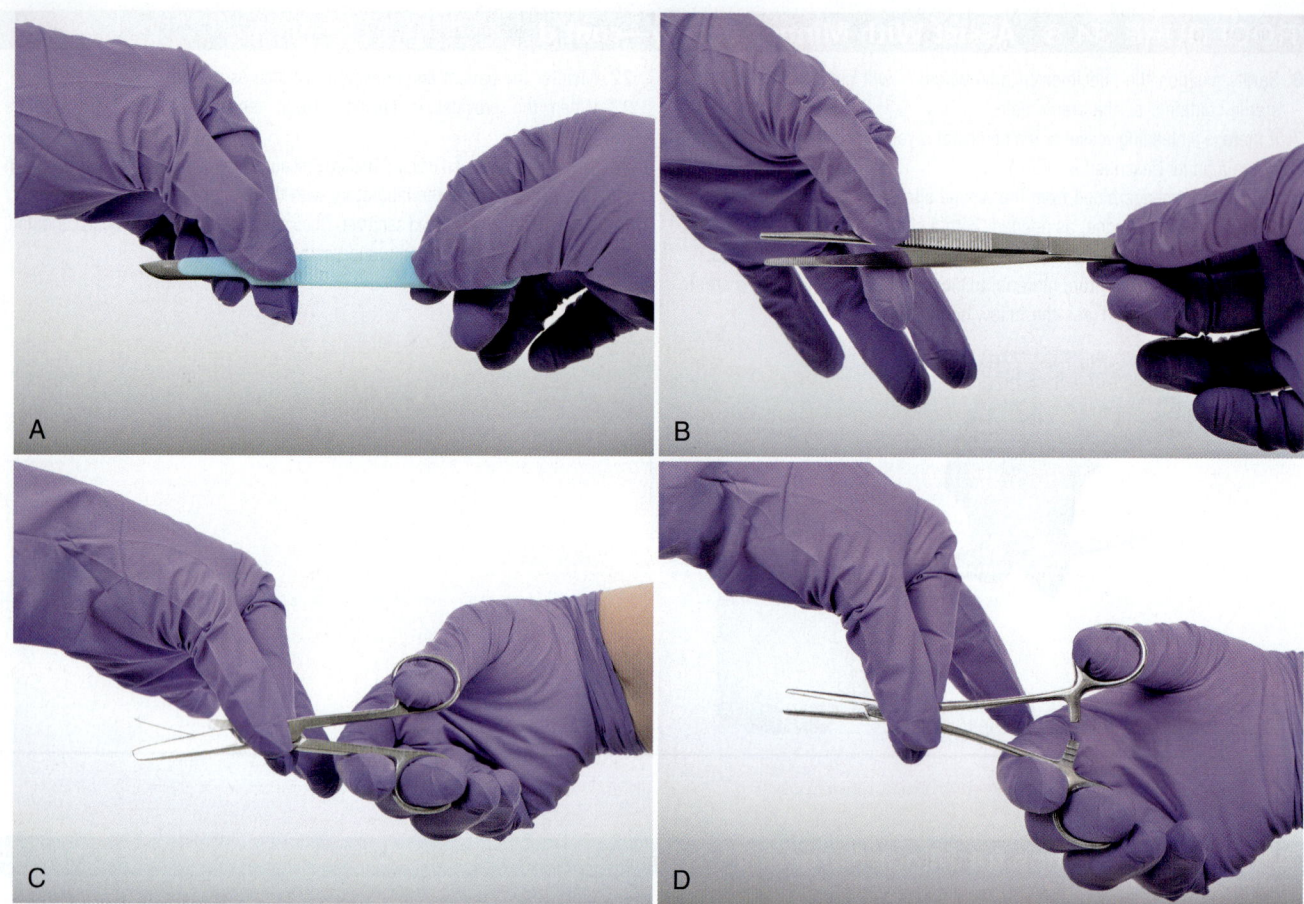

FIG. 34.32 Passing sterile surgical instruments. (A) Scalpel. (B) Forceps. (C) Scissors. (D) Clamp. (From Proctor D, et al: *Kinn's The Medical Assistant*, ed 13, St Louis, 2017, Elsevier.)

with the blade down and present the handle to the provider. Hold all instruments by their tips and pass the handle ends into the provider's palm or fingers (Fig. 34.32).

> **CRITICAL THINKING 34.8**
>
> In passing the scalpel to the provider while assisting with an incision and drainage (I&D), Callie feels the blade slice through her glove. She quickly and secretly looks at it and notices a "very tiny" nick in her glove. Because this is a "dirty" procedure, she decides to say nothing and continues assisting with the procedure. Is her reasoning sound here? What is the best approach to handling this situation? Why?

Specimen collection. If a specimen is collected during a procedure, it is placed in a sterile specimen cup or basin. Do not remove the specimen from the sterile field until the provider gives the order. The provider may want to examine the specimen again during the procedure. After the procedure is complete, place the specimen in an appropriate container, label it, and send it to the laboratory for analysis.

Completing the surgical procedure. At the conclusion of the procedure, the provider begins wound closure. The techniques and methods of tissue closure vary; all of them cannot be described or illustrated here. The two basic methods of suturing are the continuous running suture and the interrupted suture, in which each knot is placed and tied one at a time, so that if one breaks, the others keep the wound closure intact (Fig. 34.33). The interrupted technique is used for most skin closures in a medical office.

The provider may prefer that the medical assistant place the needle in a needle holder and pass it, handle first. When the wound is closed, you may assist by cutting the suture and sponging the site. If an interrupted suture method is used, the first suture is placed at the midpoint of the incision. Then each side of the first suture is mentally divided in half again, and the next two sutures are placed at each of these midpoints. The rest of the sutures are placed using the same technique until the wound edges have been completely **approximated** (uh PROK suh meyt d). The provider may also choose to close a wound with surgical staples.

> **VOCABULARY**
> **approximated:** Near, close together.

After the skin closure, sterile normal saline may be poured over the wound area to cleanse it – this process is called a *wound lavage* – or the area is cleansed with an antiseptic and blotted dry using sterile dry sponges. Care must be taken not to disturb the wound edges or sutures. Next, a sterile dressing is placed over the incision (Procedure 34.9), and a bandage is applied to support the dressing.

Postoperative responsibilities. After caring for the patient, the medical assistant clears the sterile field, following Standard Precautions. Wear gloves until all contaminated materials have been properly removed and handled. Place disposable equipment and supplies in biohazard waste containers and/or sharps containers. The room should be checked for any blood spills or other contamination and disinfected appropriately.

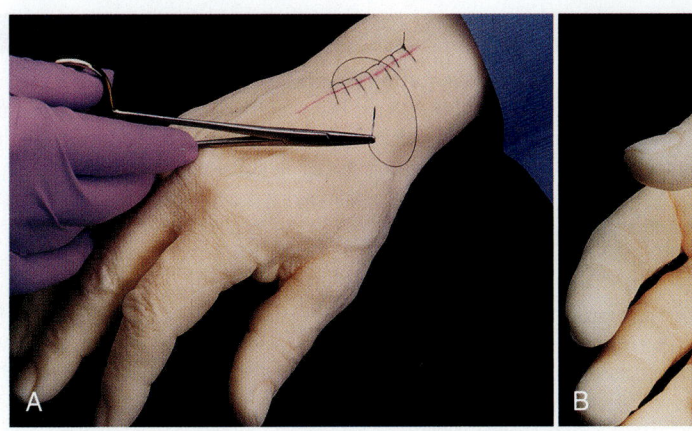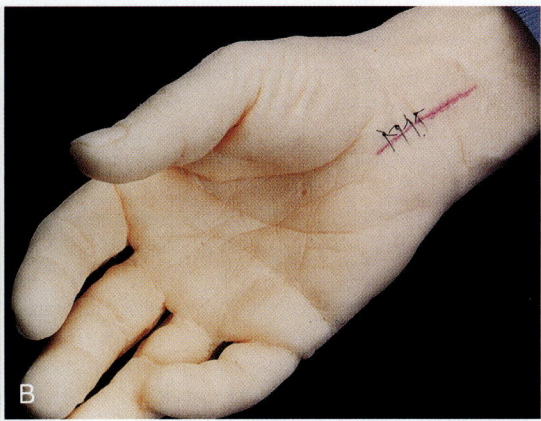

FIG. 34.33 (A) Continuous (i.e. running) suture placement. (B) Interrupted suture placement. (From Proctor D, et al: *Kinn's The Medical Assistant*, ed 13, St Louis, 2017, Elsevier.)

PROCEDURE 34.9 Apply a Sterile Dressing

Task:
Perform dressing change. Apply a sterile dressing while maintaining aseptic technique. Instruct and prepare the patient for the procedure. Explain the rationale for the procedure

Equipment and Supplies
- Gloves
- Biohazard waste container
- Sterile water or hydrogen peroxide (optional)
- Disposable ruler
- Culture swab
- Lab requisition, label, and plastic specimen bag for transport
- Sterile gloves
- Antiseptic swabs
- Sterile dressing and ABD pad
- Tape
- Mannequin with a wound
- Patient's record

Order:
Change dressing and apply a sterile dressing. Culture wound drainage.

Scenario:
Dr. Walden ordered a dressing change. You are to apply a sterile dressing after you obtain a culture of the wound drainage. As you are beginning the procedure, the patient asks "why" questions regarding PPE and the reason for the wound culture. You need to explain the rationale for wearing PPE and why a wound culture is obtained.

Directions:
Role-play the scenario with a peer. The peer will be the patient and you are the medical assistant. After the role-play, the rest of the procedure is done on a mannequin.

Procedural Steps
1. Wash hands or use hand sanitizer. Assemble supplies on Mayo stand/tray and place biohazard waste container within easy reach.
2. Greet the patient. Identify yourself. Verify the patient's identity with full name and date of birth. Verify the patient's allergies.
3. Instruct and prepare the patient for the procedure. Explain the procedure to be performed in a manner that is understood by the patient. Explain the following: what will occur, what the patient should do during the procedure, how long the procedure will take, and what the patient will sense (e.g., feel, smell, etc.). Answer any questions the patient may have on the procedure.

Scenario update: The patient questions why you need to change gloves so much during the procedure. He/She also asks why the wound culture needs be done.

4. Based on the patient's comments, explain the reason for changing your gloves during the procedure and also for the wound culture. Demonstrates empathy and appropriate nonverbal communication when addressing the patient's questions and concerns.

Scenario update: The rest of the steps can be done on a mannequin.

5. Put on gloves. Loosen tape on old bandage from edges to the middle, towards the wound. Remove bandage and dressing, one at a time. If dressing is stuck, use a small amount of sterile water or hydrogen peroxide to loosen.
6. Check for drainage on the dressing and bandage. Note the color of the drainage. Measure any drainage using a disposable ruler, then discard everything in the biohazard waste container.
7. Assess the wound. If present, count the sutures or staples. Check if they are intact. Check the wound for signs of infection.
8. If the wound is open and/or redness or drainage is present:
   a. Culture the wound using a sterile swab (if ordered). Place in a culture transfer tube. Squeeze the tube to release formalin to preserve the specimen.
   b. Concisely and accurately report the relevant information (any issues with the wound or wound closures) to the provider. Ask the provider to check the wound before re-dressing.
9. Remove gloves and place in biohazard waste container.
10. Wash hands or use hand sanitizer.
11. Open and arrange sterile supplies in the order they will be used. Apply the principles of sterile technique.
12. Put on sterile gloves. State that the nondominant hand will be nonsterile and the dominant hand will be sterile.
13. With the nondominant hand, pick up the antiseptic swab container. With the dominant hand, grasp an antiseptic swab without touching the package. Clean from center of wound to edge, use one roll of the swab and discard in waste container. Start with new swab where you left off with the previous swab. Continue until all the exudate is removed.
14. With the dominant hand, remove the sterile dressing without touching the package. Place the sterile dressing material over the wound and cover the wound completely.
15. With the dominant hand, place an ABD pad over the dressing as a bandage.

Continued

UNIT 4 Basic Clinical Procedures

PROCEDURE 34.9 Apply a Sterile Dressing—cont'd

16. Remove and discard the sterile gloves. Secure the bandage with tape.
17. Provide patient education as needed for wound care.
18. Complete the lab requisition for the culture. Put on gloves. Label the culture tube and place the culture tube in the plastic specimen bag for transport to the lab.
19. Clean up the area. Discard all biohazardous waste in biohazard waste containers. Discard all other waste in in the regular waste containers. Disinfect the tables.
20. Remove gloves and dispose of them appropriately. Wash hands or use hand sanitizer.
21. Using the patient's health record, document the following: wound appearance, number of intact sutures or staples (if present), the culture obtained, wound care performed, and the patient education provided.
22. In the written response section, discuss the implication for failing to comply with CDC regulations in healthcare settings.

Documentation Example
10/12/20•• 2:15 pm: Dressing change completed to wound on Ⓛ midforearm. Area slightly inflamed, mod amt serosanguineous drainage noted. Site cleansed and sterile dressing applied. Pt instructed on home wound care and to notify provider if drainage changes, inflammation increases, or fever occurs._____
_____Callie Casper, CMA (AAMA)

Written Response
You failed to wear gloves when changing a patient's dressing. During the procedure, you got blood on your hands. Discuss the implication for failing to comply with CDC regulations in healthcare settings. Answer the following questions:
1. How might your actions (of not wearing gloves) impact the patient's health and safety
2. How might your actions (of not wearing gloves) impact your health and safety?

BOX 34.12 Single-Assistant Preparation for Minor Surgery

1. Sanitize your hands and gather all supplies.
   - *Sterile side (Mayo tray):* Two towel packs, skin prep pack, patient drape pack, instrument pack, miscellaneous pack or packs, three glove packs, face shields, impermeable gowns
   - *Nonsterile side (side counter):* Syringes, suture material, anesthetic solutions, additional sponges, sterile dressings, bandages, transfer forceps, waste basin, sharps and biohazard waste containers, nonsterile gloves, face shields, and impermeable gowns
2. Verify that the informed consent has been signed and is in the patient's health record.
3. Identify the patient and escort him or her into the room.
4. Greet and converse with the patient.
5. Position the patient on the table.
6. Sanitize your hands.
7. Open the first towel pack.
8. Open the skin prep pack.
9. Pour the soap and antiseptic solutions.
10. Expose the site to be prepped.
11. Put on gloves and arrange prep items within the sterile field.
12. Place sterile towels at skin scrub boundaries using sterile technique.
13. Prep the patient's skin.
14. Discard skin prep materials in appropriate sharps/biohazard containers.
15. Discard gloves; sanitize your hands, following the guidelines for a surgical hand scrub (Procedure 34.4) if this procedure is part of the policy of the provider or the facility.
16. Open the table drape pack on the Mayo stand to create a sterile field.
17. Open the instrument pack or packs and transfer the instruments to the sterile field. Add the sterile syringe unit.
18. Add sterile items as requested.
    The provider joins you and converses with the patient.
19. Open the provider's glove pack (the provider now puts on gloves).
20. Open the patient drape pack (the provider now drapes the surgical site).
21. Cleanse and hold up the anesthetic vial for the provider to withdraw anesthetic with the sterile syringe (the provider now administers the anesthetic).
22. Repeat the surgical hand wash; reglove with a new glove pack.
23. Arrange the sterile field instruments and other materials for safety and in sequence; check the condition of each instrument.
24. Open the suture/needle pack per the provider's choice; load the first suture into the needle holder.
25. Place two gauze squares at the site.
26. Assist with the procedure.[a]
    - *For the provider:* Pass the instruments; maintain the field; anticipate his or her needs; and cut sutures.
    - *For the patient:* Retract tissue; sponge blood from the wound; apply the sterile bandage; and care for the specimen.
27. Help the patient sit up and dress if needed and monitor vital signs as instructed.
28. Record and prepare specimens.
29. Sanitize and disinfect the room; clear materials and discard in biohazard waste containers.
30. Document the procedure in the patient's health record.
31. Help the patient prepare to leave the office.
32. Sanitize, disinfect, and sterilize the equipment at the first available time.

[a]By law, the assistant may not clamp tissues, place sutures, or alter body tissues in any way.

After completing this process, remove the contaminated gloves and sanitize your hands (Box 34.12).

Wear gloves while disinfecting the room, including the table, Mayo stand, side and back tables, any other equipment in the room, and the floor. Used instruments must be sanitized, disinfected, and resterilized for future use.

The provider and the medical assistant both document the procedure in the patient's health record.

Postoperative instructions and care. The patient should be given time to rest after the surgery. If a sedative was administered, make sure the patient has recovered sufficiently to avoid injury after the surgery or during the trip home. If the patient was given a topical or local anesthetic, explain to him or her that the anesthesia effect will wear off and that some discomfort may be felt at the operative site. Check with the provider whether pain medication needs to be prescribed. If medication has been prescribed, review the purpose of the medication and the directions for its use with the patient and his or her companion. Make a follow-up appointment before the patient leaves the office.

Postoperative care extends for the total recovery period, not just for the time of immediate care before the patient leaves the office. Most medical assistants are responsible for teaching patients to care for themselves at home after surgery. A postoperative patient may have trouble comprehending or remembering instructions. All instructions

POSTOP INSTRUCTIONS FOR _____

☐ Elevate your arm.
☐ Elevate your leg.
☐ Limit food intake to _____.
☐ Limit activity to _____.
☐ Do not bathe or shower.
☐ Sponge bath only.
☐ Change dressing as instructed.
☐ Call the office for fever, redness, pain, swelling, or bleeding.
☐ Take _____ every 4 hours as needed for pain.
☐ Return to school/work in _____ days.
☐ Call the office tomorrow before _____ p.m.
☐ Your next appointment is on M T W Th F S _____ at _____.

FIG. 34.34 An example of preprinted postoperative patient instructions. (From Proctor D, et al: *Kinn's The Medical Assistant*, ed 13, St Louis, 2017, Elsevier.)

should be given to the patient in writing. They should be simple and easily understood by both the patient and caregivers. These instructions can be preprinted forms for each type of surgery, or a general form with checked boxes for particular postoperative instructions that apply specifically to the individual patient (Fig. 34.34).

Warning signs. Explain to the patient the importance of calling the office if any questions come up or changes occur that cause the person concern. If the patient does not call within the next 24 hours, you should call the patient. Many patients tend to "ride it out" or say they did not want to disturb you. Never allow the postoperative patient to leave the office without the provider's knowledge and approval. Tell the patient to call the office immediately if he or she notes redness around the operative site, bleeding from the wound, fever, swelling, or increasing or severe pain. The wound should be kept clean and dry, and the patient should be taught how to change the dressing, if needed.

Follow-up. If the healing process is a long one or if the wound becomes infected, the patient may return for follow-up care. If the wound requires a new dressing, follow Standard Precautions; wear gloves and other protective barriers as appropriate. If at any time you determine that the wound may be infected, stop and have the provider examine it. Generally, no bandaging material should be reused, including elastic bandage wraps.

Tape applied directly to a patient's skin is not a good dressing immobilizer. If tape is used, always keep it to a minimum. If tape is holding a dressing in place, always remove it by pulling toward the wound. If it is adhering to a hairy area of the body, lift the outer tape edge with one hand and slowly and gently separate the underlying hair and skin from the tape with the thumb of your other hand. Peel the skin from the bandage, not the bandage from the skin. Never rapidly "rip" tape from the body, because this may injure the skin. If the tape is not irritating to the patient, it may be advisable to leave the tape in place until total healing has taken place.

When the wound has healed, the provider may ask the medical assistant to remove the patient's sutures or staples. The patient must return to the facility to have the sutures/staples removed (Procedure 34.10). When removing sutures or staples, it is important for medical assistants to alert the provider to any concerns they notice with the wound healing, and to document the procedure.

Wound Care

A wound can be intentional (e.g., from a surgical incision) or accidental, and it may be open or closed (Fig. 34.35). An open wound has an outward opening; the skin is broken, exposing the underlying tissues. A closed or nonpenetrating wound does not have an outward opening, but the underlying tissues are damaged, as in a hematoma, contusion, or bruise. Closed wounds usually are the result of some type of blunt trauma to the body. An aseptic (i.e., clean) wound is not infected with pathogens. Septic wounds are infected with pathogens.

Open wounds may be classified according to the appearance of their openings. An incised wound has a clean edge and is made with a cutting instrument. An incised wound may be the result of surgery, an accident, or a knife wound. A lacerated wound has torn or mangled tissues and is made by a dull or blunt instrument. A penetrating or puncture wound is caused by a sharp, slender object, such as a needle or an ice pick, and passes through the skin into the underlying tissues. A perforated wound is a penetrating wound that passes through to a body organ or cavity, such as a gunshot wound.

Wound Healing. All wounds go through a healing or repair process that has four phases. **Hemostasis** (hee muh STEY sis) is the first phase. Blood vessels contract to control hemorrhage, and blood platelets form a network that acts as a glue to plug the wound. After a cascade of chemical reactions, fibrin is released into the wound and clotting begins. Fibrin continues to collect red blood cells (RBCs), and the clot dries into a scab.

The second, or inflammatory, phase focuses on destroying bacteria and removing debris. Special white blood cells (WBCs), called *macrophages*, arrive to clear away bacteria and dead tissue. Within 1 to 4 days the fibrin threads contract and pull the edges of the wound together under the scab. During this phase, edema, *erythema* (redness), heat, and pain can occur.

The third phase, *proliferation*, encompasses wound healing and new growth; this lasts 5 to 20 days. During this phase, the tissues repair themselves. New cells form, and the wound continues to contract and seal. If the wound is a clean surgical incision, complete contraction usually takes place and a **cicatrix** (SIK uh triks) forms.

> **VOCABULARY**
> **cicatrix:** Early scar tissue that appears pale, contracted, and firm.
> **hemostasis:** The stoppage of bleeding.

PROCEDURE 34.10 Remove Sutures and/or Surgical Staples

Task:
To remove sutures and/or surgical staples from a healed incision using sterile technique and without injuring the closed wound.

Equipment and Supplies
Sterile suture removal kit containing the following:
- Suture removal scissors
- Gauze
- Thumb dressing forceps
- Steri-Strips or adhesive bandage strips (e.g., Band-Aids)
- Skin antiseptic swabs (e.g., Betadine swabs)
- Surgical staple remover with 4×4-inch gauze
- Biohazardous waste/sharps container
- Sterile gloves
- Patient's record

Procedural Steps
1. Wash hands or use hand sanitizer. Assemble the necessary supplies.
2. Greet the patient. Identify yourself. Verify the patient's identity with full name and date of birth. Explain the procedure to be performed in a manner that is understood by the patient. Answer any questions the patient may have on the procedure. Instruct the person to lie or sit still during the procedure.
   Purpose: To ensure cooperation during the procedure.
3. Position the patient comfortably and support the sutured area.
4. Place dry towels under the site.
5. Check the incision line to make sure the wound edges are approximated and there are no signs of infection, such as inflammation, edema, or drainage.
   Purpose: Sutures or staples should not be removed unless the site is completely healed with the wound edges together; infection at the site will interfere with the healing process; removing sutures or staples before the site is completely healed may result in the wound edge separating.
6. Put on gloves. Using antiseptic swabs, cleanse the wound to remove exudate and destroy microorganisms around the sutures or staples. Clean the site from the inside out, starting at the top of the wound and working your way down. Use a new swab if the step must be repeated. Remove gloves and discard.
   Purpose: Dried exudate on sutures or staples may make removing them without traumatizing the wound more difficult. Cleansing the wound reduces the possibility of wound infection.
7. Open the suture or staple removal pack while maintaining the sterility of the contents.
8. Place sterile gauze next to the wound site.
   Purpose: To receive the removed sutures or staples.
9. Put on sterile gloves.
10. Remove the sutures or staples.

To Remove Sutures
a. Grasp the knot of the suture with the dressing forceps without pulling.
b. Cut the suture at skin level.
c. Lift, do not pull, the suture toward the incision and out with the dressing forceps.
d. Place the suture on the sterile gauze sponge and check that the entire suture strand has been removed.
   Purpose: Suture fragments left in a wound may cause irritation and/or infection and may prolong the healing process.
e. If any bleeding occurs, blot the area with a sterile gauze sponge before continuing.
f. Continue in the same manner until all sutures have been removed.

To Remove Staples
a. Gently place the bottom jaw of the staple remover under the first staple (see the following figure).
b. Tightly squeeze the staple handles together.
c. Carefully tilt the staple remover upward until the staple lifts out of the wound.
d. Place the removed staple on a 4×4-inch gauze square.
e. Continue the process until all staples have been removed.

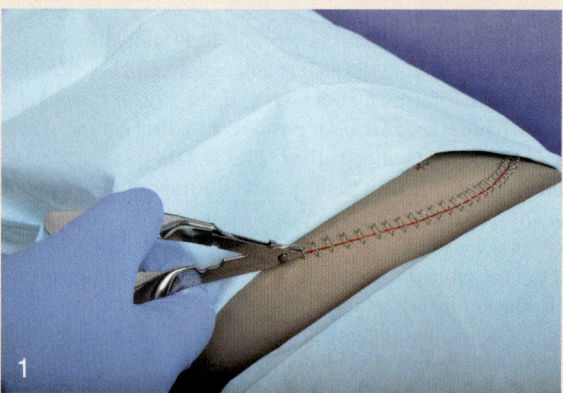

11. Remove the gauze holding the sutures or staples. Dispose of sutures in the biohazardous waste container. Dispose of staples in the biohazardous sharps container.
12. The provider may apply or may have you apply Steri-Strips or an adhesive bandage strip for added support, strength, and protection.
13. Instruct the patient to keep the wound edges clean and dry and not to place excessive strain on the area.
14. Document the procedure, wound condition, number of sutures or staples removed, whether a dressing or bandage was applied, and the instructions on wound care given to the patient.
    Purpose: A procedure that is not documented was not done.

Documentation Example
07/30/20•• 10:20 am: Pt in for suture removal. The edges of the wound are well approximated with 5 intact sutures. There is no sign of infection. The site was cleaned with Betadine and 5 sutures were removed. Pt instructed on home wound care and to notify provider if drainage changes, inflammation increases, or fever occurs_____Callie Casper, CMA (AAMA)

The final phase, the *remodeling* phase, extends from day 21 onward. Clean, shallow wounds may contract in the first two stages; large or mangled wounds require the time and cellular activity of this third phase to build a bridge of new tissue to close the gap of the wound. The cells produce a fibrous protein substance called *collagen* (i.e., connective tissue) that gives the wounded tissues strength and forms scar tissue. Scar tissue is not true skin; it usually is very strong, but it lacks the elasticity of normal skin tissue. There is no blood supply or nerves in scar tissue.

Several factors influence the healing process. People who are young, in good general health, and have adequate nutrition heal more rapidly. Adequate protection and rest of the injured area also enhance the healing process. Destruction or reinjury during the second phase can delay healing and increase scarring. Wounds are susceptible to infection because

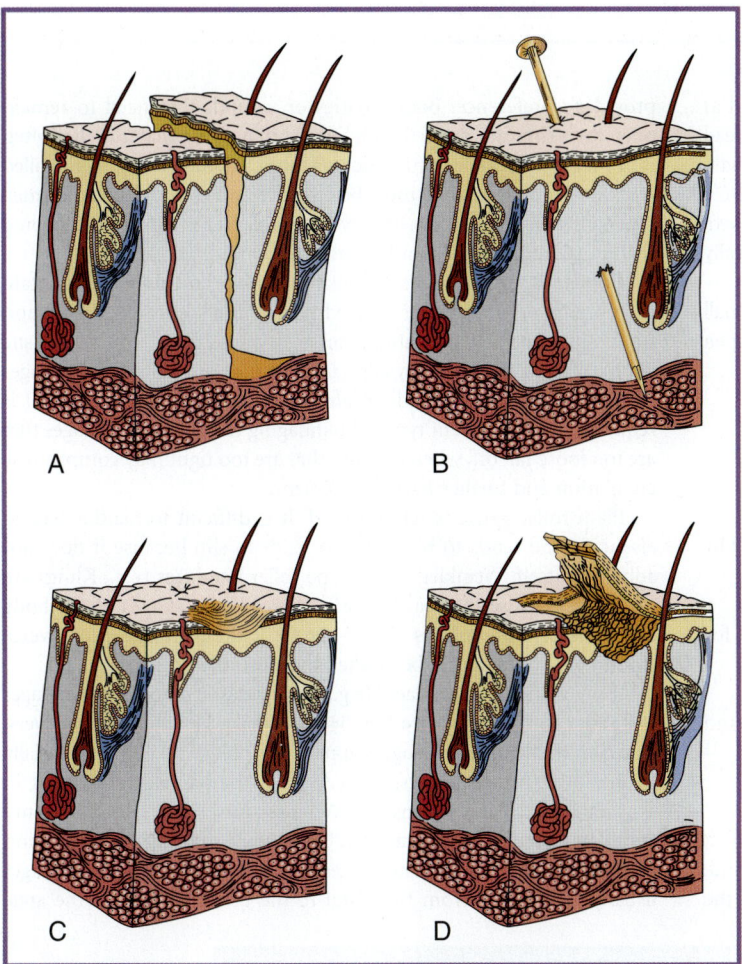
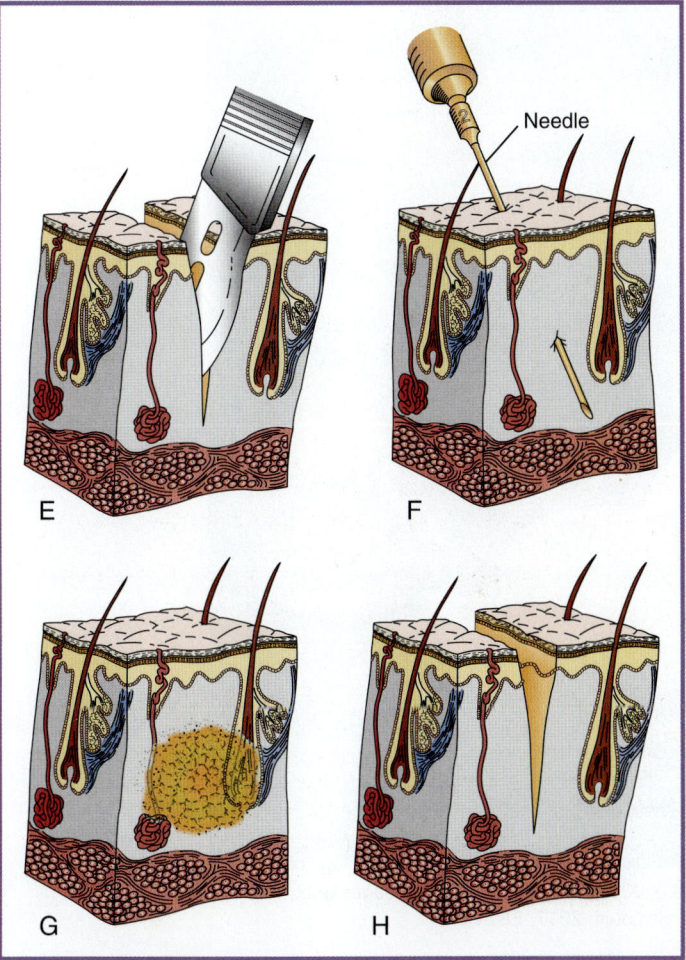

FIG. 34.35 Types of wounds. (A) Laceration – a jagged, irregular breaking or tearing of tissues, usually caused by blunt trauma. (B) Puncture – piercing of the skin by a pointed object, such as a pin, nail, splinter, or bullet. (C) Abrasion – a superficial wound made by scraping of the skin. (D) Avulsion – tissue forcibly torn or separated, caused by accidents. (E) Surgical incision – a neat, clean cut. (F) Hypodermic puncture – an injection under the skin. (G) Contusion – a closed, nonpenetrating wound in which blood from broken vessels accumulates in tissues. (H) Incision – a neat, clean cut from sharp objects, such as glass, knives, or metal. (From Proctor D, et al: *Kinn's The Medical Assistant*, ed 13, St Louis, 2017, Elsevier.)

the normal skin barrier is broken. If debris is present in a wound as the result of the breakdown of various cellular components, this dead (i.e., necrotic) tissue acts as a culture medium for bacterial growth. Suppuration (i.e., pus) contains necrotic tissue, bacteria, dead WBCs, and other products of tissue breakdown. Necrotic tissue must be removed; the removal of debris is called *débridement,* which may occur naturally or may be performed surgically.

Sometimes the provider may prefer no dressing or bandage on small wounds. This is called *open wound healing.* Some advantages to open wound healing are:
- Air can circulate freely around the wound.
- The wound is not irritated or rubbed by a dressing.
- The wound stays dry, which inhibits bacterial growth, reducing the chance of infection.
- Sutures stay dry and hold together better.
- Any preexisting infection remains localized and is not spread by the dressing or bandage.

Dressings. A dressing is a sterile covering placed over a wound for the purposes of:
- Protecting the wound from injury and contamination
- Maintaining constant pressure to minimize bleeding and swelling
- Holding the wound edges together
- Absorbing drainage and secretions

A dressing usually consists of a strip of lubricated mesh gauze, a nonstick Telfa pad, or a clear dressing placed over a sutured wound. Gauze may be placed over nonadhering material, depending on the provider's preference. Body cavities or wounds that need to remain open for a time are dressed with long, thin packing material that often is impregnated with an antiseptic or a lubricant; this sometimes is called *packing.* A good dressing must be effective and comfortable and must remain in place. If the dressing covers a hairless area, it may be anchored with tape, but no tape should touch the wound.

Bandages. Bandages hold dressings in place and also help maintain even pressure, support the affected part, and help protect the wound from injury and contamination. Bandages can be gauze, cloth, or elastic cloth rolls and are bound by clips, tape, or ties. Dressings and bandages frequently appear easy and simple to apply; however, special skill is required to use different types of bandaging techniques. Bandages that are too loose fall off, whereas those that are too tight may compromise circulation and further harm the patient.

Plain roller gauze is seldom used. It is difficult to handle, has no elasticity, and tends to bind. It also tends to slip because it does not adhere to itself. Wrinkled crepe–type roller bandages (e.g., Kling) are preferred because they easily conform to various shapes of the body and adhere to themselves (Fig. 34.36A). If the bandage is to cover a wound, it should always be applied over a sterile dressing.

Plain elastic cloth bandages (e.g., Ace) or elastic roller cloth bandages with adhesive backing (see Fig. 34.36B) make flexible, secure covers. When an elastic roller bandage is applied as a pressure bandage, especially to the lower limbs, it is essential to keep the bandage consistent in spacing and tension to ensure even pressure. Even, gentle pressure stimulates circulation and healing. Uneven pressure causes constriction points that can create pressure sores, ulcers, or edema. Roller bandages usually are applied from the distal to the proximal part of the area,

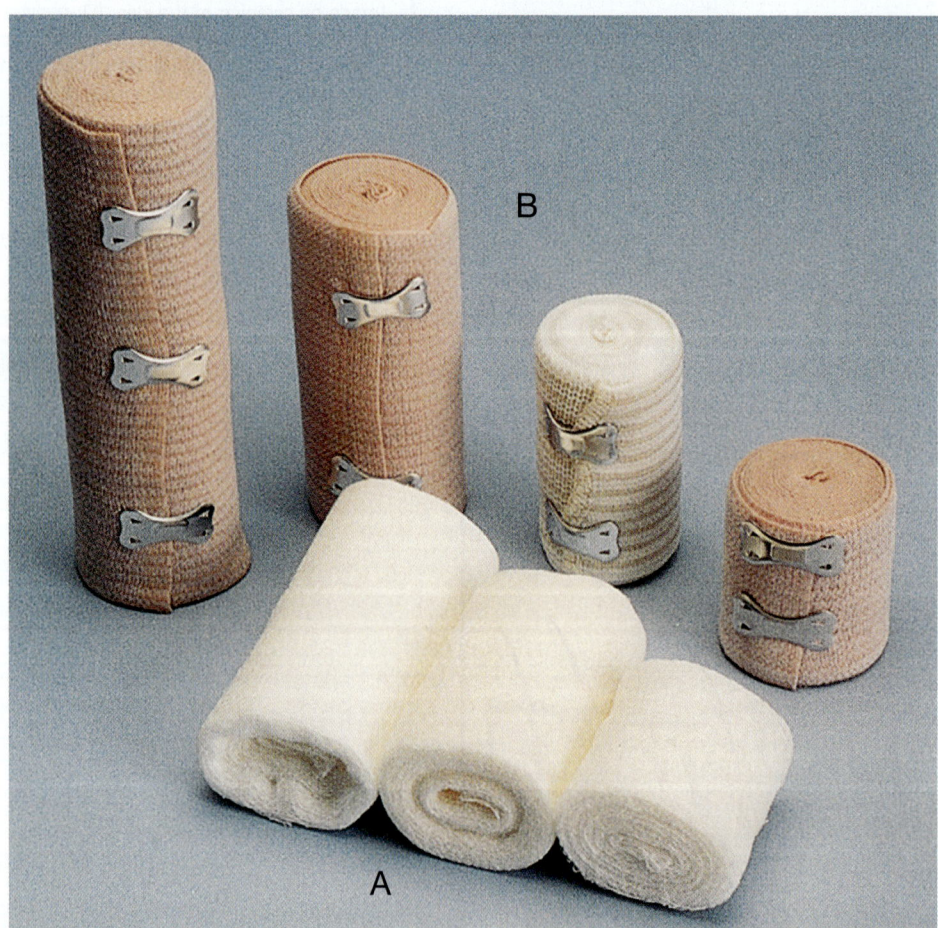

FIG. 34.36 (A) Wrinkled crepe–type roller bandages (e.g., Kling). (B) Elastic roller bandages (e.g., Ace). (From Proctor D, et al: *Kinn's The Medical Assistant,* ed 13, St Louis, 2017, Elsevier.)

BOX 34.13   Remember: CSMT When Bandaging

When applying bandages, you should assess the following:
- **C**olor: Should be the same as the opposite extremity; report any bluish or white fingers or toes
- **S**ensation: Should be able to feel fingers/toes; report any numbness
- **M**ovement: Should be able to move fingers/toes
- **T**emperature: Should be the same as the opposite extremity; report any cool/cold fingers/toes

because they are more even and snug if they are wrapped from a smaller to a larger circumference. Elevate the limb while you are bandaging and work with the roller facing upward, close to the patient's skin. Elastic bandages are excellent for bandaging the hand and wrist and the foot and ankle (Box 34.13).

Seamless tubular gauze bandage, with or without elastic, is a superior material for covering round, narrow surfaces such as fingers or toes. It can be used as a dressing if the gauze material is sterile; it can also be used as a bandage. A tubular gauze bandage is applied with a cage-like applicator (Fig. 34.37). Work with the open circle of the applicator toward the patient. Hold the applicator in the dominant hand and control the tension flow with your fingers as the applicator is gradually rotated and the material slides off. Tubular dressing may be applied with or without slight pressure. Beyond the tip of the bandaged part, give the applicator a full half-turn, place the applicator again over the part, and repeat the process, being careful not to create a tourniquet effect when you reverse the applicator. When the desired thickness of the bandage is reached, cut the gauze and anchor the final gauze application with tape or by tying at the wrist.

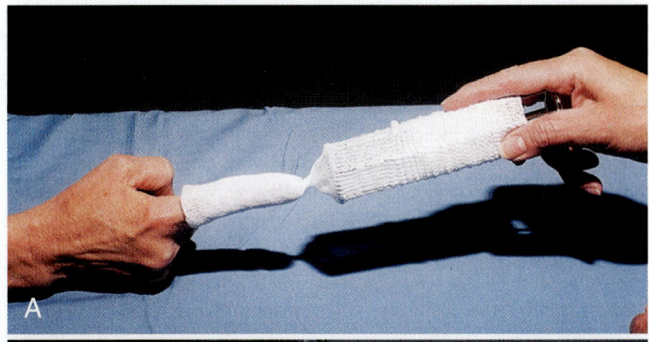
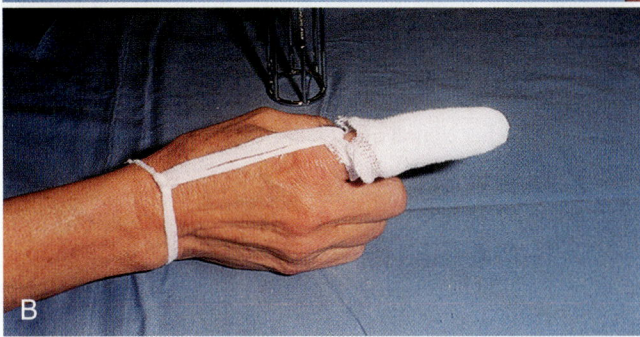

FIG. 34.37 (A) Tube gauze is applied with even tension and is twisted at the fingertip before the next layer is applied. (B) Tube gauze bandage has been applied and secured by tying at the wrist. (From Proctor D, et al: *Kinn's The Medical Assistant*, ed 13, St Louis, 2017, Elsevier.)

EXCEPTIONAL CUSTOMER SERVICE

A medical assistant can help the patient in many ways. The best time to instruct your patient in aseptic techniques to be used at home is while you are performing an aseptic procedure. For example:
- While sanitizing your hands before a procedure or examination, explain to the patient that hands should be washed before meals; after sneezing, coughing, or nose blowing; after using the bathroom; before and after changing a dressing or bandage; and after changing an infant's diaper.
- Instruct the patient about the differences between sterile and clean dressings and bandages. Show the person step by step how to change a dressing properly and then how to dispose of the contaminated items.

A medical assistant's duty may include calling the patient the day before surgery to confirm the scheduled surgical procedure and appointment time. Explaining the procedure and what to expect during and after surgery prepares the patient and helps calm the person's fears or concerns. Lying still during surgery is important, and eating a light meal the night before should be encouraged. Bathing before coming to the office helps reduce the number of bacteria on the skin, and comfortable, loose clothing should be worn. Sometimes in the course of general conversation, the medical assistant can pick up hints of concerns the patient may have and can direct the conversation into a discussion of these concerns.

Patients should be informed that they may need someone to accompany them home. A bandage is applied after surgery, and it must be kept clean and dry. The patient may have some pain, and the provider probably will prescribe some type of analgesic. After the procedure is complete, make sure the patient makes an appointment for a return visit and examination. Patients should also be encouraged to call the office immediately if they suspect an infection or have a sudden increase in pain at the surgical site.

CLOSING COMMENTS

Assisting with minor surgery can be challenging and rewarding. There are many things to remember, but the key piece is to always maintain sterile technique. Whether it is in handling instruments, setting up trays, or assisting the provider, sterile technique must be followed to protect our patients.

CHAPTER REVIEW

In this chapter we started out by discussing what is needed to set up for minor surgery. A medical assistant must know the basic instruments that are used for the various procedures that are performed in an ambulatory care facility. You must also know how to handle the instruments after they have been used.

Sanitizing instruments involves washing them with a low-sudsing detergent to remove organic matter and to reduce the number of microorganisms. This is the first step in the sterilization process. If the instruments are not sanitized well, sterilization may not occur.

After the instruments have been sanitized, they must be prepared for the autoclave. They should be wrapped with the appropriate material and then loaded properly into the autoclave. You must be familiar with how the autoclave in your healthcare facility works. It is important to check the sterilization indicators when removing packs from the autoclave. It is also important to perform all quality assurance measures to ensure that the autoclave is functioning properly.

Various types of surgical procedures and the equipment needed for each were discussed. The more you work with your provider, the more comfortable you will be with each of the procedures. When assisting the provider, you must maintain sterile technique. Nonsterile items should never pass over the sterile field. If this does happen, you should admit it so that things can be made sterile again.

The last section of this chapter discussed the phases of wound healing. It is important for medical assistants and their patients to understand what is happening with the wound and the care that must be taken during each phase.

Dressings and bandages are often applied after a minor office procedure. Dressings are considered sterile and are applied directly to the wound. Bandages can be used to hold dressings in place. When applying bandages, it is important to start at the proximal point and work towards the distal point. After applying the bandage, the medical assistant should assess using CSMT.

SCENARIO WRAP-UP

Callie is finding her clinical medical assisting position at the Walden-Martin Family Medicine Clinic rewarding, exciting, and challenging. She enjoys coming to work every day and has learned all aspects of her position much more quickly than most of her peers. Callie frequently reads the latest information on new developments in minor surgery practice. Her concern for her patients' well-being makes her stand out, and the providers constantly get positive comments on her level of professionalism.

Callie has made a few errors in sterile technique since starting the clinical assistant position, but she has learned from each situation and has never covered up a mistake. Whenever she realized that she did not follow procedure, she has discussed the issue with her supervisor and with Dr. Perez. In this way, errors can be corrected, if possible, and she most likely will not make the same or similar mistakes again.

Callie is a team player who consistently tries to anticipate the needs of the provider and patient both before and during surgery. Her cooperative, supportive manner is appreciated by everyone on the clinical staff.

35

Patient Coaching With Health Promotion

LEARNING OBJECTIVES

1. Describe the medical assistant's role as a coach.
2. Discuss the stages of grief, as well as how the health belief model helps to explain what factors influence a person's health beliefs and practices.
3. Describe the three domains of learning.
4. Explain how a medical assistant can adapt coaching to the patient.
5. Describe the teaching-learning process.
6. Discuss how a medical assistant can coach on disease prevention.
7. Do the following related to coaching on health maintenance and wellness:
   - Describe how a medical assistant can coach on health maintenance and wellness.
   - Explain the different types of self-exams and screenings.
   - Coach patients on how to perform a breast self-exam and a testicular self-exam.
   - Perform a monofilament foot exam.
8. Do the following related to coaching on diagnostic procedures and treatment plans:
   - Describe how a medical assistant can coach on diagnostic procedures and treatment plans.
   - Apply a cold pack.
   - Coach a patient to use axillary crutches, a walker, and a cane.
   - Describe teaching required for casts, splints, cold and hot therapy, and assistive devices.
9. Describe care coordination and patient navigation, develop a list of community resources, and facilitate referrals.

CHAPTER OUTLINE

1. Opening Scenario, 800
2. You Will Learn, 800
3. Introduction, 800
4. Coaching, 800
5. Making Changes for Health, 801
   a. Stages of Grief, 801
   b. Health Belief Model, 801
6. Basics of Teaching and Learning, 802
   a. Domains of Learning, 802
      i. *Cognitive Domain, 802*
      ii. *Psychomotor Domain, 802*
      iii. *Affective Domain, 802*
   b. Adapting Coaching to the Patient, 802
      i. *Developmental Level, 802*
      ii. *Cultural Diversity, 803*
      iii. *Communication Barriers, 806*
   c. Teaching-Learning Process, 806
7. **Coaching on Disease Prevention, 806**
8. **Coaching on Health Maintenance and Wellness, 809**
   a. Self-Exams, 809
      i. *Breast Self-Exam, 809*
      ii. *Testicular Self-Exam, 810*
      iii. *Skin Self-Exam, 810*
      iv. *Oral Cancer Self-Exam, 812*
   b. Regular Screenings, 812
   c. One-Time Screenings, 814
   d. Additional Screenings, 815
9. **Coaching on Diagnostic Tests, 817**
10. **Coaching on Treatment Plans, 817**
    a. Medication Administration at Home, 818
    b. Casts and Splints, 818
    c. Cold and Hot Therapy, 820
       i. *Cold Therapy, 820*
       ii. *Heat Therapy, 820*
    d. Ultrasound Therapy, 821
    e. RICE Therapy, 822
    f. Exercise Therapy, 823
       i. *Electrical Muscle Stimulation, 823*
    g. Complementary Therapies, 823
       i. *Massage Therapy, 823*
       ii. *Chiropractic Care, 823*
       iii. *Acupressure and Acupuncture, 823*
    h. Assistive Devices, 823
       i. *Crutches, 824*
       ii. *Walkers, 825*
       iii. *Canes, 828*
       iv. *Wheelchairs, 828*
11. **Care Coordination, 828**
12. **Closing Comments, 831**
13. **Chapter Review, 831**
14. **Scenario Wrap-Up, 832**

OPENING SCENARIO

Suzanne Peterson, a certified medical assistant (CMA) through the American Association of Medical Assistants (AAMA), has worked for Walden-Martin Family Medical (WMFM) Clinic for 3 years. She had prior experience at a busy urgent care clinic. She enjoys working in a family practice environment. Her favorite part of her job is working with patients. She likes coaching patients on health practices and on the treatment plans. She feels that it is very important for patients to understand how to self-manage their conditions and to know when to contact their providers.

Over the years, Suzanne has seen the role of the medical assistant expand. She has learned the importance of screening patients during the initial interview. The information that she enters into the electronic health record is then used to collect data on how well the clinic provides patient care. She has also learned the importance of patient care coordinators. She hopes WMFM Clinic implements a care coordinator program soon.

YOU WILL LEARN

1. To apply the basics of teaching and learning, including the domains of learning and how to adapt coaching to patients.
2. To perform common coaching as required for disease prevention, including cough hygiene, nicotine cessation, and vaccinations.
3. To perform coaching as required for health maintenance, including self-exams and screenings.
4. To perform coaching as required for common diagnostic tests.
5. To perform coaching as required for treatment plans, including medication administration and the use of casts, splints, cold and hot therapies, assistive devices, and other therapies.
6. To coordinate care, navigate patients, and make community resource referrals.

INTRODUCTION

Healthcare is changing, and the role of the medical assistant is changing too. Some of the current challenges in healthcare include the following:
- Pressure to reduce cost
- Shorter primary care provider visits, yet an increased need for data collection to incorporate patient interviews and outcome measurements (e.g., test results)
- Patients leaving the facility not understanding what they were told
- An unwillingness on the part of patients to adhere to treatment plans (e.g., not taking medication or not taking it correctly, not making lifestyle changes that would improve their health)

Many experts have researched ways to decrease these challenges. Several studies have examined patient medication **adherence** (ad HEER uh ns) or **compliance** (kuhm PLIE uhns). *Medication adherence* means patients are taking the right dose at the right times as prescribed by the provider. Research has shown that medication adherence with chronic diseases is low. This leads to the progression of the disease and more medical visits for the patient. Ultimately, nonadherence to medication is increasing the cost of healthcare.

Why is it that patients do not take their medication correctly? This question has been a focus of many studies. Common reasons include the following:
- Forgetfulness
- Confusion on how to take it
- Side effects, cost of the medication
- Feeling it is not helping

Research has shown that many patients are confused after seeing their providers. Patients do not always understand the treatment plan designed to manage their conditions. Confusion about medication and home care is prevalent. Many patients are not able to manage their disease adequately between provider visits; thus their condition worsens. To solve this problem, ambulatory care facilitates are moving toward coaching and care coordination. This chapter focuses on the medical assistant's role in coaching and care coordination.

> **VOCABULARY**
> **adherence:** The act of sticking to something.
> **cessation**: A bringing to an end.
> **compliance**: The act of following through on a request or demand. Patient compliance sounds negative, thus patient adherence is now being used.

COACHING

Coaching provides patients with skills, knowledge, support, and confidence to manage their disease between provider visits. One study found that coaching by medical assistants increased the patients' compliance to medication regimens and lifestyle changes. Coaching is extremely valuable for patients. The medical assistant can coach patients in many areas:

- *Disease prevention:* Provide patients with information on preventing the disease or the spread of disease. Medical assistants can provide information on hygiene practices, recommended vaccines, and nicotine **cessation** (se SAY shuhn).
- *Health maintenance:* Provide patients with information on routine screenings and show patients how to do self-exams (e.g., foot, breast, and oral self-exams).
- *Diagnostic tests*: Instruct patients prior to diagnostic tests. This can include special preparation (e.g., fasting and bowel cleansing preparations).
- *Treatment plans*: Instruct patients on home cares and follow-ups as ordered by the provider. Research has shown that coaching can help patients understand information from the visit. It can ensure patients understand how they need to proceed and addresses any concerns before patients leave the facility. Coaching educates patients on self-management of diseases, thus increasing compliance to the treatment plans.
- *Specific needs:* Patients have unique concerns. These can include personal, family, social, financial, and culture-related issues. By listening and asking questions, the medical assistant can help address their specific needs. By closely working with the patient, the medical assistant can provide emotional support and create a bond with the patient. This bond helps the patient feel comfortable. With encouragement, the patient may be more willing to call the medical assistant with questions and concerns between visits.
- *Community resources*: By listening to patients and by asking questions, the medical assistant can identify patients' unique needs. Patients have many needs that impact their health. For instance, if a patient has a limited income, does the patient purchase the prescribed medication, or food? Community resources exist to address many needs, including low-cost medications, food banks, transportation, medical supplies, assisted living, and so on.

This chapter provides information on specific aspects of patient education required for these coaching areas. But first, let's examine health beliefs and practices and how to adapt education to patients' needs.

MAKING CHANGES FOR HEALTH

Often, healthcare professionals see patients who do not comply with the treatment plan. They may not take the prescribed medication, or maybe they do not make the recommended lifestyle changes. If the diagnosis is life threatening or life changing, grief and loss can occur. Other times, patients may not perceive the change as necessary. The following sections examine theories that may explain why patients do not comply to the treatment plan.

Stages of Grief

Elizabeth Kübler-Ross studied people's reactions to dying. She found that people experienced similar stages. Over the years, these stages have been applied to grief and loss. When a patient and the family get a life-threatening or life-changing diagnosis, they can feel grief and loss. People go through the stages of grief in their own way and at their own pace (Table 35.1). This process can take weeks to months. Patients may not be open to making the recommended changes. Healthcare professionals may view this as the patient not wanting to comply with the treatment plan. Sometimes a patient has to accept a diagnosis before compliance occurs. It is important for the medical assistant to adapt interactions to help with the stages of grief.

> **CRITICAL THINKING 35.1**
>
> Suzanne has seen many patients dealing with grief. Why might a patient who is grieving not adhere to a treatment plan?

Health Belief Model

The health belief model helps explain what factors influence a person's health belief and practices. The first part of this model deals with a person's perception of his or her chance of developing a disease. Some examples include the following:

- Jess is in her 20s and has lost her mother, sister, and grandmother to breast cancer. She feels her chance of developing breast cancer is significant.
- Sam has an older brother with heart disease that is being managed by medication, diet, and exercise. Sam blames the disease on his brother's stressful job. Sam does not have a stressful job, so he feels he will not get heart disease. Even though Sam receives education on a heart-healthy lifestyle, he ignores the information.

The second part of this model deals with a person's perception of the severity of the disease. A person's perception is influenced by personal, social, and environmental factors (Box 35.1). In the prior example, Jess has lost three family members to breast cancer. She perceives breast cancer as being a severe disease. Sam, on the other hand, may not perceive the severity of heart disease, because his brother's heart disease is being managed.

The third part of the model focuses on whether the person will take preventive action. A person weighs the benefits and barriers of taking the preventive actions. For example, Jess may decide to have a double mastectomy as a preventive strategy. For many it may seem severe, but for Jess, she is willing to take such a preventive action. Sam, on the other hand, may not see the benefit of following a heart-healthy lifestyle. He may feel that he has to "give up" his current lifestyle and make changes.

Because a medical assistant coaches patients on preventive actions, it is important to remember the model. Start with identifying if the person perceives he or she is at risk for a disease. Exploring the patient's beliefs and educating the patient on the facts while getting rid of the myths can be helpful. Discussing the severity of the disease or what the disease can lead to is the next important step. Finally, helping to decrease the barriers and helping the person see the benefits of the preventive action is important.

> **CRITICAL THINKING 35.2**
>
> Suzanne has had patients state they do not want to give up their lifestyle and follow the provider's recommendations for better health. How might a medical assistant address this issue with a patient?

TABLE 35.1 Stages of Grief and Dying

Stage	Description	Adaptive Interactions
Denial	Refuses to accept the fact (i.e., diagnosis or prognosis). May refuse to discuss the diagnosis. May not remember the health coaching. Denial is a defense mechanism that allows the person to ignore what is happening.	Provide handouts that explain the disease and treatment. Encourage family member(s) support with the treatment. Provide online and community resources (i.e., support groups).
Anger	Anger can be directed at self or others. Anger can surface at unrelated times and be directed toward unrelated issues.	Use therapeutic communication techniques (e.g., reflection) to acknowledge the patient's feelings about the issue. Recognize the real cause of the anger.
Bargaining	Attempts to bargain with the higher power the person believes in (i.e., God). Sometimes the patient will bargain with the provider to make lifestyle changes at a later time.	Work with the healthcare team regarding the bargaining requests. Help provide opportunities where the patient can make decisions.
Depression	People feel sadness, fear, and uncertainty. They may grieve the loss of their health or independence, or they may dread the change that is occurring.	Encourage the use of community and healthcare resources to help ease the change process for the patient and family members.
Acceptance	Has come to terms with situation.	Provide coaching on aspects of the disease and self-care management.

> **BOX 35.1 Influencing Factors**
>
> - Personal factors (e.g., age, gender, race, employment)
> - Social factors (e.g., peers, personality, family)
> - Perceived threats of the disease
> - Cues to action (e.g., mass media campaigns, social media, advice from family, friends, and healthcare providers and professionals)

BASICS OF TEACHING AND LEARNING

Domains of Learning

Learning is the process of gaining new knowledge or skills through instruction, experience, or study. We learn new information in three different ways or *domains*: cognitive, psychomotor, and affective. These domains are discussed in the coming sections.

Cognitive Domain. The *cognitive domain* of learning involves mental processes of recall, application, and evaluation. We learn new information by listening to what is said and by reading written words. Many experts believe we have three ways to store memories:

- *Sensory stage*: For a memory to be created, we must pick up something from our senses (e.g., touch, hearing, sight). Our senses are constantly picking up perceptions. Many will be forgotten in a split second. We will pay attention to just a few, and they will move to the short-term memory. The deciding factor between what is forgotten and what moves into the short-term memory is based on its importance to us.
- *Short-term memory*: This is our temporary working memory. If you do nothing with the memory, it will fade within 30 seconds. The short-term memory can only handle about seven units of information at once. By chunking information into meaningful units or attaching it to something we already know, we can increase the amount in our short-term memory.
- *Long-term memory*: The more we use short-term memories, the quicker they enter our long-term memory. We can add endless memories to our long-term memory, but without use (recall) those memories can fade.

Our goal for patient education is to put the information into patients' long-term memory. Not everything we tell the patient will be picked up and remembered. We hope the important information will be. The following tips can be used to help patients remember critical information:

- *Present the information at an appropriate level for the patient.* Most studies show that patient education literature should be at a sixth-grade reading level. According to medlineplus.gov, patient educational materials should be between a seventh- and eighth-grade reading level. If the patient's primary language is not English, then a lower reading level is needed.
- *Build on the patient's prior knowledge about the topic.* Start by finding out what the patient knows about the topic. Clarify any inaccurate information. Then provide new information that builds on the existing knowledge.
- *Present information in small chunks, in a clear well-organized manner.* Do not overwhelm the patient; keep to the facts and keep it simple. For complex topics, meeting with the patient over several days may help the patient to retain the information.
- *Provide the information in two different ways* (e.g., verbally discuss it and provide a written handout) (Fig. 35.1).
- *Tell the patient "this is important to remember" and repeat important information several times during the session.* Be aware that if everything is "important to remember" nothing will be remembered. Do not over use this strategy.
- *Have the patient teach back the information you provided.* This allows you to check what the patient recalls and if it is accurate. Teaching back also helps the patient remember the information even more.

Table 35.2 provides strategies to use for the cognitive domain. The *barriers* or reasons why learning does not occur effectively are also listed. These barriers are important for the medical assistant to limit if possible.

Psychomotor Domain. The *psychomotor domain* is the "doing" domain. We learn new skills and procedures by watching demonstrations and assisting with something. Many people would prefer to attempt a skill versus reading about it or discussing it. They learn best through the psychomotor domain. Table 35.2 provides some barriers to the psychomotor domain.

Some tips to help patients remember critical information include the following:

- Provide written step-by-step directions for the patient to follow and then take home.
- Give timely feedback on the person's performance.
- Have the patient "teach back" the skill to check for accuracy.
- Repeated practice doing the skill helps with recall and retention of the steps.
- Make sure to use the equipment and supplies the patient will be using at home.

Affective Domain. The *affective domain* is the "feeling" domain. It includes our feelings, emotions, values, and attitudes. Our emotions and values are very important. They impact our motivation, confidence, and priorities. When our personal values conflict with the new information presented, a barrier to learning can occur. Pain is another example of an affective barrier. If you are instructing a patient on wound care and he is in pain, he may not remember what you said. Additional barriers to the affective domain are listed in Table 35.2.

Make sure that you address (as much as you can) any affective domain barriers prior to educating a patient. If another family member accompanied the patient, it can be helpful to instruct both the patient and the family member (Fig. 35.4). Written home instructions should also be given.

Adapting Coaching to the Patient

When coaching patients, it is important to recognize that patients are individuals. One way of presenting new information to a patient may not work for another patient. It is important for the medical assistant to consider the barriers to learning and possible ways to help the patient overcome those barriers. It is also important for the medical assistant to remember the patient's developmental level and possible cultural diversity issues that may impact learning.

Developmental Level. As we grow and develop, our thought processes and behaviors change. We learn differently. We can understand more complex concepts than when we were younger. It is important for the medical assistant to consider the person's developmental level when

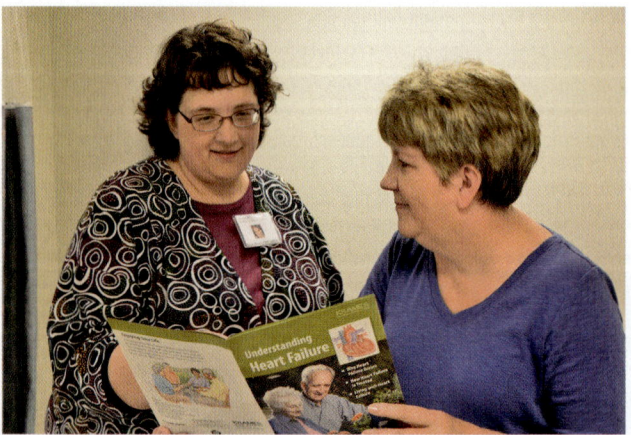

FIG. 35.1 Provide patients with handouts to take home.

CHAPTER 35 Patient Coaching With Health Promotion

TABLE 35.2 Strategies to Use and Barriers for the Three Domains of Learning

Domains	Involves	Teaching Strategies to Use	Barriers to Learning	Strategies to Adapt to Barriers
Cognitive	Learning new concepts and information	Discussion, written information, DVDs, computer instruction	Memory or cognition issues; language barriers	Keep it simple. Provide easy-to-read handouts. Use an interpreter and provide handouts in the patient's primary language if possible.
Psychomotor	Learning new skill or procedure	Demonstration and return demonstration (Fig. 35.2)	Tremors and paralysis; sensory limitations (e.g., visual impairment, hearing impairment)	Use adaptive equipment like a magnifying glass and a magnifier for syringes (Fig. 35.3).
Affective	A change in attitude or emotions that will influence the person's behavior	Discussion, role-play, and simulations	Anxiety, denial, pain, fatigue, or stress, cultural customs, previous experience, and poor coping skills	Provide analgesics as ordered by the provider, help to minimize barriers, provide home instructions, and include additional family member(s) if possible.

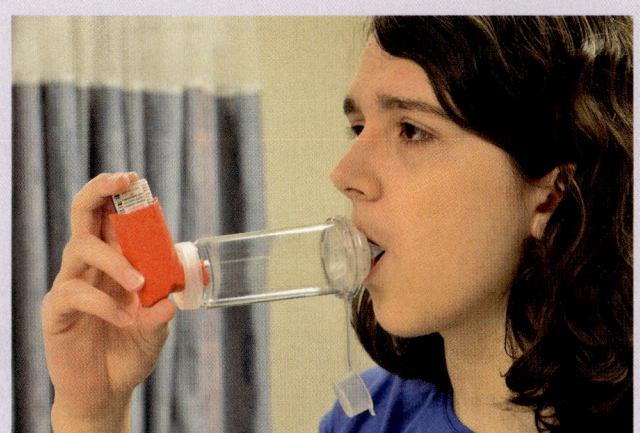

FIG. 35.2 Have patients do a return demonstration.

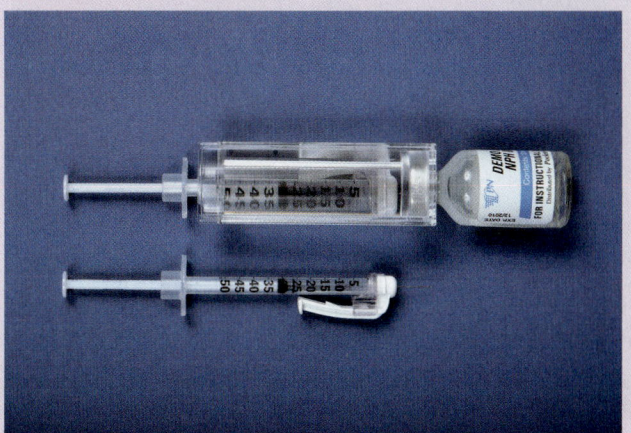

FIG. 35.3 Syringe magnifiers are used by people with visual impairments. The magnifiers increase the size of the calibration markings on the syringes.

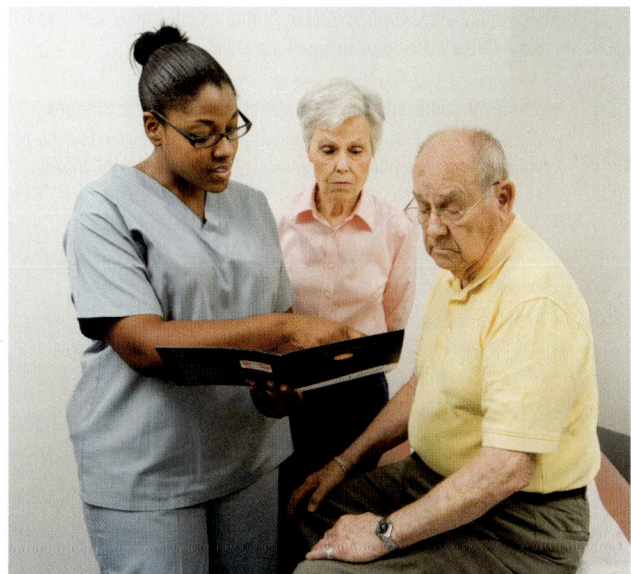

FIG. 35.4 Teaching the family member along with the patient can provide the patient with more support. (From Proctor D, et al: *Kinn's The Medical Assistant*, ed 13, St. Louis, 2017, Elsevier.)

coaching. For instance, young children are concrete thinkers. What you say is what they believe you will do. "I am going to take your blood pressure." Two-year-old children would have no idea what you are going to do. If you say, I am going to give your arm a hug, then they may have a better understanding of what you are going to do. Coaching techniques you use for teens will be different from those you use with older adults (Fig. 35.5). Also, referencing materials as you talk can be helpful to the patient.

Erikson's psychosocial developmental stages can be useful when considering the developmental level of patients. Understanding the goal of each stage can help a medical assistant to coach patients in that age group. Table 35.3 provides coaching tips based on the developmental stages.

> **CRITICAL THINKING 35.3**
>
> In the family practice environment, Suzanne sees patients of all ages. Explain why the methods she uses with 2-year-old children should differ from those she uses when working with teens. What strategies could she use when coaching both of these populations?

Cultural Diversity. *Culture* is the set of behaviors, ideas, and customs shared by a specific group of people, which distinguishes the members from other people. Some characteristics of a culture group may include its language, religious beliefs, geographic origin, ethnicity, history, sexual orientation, and socioeconomic class. Culture can be learned from prior generations and passed on to future generations. It is dynamic and evolving. Our culture frames and shapes how we feel about our health and the world around us. Box 35.2 list factors that are impacted by a person's culture and that healthcare professionals should consider.

In the United States, disease conditions are seen as more of a scientific situation. Science plays a major role in medicine. Many other cultures take more of a *holistic* (hoe LIS tik) approach. A holistic view focuses on the interrelationship among the physical, mental, social, and spiritual aspects of the person's life. A holistic approach is broader than a scientific approach to health and illness.

Many cultures have similar practices:
- *Coining* and *spooning*: rubbing a silver coin or spoon vigorously on the skin. These practices leave red marks on the skin. Do not confuse the marks with signs of abuse.

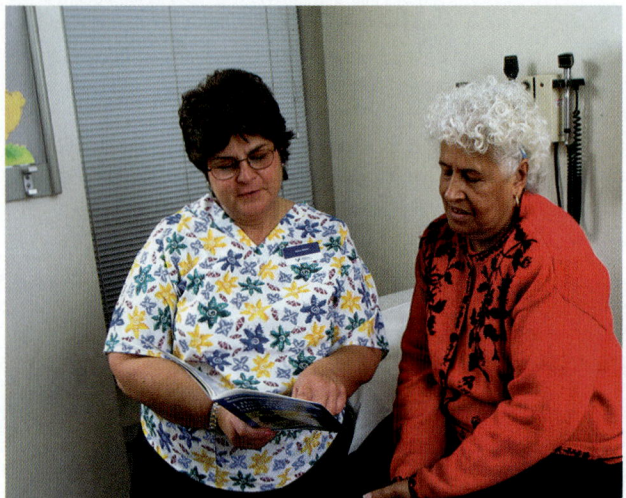

FIG. 35.5 When coaching a patient, make sure to be at the patient's level. Referencing materials as you talk can be helpful to the patient. (From Proctor D, et al: *Kinn's The Medical Assistant*, ed 13, St. Louis, 2017, Elsevier.)

> **BOX 35.2 Factors Impacted by a Person's Culture**
>
> - Role of the family and community (Who makes the healthcare decisions? Who pays for the healthcare? Who needs to be present during healthcare discussions?)
> - Religion (What are the beliefs about illness? Will the person's religious beliefs impact adherence to the treatment?)
> - Views on health, wellness, death, and dying
> - Views on complementary therapies (e.g., chiropractic care, massage) *and alternative therapies* (other practices used in place of conventional medicine)
> - Views on gender roles and relationships
> - Beliefs related to food, diet, illness and health
> - Beliefs regarding sexuality, fertility, and childbirth

TABLE 35.3 Erikson's Psychosocial Development Stages With Coaching Tips

Erikson's Psychosocial Development Stages	Goals of Stage	Coaching Tips
Trust versus mistrust (age range: 0–1.5 years [infancy])	Must develop trust, with the ability to mistrust should the need arise.	Use a calm soothing voice, hold child securely. Involve the parent(s) as much as possible. Keep routines consistent as much as possible (if it is time for the infant to eat, allow the child to eat unless eating/drinking is restricted for a medical reason).
Autonomy versus shame and doubt (age range: 1.5–3 years [toddler])	Must explore and manipulate things in their "world" to develop autonomy and self-esteem.	Use simple, familiar words. Allow child to handle equipment and make choices. Use play to teach the child.
Initiative versus guilt (age range: 3–6 years [preschool])	Encourage to try new activities. Must assume responsibilities and learn new skills. Will make child feel purposeful and increase self-esteem.	Use familiar words and simple explanations and demonstrations. Allow the child to handle equipment and make choices. Explain a procedure as the child would sense it (e.g., how it feels, looks).
Industry versus inferiority (age range: 6–12 years [school age])	Must seek to finish tasks. Recognition for accomplishments is important.	Use engaging simple tools to communicate information (DVDs, gaming software, pamphlets). Encourage discussion, questions, and making choices. Use concrete terms (with pictures and diagrams) when explaining procedures.
Identity versus role confusion (age range: 12–18 years [adolescence])	To know whom you are as a person and how you fit into the world around you. Creates a meaningful self-image.	Provide privacy and independence. Encourage responsible decision making. Encourage discussion and questions. Address how a procedure might affect the adolescent's appearance. Promote honest discussion about lifestyle issues.
Intimacy versus isolation (age range: 18–25 years [young adult])	Can vary. Develops friendships; takes on commitments.	Identify motivating factors. Find out what they know about the topic; correct any inaccuracies. Build on prior information. Listen to their concerns and provide resources as needed.
Generativity versus stagnation (age range: about 25–60 years [middle adulthood])	Achieve a balance between the concern for the next generation (having a family) and being self-absorbed.	
Ego integrity versus despair (age range: 60 and older [late adulthood])	Reflect on one's life and come to terms with it instead of regretting the past.	Communicate with dignity and respect. Use simpler language. Speak clearly. Allow time to respond. Find out what they know about the topic; correct any inaccuracies. Build on prior information. Listen to their concerns and provide resources as needed.

- *Cupping*: applying suction to the skin, which can leave marks. Do not confuse these marks as signs of abuse.
- *Acupressure*: applying firm pressure on specific points on the body.
- *Acupuncture*: inserting fine needles into *acupuncture points* (specific sites on the body).

It is important to remember that not every member of the same culture has the same health beliefs. Differences are typically seen between the generations (Fig. 35.6). Box 35.3 provides some general health differences for different cultures. The healthcare professional should not assume patients have specific health beliefs. Being aware of possible cultural beliefs and practices of a group is important. It can help the medical assistant ask related questions to identify a patient's beliefs and practices.

CRITICAL THINKING 35.4

In the family practice environment, Suzanne sees patients from a variety of cultures. If you worked in a similar place, what would you do if you noticed red circles on a child's back? You are unsure as to what caused the circles.

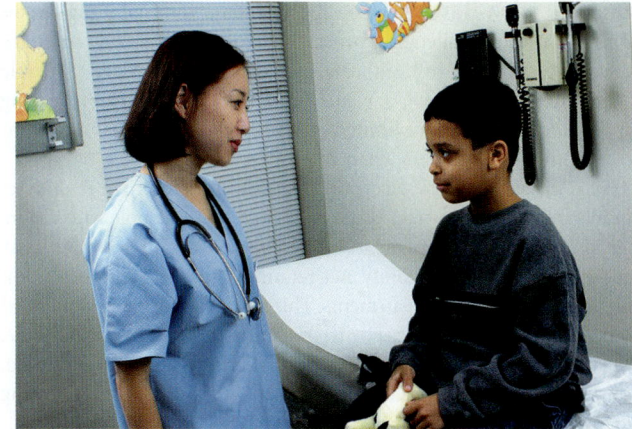

FIG. 35.6 Patients come from a variety of backgrounds and cultures. (From Proctor D, et al: *Kinn's The Medical Assistant*, ed 13, St. Louis, 2017, Elsevier.)

BOX 35.3 Cultural Differences

African Americans
- Extended family and church play important roles.
- May have a key family member that must be consulted on healthcare decisions.
- Older members may look at their health as being up to God's will, though younger members seek health screening and treatments as needed.

Cambodians
- Good health means the person is balanced; believe in the balance of hot and cold.
- Illness may be seen as punishment for sins in a past life.
- Typically use traditional healing practices before seeking conventional medicine. May use herbs, cupping and coining, acupuncture and acupressure.
- They may not be interested in preventive care and screenings.

Chinese
- May use acupuncture, massage, and herbs, seeking care from traditional practitioners for less severe illnesses.
- Respectful of elders, teachers, and healthcare professionals. May impact how a person interacts and discusses health topics with the healthcare professional. The person may not ask questions or discuss concerns.

Hispanics/Latinos
- May have strong family and religious beliefs. Family is respected and plays an important role. May view an illness as God's will.
- May use home remedies or folk healer's advice over conventional medicine.
- Sickness is caused from a person having too much heat or cold. Foods and herbs are used to bring back the balance. (Heat and cold are not temperature related.) Cold diseases have more unseen symptoms like a chest cold and earache. Hot diseases have more visible symptoms like vomiting, fever, and sore throat.
- Males often answer questions and give consent. Make sure to address the patient also. Friendliness and respectfulness is very important.

Hmong
- Lack words in native language for medical terms and some body organs.
- May seek care from folk medicine doctors and shaman.
- Herbs, massage, coining or spooning, and cupping can be used.
- Accessories may be worn around wrists, necks, or ankles for health or religious reasons.

- Respecting older family members is very important. Often oldest male in the family is the decision maker. Extended family is very important.
- Eye contact is considered rude.
- Touching the head of a child is not accepted. The head is considered sacred.

Native Americans
- May place a lot of value on family and spiritual beliefs
- State of health occurs when living in total harmony with nature. Illness is the imbalance between the person and nature.
- May use a traditional tribal medicine person.
- Often avoid direct eye contact out of respect and concern for the loss of one's soul.

Russians
- May view healthcare with some mistrust, based on past experience.
- May not be used to asking questions and participating in a discussion with a provider.
- Some practice home remedies and bonki. *Bonki* is practiced by pressing glass cups against the person's shoulders to ease the symptoms. Bruising can occur, which should not be confused with abuse.
- Family likes to receive news about patient's condition and prognosis and may not give bad news to the patient. This lessens the person's anxieties and promotes calmness.

Somali
- Believe that individuals do not prevent illness, which is only done through prayer and living a life according to their religion.
- Use traditional spiritual healers.
- May not take medication if they feel healthy.
- Healthcare decisions are made by the family, and the father gives consent for procedures.
- Male and female circumcisions are performed; being uncircumcised means the person is unclean.

Vietnamese
- Illness is often explained by mystical beliefs.
- Health is the balance between the hot and cold poles that govern the bodily functions.
- Use alternative therapies such as acupuncture, coining, spooning, and cupping.

Communication Barriers. Coaching patients with communication barriers can be a challenging process. Hearing, vision, and language barriers are common in healthcare. It is estimated that 2% of people in the United States have a visual impairment, 3% have a hearing impairment, and 9% have limited English proficiency. It is important to overcome these barriers when coaching patients.

For healthcare agencies accepting federal funds, the Civil Rights Act requires that all patients have equal access to services. People with vision, hearing, or speech impairments use different ways to communicate. The Americans with Disability Act requires effective communication with patients who have impairments. This may mean offering a qualified medical interpreter or other interpretation services free of charge. Large-print materials and written instructions are also required. Translated written materials are needed for non-English-speaking patients.

Boxes 35.4 to 35.6 provide tips for communicating with patients. It is important to listen to patients concerning what works best for them.

BOX 35.4 Tips for Communicating With Patients Who Have Impaired Hearing

- Face the person when speaking.
- Determine if the person has better hearing in one ear over the other. Position yourself so your voice is close to that side.
- If the patient has a hearing aid, encourage the patient to use it.
- Use a low-pitched voice, and speak clearly, slowly, and distinctly. Pause between sentences or phrases. Speak naturally; do not shout. Limit medical terms.
- Say the person's name before you begin a conversation.
- Keep your hands away from your face when talking.
- If an interpreter is present, look at the patient, not the interpreter.
- Limit extra noises in the environment.
- Attempt to rephrase or find a different way to say something if the patient has difficulty understanding a phrase.
- Provide important information in writing.
- Have the person repeat back important information.

BOX 35.5 Tips for Communicating With Patients Who Have Impaired Vision

- Ensure the room has adequate light. Avoid having the patient look toward the light source directly.
- Make sure the patient is wearing glasses or contacts if needed.
- Provide the patient with large-print directions or brochures.

BOX 35.6 Tips for Communicating With Patients Who Have Language Barriers

- Address the patient by his or her last name (e.g., Mrs. Martinez, Mr. Nguyen).
- Be respectful and courteous.
- Use simple phrases. If medical terminology must be used, make sure to define it for patients.
- Use an interpreter or an interpretation service. Focus on the patient and not on the interpreter.
- Use translated materials.
- Pictures and models can be helpful during the coaching session.

Teaching-Learning Process

Teaching opportunities vary greatly in ambulatory care. Sometimes a patient wants to know what a certain medication is for. Other times, the medical assistant needs to coach a patient on a diagnostic test.

Always take a moment to look over any information you provide to patients. Make sure you know the content before you review it with the patient. Providing information that conflicts with the handout will confuse the patient.

The medical assistant should start the coaching process by finding out what the patient knows about the topic. A simple way to do this is by asking a few questions like "Have you had an ultrasound before? If so, what do you remember about it?" This helps the medical assistant identify what the patient knows. From there the medical assistant can begin teaching.

Other coaching sessions will be lengthy because more complex topics are being taught. These coaching sessions should be well planned so the time is used efficiently. Using the teaching-learning process requires the following steps:

1. Assessing the learning needs
2. Determining teaching priorities
3. Planning the teaching process
4. Implementing the teaching process
5. Evaluating the patient's learning
6. Documenting the teaching-learning process

Table 35.4 describes the teaching-learning process. Box 35.7 provides tips on patient education materials used during the teaching-learning process.

COACHING ON DISEASE PREVENTION

Medical assistants coach patients of all ages on disease prevention. It is important to help patients understand ways to prevent diseases in their lives (Procedure 35.1). Common disease prevention coaching by age group includes the following:

- School-age children: teaching about handwashing and cough etiquette (Box 35.8).
- Teens and adults: teaching about ways to prevent sexually transmitted infections (STIs) and the risks of using cigarettes, tobacco, and e-cigarettes (Boxes 35.9 and 35.10).
- All age groups: coaching patients and parents on the vaccines recommended for that specific age (see Procedure 35.1). Childhood immunization schedules can be found on the website for the Centers

BOX 35.7 Tips on Patient Education Materials

Guidelines to follow if you are responsible for developing or ordering educational supplies include:

- The material should be written in lay language at a sixth- to eighth-grade level to promote understanding.
- Good pictures can help patients understand the information.
- Information should be well organized and clearly described.
- All material should be checked for accuracy. (Providers will request to approve the information ahead of time.)
- Handouts should be attractive and professional.
- Copies should be available in languages other than English when possible and in large print for visually impaired clients.
- Do not use disease information literature from medical and pharmaceutical companies that includes advertising of their products. (This type of information can create confusion if the patient is not using the product advertised.)

TABLE 35.4 Teaching-Learning Process

Step	Description
1. Assess the learning needs	The first step is to assess: What does the patient need to learn? How ready is the patient for learning? What are the patient's motivations and concerns? What is the patient's learning style? It is important to identify the patient's *learning goals* or the main reason for learning the content.
2. Determine teaching priorities	It is important to prioritize what the patient needs to learn first. When there is a lot of content to learn, the medical assistant must prioritize the most important topics and address those. Other topics will be addressed on another day. To determine the priorities, ask what information does the patient need to maintain his or her health until the next meeting?
3. Plan the teaching	When planning, determine what teaching aids and strategies will be used. *Teaching aids* are materials that will be used. These can include brochures, online resources, health-related apps, DVDs, posters, models, and drawings. Be sure to consider the patient's individual needs (e.g., primary language, developmental level, barriers to learning). For patients with lower reading levels or English as a secondary language, using more pictures can be helpful. *Teaching strategies* are ways the information will be given. For skills, demonstration and role-play with demonstration are effective strategies. Discussion, DVDs, and internet sites can be helpful for teaching about a disease, diagnostic tests, or treatment. The teaching strategies and aids used must be appropriate for the content being taught. For instance, demonstrating how to give an injection and having the patient give a return demonstration will be more useful than just discussing the steps of giving an injection.
4. Implement the teaching	It is important to start with the basics and build from there. Keep the information simple, focused, and appropriate for the individual patient. Reinforce important information. If teaching a skill, make sure to have the equipment available that the patient will use at home. This will promote the patient's comfort with the task.
5. Evaluate the learning	After teaching important points, have the patient summarize what you stated. Keeping the patient involved will help him or her to retain more information. Throughout the teaching session, make sure to ask the patient for feedback on if he or she understands what you are discussing. Instead of just saying, "Do you understand?" Ask specific questions to evaluate the patient's learning—for example, "What are four symptoms of low blood sugar?" Summarize the important points at the end of the teaching session. Answer any questions the patient may have. Identify areas were the patient needs more information. If there will be more than one session, summarize what will occur during the next meeting.
6. Document the teaching and learning	It is important to document the content taught to the patient, how the patient responded, evidence that the patient learned the content, handouts given, and any plans for follow-up. Make sure to include the provider's name and any adaptations you made to individualize the teaching/learning experience. Evidence may include statements such as "Pt safely and accurately walked 20 feet using the walker." "Pt stated six signs and symptoms of hypoglycemia."

BOX 35.8 Cough Etiquette

- When coughing or sneezing, turn away from others and cover your mouth and nose with a tissue. If a tissue is not available, cough or sneeze into your elbow or upper sleeve.
- Discard the tissue in the nearest waste container.
- Sanitize hands with an alcohol-based hand rub or wash hands.

BOX 35.9 How to Prevent Sexually Transmitted Infections

- Abstinence (not having any type of sex) is the most reliable way to prevent STIs.
- Long-term mutual monogamy (an agreement to be sexually active with just one person) with an uninfected partner is also a reliable way to prevent STIs.
- Decreasing the number of partners decreases the risk. All partners need to be tested.
- Use latex condoms, though they are not 100% effective.
- Avoid sharing underwear and towels.
- Wash after intercourse.
- Avoid anyone with a genital rash, sore, discharge, or other symptoms.
- Get vaccinated for hepatitis B and human papilloma virus (HPV).

for Disease Control and Prevention (CDC), https://www.cdc.gov/vaccines/schedules/downloads/child/0-18yrs-child-combined-schedule.pdf (also see Chapter 32). Common adult vaccines usually include the following:
- Influenza: yearly
- Tetanus and diphtheria (Td): every 10 years and substitute tetanus, diphtheria, and acellular pertussis vaccine (Tdap) once.
- Herpes zoster vaccine (HZV): one dose after age 60.
- 13-valent pneumococcal conjugate vaccine (PCV13): one dose usually after age 65, unless given before based on the patient's health.
- 23-valent pneumococcal polysaccharide vaccine (PPSV23 or PPSV): one to two doses depending on patient's health
- Additional vaccines can be given based on the situation (e.g., traveling or job related); adulthood immunization schedules can

be found on the CDC's website, https://www.cdc.gov/vaccines/schedules/downloads/adult/adult-combined-schedule.pdf

CRITICAL THINKING 35.5

Suzanne has seen many patients who smoke. Describe how a medical assistant should discuss cessation with a patient who uses nicotine.

PROCEDURE 35.1 Coach a Patient on Disease Prevention

Tasks
Coach a patient on the recommended vaccinations for his or her age. Adapt coaching for the patient's communication barrier and developmental life stage. Document the coaching in the patient's health record.

Equipment and Supplies
- Vaccine Information Statements (VIS) (available at http://www.immunize.org/vis/)
- Patient's health record

Scenario
You are working with Dr. David Kahn. You need to room Charles Johnson (date of birth [DOB]: 03/03/1958), and his record indicates he has not been seen in several years. Charles has significant hearing loss, and he communicates by signing. His wife interprets for him. You look in his health record and see that he is due for influenza, Td, and herpes zoster (HZV) (shingles) immunizations. Per the provider's request (order), you need to coach adult patients on potential vaccines they are due for during the initial rooming process.

Directions
Role-play this scenario with two peers.

Procedural Steps
1. Wash hands or use hand sanitizer.
   Purpose: Hand sanitization is an important step for infection control.
2. Greet the patient. Identify yourself. Verify the patient's identity with full name and date of birth. Explain what you will be doing.
   Purpose: It is important to identify the patient in two different ways to ensure that you have the correct patient. Explaining the procedure can make the patient feel more comfortable and helps to reduce anxiety.
3. Arrange the chairs so the patient can see both you and the person signing. Speak slowly. Pause as needed to allow person signing to finish with the last statement. Look at the patient when communicating.
   Purpose: The medical assistant must focus the patient and not the person signing or the interpreter. Speaking slowly and pausing allows the person to sign what you are saying.
4. Use simpler language when talking. Speak clearly. Communicate with dignity and respect. Allow time for the patient to respond. Listen to the patient's concerns.
   Purpose: When working with older patients, it is important to treat them with respect and dignity. Listening is important.
5. Ask the patient if he has received vaccines somewhere else over the past few years.
   Purpose: It is important to verify that the health record is accurate.

Scenario Update
The patient has not seen any healthcare providers over the past few years. The only vaccines received were given at this facility.
6. Describe the vaccines that are due. Use the VIS for each vaccine as you coach the patient on the purpose of the vaccine.
   Purpose: The VIS is written for patients and describes the vaccine, disease(s) it prevents, and adverse reactions (side effects).

Scenario Update
The patient knows the shingles vaccine is not covered and costs more than $200. He refuses the shingles vaccines, and he does not believe in getting the influenza vaccine. He is interested in getting the Td vaccine.
7. Ask the patient which vaccines he is interested in getting. If he refuses, be respectful of his choice. Any reason he gives for the refusal should be communicated to the provider.
   Purpose: Patients have the right to refuse. Any treatment refused must be communicated to the provider.
8. Document the coaching in the patient's health record. Include the provider's name, what was taught, how the patient responded and any vaccines refused.
   Purpose: It is important to document the procedure in the health record to show it was done.

07/16/20XX 1305 Per Dr. Kahn's order, instructed pt on the HZV, influenza, and Td vaccines. Pt stated he was not interested in the influenza vaccine or the HZV. He also stated his insurance wouldn't cover the HZV and he didn't have the money to pay for it. He is interested in receiving the Td vaccine. Reviewed the Td VIS (07/15/20XX) with the patient. Pt stated he understood and would call if he had any issues. Due to pt's hearing impairment, pt's wife interpreted for pt during the visit. Suzanne Peterson CMA (AAMA)

BOX 35.10 Health Risks Associated With Cigarettes, Smokeless Tobacco, and E-Cigarettes

Tobacco smoke contains more than 7000 chemicals, of which 250 are harmful and at least 69 can cause cancer. One in five deaths are related to smoking. According to the Centers for Disease Control and Prevention (CDC), smokers are more likely to develop heart disease, lung cancer, and strokes. Smoking can cause problems in all parts of the body. (See Chapter 11.)

Secondhand smoke causes lung cancer, strokes, low-birth-weight babies, and heart disease. Children exposed to secondhand smoke have increased risks of sudden infant death syndrome (SIDS), ear infections, bronchitis, pneumonia, colds, and asthma.

Quitting has numerous health advantages for the smoker:
- Blood pressure and heart rate begin to return to normal.
- Within a few hours, carbon monoxide levels in the blood decline.
- Within a few weeks, circulation improves and abnormal respiratory systems (e.g., cough, wheezing) decrease.
- One year after quitting smoking, the cardiovascular risks decrease sharply.
- Two to 5 years after quitting, risk for stroke returns to nonsmoker level.
- Five years after quitting, the risk of cancer of the esophagus, bladder, throat, and mouth is cut in half.
- Ten years after quitting, the lung cancer risk decreases by 50%.

The CDC reports that at least 28 cancer-causing chemicals have been found in smokeless tobacco (e.g., chew and dip). Smokeless tobacco can cause cancer of the mouth, pancreas, and esophagus.

According to the U.S. surgeon general, e-cigarettes heat liquids to form an aerosol that is then inhaled. Many people call this vaping. The liquids typically contain nicotine, flavorings, and other additives. E-cigarettes are considered tobacco products because they contain nicotine that comes from tobacco. The nicotine makes e-cigarettes addictive. The additives can pose health risks.

There are many resources available to help smokers quit, including online resources (Smokefree.gov) and the National Cancer Institute's Smoking Quitline. Local resources are usually available. Healthcare providers can discuss medications that can be helpful.

From the Centers for Disease Control and Prevention (CDC), https://www.cdc.gov/tobacco/infographics/health-effects/index.htm#smoking-risks. Know the Risks, https://e-cigarettes.surgeongeneral.gov/.

COACHING ON HEALTH MAINTENANCE AND WELLNESS

Often with health maintenance and wellness, the provider establishes standing orders for specific education to be given based on the patient's history or age. When the medical assistant rooms a patient, a health history is obtained, and screening questions are asked. Based on the patient's answers, the medical assistant may need to provide coaching on specific topics per the provider's standing orders. For instance, a patient states she smokes 1 pack of cigarettes daily. The provider's standing order for smokers requires the medical assistant to provide information on the hazards of tobacco use and resources for quitting. Another example would be a patient who is turning 50. Since colon cancer screenings typically start at age 50, the provider's standing order would be to provide this information to the patient.

The following sections discuss self-exams that can be taught to patients and the screenings that are commonly done. The medical assistant completes some screenings, whereas others require the medical assistant to educate the patient on the tests to be performed.

Self-Exams

The purpose of self-exams is to identify changes in one's body. Sometimes these changes can be the first sign of a disease. Self-exams are typically done monthly. To help maintain a person's health, the early diagnosis of a disease like cancer is important.

Breast Self-Exam. Breast cancer can affect both females and males, though males are at a lower risk. Breast cancer is the second most common cancer in females after skin cancer. The risk of breast cancer increases with age. About one in eight women will have invasive breast cancer. Typically, the survival rate is higher the earlier the cancer is diagnosed.

According to the American Cancer Society, research has not shown a benefit for patient or provider breast exams when women are also getting mammograms. It is recommended for women with an average risk of breast cancer to start having yearly mammograms between ages 45 and 50.

It is important for all women to know what is normal with their breasts. Any abnormality should be reported to their provider (Box 35.11). Some providers still recommend a monthly breast self-exam (BSE) to be done after the menses. Procedure 35.2 describes how to perform a BSE. It is helpful for the medical assistant to provide the patient with a brochure showing the technique. It is also recommended to show the technique on a model (Fig. 35.7). If possible, the patient should demonstrate the technique back to the medical assistant. This practice helps the medical assistant determine if the patient understood the coaching.

BOX 35.11 Warning Signs of Breast Cancer

- Change in the skin (redness, warmth, darkening of the color, dimpling, puckering)
- Lump or hard area inside the breast or in the axilla area
- Change in the size or shape of the breast
- Change in the nipple (inverted or pulling in appearance; rash, sore, or drainage)
- Pain that does not go away

PROCEDURE 35.2   Coach a Patient on Breast Self-Exam

Tasks
Coach a patient to do a breast self-exam (BSE) while considering the patient's cultural beliefs and developmental life stage. Document your teaching in the patient's health record.

Equipment and Supplies
- Breast self-examination brochure (optional)
- Breast model
- Provider's order
- Patient's health record

Scenario
You are working with Dr. David Kahn. He has ordered you to show Binh, a 17-year-old Vietnamese patient, how to do a breast self-exam. She has a strong family history of breast cancer. The patient can fluently speak and understand English.

Procedural Steps
1. Wash hands or use hand sanitizer.
   Purpose: Hand sanitization is an important step for infection control.
2. Read the provider's order. Assemble the equipment.
   Purpose: It is important to know the provider's order before starting the procedure.
3. Greet the patient. Identify yourself. Verify the patient's identity with full name and date of birth. Explain the procedure to be performed in a manner that the patient understands. Answer any questions the patient may have about the procedure.
   Purpose: It is important to identify the patient in two different ways to ensure that you have the correct patient. Explaining the procedure can make the patient feel more comfortable and helps to reduce anxiety.
4. Provide privacy and independence during the session. Encourage the patient to ask questions and discuss her concerns.
   Purpose: It is important to adapt the coaching to the patient's developmental stage. Privacy and independence are important to someone who is 17. Encouraging questions and discussions is also effective.
5. Ask the patient if she is familiar with breast self-examinations. Ask about her thoughts on illness and if she does alternative therapies. Explain the importance of doing a self-exam.
   Purpose: In the Vietnamese culture, illness is often explained by mystical beliefs. Asking the patient her thoughts might be helpful for the medical assistant during the coaching session.
6. Explain to the patient that she will need to undress and look at her breast in the mirror to identify any changes. Let her know that she will need to check to see if they are the usual size, shape, and color. She should also look for swelling, redness, rash, dimpling, puckering, or bulging of the skin. She should check to see if the nipple position or appearance has changed. Finally, she should check to see if any fluid is coming from the nipple by placing her thumb and index finger on the tissue by the nipple and pulling outward toward the end of the nipple (Fig. 1).
   Purpose: Changes in the appearance may indicate an issue.
7. Instruct the patient that she needs to change positions and continue to check the appearance of the breasts. She needs to place her hands on her hips and press down. This tightens the chest muscle under the breasts. While in this position, she should turn from side to side to see the outer

Continued

PROCEDURE 35.2   Coach a Patient on Breast Self-Exam—cont'd

part of the breasts. Instruct her to clasp her hands behind her head or raise her arms and look at the outer part of the breasts again (Fig. 2).

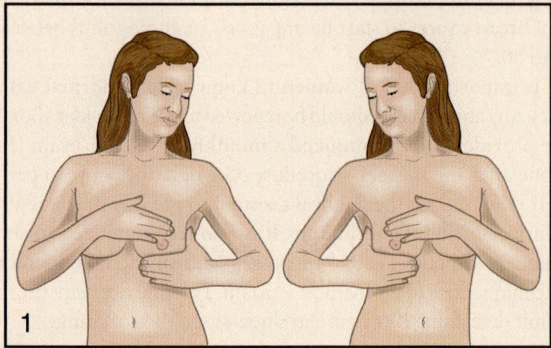

Purpose: Sometimes changing the arm position may cause an abnormality to appear.

8. Instruct the patient to bend forward and roll her shoulders and elbows forward while tightening her chest muscles. While in this position, she can check for changes in the shape of the breasts.
   Purpose: Abnormalities may be seen in this position.
9. Instruct the patient to palpate the breast using one of the two techniques. Use the model as you explain the technique.
   a. *Lying down technique*: Instruct the patient to check the breast while lying down. Have her do the following: Tuck a small pillow under the side being checked. Tuck one arm under the head, and with the other hand check the opposite breast (e.g., right hand checks the left breast). Use the first two or three finger pads. With fingers together, use a circular motion and a firm, smooth touch to check the entire breast. Start at the top outer breast tissue and move around the breast in a circular pattern. When the top of the breast is reached again, move in 1 inch toward the nipple and complete another circle around the breast. Repeat until the entire breast from the armpit to the cleavage is checked. Then place fingers flat on the nipple and feel for any changes beneath the nipple. Repeat these steps on the other breast.
   b. *Shower technique*: Place the right hand on the right hip. With a soapy left hand, feel for changes in the right axilla area. Use 2 or 3 finger pads to press on the breast. Move in an up and down pattern over the breast tissue. Make sure to cover from the bra line to the collarbone. Repeat on the opposite side.

Purpose: This position allows the patient to check the entire breast. The entire breast including under the arm and up to the collarbone needs to be checked for changes.

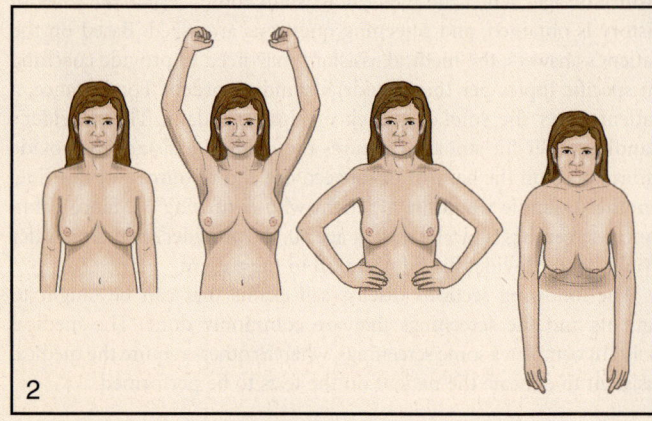

10. Have the patient select a technique that she will use. Encourage the patient to demonstrate the technique on the breast model. Coach the patient on ways to improve the exam if needed.
    Purpose: It is important to have the patient demonstrate the skill to check the accuracy her technique.
11. Answer any questions the patient may have. Provide the patient with a brochure to take home (optional).
    Purpose: It is important to answer any questions the patient has and if possible provide her with a brochure to take home.
12. Document the patient education in the patient's health record. Include the provider's name, the order, what was taught, how the patient responded, how the patient did the demonstration, and any handouts provided.
    Purpose: It is important to document the patient education in the health record to show it was done.

07/19/20XX 1505 Per Dr. Kahn's order, instructed pt on the BSE. Instructed the patient on how to check for changes in the breast. Explained the lying and showering techniques. Pt opted for the showering technique. She demonstrated how to palpate the breast tissue correctly using a breast model. All her questions were answered. Provided her with the "BSE" brochure and encouraged her to perform it monthly. Suzanne Peterson CMA (AAMA)

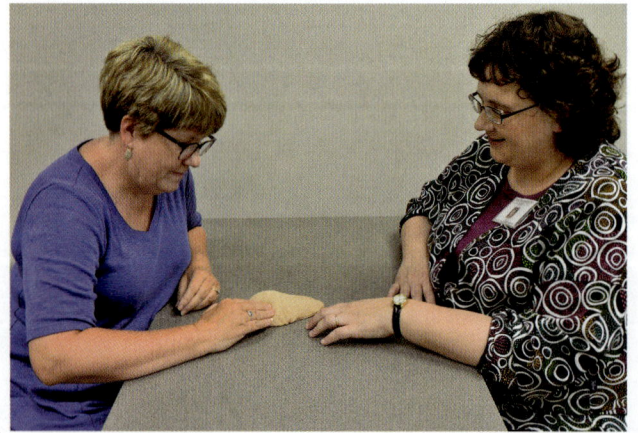

FIG. 35.7 Coaching a patient regarding the breast self-exam.

Testicular Self-Exam. According to the American Cancer Society, males at any age can develop testicular cancer. About 50% of those diagnosed are between 20 and 34 years of age. It is estimated that 1 in 263 males will get testicular cancer. If the cancer is found early (before it has spread), there is a good chance of a cure. Box 35.12 lists symptoms of testicular cancer.

The American Cancer Society recommends that providers perform a testicular exam as part of a routine physical exam. Some providers recommend that after puberty (around age 15) males should do a monthly testicular self-exam (TSE) after a shower (Procedure 35.3). Again, it is helpful for the patient to have a brochure and to practice the technique on a model during the coaching session.

Skin Self-Exam. Skin cancer is the most common type of cancer in the United States. The three most common types of skin cancer are basal cell, squamous cell, and melanoma. Basal cell and squamous cell

CHAPTER 35   Patient Coaching With Health Promotion

PROCEDURE 35.3   Coach a Patient on Testicular Self-Exam

Tasks
Coach a patient to do a testicular self-exam (TSE) while considering the patient's developmental life stage. Document your teaching in the patient's health record.

Equipment and Supplies
- Testicular self-examination brochure (optional)
- Testicular model
- Provider's order
- Patient's health record

Scenario
You are working with Dr. David Kahn. He has ordered you to provide Truong Tran (DOB: 05/30/1991) with TSE coaching.

Procedural Steps
1. Wash hands or use hand sanitizer.
   Purpose: Hand sanitization is an important step for infection control.
2. Read the provider's order. Assemble the equipment.
   Purpose: It is important to know the provider's order before starting the procedure.
3. Greet the patient. Identify yourself. Verify the patient's identity with full name and date of birth. Explain the procedure to be performed in a manner that the patient understands. Answer any questions the patient may have about the procedure.
   Purpose: It is important to identify the patient in two different ways to ensure that you have the correct patient. Explaining the procedure can make the patient feel more comfortable and helps to reduce anxiety.
4. Ask the patient what he knows about the self-exam. Clarify any inaccuracies. Build on the patient's prior knowledge of the topic during the session. Identify the patient's motivating factor for learning about the self-exam. Listen to the patient's concerns.
   Purpose: It is important to adapt the coaching to the patient's developmental stage. Because of the patient's age, identifying motivating factors is important.
5. Explain to the patient that the best time to do the self-exam is after a warm shower or bath.
   Purpose: The scrotal skin is more relaxed.
6. Demonstrate on the model while discussing the technique. Instruct the patient to examine each testicle gently with both hands. Roll the testicle between the thumb and fingers (Fig. 1). Show the patient the epididymis, the soft curved structure behind and on top of the testicle (Fig. 2). Then show the patient how to examine the vas deferens, which is the tube that runs up the epididymis (Fig. 3).
   Purpose: This allows the person to do a better self-exam.

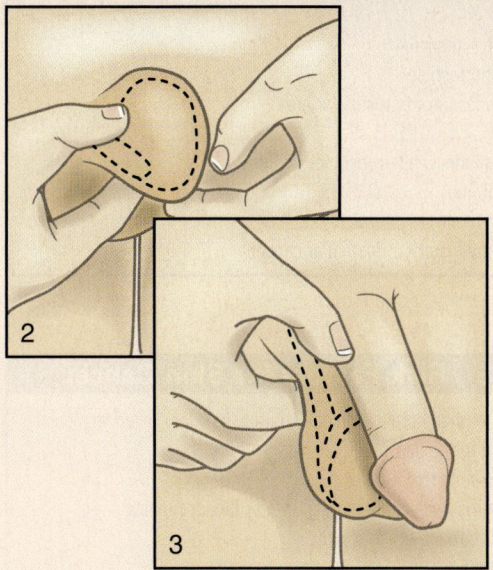

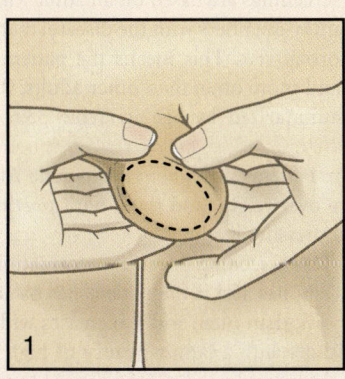

7. Instruct the patient to feel for any abnormalities and lumps. These could be painless or painful. Instruct the person to look for changes in the size, texture, or shape.
   Purpose: Any changes should be reported to the provider for possible follow-up.
8. Have the patient demonstrate the technique on the model. Coach the patient on ways to improve the exam if needed.
   Purpose: It is important to have the patient demonstrate the teaching to check for accuracy of technique and correct understanding.
9. Answer any questions the patient may have. Provide the patient with a brochure to take home (optional).
   Purpose: It is important to answer any questions the patient has and if possible provide him with a brochure to take home.
10. Document the patient education in the patient's health record. Include the provider's name, the order, what was taught, how the patient responded, how the patient did the demonstration, and any handouts provided.
    Purpose: It is important to document the patient education in the health record to show it was done.

07/19/20XX 1505 Per Dr. Kahn's order, instructed pt on TSE. Instructed the patient on how to check for changes in the testes. Explained the technique and encouraged the patient to do monthly checks after a warm shower/bath. Pt provided an accurate return demonstration. His questions were answered. Gave pt the "TSE" brochure. Suzanne Peterson CMA (AAMA)

BOX 35.12 Testicular Cancer

Symptoms:
- Painful or swollen testicle
- Lump on or in the testicle
- Feeling of heaviness in the testicular area

Risk factors:
- Cryptorchidism (undescended testicle)
- Klinefelter syndrome
- Caucasian
- Personal or family history of testicular cancer

BOX 35.13 Risk Factors for Skin Cancer

- Skin that is lighter than normal skin color; burns, freckles, or reddens easily; becomes painful in the sun
- Family or personal history of skin cancer
- History of sunburns (especially early in life) or indoor tanning
- Exposure to sun through work or play
- Green or blue eyes
- Red or blond hair
- Certain types and a large number of moles

TABLE 35.5 Early Warning Signs of Malignant Melanoma: ABCDE Rule

Asymmetry	One half of the mole does not match the other half.
Border	The edges of the mole are blurred or irregular.
Color	The mole is not the same color throughout and has shades of tan, brown, black, red, white, or blue
Diameter	The mole is larger than 6 mm, about the size of a pencil eraser or pea; but it could be smaller.
Evolving	The mole changes over time.

BOX 35.14 Symptoms of Oral Cancer

- White or red patches in the mouth or on the gums, tongue, or lips.
- Numbness or pain in the mouth; pain with chewing or talking
- Long-term hoarseness or sore throat
- Swelling in the jaw area or constant earache
- Bleeding in the mouth or a long-term sore
- Feeling of a lump or something stuck in the throat

---

carcinomas are curable. Melanoma is more dangerous and can cause death. These three types of skin cancers are caused by overexposure to ultraviolet (UV) light. UV exposure comes from the sun, tanning beds, and sun lamps. UV rays are an invisible kind of radiation that penetrates and changes skin cells.

Certain people have more risk than others for skin cancer (Box 35.13). Experts recommend monthly skin self-exams. It is important to watch for changes in moles. To remember how moles may change, use the ABCDE rule (Table 35.5). Any change in moles, including in the size, shape, color, elevation, or symptom (e.g., bleeding, itching, or crusting), should be reported immediately (Fig. 35.8).

When doing the monthly skin check, start at the scalp and work toward the soles of the feet. Use mirrors to exam the back of the ears and the back. Many people miss mole changes on the back of their ears. When examining hands and feet, make sure to check between the fingers and toes as well as the nail beds. Check all skin surfaces. Document the location of the moles and their appearances. Any changes seen or any suspicious-looking mole should be reported to the provider immediately.

Oral Cancer Self-Exam. Oral cancer includes cancer of the lips, tongue, throat, salivary glands, pharynx, larynx, and sinuses. Most oral cancers occur after age 40. It is estimated that more than 40,000 new cases of oral cancer are diagnosed yearly with almost 9000 related deaths. Early detection is important for oral cancer (Box 35.14). Here are some facts about oral cancer:
- Men get oral cancer twice as often as women.
- Using tobacco, drinking alcohol, or having oral human papilloma virus (HPV) are risk factors for oral cancer.
- About 25% of those with oral cancer had no risks.

Oral cancer screening is routinely done by the dentist and should occur every 6 months. It is important for people to do a monthly oral cancer self-exam. Any changes in appearance or sores that do not heal should be reported to the dentist immediately. According to the American Dental Hygienists Association, an oral cancer self-exam consists of looking for lumps and color changes and then feeling for lumps and swelling. To do an oral cancer self-exam, follow these steps:
- Check the head and neck for lumps, bumps, or swelling. Is one side of the face larger than the other?
- Check the skin on the face for changes. Is there a color change? Are there sores, moles, or growths?
- Check for any lumps or tenderness in the neck.
- Check the upper and lower lip for sores and color changes. After the visual inspection, feel for any changes in texture or lumps.
- Check the inner cheek for any color changes (red, white, or dark patches). Then palpate the cheeks with a thumb on the outside and a finger inside. Are any lumps found?
- Check the roof of the mouth for lumps and color changes. Feel for any lumps.
- Check the floor of the mouth using your tongue for any lumps or color changes. Examine all angles. Feel the tongue with a finger for any lumps or tenderness.

Regular Screenings

Medical assistants in primary care typically need to talk with patients about the recommended regular screenings for different diseases. Suggested times for screenings are based on an adult with an average risk. If a patient has family members with the disease, that person may have a higher than normal risk. This means the patient may need to be screened earlier and more often than other adults. Regular preventive screenings are summarized by age in Table 35.6 and include the following:

- *Blood pressure*: Patients at higher risk include African Americans, those who are overweight, and those with previously higher than normal blood pressure readings.
- *Bone density*: This screening provides information on the strength of the patient's bones and if the patient has osteoporosis. Women have a higher risk than men, and it increases with age.
- *Cholesterol*: Adults with a family history of high cholesterol levels or have high cholesterol need more frequent testing.
- *Colorectal cancer screening*: The stool screenings start at age 45 and are done every 1 or 3 years depending on the test (Table 35.7). After age 75, it is up to the patient and the provider.

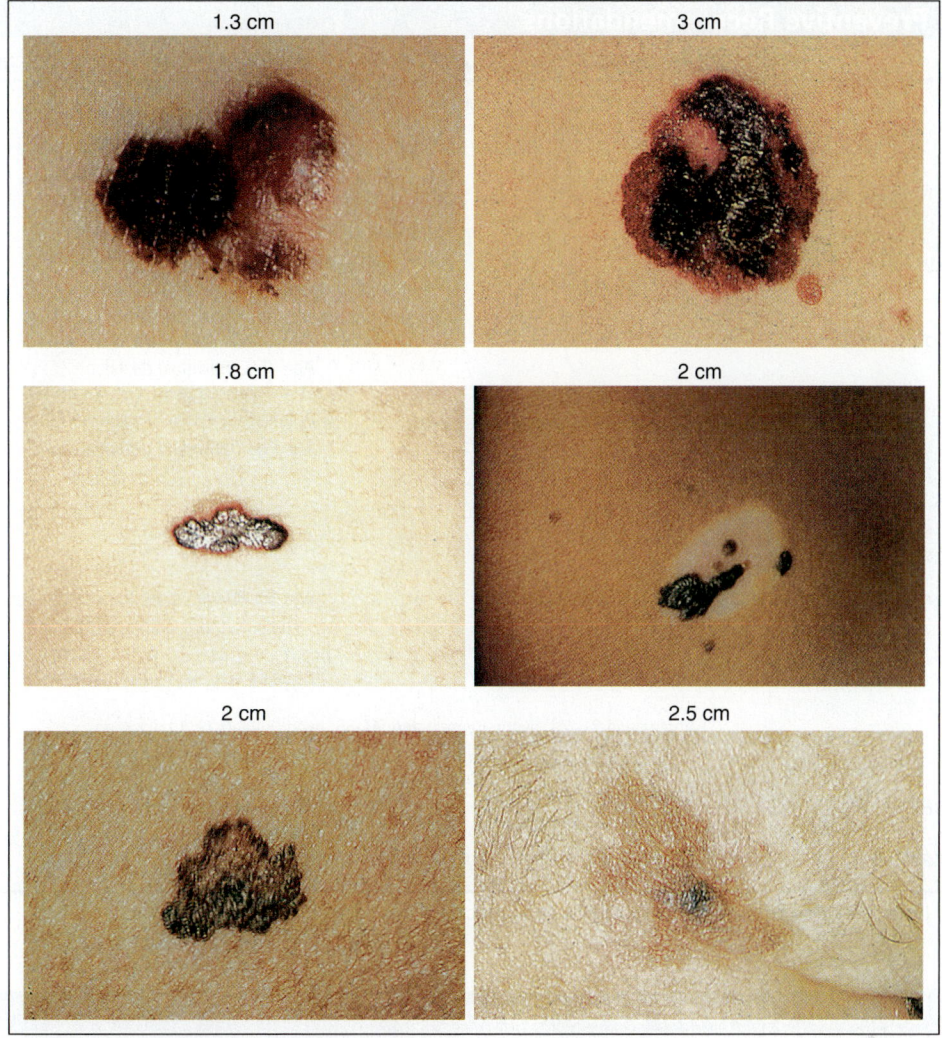

FIG. 35.8 Malignant melanomas. Note the presence of the ABCDE characteristics. (From Rothrock J: *Alexander's Care of the Patient in Surgery*, ed 14, St Louis, 2011, Mosby.)

- *Dental exam*: The American Dental Association recommends a dental exam and cleaning yearly. Dental health can impact the overall health of the body.
- *Dilated eye exam*: It is important to have a dilated eye exam if a person has a risk of eye disease (e.g., glaucoma). The CDC recommends the dilated eye exams for the following individuals:
  - Patients with diabetes (recommended annually)
  - African American patients age 40 years and older (recommended every 2 years)
  - Patients older than 60 years of age (recommended every 2 years)
  - Patients with a family history of glaucoma (recommended every 2 years)
- *Lung cancer screening*: Patients who are 55 to 80 years old, have a history of heavy smoking, and are currently smoking or quit in the previous 15 years should be screened for lung cancer. (Heavy smoking means smoking one pack of cigarettes a day for 30 years or two packs for 15 years.)
- *Mammograms*: This x-ray of the breasts helps to identify breast cancer. Some providers may suggest mammograms for females starting between ages 45 to 50. The recommendation is for females age 50 to 74 to have a mammogram every 2 years.
- *Pap test*: This test is used to identify cervical cancer.
- *Prostate cancer*: Risk factors include being 50 years old or older, being African American, exposure to Agent Orange, and having a father, brother, or son who had prostate cancer. No specific test exists for prostate cancer. The digital rectal exam (DRE) and the prostate-specific antigen (PSA) test are used. The provider may offer either test after age 50. Frequency is based on the patient's history.
- *Type 2 diabetes mellitus*: Adults should be screened every three years or sooner depending on their medical history.

> **MEDICAL TERMINOLOGY**
> **endo-** within, inner
> **-scopy**: process of viewing

> **CRITICAL THINKING 35.6**
> Suzanne has seen more providers ordering the fecal immunochemical test (FIT) over the guaiac fecal occult blood test. What are the advantages of the FIT test?

TABLE 35.6 Preventive Recommendations

	Age 18–39	Age 40–44	Age 45–64	Age 65+
Blood Pressure	Every 3–5 years	Annually		
Bone Density				Females: every 2 years
Cholesterol	Every 5 years			
Fecal Stool Tests (gFOBT, FIT)			Age 45–75; annually Age 75+: individual decision	
Stool DNA Test (Cologuard)			Age 45–75; every 3 years Age 75+: individual decision	
Colonoscopy			Age 45–75; every 10 years Age 75+: individual decision	
Dental Exam	Annually			
Dilated Eye Exam			Age 60+: every 2 years	
Lung Cancer Screening			Age 55–80 who meet the criteria: annual low-dose computed tomography (LDCT)	
Mammogram			Females age 50–74: every 2 years	
Pap Test	Females age 21–29: every 3 years; age 30–65: every 3 years or if having an HPV test then every 5 years.			Individual decision
Prostate Cancer (DRE or PSA test)			Males: age 50+: individual decision	
Type 2 Diabetes Mellitus	Every 3 years or more frequent if patient has hypertension or obesity			

From Healthfinder.gov, https://healthfinder.gov/HealthTopics/Category/doctor-visits.

TABLE 35.7 Common Colorectal Cancer Screenings

Test	Description	Testing Frequency
Guaiac fecal occult blood test (gFOBT)	Stool samples are collected by the patient and returned to the medical laboratory for testing. This test detects blood in the stool. Many foods can create false positives, thus a patient must follow the dietary limitations prior to testing.	From age 45 to 75 years old: every year From 75 to 85 years old: individual decision based on health of the person and prior screening history
Fecal Immunochemical Test (FIT)	Stool samples are collected by the patient and returned to the medical laboratory for testing. Uses antibodies to detect human hemoglobin protein. No dietary restrictions are required.	
Cologuard Stool DNA test (FIT-DNA)	Stool samples are collected by the patient and returned to a specific medical laboratory for testing. A computer analysis is done to determine if blood is present. It also looks at the DNA in the stool to determine if cancer or precancerous cells are present. Positive results should require a colonoscopy. No patient preparation is required.	Every 3 years Used in place of the gFOBT and FIT
Colonoscopy	An endoscope is inserted through the anus and used to visualize the colon. Requires patient dietary and colon preparation.	Every 10 years

One-Time Screenings

People are recommended to have the following screenings at least once, unless a person's risk is greater than average:

- *Abdominal aortic aneurysm*: Males between 65 to 75 years of age who have smoked at one time in their lives should receive this screening. This population has the highest risk of having an abdominal aortic aneurysm (AAA).
- *Human immunodeficiency virus (HIV) screen (blood test)*: People 15 to 65 years old need to get an HIV test at least once in their lifetime. All pregnant women need to be tested. People with a high risk for HIV should have annual testing, if not more often. High-risk factors include multiple sexual partners, sexual partners who have or may have HIV, use injectable illegal drugs, and so on.

- *Hepatitis C*: This condition is passed through blood from an infected person. A person with risk factors should be tested. Risk factors for hepatitis C include the following:
  - Born between 1945 and 1965
  - History of a blood transfusion or organ transplant before 1992
  - Used injected illegal drugs
  - Have chronic liver disease, HIV, or AIDS

Additional Screenings

When rooming patients, medical assistants have to perform different screenings. Either the patient's age or the patient's responses will trigger the need for the screening. The screenings have increased throughout the years. This is due to increased data collection requirements and focusing on prevention and quality patient care. Common screenings include the following:

- *Alcohol misuse screening*: Drinking in moderation means that females have no more than one drink a day and males have no more than two drinks per day. (A drink is classified as a 12-oz bottle of beer, a 5-oz glass of wine, or a 1.5-oz shot of liquor.) Drinking more than the recommended daily amount may lead to health issues.
- *Nicotine or tobacco screening*: Various tools are used. Tools typically focus on whether or not tobacco products are used, how much is used per day, history of use, and quitting behaviors (e.g., strategies used in the past or thoughts of quitting).
- *Drug abuse screening*: Various tools are used. Tools focus on prescription drug use for nonmedical reasons and illegal drug use. Tools are designed differently, but it is important to identify any history of or recent drug abuse. Box 35.15 lists common signs of drug abuse.
- *Intimate partner violence screening*: This screen covers domestic abuse. It is important to remember that both males and females can be the victims of domestic abuse. Many psychological and health problems come from violence, including substance abuse, obesity, depression, brain trauma, pregnancy complications, and chronic pain. Intimate partner violence includes controlling behaviors, physical abuse, sexual abuse, and emotional or verbal abuse.
- *Elderly safety screening*: These screening tools focus on how safe the older person feels at home. The tools screen for abuse and neglect. Box 35.16 provides types and symptoms of elder abuse and neglect.
- *Functional status screening*: Several tools are available for primary care providers to use for older patients. By using a functional status screening tool, the provider obtains information on the patient, such as the following:
  - Physical functions with daily activities (e.g., grooming, bathing, walking, and eating)
  - Psychological health (e.g., mood and anxiety)
  - Role function (e.g., employed or volunteer)
  - Social function (e.g., interacting with others or isolating self)
- *Depression screening*: Several tools are used to screen for depression. The screening tools ask questions related to moods, thoughts, and feelings. The number of questions will vary depending on the tools. For instance, the Patient Health Questionnaire–2 (PHQ-2) asks two questions that focus on the frequency of depressed mood and anhedonia (AN hee DOE nee ah) over the previous 2 weeks. If the patient screens positive, then the Patient Health Questionnaire–9 (PHQ-9) is given to see if the patient meets the criteria for a depressive disorder (Fig. 35.9). (The first two questions of the PHQ-9 are the two questions on the PHQ-2 tool.)
- *Peripheral neuropathy screening*: Screening questions focus on loss of feeling or a "pins and needles" sensation in the feet and hands. Besides asking the patient screening questions, the medical assistant may also need to do a monofilament foot test (Procedure 35.4). This time can present a great opportunity to coach patients on foot care (Box 35.17). Proper foot care can help to limit foot sores and identify suspicious areas sooner.

> **VOCABULARY**
> **anhedonia**: The inability to feel or experience pleasure during a pleasurable activity.

BOX 35.15 Common Signs of Drug Abuse

- Poor hygiene
- Loss of interest in favorite things
- Very energetic, talking fast, very sociable
- Tired, sad, nervous, agitated, and bad moods
- Eating and sleeping patterns change
- Missing school, work, or appointments
- Spending money excessively
- Slowed reaction time, paranoid thinking

BOX 35.16 Types and Signs of Elder Abuse and Neglect

- *Physical abuse*: fractures, rope marks, cuts, bruising, dislocations, broken glasses, giving too little or too much medication, bleeding, and sudden changes in the person's personality or behavior
- *Sexual abuse*: unexplained sexually transmitted infections, bruising in the genital region, and reports from the older person
- *Emotional abuse*: not communicating, withdrawn, agitated, and symptoms that mimic dementia
- *Neglect*: malnutrition, dehydration, lack of proper living conditions, and failing to treat health problems
- *Abandonment*: leaving the person in a public place
- *Financial abuse*: stealing from the older person, forging signatures on financial transactions, and any other illegal action that represents a financial loss for the older person

---

BOX 35.17 Foot Care for Patients With Neuropathy

The medical assistant can coach the patient on proper foot care. It is important for patients to check their feet daily and also to care for their feet daily. The following points should be reinforced with patients who have neuropathy:

- Check shoes for damaged areas or stones before putting them on. Wear good-fitting shoes at all times to protect feet.
- Check feet when taking off shoes. Look at all sides of the feet and between the toes. Check for redness, blisters, swelling, sores, and so forth.
- Keep nails trimmed to a proper length.
- Wash feet every day with lukewarm water and soap. Dry well with a soft towel. Use lotion, lanolin, or oil on dry skin, but do not put it between toes as this could cause an infection.
- Seek medical care immediately for foot sores.
- Avoid putting pressure for long periods of time on areas with nerve damage.
- Use an elbow instead of the toes or hands to check the bathwater temperature.

PATIENT HEALTH QUESTIONNAIRE-9 (PHQ-9)

Over the last 2 weeks, how often have you been bothered by any of the following problems?
(Use "✓" to indicate your answer)

Problem	Not at all	Several days	More than half the days	Nearly every day
1. Little interest or pleasure in doing things	0	1	2	3
2. Feeling down, depressed, or hopeless	0	1	2	3
3. Trouble falling or staying asleep, or sleeping too much	0	1	2	3
4. Feeling tired or having little energy	0	1	2	3
5. Poor appetite or overeating	0	1	2	3
6. Feeling bad about yourself — or that you are a failure or have let yourself or your family down	0	1	2	3
7. Trouble concentrating on things, such as reading the newspaper or watching television	0	1	2	3
8. Moving or speaking so slowly that other people could have noticed? Or the opposite — being so fidgety or restless that you have been moving around a lot more than usual	0	1	2	3
9. Thoughts that you would be better off dead or of hurting yourself in some way	0	1	2	3

For office coding 0 + _____ + _____ + _____
=Total Score: _____

If you checked off any problems, how difficult have these problems made it for you to do your work, take care of things at home, or get along with other people?

Not difficult at all ☐   Somewhat difficult ☐   Very difficult ☐   Extremely difficult ☐

FIG. 35.9 Example of a depression screening tool: Patient Health Questionnaire–9 (PHQ-9).

PROCEDURE 35.4 Perform a Monofilament Foot Exam

Tasks
Perform a monofilament foot exam to screen for peripheral neuropathy. Give health maintenance coaching by providing foot care instructions. Document test results in the patient's health record.

Equipment and Supplies
- 10-g monofilament tool
- Gloves
- Paper towel
- Provider's order or standing order
- Patient's health record

Procedural Steps
1. Wash hands or use hand sanitizer.
   Purpose: Hand sanitization is an important step for infection control.
2. Read the provider's order. Assemble the equipment.
   Purpose: It is important to know the provider's order before starting the procedure.
3. Greet the patient. Identify yourself. Verify the patient's identity with full name and date of birth. Explain the procedure to be performed in a manner that the patient understands. Answer any questions the patient may have about the procedure.
   Purpose: It is important to identify the patient in two different ways to ensure that you have the correct patient. Explaining the procedure can make the patient feel more comfortable and helps to reduce anxiety.
4. Ask the patient to remove socks and shoes and rest the feet on the paper towel. The paper towel should be placed under the person's feet either on the floor or on the exam table step.
   Purpose: This prepares the patient for the test.
5. Using your hand, demonstrate that the monofilament is flexible and not sharp. Also demonstrate the monofilament on the patient's hand. Put gloves on.
   Purpose: This alleviates the patient's anxiety. Demonstrating on the patient's hand allows the patient to know how it feels.
6. Instruct the patient to close his or her eyes. Tell the patient to say "yes" when he or she feels the monofilament on the foot.
   Purpose: The patient's eyes must be closed for this test to be accurate.
7. Start with the great toe and place the monofilament perpendicular to the skin. Press the monofilament until it bends, hold for 1 second, and release (Fig. 1). Pause to give the patient an opportunity to confirm it was felt. A confirmation is a positive or normal response. The test result is abnormal if the patient cannot feel in one area.
   Purpose: It is important to hold the monofilament for 1 second for accurate results.

PROCEDURE 35.4 Perform a Monofilament Foot Exam—cont'd

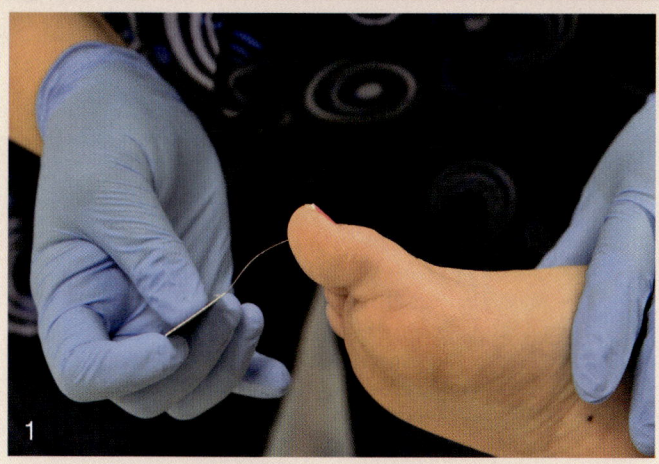

1

8. Do not cue the patient if no confirmation is given. Just move to the next location. Randomly test 9 to 12 locations on the anterior and posterior side of each foot or as the provider indicates (Fig. 2). If a patient does not feel the site, check it three times randomly. Make sure to space out testing times (e.g., the time between each check).
   Purpose: If the test is done in a rhythmic way, the patient may confirm the feeling without really feeling the test.

9. Discard supplies in the waste container. Remove gloves and wash hands.
   Purpose: Washing hands is important for infection control.

10. Coach patient on proper foot care to prevent sores. Include when to check feet, what to look for, and how to care for feet daily. Suspicious areas need to be watched carefully and reported to the provider if they do not return to normal.
    Purpose: Carefully monitoring can help prevent serious foot sores.

11. Document the test results in the patient's health record. Include the provider's name, the order, and the results of the test. For the test, the first number indicates the total number of sites felt, and the last number indicates the total times done. Indicate all sites where the patient did not feel the test. Include any teaching done.
    Purpose: It is important to document the patient education in the health record to show it was done.

07/19/20XX 1625 Per Dr. Kahn's order, performed a monofilament exam on both feet. Right foot 9/12 and left foot 12/12. Right posterior great toe 0/3. Pt coached on foot care. Stressed daily foot care and inspections. Pt listed the foot care he needs to do daily. He indicated what and where on his feet he needs to examine daily. All his questions were answered. The "Feet Guide for Neuropathy" brochure was given to the patient ——————
—Suzanne Peterson CMA (AAMA)

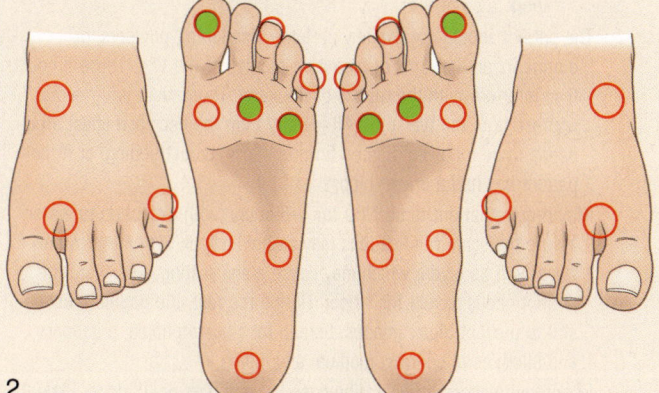

2

COACHING ON DIAGNOSTIC TESTS

It is important for the medical assistant to provide the necessary teaching for diagnostic and laboratory tests ordered for patients. For tests to be completed, the patient needs to be prepared. Some tests require fasting, whereas others do not. The medical assistant needs to provide answers to these questions:
- What is the test?
- Where does the patient need to go for the test? When is the test scheduled?
- Does the test require fasting? If so, for how long? If no foods or beverages can be consumed, does this include water?
- Should patients continue or stop taking their medications? This may require a discussion with the provider.

> **MEDICAL TERMINOLOGY**
> **bi/o:** life, living
> **hem/o:** blood
> **-occult:** secret or hidden

> **CRITICAL THINKING 35.7**
> Sometimes Suzanne has a patient who refuses to follow the preparation steps for a diagnostic test. How might you handle this situation?

It is important to give patients the correct answers. Table 35.8 provides information on common imaging procedures. Table 35.9 summarizes several medical laboratory tests. Remember, patient preparation may vary based on the facility.

COACHING ON TREATMENT PLANS

Many facilities have the medical assistants meet with the patients after the providers finish. The medical assistants review the treatment plan with the patients. They answer any questions, explore any issues the patients may have, and provide additional instructions. As mentioned, this type of coaching has been shown to increase patients' compliance to the treatment plans. Additionally, it provides patients with a lifeline should they have questions or concerns at home.

TABLE 35.8 Common Patient Instructions for Imaging Procedures

Imaging Procedure	Description	Common Patient Instructions
X-ray	X-ray particles pass through the body, and an image is recorded. Many different types of x-rays.	Provide overview of test and why it is being done. Screen for pregnancy. X-rays are painless, though some body positions may be uncomfortable. Patients may be asked to hold their breath during the procedure to get a clear x-ray.
Computed tomography scan (CT scan, CAT scan)	Uses x-rays to create pictures of cross sections of the body. Several types of CT scans exist; each may have different preparations. Patient will lie on a narrow table that slides into the center of the CT scanner. The x-ray beam will rotate around the patient, creating separate images (slices) of the body.	Provide overview of test and why it is being done. May require an intravenous (IV) or oral contrast medium. If so, • Check allergies (contrast medium and iodine). • Check if patient has kidney disease or is on dialysis. • Nothing by mouth (NPO) for 4–6 hours before test. • Address if medications need to be stopped. • IV contrast medium may cause a slight burning feeling and a metallic taste in the mouth; flushing can occur.
Magnetic resonance imaging (MRI)	Uses powerful magnets and radio waves to create the images of the body. Does not use radiation. Several types of MRIs exist; may have different preparations. Patient will lie on a table. The machine makes loud noises. No metal is allowed in the room.	Provide overview of test and why it is being done. May require contrast (see CT scan contrast medium information). • May require being NPO for 4–6 hours • Must identify if patient is *claustrophobic* (afraid or anxious of close spaces). • Due to strong magnets, must screen for artificial heart valves, brain aneurysm clips, heart pacemaker or defibrillator, cochlear (inner ear) implants, recent artificial joint, vascular stents, or history of working with metal. • Must remove all metal from patient including removable dental work (e.g., plates).
Mammography	An x-ray picture of the breasts, used to find tumors. The breast will be compressed on a flat surface for the x-ray.	The patient should not use any perfume, deodorant, powders, or ointments on the arms or breast on the day of the test. These products may interfere with the results of the x-ray. The patient will need to undress from the waist up. All jewelry from the neck and chest area needs to be removed. Screen for pregnancy, breastfeeding, or if the patient has had a breast biopsy.
Positron emission tomography (PET) scan	Imagining test that uses an IV radioactive substance (tracer) to identify disease in the organs and tissues. Patient will lie on a table that slides into the tunnel shaped PET scanner.	May require patient to be NPO for 4–6 hours (with exception to water) before the scan. Medications may be held (check with the provider). IV tracer will be given, which may cause a sharp sting. Afterward the patient needs to rest for 1 hour. During the test, the patient must lie still to prevent blurry images. Screen for claustrophobia, pregnancy, and allergies to contrast medium and iodine.
Ultrasound (US)	Uses high-frequency sound waves to create the image of the organs and structures.	May require special preparation based on the type of US done. Patient will need to expose the area. A clear, water-based gel is applied to the skin, and a transducer (handheld probe) moves over the area.

Medical assistants coach patients on treatments to do at home. These could include taking medications, caring for casts and splints, applying hot or cold therapy, and using assistive devices. Besides these treatments, the medical assistant may also need to help coordinate the patient's care for additional treatments such as physical, occupational, or massage therapies. This section focuses on common treatments and important information for patients to know.

Medication Administration at Home

It is important for patients to know how to take medications at home. This includes when to take medications and how to take them. Do the medications need to be taken on an empty stomach? Can they be taken with the other medications? Do they need to be taken at bedtime? Some patients are on a lot of medications. It is important that the medications are taken correctly.

When updating the patient's current medications list, it is common to find discrepancies. The patient can be taking the medication differently than how it was ordered. Any discrepancy found needs to be communicated to the provider. The medical assistant may coach the patient on the proper ways to take medication. Sometimes the medical assistant may need to help patients find ways to remember to take medications. Many patients use medication boxes that they, a family member, or a pharmacy set up. The boxes typically are arranged for 7 days a week with one or more boxes per day (Fig. 35.10). The medications are placed in each box based on the administration time. Some have boxes for morning, noon, and night medications.

If patients are receiving injections at home, they will need to know how to safely dispose of the needles. Patients can dispose of needles in biohazard sharps containers. These containers are available at local pharmacies and medical supply stores. An internet search can identify local sites that take biohazard sharps containers from patients. Some drug companies have mail-back programs for specific medications. (For more information, visit https://safeneedledisposal.org.) Box 35.18 describes how patients can discard medications at home.

Casts and Splints

Splints and casts are applied to immobilize joints and bones after injury or surgery. A *splint* consists of a strip of rigid material that immobilizes

TABLE 35.9 Patient Instructions for Common Medical Laboratory Tests

Medical Laboratory Test	Use	Common Patient Preparation
Creatinine	Used to monitor kidney health and disease.	May need to fast overnight. May need to refrain from eating meat for a period of time, as it could increase the creatinine level.
Guaiac fecal occult blood test (gFOBT)	Fecal specimen exam to detect occult or hidden blood, which may indicate gastrointestinal (GI) bleeding. Intestinal bleeding may be an indicator of colon cancer.	Seven days prior to the test: • Stop taking aspirin and nonsteroidal anti-inflammatory medications (e.g., ibuprofen, naproxen, and indomethacin). • Do not take vitamin C supplements. Three days before the test: • Do not eat red meat and raw fruits or vegetables (like horseradish, turnips, broccoli, melons, and radishes). Stool samples are collected over several days, and cards are prepared and sent to the laboratory.
Fecal immunochemical test (FIT)	Fecal specimen exam to detect human hemoglobin protein, which may indicate GI bleeding.	No preparation required. Stool sample is collected by the patient and sent to the laboratory.
Cologuard stool DNA test (FIT-DNA)	Used to detect blood in the stool. Computer analysis looks at the DNA in the stool, checking for cancer and precancerous cells.	Stool sample is collected by the patient and returned to a specific medical laboratory for testing.
Glucose tests	Used to determine the blood glucose level.	For a fasting glucose test, the patient needs to be NPO (with exception to water) for at least 8 hours. Other glucose tests may require fasting and eating at specific times.
Lipid profile	Used to monitor cholesterol levels and treatment.	May require NPO (with exception to water) prior to the test.
Pap test	Used to screen for cervical cancers and some uterine or vaginal infections.	Do not schedule the test during the menstrual period. For 48 hours prior to the test: • Refrain from sexual intercourse. • Do not use vaginal creams or foams. For 24 hours prior to the test: • Do not douche or tub bathe.

an extremity. It provides partial protection while the site heals. The splint can be adjusted as the swelling changes. Ready-made splints and custom-designed splints are used in the ambulatory care environment. Ready-made splints usually have Velcro straps, which assist when taking off or putting on the splints. Custom-designed splints are used with elastic bandages. Casts provide additional protection to the injured area. Casts are made from fiberglass or plaster. Table 35.10 describes the advantages of both types of casts. The medical assistant can help the provider apply the cast and the custom-designed splints. The medical assistant can remove casts.

It is important for the patient to learn how to care for the cast:
- Cover the cast with a plastic bag prior to bathing or showering. If the cast gets wet, use a hair dryer on a cool setting to dry a fiberglass

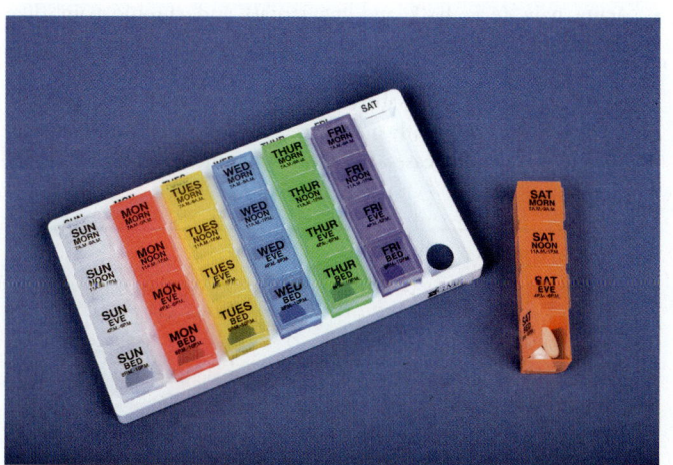

FIG. 35.10 Daily medication boxes can help patients remember to take their medications.

BOX 35.18 Discarding Medications at Home

It is important to encourage patients to discard expired, unwanted, or unused medications. This will help prevent misuse and theft. To get rid of controlled substances, take the medications in their original prescription bottles to a medicine take-back facility. Usually, Drug Enforcement Administration (DEA) representatives are available to take control of the controlled substances. Another option is to contact a DEA-authorized collector. The DEA's website has more information on both programs (https://www.deadiversion.usdoj.gov).

If these programs are not available, some medications are labeled with specific disposal instructions. Many times the label recommends flushing controlled substances down the sink or toilet. The website for Food and Drug Administration (FDA) contains a complete list of medications that can be discarded by flushing (www.fda.gov).

If the label does not indicate flushing, then mix the medications in an unpalatable substance (dirt, used coffee grounds, or kitty litter). Place the mixture in a plastic bag. Seal and throw in the household trash. Make sure all personal information and the prescription number have been scratched out on empty pill bottles.

TABLE 35.10 Advantages of Both Types of Casts

Fiberglass Casts	Plaster Casts
Weighs less than plaster	Cheaper than fiberglass
More durable and porous, allowing air flow	Easier to shape
Can be used during x-rays	
Colorful	

TABLE 35.11 CSMT Normal and Abnormal Findings

	Normal	Abnormal
Color	Color of extremity and nail beds should match the opposite extremity. Should be pink.	Pale or bluish skin.
Sensation	Normal sensation. Should be able to feel light touch on the fingers or toes.	Increased pain, burning, or stinging; "asleep" feeling or pins-and-needles sensation or numbness. Unable to feel light touch.
Motion	Movement of toes and fingers are normal. There should be no swelling.	Unable to move toes or fingers on the casted side. Swelling on injured side.
Temperature	Temperature matches the opposite extremity. Should be warm.	Cold or cooler than the opposite extremity.

BOX 35.19 Those at Risk for Tissue Injury

These patients are at higher risk for tissue injury with hot or cold applications:
- Younger children because of their thinner skin.
- Older adults due to their decreased sensitivity to pain.
- People with impaired circulation (e.g., those with peripheral vascular diseases and diabetes mellitus).
- People with altered sensitivity (e.g., those who are confused or have neurologic disorders including diabetic neuropathy and spinal cord damage).
- Those who have the application placed on an open wound, broken skin, or stoma. This tissue is more sensitive.
- Those who have the applications placed on edematous or scarred areas. Scars and edema reduce sensitivity.

---

cast. If the cast does not dry or if it becomes smelly or moldy, contact the provider.
- Avoid putting weight or pressure on the cast.
- Do not put anything inside the cast including sharp objects, powder, or lotion.
- A metal file can be used to smooth down rough sections of a fiberglass cast.
- A sling can be used to help support a casted arm.

It is also important to treat the recent injury, if applicable. The extremity should be elevated and iced to minimize swelling. If the extremity swells too much for the size of the cast, compartment syndrome can occur. The swelling of the casted extremity can cause damage to the muscles, blood vessels, and nerves. The damage can be permanent if not treated. It is important to teach patients about checking the color, sensation, motion, and temperature (CSMT) of the casted extremity. Table 35.11 describes CSMT normal and abnormal findings. Any suspicious abnormal findings should be reported to the provider immediately.

Cold and Hot Therapy

Cold and hot are therapeutic *modalities* (moe DAL i tee) or treatments used for orthopedic injuries and infections. The applications can be dry or moist. Dry means no moisture is left on the skin; whereas moist leaves moisture on the skin. Dry applications tend to pull moisture out of the skin. Moist applications tend to increase tissue elasticity and penetrate the heat or cold deeper into the tissues.

In some facilities, it is a common practice to provide an ice pack to a patient who comes in with a recent injury. When using hot or cold applications, the medical assistant should ask the patient if it feels too hot or too cold. The medical assistant should monitor the area being treated. Some patients are more prone to tissue injury (Box 35.19). Prolonged erythema or paleness, pain, swelling, and blisters should be reported to the physician.

Many times, the medical assistant must coach patients on the use of hot and cold applications. It is important to address the following:
- Know what supplies are required and where they can be purchased.
- Use a protective covering between the skin and the application.
- Never fall asleep with an application on the skin.
- Never place an application over metal jewelry.
- Know the length of time for each application, the number of times a day ordered, and the number of days for treatment.
- Hot and cold therapy should be applied for 15 to 20 minutes. Additional time can harm the tissues.
- After the session, remove the application. Allow the skin to return to the normal temperature before applying again.

Cold Therapy. Cold therapy is typically used for sprains, strains, fractures, joint injuries, shin splints, and other injuries. A cold application causes vasoconstriction (VAY zoe kahn strik shuhn), which reduces blood flow to the area. As a result, tissue metabolism decreases, less oxygen is used, and less waste accumulates. The nerve endings in the area become numb. The blood viscosity increases, which causes clotting. Cold therapy helps to reduce pain and inflammation and prevents *edema* (swelling) in the area. Table 35.12 describes common types of cold applications. Procedure 35.5 describes how to apply a cold pack.

Heat Therapy. Heat therapy can be used to relieve the following:
- Acute pain (e.g., back and menstrual) and chronic pain (like arthritis)
- Sinus congestion
- Infection (e.g., localized abscesses)

Heat therapy can help with muscle relaxation. It can produce local vasodilation, which increases circulation. The increased blood supply

---

VOCABULARY

compartment syndrome: A serious condition that involves increased pressure, usually in the muscles; which leads to compromised blood flow and muscle and nerve damage.

vasoconstriction: Contraction of the muscles causing the narrowing of the inside tube of the vessel.

stoma: A temporary or permanent surgically created opening used for drainage (i.e., urine, stool).

TABLE 35.12 Types of Cold Applications

Type	Dry or Moist	Description	Uses
Cold compress	Moist	Washcloth or other soft cloth is wet by a cold solution (e.g., water) and applied to the skin.	Usually used on the face and forehead for discomfort and pain.
Chemical cold pack	Dry	Comes in a variety of sizes. Stored at room temperature. Contains inner areas of a dry chemical and water. When activated, the water and chemical mix creates coldness.	Used to decrease inflammation, prevent edema, reduce bleeding, and decrease pain.
Ice bag	Dry	A bag with cubes or pieces of ice.	A towel or protective covering needs to be placed between the skin and the pack or bag. This protects the skin from a burn or from the cold.
Gel pack	Dry	Aqueous gel that freezes. Reusable. Stored in freezer (Fig. 35.11).	
Bead pack	Dry	Little beads of gel conform to the site even when frozen. Similar to a frozen bag of peas. Reusable. Stored in freezer (see Fig. 35.11).	

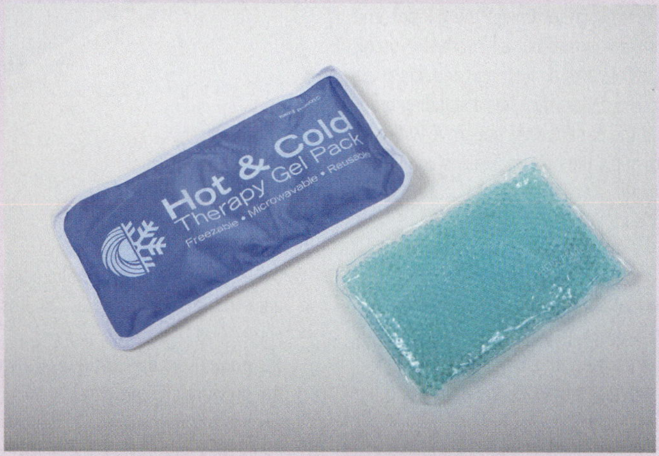

FIG. 35.11 Cold and hot gel and bead packs.

to a local area helps to absorb the extra fluid (from edema). Table 35.13 discusses the types of hot applications. Additional types of heat therapy will be discussed.

Paraffin bath therapy. Paraffin provides deep heat therapy. The heat can reduce pain and tenderness. It has been found to maintain muscle strength and increase mobility. Paraffin therapy is a common treatment for arthritis and other conditions that cause pain and stiffness.

A paraffin bath uses melted paraffin and mineral oil warmed to about 125°F. The patient bathes a foot or hand in the bath. Once the extremity is coated, the patient should lift it out and let it dry for a few seconds (Fig. 35.12). This process is repeated until the patient has 10 to 12 layers of wax built up on the extremity. The foot or hand is then wrapped in plastic and then a towel to retain the moisture and heat. After 20 minutes, it is unwrapped and the wax is removed.

Heat lamp therapy. Infrared heat lamps are red-colored near-infrared bulbs. The rays penetrate the body, killing pathogens and healing tissue. Pathogens such as bacteria, viruses, and parasites cannot withstand heat. These pathogens can be killed with infrared heat lamps. Red infrared heat lamp therapy can also improve circulation and oxygenation of tissues. This therapy may help wounds heal faster.

Ultrasound Therapy

Ultrasound therapy has been used for a long time to treat pain and promote healing. The ultrasound transducer head produces sound waves. Ultrasound gel is applied to the skin. As the transducer head is moved over the skin, the gel helps with the transmission of sound waves into

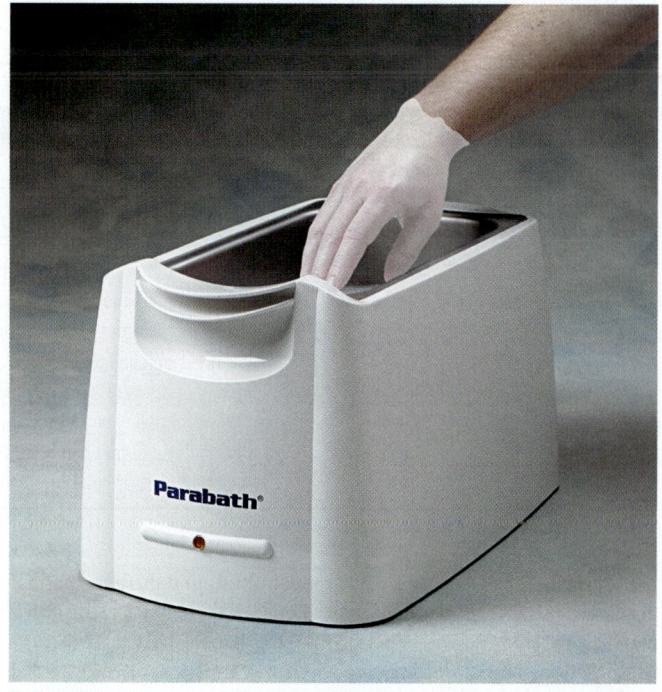

FIG. 35.12 A paraffin bath. (From Proctor D, et al: *Kinn's The Medical Assistant,* ed 13, St. Louis, 2017, Elsevier.)

PROCEDURE 35.5 Apply a Cold Pack

Tasks
Apply a cold pack (chemical, gel, or bead) to a body area to reduce pain and prevent further swelling per treatment plan. Document the procedure in the patient's health record.

Equipment and Supplies
- Cold pack (chemical, gel, or bead)
- Towel or another type of protective covering for the cold pack
- Provider's order or standing order for orthopedic injuries
- Patient's health record

Scenario
You are working with Dr. David Kahn. Johnny Parker (DOB: 06/15/2010) arrives holding his arm and crying. Another medical assistant brings the patient and parent to the exam room. The medical assistant comes out and updates you on Johnny. His parent states that Johnny fell off his bike an hour ago and has since been complaining of pain in his right wrist. The department has a standing order to apply a cold pack to orthopedic injuries if the patient does not arrive with one in place. The medical assistant asks you to apply the cold pack as he completes the vital signs and medical history on Johnny.

Procedural Steps
1. Wash hands or use hand sanitizer.
   Purpose: Hand sanitization is an important step for infection control.
2. Read the standing order or the provider's order. Assemble the equipment. If using a chemical cold pack, activate the pack by squeezing it.
   Purpose: It is important to know the provider's order or the standing order before starting the procedure.
3. Greet the patient. Identify yourself. Verify the patient's identity with full name and date of birth. Explain the procedure to be performed in a manner that the patient understands. Answer any questions the patient may have about the procedure.
   Purpose: It is important to identify the patient in two different ways to ensure that you have the correct patient. Explaining the procedure can make the patient feel more comfortable and helps to reduce anxiety.
4. Cover the cold pack with a towel or protective covering.
   Purpose: The cold pack must never be put directly on the skin. Place a towel or protective covering between the cold pack and the skin to prevent injuries.
5. Assist the patient to position the cold pack over the injured area (Fig. 1).
   Purpose: Some patients like to place the cold pack themselves on the injured area.

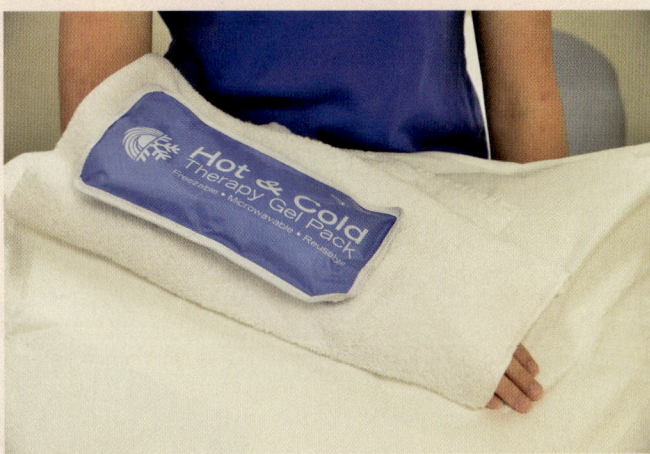

6. Coach patient on the use of a cold pack. Advise the patient to leave the cold pack in place for 15 to 20 minutes or until the area feels numb, whichever comes first.
   Purpose: Cold applications are typically applied for 15 to 20 minutes or per the provider's order.
7. Document the procedure in the patient's health record. Include the provider's name, the order, what was taught, and how the patient responded.
   Purpose: It is important to document the procedure in the health record to show it was done.
   07/19/20XX 1505 Pt arrived holding right wrist and complaining of pain. Parent stated that he fell off his bike about 1 hour ago. Per Dr. Kahn's standing order, applied cold pack to pt's right wrist. Instructed pt and parent to keep the cold pack (covered with a towel) on the wrist for 15–20 minutes. Parent stated she would remove it at that time. Suzanne Peterson CMA (AAMA)

TABLE 35.13 Types of Hot Applications

Type	Dry or Moist	Description	Uses
Hot soak/whirlpool bath	Moist	Part of the body is submerged into warm water or a warm medicated solution. Should be warmed to 105°–110°F.	Used to cleanse wounds. Helps to ease discomfort.
Hot compress	Moist	Washcloth or other soft cloth is wet by a hot solution (e.g., water) and applied to the skin.	Can be used on many places on the body including the face and eyes.
Heating pad	Dry	Electric pad that warms. Inspect for safety purposes.	Used for spasms and pain.
Chemical hot pack	Dry	Comes in a variety of sizes. Stored at room temperature. Contains inner areas of a dry chemical and water. When activated, the water and chemical mix, creating heat for a period of time.	Must be covered with a towel or protective covering.
Gel pack	Dry	Aqueous gel that can be microwaved. Reusable (see Fig. 35.11).	
Bead pack	Dry	Little beads of gel that can be microwaved. Reusable (see Fig. 35.11).	

the soft tissue. There are two main types of ultrasound therapy: thermal and mechanical. The main difference between these types is the speed at which the sound waves penetrate the soft tissue. Ultrasound therapy must be done by a trained therapist. This treatment is often provided in chiropractic, sports medicine, physical therapy, and occupational therapy facilities.

RICE Therapy

For orthopedic injuries, RICE is commonly ordered as a treatment for usually the first 48 to 72 hours. After 72 hours, moist heat is prescribed for ankle sprains. RICE stands for rest, ice, compression, and elevation:
- *Rest:* Reduce activities for a period of time. Crutches can help an injured leg/ankle rest.

- *Ice*: Apply a cold pack to the injured area for 15 to 20 minutes, 4 to 8 times daily. Always use a protective covering between the cold pack and the skin to prevent a cold injury or frostbite.
- *Compression*: Use elastic wraps or splits to reduce swelling. It is important to monitor the CSMT of a wrapped extremity.
- *Elevation*: Elevate the injured extremity higher than the level of the heart, to help decrease swelling.

Exercise Therapy

Often patients are encouraged to exercise to maintain their strength and joint mobility. For patients recovering from surgery (e.g., orthopedic, cardiac), they may need to see a physical therapist or an occupational therapist. These therapists work with patients to regain their mobility and strength. Range-of-motion, isometric, and isotonic exercises are encouraged to maintain strength, flexibility, and mobility.

Range of motion (ROM) means the normal movement allowed by the joint. ROM exercises help to maintain flexibility and joint mobility. Patients are encouraged to do ROM exercises to reduce stiffness. For patients who have had a stroke or other trauma that impacts movement, ROM exercises are critical to prevent joints from freezing up. Frozen joints have limited to no movement. It is important to exercise joints each day. *Active ROM exercises* are done by the patient, whereas *passive ROM exercises* are done by a caregiver or therapist.

Isometric (i so MEH trick) contractions do not change the muscle length, but they do increase the muscle tension. Pushing against the wall causes isometric contractions. *Isotonic* (i so TON ick) contractions cause movement at a joint. The muscle usually shortens and thickens. Examples of isotonic contractions occur with walking, lifting weights, and running.

Electrical Muscle Stimulation. A transcutaneous electrical nerve stimulation (TENS) unit is used for pain relief (Fig. 35.13). Electrodes are placed on the skin in specific locations. The adjustable low-voltage machine sends electrical current through disposable gel electrodes into the skin. The current stimulates specific nerves, producing a tingling or massaging sensation that reduces pain. TENS units have been used for passive exercise of muscles when a patient cannot exercise the extremity (e.g., due to injury or stroke). The electrical stimulation can prevent atrophy of normal muscles. TENS units are also used to treat the pain from muscle, joint, or other orthopedic conditions.

> **VOCABULARY**
> **electrodes:** Adhesive patches that conduct electricity from the body to the machine wires (e.g., ECG and transcutaneous electrical nerve stimulation [TENS] unit).

Complementary Therapies

Complementary therapies are used together with conventional medicine. For instance, massage and chiropractic care are considered complementary therapies. Sometimes people will use the term *alternative*, but that means the therapy is being used instead of conventional medicine. Most patients using complementary therapies will also see their healthcare provider.

Massage Therapy. Massage ranges from light stroking to deep rubbing. Pressure is applied to a person's skin and muscles. Studies have shown that massage reduces stress, pain, and muscle tension. Massage is performed by massage therapists, who are specially trained in the procedures. There are several types of massage:
- *Deep massage*: Used to help with muscle damage from injuries. Slower more forceful massage is done to the muscles and connective tissues (e.g., tendons and ligaments).

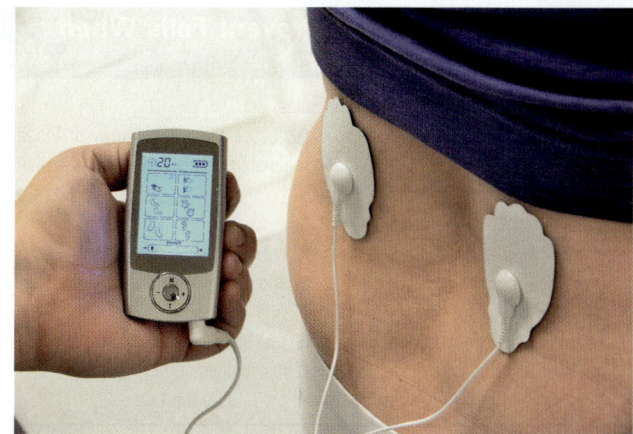

FIG. 35.13 A transcutaneous electrical nerve stimulation (TENS) unit.

- *Swedish massage*: Used to relax a person. Involves a gentle massage of long strokes and deep circular movements that can energize the individual.
- *Sports massage*: Used on athletes to help prevent or treat injuries. The technique is similar to the Swedish massage.
- *Trigger point massage*: Used to help with muscle damage from injury or overuse. Involves a focused massage on tight muscles.

Chiropractic Care. Chiropractic care focuses on the relationship between the spine and the function of the body. The goal is to correct alignment problems and thereby alleviate pain, improve function, and support the body's natural ability to heal itself. Spinal manipulation has been shown to be beneficial for low back pain, headaches, neck pain, whiplash-associated disorders, and upper and lower extremity joint conditions.

Chiropractic doctors have at least 4 years of additional training beyond a bachelor's degree. The training includes both classroom and direct patient care. The doctors must pass the national licensing exam. State law regulates their practice, and many state boards require continuing education to maintain the license.

Acupressure and Acupuncture. Both acupressure and acupuncture have been practiced for thousands of years. Acupressure involves applying firm pressure on specific points on the body. Acupuncture involves inserting fine needles into *acupuncture points* (specific sites on the body). The needles may be removed quickly or left in for longer periods of time. Acupressure and acupuncture are used to treat a wide range of symptoms including pain, nausea, neuropathy, anxiety, depression, and sleep disturbance.

Assistive Devices

An *assistive device* is used to help a person perform a specific task, such as walking. Crutches, walkers, canes, and wheelchairs are considered assistive devices. Many times these assistive devices can be purchased at pharmacies and medical supply stores. The medical assistant should know how to adjust the device to fit the patient. Medical assistants may also coach patients on the proper use of the assistive device. Improper use of assistive devices can lead to falls and injuries (Box 35.20).

> **CRITICAL THINKING 35.8**
> Suzanne has had to teach patients about assistive devices. She discusses ways to prevent falls and how to transfer between different positions. Why are both of these topics important to address?

BOX 35.20 Ways to Prevent Falls When Using Assistive Devices

- Wear shoes with rubber or nonskid soles.
- Remove items in the walkway that can cause falls (e.g., throw or loose rugs, cords, and clutter). Small indoor animals may also cause falls if they are near the person's feet.
- Make sure that floors are clean and dry.
- When sitting, back up until the seat touches the back of the legs. With a free hand, grab the seat or armrest and lower yourself into the chair or onto the toilet.
- To stand, scoot forward in the chair and use the free hand to push up from the seat to stand up. Make sure to get your balance before moving.
- Consider adding handrails inside of the tub and by the toilet.

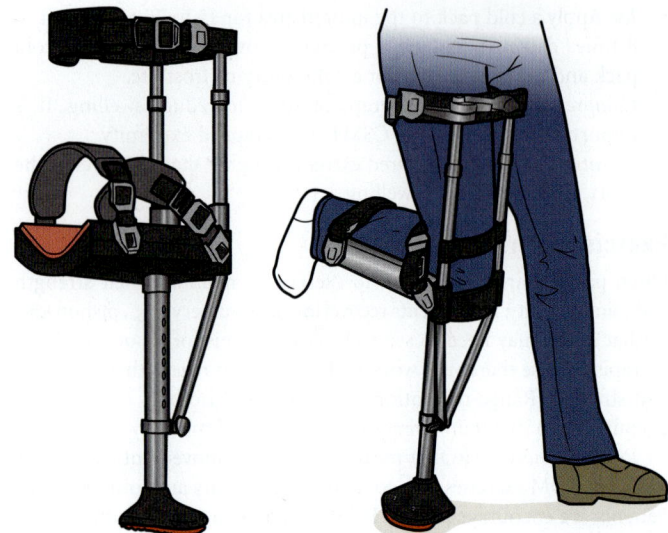

FIG. 35.15 A hands-free crutch.

BOX 35.21 To Fit Axillary Crutches

The patient must be wearing shoes. Have patient stand straight up. Fit the crutches so they are 1 to 1½ inches (about 2 finger-widths) below the armpit. The crutch should be about 4 to 6 inches to the side and front of each foot. Handgrips must be near the wrist and even with the top of the hip line. When the hands are on the handgrip, the elbow should be bent 15 to 30 degrees.

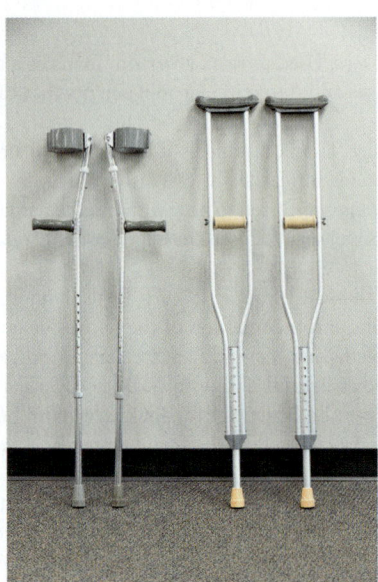

FIG. 35.14 *(From left to right)* Forearm crutches (also called Lofstrand or elbow crutches) and axillary crutches.

Crutches. Crutches are used to help a person walk. Crutches can be made out of aluminum or wood. They need to be adjusted for the patient's size. Crutches come in a variety of sizes to fit young children and adults. Over the years, many types of crutches have been developed. The more common crutches include the following:

- *Axillary crutches*: Most common type; used when recovering from a foot, ankle, or leg injury or surgery (Fig. 35.14).
- *Forearm crutches*: Also called Lofstrand or elbow crutches; require more upper body strength. An open elbow cuff fits around the patient's forearm (see Fig. 35.14). These crutches help with proper posture and body mechanics.
- *Extension crutches*: Also called Canadian crutches. These combine the underarm crutch with an elbow cuff, which provides extra support for the patient.
- *Platform crutches*: Also called triceps crutches. These have padded armrests with handgrips. These crutches are used when patients cannot straighten their arms to hold the handgrip of the crutch.
- *Hands-free crutch*: Straps to the thigh and a platform supports the lower leg (Fig. 35.15).

Using axillary crutches. Axillary crutches need to be fitted correctly to allow for good body mechanics and to decrease the risk of injury (Box 35.21). *Crutch palsy* can occur with poorly fitted crutches or if the patient rests on the top of the crutches while walking. The axillary nerves can be temporarily or permanently damaged. This can cause loss of hand strength and weakening of the wrist and forearm muscles.

Providers will indicate the type of crutch, along with any limitations. Common limitations with crutches include the following:

- *Weight bearing as tolerated*: Patients can place more than half of their body weight on their "bad" or affected extremity if it is not painful.
- *Partial weight bearing*: The provider will indicate how much weight can be placed on the affected extremity.
- *Toe-touch weight bearing*: Patients can touch the ground with their toes on the affected side. The toe-touch helps with balance. No weight bearing is allowed on the affected extremity.
- *Non weight bearing*: Patients cannot put weight on their affected extremity. This type of limitation would require the three-point crutch gait.

There are several *gaits* or ways to walk with crutches. The provider may also order the gait. The gait depends on whether the patient can put weight on the affected extremity. The following are common gaits:

- *Two-point crutch gait*: Mimics normal walking. The patient must be able to put some weight on both legs. From the **tripod position** (starting position) use this sequence: move the right crutch with left foot forward and then move the left crutch with the right foot forward. There are two individual movements with this gait. Repeat this pattern (Fig. 35.16A).
- *Four-point crutch gait*: Must be able to put some weight on both legs. This gait is slower, but safer for those with generalized weakness. From the tripod position use this sequence: move the right crutch forward, then the left foot forward, followed by the left crutch forward, and lastly bring the right foot forward. There are four individual movements with this gait. Repeat this pattern (Fig. 35.16B).

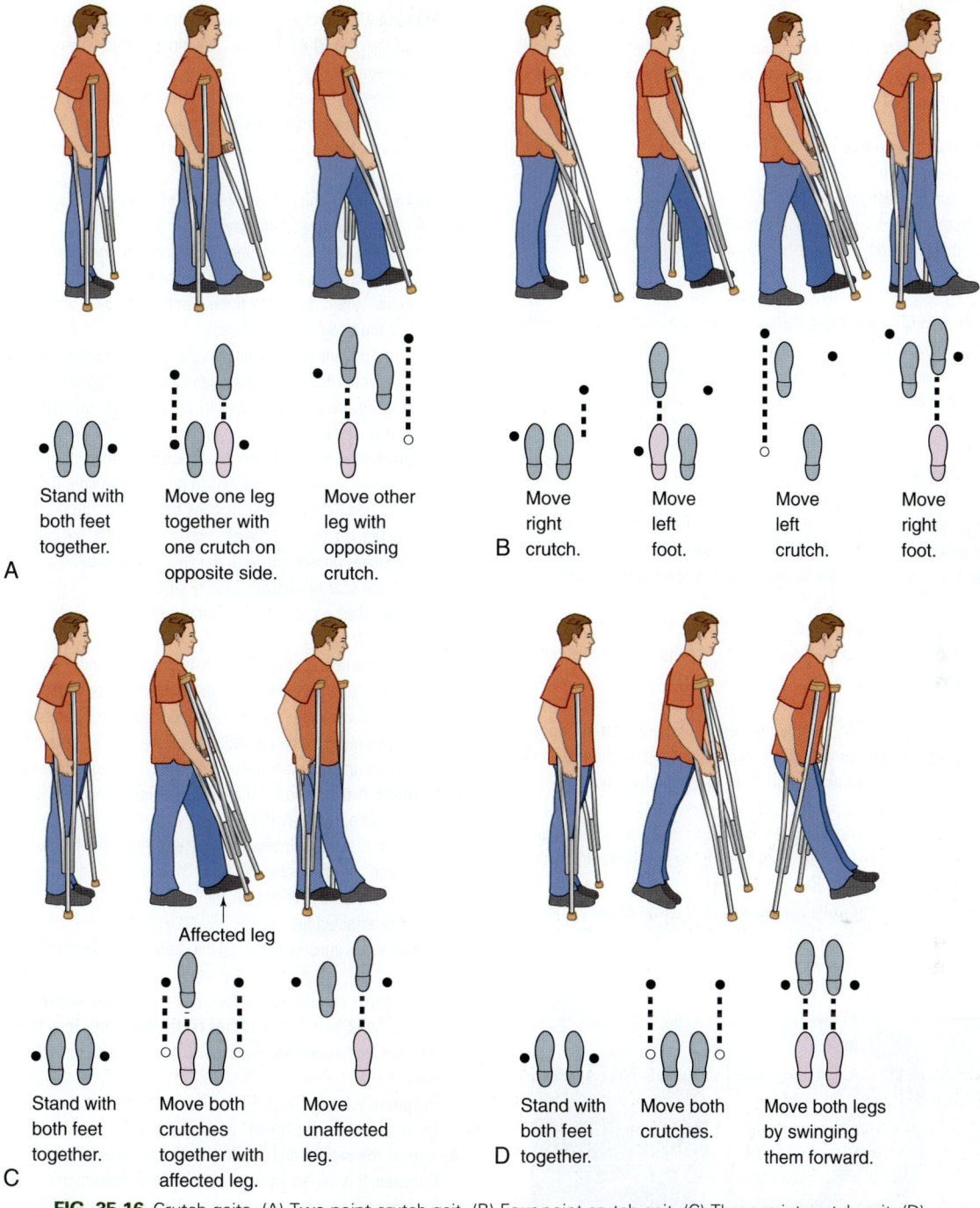

FIG. 35.16 Crutch gaits. (A) Two-point crutch gait. (B) Four-point crutch gait. (C) Three-point crutch gait. (D) Swing through gait. (From Proctor D, et al: *Kinn's The Medical Assistant*, ed 13, St. Louis, 2017, Elsevier.)

- *Three-point crutch gait*: Used when partial weight bearing or non weight bearing is indicated. From the tripod position, use this sequence: Move both crutches and the affected leg forward, then move the "good" or unaffected leg forward. Repeat this pattern (Fig. 35.16C and Procedure 35.6).
- *Swing to crutch gait*: Must be able to put some weight on both legs. From the tripod position, use this sequence: move both crutches forward, then swing the body so the feet are *even with* the line of the crutches. Repeat this pattern.
- *Swing through crutch gait*: Must be able to put some weight on both legs. From the tripod position, use this sequence: move both crutches forward, then swing the body so the feet land *in front* of the line of the crutches. Repeat this pattern (Fig. 35.16D).

> **VOCABULARY**
> **tripod position**: The standing position when using crutches; crutch tips are 4 to 6 inches to the side and front of each foot.

Walkers. Some patients use walkers after surgery. Many older adults use walkers for help with balance and support. Walkers provide more support than canes (Box 35.22). A walker's wide base helps stabilize

PROCEDURE 35.6   Coach a Patient to Use Axillary Crutches

Tasks
Fit crutches to the patient. Coach the patient to use crutches properly while considering the patient's developmental life stage. Document your teaching in the patient's health record.

Equipment and Supplies
- Axillary crutches
- Handout on crutch walking (optional)
- Provider's order
- Patient's health record

Scenario
You are working with Dr. David Kahn. He has ordered you to teach Daniel Miller (DOB: 3/21/2012) how to use axillary crutches. Daniel broke his left leg, and his treatment plan requires that he not bear weight on the left leg for 6 weeks. Daniel's bedroom is on the second floor, so he has to learn how to use crutches on the stairs also.

Procedural Steps

1. Wash hands or use hand sanitizer.
   Purpose: Hand sanitization is an important step for infection control.
2. Read the provider's order. Assemble the equipment.
   Purpose: It is important to know the provider's order before starting the procedure.
3. Greet the patient. Identify yourself. Verify the patient's identity with full name and date of birth. Explain the procedure to be performed in a manner that the patient understands. Answer any questions the patient may have about the procedure.
   Purpose: It is important to identify the patient in two different ways to ensure that you have the correct patient. Explaining the procedure can make the patient feel more comfortable and helps to reduce anxiety.
4. Ensure the patient is wearing shoes, and ask the patient to stand up straight. Assist as needed. Fit the crutches to the patient so they are 1 to 1½ inches (about 2 finger-widths) below the armpit (Fig. 1). The crutch should be about 4 to 6 inches to the side and front of each foot.
   Purpose: Pressure in the axilla can cause crutch palsy. Adjust the length on the crutches as needed.

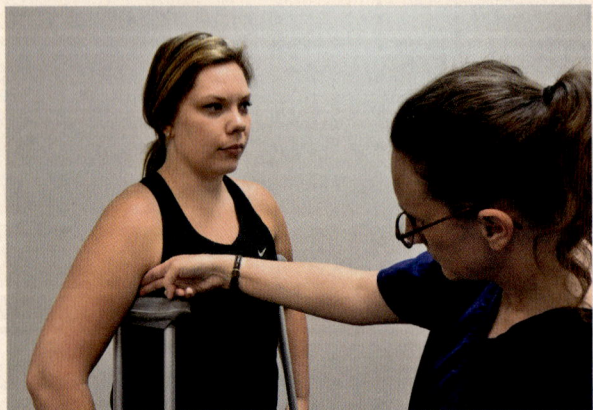

5. Adjust the handgrips so they are near the patient's wrist and even with the top of the hip line. This should allow for a 15- to 30-degree bend in the elbow when the patient's hands are on the handgrip.
   Purpose: This position allows for the most strength with the hands.
6. Coach the patient using strategies appropriate for the patient's developmental stage. Encourage discussion and questions. Use concrete terms when explaining the procedure. Show simple pictures.
   Purpose: Coaching a child requires strategies that are simple and concrete. Encourage the child to ask questions, which helps to clear up any misconceptions.
7. Using age-appropriate language, instruct the patient to keep the injured leg as relaxed as possible. The knee should be slightly bent, and the patient should look forward when walking. Instruct the patient not to bear weight on the axilla.
   Purpose: For a child, it is important to keep your language simple and to demonstrate what you are saying.
8. Have the patient start in the tripod position and then move the crutches about 12 inches in front of his or her body (or less for a child).
   Purpose: When doing the three-point crutch gait, placing the crutches in front of the body is the first step.
9. Have the patient put his/her weight on the crutches and move the body forward. Finish the step by having the patient swing the "good" or unaffected leg forward. Do not place weight on the "bad" or affected leg. Continue with these steps.
   Purpose: Placing weight on the affected extremity may harm the leg.
10. *To sit down:* Instruct the patient to do the following: Back up to the chair, toilet, or bed until the seat touches the back of the legs. Move the "bad" or affected leg forward, balancing on the "good" or unaffected leg. Hold both crutches on the side with the "bad" or affected leg. Use the free hand to grab the seat or armrest. Slowly sit down.
    Purpose: Backing up until the seat touches the back of the legs is important to prevent falls.
11. *To stand up:* Instruct the patient to do the following: Move toward the front of the seat and move the "bad" or affected leg forward. Hold both crutches on the side with the "bad" or affected leg. Use the free hand to push up from the seat to stand up. Balance on the "good" or unaffected leg while placing a crutch in each hand. Balance is needed before moving.
    Purpose: If the person is unstable, the risk of falling is greater. Stand still until balance is achieved.
12. *To go up the stairs:* Instruct the patient to do the following: Step up with the "good" or unaffected leg first. Then bring the crutches up, one in each arm. Finally place weight on the "good" or unaffected leg and bring the "bad" or affected leg up.
    Purpose: It is important to go up the stairs, start with the "good" or unaffected leg.
13. *To go down stairs:* Instruct the patient to do the following: With a crutch in each hand, place the crutches on the first step. Then move the "bad" or affected leg forward and down. Lastly, follow with the "good" or unaffected leg.
    Purpose: When going down stairs, the crutches then the "bad" or affected leg come before the "good" or unaffected leg.
14. Instruct the patient and family on ways to prevent falls.
    Purpose: It is important to also educate the patient on how to prevent falls.
15. Document the patient education in the patient's health record. Include the provider's name, the order, what was taught, how the patient responded, how the patient did the demonstration, and any handouts provided.
    Purpose: It is important to document the patient education in the health record to show it was done.

07/21/20XX 1423 Per Dr. Kahn's order, pt fitted with crutches and taught with his mother on the 3-point crutch gait. They were told of the non-weight-bearing limitation on the left leg × 6 wks. Pt was able to correctly walk 20 feet using the 3-point gait. He was able to walk up and down the stairs safely with crutches. Pt was also taught to sit down and get up from a chair. Pt demonstrated the techniques correctly. Pt's mother was given the crutch booklet. All their questions were answered, and mother was given a follow-up number for additional questions ———————— Suzanne Peterson CMA (AAMA)

BOX 35.22 Examples of Options for Walkers

Some walkers can have additional options that include a seat, basket, food tray, and platform walker attachment (Fig. 35.17). The platform attachment is designed for a patient who has limited strength and cannot grip the walker. An adjustable strap secures the patient's forearm onto the padded section of the attachment.

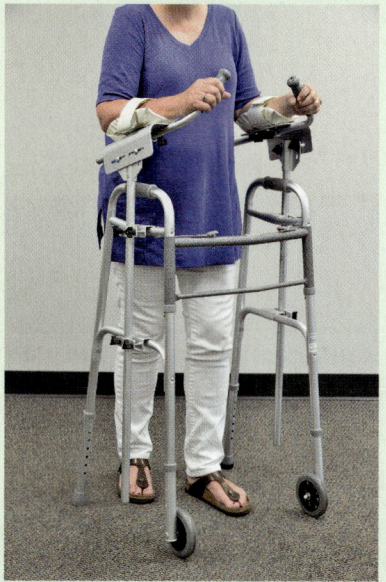

FIG. 35.17 The platform walker attachment is designed for patients who are unable to grip the walker. This walker has two platform attachments.

BOX 35.23 To Fit a Standard Walker

The patient must be wearing shoes. Have the patient step into the walker. Relax the arms at the side of the body. The top of the walker grip should be near the crease in the wrist and even with the top of the hip line. With the shoulders relaxed and the hands on the grips, the elbows should be bent 15 degrees.

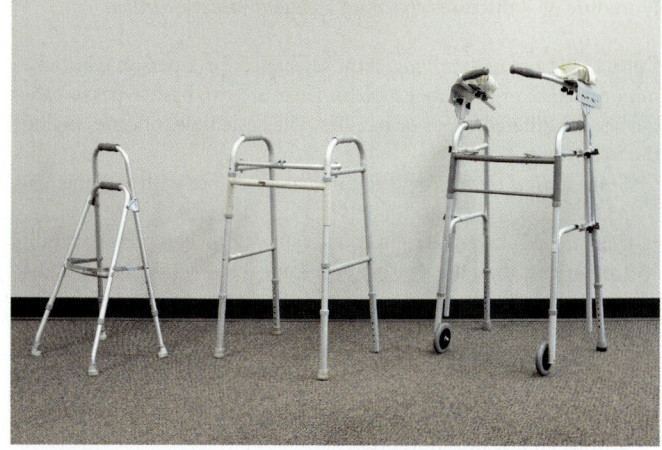

FIG. 35.18 *(From left to right)* A hemi walker, standard walker, and two-wheel walker with platform walker attachments.

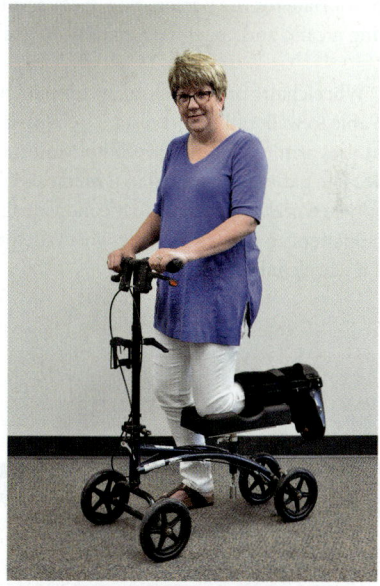

FIG. 35.19 Knee walker.

the gait of the patient and can support up to 50% of the body weight. Walkers are made of aluminum and can easily be adjusted to fit an individual (Box 35.23). They are lightweight and several types can fold flat for storage and travel. Several types of walkers are available:

- *Standard walker*: A very common walker; has four nonskid, rubber-tipped legs (Fig. 35.18). A person needs to pick up the walker with every completed step. Sometimes tennis balls are inserted over the feet to help move the walker easily across the floor.
- *Two-wheel walker*: Resembles the standard walker, but the front two legs have wheels. This type of walker is for those who need some help but not constant weight-bearing help (see Fig. 35.18).
- *Three-wheel walker* and *four-wheel walker*: Also called a *rollator*. Each leg has a wheel, and many rollators have brakes by the handles. Some models have a seat and a basket. These walkers are for people who do not need to lean on a walker for balance.
- *Knee walker*: A foot-propelled scooter that has platform to rest a knee and lower leg (Fig. 35.19). This is commonly used instead of axillary crutches for leg or foot conditions.
- *Hemi walker*: Also called a one-hand walker. These walkers are used by patients who can only grasp the walker with one hand due to a stroke or arm/hand amputation (Fig. 35.20).

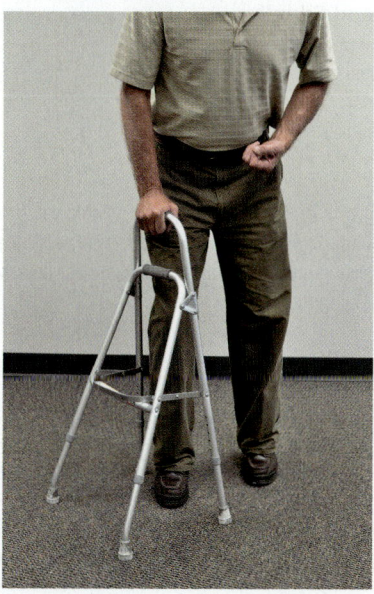

FIG. 35.20 A hemi walker is also called a one-hand walker.

Procedure 35.7 discusses coaching a patient to use a walker.

Canes. A cane can provide extra assistance for a person who has a minor balance or stability problem. There are two basic types of canes but several different grips or handles. The basic types of canes include the following:
- *Single-tipped cane*: Provides minimal assistance with walking (Fig. 35.21).
- *Four-tipped cane*: Also called quad cane. It provides greater stability for patients than the single-tipped cane (see Fig. 35.21).

The grip or handle can come in several styles. Some of the more common handles include the following:
- *Offset handle*: Usually used if the person has an issue that impacts mobility (see Fig. 35.21).
- *Tourist handle*: Very popular and the handle can be placed on the arm when it is not in use (see Fig. 35.21).
- *Orthopedic handle*: Has an easy to grip design and provides more hand comfort.

Tingling, numbness, or pain in the hand and fingers may indicate the handle is not appropriate for the person. Box 35.24 and Procedure 35.8 discuss measuring a cane and coaching a patient to use a cane.

Wheelchairs. Wheelchairs provide mobility for patients who cannot walk or who are able to walk only short distances. With a regular wheelchair, the patient uses arm muscles for mobility. Motorized wheelchairs are also available. The patient is referred to a medical equipment store, where the appropriate wheelchair is fitted to the individual. It is important to encourage the patient to always lock the wheels before transferring into and out of a wheelchair.

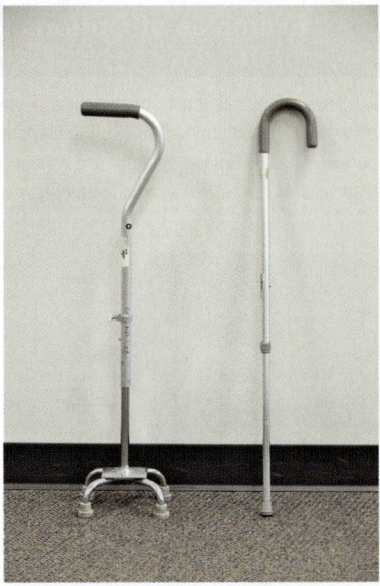

FIG. 35.21 *(From left to right)* A four-tipped cane with an offset handle and a single-tipped cane with a tourist handle.

CARE COORDINATION

Care coordination provides personalized patient- and family-centered care in a team-based environment (Box 35.25). It ensures the patient's needs and preferences for healthcare services are met. The care

---

PROCEDURE 35.7 Coach a Patient to Use a Walker

Tasks
Fit a standard walker to the patient. Coach patient to use a standard walker properly while considering the patient's communication barrier and developmental life stage. Document teaching in the patient's health record.

Equipment and Supplies
- Standard walker
- Walker handout (optional)
- Provider's order
- Patient's health record

Scenario
You are working with Dr. David Kahn. He has ordered you to teach Jana Green (DOB: 5/1/1936) how to use a standard walker. Jana needs the walker for extra stability. She has a hearing impairment. She can hear best with her right ear. She has no hearing in the left ear.

Procedural Steps
1. Wash hands or use hand sanitizer.
   Purpose: Hand sanitization is an important step for infection control.
2. Read the provider's order. Assemble the equipment.
   Purpose: It is important to know the provider's order before starting the procedure.
3. Greet the patient. Identify yourself. Verify the patient's identity with full name and date of birth. Explain the procedure to be performed in a manner that the patient understands. Answer any questions the patient may have about the procedure.
   Purpose: It is important to identify the patient in two different ways to ensure that you have the correct patient. Explaining the procedure can make the patient feel more comfortable and helps to reduce anxiety.
4. Face the person when speaking. Position yourself so your voice is directed toward the patient's good ear. Use a low-pitched voice and speak clearly, slowly, and distinctly. Speak naturally. Limit medical terminology as you speak.
   Purpose: It is important to speak naturally and do not shout. Listen to the patient, and follow what he or she states works the best with the impairment.
5. Use simpler language when talking. Speak clearly. Communicate with dignity and respect. Allow time for the patient to respond. Listen to the patient's concerns.
   Purpose: When working with older patients, it is important to show respect and to value their dignity. Listening is important.
6. Ensure the patient is wearing shoes, and ask the patient to step into the walker. The top of the walker grip should be even with the top of the hip line and near the crease in the wrist, when the arms are at the side of the body. Adjust as needed. Keeping the shoulders relaxed and the hands on the grips will ensure the elbows are bent at a 15-degree angle (Fig. 1).
   Purpose: For body mechanics, it is important to have the walker adjusted to fit the person. Using a walker that is too tall or too short can cause stress

PROCEDURE 35.7 Coach a Patient to Use a Walker—cont'd

on the upper shoulders and back. A person should not lean over to walk, as this increases the risk of falls.

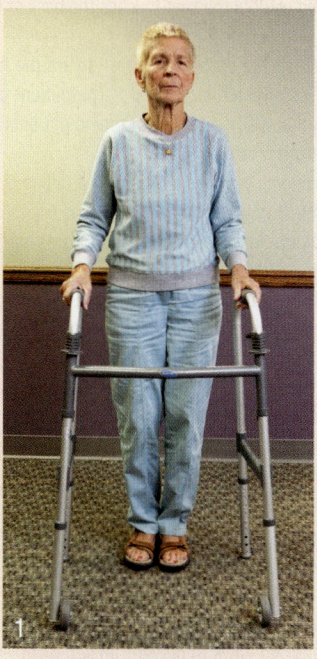

7. Have the patient place the walker one step ahead of his or her body. Instruct the patient to use the "bad" or affected leg to step into the walker. The patient should not touch the front bar with the leg. Have the patient step forward with his or her other leg to complete the step. The patient will continue with this pattern while holding up the head and looking forward.
Purpose: Being too close to the front bar can impact the patient's stability.

8. *To sit down:* Instruct the patient to back up to the chair, toilet, or bed until the seat touches the back of the legs. The patient can then use one hand to grab the seat or armrest and slowly sit down.
Purpose: Backing up until the seat touches the back of the legs is important to prevent falls.

9. *To stand up:* Instruct the patient to move toward the front of the seat. Have the walker in front of the person. Have the patient use one hand to push up from the seat to stand up and then place hands on the walker. Remind patients to make sure they have their balance before moving.
Purpose: If the person is unstable, the risk of falling is greater. It is important to stand still until balance is achieved.

10. Instruct the patient on ways to prevent falls. The walker should never be used on stairs or an escalator. If using a bag on the front of the walker, make sure not to overload it. Make sure to place all four legs on the ground before moving into the walker.
Purpose: It is important to educate the patient on how to prevent falls. Too much weight in the front of the walker may cause it to tilt and the patient to fall.

11. Document the patient education in the patient's health record. Include the provider's name, the order, what was taught, how the patient responded, how the patient did the demonstration, and any handouts provided.
Purpose: It is important to document the patient education in the health record to show it was done.

07/21/20XX 1423 Per Dr. Kahn's order, patient was fitted with a walker and instructed how to use it. Pt was able to walk using the walker correctly. Pt was also able to sit and stand while using the walker. Pt demonstrated techniques correctly and safely. Coached patient on safety issues with the walker and how to decrease the risk of falls. Pt was able to verbalize four ways to prevent falls when using the walker. All the pt's questions were answered. Pt was given the walker booklet to take home. Suzanne Peterson CMA (AAMA)

BOX 35.24 To Fit a Cane

The patient must be wearing shoes. Relax the arms at the side of the body. The top of the cane should be near the crease in the wrist. With the shoulders relaxed and the hand on the cane, the elbow should be bent 15 degrees.

BOX 35.25 Advantages of Care Coordination

- Greater efficiency with providing patient care
- Reduced costs
- Greater patient care
- Individualized patient guidance and services
- Encourages patients to focus on goals and self-management
- Decreases hospital emergency department visits and readmissions

coordinator communicates between the patient and healthcare team. Care coordinators ensure patients get timely care and do not fall through the cracks. In the ambulatory care setting, care coordination can be set up in different ways. It has been shown to be successful in primary and specialty care areas. The overall goals include:

- Help patients understand why and what services are needed
- Schedule and sequence appointments
- Provide instructions and directions to patients
- Ensure that test results are available to the providers during patient appointments
- Communicate patient needs and concerns to providers

A **patient navigator** (also called patient advocate) has been described as a type of care coordinator. The navigator program was established at the Harlem Hospital Center in 1990. The goal was to assist cancer patients in accessing quality healthcare. Based on the success of patient navigators, the Patient Navigator, Outreach and Chronic Disease Prevention Act of 2005 funded additional positions. Today, patient navigators typically guide chronically ill patients through the healthcare system. They identify patients' financial, cultural, physical, and emotional barriers. Then, they work closely with the healthcare team and the patients to ensure barriers are eliminated and patients get timely care.

> **VOCABULARY**
> **patient navigator**: A person who identifies patients' barriers, works closely with the healthcare team and patients, and guides the patients through the healthcare system; may also be called a patient advocate.

PROCEDURE 35.8 Coach a Patient to Use a Cane

Tasks
Fit a cane to a patient. Coach the patient to use a cane. Document teaching in the patient's health record.

Equipment and Supplies
- Cane
- Handout on cane walking (optional)
- Provider's order
- Patient's health record

Scenario
You are working with Dr. David Kahn. He has ordered you to teach Ella Rainwater (DOB: 7/11/1959) how to use a cane. Ella has left side weakness.

Procedural Steps

1. Wash hands or use hand sanitizer.
   Purpose: Hand sanitization is an important step for infection control.
2. Read the provider's order. Assemble the equipment.
   Purpose: It is important to know the provider's order before starting the procedure.
3. Greet the patient. Identify yourself. Verify the patient's identity with full name and date of birth. Explain the procedure to be performed in a manner that the patient understands. Answer any questions the patient may have about the procedure.
   Purpose: It is important to identify the patient in two different ways to ensure that you have the correct patient. Explaining the procedure can make the patient feel more comfortable and helps to reduce anxiety.
4. Ensure the patient is wearing shoes. The top of the cane should be near the crease in the wrist, when the arms are at the side of the body. Adjust as needed. With the patient's shoulders relaxed and hand on the cane, ensure the elbow is bent at a 15-degree angle.
   Purpose: For body mechanics, it is important to have the cane fitted correctly.
5. Instruct the patient to hold the cane on the "good" or unaffected side. The patient should take a step moving the "bad" or affected leg and the cane forward at the same time and then step forward with the "good" leg. Instruct the patient to lean on the cane as needed.
   Purpose: The cane is held on the "good" or unaffected side so it can provide added support to the opposite leg.
6. *To sit down:* Instruct the patient to back up to the chair, toilet, or bed until the seat touches the back of the legs. The patient can then use a hand to grab the seat or armrest and slowly sit down.
   Purpose: Backing up until the seat touches the back of the legs is important to prevent falls.
7. *To stand up:* Instruct the patient to move toward the front of the seat and move the "bad" or affected leg forward. The patient can then use a hand to push up from the seat to stand up. Remind patients to make sure to get their balance before moving.
   Purpose: If the person is unstable, the risk of falling is greater. Instruct the patient to stand still until balance is achieved.
8. *To go up the stairs:* Instruct the patient to step up with the "good" or unaffected leg first while holding onto the rail. Then the patient should bring up the "bad" or affected leg to the same step. If there is no handrail, the cane and the "bad" leg should be placed on the stair at the same time.
   Purpose: It is important to go up the stairs, starting with the "good" or unaffected leg.
9. *To go down stairs:* Instruct the patient to hold onto the rail and move the "bad" or affected leg down first. Then the patient should place the "good" or unaffected leg on the same step as the "bad" leg. When there is no handrail, instruct the patient to place the cane on the lower step, then place the "bad" or affected leg, and lastly place the "good" or unaffected leg next to the "bad" or affected leg.
   Purpose: When going down stairs, the cane and then the "bad" leg come down first, followed by the "good" leg.
10. Instruct the patient on ways to prevent falls.
    Purpose: It is important to also educate the patient on how to prevent falls.
11. Document the patient education in the patient's health record. Include the provider's name, the order, what was taught, how the patient responded, how the patient did the demonstration, and any handouts provided.
    Purpose: It is important to document the patient education in the health record to show it was done.

07/25/20XX 1105 Per Dr. Kahn's order, pt was fitted with a cane and was instructed on walking with a cane, doing stairs, and sitting/standing. Pt was able to walk about 30 feet with a cane correctly. Pt was able to safely walk up and down and sit/stand while using the cane. Pt's questions were answered. Pt was given the "Using a Cane" booklet. Suzanne Peterson CMA (AAMA)

BOX 35.26 Possible Areas Involved With Care Coordination

- Interview patients to identify their needs and barriers to wellness and healthcare.
- Provide patients with resources based on their needs and barriers.
- Schedule and sequence appointments.
- Make sure the required information is communicated to and from specialty departments.
- Assist with reducing language barriers by identifying bilingual providers and translators.
- Discuss special needs patients have with their healthcare team.
- Identify community resources, which may include the following:
  - Transportation and medical equipment
  - Adult daycare, assistive living, and long-term care
  - Educational programs and support groups
  - Low-cost medication programs
  - Low-cost preventive screening and immunizations

In the ambulatory care setting, medical assistants can be care coordinators. A person must have strong interpersonal skills to be successful as a care coordinator. The medical assistant must listen to the patient and family to identify their needs and concerns. The care coordinator must be compassionate, yet provide firm guidance with patients who are difficult. Box 35.26 describes the possible areas involved with care coordination. Procedure 35.9 describes the process of creating a current list of community resources and referring patients or family members.

EXCEPTIONAL CUSTOMER SERVICE

Just by the design, care coordination helps provide patients with individual assistance. Patients who feel well cared for and who feel comfortable talking with their healthcare team stay with their provider. It is estimated that care coordination will increase in popularity in the coming years. This model of care will also promote exceptional customer service in healthcare.

CHAPTER 35 Patient Coaching With Health Promotion

PROCEDURE 35.9 Develop a List of Community Resources and Facilitate Referrals

Tasks

As a patient navigator, develop a current list of community resources that meet the patient's healthcare needs. Discuss the resources with the patient and facilitate referrals to the chosen resources.

Equipment and Supplies

- Computer (with internet) or a telephone book
- Paper and pen
- Community Resource Referral Form or referral form
- Patient's health record

Scenario 1

Robert Caudill (DOB: 10/31/1940) was just diagnosed with dementia. He currently lives with his daughter, Ruby, who works full time. Ruby is feeling overwhelmed with being his only caregiver and realizes that she needs to find someone to care for her father while she is working.

Scenario 2

Leslie Green just tested positive for pregnancy. She is still a teenager and does not feel that she has a support system to help her make decisions.

Scenario 3

Ella Rainwater's husband of 30 years died suddenly 1 month ago. Ella (DOB: 07/11/1959) stated that she feels alone and has no one to talk to. Her daughter feels that she needs the support of others who have gone through the same thing.

Directions

Role-play these scenarios with two peers.

Procedural Steps

1. Using the scenarios, identify the possible types of community resources that would assist each patient or family. Identify three different types of resources (e.g., medical equipment, support group) that would meet each patient's needs.
   Purpose: A variety of community resources are available for patients and families who are dealing with chronic illnesses and death. The types of resources range from daycare, meals, transportation, medical equipment, assistive living, support groups, and reduced costs for medications.

2. Using the internet or the phone book, identify two local resources for each of the three kinds of resources (i.e., find two assistive living resources, two medical equipment suppliers, etc.). Make a list of six resources for the patient and family. Include the following:
   a. Organization's name
   b. Address and contact information
   c. Summary of the services provided
   d. Cost and other relevant information
   Purpose: As the patient navigator or care coordinator, it is important for you to provide patients and families with the contact information for various community resources. This information can help the family find the best solution for the situation.

3. *Role-play the scenario indicated by the instructor.* Provide the patient or family member with the list of six resources. Describe the services offered and any costs.

4. Allow the patient or family member time to review the services. Answer any questions.
   Purpose: Complete the referral form to facilitate the referral to community resources.

5. Use professional, tactful verbal and nonverbal communication as you work with the patient or family member.
   Purpose: Patients and family members are more apt to respond positively to assistance if the medical assistant's communication is professional, empathic, and tactful. Talking down to patients or acting superior are unprofessional behaviors that negatively impact the working relationship with patients.

6. *Role-play making the community referrals:* Have the patient or family member decide on two or more services they are interested in. Complete the referral document. Have the patient provide any additional information required on the form. Call the community resource agency, and provide the referral information to the representative (a peer).
   Note: Some community referrals (e.g., support groups) will require the patient to make contact and not the healthcare professional.
   Purpose: The referral document is used by many organizations to capture the patient's preferences and to help process the referral.

7. Document the patient education and the referrals in the health record.
   Purpose: It is important to document all patient interactions and referrals in the health record.

CLOSING COMMENTS

It is an exciting time to become a medical assistant. The medical assistant's role is changing to meet healthcare needs. Studies have shown that medical assistants play an important role in coaching and helping patients comply with treatment and lifestyle changes. It is important for the medical assistant to coach the patient in a manner that helps the patient understand and retain the information. Adapting the coaching to the patient's communication barriers, developmental stage, and cultural practices will help the patient complete with the treatment plan.

CHAPTER REVIEW

This chapter focused on coaching patients and coordinating care. It is helpful for the medical assistant to understand why patients may not always comply with the treatment plan. When a patient is diagnosed with a life-changing condition, the person can experience grief. It may take some time before the person complies with the recommended treatments. In other situations, the health belief model helps healthcare professionals understand why a person may or may not make the recommended lifestyle changes. Factors including the perceived risks and severity of the disease, along with the barriers and the benefits of prevention impact the compliance.

There are three domains of learning: cognitive, psychomotor, and affective. For each domain, specific teaching strategies are used. For instance, the psychomotor domain includes learning new skills. Demonstration and return demonstration are teaching strategies that can be used for this domain. Along with the domains come barriers to learning. These barriers must be overcome or the medical assistant must adapt to these barriers to help the patient learn the content.

Besides adapting coaching for the barriers to learning, a medical assistant must also consider the patient's developmental level and cultural diversity. Erikson's psychosocial developmental stages help a medical assistant understand the developmental goals for different ages. Specific coaching techniques can be used to teach patients of different developmental stages. Cultural diversity is all around us. Knowing general cultural practices for the populations typically seen in the ambulatory care setting is important. Adapting coaching to meet a person's cultural practice will increase the compliance with the treatment plan. For this to occur, the medical assistant must be open and respectful with the patient. It is important for the medical assistant to ask questions and then help the patient incorporate the changes into his or her lifestyle.

Medical assistants can provide coaching to patients in these areas:
- *Coaching on disease prevention*: Examples include discussing good hygiene practices, recommended vaccinations, preventing STIs, and nicotine (tobacco) cessation.
- *Coaching on health maintenance and wellness*: Examples include self-exams and information related to specific screenings.
- *Coaching on diagnostic tests*: Patients need to be aware of what to expect and how to prepare for tests.
- *Coaching on treatment plans*: Patients need to be instructed on home medication administration, therapies, and assistive devices. Proper coaching will help patients adhere to the treatment plan.
- *Coaching on community and healthcare resources:* Through care coordination or healthcare navigation, the medical assistant has the opportunity to provide information about community resources that will help the patient. The medical assistant can also help the patient to navigate through the maze of healthcare services required. It is important to listen and ask questions to identify where the patient needs extra assistance and support. Knowing about the community resources will then allow the medical assistant to match the patient's needs to the resources. Providing this information to the patient, allowing the patient to decide what resources would be helpful, and then assisting with referrals as needed are all part of care coordination.

SCENARIO WRAP-UP

During Suzanne's yearly review with her supervisor, she mentioned that she was interested in becoming a care coordinator. She and the supervisor discussed how the program might assist the providers and patients. Suzanne agreed to research the role and bring a proposal to her supervisor in the coming weeks. The supervisor would then take it to the provider meeting and discuss the care model with all of the WMFM providers. Both were excited to pursue new changes in the practice and continue to provide patients with the best possible care.

36

Patient Coaching With Nutrition

LEARNING OBJECTIVES

1. Describe metabolism.
2. Describe dietary nutrients including carbohydrates, protein, fat, minerals and electrolytes, vitamins, water, and fiber. Also, define the function of dietary supplements.
3. Explain current dietary guidelines.
4. Describe how to read a food label.
5. Do the following related to medically ordered diets:
   - Describe the different types of medically ordered diets.
   - Identify the special dietary needs for weight control, diabetes, cardiovascular disease, and hypertension.
   - Identify the special dietary needs for those with food allergies, celiac disease, and lactose intolerance.
6. Identify special dietary needs for those with various conditions, including pregnancy and lactation, epilepsy, HIV and AIDS, and cancer.
7. Describe eating disorders.
8. Instruct a patient on dietary changes while demonstrating awareness of others' concerns.

CHAPTER OUTLINE

1. **Opening Scenario,** 834
2. **You Will Learn,** 834
3. **Introduction,** 834
4. **Metabolism,** 834
5. **Dietary Nutrients,** 834
   a. Carbohydrates, 835
      i. *Glycemic Index,* 836
   b. Protein, 836
   c. Fat, 837
   d. Minerals and Electrolytes, 837
   e. Vitamins, 838
   f. Water, 838
6. **Dietary Guidelines,** 840
   a. MyPlate, 840
   b. Dietary Guidelines, 840
7. **Reading Food Labels,** 840
8. **Medically Ordered Diets,** 842
   a. Clear Liquid Diet, 842
   b. Full Liquid Diet, 842
   c. Soft and Mechanical Soft Diet, 842
   d. Bland Diet, 843
   e. Weight Control Diet, 843
   f. Diabetic Eating Plans, 843
   g. Low-Sodium Diet, 845
      i. *Dietary Approaches to Stop Hypertension,* 845
   h. Heart-Healthy Diet, 845
   i. Low-Protein Diet, 846
   j. High- and Low-Fiber Diets, 846
   k. Elimination Diet and Food Allergies, 846
      i. *Gluten-Free Diet,* 847
   l. Lactose-Intolerance Diet, 847
9. **Nutritional Needs for Various Populations,** 847
   a. Pregnancy and Lactation, 847
   b. Epilepsy, 847
   c. HIV and AIDs, 847
   d. Cancer, 847
10. **Eating Disorders,** 848
    a. Anorexia Nervosa, 848
    b. Binge Eating Disorder, 849
    c. Bulimia Nervosa, 849
11. **Instructing Patients on Dietary Changes,** 849
    a. Awareness of Others' Concerns, 849
12. **Closing Comments,** 851
13. **Chapter Review,** 851
14. **Scenario Wrap-Up,** 852

OPENING SCENARIO

Kayla Smith, registered medical assistant (RMA), has been working at Walden-Martin Family Medical (WMFM) Clinic for 4 years. She enjoys working with the patients and the providers. Her supervisor is impressed with Kayla's motivation, patient care skills, and attention to detail. Kayla was asked to mentor Tim Brown, a medical assistant student from a local college.

Tim has finished his courses and is now completing his practicum at the clinic. Tim has an interest in nutrition, as his mother is a registered dietitian. He is eager to see how Kayla works with patients who have dietary changes. He hopes he will have the opportunity to observe her and then assist with the teaching process before doing it by himself.

YOU WILL LEARN

1. To identify dietary nutrients including carbohydrates, fat, protein, minerals/electrolytes, vitamins, fiber, and water.
2. To describe the function of dietary supplements.
3. To distinguish the special dietary needs of those with diabetes, cardiovascular disease, hypertension, cancer, and lactose sensitivity.
4. To identify the special dietary needs for a person with allergies or celiac disease.
5. To instruct a patient according to the patient's special dietary needs.
6. To show awareness of a patient's concerns regarding a dietary change.

INTRODUCTION

Nutrition is a field of study that examines the substances in food that help us grow and stay healthy. Nutrition can also be defined as the intake of food for the body's dietary needs. It is important to eat a healthy and balanced diet. *Nutrients* are the chemicals in food that the body uses for energy, growth, and development. Nutrients include water, protein, carbohydrate, fat, vitamins, and minerals.

A medical assistant helps the provider by instructing patients on dietary changes. It is important to be aware of nutrients and different types of diets commonly ordered in the ambulatory care environment. This chapter discusses *metabolism* (me TAB oh lizm) and nutrients essential for growth and development. Dietary requirements along with medically ordered diets are also discussed.

METABOLISM

Metabolism is the process the body uses to obtain or make energy from the food eaten. Metabolism has two phases:
- *Catabolism* (kah TAB oh lizm): the process of breaking down molecules into smaller molecules resulting in energy being released
- *Anabolism* (ah NAB oh lizm): the process of smaller molecules being used to build larger molecules with the use of energy

For example, you eat a piece of chocolate candy with peanuts. It is broken down by enzymes (EN zimes) in the intestines. The enzymes break down the proteins into amino (ah ME noe) acids, the fats into fatty acids, and the complex *carbohydrates* (KAAR bow hye drate) into simple sugars (e.g., glucose). These substances are absorbed by the blood and brought to the cells. In the cells, other enzymes catabolize or break down these substances, and energy is released. This is catabolism. The energy released can be used or stored by the body. The small molecules created from catabolism are used to create larger molecules as the body repairs tissues and performs other functions. This process requires energy and is called *anabolism*. Every action of the body, involuntary or voluntary, requires energy.

> **VOCABULARY**
> **amino acids**: Released during the digestion of protein foods in the intestines; carried by the blood to cells, where they are used to make proteins. Used for growth, maintenance, and repair of cells; they also transport nutrients.
> **enzymes**: Special proteins that speed up the chemical reaction in the body.
> **fatty acids**: Result when fats are broken down; used by the body for energy and tissue development.
> **glucose**: Results when carbohydrates are broken down; main sugar found in the blood and used as the main source of energy.
> **metabolism**: The chemical process that occurs within a living organism to maintain life.

Many times metabolism is thought of as what influences our bodies to gain or lose weight. This is where calories come in. A *calorie* is a unit that measures how much energy is in a particular food. A chocolate bar has more calories than an apple. So the candy provides more energy to our body than the apple. People use calories or the energy at different rates. Some people eat a lot of food and do not put on any weight, whereas others feel they look at food and gain weight. The number of calories a person burns each day is affected by the following factors:
- How much the person exercises
- The amount of fat and muscle on the person's body
- The person's *basal metabolic rate (BMR)*, or the rate the body burns calories while the person is at rest

BMR can play a role in a person's tendency to gain weight. For example, two people eat and exercise the same amount, but they have two different BMRs (Box 36.1). The person with the lower BMR would have greater tendency to gain more weight. Remember, the body stores unused calories as fat.

DIETARY NUTRIENTS

Nutrients in food, such as carbohydrates, can provide energy. Nutrients can also supply materials to build and repair tissues (e.g., proteins and amino acids). Lastly, nutrients can regulate metabolic processes. Some nutrients have only one purpose, whereas others have several jobs in

> **BOX 36.1 Variables That Impact Basal Metabolic Rate (BMR)**
> - *Genetics*: Some people are born with a higher metabolism.
> - *Gender*: Males have a higher density of lean muscle mass with a lower body fat percentage. This causes a higher BMR.
> - *Age*: BMR decreases with age.
> - *Weight*: The heavier an individual, the higher the BMR.
> - *Body surface area*: This relates to a person's height and weight. The larger the body surface area, the higher the BMR.
> - *Body fat percentage*: The lower a person's body fat percentage, the higher his or her BMR.
> - *Diet*: Starvation and low-calorie diets can decrease the BMR.
> - *Body temperature*: A higher body temperature results in an increased BMR.
> - *External temperature*: The colder the external temperature, the more the body has to provide additional heat to maintain the body's temperature. This increases the BMR.
> - *Thyroxin*: Produced by the thyroid gland, thyroxin can increase the BMR.
> - *Exercise and lean muscle tissue*: Exercise will create lean muscle tissue, which increases the BMR.
> - *Drugs*: Certain drugs, like caffeine, can increase the BMR.

the body. A combination of different foods is necessary to promote health. With a little planning, all the body's needs can be met by a well-balanced diet.

Nutrients can be classified into two different groups. *Essential nutrients* cannot be made by the body and must be in the food eaten. *Nonessential nutrients* are created by the body and do not need to be in food. For example, vitamin D is created from sun exposure on the skin. Foods can also be described as *non-nutrient rich*. This means they lack vitamins, minerals, and fiber. They provide "empty calories" and can cause people to gain weight. Many carbohydrate-rich foods, like desserts, are non-nutrient-rich.

Carbohydrates

Carbohydrate (KAAR bow hye drate) is a nutrient found in our diet. Carbohydrates are used for energy and to regulate protein and fat metabolism. This nutrient encompasses a broad range of simple sugars, starches, and fiber (Table 36.1).

There are many types of simple sugars:
- White sugar (also called sucrose)
- Fructose and glucose found in fruits and vegetables
- Other sugars used in foods, such as corn syrup, high-fructose corn syrup, honey, and lactose (milk sugar)

During digestion, most sugars (except lactose) break down into fructose and glucose. Lactose breaks down into glucose and galactose. Simple sugars are rapidly absorbed and quickly increase blood glucose levels. They provide a quick source of energy.

Starches are called complex carbohydrates. Examples of complex carbohydrates include whole grains, potatoes, pumpkins, squash, beets, lentils, and quinoa (KEEN waah) seeds (Box 36.2). They are digested in the intestine before being absorbed. Complex carbohydrates break down into simple sugars and become a source of energy.

The glucose from the simple sugar and starches increases the blood glucose level. With the help of **insulin** (IN suh lin), glucose is moved out of the bloodstream and into cells; it is then used for energy. Some glucose is stored in the liver and muscles as glycogen. The body uses the stored glycogen between meals and during strenuous exercise. As the blood glucose levels start to drop, **glucagon** works on the liver to release the stored glycogen. Glycogen is released back into the blood and increases the blood glucose levels.

Fiber is different than simple sugars and starches. It can't be digested by the body and thus it doesn't raise the blood glucose level. Fiber passes through the digestive tract. It is called "roughage" and adds bulk to the stool. Fiber can come from food or supplements (Box 36.3). There are two types of fiber:
- *Soluble fiber* dissolves in water and forms a gel-like substance. Soluble fiber helps soften the stool, slows the absorption of sugar, and binds to fatty acids.
- *Insoluble fiber* bulks up the stool and helps to prevent constipation.

It is important to remember that excessive carbohydrates can be converted into fat. Box 36.4 describes good carbohydrate dietary choices.

> **VOCABULARY**
> **glucagon**: A hormone produced by the alpha cells in the pancreas; works on the liver to release glycogen and thereby prevent dangerously low blood glucose levels.
> **insulin**: A hormone produced by the beta cells in the pancreas; moves glucose into the cells so it can be used for energy.

> **BOX 36.2 Whole Grains and Refined Grains**
>
> Foods made from wheat, oats, cornmeal, rice, and barley are grain products. Grains are divided into whole grains and refined grains:
> - *Whole grains*: Use the entire grain kernel (e.g., bran, germ, and endosperm); include whole-wheat flour, cracked wheat (bulgur), whole cornmeal, oatmeal, and brown rice.
> - *Refined grains*: Are milled, and the bran and germ is removed to create a finer texture and longer shelf life. Examples include white flour, de-germed cornmeal, white rice, and white bread. During the milling process, dietary fiber, iron, and many B vitamins are removed. For this reason, most refined grains are *enriched*. This means certain B vitamins and iron are added back to the grains. Fiber is not added back into the product.

TABLE 36.1 Sources of Carbohydrates

Main Types	FOUND IN THESE FOODS		Uses
	Nutrient Rich	Non-Nutrient Rich	
Simple sugars	Fruits Milk, milk products	Desserts (cookies, cakes) Candy, soda Syrups, sugar, honey, and molasses	Quick source of energy
Starches (or complex carbohydrates)	Legumes (LEG yooms) (split pea, beans [kidney, black, garbanzo, and pinto]) Starchy vegetables (corn, green peas, and potatoes) Whole grains (oats, barley, quinoa seeds, and brown rice)	White bread and crackers White rice	Source of energy
Fiber — Soluble	Legumes, oats, barley, fruits (avocados, apples, citrus fruits), carrots, and psyllium	Processed and refined goods	Softens stool; lowers blood glucose level by slowing sugar absorption; lowers low-density lipoprotein (LDL, or bad cholesterol) levels by binding to fatty acids
Fiber — Insoluble	Whole grains (whole wheat and brown rice), vegetables (corn, broccoli, green beans, cauliflower, and potato with skins), nuts and seeds, popcorn, and prunes	Processed and refined goods	Increases the bulk of the stool (helps with constipation)

BOX 36.3 Fiber Supplements

Fiber supplements are usually taken to decrease constipation. They can help a person be "regular". The active ingredient in the supplements can vary between natural and synthetic soluble fiber. Consider the following:
- *Metamucil* (MET ah myoo sil) contains *psyllium* (SIL ee uhm) husk, a natural substance.
- Citrucel contains *methylcellulose* (METH ahl sel yuh lose), a semisynthetic substance.
- Fibercon contains calcium *polycarbophil* (pol ee KAHR bow fil), a synthetic ingredient.

It is important to drink plenty of water when taking fiber supplements. Some fiber supplements have been shown to lower blood pressure, blood glucose, and the risk of heart disease.

BOX 36.4 Smart Carbohydrate Choices

- Eat a variety of whole grains, fruits, vegetables, legumes, and low-fat or nonfat dairy products.
- At least half of all grains eaten should be whole grains.
- Limit processed foods in your diet, especially those with added sugar, salt, and fat.
- Eat enriched refined grains, if eating refined grains.

TABLE 36.2 Glycemic Index (GI) for Foods

Per Serving	GI	Per Serving	GI
Bagel, white frozen	72	Skim milk	32
Bread, whole wheat	71	Apple	39
Tortilla, wheat	30	Banana	62
Gatorade	78	Watermelon	72
Instant oatmeal	83	Peanuts	7

CRITICAL THINKING 36.1

Kayla wants to help Tim review carbohydrates. She asks him to list two foods from each category: simple sugars, starches, and fiber. How would you answer this question?

BOX 36.5 Protein and Disease

Protein malnutrition is seen around the world. This can lead to *kwashiorkor* (KWAH shee ohr kohr). A lack of dietary protein can cause growth failure, loss of muscle mass, anemia, edema and potbelly, skin depigmentation and hair loss, weakening of the circulatory and respiratory systems, decreased immunity, and death.

BOX 36.6 Smart Protein Choices

- Choose lean or low-fat meat and poultry.
- Eat seafood rich in omega-3 fatty acids, such as salmon, trout, herring, Pacific oysters, and Atlantic and Pacific mackerel (see Box 36.7).
- Limit processed meats (e.g., ham, sausage, and deli meats), which contain added salt (sodium).
- Eat unsalted nuts and seeds to keep sodium intake low.

BOX 36.7 Omega-3 Fatty Acids

Omega-3 fatty acids are a group of polyunsaturated fatty acids found in fish (e.g., salmon, herring, halibut, and mackerel) and some nuts and seeds. These fatty acids play a role in reducing blood cholesterol, heart disease risk, inflammation, and depression. Omega-3 fatty acids also increase the effectiveness of antiinflammatory and antidepressant drugs.

Glycemic Index. The *glycemic* (glie SEE mik) index (GI) is a numeric index used to indicate how much a carbohydrate food increases the blood glucose level. The foods are ranked from 0 to 100. Carbohydrates that are rapidly digested, absorbed, and considerably increase the blood glucose level are considered high GI foods (≥70). Low GI foods (≤55) produce a smaller change in the blood glucose level. The goal is to eat more low GI foods to decrease the risk of type 2 diabetes mellitus and heart disease. Low GI foods can also help one to maintain weight loss. Table 36.2 provides examples of the GI of some common foods.

Protein

Protein (PROE teen) is a nutrient in our diet. Proteins are broken down into amino acids. Amino acids can be used as a source of energy in the absence of carbohydrates. They are used to make proteins to help the body do the following:
- Break down food (e.g., enzymes)
- Grow and repair body tissues (e.g., connective tissue, hair, nails, muscles)
- Perform other functions (e.g., those related to hemoglobin, antibodies, and hormones)

Protein and amino acids are considered the building blocks of life. The body needs several amino acids in large enough amounts to maintain good health (Box 36.5). Amino acids are classified into three groups:
- *Essential amino acids*: Cannot be made by the body, thus must come from food eaten throughout the day
- *Nonessential amino acids*: Can be made by the body from essential amino acids or in the normal breakdown of proteins
- *Conditional amino acids*: Usually not essential, except in times of illness and stress

Foods that have all the essential amino acids to support the body are called *complete proteins*. Foods that are considered complete proteins are fish, meat, poultry, dairy products, quinoa seeds, buckwheat, chia (chee ah) seeds, and eggs. Foods that do not contain all the essential amino acids are called *incomplete proteins*. Nuts, legumes, grains, and vegetables are examples of incomplete proteins. Box 36.6 and Box 36.7 describe good food choices for dietary protein.

MEDICAL TERMINOLOGY
anti-: against
glyc/o: sugar, glucose
mal-: bad, poor
poly-: many, much, excessive, frequent

> **CRITICAL THINKING 36.2**
> Kayla wants to help Tim review proteins. She asks Tim to list six foods that contain proteins. How would you answer this question?

> **CRITICAL THINKING 36.3**
> Kayla wants to help Tim review the three types of fats. She asks Tim to describe unsaturated fats, saturated fats, and trans fatty acids. How would you answer this question?

Fat

Fat is an important nutrient in our diet. Fats provide 9 calories per gram; whereas carbohydrates and proteins provide only 4 calories per gram. The body uses fat for the following:
- A source of energy. If glucose is not available for energy, the body will break down fat and the resulting ketones are used for energy.
- Healthy skin and hair.
- Vitamin absorption. Vitamins A, D, E, and K are fat soluble.
- Insulation (cushion) for organs and keeps our body warm.
- Brain development, controlling inflammation, and blood clotting. Linoleic and linolenic acid, which are essential fatty acids, are used for these processes.

Fat is required in the diet. Table 36.3 describes the types of fats found in foods. Diets low in fats can cause cold sensitivity, increased infections, and amenorrhea in women. Long-term fat deficiency can lead to metabolic problems and fat-soluble vitamin deficiency.

Triglycerides are another type of fat in the body. Our livers make triglycerides from the calories we do not use. Triglycerides are also found in foods. Box 36.8 discusses the risks associated with high triglycerides and ways to lower the level.

Cholesterol (koh LES the rohl) is a waxy, fat-like substance. It is used to make hormones, vitamin D, bile acids, and cell membranes. Cholesterol is created in the liver and dietary cholesterol comes from animal foods (egg yolks, meat, shellfish, and cheese). Cholesterol is carried in the blood by the following lipoproteins:
- *High-density lipoprotein* (HDL): Considered "good" cholesterol. It helps move the cholesterol from the tissues to the liver. The liver helps remove cholesterol from the body. A low level of HDL increases the risk of heart disease.
- *Low-density lipoprotein* (LDL): Considered "bad" cholesterol. It moves cholesterol to tissues including arteries. Most of the cholesterol in the blood is in LDL. The greater the LDL level in the blood, the greater the risk for heart disease. LDL can be lowered through diet, exercise, and medications. Using unsaturated fats can help lower one's LDL levels.

> **MEDICAL TERMINOLOGY**
> **lip/o:** fat

Minerals and Electrolytes

Minerals are naturally occurring inorganic substances (e.g., iron, zinc, and calcium). Minerals needed by the body are divided into two categories: major and trace. *Major minerals* or macrominerals are needed in larger amounts. *Trace minerals*, or microminerals, are needed in smaller amounts in the body.

Electrolytes are minerals in the body fluid that have an electrical charge. They are found in the blood, urine, and other body fluids. Electrolytes come from the foods we eat and fluids we drink (Table 36.4). Too little or too much water in our body, vomiting, diarrhea, sweating, and kidney problems can change our electrolyte levels. A provider will order laboratory tests to measure a patient's electrolyte levels.

> **VOCABULARY**
> **antioxidant:** Synthetic or natural substances found in food and supplements; may prevent or delay some types of cell damage.

> **CRITICAL THINKING 36.4**
> Kayla asks Tim how he would explain the difference between minerals and electrolytes. How would you respond?

> **BOX 36.8 Triglycerides**
>
> Triglycerides are stored in the fat cells and have the following characteristics:
> - Are used for energy when carbohydrates are limited
> - Absorb vitamins and other nutrients
> - Contain essential fatty acids, which are important for growth and development.
>
> A person's triglyceride level is usually checked with the cholesterol levels. High triglyceride levels increase one's risk for heart disease and stroke. There are other reasons for high triglyceride levels including poorly controlled type 2 diabetes mellitus, liver disease, kidney disease, and hypothyroidism.
>
> The best ways to lower the triglyceride level is to do the following:
> - Cut back on calories and lose weight.
> - Avoid sugary and refined food; choose monounsaturated fats over saturated fats.
> - Limit the amount of alcohol consumed, and exercise daily.
> - Medications can also be ordered to help decrease the triglyceride level.

TABLE 36.3 Types of Fats

Type	Description	Impact on Cholesterol	Found in
Saturated fats	Solid at room temperature	Increase the LDL level	Butter, cheese, whole milk, ice cream, cream, fatty meats; processed coconut oil, palm oil
Unsaturated fats	Liquid at room temperature; two kinds: monounsaturated and polyunsaturated	Decrease the LDL level	Monounsaturated: olive and canola oil Polyunsaturated: safflower, sunflower, corn, and soy oil
Trans fatty acids	Also called hydrogenated fats and trans fats; created when hydrogen is added to vegetable oils during food manufacturing	Increase LDL and decrease HDL levels	Foods made with hydrogenated and partially hydrogenated oils; margarine, commercially prepared baked goods

TABLE 36.4 Examples of Major and Trace Minerals

Category	Mineral	Role in the Body	Found in
Major minerals (macrominerals)	Calcium	For healthy teeth and bones; muscle and nerve function, blood clotting, blood pressure regulation, immune system health	Milk products, canned fish (e.g., salmon), fortified soy milk, greens (e.g., broccoli), legumes
	Potassium	For proper muscle and nerve function, fluid balance	Milk, fresh fruits and vegetables, whole grains, legumes, meats
	Sodium		Table salt, processed foods, condiments
	Chloride	For proper fluid balance; stomach acid	Table salt, processed foods, tomatoes, celery, and olives
	Phosphorus	For healthy teeth and bones; important in the acid-base balance system	Meat, poultry, fish, eggs, milk, processed foods, soda pop
	Sulfur	Found in body proteins	Meats, poultry, fish, eggs, legumes, nuts
	Magnesium	Needed to make proteins; for muscle and nerve function and immune system health	Nuts, legumes, seeds, seafood, chocolate, and leafy green vegetables
Trace minerals (microminerals)	Iron	Part of hemoglobin found in the red blood cell, used for energy metabolism	Meats, fish, poultry, shellfish, egg yolks, legumes, dark leafy greens, iron-enriched or fortified foods
	Zinc	Used for making proteins, taste perception, wound healing, immune system health, production of sperm, normal growth	Vegetables, poultry, fish, meats
	Iodine	Found in thyroid hormone, which is involved with metabolism, growth, and development	Seafood, iodized salt, milk products
	Selenium	Antioxidant (AN tee ok si dahnt)	Seafood, grains, and meats
	Fluoride	Involved with healthy teeth and bones	Fish, tea, and drinking water
	Chromium	Used in the metabolism of carbohydrates and fats; also aids in insulin action and glucose metabolism	Brewer's yeast, beef, liver, eggs, chicken, wheat germ, potatoes
	Copper	Helps to form red blood cells; involved with keeping the blood vessels, nerves, immune system, and bones healthy; aids in iron absorption	Shellfish, whole grains, beans, nuts, liver, dark leafy greens, dried fruits, yeast, and cocoa

BOX 36.9 Antioxidants

When our body uses oxygen to burn food for energy, free radicals are formed. Free radicals are also formed due to environmental influences (e.g., water and air pollution, cigarette smoke, fried foods). Excessive free radicals can impact our health by attacking cells' DNA and blood vessels. This increases the risk for cardiovascular disease, strokes, arthritis, cataracts, and other degenerative diseases.

Antioxidants protect cells from free radicals and limit the damage free radicals can do to the cells. Antioxidants are powerful and beneficial for us. Antioxidants include vitamins A, C, and E, beta-carotene, lycopene, lutein, and selenium.

MEDICAL TERMINOLOGY
an-: no, not, without
cheil/o: lip
-emia: blood condition
gloss/o: tongue
hem/o: blood
-itis: inflammation
-lytic: pertaining to destruction

CRITICAL THINKING 36.5

Kayla and Tim are working with Maude Crawford. They are reviewing her medication lists. Tim asks if she takes any vitamins and minerals. Maude asks, "Why do I need a vitamin supplement?" How would you answer this question?

Vitamins

Vitamins are organic substances needed by the body in very small amounts for specific roles. There are 13 vitamins required by the body. It is important to get the recommended dietary allowance (RDA) of each vitamin. A deficit of a vitamin can lead to disease.

Vitamins are either water soluble or fat soluble (Table 36.5). Water-soluble vitamins dissolve in water. These include vitamins B and C. Any unused water-soluble vitamins leave the body through the urine. Vitamin B_{12} is an exception, because the liver stores the vitamin for years. Water-soluble vitamins need to be taken in daily. Fat-soluble vitamins are vitamins A, D, E, and K. These vitamins are absorbed more easily with the presence of fat in the diet. They can build up in the body, so typically supplements are not needed (Boxes 36.9 and 36.10).

VOCABULARY
recommended dietary allowance (RDA): Average daily level of food intake needed to meet the nutrient requirements of most healthy people.

Water

Drinking water every day is important for a person's health. Water is the basis for the fluids in the body. It makes up more than two-thirds of the body's weight. Without water, we would become dehydrated and die within a few days. All cells and organs need water to function and survive. Water plays important roles in the body, including the following:
- Keeps the body temperature normal with perspiration
- Lubricates and cushions joints (e.g., saliva, fluid around joints)
- Helps to prevent and relieve constipation by moving food through the intestines
- Protects the spinal cord, brain, and other sensitive tissues
- Gets rid of waste products in the body through urine, sweat, and stool

Our need for water increases in hot weather, when we are more active, or when we have a fever, diarrhea, or vomiting. The recommended

TABLE 36.5 Fat- and Water-Soluble Vitamins

Category	Vitamin	Recommended Dietary Allowance for Adults	Role in the Body	Found in	Deficiency Causes	Toxic?
Fat-soluble vitamins	Vitamin A	700–900 mcg	Antioxidant; helps form and maintain healthy teeth, bones, mucus membranes, soft tissue, and skin.	Dark-colored fruits and leafy vegetables, egg yolks, fortified milk products, liver, beef, fish	Night blindness	Yes, can cause liver toxicity
	Vitamin D	15–20 mcg	Bone-growth; made by the body after being in the sun	Fatty fish (e.g., salmon, herring), fish liver oils, fortified cereals, fortified milk products	Bone pain, muscle weakness	Yes, hypercalcemia (HYE per kal see mee ah) (elevated blood calcium levels) and kidney problems
	Vitamin E (tocopherol [toe KOF eh role])	15 mg	Antioxidant; helps form red blood cells and use vitamin K	Avocado, dark green and dark leafy vegetables (e.g., spinach, broccoli, and asparagus); safflower, corn, and sunflower oil; papaya, mango, wheat germ, seeds, nuts	Hemolytic (hee moh LIH tick) anemia, neurologic deficits	Yes, hemorrhagic toxicity can occur with supplement use
	Vitamin K	90–120 mcg	Blood clotting; made in the intestine	Cabbage, cauliflower, cereals, dark green and dark leafy vegetables, fish, liver, eggs, beef	Bleeding	No toxic effects reported
Water-soluble vitamin	Thiamine (THY ah min) (vitamin B_1)	1.1–1.2 mg	Used for nervous system, muscle function, and carbohydrate metabolism	Egg, enriched flour, lean meats, legumes, nuts, seeds, organ meats, peas, whole grains	Beriberi (BER ee ber ee) usually in alcoholics	No toxic effects reported
	Riboflavin (RYE bow flae vin) (vitamin B_2)	1.1–1.3 mg	Works with other B vitamins; important for growth and red blood cell production	Milk, mushrooms, spinach, almonds, lamb	Riboflavin deficiency	No toxic effects reported
	Niacin (NYE ah sin) (vitamin B_3)	14–16 mg	Used in digestive process, and skin and nerve functions; treats low HDL and high LDL cholesterol and triglyceride levels	Avocado, eggs, enriched breads and cereals, lean meats, fish, poultry, legumes, nuts, and potato	Pellagra (pah LAG rah), digestive issues	Niacin-containing supplements should be taken as provider indicates
	Pantothenic acid (PAN toh then ik) (vitamin B_5)	5 mg	Involved with metabolism, hormone and cholesterol production, and needed for growth	Avocado, broccoli, egg yolks, legumes, milk, yeast, organ meats, potatoes, and whole grains	Vitamin B_5 deficiency	No toxic effects reported
	Pyridoxine (PIR i dok seen) (vitamin B_6)	1.3–1.7 mg	Helps form red blood cells and maintain brain function; also used for protein metabolism	Avocado, banana, legumes, meat, nuts, poultry, and whole grains	Cracks around mouth, depression, rash	No toxic effects reported
	Biotin (BYE oh tin) (vitamin B_7)	30 mcg	Used for fat and carbohydrate metabolism; also used in the production of hormones and cholesterol	Chocolate, legumes, milk, nuts, organ meats (e.g., liver, kidney) pork, egg yolk, and yeast	Hair loss, cheilitis (kye LYE tis), glossitis (glah SYE tis)	No toxic effects reported
	Folate (FOH late) (vitamin B_9, folic acid)	400 mcg	Works with vitamin B_{12} to help form blood cells; important in pregnancy to prevent spina bifida	Asparagus, broccoli, beets, brewer's yeast, legumes, enriched breads and cereals, green leafy vegetables, oranges, peanut butter	Anemia, diarrhea	Caution with high doses, limited data on toxicity
	Cobalamin (KOE bal ah min) (vitamin B_{12})	2.4 mcg	Important for protein metabolism, the formation of red blood cells, and the maintenance of the central nervous system	Meat, eggs, fortified foods, milk products, organ meats, poultry, and shellfish	Pernicious (pur NIH shush) anemia, confusion	No toxic effects reported
	Vitamin C (ascorbic [ah SKOOR bik] acid)	75–90 mg	Antioxidant; promotes healthy gums and teeth; helps absorb iron; maintains healthy tissue and promotes wound healing	Citrus fruits, tomatoes, broccoli, cabbage, cauliflower, potatoes, spinach, strawberries	Scurvy (SKUHR vee)	Kidney stones, excess iron absorption, gastrointestinal disturbances

mcg, micrograms; *mg*, milligrams; *RDA*, recommended daily allowance.
Some information from the table was obtained from the Vitamins
Food and Nutrition Board, Institute of Medicine, National Academies, https://www.nal.usda.gov/sites/default/files/fnic_uploads//DRI_Vitamins.pdf.

BOX 36.10 Function of Dietary Supplements

Dietary supplements are oral products that contain a "dietary ingredient." This ingredient can include a vitamin, mineral, amino acid, herb, or another substance that can supplement a person's diet. Dietary supplements come in many forms including tablets, powders, energy bars, and liquids. Federal law does not require a dietary supplement to be proven safe or the claim truthful before it appears on the market. The Food and Drug Administration (FDA) monitors the safety of such products after they are on the market.

The function of dietary supplements is to provide nutrients that are not obtained in the foods we eat and drink. Some examples of uses of dietary supplements include the following:
- Calcium and vitamin D for bone health and low vitamin D levels
- Folic acid in pregnancy to prevent spina bifida
- Iron for low iron levels
- Fiber for constipation

Before starting a dietary supplement, it is important to talk with the provider. Some medications may interact with dietary supplements. Some dietary supplements may work against medications. For instance, taking vitamin K promotes blood clotting, and Coumadin (warfarin) delays blood clotting.

BOX 36.11 Water and Diseases

Some patients are placed on fluid restrictions. This means they can only have a certain amount of fluids a day. The provider will indicate the maximum amount of fluids to be consumed daily. It is important to limit fluids that act like a diuretic (e.g., alcohol and caffeinated beverages) because they pull fluid from the body and increase the risk of dehydration. Conditions that may require fluid restrictions include the following:
- Heart problems including congestive heart failure
- Kidney problems, such as those that might affect patients on dialysis and those with end stage renal disease
- Adrenal insufficiency and corticosteroid treatment

Some diseases and conditions require more fluids/water to be consumed. People with postural orthostatic tachycardia syndrome (POTS) need to drink at least 2 to 3 liters of water a day to maintain their blood pressure. Other conditions, such as diabetes insipidus, diabetes mellitus, and Addison disease, may cause patients to excrete more urine and thus put them more at risk for dehydration.

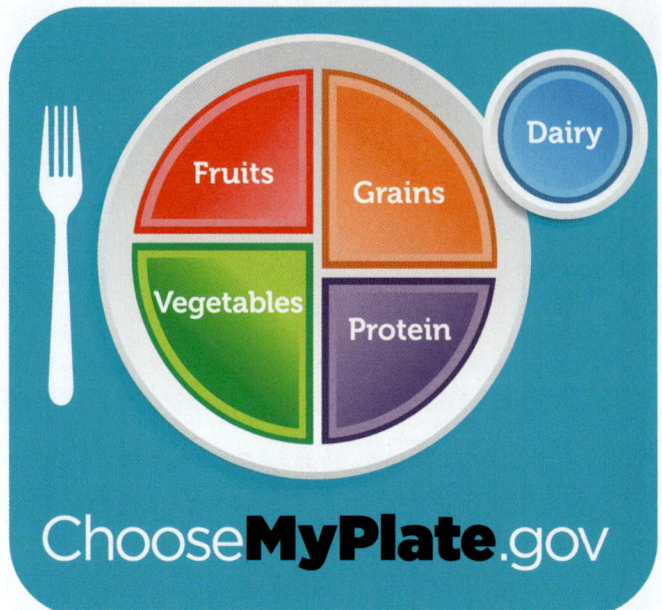

FIG. 36.1 Choose MyPlate. (From the US Department of Agriculture, www.choosemyplate.gov.)

daily intake of water for healthy men is about 13 cups, 9 cups for women. The individual need for water is based on a person's weight, age, activity level, and certain medical conditions (Box 36.11).

DIETARY GUIDELINES

For over a century, the U.S. Department of Agriculture (USDA) has provided food guides to the public. Some of the more recent guides include the following:
- 1992: Food Guide Pyramid, which showed the five basic food groups, with fats and sugars making up the tip of the pyramid
- 2005: MyPyramid Food Guidance System, which continued with the pyramid design but added physical activity and oils
- 2011: MyPlate, which was introduced along with the 2010 Dietary Guidelines for Americans

MyPlate

MyPlate focuses on making healthy food choices because everything eaten matters (Fig. 36.1). Some of the key messages with these dietary guidelines include the following:

- Fill half the plate with fruits and vegetables. Vary the color and type of fruits and vegetables.
- Make half of the grains each day whole grains.
- Vary the types of proteins eaten.
- Move to low-fat or fat-free milk and yogurt.
- Drink and eat less saturated fat, sodium, and added sugars.

MyPlate consists of five food groups along with oil (Table 36.6). Oil contains required nutrients, so the USDA addresses it. Oil is usually consumed in nuts, fish, cooking oil, and salad dressing. Most children need between 3 to 6 teaspoons, and adults need from 5 to 7 teaspoons depending on gender and age.

The MyPlate website (www.choosemyplate.gov) offers numerous resources for individuals and professionals. Online resources, including a food and exercise tracker (SuperTracker), are available for use. Tip sheets, food plans, and other resources provide additional information. MyPlate is very flexible for cultural foods.

Dietary Guidelines

The USDA publishes dietary guidelines every 5 years. The guidelines are for individuals 2 years and older. The focus is on disease prevention and health promotion. The current dietary guidelines focus on overall eating patterns, health, and the risk of chronic disease.

Key recommendations from the 2015–2020 Dietary Guidelines for Americans include those listed with the MyPlate as well as the following:
- Limit foods with saturated and trans fats, added sugars, and sodium.
  - Less than 10% of daily calories should come from saturated fats (e.g., butter, whole milk, fatty meats, coconut oil, and palm oil).
  - Individuals age 14 and older should consume fewer than 2300 milligrams (mg) of sodium a day.
- Limit the alcohol consumed to one drink per day for women and two drinks for adult men.
- Incorporate physical activity (e.g., aerobic, muscle-strengthening, and bone-strengthening activities) into the week.

READING FOOD LABELS

Knowing how to read a food label is important when making healthy food selections. The food label contains the nutritional information

CHAPTER 36 Patient Coaching With Nutrition

TABLE 36.6 Food Groups With Serving Amounts for MyPlate

Food Group	What Counts?	Children 2–8[a]	Children 9–18[a]	Women 19–51+[a]	Men 19–51+[a]
Diary	1-cup equivalent: 1 cup milk, yogurt, soymilk, almond milk, coconut milk 1½ oz natural cheese 2 oz processed cheese	2–2½ cups	3 cups	3 cups	3 cups
Proteins	1-oz equivalent: 1 oz meat, poultry, or fish ¼ cup cooked beans 1 egg 1 tablespoon peanut butter ½ oz nuts or seeds	2–4 oz	5–6½ oz	5–5½ oz	5½–6½ oz
Vegetables	1-cup equivalent: 1 cup raw or cooked vegetables or vegetable juice 2 cups raw leafy greens	½ cups	2–3 cups	2–2½ cups	2½–3 cups
Fruits	1-cup equivalent: 1 cup fruit or 100% fruit juice ½ cup dried fruit	1–1½ cups	1½–2 cups	1½–2 cups	2 cups
Grains	1-oz equivalent: 1 slice of bread 1 cup dry cereal ½ cup cooked rice, pasta, or cereal (at least half should be whole grains)	3–5 oz	5–8 oz	5–6 oz	6–8 oz

[a]Amount required is based on gender, age, and the amount of exercise. Ranges are indicated above, for more specific information, go to www.choosemyplate.gov.

Nutrition Facts
2 servings per container
Serving size 1 1/2 cup (208g)

Amount per serving
Calories 240

	% Daily Value*
Total Fat 4g	5%
Saturated Fat 1.5g	8%
Trans Fat 0g	
Cholesterol 5mg	2%
Sodium 430mg	19%
Total Carbohydrate 46g	17%
Dietary Fiber 7g	25%
Total Sugars 4g	
Includes 2g Added Sugars	4%
Protein 11g	
Vitamin D 2mcg	10%
Calcium 260mg	20%
Iron 6mg	35%
Potassium 240mg	6%

* The % Daily Value (DV) tells you how much a nutrient in a serving of food contributes to a daily diet. 2,000 calories a day is used for general nutrition advice.

FIG. 36.2 Nutrition facts. (From the Food and Drug Administration, https://www.fda.gov/Food/IngredientsPackagingLabeling/LabelingNutrition/ucm537159.htm.)

Food Label #1	Food Label #2
Ingredients: semolina (wheat), durum flour (wheat), eggs, partially hydrogenated oil, niacin, ferrous sulfate, thiamin mononitrate, riboflavin. **Contains:** Wheat, Eggs. Manufactured in a facility that uses tree nuts and eggs.	**Ingredients:** grapes, corn syrup, high fructose corn syrup, fruit pectin, and citric acid.

FIG. 36.3 Ingredient list on food labels.

and the ingredient list. The government has required food manufacturers to include certain information on the food label. The amounts for "Trans Fat" and "Added Sugars" are some of the newer additions to the food label.

Food labels provide nutritional facts. This information is presented in both the quantity (e.g., gram [g] or milligram [mg]) and as a percentage. The percentage reflects the *% Daily Value (DV)*. This is the percentage of the nutrient in a single serving in terms of the daily recommended amount based on a 2000-calorie diet. You will see this description at the bottom of the list of nutrition facts. Remember that if you are eating fewer than 2000 calories daily, these percentages will be different for you.

When reading the nutrition facts (Fig. 36.2), start at the top and work down:
- Check the calories per serving. If you eat the entire container and it consists of two servings, you need to double the calories.
- Check the amount of fat. Limit the saturated fat intake and avoid trans fats.
- The amounts listed for cholesterol, sodium, total carbohydrates, and added sugars are also numbers to consider. Choose foods with low amounts of these nutrients.
- Examine the dietary fiber, protein, vitamin D, calcium, iron, and potassium. Make sure you are getting enough of these beneficial nutrients.

Ingredient lists on foods are also important to understand (Fig. 36.3). The ingredients are listed in descending order, starting with the

one that weighs the most and ending with the one that weighs the least. There are several reasons why a person may look at the ingredient list:
- To look for trans fats: Even if the nutrition information indicates 0 grams trans fats, the product may still contain less than 0.5 grams of trans fats per serving. Look for ingredients like "hydrogenated" or "partially hydrogenated oil." This indicates the presence of trans fats. So even if the nutrition information indicates 0 grams of trans fats, you may quickly reach your daily limit if you eat more than one serving.
- To avoid certain ingredients: Some people try to avoid ingredients like high fructose corn syrup and certain food colorings.
- To identify allergens: More than 160 foods have been found to be allergens. The government has identified eight allergies that make up about 90% of all food allergy reactions. Laws regulating food labeling require manufacturers to indicate if any of these top allergens are in the food product. Advisory statements like "may contain peanuts" or "made in a factory that also process tree nuts" are optional and not required by law. (More information on allergens will be presented later in the chapter.)

MEDICALLY ORDERED DIETS

Patients may need to change their diet for a variety of reasons:
- Preparation for a procedure
- Dental problems
- Illness
- A condition that requires dietary changes (e.g., allergy and hypertension)

If the dietary change is also a lifestyle change (e.g., for diabetes or hypertension), the provider may refer the patient to a **registered dietitian** (die eh TISH an). The registered dietitian can provide in-depth **coaching** and counseling on dietary changes.

For other dietary changes or to review a person's knowledge of a specific diet, the medical assistant may be involved. When the provider orders a specific test or a particular diet, the medical assistant may need to coach the patient on the new diet. As with other coaching, it is important for the medical assistant to provide the patient with a reference handout to take home. This will help guide the patient on the dietary changes. Learning about different medically ordered diets is important for the medical assistant.

Clear Liquid Diet

A clear liquid diet is made up of foods and beverages that are liquid at room temperature. Clear means you need to see through the liquids. Clear liquid diets are ordered for only a short time because they do not contain adequate nutrition.

Table 36.7 lists the medical reasons to be on a clear liquid diet. If a person is undergoing an intestinal procedure, red or pink clear liquids are not allowed because they could be mistaken for blood in the intestine.

VOCABULARY
coaching: Providing information in a supportive environment that allows people to grow, change, or improve their situation.
registered dietitian: A credentialed healthcare professional who is trained in nutrition and is able to apply the information to the dietary needs of healthy and ill patients.
regular diet: The food and drink a person typically consumes when there are no dietary limitations.

TABLE 36.7 Clear Liquid Diet

Reasons for a Clear Liquid Diet	Foods Included on a Clear Liquid Diet
Diarrhea	Water
Vomiting	Popsicles and juice without pulp
Nausea	Soup broth
Immediately after surgery	Gelatin (Jell-O)
Preparation for intestinal procedure	Tea, coffee, sport drinks, and clear soda

TABLE 36.8 Full Liquid Diet

Reasons for a Full Liquid Diet	Foods Included on a Full Liquid Diet
Before or after surgery	Clear liquids (see clear liquid diet)
Difficulty chewing or swallowing	Strained creamy soups
Preparation for tests or procedures	Milk, milkshakes, pudding, custard and ice cream
	Liquid supplements
	Sugar, honey, syrups, butter, margarine

Full Liquid Diet

A full liquid diet is made up of foods and beverages that are liquid at room temperature. Unlike the clear liquid diet, the full liquid diet includes milk products. This diet is a step above a clear liquid diet and below a **regular diet**. Some providers will allow cooked, refined cereals (e.g., cream of rice), baby food strained meats, and potatoes pureed in soup on a full liquid diet.

Full liquid diets are ordered for only a short time because they do not contain adequate nutrition. Table 36.8 lists the medical reasons to be on a full liquid diet.

CRITICAL THINKING 36.6

Kayla and Tim are working with Janine Butler. Janine needs to undergo an intestinal procedure and needs to be on clear liquids for two days. Janine states, "I was on a full liquid diet last year for a procedure. What is the difference between a clear liquid diet and a full liquid diet?" How would you answer this question?

Soft and Mechanical Soft Diet

A soft diet is a transition between a liquid diet and a regular diet. The foods on this diet are soft in texture, low in fiber, and easy for a person to digest. The soft diet eliminates food that is hard to chew and swallow (Table 36.9).

This diet is used for patients recovering from surgery or a lengthy illness. It can also be used for people with chewing or swallowing problems due to illness or dental issues.

Mechanical soft diets consist of foods that have been prepared for easier chewing and swallowing using household tools (e.g., grinder, blender, and knife). Typically, there are no limitations (e.g., spicy, gassy, and fried) to mechanical soft diets. Mechanical soft diets are used for the following groups:

TABLE 36.9 Soft Diet

Foods Eliminated	Foods Included on a Soft Diet
Raw fruits and vegetables Chewy or crispy breads Tough meats Broccoli and cauliflower Fried, greasy foods Highly seasoned or spicy foods Nuts and seeds	Grains: soft breads, crackers, white rice, pasta Fruits and vegetables: soft cooked, canned (no skin) Milk products: milk, yogurt, cottage cheese, ice cream, pudding Protein: tender meat, poultry, and fish; eggs, tofu, smooth peanut butter

- Those recovering from head, neck, or mouth surgery
- Those who have difficulty swallowing (*dysphagia* [dis FAY jee ah]), poor fitting dentures, no teeth
- Those who are too ill to chew

MEDICAL TERMINOLOGY
dys-: difficult, bad
-phagia: condition of swallowing, eating

Bland Diet

A bland diet includes foods that are soft and low in fiber. This diet eliminates foods that are spicy, fried, or raw and beverages that contain caffeine or alcohol. Citrus juices and foods may also be eliminated. The foods included in a bland diet are similar to those incorporated into a soft diet.

A bland diet is ordered to help treat gastroesophageal reflux disease (GERD), ulcers, nausea and vomiting, diarrhea, and gas. It can also be used after stomach or intestinal surgery.

Weight Control Diet

When trying to achieve or maintain a healthy weight, a person needs to find the balance between the number of calories eaten and the number used. Extra calories eaten and not used will result in a weight gain. For people to lose 1 to 2 pounds per week, they need to reduce their calorie intake by 500 to 1000 calories a day. Identifying the calories consumed is an important step in achieving a healthy weight. Food diaries, apps, and trackers are available to help gauge food intake and activity.

Nutritional tips for patients trying to achieve a healthy weight include the following:
- Commit to a lifestyle change. Identify resources for information and support.
- Track foods eaten and beverages drank, along with physical exercise.
- Set realistic goals, knowing that slips will occur.
- Eat healthy meals. They should be low in saturated fat, trans fat, cholesterol, salt, and added sugar. Eat lean meats, fish, poultry, beans, eggs, and nuts. Include fruits (especially whole fruits), vegetables, whole grains, and fat-free or low-fat milk products.
- Control portion sizes. *Portion size* is the amount of food we eat. *Serving size* is a standard measurement of food (e.g., 1 cup or 1 oz). Many foods that come as a single portion actually contain multiple servings. For instance, a serving size of potato chips is 1 oz. The 3-oz potato chip bag is a single portion, but three servings. Another example is bread. You use two pieces of bread for a sandwich (portion size), but a serving is one slice. Most people overestimate serving sizes (Box 36.12). It is best to measure the food or use a quick estimate method (Table 36.10).

TABLE 36.10 Quick Methods to Estimate Portion Size

Amount of Food	Size of
3 oz of chicken and lean beef	Deck of cards
1 medium potato	A computer mouse
½ cup cooked pasta	Tennis ball
1 oz of cheese	Two dice
1 medium size fruit	Tennis ball
1 cup fruit or cooked vegetables	Baseball
1 oz of nuts	Handful
1 oz of chips or pretzels	Two handfuls (13–16 chips)
1 cup	Woman's fist
1 tablespoon (tbs)	First joint of thumb
1 teaspoon (tsp)	Fingertip

BOX 36.12 Portion Size and Obesity

In some cases, portion sizes and serving sizes are the same. Over the years many portion sizes have changed. Some experts attribute the growing obesity epidemic in the United States to be related to it. In the 1950s the dinner plate was 9 inches, and today its 11 to 12 inches in diameter. Some restaurants use even larger plates. With the plate change, the average portion of food as also increased. Restaurants have increased the amount of food they give, and more Americans are eating out. With the increase in portions, *portion distortion* is occurring. The size of restaurant portions is causing Americans to rethink what the "normal" portions of food should be. Here are some examples of portion changes since the 1990s:

- Bagels have increased by 3 inches and added 210 calories.
- Muffins have increased by 3.5 oz and 290 calories.
- Cheeseburgers have increased in size and added almost 260 calories.
- Soda size has increased by 13.5 oz and almost 170 calories.

As these examples show, the increase in portion sizes has led to an increase in the number of calories. Remember, the calories consumed and not used turn into fat.

Information from the National Heart, Lung, and Blood Institute, https://www.nhlbi.nih.gov/health/educational/wecan/eat-right/distortion.htm.

CRITICAL THINKING 36.7

Kayla and Tim are working with Amma Patel. Kayla is explaining the weight-controlled diet that Dr. Perez ordered for Amma. They are discussing serving size and portions. Amma states she is confused by the difference. How might you explain the difference between these two concepts? Provide an example for Amma.

Diabetic Eating Plans

People with diabetes need to monitor their carbohydrate intake. Remember that carbohydrates are broken down into glucose in the body. Insulin moves the glucose from the blood into the cells. For people with diabetes, the body either does not make enough insulin or does not respond to the insulin produced. As a result, their blood glucose levels are high. In the absence of insulin, the body metabolizes fat and uses the ketones for energy. Ketones build up in the body. (Too many ketones can lead to ketoacidosis, a life-threatening condition.) Table 36.11 indicates the treatments for type 1 and type 2 diabetes.

Over the years, several different diabetic eating plans have been created for people with diabetes mellitus. You may hear of patients being on diet plans like the exchange list system. This diet plan grouped similar foods that had the same amount of carbohydrate, protein, fat, and calories. Each food item had a measurement (e.g., 1 cup) to indicate how much could be eaten for that exchange. Three main groups were given in the plan: carbohydrate, meat, and fat.

The American Diabetes Association (www.diabetes.org) encourages the following diabetes meal plans: the glycemic index approach, the "Create Your Plate" method, and carb counting. The glycemic index (GI) was explained earlier in this chapter. Eating lower GI foods helps one to maintain a more stable blood glucose level.

The "Create Your Plate" method uses a 9-inch dinner plate (Fig. 36.4). To follow this meal plan, do the following:
- Fill half of the plate with nonstarchy vegetables (e.g., beans, broccoli, carrots, salad greens, and peppers).
- Split the remaining unfilled side of the plate in half. One small half is filled with a protein (e.g., lean meat, poultry, and fish).

TABLE 36.11 Treatments for Diabetes Mellitus

	Type 1	Type 2
Age of Onset	Any age, usually appears in childhood	Usually after age 45; becoming more common with children and younger adults; usually being overweight is the primary risk factor
Insulin	Pancreas is not producing insulin	Insulin is being produced, but may not be enough; also the cells may be resistant to insulin produced
Treatments	Insulin Carbohydrate counting and healthy eating Frequent blood glucose monitoring Regular exercise	Healthy eating Regular exercise Diabetes medications (injectables and pills or insulin) if needed Blood glucose monitoring

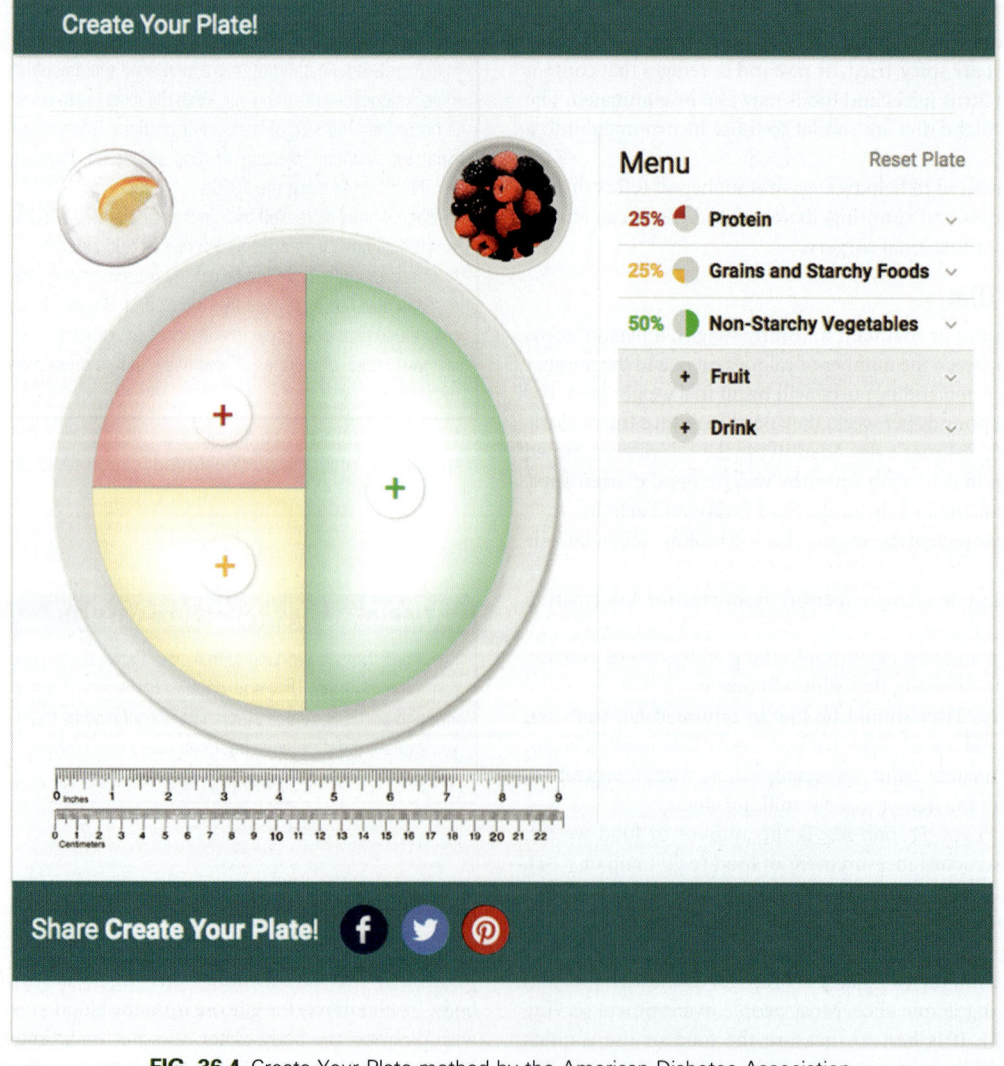

FIG. 36.4 Create Your Plate method by the American Diabetes Association.

- The other small half is filled with a grain and starch vegetable (e.g., brown rice, potato, squash, green peas, and corn).
- Complete the meal with a serving of fruit, a serving of dairy (milk product), and a non-sweetened beverage.

Carb counting, or carbohydrate counting, is a meal planning tool used by people with diabetes mellitus. Using this method, a person keeps track of the amount of carbohydrates eaten each day. Carbohydrates are measured in grams. This system may give some people better control of their diabetes, but it is a learning process. The person needs to identify which foods contain carbohydrates and how to estimate the number of grams. The total grams are calculated over the day. Some people with type 1 diabetes may need to adjust the amount of insulin they take for a specific meal based on the number of carbohydrates they will consume.

Low-Sodium Diet

Sodium is essential to our bodies because it helps to regulate fluid balance. The Food and Drug Administration (FDA) recommends that healthy adults consume no more than 2300 milligrams (mg) of sodium per day. Patients with high blood pressure, heart disease, or kidney disease are usually on reduced sodium diets. Excessive sodium in a person's diet can lead to increased blood pressure, thus increasing the risk for heart disease and stroke.

If a patient is on a reduced sodium diet, the provider will usually refer him or her to a registered dietitian. The dietitian will help educate the individual on the sources of sodium (Box 36.13). Typically, alternative lower sodium foods are discussed. Reading labels is also an important skill for those on reduced sodium diets.

Dietary Approaches to Stop Hypertension. Dietary Approaches to Stop Hypertension (DASH) is a flexible eating plan recommended for those with hypertension and cardiovascular disease. The goal of the plan is to reduce the blood pressure and the LDL and triglyceride levels. Table 36.12 indicates foods included and omitted on the DASH eating plan.

> **CRITICAL THINKING 36.8**
>
> Kayla and Tim are working with Al Neviaser, who has hypertension. Dr. Martin has ordered the DASH eating plan instructions for Mr. Neviaser. Tim explains to Mr. Neviaser that high salt foods makes the blood "salty" and more water is needed in the bloodstream to bring the "salty" level down. The extra water in the blood increases the blood pressure. Mr. Neviaser asks which foods he should stay away from. Give 10 foods that are high in salt (sodium).

Heart-Healthy Diet

The diet and lifestyle recommendations of the American Heart Association (AHA) closely resemble the DASH diet and the MyPlate guidelines.

> **BOX 36.13 Foods High in Sodium**
>
> - Processed meats (e.g., deli, bacon, frankfurters, and sausage)
> - Frozen dinners and ready-to-eat cereals
> - Canned foods (e.g., soups, vegetables, and vegetable juice)
> - Salted nuts and peanut butter
> - Buttermilk, cheese, and processed cheese products
> - Quick breads and salted crackers
> - Prepackaged mixes for potatoes, rice, and pasta
> - Olives, pickles, sauerkraut, pickled vegetables, and spaghetti sauce
> - Soy sauce, seasoning salt, marinades, ketchup, mustard, and salad dressings
> - Instant puddings and cakes
> - Chips and pretzels

The AHA incorporates a focus on exercise, along with a healthy diet. The following are the AHA's recommendations:

- Limit sugary drinks and sweets. Limit salty or highly processed foods.
- Read labels and select products with the lowest amounts of sodium, added sugar, and saturated fats. Eat fewer than 2400 mg of sodium a day to lower blood pressure. To lower the blood pressure even further, sodium can be reduced to 1500 or 1000 mg per day.
- Be physically active. Balance the calories you burn during exercise with the calories you consume to maintain your weight. Include 150 minutes of moderate physical activity or 75 minutes of vigorous physical activity or a combination of both each week. Break up exercise into 10-minute sessions if needed. To lower blood pressure or cholesterol, 40 minutes of aerobic exercise of moderate to vigorous intensity three to four times a week is recommended.
- Drink alcohol in moderation. Women should have only one drink and men should have only two drinks per day.
- Table 36.13 lists the adult servings for each food group. These are based on a 2000-calorie per day diet.

TABLE 36.12 Dietary Approaches to Stop Hypertension (DASH) Eating Plan

Included in the DASH Plan	Omitted or Limited in the DASH Plan
Fruits and vegetables	Foods high in saturated fat, total fat, and cholesterol
Low-fat or fat-free dairy foods	Red meats
Whole grains	Sugar-sweetened beverages and sweets
Poultry and fish	High-salt (sodium) foods
Beans, nuts, and vegetable oils	Full-fat dairy foods
Foods high in potassium, calcium, magnesium, protein, and fiber	Tropical oils (coconut, palm, kernel, and palm oil)
Foods low in salt (sodium)	

TABLE 36.13 American Heart Association's Eating Healthy Recommendations

Food Group	Daily Amounts	Healthy Recommendations
Diary	3 servings or 3 cups	Use low-fat (1%) and fat-free options
Proteins	2 servings or 5.5 oz	Eat fish, skinless poultry, lean and extra lean meat, nuts, seeds, beans, and legumes; limit fatty or processed meats and red meats
Vegetables	5 servings or 1.5–2.5 cups	Eat a variety of vegetables
Fruits	4 servings or 1–2 cups	Eat a variety of fruits
Grains	3–6 servings or 3–6 oz	Eat whole grains for at least half of the daily servings
Oils	3 tablespoons	Use polyunsaturated and monounsaturated oils; avoid hydrogenated oils and tropical oils

Information for these recommendations came from the American Heart Association, https://healthyforgood.heart.org/eat-smart/infographics/what-is-a-healthy-diet-recommended-serving-infographic.

Low-Protein Diet

The body uses protein for tissue repair, growth, healing, and the ability to fight infection. When protein is broken down in the body, the waste products (e.g., urea and ammonia) are eliminated in the urine. People with liver and kidney disease are often prescribed a low-protein diet. They limit or restrict foods that contain high amounts of protein (Table 36.14). Their bodies cannot clear the protein waste products. They can have nausea, headaches, fatigue, and a bad taste in the mouth. Eating a low-protein diet helps to prevent worsening of their disease. Remember, protein cannot be eliminated from the diet. It plays an essential role in the body.

High- and Low-Fiber Diets

A prior section of the chapter discussed fiber as a carbohydrate. The provider may order a low-fiber or restricted-fiber diet. This type of diet limits the type of vegetables, grains, and fruits eaten. Limiting fiber and the residue (e.g., peels, nuts, and seeds) makes the stools smaller and lessens the irritation on the intestinal lining. The provider can also order a high-fiber diet. This diet adds more bulk to the stools, thus helping with constipation issues. Table 36.15 lists the reasons for both high- and low-fiber diets.

Elimination Diet and Food Allergies

A food allergy occurs when the immune system overreacts to a protein in the food. The immune system makes IgE antibody in response to the protein. This causes the person to quickly experience the allergy symptoms. Symptoms may include itching, hives, nausea and vomiting, diarrhea, difficulty breathing (e.g., tightness in the throat, coughing, wheezing) or anaphylaxis (AN ah fah lak sis).

As earlier indicated, eight allergies make up about 90% of the food allergy reactions. It is important to realize that parts of these foods are used in other foods (Box 36.14). For instance, milk proteins (e.g., whey and casein) and milk sugar, lactose, appear in some surprising food and nonfood products. Some examples include chicken broth, deli meats, hot dogs, French fries, shampoo, and dry powder medication inhalers (e.g., Advair Diskus, Flovent Diskus, and Serevent Diskus). Reading ingredient lists is critical for those with allergies.

When people suspect a food allergy, the elimination diet can be used. People remove the suspicious foods from their diet. They may need to track what they eat and how they feel. Slowly they add the suspicious foods back into their diet, one food at a time. This process helps identify the allergen. In some cases, a cross-reactivity may occur and the person will have additional food allergies. Box 36.15 discusses cross-reactivity and oral allergy syndrome. An allergist can help one to identify additional food and environmental allergies.

VOCABULARY

anaphylaxis: A rapidly progressing, life-threatening allergic reaction; characterized by hives, swelling of the mouth and airway, difficulty breathing, wheezing, and loss of consciousness.

MEDICAL TERMINOLOGY

diverticul/o: diverticulum
-itis: inflammation

TABLE 36.14 Foods With High, Small, and Trace Amounts of Protein

High Amounts	Small Amounts	Trace Amounts
Milk products (e.g., yogurt and cheese)	Vegetables	Fruits
Peanut butter	Starches (e.g., breads, cereals, and pastas.	Sugars
Meat, fish, and poultry		Fats
Eggs		

TABLE 36.15 Reasons for Low- and High-Fiber Diets

Reasons for Low-Fiber Diet	Reasons for High-Fiber Diet
Narrowing of the intestine due to a tumor	Decreases constipation and may lower the risk of hemorrhoids
During a flare-up of an intestinal disease (e.g., irritable bowel syndrome, Crohn's disease, and diverticulitis)	Lowers cholesterol levels
After intestinal surgery	Helps control blood glucose levels
Prior to an intestinal procedure (e.g., radiation and colonoscopy)	Used for weight loss

---

BOX 36.14 Top Eight Food Allergens

These eight food allergens can be hiding in ingredient lists under other names. Some examples are listed here:

- Milk (e.g., cream, casein, ghee, galactose, lactalbumin, lactose, and whey)
- Eggs (e.g., albumin, eggnog, ovalbumin, and ovomucin)
- Fish (e.g., cod, bass, flounder)
- Crustacean shellfish (e.g., crab, lobster, shrimp)
- Tree nuts (e.g., almonds, cashews, filberts, hazelnuts, marzipan, nut meal)
- Peanuts (e.g., peanut butter, peanut flour)
- Wheat (e.g., emmer, einkorn, durum, kamut, modified wheat starch, wheat bran, wheat germ)
- Soybeans (e.g., edamame, miso, soya, tempeh, tofu)

BOX 36.15 Cross-Reactivity With Allergens

Another issue faced by those with food allergies is cross-reactivity. This means that the protein in the allergic food is similar to other foods. The person's immune system cannot tell the proteins apart and thus reacts to similar foods. Cross-reactivity can occur with foods and nonfood items. For instance, a person with a latex allergy could also be allergic to avocados, bananas, chestnut, and kiwi.

Oral allergy syndrome (also called pollen-food syndrome) is caused by cross-reacting allergens found in pollens, raw foods, and tree nuts. Symptoms include itchy mouth and ears, scratchy throat, and swollen lips, mouth, tongue, and throat. Typically, the symptoms disappear when the food is out of the mouth. Some common cross-reactions include the following:

- Ragweed pollen: cucumber, banana, melons, potatoes, and zucchini
- Grass pollen: celery, melons, oranges, peaches, and tomato
- Birch pollen: pitted fruit (e.g., plum, pear, peach, and apple), kiwi, carrot, celery, almond, and hazelnut

BOX 36.16 Food to Avoid on a Gluten-Free Diet

- Barley and malt products (e.g., flavoring and vinegar)
- Rye
- Triticale (wheat and rye crossbred hybrid)
- Wheat (e.g., durum flour, farina, graham flour, spelt, semolina, and kamut)

Gluten-Free Diet. People with celiac disease are put on a gluten-free diet. Gluten is a protein found in wheat, barley, and rye (Box 36.16). It is commonly found in breads, cereals, pastas, cakes, cookies, and other foods. Gluten causes inflammation in the small intestine of people with celiac disease. Removing gluten from the diet helps to control the symptoms.

The FDA regulates the gluten-free food labeling claim. This is a voluntary claim that manufacturers may opt to use. If they use the label, they are accountable for using the claim in a truthful way.

Lactose-Intolerance Diet

Lactose intolerance, or sensitivity, is not an allergy. Lactose is the main sugar found in dairy products. Lactose is broken down by lactase, an enzyme created by the small intestine. If a person's small intestine does not produce enough lactase, the lactose moves into the large intestine. The bacteria in the large intestine break down the lactose, causing bloating, cramps, diarrhea, nausea, and gas. Treatment for lactose intolerance or sensitivity involves avoiding milk products or using an oral enzyme replacement supplement.

NUTRITIONAL NEEDS FOR VARIOUS POPULATIONS

Nutritional needs change throughout life. Our needs for calories, vitamins, minerals, and protein change as we grow and develop. With pregnancy and breastfeeding, the needs increase. With disease conditions, the needs change. We have already discussed different diets and conditions treated with those eating plans. Table 36.16 describes the nutritional needs by age groups.

Pregnancy and Lactation

During pregnancy, it is important to eat a healthy diet. The first trimester can be difficult with nutrition. Depending on the mother's morning sickness, eating a balanced diet can be tricky. Many providers recommend eating small, frequent meals to combat morning sickness. Dry crackers and toast are also encouraged. Eating low-odor protein foods can also help. Avoiding triggers such as spicy foods and certain smells are important in managing morning sickness.

Providers usually recommend a daily prenatal vitamin and mineral supplement to ensure adequate folic acid and prevent spina bifida. Consuming alcohol during pregnancy is not recommended. Despite the saying "eating for two," the daily caloric intake only needs to increase by 300 calories for the second and third trimester of most pregnancies.

With lactation or breastfeeding, the mother needs to eat a healthy diet, and a vitamin supplement may be recommended. It is important to get adequate vitamins and minerals, which are passed to the baby in the breast milk. The mother also needs to drink additional water to maintain her milk volume.

Epilepsy

Some patients with epilepsy follow a ketogenic diet. This diet consists of very low-carbohydrate, high-fat, and adequate protein foods. Some people have also used this type of diet to lose weight. Without carbohydrates, the body metabolizes fat, and the ketones are used for energy.

TABLE 36.16 Nutritional Needs by Age Groups

Age	Nutritional Needs
Infancy to 2 years	Birth to 6 months of age: Breast milk or formula is given. If an infant cannot tolerate milk-based formulas, other types of formulas are available including soy formula. Some formulas are available by prescription only. Six months of age: The child is started on soft, pureed solid foods. Usually, infant cereals, fruits, and vegetables are first introduced. One year of age: The child is transitioned to whole milk, and pureed foods are gradually replaced with easy-to-eat foods. It is important to offer foods from each food group.
2 to 12 years	Age 2: The child should eat several dairy products, fruits, vegetables, meats, breads, pasta, cereals, and beans. As the child grows and develops, more foods can be added to his or her diet. Portion sizes also grow.
12 to adulthood	Adolescents experience rapid growth periods, which require more energy. Teens may need encouragement to consume dairy products (e.g., milk) instead of soda. The growth spurts require calcium for strong bones. Females who have started their menses should eat foods high in iron to replace the iron lost in menstrual blood.
Older adults	As a person grows older, the metabolism decreases, and the caloric needs also decrease. Special nutritional concerns of the older adult include the following: • Difficulty chewing and swallowing, which can be related to poor-fitting dentures. • Decrease in eating due to changes in their senses (e.g., taste, smell) • Lack of a well-balanced diet (e.g., limited income, loneliness, and lack of initiative to cook for oneself)

It is important to monitor kidney function when a person is on a ketogenic diet.

HIV and AIDS

When a person has HIV or AIDS, it is important to eat a well-balanced diet. Making sure the immune system is nutritionally supported is critical. People with this disease can struggle with several issues including nausea, diarrhea, constipation, and poor appetite. The provider may order medications to help with the nausea. Drinking extra fluids will help with both diarrhea and constipation issues. Restricting milk products with diarrhea and pushing fiber with constipation can help. A poor appetite can cause weight and nutrient loss. Frequent small meals, nutritional supplements, and light exercise may help. A provider may encourage a daily vitamin and mineral supplement. With unintended weight loss, additional "healthy" calories should be added to the diet.

Cancer

Patients undergoing radiation and chemotherapy can experience issues that impact eating. The treatments can harm fast-growing cells in the lining of the mouth, lips, and intestinal tract. Patients may have mouth sores that cause pain and swallowing problems. Taste and smell changes can occur. The treatments can cause appetite changes, diarrhea or constipation, fatigue, dry mouth, nausea, vomiting, and weight gain or loss. Good nutrition is critical for people to regain their strength and to heal after the treatments. A registered dietitian is commonly involved with the team of healthcare professionals caring for patients undergoing treatment.

Nutritional tips for patients undergoing cancer treatments include the following:
- Eat a soft, bland diet.
- Eat six to eight small meals a day instead of three meals. Attempt to eat high-calorie, high-protein snacks (e.g., hard-cooked eggs, peanut butter, nuts, supplements, trail mix, and canned chicken).
- Take only sips of liquids during meals. Drink most of the liquids between meals. Drink 8 to 10 cups of liquid a day to prevent constipation. Water, prune juice, and warm liquids are helpful.
- To reduce mouth dryness and sores, limit caffeine and alcohol; keep the mouth clean using water or a mild mouth rinse; avoid tart, acidic or salty foods; eat lukewarm, cold, soft, and creamy foods; and use anesthetic rinses prior to eating.
- Avoid foods with strong odors and food that are overly sweet, spicy, greasy, or fried.
- Eat small bites and chew the food well. Eat dry foods (e.g., crackers, toast).
- In addition, use a straw, small spoon, and puree food as needed. Suck on hard candies and ice chips to soothe the mouth and prevent mouth dryness.

CRITICAL THINKING 36.9

Kayla and Tim are working with Noemi Rodriguez, who is currently undergoing chemotherapy. She was not able to see her oncologist today, and she had a very sore mouth after the last treatment. Dr. Martin has seen her and wants Kayla to give her some nutritional tips. What might Kayla say to Noemi?

EATING DISORDERS

Eating disorders affect people of both genders. The rate of eating disorders in females is 2.5 times greater than it is in males. Eating disorders typically appear during the teen years or young adulthood, but they can start earlier or later in life.

Eating disorders are real, treatable illnesses. They typically coexist with other illnesses including substance abuse, anxiety disorders, and depression. Eating disorders, especially anorexia, can be life threatening without treatment.

Anorexia Nervosa

Anorexia nervosa (an oh RECKS see ah nur VOH sah) is a psychiatric eating disorder that causes people to lose more weight than what is healthy (Fig. 36.5). Individuals with this disorder have an intense fear of gaining weight. Often it starts during the preteen to teen years. It is more prevalent with females. Risk factors for anorexia nervosa include the following:
- A history of anxiety disorder or eating problems as a child
- Worry about weight and shape of their body; negative self-image
- An exaggerated focus on rules and trying to be perfect

Box 36.17 lists the symptoms of anorexia nervosa. The provider will order extensive laboratory tests to look at thyroid, liver, and kidney function. An electrocardiogram and bone density test may also be ordered. Treatment focuses on helping these patients recognize they

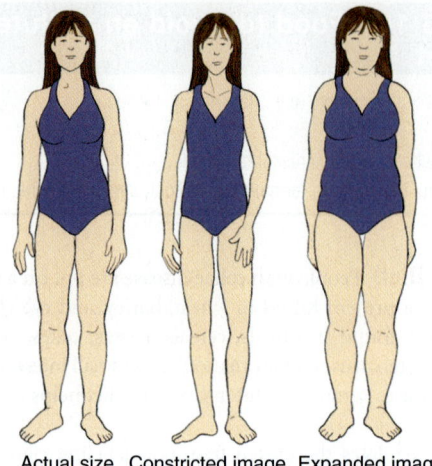

Actual size   Constricted image   Expanded image
                (−20%)   (+20%)

FIG. 36.5 The perception of body shape and size can be evaluated with the use of special computer drawing programs that allow a subject to distort (increase or decrease) the width of a picture of a person's body by as much as 20%. Subjects with anorexia consistently adjusted their own body picture to a size 20% larger than its true form, which suggests that they have a major problem with the perception of self-image. (From Stuart GW, Laraia MT: *Principles and Practice of Psychiatric Nursing*, ed 9, St. Louis, 2009, Mosby.)

BOX 36.17 Symptoms of Anorexia Nervosa

- Underweight, intense fear of gaining weight
- Very distorted body image (see Fig. 36.5)
- Severely limit the amount of food they eat
- Exercising all the time
- Going to the bathroom right after meals, vomiting secretly after eating
- Refusing to eat around others
- Using diuretics, laxatives, or diet pills
- Blotchy or yellow dry skin, covered with fine hair
- Confused, poor memory or judgment, slow thinking, depression
- Dry mouth
- Extreme sensitivity to cold
- Thinning of bones (osteoporosis)
- Wasting away of muscle
- Loss of body fat

MEDICAL TERMINOLOGY

an-: without
-ia: condition
orex/o: appetite

CRITICAL THINKING 36.10

Kayla and Tim are working with Celia Tapia, who is being seen for anorexia nervosa. She was diagnosed 10 months ago. When Kayla had to obtain Celia's weight, she had Celia step backward on the scale, so her back was to the digital reading. During the rooming process, Kayla never told Celia her weight. Based on what you know about anorexia nervosa, why does the medical assistant not share the patient's weight with her?

have an illness. Many types of treatments are available, though compliance with treatment is difficult. It is common for the disease to return.

Binge Eating Disorder

Binge eating disorder occurs when people regularly eat unusually large amounts of food in a short amount of time. They feel out of control, unable to manage what or how much they eat. A person may have binge eating disorder if this behavior occurs weekly for 3 months. It is the most common eating disorder. It impacts young women and middle age men. The exact cause is unknown, but the following may be related:
- Genetics (having a family member with an eating disorder)
- Changes in brain chemicals; depression or other negative emotions
- Unhealthy dieting

Bulimia Nervosa

Bulimia nervosa (boo LIM ee ah nur VOH sah) is also called bulimia. It is an eating disorder that causes overeating that leads to self-disgust. This is followed by vomiting, laxative use, or excessive exercise to prevent weight gain. Bulimia may also occur with anorexia nervosa. More women than men have bulimia. It is more common in teens and young women.

People with bulimia are usually at a normal weight, though they feel overweight. Symptoms that others see include the following:
- Excessive exercising
- Eating large amounts of food or buying large amounts of food that disappear right away
- Trips to the bathroom after meals
- Discarded boxes from laxatives, diet pills, emetics to induce vomiting, or diuretics.

Box 36.18 list the signs of bulimia found during the physical exam. Treatment is usually on an outpatient basis unless the individual has a coexisting diagnosis. Support groups, counseling, and medications can be helpful.

INSTRUCTING PATIENTS ON DIETARY CHANGES

When a patient needs a dietary change, the provider will give the order to the medical assistant. The provider will tell the medical assistant what type of diet the patient needs to be on. If the diet is only for a short period of time, the provider will indicate the time period. Sometimes the dietary change is related to a procedure. The provider will order the diagnostic procedure, and the medical assistant should be knowledgeable about the dietary changes required for that procedure.

Before meeting with the patient, it is important for the medical assistant to gather any brochures or information needed. Remember, it is a good idea to send the patient home with written instructions on dietary changes. If the patient does not understand English, use an interpreter service and make sure brochures are in the patient's primary language.

Lastly, before meeting with the patient, the medical assistant should look over the brochure. It is important to be knowledgeable about the content you are explaining to the patient. Reading the brochure aloud as a way of instructing the patient is not professional. The patient may feel you do not know what you are talking about.

> **BOX 36.18 Signs of Bulimia**
>
> - Broken blood vessels in the eyes (this occurs from the strain of vomiting)
> - Dry mouth, pouch-lick look to the cheeks
> - Rashes and pimples
> - Small cuts and calluses on the tops of fingers (from inducing vomiting)
> - Dehydration and electrolyte imbalance

When a medical assistant instructs a patient on a dietary change, it is important to know why people eat what they do and to understand how cultural dietary traditions relate to illness, as described in the following section. Box 36.19 provides a review of communication techniques and nonverbal behaviors that can show awareness of a patient's concerns. Procedure 36.1 details the process of coaching a patient regarding a dietary change.

Awareness of Others' Concerns

When working with patients regarding a dietary change, it is important to understand the factors that can impact what we eat:
- *Cost*: How much money we have impacts what foods we purchase. It can be expensive to purchase fresh fruits and vegetables, fish, and lean cuts of meat. Less expensive options are available, but they may not have the same taste or appeal.
- *Convenience*: With busy lifestyles, people sometimes choose what is easiest and quickest. This usually includes eating out or take-home meals.

> **BOX 36.19 Showing Awareness of a Patient's Concerns**
>
> Being aware means being alert and understanding what you are perceiving. When working with patients, we first need to be aware of the patient's concerns before we can show that we are aware. It is important to be accurate in our perception of the patient's concerns. If our perceptions are incorrect, we could say or behave in a way that is insensitive to the patient.
>
> Chapter 15 discusses therapeutic communication techniques. Let's review a few ways a medical assistant can show awareness of the patient's concerns:
>
> - *Reflection*: The medical assistant puts words to the patient's emotional reaction, which acknowledges the person's feelings—for example, "It sounds like you are unsure of this new way of eating."
> - *Restatement or paraphrasing*: The medical assistant rewords or rephrases a patient statement to check the meaning and interpretation. This shows you are listening and understanding the patient. You might say, for example, "What I am hearing is that you really like your family traditions for holiday meals."
> - *Summarizing*: This allows the medical assistant to recap and review what was said—for example, "If I understand how you feel about this new eating plan…"
>
> Remember that a medical assistant can also show awareness by using positive and open, nonverbal behaviors. These nonverbal behaviors could be used when working with a patient on a dietary change:
>
> - *Position:* The medical assistant should be at the level of the other person and angled toward the patient. For example, if the patient is sitting, then the medical assistant should be sitting also.
> - *Arms and posture*: The medical assistant should be poised with his or her arms to the side. This is an open, positive nonverbal behavior that shows interest in the other person.
> - *Facial expression*: The medical assistant should be smiling. Refrain from rolling your eyes, yawning, or frowning. These can be perceived as being bored or rude.
> - *Gestures and touch*: The medical assistant should use small gestures and an appropriate light touch on the hand of the patient, depending on the situation.
> - *Mannerisms*: The medical assistant should focus on the patient. It is not appropriate to look at your watch, phone, or the clock. This gives the patient the feeling you are bored or impatient.

PROCEDURE 36.1   Instruct a Patient on a Dietary Change

Tasks
Instruct a patient according to a patient's special dietary needs. Show awareness of the patient's concerns regarding the dietary change. Document in the health record.

Scenario
You are working with Dr. Angela Perez, a family practice provider. She just finished seeing Al Neviaser (date of birth [DOB]: 6/21/1968). Dr. Perez orders for heart-healthy diet instructions to be given to the patient.

Equipment and Supplies
- Patient's health record
- Heart-healthy diet brochure

Procedural Steps
1. Using the scenario, role-play the situation with a peer. Assemble supplies needed for the provider's order. Ensure that the patient can read and understand the written materials. Verify the order if you have any questions.
   Purpose: Using written materials is helpful when instructing a patient on a dietary change.
2. Greet the patient. Identify yourself. Verify the patient's identity with full name and date of birth. Explain the order from the provider. Answer any questions the patient may have about the procedure.
   Purpose: It is important to identify the patient in two different ways to ensure that you have the correct patient. Explaining the order can make the patient feel more comfortable and helps to reduce anxiety.
3. Position yourself at the same level as the patient. Angle yourself toward the patient. Have a poised position.
   Purpose: This position shows positive nonverbal behaviors to the patient. Being at the same level as the patient and angling toward the patient shows openness.
4. Accurately instruct the patient on the new diet. Use the written materials as you discuss the new eating plan.
   Purpose: The information taught to the patient should match what is in the written materials. Any inaccuracies will confuse the patient.
5. Use words that the patient can understand. Refrain from jargon and medical terminology. Use professional verbal and nonverbal communication.
   Purpose: Jargon and medical terminology can confuse patients. Unprofessional nonverbal behaviors like rolling your eyes, checking the clock, or yawning are disrespectful to the patient.

Scenario Update
After going over the heart-healthy eating plan, Mr. Neviaser states he is not sure this diet is for him. He likes his red meat and does not like to eat fish. He does not have a lot of money to buy expensive fresh fruits and vegetables.

6. Using therapeutic communication techniques (e.g., reflection, restatement, and summarizing), show the patient you are aware of his concerns.
   Purpose: By using therapeutic communication techniques, the medical assistant can show awareness of the patient's concerns.
7. Based on the patient's concerns, provide food alternatives that would meet the eating plan requirements.
   Purpose: The medical assistant can show awareness of the patient's concerns by providing alternative food choices that would meet the patient's requirements.
8. Evaluate the patient's understanding of the teaching by asking the patient to summarize the eating plan or describe a day's worth of meals. Answer any questions the patient may have.
   Purpose: It is important to check the patient's understanding of what was taught. Having the patient provide information back to the medical assistant is a better evaluation of understanding than asking, "Do you understand?"
9. Document the instruction in the patient's health record. Include the order, instruction given, written materials provided, and the patient's feedback.
   Purpose: Documenting indicates the instruction was provided to the patient. 11/04/20XX 0923 Per Dr. Perez's order, the pt and his wife were instructed on a heart-healthy diet. Pt indicated he did not eat fish and was concerned about the cost of fresh foods. Alternative healthy proteins and inexpensive food options were discussed with the patient. The pt and his wife were able to describe a day's worth of heart-healthy meals. Pt was encouraged to call with any additional questions. _____ Kayla Smith RMA

- *Background*: Our background can influence the foods we eat. Some cultures have healthier diets than others (Box 36.20). It can be helpful for people to modify cultural dishes by cutting the salt, fat, and sugar, without giving up the taste.
- *Emotional comfort*: Some people may eat when they are happy or when they are sad. Usually under these conditions, the food choices are not the healthiest. Some people stop eating when they are emotional.
- *Routine*: People eat what they always eat out of habit, personal preference, and availability. People may also eat with certain activities, like viewing a sports event, driving, or watching television. These habits are difficult to break.

It is important for the medical assistant to get to know what the patient is eating and why. This helps when coaching a patient on a dietary change. For instance, knowing your patient has a limited food budget is helpful when coaching him or her on healthier choices. You might be able to share ideas on healthy foods that are less costly or places to shop that are cheaper.

As medical assistants work with patients from various cultures, it is important to know more about those cultures. Many cultures have dietary traditions that influence how they respond to illness. In some cultures, food is considered a cure for illness. For instance, in the Asian culture when people are sick, they are out of balance in that

BOX 36.20   Cultural Diets

- Asian diets include whole grains (e.g., millet and rice), fruits, vegetables, legumes, nuts, and seeds. Fats are derived largely from vegetable oils (peanut or sesame oils). Dairy products are not traditionally eaten. Protein sources include broiled or stir-fried fish and seafood, egg whites, tofu, and nuts.
- Latin American diets include food from plant sources at each meal. This can include maize (corn), potatoes, fruits, vegetables, whole grains, beans, and nuts. Poultry, fish, and dairy typically are consumed daily. Meat and eggs are eaten weekly.
- Mediterranean diets include whole grains, fresh fruits and vegetables, and all types of legumes (e.g., beans, lentils, and peas) daily. Olive oil is used. Fish, poultry, and eggs are consumed weekly and meat monthly.
- Mexican diets include corn or flour tortillas, cabbage, legumes, squash, tomatoes, corn, and potatoes daily. Cheeses are eaten, but milk is not regularly consumed. Protein sources typically are fish, beef, poultry, lamb, and many types of beans.

they have too much heat or cold. To correct this balance, the person needs to eat foods of the opposite quality. It is important to be sensitive to these cultural practices. If the dietary change conflicts with the cultural practice, it is important to talk with the provider. A referral to a registered dietitian may provide the patient with extra support and information.

> ### CRITICAL THINKING 36.11
> Kayla and Tim are working with Amma Patel. She has returned for a follow-up visit regarding her new weight-controlled eating plan. Amma is struggling with the diet and with the need to give up her old eating habits. How can Kayla demonstrate her awareness of Amma's concerns regarding a dietary change?

CLOSING COMMENTS

Good nutrition is important for a person's health and well-being. For many people, changing their diet can be difficult and uncomfortable. It is important for the medical assistant to be sensitive to the change that the patient is asking about. Educating the patient about the benefits of making a dietary change may make the transition easier. Compliance with the diet increases if the person meets certain conditions:
- Can modify special foods and not give them up completely
- Has support from family and friends
- Can slowly transition to the new diet, though this might not always be possible

The medical assistant is an important team member when there is a need to help patients transition to a new diet. It is important for the medical assistant to be familiar with the dietary changes required for common procedures and diagnoses.

> ### EXCEPTIONAL CUSTOMER SERVICE
> When working with patients who are making dietary changes, it is important to be respectful of the patient. It is easy to tell a patient what to eat and what not eat, but that might not be the best way to approach the situation. A medical assistant may want to start by finding out the patient's favorite foods. What foods does the patient typically eat at meals? Are any health beliefs related to that food? Learning about the patient's diet can then help the medical assistant coach the patient.
>
> If the medical assistant feels the patient needs additional dietary support, talking with the provider is important. The provider can refer the patient to a registered dietitian for additional assistance.

CHAPTER REVIEW

This chapter discussed nutrition and metabolism. Catabolism releases energy as the molecules are broken into smaller molecules. Anabolism uses energy to build larger molecules from smaller molecules. Nutrients include the following:
- Carbohydrates are used for energy and to regulate protein and fat metabolism. Simple sugars, starches, and fiber are carbohydrates. Desserts, milk products, breads, and fruits are some examples of carbohydrates. The glycemic index is a numeric index used to indicate how much a carbohydrate increases the blood glucose level.
- Proteins break down into amino acids; both are considered building blocks for the body. Essential amino acids must come from food eaten, whereas nonessential amino acids are made in the body. Meat, poultry, dairy products, eggs, and nuts are sources of protein.
- Fat provides a source of energy when carbohydrates are not available. Saturated fats are solid at room temperature and should be limited in the diet. Unsaturated fats are liquid at room temperature. Monounsaturated and polyunsaturated fats are two types of unsaturated fats. Trans fatty acids or trans fats are created during the food manufacturing process. They are considered unhealthy.
- Minerals in the body are called electrolytes. Some examples include calcium, potassium, sodium, sulfur, iron, and iodine.
- Vitamins can be either fat or water soluble. Vitamins A, D, E, and K are fat soluble, and B vitamins and vitamin C are water soluble. A deficit of a vitamin can lead to a disease.
- Water is the basis for the fluids in the body. Our bodies need water to function and survive.

Eating a well-balanced diet, low in saturated fat, trans fats, added sugars, and sodium, will help a person to get all the required nutrients.

There are many medically ordered diets that patients may be put on. Here are the diets that were discussed in this chapter:
- *Clear liquid diet*: Made up of foods and beverages that turn to liquid at room temperature.
- *Full liquid diet*: Made up of clear liquids and milk products.
- *Soft and mechanical soft diet*: Made up of foods soft in texture, low in fiber, and easy to digest. Mechanical soft diets are prepared for easier chewing.
- *Bland diet*: Consists of foods that are soft and low in fiber and eliminates foods that are spicy, fried, and raw. Citrus foods, caffeine, and alcohol are eliminated.
- *Weight control diet*: Can help people lose or maintain weight. Control of portion sizes is very important on the weight control diet.
- *Diabetic eating plans*: Used for people with diabetes, who need to monitor their carbohydrate intake. There are several diabetic eating plans, including the glycemic index approach, the "Create Your Plate" method, and carb counting.
- *Low-sodium diet*: Helps to lower the blood pressure and also used to address kidney disease. DASH is used for hypertension and cardiovascular disease.
- *Heart-healthy diet*: Consists of limiting sugary, salty, and highly processed foods. Limiting the consumption of saturated fats, trans fats, and added sugar is also important.
- *Low-protein diet*: Used for people with liver and kidney disease.
- *High- and low-fiber diets*: Limit or add fiber to the diet. A high-fiber diet helps with constipation and weight loss. Low-fiber diets are used during a flare-up of an intestinal disease.
- *Elimination diet*: Removes suspicious allergens from the diet. Slowly they are reintroduced to find the allergens.
- *Gluten-free diet*: Used for people with celiac disease. Wheat, barley, and rye foods are removed from the diet.
- *Lactose-intolerance diet*: Involves avoiding milk products or using oral enzyme replacement supplements.

Nutrient needs vary throughout the population and with different disease processes. For some situations, the provider may recommend dietary supplements to ensure that adequate vitamins and minerals are consumed.

SCENARIO WRAP-UP

Tim really enjoyed working with Kayla for his practicum. He learned a lot from her as she worked with patients. His favorite part of the experience was the patient education, in which he was able to observe and participate. Kayla also learned from Tim during the experience. Because of his interest in nutrition, Tim was able to share with Kayla what he knew about current dietary trends.

Tim hopes to obtain a medical assistant job in a practice like the one where he did his practicum. He feels that the family practice environment will allow him to use many of the skills he learned in school. He will also have a lot of experience talking to patients about dietary changes.

37

Pharmacology Basics

LEARNING OBJECTIVES

1. Describe the sources and uses of drugs.
2. Describe pharmacokinetics, including absorption, distribution, metabolism, and excretion.
3. Discuss drug action, including the factors that influence drug action, the therapeutic effects of drugs, and the adverse reactions of drugs.
4. Explain drug legislation that is important in the ambulatory care setting.
5. List and describe the four types of drug names.
6. Do the following related to drug reference information:
   - Describe various methods to access drug reference information.
   - Identify the classifications of medications, including the indications for use, desired effects, side effects, and adverse reactions.
   - Discuss the terminology used in drug reference information.
7. Do the following related to types of medication orders:
   - Discuss types of medication orders.
   - List the four parts of a prescription.
   - List the types of information that all prescriptions need to include.
   - Prepare prescriptions using prescription refill procedures.
   - List and discuss commonly approved abbreviations.
   - Describe common requirements for scheduled substances.
8. Discuss over-the-counter (OTC) medications and herbal products.
9. Discuss and utilize basic math guidelines, including how to round numbers and how to use roman numerals.
10. Do the following related to measurement systems and temperature conversion:
    - Define basic units of measure in the household system and the metric system.
    - Convert among measurement systems.
    - Convert between Fahrenheit and Celsius temperatures.
11. Perform pharmacology calculations, such as total number of tablets needed, tablets per dose, liquid medication doses, and pediatric doses.

CHAPTER OUTLINE

1. Opening Scenario, 854
2. You Will Learn, 854
3. Introduction, 854
4. Pharmacology Basics, 854
   a. Sources of Drugs, 854
   b. Uses of Drugs, 854
   c. Pharmacokinetics, 854
      i. *Absorption,* 855
      ii. *Distribution,* 855
      iii. *Metabolism,* 856
      iv. *Excretion,* 856
   d. Drug Action, 856
      i. *Factors Influencing Drug Action,* 856
      ii. *Therapeutic Effects,* 857
      iii. *Adverse Reactions,* 857
5. Drug Legislation and the Ambulatory Care Setting, 857
   a. Food, Drug, and Cosmetic Act, 858
   b. Controlled Substances Act, 858
      i. *Compliance With the Controlled Substance Act,* 858
6. Drug Names, 859
7. Drug Reference Information, 860
   a. Drug Classification, 860
   b. Drug Terminology, 861
8. Types of Medication Orders, 862
   a. Prescriptions, 867
      i. *Medical Assistant's Role,* 867
      ii. *Controlled Substance Prescriptions,* 871
9. Over-the-Counter Medications and Herbal Products, 871
10. Math for Medications, 871
    a. Math Guidelines, 872
       i. *Rounding Numbers,* 872
       ii. *Roman Numerals,* 874
    b. Measurement Systems, 874
       i. *Household System,* 874
       ii. *Metric System,* 874
    c. Temperature Conversion, 876
    d. Total Number of Tablets Needed, 876
    e. Tablets per Dose, 877
    f. Liquid Medication Doses, 879
       i. *When Units Do Not Match,* 879
       ii. *Solutions,* 879
       iii. *Pediatric Doses,* 879
11. Closing Comments, 883
12. Chapter Review, 883
13. Scenario Wrap-Up, 883

OPENING SCENARIO

Gabe Garcia, a certified medical assistant (CMA) through the American Association of Medical Assistants (AAMA), has worked for Walden-Martin Family Medical (WMFM) Clinic for 7 years. He was hired right after he completed his medical assistant program. Gabe was asked to be Mark Allen's mentor for practicum. Mark has just completed all of his medical assistant courses at the local college and now needs 160 hours of practicum. He is excited to be working with Gabe.

Gabe works with several of the WMFM providers. He spends 1 to 2 hours a day working with prescription refills. Gabe also rooms patients, obtains their vital signs and history, and assists with injections. Mark will have a lot of great experiences with Gabe.

YOU WILL LEARN

1. To identify the basics of drugs, including the sources, uses, pharmacokinetics, and action.
2. To describe drug legislation and how it impacts the medical assistant practice.
3. To list the four names a drug could have.
4. To describe common drug classifications and reference information terminology.
5. To prepare prescriptions for the provider to sign.
6. To solve medication-related math problems.

INTRODUCTION

Pharmacology (FAHR mah kol oh jee) is the study of the properties, actions, and uses of drugs. A *drug* is a chemical substance used to cure, treat, prevent, or diagnose disease. In the ambulatory care setting, medical assistants deal with medication, from history taking to administering medications. Medical assistants must have a general understanding of the classification of drugs. They need to know how to pronounce the medication names. They must know how to give medications, typical side effects, and the dose to give. New medications are continually being developed and released for patient treatment. Thus medical assistants must stay updated on medications.

> **VOCABULARY**
> **side effects**: Unpleasant effects of a drug in addition to the desired or therapeutic effect.

PHARMACOLOGY BASICS

Medications have been around for a long time. The first medications came from natural products found in our ancestors' living environment. Today, with advancing technology, most medications are created in a laboratory setting. These sources and others will be explained along with the uses of medications.

In addition, a basic description of how medication enters, moves through, and exits the body will be given. This knowledge will help the medical assistant identify patients who may be at risk for medication issues because of their age or their disease process.

Sources of Drugs

Drugs are either created from natural sources or made synthetically in a laboratory. Plants, animals, minerals, and microbiological sources are all natural sources of drugs.

Plants are the oldest source of drugs. Our ancestors found that different plants helped with different symptoms. Leaves, bark, stems, roots, and fruits have been used in medicinal preparations through the years. Some examples of medicinal plant sources include the following:

- *Digitalis* (DIJ i tal is) (a heart medication) comes from the purple foxglove flower.
- Nicotine comes from the tobacco leaves.
- *Quinidine* (KWIN i deen) (antimalarial medications) comes from the *cinchona* (sing KOE nah) bark.

Animals are also a source of medications. Natural substances are extracted from animal tissues and organs. *Heparin* (HEP ah rin) comes from pig intestines. It is an *anticoagulant* (AN tie koe ag yuh lahnt), which is used to prevent blood clots. Lanolin is found in topical preparations used to protect the skin. It comes from the sebaceous glands of sheep. Other medications are developed with lactose and gelatin, which are from animals.

Minerals and microbiological substances are other natural sources of medications. Examples of minerals include the following:

- Iron is used to treat iron-deficiency anemia.
- Iodine is an antiseptic.
- Zinc is used as a supplement. It is also found in topical pastes for wounds.

One microbiological source is *Penicillium chrysogenum*. This is a fungus that creates penicillin.

Many medications originated in nature but have been recreated in the laboratory setting. For instance, insulin initially came from cattle and pigs. Many people developed allergies to the insulin. Now synthetic insulin is widely used. Biotechnology and genetic engineering techniques are continually being used to create new medications. With the help of technologic advances, individualized medications are also being produced. (Individualized medications will be discussed later in the chapter.) Synthetic medications are cheaper to produce because they are created in mass volumes. The quality of synthetic medications can also be controlled.

Uses of Drugs

When studying medications, it is important to identify the uses of drugs. Why are they being prescribed? What do they do in the body? Table 37.1 lists the eight common uses of drugs. Some medications may have more than one use.

> **MEDICAL TERMINOLOGY**
> **hypo-**: deficient
> **-ism**: condition
> **thyroid/o**: thyroid gland

> **CRITICAL THINKING 37.1**
> Gabe and Mark were discussing the basics of pharmacology and the eight uses of medications. Gabe asked Mark which use would include taking an antihistamine for allergy symptoms. How would you answer this question?

Pharmacokinetics

Pharmacokinetics (FAHR mah koe ki net iks) is the study of drug absorption, distribution, metabolism, and excretion in the body. Through pharmacokinetics, we understand when a medication starts to work in the body. We know how it moves through the body and which organs metabolize and excrete the drug from the body. Some of the patients you will be working with will have greater risks of side effects and toxicity. Understanding the basics of pharmacokinetics will help you identify those at greater risk for problems.

TABLE 37.1 Uses of Drugs

Use	Description
Prevention	Drugs used to prevent diseases. Example: vaccines are given and the body creates antibodies to protect against specific diseases.
Treatment	Drugs that relieve the symptoms while the body fights off the disease. Example: acetaminophen (a set a MEE noe fen) brings down a fever, while the body fights off the viral infection.
Diagnosis	Drugs used to diagnose or monitor a condition. Example: contrast medium (radiopaque dye) is given to highlight organs on x-rays.
Cure	Drugs that eliminate the disease. Example: amoxicillin (ah mox i SIL in) is used to cure strep throat.
Contraceptive	Drugs used to prevent pregnancy. Example: Depo-Provera (DEP oh proe VER ah) is a injectable contraceptive medication.
Health maintenance	Medications used to maintain or enhance health. Examples: vitamins and minerals.
Palliative (PAL ee ah tiv)	Drugs that do not cure or treat the disease, but improve the quality of life. Example: Morphine (MOR feen) is a pain medication that is commonly used by patients with cancer.
Replacement	Drugs that provide the patient with a substance needed to maintain health. Example: levothyroxine (lee voe thye ROX een) is used for patients with hypothyroidism.

VOCABULARY
toxicity: The harmful and deadly effect of a medication that can develop due to the buildup of medication or by-products in the body.

TABLE 37.2 Routes of Medication Administration

Route of Medication	Description
Oral (po)	Medications taken by mouth.
Sublingual (SL) (sub LIN gwal)	Placed under the tongue to dissolve; absorbs quickly into the bloodstream.
Buccal (BUCK uhl)	Placed in the cheek by the gums to dissolve and absorb quickly.
Intramuscular (IM)	Injected into the muscle. The greater the blood vessels in the muscle, the quicker the absorption.
Subcutaneous (subcut)	Injected just below the skin; moves into the capillaries or the lymphatic vessels and is brought to the bloodstream. This process is slower than the absorption of intramuscular drugs.
Intravenous (IV)	Injected directly in the bloodstream. Has the fastest absorption rate.

BOX 37.1 Routes Impact the Dose

Oral medications are absorbed in the stomach or in the intestines. The blood containing the absorbed digestive nutrients and drugs passes through the hepatic portal vein and the liver before it circulates to the rest of the body. In the liver, some of the drugs are chemically altered. Some of the active drug is lost during this first pass through the liver. This decreases the amount of drug in the circulating blood that can be used.

For instance, a person is having an allergic reaction and needs Benadryl. If taken orally, the person takes 50 mg. If taken intravenously, 10 mg may be given. This is because all 10 mg gets into the bloodstream, whereas some of the 50 mg is lost as it passes through the liver before circulating through the body. It is important for a medical assistant to realize that doses (e.g., 10 mg) may vary based on the route used to give the medication.

Absorption. Drugs can be administered many ways. *Route* is the means by which a drug enters the body. Where a drug enters the body is also considered the *site of administration* (Table 37.2). (Additional routes will be discussed in the Chapter 38.)

Absorption is the movement of drug from the site of administration to the bloodstream. The rate of absorption is influenced by the following factors:

- *Route*: Oral medications need to pass through the gastrointestinal (GI) tract. This takes time. Intravenous (IV) medications are directly administered into the bloodstream. IV medications have virtually no absorption time. They start working faster than drugs given by other routes.
- *Blood flow to the absorption area*: Medication given by the sublingual and buccal routes are absorbed quickly into the bloodstream. These sites are rich with blood vessels. Intramuscular (IM) medications absorb quicker than subcutaneous medications. The muscle tissue has more blood vessels than the subcutaneous tissue.
- *Ability of the medication to be absorbed*: Liquid medications are easier to absorb than solid medications. Solid medications need to be broken down before they absorb. Acidic medications are absorbed in the stomach. Base (or alkaline) medications are absorbed in the intestines.
- *Conditions at the site of the absorption*: Some medications must be taken with food. This can slow the absorption of the medication. Some medications taken on an empty stomach can be absorbed

faster. The intestines provide more surface area than the stomach for the absorption of medications.

MEDICAL TERMINOLOGY
-al, -ar, -ous: pertaining to
bucc/o: cheek
cutane/o: skin
intra-: within
lingu/o: tongue
muscul/o: muscle
sub-: under
ven/o: vein

Distribution. Once the drug is absorbed into the blood, it rapidly circulates through the body (unless it has to go through the liver) (Box 37.1). During this time, the drug is brought to the body tissues. The movement of absorbed drug from the blood to the body tissues is called *distribution*. The speed of the drug's movement from the blood to the tissues varies greatly. Some drugs bind with proteins in the blood and move slowly into tissues. Some drugs accumulate in certain tissues. These tissues act as *reservoirs*, slowly releasing the drug into the bloodstream and keeping the blood levels from decreasing too rapidly. This process prolongs the effect of the drug. Circulation issues (e.g., peripheral artery disease) can also slow the distribution of medication.

For the medication to move into certain organs, it must be able to pass through the tissues. The blood-brain barrier only allows certain fat-soluble medications to pass into the cerebrospinal fluid and the brain. In comparison, the placental membrane allows most drugs to pass through from the mother to the baby in utero. This is why only certain medications are prescribed during pregnancy.

Metabolism. *Metabolism* is a series of chemical processes whereby enzymes change drugs in the body. Metabolism is necessary so that medications can be cleared from the body. Active forms of drugs may be converted into water-soluble compounds, which are eventually excreted. Prodrugs can be changed into active forms of drugs (Box 37.2).

Most drug metabolism occurs in the liver. Younger children, older adults, and those with liver disease may have issues metabolizing medications. These populations could be at risk for drug toxicity. To prevent toxicity, the dose of medication is adjusted for at-risk populations.

> **MEDICAL TERMINOLOGY**
> **col/o**: colon
> **-itis**: inflammation
> **pro**: before, forward

Excretion. The *metabolites* (muh TAB uh lahyt) are excreted from the body, much like other waste products. Most drugs are excreted through the large intestine and kidneys. The large intestine excretes the undigested drug products in the stool. The kidneys excrete metabolites in the urine. Waived urine drug screening tests can detect certain metabolites.

Drugs can also be excreted in breast milk. This is critical information to have when a mother is breastfeeding her baby. As with pregnancy, only a limited amount of drugs is safe with breastfeeding. Most drug references indicate if medications pass into the breast milk. Other ways drugs can be excreted are through sweat, exhaled air, and saliva.

Young children, older adults, and those with kidney disease are at risk for the buildup of metabolic drug by-products in the body. These populations are at greater risk for symptoms of toxicity.

> **VOCABULARY**
> **metabolites**: By-products of drug metabolism.

Drug Action

Drugs are chemicals that can cause changes in the cells. There are four main drug actions:

- *Depressing*: slows down the cell's activity. For example, narcotic medications decrease the activity in the brain's respiratory center. This action slows the respiration rate.
- *Stimulating*: increases the cell's activity. For instance, caffeine increases brain activity.
- *Destroying*: kills cells or disrupts parts of cells. For example, chemotherapy medications destroy cancer cells.
- *Replacing substances*: substances required by the body can be given as medications. For instance, patients with type 1 diabetes mellitus take insulin.

Factors Influencing Drug Action. One might think that a drug works the same for everyone. This is not so. Personal characteristics can cause minor differences in how a drug works from one person to another (Box 37.3). Many factors influence drug action. Table 37.3 lists some examples.

BOX 37.2 Prodrugs

Prodrugs (PROE drugs) are medications that are administered in an inactive form. Through the normal metabolic processes, the medication is changed into an active form of a drug. The liver and the intestines are sites that can convert prodrugs to active forms of drugs. For instance *sulfasalazine* (sul fa SAL a zeen) (Azulfidine) is an antiinflammatory drug that is used to treat ulcerative colitis. It is also a prodrug. It is ingested in an inactive form. Bacteria in the colon change the drug into an active drug that is used by the body.

BOX 37.3 Pharmacogenomics Testing

Most medications are dosed as "one size fits all." Each person's genetic makeup impacts how that person responds to medications. *Pharmacogenomics* (FAAHR mah koe jah noe miks) is the study of how genetic factors influence a person's metabolic response to a specific medication. It can also be called *pharmacogenetics* (FAAHR mah koe jah ne tiks).

Pharmacogenomics testing usually requires a small blood or saliva sample. The sample is analyzed to determine if a specific medication will be an effective treatment for a particular individual. Testing can determine the best dose of medication and if the person could have serious side effects from the medication. A different pharmacogenomics test is required for each medication. Pharmacogenomics is largely used in cancer treatments, but it is becoming more common in other areas of medicine.

TABLE 37.3 Examples of Factors That Influence Drug Action

Factors	Description
Age	Infants and older adults have problems metabolizing and excreting medications. Their liver and kidneys are less effective. This can lead to possible drug accumulation and toxicity.
Body size	A person's size impacts the amount of drug needed. Children's dosages are calculated based on body weight. Thinner people require less medication than heavier people.
Gender	Women have a higher proportion of body fat. Hormonal differences can impact metabolism. Women can react differently to some medications compared with men.
Genetics	Genetic makeup can impact how a person responds to drugs (Box 37.3).
Diseases	Poor circulation, liver disease, and kidney disease can alter drug action.
Diet	Certain foods can impact a drug's action. For instance, milk products can decrease the effects of tetracycline (tet ra SYE kleen) (an antibiotic).
Drug dosage and route and timing of administration	The greater the amount of drug taken, the greater the effect will be. The route will also impact drug action. Drugs absorb, distribute, and metabolize differently based on the administration route. Some drugs work better when taken with food, whereas others do not.
Mental state	People with positive attitudes tend to do better than those with negative attitudes.
Environmental temperature	In hot weather, heat relaxes blood vessels. This can speed up the distribution of medication, thus speeding up the drug action.

Therapeutic Effects. Each medication has one or more *therapeutic effects* or desired effects. This is the intended action of the medication. For instance, the therapeutic effect of a pain reliever is to decrease pain. Sometimes multiple doses are needed to achieve the therapeutic effect. Other times just one dose of medication can achieve the therapeutic effect. For some medications, the provider may prescribe a higher initial dose, called a *loading dose*. This helps to quickly increase the medication level in the blood. A loading dose helps the person achieve the **therapeutic range** sooner. If the person's blood levels go beyond the therapeutic range, then the person usually experiences toxicity.

Adverse Reactions. Many times, when a medication is correctly administered, the therapeutic effect occurs. However, sometimes issues arise, and the person has problems with the medication. The person can experience an unexpected or life-threatening reaction, which is called an *adverse reaction*. Table 37.4 lists common adverse reactions.

Many experts and drug reference information will include side effects with adverse reactions. They may divide these into mild, moderate, and severe reactions. The side effects usually fall in the mild category. Severe adverse reactions are those that can cause disability, hospitalization, death, or birth defects.

Other reference information separates adverse reactions/events and side effects. Adverse reactions or events would be those that are life threatening and may cause disability or birth defects. Side effects would be unpleasant effects of the drug, in addition to the desired or therapeutic effect. They can be harmless or may cause injury. The most common side effects include symptoms of GI distress such as nausea, vomiting, constipation, and diarrhea.

DRUG LEGISLATION AND THE AMBULATORY CARE SETTING

In the ambulatory care environment, medications can be prescribed, administered, and dispensed (Table 37.5). Federal and state legislation govern these three activities. We will examine the laws, the agencies responsible for overseeing the laws, and the impact on medical assistants.

CRITICAL THINKING 37.2

Gabe and Mark were discussing therapeutic effect and loading dose. Gabe shared that patients sometimes get confused on how much medication to take when they are given two amounts, a loading dose and the regular amount. How might a healthcare professional instruct a patient who needs to take a loading dose?

VOCABULARY
addiction: A disease that occurs when a person cannot stop or limit the use of a drug, even after negative consequences have been experienced.
psychiatrists: Medical doctors who have been specially trained to diagnose and treat patients with mental, emotional, and behavioral conditions.
therapeutic range: Is reached when blood concentrations of a medication are high enough for the therapeutic effect to occur.

TABLE 37.4 Common Adverse Reactions

Adverse Reaction	Description
Allergy	Drug allergy occurs when a person develops antibodies against a specific drug. When the drug is taken, the antibodies attack the antigens from the drug. Tissues are damaged during this process, and histamines are released. Histamines cause the allergic reactions.
Anaphylaxis (AN ah fi LAK sis)	Extreme hypersensitivity to a specific drug (antigen) can cause life-threatening symptoms including swelling of the mouth and airway, difficulty breathing, wheezing, loss of consciousness, and death.
Idiosyncrasy (ID ee oh sing kreh see)	A peculiar response to a certain drug. For instance, Benadryl causes drowsiness. When it is given to children, they often get extremely agitated.
Cumulative effect	For medications taken routinely, often the prior dose is not completely metabolized and excreted before the next dose is given. This can lead to a buildup of medication or by-products that can produce toxic effects.
Toxicity	The harmful and possibly deadly effects of the medication that can develop due to the buildup of medication or by-products in the body. People with liver or kidney disease, young children, older adults, and those who overdose are at risk for toxicity.
Drug interactions	When two or more drugs are taken, sometimes a drug-drug interaction can occur. The interactions can be helpful or harmful. Three types of drug interactions can occur: • *Antagonism* (an TAG o nizm): one drug decreases or blocks the effect of another drug. Example: Naloxone is given for narcotic overdosage. • *Synergism* (SIN er jizm): the combined effect of two drugs used together is greater than the sum of each drug's effect (e.g., 1 + 1 > 2). Example of a harmful interaction: alcohol has a synergistic effect on antidepressants. • *Potentiation* (poe ten shee AE shun): a type of synergism; one drug increases the effect of the second drug. With L-dopa and carbidopa, one drug has no effect but increases the effect of the other drug (e.g., 0 + 1 > 1).
Tolerance	The need for a larger dose to get the same therapeutic or desired effect. Tolerance can be seen when taking narcotic pain medications and anticonvulsants (for seizures).
Drug dependence	Strong psychological or physical need to take a certain drug. Withdrawal symptoms can be experienced when a person stops using a drug. Drug dependence can occur with or without **addiction**.

TABLE 37.5 Medication Activities in the Ambulatory Care Setting

Activities	Description	Examples of Who Can Perform the Activity
Prescribe	To order a medication as a treatment for a condition.	Doctors (MD, DO, dentists, and psychiatrists) and advance practice professionals including physician assistants (PAs), nurse practitioner (NPs), and certified nurse midwives (CNMs) (State prescribing laws can vary for advance practice professionals.)
Administer	To give a prescribed dose of medication to a patient.	Medical assistants or nurses (State laws related to medication administration by medical assistants can vary.)
Dispense	To give a supply of medication that the patient will take at a later time.	Pharmacists

TABLE 37.6 Some Areas That Are Covered by the Food and Drug Administration

Areas	Examples
Foods	Dietary supplements, bottled water, food additives, infant formula, and other food products
Drugs	Prescription drugs (brand-name and generic) and nonprescription (over-the-counter) drugs
Biologics	Vaccines, blood and blood products
Medical devices	Medical equipment (from simple [tongue depressor] to complex [heart pacemaker]), dental devices, surgical implants

CRITICAL THINKING 37.3

At WMFM, pharmaceutical representatives drop off sample medications that are given to patients. Usually, the provider will give a few days' worth of samples to a patient to ensure the patient is tolerating the medication. If the patient has no issues, then he or she gets the prescription filled. Mark had seen the provider bag up a few samples and attach directions to the bag. The provider gave the bag to Gabe and asked him to give it to the patient. Mark asked Gabe, "Who is dispensing the medication?" How would you answer this question?

Food, Drug, and Cosmetic Act

The Food, Drug, and Cosmetic Act is enforced by the Food and Drug Administration (FDA). The FDA is a federal agency in the Department of Health and Human Services (HHS). The FDA is responsible for the safety, effectiveness, security, and quality of drugs, cosmetics, and food (Table 37.6). Manufacturers must submit applications for new products to the FDA. Manufacturers must provide adequate data to show the safety and effectiveness of the product. The FDA must determine if drugs, devices, and products are safe and effective. Once this is determined, then the product is released to the general public.

The FDA monitors the safety of products released to the market. The FDA Adverse Event Reporting System (FAERS) is a computerized database that helps the FDA monitor drugs. It contains reports of adverse events reported to the FDA. MedWatch is the FDA's reporting program. It provides information on products overseen by the FDA. MedWatch is available to healthcare professionals (www.fda.gov/safety/medwatch/).

If the FDA determines a medication is unsafe, it will recall the medication. The medical assistant should remove any recalled medications from the stock and sample cabinets. (*Sample medications* come from pharmaceutical companies and are used for patients.) Concerned patients may contact their providers. The provider will determine what action to take for each patient.

Controlled Substances Act

The Controlled Substances Act (CSA) Title II of the Comprehensive Drug Abuse Prevention and Control Act of 1970 is a federal law. The Drug Enforcement Agency (DEA) is a federal law enforcement agency under the U.S. Department of Justice. The DEA enforces the CSA. The DEA oversees the manufacturing, importation, possession, use, and distribution of illegal and legal controlled substances.

Under the CSA, controlled substances are divided into five schedules. These schedules are arranged from the greatest to least abuse potential (Table 37.7). State statutes also address procedures related to scheduled medications. It is important for the medical assistant to know the schedule of commonly ordered medications. Some controlled substance prescriptions are handled differently. This will be discussed later in the chapter.

Compliance With the Controlled Substance Act. Providers prescribing controlled substances need a DEA registration number. Each provider has a unique number. The DEA number is good for 3 years. The medical assistant may need to assist the provider in renewing or obtaining a DEA number. This can be done at the DEA website at www.deadiversion.usdoj.gov. Additional state requirements may be needed before a provider can prescribe controlled substances.

Controlled substances have a paper trail. This record starts with the manufacturer and ends when the medication is dispensed or administered. In some healthcare facilities, the in-house pharmacy handles the controlled substances that are administered. The provider gives the medical assistant a prescription for a patient. The medical assistant gives the pharmacist the prescription and, in return, gets the medication. (Please note that some state laws do not allow medical assistants to administer controlled substances.) With this scenario, the pharmacist is responsible for tracking the paperwork for the controlled substances.

In healthcare facilities without pharmacies, providers must take the responsibility of ordering controlled substances from the manufacturer. The medical assistant must help the provider comply with the Controlled Substance Act. The following sections will discuss common compliance activities.

Storage. All controlled substances must be adequately safeguarded (Box 37.4). They need to be kept in a locked cabinet or safe of substantial construction. Keys should be placed in a locked area accessible only to authorized persons. Controlled substances should be kept in their original containers. Medications with different lot numbers or expiration dates should not be combined or repackaged.

Inventory records. It is important to keep an ongoing log of controlled substances received from manufacturers and administered to patients. Medications are tracked by the manufacturer, lot number, and expiration date. This information is found on the package. When a patient needs a controlled substance, the medical assistant must complete the log. The log typically requires the following:

- The medication information (name, dose, lot number, and expiration date)

TABLE 37.7 Schedule of Controlled Substances

Schedule	Psychological and Physical Dependence	Examples
I	Highest potential for abuse; drugs with no currently accepted medical use	• Heroin, lysergic acid diethylamide (LSD), ecstasy
II/IIN (C–II)	High level of abuse; can lead to severe psychological or physical dependence	• Schedule II narcotics: oxycodone (OxyContin, Percocet), fentanyl (Duragesic), codeine, morphine • Schedule IIN stimulants: amphetamine (Adderall), methamphetamine (Desoxyn), methylphenidate (Concerta, Ritalin LA)
III/III N (C–III)	Moderate to low physical dependence or high psychological dependence	• Schedule III narcotics: acetaminophen with codeine (Tylenol #2 or #3), buprenorphine (Suboxone) • Schedule III N non-narcotics: ketamine, anabolic steroids (e.g., Depo-Testosterone)
IV (C–IV)	Low potential for abuse relative to substances in Schedule III	• Schedule IV substances: alprazolam (Xanax), clonazepam (Klonopin), diazepam (Valium), lorazepam (Ativan)
V (C–V)	Lowest potential for abuse relative to substances listed in Schedule IV; contains limited quantities of certain narcotics	• Schedule V substances: Robitussin AC, ezogabine (Potiga)

BOX 37.4 Storage of Medications

- Store controlled substances in a different location than nonnarcotic medications.
- Refer to package inserts for specific storage information.
- Store medications in a cool, dry location. Keep medications away from the light, heat, or moisture.
- For refrigerated and frozen medications, keep temperature logs to ensure the appropriate temperature range is maintained.
- Keep *stock medications* (purchased by department) separated from *sample medications* (given from pharmaceutical manufacturers for patients).
- Keep medications out of exam rooms. Lock medication cabinets at the end of the day.
- For information on vaccine storage, refer to Chapter 22.

BOX 37.5 Discarding Medications in the Healthcare Facility

Discard medication that is expired, contaminated, unlabeled, or opened and not used. Some healthcare facilities have medication discarding programs to prevent medications from entering the city's water supply. Remember, if the medication is a controlled substance, two authorized employees must sign a waste log before the medication is discarded. Both employees must witness the disposal.

To discard medication, follow these steps if the facility has no other procedures in place:

- Return expired controlled substances to the place from which they were received (e.g., manufacturer), accompanied with the proper paperwork.
- Flush liquids down the sink.
- Flush pills down the toilet.
- Mix powdered medications with water and flush them down the toilet.
- Flush fluid in syringes down the sink, and discard the syringe in a biohazardous sharps container.

- The ordering provider's name
- Information on the patient receiving the medication (name, date of birth, address, health record number, etc.)
- The name or initials of the person administering the medication

The log must be kept separate from the patient's health record. The medication must also be documented in the patient's health record after it is administered.

Periodically *reconciling* of the log with the actual inventory count is important to identify missing medication. An inventory of all controlled substances must be done at least annually, unless required more often by law. Some states have special requirements for the inventory. It is important for the medical assistant to be knowledgeable about the special state requirements. The controlled substance inventory and log records need to be kept for 2 years. The records may be inspected by individuals authorized by the attorney general.

> **VOCABULARY**
> **reconciling:** Comparing a document with another document to ensure that they are consistent.

Drug destruction. Expired controlled substances are returned to the place from where they were received. For example, controlled substances that were sent by the manufacturer must be returned to the manufacturer along with the required paperwork.

Sometimes a controlled substance must be destroyed in the healthcare facility. Such situations include the following:

- Only part of the medication is used for the patient and the extra amount must be destroyed.
- The patient refuses the medication after it has been opened and prepared.
- The medication was accidentally contaminated before it was administered.

In these situations, the destruction of the controlled substance must be made in the presence of two authorized persons (e.g., medical assistants, nurses). An entry on the waste log must be made. The following information needs be included: the date, drug name and strength, quantity, reason for destruction and signatures of both persons. Box 37.5 describes how to discard medications in the healthcare facility.

Theft and diversion reporting. Diversion of controlled substances means using the medication for personal reasons (Box 37.6). If a medical assistant identifies that controlled substances are missing, it is important to notify the provider and supervisor. Many states and the DEA require any theft or loss to be reported to them within a given period of time. A report must be completed and filed by the deadline.

DRUG NAMES

A single drug may have up to four names: chemical, generic, official, and brand. The drug is known by its chemical name until it receives

BOX 37.6 Medical Assistant's Role in Preventing Drug Abuse

By following these guidelines, the medical assistant can help prevent drug abuse:
- Carefully monitor patients who repeatedly call for prescription refills of controlled substances. Be aware that some patients will give aliases (false names).
- Request health records from other facilities for patients who report previous prescriptions for scheduled drugs.
- If the facility uses paper prescription pads, keep blank pads in a locked cabinet. They should be stored away from patient treatment areas.
- Never use prescription pads for notepads. Never use preprinted or presigned forms.
- Secure computers used for electronic health record (EHR) documentation to prevent patient access to prescription generation.
- Keep only a limited supply of controlled substances on hand.
- Keep accurate, complete records of controlled substances dispensed on site. Patients' records should contain information on prescribed and administered controlled substances.

BOX 37.7 Generics Versus Brands Medications

If you ever walk through the pain medication aisle at a local store, you will see many bottles of ibuprofen products. The expensive products are name brands and the inexpensive products are generic brands.

The company that initially created the medication will market it using a brand name. That company has sole rights to manufacture the medication until the patent expires. During this time, it is not uncommon for the price to be expensive. The manufacturer may have spent years developing the medication before it went to market. Once the patent expires, other companies may create their own version of the medication. Some will market the medication under a brand name and others will use generic names.

When a company creates a medication, the company determines the appearance of the medication (e.g., color, size, and shape). It also comes up with the nonactive ingredients or additives. This might be a color, sweetener, flavor, fillers, binders, and so on. For the active ingredient, the medication (i.e., ibuprofen), the company must comply with the FDA's regulations. The active ingredient must be of the same quality, purity, and amount as any other FDA-approved ibuprofen product of the same strength.

Most people do not notice a difference between generic and brand name medications. Other people do notice a difference. Their bodies may react to the nonactive ingredients differently. This can impact their treatment of certain conditions. The provider can indicate if a generic medication can be used for prescriptions. This is important to keep in mind if you are assisting a provider by preparing prescriptions.

the FDA approval. The medical assistant should be familiar with the brand and generic names of common medications (Box 37.7).
- *Chemical name:* represents the drug's exact chemical formula. For example, the chemical name of *ibuprofen* (eye BYOO proe fen) is 2-(4-isobutylphenyl) propanoic acid.
- *Generic name:* assigned by the U.S. Adopted Names (USAN) Council. Similar medications are given similar-sounding generic names. All drugs need to have the generic name on the packaging. For example, ibuprofen is a generic name.
- *Official name*: used to list the medication in the United States Pharmacopeia and the National Formulary (USP–NF). This book provides the standards (strength, purity, etc.) for drugs in the United States. In many cases, the official name is the same as the generic name. For example, ibuprofen is also the drug's official name.
- *Brand name:* also called trade name. The manufacturer assigns and registers the medication name. No other company can use that name. Usually the brand name begins with a capital letter and is followed by the registered sign (®). For example, brand names of ibuprofen include Advil and Motrin.

CRITICAL THINKING 37.4

Mark and Gabe were working with Janine Butler, a patient being seen for hypertension. While they were reviewing Janine's current medication list, she asked them what the difference was between generic and brand name medication. How might you answer this question?

DRUG REFERENCE INFORMATION

A medical assistant is obligated to become familiar with the drugs that are most frequently prescribed in the department. It is essential to know their indications, adverse reactions, administration routes, dosage, and storage. Using drug reference information can help the medical assistant learn about drugs. In the ambulatory care environment, drug reference information is available in both print and digital form.

With each drug (including drug samples and stock medications), the manufacturer includes a package insert. The package insert provides information about the medication, side effects, administration techniques, dosages, storage, and so on.

Drug handbooks provide condensed, more common information on the drugs. Many of these books are organized by the generic names of drugs.

An old classic, the Physician Desk Reference (PDR), was a very large book that contained a comprehensive collection of package insert information. After publishing the 2017 version (the 71st edition), the company stopped printing the PDR. The drug reference information is available through its digital online products (Prescribers' Digital Reference [PDR]), its app, and other products that integrate with electronic health records. More information can be found on the website (www.pdr.net).

The digital drug reference information has a huge advantage over print information. It can be updated quickly and easily compared with print information. With new medications being released to the public regularly, many providers prefer updated drug reference information. The market for digital drug information has grown over the years. Digital drug reference information is available online, through apps, and with electronic health records:
- Online drug reference information is available from many sites. It is important for the medical assistant to use reliable websites. Governmental websites (e.g., medlineplus.gov and www.fda.gov) contain updated, reliable information. Sites that patients use may contain older information and can include medications that are not available in the United States.
- When selecting an app for drug reference information, be sure it is routinely updated. Read the reviews, and research the company providing the information. Only use reputable apps for drug reference information.
- Many electronic health record software programs can incorporate drug reference information. This makes it easy for healthcare professionals to look up drug information.

Drug Classification

Drugs are grouped by classification or class. It is important for a medical assistant to be aware of the class of drugs. For instance, patients will ask why they are taking a specific medication. The medical assistant should know if the medication is for hypertension, diabetes treatment, and the like. Table 37.8 provides a list of classifications of medications with descriptions. (Appendix D, Medication Classification, provides additional classification information. The appendix includes indications for use, desired effects, side effects, adverse reactions, and common generic and trade names of medications.)

Drug Terminology

Regardless of how drug reference information is obtained, it is important for the medical assistant to understand the different sections. The following sections are typically found in drug reference information:

TABLE 37.8 Examples of Medication Classifications

Classification	Pronunciation	Description
Analgesic	(AN ahl jee zik)	Relieves pain
Anesthetic	(an es THET ik)	Produces local or general anesthesia
Antacid	(ant AS id)	Neutralizes stomach acid
Anti-Alzheimer	(AN tie AWLTZ hye mer) (Note: anti- can be [AN tie] or [AN tee])	Treats dementia (Alzheimer)
Antianxiety	(AN tie ang ZIE e tee)	Reduces anxiety and tension
Antiarrhythmic	(AN tie ah RITH mik)	Treats heart arrhythmias
Antibiotic	(AN ti bye OT ik)	Treats bacterial infections
Anticholinergic	(AN tie koe leh nuhr jik)	Reduces smooth muscle spasms
Anticoagulant	(AN tie koe ag yuh lahnt)	Decreases blood clotting ability
Anticonvulsant	(AN tie kohn vul sahnt)	Reduces the frequency and severity of seizures
Antidepressant	(AN tie di PRES ahnt)	Treats depression
Antiemetic	(AN tie e MET ik)	Reduces nausea and vomiting
Antifungal	(AN tie FUNG gal)	Treats fungal infections
Antigout	(AN tie GOUT)	Reduces the uric acid in the body
Antihistamine	(AN tie HIS tah meen [-min])	Relieves allergies by blocking the histamine action
Antihyperglycemic	(AN tie HYE per glye SEE mik)	Reduces blood glucose level
Antihypertensive	(AN tie hye pehr ten siv)	Lowers blood pressure
Antiinflammatory	(AN tie in FLAM ah tohr ee)	Reduces inflammation
Antimigraine	(AN tie MYE grain)	Treats or prevents migraine headaches
Antineoplastic	(AN tie NEE oh plaz tik)	Slows or stops the growth of cancer cells
Antiplatelet	(AN tie PLATE lit)	Prevents the function of platelets (formation of clots)
Antipsychotic	(AN tie sye KOT ik)	Alters the chemical actions in the brain
Antitussive	(AN tie TUS iv)	Suppresses coughs
Antiviral	(AN tie VIE rahl)	Treats viral infections
Bronchodilator	(BRONG koe die lay tohr)	Relaxes the smooth muscles of the bronchi
Cholesterol-lowering agent	(koh LES the rohl)	Reduces low-density lipoprotein and triglycerides in the blood while increasing the high-density lipoprotein
Contraceptive	(KON trah SEP tiv)	Inhibits conception (prevents pregnancy)
Corticosteroid	(KOHR ti koe STER oid)	Reduces inflammation
Decongestant	(DEE kohn JES tahnt)	Relieves nasal and sinus congestion
Diuretic	(DYE uh RET ik)	Increases urinary output and lowers blood pressure
Electrolyte	(ih LEK troh lite)	Maintains normal electrolyte level and proper functioning of the body systems
Erectile dysfunction agent	(ee REK tile)	Facilitates an erection
Expectorant	(ik SPEK tohr ahnt)	Thins bronchial secretions, making it easier to cough up the mucus
Hematopoietic	(HEE mah toe poi EE tik)	Promotes blood cell production
Hemostatic	(HEE moh STAT ik)	Clots blood
Hormone replacement	(HOHR mone)	Replaces hormones or compensates for hormone deficiencies
Laxative	(LAK sah tiv)	Promotes stools
Leukotriene receptor antagonist	(LOO koh TRY een, an TAG ah nist)	Blocks the action of substances that cause asthma and allergic rhinitis
Miotic	(mye OT ik)	Drains excessive fluid from the eye, used for glaucoma
Muscle relaxant	(re LAK sahnt)	Decreases pain
Mydriatic	(MID ree at ik)	Dilates the pupil, used for ophthalmic procedures
Osteoporosis agent	(OS tee oh poh roe sis)	Promotes bone mineral density, used to treat osteoporosis
Proton-pump inhibitor	(PROE ton, in HIB i tohr)	Decreases the acid produced in the stomach
Sedative-hypnotic	(SED ah tiv, hip NOT ik)	Slows brain activity, allowing sleep
Stimulant	(STIM yuh lahnt)	Stimulates the brain and body, makes the person more alert
Tumor-necrosis factor (TNF) inhibitor	(neh KROE sis)	Blocks the action of TNF, preventing inflammation in autoimmune disorders

- *Names:* usually the generic name is listed with the trade names. Some references may indicate if the trade name found in the United States or Canada.
- *Description:* describes the medication and its general use.
- *Boxed warning:* also referred to as a "black box warning." It addresses serious or life-threatening risks. This information also appears on the drug's label.
- *Dosage:* specifies the route, dose, and timing of the medication; usually corresponds to an indication (disease or condition). May provide information on doses for different age ranges. *Maximum dosage* indicates the greatest amount of medication a person should have within a 24-hour period.
- *Indication:* conditions or diseases for which the drug is used.
- *Dosage considerations:* indicates recommended changes in dosages for special populations (e.g., patients with hepatic impairment, renal impairment).
- *How supplied:* lists the **form** (e.g., chewable tablets, capsules) and the strength (e.g., 250 mg).
- *Administration:* provides information on how the medication should be administered. Includes important administration techniques such as information on shaking the medication, if it needs to be taken with food, and so on.
- *Contraindications* (KON trah IN di KAY shuns): reasons or conditions that make administration of the drug improper or undesirable. For example, aspirin is contraindicated in patients with GI bleeding.
- *Precautions:* indicates necessary actions or special cares that need to be taken when the patient is on the medication. May include information on laboratory tests, special populations (children and geriatric), pregnancy, breastfeeding, and so on (Box 37.8).
- *Adverse reactions:* also called side effects in some information. This section describes known undesirable experiences associated with the medication. Reactions may be divided into severe (life threatening, serious reactions), moderate, and mild.
- *Interactions:* includes medications, foods, and beverages that interact with the medication. These products may either increase or decrease the medication levels in the blood. They may also increase the risk of adverse reactions if taken together.
- *Action:* How the drug provides therapeutic results in the body, or the use of the drug.
- *Pharmacokinetics:* provides information on the absorption, distribution, metabolism, and excretion of the medication. Information on when the drug is at its highest level in the body or when the drug starts working may be included (Table 37.9).

> **VOCABULARY**
>
> **form**: Physical characteristics of a medication (e.g., tablet and suspension).

> **CRITICAL THINKING 37.5**
>
> Gabe mentioned to Mark that he learned that the FDA had changed the pregnancy risk categories. Mark had not heard about this. Gabe further explained why. Describe why the new changes will provide more information to providers and patients.

Table 37.10 provides drug information on the top 50 commonly prescribed medications. Please use drug reference information for additional information on these products.

TYPES OF MEDICATION ORDERS

A *medication order* refers to directions given by a provider for a specific medication to be administered to a patient. The medical assistant receives the information from the provider. The provider must give the following information:

- Patient's name and health record number or date of birth (DOB) (e.g., "Noemi Rodriguez DOB 11/04/1971")
- Medication name, dose, and route (e.g., "Tylenol 1 g po")

The provider can give the order over the phone or in person. This type of order is called a *verbal order*. It is important for the medical assistant to write down the order and read it back to the provider. This process ensures the order was heard and recorded correctly. The provider can also give the medical assistant a *written order*. Usually, these are written on a prescription pad or in an electronic message. A written order only needs clarification from the provider if the medical assistant cannot read the order or has a question.

> **BOX 37.8 Pregnancy and Lactation Labeling Final Rule**
>
> Since 1979 the FDA has enforced the use of pregnancy risk categories. The A, B, C, D, and X categories indicate the risk to the baby in utero. In 2015 the Pregnancy and Lactation Labeling Rule (PLLR) replaced the pregnancy risk letter categories with more comprehensive information. The goal is to provide the provider and patient with pregnancy and lactation information. This information can be used when discussing the risks versus the benefits of a medication. The FDA created the new system to help with patient-specific counseling and informed decision making for pregnant and breastfeeding mothers who need medication therapies. The system consists of three subcategories with detailed information about the following:
>
> - *Pregnancy:* includes information on the risks during pregnancy for the mother and baby, as well as data on the risk of adverse developmental outcomes.
> - *Lactation:* includes information on the presence of the drug in breast milk, the effects on a breast-fed child, and the impact on milk production.
> - *Females and males of reproductive potential:* includes information about when pregnancy testing or contraception is required during drug therapy and data that suggests drug-associated fertility effects.

TABLE 37.9 Common Drug Action Timing Terms	
Term	**Once the Drug Is Administered:**
Biologic half-life	Time it takes half of the drug to be metabolized or eliminated by normal biologic processes
Onset	The time it takes for the drug to produce a response
Peak	The time it takes for the drug to reach its greatest effective concentration in the blood
Duration	The time during which the drug is present in the blood at great enough levels to produce a response

Text continued on p. 868

TABLE 37.10 Information on Commonly Prescribed Medications

Generic Name	Brand/Trade Name(s)	Class/Schedule	Medication Information
hydrocodone/ acetaminophen (APAP) (hye droe KOE done, a set a MEE noe fen)	Vicodin (vye KOE din) Norco (NOHR koe) Lortab (LORE tab)	Analgesics (Narcotic [opioids]) C-II	*Indication:* moderate to severe pain *Desired effects/action:* changes the way the brain and nervous system respond to pain *Side effects:* GI intolerance, difficulty urinating, anxiety, fuzzy thinking *Adverse reaction:* slowed breathing, chest tightness
oxycodone/ acetaminophen (APAP) (ox i KOE done, a set a MEE noe fen)	Percocet (PER koe set) Oxycet (OKS ee set) Roxicet (ROKS i set)	Analgesics (Narcotic [opioids]) C-II	*Indication:* moderate to severe pain *Desired effects/action:* changes the way the brain and nervous system respond to pain *Side effects:* GI intolerance, flushing, headache, mood changes *Adverse reaction:* slowed breathing, angina, hypersensitivity, seizures
tramadol (TRAH mah dole)	Ultram (UHL tram) Conzip (KON zip)	Analgesics (Narcotic [opioids]) C-II	*Indication:* moderate to severe pain *Desired effects/action:* changes the way the brain and nervous system respond to pain *Side effects:* GI intolerance, difficulty sleeping, change in mood, dry mouth *Adverse reaction:* hallucination, agitation, hypersensitivity, arrhythmias
memantine (meh MAN teen)	Namenda (NAH men dah)	Anti-Alzheimer	*Indication:* Alzheimer *Desired effects/action:* decreases the brain chemicals that cause the dementia *Side effects:* GI intolerance, edema, weight loss, dizziness, anxiety, aggression *Adverse reaction:* angina, seizures, hypertension
alprazolam (al PRAY zoe lam)	Xanax (ZAN aks)	Antianxiety (Benzodiazepines) C-IV	*Indication:* anxiety and panic disorders *Desired effects/action:* decreases abnormal excitement in the brain *Side effects:* drowsiness, headache, dizziness, GI intolerance, dry mouth, weight changes *Adverse reaction:* seizures, jaundice, depression, memory problems
clonazepam (kloe NA ze pam)	Klonopin (CLON uhh pin)	Antianxiety (Benzodiazepines) C-IV	*Indication:* seizures, panic attacks *Desired effects/action:* decreases abnormal excitement in the brain *Side effects:* drowsiness, coordination problems, joint pain, blurred vision, changes in sex drive *Adverse reaction:* hypersensitivity
diazepam (dye AHZ eh pam)	Valium (vah LEE uhm)	Antianxiety (Benzodiazepines) C-IV	*Indication:* relieves anxiety, muscle spasms, and seizures *Desired effects/action:* *Side effects:* GI intolerance, weakness, tiredness, drowsiness, dry mouth *Adverse reaction:* restlessness, frequent urination, blurred vision
digoxin (di JOX in)	Lanoxin (lan OKS in) Digitek (DIJ i tek) Cardoxin (kar dox in)	Antiarrhythmics	*Indication:* congestive heart failure (CHF), atrial fibrillation *Desired effects/action:* helps the heart work better, controls heart rate *Side effects:* dizziness, drowsiness, visual changes (blurred, yellow), arrhythmias *Adverse reaction:* swelling of hands and feet, unusual weight gain, difficulty breathing *Assessment:* take apical pulse, hold if <60 in adults, <70 in children, and <90 in infants
cephalexin (sef a LEX in)	Keflex (KEF leks)	Antibiotics (Cephalosporin)	*Indication:* bacterial infections (e.g., urinary tract, ear, and pneumonia) *Desired effects/action:* stops bacteria growth *Side effects:* GI intolerance, agitation, confusion, headache *Adverse reaction:* hypersensitivity, watery or bloody stools, hallucinations
azithromycin (az ith roe MYE sin)	Zithromax (zith ROW maks) Zithromax Z-Paks (zith ROW maks ZEE paks) Zmak (ZEE mak)	Antibiotics (Macrolide)	*Indication:* bacterial infections (e.g., sexually transmitted infections, bronchitis, and pneumonia) *Desired effects/action:* stops bacteria growth *Side effects:* GI intolerance, headache *Adverse reaction:* hypersensitivity, mouth sores, arrhythmias, jaundice, dark-colored urine
amoxicillin (ah mox i SIL in)	Amoxil (ah MUHHS il) Moxtag (MUHHS tag)	Antibiotics (Penicillin)	*Indication:* bacterial infections (e.g., pneumonia, gonorrhea, ear, and throat) *Desired effects/action:* stops the bacteria growth *Side effects:* GI intolerance *Adverse reaction:* hypersensitivity, seizures, jaundice

Continued

TABLE 37.10 Information on Commonly Prescribed Medications—cont'd

Generic Name	Brand/Trade Name(s)	Class/Schedule	Medication Information
warfarin (WAR far in)	Coumadin (COU mah din)	Anticoagulants	*Indication:* prevents blood clots from forming *Desired effects/action:* decreases clotting ability of the blood *Side effects:* GI intolerance, loss of hair, chills *Adverse reaction:* hypersensitivity, infection, angina, jaundice, bleeding
gabapentin (GAH bah pen tin)	Neurontin (NOOR on tin) Horizant (huhh RI zant)	Anticonvulsants	*Indication:* seizures, postherpetic neuralgia, restless legs syndrome (RLS) *Desired effects/action:* decreases abnormal excitement in the brain; decreases seizures *Side effects:* drowsiness, blurred vision, anxiety, memory problems, weakness, GI intolerance *Adverse reaction:* hypersensitivity, seizures
duloxetine (doo LOX e teen)	Cymbalta (sim-BAL tuh)	Antidepressant (Selective serotonin and norepinephrine reuptake inhibitors [SNRIs])	*Indication:* major depressive disorder, generalized anxiety disorder, diabetic peripheral neuropathy, fibromyalgia, chronic pain *Desired effects/action:* increases the amounts of serotonin and norepinephrine in the brain; helps to maintain mental balance and stop pain signals in the brain *Side effects:* orthostatic hypotension *Adverse reaction:* suicidal thoughts, hepatotoxicity, seizures, glaucoma, hyponatremia
citalopram (sye TAL oh pram)	Celexa (seh LEK suh)	Antidepressant (Selective serotonin reuptake inhibitors [SSRIs])	*Indication:* depression *Desired effects/action:* increases the amount of serotonin in the brain; helps to maintain mental balance *Side effects:* GI intolerance, frequent urination, weakness, joint pain, weight loss *Adverse reaction:* angina, shortness of breath, arrhythmias, hallucinating, coma, hypersensitivity, confusion, seizures, suicidal thoughts
escitalopram (es sye TAL oh pram)	Lexapro (LEK suh proh)	Antidepressant (Selective serotonin reuptake inhibitors [SSRIs])	*Indication:* depression, generalized anxiety disorder (GAD) *Desired effects/action:* increases the amount of serotonin in the brain; helps to maintain mental balance *Side effects:* GI intolerance, increased sweating, change in sex drive, flulike symptoms *Adverse reaction:* unusual excitement, hallucinations, confusion, arrhythmias, severe muscle stiffness, suicidal thoughts
sertraline (SER tra leen)	Zoloft (ZOH loft)	Antidepressant (Selective serotonin reuptake inhibitors [SSRIs])	*Indication:* depression, obsessive-compulsive disorder (OCD), panic attacks, posttraumatic stress disorder (PTSD) *Desired effects/action:* increases the amount of serotonin in the brain; helps to maintain mental balance *Side effects:* GI intolerance, weight changes, difficulty falling asleep, change in sex drive, excessive sweating *Adverse reaction:* seizures, abnormal bleeding, arrhythmias, hypersensitivity, suicidal thoughts
trazodone (TRAZ oh done)	Oleptro (oh LEP troh)	Antidepressant (Serotonin modulators)	*Indication:* depression *Desired effects/action:* increases the amount of serotonin; helps to maintain mental balance *Side effects:* GI intolerance, weakness, headache, confusion, sweating, decreased coordination *Adverse reaction:* angina, fainting, seizures, coma, arrhythmias, suicidal thoughts
promethazine (prow METH ah zeen)	Promethegan (prow METH ee gan)	Antihistamines	*Indication:* allergies, allergic conjunctivitis, anaphylaxis, sedation for procedures, motion sickness *Desired effects/action:* blocks histamine action *Side effects:* drowsiness, difficulty sleeping, ringing in ears, blurred vision, GI intolerance *Adverse reaction:* wheezing, slowed breathing, sweating, stiff muscles, decreased alertness
metformin (met FOR min)	Glucophage (gloo koe FAJE) Fortamet (for TAY met) Glumetza (gloo MET zah) Riomet (REE oh met)	Antihyperglycemics	*Indication:* type 2 diabetes mellitus *Desired effects/action:* decreases glucose absorption and increases body's response to insulin; controls the blood glucose level *Side effects:* GI intolerance, metallic taste in the mouth, flushing of the skin, nail changes *Adverse reaction:* angina, rash

TABLE 37.10 Information on Commonly Prescribed Medications—cont'd

Generic Name	Brand/Trade Name(s)	Class/Schedule	Medication Information
valsartan (val SAR tan)	Diovan (die OH van)	Antihypertensive (Angiotensin II receptor antagonists)	*Indication:* hypertension, heart failure, postmyocardial infarction (MI) *Desired effects/action:* prevents vasoconstriction, which lowers the blood pressure *Side effects:* headache, dizziness, flu symptoms, GI intolerance, blurred vision, mild itching *Adverse reaction:* hyperkalemia, arrhythmias
benazepril (ben AY ze pril)	Lotensin (LOW ten sin)	Antihypertensive (Angiotensin-converting enzyme [ACE] inhibitors)	*Indication:* hypertension *Desired effects/action:* causes vasodilation, decreasing the blood pressure *Side effects:* cough, drowsiness, headache *Adverse reaction:* jaundice, difficulty breathing, lightheadedness, swelling, hoarseness
lisinopril (lyse IN oh pril)	(no brand names)	Antihypertensive (Angiotensin-converting enzyme [ACE] inhibitors)	*Indication:* hypertension, heart failure *Desired effects/action:* causes vasodilation, decreasing the blood pressure *Side effects:* cough, dizziness, tiredness, GI intolerance, rash *Adverse reaction:* angina, lightheadedness, difficulty swallowing, hypersensitivity
atenolol (ah TEN oh lole)	Tenormin (TEN ore min)	Antihypertensive (Beta blockers)	*Indication:* hypertension, angina *Desired effects/action:* relaxes blood vessels and slows the heart rate, thus improving blood flow and decreases blood pressure *Side effects:* dizziness, tiredness, depression, GI intolerance *Adverse reaction:* shortness of breath, swelling of legs and hands, weight gain, fainting
metoprolol (me TOE proe lole)	Lopressor (low PRES sohr)	Antihypertensive (Beta blockers)	*Indication:* hypertension, angina *Desired effects/action:* relaxes blood vessels and slows the heart rate, thus improving blood flow and decreases blood pressure *Side effects:* dizziness, tiredness, depression, GI intolerance *Adverse reaction:* hypersensitivity, weight gain, arrhythmias
carvedilol (KAR ve dil ol)	Coreg (CORE ehg)	Antihypertensive (Beta blockers)	*Indication:* heart failure, hypertension *Desired effects/action:* relaxes blood vessels and slows the heart rate, thus improving blood flow and decreases blood pressure *Side effects:* hyperglycemia, tiredness, weakness, dizziness, visual changes, joint pain, difficulty sleeping *Adverse reaction:* shortness of breath, swelling of arms and legs, arrhythmias
amlodipine (am LOE di peen)	Norvasc (NOR vask)	Antihypertensive (Calcium channel blockers)	*Indication:* hypertension, angina *Desired effects/action:* relaxes the vessels so the heart does not have to pump as hard *Side effects:* GI intolerance, headache, swelling of legs and arms, tiredness, flushing *Adverse reaction:* more frequent or severe angina, fainting, arrhythmias
ibuprofen (eye BYOO proe fen)	Advil (AD vil) Motrin (MOE trin) Midol (MYE dohl)	Antiinflammatory drugs (Nonsteroidal [NSAIDs])	*Indication for use:* osteoarthritis, rheumatoid arthritis, fever, pain *Desired effects/action:* stops the body's production of substances that causes pain, fever, and inflammation *Side effects:* GI intolerance, ringing in the ear *Adverse reaction:* weight gain, hypersensitivity, hoarseness, jaundice, bloody urine, stiff neck
clopidogrel (kloh PID oh grel)	Plavix (PLAH viks)	Antiplatelets	*Indication:* used to prevent clots after a stroke, heart attack, or severe angina *Desired effects/action:* prevents platelets from collecting and forming clots *Side effects:* excessive tiredness, GI intolerance, nosebleed, dizziness *Adverse reaction:* hypersensitivity, bloody and tarry stools, coffee grounds–looking emesis, blood in urine, visual changes
aripiprazole (ay ri PIP ray zole)	Abilify (a BIL i fie)	Antipsychotics (atypical)	*Indication:* schizophrenia, bipolar disorder, major depressive disorder, Tourette disorder *Desired effects/action:* Changes the actions of chemicals in the brain *Side effects:* GI intolerance, insomnia, headache, anxiety, trouble swallowing *Adverse reaction:* suicidal thoughts, stroke, compulsive behaviors, orthostatic hypotension, tardive dyskinesia
quetiapine (kwe TYE a peen)	Seroquel (SER oh kwell)	Antipsychotics (atypical)	*Indication:* schizophrenia, bipolar disorder *Desired effects/action:* changes the activity of certain substances in the brain *Side effects:* drowsiness, pain in joints, weakness, GI intolerance, difficulty concentrating and speaking *Adverse reaction:* seizures, visual changes, uncontrollable movements, arrhythmias

Continued

TABLE 37.10 Information on Commonly Prescribed Medications—cont'd

Generic Name	Brand/Trade Name(s)	Class/Schedule	Medication Information
tiotropium (tee oh TRO pee um)	Spiriva (SPIR ee vah)	Bronchodilators	*Indication:* chronic obstructive pulmonary disease (COPD) *Desired effects/action:* prevent bronchospasms *Side effects:* dry mouth, GI intolerance, nosebleed, muscle pain, cold symptoms *Adverse reaction:* hypersensitivity reaction, paradoxical bronchospasm, glaucoma, urinary retention
albuterol (al BYOO ter ole)	Ventolin HFA (ven TOE lin) Proventil HFA (PRO ven til) Proair (PRO air)	Bronchodilators	*Indication:* bronchospasm (e.g., asthma) *Desired effects/action:* relaxes bronchial muscles and increases air flow to lungs *Side effects:* headache, dizziness, insomnia, cough, sort throat, nausea, vomiting, dry mouth *Adverse reaction:* paradoxical bronchospasm, cardiovascular effects, hypersensitivity, hypokalemia
atorvastatin (a TORE va sta tin)	Lipitor (LIP-ih-tore)	Cholesterol-lowering agent	*Indication:* hyperlipidemia, hypertriglyceridemia *Desired effects/action:* slows production of cholesterol in the body; decreases LDH and triglycerides; increases HDL *Side effects:* GI intolerance, joint pain, memory loss, confusion *Adverse reaction:* muscle pain, lack of energy, angina, weakness, hypersensitivity, dark colored urine, jaundice
rosuvastatin (roe soo vah STAT in)	Crestor (CRESS tor)	Cholesterol-lowering agent	*Indication:* hyperlipidemia, hypertriglyceridemia *Desired effects/action:* slows production of cholesterol in the body; decreases LDH and triglycerides; increases HDL *Side effects:* headache, depression, muscle and joint pain, insomnia, GI intolerance *Adverse reaction:* muscle damage leading to acute renal failure and liver damage
simvastatin (SIM va stat in)	Zocor (ZOE kore)	Cholesterol-lowering agent	*Indication:* hyperlipidemia, hypertriglyceridemia *Desired effects/action:* slows production of cholesterol in the body; decreases LDH and triglycerides; increases HDL *Side effects:* GI intolerance, memory loss, confusion, headache *Adverse reaction:* muscle pain, dark red urine, lack of energy, jaundice, hypersensitivity
methylprednisolone (meth ill pred NISS oh lone)	Medrol (meh DROL)	Corticosteroid (oral)	*Indication:* arthritis, certain cancers, allergies, asthma *Desired effects/action:* relieves inflammation symptoms *Side effects:* GI intolerance, increased hair growth, insomnia, acne *Adverse reaction:* swollen face and legs, visual problems, infection, black or tarry stool
fluticasone (floo TIK a sone)	Flonase nasal spray (FLOW nase) Flovent HFA (FLOW vent) Flovent Diskus (FLOW vent DISK us)	Corticosteroid (Nasal and inhaled)	*Indication:* hay fever, allergies (nasal spray); asthma (inhaled) *Desired effects/action:* decreases inflammation and allergy reaction *Side effects:* headache, dryness in mouth, hoarseness or deepened voice *Adverse reaction:* reduced bone marrow density, immunosuppression, adrenal suppression, glaucoma, cataracts, hypersensitivity in individuals with milk allergy (Diskus)
furosemide (fyoor OH se mide)	Lasix (LAY siks)	Diuretics	*Indication:* hypertension *Desired effects/action:* causes the kidneys to increase the excretion of water and salt *Side effects:* frequent urination, blurred vision, headache, constipation, diarrhea *Adverse reaction:* ringing in the ears, loss of hearing, blisters, jaundice, hypersensitivity
hydrochlorothiazide (HCTZ) (hye droe klor oh THYE a zide)	Microzide (MYE kroe zide) Oretic (ORE eh tik)	Diuretics	*Indication:* hypertension *Desired effects/action:* causes the kidneys to increase the excretion of water and salt *Side effects:* frequent urination, diarrhea, loss of appetite, headache, hair loss *Adverse reaction:* joint pain, unusual bleeding, hypersensitivity, visual change
potassium (poe TASS i um)	K-Tab (KAY tab) Klor-Con (KLOHR kuhhn) K-Dur (KAY duhr) Micro-K (MYE krow kay)	Electrolyte	*Indication:* mineral supplement needed for certain diseases and medications (e.g., diuretic) *Desired effects/action:* proper functioning of the body systems *Side effects:* GI intolerance *Adverse reaction:* confusion, listlessness, gray skin, black stools

TABLE 37.10 Information on Commonly Prescribed Medications—cont'd

Generic Name	Brand/Trade Name(s)	Class/Schedule	Medication Information
levothyroxine (lee voe thye ROX een)	Synthroid (SIN throid) Levothroid (LEE voe throid) Levoxyl (LEV ok sil)	Hormone replacement (Thyroid hormone)	*Indication:* hypothyroidism, pituitary TSH suppression *Desired effects/action:* replacement hormone; regulates body's energy and metabolism *Side effects:* reversible hair loss, dry skin, GI intolerance, headache, nervousness *Adverse reaction:* cardiac arrhythmias, angina, myocardial infarction, heart failure
montelukast (mon te LOO kast)	Singulair (SING u lair)	Leukotriene receptor antagonists	*Indication:* asthma, exercise-induced bronchospasms *Desired effects/action:* blocks the action of substances that cause asthma and allergic rhinitis *Side effects:* headache, dizziness, heartburn, stomach pain, tiredness *Adverse reaction:* hypersensitivity, numbness in arms and legs, swelling of the sinuses
carisoprodol (kar eye soe PROE dole)	Soma (SOW mah)	Muscle relaxant C-IV	*Indication:* painful musculoskeletal conditions (e.g., strains, sprains, muscle injuries) *Desired effects/action:* decreases pain *Side effects:* drowsiness, clumsiness, tachycardia, GI intolerance *Adverse reaction:* difficulty breathing, fever, weakness, burning in the eyes, seizures
cyclobenzaprine (sye kloe BEN za preen)	Flexeril (FLEKS er il)	Muscle relaxant	*Indication:* painful musculoskeletal conditions (e.g., strains, sprains, muscle injuries) *Desired effects/action:* works on the brain and nervous system to allow muscle relaxation *Side effects:* GI intolerance, extreme tiredness, dry mouth *Adverse reaction:* hypersensitivity, angina
esomeprazole (es oh ME pray zol)	Nexium (neks EE uhm)	Proton-pump inhibitors	*Indication:* Gastroesophageal reflex disease (GERD), erosive esophagitis, *Helicobacter pylori* ulcers *Desired effects/action:* Decreases the amount of stomach acid *Side effects:* headache, drowsy, dry mouth, GI intolerance *Adverse reaction:* acute interstitial nephritis, *C. difficile*, bone fracture, systemic lupus erythematosus, cyanocobalamin (Vitamin B_{12}) deficiency, hypomagnesemia
omeprazole (oh MEE pray zol)	Prilosec (PRY low sek)	Proton-pump inhibitors	*Indication:* gastroesophageal reflux disease (GERD), ulcers, H. pylori *Desired effects/action:* decreases stomach acid *Side effects:* GI intolerance, headache *Adverse reaction:* hypersensitivity, dizziness, arrhythmias, muscle spasm
zolpidem (ZOL pi dem)	Ambien (am bee ehn) Edluar (ED loo ahr) Zolpimist (ZOL pi mist)	Sedative-hypnotics C-IV	*Indication:* insomnia *Desired effects/action:* slows activity in the brain allowing sleep *Side effects:* drowsiness, headache, dizziness, drugged feeling, unsteady walking, GI intolerance *Adverse reaction:* jaundice, hypersensitivity, light-colored stools, angina, blurred vision
methylphenidate (meth il FEN i date)	Concerta (con SERT ah) Ritalin LA (RIT ah lin el aye)	Stimulants C-II	*Indication:* attention deficit hyperactivity disorder (ADHD), narcolepsy *Desired effects/action:* changes certain substances in the brain, allowing a person to concentrate and focus *Side effects:* nervousness, difficulty falling asleep, GI intolerance, restlessness, muscle tightness *Adverse reaction:* angina, arrhythmias, seizure, blurred vision

Besides describing medication orders by how they are given to the medical assistant, they can also be described by the type of order. Table 37.11 describes types of medication orders.

Prescriptions

A *prescription* is a written order by a provider to the pharmacist. It tells the pharmacist what medication and how much should be dispensed to the patient. There are four parts to a prescription: superscription, inscription, signature, and subscription. Fig. 37.1 describes the four parts of a prescription.

Medical Assistant's Role. In some ambulatory care facilities, medical assistants prepare prescriptions for providers to sign. Some scenarios may include the following:

- A patient may request refills while the medical assistant is rooming the patient. The medical assistant may prepare the prescriptions so the provider just needs to sign for the refills.
- A patient may call the department and request a refill on a medication. Using a medication refill protocol, the medical assistant needs to see if the patient can get a refill (Fig. 37.2). If the patient can, then the medical assistant prepares the prescription and has the provider sign it.

The prescription must be written in ink or be computer generated. A medical assistant can prepare prescriptions for the provider to sign. The provider is responsible for ensuring the prescription meets the federal and state laws and regulations. All prescriptions need to include the following:

- Date of issue (when it was written)
- Patient information (name and address is required; date of birth is helpful)

TABLE 37.11

Type of Order	Description	Examples
Routine order	Medication taken at a regular interval until it is canceled or expired. (Most non-narcotic routine orders expire in 12 months.)	"Vitamin B_{12} 100 mcg IM monthly." "Synthroid 75 mcg qam po."
Standing order	Order applies to all patients who meet specific criteria. For departments, usually all providers agree collectively on standing orders and sign the order.	"For patients 18 years and older, with no allergy to acetaminophen and who have a temperature of 103°F or higher: give acetaminophen 650 mg po × 1 dose."
PRN order	Medication that is given on an "as needed" basis for specific signs and symptoms. (It is important to indicate these symptoms when documenting the administered medication in the patient's health record.)	"Acetaminophen 325 mg, 2 tabs po q 4–6 hr prn pain."
Single (or one-time) order	Medication is administered one time.	"Acetaminophen 650 mg po × 1 dose"
Stat order	Medication is administered one time right now.	"EpiPen 0.3 mg IM stat."

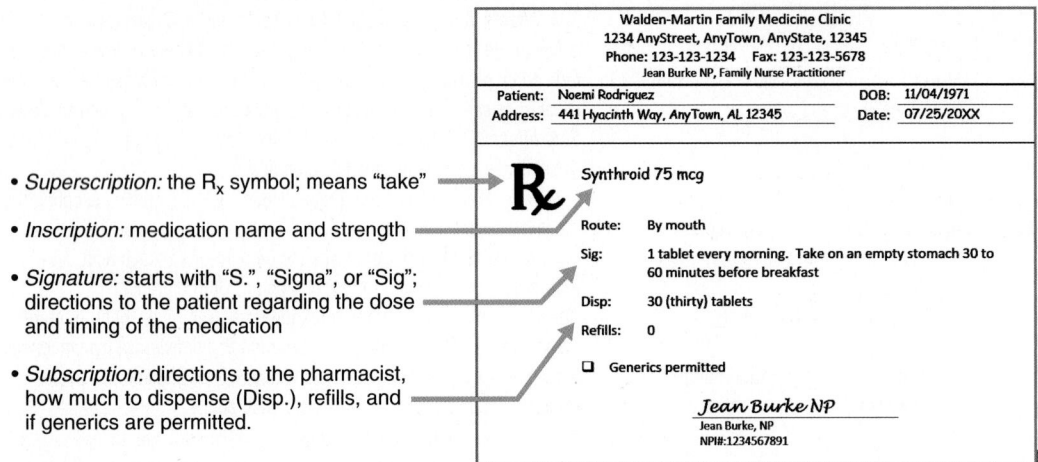

- *Superscription:* the R_x symbol; means "take"
- *Inscription:* medication name and strength
- *Signature:* starts with "S.", "Signa", or "Sig"; directions to the patient regarding the dose and timing of the medication
- *Subscription:* directions to the pharmacist, how much to dispense (Disp.), refills, and if generics are permitted.

FIG. 37.1 Parts of a prescription.

Prescription Refill Protocol
Walden-Martin Family Medicine Clinic

Description: A Certified Medical Assistant (CMA) can refill current hypertensive medications that fall within the guidelines of this protocol.

Step 1	Step 2	
For medications to be refilled, the following points need to be addressed.	Qualifying Medications	Prescription Refill
• Has the person seen the provider within the last year? • Is the prescription for a hypertensive, hyperlipidemia, or hyperthyroidism medication, a current prescription? • Is the person free of concerns or complications due to the medication? • Is it time for a refill? (The medical assistant must verify that it is time for a refill.) If the answers to the above questions are all YES, then proceed to Step 2. If any of the answers to the above questions are NO, then schedule the person for an appointment with the provider	amlodipine amlodipine/benazepril atenolol atenolol/Chlorthalidone benazepril captopril diltiazem enalapril felodipine fosinopril irbesartan isradiprine lisinopril losartan nifedipine quinapril ramipril	Extend the current prescription for 6 months. Instruct patient that in 6 months: • A visit to the provider will be required • Blood pressure reading will be required • Lab work may be required

FIG. 37.2 Example of a prescription refill protocol. The medical assistant uses a protocol to determine what action to take with prescription refill requests.

- Provider's full name and address.
- Drug name (e.g., Amoxicillin)
- Drug strength (e.g., 500 mg)
- Dosage form (e.g., tablets)
- Quantity prescribed (e.g., 14 [fourteen])—writing out the number prevents people from altering the prescription. This is especially important with controlled substances.
- Directions for use (e.g., take 1 tablet q 12 hr)
- Number of refills (e.g., Refills 0)
- National Provider Identifier (NPI) and signature of provider (a manual signature is required for controlled substances)
- Indicate if a generic is acceptable

If an electronic prescription were sent to the pharmacy and a paper copy is given to the patient, the copy should indicate it is a copy ("Copy only—not valid for dispensing"). Procedure 37.1 indicates how to prepare prescriptions using a prescription refill procedure. Only facility-approved abbreviations should be used when preparing prescriptions and documenting in the patients' health records. Tables 37.12 to 37.16 provide commonly approved abbreviations.

TABLE 37.12 Abbreviations Related to Route and Medication Form

Abbreviations	Meaning
subcut	subcutaneous
ID	intradermal
IM	intramuscular
IV	intravenous
NAS	nasal
po, PO	by mouth
tinct	tincture
ung.	ointment
sol., soln	solution
cap	capsule
tab(s)	tablet(s)

CRITICAL THINKING 37.6

Mark and Gabe were working on prescription refills. A patient who just started taking a schedule 2 medication called in for a refill. He expressed that he was not happy that there were no refills on his original prescription. How might Gabe handle this type of call? What could he say to help the patient understand the situation?

VOCABULARY

National Provider Identifier (NPI): An identifier assigned by the Centers for Medicare and Medicaid Services (CMS) that classifies the healthcare provider by license and medical specialties.

PROCEDURE 37.1 Prepare a Prescription

Tasks
Prepare a prescription using a prescription refill protocol. Use approved abbreviations.

Scenario
You received a call from Noemi Rodriguez (DOB 11/04/1971). She is requesting refills on three of her prescriptions from Jean Burke, NP. She saw Jean Burke 10 months ago. Noemi has NKA. She is doing well with the prescriptions and has no concerns. You determine it is time for refills. Her prescriptions include Coumadin 5 mg, 1 tablet orally daily; Tenormin 50 mg, 1 tablet orally daily; and Plendil 5 mg, 1 tablet orally daily.

Equipment and Supplies:
- SimChart for the Medical Office (SCMO) or paper prescriptions and pen
- Prescription refill protocol (Fig. 37.2)
- Drug reference book or online resource

Procedural Steps
1. Using the scenario, look up the generic medication names using the drug reference book or online resource.
   Purpose: Generic names are typically used in the healthcare facility, though patients may give the brand name.
2. Read the prescription refill protocol. Compare the generic names to the list of medications given. Identify medications that meet the protocol.
   Purpose: All the criteria need to be met for the medical assistant to prepare prescriptions using the prescription refill protocol.
3. Prepare prescriptions for refill per the protocol using SCMO or paper prescriptions.
   a. Using SCMO: Search for the patient. Verify the date of birth before selecting the patient. On the INFO PANEL, select Phone Encounter. Complete the fields on the Create New Encounter window and save. Check the box beside the No known allergy statement on the allergy screen and save. Select Order Entry from the Record dropdown list, and select Add in the Out-of-office section (Fig. 1).
   b. Using paper prescriptions: Add in the patient's complete name, date of birth, and address.
   Purpose: Most agencies using electronic health records require medical assistants to update the allergy screen when preparing refills. Prescriptions require the patient's name and address. If the DOB is available, add this to the prescription. An electronic health record will automatically add this information when it sends the prescription to the pharmacy.
4. Using the information in the scenario, complete the prescription information on either the paper prescription or in the SCMO fields. Use only approved abbreviations.
   Purpose: All information is required on the prescription for it to be accepted by the pharmacist and filled for the patient.
5. Complete any additional prescriptions as needed by the prescription refill protocol.
   Purpose: The patient requested refills on the medications indicated. Any medications that can be refilled should have prescriptions prepared for the provider.
6. Review the prescriptions for any errors. Void the prescription and redo if needed.
   Purpose: It is important to prepare accurate prescriptions. Any errors need to be fixed before giving the prescriptions to the provider.
   Note: After the provider signs the prescriptions and depending on the facility's policy, the medical assistant may need to document the refill in the health record. This cannot be done until the provider approves the prescriptions.

Continued

PROCEDURE 37.1 Prepare a Prescription—cont'd

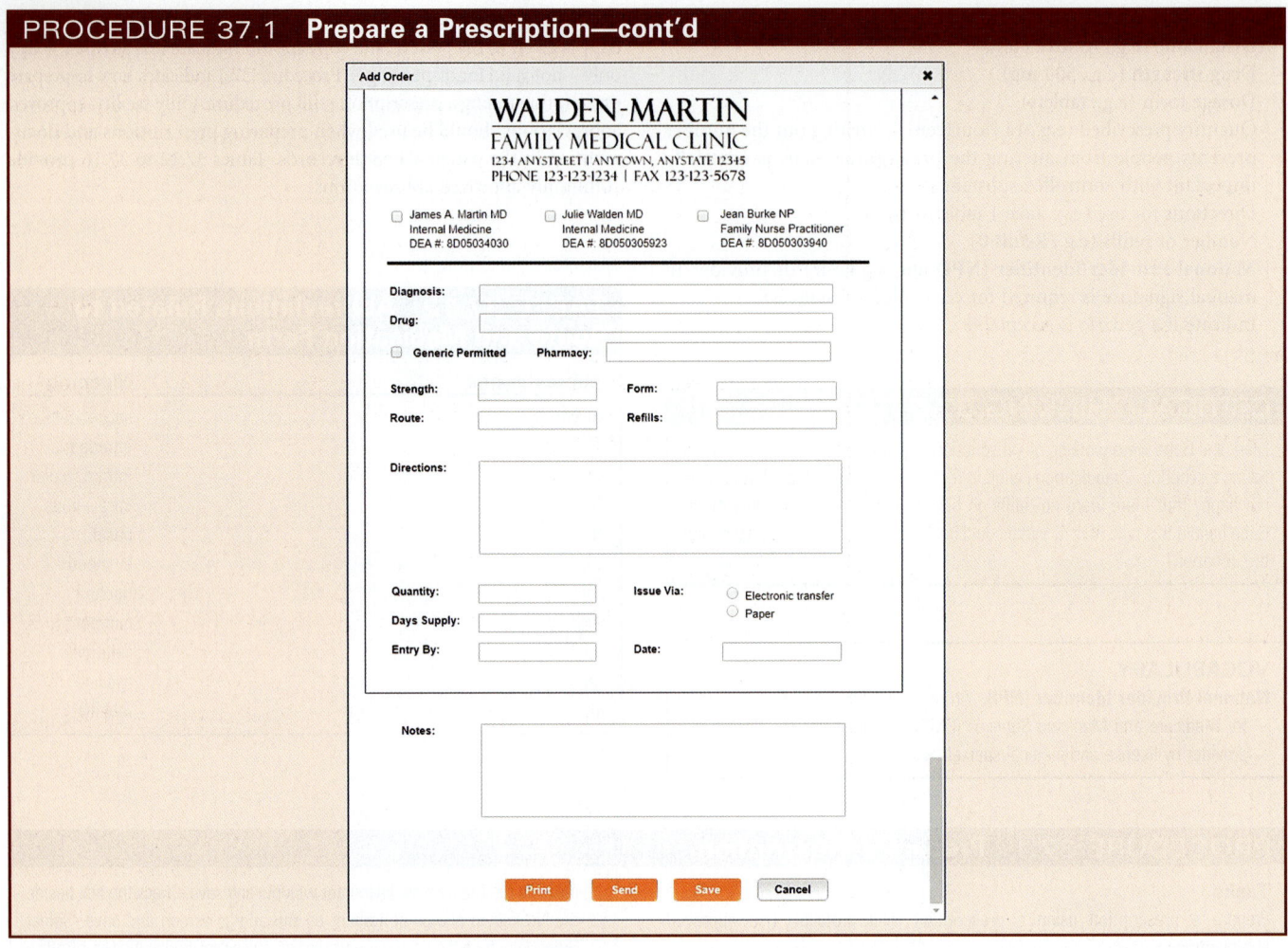

TABLE 37.13 Abbreviations Related to Measurements

Abbreviations	Meaning
C	Celsius
F	Fahrenheit
m	meter
cm	centimeter
mm	millimeter
kg	kilogram
g	gram
mg	milligram
mcg	microgram
L	liter
mL	milliliter
gr	grain
gtt(s)	drop(s)
lb	pound
fl oz	Fluid ounce
oz	ounce
pt	pint
qt	quart
Tbs, tbsp	tablespoon
tsp	teaspoon

TABLE 37.14 Abbreviations Related to Timing

Abbreviations	Meaning
ac	before meals
pc	after meals
ad lib	as desired
d	day
AM, a.m.	morning
PM, p.m.	afternoon
noc, noct	night
h, hr	hour
min	minute
$\bar{p}$	after
prn	as needed
qh	every hour
q(2,3,4,6,8)h	every (2, 3, 4, 6, 8) hours (q2h = every 2 hours)
qid	four times a day
tid	three times a day
bid	twice a day
qam	every morning
stat, STAT	immediately

Once the prescriptions are prepared, they need to be given to the provider to sign. Either the provider or the medical assistant needs to document the refills in the patient's health record. The facility's policy will indicate who is responsible for the documentation.

Controlled Substance Prescriptions. For security reasons, the provider's DEA number should only be on controlled substance prescriptions. It is not appropriate for the number to appear on non-narcotic prescriptions. The NPI is a national number that is unique to the provider. This number, not the DEA number, is used for any tracking or treatment identification purposes.

The medical assistant needs to be aware of the special requirements for controlled substances. It is important for the medical assistant to stay updated on which frequently prescribed medications are controlled substances. Table 37.17 describes common requirements for the scheduled substances.

OVER-THE-COUNTER MEDICATIONS AND HERBAL PRODUCTS

Over-the-counter (OTC) and herbal medications can impact medication treatment. It is important for the medical assistant to obtain a list of current prescription and OTC and herbal medications (Tables 37.18 and 37.19). Some patients may hesitate or not want to share the OTC and herbal medications. It is important for the medical assistant to be professional and respectful when dealing with these situations. Sometimes patients do not realize that OTC and herbal medications can interfere with other medications. By explaining this, the medical assistant may make patients more willing to share information on the OTC and herbal medications they take.

MATH FOR MEDICATIONS

All medical assistants should be able to convert between units of measure. It is also important to be able to accurately calculate medication doses. This section discusses different types of math problems that a medical assistant should be able to do. Please note that in some states, calculating medical dosages may be outside of the legal scope of practice for medical assistants. State laws vary.

TABLE 37.15 Abbreviations Related to Medications

Abbreviations	Meaning
ASA	aspirin
Fe	iron
K	potassium
MOM	milk of magnesia
NS	normal saline
NSAID	nonsteroidal antiinflammatory drug
OTC	over-the-counter (drugs)
PPD	purified protein derivative (tuberculin skin test)

TABLE 37.16 Miscellaneous Abbreviations

Abbreviations	Meaning
aa	of each (used in prescriptions)
aq	water
c̄	with
med	medicine
NKA	no known allergies
NKDA	no known drug allergies
NPO	nothing by mouth
Pt, pt	patient
qs	quantity sufficient
Rx	Take
Sig	give the following directions
s̄	without
VO	verbal order
x	times

TABLE 37.17 Special Requirements for Controlled Substances

Schedule	Prescription Specifics
I	Drugs with no currently accepted medical use.
II/IIN (C–II)	Written prescription manually signed by the provider or an electronic prescription that meets all DEA requirements for electronic prescriptions for controlled substances. No refills. In some cases the prescription can be faxed to the pharmacy. The medication cannot be dispensed until the original prescription is given to the pharmacy.
III/III N and IV (C–III, C–IV)	Call-in prescriptions, written prescriptions, and electronic prescriptions are allowed. Faxed prescriptions must be manually signed by the provider prior to faxing. Prescription good for 6 months No more than five refills are allowed.
V (C–V)	Phoned prescriptions, written prescriptions, e-prescriptions, and faxed prescriptions allowed. Prescription is good for 12 months (like non-narcotic prescriptions). Refill quantity is up to the provider.

Math Guidelines

When calculating medication dosages, it is important to verify the amount with a coworker or the provider. Many times the provider will give you the amount to draw up, but sometimes the medical assistant must perform calculations.

With medications, it is important to be accurate in calculating and also documenting amounts. Table 37.20 provides a few healthcare rules with writing numbers.

Rounding Numbers. When calculating answers, sometimes our numbers need to be rounded. Let's review the steps in rounding.

1. Find the place value where you want to end up. (We want our answer to be to the nearest tenth, or one place after the decimal point; see Fig. 37.3.)
2. Look at the number to the right of the place value. In Fig. 37.3, 5 sits in the hundredth place. When rounding, remember the following:
   - 4 or below: drop the number(s) to the right of the place value
   - 5 or above: add 1 to the rounded place value and drop the number(s) to the right of the place value

This means that because a 5 is in the hundredth place, add 1 to the 3. Drop the 5 and 7. Your answer is 751.4. Box 37.9 provides additional practice problems.

TABLE 37.18 Common Over-the-Counter (OTC) Medications

OTC Medication	Classification	Indication and Desired Effect	Adverse Reactions	Drug Interactions
• Aspirin (AS pir in) (ASA) • Ibuprofen (Advil, Motrin) • Naproxen (na PROX en) (Aleve, Naprosyn)	Analgesics (nonsteroidal antiinflammatory drugs [NSAIDs])	Inflammation and pain relief	GI bleeding, compromised renal function, tinnitus, diarrhea, and nausea	Antihypertensives, hyperglycemics, sulfa antibiotics, diuretics
Acetaminophen (a set a MEE noe fen) (Tylenol)	Analgesic, antipyretic	Relief of pain and fever	Liver damage	Warfarin
Pseudoephedrine (soo doe e FED rin) (Sudafed)	Decongestant	Relief nasal congestion caused by colds, allergies, and hay fever	Hypertension, vasospasm, arrhythmia, cerebrovascular accident	Antidepressant–monamine oxidase inhibitors (MAOIs)
Diphenhydramine (dye fen HYE dra meen) (Benadryl)	Antihistamine	Cough, cold, allergy, and insomnia	Drowsiness, confusion, hallucinations, delirium	
Dextromethorphan (dex troe meth OR fan) (Benylin and many DM cough and cold formulas) Robitussin	Antitussive	Suppression of cough reflex	Dizziness, lethargy, nausea	Antidepressant–monamine oxidase inhibitors (MAOIs)

TABLE 37.19 Commonly Used Herbal Products

Name	Uses	Side Effects and Cautions
Acai	Weight loss and antiaging; antioxidant.	Little scientific information about the safety of acai; no scientific evidence to support use for any health-related purpose; might affect magnetic resonance imaging (MRI) results.
Aloe vera	Aloe gel is used for burns, frostbit, psoriasis, and cold sores. It can also be taken orally for osteoarthritis, bowel diseases, and fever.	Topical use of aloe gel is likely to be safe. More studies are needed to determine the safety of oral preparations. People with diabetes should be cautioned against using aloe, as it may lower blood glucose levels.
Black cohosh	Relieve symptoms of menopause; treat menstrual irregularities and premenstrual syndrome; induce labor.	Headaches, gastric complaints, heaviness in the legs, weight problems; safety unknown for pregnant women or those with breast cancer.
Echinacea	Treat or prevent colds, flu, and other infections; believed to stimulate the immune system.	Most studies indicate echinacea does not appear to prevent colds or other infections; some people experience allergic reactions, including rashes, increased asthma, and anaphylaxis; gastrointestinal (GI) side effects.
Flaxseed	Flaxseed and flaxseed oil are used for constipation, diabetes, high cholesterol levels, cancer, and other conditions.	Few reported side effects; contains soluble fiber and is an effective laxative; both flaxseed and flaxseed oil can cause diarrhea. It is not recommended during pregnancy.

TABLE 37.19 Commonly Used Herbal Products—cont'd

Name	Uses	Side Effects and Cautions
Garlic	Treat high cholesterol, heart disease, hypertension; prevent certain types of cancer, including stomach and colon cancer.	Some evidence indicates garlic can slightly lower blood cholesterol levels and may slow development of atherosclerosis; side effects include breath and body odor, heartburn, GI upset, and allergic reactions; acts as a mild anticoagulant (similar to aspirin); may increase the risk of bleeding; interferes with effectiveness of saquinavir, a drug used to treat human immunodeficiency virus (HIV) infection.
Ginger	Alleviate nausea associated with postoperative state, motion sickness, chemotherapy, and pregnancy; used for rheumatoid arthritis, osteoarthritis, and joint and muscle pain.	Short-term use can safely relieve pregnancy-related nausea and vomiting; also may help with chemotherapy nausea and vomiting. Side effects most often reported are gas, bloating, heartburn, and nausea.
Asian ginseng	Support overall health and boost immune system; improve mental and physical performance; treat erectile dysfunction, hepatitis C, and menopause symptoms; lower blood glucose and control blood pressure.	Limited information available, more studies needed. May affect blood glucose levels and blood pressure; thus patients should discuss this with their provider. May interact with certain medications like anticoagulants.
Ginkgo biloba (GING koe BIL oh bah)	No conclusive evidence that it helps any health condition.	Side effects may include headache, stomach upset, and allergic skin reactions. Ginkgo may increase the risk of bleeding with pregnancy and those on anticoagulants.
Green tea	Improve mental alertness, relieve digestive symptoms and headaches, promote weight loss; may have protective effects against heart disease and cancer.	Safe in moderate amounts; possible complications include liver problems with concentrated green tea extracts but not when used as a beverage. A specific green tea extract ointment is a prescription drug used for treating genital warts.
St. John's wort (wohrt)	Treat mental disorders and nerve pain; kidney and lung diseases, insomnia, and wounds.	Some scientific evidence shows it helps treat mild to moderate depression; not effective in treating major depression. Side effects include photophobia (increased sensitivity to sunlight), anxiety, dry mouth, dizziness, GI symptoms, fatigue, headache, and sexual dysfunction. Can cause life-threatening reactions with certain medications. Drugs that can be affected include the following: • Antidepressants • Birth control pills • Cyclosporine (prevents rejection of transplants) • Digoxin (heart medication) • Some HIV and cancer medications • Warfarin and related anticoagulants

Modified from the National Center for Complementary and Alternative Medicine. https://nccih.nih.gov/health/herbsataglance.htm.

TABLE 37.20 Healthcare Rules When Writing Numbers

Rules to Follow	Correct Examples	Incorrect Examples
1. Follow the number with the correct abbreviation for the unit of measure. Leave a space between the number and the abbreviation. Do not use a period with the abbreviations.	2 mg 10 mL 2 tabs	mg2 mL 10 2 tabs.
2. Write a fraction of a dose as a decimal.	0.5 mg	½ mg
3. If the dose is less than 1, place a zero to the left of the decimal point. This reduces the risk of misreading the dose as a whole number.	0.75 mcg 0.2 mL	.75 mcg .2 mL
4. Do not place a decimal point and a zero after a whole number. This risks misreading and giving 10 times the dose.	2 mL 2.3 mL	2.0 mL 2.30 mL

Hundred	Ten	One	.	Tenth	Hundredth	Thousandth
7	5	1	.	3	5	7

FIG. 37.3 Place value.

UNIT 5 Advanced Clinical Procedures

> ✳ **STUDY TIP**
> Think of the numbers after the decimal point as being houses on a road. Just look at the next-door neighbor to make the decision if you need to round up by one or keep the number. Don't be a noisy neighbor and look down the street!

BOX 37.9 Math Practice: Rounding

Directions: Round the following numbers to the nearest tenth. Write out as you would for a medication dose with a zero before the decimal point if the answer is less than 1 and no trailing zeros.

1. 2.467 = _____
2. .358 = _____
3. .98 = _____
4. 4.65 = _____
5. 45.234 = _____
6. 7.788 = _____

Roman Numerals. Sometimes a number might be written using Roman numerals (Box 37.10). It is good for a medical assistant to be familiar with the Roman numeral system. If they are used in healthcare, you will see them written in small letters. Sometimes a line may be written above the Roman numeral.

> ✳ **STUDY TIP**
> Sometimes the Roman numerals for 5 and 10 can be confusing. Remember that FIVE has a "V." The Roman numeral for five is "v."

BOX 37.10 Roman Numerals

i = 1 vi = 6	$\overline{ss}$ = ½ or 0.5	**Examples:**
ii = 2 vii = 7	(for "ss": write out "one-half" in	vss = 5½ or 5.5
iii = 3 viii = 8	documentation notes to avoid errors)	iiiss = 3½ or 3.5
iv = 4 ix = 9		
v = 5 x = 10		

TABLE 37.21 Household Abbreviations

Abbreviations	Meaning
gtt, gtts	drop, drops
tsp	teaspoon
Tbs or tbsp	tablespoon
fl oz	fluid ounce
oz	ounce
qt	quart
pt	pint
lb	pound

BOX 37.11 Household and Metric Equivalents

Weight	Liquids	
2.2 lb = 1 kg	3 tsp = 1 Tbs	1 Tbs = 15 mL
16 oz = 1 lb	1 oz = 30 mL	1 oz = 2 Tbs
	1 tsp = 5 mL	1 oz = 6 tsp

BOX 37.12 Math Practice: Household and Metric Systems

Directions: Solve the following problems. Round your answers to the nearest tenth.

1. 11 oz = _____ lb
2. 90 mL = _____ oz
3. 8 tsp = _____ mL
4. 20 Tbs = _____ mL
5. 5.5 oz = _____ Tbs
6. 4 oz = _____ tsp
7. 23 lb = _____ kg
8. 28 kg = _____ lb
9. 56 oz = _____ lb

Measurement Systems

In healthcare, both the household and metric systems are used. For instance, we weigh patients in pounds and tell a mother to give her son 1 teaspoon of medication before meals. Using the metric system is more accurate. The provider will use a child's weight in kilograms (kg) to calculate a medication dosage. The pharmacist will show the mother that 1 teaspoon is really 5 mL on the oral syringe. The oral syringe and plastic medicine cup are more accurate for medications than the spoons used in the kitchen.

Household System. Sometimes we need to move within the household system as we solve problems. Other times we need to use both the metric and household measurement systems. Table 37.21 provides household measurement abbreviations. Box 37.11 provides the household and metric equivalents. There are many ways to set up problems when calculating between household and metric equivalents. The proportion method is one of the easiest methods (Fig. 37.4). This method is easy if you remember three things:

1. *Keep the information separate.* The problem information is on one side of the equal sign and the equivalent information is on the other side.
2. *Keep the labels in the same place.* The labels should be in the exact same location on both sides of the equal sign.
3. *Cross-multiply in the direction of the two numbers, then divide by the remaining number.* You have your answer!

Box 37.12 provides practice household and metric system problems.

Metric System. The metric system is commonly used in healthcare. We use the metric system when measuring medications and wounds. A medical assistant should know how to use the metric system. Note these standards when using the metric system:

- Weight is measured in grams (g).
- Volume is measured in liters (L).
- Length is measured in meters (m).

Gram, liter, and *meter* are called the root words. *Prefixes* are added to the front of the root word to indicate the size of the unit. Fig. 37.5 lists the prefixes that can be added to the root words. Only those prefixes routinely used in healthcare are given, along with common equivalents (Table 37.22). Remember that a person cannot move from base unit to base unit (i.e., gram to liter or meter to gram). A person can only move within a base unit (i.e., centimeter to millimeter).

CHAPTER 37 Pharmacology Basics

Problem:	15 Tbs = _____ mL	
Step 1:	Turn the problem into a fraction. It doesn't matter which number goes on the top or bottom, just keep the label with the number. Use X for the unknown (the blank line)	**PROBLEM** $\dfrac{15 \text{ Tbs}}{x \text{ mL}}$
Step 2:	Add an equal sign and make a fraction on the opposite side. Fill in the labels. The labels need to be in identical locations on both sides of the equal sign.	**PROBLEM** **EQUIVALENT** $\dfrac{15 \text{ Tbs}}{x \text{ mL}} = \dfrac{\text{Tbs}}{\text{mL}}$
Step 3:	Using Box 37-11, find the equivalent for Tbs and tsp. Fill in the numbers in the equivalent fraction. Make sure to put the right number in front of the correct label.	**PROBLEM** **EQUIVALENT** $\dfrac{15 \text{ Tbs}}{x \text{ mL}} = \dfrac{1 \text{ Tbs}}{15 \text{ mL}}$
Step 4:	Now solve for the unknown. Using a calculator: Multiply in the diagonal direction of the two numbers (15 × 15) and then divide by the number in the other direction (1) and the answer is X.	**PROBLEM** **EQUIVALENT** $\dfrac{15 \text{ Tbs}}{x \text{ mL}} = \dfrac{1 \text{ Tbs}}{15 \text{ mL}}$ 15 × 15 = __225__ / 1 = __225__
	To solve without a calculator: multiply diagonally and solve for X. The answer is 225 mL. *Always make sure to label your answer.*	15 × 15 = 1x 255 = 1x $\dfrac{225}{1} = \dfrac{1x}{1}$ 225 = x

FIG. 37.4 Solving household and metric problems.

Size of the unit of measure	Prefixes	Size	Or another way to look at it!	
LARGE ↓ **SMALL**	Kilo (k)	1000 base units	1 kilo = 1000 base units (Example: 1 kg = 1000 g)	Larger than the base unit
	BASE UNITS (Meter, Liter or Gram)			
	Centi (c)	0.01 unit	100 centi = 1 base unit (Example: 100 cm = 1 m)	Smaller than the base unit
	Milli (m)	0.001	1000 milli = 1 base unit (Example: 1,000 mL = 1 L)	
	Micro (mc)	0.000001	1,000,000 micro = 1 base unit (Example: 1,000,000 mcg = 1g)	

FIG. 37.5 Prefixes of metric measurement.

TABLE 37.22 Metric Measurements Used in Healthcare

	Volume	Length	Weight
Units of Measure With Abbreviations	Liter (L) Milliliter (mL or ml) [Note: 1 cc = 1 mL] Cubic centimeter (cc)]	Meter (m) Centimeter (cm) Millimeter (mm)	Gram (g) Kilogram (kg) Milligram (mg) Microgram (mcg)
Equivalents Commonly Used	1 L = 1000 mL 1 L = 1000 cc 1 mL = 1 cc (To avoid errors in documentation, use mL instead of cc.)	1 m = 100 cm 1 m = 1000 mm 1 cm = 10 mm	1 g = 1000 mg 1 g = 1,000,000 mcg 1 kg = 1000 g 1 mg = 1000 mcg

Problem:	17 g = _____ mg		
Step 1:	Turn the problem into a fraction. It doesn't matter which number goes on the top or bottom, just keep the label with the number. Use X for the unknown (the blank line)	**PROBLEM** $\frac{17 \text{ g}}{x \text{ mg}}$	
Step 2:	Add an equal sign and make a fraction on the opposite side. Fill in the labels. The labels need to be in identical locations on both sides of the equal sign.	**PROBLEM** $\frac{17 \text{ g}}{x \text{ mg}}$ =	**EQUIVALENT** $\frac{\text{g}}{\text{mg}}$
Step 3:	Using Table 37-20, find the equivalent for gram (g) and milligram (mg). Fill in the numbers in the equivalent fraction. Make sure to put the right number in front of the correct label.	**PROBLEM** $\frac{17 \text{ g}}{x \text{ mg}}$ =	**EQUIVALENT** $\frac{1 \text{ g}}{1000 \text{ mg}}$
Step 4:	Now solve for the unknown. Using a calculator: Multiply in the diagonal direction of the two numbers (17 × 1000) and then divide by the number in the other direction (1) and the answer is X.	**PROBLEM** $\frac{17 \text{ g}}{x \text{ mg}}$ = 17 × 1000 = 17,000 / 1 = 17,000	**EQUIVALENT** $\frac{1 \text{ g}}{1000 \text{ mg}}$
	To solve without a calculator: multiply diagonally and solve for X.	17 × 1000 = 1x 17,000 = 1x $\frac{17,000}{1} = \frac{1x}{1}$	
	The answer is 17,000 mg. *Always make sure to label your answer.*	17,000 = x	

FIG. 37.6 Solving a metric system problem.

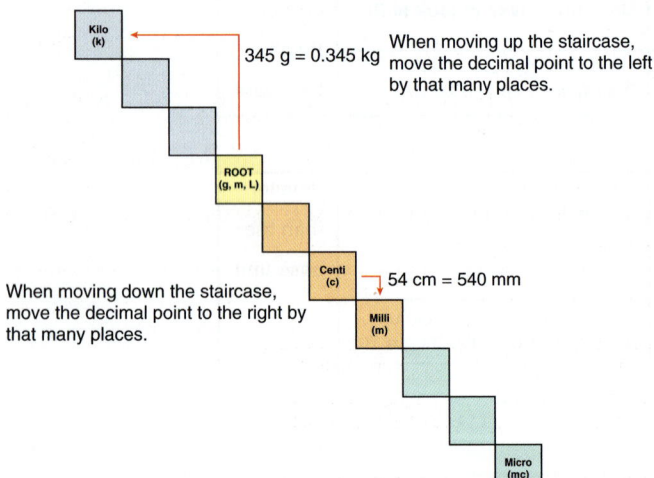

FIG. 37.7 Memory tool for solving metric problems.

BOX 37.13 Math Practice: Metric System

Directions: Solve the following problems. Do not round your answers.

1. 21 mL = _____ cc   2. 1.2 L = _____ cc   3. 2450 mL = _____ L
4. 2300 mm = _____ m   5. 87 cm = _____ mm   6. 458 cm = _____ m
7. 2.3 g = _____ mg   8. 1.3 kg = _____ g   9. 230 mcg = _____ mg

BOX 37.14 Math Practice: Temperature Conversions

Directions: Solve the following problems. Round your answers to the nearest tenth.

1. 93.3°F = _____ °C   2. 42.9°F = _____ °C   3. 53°F = _____ °C
4. 103°C = _____ °F   5. 39.9°C = _____ °F   6. 88.2°C = _____ °F

There are many ways to solve metric system problems. Solving metric problems using the proportion method is shown in Fig. 37.6. Fig. 37.7 provides a memory tool for solving metric problems. Box 37.13 provides practice metric system problems.

Temperature Conversion

Fahrenheit (°F) and Celsius (°C) are used in healthcare. A medical assistant should be able to convert between these two units of measure. Figs. 37.8 and 37.9 illustrate how to convert between a Fahrenheit and a Celsius temperature. To remember the steps for temperature conversion, use the memory tool presented in Fig. 37.10. Box 37.14 provides practice problems for converting Fahrenheit and Celsius temperatures.

Total Number of Tablets Needed

It is not uncommon for patients to call their provider requesting enough medication for a trip. It is important for the medical assistant to be able to calculate how many tablets a patient needs for a period of time.

Fig. 37.11 shows a medication order. The first part shows the name of the medication along with the tablet size (strength of each tablet). The last part of the order shows how many tablets to take (*dose*) and how many time to take it during the day. It also shows how long to take the medication. Fig. 37.12 shows how to solve this type of problem. Box 37.15 provides additional practice problems.

Tablets per Dose

It is common for the provider to give medication orders without a tablet amount. For instance, the provider ordered "Tylenol 975 mg po." The medical assistant must figure out how many tablets to give to the patient. To start, figure out the number of milligrams in each tablet,

Problem:	102 °F = _____ °C	
Step 1:	Subtract 32 from the Fahrenheit temperature.	102 − 32 = 70
Step 2:	Divide the answer by 1.8 and round to the nearest tenth.	70 / 1.8 = 38.88889 Answer: 38.9 °C

FIG. 37.8 Change from Fahrenheit to Celsius.

Problem:	25 °C = _____ °F	
Step 1:	Multiple the Celsius number by 1.8	25 x 1.8 = 45
Step 2:	Add 32 to the answer.	45 + 32 = 77 Answer: 77 °F

FIG. 37.9 Change from Celsius to Fahrenheit.

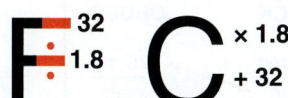

FIG. 37.10 Memory tool for temperature conversions.

Amoxicillin 500 mg, 1 tab tid po x 10 days

Medication name and size of the tablet	Daily dose (amount and timing) and number of days

FIG. 37.11 Medication order.

BOX 37.15 Math Practice: Number of Tablets Needed

Directions: Calculate the number of tablets the patient will need for the entire time.

1. Prescription: XYZ medication 200 mg, 5 tabs tid × 6 days. How many tablets will the patient need?
2. Prescription: XYZ medication 250 mg, 3 tabs qid × 14 days. How many tablets will the patient need?
3. Prescription: XYZ medication 50 mg, 4 tabs bid × 10 days. How many tablets will the patient need?
4. Prescription: XYZ medication 70 mg, 4 tabs tid × 13 days. How many tablets will the patient need?

Problem:	Prescription: Amoxicillin 500 mg, 1 tab tid po × 10 days. How many tablets would the patient need?	
Step 1:	Figure out the number of tablets per dose. (Use the abbreviation list if you need to.)	1 tab means 1 tablet
Step 2:	Figure out the number of tablets taken throughout the day. Do this by multiplying the number of tablets per dose (1 tablet) by the number of times the medication is taken during the day (tid means 3 times a day).	1 tablet per dose × 3 times a day (tid) 3 tablets per day
Step 3:	Figure out the number of tablets needed. Multiple the number of tablets per day by the number of days. The answer is 30 tablets.	3 tablets per day × 10 days 30 tablets needed

FIG. 37.12 Calculate the number of tablets needed.

which will be indicated on the label of the stock medication. Once the tablet size is identified, then the medical assistant can calculate the number of tablets required.

There are several ways to solve this type of problem. Two methods will be shown. Fig. 37.13 shows the proportion method, but it may help to remember it as the "stock and order" method. The second method shows the formula method (Fig. 37.14). Box 37.16 provides additional practice problems. Box 37.17 provides tips for double-checking your answers.

> **VOCABULARY**
>
> **scored tablet**: A tablet with a groove on the surface, used for splitting it in half.

Setting Up the Problem	Make sure to put the stock information on one side of the equal sign and the order information on the other. It doesn't matter which side you put the information.	
Problem:	Order: Tylenol 975 mg po Stock: Tylenol 325 mg per tablet How many tablets should be given?	
Step 1:	Put the stock information into a fraction. It doesn't matter the location of the numbers. Make sure to add the labels. (Remember: 325 mg per tablet really means 325 mg in each tablet.)	**STOCK** $\dfrac{325 \text{ mg}}{1 \text{ tab}}$
Step 2:	Add an equal sign and make a fraction on the opposite side. Fill in the labels. The labels need to be in identical locations on both sides of the equal sign.	**STOCK** **ORDER** $\dfrac{325 \text{ mg}}{1 \text{ tab}} = \dfrac{\text{mg}}{\text{tab}}$
Step 3:	Fill in the order information. You do not know the number of tablets, so that is the unknown (X).	**STOCK** **ORDER** $\dfrac{325 \text{ mg}}{1 \text{ tab}} = \dfrac{975 \text{ mg}}{x \text{ tab}}$
Step 4:	Now solve for the unknown. Using a calculator: Multiply in the diagonal direction of the two numbers (1 × 975) and then divide by the number in the other direction (325) and the answer is X.	**STOCK** **ORDER** $\dfrac{325 \text{ mg}}{1 \text{ tab}} = \dfrac{975 \text{ mg}}{x \text{ tab}}$ 1 × 975 = $\underline{975}$ / 325 = $\underline{3}$
	To solve without a calculator: multiply diagonally and solve for X.	1 × 975 = 325x 975 = 325x $\dfrac{975}{325} = \dfrac{325x}{325}$ 3 = x
	The answer is 3 tablets.	

FIG. 37.13 Method 1—Stock and order (proportion) method: Calculate the number of tablets per dose.

Setting Up the Problem	This method uses a formula that needs to be memorized: $\dfrac{D \text{ (desired)}}{H \text{ (on hand)}} \times V \text{ (vehicle – tablet or liquid)}$	
Problem:	Order: Tylenol 975 mg po Stock: Tylenol 325 mg per tablet How many tablets should be given?	
Step 1:	D is 975 mg H is 325 mg V is 1 tablet	$\dfrac{975 \text{ mg}}{325 \text{ mg}} \times 1 \text{ tablet}$
Step 2:	Multiply the problem. Then divide 975 by 325 to figure out the tablet amount.	$\dfrac{975 \text{ mg}}{325 \text{ mg}} \times 1 \text{ tablet} = \dfrac{975}{325}$
	The answer is 3 tablets.	Answer: 3 tablets

FIG. 37.14 Method 2—Formula method: Calculate the number of tablets per dose.

BOX 37.16 Math Practice: Tablets per Dose

Directions: Calculate the number of tablets to give.
1. Order: ABC 120 mg po; stock: ABC 80-mg po scored tablet. How many tablets should be given?
2. Order: ABC 150 mg po; stock: ABC 30-mg po scored tablet. How many tablets should be given?
3. Order: ABC 105 mg po; stock: ABC 30-mg po scored tablet. How many tablets should be given?
4. Order: ABC 65 mg po; stock: ABC 130-mg po scored tablet. How many tablets should be given?

BOX 37.18 Math Practice: Liquid Medication Doses

Directions: Solve the following problems. Round your answers to the nearest tenth.
1. Order: ABC 3200 units
   Stock: ABC 2800 units/mL
   How many milliliters will you give?
2. Order: ABC 230 units
   Stock: ABC 120 units/mL
   How many milliliters will you give?
3. Order: ABC 10 mg
   Stock: ABC 25 mg/3 mL
   How many milliliters will you give?
4. Order: ABC 45 mg
   Stock: ABC 125 mg/mL
   How many milliliters will you give?
5. Order: ABC 120 mg
   Stock: ABC 280 mg/mL
   How many milliliters will you give?
6. Order: ABC 500 mg
   Stock: ABC 1200 mg/2 mL
   How many milliliters will you give?

BOX 37.17 Double-Check Your Answers

It is important to double-check your answers. Remember the following:
- If the order is larger than the stock tablet, then you will be giving more than 1 tablet.
- If the order is smaller than the stock tablet amount, then you will be giving less than a tablet.

Liquid Medication Doses

When preparing a liquid medication, you will see two different units of measure on a bottle:
- Units, g, mg, or mcg: relates to the weight of the powdered medication (that is mixed in the liquid)
- cc or mL: relates to the volume of liquid that the powdered medication comes in

For instance, a bottle label states "50 mg/2 mL." This means that there are 50 mg of powdered medication mixed into 2 mL of liquid. If you want 50 mg of medication, then you would need to use 2 mL of liquid. Another example is 1500 mg/mL. This means that there are 1500 mg of powdered medicine in each mL of liquid. Remember that sometimes 1 mL is indicated by just "mL."

There are several ways to solve this type of problem. Two methods will be shown. Fig. 37.15 shows the stock and order (proportion) method, and Fig. 37.16 will uses the formula method. Box 37.18 provides additional practice problems.

When Units Do Not Match. Sometimes the units of weight on the label do not match the order. For instance, the provider may want "ABC 500 mg" to be given. The stock vial indicates "1 g/mL." This might be confusing. Remember that two of the labels need to match before you can solve the problem. Follow these steps:
- Identify similar labels. Using the example, notice that two of the three labels use grams (mg and g).
- Change the grams into milligrams. There are many ways to do this. You can refer back to "Solving a metric system problem" if you need to. Remember that 1 g = 1000 mg. Rewrite the problem so it reads: Order: ABC 500 mg Stock: 1000 mg/mL.
- Now solve the problem using the previous method ("Calculating liquid medication doses").

Box 37.19 provides some practice problems.

Solutions. In the ambulatory care environment, a medical assistant may find that topical anesthetics used for minor surgeries come in a solution. For instance, a provider asks you to get the strongest *Xylocaine* (ZIE lah kane) vial in the cabinet. You see a 1% and a 2% vial. What does this mean?

When the manufacturer made the medication, the "recipe" called for powdered drug to be mixed with a liquid:
- A 1% solution means: 1000 mg of powdered drug mixed in 100 mL of liquid.
- A 2% solution means: 2000 mg of powdered drug mixed in 100 mL of liquid.

(The 100 mL of liquid always remains regardless of the number in front of the percentage sign.) Going back to the provider's request, you would give the provider the 2% vial, as it is the strongest solution available.

Pediatric Doses. As with all medication calculations, it is important to be accurate for the safety of the patient. It is recommended that two people calculate a pediatric dose just to be sure of the accuracy.

Medication dosages for children are typically based on the child's weight. For this type of problem, the medical assistant needs the child's weight, the drug order, and the information on the stock medication label (Box 37.20). Let's look at the information. Notice the patient's weight is in pounds. The order is 0.1 mg per every kilogram of weight. The unit of measure for weight is different, one being pounds and the other kilograms.
- The first step is to switch the patient's weight to kilograms. This goes back to converting between the household and metric systems.
- The second step is to figure out the number of milligrams of medication the child needs. Imagine this scenario: a person tells you, you can have 2 chocolate bars for each kilogram you weigh. How would you figure it out? A simple way is to multiply 2 by the number of kilograms you weigh ($68 \times 2 = 136$ bars). You can use this same method to calculate the medication order.
- The final step is to calculate the liquid medication dose or the number of milliliters you will give. This was done in the prior section.

Fig. 37.17 shows the steps for solving this type of problem. You can modify the steps and use the formula method if you like. Box 37.21 provides additional practice problems. Procedure 37.2 provides additional practice examples.

Setting Up the Problem	Make sure the label information is on the stock side of the formula. The order is on the opposite side. Remember labels need to be in the same location on both sides of the equal sign.
Problem:	Order: ABC medication 1500 mg Stock: ABC medication 1300 mg / 2 mL How many mL(s) will you give?
Step 1:	Put the stock information into a fraction. It doesn't matter the location of the numbers. Make sure to add the labels. STOCK $\dfrac{1300 \text{ mg}}{2 \text{ mL}}$
Step 2:	Put the order information on the other side. Make sure the labels are in the exact same location. STOCK ORDER $\dfrac{1300 \text{ mg}}{2 \text{ mL}} = \dfrac{1500 \text{ mg}}{x \text{ mL}}$
Step 3:	Now solve for the unknown. Using a calculator: Multiply in the diagonal direction of the two numbers (2 × 1500) and then divide by the number in the other direction (1300). Round your answer to the nearest tenth. STOCK ORDER $\dfrac{1300 \text{ mg}}{2 \text{ mL}} = \dfrac{1500 \text{ mg}}{x \text{ mL}}$ 2 × 1500 = 3000 / 1300 = 2.3 mL You would give 2.3 mL of ABC medication.
	To solve without a calculator: multiply diagonally and solve for X. Round your answer to the nearest tenth. $1300x = 1500 \times 2$ $1300x = 3000$ $\dfrac{1300x}{1300} = \dfrac{3000}{1300}$ $x = 2.3 \text{ mL}$

FIG. 37.15 Method 1—Stock and order (proportion) method: Calculate liquid medication doses.

Setting Up the Problem	This method uses a formula that needs to be memorized: $\dfrac{D \text{ (desired)}}{H \text{ (on hand)}} \times V \text{ (vehicle – tablet or liquid)}$
Problem:	Order: ABC medication 1500 mg Stock: ABC medication 1300 / 2 mL How much medication (in mL) should be given?
Step 1:	D is 1500 mg H is 1300 mg V is 2 mL $\dfrac{1500 \text{ mg}}{1300 \text{ mg}} \times 2 \text{ mL}$
Step 2:	Multiply the problem. Then divide 3000 by 1300 to figure out the amount. Round the answer to the nearest tenth. $\dfrac{1500 \text{ mg}}{1300 \text{ mg}} \times 2 \text{ mL} = \dfrac{3000}{1300}$ You would give 2.3 mL of ABC medication.

FIG. 37.16 Method 2—Formula method: Calculate liquid medication doses.

BOX 37.19 Math Practice: When Units Do Not Match

Directions: Solve the following problems. Round your answers to the nearest tenth.

1. Order: ABC 2500 mg
   Stock: ABC 2.8 g/2 mL
   How many milliliters will you give?
2. Order: ABC 1800 mg
   Stock: ABC 2 g/mL
   How many milliliters will you give?
3. Order: ABC 1.2 g
   Stock: ABC 2500 mg/2 mL
   How many milliliters will you give?
4. Order: ABC 450 mg
   Stock: ABC 1.2 g/2 mL
   How many milliliters will you give?
5. Order: ABC 420 mg
   Stock: ABC 1 g/2 mL
   How many milliliters will you give?
6. Order: ABC 750 mg
   Stock: ABC 1.2 g/2 mL
   How many milliliters will you give?
7. Order: ABC 650 mg
   Stock: ABC 1.8 g/3 mL
   How many milliliters will you give?
8. Order: ABC 400 mg
   Stock: ABC 3 g/2 mL
   How many milliliters will you give?

BOX 37.20 Example of Information

Patient's wt: 33 lb
Order: ABC medication 0.1 mg/kg
Stock: ABC medication 1 mg/mL

BOX 37.21 Math Practice: Pediatric Medication

Directions: Round to the nearest thousandth while solving, and then round your answer to the nearest tenth.

1. Patient's weight: 40 lb
   Order: ABC medication 0.3 mg/kg
   Stock: ABC medication 2 mg/mL
   How many milliliters will you give?
2. Patient's weight: 58 lb
   Order: ABC medication 0.8 mg/kg
   Stock: ABC medication 60 mg/2 mL
   How many milliliters will you give?
3. Patient's weight: 145 lb
   Order: ABC medication 2 mg/kg
   Stock: ABC medication 80 mg/mL
   How many milliliters will you give?
4. Patient's weight: 31 lb
   Order: ABC medication 0.3 mg/kg
   Stock: ABC medication 2 mg/mL
   How many milliliters will you give?
5. Patient's weight: 60 lb
   Order: ABC medication 0.8 mg/kg
   Stock: ABC medication 50 mg/2 mL
   How many milliliters will you give?
6. Patient's weight: 86 lb
   Order: ABC medication 1.5 mg/kg
   Stock: ABC medication 80 mg/2 mL
   How many milliliters will you give?

PROCEDURE 37.2 Calculate Medication Dosages

Tasks
Calculate oral and injectable medication dosages.

Orders
Order 1: Dr. Martin orders ABC medication 135 mg. Stock bottle reads: 45 mg score tablets
Order 2: Dr. Martin orders ABC medication 650 mg. Stock bottle reads: 1300 mg score tablets
Order 3: Dr. Martin orders XYZ medication 430 mg IM. Stock bottle reads: 1000 mg / 2 mL
Order 4: Dr. Martin orders XYZ medication 680 mg IM. Stock bottle reads: 1200 mg / mL
Order 5: Dr. Martin orders MNO medication 3 mg / kg IM. Child weighs 53 pounds. Stock bottle reads: 125 mg / mL
Order 6: Dr. Martin orders MNO medication 5 mg / kg IM. Child weighs 71 pounds. Stock bottle reads: 225 mg / mL

Equipment and Supplies:
- Provider's order
- Paper and pencil
- Calculator (optional per instructor)

Procedural Steps
Using Order 1, calculate the number of tablets to give the patient. Label your answer.
Purpose: It is important to label your answer to avoid any mistakes in the dosage.
Using Order 2, calculate the number of tablets to give the patient. Label your answer.
Using Order 3, calculate the amount of mL to give the patient. Round your answer to the nearest tenth. Label your answer.
Purpose: Most injections are measured in tenths of a mL.
Using Order 4, calculate the amount of mL to give the patient. Round your answer to the nearest tenth. Label your answer.
Using Order 5, calculate the amount of mL to give the patient. Round your answer to the nearest tenth. Label your answer.
Note: When working through the problem, round your answer two places beyond your answer. In this situation, round your answers as you work to the thousandth place (or three places after the decimal point).
Using Order 6, calculate the amount of mL to give the patient. Round your answer to the nearest tenth. Label your answer.
Double check your answers to ensure the correct dose will be given.
Purpose: When calculating medications, it is important to recheck the work to ensure your answer is correct.

Setting Up the Problem:	There are three main steps to this problem. When you complete a step, round two places beyond your answer. For instance, if your answer is to be in tenths, then during the problem, round to the thousandth (3 places after the decimal). This will ensure accuracy in the answer.		
Problem:	Patient's weight: 33 lb Order: ABC medication 0.1 mg/kg Stock: ABC medication 1 mg/mL How many mL(s) will you give?		
Step 1:	Move the patient's weight into kg. 33 lb = _____ kg This can be done several ways. Use your favorite method or follow the example on the right.	PROBLEM $\dfrac{33\ lb}{x\ kg}$	EQUIVALENT $= \dfrac{2.2\ lb}{1\ kg}$
	Now solve for the unknown. Using a calculator: Multiply in the diagonal direction of the two numbers (33 × 1) and then divide by the number in the other direction (2.2). Round your answer to the nearest thousandth (if needed).	PROBLEM $\dfrac{33\ lb}{x\ kg}$ 33 × 1 = 33 / 2.2 = 15 kg	EQUIVALENT $= \dfrac{2.2\ lb}{1\ kg}$
	To solve without a calculator: multiply diagonally and solve for X. Round your answer to the nearest thousandth (if needed)	$33 \times 1 = 2.2x$ $33 = 2.2x$ $\dfrac{33}{2.2} = \dfrac{2.2x}{2.2}$ $15 = x$	
	Tip: Cross out the pounds in the problem and add in your new information (15 kg).	**Updated weight: 15 kg**	
Step 2:	Calculate the number of mg of medication needed. Again, there are several ways. The easiest is to multiple the weight by the order (15 kg x 0.1 mg) or you can set it up like indicated on the right and solve like prior problems. Since this is in the middle of the problem, round to the nearest thousandth (if needed).	ORDER $\dfrac{0.1\ mg}{1\ kg}$ 0.1 × 15 = 1.5 / 1 = 1.5 mg	UPDATED $= \dfrac{x\ mg}{15\ kg}$
	Tip: Cross out the order information in the problem and add in your new information (1.5 mg).	**Updated order: ABC medication 1.5 mg**	
Step 3:	Calculate the liquid medication dose. Put the stock information into a fraction. Put the order information on the other side. Make sure the labels are in the exact same location.	STOCK $\dfrac{1\ mg}{1\ mL}$	ORDER $= \dfrac{1.5\ mg}{x\ mL}$
Step 4:	Now solve for the unknown. Using a calculator: Multiply in the diagonal direction of the two numbers (1 × 1.5) and then divide by the number in the other direction (1). Round your answer to the nearest tenth (if needed).	STOCK $\dfrac{1\ mg}{1\ mL}$ 0.1 × 1.5 = 1.5 / 1 = 1.5 mL You would give 1.5 mL of ABC medication.	ORDER $= \dfrac{1.5\ mg}{x\ mL}$
	To solve without a calculator: multiply diagonally and solve for X. Round your answer to the nearest tenth.	$1x = 1 \times 1.5$ $1x = 1.5$ $\dfrac{1x}{1} = \dfrac{1.5}{1}$ $x = 1.5\ mL$	

FIG. 37.17 Stock and order (proportion) method: Calculate pediatric medication.

CLOSING COMMENTS

Working with medications is an important responsibility for the medical assistant. It is critical for the medical assistant to be knowledgeable about the medication. Knowing the actions, normal dose, and common side effects is important. It is your professional obligation to know about all of the drugs you administer. If you do not know the drug, then you cannot administer it until you do. Drug reference materials are important resources for all healthcare professionals. Learning how to find what you need to know is important. Medical assistants need to anticipate using drug reference materials often.

For the medical assistant, learning about new medications will be a career-long pursuit. Changes in the pharmacology aspect of healthcare are constant. It is important for medical assistants to stay on top of changes in their practice area. This will be especially important when working with patients and prescription refills.

> **EXCEPTIONAL CUSTOMER SERVICE**
>
> When working with prescription refills, it is important for the medical assistant to process the refill in a timely fashion. If the medical assistant procrastinates and does not process the refill, the patient may not have the medication when she or he needs it. Some medications need to be taken on a daily basis. If a dose is skipped, the patient may have serious consequences.
>
> It is also important that the medical assistant honors what that patient was told. If the patient is told that the medication will be sent to a pharmacy by a specific time, it is important for the medical assistant to ensure this is done. If the medication is held up for some reason, the medical assistant should notify the patient about the delay.

CHAPTER REVIEW

This chapter covered the drug basics, including the sources, uses, and pharmacokinetics. The sources of drugs include natural and synthetic. Natural sources include plants, animals, minerals, and microbiologic courses. Synthetic medications are created in a laboratory setting. Medications are used for prevention, treatment, diagnosis, cure, contraception, health maintenance, palliative care, and replacement. Pharmacokinetics involves drug absorption, distribution, metabolism, and excretion. The very young, older adults, and those with kidney and liver disease are at risk for drug toxicity. Too much medication or metabolites in the body can cause harmful effects.

Drug action is influenced by many factors, including age, size, gender, disease, and diet. For the therapeutic or desired effect to occur, medication levels in the blood must be in the therapeutic range. If the level is beyond the therapeutic range, the person can experience symptoms of toxicity.

The Food, Drug, and Cosmetic Act enforced by the FDA and the Controlled Substance Act imposed by the DEA impact the healthcare setting. The medical assistant is responsible for removing any recalled medications from the department. Compliance with the CSA is the responsibility of the medical assistant and the provider. The medical assistant needs to follow the storage, tracking, destruction, and theft reporting rules for controlled substances.

This chapter also covered the four names for medications: the chemical, generic, official, and brand names. Drug reference materials are critical for learning about medications. Terminology commonly found in reference information was discussed. Using drug reference information is common when preparing prescriptions for the provider to sign. Remember, it is not within the medical assistant's scope of practice to order (sign) prescriptions. This falls within the provider's scope of practice. The provider is responsible for the accuracy of the prescription and for ensuring that it meets the state and federal laws.

The final part of the chapter covered common math problems that a medical assistant should be able to solve. The scope of practice for medical assistants may vary by state when it comes to calculating drug dosages. Regardless, being proficient at math for medications is important for a medical assistant.

SCENARIO WRAP-UP

Mark is enjoying working with Gabe. He is amazed at how much Gabe knows about medications that the providers commonly prescribe. Mark feels that he will never be as fluent with the medications as Gabe is. He even mentioned this to Gabe. His mentor laughed and said he felt the same way during his own practicum. Over the years, he has used drug reference materials to help him learn about medications. He has a practice of looking up medications he does not know. This helped him become more fluent. He assured Mark, that if he was willing to read up on medications, he too will be fluent with them.

Mark is looking forward to administering medications with Gabe. Now that he understands how to use the drug reference materials, he will be working hard to learn the medications he encounters.

38

Administering Medication

LEARNING OBJECTIVES

1. Verify and discuss the rules of medication administration.
2. Discuss the various types of medication forms.
3. Administer oral medications.
4. Describe and demonstrate other routes of medications: sublingual, buccal, transdermal, inhalation, topical, irrigation, and parenteral.
5. Discuss types and parts of needles and syringes.
6. Prepare and administer parenteral (excluding intravenous [IV]) medications.
7. Prepare and administer intradermal injections. Also, discuss allergy testing.
8. Prepare and administer subcutaneous injections.
9. Prepare and administer intramuscular injections.
10. Monitor intravenous therapy.

CHAPTER OUTLINE

1. **Opening Scenario, 885**
2. **You Will Learn, 885**
3. **Introduction, 885**
4. **Nine Rules of Medication Administration, 885**
    a. Right Medication, 885
    b. Right Dose, 885
    c. Right Route, 886
    d. Right Time, 886
    e. Right Patient, 886
    f. Right Education, 887
    g. Right to Refuse, 887
    h. Right Technique, 887
    i. Right Documentation, 887
5. **Forms of Medications, 887**
6. **Routes of Medications, 889**
    a. Oral Route, 890
    b. Sublingual and Buccal Routes, 890
    c. Transdermal Route, 890
    d. Inhalation Route, 892
    e. Topical Routes, 892
        i. *Vaginal Route, 893*
        ii. *Rectal Route, 893*
        iii. *Nasal Route, 893*
        iv. *Ocular Route, 893*
        v. *Otic Route, 893*
    f. Irrigation Route, 893
    g. Parenteral Route, 896
7. **Needles and Syringes, 899**
    a. Hypodermic Needles, 899
        i. *Gauge and Length, 899*
        ii. *Safety Needles, 900*
    b. Hypodermic Syringes, 900
    c. Working with the Needle and Syringe, 900
        i. *Uncapping and Recapping Needles, 903*
        ii. *Switching Needles, 903*
8. **Preparing Parenteral Medication, 904**
    a. Using an Ampule, 904
    b. Using a Prefilled Sterile Cartridge, 906
    c. Specialty Syringe Units, 906
    d. Using a Vial, 908
    e. Reconstituting Powdered Medication, 909
    f. Mixing Insulins, 913
9. **Giving Parenteral Medications, 914**
    a. Guidelines for Parenteral Medications, 915
    b. Special Situations, 915
10. **Intradermal Injections, 915**
    a. Tuberculin Testing, 917
        i. *Two-Step Testing, 921*
        ii. *Blood Tuberculin Tests, 921*
    b. Allergy Testing, 921
11. **Subcutaneous Injections, 922**
    a. Administration Techniques, 922
        i. *Aspiration, 922*
    b. Subcutaneous Sites, 924
12. **Intramuscular Injections, 926**
    a. Administration Techniques, 926
        i. *Aspiration, 926*
        ii. *Air Lock Technique, 927*
        iii. *Z-track Technique, 927*
    b. Intramuscular Sites, 927
        i. *Deltoid Site, 927*
        ii. *Vastus Lateralis Site, 928*
        iii. *Ventrogluteal Site, 928*
13. **Monitoring Intravenous Therapy, 931**
14. **Closing Comments, 932**
15. **Chapter Review, 932**

CHAPTER 38 Administering Medication

OPENING SCENARIO

Gabe Garcia, CMA (AAMA), has worked for the Walden-Martin Family Medical (WMFM) Clinic for 7 years. He is currently Mark Allen's mentor for practicum. Mark has been working with Gabe for a couple of days. He has learned how Gabe handles prescriptions from the providers. As Mark advances in his practicum, he will be working with Gabe to administer medications to patients. Mark enjoyed practicing injections on his peers in school and looks forward to improving his skills during practicum.

YOU WILL LEARN

- The Nine Rules of Medication Administration.
- The forms and routes of medications commonly used in the ambulatory care setting.
- To handle syringes and needles, including uncapping, recapping, and switching needles.
- To prepare parenteral medications, including using an ampule, prefilled sterile cartridge, and vials; also, reconstituting medication and mixing insulins.
- The types of tuberculin testing and allergy testing.
- Administration techniques for intradermal, subcutaneous, and intramuscular injections.
- To locate the sites for intradermal, subcutaneous, and intramuscular injections.
- To administer intradermal, subcutaneous, and intramuscular injections.

INTRODUCTION

In the prior chapter, you learned the basics of pharmacology. Using drug reference information and solving pharmacology-related math problems were discussed. You will use these skills when administering medications. In this chapter, administration safety techniques will be discussed, along with medication forms and routes. The techniques of preparing and administering medications will be the primary focus.

It is important to remember that medications can cause serious harm to patients. It is critical to pay attention to the details when you prepare and administer medications. Preventing errors and providing superior patient care are goals each time medication is given. Administering medication is an important responsibility for healthcare professionals.

State laws vary on medical assistants administering medications. In some situations, the state law allows medical assistants to administer medications, but the facility's policies do not. It is important for medical assistants to know their state's laws and the facility's policies on medication administration.

NINE RULES OF MEDICATION ADMINISTRATION

Throughout this chapter, administration procedures for various routes will be given. Before learning how to give medications, it is important to understand the medication safety rules.

Over the years the guidelines have grown to include additional steps to address patient education and rights.

Each time you prepare and give medication, it is important that you follow the Nine Rules of Medication Administration. These rules are designed to help you look at the details and avoid making errors during the procedure (Fig. 38.1).

Right Medication

A prescription (or an order) from a provider is required before a medication can be given. As the prior chapter discussed, orders can be written or verbal. For all verbal orders, make sure to write down the order and read it back to the provider. This helps to ensure the accuracy of the order. The order needs to include several things, including the medication's name and **form**.

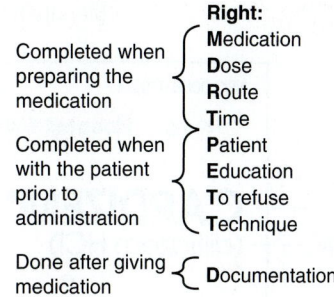

FIG. 38.1 Mnemonic for the Nine Rules of Medication Administration.

> **VOCABULARY**
> **form:** Physical characteristics of a medication (e.g., tablet, suspension).

With the order in hand, the medical assistant must prepare the medication. This requires finding the correct medication. Fig. 38.2 shows two drug labels. Drug labels look different from one manufacturer to another. Sometimes the brand name will appear on the label (e.g., Cardizem) with the generic name. Some labels will only have the generic name listed (e.g., cephalexin [sef a LEX in]). Use drug reference information if you are not familiar with the medication listed on the prescription. Sometimes the provider will give a brand name, but the stock medication will indicate only a generic name. Make sure you have the correct medication.

Having the correct medication also includes the right form. Fig. 38.2 shows labels with two different forms of medications. Cardizem is in tablet form, and cephalexin is in liquid form. (More information on forms of medications will be given later in the chapter.)

You will need to check the medication order against the label three times during the preparation process to ensure that you have the correct name and form of medication. You check the label:

- When you get the medication from the storage area (e.g., cabinet, freezer, and refrigerator.).
- Before preparing the medication
- Before you return the medication to the cabinet or refrigerator

It is important that you do an activity between each check. For instance, after you do the first check, assemble the supplies you need to prepare the medication. Then do the second check. As you clean up your area, you do the third check. Too often we reach for something based on the color, size, or location of the object. We may look at the label and think we see what we want to see. Checking the label three times, with activities between, helps to ensure that you have the right medication.

Right Dose

The dose of medication is on the order. The provider may have written the order in two different ways, even though the amount is the same:

- acetaminophen (a set a MEE noc fen) 500 mg, 2 tabs po × 1 dose
- acetaminophen 1000 mg po × 1 dose

The first one shows the tablet strength (e.g., 500 mg) and the number of tablets (e.g., 2) to give. If the stock medication comes in 500 mg tablets, the medical assistant has no calculations to do. The second order just shows the number of milligrams to give (e.g., 1000 mg). The medical assistant would need to calculate how many tablets to give. (This was discussed in Chapter 37.)

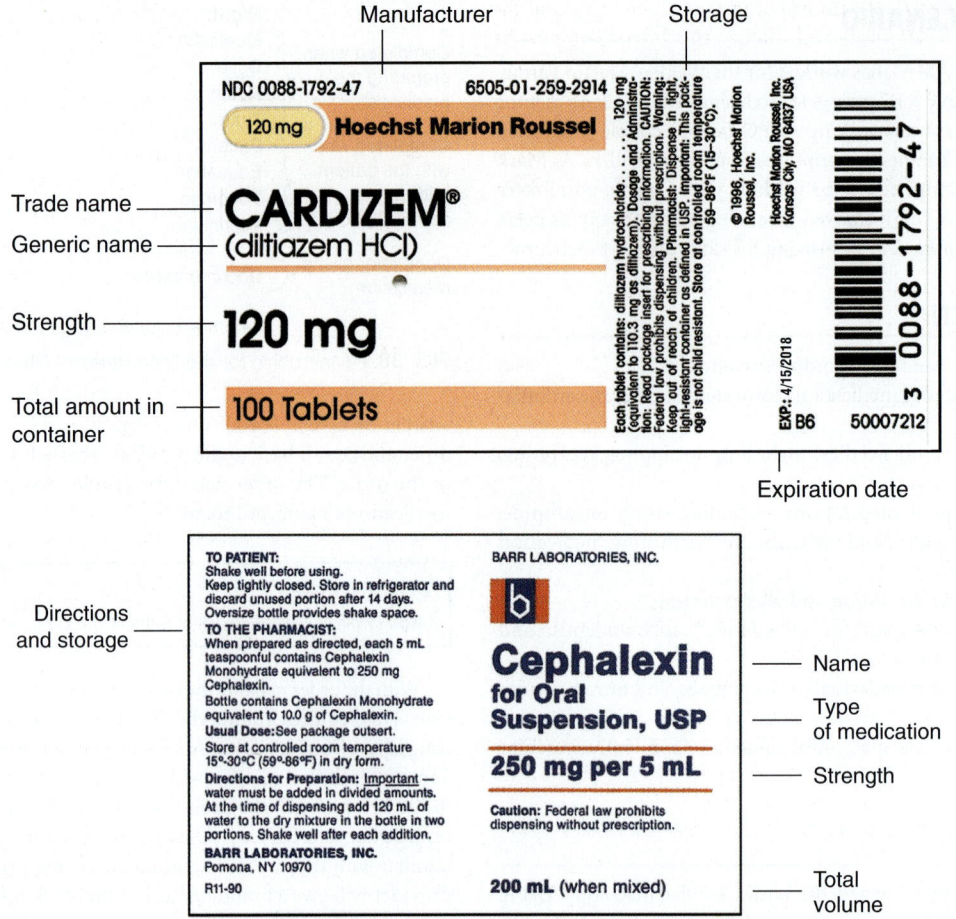

FIG. 38.2 Drug labels. (From Brown M, Mulholland JM: *Drug Calculations: Process and Problems for Clinical Practice*, ed 9, St Louis, 2012, Mosby.)

Right Route

Besides checking the label for the name and form, it is also important to check the *route*. The route of the medication must match the provider's order. The route for cephalexin is oral (see Fig. 38.2). The route should be checked, along with the name and form, three times before the medication is given.

> **VOCABULARY**
> **route:** The means by which a drug enters the body.

Right Time

Medications need to be given at the right time. For most medication orders, the time is part of the order. Some orders are stat, whereas others are every month. Vaccines are a little different. Timing for vaccines may not be written on the provider's order, but the medical assistant should ensure that it is the correct time for a vaccine to be given (Box 38.1). The medical assistant will need to review the patient's vaccination history and the person's age. Using immunization schedules or the immunization tables in electronic health records (EHR), the medical assistant can determine what vaccines are due.

Right Patient

Before giving the medication to the patient, it is important to correctly identify the patient. Ask the patient or parent/guardian to state his or her full name and date of birth. Some agencies will require patients to

> **BOX 38.1 Timing of Vaccines**
>
> There are two main types of vaccines available:
> - *Live virus vaccines*: The microorganism is alive but *attenuated* (weakened) in the laboratory. Vaccine examples include MMR (measles, mumps, and rubella), varicella (chickenpox), zoster (shingles), and yellow fever.
> - *Inactivated vaccines*: The microorganism is dead. This type includes *toxoid vaccines* made from modified toxins of microorganisms (e.g., diphtheria and tetanus).
>
> When vaccines are given, the immunization schedule must be followed. The immunization schedule indicates the person's age and the timing between doses. Vaccination too early or before a specific age will result in the patient having to be revaccinated.
>
> Vaccinations are postponed when patients have a moderate or severe acute illness. Specific vaccines are not given if a person has a severe allergic reaction to a vaccine component, to latex, or to a prior dose. Patients may not receive a live virus vaccine if they:
> - Were vaccinated with another live virus vaccine less than 28 days ago
> - Are pregnant or may be pregnant in the next month. The human papillomavirus (HPV) vaccine is also contraindicated with pregnancy.
> - Are immunocompromised (e.g., cancer, leukemia, HIV/AIDS)
> - Are receiving chemotherapy or high-dose steroid therapy
> - Had recently received a blood transfusion, immune (gamma) globulin, or antiviral medication
>
> Consult the CDC website for information on vaccine schedules and catch-up schedules: https://www.cdc.gov/vaccines/index.html. The CDC also has a free app available for vaccine information.

spell their last names. Verify the information against the order and the patient's health record. All three must match. Any differences must be resolved before the medication is given.

In some agencies, patients are given identification bracelets that are scanned before medication is given. The medication is also scanned. An automatic entry is made in the EHR. This is a common practice in hospitals. This practice is starting to be seen in ambulatory care facilities. The identification process with bracelets still requires asking the patient's name and date of birth. The information is checked against the bracelet and the order.

> **CRITICAL THINKING BOX 38.1**
>
> Gabe is introducing Mark to the facility's medication procedures. Gabe encourages Mark to have the patients give their complete name and date of birth. He also tells Mark it is a good idea to have the patients spell their last names. Why is spelling the last name an important safety check?

Right Education

Before administering the medication to the patient, the medical assistant must:

1. Give the name of the medication and who ordered it. For example: "Dr. Martin ordered acetaminophen for your fever."
2. Explain the desired effect or action of the medication. For example: "The acetaminophen will bring down your fever."
3. Describe common side effects of the medication. For example: "The acetaminophen may cause nausea, rash, and a headache."
4. Verify the patient's allergies.

If the patient is receiving a vaccination, the facility may require a questionnaire to be completed. The medical assistant may need to give a Vaccine Information Statement (VIS) prior to administering the vaccine. If the patient cannot read, the medical assistant should review the VIS with the patient. The VIS provides important information to the patient about the vaccine and common and uncommon side effects (Box 38.2). VISs in other languages are available online.

> **CRITICAL THINKING BOX 38.2**
>
> Part of the WMFM Clinic's policy is to explain to patients what was ordered and why they are getting it. Why is it important to tell patients the name of a medication or procedure and the reason they are getting it? How might this add to exceptional customer service?

Right to Refuse

The patient or the parent (or the person legally responsible for the patient) has a right to refuse any medication. If a patient refuses the medication, the medical assistant should respect the patient's wishes. Don't pressure the patient. Notify the provider that the ordered medication was refused and the reason if it was shared. Document the refusal of the medication and the provider who was informed. The provider will talk with the patient regarding other options.

Right Technique

When giving the medication, the medical assistant must give it in the right way. This may include an assessment before the medication is administered. Examples of right technique include:

- Obtain vital signs before giving specific medication. For instance, digoxin must be held if an adult's pulse is under 60.

> **BOX 38.2 Vaccine Information Statement (VIS)**
>
> The Vaccine Information Statement was created by the Centers for Disease Control and Prevention (CDC). A VIS provides information to the patient or to the guardian/parent on the benefits and risks of the vaccine. The National Childhood Vaccine Injury Act requires that all patients (or parents/guardians) get the appropriate VIS prior to every dose of vaccine administered, regardless of the age of the patient. The specific list of vaccines that require the VIS are listed on the CDC's website at https://www.cdc.gov/vaccines/hcp/vis/about/facts-vis.html
>
> The VIS can be displayed on a computer screen or as a laminated copy that can be read by the patient prior to administration of the vaccine. Copies of the VIS can be given to the patient or parent/guardian to take home. The provider must offer the information; however, the patient or parent/guardian has the right to decline to take the document. (VISs can be downloaded in about 40 different languages for patients who do not speak English.)
>
> Besides giving the patient or parent/guardian the VIS prior to the vaccination, the medical assistant must document the following in the patient's health record:
> - The edition date of the VIS. This is found on the back of the document in the bottom right corner. Make sure to have the latest edition of the VIS.
> - The date the VIS was provided, and the date the vaccine was administered (usually the two are done on the same day).
> - The office address, name, and title of the person who administered the vaccine.
> - The vaccine's manufacturer and lot number.

From the Centers for Disease Control and Prevention (CDC): https://www.cdc.gov/vaccines/hcp/vis/about/facts-vis.html. Accessed April 6, 2018.

- Obtain information about the patient's pain level before giving an analgesic medication. The medical assistant can ask the patient to rate the pain using a 0–10 scale. Zero is no pain and 10 is the worse pain ever. Another pain assessment tool is the Wong-Baker FACES Pain Rating Scale (Fig. 38.3). The medical assistant should explain the scale to patients. Then patients can state how they feel. This scale works well for children.
- Some medications must be taken with food and others with a full glass of water. Medications that need to be taken on an empty stomach need to be taken 1 hour before meals or 2 hours after meals.

Information regarding the techniques to use when administering the medication can be found in drug reference information.

Right Documentation

After giving a medication, the medical assistant must document it in the patient's health record. If the medication is not documented, it appears it wasn't given. The documentation will vary based on what the patient received. Some documentation is done in narrative form, whereas vaccines are documented on paper or in electronic vaccination forms. Box 38.3 identifies the elements that should be in the documentation.

FORMS OF MEDICATIONS

The form is the physical characteristics of the medication. Forms can be grouped into solids, semisolids, and liquids. Solid and semisolid medications are commonly prescribed and found in over-the-counter (OTC) products. Table 38.1 provides examples of solid and semisolid

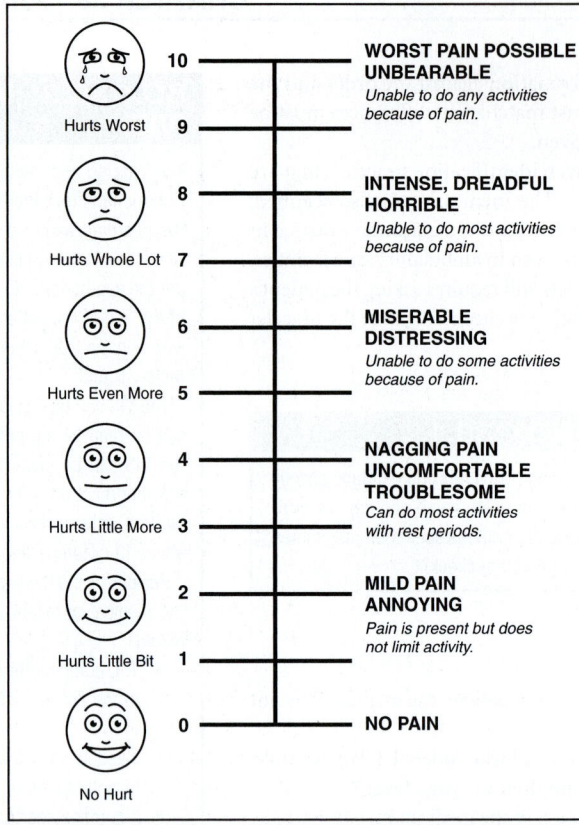

FIG. 38.3 Wong-Baker FACES Pain Rating Scale.

BOX 38.3 Medication Documentation Elements

- Provider ordering the medication
- Assessment done (e.g., vital signs or pain level)
- Allergies
- Teaching/instructions given to patient (includes edition date of the Vaccine Information Statement [VIS])
- Name of medication (acetaminophen)
- Dose given (e.g., 650 mg)
- Route given (e.g., po)
- Lot number (usually only required for vaccines and controlled substances)
- Expiration date (usually only required for vaccines and controlled substances)
- Manufacturer (usually only required for vaccines and controlled substances)
- How patient tolerated the medication
- Additional information as needed (e.g., patient is resting on exam table)
- Signature if note is handwritten (an electronic health record [EHR] uses automatic signatures for documentation entries)

BOX 38.4 Crushing Medications

Children, older adults, and others may have problems swallowing solid medications. Crushing medications is sometimes an option. The medication should be placed in a small amount of food or liquid (e.g., pudding or jam). It is important to eat or drink all the food or liquid to get the entire dose of medication.

Solid medications typically have an unpleasant taste. It is important to share with parents that children sometimes shy away from foods with an unpleasant taste. For instance, if a parent mixes the medication with the milk in a bottle, the baby may not want to drink the milk. This can be a problem if the baby drinks only milk.

Medications that cannot be crushed include:

- Slow- or extended-release tablets: Crushing, chewing, or cutting the tablet can cause a person to get the dose faster than he or she should, resulting in an overdose.
- Enteric-coated tablets: Crushing, chewing, or cutting the tablet causes the protective nature of the coating to be lost. The person could have more stomach distress.

BOX 38.5 Examples of Acronyms for Slow-Release Tablets

CD – controlled delivery
CR – controlled release
DR – delayed release
ER – extended release
LA – long acting
SA – sustained action
SR – sustained release
TD – time delay
TR – time release
XL – extended release
XR – extended release

BOX 38.6 Alcohol in Medications

Several forms of liquid medications contain alcohol. This is a concern for patients who are recovering alcoholics or have other health issues, such as diabetes. An internet search can provide lists of medications with their alcohol content. The drug reference information also provides information on the ingredients.

If a patient mentions that he or she is a recovering alcoholic, it is important for the medical assistant first to acknowledge the person's accomplishment. Then the medical assistant should communicate the information to the provider. This may make a difference in what medication the provider gives to the patient. Giving a patient a medication with alcohol may be harmful to the patient's success and health.

TABLE 38.1 Examples of Solid and Semisolid Medication Forms

Form	Description
Tablet	Solid form of medication formed by compressed powdered medication; may be coated. Can come in various sizes and shapes (Fig. 38.4).
Chewable tablet	Designed to be chewed prior to swallowing (see Fig. 38.4). Example: chewable vitamin
Caplet (KAP lit)	Coated, oval medication tablet (see Fig. 38.4).
Capsule (KAP sul)	Medication in a hard or soft gelatin shell (see Fig. 38.4).
Scored tablet	A notched tablet which can be split in half with a pill cutter (or splitter) (see Fig. 38.4; also Fig. 38.5).
Enteric coated tablets or capsules (en TER ik)	Coated to pass through the acidic environment of the stomach. Breaks down in the base environment of the intestines. Do not crush, cut, or chew these tablets, or the protective property will be lost.
Buffered	A solid medication containing the active medication and an antacid. The antacid lowers the pH in the stomach, neutralizing the acid and thereby reducing stomach irritation. Example: buffered aspirin
Fast dissolving tablet or film strip	Also called *oral disintegrating tablets*. Solid form of medicine that is placed on the tongue (or by the cheek [buccal]) and breaks down rapidly in the presence of saliva. Example: Belbuca
Extended release tablet or capsule	Designed to break down over time. Do not crush, chew, or cut tablet as this may cause an overdose. Many acronyms (see Box 38.5). Example: Calan SR
Effervescent tablet	Contains an acid substance and carbonate or bicarbonate. When placed in water, it releases carbon dioxide, creating a pleasant-tasting carbonated drink. Example: K-Lyte Effervescent Tablets
lozenge (troche) (LOZ enj, TROE kee)	Flat, round form containing active medication and a sweetened flavoring; dissolves on the tongue. Used for local treatment of the mouth and throat. Example: cough drop
Powder	Nonpotent powdered medication that must be mixed with a liquid before it can be taken. Example: MiraLAX
Ointment and **paste**	Semisolid, greasy drug preparations that are applied to the skin, rectum, or nasal mucosa. Pastes are thicker and less penetrating than ointments. Example: Nystatin Ointment
Cream	Semisolid drug preparation made of active medication, oil, and water. Example: Nystatin Cream
Suppository and **pessary** (su POZ I tore ee, PES ah ree)	Active medication mixed in an oil base (e.g., cocoa butter). Solid at room temperature but melts at body temperature. Suppositories are typically shaped like a small torpedo and used in the rectum, urethra, or vagina. Pessaries are vaginal suppositories. Example: Dulcolax suppository

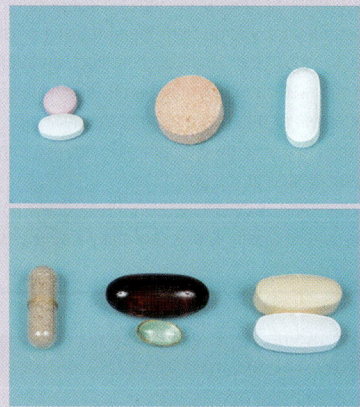

FIG. 38.4 Left to right: Top row – tablets, chewable, and caplet. Bottom row – hard-shelled capsule, soft-shelled capsules, and scored caplets.

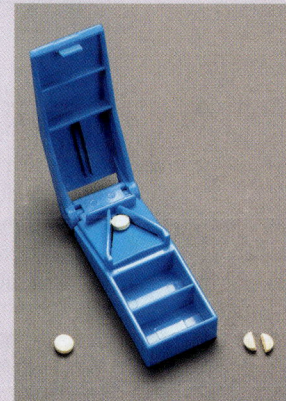

FIG. 38.5 Pill cutter or splitter. (From Proctor D, et al: *Kinn's The Medical Assistant*, ed 13, St Louis, 2017, Elsevier.)

medication forms. New drug delivery systems or drug forms have been approved by the U.S. Food and Drug Administration (FDA) in the past few years. This has helped to provide additional options to those who cannot swallow pills. It is common for patients or parents to have concerns about swallowing pills. Box 38.4 discusses crushing solid medications. Box 38.5 lists examples of slow-release tablet acronyms.

Liquid and semiliquid medications have various uses. They can be swallowed, rubbed on the skin, or instilled in the nose, eyes, or ears. Liquid medications are easily taken by children, older adults, and those with swallowing problems. With liquid medications, the active medication is mixed with water, alcohol, or both (Box 38.6). If the active medication dissolves in the liquid, the medication is a *solution*. If the active medication does not dissolve and becomes suspended in the liquid, it is called a *suspension*. Over time the suspended drug will settle to the bottom of the container. It is important to shake suspensions before pouring the medication. Table 38.2 describes examples of solutions and suspensions.

ROUTES OF MEDICATIONS

For drug administration, the route is how a drug enters the body. As discussed in the prior chapter, the dose of medication can differ based on the route. The following sections will discuss common routes of medication. There are many other routes that are not commonly used in the ambulatory care environment.

Oral Route

Medications taken by the oral route (po) are medications we take by mouth. Special administration techniques may be required for oral medications. These may include:
- Oral medications that coat the mouth or throat should not be immediately followed with water.
- Oral medications that require water for swallowing require more than a sip. Some medications require a glass of water after taking the medication.
- A straw should be used for liquid medications that stain the teeth.
- Liquid medications should be measured only with a plastic medication cup or an oral medication syringe. Household measuring devices, such as spoons, are not accurate.

It is important to notify the provider if the patient is unable to take the medication due to nausea, vomiting, or problems swallowing. Do not attempt to see if the patient can swallow the pill. It is better to talk with provider if the patient is concerned. Remember some medications can be crushed safely, whereas others cannot. Procedure 38.1 describes the steps to administer solid and liquid medications.

CRITICAL THINKING BOX 38.3

Gabe and Mark are working with Charles Johnson, who has a temperature of 103.4° F. The provider orders acetaminophen 500 mg, 2 tabs po for the patient. Mr. Johnson tells Gabe and Mark that he can't swallow pills. Can they give him liquid acetaminophen, or must they talk with the provider first about the situation?

Sublingual and Buccal Routes

Sublingual (sub LING gwehl) (SL) medications are placed under the tongue. *Buccal* (BUK ahl) medications are placed between the cheek and the gums. Both mucous membrane areas are rich in blood vessels. The medication is absorbed very rapidly into the bloodstream.

Patients should not eat or smoke prior to taking SL and buccal medications. Patients should not chew or swallow SL or buccal medications. Water can be taken prior to the medication to wet the mouth. No liquids can be taken until the medication has dissolved. Patients should alternate cheeks used for buccal medication to avoid mucosal irritation.

Transdermal Route

Transdermal (trans DUHR mahl) *medications* are placed on the skin and absorbed into the bloodstream. Transdermal medications are different than topical medications, which provide a **local** action. Transdermal medications provide a **systemic** action. The transdermal drug delivery system uses patches that adhere to the skin (Fig. 38.6). Medication in the patch is slowly absorbed through the skin. Depending on the medication, the patch may be worn for a part of a day to many days. Box 38.7 describes how to replace a transdermal patch.

VOCABULARY
local: Affecting the area where applied.
systemic: Affecting the entire body.

MEDICAL TERMINOLOGY
-al: pertaining to
sub-: under
trans-: through

BOX 38.7 Replacing Transdermal Patches

When replacing a patch or teaching a patient to use transdermal patches, follow these steps:
- Write the date and time on the new patch.
- Wear disposable gloves if changing a patch on another person.
- Remove the old patch. Fold the sticky sides together and discard. If the old patch is not removed, the person may be at risk for an overdose.
- Remove any residual medication from the skin using a tissue.
- Decide where to apply the new patch. Select a different location. Depending on the medication, it may be on the shoulder, back, upper arm, lower abdomen, or hip. Clean and dry the new site.
- Remove the protective liner on the patch. Do not use torn patches. Do not touch the sticky side of the patch.
- Place the patch's sticky side on the skin. Press down on the patch to ensure it adheres to the skin. Make sure the patch is smooth, without folds.

TABLE 38.2 Examples of Solutions and Suspensions

Type	Form	Description
Solutions	Tincture (TINGK chur)	Very potent solution of alcohol or alcohol and water and the active medicine. Example: iodine tincture
	Fluid extract (floo id EK strakt)	Alcoholic plant source extractions; very concentrated and more potent than tinctures. Example: belladonna fluid extract
	Spirit	An alcoholic solution with substances that easily evaporate. Example: aromatic ammonia spirit
	Elixir (ee LIK sir)	Clear sweetened liquid preparation that contains alcohol. Example: digoxin elixir
	Syrup	A sugar and water solution that contains flavoring and medicinal substance. Example: cough syrup (some syrups contain alcohol)
Suspensions	Emulsion (ee MUL shun)	A suspension of oil and water. Example: ophthalmic cyclosporine
	Gel and magma (MAG mah)	Suspensions consisting of minerals and water. Gels are semisolids and contain finer particles than magmas. The minerals settle out with standing. Shake before using. Example: milk of magnesia
	Liniment (LIN uh mehnt)	A suspension that is rubbed on the skin; used to reduce pain and stiffness. Example: Ben-Gay
	Lotion	A water-based suspension that is applied to the skin. Example: calamine lotion
	Aerosol (ahr ah SOL)	A suspension of medication in a gas, usually used for respiratory or sinus conditions. Example: albuterol (al BYOO ter ole) metered-dose inhaler

CHAPTER 38 Administering Medication

PROCEDURE 38.1 Administer Oral Medications

Tasks
Calculate the dose to give. Prepare a liquid and a solid medication and administer medications to a patient. Document medication administration.

Equipment and Supplies
- Provider's orders
- Patient's health record
- Drug reference information
- Liquid medication and a solid medication (use drug labels in Fig. 38.2)
- Paper cup
- Plastic medication cup
- Marker
- Medication tray
- Glass of water

Orders
Diltiazem 240 mg po and Cephalexin Oral Suspension 375 mg po.

Procedural Steps

1. Using the drug reference information and the orders, review the information on the medications.
   Purpose: The medical assistant must know about the medication that is being given.
2. Using the orders and the labels in Fig. 38.2, calculate the amount of medication you need to give. Verify the right doses with the instructor. Verify if it is the right time for the order, if that applies.
   Purpose: The orders do not specify the number of tablets or the amount of liquid (mL) to give. The medical assistant must calculate both. It is important to check your answer with a peer in the workplace before preparing the medication. This is how to ensure that the right dose is being given.
3. Wash your hands or use hand sanitizer. Select the right medications from the storage area. Check each medication label against the order. Check for the right name, form, and route. Check the expiration date to make sure the drug is not expired.
   Purpose: It is important to do the first check of the label when getting medications from the cabinet. Do not administer expired medications.
4. Assemble the supplies required to prepare the medications. Using the marker, write the medication name and dose on the appropriate cups (Fig. 1).
   Purpose: The paper cup will be used for the tablets, and the plastic cup will be used for the liquid. Make sure not to write over the measurement markings on the plastic cup. Labeling the cups is a safety measure. All medications prepared need to be labeled. Writing an assessment reminder on the cup is optional and can be helpful when the medical assistant needs to do an assessment (e.g., blood pressure) prior to the administration.

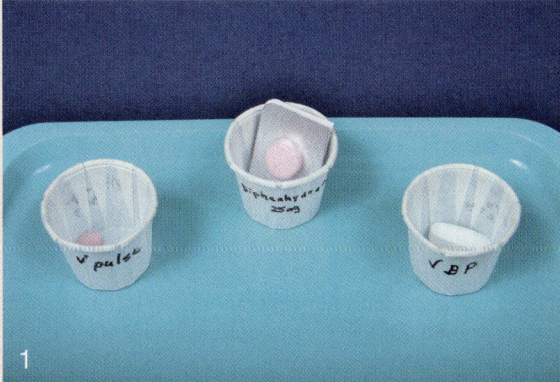

5. Perform the second medication check. Check each medication label against the order. Check for the right name, form, and route.

   Purpose: It is important to do the second check of the label before pouring the medications into the cups.
6. For the solid medication: Remove the cover of the container and hold it so the inside is facing up. Carefully pour the correct number of tablets into the cover. If you pour too many into the cover, pour the extra tablets back into the bottle. When you have the correct number of tablets in the cover, pour them from the cover into the paper cup. Place the cover on the container. Make sure not to contaminate the inside of the container or the cover.
   Purpose: Inside the medication container and the cover are sterile. You can pour the tablets back and forth between these two sites until you have the correct number of tablets in the cover. Once you pour the tablets into the paper cup, they are no longer sterile. They cannot be put back into the sterile medication container. If using *unit dose* (individual packaged tablets [blister packs]), tear off the number of tablets needed and place in the paper cup. Do not open until you are with the patient. If the patient refuses the medication, the unopened unit dose medications can be returned to the original box.
7. For liquid medication:
   a. Place the plastic medication cup on a high, even surface. Uncover the bottle and place the cover on the counter, making sure the inside is facing up. Place your palm over the medication label. Position yourself so you are eye level with the medication cup (Fig. 2).
   Purpose: The cup needs to be on an even surface. Read the amount at eye level to ensure the accuracy of the measurement. Palming the label keeps the label clean as you pour the medication.

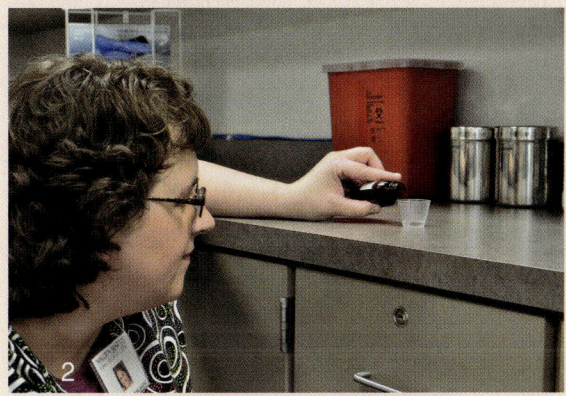

   b. Pour the medication into the cup until the lowest point of the meniscus is at the measurement needed (Fig. 3).
   Purpose: When liquid is poured into a container, it is higher at the edges than the middle. This is called the *meniscus* (meh NIS kuhs). The liquid must be measured at the lowest point of the meniscus.

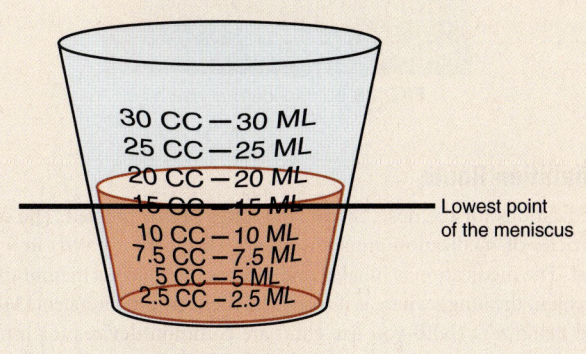

Continued

PROCEDURE 38.1 Administer Oral Medications—cont'd

   c. If too much medication is poured into the cup, flush the extra down the sink. Replace the cover on the bottle without contaminating the inside of the cover or bottle.

   Purpose: Any extra medication in the cup cannot be poured back into the sterile medication bottle. The medication in the bottle and the inside cover need to remain sterile.

8. Place the medication cups on the medication tray. Clean up the area.
   Purpose: It is important for the medical assistant to clean up the work area.
9. Perform the third medication check. Check each medication label against the order. Check for the right name, form, and route. Verify that the amount of medication in each cup is correct according to the order.
   Purpose: It is important to do the third check of the label before placing the medications back into the cabinet.
10. Prior to entering the exam room, knock on the door and give it a moment. Greet the patient. Identify yourself. Verify the patient's identity with full name and date of birth. Make sure the patient's information matches the order and the record. Explain what you are going to do.
    Purpose: It is important to identify the patient in two different ways to ensure that you have the correct patient. Explaining the procedure can make the patient feel more comfortable and helps to reduce anxiety.
11. Provide the right education to the patient. Explain the medication ordered, the desired effect, and common side effects, and identify the provider who ordered it. Answer any questions the patient may have. Use language the patient can understand. Ask the patient if he or she has any allergies. If the patient refuses the medication, notify the provider.

Purpose: The patient needs to be aware of what you are giving, the action, side effects, and who ordered it. It is also important to double-check the patient's allergies before administering the medication.

12. Perform the right technique. Do any assessments required prior to giving the medication. If the patient can have water with the medication, have water available.
    Purpose: Some medications require assessments prior to administration.
13. Allow the patient to take the medication in his or her hand or to use the cup. Stay with the patient until the medication has been taken.
    Purpose: The medical assistant needs to ensure that the medication is taken.
14. Document the procedure in the health record. Include assessments done; allergies; teaching or instructions provided; the provider who ordered the medication; the medication's name, dose, and route; and how the patient tolerated the medication. For vaccines and controlled substances, add the lot number, expiration date, and manufacturer's number.
    Purpose: The medications given need to be documented to indicate that they were given.

Documentation Example
10/30/20XX 0936 BP 162/92 left arm, sitting. NKA. Per Dr. Martin's order, administered Diltiazem 120 mg, 2 tabs po and cephalexin suspension 250 mg/5 mL, 375 mg po. Medication action and side effects discussed with patient prior to administration. Pt had no questions and verbalized understanding. Pt tolerated the medications without problems._____Gabe Garcia CMA (AAMA)

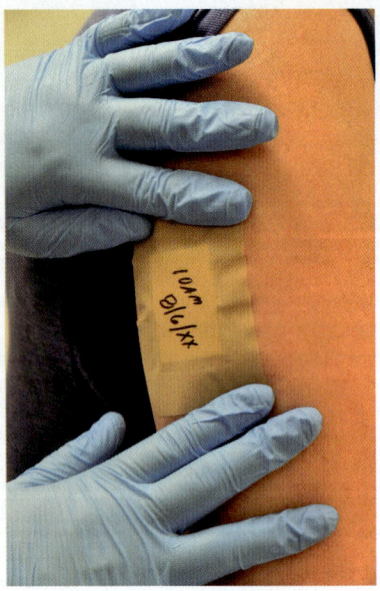

FIG. 38.6 Transdermal patch.

BOX 38.8 Applying Topical Medication to the Skin

When the medical assistant applies a topical medication to a patient's skin, it is important to do the following:
- Wear gloves.
- Use a sterile applicator (tongue blade or swab) to remove medication from the container. To keep the container sterile, a new sterile applicator must be used each time.
- Rub creams gently into the skin.
- Pat lotions onto the skin.
- Liniments must be rubbed into the skin.
- Apply ointments using a sterile applicator.
- For aerosol topical sprays, hold the bottle 3 to 6 inches from the skin and spray.

Inhalation Route

Medications for the nose, throat, and lungs can be inhaled. The small particles of medication are aerosolized (AR oh sol eye zed) in a fine mist. The medication is inhaled and reaches the mucous membrane or alveoli in the lungs, where is it absorbed. Metered-dose inhalers (MDIs) and nebulizers (NEB you lize ehrs) are common devices for inhaled drugs. (Chapter 39 discusses MDIs and nebulizers.)

Topical Routes

Applying a drug to a mucous membrane or skin is considered the *topical route*. Absorption through the mucous membrane is usually faster than the skin. Topical medications provide a local effect. Topical drugs include medications that are:
- Applied to the skin (Box 38.8)
- Inserted into the vagina, rectum, and bladder

- *Instilled* (poured medication drop by drop) into the eyes, ears, and nose
- Mixed in a large volume of water or sterile fluid and used to *irrigate* (flush) the eyes, ears, nose, bladder, rectum, or vagina

Vaginal Route. The vaginal route is used to insert suppositories, tablets, creams, and foams into the vagina. Typically, vaginal medications are used to treat local infections. Most medications can be inserted using the accompanying applicator. If no applicator is available, the patient should insert medications like suppositories, using a finger (Box 38.9). Vaginal instillation is most effective if the patient remains lying down after administration to prevent leakage. Many medications are intended to be used at bedtime. The patient may need to wear a pad to absorb drainage.

Rectal Route. Rectal medications are inserted into the rectum. Suppositories and enemas are the most common forms of rectal medication. The medication is absorbed slowly and irregularly through the rectal mucous membrane. This route is useful when a patient cannot tolerate oral medications or if the patient is constipated. Box 38.9 describes how to give rectal suppositories. It is important to give both the enema and suppository time to work before the person uses the bathroom.

> **BOX 38.9 Inserting Suppositories**
>
> Sometimes a medical assistant needs to teach a patient about inserting suppositories. It is helpful for the patient to know what supplies are needed and where the supplies can be purchased. Supplies required include the suppository, disposable gloves, and water-soluble jelly (K-Y Jelly). Encourage the patient to review the storage directions for the suppositories.
> The following tips are helpful for inserting a suppository:
> - Remove the wrapping from the suppository.
> - Lubricate the pointed part of the suppository with water-soluble jelly.
> - For rectal suppositories: Place the person in the Sims position (side-lying, with the knee drawn up toward the chest).
> - Carefully insert the suppository pointed side first.
> - For adults and older children: Use the gloved index finger to push the medication in. Both vaginal and rectal suppositories should be inserted about 3 to 4 inches. Have the person slowly breathe to help with the discomfort.
> - For small children: Use the gloved little finger to insert the medication. Rectal suppositories should be advanced about 2 inches.

> **CRITICAL THINKING BOX 38.4**
>
> Gabe and Mark are working with Jana Green. She needs to have an intestinal procedure performed. To prepare she needs to give herself an enema at home prior to the procedure. Why is it important for Gabe and Mark to provide her with the information on how to do the procedure and where to purchase the supplies?

Nasal Route. Drugs given via the nasal route are breathed in through the nose. The medication is absorbed through the nasal mucous membrane. The medication can have local or systemic effects. If the medical assistant is administering the nasal medication, it is important to wear gloves. Patients should blow their nose prior to receiving the medication. They should sit in an upright position. The patient should sniff when the medication is given. Intranasal medications should be charted as "intranasal" or "NAS."

Ocular Route. Medication may be instilled into the eye to treat an infection, soothe irritation, anesthetize the eye, or dilate the pupils before examination or treatment. Ophthalmic (of THAL mik) medications are available in different forms. Liquid drops usually are supplied in small squeeze bottles. The tip allows one drop at a time to be administered. Other bottles may have a dropper that is used to administer the medication. Eye ointments comes in small metal or plastic tubes. The tip allows a small ribbon of ointment to be administered along the inner lower eye lid margin (Procedure 38.2).

When instilling eye medications, avoid injuring the eye. Do not touch the eye with the tip or applicator. Always keep the tip or applicator sterile. If it gets contaminated, discard the container.

Otic Route. Ear conditions can cause pain and make hearing difficult. Medication may be instilled into the ear to treat infection or inflammation, or to soften ear cerumen. Procedure 38.3 describes how to administer ear drops. It is important to ensure that the ear drops get into the external canal.

Irrigation Route

Per the FDA, irrigation is also a route of administration. *Irrigation* means to bathe or flush open wounds or body cavities. Irrigation can be used to remove foreign bodies or debris. It can also be used to bathe the area with medication. Wound, eye, and ear irrigations are commonly seen in ambulatory care settings.

Eye irrigation is done to remove foreign bodies or to flush irritants (e.g., chemicals) from the eye (Procedure 38.4). Irrigation equipment can vary and may include:
- Normal saline intravenous (IV) bag and tubing
- Prepackaged eye irrigation
- Bulb syringe
- Sterile normal saline fluid

Irrigation of the external auditory canal is done to:
- Remove excessive or impacted cerumen (Procedure 38.5)
- Remove a foreign body (contraindicated if the item will absorb fluid [e.g., bean, pea, or corn kernel])
- Treat the inflamed ear with an antiseptic solution

Often ear drops are used to soften impacted cerumen. Softening the cerumen usually means that less time will be needed for irrigating, which lessens the patient's discomfort.

Irrigation of the ear can be difficult for some patients to experience. Use sterile irrigation fluid to decrease the risk of infection. Warm the fluid to the body temperature. Studies have shown that lukewarm fluid is better tolerated than room temperature fluid. Monitor the patient during the procedure. Should the patient have problems, stop the procedure, and talk with the provider. Ear irrigation should not be done if the tympanic membrane is perforated or if an infection or tympanic tube is present.

> **VOCABULARY**
>
> **canthus**: The angular junction of the eyelids at either corner.

PROCEDURE 38.2 Instill an Eye Medication

Tasks
Instill an eye drop or ointment and document medication administration.

Equipment and Supplies
- Provider's order
- Patient's health record
- Drug reference information
- Sterile ophthalmic eye drops or ointment
- Sterile gauze
- Gloves

Order 1
Atropine Sulfate Ophthalmic Solution 1% 1 drop in both eyes.

Order 2
Neosporin Ophthalmic Ointment to left eye.

Procedural Steps

1. Wash your hands or use hand sanitizer.
   Purpose: Hand sanitization is an important step for infection control.
2. Select the right medication from the storage area. Check the medication label against the order. Check for the right name, form, and route. Check the expiration date to make sure the drug is not expired. Verify the right dose and the right time.
   Purpose: It is important to do the first check of the label when getting the medication from the cabinet. Do not administer expired medications.
3. Using the drug reference information and the order, review the information on the medication.
   Purpose: The medical assistant must know about the medication that is being given.
4. Perform the second medication check. Check the medication label against the order. Check for the right name, form, dose, and route.
   Purpose: It is important to do the second check of the label before proceeding with the procedure.
5. Assemble the supplies required for the procedure.
   Purpose: You need to have the supplies ready before going to the exam room.
6. Perform the third medication check. Check each medication label against the order. Check for the right name, form, dose, and route.
   Purpose: It is important to do the third check of the label before seeing the patient.
7. Prior to entering the exam room, knock on the door and give it a moment. Greet the patient. Identify yourself. Verify the patient's identity with full name and date of birth. Make sure the patient's information matches the order and the record. Explain what you are going to do.
   Purpose: It is important to identify the patient in two different ways to ensure that you have the correct patient. Explaining the procedure can make the patient feel more comfortable and helps to reduce anxiety.
8. Provide the right education to the patient. Explain the medication ordered, the desired effect, common side effects, and identify the provider who ordered it. Answer any questions the patient may have. Use language the patient can understand. Ask the patient if he or she has any allergies. If the patient refuses the medication, notify the provider.
   Purpose: The patient needs to be aware of what you are giving, its action, side effects, and who ordered it. It is also important to double-check the patient's allergies before administering the medication.
9. Assist the patient into a sitting or supine position. Ask the patient to tilt the head backwards and look up.
   Purpose: These positions allow the medical assistant to instill the medication.
10. Put on gloves. If crusting or draining is present on the eyelid, gently wash the area from the inner to outer **canthus** (KAN thus) (Fig. 1). Discard the gauze after each wipe. Dry the area.
    Purpose: Gloves are used for infection control purposes. Washing and drying the eye prepares the area for the medication.

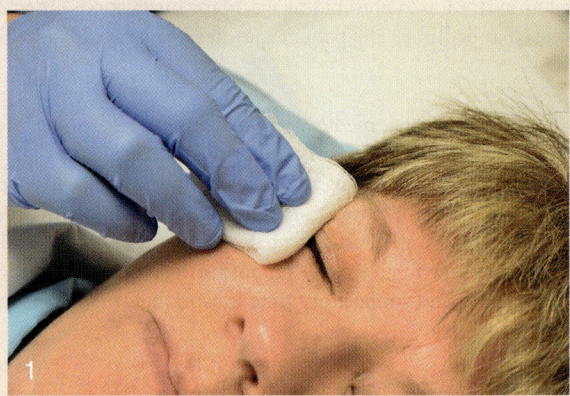

11. Perform the right technique. With your nondominant hand holding a sterile gauze, pull the lower conjunctival sac downward, creating a pocket for the medication (Fig. 2). Instruct the patient to look up.
    a. *For eye drops:* With your dominant hand, hold the bottle or the dropper ¾ inch away from the conjunctival sac. Drop the required number of drops into the pocket (see Fig. 2). If the drop misses the eye or the patient blinks, wipe the liquid on the skin and repeat the drop. Have the person keep the eye closed for 2 to 3 minutes after the administration of the drop. Have the person gently press against the inner corner of the eye and the nose bone for 2 to 3 minutes.
    Purpose: Pressing in the corner after the drops keeps the medication from draining into the tear ducts and nose. This helps to reduce the systemic effects of the medication.

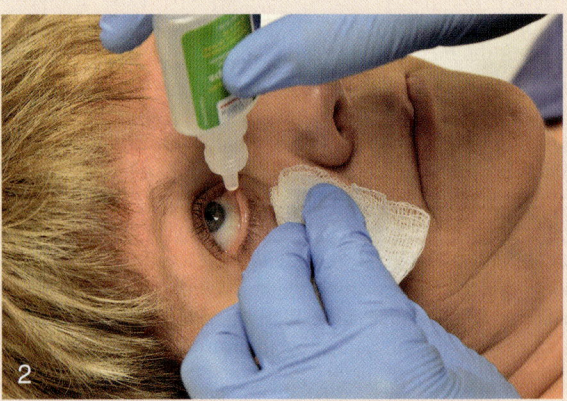

PROCEDURE 38.2   Instill an Eye Medication—cont'd

b. *For eye ointment:* With the dominant hand, hold the ointment container above the lower lid. Working from inner to outer canthus, apply a small strip (about ½ inch) of ointment along the inner lower lid margin (Fig. 3). Have the patient close the eye for 1 to 2 minutes to allow the medication to be absorbed. Wipe up any extra ointment from the eyelid.
Purpose: Rubbing the eyelid after administering the ointment helps to spread the medication over the eye.

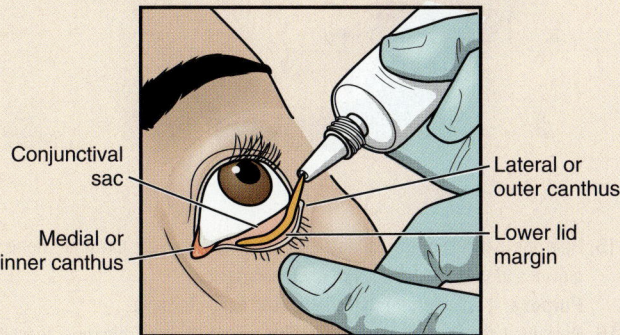

12. Help the patient into a comfortable position. Clean up the area. Remove gloves and wash your hands or use a hand sanitizer.
Purpose: It is important that the patient is comfortable.
13. Document the procedure in the health record. Include allergies, teaching or instructions provided, the provider who ordered the medication, the medication's name, dose, and route, and how the patient tolerated the medication.
Purpose: The medication given needs to be documented to indicate it was given.

Documentation Example
10/30/20XX 1136 NKA. Per Dr. Martin's order, administered Neosporin Ophthalmic Ointment to left eye. Medication action and side effects discussed with patient prior to administration. Pt had no questions and verbalized understanding. Pt tolerated the medication without problems._____Gabe Garcia, CMA (AAMA)

PROCEDURE 38.3   Instill Ear Drops

Tasks
Instill ear drops and document medication administration.

Equipment and Supplies
- Provider's order
- Patient's health record
- Drug reference information
- Otic drops
- Gauze
- Gloves

Order
Ciprodex Otic 0.1% 4 drops in left ear.

Procedural Steps
1. Wash your hands or use hand sanitizer.
Purpose: Hand sanitization is an important step for infection control.
2. Select the right medication from the storage area. Check the medication label against the order. Check for the right name, form, and route. Check the expiration date to make sure the drug is not expired. Verify the right dose and the right time.
Purpose: It is important to do the first check of the label when getting medications from the cabinet. Do not administer expired medications.
3. Using the drug reference information and the order, review the information on the medication.
Purpose: The medical assistant must know about the medication that is being given.
4. Perform the second medication check. Check the medication label against the order. Check for the right name, form, dose, and route.
Purpose: It is important to do the second check of the label before proceeding with the procedure.
5. Assemble the supplies required for the procedure.
Purpose: You need to have the supplies ready before going to the exam room.
6. Perform the third medication check. Check the medication label against the order. Check for the right name, form, dose, and route.
Purpose: It is important to do the third check of the label before seeing the patient.
7. Prior to entering the exam room, knock on the door and give it a moment. Greet the patient. Identify yourself. Verify the patient's identity with full name and date of birth. Make sure the patient's information matches the order and the record. Explain what you are going to do.
Purpose: It is important to identify the patient in two different ways to ensure that you have the correct patient. Explaining the procedure can make the patient feel more comfortable and helps to reduce anxiety.
8. Provide the right education to the patient. Explain the medication ordered, the desired effect, and common side effects, and identify the provider who ordered it. Answer any questions the patient may have. Use language the patient can understand. Ask the patient if he or she has any allergies. If the patient refuses the medication, notify the provider.
Purpose: The patient needs to be aware of what you are giving, its action and side effects, and who ordered it. It is also important to double-check the patient's allergies before administering the medication.
9. Assist the patient into a sitting position, or into a side-lying position on the unaffected side.
Purpose: These positions allow the medical assistant to instill the medication.
10. Warm the medication bottle with your hands if needed. The drops should be at room temperature. Shake the medication if needed. Put on gloves.
Purpose: If the drops are too hot or too cold, the patient may experience nausea and vertigo. Gloves are used for infection control purposes.
11. Perform the right technique. Have the patient tilt his or her head so the affected ear is upward. If cerumen or drainage is blocking the canal, gently remove it with a cotton-tipped applicator.
Purpose: The canal must be opened to instill the drops.

Continued

PROCEDURE 38.3 Instill Ear Drops—cont'd

12. Remove the cover of the bottle. With your nondominant hand, gently pull the pinna up and back if the patient is older than age 3. This straightens the external auditory canal. For patients younger than 3, pull the pinna down and back.
    Purpose: Straightening the canal allows the medication to flow down it.
13. Hold the dropper firmly in your dominant hand. Place the tip of the dropper about ½ inch above the ear canal (Fig. 1). Be sure not to contaminate the dropper by touching it to the patient. Carefully drop the required number of drops in the patient's ear. Replace the cover.
    Purpose: If the bottle tip gets contaminated, the bottle needs to be discarded.

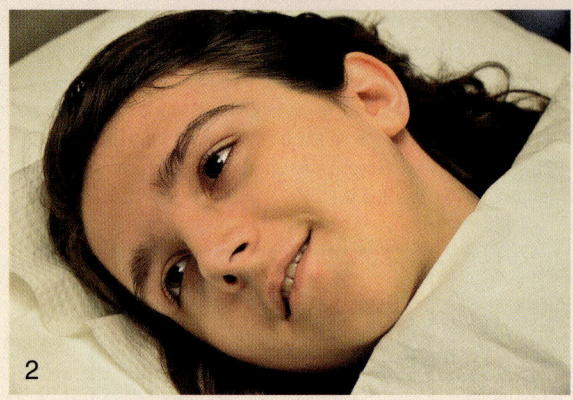

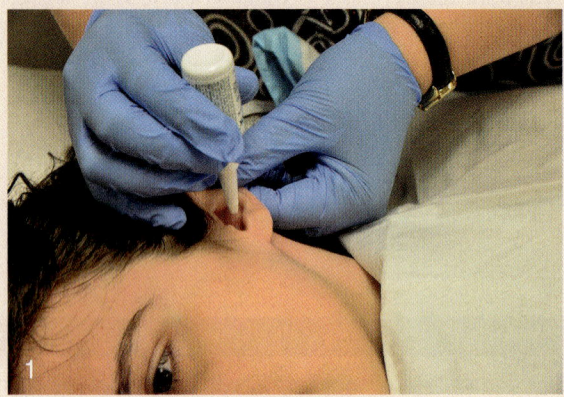

14. Have the patient keep the ear facing up for 3 to 5 minutes, depending on the medications (Fig. 2).
    Purpose: This allows the medication to move throughout the canal.
15. Help the patient into a comfortable position. Clean up the area. Remove gloves and wash your hands or use hand sanitizer.
    Purpose: It is important that the patient is comfortable.
16. Document the procedure in the health record. Include allergies, teaching or instructions provided, the provider who ordered the medication, the medication's name, dose, and route, and how the patient tolerated the medication.
    Purpose: The medication given needs to be documented to indicate it was given.

Documentation Example
11/02/20XX 1526 NKA. Per Dr. Martin's order, administered Ciprodex 0.1% 4 gtts to left ear. Pt kept left ear facing up for 5 minutes. Medication action and side effects discussed with patient prior to administration. Pt had no questions and verbalized understanding. Pt experienced slight dizziness when drops were instilled. Dizziness went away within a few minutes. Pt states he is feeling fine._____Gabe Garcia CMA (AAMA)

There are several ear irrigation systems on the market. Ear irrigation equipment can include:
- A large syringe and a container of fluid; it is important to regulate the flow of solution into the ear. Too much air or solution from the syringe can cause discomfort for the patient.
- Systems that connect to a faucet and have flow regulators.
- A spray bottle system – the Elephant Ear Wash System and similar systems are economical and safe (Fig. 38.7).

CRITICAL THINKING BOX 38.5
Aaron Jackson comes in with a dried pea stuck in his ear. Mark is excited to do an ear irrigation, but Gabe tells Mark that the provider may not order irrigation. Why might irrigation not be ordered for foreign bodies that can absorb fluid?

Parenteral Route
The *parenteral* (pa REN tehr ahl) *route* involves administration by infusion, injection, or implantation. In the ambulatory care environment,

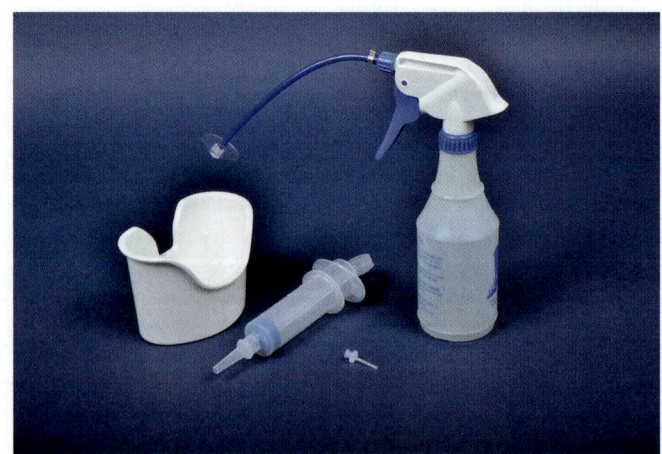

FIG. 38.7 Left to right: Ear basin, large syringe, and the spray bottle system (disposable tip and spray bottle).

PROCEDURE 38.4 Irrigate a Patient's Eye

Tasks
Irrigate a patient's eye and document patient care.

Equipment and Supplies
- Provider's order
- Patient's health record
- Drug reference information
- Sterile ophthalmic irrigation solution and supplies
- Disposable waterproof pad and towels
- Basin
- Sterile gauze
- Gloves

Order
Irrigate right eye with 1 L Normal Saline.

Procedural Steps

1. Wash your hands or use hand sanitizer.
   Purpose: Hand sanitization is an important step for infection control.
2. Select the right medication (fluid) from the storage area. Check the medication label against the order. Check for the right name, form, and route. Check the expiration date to make sure the fluid is not expired. Verify the right dose and the right time.
   Purpose: It is important to do the first check of the label when getting medications from the cabinet. Do not administer expired medications or fluids.
3. Using the drug reference information and the order, review the information on the medication.
   Purpose: The medical assistant must know about the medication that is being given.
4. Perform the second medication check. Check the medication label against the order. Check for the right name, form, dose, and route.
   Purpose: It is important to do the second check of the label before proceeding with the procedure.
5. Assemble the supplies required for the procedure.
   Purpose: You need to have the supplies ready before going to the exam room.
6. Perform the third medication check. Check the medication label against the order. Check for the right name, form, dose, and route.
   Purpose: It is important to do the third check of the label before seeing the patient.
7. Prior to entering the exam room, knock on the door and give it a moment. Greet the patient. Identify yourself. Verify the patient's identity with full name and date of birth. Make sure the patient's information matches the order and the record. Explain what you are going to do.
   Purpose: It is important to identify the patient in two different ways to ensure that you have the correct patient. Explaining the procedure can make the patient feel more comfortable and helps to reduce anxiety.
8. Provide the right education to the patient. Explain the procedure ordered, the desired effect, and common side effects, and identify the provider who ordered it. Answer any questions the patient may have. Use language the patient can understand. Ask the patient if he or she has any allergies. If the patient refuses the procedure, notify the provider.
   Purpose: The patient needs to be aware of the procedure you will be performing, its action and side effects, and who ordered it. It is also important to double-check the patient's allergies before starting the procedure.
9. Using room temperature fluid, set up the equipment. If using an intravenous (IV) bag, prime or run fluid through the tubing. If using a prepackaged solution, remove the cover. If using a bulb syringe, pour the required fluid into a basin – remember to palm the label. Draw the solution into the bulb syringe.
   Purpose: Having the fluid ready for the irrigation is important before you hold the eye open.
10. Assist the patient into a sitting or supine position. Have the patient remove glasses or contact lens. Ask the patient to turn the head towards the side of the affected eye. Place the disposable waterproof pad over the patient's neck and shoulder. Place or have the patient hold the drainage basin next to the affected eye.
    Purpose: Protecting the unaffected eye from the solution is important so it does not also get contaminated. The basin will collect the irrigation fluid from the eye.
11. Put on gloves. Moisten a gauze pad with the irrigation fluid. Using the gauze, clean the eyelid from the inner to outer canthus (Fig. 1). Discard the gauze after each wipe.
    Purpose: Debris on the eyelid must be removed before the irrigation can be done.

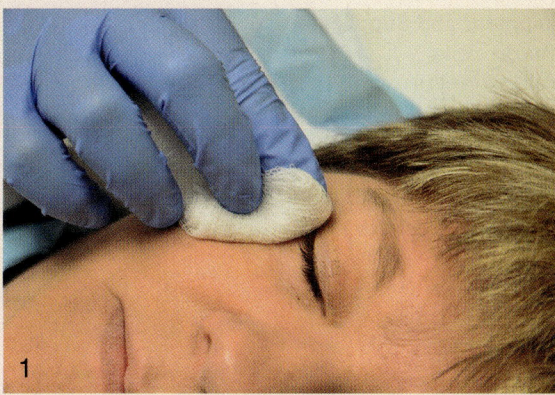
1

12. Perform the right technique. With your nondominant hand, separate and hold the eyelids using the index finger and thumb. With the dominant hand, hold the irrigation equipment on or near the bridge of the nose (Fig. 2).
    Purpose: Using the nose to help steady the irrigation will help to provide a steady flow of fluid going into the eye.

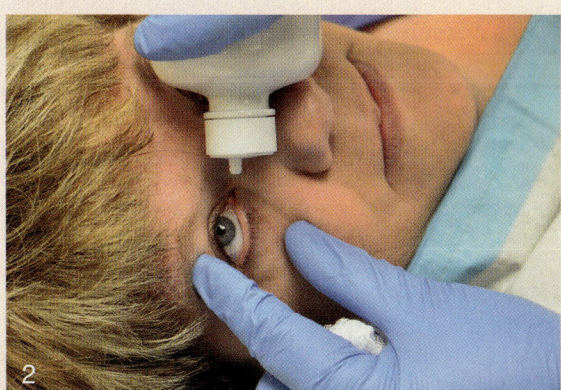
2

13. Direct the solution towards the lower conjunctiva of the inner canthus. Allow a steady flow of solution to slowly flush the eye from the inner to the outer canthus. Do not touch the tip of the irrigation equipment to the eye.
    Purpose: Touching the eye with the irrigation equipment could lead to an eye injury.
14. Continue until the ordered amount of fluid has flushed the eye. Dry the eyelid with sterile gauze, moving from the inner to outer canthus.
    Purpose: It is important to follow the exact order of the provider.
15. Help the patient into a comfortable position. Clean up the area. Remove gloves and wash your hands or use hand sanitizer.
    Purpose: It is important that the patient is comfortable.

Continued

PROCEDURE 38.4   Irrigate a Patient's Eye—cont'd

16. Document the procedure in the health record. Include allergies, teaching or instructions provided, the provider who ordered the irrigation, the fluid used for the irrigation, the amount used, the site, and how the patient tolerated the procedure.
    Purpose: The irrigation performed needs to be documented to indicate that it was done.

Documentation Example
10/30/20XX 1440 NKA. Per Dr. Martin's order, irrigated right eye with 1 liter of normal saline IV fluid. Purpose of irrigation and side effects discussed with patient prior to procedure. Pt had no questions and verbalized understanding. Pt tolerated the procedure without problems._____Gabe Garcia CMA (AAMA)

PROCEDURE 38.5   Irrigate a Patient's Ear

Tasks
Irrigate a patient's ear and document patient care.

Equipment and Supplies
- Provider's order
- Patient's health record
- Ear wash basin
- Elephant ear wash system (or other ear wash system)
- Disposable waterproof pad and towels
- Thermometer (optional)
- Otoscope and disposable speculum (optional)
- Gauze
- Gloves
- Sterile water or saline
- Waste container

Order
Irrigate left ear with warm sterile water.

Procedural Steps
1. Wash your hands or use hand sanitizer.
   Purpose: Hand sanitization is an important step for infection control.
2. Select the right medication (fluid) from the storage area. Check the medication label against the order. Check for the right name and route; check the expiration date.
   Purpose: It is important to do the first check of the label when getting the medications from the cabinet.
3. Assemble the equipment and supplies needed. Perform the second medication check. Check the medication (fluid) name and route against the order.
   Purpose: You need to have the supplies ready before going to the exam room.
4. Clean up the work area and perform the third medication check. Check the medication (fluid) name and route against the order.
   Purpose: It is important to do three checks before using the fluid.
5. Prior to entering the exam room, knock on the door and give it a moment. Greet the patient. Identify yourself. Verify the patient's identity with full name and date of birth. Make sure the patient's information matches the order and the record. Explain what you are going to do.
   Purpose: It is important to identify the patient in two different ways to ensure that you have the correct patient. Explaining the procedure can make the patient feel more comfortable and helps to reduce anxiety.
6. Provide the right education to the patient. Explain the procedure ordered, the desired effect, and common side effects of ear irrigations; also identify the provider who ordered the procedure. Answer any questions the patient may have. Use language the patient can understand. If the patient refuses the procedure, notify the provider.
   Purpose: The patient needs to be aware of the procedure you will be performing, its action and side effects, and who ordered it.
7. Prepare the equipment. Warm the irrigating solution to body temperature (98.6°F [check with a thermometer]) or until it is lukewarm. Lukewarm is neither hot nor cold. Fill the spray bottle with the fluid. Attach the disposable tip to the nozzle on the hose. If another type of ear wash system is being used, prepare the equipment and the fluid.
   Purpose: Having the fluid ready for the irrigation is important before holding the ear. Sterile irrigating fluid is recommended.
8. Assist the patient into a sitting position. Wrap a waterproof pad around the person's shoulder, protecting the clothing. Have a towel available for the patient if needed. Have the patient tilt his or her head towards the affected ear. Have the patient hold the ear wash basin under the affect ear.
   Purpose: It is important to protect the patient's clothing from the irrigating fluid.
9. Put on gloves. Using gauze, wipe any debris from the outer ear.
   Purpose: Debris on the outer ear must be removed before the irrigation can be done.
10. Insert the disposable tip gently into the ear (Fig. 1). Do not insert it too far because it could injure the canal. If possible, gently pull the pinna up and back if the patient is older than age 3. For patients younger than 3, pull the pinna down and back.
    Purpose: If using the spray bottle irrigation system, you will not be able to pull the pinna. One hand is holding the tip, and the other hand is squeezing the trigger. Other systems may allow you a free hand to position the pinna to open the canal.

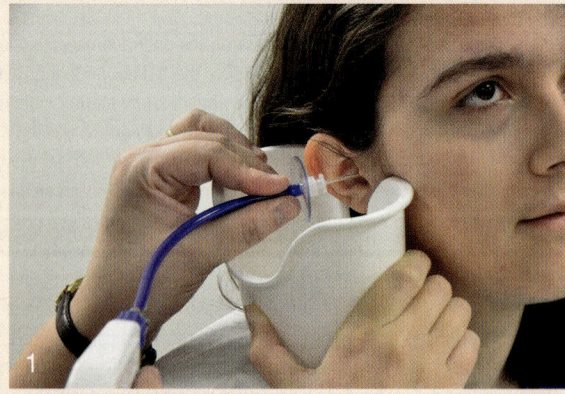

1

11. Keeping the tubing straight, spray the fluid into the ear canal. Aim the fluid towards the top of the ear canal.
    Purpose: Aiming the fluid towards the top of the canal helps prevent injury to the tympanic membrane. It can also make the procedure more comfortable for the patient.

CHAPTER 38 Administering Medication

PROCEDURE 38.5 Irrigate a Patient's Ear—cont'd

12. Continue irrigating until the solution is used up, the maximum time has been reached, the desired result is achieved, or the patient has problems with the procedure. Empty the ear wash basin when it fills. Observe the fluid for any substances (i.e., cerumen).
    Purpose: The provider's order or the facility's procedures will indicate the amount of irrigation fluid to use or when to stop the irrigation.
13. Dry the outside of the ear with gauze. If the facility's procedure indicates, use an otoscope to observe the canal. Attach the speculum to the otoscope. Straighten the ear canal by pulling in the appropriate direction on the pinna. Gently insert the otoscope and observe the canal.
    Purpose: Observing the canal helps you check the results of the irrigation.
14. Place a clean, absorbent towel on the examination table. Have the patient rest quietly with the head turned to the irrigated side while you wait for the provider to return to check the affected ear.
    Purpose: This allows the fluid in the canal to drain out.
15. Clean up the work area. Remove your gloves and dispose in the waste container. Sanitize your hands.
    Purpose: Hand sanitization is an important step for infection control.
16. Document the procedure in the health record. Include teaching or instructions provided, the provider who ordered the irrigation, the fluid used for the irrigation, the amount used, the site, and how the patient tolerated the procedure.
    Purpose: The irrigation performed needs to be documented to indicate that it was done.

Documentation Example
11/04/20XX 1540 Per Dr. Martin's order, irrigated left ear with lukewarm sterile water for 15 min. Flushed out moderate amount of brown cerumen. Pt had slight dizziness initially with irrigation, which resolved quickly. Pt rested on exam table._____ Gabe Garcia CMA (AAMA)

---

injections and infusions are common. Vaccine administration in primary care settings (e.g., family practice and internal medicine) is a frequent duty of medical assistants. Types of injections performed by medical assistants include:
- *Intramuscular* (IM): Administration within a muscle
- *Subcutaneous* (subcut): Administration beneath the skin
- *Intradermal* (ID): Administration within the dermis

The rest of the chapter will focus on the parenteral route. The following topics will be discussed: injection supplies, medication preparation, site location, and medication administration. The chapter will conclude with a discussion on intravenous (IV) infusions and the role of the medical assistant. An intravenous infusion means fluid and medications are administered into a vein.

FIG. 38.8 Parts of a hypodermic needle. (From Proctor D, et al: *Kinn's The Medical Assistant*, ed 13, St Louis, 2017, Elsevier.)

- *Bevel*: Slanted end of the shaft
- *Lumen* (LOO muh n): Hollow space inside the needle; the size is indicated by the *gauge* (geyj) number.

Gauge and Length. Each needle has two measurements: the gauge (G) and the length. The lumen size is indicated by the gauge (G) and is given a numeric value. The higher the gauge number, the smaller the lumen. The thickness of the needle wall increases along with the lumen size. This means that an 18 gauge (G) needle makes a larger hole than a 25 G needle. The 18 G needle has a thicker wall than the 25 G needle. As the gauge number increases, the needles bend easier. Thicker-walled needles (smaller gauge numbers) are used for deeper injections. Thinner-walled needles (larger gauge numbers) are used for more superficial injections.

The medication's **viscosity** (vi SKOS I tee) is also an important factor when selecting the gauge of the needle. A medication with a syrupy thickness (high viscosity) would be harder to push out of a needle compared to a medication as thin as water. Using a finer lumen needle (a larger gauge number) would be more appropriate for watery medications. Using a wider lumen needle (smaller gauge number) would be better for thicker medications.

The needle length refers to the length of the shaft. The needle length is dependent on the type of injection given and the size of the patient. The length of the needle for an intradermal injection is smaller than

> **MEDICAL TERMINOLOGY**
> **derm/o, cutane/o:** skin
> **hypo:** under
> **-ic:** pertaining to
> **intra-:** within
> **muscul/o:** muscle
> **-ous, -al:** pertaining to
> **ven/o:** vein

NEEDLES AND SYRINGES
Hypodermic Needles
A hypodermic needle attaches to a hypodermic syringe. Hypodermic needles come with syringes or are packaged separately. It is important for the medical assistant to know the parts of the needle (Fig. 38.8). The entire needle needs to remain sterile for the injection.
- *Hub*: Attaches or screws onto the syringe
- *Hilt*: Where the needle attaches

> **VOCABULARY**
> **viscosity:** Resistance to flow; the thicker the liquid, the higher the viscosity.

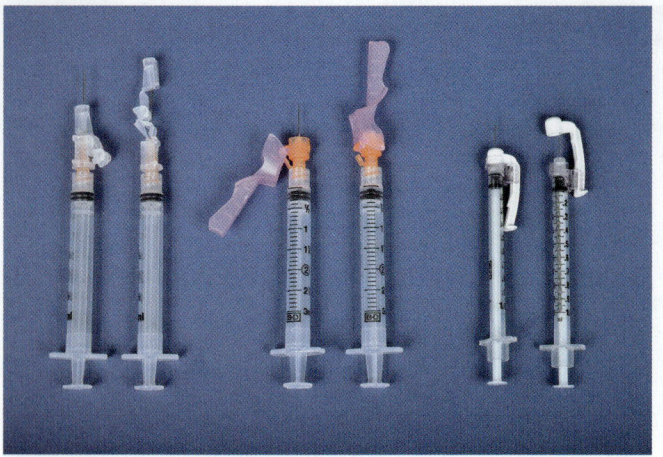

FIG. 38.9 Protective sheaths and hinged needle shields must be activated by the healthcare professional. Each type of needle is shown before the injection and after the safety device has been activated.

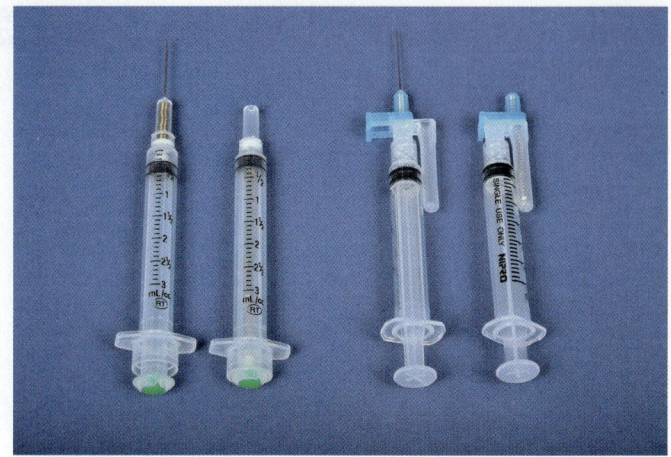

FIG. 38.10 With retractable needles, the needle is retracted into the syringe or another chamber. Each type of needle is shown before the injection and after the needle has been retracted.

that used for an intramuscular injection. The length of an intramuscular injection needle for a 300-pound person would be longer than that for a 100-pound person. Knowing the length and gauge required for an injection are important for the medical assistant.

Safety Needles. Due to the Needlestick Safety and Prevention Act, safety needles are common in the ambulatory care setting. Safety needles are designed to reduce the risk of needlesticks after an injection. A *passive safety needle* is designed so that the needle is automatically covered after the injection. Passive safety needles are currently used with insulin pens. It is forecasted that in the next few years, more passive safety needles will be available. An *active safety needle* requires the healthcare professional to activate the safety device. These are most common for injections. Current active safety needles fall into two groups:
- *Protective sheaths* and *hinged needle shields*: The safety device is a sleeve over the syringe barrel or a hinged needle shield (Fig. 38.9). These devices are moved over the needle after the injection. Once in place, the needle cannot be uncovered. The risk of needlesticks decreases if the safety device is activated with the hand holding the syringe.
- *Retractable needles*: After the injection, the healthcare professional activates a device that retracts the needle either into the syringe or into another chamber (Fig. 38.10).

Hypodermic Syringes

Hypodermic syringes attach to needles and hold the medication for the injection. They come in many different sizes (e.g., 1, 3, 5, 6, 10, and 12 mL), but usually the facility only stocks three or four sizes (Fig. 38.11). Fig. 38.12 shows the parts of the syringe. Syringes can have either a Luer Lok tip or a slip tip (Fig. 38.13). Calibration marks are on the barrel of the syringe. It is important for the medical assistant to be able to read medication amounts in syringes. Box 38.10 discusses reading syringes.

Working With the Needle and Syringe

Syringes come packaged different ways:
- A syringe can be packaged by itself. A needle must be added to the syringe when giving an injection.
- A syringe may be packaged with a needle. The unit must be assembled.
- A syringe and needle unit may come preassembled. Always tighten the needle on the syringe before using the unit.

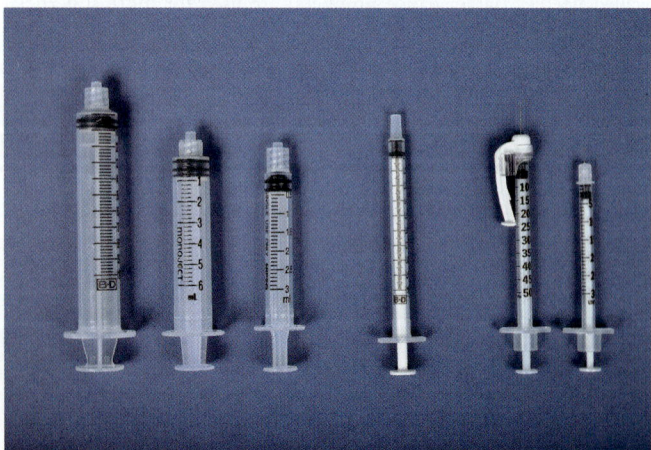

FIG. 38.11 Syringes come in various sizes. Some come with the needles attached.

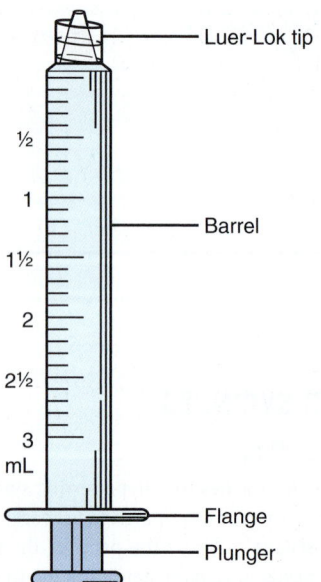

FIG. 38.12 Parts of a syringe. (From Proctor D, et al: *Kinn's The Medical Assistant*, ed 13, St Louis, 2017, Elsevier.)

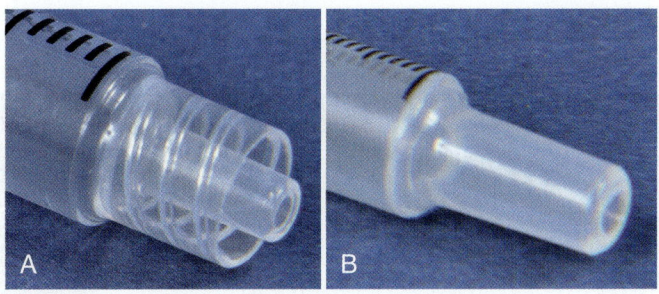

FIG. 38.13 (A) Luer Lok. (B) Slip tip.

BOX 38.10 Reading Syringes

Syringes have calibrations printed on the barrel. These markings help you read how much medication is in the syringe. Look at Fig. 1. You will notice that some of the lines are longer and/or darker than others. That helps you determine either a full or half of a milliliter (mL).

The first step in reading the amount is to look at the calibrations and determine how many lines make up 1 mL (cc). Start by counting the lines under 1 mL and count the 2 mL line. Fig. 1 shows the calibrations for 3 mL syringes. Using this figure, how many lines make up 1 mL? You should have counted 10 lines. This means that each line is worth 0.1 mL.

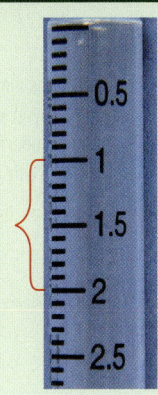

Fig. 2 represents the calibration markings found on 5, 6, 10 and 12 mL syringes. How many lines make up 1 mL? You should have counted 5. This means that each line is worth 0.2 mL. Syringes with this type of calibration can only measure even amounts of medication (i.e., 1.2, 2, 3.6 mL).

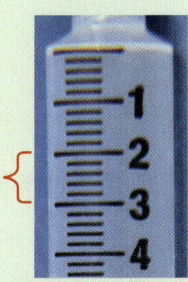

Fig. 3 represents the calibration markings found on 1 mL or intradermal syringes. What is different about the calibrations on this syringe? Did you notice that the numbers are in tenths (e.g., .1, .2)? This syringe is calibrated to the hundredth, or two places after the decimal point. To figure out how much each line is worth, count the lines for 0.1 mL. What did you get? You should have counted 10 lines. Each line is worth 0.01 mL.

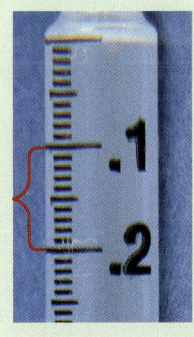

A trick to figure out the amount: Start at the top. The very top line with no amount is 0.00 (Fig. 4). Count each line down: 0.01, 0.02, and so on. You can also do this for lines after a marked amount. For instance, think of 0.1 as 0.10, and the next line as 0.11 mL. What is the amount for A and B in Fig. 4?

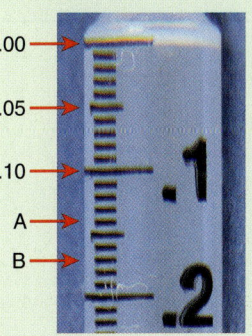

Continued

BOX 38.10   Reading Syringes—cont'd

Fig. 5 shows the calibrations on syringes typically used for irrigations. These syringes can hold large amounts (e.g., 20, 50 or 60 mL). When you look at this syringe, you will notice that full numbers are indicated on the side (e.g., 5, 10, 15). In between each of these numbers are four lines. Thus, you could start counting at the 5 line, and the one below would be 6, 7, etc. Each line is worth 1 mL.

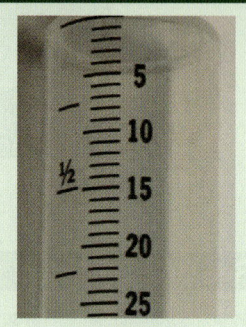

Fig. 6 represents the calibrations found on insulin syringes. Insulin is measured in units, not mL. If you look at this syringe, you will notice 5, 10, 15, and 20. There are four little lines between these numbers. If you start counting at 10, you will see that each line is worth 1 unit. With insulin, the dose is always a full unit (e.g., 32, 45, 67).

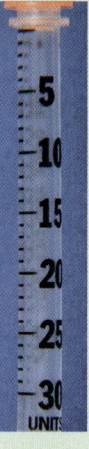

The rubber stopper on the plunger indicates the amount in the syringe. Some rubber stoppers are pointed (Fig. 7), and others are flat (Fig. 8). The measuring mark is where the rubber stopper touches the barrel (see the red arrows in Figs. 7 and 8).

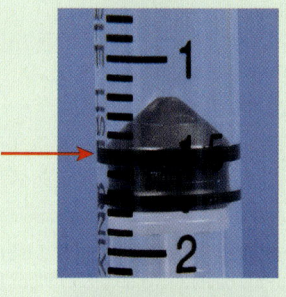

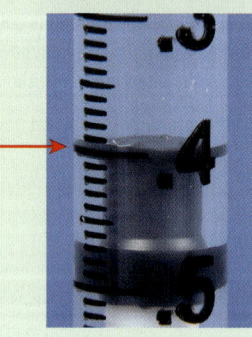

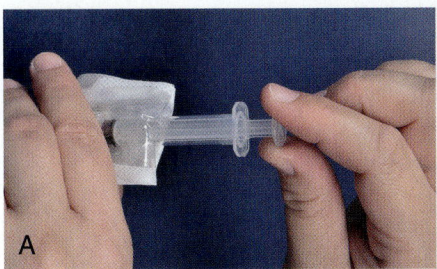 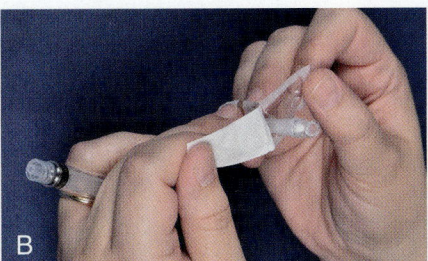 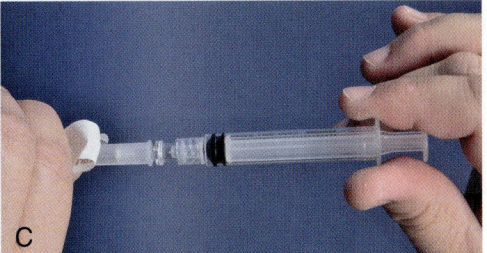

FIG. 38.14 (A) When removing the syringe from the packaging, just touch the flange or barrel. (B) Place the syringe between your fingers with the tip face away from your fingers. Then open the needle package. (C) Hold down the packaging flaps to prevent contamination of the needle. Attach the syringe.

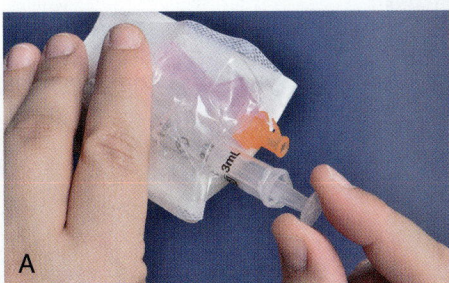 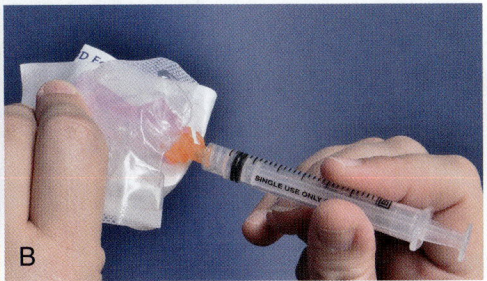

FIG. 38.15 (A) Remove the syringe without touching the needle. (B) Continue to hold down the packaging flaps and attach the needle to the syringe.

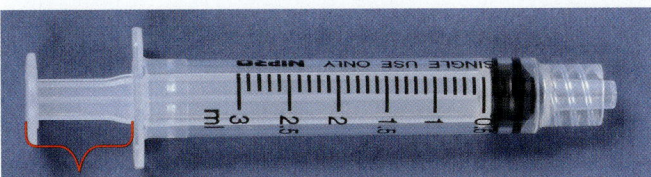

FIG. 38.16 Touch only the part of the plunger that is outside of the barrel.

We will discuss how to assemble the needle and syringe. The needle and syringe can be assembled with clean, ungloved hands.

When a syringe is packaged by itself, first open the syringe. When removing the syringe from the packaging, it is important not to touch the syringe tip to anything (Fig. 38.14A). The tip needs to remain sterile since it attaches to the needle. The syringe should be held until the needle is attached. As you are holding the syringe, use your fingers to open the needle package (Fig. 38.14B). It is important hold down the packaging flaps to prevent contaminating the needle. Attach the syringe to the needle and lift the needle out of the package (Fig. 38.14C). The needle and syringe unit can be placed on the counter. The needle cover should remain on to protect the sterility of the needle.

When the needle and syringe are packaged together, yet not assembled, carefully open the packaging. Hold down the packaging flaps. Angle the contents so the syringe can be grasped without going over or touching the needle (Fig. 38.15A). Remove the syringe and then attach it to the needle (Fig. 38.15B). Remove the needle from the packaging. Once the syringe and needle are assembled, the unit can be placed on the counter.

When working with the plunger, only touch the section that remains outside of the syringe when the plunger is completely pushed in (Fig. 38.16). Touching the plunger that goes inside the barrel could potentially contaminate the medication.

Uncapping and Recapping Needles. Never recap a needle that has been used on a patient. Needles can be recapped until they are used on a patient. As you prepare medication, you will need to uncap and recap the needle. It is important to maintain the sterility of the needle. If there is any doubt, consider the needle contaminated and replace it with a new one.

- **To uncap:** Hold the cover between the fingers of your nondominant hand. Hold the syringe with the fingers and thumb of your dominant hand. Pull your hands apart horizontally (side-to-side) in a smooth continuous motion (Fig. 38.17A).
- **To recap:** Use the one-handed scoop technique. Place the cover on a firm, flat surface. If the cover rolls, place a finger of your nondominant hand at the far end of the cover. This will keep the cover in place. Carefully insert the needle into the cover. If the needle touches the outside surface of the cover or any other surface, it is contaminated. Scoop up the cover and secure the cover onto the needle (Fig. 38.17B).

Switching Needles. When switching needles, it is important not to give yourself a needlestick and to protect the sterility of the new needle. There are several methods used to switch needles. One method includes opening the new needle package. Hold the packaging flaps down with the index finger and thumb of your nondominant hand. With your dominant hand, place the syringe with the covered needle between the middle and ring fingers of your nondominant hand (Fig. 38.18A). Firmly grasp the covered needle in your palm. The syringe should be above the top of your hand. With your dominant hand, remove the syringe from the old needle and attach it to the new needle (Fig. 38.18B and C). Your nondominant hand should be holding both needles during the entire time. Discard the old needle into the biohazard sharps container.

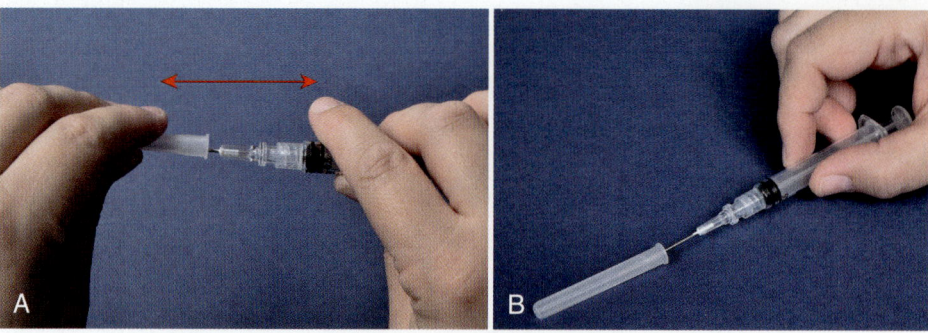

FIG. 38.17 (A) Uncapping a needle. (B) One-handed scoop technique.

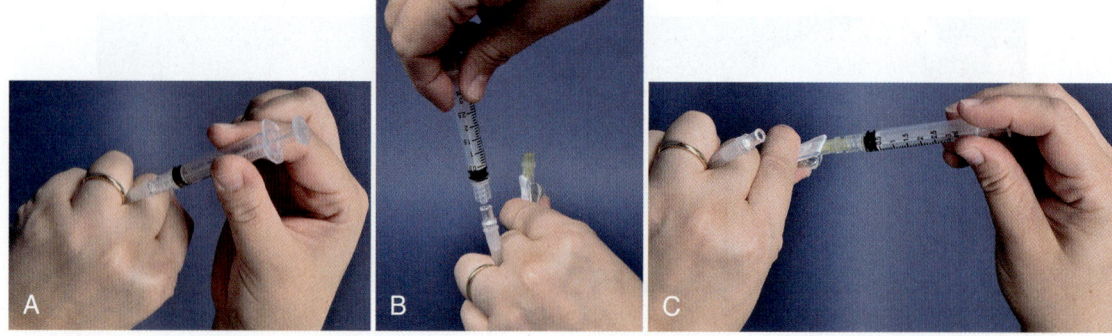

FIG. 38.18 (A) Place the syringe unit between the fingers of your nondominant hand and firmly grasp the covered needle. (B) Hold the old covered needle securely as you detach it from the syringe. (C) Attach the new needle while holding the old needle between your fingers.

PREPARING PARENTERAL MEDICATION

As with all medication preparation, it is important to be in a well-lit room and to be free from distraction. The medical assistant must be focused on the procedure to reduce the risk of errors. For all parenteral medications:
- If the medication looks abnormal in color or clarity, discard the medication.
- Some medications will have **precipitate** (pri SIP i tate) at the bottom of the vial. If this is normal for that medication, make sure to mix it prior to withdrawing medications. If the precipitate is abnormal, a chemical reaction may have occurred. The vial needs to be discarded.
- If the medication has expired, discard it.
- If the medication is no longer sterile, discard it.

Using an Ampule

Ampules (AM pools) contain a single dose of medication. They may contain more than what is needed for the patient. The extra medication is wasted. Medications in ampules react to other substances and require the all-glass environment to remain stable. An ampule has a prescored neck, which is snapped off during the preparation process. An ampule opener or breaker is a safety device used to snap off the top of the ampule (Fig. 38.19). A filter needle on a syringe is used to **aspirate** (AS pi rate) the medication into the syringe. This needle has a small filter that catches glass particles before they enter the syringe barrel. The filter needle must be removed before the injection is given to the patient. Procedure 38.6 describes the steps of preparing medication using an ampule.

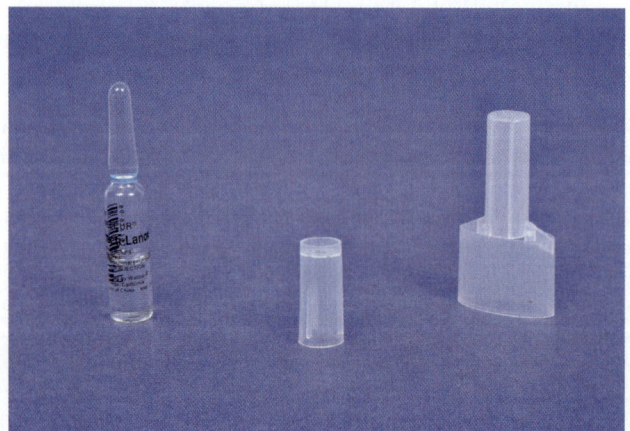

FIG. 38.19 An ampule with two different ampule openers/breakers. (From Proctor D, et al: *Kinn's The Medical Assistant*, ed 13, St Louis, 2017, Elsevier.)

> **VOCABULARY**
> **aspirate:** To withdraw fluid using suction.
> **precipitate:** Solid particles that settle out of a liquid.

PROCEDURE 38.6   Prepare Medication From an Ampule

Task
Prepare medication from an ampule.

Equipment and Supplies
- Provider's order
- Ampule of medication
- Gauze or ampule breaker
- Alcohol wipes
- Filter needle and hypodermic safety needle
- 3 mL syringe
- Biohazard sharps container
- Waste container
- Drug reference information
- Marker

Order
0.9% Sodium Chloride 0.7 mL IM

Procedural Steps

1. Wash your hands or use hand sanitizer. Using the drug reference information and the order, review the information on the medication if needed. Clarify any questions you have with the provider.
   Purpose: Hand sanitization is an important step for infection control. It is important to be knowledgeable about the medication you are giving.
2. Select the right medication from the storage area. Check the medication label against the order. Check for the right name, form, and route. Check the expiration date to make sure the drug is not expired. Verify the right dose and the right time.
   Purpose: It is important to do the first check of the label when getting medications from the cabinet. Do not administer expired medications.
3. Assemble the supplies required for the procedure.
   Purpose: Remember to split up the three medication checks with activities between each check.
4. Perform the second medication check. Check the medication label against the order. Check for the right name, form, dose, and route.
   Purpose: It is important to do the second check of the label before proceeding with the procedure.
5. Attach the filter needle to the syringe without contaminating the unit. Using a marker, label the syringe with the medication name.
   Purpose: You will use the filter needle first during the procedure.
6. Gently tap the medication from the head of the ampule or hold the ampule securely, upright in your hand (Fig. 1). Quickly move your hand downward. After all the medication has drained into the body of the ampule, wipe the neck with an alcohol wipe.
   Purpose: Any medication left in the head will be lost after it is snapped off. Tapping or quickly bringing the ampule down will drain the medication into the body.
7. Place the ampule breaker over the head of the ampule (following the directions from the manufacturer) or wrap the neck with gauze (Figs. 2 and 3). Hold the body with your nondominant hand. With your dominant hand, firmly hold the head (or breaker) between your first two fingers and thumb. Quickly snap off the head of the ampule, making sure it breaks away from your body and others (Fig. 4).
   Purpose: It is important to protect your fingers from the broken glass.

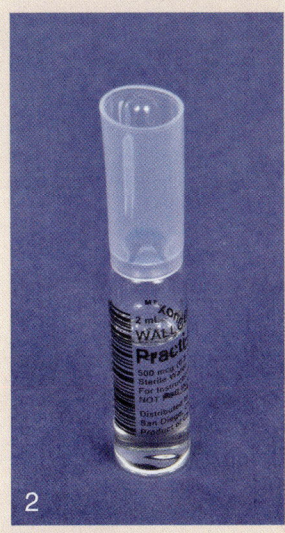

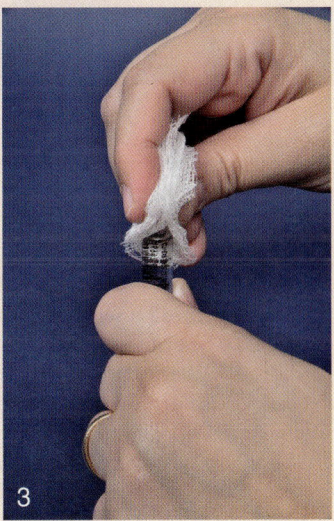

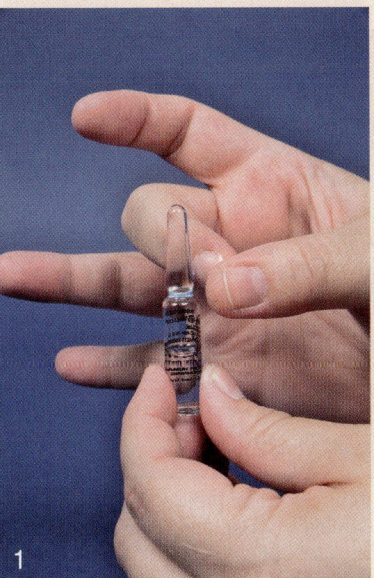

Continued

PROCEDURE 38.6 Prepare Medication From an Ampule—cont'd

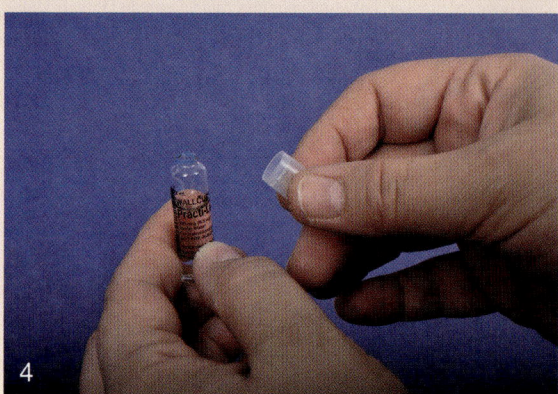

8. Discard the breaker or gauze with the ampule head in a biohazard sharps container (Fig. 5).
   Purpose: It is important to discard the head immediately to protect yourself.

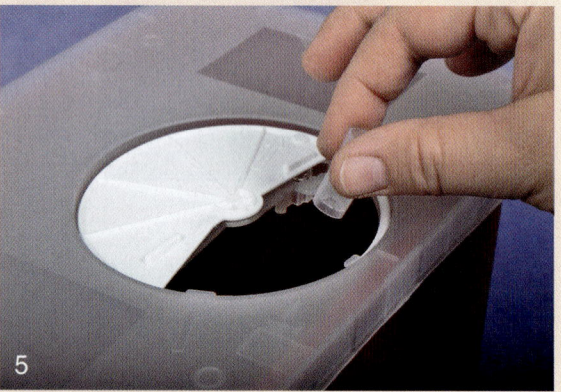

9. Place the ampule on a flat surface. Uncover the filter needle and insert the needle into the ampule without contaminating the needle. Keeping the bevel in the medication, pull the plunger upward, aspirating the medication into the syringe. Tilt the ampule as you remove all the medication.
   Purpose: Keeping the bevel in the medication will prevent air being aspirated into the syringe.
10. Recap the needle using the one-hand scoop technique. Perform the third medication check. Check the medication label against the order. Check for the right name, form, and route. Discard the ampule in the biohazard sharps container.
    Purpose: It is important to do the third check of the label before seeing the patient.
11. Remove the filter needle and attach a new needle without contaminating the unit. Discard the filter needle in the biohazard sharps container.
    Purpose: The filter needle needs to be removed before the injection is given.
12. Hold the syringe in a vertical position with the uncapped needle pointed upward. Tap the barrel carefully with the fingertips or a pen to move the air bubbles up to the top of the barrel. Once all the air bubbles are at the top, push the plunger slowly to the correct calibration marking for the ordered dose. Recap the needle.
    Purpose: The air needs to be at the top of the syringe before you measure the correct amount of medication.
13. Double-check the dose of medication measured against the order. Make sure no air bubbles are in the syringe.
    Purpose: Air bubbles take up space. If air bubbles are present, then the correct dose will not be given.
14. Maintain sterility of the medication and the needle throughout the procedure.
    Purpose: The needle and medication need to be sterile for the injection.
15. Clean up the work area. Packaging and other waste should be discarded in the waste container.
    Purpose: It is professional to clean up after yourself. Never fill a biohazard sharps container with uncontaminated waste (e.g., packaging).

Using a Prefilled Sterile Cartridge

A prefilled, sterile cartridge comes filled with a single dose of medication. It is not uncommon that the medication in the syringe is more than what the provider ordered. The cartridge may come with or without a needle. A safety needle can be attached to the Luer Lok on the prefilled cartridge. A reusable cartridge holder (e.g., Carpuject or Tubex) is needed to give the medication (Fig. 38.20). The medical assistant must assemble the cartridge and the reusable cartridge holder prior to administering the medication. Procedure 38.7 describes how to use a Carpuject holder and prepare the medication.

Specialty Syringe Units

Specialty syringe units are designed for patients to give themselves medication. Different types of syringe units are available. Fig. 38.21 shows an insulin pen. The dose of insulin required can be set by the dial. The patient needs to change the needle with each dose. Insulin pens cannot be shared between patients.

The EpiPen and other epinephrine pens are automatic injector systems (Fig. 38.22). The pens are dosed for adults or children. People at risk for anaphylactic reactions (e.g., from food allergens, bee stings) should carry epinephrine pen(s) to prevent a fatal reaction. Simulators can accompany some of the injector systems. These are useful when teaching patients how to give their own injections.

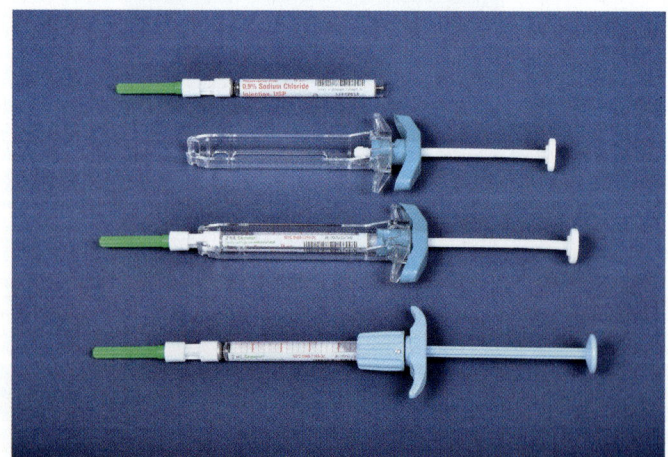

FIG. 38.20 Top to bottom: Prefilled syringe, Carpuject holder, prefilled syringe in a Carpuject holder, and a prefilled syringe in a Tubex cartridge holder.

CHAPTER 38 Administering Medication

PROCEDURE 38.7 Prepare Medication Using a Prefilled Sterile Cartridge

Tasks
Prepare medication using a prefilled sterile cartridge. Discard a prefilled sterile cartridge with a reusable holder.

Equipment and Supplies
- Provider's order
- Prefilled sterile cartridge
- Hypodermic safety needle (if needed)
- Carpuject cartridge holder
- Biohazard sharps container
- Waste container
- Drug reference information

Order
0.9% Sodium Chloride 1.6 mL IM

Procedural Steps

1. Wash your hands or use hand sanitizer. Using the drug reference information and the order, review the information on the medication if needed. Clarify any questions you have with the provider.
   Purpose: Hand sanitization is an important step for infection control. It is important to be knowledgeable about the medication you are giving.

2. Select the right medication from the storage area. Check the medication label against the order. Check for the right name, form, and route. Check the expiration date to make sure the drug is not expired. Verify the right dose and the right time.
   Purpose: It is important to do the first check of the label when getting the medication from the cabinet. Do not administer expired medications.

3. Assemble the supplies required for the procedure.
   Purpose: Remember to split up the three medication checks with activities between each check.

4. Perform the second medication check. Check the medication label against the order. Check for the right name, form, dose, and route.
   Purpose: It is important to do the second check of the label before proceeding with the procedure.

5. Break the seal. With one hand on the needle cover and the other on the barrel of the prefilled cartridge, move your hands together until you hear a pop. If needed, remove the cover on the cartridge and attach a covered needle.
   Purpose: This breaks the seal in the cartridge.

6. Hold the Carpuject holder so the opening (for the barrel) is facing up. Pull the plunger rod out until it clicks. Turn the blue lock until it clicks. This should increase the space between the blue lock and the flange (Fig. 1).

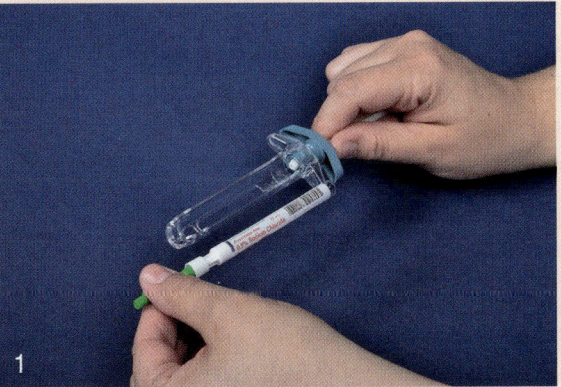

   Purpose: The Carpuject holder needs to be opened before the cartridge can be placed in it.

7. Insert the cartridge into the Carpuject holder (Fig. 2). To secure the cartridge, turn the blue lock on the Carpuject holder until it clicks. The space between the blue lock and the flange should decrease. Turn the white plunger rod until it screws onto the rubber stopper (Fig. 3).
   Purpose: The cartridge must be secured in the Carpuject holder.

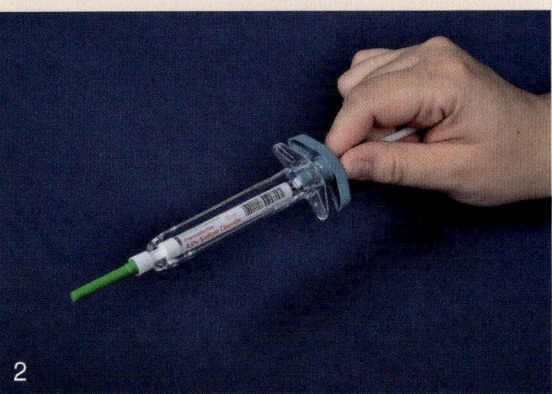

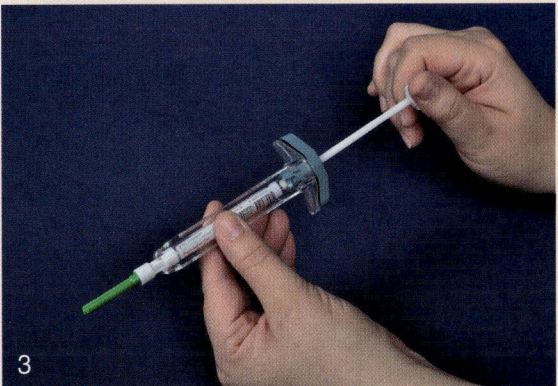

8. Remove the cover. Hold the syringe unit in a vertical position with the uncapped needle or tip pointed upward. Tap the barrel carefully with the fingertips or a pen to move the air bubbles up to the top of the barrel. Once all the air bubbles are at the top, push the plunger slowly to the correct calibration marking for the ordered dose.
   Purpose: The air needs to be at the top of the syringe before you measure the correct amount of medication.

9. Recap the needle using the one-hand scoop technique. Perform the third medication check. Check the medication label against the order. Check for the right name, form, and route.
   Purpose: It is important to do the third check of the label before seeing the patient.

10. Double-check the dose of medication measured against the order. Make sure no air bubbles are in the syringe.
    Purpose: Air bubbles take up space. If air bubbles are present, then the correct dose will not be given.

11. Maintain sterility of the medication and the needle throughout the procedure.
    Purpose: The needle and medication need to be sterile for the injection.

Continued

UNIT 5 Advanced Clinical Procedures

PROCEDURE 38.7 Prepare Medication Using a Prefilled Sterile Cartridge—cont'd

12. After giving the injection, unscrew the plunger rod and pull out until it clicks. Turn the blue lock until it clicks. The space between the blue lock and the flange should increase in size.
    Purpose: The Carpuject holder needs to be opened to remove the used cartridge.
13. Carefully invert the Carpuject holder over a biohazard sharps container to discard the cartridge (Fig. 4). Hold the Carpuject holder firmly so it does not end up in the sharps container.
    Purpose: Only the cartridge should be discarded.
14. Disinfect the Carpuject holder. Clean up the work area. Waste should be put in the waste container.
    Purpose: Disinfection is an important step for infection control.

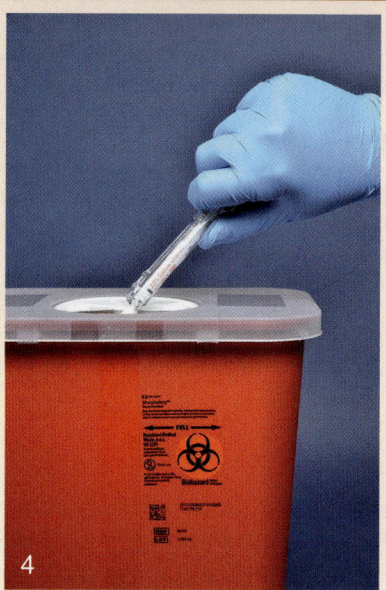

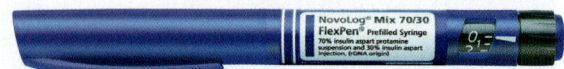

FIG. 38.21 NovoPen. (From Proctor D, et al: *Kinn's The Medical Assistant*, ed 13, St Louis, 2017, Elsevier.)

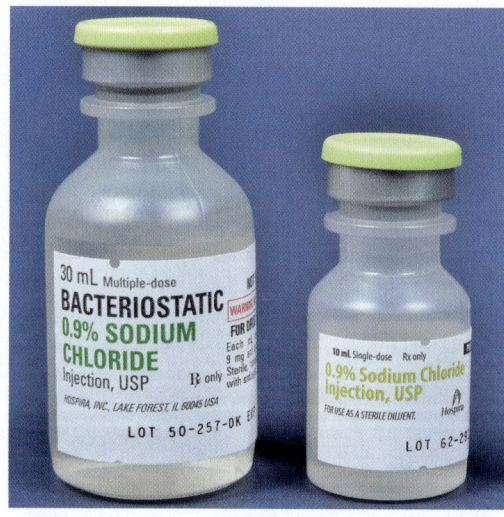

FIG. 38.23 Multiple-dose and single-dose vials.

Using a Vial

Vials are plastic or glass containers with a rubber stopper that is covered by a cap. Vials contain powdered or liquid medications. Liquid medication is more common. The liquid can be parenteral medications, sterile normal saline (0.9% sodium chloride), or sterile water. Vials come in single-dose or multidose (Fig. 38.23). Single-dose or single-use vials are only good for a single patient and a single injection procedure. If the vial needs to be entered more than once for a single patient as part of a single procedure, then a new needle and syringe must be used. Discard the vial after the procedure. Single-dose vials do not contain any ingredients that would prohibit microorganism growth. Thus, they are only good for a single use.

Multidose vials contain many doses of medication. The label will clearly state that the vial is a multidose vial. These vials contain an

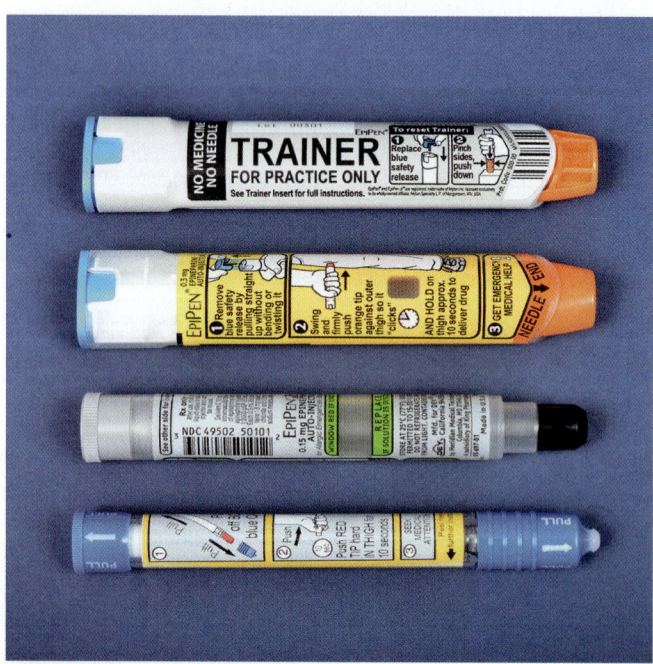

FIG. 38.22 Top to bottom: EpiPen trainer, Epipen for older children and adults, EpiPen Jr for children, and a generic epinephrine pen.

antimicrobial preservative that prevents the growth of bacteria. The preservative does not help protect the fluid against viruses and other sources of contamination if safe injection practices are not followed. When multidose vials are opened (cap is removed or the stopper is punctured), they are only good for 28 days (unless the manufacturer states otherwise). The new expiration date should be written on the label. If the manufacturer's expiration date is shorter than the 28 days, then the sooner date must be used.

Each time the multidose vial is entered, the rubber stopper must be disinfected, and a sterile needle and syringe must be used. The vial is under pressure. You need to add air into the vial before you draw out the amount of liquid you need. The amount of air added should equal the amount of liquid you draw out. Always make sure you have the correct amount of medication in your syringe before you withdraw the needle.

Never inject unneeded medication back into the vial once the needle has been removed from the vial. Procedure 38.8 describes how to prepare medication from a vial.

Reconstituting Powdered Medication

As previously mentioned, vials can contain powdered medication. A powdered medication needs to be mixed with a **diluent** (DIL yoo ehnt). Typically, sterile normal saline or sterile water is used as a diluent,

> **VOCABULARY**
> **diluent:** A liquid substance that dilutes or lessens the strength of a solution or mixture.

PROCEDURE 38.8 Prepare Medication From a Vial

Task
Prepare medication from a vial.

Equipment and Supplies
- Provider's order
- Vial of medication
- Alcohol wipes
- Hypodermic safety needle and 3 mL syringe or needle/syringe unit
- Biohazard sharps container
- Waste container
- Drug reference information
- Marker

Order
0.9% Sodium Chloride 1.2 mL IM

Procedural Steps

1. Wash your hands or use hand sanitizer. Using the drug reference information and the order, review the information on the medication if needed. Clarify any questions you have with the provider.
   Purpose: Hand sanitization is an important step for infection control. It is important to be knowledgeable about the medication you are giving.
2. Select the right medication from the storage area. Check the medication label against the order. Check for the right name, form, and route. Check the expiration date to make sure the drug is not expired. Verify the right dose and the right time.
   Purpose: It is important to do the first check of the label when getting medications from the cabinet. Do not administer expired medications.
3. Assemble the supplies required for the procedure.
   Purpose: Remember to split up the three medication checks with activities between each check.
4. Perform the second medication check. Check the medication label against the order. Check for the right name, form, dose, and route.
   Purpose: It is important to do the second check of the label before proceeding with the procedure.
5. Open the syringe and needle. Tighten the preassembled syringe and needle unit or attach the needle to the syringe. Using a marker, label the syringe with the medication name.
   Purpose: Labeling the medication is critical for medication safety.
6. Mix the medication by rolling it with your hands if needed (Fig. 1). Remove the cap on the vial (if present). Clean the rubber stopper with an alcohol wipe (Fig. 2). Let the stopper dry.

Purpose: The rubber stopper must be disinfected each time you enter the vial with a needle.

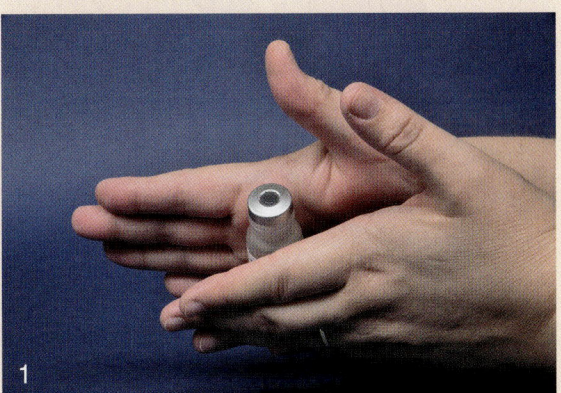

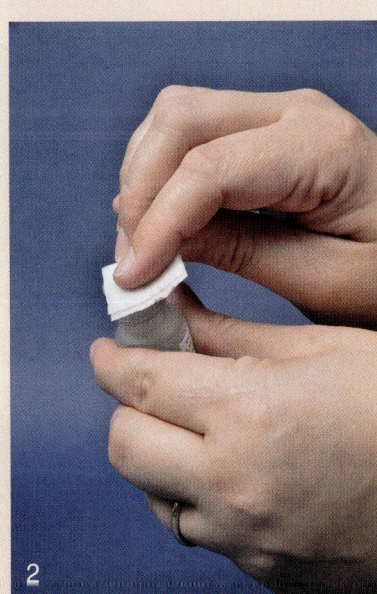

7. With the syringe in a vertical position, pull the syringe plunger down. Draw up an amount of air equal to the amount of medication ordered.
   Purpose: The vial is under pressure. When fluid is taken out, air must be added in. Not enough replaced air makes it difficult to withdraw the

Continued

PROCEDURE 38.8   Prepare Medication From a Vial—cont'd

medication. Too much air causes the pressure to increase in the vial. The extra pressure causes the medication to be forced into the syringe without the plunger being pulled.

8. Hold the vial firmly against a flat surface. Insert the needle into the center of the dried rubber stopper. Inject the aspirated air above the fluid in the vial (Fig. 3).
   Purpose: Adding the air into the fluid will increase the bubbles.

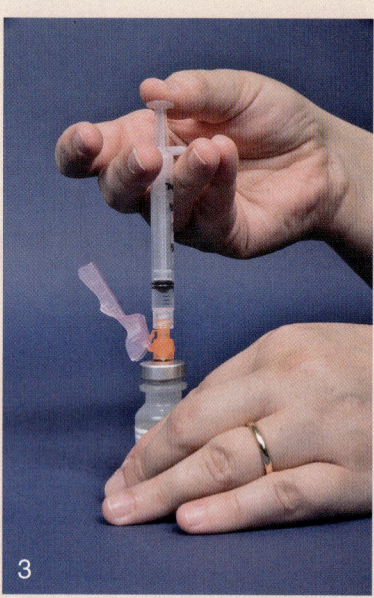

9. With the palm of your nondominant hand facing upward, grasp the vial between your middle and index fingers. Keeping the syringe unit in the vial, pick up and invert them. Use your thumb and the ring and little fingers of your nondominant hand to stabilize the syringe in the vial (Fig. 4).
   Purpose: It is important to stabilize the syringe, so the needle does not bend.

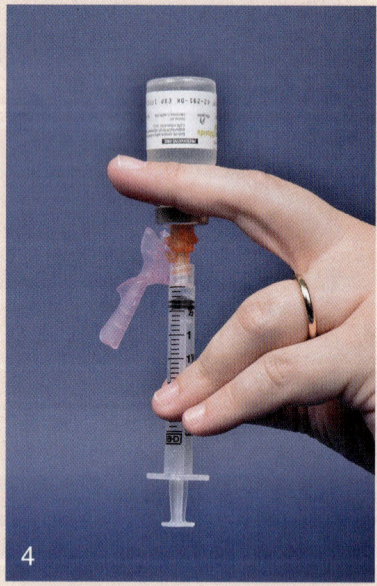

10. With the syringe at eye level, pull the plunger down using your dominant hand. Fill the syringe with more medication than what was ordered (Fig. 5).
    Purpose: Air bubbles will need to be ejected back into the vial. The extra medication helps with this process.

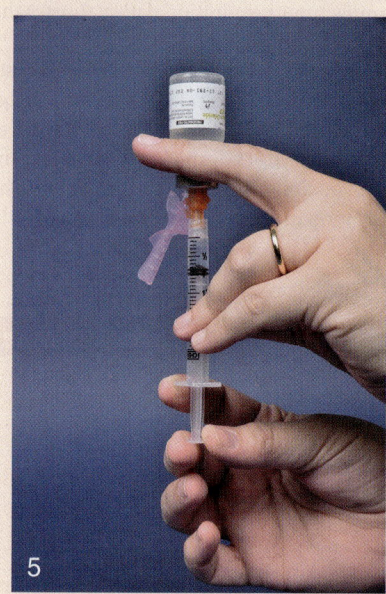

11. Continue to hold the vial/needle/syringe unit in a vertical position (with the needle pointing upward) with your nondominant hand. With your dominant hand, either use your fingers or a pen to tap the bubbles to the top of the barrel.
    Purpose: Bubbles rise to the top. With the syringe pointing straight up, the bubbles tend to move to the top of the barrel near the needle.

12. Once all the air bubbles are at the top, push the plunger slowly to the correct calibration marking for the ordered dose.
    Purpose: The air needs to be at the top of the syringe before you measure the correct amount of medication.

13. Double-check that no air bubbles are in the syringe and the right dose was measured. If everything is correct, remove the vial from the syringe/needle unit.
    Purpose: Air bubbles take up space. If air bubbles are present, then the correct dose will not be given.

14. Use the one-hand scoop technique to cover the needle. Perform the third medication check. Check each medication label against the order. Check for the right name, form, and route.
    Purpose: It is important to do the third check of the label before seeing the patient.

15. Maintain sterility of the medication and the needle throughout the procedure.
    Purpose: The needle and medication need to be sterile for the injection.

16. Clean up the work area.
    Purpose: It is professional to clean up after yourself.

although other medications may also be used (per the provider's order and the manufacturer's directions). The most common powdered medications in primary care are live virus vaccines. These need to be reconstituted (ree KON sti toot ed) (Procedure 38.9).

If the vial is a multidose vial, it is important to write the expiration date on the label. The expiration date for reconstituted medications will vary. See the manufacturer's insert for the length of time that the medication will remain stable after reconstitution. Besides the expiration date, include your initials and the fluid that was used to reconstitute the medication. These three pieces of information need to be on the multidose label.

There are four major steps in reconstituting powdered medication and withdrawing a dose of the medication (Fig. 38.24). The process includes:

- Step 1: Remove air from the powdered medication vial and put air into the diluent vial.
- Step 2: Withdraw liquid from the diluent vial and add it to the powdered medication vial.
- Step 3: Mix the liquid with the powdered medication.
- Step 4: Add in air and withdraw the dose needed.

> **VOCABULARY**
> **reconstituted:** A dried substance (powder) that has been restored to a fluid form, so it can be injected.

PROCEDURE 38.9 Reconstitute Powdered Medication

Tasks
Reconstitute powdered medication and prepare the dose of medication.

Equipment and Supplies
- Provider's order
- Vial of powdered medication
- Vial of diluent
- Alcohol wipes
- 2 hypodermic syringes (a 3 mL and a larger syringe)
- 2 hypodermic needles (including a safety needle)
- Biohazard sharps container
- Waste container
- Drug reference information

Order
(Powdered medication name) 0.5 mL IM

Procedural Steps
1. Wash your hands or use hand sanitizer. Using the drug reference information and the order, review the information on the medication if needed. Clarify any questions you have with the provider.
   Purpose: Hand sanitization is an important step for infection control. It is important to be knowledgeable about the medication you are giving.
2. Select the right medication from the storage area. Check the medication label against the order. Check for the right name, form, and route. Check the expiration date to make sure the vials are not expired. Verify the right dose and the right time. Read the medication label to determine the correct diluent. Obtain the diluent and check the name, route, and expiration date.
   Purpose: It is important to do the first check of the label when getting the medications from the cabinet. The label of the powdered medication will indicate the diluent to use. The diluent label must also be checked.
3. Assemble the supplies required for the procedure. If needed, calculate the dose of medication required.
   Purpose: Remember to split up the three medication checks with activities between each check.
4. Perform the second medication check. Check the medication labels against the order and directions for reconstituting the powder. Check for the right name, form, and route.
   Purpose: It is important to do the second check of the label before proceeding with the procedure.
5. Open and assemble the syringes and needles. If needed, attach the needles to the syringes without contaminating the units.
   Purpose: It is important to keep the needle sterile. If contamination occurs, discard the equipment, and start over.
6. Remove the caps on the vials. Clean the rubber stoppers with an alcohol wipe. Let the stoppers dry.
   Purpose: The rubber stopper must be disinfected each time you enter the vial with a needle.
7. With the powdered medication vial on a firm surface, insert the needle of the largest volume syringe unit. Make sure the tip stays out of the powder. Pull back on the plunger and withdraw air equal to the amount of diluent that must be added. Pull the needle/syringe out of the stopper.
   Purpose: The vial is under pressure. When liquid is put in, the same volume of air must be removed to keep the pressure equal.
8. Using the syringe with the aspirated air (equal to the amount of diluent needed), insert the needle into the center of the dried rubber stopper of the diluent vial. Push the air into the vial, but do not force the air into the vial. Make sure the needle is not in the fluid.
   Purpose: Adding the air into the fluid will increase the bubbles. Forcing the air into the vial may cause the vial to have too much pressure.
9. With the palm of your nondominant hand facing upward, grasp the vial between your middle and index fingers. Keeping the syringe unit in the vial, pick up and invert them. Use your thumb and the ring and little fingers of your nondominant hand to stabilize the syringe in the vial. Pull down on the plunger until you have more diluent than what you need.
   Purpose: It is important to stabilize the syringe, so the needle does not bend.
10. Continue to hold the vial/needle/syringe unit in a vertical position (with the needle pointing upward) with your nondominant hand. With your dominant hand, either use your fingers or a pen to tap the bubbles to the top of the barrel.
    Purpose: Bubbles rise to the top. With the syringe pointing straight up, the bubbles tend to move to the top of the barrel near the needle.
11. Once all the air bubbles are at the top, push the plunger slowly to the correct calibration marking for the ordered dose. Keep the syringe at eye level.
    Purpose: The air needs to be at the top of the syringe before you measure the correct amount of medication.
12. Double-check that no air bubbles are in the syringe and the right dose was measured. If everything is correct, remove the vial from the syringe/needle unit.
    Purpose: Air bubbles take up space. If air bubbles are present, then the correct dose will not be given.

Continued

PROCEDURE 38.9 Reconstitute Powdered Medication—cont'd

13. Using an alcohol wipe, clean the rubber stopper of the powdered medication vial. With the vial flat on a hard surface, insert the needle into the dried stopper. Push the diluent into the vial. If resistance is met, take your finger off the plunger, and allow air to fill in the syringe. Gradually work all the diluent into the vial. Withdraw the needle from the vial and discard the needle and syringe in the biohazard sharps container.
    Purpose: Forcing the diluent into the vial may cause the vial to "explode" at the weakest point.
14. Gently mix the vial by rolling it in your palms. Mix the medication until all the powder is dissolved.
    Purpose: The powder needs to be totally dissolved so the correct dose is given.
15. Clean the rubber stopper of the powdered medication vial with an alcohol wipe. Let the stopper dry. With the second syringe in a vertical position, pull the syringe plunger down. Draw up an amount of air equal to the amount of medication ordered.
    Purpose: Think of this step as starting over. Air needs to be inserted into the diluted powder vial to draw up the correct amount of medication.
16. Hold the vial firmly against a flat surface. Insert the needle into the center of the dried rubber stopper. Inject the aspirated air above the fluid in the vial.
    Purpose: Adding the air into the fluid will increase the bubbles.
17. With the palm of your nondominant hand facing upward, grasp the vial between your middle and index fingers. Keeping the syringe unit in the vial, pick up and invert them. Use your thumb and the ring and little fingers of your nondominant hand to stabilize the syringe in the vial.
    Purpose: It is important to stabilize the syringe, so the needle does not bend.
18. With the syringe at eye level, pull the plunger down using your dominant hand. Fill the syringe with more medication than what was ordered.
    Purpose: Air bubbles will need to be ejected back into the vial. The extra medication helps with this process.
19. Continue to hold the vial/needle/syringe unit in a vertical position (with the needle pointing upward) with your nondominant hand. With your dominant hand, either use your fingers or a pen to tap the bubbles to the top of the barrel.
    Purpose: Bubbles rise to the top. With the syringe pointing straight up, the bubbles tend to move to the top of the barrel near the needle.
20. Once all the air bubbles are at the top, push the plunger slowly to the correct calibration marking for the ordered dose.
    Purpose: The air needs to be at the top of the syringe before you measure the correct amount of medication.
21. Double-check that no air bubbles are in the syringe and the right dose was measured. If everything is correct, remove the vial from the syringe/needle unit.
    Purpose: Air bubbles take up space. If air bubbles are present, then the correct dose will not be given.
22. Use the one-hand scoop technique to cover the needle. Perform the third medication check. Check each medication label against the order. Check for the right name, form, and route.
    Purpose: It is important to do the third check of the label before seeing the patient.
23. Maintain sterility of the medication and the needle throughout the procedure.
    Purpose: The needle and medication need to be sterile for the injection.
24. If the medication is in a multidose vial, label the vial with the expiration date, diluent added, and your initials. Clean up the work area. Put the packaging and other waste in the waste container. Discard the vial(s) in the biohazard waste container.
    Purpose: It is professional to clean up after yourself.

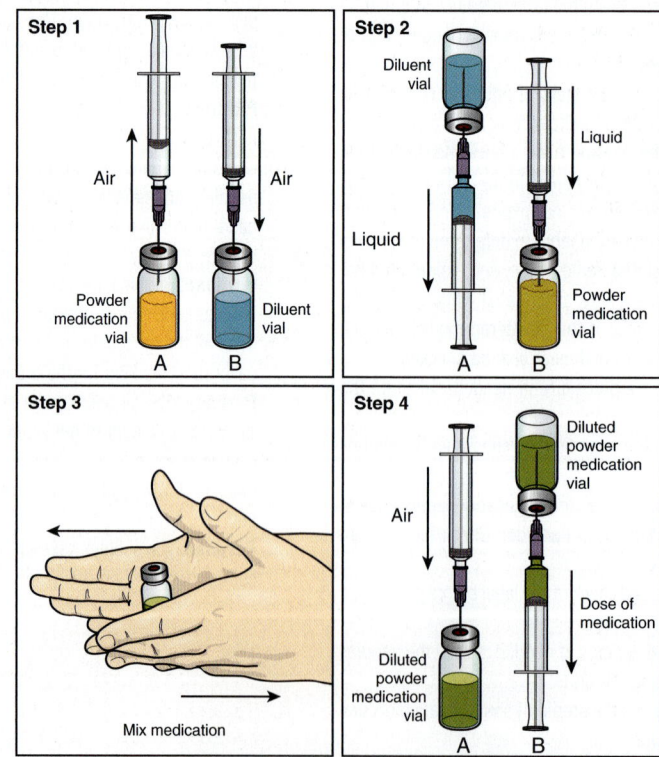

FIG. 38.24 Steps for reconstituting medication and withdrawing a dose of medication.

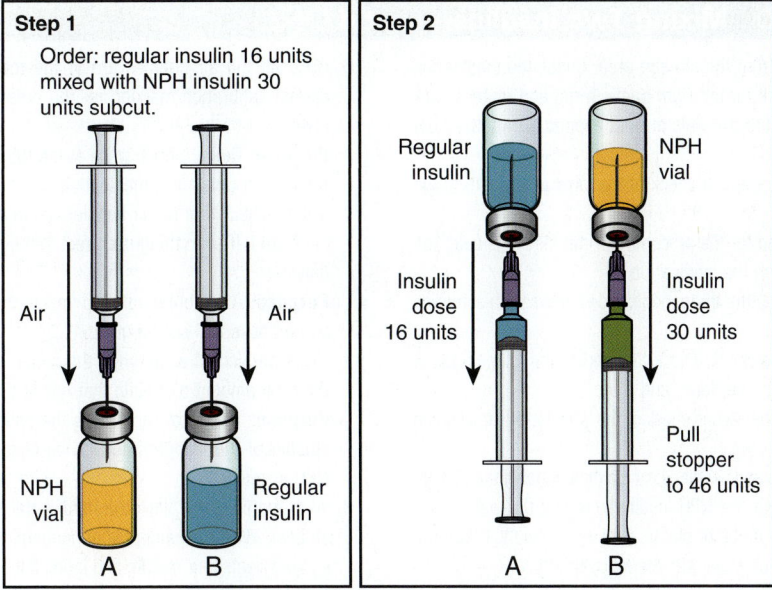

FIG. 38.25 Mixing two insulins.

Mixing Insulins

Patients with diabetes may use insulin to help manage their disease. Taking insulin requires about four injections a day. Some patients may need two different insulins at the same time. Many premixed insulins are available for patients. However, for some individuals the premixed insulins are not an option, and they must mix the two insulins in one syringe. During this combination process, it is important that the vials do not get contaminated with another type of insulin. If by chance contamination occurs, it is better for the rapid-acting or short-acting insulin (Regular insulin) to be mixed in the intermediate-acting insulin vial (e.g., NPH insulin). This means that Regular insulin must be drawn up in the syringe first and then NPH is added (Fig. 38.25). Procedure 38.10 describes the steps for mixing two insulins in one syringe.

Depending on the state's laws and the facility's policies, administering insulin may be within the medical assistant's scope of practice. Understanding how to mix two insulins in the same syringe is important. Not all insulins can be mixed. Use drug reference information to ensure that the two insulins ordered can be mixed.

As discussed earlier in the chapter, insulin is measured in units. Special insulin syringes are available to measure small or large insulin dosages. Insulin is typically stored in the refrigerator and should be warmed to room temperature prior to administration. Cloudy insulins (e.g., NPH) are suspensions and need to be mixed before drawing up the insulin. Mix cloudy insulins by gently rolling the vial between your hands. Clear insulin (e.g., Regular insulin) does not need to be mixed or rolled in your hand.

Patients receiving insulin must rotate their injection sites. This prevents tissue damage and absorption issues with the insulin. It might be helpful for patients to mark the site of the last injection with a spot bandage or a piece of tape. The easiest way to rotate sites is to give subsequent injections in a circular pattern around the first injection site in a specific location. The goal is to avoid using the same location again for another month.

CRITICAL THINKING BOX 38.6

Mark struggles to remember the order for drawing up insulin. What might be a few good ways to remember the process of drawing up two insulins in the same syringe?

PROCEDURE 38.10 Mixing Two Insulins

Task
Mixing two insulins in one syringe.

Equipment and Supplies
- Provider's order
- Regular insulin vial
- NPH insulin vial
- Alcohol wipes
- Insulin needle and syringe unit
- Biohazard sharps container
- Waste container
- Drug reference information
- Marker

Order
Regular insulin 16 units mixed with NPH insulin 30 units subcut.

Procedural Steps
1. Wash your hands or use hand sanitizer. Using the drug reference information and the order, review the information on the medication if needed. Clarify any questions you have with the provider.
   Purpose: Hand sanitization is an important step for infection control. It is important to be knowledgeable about the medication you are giving.

PROCEDURE 38.10 Mixing Two Insulins—cont'd

2. Select the right medications from the storage area. Check the medication labels against the order. Check for the right name, form, and route. Check the expiration date to make sure the vials are not expired. Verify the right dose and the right time.
   Purpose: It is important to do the first check of the label when getting the medications from the cabinet.
3. Assemble the supplies required for the procedure. If the insulin is cold, roll the vials in your hands to warm the medication.
   Purpose: Remember to split up the three medication checks with activities between each check.
4. Perform the second medication check. Check the medication labels against the order. Check for the right name, form, and route.
   Purpose: It is important to do the second check of the label before proceeding with the procedure.
5. Open and assemble the syringe and needle. Using a marker, label the syringe with the medication name. Mix the NPH insulin by rolling the vial in your hands. If present, remove the metal or plastic caps on the vials. Clean the rubber stoppers with an alcohol wipe. Let the stoppers dry.
   Purpose: The rubber stopper must be disinfected each time you enter the vials with a needle.
6. With the syringe in a vertical position, pull the syringe plunger down. Draw up an amount of air equal to the amount of NPH insulin ordered. With the NPH vial on a firm surface, insert the needle in the rubber stopper. Inject the air into the NPH vial, keeping the needle tip out of the medication. Withdraw the needle from the stopper.
   Purpose: The vial is under pressure. Adding air is required before removing medication.
7. With the syringe in a vertical position, pull the syringe plunger down. Draw up an amount of air equal to the amount of Regular insulin ordered. With the Regular vial on a firm surface, insert the needle into the rubber stopper. Inject the air into the Regular vial, keeping the needle tip out of the medication.
   Purpose: The vial is under pressure. Adding air is required before removing medication.
8. With the palm of your nondominant hand facing upward, grasp the vial between your middle and index fingers. Keeping the syringe unit in the vial, pick up and invert them. Use your thumb, ring, and little fingers of your nondominant hand to stabilize the syringe in the vial. Pull down on the plunger until you have more Regular insulin than what you need.
   Purpose: It is important to stabilize the syringe, so the needle does not bend.
9. Continue to hold the vial/needle/syringe unit in a vertical position (with the needle pointing upward) with your nondominant hand. With your dominant hand, either use your fingers or a pen to tap the bubbles to the top of the barrel.
   Purpose: Bubbles rise to the top. With the syringe pointing straight up, the bubbles tend to move to the top of the barrel near the needle.
10. Once all the air bubbles are at the top, push the plunger slowly to the correct calibration marking for the ordered dose. Keep the syringe at eye level.
    Purpose: The air needs to be at the top of the syringe before you measure the correct amount of medication.
11. Double-check that no air bubbles are in the syringe and the right dose was measured. If everything is correct, remove the vial from the syringe/needle unit.
    Purpose: Air bubbles take up space. If air bubbles are present, then the correct dose will not be given.
12. Using an alcohol wipe, wipe the rubber stopper of the NPH vial. Calculate the total amount of insulin that needs to be given.
    Purpose: This total represents the calibration marking where the rubber stopper of the plunger needs to be pulled down to when withdrawing the NPH insulin.
13. With the NPH vial flat on a hard surface, insert the needle into the dried stopper. With the palm of your nondominant hand facing upward, grasp the vial between your middle and index fingers. Keeping the syringe unit in the vial, pick up and invert them. Use your thumb and the ring and little fingers of your nondominant hand to stabilize the syringe in the vial. Pull down on the plunger until the rubber stopper reaches the calibration mark required. Do not withdraw any extra NPH insulin.
    Purpose: If any additional NPH insulin is drawn up, the syringe must be discarded in the biohazard sharps container. No insulin can be injected into the NPH vial.
14. Double-check that no air bubbles are in the syringe and the right dose was measured. If everything is correct, remove the vial from the syringe/needle unit.
    Purpose: Air bubbles take up space. If air bubbles are present, discard the syringe and start over.
15. Use the one-hand scoop technique to cover the needle. Perform the third medication check. Check each medication label against the order. Check for the right name, form, and route.
    Purpose: It is important to do the third check of the label before seeing the patient.
16. Maintain sterility of the medication and the needle throughout the procedure.
    Purpose: The needle and medication need to be sterile for the injection.
17. Clean up the work area. Put the packaging and other waste in the waste container. Place the insulin vials back in their storage location.
    Purpose: It is professional to clean up after yourself.

GIVING PARENTERAL MEDICATIONS

Some medications can be given by several routes. Other medications can only be given by injection. Parenteral medication administration has several advantages:
- It is useful when the patient has gastrointestinal distress or is unconscious.
- It offers good absorption compared to other routes, such as the oral route.
- The *onset* (time medication starts working) is more rapid than with other routes.
- Some types of parenteral medications have a longer *duration time* (time it works in the body).

Disadvantages of parenteral medication administration include:
- Pain with the injection
- Risk for infection due to the injection
- Unpredictable absorption rate for those with poor circulation (e.g., patients with peripheral artery disease, diabetes, obesity, or Raynaud's disease)

When it comes to giving injections, over time you will gain confidence and it will become easy. Always:
- Follow the Nine Rules of Medication Administration.
- Check the medication's label against the order three times.
- Know about the medication you are giving (what is it, why is it being ordered, how is it given, and what are the common side effects).
- Label all syringes with the name of the medication they contain.
- Follow medical asepsis and the Bloodborne Pathogens Standard established by the Occupational Safety and Health Administration (OSHA).
- Ensure that the needle is not directed at your hand holding the patient, when giving an injection. Slight movement may cause a needlestick.

Following these guidelines will help you to perform injections safely and protect your patient from medication errors.

Guidelines for Parenteral Medications

Prepare and store medications in a separate area, away from the exam rooms. Medications can be prepared without the use of gloves. Ensure that all needles are tightly covered and placed on a tray when carrying them to the exam room. Never transport medication in your pockets. Bring only one patient's medication at a time to avoid confusion and error.

When selecting an injection site:
- Never give an injection near bones or blood vessels.
- Avoid scar tissue, a change in skin pigmentation or texture, or abnormal growth (e.g., mole or wart).
- Avoid abrasions, lesions, wounds, bruises, and edematous (i DEM ah tahs) areas.
- The site should large enough to hold the amount of medication injected.
- Avoid sites recently used (within the last month).

According to the Immunization Action Coalition (www.immunize.org), it is safe to give subcut and IM vaccines into a tattoo. However, it is not a good idea to inject into a newly tattooed area. If you must inject in a tattooed area, attempt to use a lighter pigmented area. All injections pose the risk of a reaction or an infection at the injection site. Dark pigments may mask a reaction or an infection.

To minimize pain with injections, insert subcut and IM needles swiftly. Inject the medication at the rate of 10 seconds per 1 mL to avoid unnecessary discomfort. Remove the needle quickly, using the same angle as the entry. Other ways used to reduce pain and anxiety are discussed in Box 38.11.

CRITICAL THINKING BOX 38.7

Gabe talks with Mark about distractions to use when giving IM injections. He mentions having patients wiggle their toes or move their fingers when giving an injection on that extremity. He explains that he tells the patient about the movement prior to starting the injection. Gabe reminds the patient when he is aspirating, just prior to injecting the medication. What might be the benefit of reminding the patient when aspirating?

Special Situations

Even if the procedure was done correctly, sometimes things can go wrong. It is important for the medical assistant to know what to do in those situations.

If a needle breaks during an injection or if the needle separates from the syringe, pull out the needle, if it is visible. Discard the needle in the biohazard sharps container. If the needle breaks off and it is not visible, mark the spot with a pen and yell for help. If the injection was given in the arm, place a tourniquet above the spot to prevent the needle from moving in the body. Notify the provider immediately.

With intramuscular injections, sometimes the bone can be hit during the procedure. If this occurs, pull the needle out about a $\frac{1}{4}$ inch and give the medication.

With any medication, a patient can experience an anaphylactic reaction. *Anaphylaxis* (AN ah fi LAK sis) is a severe allergic reaction that can be life-threatening. Having the patient wait 15 minutes after an injection allows you to monitor the patient for unusual symptoms (Box 38.12). If the patient is experiencing any unusual symptoms, it is important to tell the provider immediately. The first-line medication for anaphylaxis is epinephrine.

INTRADERMAL INJECTIONS

Intradermal (ID) injections are given just under the epidermis (Fig. 38.29). Fig. 38.30 show sites recommended for intradermal injections. In ambulatory care, the following intradermal injections may be given:
- Mantoux tuberculin test (TST)
- Intradermal flu vaccine (e.g., Fluzone Intradermal) (Box 38.13)
- Allergy testing

Table 38.3 contains a quick summary of intradermal injection information.

TABLE 38.3 Quick Summary of Intradermal Injections

Syringe used	1 mL (tuberculin syringe)
Needle size	$\frac{1}{4}$ to $\frac{5}{8}$ inch; 25-27 gauge
Angle of entry	5–15 degrees with bevel facing upward
Maximum volume	0.1 mL
Common sites	Forearm, upper arm, and back
Additional sites	Separate by at least 2 inches
Patient position	Sitting with arm extended
Administration	Pull skin taut at injection site

BOX 38.11 Techniques to Help Reduce Pain and Anxiety With Injections

Techniques that can be used to help reduce a patient's pain and anxiety about injections include:

- Giving a sugar-coated pacifier or sugar water (must be ordered by the provider), which helps to soothe children under age 1 year after injections.
- Applying a topical anesthetic skin refrigerant (e.g., Pain Ease), which works immediately (Figs. 38.26 and 38.27).
- Applying a topical anesthetic (e.g., EMLA cream) at the injection site, which works in about 30 to 40 minutes.
- Talking with the patients to distract them from the procedure.
- Having patients move their toes or fingers on the extremity used when an IM injection is given. (Have patients "play the piano" with their fingers when giving a deltoid injection.)
- Using products that provide cold and vibration sensations (e.g., Buzzy), which overwhelm the nerves affected by the injection (Fig. 38.28).
- Administering the most painful injection last.

BOX 38.12 Signs and Symptoms of Anaphylaxis

- Warm feeling, flushing
- Shortness of breath
- Dyspnea (DISP nee uh) (difficulty breathing), wheezing
- Throat tightening, difficulty swallowing
- Cough
- Anxiety
- Pain or cramping
- Vomiting or diarrhea
- Loss of consciousness
- Shock
- Palpitations, dizziness

BOX 38.13 Intradermal Flu Vaccine

Currently, the intradermal flu vaccine is the only intradermal vaccine. Fluzone Intradermal contains less antigen than the IM flu vaccines and is approved for use for adults age 18 to 64-years-old. Fluzone Intradermal uses a nontraditional ID site. The vaccine is given in the IM deltoid area, though it goes in the epidermis and not in the muscle like IM injections.

The vaccine comes in a prefilled microinjection syringe containing 0.1 mL of medication. The syringe contains a 30 G microneedle.

After preparing the site, hold the syringe between the thumb and middle finger of your dominant hand. With a quick, short motion, insert the needle at a 90-degree angle. Do not aspirate. Push the plunger and then remove the syringe. If the syringe comes with a needle shield, push firmly on the plunger to activate it.

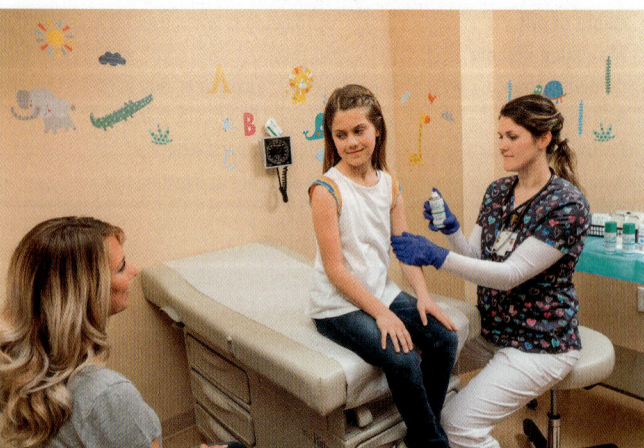

FIG. 38.26 Topical anesthetic skin refrigerant spray. (Courtesy Gebauer-Tri-Point-Medical, Cleveland, OH.)

GEBAUER'S PAIN EASE®
MEDIUM STREAM SPRAY AND MIST SPRAY

CAUTION: Federal law restricts this device to sale by or on the order of a licensed healthcare practitioner.

Hold the can upright while spraying.

INDICATIONS FOR USE: Gebauer's Pain Ease Medium Stream Spray and Mist Spray are vapocoolants (skin refrigerants) intended for topical application to skin, intact mucous membranes (oral cavity, nasal passage ways and the lips) and minor open wounds. Pain Ease instantly controls pain associated with injections (venipuncture, IV starts, cosmetic procedures), minor surgical procedures (such as lancing boils, incisions, drainage of small abscesses and sutures) and the temporary relief of minor sports injuries (sprains, bruising, cuts and abrasions).

PRECAUTIONS:
1. Do not spray in the eyes.
2. Do not use this product on persons with poor circulation or insensitive skin.
3. When used to produce local freezing of tissues, adjacent skin areas should be protected by an application of petroleum.
4. The freezing and thawing process may be painful, and freezing may lower local resistance to infection and delay healing.
5. Over application of the product might cause frostbite and/or alter skin pigmentation.
6. Do not use on large areas of damaged skin, puncture wounds, animal bites or serious wounds.
7. Apply only to intact mucous membranes.
8. Do not use on genital mucous membranes.

ADVERSE REACTIONS: Freezing can occasionally alter skin pigmentation.

CONTRAINDICATIONS: Pain Ease is contraindicated in individuals with a history of hypersensitivity to 1,1,1,3,3-Pentafluoropropane and 1,1,1,2-Tetrafluoroethane. If skin irritation develops, discontinue use.

WARNINGS:
For external use only. Contents under pressure.
For use on minor open wounds only.
For use on intact mucous membranes only.
KEEP OUT OF THE REACH OF CHILDREN

INSTRUCTIONS: Press the actuator button firmly, allowing Pain Ease to spray from the can.

PRE-INJECTION & MINOR SURGICAL TOPICAL ANESTHESIA: Have all necessary equipment ready and prepare the procedure site per facility's protocol. Hold the can upright, 3 to 7 inches (8 to 18cm) from the procedure site, about a can's length away. Spray steadily 4 to 10 seconds or until the skin begins turning white, whichever comes first. Do not spray longer than 10 seconds. After spraying the site, immediately perform the procedure. The anesthetic effect of Pain Ease lasts about one minute. Reapply if necessary.

*Apply petrolatum to protect the adjacent area for minor surgical procedures.

TEMPORARY RELIEF OF MINOR SPORTS INJURIES: The pain of bruises, contusions, swelling, minor sprains, cuts and abrasions may be controlled with Pain Ease. The amount of cooling depends on the dosage. Dosage varies with duration of application. The smallest dose needed to produce the desired effect should be used. The anesthetic effect of Pain Ease lasts about one minute. This time interval is usually sufficient to help reduce or relieve the initial trauma of the injury. Hold the can upright, 3 to 7 inches (8 to 18 cm) from the target area, about a can's length away. Spray steadily 4 to 10 seconds or until the skin begins turning white, whichever comes first. Do not spray longer than 10 seconds. Reapply if necessary.

CONTENTS: 1,1,1,3,3-Pentafluoropropane and 1,1,1,2-Tetrafluoroethane

STORAGE: Do not puncture or incinerate container. Do not expose to heat or store at temperatures above 50°C (120°F).

DISPOSAL: Dispose of in accordance with local and national regulations.

HOW SUPPLIED: Aerosol Can

Gebauer's Pain Ease® Medium Stream Spray
3.5 fl. oz. (103.5mL) - P/N 0386-0008-03
1.0 fl. oz. (30mL) - P/N 0386-0008-04

Gebauer's Pain Ease® Mist Spray
3.5 fl. oz. (103.5mL) - P/N 0386-0008-02
1.0 fl. oz. (30mL) - P/N 0386-0008-01

For more information about this product contact Gebauer Company.

Manufactured by:
Gebauer Company
Cleveland, OH 44128
1-800-321-9348
www.Gebauer.com
Products Made in the U.S.A
©2015 Gebauer Company, Rev 06/15

FIG. 38.27 Package insert for Pain Ease, a vapocoolant (skin refrigerant). (Courtesy Gebauer-Tri-Point-Medical, Cleveland, OH.)

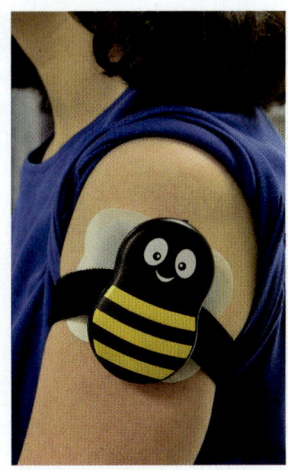

FIG. 38.28 Buzzy helps reduce pain naturally by overwhelming the nerves with vibration and cold sensations.

Tuberculin Testing

There are two types of tuberculin tests approved by the FDA: the skin test and the blood test. The Mantoux tuberculin skin test (TST) is used to determine whether a patient is infected with *Mycobacterium tuberculosis*. It is important for the medical assistant to be knowledgeable about and skilled at administering and reading the test.

To perform the TST, tuberculin purified protein derivative (PPD) 0.1 mL is given ID into the inner surface of the forearm (Procedure 38.11). A tuberculin syringe and needle, with the bevel facing upward, is used to slowly inject the PPD, creating a wheal. A *wheal* is a tense, pale elevation of the skin. The wheal must measure 6 to 10 mm in diameter, or the test must be repeated.

The patient returns within 48 to 72 hours to have the test read. Reading before or after this time invalidates the results. When reading the test, palpate the site to check for a raised, hardened area, called an *induration* (IN duh RAY shuhn). If an induration is felt, measure the raised area across the forearm (perpendicular to the bone). The erythema (redness) is not measured. The diameter of the induration is read in millimeters (mm) and must be noted in the health record. The medical assistant can never state that the test result is positive or negative. The provider uses the test results and the patient history to determine if the patient has tuberculosis (TB). A TST reading between 5 and 15 mm can be positive for different populations. Table 38.4 describes the different populations.

At times the TST reading may be incorrect. A false-positive reaction means the person reacted to the test even though no *M. tuberculosis* is present (Box 38.14). A false-negative reaction means the person may

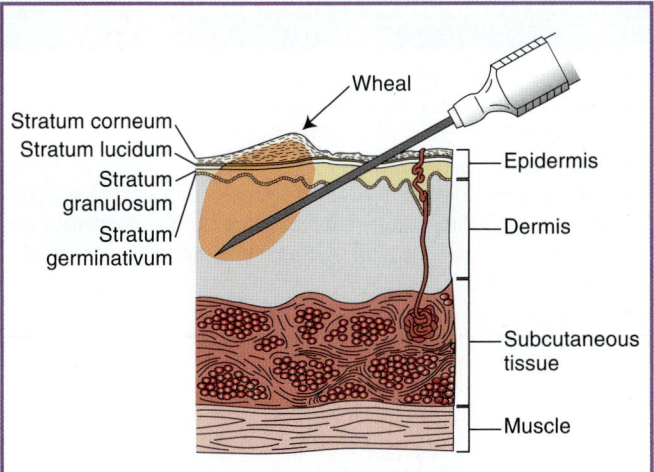

FIG. 38.29 The intradermal (ID) injection is administered just under the epidermis. Because the drug is dispersed in an area where many nerves are present, it causes momentary burning or stinging. Small amounts of medication are injected. (From Proctor D, et al: *Kinn's The Medical Assistant*, ed 13, St Louis, 2017, Elsevier.)

BOX 38.14 Reasons for False-Positive Reactions With Mantoux Tuberculin Skin Tests

- Lung infection with nontuberculous mycobacteria (NTM). This organism is found in the water and soil and is inhaled.
- Previous vaccination with bacillus Calmette-Guérin (BCG) vaccine. Many foreign-born patients from countries with a high risk of TB may have received BCG abroad. The BCG vaccine has been approved by the U.S. Food and Drug Administration (FDA), but it is used in very limited situations.
- Incorrect administration or reading of the TST.

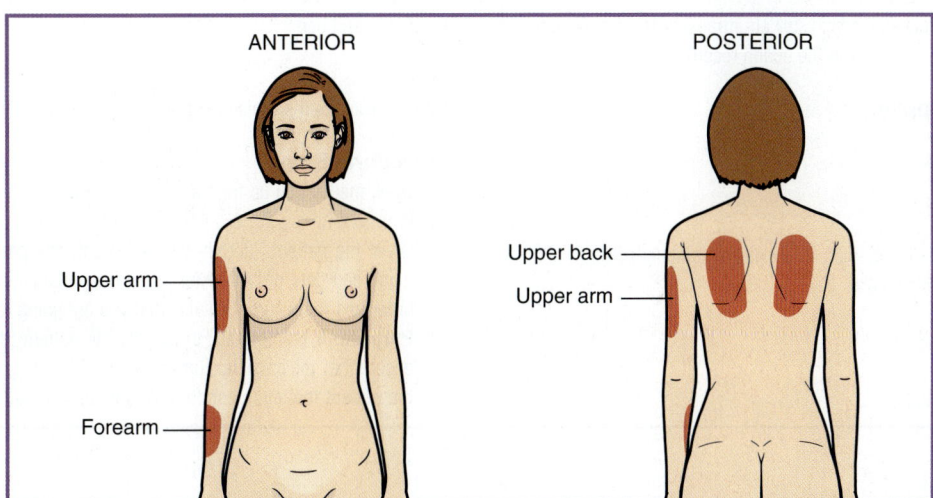

FIG. 38.30 Sites recommended for intradermal injections.

TABLE 38.4 Tuberculin Skin Reaction Categories

Induration ≥5 mm considered positive in patients with:	Induration ≥10 mm considered positive in patients with:	Induration ≥15 mm considered positive in patients with:
• Human immunodeficiency virus (HIV) infection • Organ transplant • Immunosuppression • Recent contact with a person with tuberculosis (TB) • Fibrotic changes on a chest x-ray consistent with prior TB	• Recent immigrants (<5 years) from high-risk areas • Injection drug users • People living or working in high-risk areas (e.g., living in a group setting [jail, nursing home]; employees in a clinical position with a high risk of TB exposure) • Children < 4 years of age or children exposed to high-risk adults	• No known risk for TB

From Centers for Disease Control and Prevention (CDC): https://www.cdc.gov/tb/publications/factsheets/testing/skintesting.htm. Accessed July 14, 2017.

---

not have reacted to the test even though the patient is infected with *M. tuberculosis* (Box 38.15).

The TST can be given to most patients, including infants, pregnant women, patients infected with the human immunodeficiency virus (HIV), and those vaccinated with bacille Calmette-Guérin (BCG). Patients with a history of BCG vaccination may have a positive reaction to the TST. If a patient mentions a history of receiving BCG vaccine, it is important for the medical assistant to inform the provider before performing the skin test. The provider may opt to have the patient undergo the blood test instead.

The TST is contraindicated in patients who had:
- A severe reaction to a past TST (e.g., necrosis, ulcers, blisters, or anaphylaxis)
- A history of a positive TST result
- A live virus vaccine less than 4 to 6 weeks ago. A TST and a live virus vaccine can be given on the same day, or the TST can be given 4 to 6 weeks after the vaccine.

> **BOX 38.15 Reasons for False-Negative Result With Mantoux Tuberculin Skin Tests**
>
> - Weakened immune system
> - Exposure to TB infection within previous 8 to 10 weeks
> - Very old TB infection
> - Patient less than 6 months old
> - Recently received a live virus vaccine (e.g., measles, yellow fever, chickenpox), or had a viral infection (e.g., influenza), or received corticosteroids or immunosuppressive medications. A false reaction may occur up to 5 to 6 weeks afterwards.
> - Incorrect administration or reading of TST

PROCEDURE 38.11 Administer an Intradermal Injection

Tasks
Prepare medication from a vial, administer an intradermal injection, read the tuberculin skin test, and document in the health record.

Equipment and Supplies
- Provider's order
- Patient's health record
- Vial of medication
- Alcohol wipes
- 1 mL syringe with ¼- to ⅝-inch, 25-27 gauge safety needle
- Bandage (if per facility's policy)
- Medication tray
- Biohazard sharps container
- Waste container
- Drug reference information
- Gloves
- Marker and pen

Order
Tuberculin purified protein derivative (PPD) (5 tuberculin units) 0.1 mL ID.

Procedural Steps
1. Draw medication up from a vial (see Procedure 38.8).
2. Prior to entering the exam room, knock on the door and give it a moment. Greet the patient. Identify yourself. Verify the patient's identity with full name and date of birth. Make sure the patient's information matches the order and the record. Explain what you are going to do.
   Purpose: It is important to identify the patient in two different ways to ensure that you have the correct patient. Explaining the procedure can make the patient feel more comfortable and helps to reduce anxiety.

CHAPTER 38 Administering Medication

PROCEDURE 38.11 Administer an Intradermal Injection—cont'd

3. Provide the right education to the patient. Explain the medication ordered, the desired effect, and common side effects; also identify the provider who ordered it. Answer any questions the patient may have. Use language the patient can understand. Ask the patient if he or she has any allergies. If the patient refuses the medication, notify the provider.
   Purpose: The patient needs to be aware of what you are giving, its action and side effects, and who ordered it. It is also important to double-check the patient's allergies before administering the medication.
4. Perform the right technique. Ask the patient:
   - Can you return in 48 to 72 hours for the reading?
   - Have you ever had BCG?
   - Have you ever had a TB skin test? If yes, did you have a reaction to it?

   Purpose: These questions are important to determine if the patient should get the test or if the medical assistant should talk with the provider.
5. Use hand sanitizer and put on gloves.
   Purpose: Hand sanitization is an important step for infection control.
6. Have the patient extend a forearm with the palm facing upward. Identify an appropriate site for an injection. The site should be 2 to 4 inches below the elbow. Loosen the cap on the needle, but still protect the needle from contamination. Open the alcohol wipes.
   Purpose: The site should be free from veins, scars, wounds, abrasions, etc. If the person has a reaction, having the site away from the elbow doesn't limit its motion. Loosening the cap prior to starting allows you to remove the cap with one hand during the procedure.
7. Place your nondominant hand to the side of the site, pulling the skin taut (Fig. 1). Option: Place your nondominant hand on the back of the patient's forearm, pulling the skin taut (Fig. 2).
   Purpose: The skin needs to be taut to insert the needle.
8. Cleanse the site with an alcohol wipe using a circular motion. Move from the center outward, using some friction to help clean the site. Create about a 2-inch circle at the site. Let the site dry while continuing to hold the area.
   Purpose: Cleaning from the inside to the outside prevents contamination of the cleaned area. Avoid waving over or blowing on the alcohol, which contaminates the site.
9. Pick up the syringe and tip it to remove the cover. Grasp the syringe in your dominant hand, using your thumb and index finger. Make sure to have no fingers under the syringe. Ensure that the bevel is up.
   Purpose: The syringe needs to be lowered to the skin after it is inserted. Having fingers under the syringe changes the angle and can affect the administration.
10. At a 5- to 15-degree angle, slowly insert the needle until the bevel is covered with skin (Fig. 3). Carefully lower the syringe to the skin and hold it steady with your dominant hand (Fig. 4).
    Purpose: If a greater angle is used or if more of the needle is inserted, the injection may be given deeper than it should be. Holding the syringe against the skin helps support it during the injection.

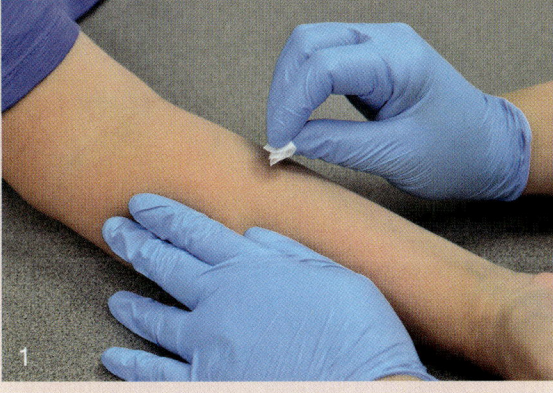

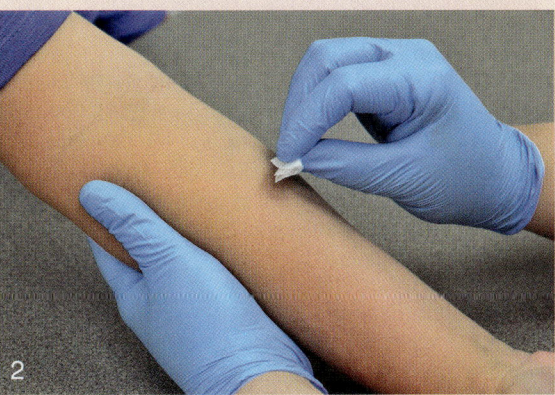

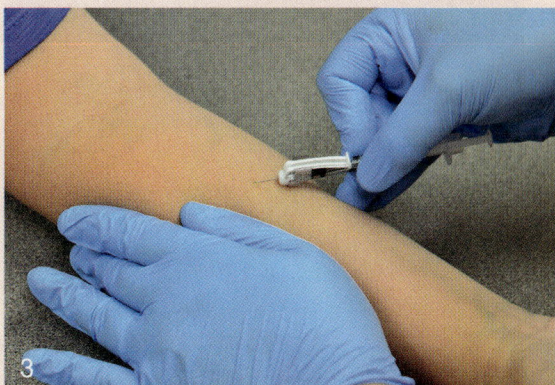

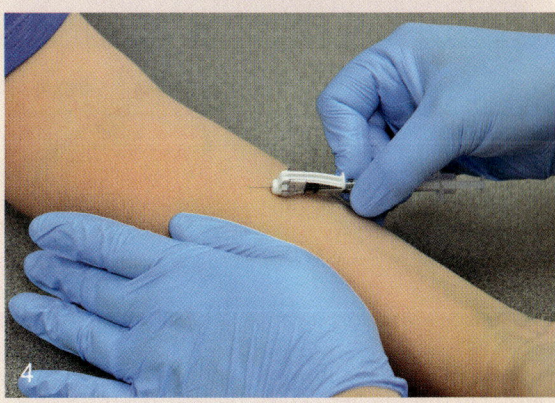

Continued

PROCEDURE 38.11   Administer an Intradermal Injection—cont'd

11. Carefully move your nondominant hand to the plunger. Slowly and steadily inject the medication by pressing on the plunger (Fig. 5). If a 6 to 10 mm wheal does not appear, repeat the test at least 2 inches from the site (Fig. 6).
    Purpose: Any movement of the needle/syringe can dislodge the needle from the site.

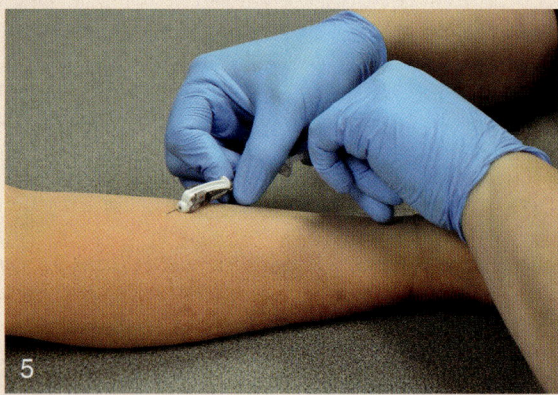

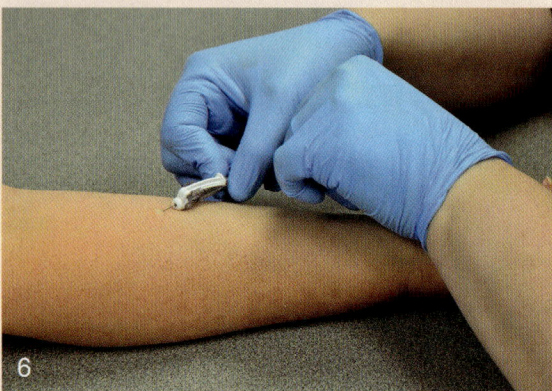

12. Double-check the barrel of the syringe to make sure all the medication was administered. Withdraw the needle. Activate the needle's safety device with one hand.
    Purpose: It is important to administer all the medication. Using more than one hand to activate the safety device increases the risk for needlestick injuries.
13. Discard the needle/syringe in a biohazard sharps container. Make sure to put the needle in first.
    Purpose: Safely discarding the needle/syringe will help prevent needlestick injuries.
14. Do not massage the area. Per the facility's policy, if the person has a light-colored shirt with long sleeves, offer a bandage. Place the bandage on very loosely to just absorb any blood from the site.
    Purpose: It is very important that the bandage not be put on snugly, because some of the medication could be lost at the site. If a bandage is used, it needs to be very loosely applied. Some agencies will not allow the use of a bandage.
15. Observe the patient for any adverse reactions. Clean up the area. Discard the waste in the waste container. Sanitize your hands.
    Purpose: It is important to monitor the patient and clean up the work area.
16. Document the procedure in the health record. Include assessments done, allergies, teaching or instructions provided, the medication name, dose, and route, the provider who ordered the medication, and how the patient tolerated the medication. Also include the manufacturer, the lot number, and the expiration date of the vial.
    Purpose: Medications given need to be documented to indicate they were given.

Scenario Update
The patient returns for the reading.

17. Check the health record to identify the location of the test. Greet the patient. Identify yourself. Verify the patient's identity with full name and date of birth. Make sure the patient's information matches the order and the record. Explain what you are going to do.
    Purpose: It is important to identify the patient in two different ways to ensure that you have the correct patient. Explaining the procedure can make the patient feel more comfortable and helps to reduce anxiety.
18. Palpate the site for an induration. If an induration is felt, ask the patient if you can write on his or her arm. Using a ball point pen, draw a line towards the induration from the outer edge of the arm. Repeat on the other side (Fig. 7). *Option:* Palpate the induration to find edge and mark edge, and then mark the edge with a pen. Repeat on the other side. Using a millimeter ruler, accurately measure the distance between the two points.
    Purpose: The ball point pen will stop at the edge of the induration. This provides you with two visible points to measure the size of the induration.

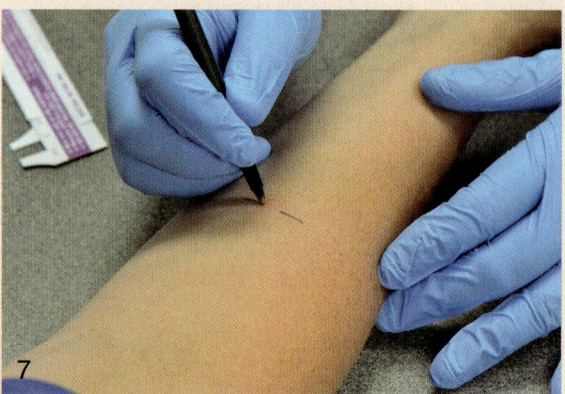

19. Document the reading in the patient's health record. Include the reason for the patient's visit, the test site, the size of the induration in millimeters, and the provider notified.
    Purpose: The medical assistant must document the size of the induration if one is present. If no induration is present, then document 0 mm. The provider will determine if the test is negative or positive.

Documentation Example 1
11/1/20XX 0805 NKA. No prior history of TST. Per Dr. Martin's order, administered: Tuberculin purified protein derivative (PPD) 0.1 mL (5 tuberculin units) ID left forearm. (Vial: ABC Manufacturer, Lot#1345, Expires 10/20XX). Pt tolerated test without a problem. Test side effects discussed with pt prior to administration. Pt instructed to return between 48 and 72 hours, and follow-up appointment was made. Pt had no questions and verbalized understanding of instructions._____Gabe Garcia CMA (AAMA)

Documentation Example 2
11/3/20XX 1005 Pt returned for TST reading. Left forearm induration measured 4 mm. Dr. Martin was notified._____Gabe Garcia CMA (AAMA)

Two-Step Testing. In some patients who have had a TB infection, the body "forgets" to react to the TST. This can occur if the infection was many years ago. The initial TST may be negative, and the person may have a false-negative reaction. Receiving a second TST can help the body "remember" the infection, thus causing a more accurate (positive) reading. This is called the *booster effect* or *booster phenomenon*. The second TST can be done 1 to 3 weeks after the initial test was read.

New residents in long-term care facilities (e.g., nursing homes) usually have a two-step TST done. Healthcare students and professionals also need to have a two-step TST. Once the two-step TST is completed, they need yearly TSTs. If the time since the last TST exceeds 1 year, they may need to complete another two-step TST. Fig. 38.31 shows what occurs if the initial test result is positive or negative.

> **CRITICAL THINKING BOX 38.8**
>
> Gabe and Mark are working with Julia Berkley, who has come in for a physical prior to starting college. She is going into health care, and her paperwork indicates that she needs a two-step TB skin test. Julia asks what this means. How might you explain a two-step TB skin test?

Blood Tuberculin Tests. The FDA has approved two blood tuberculin tests: the QuantiFERON-TB Gold In-Tube test (QFT-GIT) and the T-SPOT TB test (T-Spot). If a patient has had the BCG vaccine or is unable to return for the skin test reading, the blood test is preferred. The blood test replaces the skin test. A healthcare professional or student only needs one blood test initially, unlike the two-step skin test. After the initial test, a yearly skin or blood tuberculin test is required.

After the medical assistant draws a patient's blood, it is sent to the laboratory for analysis. The error rate with a blood test is much lower than with the palpated, measured reading of the TST. If the TB blood test result is:

- Positive: The person has been infected with TB. The provider will order additional tests to determine if the person has latent TB infection or TB disease. (See Chapter 11 for more information on these two diseases.)
- Negative: It is unlikely the person has TB.

Allergy Testing

Allergy testing is done to identify a patient's food, medication (e.g., penicillin), or environmental allergies. It is important that the patient prepare for the test (Box 38.16). After meeting with the patient and reviewing the allergy symptoms and medical history, the provider will determine what allergies should be tested. There are three direct skin tests commonly used:

- *Skin prick test*: Involves placing a small amount of the allergen on the skin (forearm, upper arm, or back). The skin is pricked, and the allergen goes under the surface. Several allergens can be tested at the same time. Once the test is given, the patient is monitored. After 15 to 20 minutes the medical assistant measures the erythema (redness) and the induration at each site.
- *Intradermal skin test*: Involves giving small amounts of the allergen using the intradermal route. This is used for bee venom and penicillin allergy testing. It can also be used if the skin prick test was negative and the provider still believes the patient has the allergy.
- *Patch test*: Involves taping possible allergens to the skin for 48 hours (Fig. 38.32). The test results are measured in 72 to 96 hours.

Typical direct skin test guidelines are discussed in Box 38.17.

Sometimes the provider will order a blood test for certain allergens instead of doing the direct skin test. A serum antibody test (blood test) is required. Specific immunoglobulin E antibodies are increased in people with allergies. In the past the tests were called RASTs (radioallergosorbent test). The RASTs used radioactivity to detect the antibodies, but current tests do not. A multiple-antigen simultaneous test (MAST) is a blood test that can examine multiple antigens at the same time. The blood tests are not affected by antihistamines taken by the patient, unlike the skin tests. The results are available in a few days.

> **BOX 38.16 Patient Education Prior to Allergy Testing**
>
> Prior to the appointment, it is important that patients stop medications that may mask or hide allergies. Typically, guidelines include:
>
> - Stop long-acting antihistamines for 5 days before the testing. Examples include cetirizine (se TI ra zeen) (Zyrtec), desloratadine (des lor AT a deen) (Clarinex), fexofenadine (fex oh FEN a deen) (Allegra), and loratadine (lor AT a deen) (Claritin, Alavert).
> - Stop all over-the-counter (OTC) cold, sleep, and allergy medications; prescribed allergy medication; and specific acid reflux medications 3 days before testing. Examples include diphenhydramine (dye fen HYE dra meen) (Benadryl), meclizine, (MEK li zeen), famotidine (fa MOE ti deen) (Pepcid), and ranitidine (ra NI ti deen) (Zantac).

> **BOX 38.17 Direct Allergy Testing Guidelines**
>
> - Select an appropriate testing site. Sites should be at least 1 inch apart so reactions are independent from each other. Mark sites with pen to indicate allergen.
> - Put on gloves and cleanse sites with an alcohol wipe prior to the test.
> - Measure sites after the proper waiting time. Document both the erythema and the induration.
> - Monitor the patient for 30 minutes after administration of the tests for severe allergy reactions.
> - After the testing, the pen marks can be removed with alcohol wipes. Per the provider's order, apply diphenhydramine cream to the test sites. This will reduce the erythema, itchiness, and indurations.
> - A positive and negative control test will also be done with the direct skin test to ensure the accuracy of the results. The negative test usually uses normal saline. Some patients will have a minor reaction at the injection site due to the needle entry. The positive test usually uses a histamine that should cause a 3 mm induration reaction with surrounding erythema.

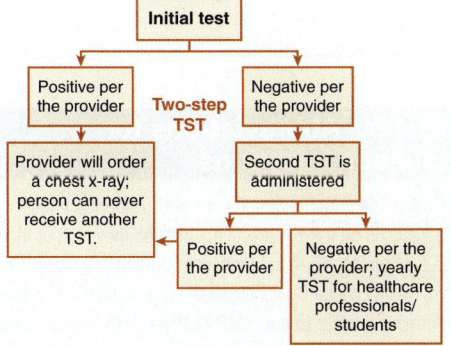

FIG. 38.31 The process with two-step TST test.

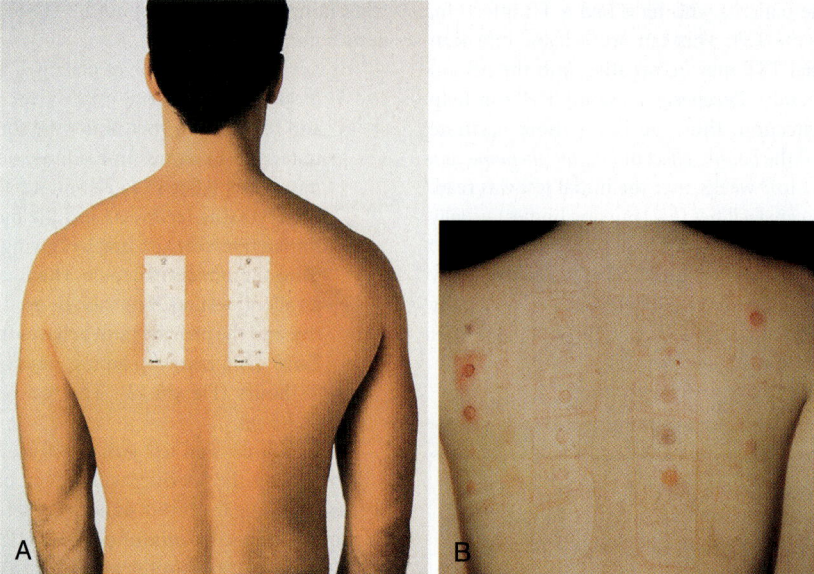

FIG. 38.32 (A) For the allergen patch test, a patch impregnated with individual allergens is applied to the patient's back. (B) Positive allergy reactions of varying intensity. (From Habif TP: *Clinical Dermatology*, ed 5, St Louis, 2010, Mosby.)

SUBCUTANEOUS INJECTIONS

Subcutaneous (subcut) injections involve placing medication into the subcutaneous layer, under the dermis (Fig. 38.33 and Box 38.18). The subcutaneous layer has fewer blood vessels than the muscles. The medication absorbs slower in the subcutaneous layer compared to medications injected into the muscles. The patient may complain of discomfort or pain with a subcutaneous injection. Subcutaneous tissue contains pain receptors. Table 38.5 contains a quick summary of subcutaneous injection information. Common medications given via the subcutaneous route include:

- Several vaccines, for example: measles-mumps-rubella (MMR), varicella, shingles, and polio
- Enoxaparin (Lovenox) and heparin
- Insulin

Administration Techniques

When a subcut injection is given, the angle depends on the needle length. If a ⅝-inch needle is used, then the medical assistant should use a 45-degree angle. If a ½-inch needle is used, then a 90-degree angle should be used. It is important to pinch up the tissue with the index finger and thumb of the nondominant hand. This ensures that the injection is given into the subcutaneous tissue.

Aspiration. Aspiration is used to check if the needle is in a blood vessel. This is done once before the medication is given. (The aspiration technique will be discussed in detail in the IM section, later in the chapter.) With subcut injections, the aspiration should be done if the medication manufacturer recommends it. It should also be done if it is part of the facility's policy.

Insulin, which is given subcut, is not aspirated. Subcut immunizations do not need to be aspirated, per the Centers for Disease Control and Prevention (CDC). Anticoagulants (AN tee koe ag yuh lahnts), such as enoxaparin (Lovenox) (Box 38.19) and heparin, are administered in the abdomen. They are not aspirated, per the manufacturers. Hold pressure to the site after the injection until the bleeding has stopped.

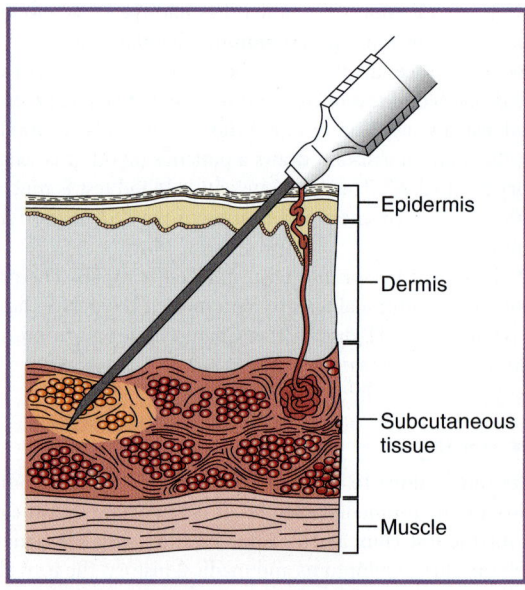

FIG. 38.33 The subcutaneous (subcut) injection is administered in the subcutaneous layer. This method is used for small amounts of nonirritating medications in aqueous solution. (From Proctor D, et al: *Kinn's The Medical Assistant*, ed 13, St Louis, 2017, Elsevier.)

> **BOX 38.18 Abbreviations for Subcutaneous Injections**
>
> There have been many abbreviations for subcutaneous injections over the years. Some may still be used in practice, although they are not recommended. The Institute for Safe Medication Practices (ISMP) discourages the use of: SC, SQ, and sub q. Healthcare professionals should use "subcut" or "subcutaneously." For more information, refer to the ISMP website: http://www.ismp.org/tools/errorproneabbreviations.pdf.

CHAPTER 38 Administering Medication

TABLE 38.5 Quick Summary of Subcutaneous (Subcut) Injections

Syringe used	3 mL most common; 1 mL could be used
Needle size and angle of entry	25 gauge; ½ inch with a 90 degree angle of entry, or ⅝ inch with a 45 degree angle of entry. The bevel position doesn't matter.
Maximum volume	0.5–1.5 mL (0.5 mL in children)
Common sites	Lower abdomen, anterior thigh, and upper outer arm (see Fig. 38.34)
Sites for vaccines	<1 yr: anterior thigh >1 yr: upper outer arm or anterior thigh
Additional sites	Separate sites by 1 inch
Patient position	Sitting
Administration technique	Pinch site. If 2 inches of tissue can be pinched, insert the needle at a 90-degree angle. If 1 inch of tissue can be pinched, insert the needle at a 45-degree angle. Rotate sites.

BOX 38.19 Special Considerations When Giving Enoxaparin

When administering enoxaparin (Lovenox), follow these instructions:
- Make sure the drug is clear and colorless or pale yellow.
- Do not push any air or drug out of the syringe before giving the injection unless your healthcare provider tells you to. The air allows the medication to enter slower, reducing the risk of bruising.
- Using your finger and thumb, pinch a fold of skin 1 to 2 inches away from the umbilicus in the lower abdomen. Push the entire needle into the skin. Press down on the syringe plunger and inject the medication. Hold the pinched skin the entire time during the injection. Remove the needle. Do not rub or massage the site after the injection.

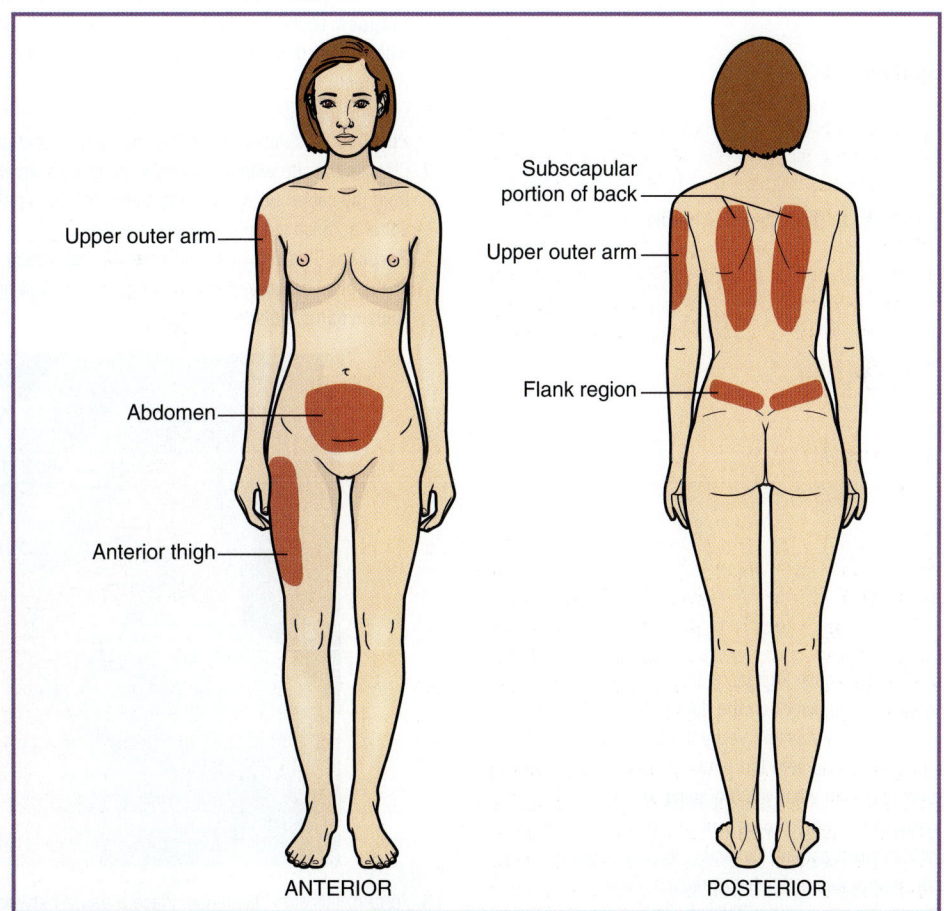

FIG. 38.34 The subcutaneous (subcut) injection sites commonly used include the outer posterior aspect of the upper arm, the lower abdomen, and the anterior aspect of the thigh. The subscapular portion of the back and the flank region are other subcut sites.

Subcutaneous Sites

Typically, three subcut sites are used in ambulatory care:
- **Abdominal site:** Have the patient remove the clothing in that area. Provide a drape sheet if needed to protect the patient's modesty. The site is located below the costal margins to the iliac crests. Stay 2 inches away from the umbilicus. It is important to stay away from the waistline and any scars. The patient may have more discomfort if the injection is given at the waistline due to the rubbing of clothing.
- **Outer posterior aspect of the upper arm:** Expose the arm. The outer posterior site extends from 3 inches above the elbow to about 3 fingerbreadths below the acromion process. It is important to stay away from the shoulder area.
- **Anterior aspect of the thigh:** Place one hand above the knee and the other hand below the greater trochanter. The site is the middle one third of the thigh. The site extends from the front midline to the back midline, wrapping around the outer thigh. Usually only the middle one third – from the front midline to the outer thigh – is used. Injections are not done on the back of the leg, because sitting would irritate the injection site.

Procedure 38.12 describes the steps in giving a subcutaneous injection.

PROCEDURE 38.12 Administer a Subcutaneous Injection

Tasks
Prepare medication from a vial, administer a subcutaneous injection, and document the medication administration in the health record.

Scenario
Dr. Martin ordered polio vaccine (IPV) 0.5 mL subcut for Johnny Parker (DOB 06/15/2010). (Vial information: ABC Manufacturer, Lot #1234, expires 1 year from today)

Equipment and Supplies
- Provider's order
- Patient's health record
- Vial of medication
- Alcohol wipes
- 3 mL syringe with $\frac{5}{8}$-inch or $\frac{1}{2}$-inch, 25-gauge needle
- Gauze
- Bandage
- Medication tray
- Gloves
- Biohazard sharps container
- Waste container
- Drug reference information
- VIS for polio vaccine (IPV) (optional)
- Gloves
- Marker

Order
Polio vaccine (IPV) 0.5 mL subcut.

Procedural Steps
1. Draw medication up from a vial (see Procedure 38.8 or 38.9).
2. Prior to entering the exam room, knock on the door and give it a moment. Greet the parent/patient. Identify yourself. Verify the patient's identity with full name and date of birth. Make sure the patient's information matches the order and the record. Explain what you are going to do.
   Purpose: It is important to identify the patient in two different ways to ensure that you have the correct patient. Explaining the procedure can make the patient feel more comfortable and helps to reduce anxiety.
3. Provide the right education to the parent/patient. Explain the medication ordered, the desired effect, and common side effects; also identify the provider who ordered it. Answer any questions the patient may have. Use language the patient can understand. Ask the patient if he or she has any allergies. If the patient refuses the medication, notify the provider.
   Purpose: The patient needs to be aware of what you are giving, its action and side effects, and who ordered it. It is also important to double-check the patient's allergies before administering the medication.
4. Use hand sanitizer and put on gloves.
   Purpose: Hand sanitization is an important step for infection control.
5. Loosen the cap on the needle, but still protect the needle from contamination. Open the alcohol wipes. Have gauze and a bandage available.
   Purpose: Loosening the cap prior to starting allows you to remove the cap with one hand during the procedure. You should never remove the cap with your teeth.
6. Find the injection site.
   Purpose: It is important to find the correct location for the injection.
7. Cleanse the site with an alcohol wipe using a circular motion (Fig. 1). Move from the center outward, using some friction to help clean the site. Create about a 2-inch circle at the site. Let the site dry.
   Purpose: Cleaning from the inside to the outside prevents contamination of the cleaned area. Avoid waving over or blowing on the alcohol, which contaminates the site.

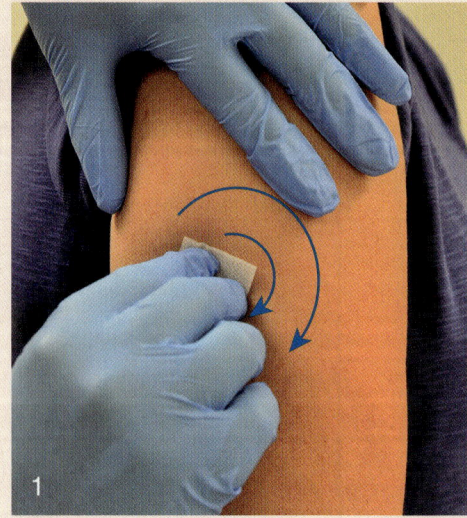

8. Perform the right technique. Place a gauze between the index and middle fingers of your nondominant hand. With that hand, use your index finger and thumb to pinch up at the cleansed area.
   Purpose: The site needs to be pinched for a subcut injection.
9. Pick up the syringe and tip it to remove the cover. Hold the syringe between the thumb and index finger of your dominant hand (Fig. 2). Quickly and smoothly insert the needle into the site using at a 45- or 90-degree angle, depending on the needle size. Insert the entire needle. Make sure the needle

CHAPTER 38 Administering Medication

PROCEDURE 38.12 Administer a Subcutaneous Injection—cont'd

tip is not pointed towards your nondominant hand. Make sure the needle is not pointed towards your mondominant hand.

Purpose: Ensuring that the tip is not pointed towards your hand will lessen the needlestick risk. Aspiration for subcut injections is based on the facility's policy and the recommendation from the manufacturer.

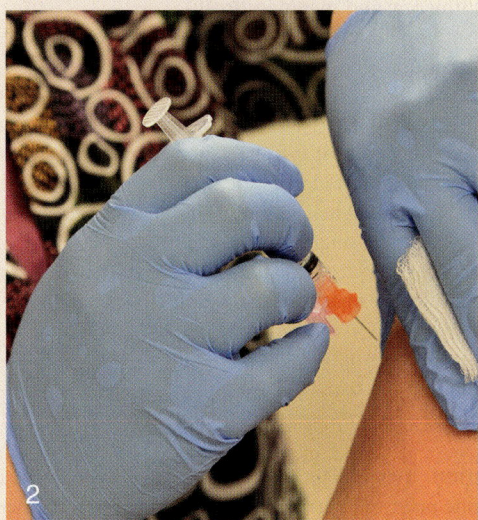

10. *One-hand option:* Continue to pinch the site. Securely grasp the syringe between your fingers of your dominant hand. With your dominant hand, aspirate if required, and then push the plunger to inject the medication. *Two-hand option:* Release the pinch and with the nondominant hand, aspirate if required, and then push the plunger to inject the medication.

    Purpose: Follow the facility's policy on whether to use the one- or two-hand option.

11. Inject the medication at a rate of 1 mL over 10 seconds. Ensure that all the medication has been injected before pulling out the needle at the same angle used for entry. Release the pinch if using the one-hand option.

    Purpose: Injecting the medication too slowly or to quickly can be uncomfortable for the patient.

12. Activate the needle's safety device with one hand while using the other hand to cover the site with gauze. Gently apply pressure at the site to stop any bleeding. Apply a bandage if the patient requests it.

    Purpose: Ask the patient if he or she would like a bandage if the site has stopped bleeding. Remember that some bandages may contain latex, which can be an allergen to some people. Some people may be allergic to the adhesive.

13. Discard the needle/syringe in a biohazard sharps container. Make sure the needle goes into the sharps container first.

    Purpose: Safely discarding the needle/syringe will help prevent needlestick injuries.

14. Observe the patient for any adverse reactions. Clean up the area. Discard the waste in the waste container. Sanitize your hands.

    Purpose: It is important to monitor the patient and to clean up the work area.

15. Document the procedure in the health record. Include assessments done, allergies, teaching or instructions provided, the provider who ordered the medication, the medication's name, dose, and route, and how the patient tolerated the medication. Also include the manufacturer, the lot number, and the expiration date for vaccines and controlled substances. Fig. 3 shows the documentation using an electronic health record.

    Purpose: Medications given need to be documented to indicate they were given.

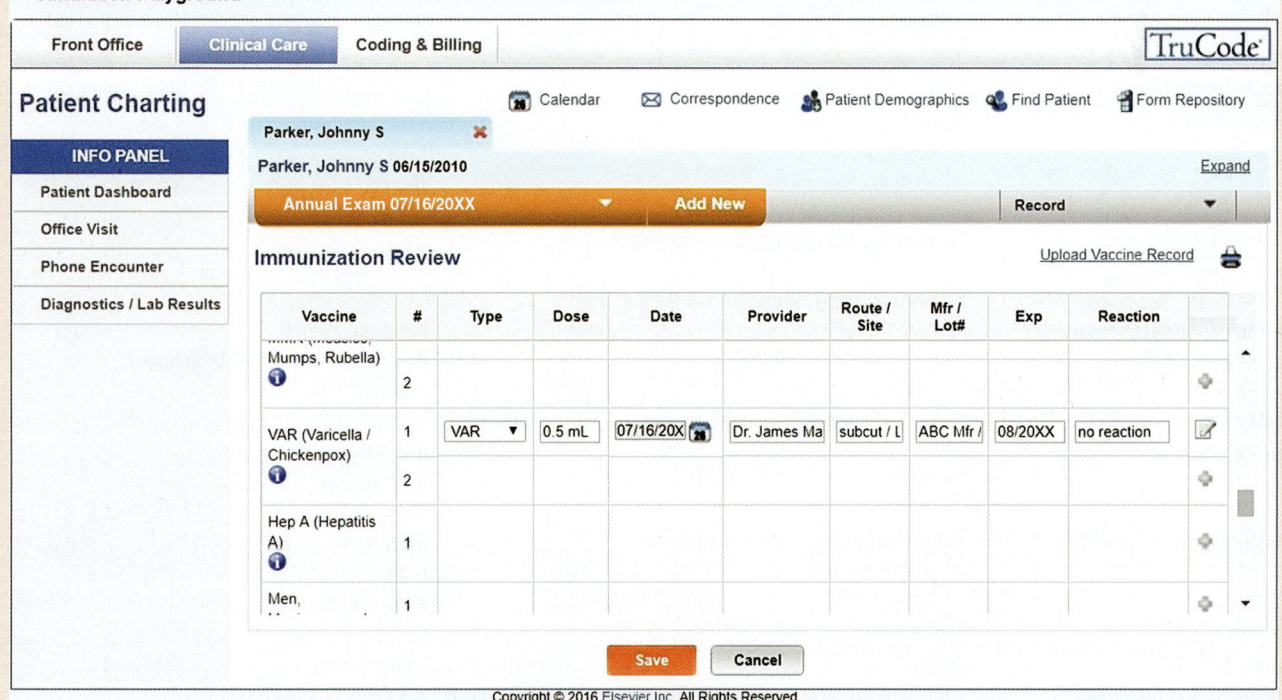

INTRAMUSCULAR INJECTIONS

Intramuscular injections involve placing medication into the muscle (Fig. 38.35). There are more blood vessels in the muscles; thus, absorption is faster than in the subcutaneous layer. For medications given by IM injection, *aqueous* (watery) medications should be given with a higher gauge needle than that used for oil-based medications. Table 38.6 contains a quick summary of intramuscular injection information. Common medications given via the intramuscular route include:
- Several vaccines, for example: Hepatitis A and B; tetanus-diphtheria (dif THEHR ee ah) (Td), or with pertussis (per TUS is) (Tdap); influenza; and meningococcal
- Antibiotics and medroxyprogesterone (me DROX ee proe JES te rone) (Depo-Provera)

Administration Techniques

As with all injections, it is important to do the procedure safely. The medical assistant must identify the correct site and follow the guidelines for medical asepsis. When administering an IM injection, it is important to use a 90-degree angle for entry. The skin should be flattened or stretched over the site with the nondominant hand. Administration techniques for IM injections consist of:
- Being safe
- Minimizing pain
- Finding the correct site

The follow sections will address these three goals.

Aspiration. When giving an intramuscular injection, it is important to aspirate prior to injecting the medication. Once the needle is in the site, the medical assistant should pull back on the plunger for 5 seconds and check the barrel of the syringe. Lack of blood in the barrel means the needle is not in a blood vessel – it is safe to inject the medication. If blood appears in the barrel, remove the needle, discard the syringe, and restart the procedure. Immunizations do not need to be aspirated, per the CDC.

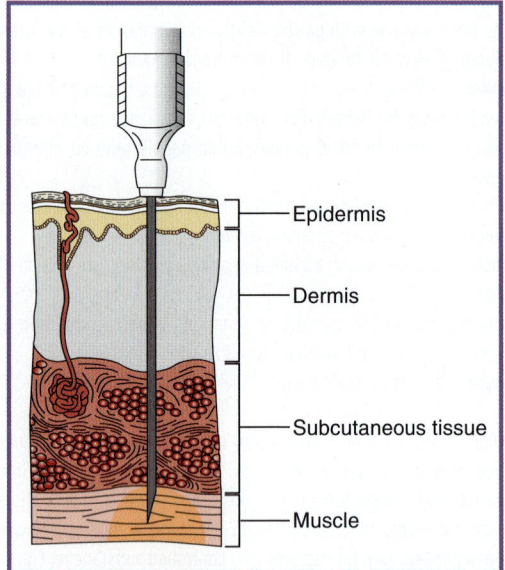

FIG. 38.35 Anatomical illustration of the intramuscular (IM) injection. Note that the needle is inserted at a 90-degree angle, which deposits the medication into the large central part of the muscle. (From Proctor D, et al: *Kinn's The Medical Assistant*, ed 13, St Louis, 2017, Elsevier.)

TABLE 38.6 Quick Summary of Intramuscular (IM) Injections

	Deltoid	Vastus Lateralis	Ventrogluteal
Syringe used	3 mL		

Needle length (determined by the patient's size)	1–11 yr: ⅝–1 inch
	Adults: ⅝–1½ inch
	By weight:
	    <130 lb: ⅝ inch
	    130–152 lb: 1 inch
	    Females 152–200 lb/males 152–260 lb: 1–1½ inch
	    Females >200 lb/males >260 lb: 1½ inch
		0–28 days: ⅝ inch
		1–12 mo: 1 inch
		1–18 yr: 1–1¼ inch
		18+ yr: 1–1½ inch
			Birth–28 days: ⅝ inch
			1 mo–12 yr: 1 inch
			12+ yr: 1–1½ inch

Needle gauge (G) (determined by the medication)	22-25 G	Children: 22-25 G Adults: **oil-base**: 18-21 G; **aqueous**: 20-25 G	
Angle of entry	90 degrees (bevel doesn't matter)		
Maximum volume	1 mL for teens and adults	Birth–1 yr: 1 mL 1–11 yr: 2 mL 12+ yr: 3 mL	
Sites for vaccines per CDC	1–3 yr: Only if muscle mass is adequate 3+ yr: Can be used	Birth–1 yr: required 1–3 yr: Preferred 3+ yr: Can be used	
Additional sites	Separate sites by 1 inch		
Patient position	Sitting	Sitting, supine	Side lying
Administration technique	Stretch the skin over the injection site. Use a 90 degree angle of entry.		
Possible complications	Necrosis, hematoma, ecchymosis (bruising), abscess, pain, and vascular and nerve injuries		

Air Lock Technique. When an IM injection is given, the air lock technique can be used. Remove the bubbles in the syringe and measure the exact amount of medication needed. Once these steps have been done, add 0.2 to 0.5 mL of air into the syringe. This is the known as the *air lock technique*. When the IM injection is given, the medication is pushed in first, followed by the air. When the needle is withdrawn, the air creates a "lock," keeping the medication in the muscle. The air fills in the needle hole. The air lock prevents the irritating medication from tracking back up the tissues to the skin, creating pain for the patient.

Z-Track Technique. The Z-track technique is another injection method that can reduce pain and discomfort for the patient. Like the air lock technique, this method prevents the medication from tracking back through the subcutaneous tissue. The medication is sealed in the muscle, thus minimizing discomfort for the patient.

The Z-track technique should be used for irritating medications. The ventrogluteal site is the recommended site for injections of irritating medications. For the Z-track technique, the skin is pulled laterally with the medical assistant's nondominant hand. The site is cleansed, and the injection is given (Fig. 38.36A and B). As the needle is withdrawn, the skin is released (Fig. 38.36C).

Intramuscular Sites

Deltoid Site. The deltoid is a triangular-shaped muscle located near the shoulder and upper arm. This muscle site is used to give a small volume of aqueous medications, such as vitamin B_{12} and vaccines. The CDC recommends this site be used when vaccines are given to teens and adults. To find the site, expose the upper arm. Make sure the sleeve does not act as a tourniquet. If the sleeve is tight, have the patient slip the arm out of the shirt.

Palpate the acromion process (Fig. 38.37). Place a finger on the acromion process and then 2 fingers below that. The top of the site is

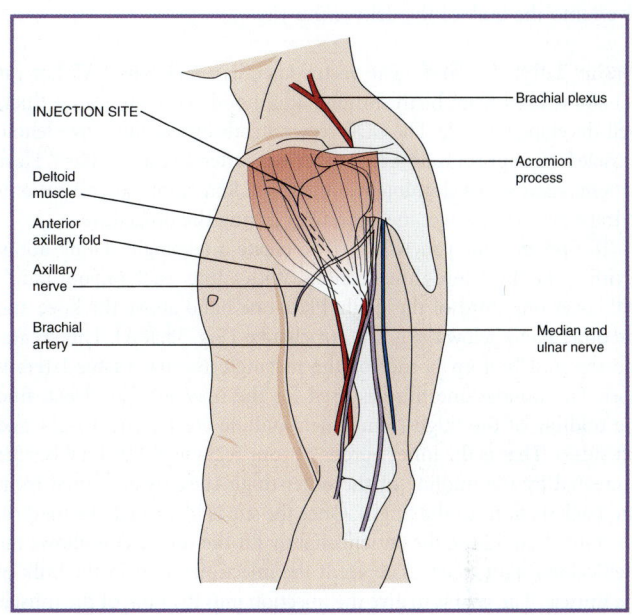

FIG. 38.37 Deltoid site. (From Proctor D, et al: *Kinn's The Medical Assistant*, ed 13, St Louis, 2017, Elsevier.)

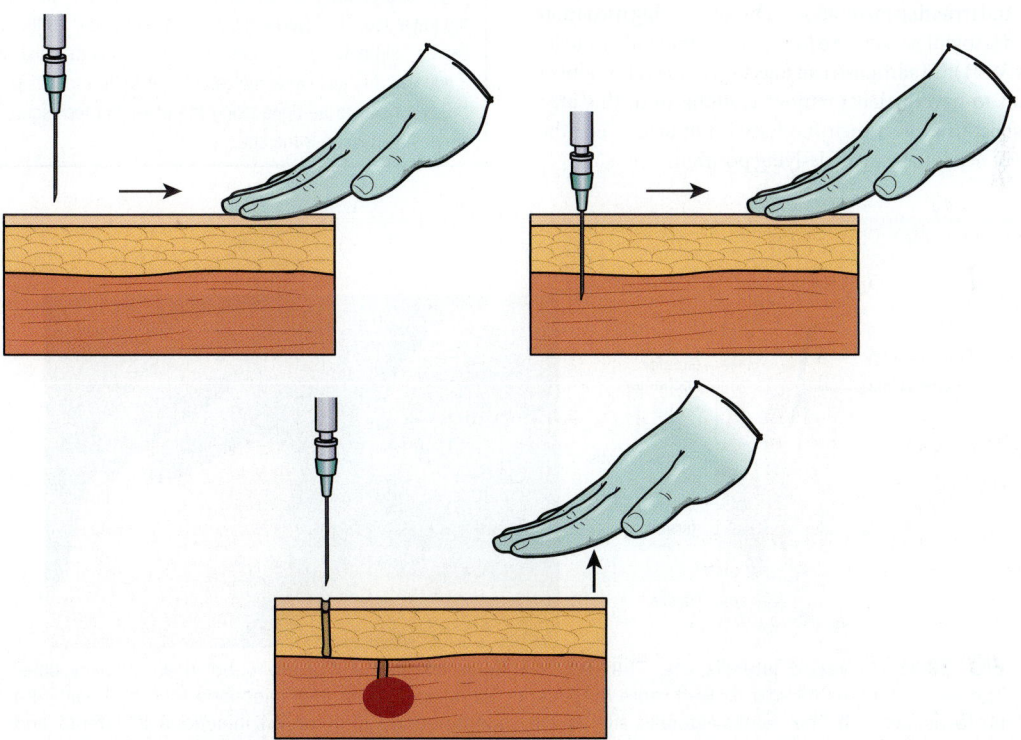

FIG. 38.36 Z-track technique. (A) Displace and then cleanse the skin. (B) Inject the medication. (C) Release the skin and pull the needle out at the same time. The medication is locked in the muscle.

1 to 2 inches (or 2 fingerbreadths) below the acromion process. The bottom of the site is at the anterior axillary fold (top of the axilla). The injection site should be somewhere between the top and the bottom of the site. Once the medical assistant finds the site, it is a good idea to have the patient lift his or her arm. The medical assistant can find the bulk (biggest part) of the deltoid muscle. The injection should be given into the bulk of the deltoid muscle.

Vastus Lateralis Site. The vastus lateralis (VAS tuhs LAT her ray lis) site is used from birth through adulthood. This site uses a thick, well-developed muscle. The CDC recommends this site until the deltoid muscle is the appropriate size for vaccines (after 1 year or older). Have patients remove the clothing over the thigh. Remember to give patients a drape sheet to protect their modesty during the procedure.

To find the site, you will need to create a rectangle. Think about dividing the thigh into three sections. With adults, each of your hands will cover one third of the thigh. Place one hand above the knee and the other hand below the greater trochanter (Fig. 38.38A). This creates the top and bottom border of the rectangle (or the vastus lateralis site). The middle one third is used for the injection site. Next, find the midline of the thigh (remember, midline creates equal right and left sides). That is the inner border of your rectangle. The final border is created by the midline of the outer thigh (i.e., creates equal front and back sections of the thigh). Once the site is identified, the medical assistant should have the patient slightly lift the thigh. This allows the medical assistant to check to see if the injection site is in the bulk of the muscle. The goal is to give the injection into the bulk of the muscle (Fig. 38.38B). Procedure 38.13 describes the procedure for giving an intramuscular injection. Box 38.20 describes giving injections to small children.

Ventrogluteal Site. The ventrogluteal site is an excellent site for oil-based medications and irritating medications. This site is being used more often, because the dorsogluteal site is no longer a recommended site for IM injections (Box 38.21). To administer an injection in the ventrogluteal site, it is important to have patients remove clothing from this area. Offering a drape sheet to protect their modesty is important. For this injection, the patient needs to be in a side-lying position.

The most complex part of using the ventrogluteal site is to ensure that the correct hand is used to find the site. Remember to use the hand opposite the injection site. For instance, if the injection site is on the patient's left side, then use your right hand. Follow these steps to find the site:
- Place the palm of your hand on the patient's greater trochanter (Fig. 38.39).
- Your fingers need to point towards the patient's head, and your thumb to the patient's groin. (If your thumb is facing the patient's back side, you are using the wrong hand!)
- Place your index finger on the anterior superior iliac spine. If your fingers are short or if the patient is tall, point your index finger towards the anterior superior iliac spine.
- Move your middle finger back along the iliac crest towards the patient's buttock.

The positioning of your index and middle fingers forms a triangle. The injection point is at the center of the triangle. Remember, if you are giving an irritating medication, use the Z-track method to help reduce pain. Procedure 38.14 describes the steps of the Z-track technique.

> **BOX 38.20 Giving Injections to Small Children**
>
> For injections given to small children, the subcutaneous (subcut) and intramuscular (IM) sites in the thigh are in the same location. It is helpful to have the parent/guardian hold the child's upper body and hands (however, the medical assistant should anticipate that the adult may not hold securely). If another staff member is available, having him or her hold the lower extremities is helpful. Many times children may need more than one injection. For this scenario, it is helpful to have two medical assistants each give an injection at the same time.
>
> The medical assistant should hold the joint above the injection site and hold the lower leg. The lower leg can be carefully bent off the table. The lower leg can be held between the side of the table and the medical assistant's body. If you use this technique, be careful not to hurt the child's leg. Injections for children need to be done using the one-hand technique, because the other hand is holding near the site.

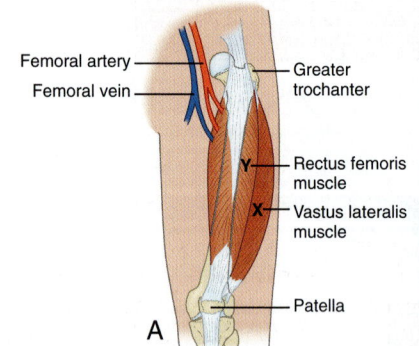
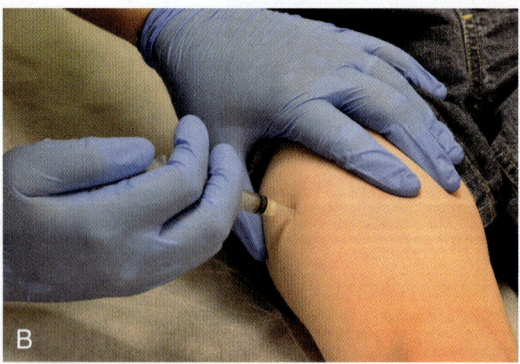

FIG. 38.38 (A) Vastus lateralis site. The vastus lateralis muscle is typically used in ambulatory care. The rectus femoris muscle is used more by patients for intramuscular (IM) injections than by healthcare professionals. (B) The vastus lateralis site is the recommended site for IM injections in infants and young children. (From Proctor D, et al: *Kinn's The Medical Assistant*, ed 13, St Louis, 2017, Elsevier.)

PROCEDURE 38.13 Administer an Intramuscular Injection

Tasks
Prepare medication from a vial, administer an intramuscular injection, and document the medication administration in the health record.

Scenario
Dr. Martin ordered Influenza vaccine (IIV) 0.5 mL IM for Erma Willis (DOB 12/09/1947). (Vial information: MN Manufacturer, Lot #7845, expires 1 year from today).

Equipment and Supplies
- Provider's order
- Patient's health record
- Vial of medication
- Alcohol wipes
- 3 mL syringe
- 22-25 gauge, 1–1½-inch needle
- Gauze
- Bandage
- Medication tray
- Biohazard sharps container
- Waste container
- Drug reference information
- VIS for influenza vaccine (optional)
- Gloves
- Marker

Order
Influenza vaccine (IIV) 0.5 mL IM.

Procedural Steps

1. Draw medication up from a vial (see Procedure 38.8).
2. Prior to entering the exam room, knock on the door and give it a moment. Greet the patient. Identify yourself. Verify the patient's identity with full name and date of birth. Make sure the patient's information matches the order and the record. Explain what you are going to do.
   Purpose: It is important to identify the patient in two different ways to ensure that you have the correct patient. Explaining the procedure can make the patient feel more comfortable and helps to reduce anxiety.
3. Provide the right education to the patient. Explain the medication ordered, the desired effect, and common side effects; also identify the provider who ordered the medication. Answer any questions the patient may have. Use language the patient can understand. Ask the patient if he or she has any allergies. If the patient refuses the medication, notify the provider.
   Purpose: The patient needs to be aware of what you are giving, its action and side effects, and who ordered it. It is also important to double-check the patient's allergies before administering the medication.
4. Use hand sanitizer and put on gloves.
   Purpose: Hand sanitization is an important step for infection control.
5. Loosen the cap on the needle, but still protect the needle from contamination. Open the alcohol wipes. Have gauze and a bandage available.
   Purpose: Loosening the cap prior to starting allows you to remove the cap with one hand during the procedure. You should never remove the cap with your teeth.
6. Find the site using the landmarks.
   Purpose: It is important to find the correct location for the injection.
7. Cleanse the site with an alcohol wipe using a circular motion. Move from the center outward, using some friction to help clean the site. Create about a 2-inch circle at the site. Let the site dry.
   Purpose: Cleaning from the inside to the outside prevents contamination of the cleaned area. Avoid waving over or blowing on the alcohol, which contaminates the site.
8. Perform the right technique. Place a gauze between the index and middle fingers of your nondominant hand. With that hand, stretch or flatten the site. Hold the site.
   Purpose: The site needs to be flattened or stretched for an intramuscular injection.
9. Pick up the syringe and tip it to remove the cover. Hold the syringe like a dart with your dominant hand (Fig. 1). Quickly and smoothly insert the needle into the site at a 90-degree angle. Insert the entire needle.
   Purpose: Inserting the needle quickly is important to minimize pain.

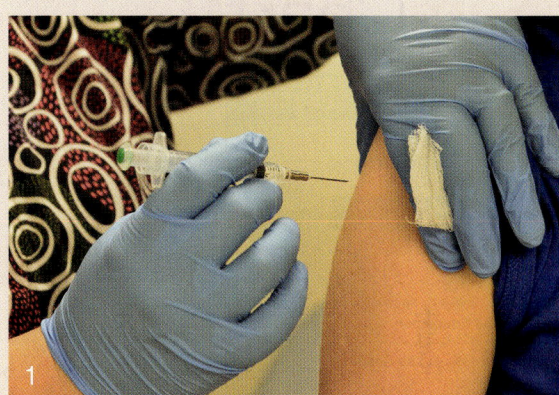

10. *One-hand option:* Continue to hold the site. Securely grasp the syringe between the fingers of your dominant hand. Place your thumb under the plunger edge and push the plunger out farther to aspirate (Fig. 2). *Two-hand option:* Move the nondominant hand to the plunger. Pull the plunger out farther to aspirate.
    Purpose: It is important to aspirate before giving an IM injection. Follow the facility's policy on whether to use the one- or two-hand option.

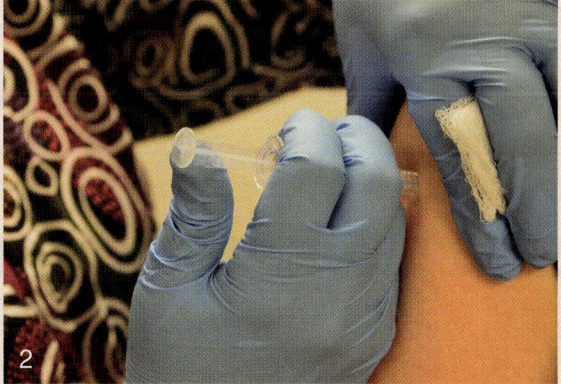

11. Aspirate for 5 seconds and check the barrel for blood. If blood is seen, pull out the needle and discard. Restart the procedure. If no blood is seen, inject the medication at a rate of about 10 seconds per milliliter. Ensure that all the medication has been injected before pulling out the needle at the same angle used for entry.
    Purpose: It is important not to give the injection if the needle is in the bloodstream.

Continued

PROCEDURE 38.13 Administer an Intramuscular Injection—cont'd

12. Activate the needle's safety device with one hand while using the other hand to cover the site with gauze. Gently apply pressure at the site to stop any bleeding. Apply a bandage if the patient requests it.
    Purpose: Ask the patient if he or she would like a bandage if the site has stopped bleeding. Remember that some bandages may contain latex, which can be an allergen to some people. Some people may be allergic to the adhesive.
13. Discard the needle/syringe in a biohazard sharps container. Make sure to put the needle in first.
    Purpose: Safely discarding the needle/syringe will help prevent needlestick injuries.
14. Observe the patient for any adverse reactions. Clean up the area. Discard the waste in the waste container. Sanitize your hands.
    Purpose: It is important to monitor the patient and clean up the work area.
15. Document the procedure in the health record. Include assessments done, allergies, teaching or instructions provided, the provider who ordered the medication, the medication's name, dose, and route, and how the patient tolerated the medication. Also include the manufacturer, lot number, and expiration date for vaccines and controlled substances. Fig. 3 shows the documentation using an electronic health record.
    Purpose: Medications given need to be documented to indicate they were given.

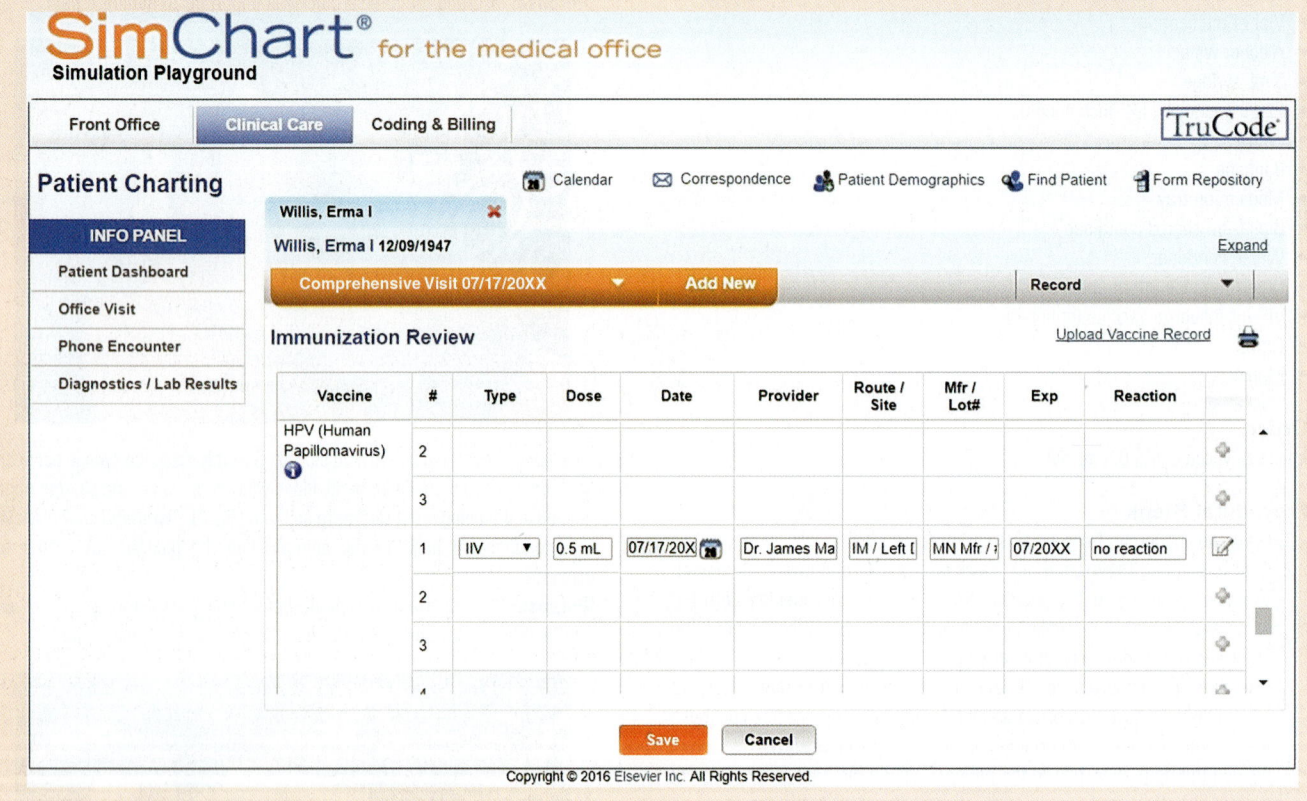

BOX 38.21 Dorsogluteal Site

The dorsogluteal site was a very common intramuscular (IM) site for irritating medications. However, the dorsogluteal site is near the sciatic nerve and large blood vessels. Over the years, many patients developed complications because of dorsogluteal injections. Agencies have had to defend lawsuits related to dorsogluteal injection complications.

Current evidence has demonstrated that dorsogluteal sites pose a high risk for injury. The current recommendation is that the dorsogluteal site should not be used. The ventrogluteal site is ideal for the medications that were always given in the dorsogluteal site. Many healthcare professions have moved away from teaching the dorsogluteal site since the recommendation became public.

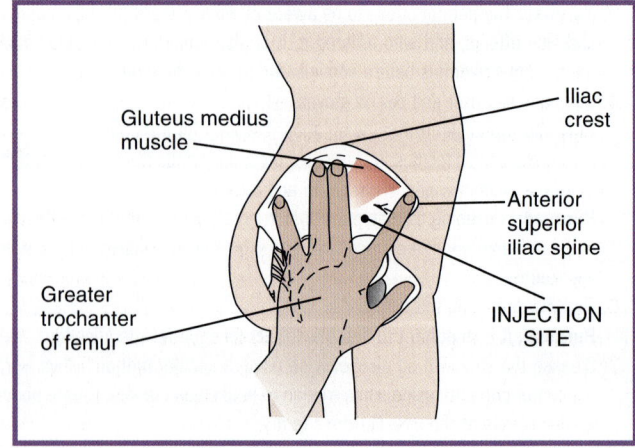

FIG. 38.39 Ventrogluteal site.

CHAPTER 38   Administering Medication

MONITORING INTRAVENOUS THERAPY

Intravenous therapy is performed by nurses in ambulatory care facilities. IVs can be used to deliver medication and fluids. A needle inside a catheter is used to start the IV. The needle is removed, and the catheter is hooked up to the IV tubing that runs from the insertion site to the IV bag. The nurse must start the IV, adjust the flow, and monitor the patient during the procedure.

The medical assistant's role with IVs includes scheduling a patient for an IV infusion. It is important to schedule the IV infusion at the appropriate time. Sometimes the patient may need to come in for an IV medication that is scheduled every so many hours. It is important to keep the patient on schedule with the medication.

Sometimes the clinical medical assistant may assist the nurse with checking on the patient. The medical assistant should be aware of common problems that can arise with IVs. The nurse needs to be notified of any problems immediately. Common concerns with IV therapy include:
- Edema (swelling) or increasing pain at the IV insertion site
- Blood moving up the IV tubing
- An almost-empty bag of fluids
- A patient who is having difficulty breathing or who has increased audible wheezing

---

PROCEDURE 38.14   Administer an Intramuscular Injection Using the Z-Track Technique

Task
Prepare medication from a vial, administer an intramuscular injection, and document the medication administration in the health record.

Scenario
Dr. Martin orders Iron Dextran 0.5 mL IM for Erma Willis (DOB 12/09/1947). (Vial information: FE Manufacturer, Lot #625, expires 1 year from today)

Equipment and Supplies
- Provider's order
- Patient's health record
- Vial of medication
- Alcohol wipes
- 3 mL syringe
- 22-25 gauge, 1–1½-inch needle
- Gauze
- Bandage
- Medication tray
- Biohazard sharps container
- Waste container
- Drug reference information
- Gloves
- Marker

Provider's Order
Iron Dextran 0.5 mL IM

Procedural Steps

1. Draw medication up from a vial (see Procedure 38.8).
2. Prior to entering the exam room, knock on the door and give it a moment. Greet the patient. Identify yourself. Verify the patient's identity with full name and date of birth. Make sure the patient's information matches the order and the record. Explain what you are going to do.
   Purpose: It is important to identify the patient in two different ways to ensure that you have the correct patient. Explaining the procedure can make the patient feel more comfortable and helps to reduce anxiety.
3. Provide the right education to the patient. Explain the medication ordered, the desired effect, and common side effects; also identify the provider who ordered the medication. Answer any questions the patient may have. Use language the patient can understand. Ask the patient if he or she has any allergies. If the patient refuses the medication, notify the provider.
   Purpose: The patient needs to be aware of what you are giving, its action and side effects, and who ordered it. It is also important to double-check the patient's allergies before administering the medication.
4. Use hand sanitizer and put on gloves.
   Purpose: Hand sanitization is an important step for infection control.
5. Loosen the cap on the needle, but still protect the needle from contamination. Open the alcohol wipes. Have gauze and a bandage available.
   Purpose: Loosening the cap prior to starting allows you to remove the cap with one hand during the procedure. You should never remove the cap with your teeth.
6. Find the site using the landmarks.
   Purpose: It is important to find the correct site.
7. Perform the right technique. Place a gauze between the index and middle fingers of your nondominant hand. With that hand, displace the tissue.
   Purpose: The tissue needs to be displaced before you cleanse the site.
8. Cleanse the site with an alcohol wipe using a circular motion. Move from the center outward, using some friction to help clean the site. Create about a 2-inch circle at the site. Let the site dry while continuing to hold the area.
   Purpose: Cleaning from the inside to the outside prevents contamination of the cleaned area. Avoid waving over or blowing on the alcohol, which contaminates the site.
9. Pick up the syringe and tip it to remove the cover. Hold the syringe like a dart with your dominant hand. Quickly and smoothly insert the needle into the site at a 90-degree angle. Insert the entire needle.
   Purpose: Inserting the needle quickly is important to minimize pain.
10. Continue to hold the site. Securely grasp the syringe between the fingers of your dominant hand. Place your thumb under the plunger edge and push the plunger out farther to aspirate.
    Purpose: It is important to aspirate before giving an IM injection. Follow the facility's policy on whether to use the one- or two-hand option.
11. Aspirate for 5 seconds and check the barrel for blood. If blood is seen, pull out the needle and discard. Restart the procedure. If no blood is seen, inject the medication at a rate of about 10 seconds per mL. Ensure that all the medication has been injected. Wait 10 seconds before withdrawing the needle and letting go with your nondominant hand.
    Purpose: It is important not to give the injection if the needle is in the bloodstream. Waiting 10 seconds allows the medication to start absorbing.
12. Activate the needle's safety device with one hand while using the other hand to cover the site with gauze. Gently apply pressure at the site to stop any bleeding. Apply a bandage if the patient requests it.

Continued

PROCEDURE 38.14 Administer an Intramuscular Injection Using the Z-Track Technique—cont'd

Purpose: Ask the patient if he or she would like a bandage if the site has stopped bleeding. Remember that some bandages may contain latex, which can be an allergen to some people. Some people may be allergic to the adhesive.

13. Discard the needle/syringe in a biohazard sharps container. Make sure to put the needle in first.
    Purpose: Safely discarding the needle/syringe will help prevent needlestick injuries.
14. Observe the patient for any adverse reactions. Clean up the area. Discard the waste in the waste container. Sanitize your hands.
    Purpose: It is important to monitor the patient and also clean up the work area.

15. Document the procedure in the health record. Include assessments done, allergies, teaching or instructions provided, the provider who ordered the medication, the medication's name, dose, and route, and how the patient tolerated the medication. Also include the manufacturer, lot number, and expiration date for vaccines and controlled substances.
    Purpose: Medications given need to be documented to indicate they were given.

Documentation Example
11/1/20XX 1420 NKA. Per Dr. Martin's order, administered Iron Dextran 0.5 mL IM in left ventrogluteal site using Z-track method. Pt stated she had pain initially but is feeling better. Side effects were discussed with pt prior to administration. Pt had no questions and verbalized understanding of instructions._____Gabe Garcia CMA (AAMA)

CLOSING COMMENTS

The medical assistant has an important role in administering medications. Paying attention to details is critical. If a medication error occurs, the medical assistant must act immediately. It is important to immediately notify the provider. The provider will identify what steps need to be taken. The medical assistant needs to also complete an incident report. (Incident reports are discussed in Chapter 17). The supervisor needs to also be notified. In most cases the supervisor will ensure that the patient is not charged for the medication given in error. The supervisor may also need to complete a state or federal report on the medication error.

EXCEPTIONAL CUSTOMER SERVICE

The medical assistant can provide exceptional customer service by paying attention to details when administering medications. Teaching patients prior to the administration and monitoring patients for side effects are important. Any questions or concerns the medical assistant has should be discussed with the provider.

CHAPTER REVIEW

This chapter covered the Nine Rules of Medication Administration: the right medication, dose, route, time, patient, education, technique, and documentation, and the right to refuse. Comparing the label with the order three times is important before giving the medication.

The form is the physical characteristics of a medication, and the route is how the medication gets into the body. Routes discussed include oral, sublingual (under the tongue), buccal (in the cheek), transdermal, inhalation, topical (e.g., vaginal, rectal, nasal, ocular, and otic), irrigation, and parenteral.

The gauge and length of needles are important considerations when giving injections. The gauge is selected based on the thickness of the medication. The length is based on the size of the patient and the type of injection. Safety needles help prevent needlesticks. Most safety needles require the medical assistant to activate the safety device after the injection.

When you are preparing medication using an ampule, it is important to use a filter needle to withdraw the medication. Single-dose or multidose vials are available. It is important to add the expiration date to the multidose vials. Reconstituting powdered medications requires the correct diluent, as indicated by the manufacturer. All the medication powder needs to be dissolved before the dose can be withdrawn. When you measure medications, it is important to get the bubbles (air) out of the syringe before measuring the correct dose.

Common intradermal sites include the forearm, upper arm, and back. TST and allergy tests are common ID injections. Tuberculosis testing can include either a skin test or a blood test. The two-step TST helps to ensure that the test results are accurate. The advantage of the blood test is that the patient does not need to return for the TST reading in 48 to 72 hours. Also, it replaces the two-step TST.

Insulin and several vaccines are given by a subcut injection. The subcutaneous sites include the abdomen, posterior outer upper arm, and middle third of the thigh. Subcut injections absorb slower than IM injections.

The deltoid, vastus lateralis, and ventrogluteal muscles are the common sites used for IM injections. The Z-track technique can be added to the procedure to help minimize discomfort with irritating medications. The air lock technique can also be used. It is important to aspirate prior to injecting the medication.

SCENARIO WRAP-UP

Gabe and Mark continued to work together for the remaining weeks of practicum. Mark had the opportunity to give several TSTs. He was able to do subcut and IM injections also. Mark learned the importance of distracting patients during injections; they seemed to tolerate the injection much better.

One of the other medical assistants had a medication error. The medication was given to the wrong patient. This error really impressed on Mark the importance of the nine rules of medication administration. He is adamant that he will never forget to follow each rule each time he gives medications. He doesn't want to deal with a medication error.

39

Cardiopulmonary Procedures

LEARNING OBJECTIVES

1. Review the structures and functionality of the cardiovascular system.
2. Use correct electrocardiography (ECG) terminology, discuss ECG waves and segments, and describe ECG intervals.
3. Describe the medical assistant's role in a resting 12-lead ECG. Also, list and discuss bipolar (standard) leads, augmented leads, and chest (precordial) leads.
4. Describe ECG supplies and equipment.
5. Prepare a patient for an ECG, and obtain an electrocardiogram.
6. Troubleshoot artifacts in an ECG.
7. Evaluate an ECG tracing.
8. Identify abnormal rhythms in an ECG tracing.
9. Discuss additional ECG testing, including exercise stress tests, nuclear stress tests, Holter monitors, cardiac event recorders, implantable loop recorders, transtelephonic monitoring, and portable handheld ECG monitors.
10. Discuss the respiratory system, measure the peak flow rate, and perform spirometry.
11. Describe pulmonary treatments, including metered-dose inhalers, nebulizer treatments, and oxygen therapy.

CHAPTER OUTLINE

1. **Opening Scenario**, 934
2. **You Will Learn**, 934
3. **Introduction**, 934
4. **Cardiovascular System Review**, 934
    a. Heart Structure, 934
    b. Blood Flow, 935
    c. Heart's Conduction System, 936
5. **ECG Tracing**, 937
    a. ECG Terminology, 937
    b. ECG Waves and Segments, 937
    c. ECG Intervals, 938
6. **12-Lead ECG**, 939
    a. Bipolar (or Standard) Leads, 939
    b. Augmented Leads, 939
    c. Chest (or Precordial) Leads, 939
7. **ECG Supplies and Equipment**, 939
    a. Thermal ECG Paper, 940
    b. Electrodes, 941
    c. Electrocardiograph, 941
        i. *Settings and Calibration*, 942
8. **ECG Procedure**, 942
    a. Patient Preparation, 942
    b. Applying Electrodes and Lead Wires, 945
    c. Running the ECG Tracing, 946
    d. Troubleshooting Artifact, 947
        i. *Wandering Baseline*, 947
        ii. *Somatic Tremor*, 947
        iii. *AC Interference*, 947
        iv. *Interrupted Baseline*, 948
    e. Evaluating an ECG Tracing, 948
        i. *Rate*, 948
        ii. *Rhythm*, 948
        iii. *Analyzing an ECG Tracing*, 948
    f. Identifying an Abnormal Rhythm, 948
        i. *Sinus Arrhythmias*, 948
        ii. *Atrial Arrhythmias*, 948
        ii. *Heart Block*, 949
        iv. *Ventricular Arrhythmias*, 949
        v. *Implantable Device Rhythms*, 950
    g. Finishing the ECG, 950
9. **Additional ECG Testing**, 951
    a. Exercise Stress Test, 951
    b. Nuclear Stress Test, 952
    c. Holter Monitor, 952
    d. Cardiac Event Recorder, 952
    e. Implantable Loop Recorder, 953
    f. Transtelephonic Monitoring, 954
    g. Portable Handheld ECG Monitors, 954
10. **Respiratory System**, 954
    a. Pulmonary Function Tests, 954
        i. *Peak Flow Rate*, 955
        ii. *Spirometry*, 955
    b. Pulmonary Treatments, 956
        i. *Metered-Dose Inhalers*, 956
        ii. *Nebulizer Treatment*, 958
        iii. *Oxygen Therapy*, 958
11. **Closing Comments**, 962
12. **Chapter Review**, 962

OPENING SCENARIO

Renee Thomas, CMA (AAMA), is a Certified Medical Assistant at Walden-Martin Family Medical (WMFM) Clinic. According to her manager, over the time that she has been with WMFM Clinic, she has excelled. Because of Renee's professionalism and attention to detail, her manager, Sue, has asked her to mentor a new medical assistant, Eva Ning.

Eva Ning, RMA, just graduated from a local medical assistant program. She really enjoyed the hands-on learning with the skills. Now that she has graduated, she looks forward to learning on the job.

Eva and Renee will spend a month with each provider. This month they are working with Dr. David Kahn, who sees many older patients. Renee tells Eva that they will be doing a lot of cardiopulmonary tests and treatments. Eva looks forward to learning from Renee and Dr. Kahn.

YOU WILL LEARN

- To describe the components of the ECG tracing.
- To obtain a clear ECG and to reduce artifacts in a tracing.
- To describe other types of ECG tests.
- To perform pulmonary testing procedures, including peak flow reading and spirometry.
- To perform pulmonary treatments, including nebulizer treatments and oxygen therapy.

INTRODUCTION

Heart disease is the leading cause of death in the United States. Medical assistants in primary and specialty areas often care for patients with heart disorders. All medical assistants must:
- Understand the cardiovascular system
- Recognize early symptoms of potential disorders
- Coach patients on cardiopulmonary tests and treatments ordered by providers
- Accurately perform cardiopulmonary tests
- Identify and troubleshoot problems when performing tests

The heart is a complex organ. Electrical impulses move through the heart, and the cells react by contracting. The contracting cells result in contraction of the chambers. The contractions cause the blood to move through the heart and out to the arteries. To monitor the heart's function, both the electrical and mechanical activities of the heart can be assessed. When a provider needs to assess the electrical activity of the heart, an electrocardiogram (ee leck troh kar dee AH gram) is commonly ordered.

Electrocardiography is a painless test. Electrodes are placed on the body, and wires connect the electrodes to the ECG machine (*electrocardiograph*). The electrical impulse from the heart makes its way to the surface of the skin. Think of what occurs when you throw a rock into a lake. Waves are created, and they eventually make their way to the shore. The electricity from the heart eventually makes its way to the surface of the skin. The electrodes pick up the electricity, and the electricity moves into the machine. The electrocardiograph creates a record of the impulses, which is called an *electrocardiogram* (ECG, EKG).

A medical assistant performs the electrocardiography. The provider reads and interprets the ECG to identify any abnormalities in the electrical conduction in the heart. It is important for the medical assistant to:
- Know the normal function of the heart
- Perform the procedure accurately
- Identify problems during the ECG procedure and take appropriate actions

Besides ECGs, the medical assistant is responsible for pulmonary testing, including measuring the peak flow rate and performing spirometry (spi ROM e tree) testing. The medical assistant can administer nebulizer treatments and oxygen therapy, as ordered by the provider.

In this chapter, ECGs, pulmonary tests, and pulmonary treatments are discussed. The chapter begins with a review of the cardiovascular system. The components of the ECG and the process of obtaining an ECG follow the review. The chapter concludes with a discussion about pulmonary testing and treatments.

CARDIOVASCULAR SYSTEM REVIEW

Heart Structure

The heart is divided into four chambers. Two atrial chambers receive the blood from the body. Two ventricular chambers pump blood out to the body. The septum (SEP tum) divides the right and left sides of the heart.

The tricuspid (try KUSS pid) valve is found between the right atrium and the right ventricle (Fig. 39.1). The pulmonary valve is between the right ventricle and the pulmonary artery. The bicuspid (bye KUSS pid), or mitral (MYE trul), valve is found between the left atrium and left ventricle. The aortic (AE ore tik) valve is between the left ventricle and the aorta. When the valves open, blood moves to the next chamber, or out of the heart through the arteries. The mechanical action of the heart and valves can be assessed by echocardiography (eck oh kar dee AH gruh fee) (ECHO).

The heart wall has three layers: the epicardium (eh pee KAR dee um), the myocardium (mye oh KAR dee um), and the endocardium (en doh KAR dee um). Cardiac muscle fibers in the myocardium are electrically linked together, forming "one unit." A myocardial cell forms a strong connection to the next cells through special junctions called *intercalated discs*. These discs allow electricity to flow freely from one cell to the next. The intercalated discs are responsible for the cell-to-cell communication that is required for coordinated muscle contraction. The intercalated discs help the muscle fibers form one unit that contracts all at once, instead of a little at a time. The one-unit approach is important, because the atria and ventricles need to contract in an appropriately timed and coordinated effort.

VOCABULARY

echocardiography: The use of ultrasonic waves directed through the heart to study the structure and motion of the heart. The visual record produced is called an *echocardiogram*.

electrocardiogram (ECG, EKG): A record or recording of electrical impulses of the heart as produced by an electrocardiograph.

electrodes: Adhesive patches that conduct electricity from the body to the ECG machine wires.

MEDICAL TERMINOLOGY

atri/o: atrium
atrium (singular), **atria** (plural)
cardi/o: heart
echo-: sound
electr/o: electricity

-gram: record, recording
-graphy: process of recording
sept/o: septum
septum (singular), **septa** (plural)
ventricul/o: ventricle

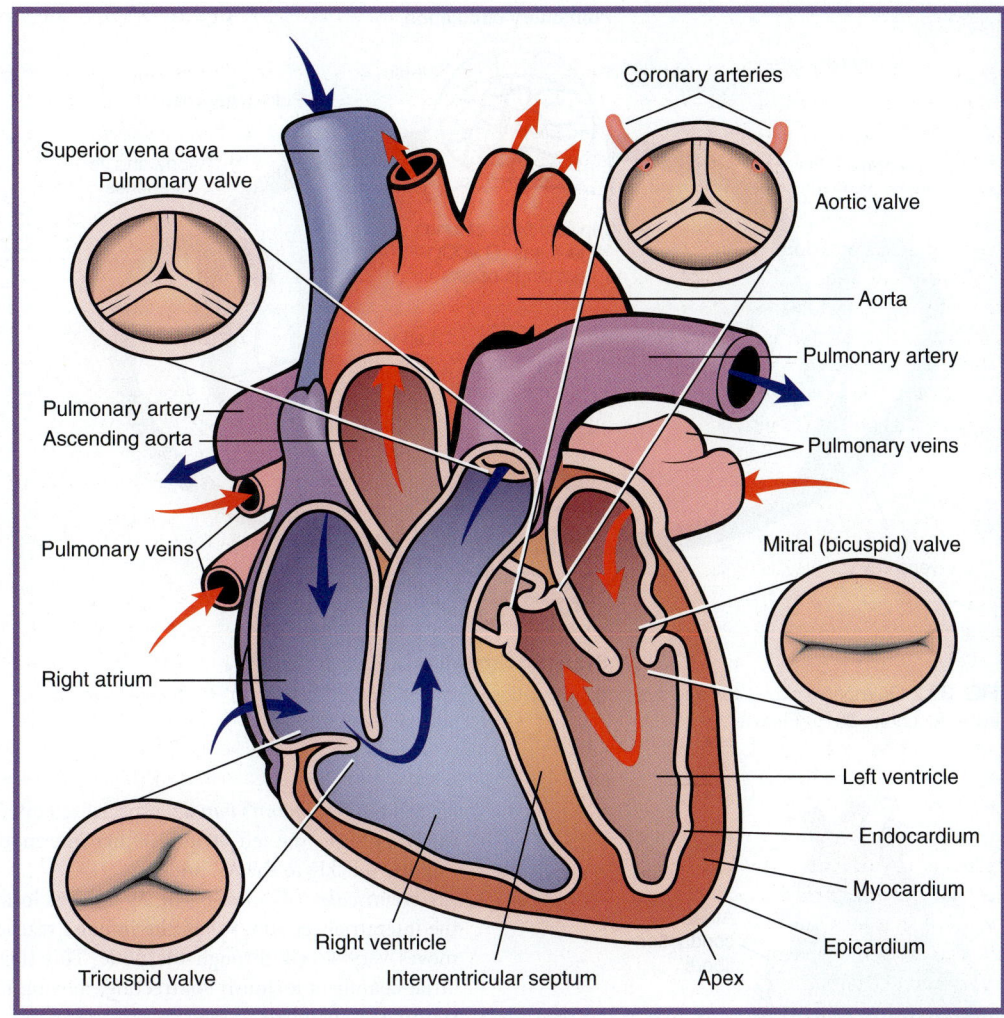

FIG. 39.1 Chambers and valves of the heart. (From Damjanov I: *Pathology for the Health-Related Professions*, ed 4, St Louis, 2012, Saunders.)

Blood Flow

The right atrium receives deoxygenated blood from the following structures:
- Superior vena cava (blood comes from the head, neck, and upper extremities)
- Inferior vena cava (blood comes from the thorax, abdomen, pelvis, and lower extremities)
- Coronary sinus (blood from the coronary veins)

When the right atrial chamber contracts, the tricuspid valve (atrioventricular [AV] valve) opens. Blood empties from the right atrium into the right ventricle. When the ventricles contract, the deoxygenated blood in the right ventricle passes through the opened pulmonary valve (semilunar [SL] valve) and moves into the pulmonary artery. The pulmonary artery brings the blood to the lungs. In the lungs, the blood picks up oxygen (O_2) and gives up carbon dioxide (CO_2). The pulmonary vein brings the oxygenated blood back to the left atrium. When the left atrial chamber contracts, the blood is pushed past the opened mitral (or bicuspid) valve (AV valve). The blood empties into the left ventricle. When the ventricles contract, the blood in the left ventricle moves through the opened aortic valve (SL valve) and into the aorta. The aorta transports oxygenated blood to the body. The first arteries to split off the aorta are the left and right coronary arteries. These arteries bring the oxygenated blood to the heart muscles (Fig. 39.2).

A complete heartbeat, or *cardiac cycle,* can be divided into diastole (di AS toe lee) and systole (SIS toe lee) phases. During the *diastole* phase, the heart is at rest and the atria fill with blood. The *systole* phase occurs when the heart is contracting.

MEDICAL TERMINOLOGY
endocardi/o: endocardium
myocardi/o: myocardium
epi-: above, on top of

CRITICAL THINKING BOX 39.1
Renee wanted to help Eva review the cardiovascular structures before they saw their first patient of the day. She asks Eva to describe the blood flow through the heart, starting with the superior vena cava and the inferior vena cava. If you were Eva, what would be your answer?

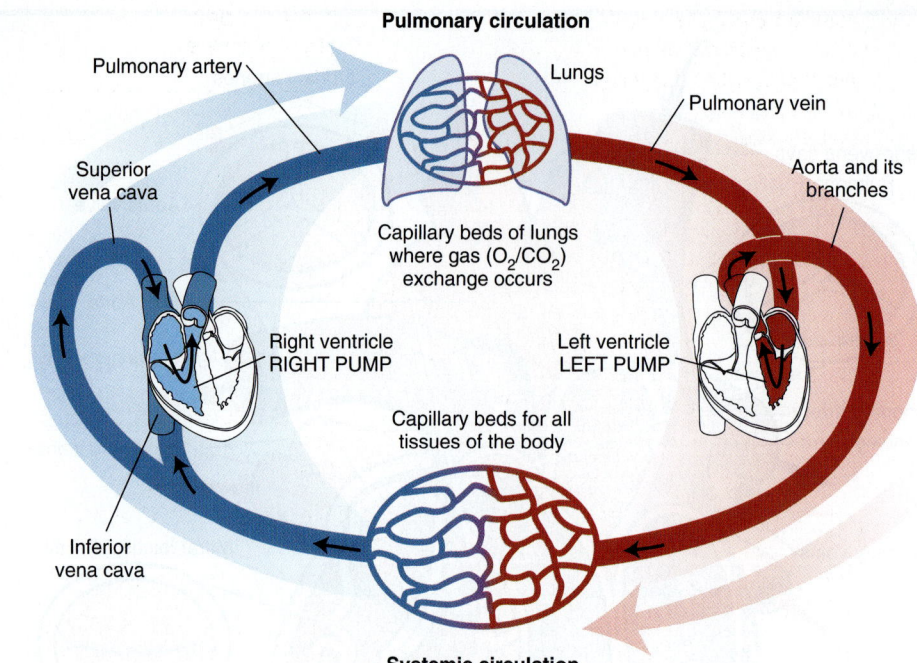

FIG. 39.2 Pulmonary circulation and systemic circulation. (From Shiland B: *Mastering Healthcare Terminology*, ed 5, St Louis, 2015, Elsevier.)

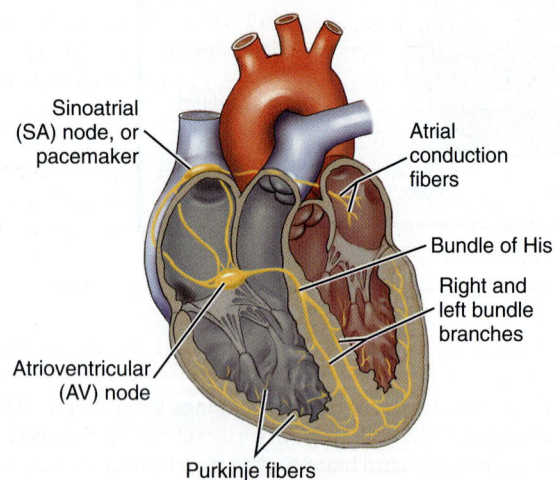

FIG. 39.3 Electrical conduction pathway of the heart. (From Shiland B: *Mastering Healthcare Terminology*, ed 5, St Louis, 2015, Elsevier.)

Heart's Conduction System

The electrical cells make up the conduction system of the heart. These cells are found throughout the myocardium. They can respond to and transmit electrical impulses to neighboring cells. The conduction system is composed of five structures:

1. *Sinoatrial* (SIE noe ae tree el) (SA) *node:* The SA node is called the "pacemaker of the heart" (Fig. 39.3). It is located in the posterior superior wall of the right atrium. The cardiac cells in the SA node generate the impulse. An impulse from the SA node starts each heartbeat. When the SA node discharges the impulse, it travels in many directions through the heart muscle. Nearby atrial cardiac cells slowly pick up the impulse. The impulse also moves quickly across special bands of tissue called *intermodal tracts* (in ter mohd ahl trakts). *Bachmann's bundle*, a specialized intermodal tract, takes the impulse to the left atrium. Other intermodal tracts take the impulse quickly to the AV node.
2. *Atrioventricular (AV) node:* The AV node is located at the base of the interatrial septum. When the impulse reaches the AV node, it moves very slowly through the node. This slowdown allows the atrial chambers to finish contracting, moving the blood into the ventricular chambers.
3. *Bundle of His* (or *AV bundle*): The bundle of His is located in the upper interventricular septum. When the impulse leaves the AV node, it moves to the bundle of His.
4. *Right and left bundle branches:* The bundle branches are located in the lower interventricular septum. After the impulse passes through the bundle of His, it enters the right and left bundle branches. The right bundle branch brings the impulse to the right ventricle. The left bundle branch brings the impulse to the left ventricle.
5. *Purkinje* (pur KIN jee) *fibers*: The bundle branches split into many Purkinje fibers. The Purkinje fibers transmit the impulse quickly and efficiently to the ventricular cardiac cells. This helps the ventricular chambers to contract.

The cardiac cells cycle through three states, or steps, in the same sequence for each impulse.

1. *Polarized state*: Before the impulse hits the cardiac cell, the cell is in the resting state, or *resting potential*. The inside of the cardiac cell is negatively charge. Outside of the cell is positively charged. There is no electrical activity seen on the ECG during the polarized state.
2. *Depolarized state*: When the impulse hits the cardiac cell, large amounts of positively charged sodium ions (AHY ons) move into the cell. A small amount of potassium ions moves outside of the cell. The

> **VOCABULARY**
>
> **ion**: An electrically charged atom, or the smallest component of an element,

movement of sodium and potassium changes the cell's charge to positive. The change, also called *action potential*, allows the impulse to move through the cell. *Depolarization* (when the impulse hits the cell) causes electrical activity on the ECG.

3. *Repolarized state*: After the impulse passes over the cell, the sodium and potassium ions move back to their original locations. This causes the cell's charge to change back to a negative charge. This recovery phase is called the *repolarized state*. Electrical activity (less than the depolarized state) can be recorded during the repolarized state.

Remember that the impulse occurs first. Very soon after the impulse occurs, the contraction starts. These are two very distinct activities yet appear very closely together. The electrical activity from the depolarized state and the repolarized state is recorded on the ECG. The contractions are mechanical actions and are not recorded on the ECG. An ECHO can be used to gather information on the mechanical action of the heart.

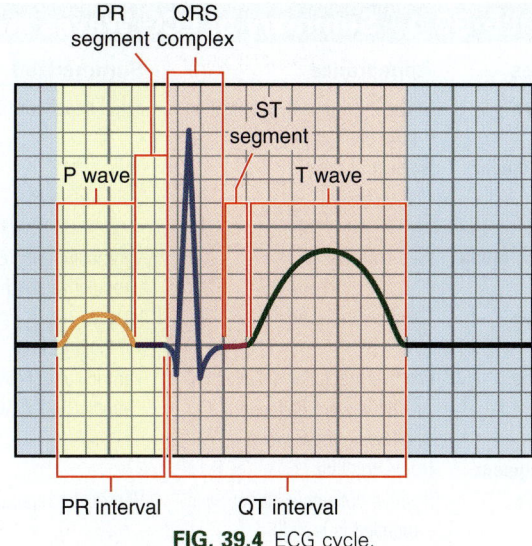

FIG. 39.4 ECG cycle.

> ### STUDY TIP
> Think of the three states as:
> - Polarized state – resting state
> - Depolarized state – discharge (impulse) state
> - Repolarized state – recovery state
>
> Remember when discussing these three states that the cardiac chamber comes before the word (e.g., atrial polarization).

> ### STUDY TIP
> Remember that the electrocardiogram (ECG) measures the electrical activity, and the echocardiography (ECHO) assesses the mechanical action (e.g., valves opening and closing).

> ### CRITICAL THINKING BOX 39.2
> Renee, knowing they have ECGs scheduled for today, asks Eva to list the conduction system in order and briefly describe polarization, depolarization, and repolarization. How might Eva answer this question?

ECG TRACING

The medical assistant performs the ECG procedure. The ECG is read or interpreted by the provider. It is important for the medical assistant to understand the components of the ECG tracing. A medical assistant must be able to identify **artifact** in the recording. If artifact is seen, corrective action needs to be taken to get a clear ECG tracing. The medical assistant will also need to know how to identify life-threatening rhythms. When these are seen, it is important that the medical assistants get immediate help. Artifact and life-threatening rhythms will be discussed later in the chapter.

> **VOCABULARY**
> **artifact:** A substance, structure, or event that does not naturally occur in a situation. Examples include interference, or electrical "garbage," on an ECG, or crystals, lint, or contamination of a staining technique.

ECG Terminology

To understand the ECG tracing, it is important to understand the common terminology used:
- *Isoelectric line*: A straight line; represents a period of time with no electrical activity. Also called the *baseline*.
- *Deflection*: Any movement away from the baseline in the tracing. The deflections reflect the heart's electrical flow. Upward movement is called a *positive deflection*. Downward movement is a *negative deflection*.
- *Wave*: A deflection from the baseline
- *Complex*: A form made up of many waves (e.g., QRS complex)
- *Segment*: A part of a line between two points (e.g., the ST segment starts at the end of the S wave and ends at the start of the T wave.)
- *Interval*: A period of time between two points or events. During an interval, many waves can occur.

Each deflection in the ECG tracing corresponds to a part of the cardiac cycle. The ECG cycle consists of waveforms that are labeled: P, Q, R, S, T, and U. The Q, R, and S waves are usually grouped together and called the *QRS complex* (Fig. 39.4). In the next section, each part of the ECG is discussed in more detail.

ECG Waves and Segments

The *P wave* is the first deflection in the tracing. It is created from the electrical impulses moving through the right and left atria. The P wave appears as a small, rounded hill. The first part of the P wave reflects the impulse moving from the SA node to the AV node in the right atrium. The second part of the P wave reflects the impulse in the left atrial chamber. Electricity given off when the atrial cells are depolarized creates the P wave. Thus, the P wave represents *atrial depolarization*. During the P wave, the atrial chambers contract and the blood moves into the ventricles (Table 39.1).

The *PR segment* follows the P wave and appears as an isoelectric line. The electrical impulse moves slowly through the AV node. This electricity is not picked up on the ECG tracing. The PR segment is the time between the end of the atrial depolarization and the start of the ventricular depolarization. During the PR segment, the atrial chambers finish contracting.

The *QRS complex* is the next wave in the tracing. The impulse moves from the AV node through the remaining conduction system structures.

TABLE 39.1 Summary of ECG Waves and Segments

Waves	Appearance	Summarized	Conduction System	Mechanical Action
P wave	Small "hill" (positive deflection seen on lead II)	Atrial depolarization	Impulse moves from the SA node (pacemaker) to the AV node.	Atrial chambers contract; blood moves into the ventricles.
PR segment	Isoelectric line		Impulse moves slowly through AV node; electricity is not picked up on tracing.	
QRS complex	(See below)	Ventricular depolarization; atrial repolarization (hidden)	AV node to the bundle of His to the right and left bundle branches to the Purkinje fibers.	Ventricular chambers contract, pushing blood out of the heart.
Q wave	Negative deflection	Interventricular septal depolarization		
R wave	Positive triangular deflection	Ventricular depolarization; atrial repolarization (hidden)		
S wave	Any downward deflection following the R wave			
ST segment	Isoelectric line			
T wave	Positive deflection (upright and rounded in lead II)	Ventricular repolarization		
U wave	Usually not seen.	Purkinje fibers are repolarized		

AV, Atrioventricular; *SA,* sinoatrial.

The electricity given off from the impulse moving down the septum and around the outer walls of the ventricles creates the QRS complex. The electricity from the activity in the ventricles masks the repolarization electricity given off from the atrial cells as they recover. The QRS complex activity can be summarized as ventricular depolarization and atrial repolarization. During the QRS complex, the ventricles start contracting and the blood moves into the arteries.

Each wave in the QRS complex is different. The Q wave is a negative deflection and represents interventricular septal depolarization. The large, triangular-shaped R wave reflects the depolarization of most of the ventricular walls. The S wave is the final depolarization of the ventricular walls. Not all of these three waves may be seen. The positive and negative deflections of these waves can be different in the 12 *leads,* or pictures.

STUDY TIP

Summary of the Tracing
- P wave: Atrial depolarization (the impulse moves through the atria)
- QRS complex: Ventricular depolarization (the impulse moves through the ventricles) and atrial repolarization (atrial cells are in a recovery state)
- T wave: Ventricular repolarization (ventricular cells are in a recovery state)
The atria are always one stage ahead of the ventricles until both are in the polarized state. For instance, atrial polarization occurs with ventricular repolarization.

The *ST segment* follows the last wave in the QRS complex and ends at the start of the T wave. The *J point* is the point where the QRS complex ends and the ST segment starts. The ST segment is an isoelectric line. There is no electrical activity in the heart during this segment. (Remember, the impulse moving through the conduction system finished in the QRS complex.) During the ST segment, the ventricles finish contracting.

Repolarization causes electrical activity that creates the remaining waves. The *T wave* follows the ST segment and appears as a smooth, rounded, asymmetric waveform. The electrical activity from ventricular repolarization creates the T wave.

The *U wave* may follow the T wave, but in many cases it is not seen. The U wave is created from the repolarization of the Purkinje fibers. A U wave may also appear if the patient has hypercalcemia, hypokalemia, or digoxin toxicity.

CRITICAL THINKING BOX 39.3

Before doing the ECGs scheduled for today, Renee reviews the waveforms with Eva. She asks Eva the following questions regarding the ECG tracing:
- What shows atrial depolarization?
- What shows ventricular depolarization?
- What shows ventricular repolarization?

ECG Intervals

An *interval* is a period of time from a start point to an end point. It is not a wave. If you need to define what occurs during an interval, you would simply summarize the activities that happen for each wave and segment during the interval period of time.

The *PR interval* starts at the beginning of the P wave and ends at the start of the Q wave. It represents atrial depolarization. The *QT interval* starts at the beginning of the Q wave and extends to the end of the T wave. During the QT interval, the atrial chambers move from repolarization to the polarized state. The ventricular chambers depolarize and then move into the repolarized state.

CRITICAL THINKING BOX 39.4

Eva is confused about the PR interval and the QT interval. How might Renee describe these two intervals?

STUDY TIP

Remember, an interval is a period of time. You can summarize what occurs for each of these intervals by thinking about what occurs between these two points in time. Do not confuse the PR interval with the PR segment. They are two very different things.

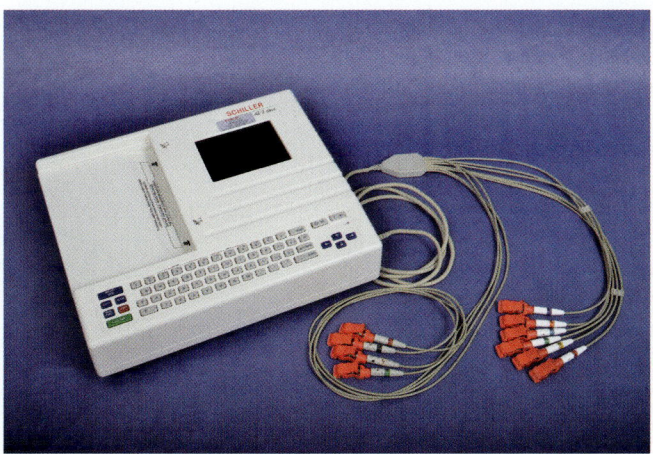

FIG. 39.5 ECG machine. (From Proctor D, et al: *Kinn's The Medical Assistant*, ed 13, St Louis, 2017, Elsevier.)

12-LEAD ECG

One of the most common ECG procedures in the ambulatory care setting is a resting 12-lead ECG. The medical assistant is responsible for:
- Assembling the supplies and equipment needed
- Preparing the patient for the test
- Performing the test

Before the medical assistant finishes the procedure, the ECG tracing must be examined for artifact. If any artifact is present on the tracing, the medical assistant must problem-solve the situation. Ultimately, the goal is to give the provider a clear ECG.

For a resting 12-lead ECG, the patient rests on the exam table. Ten electrodes are placed on the body. Lead wires attach to the electrodes and connect to the ECG machine (electrocardiograph). The 10 electrodes and lead wires pick up the electrical impulse from the surface of the body and carry it to the ECG machine (Fig. 39.5). The machine creates a tracing of 12 leads, or pictures.

A more in-depth discussion of electrode placement and artifact will occur later in the chapter. For now, it is important to have an idea of where the electrodes are placed on the body. An electrode is placed on each of the arms and legs. The right leg electrode is considered the ground electrode and is required for a clear ECG tracing. Six electrodes are placed on the chest.

Using the 10 electrodes and lead wires, the ECG machine creates 12 images, or pictures, that are called leads. Each lead picture looks different. Think of a photographer moving around a person, taking 12 pictures. Each picture looks different because of the change of the photographer's angle. For each lead, the picture is created differently. It is important for the medical assistant to know what electrodes and lead wires create the leads when troubleshooting unclear tracings. The three types of leads – bipolar, augmented, and precordial – are discussed in the following sections.

> ### CRITICAL THINKING BOX 39.5
> Robert Caudill is scheduled for an ECG today. When he arrives, Eva discusses the procedure. Robert asks what "12 lead" stands for. How might Eva describe this term to Robert?

Bipolar (or Standard) Leads

The **bipolar** (standard) leads are named leads I, II, and III. They use the arm electrodes and the left leg electrode to create pictures of the vertical (or frontal) plane of the heart. (Remember, the right electrode is used as a ground and is important for all leads.)

The bipolar leads are created from a measurement of current traveling from a negative pole to the positive pole (Fig. 39.6):
- Lead I: Right arm (RA) to left arm (LA)
- Lead II: Right arm (RA) to left leg (LL)
- Lead III: Left leg (LL) to left arm (LA)

If you join the end points (positive poles) of these three leads, you get a triangle. This triangle is known as *Einthoven's triangle.*

It is important to know which two electrodes create each lead when troubleshooting problems with the ECG tracing. If a lead has artifact, the medical assistant must check the two electrodes and the lead wires that create the lead.

> ### CRITICAL THINKING BOX 39.6
> As Eva and Renee perform an ECG, they find artifact on a few leads. For the following leads, which electrodes should be checked in each situation?
> - Lead II is unclear.
> - Lead I and III are unclear.
> - Lead II and III are unclear.

Augmented Leads

Augmented leads also provide information on the vertical (frontal) plane of the heart. These **unipolar** leads are *augmented* or increased in size on the tracing. Augmented leads use the right arm (RA), left arm (LA), and left leg (LL) electrodes.

Each augmented lead uses all three extremity electrodes (RA, LA, and LL) to create the picture. Midpoint between two of the electrodes is the negative pole. The current is measured as it moves from the negative pole to the positive pole (Table 39.2).

If the medical assistant identifies artifact on an augmented voltage - right arm (aVR) lead, all three electrodes and lead wires should be checked. (Check the RA, LA, and LL electrode and lead wires.)

Chest (or Precordial) Leads

The chest (precordial) leads are also unipolar leads. Each is a positive pole. The precordial leads provide information on the horizontal (front to back) plane of the heart. The six precordial leads are labeled V_1, V_2, V_3, V_4, V_5, and V_6 (Fig. 39.7).

The six leads are numbered the same as the precordial lead wires (i.e., V_1 through V_6). If one of the leads is unclear, the medical assistant should refer to the related lead wire and electrode. For instance, with artifact on V_4, the medical assistant will check the V_4 electrode and lead wire.

ECG SUPPLIES AND EQUIPMENT

The medical assistant needs to be familiar with the supplies and equipment used for ECGs. It is important to monitor the expiration dates of ECG supplies. Using expired supplies can cause unclear ECG tracings.

> ### VOCABULARY
> **bipolar**: Having two poles or electrical charges.
> **unipolar**: Having one pole or electrical charge.

UNIT 5 Advanced Clinical Procedures

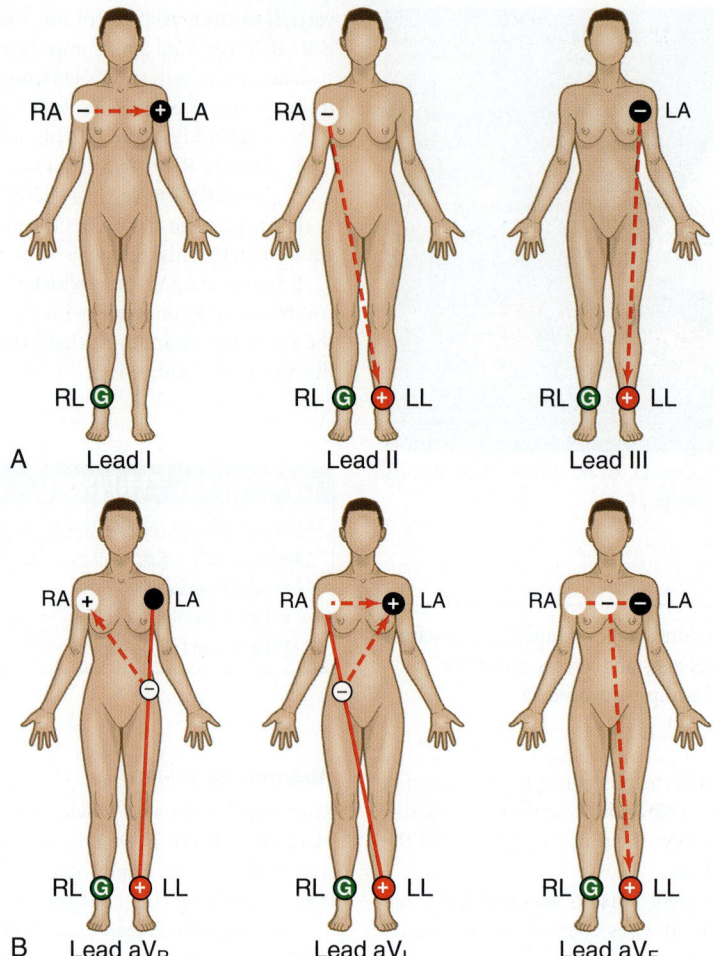

FIG. 39.6 Bipolar or standard (A) and augmented (B) limb leads. (From Proctor D, et al: *Kinn's The Medical Assistant*, ed 13, St Louis, 2017, Elsevier.)

TABLE 39.2 Augmented Voltage Leads

Lead	Measures Current Travel Toward Positive Pole
aVR (augmented voltage – right arm)	Right arm
aVL (augmented voltage – left arm)	Left arm
aVF (augmented voltage – left leg [foot])	Left leg

BOX 39.1 Handling Tips for Thermal ECG Paper

- Store in a dry, cool, dark location.
- Do not expose to heat, bright light, or ultraviolet (UV) light source.
- Do not expose to alcohol, adhesives, cleaners, or solvents.
- Do not store with vinyl, shrink wrap, or plastics.

VOCABULARY

caliper: A pocket-sized tool used for measuring the height and width of the ECG waves and intervals.

Thermal ECG Paper

ECG machines with printers use special ECG paper. The paper can be either Z-fold paper or 8.25 × 11-inch paper. A special heat-sensitive coating on the paper allows the tracing to be "burnt" onto the paper. Box 39.1 presents tips on handling the ECG paper.

The ECG paper is universally created with small and large boxes. A small box is 1 × 1 mm and the large box is 5 × 5 mm. The large box is made up of 25 small boxes (5 rows and 5 columns) (Fig. 39.8). It has a thicker border than the small boxes. When the provider analyzes the tracing, the height and the width of the wave forms are measured with a caliper (KAL uh per) (Fig. 39.9). The small and large boxes can help in the interpreting process.

The vertical lines measure the amplitude, or *voltage*, of the waveforms. Each small box is 0.1 mV (millivolt), and each large box is 0.5 mV. To determine the amplitude, count the small boxes vertically, starting at the baseline to the highest/lowest point of the wave.

The horizontal lines measure the time. When the paper speed (*chart speed*) is set at 25 mm/second, each small box is 0.04 second and each large box equals 0.2 second. To determine the width and time of the waveform, count the small boxes horizontally from the start to the finish of the wave. Multiply the number of small boxes by 0.04 to find the time.

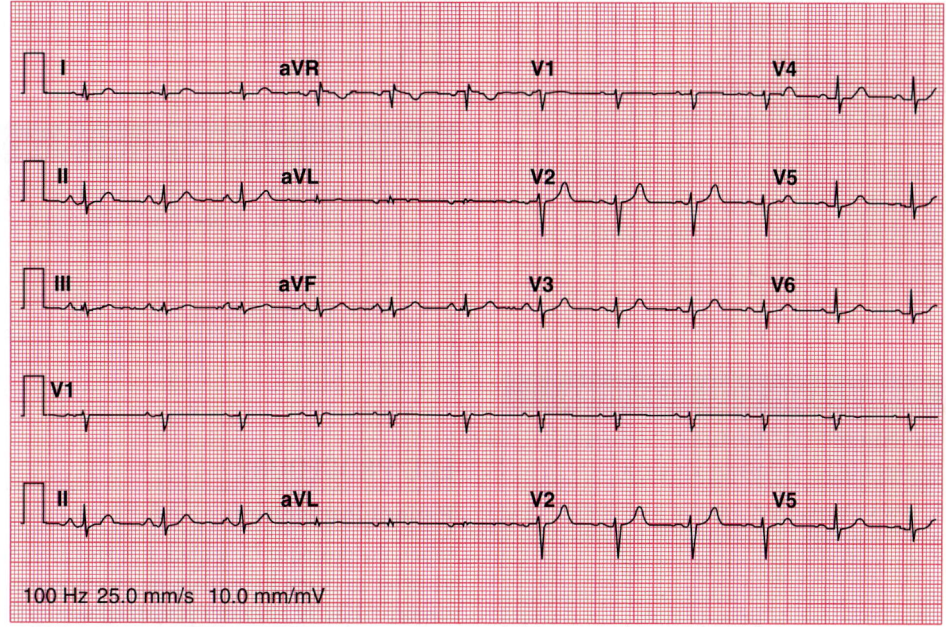

FIG. 39.7 A 12-lead ECG showing a normal sinus rhythm. (From Phalen T, Aehlert BJ: *The 12-lead ECG in Acute Coronary Syndromes*, ed 3, St Louis, 2012, Mosby.)

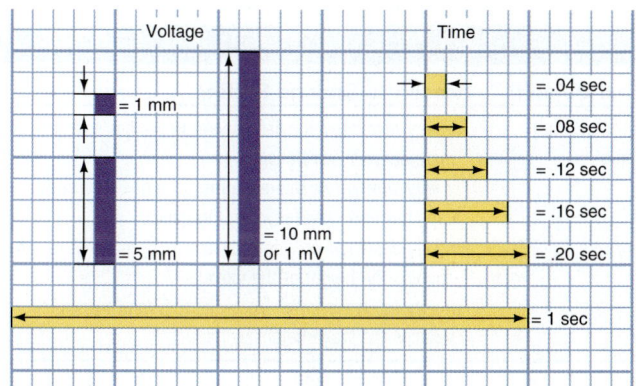

FIG. 39.8 ECG paper. (From Proctor D, et al: *Kinn's The Medical Assistant*, ed 13, St Louis, 2017, Elsevier.)

Electrodes

Electrodes are single-use disposable adhesive tabs that are placed on the skin. The skin is a poor conductor of electricity. The electrodes contain an electrolyte gel that helps pick up the electrical impulses. As the impulses make their way to the surface of the body, the electrolyte gel helps to conduct the impulses into the lead wires. For a resting 12-lead ECG, the most common type of electrode is the tab variety (Fig. 39.10A.). The snap electrode is used more often for exercise stress tests and in hospital settings (Fig. 39.10B.).

It is important to check the expiration date of the electrodes. If they are expired, the gel may be dried out and the conduction will be poor. Many operators' manuals for ECG machines recommend not mixing different manufacturers' electrodes.

Electrocardiograph

The lead wires may have a snap or a clip (also called an *alligator clip*; patient end adaptor) that attaches to the electrode. The lead wires merge into the patient cable that takes the electrical impulses to the electrocardiograph (ECG machine). In the machine, the impulses pass through an amplifier, which magnifies the impulses. A digital converter changes the analog signal into a digital signal. The digital signal can be printed on special ECG paper, which will be discussed in the next section.

The features of ECG machines can vary greatly. The two types of ECG devices in ambulatory healthcare facilities include the box model and the computer-based ECG (Table 39.3). The computer-based ECG can use its own computer device with preloaded software, or a facility can purchase software to add to any laptop computer. With the advancement in technology, specialists and providers can be sent the ECG via Bluetooth or Wi-Fi. ECGs can be sent to wireless or remote printers or computer systems. They can also be uploaded into an electronic health record (EHR).

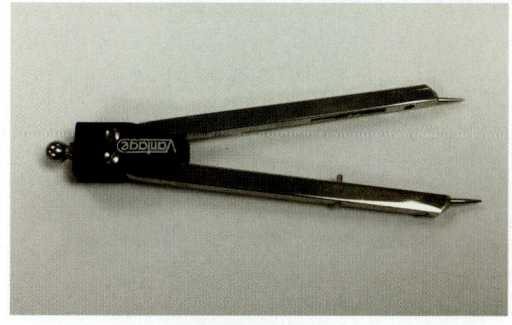

FIG. 39.9 Caliper.

Settings and Calibration. ECG machines have settings that can be useful for obtaining a tracing. Many machines have filters to block disturbances. Filters can help to create a clearer tracing. Refer to the operator's manual when changing settings. Table 39.4 presents common settings. It is important to indicate on the tracing if any of the default settings were changed. Changes to the default settings will affect how the provider measures and interprets the tracing.

Most ECG machines automatically complete a self-test when the machine is turned on. Typically, the self-test examines the battery and the memory. Like many machines used in the healthcare setting, the ECG machine needs to be calibrated daily or per the facility's policy. The calibration results should be documented on the log flow sheet. (Additional information on maintenance of the electrocardiograph is presented in Box 39.2.)

When ECG machines are calibrated, the sensitivity, or gain, should to be checked. The machines usually print a calibration marking either at the beginning or at the end of the tracing. This marking is called the *standardization mark*. If the machine is set at 10 mm/mV, the standardization mark will be an upward rectangle that is 10 small boxes tall. If the gain is doubled, then the standardization mark also will be doubled in size (Fig. 39.11).

> ### CRITICAL THINKING BOX 39.7
> The next day, Eva prepares to do an ECG on Charles Johnson. She turns on the machine to check to see if it has been set up correct. She sees the following:
> - Chart speed: 10 mm/s
> - Gain: 10 mm/mV
>
> Which of these settings is normal and which needs to be changed prior to the next ECG?

ECG PROCEDURE

Patient Preparation

When the procedure is started, it is always important for the medical assistant to coach the patient on the procedure and the preparation required. Box 39.3 reviews patient education for the ECG procedure. The patient needs to remove all clothing above the waist and wear a gown that opens in the front. Cloth gowns or paper capes can be used.

TABLE 39.3 Features on ECG Machines

Box Model ECG Machine	Computer-Based ECG	Features Commonly Seen on Both
• LCD screen	• Touch screen • Stress testing features	• Interpretive software to assist provider when reading tracing • Bluetooth or Wi-Fi capacity • Thermal printer • Spirometer

TABLE 39.4 Common ECG Settings

Setting	Description	Normal Default	Reason to Change Setting
Chart speed	Regulates the speed of the paper during the recording. *Example:* 25 mm/s means 25 millimeters (25 small blocks) of tracing is printed in 1 second.	25 mm/s (second)	*For very fast rates:* Increase speed to 50 mm/s to get more defined waveforms. *For very slow rates:* Decrease rate to 5 or 10 mm/s to capture more waveforms on the paper.
Gain or sensitivity	Regulates the height (amplitude) of the tracing. *Example:* 10 mm/mV means 1 mV (millivolt) of electricity causes the recorder to move up 10 millimeters (10 small blocks).	10 mm/mV	*For very short waveforms:* Increase to 20 mm/mV, which doubles the height of the waves. *For very tall waveforms:* Decrease to 5 mm/mV, which reduces the wave height by half.

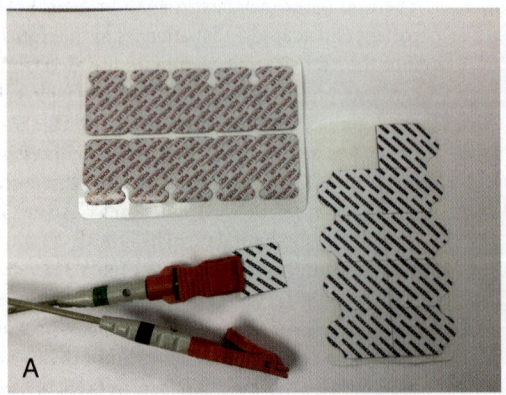 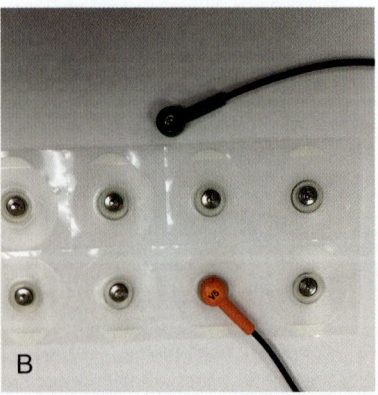

FIG. 39.10 (A) The appearance of tab electrodes can vary, depending on the manufacturer. Alligator clips on the lead wires attach to the tab electrodes. (B) Snap electrodes use the snap adaptors on the lead wires.

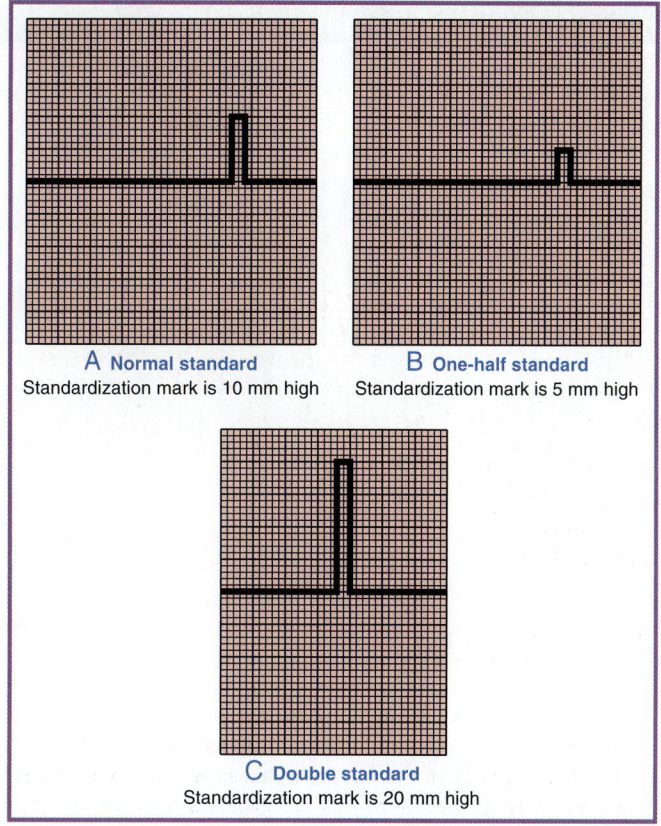

FIG. 39.11 Sensitivity standards. (From Proctor D, et al: *Kinn's The Medical Assistant*, ed 13, St Louis, 2017, Elsevier.)

BOX 39.2 Maintenance of the Electrocardiograph

- The lead wires are not disposable; clean as indicated in the operator's manual.
- Handle the lead wires and patient cable with care. They should be stored in a loose coil. Tight coils or bending of the wires and cable can result in breakage of the fine wires inside the unit. This will cause artifact on the ECG and requires replacement of the cable.
- Clean the tracing stylus and the machine casing as indicated in the operator's manual.

BOX 39.3 Patient Education With ECGs

The medical assistant should prepare the patient for an ECG by explaining that:
- Ten electrodes and wires are placed on the body.
- The machine will take 12 pictures of the electrical activity of the heart.
- The procedure is painless.
- The patient must be still and not talk during the time the pictures are being made (during the actual tracing).
- The patient should not use his or her cell phone or other electronic device during the procedure.
- The provider will need to look at the ECG pictures and then the patient will be notified of the results. (Remember, the medical assistant cannot tell the patient if it is normal or abnormal.)

An electrode must be placed on each lower leg, so tights or pantyhose also must be removed. Socks and pants can be moved to allow application of the electrodes, so they can usually stay on (Procedure 39.1).

The patient should be in the supine position on the exam table. A pillow can be placed under the patient's head. The patient's legs and arms need to be supported on the table. It is important for the patient to be relaxed and comfortable during the procedure. If the patient is having chest pain or problems breathing, the head of the exam table may be elevated. Any change of position from the supine position must be noted on the ECG tracing. Any position change can create a change on the leads (pictures). The provider needs to be aware of it when reading the tracing.

Before placing the electrodes on the skin, it is important to prepare the skin. This helps the electrodes adhere and minimizes artifact, thus producing an accurate tracing. There are several techniques used to prepare the skin:
- Wipe the area with an alcohol pad to clean it. This helps to remove sweat and lotion that may prevent the electrodes from adhering to the skin.

PROCEDURE 39.1 Perform Electrocardiography

Tasks:
Perform electrocardiography and routine maintenance on the machine. Document the procedure in the patient's health record.

Equipment and Supplies
- ECG machine
- Disposable electrodes
- ECG paper
- Alcohol pads
- Razor (optional)
- Gauze pads (optional)
- Patient gown or paper cape
- Tissue
- Disinfecting wipes
- Gloves
- Trash container
- Patient's health record

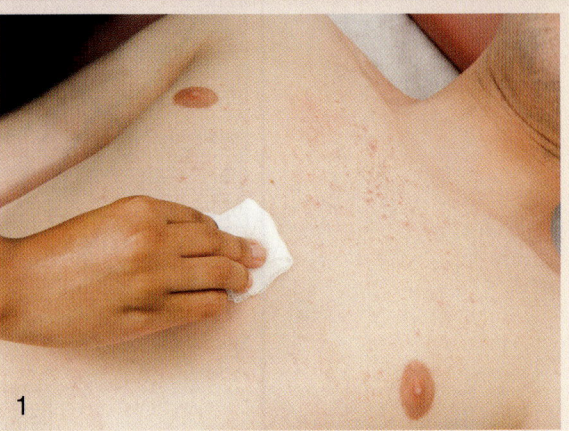

Procedural Steps
1. Wash hands or use hand sanitizer.
   Purpose: Hand sanitization is an important step for infection control.
2. Assemble equipment and supplies needed for the ECG procedure. Plug in and turn on the ECG machine. Verify that the standardization and chart/paper speed are correct.
   Purpose: Having the equipment ready helps reduce the patient's wait time.
3. Greet the patient. Identify yourself. Verify the patient's identity with full name and date of birth. Explain the procedure in a manner that is understood by the patient. Answer any questions the patient may have on the procedure.
   Purpose: It is important to identify the patient in two different ways to ensure that you have the correct patient. Explaining the procedure can make the patient feel more comfortable and helps to reduce anxiety.
4. Ask the patient to remove all clothing from the waist up, including undergarments, and put on the gown/cape so that the opening is in the front. Ask the patient if assistance is needed. If so, help. If not, leave the room and allow the patient time to change. When reentering the room, provide a courtesy knock on the door.
   Purpose: The patient needs to be undressed from the waist up for you to place the electrodes. Patients require privacy to change.
5. Assist the patient into a comfortable supine position on the exam table. Provide support for the legs and arms.
   Purpose: To reduce artifact on the tracing, the patient must be comfortable and the extremities need to be supported.
6. Identify the locations for the ECG electrodes on the chest. Prepare the skin. If the patient has a hairy chest, get the person's permission prior to shaving the areas (optional). Wipe each spot with alcohol and allow it to dry. Fold the gauze pad over your index finger and briskly rub the site to abrade the skin (optional) (Fig. 1).
   Purpose: The alcohol will prepare the skin and help the electrode adhere to the skin.
7. Correctly apply the six chest electrodes. If tab electrodes are used, the tabs should be pointed toward the waist.
   Purpose: Having the tabs face the core of the body will help reduce the tension on the lead wires when they are attached.
8. Identify the locations for the ECG electrodes on the extremities. Refer to the operating manual for arm electrode position if needed. Wipe each spot with alcohol and allow it to dry. Correctly apply the four limb electrodes to nonbony areas. If tab electrodes are used, the lower leg tabs should point toward the waist. The arm/wrist tabs should be pointed toward the fingers.
   Purpose: The alcohol will prepare the skin and help the electrode adhere to the skin.
9. Attach the correct lead wire to each of the electrodes (Fig. 2). The wires should follow the natural contour of the body and not overlap.
   Purpose: Overlapping wires can cause artifact.

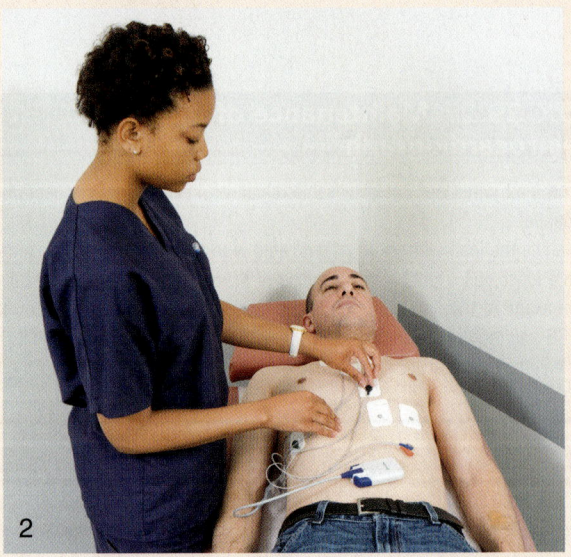

PROCEDURE 39.1 Perform Electrocardiography—cont'd

10. Enter the patient's data into the ECG machine. Identify any changes with the default settings, electrode position, or patient's position.
    Purpose: The ECG tracing needs to be labeled with the patient's identifying information. The provider must be aware of any changes in the procedure. Electrode position changes, chart/paper speed, etc., can change the appearance of the tracing.
11. Double-check that the lead wires are in the correct position and are attached to the electrodes. Make sure each electrode is attached to the skin. Take any corrective action necessary.
    Purpose: The lead wires and electrodes must be in the correct spot and attached for the tracing to be accurate.
12. Instruct the patient to lie still and not to talk during the tracing.
    Purpose: Talking and moving during the tracing will create artifact.
13. Verify that the filter(s) are on. Check the leads on the screen or monitor. Take any corrective action necessary. Run the tracing when the leads look clear and without artifact.
    Purpose: The filters will minimize the artifact. Checking the appearance of the leads helps to identify if corrective action is needed to minimize artifact.
14. Check the tracing for clarity and abnormal life-threatening rhythms. If artifact is present, take corrective action to minimize artifact and run another tracing.
    Purpose: The provider will need a clear tracing. Life-threatening rhythms need to be identified and the provider needs to be told immediately.
15. Disconnect the lead wires and remove the electrodes. Wipe any reside from the patient's skin. Wash your hands and instruct the patient to get dressed. Ask the patient if assistance is needed. If so, help the patient to dress.
    Purpose: The medical assistant must be the one to remove the wires and electrodes.
16. Provide the patient with information about following up with the provider. Complete any necessary actions with the ECG (e.g., upload to the electronic health record, mount and route to the provider).
    Purpose: After tests, patients will want to know what the results are. The provider will need to read the tracing before any results are given to the patient.
17. Document accurately in the patient's health record. When documenting, indicate the provider ordering the test, what test was performed, how the patient tolerated the test, and what you did with the ECG tracing. You can also add any instructions you provided to the patient regarding follow-up.
    Purpose: Indicating who ordered the test and what was done is important for insurance reimbursement and for legal reasons.

Routine Machine Maintenance: Adding Paper
18. Review the operator's manual on how to change the paper. Gather the new ream of ECG paper (or roll).
    Purpose: The operator's manual will indicate how the paper should be added to the machine.
19. Open the machine. Remove the remaining paper and add the new paper per the steps in the manual.
    Purpose: It is important to remove the last few sheets of the old paper to make room for the new ream.
20. Put on gloves and disinfect the lead wires per the operator's manual. Disinfect the exam table. Clean up the work area. Remove the gloves. Wash your hands.
    Purpose: For infection control purposes, it is important to disinfect the lead wires and exam table between each use.

Documentation Example
08/06/20XX 1423 Per Dr. James Martin's order, a resting 12-lead ECG was performed. Pt tolerated the procedure well. Pt was instructed to call the clinic tomorrow for the ECG results. The ECG tracing was routed to Dr. Martin.____
_____Eva Ning, RMA

- Use a razor to shave chest hair. Obtain the patient's verbal consent before shaving the chest.
- Gently abrade the skin, using a gauze sponge, special gel, or special fine sandpaper tape (Fig. 39.12).

Applying Electrodes and Lead Wires

Apply electrodes to both arms and legs. The electrodes on the lower legs should be placed on the inner side, just above the ankles. If tab electrodes are used, have the tabs on the leg electrodes point toward the center of the person. All the other tabs can be facing the feet.

The placement of the arm electrodes may vary, depending on the ECG machine and manufacturer. For instance, many Schiller ECG machines indicate that the electrodes should be placed just above the wrists. Other machines indicate placement on the upper arms. Check the operator's manual for correct placement of the arm electrodes. Table 39.5 describes where to place the electrodes on the limbs and the chest (Fig. 39.13).

The lead wires are typically color coded and include an abbreviation on each wire. Colors may vary from manufacturer to manufacturer. It is important to know and to use the abbreviations. One of the most common errors is to mix up the right and left limb lead wires. This can cause abnormal leads (pictures) and result in additional patient workup before the mistake is discovered. It is important to always double-check the placement of the lead wires.

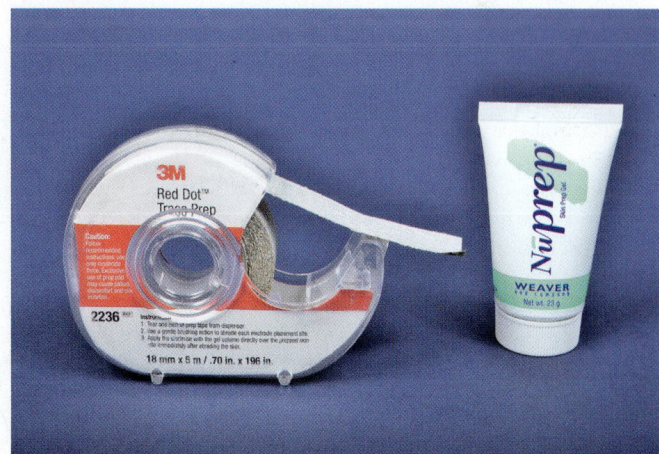

FIG. 39.12 Special fine sandpaper tape and Nuprep Skin Prep Gel are used to abrade the skin. This provides a better ECG tracing.

In some cases, the electrodes may need to be placed in alternative locations. Table 39.6 identifies special situations. It is important to note on the ECG tracing any electrode placement deviation from the normal location. The provider reading the tracing needs to take the placement into consideration.

Running the ECG Tracing

Once the lead wires are attached to the electrodes, the medical assistant enters the patient information into the ECG machine. In some facilities this may be done prior to bringing the patient into the room for the ECG. Typically, the patient's name, date of birth, and medical record number are entered. Facilities will have additional information that they require to be entered, such as the ordering provider's name.

After the information is entered, the medical assistant should remind the patient to remain still and not to talk during the procedure. It usually takes a minute or less for the tracing to be created with a multichannel machine (Box 39.4). Talking and movement will create artifact. If the patient is cold, a blanket can be used to cover him or her.

Prior to running the tracing, double-check that all the electrodes are attached, and the lead wires are in the correct location. If the ECG machine has a screen, check the digital picture of the leads. Are they

TABLE 39.5 Electrode and Lead Wire Placement

Electrode	Lead Wire Abbreviation and Color	Placement
Right arm	RA (white)	Placed just above the wrist or upper arm indicated in the operator's manual
Left arm	LA (black)	
Right leg	RL (green)	Placed on the inner lower leg, just above the ankle
Left leg	LL (red)	
Chest V_1	V1 (red)	Fourth intercostal space at the right sternal edge
Chest V_2	V2 (yellow)	Fourth intercostal space at the left sternal edge
Chest V_3	V3 (green)	Midway between V_2 and V_4
Chest V_4	V4 (blue)	Fifth intercostal space on the mid-clavicular line
Chest V_5	V5 (orange)	Same horizontal plane as V_4 at the left anterior axillary line or the midpoint between V_4 and V_6
Chest V_6	V6 (purple)	Same horizontal plane as V_4 at the midaxillary line

TABLE 39.6 Electrode Placement in Special Situations

Condition	Electrode Placement
Dextrocardia (the heart is located on the right side of the chest)	Place chest electrodes on the right side of the chest using the same intercostal spacing and landmarks. Switch the right and left limb lead wires (e.g., LA would be attached to the right arm electrode).
Amputated limb	Place electrode on the remaining part of the limb. Place the electrode on the opposite limb in the same location.
Casted limb	Place the electrode above the cast on the limb. Place the electrode on the opposite limb in the same location.
New surgical incision or wound	Place the electrodes near the correct area, but not on the incision or wound.

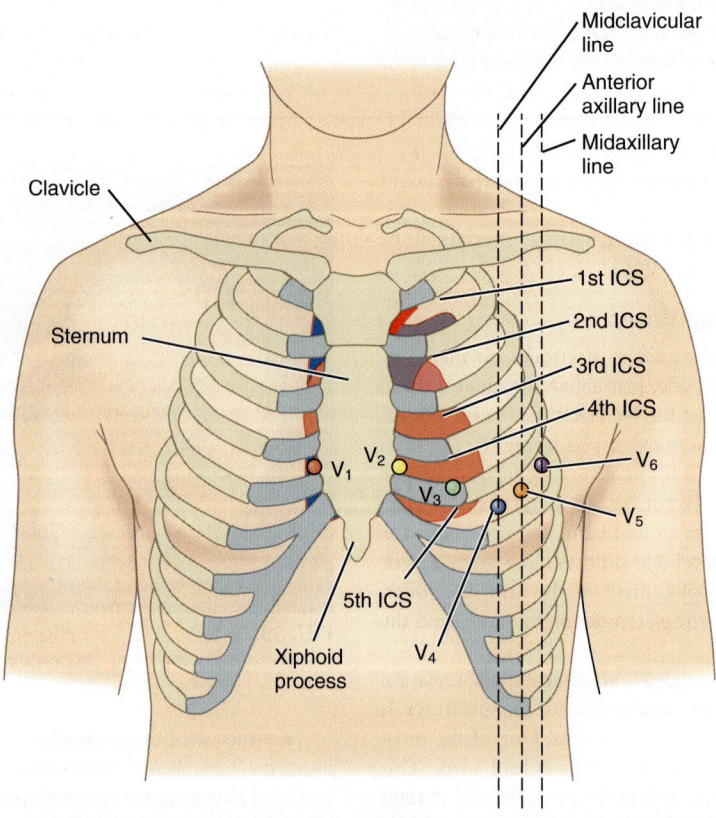

FIG. 39.13 Chest leads. *ICS*, Intercostal space. (From Proctor D, et al: *Kinn's The Medical Assistant*, ed 13, St Louis, 2017, Elsevier.)

BOX 39.4 Single- and Multiple-Channel ECG Machines

ECG machines can be single or multiple channel. In single-channel models, the machine contains one amplifier channel and one recording stylet. The single-channel machines record one lead (picture) at a time. The medical assistant must manually switch to the next lead until the procedure is done. When these machines are used, the process of recording a tracing takes 3 to 5 minutes. Single-channel machines can use paper rolls or Z-fold paper. These small strips of paper need to be mounted (see the section Finishing the ECG).

Multichannel machines monitor all 12 leads. This model has several stylets that allow for four groups of three leads to be traced every few seconds. With some machines, a fourth stylet traces one lead for the entire width of the page. Typically, the multichannel machines print the tracing on an 8.25 × 11-inch paper or Z-fold paper.

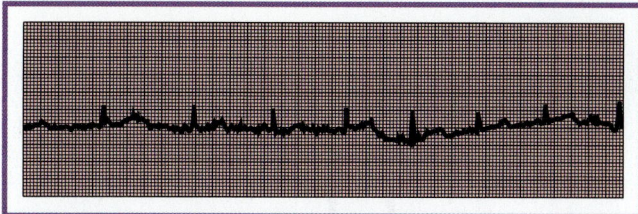

FIG. 39.15 Somatic tremor artifact. (From Proctor D, et al: *Kinn's The Medical Assistant*, ed 13, St Louis, 2017, Elsevier.)

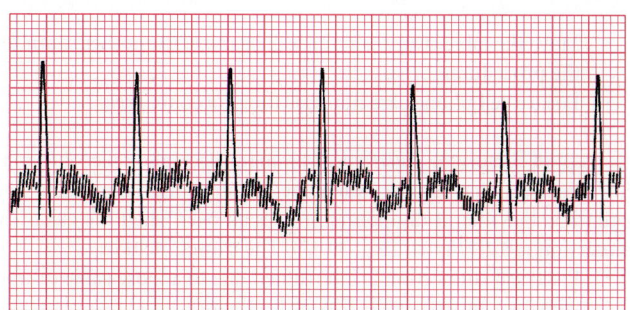

FIG. 39.16 AC interference artifact. (From Urden L, Stacy K, Lough M: *Thelan's Critical Care Nursing: Diagnosis and Management*, ed 7, St Louis, 2014, Mosby.)

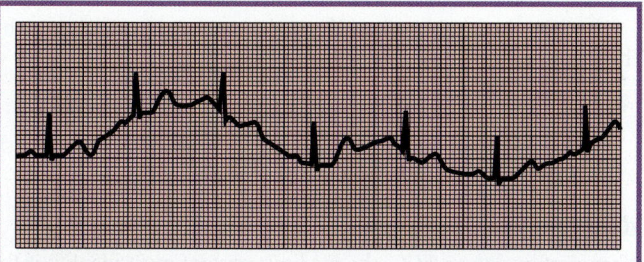

FIG. 39.14 Wandering baseline artifact. (From Proctor D, et al: *Kinn's The Medical Assistant*, ed 13, St Louis, 2017, Elsevier.)

clear (without artifact)? If not, is the filter(s) on? Are the leads (pictures) an equal distance from each other? Is the baseline horizontal, or is it moving up and down like a rollercoaster? Do not run the tracing until it is clear, and the baseline is horizontal. Problem-solve and fix the issue before running the tracing or redo the tracing if it was printed. Additional problem-solving strategies will be discussed later in this chapter. Once the tracing looks good on the screen, print it.

Troubleshooting Artifact

Artifact is signal distortion or unwanted, erratic movement of the stylus caused by outside interference. The medical assistant needs to identify the type of artifact and then take actions to prevent the artifact. The leads can be viewed on the screen or after printing the ECG tracing. Carefully look for artifact. The following sections discuss the appearance and causes of the common types of artifact and ways to prevent them.

Wandering Baseline. *Wandering baseline* artifact is an upward and downward movement of the waveform (Fig. 39.14). The isoelectric lines shift locations. This artifact can be caused from:
- Poor skin preparation: Patient has oily skin or used lotion. The electrodes are falling off.
- Old electrodes: The electrodes are dirty or expired; or the gel on the electrodes is dried.
- Placement of electrodes: If electrodes are placed on bony areas.
- Movement: The movement of breathing can also be the cause of this artifact.

The medical assistant should:
- Clean the skin with alcohol and allow it to dry. Slightly abrade the skin with a gauze pad or fine sandpaper tape to help the electrodes stick to the skin.
- Replace the electrode with a new one. Ensure the electrodes are not expired and the gel is not dried.
- Make sure all electrodes and lead wires are firmly attached.
- Make sure the baseline filter is turned on (if it is a feature of the machine).

Somatic Tremor. *Somatic tremor* artifact appears as jagged peaks with irregular heights and spacing (Fig. 39.15). The causes include:
- Involuntary movement: Tremors from disease conditions (e.g., Parkinson's disease), shivering due to coldness
- Voluntary movement: Talking, chewing gum, supporting arms or legs because table is too small for the person

The medical assistant should:
- Help the patient relax. Cover the patient with a blanket if he or she is cold.
- Remind the patient to not move or talk during the tracing.
- Watch to see if there is a pattern with involuntary movements. Take the tracing when the movements lessen.
- Use a larger exam table for the procedure.
- If the machine has a muscle tremor filter, make sure it is turned on.

AC Interference. *AC interference* artifact appears as a series of small spikes that creates a thick-looking tracing. (Fig. 39.16). The causes include:
- Electrical interference: Too many electrical devices in the area; patient cable and lead wires are wrapped closely together; electrical cord is under the exam table; and electrical outlet is improperly grounded. A cell phone in a patient's pocket may also cause interference.

The medical assistant should:
- Unplug the ECG machine.
- Unplug or remove nearby electrical devices (e.g., laptops, pagers, cell phones).
- Separate the lead wires so they do not overlap.

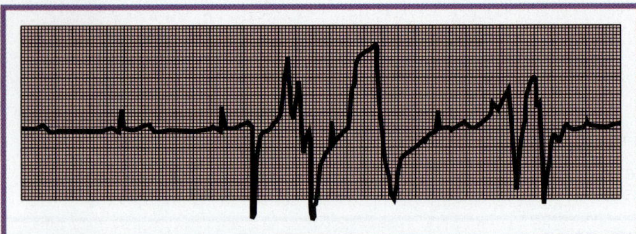

FIG. 39.17 Interrupted baseline artifact. (From Proctor D, et al: *Kinn's The Medical Assistant*, ed 13, St Louis, 2017, Elsevier.)

- Move the table away from the wall or move to another room for the procedure.
- Ensure cell phones are not near the procedure area.

Interrupted Baseline. *Interrupted baseline* artifact (also called intermittent signal artifact) occurs when the tracing looks normal at the beginning, but then it disappears or goes all over when the electrical connection is interrupted (Fig. 39.17). The causes include:
- Electrical connection is interrupted due to a loose cable or lead wire, or a broken cable, clip, or lead wire.

The medical assistant should:
- Check that all electrodes and lead wires are attached.
- If a broken wire is suspected, a new cable will be needed.

> **CRITICAL THINKING BOX 39.8**
> While Eva is performing Charles Johnson's 12-lead ECG, she notices that the tracing line looks thick. On closer inspection she finds that there are small, spiked lines that make the tracing look like a thick line. What is occurring? How might Eva troubleshoot the problem?

Evaluating an ECG Tracing

The medical assistant must be able to determine abnormal rates and rhythm. When these occur, the medical assistant must immediately alert the provider. It is helpful to keep the patient hooked up to the ECG machine in case additional monitoring is required.

Rate. Many machines indicate the heart rate. The medical assistant can also calculate the rate from the ECG tracing. Methods used to calculate a regular heart rate when the paper speed (chart speed) is 25 mm/second include:
- *Six second method*: Count the number of P waves in a 6-second strip (30 large boxes) and multiply by 10 (least accurate method).
- *1500 method*: Count the number of small boxes between two R waves or the two P waves. Divide the number into 1500.
- *Sequence method*: Count the number of large boxes between the R waves. By memorizing the numbers in Table 39.7, you will have a quick method to calculate the heart rate.

Rhythm. The rhythm of a heartbeat is either regular or irregular. You can identify an irregular heartbeat when taking the patient's pulse. This same patient will show an irregularity when an ECG is recorded. An irregular rhythm on an ECG tracing will have time differences between cardiac cycles. With a regular rhythm, each cardiac cycle occurs the same length of time apart. To check for ventricular rhythm, you can count the boxes between two consecutive RR intervals. Atrial rhythm is determined by counting the boxes between two consecutive PP intervals. If the heart rhythm is regular, each of these interval measurements is the same.

TABLE 39.7 Sequence Method

Number of Large (5 mm) Boxes Between R Waves	Heart Rate
1	300
2	150
3	100
4	75
5	60
6	50
7	43
8	37

Analyzing an ECG Tracing. For most medical assistants, their job description states that they need to be able to perform ECGs. For some medical assistants, they may work as an ECG technician. In this position they may need to analyze an ECG tracing.

The ECG rhythm strip (lead II view) is evaluated from left to right. The following should be assessed:
- Rate: What is the rate?
- Rhythm: Is it regular or irregular?
- Appearance of the segments, waves, and intervals: Table 39.8 lists questions to consider when analyzing a tracing.

Identifying an Abnormal Rhythm

When performing an ECG, the medical assistant must identify if the patient has an **arrhythmia** (ah RITH mee ah) that requires immediate care by the provider. If the medical assistant identifies a life-threatening arrhythmia, it is important to keep the patient hooked up to the ECG machine and to immediately get the provider.

> **VOCABULARY**
> **arrhythmia:** An abnormal heart rate or rhythm.

Sinus Arrhythmias. A sinus rhythm is considered normal. The electrical activity begins in the SA node and goes through the rest of the conduction system. Atrial and ventricular depolarizations occur. With sinus arrhythmias, the electrical pathway is normal. The rate or rhythm of the heartbeat is altered. The alteration may come from the SA node firing too slowly or too quickly.
- *Sinus bradycardia*: The adult heart rate is below 60 beats per minute. This is a normal finding in well-conditioned athletes. It is abnormal in other individuals.
- *Sinus tachycardia*: The adult heart rate is above 100 beats per minute. This is normal in a person doing aerobic exercise. It is abnormal in a resting individual.

Atrial Arrhythmias. Atrial arrhythmias occur when there is a problem with the SA node starting the impulse. They can also occur due to a conduction problem in the atria.
- *Premature atrial contractions (PACs)*: Occur when the atria contract sooner than they should. The P wave can be abnormally shaped, or an extra P wave can be seen. PACs can be seen in people who smoke or consume large amounts of caffeine. An occasional PAC is not abnormal. More than six PACs in a minute is considered abnormal.
- *Atrial flutter*: Occurs when the atria contract faster than the ventricles (up to 300 beats per minute). They become out of sync with the ventricles. Extra P waves are seen with regular QRS complexes. Atrial

TABLE 39.8 Analyzing an ECG Tracing

	Normal	Questions to Address	Timing (Horizontal – Length)
P wave	Largest in lead II Upright in all leads except aVR Voltage (vertical – height): less than 2.5 small boxes (0.25 millivolts)	Is there one P wave before each QRS complex? Is each P wave a positive deflection? Are all the P waves similar in size and shape? Is there more than one P wave per cardiac cycle?	>0.11 seconds
PR interval	From start of P wave to start of QRS complex	Are the PR intervals the same size throughout the tracing?	0.12–0.2 seconds
QRS complex	Largest in lead II compared to leads III and I	Is there a QRS complex without a previous P wave?	0.06–0.12 seconds
ST segment	On the baseline	Is the ST segment lower or higher than the baseline? (Could be an indication of infarction or ischemia.)	Not usually measured
QT interval	From start of Q wave to end of T wave	Are the QT intervals the same size throughout the tracing?	0.40 seconds

---

BOX 39.5 Diseases That Can Cause Atrial Flutter

- Coronary heart disease
- Hypertension
- Cardiomyopathy
- Heart valve diseases
- Hyperthyroidism
- Pulmonary embolism
- Obstructive pulmonary disease

---

flutter can be caused by alcohol and stimulants (cocaine, caffeine, diet pills, and cold medications). It can also be caused by diseases (Box 39.5). Atrial flutter is reversed with medication to slow the heart or with *cardioversion* (electrical shock).

Heart Block. A heart block occurs when there is a disruption or slowing of the electrical impulse through the heart. Heart block can be congenital or acquired. Heart disease, surgery, or medications can cause acquired heart block. There are three types of heart block, with third degree being the most severe:
- *First-degree heart block*: The impulse slows as it moves from the atria to the ventricles. This creates a longer PR segment. First-degree heart block may not cause symptoms. It may not require treatment.
- *Second-degree heart block*: The impulse slows or is blocked as it moves into the ventricles. When blocked, there is no QRS complex after the P wave, and the ventricles do not contract. When the impulse slows, the PR segment is longer. This arrhythmia requires a pacemaker to help maintain the heart rate. Pacemakers will be discussed in a later section of this chapter.
- *Third-degree heart block*: The impulse does not reach the ventricles. As a backup system, special ventricular cells create an impulse that causes the ventricles to contract. On the ECG tracing, the P wave is faster than normal and the QRS complex is not coordinated with the P wave. This is a life-threatening arrhythmia and requires emergency treatment and a pacemaker.

Ventricular Arrhythmias. Ventricular arrhythmias are abnormalities in the ventricles. Most of the ventricular arrhythmias discussed are life-threatening rhythms.

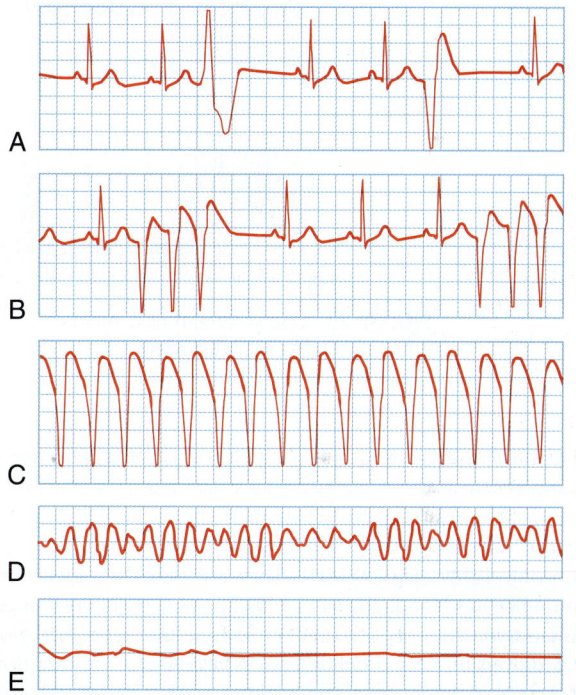

FIG. 39.18 (A) Premature ventricular contraction (PVC). (B) Three PVCs in a row. (C) Ventricular tachycardia (V-tach). (D) Ventricular fibrillation (V-fib). (E) Asystole. (From Proctor D, et al: *Kinn's The Medical Assistant*, ed 13, St Louis, 2017, Elsevier.)

- *Premature ventricular contractions (PVCs)*: Occur when the ventricles contract sooner than they should. An impulse originating in the ventricles creates this abnormality. The QRS complex appears before a P wave. The P wave can also be absent. The T wave can be abnormally shaped, and a widened QRS complex can be seen (Fig. 39.18A and B). PVCs can be caused by tobacco, alcohol, epinephrine, and anxiety. They can also be caused by hypertension, coronary artery disease, and lung disease. Infrequent PVCs can be normal. More than six PVCs in a minute is abnormal and can lead to a life-threatening condition.
- *Ventricular tachycardia (V-tach)*: Occurs when the ventricles beat at a rapid rate (up to 250 beats per minute). It may be seen with multiple PVCs in a row. It may be a short run of fast beats or may

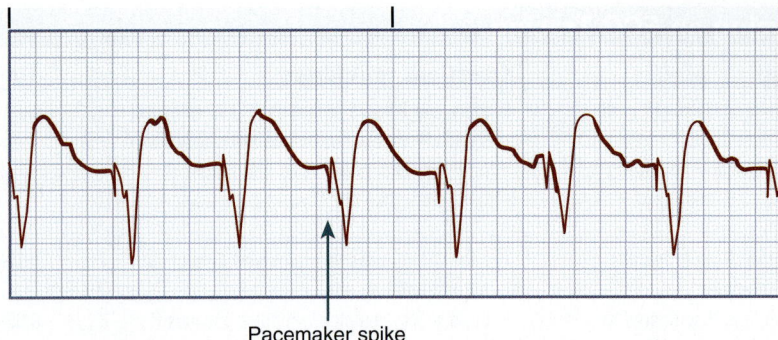

FIG. 39.19 Pacemaker rhythm strip. (From Lewis S, et al: *Medical-Surgical Nursing*, ed 9, St Louis, 2014, Mosby.)

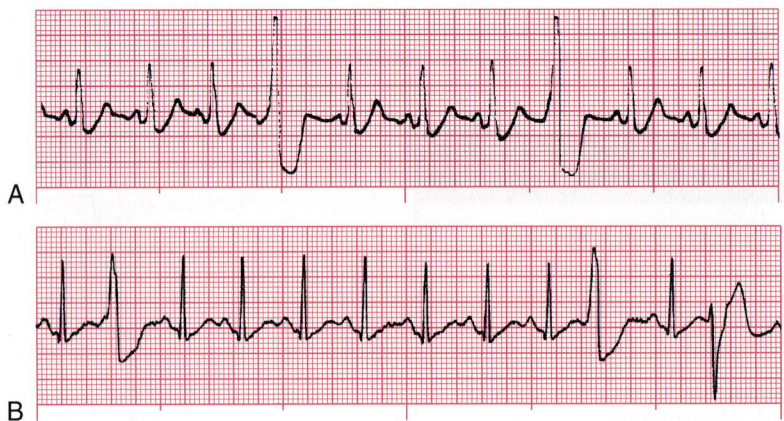

FIG. 39.20 Pacemaker and placement in the chest. (From Proctor D, et al: *Kinn's The Medical Assistant*, ed 13, St Louis, 2017, Elsevier.)

last longer than 30 seconds (Fig. 39.18C). V-tach is a life-threatening condition. If it is not reversed with drugs and/or cardioversion, it can become ventricular fibrillation.
- *Ventricular fibrillation (V-fib)*: Occurs when the ventricles quiver uncontrollably (Fig. 39.18D). They are essentially ineffective at pumping any blood. The patient has no pulse, is not breathing, and is unresponsive. This is the most critical, life-threatening arrhythmia. Cardioversion with a defibrillator is necessary to restore normal function of the electrical conduction system.
- *Asystole*: Results in the absence of a heartbeat. A flat line appears on the tracing (Fig. 39.18E).

Implantable Device Rhythms. Implantable devices (e.g., pacemaker and implantable cardioverter-defibrillator) create abnormal waveforms on the ECG tracing. A pacemaker is used to treat some types of arrhythmias. It uses low-energy electrical pulses to assist the heart to beat at a normal rate. Pacemakers can change the ECG tracing. Fig. 39.19 shows a pacemaker rhythm strip. There are two types of pacemakers:
- Temporary pacemaker: Used in an emergency until the permanent pacemaker can be placed. Also used for temporary conditions (e.g., heart attack and medication overdose).
- Permanent pacemaker: Surgically inserted into the chest or abdomen (Fig. 39.20). Patients can use technology (e.g., smart phones) to transmit their pacemaker data to their provider.

An implantable cardioverter-defibrillator (ICD) can provide low-energy electrical pulses and high-energy pulses (Fig. 39.21). The high-energy pulses can treat life-threatening arrhythmias. ICDs are surgically implanted in the chest or abdomen. The ICD is programmed to meet the needs of the patient. Some ICD functions can be checked using technology such as pacemakers. ICD batteries can last 5 to 7 years.

Finishing the ECG

If the ambulatory care facility uses an EHR system and the ECG machine interfaces with the EHR software, then follow the procedure and upload the tracing to the patient's health record. The provider will read the tracing once it is uploaded.

An ECG must be read by the provider before it is filed in the paper medical record. If the tracing was done on small strips of ECG paper, the strips need to be mounted per the facility's procedures. Special 8.5 × 10-inch paper with adhesive strips is used to stick the ECG tracing strips. Once the strips are mounted, they can be given to the provider to read. If the ECG prints on 8.5 × 10-inch paper, it does not need to be mounted. It can be given to the provider immediately.

CRITICAL THINKING BOX 39.9

The clinic uses an ECG machine that uploads the ECGs into patients' electronic health records. Based on what you have learned so far in your courses, why is this useful and efficient?

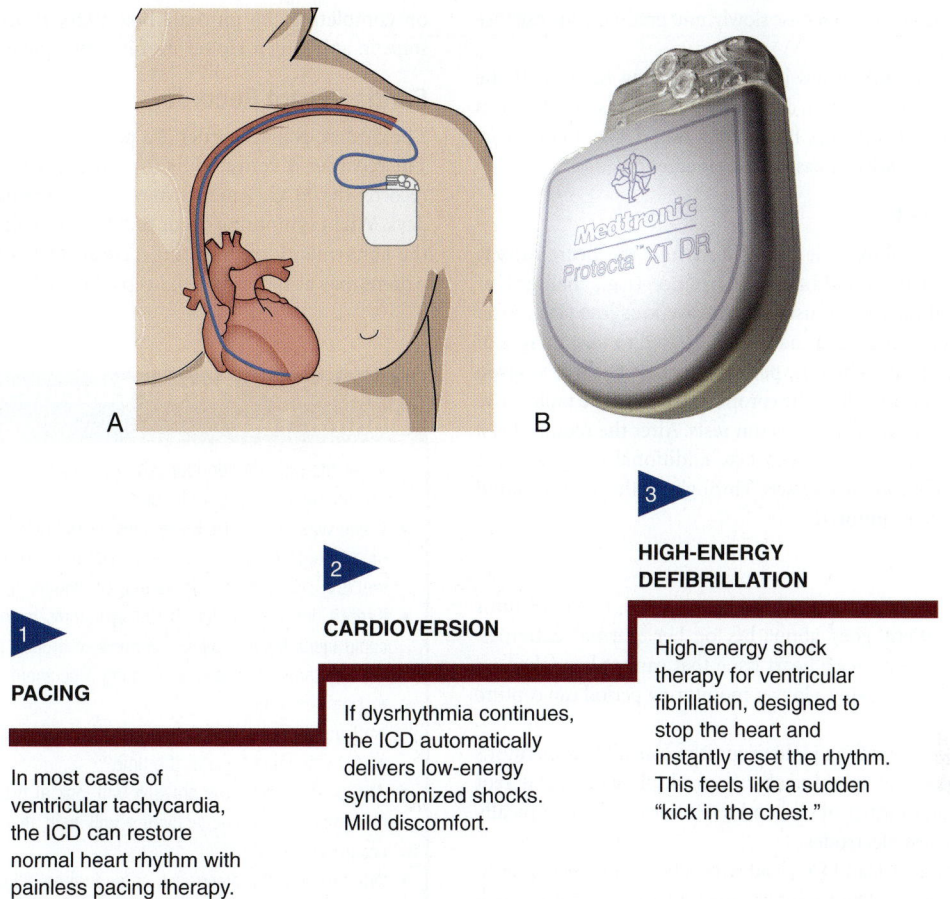

FIG. 39.21 Implanted cardioverter-defibrillator (ICD). (From Urden L, Stacy K, Lough M: *Thelan's Critical Care Nursing: Diagnosis and Management*, ed 7, St Louis, 2014, Mosby.)

ADDITIONAL ECG TESTING

Exercise Stress Test

An exercise stress test records the ECG while the patient is exercising. The patient either walks on a treadmill with an incline or uses an exercise bike (Fig. 39.22). During the test, a continual ECG is recorded, and the blood pressure is monitored.

Why the test is ordered:
- The patient is starting an exercise program.
- The patient has angina that is getting worse.
- To evaluate the patient's heart after an angioplasty or bypass surgery.
- To evaluate heart rhythm changes with the stress of exercise.

Preparation for the test:
- The patient should wear clothes and shoes for exercising.
- The provider will indicate what daily medications should be taken prior to the test.
- The patient should not take a dose of Viagra, Cialis, or Levitra for erectile dysfunction 48 hours before a stress test.
- The patient should not smoke or consume caffeine or alcohol 3 hours before the test.
- The patient signs a consent form prior to the test.

During the test:
- Electrodes and lead wires will be placed on the patient. A blood pressure cuff will be applied to the patient's arm.

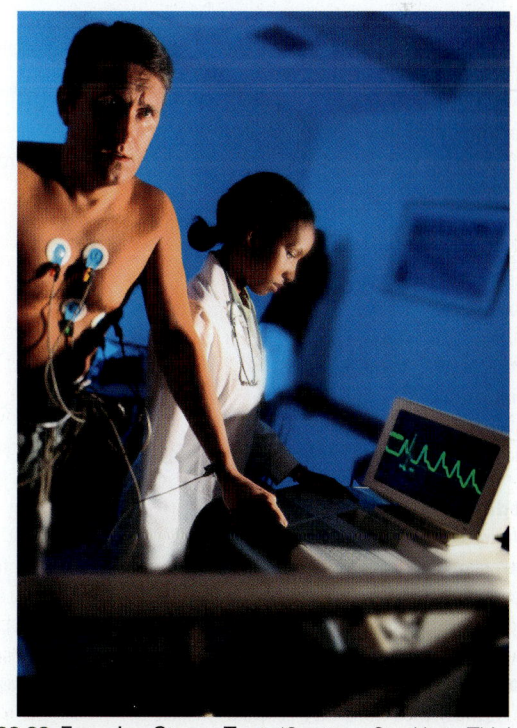

FIG. 39.22 Exercise Stress Test. (Courtesy Stockbyte/Thinkstock.)

- The patient will begin to exercise slowly, and gradually the exercise difficulty will increase.
- The provider should always be present during the test. If the patient has chest discomfort, dizziness, palpitations, or shortness of breath, the test will stop. Emergency supplies or a crash cart should be kept nearby in case of an emergency.

Nuclear Stress Test

The nuclear stress test shows the blood flow into the heart muscle during rest and activity. A radioactive substance (e.g., thallium or sestamibi) is injected into a vein using an intravenous line (IV). After 15 to 45 minutes of resting, a gamma camera is used to take images of the blood flow in the heart. Then the person either exercises or is given a vasodilating medication to dilate the coronary arteries. The radioactive substance is again injected, and the person rests. After the required rest period, the gamma camera is used to take additional images of the blood flow through the coronary vessels. Throughout the test, the blood pressure and ECG are monitored.

Holter Monitor

A Holter monitor is used to monitor the heart over a 24- to 48-hour period while the patient goes about his or her normal activities. Sometimes patients experience a heart issue that cannot be picked up on a resting 12-lead ECG. Having a longer monitoring period can capture the abnormalities.

When placing electrodes for a Holter monitor, consult the operator's manual. There are many configurations for electrode placement. Different monitors use varying number of electrodes. Holter monitors typically use three to seven chest electrodes.

As with the resting 12-lead ECG, lead wires attach the electrodes to the small Holter monitor. The monitor runs on batteries and is small enough to fit into a pocket. The patient is given a journal and instructions on completing the journal (Box 39.6). Procedure 39.2 describes the steps in applying a Holter monitor to a patient.

Cardiac Event Recorder

The cardiac event recorder is a portable, battery-powered ECG device. The recorder is activated by the patient when symptoms occur, and it records the ECG. Patients may wear a cardiac event recorder for 30 days. When symptoms occur only occasionally, it is difficult to capture the abnormality on a resting 12-lead ECG or a Holter monitor. The patient may also be asked to keep a journal, as with the Holter monitor.

BOX 39.6 Patient Education for a Holter Monitor Test

- Wear the monitor continuously. The monitor will be removed during your appointment in 24 to 48 hours.
- While wearing the Holter monitor, avoid metal detectors, large magnets, high-voltage areas, x-rays, and electric blankets. Do not get the monitor wet (e.g., no bathing, showering, or swimming).
- Keep a detailed journal of the symptoms experienced. These symptoms could include chest pain, shortness of breath, palpitations or changes in the heartbeat, dizziness, or fainting. Document:
  - Date and time
  - Symptoms experienced
  - Activity being done at the time
- At the return visit, the provider will look at the tracing for abnormalities. The journal of timed activities will help the provider identify what is occurring.
- What to do if the electrodes or lead wires fall off.
- Who to contact in case of questions or if problems occur.

PROCEDURE 39.2 Apply a Holter Monitor

Tasks:
Apply a Holter monitor and coach a patient on the procedure. Document the procedure in the patient's health record.

Equipment and Supplies
- Holter monitor and supplies (new batteries, flash memory card [if required], carrying case, and operator's manual)
- Disposable electrodes
- Razor
- Sharps container
- Alcohol pads
- Gauze pads (optional)
- Cloth nonallergenic tape (optional)
- Journal
- Trash container
- Patient's health record

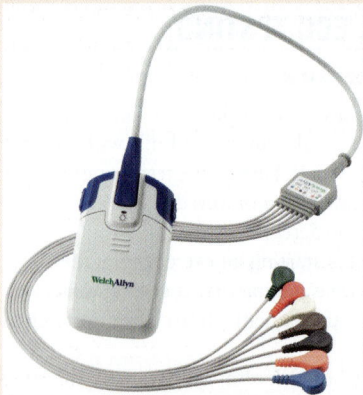

1 (Courtesy Welch Allyn, Skaneateles Falls, NY.)

Procedural Steps
1. Wash hands or use hand sanitizer.
   Purpose: Hand sanitization is an important step for infection control.
2. Assemble equipment and supplies needed for the procedure. Insert flash memory card if required. Insert new batteries into the monitor (Fig. 1). Consult the operator's manual for the required number and placement of electrodes.
   Purpose: Having the equipment ready helps reduce the patient's wait time. New batteries will ensure accurate functioning.
3. Greet the patient. Identify yourself. Verify the patient's identity with full name and date of birth. Explain the procedure in a manner that is understood by the patient. Answer any questions the patient may have on the procedure.
   Purpose: It is important to identify the patient in two different ways to ensure that you have the correct patient. Explaining the procedure can make the patient feel more comfortable and helps to reduce anxiety.

PROCEDURE 39.2 Apply a Holter Monitor—cont'd

4. Ask the patient to remove clothing from the waist up and to sit at the end of the exam table. Ask the patient if assistance is needed. If so, help. If not, leave the room and allow the patient time to change. When reentering the room, provide a courtesy knock on the door.
   Purpose: The patient needs to be undressed from the waist up for you to place the electrodes. Patients require privacy to change.
5. Identify the locations for the electrodes and prepare the skin for the electrodes. Shave the area if the patient has a hairy chest. Wipe the area with the alcohol pad and allow it to dry. Fold the gauze pad over your index finger and briskly rub the site to abrade the skin.
   Purpose: These techniques help the electrodes to better adhere to the skin, which creates a better tracing.
6. Snap the lead wire onto the electrode. Apply the electrodes to the sites as indicated by the manufacturer. Press firmly and make sure the entire electrode adheres completely to the skin (Fig. 2).
   Purpose: Secure electrode attachment is necessary to produce an accurate tracing.

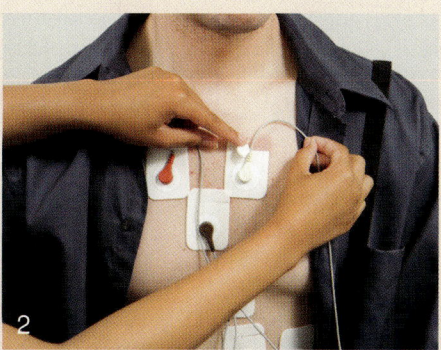

7. Loop and tape down the wires on the chest.
   Purpose: The tape will hold the wires in place and reduce the tension on the electrodes.
8. Attach the patient cable to the monitor if required. Turn on the recorder and set as indicated by the manufacturer. Enter the patient data as indicated.
   Purpose: Each manufacturer will have directions to operate the monitor.
9. Have the patient get dressed. Assist as needed.
   Purpose: Some patients may require assistance when hooked up to the monitor.
10. Coach the patient about making journal entries while wearing the monitor (Fig. 3). Provide the required patient education (see Box 39.6).
    Purpose: It is important for the patient to keep a diary of what he or she is doing. The provider will check the ECG for abnormalities and then check what the patient was doing during the event.

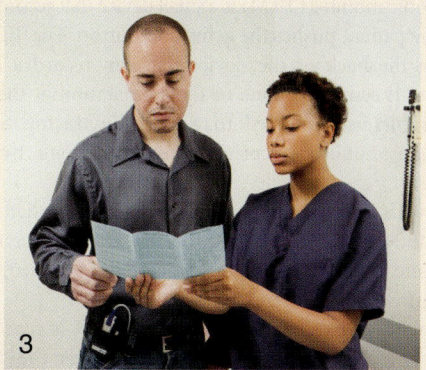

11. Assist the patient in scheduling a return appointment in 24 hours. Provide the patient with contact information should a question arise.
    Purpose: The patient will need to return in 24 hours for the monitor to be removed. Providing contact information will help reduce the patient's anxiety.
12. Document accurately in the patient's health record. Indicate the provider ordering the test, what was done, patient education provided and return appointment.
    Purpose: Indicating who ordered the test and what was done is important for insurance reimbursement and for legal reasons.

Documentation Example

08/06/20XX 1423: Per Dr. James Martin's order, a Holter monitor was applied. Pt was instructed how to complete the diary and a contact number was provided if pt has additional questions. Pt verbalized what he was to write in the diary. Appointment was made for 08/07/20XX to remove the monitor._____
_____Eva Ning, RMA

With the cardiac event recorder, the patient goes about his or her daily activities. The monitor can be removed during bathing and showering or swimming.

When patients experience symptoms, they push the recorder's activation button. An ECG is recorded and stored. The ECG can be sent to the provider via a phone or other technology. A provider will review the tracing. If there is an emergency, the patient will be called and told to go to the nearest emergency department.

There are two types of cardiac event recorders:
- Looping memory monitor (also called a *cardiac loop recorder*): A pager-sized monitor that connects to two chest electrodes by wires. The monitor continuously records the ECG. When the memory is full, it overwrites from the beginning (i.e., continues loop of recording). When a patient has symptoms, he or she activates the monitor. The ECG from prior to, during, and for a short while after the event is stored. It does not overwrite the stored ECGs.
- Symptom event monitor (also called a *post-event monitor*): Can be a handheld device or worn on the wrist. When symptoms are felt, the patient activates the monitor and places it on the chest. Small metal disks on the back of the monitor act as electrodes. The current ECG is recorded and stored. Unlike the looping memory monitor, the symptom event monitor cannot record and store the ECG prior to the symptoms.

Implantable Loop Recorder

The implantable loop record (also called a *loop recorder implant*) is a small recorder (under 2 inches) that looks like a flash drive. It is surgically implanted just under the skin in the upper left chest. It can be implanted in an ambulatory care facility.

Often the device is used for patients who have episodes of fainting, seizures, and palpitations. Other ECG tests have not been able to detect the abnormality. It also catches infrequent arrhythmias that can be missed with traditional ECG monitoring.

The device continuously records the ECG for 2 to 3 years. It records the ECG if the heart rate falls below or rises above the preset limits (set by the provider). The patient can also record the ECG if symptoms are experienced. The provider can download the saved ECG data at the next appointment.

Transtelephonic Monitoring

A transtelephonic monitor (TTM) is a small device that records a patient's ECG when the patient pushes the activation button. The TTM has four electrodes on the back of the device that can record a single lead. The ECG data is sent via phone to the base station at the provider's office. The signal is converted to a readable tracing that can be displayed on a monitor or printed out. There are two types of TTMs:
- TTM with internal memory: The ECG is recorded and stored when the patient pushes a button. The data can be transmitted by phone to the provider. This type of TTM is used for patients with infrequent arrhythmias.
- TTM with no internal memory: The TTM is placed over the heart, and the phone receiver is placed over the TTM. Once the activation button is pushed, the TTM records and immediately sends the live ECG to the provider via the phone line. The data is not saved in the device. This type of TTM is used for patients with pacemakers and internal cardioverter-defibrillators. It allows the provider to monitor the patient remotely.

Portable Handheld ECG Monitors

There are a variety of portable handheld ECG monitors on the market. Many produce a single lead. The ECG data can then be transferred to other devices using software, Bluetooth, smart phones, or USB ports. These devices are marketed to be used at home. A person can use the device and save ECG tracings. The tracings can then be reviewed by the person's provider at the next visit. The machines work differently; some having several electrode options. Finger contact, chest contact (bare skin just below the nipple), and regular chest electrodes can be used to create an ECG tracing.

> **CRITICAL THINKING BOX 39.10**
>
> Monique Jones is Eva's last patient before lunch. As Eva is gathering Monique's history, Monique mentions that she has heart palpitations. She had heard about ECG monitors that could be used at home. She was able to order one off the internet and was able to capture her palpitation spell. She is here today to show the doctor her monitor results. Eva has never heard of such a thing. How might she respond to the patient?

RESPIRATORY SYSTEM

Besides cardiac testing, pulmonary testing is also done in the ambulatory care facility. For the rest of the chapter, pulmonary testing, including measuring the peak flow rate and performing spirometry (spi ROM e tree) testing, will be examined. In addition, pulmonary treatments, including medication administration (nebulizers [NEB uh lize er] and metered-dose inhalers) and oxygen administration, will be explained.

Pulmonary Function Tests

Pulmonary function tests (PFTs) measure the patient's lung function, or how well the lungs work. Some PFTs can measure air flow, and others measure lung size. Table 39.9 reviews PFTs. The following sections provide additional information.

TABLE 39.9 Pulmonary Function Tests

Pulmonary Function Test	Measures	Procedure
Peak flow monitor	Measures the exhaled air	Handheld device used in the clinic and at home to manage chronic respiratory conditions (e.g., asthma).
Spirometry	Rate of air flow; also provides a lung size estimate	Patient breathes multiple times through a tube that is connected to a computer.
Lung volume tests	Determines lung volume	One method: Patient sits in a clear box and breathes in and out of a mouthpiece. The pressure changes in the box determine the lung volume.
Lung diffusion capacity	Determines how effectively gas travels from the lungs to the bloodstream	Patient breathes in a *tracer gas* (harmless gas), and the concentration of the gas is measured in the exhaled air.
Arterial blood gas test	Measures gases in the blood (i.e., oxygen and carbon dioxide)	Typically done in hospital settings, but may be done in clinics. Blood is taken from a wrist artery.
Pulse oximetry (ok SIM e tree)	Measures the oxygen saturation in the blood (Fig. 39.23)	A probe that is placed on the finger or on skin in other locations. (See Chapter 29 for more details.)

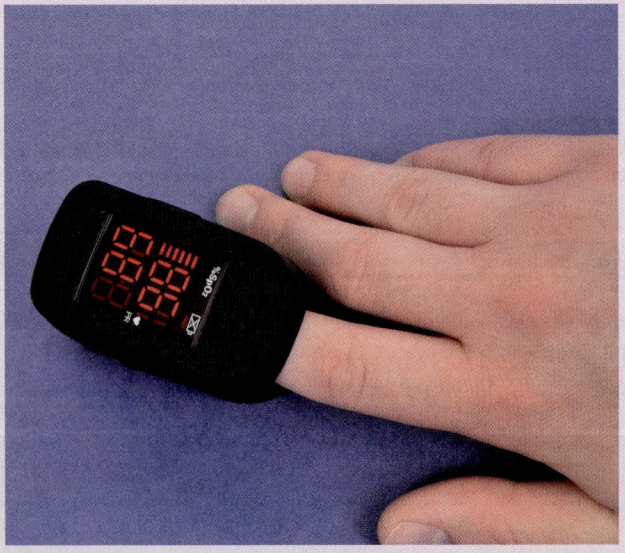

FIG 39.23 Pulse oximeter. (From Proctor D, et al: *Kinn's The Medical Assistant*, ed 13, St Louis, 2017, Elsevier.)

Peak Flow Rate. Peak flow meters can be manual or digital (Figs. 39.24 and 39.25). The peak flow meter measures the amount of air exhaled. It is used to help manage chronic diseases, such as asthma. In Chapter 11 the use of a peak flow meter was described, along with the treatment of asthma.

When a patient is performing a peak flow rate test, it is important that the medical assistant have three adequate readings. Procedure 39.3 describes the steps to measure a peak flow rate.

Spirometry. Spirometry is done to evaluate lung function as affected by respiratory, cardiac, and neuromuscular diseases. It can be ordered if the provider identifies abnormalities in the respiratory system. A spirometer can evaluate the amount of air you exhale and inhale (Fig. 39.26). It looks at how quickly the air is exhaled and the rate at which air is breathed in. Several different tests can be done with spirometry. Table 39.10 describes some of the spirometry tests.

> **MEDICAL TERMINOLOGY**
> **spir/o:** breathing
> **-metry:** process of measurement

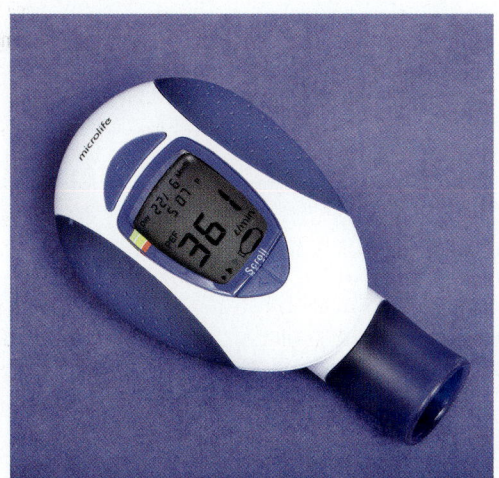

FIG. 39.24 Digital peak flow meter. (From Proctor D, et al: *Kinn's The Medical Assistant*, ed 13, St Louis, 2017, Elsevier.)

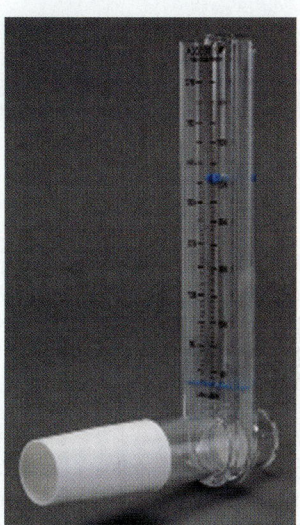

FIG. 39.25 Manual peak flow meter. (From Young AP, Proctor DB: *Kinn's The Medical Assistant*, ed 11, Philadelphia, 2011, Saunders.)

PROCEDURE 39.3 Measure the Peak Flow Rate

Tasks:
Perform a peak flow. Document the procedure in the patient's health record.

Equipment and Supplies
- Peak flow meter
- Disposable mouthpiece
- Disinfection wipes
- Gloves
- Trash container
- Paper towel or denture cup (optional)
- Patient's health record

Procedural Steps
1. Wash hands or use hand sanitizer.
   Purpose: Hand sanitization is an important step for infection control.
2. Assemble equipment and supplies needed for the peak flow procedure. Place the mouthpiece on the peak flow meter. Move the indicator to the bottom of the calibration scale (if not using a digital meter).
   Purpose: Having the equipment ready helps reduce the patient's wait time. The indicator needs to be at the bottom of the scale before the test to get an accurate reading.
3. Greet the patient. Identify yourself. Verify the patient's identity with full name and date of birth. Explain the procedure in a manner that is understood by the patient. Answer any questions the patient may have on the procedure.
   Purpose: It is important to identify the patient in two different ways to ensure that you have the correct patient. Explaining the procedure can make the patient feel more comfortable and helps to reduce anxiety.
4. Ask the patient to loosen any restrictive clothing. Gum and loose dentures should be removed from the patient's mouth. Make sure to provide a paper towel or denture cup if needed.
   Purpose: To get the most accurate results, the patient needs to be able to take a large breath in before the test. Normally, dentures can be left in the mouth, but loose-fitting dentures may affect the results of the test.
5. With the patient in the seated position, ensure that his or her feet are on the floor. The patient should sit straight up and against the back of the chair.
   Purpose: It is important for the patient to be in a position in which the lungs can fully expand.
6. Describe how the patient should do the test. "Take the deepest breath possible. Seal your lips around the mouthpiece. Blow as hard and as fast as you can." Encourage the patient to state when he or she is ready to start the test (Fig. 1).
   Purpose: Clear directions will help the patient understand what to do.

Continued

PROCEDURE 39.3 Measure the Peak Flow Rate—cont'd

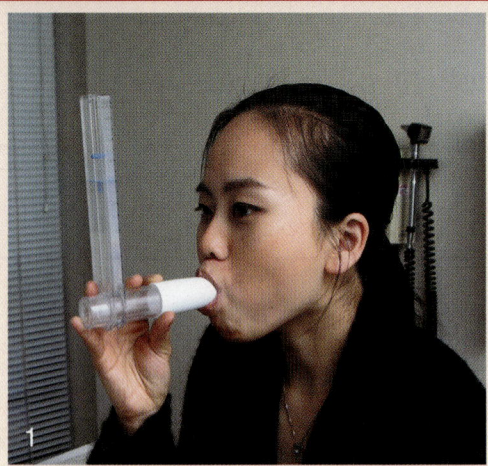

Purpose: Wearing gloves and disinfecting the peak flow meter are important for infection control.

10. Notify the provider of the readings and document the readings in the patient's health record. Indicate the provider who ordered the test, the name of the test, the results of the test, and how the patient tolerated the test.

    Purpose: Indicating who ordered the test and what was done is important for insurance reimbursement and for legal reasons.

Documentation Example

08/07/20XX 1423: Per Dr. Angela Perez's order, a peak flow was performed. Pt stated she was "a little short of breath" on the third test. Peak flow readings: 260, 230, and 200 L/min. Dr Perez was notified of results and patient's SOB complaint._____Eva Ning, RMA

7. Coach the patient during the test. After the patient has blown through the meter, read the number next to the indicator. Write the number down. Reset the indicator to the bottom of the scale (if it is not a digital meter).

    Purpose: If the patient has breathing problems, it is important to allow the patient to indicate when he or she is ready.

8. Make any adjustments as needed. Repeat the test two additional times. Write down the last two numbers.

    Purpose: Three acceptable readings are needed for the peak flow procedure.

9. Put on gloves and remove the mouthpiece. Discard the mouthpiece in the trash container. Disinfect the peak flow meter. Remove gloves wash hands or use hand sanitizer.

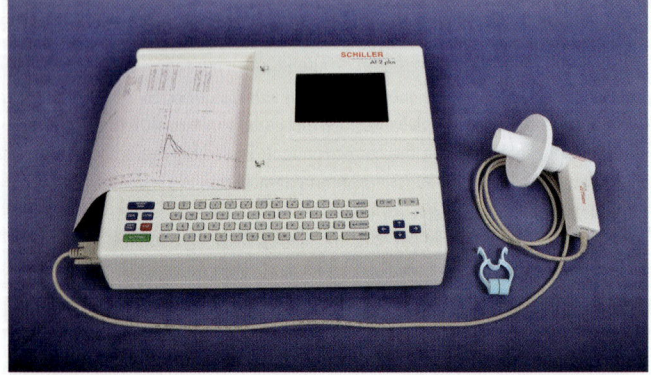

FIG. 39.26 Spirometer. (From Proctor D, et al: *Kinn's The Medical Assistant*, ed 13, St Louis, 2017, Elsevier.)

With spirometry testing, it is important that the medical assistant enter accurate patient data into the spirometer computer. Besides the patient's name, medical record number, and date of birth, the medical assistant may need to enter the person's gender, age, race, height, and weight. The patient's current height and weight need to be obtained prior to the spirometry. The computer then pulls stored data and creates a "normal" person for those characteristics. After the patient has completed the test, the computer will print out the patient's results compared to the "normal" person's results. This helps the provider identify areas of concern.

Procedure 39.4 describes the spirometry procedure. Make sure to follow the operator's manual for the machine you are using. It is important for the patient to do three adequate breaths for the spirometry. The medical assistant needs to be encouraging, yet respectful of the patient, when coaching him or her through the procedure.

Pulmonary Treatments

In the ambulatory care facility, common pulmonary treatments include medication administration and oxygen therapy. Depending on the state's statutes and the facility's policies, the medical assistant may be able to administer nebulizer treatments and oxygen therapy when ordered by the provider. The medical assistant may also instruct patients how to use metered-dose inhalers. The following sections cover metered-dose inhaler education, nebulizer treatments, and oxygen therapy.

Metered-Dose Inhalers. A metered-dose inhaler (MDI) provides aerosol medication that is breathed into the lungs. MDIs are typically ordered for conditions such as asthma and chronic obstructive pulmonary disease (COPD).

TABLE 39.10 Spirometry Tests

Spirometry Tests	Description
Expiratory reserve volume (ERV)	Maximal volume of air exhaled from the end-expiration
Functional residual capacity (FRC)	Amount of air remaining in the lungs at the end of a normal quiet respiration
Residual volume (RV)	Volume of air remaining in the lungs after a maximal exhalation
Forced vital capacity (FVC)	Maximum volume of air that can be forcefully and as rapidly as possible exhaled after taking in a full inhalation
Forced expiratory volume in 1 second (FEV_1)	Volume of air exhaled in the first second under force after a maximal inhalation
Maximum voluntary ventilation (MVV)	Maximum volume that can be exhaled per minute when breathing as rapidly and deeply as possible
Total lung capacity (TLC)	Volume of air in the lungs at maximal inhalation

CRITICAL THINKING BOX 39.11

Eva's last patient of the day is Janine Butler, who is seeing the provider because of her asthma. After the provider sees Janine, he orders a spirometry test. Eva prepares the equipment and brings Janine into the testing room. However, Janine refuses to have her height and weight measured. How might Eva explain to Janine the importance of getting an accurate height and weight?

In many cases the provider will order an MDI with a spacer. A *spacer* is a long tube that is attached to the mouthpiece of an MDI (Fig. 39.27). Spacers slow the delivery of medication from MDIs. Without a spacer, the MDI blasts the medication to the back of the throat and mouth. With inhaled corticosteroids, this can cause irritation and infections over time. When a spacer is used, the medication is blasted into the tube and over several breaths is pulled into the lungs.

In the ambulatory care facility, the medical assistant may need to provide user instructions to the patient (Box 39.7). The medical

PROCEDURE 39.4 Perform Spirometry Testing

Tasks:
Perform a spirometry test. Document the procedure in the patient's health record.

Equipment and Supplies
- Spirometry machine with paper (and operator's manual if applicable)
- Disposable mouthpiece and tubing (if applicable)
- Nose clip
- Calibration equipment
- Disinfection wipes
- Gloves
- Trash container
- Patient's health record
- Scale (if no height and weight measurement from today)

Procedural Steps

1. Wash hands or use hand sanitizer.
   Purpose: Hand sanitization is an important step for infection control.
2. Assemble equipment and supplies needed for the spirometry procedure. Calibrate the machine according to the operator's manual and the facility's procedures.
   Purpose: It is important to calibrate per the facility's procedures. Calibration ensures that the results are accurate and reliable.
3. Greet the patient. Identify yourself. Verify the patient's identity with full name and date of birth. Explain the procedure in a manner that is understood by the patient. Answer any questions the patient may have on the procedure.
   Purpose: It is important to identify the patient in two different ways to ensure that you have the correct patient. Explaining the procedure can make the patient feel more comfortable and helps to reduce anxiety.
4. Ask the patient to loosen any restrictive clothing. Have the patient remove gum and loose dentures (if applicable). Make sure to provide a paper towel or denture cup if needed.
   Purpose: To get the most accurate results, the patient needs to be able to take a large breath in before the test. Loose-fitting dentures can affect the results of the test.
5. Enter the patient's name, medical record number, age (or date of birth), race, gender, weight, and height into the machine. Enter any additional required information.
   Purpose: The information used for the spirometry calculations is: current weight, height, age, race, and gender.
6. Describe how the patient should do the test. "Take the deepest breath possible. Seal your lips around the mouthpiece. Blow as hard and as fast as you can. Blow until you empty the air from your lungs."
   Purpose: Clear directions will help the patient understand what to do.
7. Have the patient take the seated position. The patient should be sitting straight up with the feet flat on the floor and the legs uncrossed.
   Purpose: The patient may get dizzy during the test, so standing can be problematic. The seated position provides the maximum lung expansion for the test.
8. Attach the mouthpiece to the machine. Explain the purpose of the nose clip to the patient. Apply the nose clip to the patient (Fig. 1). Have the patient state when he or she is ready to start. Start the test as directed by the operator's manual.
   Purpose: The nose clip prevents air from leaking out through the nose. It provides a more accurate reading.

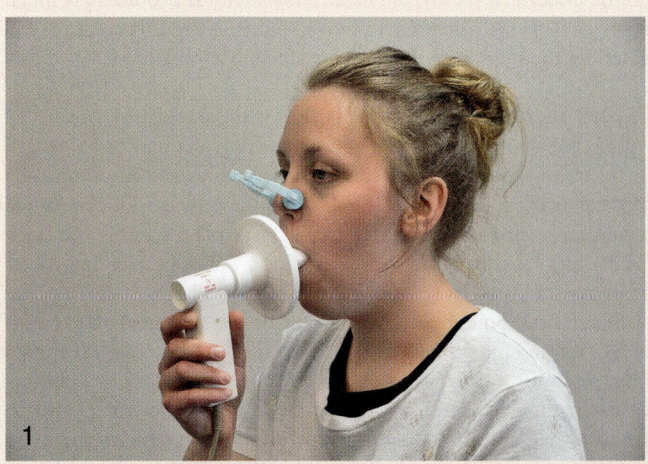

1

Continued

PROCEDURE 39.4 Perform Spirometry Testing—cont'd

9. During the test encourage the patient to empty the lungs. Repeat until three acceptable tests have been done. Allow the patient to rest between tests, if needed, and to indicate when he or she is ready for next test.
   Purpose: Usually three tests results are needed for comparison. If the patient is struggling and having difficulty breathing, check with the provider if three tests need to be done.
10. Put on gloves and remove the mouthpiece. Discard the mouthpiece in the trash container. Disinfect the spirometer as indicated in the operator's manual. Remove gloves and wash hands or use hand sanitizer.
    Purpose: Wearing gloves and disinfecting the equipment is important for infection control.
11. Document that the test was performed. Indicate the provider who ordered the test, the name of the test, how the patient tolerated the test, and what you did with the test results. Any patient instructions regarding follow-up can also be documented.

Purpose: Indicating who ordered the test and what was done is important for insurance reimbursement and for legal reasons.

Documentation Example
08/08/20XX 1423: Per Dr. James Martin's order, a spirometry test was performed. Pt stated she felt dizzy during the third attempt. The dizziness cleared within 5 minutes, and she stated she felt better. Pt was instructed to call the clinic tomorrow for the spirometry results. The spirometry results were given to Dr. Martin._____Eva Ning, RMA

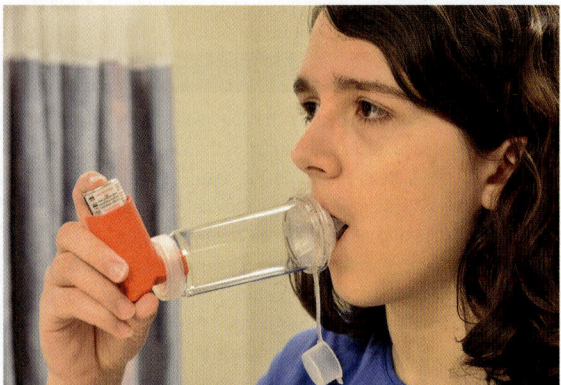

FIG. 39.27 Using a metered-dose inhaler with a spacer.

assistant should also discuss how the equipment should be cleaned (Box 39.8).

Nebulizer Treatment. Inhaled medication for asthma, COPD, and other lung diseases can be given using a nebulizer. A nebulizer treatment can be done in the ambulatory care setting and in the home. A nebulizer is a small machine that turns liquid medication into a fine spray that can be inhaled. Typically, the medication used for nebulizers is much stronger than the same medication found in a MDI. Procedure 39.5 describes the steps for administering a nebulizer treatment.

Oxygen Therapy. When a patient comes to the ambulatory care facility with a cardiac or respiratory condition, the provider may order oxygen to be administered. Oxygen should be treated as a medication. The medical assistant must get the order from the provider for how much to administer and how to administer it. Oxygen in the ambulatory care facility may be available in the room using a wall-mounted flow meter or in oxygen cylinders (portable tanks).

Room air is about 21% oxygen. Oxygen devices increase the concentration of oxygen for the patient to breathe in. Typically, a nasal cannula (Fig. 39.29) or a simple mask is used in the ambulatory care setting. Other masks that deliver higher oxygen concentrations may also be available (Fig. 39.30). Table 39.11 provides information on the more common oxygen delivery devices used in the ambulatory care setting. Procedure 39.6 presents the steps for administering oxygen.

BOX 39.7 Using a Metered-Dose Inhaler (MDI)

1. Shake the MDI 3 or 4 times. Remove the cover from the MDI's mouthpiece.
   a. If using a spacer:
      - Attach the spacer. Breathe out. Place the mouthpiece between your lips and close your lips around it.
      - Press the top of the canister on the MDI.
      - Breathe in very slowly, taking a full breath in. Some spacers will produce a whistle-like sound if you are breathing in too fast.
   b. If not using a spacer:
      - Breathe out. Place the inhaler 1 to 2 inches (about 2 finger widths) in front of your opened mouth (Fig. 39.28).
      - Press the top of the canister on the MDI.
      - Breathe in very slowly, taking a full breath in.
2. Hold your breath for 10 seconds (or count to 10) and then breathe out. If you are using inhaled, quick-relief medication (beta-agonists), wait 1 minute between puffs.
3. Repeat steps 1a or 1b and 2 until your dose is completed.

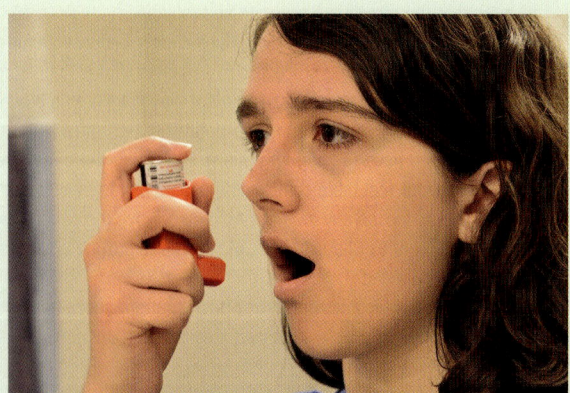

FIG. 39.28 Using a metered-dose inhaler without a spacer.

CHAPTER 39 Cardiopulmonary Procedures

BOX 39.8 Cleaning a Spacer and a Metered-Dose Inhaler

- Spacers can be taken apart, cleaned with mild soap, and then allowed to air dry.
- To clean the MDI inhaler, remove the medication canister and mouthpiece cover. Let warm water flow over the top and bottom of the MDI inhaler for about 30 seconds. Shake off and let air dry overnight. When assembling, spray twice in the air before taking a dose. Clean the MDI weekly to prevent medication from building up and blocking the dose sprayed.
- Cleaning techniques can vary with medication products. Patients should be encouraged to check the product's website for directions.

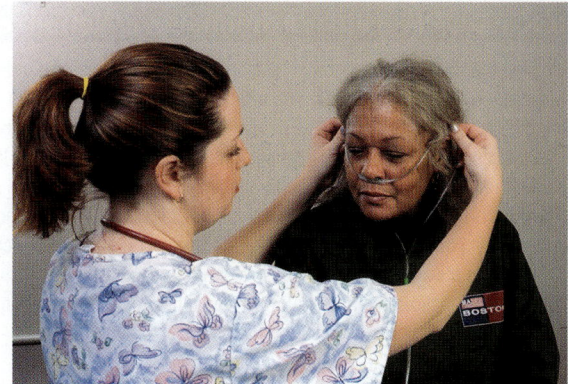

FIG. 39.29 Applying a nasal cannula. (From Proctor D, et al: *Kinn's The Medical Assistant*, ed 13, St Louis, 2017, Elsevier.)

PROCEDURE 39.5 Administer a Nebulizer Treatment

Tasks:
Administer a nebulizer treatment. Document medication administration in the patient's health record.

Equipment and Supplies
- Nebulizer machine
- Disposable nebulizer patient kit (tubing, medication cup, mouthpiece or mask, flexible tube, and tee)
- Medication as ordered
- Normal saline (as ordered or per facility's protocol)
- Provider's order
- Disinfection wipes
- Gloves
- Trash container
- Patient's health record

Order:
Levalbuterol 0.63 mg by nebulization.

Procedural Steps

1. Wash hands or use hand sanitizer. Using the drug reference information and the order, review the information on the medication if needed. Clarify any questions you have with the provider.
   Purpose: Hand sanitization is an important step for infection control. It is important to be knowledgeable about the medication you are giving.
2. Select the right medication from the storage area. Check to see if the medication is concentrated and requires normal saline to dilute it. Check the medication label (and normal saline label, if used) against the order. Check for the right name, form, and route. Check the expiration date to make sure the drug is not expired. Verify that it is the right dose and time.
   Purpose: A provider's order is required for the nebulizer treatment. The medication needs to be verified three times before it is given. The Nine Rights of Medication Administration also need to be followed.
3. Assemble equipment and supplies needed for the nebulizer treatment.
   Purpose: Having the equipment ready helps reduce the patient's wait time.
4. Perform the second medication check. Check the medication and normal saline label(s) against the order. Check for the right name, form, and route.
   Purpose: It is important to do the second check of the label(s) before pouring the medication into the medication cup.
5. Add the medication and, if required, the normal saline to the medication cup (Fig. 1). Secure the cover on the cup.
   Purpose: The medication cup holds the medication during the treatment.

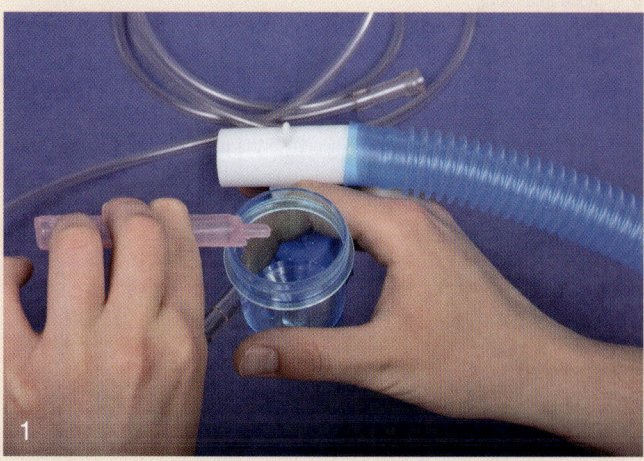

6. Perform the third medication check. Check the medication label and normal saline label (if used) against the order. Check for the right name, form, and route. Verify that the amount of medication in the cup is correct according to the order. Clean up the area.
   Purpose: It is important to do the third check of the label before giving the medication.
7. Prior to entering the exam room, knock on the door and give it a moment. Greet the patient. Identify yourself. Verify the patient's identity with full name and date of birth. Make sure the patient's information matches the order and the record. Explain what you are going to do.
   Purpose: It is important to identify the patient in two different ways to ensure that you have the correct patient. Explaining the procedure can make the patient feel more comfortable and helps to reduce anxiety.

Continued

PROCEDURE 39.5   Administer a Nebulizer Treatment—cont'd

8. Provide the right education to the patient. Explain the medication ordered, the desired effect, and common side effects; also identify the provider who ordered it. Answer any questions the patient may have. Use language the patient can understand. Ask the patient if he or she has any allergies. If the patient refuses the medication, notify the provider.
   Purpose: The patient needs to be aware of what you are giving, the action and side effects, and who ordered it. It is also important to double-check the patient's allergies before administering the medication.
9. Attach the mouthpiece (or mask). Attach the tubing to the medication cup and the machine.
   Purpose: Use a mask if ordered by the provider.
10. Perform the right technique. The patient should be sitting upright on a chair to allow for total lung expansion. Instruct the patient to hold the mouthpiece between the teeth and seal the lips around the mouthpiece. Encourage the patient to take slow, deep breaths through the mouth. The patient should hold each breath 2 to 3 seconds before exhaling.
    Purpose: Sitting upright allows for total lung expansion. If patients breathe too deeply and too fast, they will become dizzy and may hyperventilate. Holding the breath in allows the medication to disperse through the lungs.
11. Turn on the nebulizer and give the medicine cup and mouthpiece to the patient to start the treatment. Instruct the patient to put it into his or her mouth. If using a mask, position it securely and comfortably over the patient's nose and mouth.
    Purpose: It is important to make sure the mask is comfortable over the patient's face. If it is not comfortable, the patient may not tolerate the treatment.
12. Continue the treatment until the mist has stopped (approximately 10 minutes) (Fig. 2). Turn off the nebulizer. Encourage the patient to take several deep breaths and cough.
    Purpose: After the treatment, it is common that patients will need to cough. Ensure that tissue is available if the patient needs it.

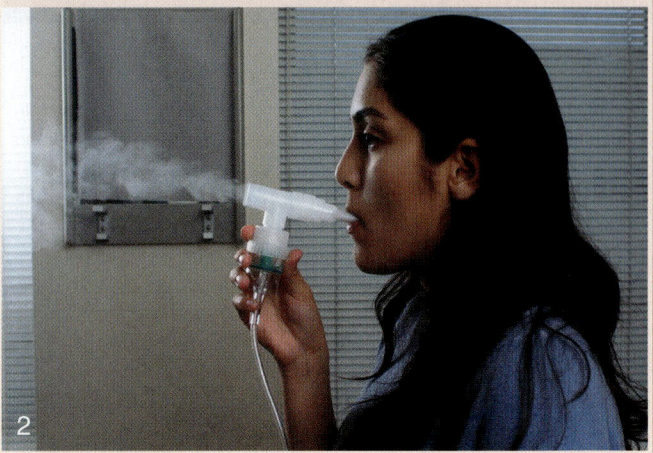

13. Put on gloves and dispose of the used supplies. Disinfect the nebulizer machine. Remove gloves and sanitize your hands.
    Purpose: To ensure infection control.
14. Document in the patient's health record: the provider ordering the treatment, what was administered, how the patient tolerated the medication, and any follow-up assessments (e.g., vital signs).
    Purpose: Documentation is the last of the Nine Rights of Medication Administration.

Documentation Example
08/06/20XX 1120: P: 76 regular, strong; R: 26 regular, shallow. Per Dr. Angela Perez's order, Levalbuterol 0.63 mg administered by nebulizer. Pt stated she felt a little shaky after the treatment and her lungs feel less tight. Pt is resting on the exam table. P: 86 regular, strong; R: 20 regular, normal. Dr. Perez notified._____Eva Ning, RMA

TABLE 39.11   Common Oxygen Delivery Devices

Type	Flow range (Liters/minute [LPM])	Oxygen Delivered	Descriptions
Nasal cannula	1–2 2–4 4–6	24%–28% 28%–34% 34%–44%	• Soft tube with prongs that are placed in the nose; make sure prongs curve downward. • A humidification device is used if flow is over 4 L/min. • Allows patient to talk, drink, and eat. • Cannot be used with upper respiratory obstructions (e.g., nasal polyps); not helpful for mouth breathers.
Mask	5–10	30%–60%	• Used for strictly mouth breathers. • Best used for short-term situations (e.g., ambulatory care). • Restrictive for communication, coughing, and eating. • Requires 5–6 L/min to avoid CO_2 accumulation in the mask.
Partial rebreathing mask	6–10	40%–70%	• Oxygen feeds into a reservoir bag attached to a mask. • About one third of expired air enters reservoir bag, and the rest exits mask through exhalation ports.
Non-rebreathing face mask	10–15	Up to about 90%	• Mask with a reservoir bag and one-way valves. • One-way valve allows patient to inhale oxygen from the reservoir bag but prevents expired air from entering bag. • Before applying to patient, occlude valve and allow reservoir bag to fill with oxygen.

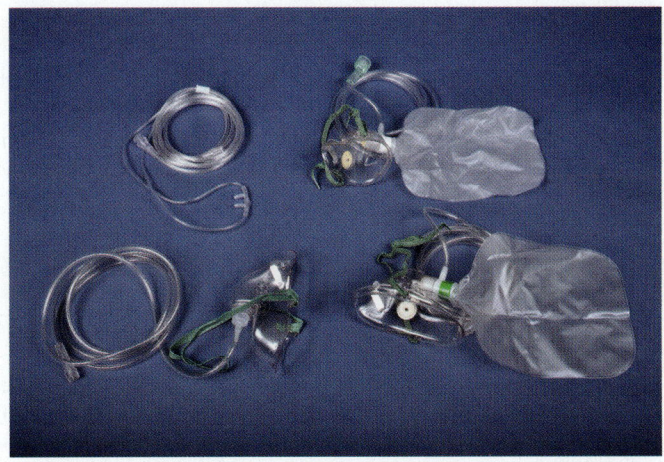

FIG. 39.30 *Top left to right:* Nasal cannula and child non-rebreather mask. Non-rebreather masks have one-way valves (e.g., yellow circle on the mask). *Bottom left to right:* Simple face mask and adult non-rebreather mask.

PROCEDURE 39.6 Administer Oxygen Per Nasal Cannula or Mask

Tasks:
Administer oxygen per nasal cannula or mask. Document in the patient's health record.

Equipment and Supplies
- Oxygen cylinder with oxygen regulator or oxygen flow meter (wall unit)
- Adult nasal cannula or simple mask
- Provider's order
- Patient's health record

Order 1:
Administer 2 L/min of oxygen per nasal cannula.

Order 2:
Administer 6 L/min of oxygen per simple mask.

Procedural Steps

1. Wash hands or use hand sanitizer.
   Purpose: Hand sanitization is an important step for infection control.
2. Assemble equipment and supplies needed for the provider's order. If an oxygen cylinder is used, identify the amount of oxygen left in the cylinder.
   Purpose: The order will include the amount to give and the device (e.g., cannula) to use for the administration. It is important to make sure the cylinder has enough oxygen for the patient.
3. Verify the order if you have any questions.
   Purpose: A provider's order is required for the oxygen administration.
4. Greet the patient. Identify yourself. Verify the patient's identity with full name and date of birth. Explain the procedure in a manner that is understood by the patient. Answer any questions the patient may have on the procedure.
   Purpose: It is important to identify the patient in two different ways to ensure that you have the correct patient. Explaining the procedure can make the patient feel more comfortable and helps to reduce anxiety.
5. Connect the nasal cannula or mask to the regulator or flow meter. Turn on the oxygen and adjust the flow rate to the correct amount per the provider's order. The ball should be centered on the number of liters ordered.
   Purpose: Oxygen needs to be flowing through the tubing before the cannula is applied to the patient.
6. Apply the mask or nasal cannula:
   a. Place the mask over the patient's nose, mouth, and chin. Place the elastic over the head. Adjust the elastic strap to tighten the mask on the face. Adjust the metal nasal bridge clamp, making sure it fits without obstructing the nose. Ensure that the mask fits tightly on the face.
   Purpose: A poorly fitting mask can cause oxygen to be directed into the eyes, causing additional problems.
   b. Insert the tips of the cannula into the nostrils. If the tips are curved, the curves face downward toward the bottom of the nose (Fig. 1). Adjust the tubing around the back of the ears and then under the chin. Encourage the patient to breathe through the nose with the mouth closed.
   Purpose: The cannula needs to be inserted correctly into the nostrils. The cannula tips may be blocked by the top of the nostrils if they are put in wrong. Breathing through the mouth when using a cannula is not as beneficial as breathing through the nose.

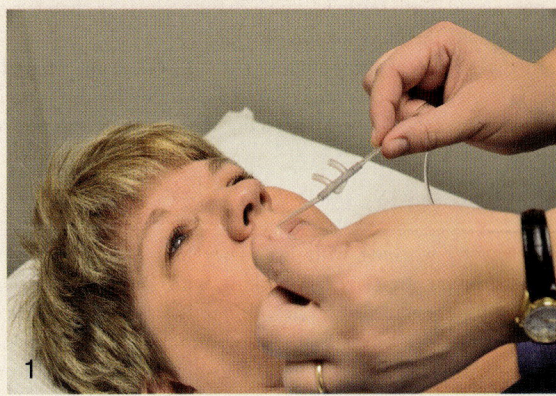

7. Make sure the patient is comfortable. Answer any questions he or she may have. Sanitize your hands.
   Purpose: Unanswered questions can cause anxiety. With breathing problems, it is important for the patient to be comfortable and calm.
8. Document the procedure. Include the ordering provider, the number of liters of oxygen administered, the device used for administering the oxygen, and the patient's condition.
   Purpose: Indicating who ordered the oxygen and what was administered is important for insurance reimbursement and for legal reasons.

Documentation Example
08/07/20XX 1540: R: 28 regular, shallow. Per Dr. Angela Perez's order, 2 L/min of oxygen administered via nasal cannula. Pt resting on exam table._____
_____Eva Ning, RMA
08/07/20XX 1555: R: 20 regular, normal. Pt stated she is "feeling better" with the oxygen and has less SOB. Dr. Angela Perez was notified._____
_____Eva Ning, RMA

CLOSING COMMENTS

In many of the ambulatory care departments, the providers will order some type of cardiopulmonary testing. Knowing how to produce a clear ECG tracing is critical. Putting the electrodes on incorrectly or switching the lead wires can lead to many problems for the patients, because they may be wrongly diagnosed with cardiac disease.

Besides knowing how to perform an ECG, the medical assistant should be knowledgeable about other ECG tests, pulmonary testing, and pulmonary treatments. The medical assistant should also be familiar with the medical terminology associated with the cardiovascular and respiratory systems.

CHAPTER REVIEW

This chapter reviewed the cardiovascular anatomy, including the heart structures, blood flow, and conduction system. The components of the ECG tracing are:

- P wave: Shows atrial depolarization; atrial chambers contract and the blood is pushed to the ventricles.
- PR segment: Isoelectric line; allows the atria to finish contracting.
- QRS complex: Shows ventricular depolarization; atrial repolarization also occurs during this time, though it is hidden. The ventricles contract, pushing blood out of the heart.
- ST segment: Isoelectric line; allows the ventricles to finish contracting.
- T wave: Ventricular repolarization and atrial polarization.

After the T wave or U wave, ventricular polarization occurs.

For a resting 12-lead ECG, three leads are bipolar, three are augmented, and the remaining six are precordial. Ten electrodes are used for the 12-lead ECG. One electrode is placed on each of the extremities, with the right leg being the ground. Six electrodes are placed on the chest. Lead wires are attached to the electrodes. If the electrocardiograph is set at 10 mm/mV, the standardization mark will be an upward rectangle that is 10 small boxes tall. The chart or paper speed should be set at 25 mm per second. Both settings can be changed, but the change needs to be indicated on the ECG for the provider.

The medical assistant should examine the ECG tracing for artifact. If artifact is seen, steps should be taken to problem-solve the situation. Then a new tracing should be run. If a life-threatening rhythm is seen on the tracing, the medical assistant needs to get the provider immediately.

There are several ECG tests besides the 12-lead ECG. Some require testing at the ambulatory care facility, whereas others monitor the ECG while the patient goes about his or her daily activities. Tests such as the Holter monitor and the cardiac event record require patients to keep a journal of their symptoms and activities.

Pulmonary function tests provide information on the function and size of the lungs. The medical assistant can perform the peak flow and spirometry tests. A medical assistant can do pulmonary treatments, including nebulizer treatments and oxygen therapy.

EXCEPTIONAL CUSTOMER SERVICE

To provide exceptional customer service, medical assistants need to:
- Provide patients with clear instructions on the cardiopulmonary procedure being done.
- Perform the procedure correctly, so the patient's results are accurate.
- Be sensitive to patients' concerns and feelings regarding cardiopulmonary diseases.
- Be respectful and empathetic when encouraging patients to breathe for spirometry tests. Remember, if the patient is short of breath or coughing due to an illness, blowing for a spirometry test can be difficult. Allow the patient to tell you when he or she is ready to do the next test.

SCENARIO WRAP-UP

Renee is enjoying working with Eva. They have seen many different cardiopulmonary tests while working with Dr. Kahn's patients. Renee has found herself learning new things. If she does not have the answers to Eva's questions about cardiopulmonary tests, she looks up the information. She finds herself learning new information as a result.

Eva is really enjoying working with Renee and Dr. Kahn. She is feeling so much better performing ECGs. Her understanding of the ECG tracing and how to resolve artifact has greatly improved. She is also feeling more confident performing cardiopulmonary testing. She is hoping to be able to work with Dr. Kahn in the future, because she enjoys ECGs so much!

40

Medical Emergencies

LEARNING OBJECTIVES

1. Discuss emergencies in healthcare settings and possible roles each team member has during an emergency.
2. Describe emergency equipment and supplies.
3. Explain first aid procedures for environmental emergencies including temperature-related emergencies, burns, poisonings, anaphylaxis, bites and stings, and foreign bodies in the eyes.
4. Discuss diabetic emergencies, and provide first aid for a patient with insulin shock.
5. Discuss musculoskeletal and neurological emergencies, and provide first aid for a patient with seizure activity.
6. Discuss respiratory emergencies, and provide first aid for a choking patient.
7. Discuss cardiovascular emergencies, and provide first aid for a patient with a bleeding wound, fracture, or syncope; a patient in shock; and a patient in need of rescue breathing or cardiopulmonary resuscitation (CPR).

CHAPTER OUTLINE

1. Opening Scenario, 963
2. You Will Learn, 963
3. Introduction, 964
4. Emergencies in Healthcare Settings, 964
5. Emergency Equipment and Supplies, 964
   a. Oxygen and Airway Supplies, 965
   b. Defibrillator, 965
   c. Medications, 967
   d. Other Supplies, 967
   e. Pediatric Supplies, 967
6. Handling Emergencies, 968
   a. Environmental Emergencies, 970
      i. *Temperature-Related Emergencies, 970*
      ii. *Burns, 970*
      iii. *Poisonings, 971*
      iv. *Anaphylaxis, 972*
      v. *Insect Bites and Stings, 973*
      vi. *Animal Bites, 974*
      vii. *Foreign Body in the Eye, 974*
   b. Diabetic Emergencies, 974
   c. Musculoskeletal Emergencies, 976
   d. Neurological Emergencies, 977
      i. *Vertigo and Dizziness, 977*
      ii. *Concussion, 978*
      iii. *Seizures, 978*
      iv. *Cerebrovascular Accident, 980*
   e. Respiratory Emergencies, 980
      i. *Hyperventilation, 980*
      ii. *Asthmatic Attack, 981*
      iii. *Choking, 981*
   f. Cardiovascular Emergencies, 982
      i. *Syncope, 982*
      ii. *Bleeding, 983*
      iii. *Shock, 983*
      iv. *Myocardial Infarction, 985*
7. Closing Comments, 989
8. Chapter Review, 989
9. Scenario Wrap-Up, 989

OPENING SCENARIO

Gabe Garcia, a certified medical assistant (CMA) through the American Association of Medical Assistants (AAMA), has worked for Walden-Martin Family Medical (WMFM) Clinic for seven years. He was hired right after he completed his medical assistant program. Gabe has learned a lot through the years. He was just promoted to a medical assistant lead position. In this new position, Gabe has additional responsibilities. He will now oversee the crash carts in the clinic, and he will train staff on emergency procedures.

The current emergency procedures need to be revised, and the crash cart procedures need updating. Gabe is excited to take over his new responsibilities. He looks forward to what he will learn in this new role.

YOU WILL LEARN

1. To handle emergencies in ambulatory care settings.
2. To use emergency equipment and supplies in ambulatory care settings.
3. To apply first aid for environmental emergencies, including cold and heat illnesses, burns, poisonings, anaphylaxis, bites, and foreign bodies in the eye.
4. To apply first aid for diabetic and musculoskeletal emergencies.
5. To apply first aid for neurological emergencies, including vertigo, concussion, seizure, and stroke.
6. To apply first aid for respiratory emergencies, including hyperventilation, asthmatic attack, and choking.

7. To apply first aid for cardiovascular emergencies, including syncope, bleeding, shock, and heart attack.

INTRODUCTION

Emergencies happen everywhere. As a medical assistant, it is important for you to know how to handle emergencies because you may need to respond to one:
- *Outside of your job, in the community.* You may be one of the first people on the scene and need to provide first aid to the victims.
- *In the healthcare setting.* You may need to provide first aid as the provider assesses the injured person. Additional treatments such as oxygen and medications are provided in the healthcare setting.
- *Over the phone.* You may need to obtain information from someone involved in an emergency and provide first aid coaching. The medical assistant asks screening questions and provides the information to the provider. The provider instructs the medical assistant as to what to tell the caller.

This chapter starts by discussing emergencies in the healthcare setting and the medical assistant's role. Next, common emergency medical equipment, supplies, and medications are explained. Lastly, emergency conditions are described, along with the first aid procedures to perform.

EMERGENCIES IN HEALTHCARE SETTINGS

Every employee in a healthcare setting should know how to get help in an emergency. This process will vary. Healthcare facilities use special phrases for emergencies. For instance, "Code Blue Urgent Care" may indicate that an emergency is occurring in Urgent Care. Sometimes the code words indicate the age of the person. For instance, "Code Pink Family Practice" may mean that an emergency is occurring in Family Practice and "pink" indicates a child.

Once the call goes out for help, staff members respond to the scene. In small settings, most members of the staff may be needed. In large facilities, only certain staff members respond. Usually, medical assistants, licensed practical nurses (LPNs), registered nurses (RNs), and providers attend the emergency. Table 40.1 indicates possible roles each team member has during an emergency.

VOCABULARY
cardiopulmonary resuscitation (CPR): The application of manual chest compressions and ventilations (also called rescue breathing) to patients who are not breathing or do not have a pulse; also known as basic life support (BLS).
code: A term used in healthcare settings to indicate an emergency situation and to summon the trained team to the scene.
standard of care: The level and type of care an ordinary, prudent healthcare professional with the same training and experience in a similar practice would have provided under a similar situation.

CRITICAL THINKING 40.1
Currently, the clinic does not have a procedure for documenting during code situations. The provider documents after the emergency. Gabe would like to discuss using a standard code form for all emergencies. A team member would be responsible for documenting during the code. Discuss the pros and cons of documenting during the code.

TABLE 40.1 Typical Roles During a Code

Team Member	Possible Roles
Provider	Assesses the patient, orders treatments and procedures, performs advanced procedures, may administer intravenous (IV) medications, and indicates when 911 needs to be called.
Nurse	Registered nurses (RNs) administer intravenous (IV) medications and fluids. Licensed practical nurses (LPNs) may do the same if permitted by the state's scope of practice. RNs and LPNs assist with treatments and procedures, perform cardiopulmonary resuscitation (ri SUS i tae shun) (CPR), call 911, and document the code activities as they occur (Box 40.1).
Clinical medical assistant	Assists with treatments and procedures, performs CPR, documents the code activities as they occur and calls 911. They may hand supplies to staff members and assist with caring for the family (moving them to a private area away from the emergency).
Administrative medical assistant	Performs CPR and hands supplies to the staff (in small agencies), calls 911, escorts the emergency responders to the patient, and assists with caring for the family.

BOX 40.1 Importance of Documentation

In a code situation, it is important that at least one team member documents everything that occurs. This is a stressful job because many things are occurring during an emergency. There are several reasons why accurate documentation is critical:
- The information is used during the code. For instance, CPR was started and the team member documented "1413 CPR initiated." As the code progresses, the provider may want to know when the CPR was started.
- Emergency responders will need to know what occurred during the code. (What medications were given? When were they given? How much was given?).
- The documentation will provide evidence if the standard of care was given to the patient. Many lawsuits have originated from emergencies. The lawyers review the documentation. They look for delays in emergency care and lack of appropriate treatment. Complete and accurate documentation may make a difference between a lawsuit surviving and being dismissed in favor of the healthcare team.

If you are new to codes and if given the option, perform a role other than documenting. Observe what occurs during a code as you complete your task. Study the code documentation form during noncode times. As you become more comfortable with codes, assist the documenter if you can. A second pair of eyes is always helpful. Lastly, become the documenter and have a seasoned team member assist you.

EMERGENCY EQUIPMENT AND SUPPLIES

The emergency supplies available at healthcare facilities will vary based on the size and location of the facility. Some practices have a small box that contains a few supplies and medications. Other practices place many crash carts throughout the building (Fig. 40.1). A *crash cart* is a rolling supply cart that contains emergency equipment.

The crash cart should be checked monthly. This can be done by the supervisor or by two qualified employees (e.g., medical assistants, LPNs,

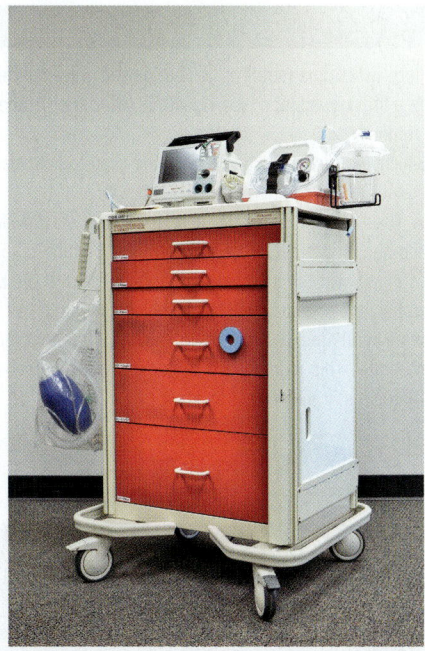

FIG. 40.1 Crash carts are used in an emergency. Having the drawers labeled allows for the speedy retrieval of supplies.

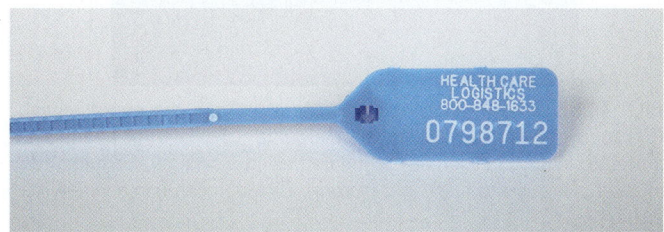

FIG. 40.2 A plastic lock is placed on the inventoried crash cart. The number is written on the inventory form for tracking purposes. These locks are easy to break in emergencies.

or RNs). Expiration dates on the supplies are checked. Old supplies are replaced with new supplies. All the equipment and supplies are inventoried. When the inventory is completed, a plastic lock (or locking tag) is placed on the cart (Fig. 40.2). The crash cart is only used in emergencies. You should never break the lock and use something from the crash cart unless it is an emergency. The plastic locks should be kept safe and only used when the cart is inventoried monthly or after an emergency. Many of the locks are numbered, and the number is written on the inventory document. Keeping the locks safe minimizes the number of people going into the crash cart for nonemergency reasons.

This section will focus on the equipment and supplies typically found on a crash cart. The medical assistant should be familiar with the supplies and their location within the crash cart.

Oxygen and Airway Supplies

Oxygen and airway supplies are common items found on crash carts. If the patient needs oxygen, the provider will order oxygen to be applied via a mask or a nasal *cannula* (CAN you lah). (Refer to Chapter 39 for additional information on oxygen delivery systems.)

If the patient has difficulty breathing or if an airway constriction maybe occurring, the provider will insert a tube in the nose or mouth to create a **patent** (PAY tent) airway.

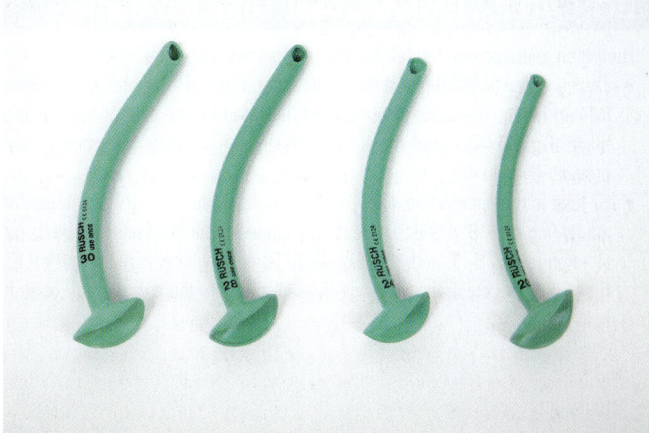

FIG. 40.3 Nasopharyngeal airways come in a variety of sizes.

- A *nasopharyngeal* (NAE zoe fah RIN jee ahl) *airway* (NPA) is also known as a nasal trumpet. It is a soft flexible tube that is inserted in the nose and provides a patent airway (Fig. 40.3).
- An **endotracheal** (EN doe TRAY kee al) **(ET) tube** is commonly used (Box 40.2). An ET tube is inserted in the trachea and provides an airway. Providers also use the following to maintain airways:
  - *Esophageal tracheal tubes*, which are placed in the trachea or esophagus
  - *Laryngeal mask airways*, which are inserted through the mouth and advanced to the hypopharynx
  - *Laryngeal tubes*, which are also inserted through the mouth and placed in the hypopharynx

> **VOCABULARY**
> **endotracheal (ET) tube**: A catheter that is inserted into the trachea through the mouth; provides a patent airway.
> **patent**: Open.

> **MEDICAL TERMINOLOGY**
> **endo-**: within
> **epiglott/o**: epiglottis
> **laryng/o**: voice box (larynx)
> **nas/o, rhin/o**: nose
> **pharyng/o**: pharynx
> **-scope**: instrument to view
> **steth/o**: chest

> **CRITICAL THINKING 40.2**
> Gabe has decided that the crash carts must be inventoried monthly. He will have two medical assistants inventory each cart. Gabe feels it is important that all medical assistants have an opportunity to inventory the crash cart at least every 4 months. Why would this be important for the medical assistants? Besides checking expiration dates, what else could they do to increase their skills and knowledge for emergencies?

Defibrillator

A *defibrillator* (dee FIB rah LAE tohr) is a device that delivers an electrical shock to the heart muscle in an attempt to restore a normal heartbeat. The defibrillator's shock causes the heart to momentarily stop. When it restarts, the hope is the heart will beat at a normal rhythm. The

BOX 40.2   Endotracheal Tube Intubation

During an endotracheal intubation, the provider will need the following:
- *Laryngoscope* (la RING goe skope) with either a curved (MacIntosh) or straight (Miller) blade. The sizes of blades are indicated on the side or back of the blade (Fig. 40.4A). Hand the laryngoscope with the blade attached to the provider (Fig. 40.4B).
- ET tube in the appropriate size. Cuffed ET tubes come in a variety of sizes for adults (e.g., 7.5, 8, and 8.5). Uncuffed ET tubes come in a variety of sizes for children (e.g., 2.5, 3, and 3.5) (Fig. 40.5). Some providers may use cuffed ET tubes on older children. A syringe is used to inflate the cuff with air once it is in place.
- Stylet (STIE let), which is a metal or flexible plastic wire inserted in the ET tube to create a firm curved tube (see Fig. 40.5). After the ET tube is in place, the stylet is removed.
- Ambu-bag, which is attached to the ET tube and used to administer room air or oxygen (Fig. 40.6).
- A stethoscope. Once the tube is in place, a team member will provide ventilation with the Ambu-bag. The provider must ensure the ET tube is in the correct location by listening over the lung field for air movement. If the ET tube is in the wrong location, the abdomen will become bloated with the air. The patient is then not being ventilated. (A provider will usually state that breath sounds are heard bilaterally. This is important to document on the code form. This verifies the ET tube is in the correct location.)

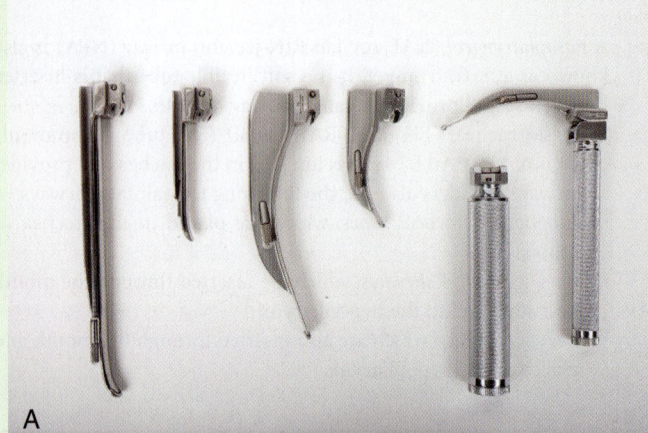

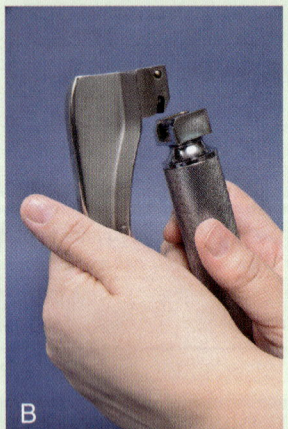

FIG. 40.4 (A) *(Left to right)* Two different sizes of straight blades and curved blades; adult laryngoscope handle and an assembled pediatric laryngoscope. A curved or straight blade must be attached to the laryngoscope handle. (B) To attach the blade, hold the blade parallel to the handle and attach.

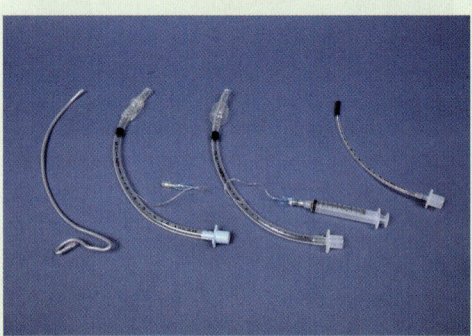

FIG. 40.5 *(Left to right)* A stylet is threaded into the endotracheal (ET) tube to help maintain the tube's curve. ET tubes for adults are cuffed (or have a balloon that is inflated using a syringe). ET tubes for children are uncuffed *(far right picture)*. ET tubes come in a variety of sizes.

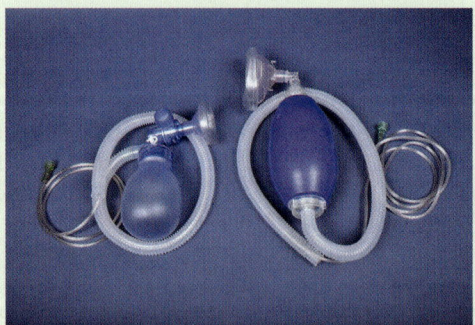

FIG. 40.6 *(Left to right)* Pediatric and adult Ambu-bags. An Ambu-bag can cover the mouth or be attached to an airway tube (e.g., endotracheal tube). Ambu-bags can come with oxygen tubing attached. The tubing can be connected to an oxygen tank. Oxygen can be administered during the ventilation.

quicker a defibrillator can be used, the better the person's chances of survival.

Typically, a defibrillator or an automated external defibrillator is used in healthcare facilities:
- A defibrillator consists of two handheld paddles that are placed on gel pads located on the patient's chest (Fig. 40.7). Gel pads are required to prevent burns. They provide better electricity conduction from the paddles to the patient. The provider indicates how many joules at which to set the machine and someone announces "All clear" to ensure no one is touching the patient. The provider pushes the button to give the shock.
- An *automated external defibrillator* (AED) is a portable, lightweight machine (Fig. 40.8). Sticky pads that contain electrodes (sensors) are attached to the patient's chest. The AED checks the heart rate and determines if a shock is required. If a shock is needed, the AED gives audible directions to the user to administer a shock.

Medications

The medications in crash carts can vary. Common medications used in emergencies are listed in Table 40.2. Most crash carts and emergency supply boxes include intravenous (IV) supplies. An IV is usually inserted in the hand, wrist, or arm of the patient. If an IV line cannot be inserted, the provider may insert an intraosseous needle that can be used to give IV fluids and medications (Fig. 40.9). The intraosseous needle can be

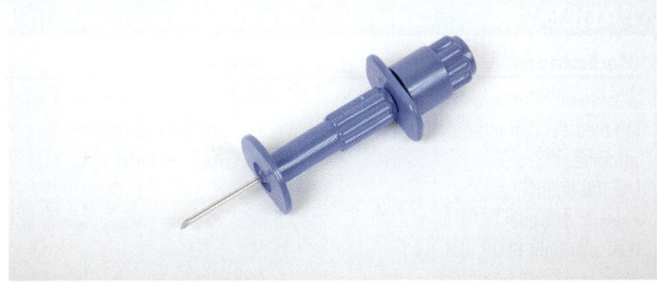

FIG. 40.9 An intraosseous needle maybe used to give IV fluids and medications in an emergency.

inserted in several locations including the humerus, tibia, and iliac crest. The provider must be specially trained to insert the intraosseous needle.

Administering IV medications is outside of the scope of the medical assistant's practice. In many states, inserting an IV and giving IV fluids are also outside of the medical assistant's scope of practice. The medical assistant may help by getting the required supplies and documenting what was given.

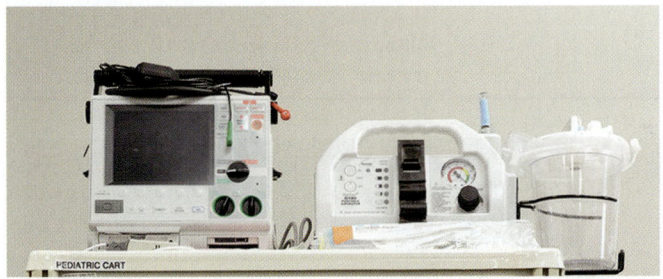

FIG. 40.7 *(Left to right)* The defibrillator usually sits on top of the crash cart. Other equipment, like a suction machine, can also be found on the top of the crash cart.

MEDICAL TERMINOLOGY	
a-: without	**hyper**: excessive, above
-ar: pertaining to	**hypo-**: under, below
brady-: slow	**-ia**: condition
calc/o: calcium	**kal/i**: potassium
-cardia: heart condition	**rhythm/o**: rhythm
-emia: blood condition	**tachy-**: rapid
gluc/o, glyc/o: glucose, sugar	**ventricul/o**: ventricle

Other Supplies

Various other supplies can be found in the crash cart. Some items not already mentioned include the following:
- Personal protective equipment like gloves; a sharps disposal container and a pocket mask
- *Algorithms* (AL guh rith uhms) or step-by-step instructions for reference
- Clipboard with documents for charting the code
- Backboard, which is placed under the patient to provide a firm surface for compressions
- Extra batteries for the laryngoscope

Pediatric Supplies

In the 1980s, James Broselow, MD, a family practice doctor working in the emergency department, got an idea for simplifying pediatric medication doses administered during emergencies. Medications for children are based on weight. Rescue personnel spent critical moments during emergencies calculating medication doses for children. Broselow's idea was to measure the child's length and come up with a suggested dose. After much research, the Broselow tape was created (Fig. 40.10A).

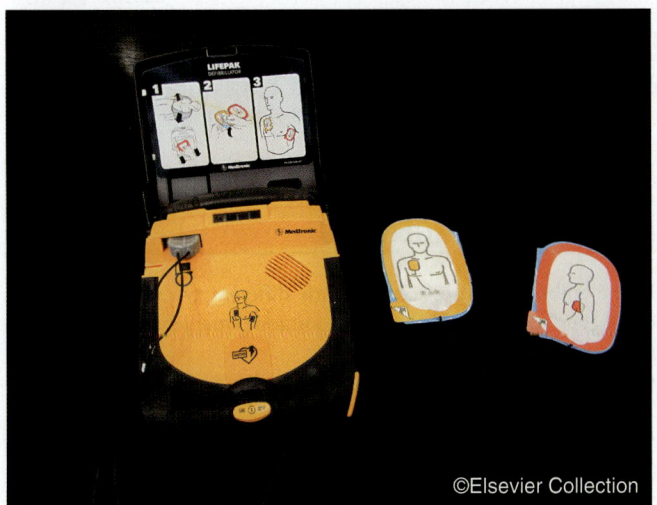

FIG. 40.8 Automated external defibrillator.

TABLE 40.2 Common Medications Used in Emergencies

Medications	Action	Used for
amiodarone (Cordarone, Pacerone) (ah mee OH dah rone)	Slows the heart rate and allows blood to fill the ventricular chambers.	Ventricular tachycardia (tack ee KAR dee ah), ventricular fibrillation (fibrill LAY shun)
atropine (AT roe peen)	Increases the heart rate.	Bradycardia (brad dee KAR dee ah)
calcium chloride (KAL see uhm KLOR ide)	Increases the calcium levels in the serum.	Hyperkalemia and *hypocalcemia* (hye poe kal SEE mee ah) (too little calcium in the blood)
diazepam (Valium) (dye AZ ee pam)	Affects the chemicals in the brain.	Seizures (see zhurs), agitation
diphenhydramine (Benadryl) (DIE fen HYE dra meen)	Antihistamine that reduces the effects of histamine	Allergic reactions, second-line drug for anaphylaxis (used after epinephrine has been given)
dopamine (Intropin) (DOE pah meen)	Increases the stimulation of the heart muscle	Hypotension, heart failure
epinephrine (Adrenalin) (EP i NEF rin)	Increases the stimulation of the heart muscle; vasoconstrictor and bronchial relaxant	Anaphylaxis, cardiac arrest, severe asthma, bronchospasms
glucagon (GLUE kah gon)	Hormone that stimulates the liver to release glucose into the blood	*Hypoglycemia* (hye poh gly SEE mee ah) (too low glucose in the blood)
lidocaine (LIE dah kane)	Helps to restore the regular heart rhythm	Ventricular arrhythmias (ah RITH mee ah)
magnesium (mag NEE zee um)	Electrolyte that helps maintain a normal heart rhythm	Arrhythmias (ah RITH mee ahs)
naloxone (Evzio, Narcan) (nal OX one)	Blocks or reverses the opioid medication effects	Opioid (narcotic) overdose
nitroglycerin (nye troe GLI ser in)	Vasodilator	Congestive heart failure, angina (an JYE nuh)
sodium bicarbonate (SOE dee uhm bye KAHR bah nate)	Decreases the pH of the serum	Metabolic acidosis, *hyperkalemia* (hye per kuh LEE mee ah) (excessive potassium in the blood)

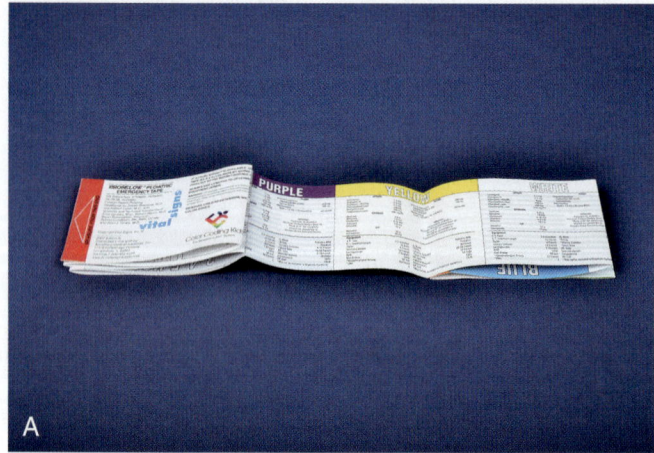
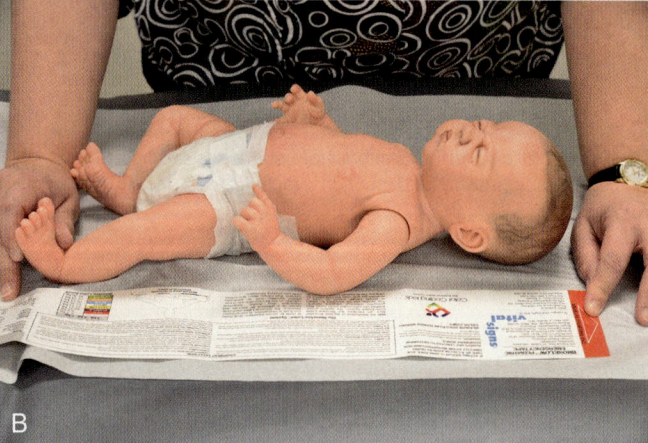

FIG. 40.10 (A) Broselow tape. (B) Measure the child with the Broselow tape. Measure from the head to the heel and identify the color by the child's heel. This is color to use during the emergency.

A healthcare professional measures a child using the tape. The tape is placed from the top of the head to the child's heel. The length is measured as a specific color (Fig. 40.10B). Based on the "color" of the child, the tape lists common medication dosages and emergency equipment sizes that should be used for that size of child. This system has sped up the response time for treating children during emergencies. It eliminates the use of reference guides and calculators for medication dosages.

Many ambulatory care settings that routinely see sick children use the Broselow tape. In addition to the tape, pediatric crash carts (Broselow ColorCode Carts) have been created (Fig. 40.11). Each color on the tape has a drawer. Each drawer contains the right sized equipment for that size of child.

HANDLING EMERGENCIES

In the ambulatory care setting, many different types of emergencies can occur. Some of the more common emergencies include the following:
- A patient who is being seen and treated has a life-threatening occurrence (e.g., an allergic reaction to a medication).
- A person (e.g., employee, visitor, or patient) has an accident or health issue that results in an emergency.
- A *walk-in patient* (a patient without an appointment) comes to the facility with a critical health issue.
- An individual calls about an emergency.

CHAPTER 40 Medical Emergencies

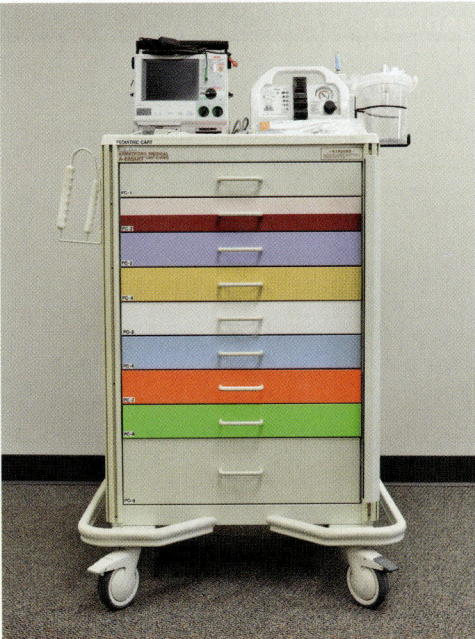

FIG. 40.11 Each drawer in the Broselow ColorCode Cart is color coded.

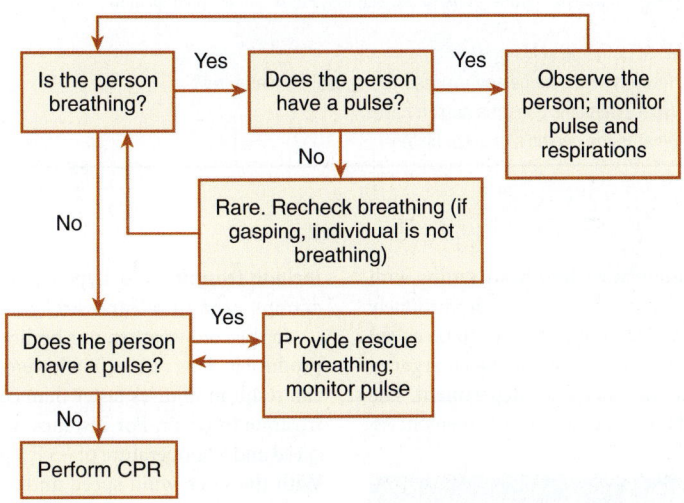

FIG. 40.12 Example of a flow map. Similar flow maps can be used when triaging or treating emergencies.

How these are handled can differ greatly among ambulatory care facilities. Box 40.3 lists some of the factors that impact how emergencies are handled. Some facilities only have minimal staff, whereas others have specific employees that respond to emergencies.

In small facilities, the medical assistant may be responsible for screening emergency calls and walk-in patients. The medical assistant must follow the facility's screening protocols. She or he cannot assess the patient or give advice. The information collected must be reported to the provider. The provider tells the medical assistant what should be done. Examples of screening questions are provided later in the chapter.

In larger facilities, registered nurses (sometimes called **triage** [tree AHZH] nurses) gather information from walk-in patients and emergency calls. Using a **triaging flow map** or triaging software, the nurse identifies how quickly the patient needs to be seen and where the patient needs to be seen (Fig. 40.12).

BOX 40.3 Factors Impacting How Emergencies Are Handled

- Facility's size and location from emergency medical services
- Available equipment and supplies
- Providers' training and scope of practice
- Number and type of clinical care employees (medical assistants, licensed practical nurses, and registered nurses) and their scopes of practice

VOCABULARY

triage: To sort out and classify the injured; used in the military and emergency settings to determine the priority of a patient to be treated.

triaging flow map: A written flow map used to make triage decision; based on answers to questions the person moves through the map until a triage decision is made.

TABLE 40.3 Cold-Related Emergencies

Condition	Frostbite	Hypothermia
Description	Occurs when the skin and body tissues are exposed to cold temperatures. Susceptible areas include cheeks, nose, ears, fingers, toes, and chin.	Core body temperature drops to below 95°F. Severe hypothermia is when the body temperature drops to 82°F, causing a life-threatening condition.
Etiology and Risk Factors	Caused by exposure to cold temperatures. Risk factors include the following: • Smoking or taking a beta-blocker medication (e.g., Atenolol) • Having diabetes or poor blood circulation • High winds, wet clothes	Caused by exposure to cold temperatures or immersion in cold water for a long period of time. Risk factors include those for frostbite; also dehydration and exhaustion.
Signs and Symptoms	Pins-and-needles sensation followed by numbness; hard, pale, cold skin; aching or lack of feeling in area; blisters.	Slurred speech; slow, swallow breathing and weak pulse; clumsy, drowsy, confused, loss of consciousness; bright red, cold skin (seen in infants).
First Aid Procedures	• Move the person to a warmer location. • Remove all wet clothing. • Observe for signs of hypothermia. • Seek medical care; if not available, then rewarm the area by soaking in warm water (104°–108°F) for 20–30 minutes. Do not rub the area. Apply sterile dressing to area. • Give the person a warm drink to replace lost fluids; do not give alcohol.	• Move the person to a warmer location. • Remove all wet clothing and cover with warm dry clothing. • Seek medical care. • Give the person a warm drink to replace lost fluids; do not give alcohol.
Possible Screening Questions	• What is the person's age? • How long was the person exposed to the cool temperatures? • What symptoms does the person have? • What is the person's medical history?	

Sometimes patients come to the ambulatory healthcare setting with life-threatening conditions. The provider sees these patients immediately and assesses their conditions. The provider will order 911 to be called if needed. Treatment is provided as the team waits for the emergency responders to transport the patient to the emergency department. The following sections explain the first aid for different types of emergencies.

> ### CRITICAL THINKING 40.3
> Gabe knows that there are times when medical assistants need to screen phone calls. This can be intimidating for new medical assistants. What procedures would Gabe put in place to help medical assistants screen emergency calls accurately yet bring down the intimidation?

Environmental Emergencies

Environmental emergencies arise from something in our environment. For instance, the outdoor temperature can cause a life-threatening condition. A bite from certain reptiles can cause death if not treated immediately. A flying piece of metal in a factory can cause blindness. Many environment-related emergencies occur, causing people to seek medical care.

Temperature-Related Emergencies. Overexposure to hot or cold temperatures can cause mild to life-threatening issues. Environmental temperatures impact the body's temperature. Cold-related conditions include frostbite and hypothermia. Heat-related conditions include cramps, exhaustion, and stroke.

In the cold weather, our bodies tend to lose heat faster than we can produce it. This results in a lowered body temperature. Uncovered skin can result in injuries faster than covered skin. It does not take long for frostbite to occur. For instance, with a 10-mile per hour (mph) wind speed and a temperature of −5°F, a person can get frostbite in 30 minutes. With the same wind speed and a temperature of −25°F, a person can get frostbite in 5 minutes.

Table 40.3 describes frostbite and hypothermia. With severe hypothermia, an individual can develop arrhythmias. Medical attention is critical. Warming a patient with hypothermia too quickly can also lead to cardiac issues and additional tissue damage. Because of this, the emergency department gradually warms all patients with hypothermia.

Heat injuries occur most often on hot, humid days. They can result in heat cramps, heat exhaustion, or heatstroke (Table 40.4). It is important to treat heat-related illnesses immediately. An untreated condition can progress to become a more severe situation. An effective way to lower the person's temperature is to apply cool, wet cloths and then fan the moist skin. This will lower the person's body temperature by the evaporation process.

Burns. Heat, freezing cold temperatures, chemicals, sunlight, radiation, and electricity can cause burns to the body tissue. Hot liquids, fires, and flammable products are the most common causes of burns. Breathing in smoke can also cause inhalation injuries. Table 40.5 describes the different degrees of burns. Providers estimate the percent of total burn

TABLE 40.4 Heat-Related Emergencies

Condition	Heat cramps	Heat exhaustion	Heat stroke
Description	Mild heat-related illness that causes muscle pains and spasms due to electrolyte imbalance. Usually occurs with strenuous activities or in those who sweat a lot.	Milder form of heat-related illness. Due to exposure to high temperatures and inadequate fluid and electrolyte replacement.	Most serious heat-related illness. Body is unable to sweat and thus cannot cool down.
Etiology and Risk Factors	Caused by prolonged heat exposure. With high humidity, the sweat, which cools the skin, does not evaporate as quickly. Risk factors include the following: • Age (older adults and children age 4 and younger) • Fever, dehydration, heart disease, poor blood circulation • Mental illness, sunburn; using alcohol • Prescription drugs (e.g., antidepressants, anticonvulsants, antipsychotics, and diuretics)		
Signs and Symptoms	• Muscle pains or spasms in the abdomen, arms, or legs.	• Heavy sweating, muscle cramps. • Cool, moist skin. • Fast, weak pulse; fast, shallow respirations. • Tired, weak, pale. • Dizzy, headache, fainting. • Nausea, vomiting.	• Body temperature over 103°F. • Red, hot, dry skin. • Rapid, strong pulse. • Dizzy, throbbing headache, nausea. • Confusion, unconsciousness.
First Aid Procedures	• Rest for several hours in a cool place. • Drink cool electrolyte (sports) beverages to replace electrolytes lost. • Do not drink caffeinated or alcoholic beverages, which can cause dehydration.	• Move to a shady or air-conditioned area and rest. • Drink cool sports beverages. • Do not drink caffeinated or alcoholic beverages. • Take a cool shower or sponge bath.	• Move the person to a shady area or air-conditioned area. • Spray or sponge the person down with cool water. • Seek medical attention immediately.
Possible Screening Questions	• What is the person's age? • How long was the person exposed to the warm temperatures? • What symptoms does the person have? What does the person's skin look like?		

surface area (%TBSA) by using the rule of nines diagram (Fig. 40.13). Table 40.6 shows the difference between the rule of nines for an adult and a child.

Poisonings. Poison can enter the body through swallowing, inhaling, injecting, or absorbing it through the skin. Boxes 40.4 and 40.5 list common poisons and provide facts about poisonings. Poison Control is a national poison resource with 55 centers around the country. This resource is available online and via a hotline (1-800-222-1222). Medical assistants should have the phone number and website available for reference. If the medical assistant receives a call regarding a poisoning, the call must be handled per the facility's protocols. Many times, the medical assistant must contact Poison Control while keeping the patient on the phone. The medical assistant then relays the information from Poison Control to the patient.

BOX 40.4 Common Poisons

- Medications (prescriptive or over the counter) taken in high doses
- Overdoses of illegal drugs
- Household products (e.g., laundry detergent, furniture polish, and cleaning products)
- Indoor and outdoor plants
- Pesticides and fertilizers
- Metals (e.g., mercury and lead)

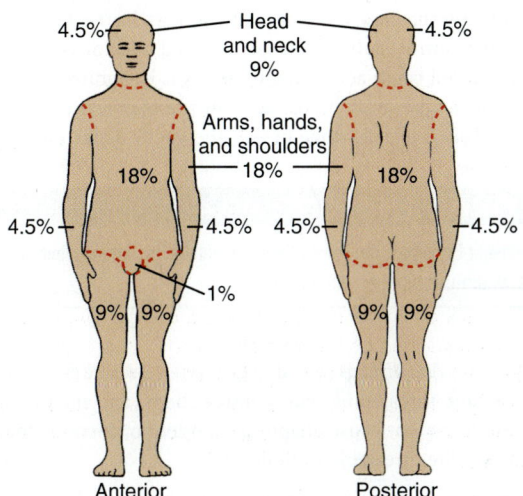

FIG. 40.13 Rule of nines for adults. (From Callen JP, Greer KE, Saller AS, et al: *Color Atlas of Dermatology*, ed 2, St. Louis, 2000, Mosby/Elsevier.)

TABLE 40.5 Types of Burns

Condition	First-degree burn	Second-degree burn	Third-degree burn	Fourth-degree burn
Also Known as	Superficial burn	Partial-thickness burn	Full-thickness burn	Deep full-thickness burn
Description	Damage to epidermis.	Damage to the epidermis and part of the dermis.	Damage to the epidermis, dermis, and subcutaneous tissue.	Damage beyond the subcutaneous tissue into the muscle and bone (not universally accepted).
Signs and Symptoms	Redness (erythema), tenderness, physical sensitivity. No scar development.	Redness, blisters, and pain. Possible scar development.	No pain because nerve endings are destroyed. Skin appears deep red, pale gray, brown, or black. Scar formation is likely.	
First Aid Procedures	For minor burns: • For unbroken skin, soak in cool water (not ice water) for at least 5 minutes. • Cover with sterile dressing. • (For second-degree burns 3 inches or larger or located on hands, feet, groin, buttock, or over a joint, treat as major burn.)		For major burns: • Seek immediate medical attention (call 911). • Do not remove burned clothing stuck to skin. • Monitor breathing. Perform rescue breathing or CPR as needed. • Raise burned body part above the heart level. • Separate burned fingers or toes with a dry, sterile dressing.	
Possible Screening Questions	• What occurred? Where was the person burned? What caused the burn? • What symptoms does the person have? What does the person's skin look like? • If affecting the face or chest, is the person experiencing any breathing issues?			

Signs and symptoms of poisoning can develop over time. They can also vary based on the poison. Some examples of symptoms include the following:
- Bluish lips, cough, difficulty breathing
- Heart palpitations, chest pain
- Confusion, dizziness, double vision, drowsiness, irritability, headache
- Nausea, vomiting, abdominal pain
- Numbness, tingling, seizures
- Unconsciousness, stupor, weakness, unusual odor

First aid includes checking and monitoring the person's airway, breathing, and pulse. If required, rescue breathing and cardiopulmonary resuscitation (CPR) are provided. Call 911 for medical help. If the person vomits, clear the airway. Monitor the person until help arrives. If poisoning is suspected, it is important to identify what the toxin is as well as how much was taken.

Do not have the person vomit unless you are instructed to do so by the Poison Control staff. If the person had swallowed a corrosive substance, it will cause additional injury as it is vomited. In this type of situation, a tube must be passed into the stomach to remove the substance. This is usually done in the emergency department.

CRITICAL THINKING 40.4
Where might Gabe post the Poison Control numbers around the clinic? Describe places where this number will be useful.

Anaphylaxis. *Anaphylaxis* (AN ah fi LAK sis) is a severe allergic reaction that can be life threatening. Food, insect stings, and medications are the top allergens that cause anaphylaxis. Allergic reactions that affect breathing are life threatening (Table 40.7).

MEDICAL TERMINOLOGY
dys-: difficult
-pnea: breathing

TABLE 40.6 Rule of Nines for Adults and Children

	Adult	Child
Head and neck	9%	18%
Front of torso	18%	18%
Back	18%	18%
Arm, hand, and shoulder	9% (LA)	9% (LA)
	9% (RA)	9% (RA)
Leg and foot	18% (LL)	13.5% (LL)
	18% (RL)	13.5% (RL)
Genital	1%	1%
Total	100%	100%

LA: left arm; RA: right arm; LL: left leg; RL: right leg

First aid for severe allergic reactions includes the following:
- Do the 3Cs (Box 40.6). Check the scene for safety. Call 911. Care for the victim.
- Give *epinephrine* (EP i NEF rin) (Epi-pen) if the person has it available (Fig. 40.14).
- Stay with the individual, and try to keep the person calm.

BOX 40.5 Poisoning Facts
- Children younger than 6 years of age make up about half of the poisoning exposures reported.
- Children ages 1 to 2 have the greatest risk of poisoning.
- Cosmetics and personal care products followed by cleaning products are the most common substances involved in childhood poison exposures.
- About 20% of adult poisonings and 40% of teen poisonings are suspected suicides.
- Analgesics followed by sedative/hypnotics/antipsychotic medications are the top substances in adult poisonings.

From Poison Control, http://www.poison.org/poison-statistics-national.

TABLE 40.7 Common Allergens and Anaphylaxis Symptoms

Common Allergens	Most Common Allergenic Foods	Anaphylaxis Symptoms
• Animal dander • Insect bites and stings (especially bee stings) • Medicines • Plants • Pollens • Foods	• Eggs • Fish • Milk • Tree nuts (hazelnuts, walnuts, almonds, Brazil nuts) • Peanuts (groundnuts) • Shellfish (crab, mussels, shrimp) • Soy • Wheat	• Warm feeling, flushing • Shortness of breath • Dyspnea (DISP nee uh) (difficulty breathing), wheezing • Throat tightening, difficulty swallowing • Cough • Anxiety • Pain or cramping • Vomiting or diarrhea • Unconsciousness • Shock • Palpitations, dizziness

BOX 40.6 The 3 Cs Are Important When a Person Responds to Emergencies

If you are the first to arrive at the scene of an emergency, it is important to do the following 3 Cs:
- **Check** the scene of the emergency. Is it safe for you? Are there any toxic or electric hazards? What occurred? How many victims are involved? Where did it occur (so you can tell the 911 dispatcher)?
- **Call 911** or the local emergency number. Provide all the details that you know.
- **Care** for the victims if it is safe to do so.

Always make sure you are safe before you assist others. If it is not safe for you, then wait for the emergency responders to arrive.

- If the person had a bee sting, scrape the stinger off the skin if it is visible. Use a fingernail or credit card to scrape it. Don't use tweezers, which can squeeze the stinger, releasing more venom.
- Monitor the individual's airway, breathing, and pulse. Perform rescue breathing or CPR if needed.
- Have the person lie flat and raise the feet 12 inches. Keep the person warm. This will help to prevent shock.

In the ambulatory care facility, if the medical assistant suspects the patient is starting to have an allergic reaction, he or she should immediately notify the provider. The provider will order epinephrine to be given and oxygen to be administered. Research has shown that epinephrine administered intramuscularly (IM) in the vastus lateralis absorbs quicker than if given IM in the deltoid or subcutaneously in the arm. If ordered, repeat every 5 to 10 minutes. Do not administer repeated injections in the same site, because **vasoconstriction** may cause tissue **necrosis** (neck KROH sis). The typical dose of epinephrine injectable solution (of 1 mg/mL) for anaphylaxis is as follows:
- Children and adults (66 lb [30 kg] or more): 0.3 to 0.5 mg (0.3–0.5 mL)

MEDICAL TERMINOLOGY
vas/o: vessel

VOCABULARY
necrosis: Tissue death.
vasoconstriction: Contraction of the muscles, causing the narrowing of the inside tube of the vessel.

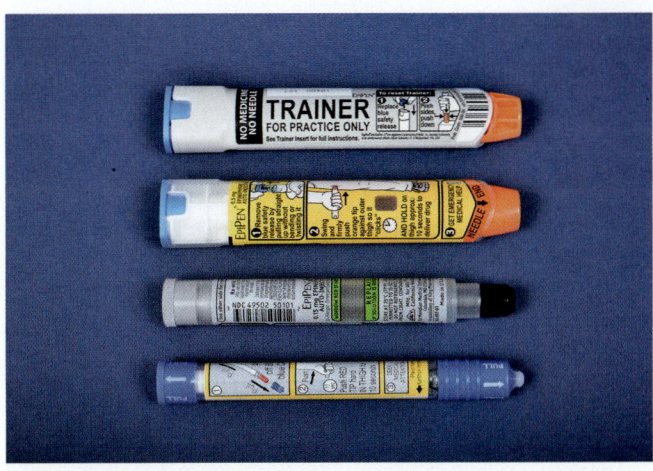

FIG. 40.14 *(Top to bottom)* Trainer that comes with the EpiPen, adult EpiPen, EpiPen Jr., and a generic adult epinephrine pen.

BOX 40.7 Screening Questions for Insect Bites and Stings
- What bit you?
- Do you have any allergies?
- How does the wound look? Describe the wound to me.
- Are you having any problems breathing? Any wheezing, shortness of breath, or difficulty breathing?
- Is there any swelling in the mouth or lips?

BOX 40.8 Removing Ticks

Ticks can spread diseases, including Rocky Mountain spotted fever, *Powassan* (pah waah sahn) virus, *Babesia* (bah BEE zhah) infection, *Lyme* (lime) disease, and *ehrlichiosis* (ahr LIK ee oh sis). If a person has a tick embedded, it needs to be removed. Wear gloves and use a fine-tipped pointed tweezer. Get as close to the head as possible. Do not squeeze the abdomen, as it may inject secretions into the person's body. Slowly pull the head out. Do not twist. Do not burn it or use petroleum jelly or nail polish. Once the tick is removed, place it in a container of rubbing alcohol to kill it. Clean the site with antiseptic soap and water. Apply an antibiotic ointment. Monitor the site for infections or other complications.

- Children (under 66 lb. [30 kg]): 0.01 mg/kg (0.01 mL/kg) with a maximum dose per injection of 0.3 mL

Insect Bites and Stings. Insect bites and stings can cause immediate skin reactions, including pain, burning, redness (*erythema* [ER i thee mah]), numbness, swelling, and itching (*pruritus* [proo RYE tuss]). In some cases, the venom can cause severe illness and death. Some people have anaphylactic reactions to stings and bites (e.g., bee stings). Anaphylaxis symptoms were addressed in the prior section. If the medical assistant receives a phone call regarding a bite or sting, it is important to gather additional information for the provider (Box 40.7). Patients may also call for advice to remove ticks (Box 40.8).

First aid for severe reactions include all the steps indicated in the anaphylaxis section. Additional steps include removing any nearby constricting items such as rings and clothing. The affected area may swell, and constricting items can cause additional problems. Box 40.9 describes the first aid for mild reactions.

BOX 40.9 First Aid for Mild Reactions

- Move to a safe location.
- Remove the stinger if it is visible.
- Wash the affected area with soap and water.
- To reduce pain and swelling, apply a cool cloth and elevate the extremity.
- For pain, apply *hydrocortisone* (HIE drah KOHR ti zone) or lidocaine cream to the area. An over-the-counter pain reliever can also be taken.
- *Calamine* (KAL ah min) lotion or a similar product can be applied to the area to decrease the pruritus (itchiness).

BOX 40.10 Screening Questions for Animal Bites

- What type of animal bit you? Do you know the animal? If so, are the shots updated?
- How does the wound look? Is it bleeding, dirty, or deep? Was it a puncture wound?
- Have you had the rabies vaccine series?
- When was your last tetanus vaccine?

CRITICAL THINKING 40.5

Gabe realized that there were no patient education pamphlets in the exam rooms. He would like to talk with his supervisor about getting brochure racks for each room. His thought was to include procedures on home emergencies/first aid for patients. If you were Gabe, describe the talking points you could make to your supervisor in favor of placing patient education materials in the exam rooms.

BOX 40.11 Animals Commonly Seen With Rabies

- Raccoons and skunks
- Bats
- Woodchucks (groundhogs)
- Foxes and coyotes
- Cats and dogs
- Cattle

TABLE 40.8 Rabies Postexposure Treatment for Nonimmunized Individuals

Medication	Purpose	Administration
Rabies immune globulin (RIG)	Antibodies specifically for rabies. Provides rapid (immediate) passive immune protection against rabies.	Dose based on weight. Administer only once between day 0 to day 7. Provider injects RIG around the bite wound if present. Remaining RIG is administered IM in the vastus lateralis or deltoid muscle (most distant from the wound). *If required, live virus vaccines (varicella, measles) must be either given with or spaced out 4 months after RIG.*
Rabies vaccine	Helps to provide long-term active immune protection against rabies.	Administer 1 mL IM in the deltoid muscle for adults and the vastus lateralis for children. Administer one each on days 0, 3, 7, and 14. A fifth dose may be recommended on day 28 for immunocompromised individuals

Animal Bites. Patients who have animal bites will typically seek care or call their providers. It is important for the medical assistant to ask some screening questions before talking with the provider (Box 40.10). Frequently, the bites are caused by domestic pets (e.g., dogs and cats). First aid for minor bites that only break the skin includes the following:

- Wash the area with soap and water.
- Apply an over-the-counter antibiotic cream. Cover the area with a clean bandage.

It is important to seek medical attention in the following situations:

- For fang punctures (like with cats): Bacteria are left deep in the puncture wound. Initially the wound may not look bad, but in a few hours the entire area could be hot and swollen.
- For bleeding wounds: Apply pressure with a clean cloth or bandage and seek help.
- For dirty or deep wounds: The person may require a tetanus vaccine booster if the last injection was given 5 or more years earlier.
- For wounds that look infected: The wound may look swollen, red, painful, or oozing.
- For questions about the rabies risk: Any wild or domestic mammal can get rabies and pass it onto people (Box 40.11).

In the ambulatory care facility, the wound is examined, cleaned, and bandaged. The medical assistant should gather information on the patient's last tetanus booster. A tetanus immunization may be given. If there is a chance of rabies exposure, the provider will discuss the treatment options. Treatment for rabies can be costly and the treatment time window is narrow. Table 40.8 describes the medications that can be given as treatment.

Foreign Body in the Eye. It is common for people with "something in their eye" to call or visit the ambulatory healthcare facility. This condition is known as a foreign body in the eye.

First aid for a foreign body in the eye is to try to irrigate it out. Washing hands before starting is important. Flush the eye with clean, warm water or with saline eye drops. Saline eye drops will be less irritating than water. If the foreign body cannot be removed through irrigation, the person should seek immediate medical care. It is important not to rub the eye, which may cause further damage.

In the ambulatory care facility, the medical assistant needs to ask the patient how the injury occurred. Further irrigation may be ordered after the provider exams the patient. It is important to check the date of the patient's last tetanus booster. The provider may order an updated tetanus booster, along with additional treatments.

Diabetic Emergencies

Diabetic emergencies occur when the person's blood glucose level is too low or too high. When a person eats carbohydrates (starches and sugars [e.g. breads, candy]), the blood glucose level increases. The pancreas makes insulin, and some people must take insulin injections. Insulin is the only thing that moves the glucose out of the blood and into the cells where it is used for energy. Without enough insulin, the blood glucose level increases. With too much insulin, the blood glucose level decreases (Table 40.9).

If the blood glucose gets too high or too low, the person can go into a diabetic coma. Permanent brain damage and death can occur. First aid for diabetic emergencies is described in Table 40.9 and Procedure 40.1.

CHAPTER 40 Medical Emergencies

TABLE 40.9 Diabetic Emergencies

Condition	Insulin shock	Diabetic ketoacidosis (DKA)
Alternative Names	Severe hypoglycemia (low blood glucose); insulin reaction	Severe hyperglycemia (high blood glucose)
Why Does It Occur?	Imbalance between insulin and the blood glucose. Too little glucose is in the blood because the individual did the following: • Took too much insulin • Ate too few carbohydrates • Engaged in too much physical activity • Drank alcohol (may occur up to 2 days after drinking)	Imbalance between insulin and the blood glucose. Too much glucose is in the blood because the individual did the following: • Took too little insulin • Ate too many carbohydrates • Is ill, has an infection, trauma or surgery. • Used an illegal drug (e.g., cocaine, Ecstasy)
Symptoms	**Hypoglycemia** • Double or blurry vision • Fast pulse, palpitations • Irritable, aggressive, nervous • Headache, unclear thinking • Shaking, tired • Sweaty, cold skin • Hunger **Severe Hypoglycemia** • Disorientation, unconsciousness • Seizures • Shock • Diabetic coma and death	**Hyperglycemia** • Thirsty, hungry, stomach pain • Nausea, vomiting • Frequent urination • Fatigue • Shortness of breath • Very dry mouth • Rapid pulse **Diabetic Ketoacidosis** • Fruity odor on breath • Diabetic coma and death
First Aid Procedures	Test blood glucose if possible. If the individual is conscious and able to swallow, give 4 oz. of fruit juice or regular (nondiet) soda or three glucose tablets. Test blood glucose every 15 minutes. If the blood glucose is under 70, give additional glucose. Continue until the glucose level is 70 or above (Procedure 40.1). If the individual is unconscious, place the patient in the **recovery position** (Fig. 40.15, Box 40.12). Call 911 and get medical help. Monitor the airway and pulse. Perform rescue breathing and CPR as needed.	Call 911 and get medical help. Monitor the airway and pulse. Perform rescue breathing and CPR as needed.
Additional Treatments	For an unconscious adult patient, glucagon 1 mL given subcutaneously or IM (Fig. 40.16). Repeat dose in 15 minutes if patient is unconscious. (Children younger than 6 years of age get 0.5 mL.) Monitor the blood glucose. Once the patient is alert and able to swallow, give additional food (e.g., sandwich).	The patient will need IV fluids, insulin, and monitoring to bring down the blood glucose level.

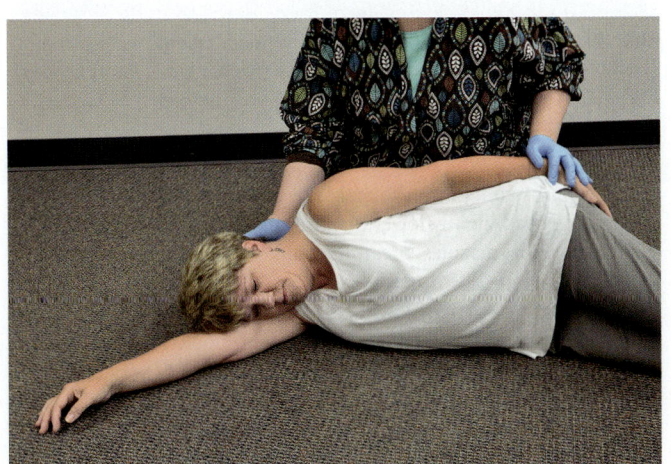

FIG. 40.15 Recovery position.

VOCABULARY

recovery position: A position on the person's side that helps to keep the airway open and clear.

BOX 40.12 How to Place a Person in the Recovery Position

- While kneeling at the person's side, place the farthest arm next to the head with the palm facing up. Take the other arm and place it next to the person's side.
- Bend the farthest leg up.
- You want to roll the person as one unit in case of head, neck, or spinal injuries. To do this, carefully slide one arm under the person's shoulder closest to you and the other under the arm and hip. Roll the person away from you and onto his or her side.
- Bend the top leg at the knee and place on top of the other knee. Place the upper arm near the person's hip.

PROCEDURE 40.1 Provide First Aid for a Patient With Insulin Shock

Tasks
Provide first aid to an individual with hypoglycemia.

Scenario
You are working with Dr. Martin, a family practice provider. Maude Crawford arrives for her appointment.

Equipment and Supplies
- Sugary drink (4-oz fruit juice or regular soda) or three glucose tablets
- Patient's health record

Procedural Steps
1. Wash hands or use hand sanitizer.
   Purpose: Hand sanitization is an important step for infection control.
2. Greet the patient. Identify yourself. Verify the patient's identity with full name and date of birth.
   Purpose: It is important to identify the patient in two different ways to ensure that you have the correct patient.

Scenario Update
Mrs. Crawford has diabetes and states that she thinks she has low blood sugar. She has blurry vision, tremors, and a headache. She asks you for something to eat. Per the facility's policy, you check her blood glucose level and it is 48 mg/dL.

3. Obtain a sugary drink or a fast-acting sugary food. Indicate how much to give to the patient.
   Purpose: Consuming a sugary food or drink will help to increase the blood glucose. Do not give a drink or food that contains fat or protein, which can slow the absorption rate.

Scenario Update
After 15 minutes, her blood glucose level is 59 mg/dL. You notify the provider while a coworker stays with the patient.

4. Describe follow-up care for the patient.
   Purpose: A blood glucose test should be done to find out how low the patient's level is. After 15 minutes of her eating/drinking the sugary food, the glucose test should be taken. If her level is below 70 mg/dL, give her additional sugary food/drink and repeat the glucose test in 15 minutes. Continue until the blood glucose level is 70 or higher.

Scenario Update
After 15 minutes, her blood glucose level is 82 mg/dL. You notified the provider.

5. Document the situation. Include the blood glucose levels, your actions, the provider notified, and the patient's response.

   10/04/20XX 1023 Pt c/o blurry vision, tremors, and a headache. She stated she thought she had low blood sugar. Four oz. of orange juice given to pt. After 15 minutes her blood glucose was 59 mg/dL. Dr. Martin notified and ordered additional orange juice and to recheck blood glucose until 70 mg/dL or more. Four oz. of orange juice given and after 15 minutes her blood glucose was 82 mg/dL. Provider notified._____Gabe Garcia CMA (AAMA)

If you come across an unresponsive person, check to see if the individual has a medical alert bracelet or necklace. (Some individuals have tattoos instead of wearing the medical alert jewelry.) The medical alert information may provide clues to what is occurring.

Musculoskeletal Emergencies

Without a diagnosis, it is hard to tell if an injury is a strain, sprain, fracture, or dislocation. It is important to always treat the injury as a fracture until the provider diagnoses the injury. A few symptoms will indicate if the injury is more severe (e.g., dislocation), including the following:
- The person has difficulty or is not able to move the extremity normally.
- The extremity is deformed.
- Bone is exposed through the skin.
- There is heavy bleeding.

If a person has any of these symptoms or the injury was related to major trauma, call 911 and get medical help. Additional first aid steps involve the following:
- For bleeding: Apply pressure to the wound with a clean cloth or sterile bandage.
- Immobilize the injured area: Do not push the bone back. Do not move the area impacted by the injury. Apply a splint beyond the joint above and the joint below the injury (Box 40.13).
- To limit swelling: Apply a cold pack to the area (Fig. 40.19A). Make sure to cover the cold pack with a towel. Do not apply the cold pack directly on the skin (Fig. 40.19B).

MEDICAL TERMINOLOGY
ket/o: ketone

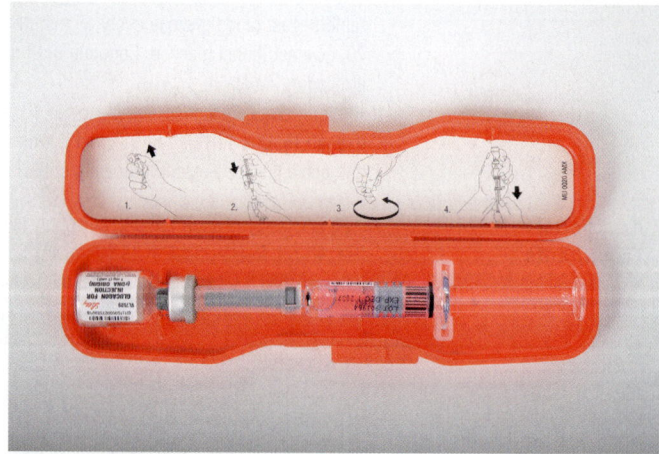

FIG. 40.16 Glucagon is given to unconscious patients with diabetes. This hormone stimulates the liver to release glucose into the bloodstream, thus increasing the blood glucose level.

- If person is going into shock: Make sure the person is lying down with the head slightly lower than the abdomen and elevate the legs. Monitor the person's breathing and pulse rate. Provide rescue breathing and CPR if needed.

Many times, patients will contact their provider regarding musculoskeletal injuries. The medical assistant should screen the patient and relay the information to the provider (Box 40.14). Typically, the provider will need to examine the patient; then an x-ray will be taken before a final diagnosis is made. Depending on the diagnosis, the medical assistant may need to help apply a splint, cast, sling, or another device. Good patient education is required. The medical assistant should coach

BOX 40.13 First Aid and Apply a Splint

- Splint the body part in the position it is in. Do not attempt to readjust the area or straighten it.
- Use a commercial splint or create a splint (Fig. 40.17). Use sticks, a board, or rolled up magazines, newspaper, or clothing as a splint.
- Make sure the splint extends below and above the injury (Fig. 40.18).
- Secure the splint with ties (e.g., belt, cloth strips).
- Check the injured area for swelling, paleness, or numbness, which may indicate the ties are on too tight. Loosen ties if needed.

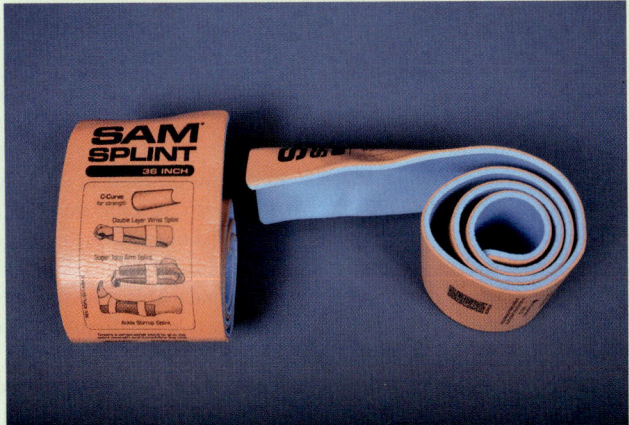

FIG. 40.17 SAM Splint is a reusable splint that can conform to the extremity impacted by the injury.

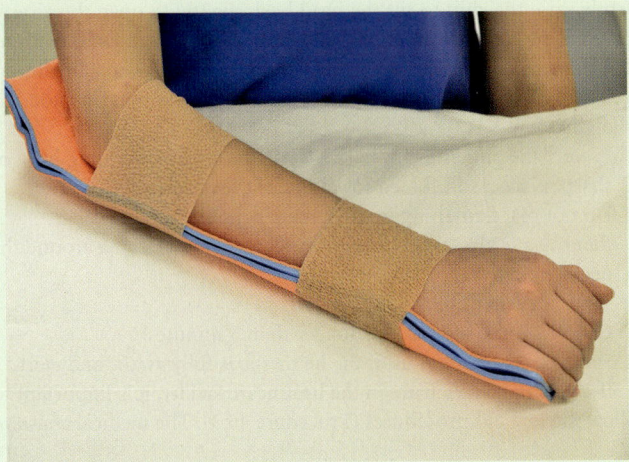

FIG. 40.18 Splint beyond the joint above and below the injury.

BOX 40.14 Screening Questions for Musculoskeletal Emergencies

- What happened?
- What does the injured body part look like? Is it deformed? Is it bleeding?
- Can the person move the injured part? Is there pain?
- How does the skin look over and near the injury?

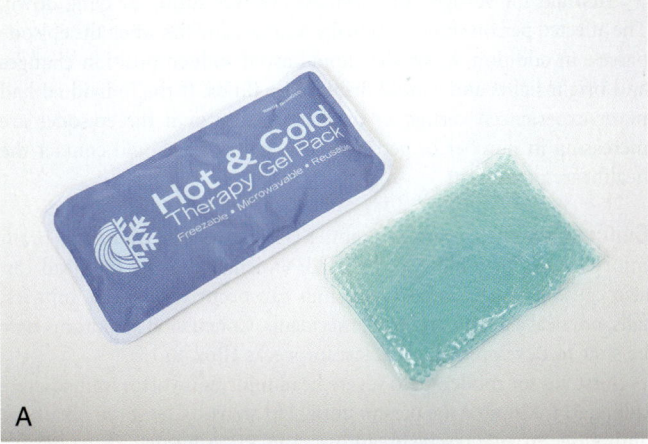

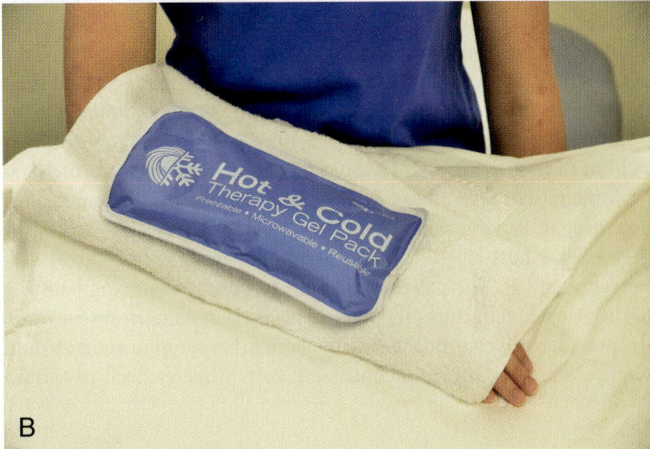

FIG. 40.19 (A) Some reusable packs can be either cold or hot packs. (B) A cold or hot pack cannot be applied directly to the skin. Place a towel between the pack and the skin.

the patient on checking the circulation on the extremity impacted. Coaching the patient on how to handle the protective device (e.g., cast, splint) while doing basic hygiene activities (e.g., showering) is important. Typically, musculoskeletal injuries require rest, ice, compression, and elevation (RICE).

Neurological Emergencies

Neurological emergencies can include minor conditions, such as dizziness, to serious conditions, like stroke. The medical assistant should know how to handle neurological emergencies.

Vertigo and Dizziness. *Vertigo* (VER ti goe) is a sensation that causes someone to feel as though everything is spinning. Peripheral vertigo is caused by an inner ear (vestibular labyrinth, semicircular canals, and vestibular nerve) issue. This issue impacts the sense of balance. Central vertigo is caused by a brainstem or cerebellum disorder. It can be caused by certain drugs (e.g., aspirin, anticonvulsants, and alcohol), migraines, multiple sclerosis, stroke, and tumors.

With dizziness, people may feel lightheaded or lose their balance. Many people get dizzy if they move too quickly from a sitting or lying position to a standing position. Their blood pressure drops, causing dizziness. People may feel like they will pass out. Usually dizziness resolves on its own, but it could be a symptom of another disorder.

First aid for vertigo and dizziness involves sitting or lying down. The affected person should gradually resume activities when the episode passes. In addition, he or she should avoid sudden position changes and bright lights and should drink more fluids. If the individual had never experienced vertigo or dizziness before or if the episodes are increasing in number or getting worse, he or she should contact the healthcare provider.

Concussion. A *concussion* (kahn KUSH ehn) is a traumatic brain injury caused by a blow to the head. Violently shaking the head can also cause a concussion. Concussions can occur with sports injuries, falls, physical assaults, and traffic accidents. Concussion symptoms may be slow to develop and could last for weeks (Box 40.15).

First aid for moderate to severe head injuries involves immediately calling 911. Monitor the person until help arrives. Check the breathing and pulse. Provide rescue breathing and CPR as needed. If the person is breathing and has a pulse, treat the condition as a spinal injury. Stabilize the head and neck by placing your hands on both sides of the person's head. Prevent any movement of the head, and keep the head in line with the spine until help arrives. If the person vomits, roll the person to the side and move the head, neck, and body as one unit. For mild head injuries, Box 40.16 lists when to seek medical treatment.

Moderate to severe head injuries are often seen in the emergency department. Patients will call or come to ambulatory care facilities if they have a possible concussion or a mild head injury (Box 40.17, Procedure 40.2). The patient may need to undergo radiologic testing to check for skull fractures and internal bleeding. If there are no fractures, the provider will educate the patient about other symptoms that would require follow-up and postconcussion care. Athletes need to refrain from playing sports until the concussion symptoms are gone. Another hit on the head can cause additional damage.

> **CRITICAL THINKING 40.6**
>
> Gabe has a 12-year-old son who plays middle school football. Before the season started, Gabe and his wife had to sign an acknowledgment form discussing concussions. What are the benefits of informing parents of school athletes about concussion symptoms?

Seizures. A *seizure* is a sudden increase of electrical activity in one or more parts of the brain. There are three major groups of seizures, including the following:

- *Generalized onset seizure*: affects both sides of the brain at the same time. Includes several types of seizures such as tonic-clonic and absent. Symptoms may include jerking, rigid or twitching muscles, and staring spells.
- *Focal onset seizure*: impacts one area of the brain. This type of seizure used to be called a partial seizure. There are two subgroups of focal onset seizures:
  - *Aware seizure*: The person is awake and alert during the seizure.
  - *Impaired awareness seizure*: The person is confused during the seizure. This type of seizure was known as a complex partial seizure.
- *Unknown onset seizure*: When the seizure began is not known.

First aid for seizures focuses on the safety of the individual. Move the person to the floor and place him or her in the recovery position. Gently raise the chin to tilt the head back slightly to open the airway. Monitor the person's breathing and pulse. Perform rescue breathing after the seizure has stopped if the patient does not resume breathing. Provide CPR if needed. Additional first aid measures include the following:

- Protect the patient from harm. Clear the area of anything hard or sharp. Place a soft folded towel under the head.
- Do not place anything in the patient's mouth.
- Remove any glasses and loosen any constrictive clothing around the neck (e.g., ties).
- Time the length of the seizure.
- Call 911 if the seizure lasts longer than 5 minutes.
- Stay with the person until the he or she is fully awake and alert.

If a person has a seizure in the healthcare facility, it is important to follow the first aid procedures (Procedure 40.3). The medical assistant

---

BOX 40.15 Symptoms of a Concussion

- Head pressure or headache
- Temporary loss of consciousness right after the incident
- Confusion, amnesia, dazed
- Dizziness, ringing in the ears
- Nausea and vomiting
- Slurred speech, delayed response to questions
- Listlessness, tiredness, sleep disturbances
- Irritability, personality changes
- Concentration and memory issues
- Taste and smell issues
- Loss of balance, unsteady gait (walk)

BOX 40.16 When to Seek Medical Care

- Loss of consciousness lasting longer than 30 seconds after the initial injury
- Repeated vomiting
- Worsening headache
- Changes in behavior or coordination (irritable, stumbling, and falling)
- Changes in orientation and speech (disoriented, confused, and slurred speech)
- Neurologic changes (seizures, visual disturbance, recurrent dizziness, difficulty with concentration, one pupil is larger than the other, or both pupils are dilated)

BOX 40.17 Screening Questions for Head Injuries

- What happened?
- Did the person lose consciousness? If so, for how long?
- Any bleeding?
- How is the person doing? Any vomiting? Are the pupils dilated, or is one larger than the other?
- Does the person remember what happened? Is the person confused or slurring his or her speech?

PROCEDURE 40.2 Incorporate Critical Thinking Skills When Performing Patient Assessment

Tasks
Use critical thinking skills while performing a patient assessment regarding a neurological emergency.

Scenario
You are working with Dr. Martin, a family practice provider. Maude Crawford's daughter called concerned about her mother. She stated that Maude fell and hit her head. She was "knocked out" for about a minute. She has been acting differently since the fall. You need to follow the "Emergency Phone Protocol" for your clinic.

Directions
Role-play the scenario with a peer. The peer will be the daughter and you will be the medical assistant. The peer can make up information regarding the scenario. Your instructor will be the provider.

WMFM Clinic – Neurological Emergency Phone Protocol
Obtain the patient's name, date of birth, signs/symptoms, and the history of the situation. After call, document situation, symptoms, and action in the patient's health record.

With the following neurological concerns, send the patient to the emergency department via the ambulance immediately.
- Seizure lasting three or more minutes
- Passing out or fainting; dizziness or weakness that doesn't go away
- Sudden or unusual headache that starts suddenly
- Unable to see or speak; sudden confusion
- Neck or spine injury
- Injuries that cause loss of feeling or inability to move
- Head injury with passing out, fainting, or confusion

With the following concerns, schedule a visit for the same day. If no appointments are available, consult the triage nurse or the provider regarding the situation.
- Headache / migraine
- Nonemergent neurological concern

Equipment and Supplies
- Patient's health record
- Paper and pen
- Emergency Phone Protocol for clinic

Procedural Steps
1. Write five questions that can be asked to obtain additional information on the patient's signs and symptoms.
   Purpose: It is important to ask open and closed-ended questions to obtain information about the patient's condition.
2. Role-play the scenario with a peer, who is the daughter. Obtain the patient's name and date of birth.
   Purpose: Obtaining the patient's information is important for any patient-related phone call.
3. Write down the patient's information obtained.
   Purpose: Writing down the information will help when you discuss the situation with the provider and when you document the call.
4. Using critical thinking skills, ask appropriate questions to obtain information about the patient's condition.
   Purpose: Thoughtful questions related to the situation and the patient's condition must be asked to gather the appropriate information.
5. Follow the protocol to determine what actions to take.
   Purpose: Protocols are approved and signed by the providers. They need to be followed by the staff.
6. Instruct the caller on what should be done.
   Purpose: The caller needs clear directions on what to do.
7. Document the call in the patient's health record. Include the caller's name, the patient's condition (e.g., signs, symptoms, and concerns), name of the protocol used, information given to the caller, and the provider who was notified.
   Purpose: Legally it is important to document all patient interaction.

PROCEDURE 40.3 Provide First Aid for a Patient With Seizure Activity

Tasks
Provide first aid to an individual having seizure activity, and document it in the health record.

Scenario
You are working with Dr. Martin, a family practice provider. Walter Biller arrives for his appointment.

Equipment and Supplies
- Watch
- Folded towel, blanket, or coat
- Patient's health record
- Gloves and other personal protective equipment (as required)

Procedural Steps
1. Wash hands or use hand sanitizer.
   Purpose: Hand sanitization is an important step for infection control.
2. Greet the patient. Identify yourself. Verify the patient's identity with full name and date of birth.
   Purpose: It is important to identify the patient in two different ways to ensure that you have the correct patient.

Scenario Update
While you are getting Mr. Biller's health history, he starts to have seizure activity.

3. Lower the patient to the floor and note the time when the seizure started. Gently raise the chin to tilt the head back slightly to open the airway.
   Purpose: The patient needs to be on the floor for his safety. It is important to time seizures.
4. Yell for help while moving the patient into the recovery position.
   Purpose: The recovery position will help to open up the person's airway. Yelling for help in the ambulatory care facility is reserved for emergencies. You need to notify the provider as soon as possible.
5. Check his pulse rate and respiration rate.
   Purpose: You need to make sure he is breathing and has a pulse. If not, rescue breathing and CPR must be started.
6. Apply gloves and other personal protective equipment as needed.
   Purpose: Wearing personal protective equipment will protect you if the patient vomits or becomes incontinent of urine or stool during the seizure.
7. Clear any hard or sharp items away from the patient. Place a soft folded towel, blanket, or coat under the patient's head.
   Purpose: It is important to protect the patient from harm.
8. Remove the patient's glasses (if on) and loosen any constrictive clothing around the neck. Stay with the person until the person is fully awake, and continue to monitor the respiration and pulse rates.
   Purpose: Tight clothing can restrict breathing.
9. Document the first aid measures you provided in the order that they occurred. In addition, document the seizure activity you witnessed, the length of episode, and the provider notified.
   Purpose: Indicating the care provided along with details of the seizure activity will help the provider.

10/05/20XX 1423 While rooming pt, he started to jerk his arms. He became unresponsive. Pt was moved to the floor and placed in the recovery position. P: 86 regular, thready; R: 18 regular, normal. Dr. Martin arrived. Pt's clothing was loosened. The seizure activity lasted for 4.5 minutes._____Gabe Garcia CMA (AAMA)

BOX 40.18   Screening Questions for Seizures

- What did the patient do during the seizure? How long was the seizure?
- Did the person lose consciousness?
- How is the patient now after the seizure?

BOX 40.19   Symptoms of Cerebrovascular Accidents

- Confusion or mental changes
- Speech difficulty (forming words, difficult to understand, or using words that do not make sense)
- Numbness of the face, arm, or leg, usually on one side of the body
- Problem seeing in one or both eyes
- Trouble walking, lack of coordination or balance, or arm weakness
- Sudden severe headache
- Facial drooping

BOX 40.20   FAST

The American Stroke Association promotes FAST to spot stroke signs and encourages calling 911:

F: Face drooping. Is one side of the face drooping or numb? Ask the person to smile to see if the smile is uneven or drooping on one side.

A: Arm weakness. Is one arm weak or numb? Raise both arms and watching for an arm to drift downward.

S: Speech difficulty. Is the person slurring his or her words? Is the person having problems speaking? Do the words not make sense, or are they hard to understand. Give the person a simple sentence to say and see if it is repeated correctly.

T: Time to call 911. If the person is showing any of these symptoms, call 911 immediately. Let the emergency responders know you think it might be a stroke. Watch the person's respiration rate and pulse rate. Do not give the person anything to eat or drink. Have the person sit upright if possible.

American Stroke Association, http://www.strokeassociation.org/STROKEORG/WarningSigns/Stroke-Warning-Signs-and-Symptoms_UCM_308528_SubHomePage.jsp.

TABLE 40.10   Signs and Symptoms of Respiratory Emergency

Skin	Unusually moist, flushed, pale, bluish, or ashen
Respirations	Slow, rapid, deep, or shallow; trouble or no breathing
Audible Breathing Sounds	Gasping, gurgling, high-pitched noises (e.g., whistling sound), wheezing
Patient Complaints	Shortness of breath, dizzy, lightheadedness, chest pain, tingling in extremities, fearful

TABLE 40.11   Causes and Symptoms of Hyperventilation

Causes	Symptoms
• Anxiety, panic attack, stress	• Dry mouth, belching, or bloating
• Bleeding, heart attack or heart failure	• Lightheadedness, weak, dizzy, difficulty concentrating
• Drugs (e.g., aspirin overdose or stimulant)	• Shortness of breath, breathlessness
• Infection, severe pain	• Chest pain, palpations
• Pregnancy	• Numbness and tingling in the arms or around the mouth
• Lung disease (e.g. COPD and asthma)	• Muscle spasms

must also notify the provider immediately. The provider may administer medications to end the seizure activity.

It is common that parents call when their child has had a seizure. Per the facility's protocol, the medical assistant may need to ask some screening questions and relay the information to the provider (Box 40.18).

Cerebrovascular Accident. A *cerebrovascular* (she ree broh VAS kyoo lur) *accident* (CVA) is also called a *stroke*. There are two types of strokes:
- *Ischemic* (I SKEE mik) *stroke*: occurs when the arterial blood flow to part of the brain is blocked. The brain cells start to die after a few minutes. This is the most common type of stroke.
- *Hemorrhagic* (HEM or aj ik) *stroke*: occurs when a weakened blood vessel ruptures.

Strokes can occur at any age, but they usually occur in older adults. The symptoms of a CVA relate to the part of the brain impacted. The individual may not have all the symptoms. Box 40.19 lists possible symptoms of CVAs.

First aid for stroke-type symptoms involves getting help (calling 911) immediately (Box 40.20). The emergency department (ED) is the best place for a patient to go. There is a small window of time where clot-dissolving medications (e.g., a tissue plasminogen activator) can be given to help the body break down the clot that is blocking the artery. If a bleeding artery has caused the stroke, the ED providers can detect this on radiologic studies.

If a patient comes to the ambulatory care facility with stroke-like symptoms, it is important for the provider to see the patient immediately. Be ready to call 911 when the provider orders you to do so. Also, monitor the patient's vital signs for changes.

> **MEDICAL TERMINOLOGY**
> **-ar**: pertaining to
> **cerebro/o**: cerebrum
> **vascul/o**: vessel

Respiratory Emergencies

Respiratory emergencies can create a number of different signs and symptoms (Table 40.10). It is important to get help immediately with respiratory emergencies. After calling 911, help the conscious individual into a comfortable position and monitor the respirations and pulse. Be ready to provide rescue breathing and CPR if required.

Common respiratory emergencies are discussed in the following sections. It is important for the medical assistant to recognize when a patient is having a respiratory emergency and get help immediately.

Hyperventilation. *Hyperventilation* or overbreathing is rapid and deep breathing. This leads to a low carbon dioxide level in the blood. It causes the feeling of breathlessness (Table 40.11). This gas imbalance creates symptoms that can mimic those of a heart attack, thus increasing one's anxiety and as well as the hyperventilation.

First aid treatments focus on raising the carbon dioxide level in the blood. This can be done by relaxing and using pursed lip breathing or slowly blowing out through the lips. A person should seek medical care if the hyperventilation episodes get worse. After diagnosing the condition, the provider may have the patient breathe slowly into a paper bag. This helps to restore the carbon dioxide and oxygen imbalances in the blood.

Asthmatic Attack. Asthma affects the airway and the lungs. It causes wheezing, breathlessness, chest tightness, and coughing. Typically it occurs at night or in the early morning hours. During an asthma attack, the airway constricts, lessening the air moving in and out of the lungs. Mucus clogs up the airway, making the airflow more difficult.

First aid actions for an asthma attack include the following:
- Helping the person into a comfortable sitting position. Usually sitting upright allows for easier breathing.
- Giving short-acting inhalers (e.g., albuterol), which will lessen the asthma attack within minutes. If the medication is not available or is not helping, call 911.

In the ambulatory healthcare setting, an asthma attack is an emergency. The provider needs to see the patient immediately. Typically, an albuterol nebulizer is ordered to relax and open the airway. It is important to monitor the pulse oximetry and vital signs.

If a patient or family member calls about an asthma attack, it is important to gather information quickly and talk with the provider (Box 40.21). If the patient is having severe respiratory distress (e.g., unable to talk or blue lips), calling 911 is critical.

BOX 40.21 Screening Questions for Asthma Attacks

- What symptoms is the person experiencing?
- Was medication given? What was the medication, and how much was administered?
- Did the medication ease the symptoms?

Choking. Choking can occur in all age groups. Most choking cases relate to swallowing large pieces of food or doing an activity (e.g., running) while eating. Other causes are denture-related issues and eating too fast. Children under 5 tend to choke on candy, grapes, and large pieces of food. They are also more likely to put nonfood items in the mouth. Plastic, balloon pieces, coins, and buttons are extremely dangerous to children. Objects smaller than 1.75 inches (the diameter of a golf ball) can be caught in the throat and cause choking. Any object caught in the throat is considered a foreign body obstruction.

First aid for choking includes asking the individual if he or she is choking. If the person can speak, then it may be a partial obstruction (Box 40.22). If the person is forcefully coughing, stand by and see if the person can clear the airway without assistance. Do not give the person any liquids until the obstruction is cleared. Procedure 40.4 describes the *abdominal thrusts* used on a conscious adult with a total airway obstruction (see Box 40.22).

Treat children older than 1 year of age the same as adults. See Box 40.23 for working with a conscious choking infant. If a person is pregnant or obese, wrap your arms around the person's chest. Place your fist in the middle of the breastbone between the nipples. Give firm, backward thrusts.

BOX 40.22 Signs of Airway Obstruction

- Partial airway obstruction
  - Forceful or weak coughing
  - Labored, noisy, or gasping breathing
  - Panicked appearance, extreme anxiety, or agitation
- Total airway obstruction
  - Clutching the throat with one or both hands
  - Unable to breathe, cry, cough, or speak
  - Bluish skin color (e.g., lips)

BOX 40.23 Conscious Choking Infant

Do the 3 Cs after gaining consent from the parent or guardians. Check the scene, call 911 (or have someone else call), and care for the infant. Hold the child with the head below the chest for the entire procedure. This allows gravity to help move the obstruction. Support the chin with your hand and the infant's body with your arm.

Have the child facing downward and give five back blows between the shoulder blades with the heel of your hand (Fig. 40.20A). Flip the infant and place two to three fingers below the nipple line on the chest. Give five chest thrusts (Fig. 40.20B). Do a mouth check, and only insert a finger to pull a loose object out. Doing a finger sweep is not recommended because it can push the item in farther. Continue until the object is out or the child becomes unconscious. If the child is unconscious, then place the child on a hard surface and begin CPR, starting with chest compressions.

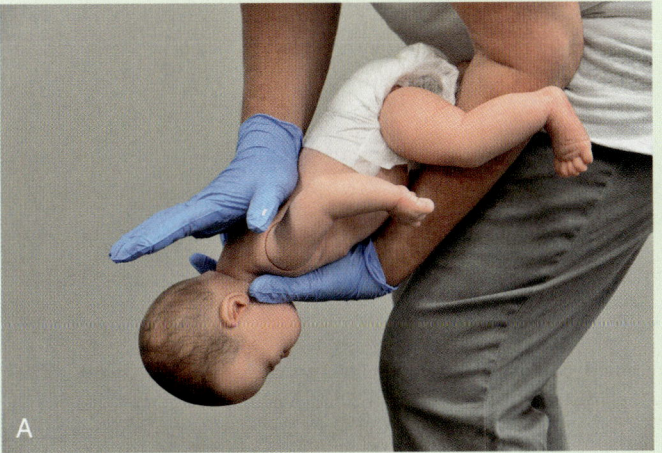
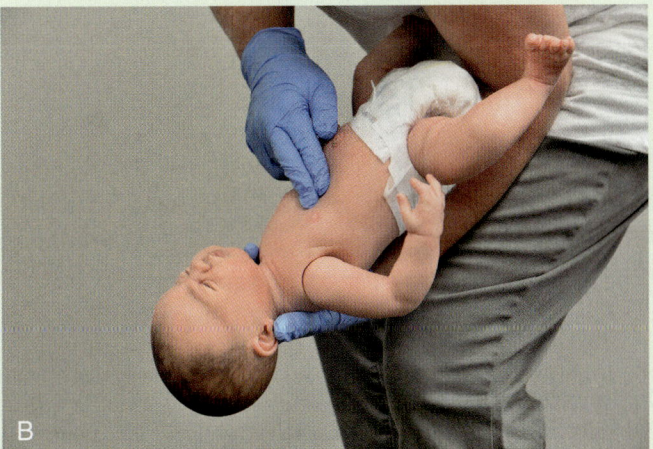

FIG. 40.20 (A) Support the infant with your arm and thigh while giving back blows. (B) Chest thrusts are administered in the same position as for cardiac compressions.

PROCEDURE 40.4   Provide First Aid for a Choking Patient

Tasks
Provide first aid to a conscious adult who is choking. Document it in the health record.

Scenario
You are working with Dr. Martin, a family practice provider. As you return from lunch, you notice that an adult visitor is having an issue. It appears that she had been eating fast food and now she is holding her neck with both hands. She appears to be panicking.

Equipment and Supplies
- Patient's health record
- Gloves
- Mannequin

Procedural Steps

1. Approach the person and ask, "Are you choking?"
   Purpose: If the person can speak and is coughing forcefully, then let her cough and try to dislodge the obstruction. If the person is not able to speak, then assist the patient.

Scenario Update
She shakes her head yes and cannot speak. She is standing.

2. Yell for help. Wear gloves if available. Stand behind the victim with your feet slightly apart. Reach your arms around the person's waist.
   Purpose: With an obstructed airway, the person may lose consciousness at any time. The rescuer must be prepared to lower the unconscious individual to the floor safely. If the person in distress is a child, the rescuer may need to kneel when providing assistance.

3. Make a fist and place it just above the person's navel. Make sure your thumb side is next to the person. Grasp the fist tightly with your other hand (Fig. 1).
   Purpose: Correct hand position is important as you do abdominal thrusts.

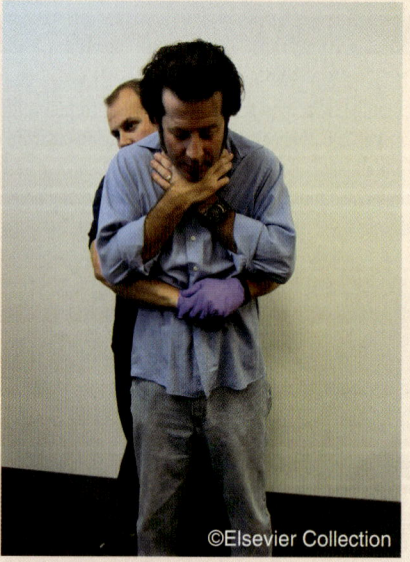
©Elsevier Collection

Scenario Update
The next steps must be done on a mannequin.

4. With the correct hand position, make quick, upward and inward thrusts with your fist. Do five abdominal thrusts before doing back blows.
   Purpose: The fist should be placed in the soft tissue of the abdomen to avoid injury to the sternum or rib cage. If the person is supine, straddle and face the person's head. Push your grasped fist upward and inward.

5. Stand behind the person and wrap one arm around the person's upper body. Position the person so he or she is bent forward with the chest parallel to the ground.
   Purpose: This position helps objects to dislodge.

6. Use the heel of your other hand to give a firm blow between the shoulder blades. Check to see if the object dislodges. If not, continue by giving another four back blows.
   Purpose: Back blows can help dislodge the item.

7. Continue to give five abdominal thrusts followed by five back blows until the object is dislodged or the person loses consciousness.
   Purpose: Repeated abdominal thrusts and back blows can help dislodge the item.
   Note: If the person faints or loses consciousness, lower the person to the floor. Call 911 (or the local emergency number) or have someone else call. Begin CPR starting with chest compressions. Check to see if the item is in the airway. Only remove it if it is loose.

Scenario Update
After two sets, she coughs out a piece of food. She can now talk.

8. Arrange for the person to be seen by the provider. Document the first aid measures you provided in the order that they occurred.
   Purpose: Indicating the care provided along with details of the situation will present the provider with a picture of what happened.
   10/06/20XX 1223 Pt was found in reception room with her hands on her throat. She appeared to be panicky. She could not speak but indicated with a nod of her head that she was choking. After being given 2 sets of back blows and abdominal thrusts, she was able to cough out some undigested food. R: 22 regular, normal. Pt is alert. She agreed to see Dr. Martin immediately._____Gabe Garcia CMA (AAMA)

Cardiovascular Emergencies

Syncope. *Syncope* (SING kuh pee) means fainting, passing out, or having a temporary loss of consciousness. When people are about to faint, they may feel dizzy, nauseous, or lightheaded. The skin may be cold and clammy. People may experience a "black out" or "white out" in their visual field. Muscle control is lost. Fainting occurs when the blood pressure drops suddenly and the blood flow to the brain is decreased. Possible reasons for fainting are listed in Box 40.24.

First aid actions for people who feel faint include having them sit and place their head between their knees (Fig. 40.21). For people who faint, position them on their back. Check their airway and make sure it is clear. Check for a pulse. If the pulse is not present, start CPR. Additional first aid measures include the following:

- Loosen any constrictive clothing.
- Raise the legs above the heart level (about 12 inches) (Fig. 40.22).
- Get help/call 911 if the person does not regain consciousness within 1 minute.

Bleeding. Bleeding can occur with and without trauma. First aid for bleeding involves stopping the bleeding and calling for help (Procedure 40.5). Nosebleeds are common in certain people. If a person has a nosebleed, have him or her sit upright and lean forward to prevent the person from swallowing the blood. Pinch the nostrils for 5 to 10 minutes, which helps to stop the bleeding. Continue to pinch the nostril until the bleeding stops. The individual should refrain from blowing the nose for several hours to prevent rebleeding.

In the ambulatory care facility, always wear gloves and the required personal protective equipment (PPE) before assisting patients. Follow these steps to stop the bleeding:
- For bleeding wounds, remove any obvious debris. Do not remove any large objects embedded in the wound.
- Place a sterile gauze or clean cloth over the wound and press firmly to control the bleeding. Do not put direct pressure over an embedded object, an eye, or displaced organs.
- For severe bleeding, help the person lie down and cover person with a blanket. This will keep the person warm and conserve body heat.
- If the bleeding seeps through the gauze, apply another layer on top of the initial gauze. Do not move the initial gauze.
- To slow the bleeding or if the bleeding is spurting from an artery:
  - Elevate the bleeding extremity above the heart level. Hold direct pressure over the site.
  - If bleeding does not stop with the elevation and direct pressure, apply pressure to the artery above the wound by pushing the artery against a bone. Continue to apply direct pressure on the wound. To see if the bleeding has stopped, slowly lift your fingers from the pressure point over the artery. Check to see if the wound is still bleeding. If bleeding, continue to apply pressure. Do not hold pressure at the pressure point for longer than 5 minutes after the bleeding stops.

Shock. Shock occurs when the body is not getting enough blood flow. The vital organs (e.g., heart, brain) do not get enough oxygen and nutrients for the cells to function properly and survive. Organ damage can occur. Shock is a life-threatening condition. There are many types of shock (Table 40.12). Box 40.25 lists the symptoms of shock. This condition requires immediate treatment for a chance of survival.

First aid actions for shock includes calling 911 immediately. Check the person for responsiveness. Monitor the airway, breathing, and pulse. If needed, perform rescue breathing and CPR. If the person is breathing and has a pulse, monitor the vital signs at least every 5 minutes. If the person does not have any injuries to the head, neck or back, or legs, raise the legs 12 inches. This helps the blood to move back to

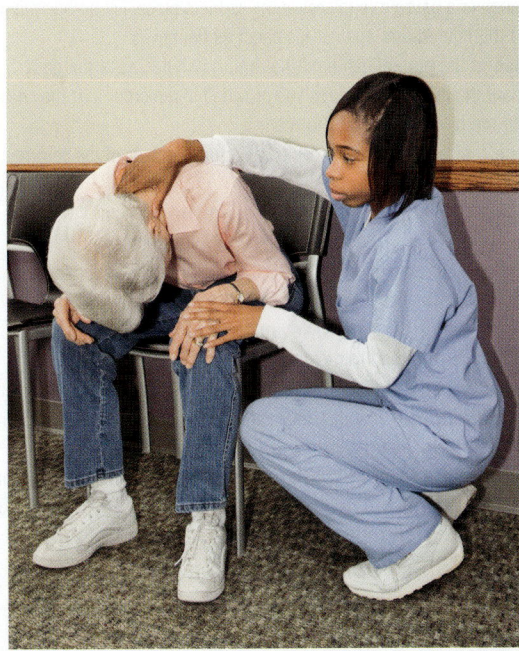

FIG. 40.21 Placing the head between the legs helps to decrease the faint feeling. (From Proctor D, et al: *Kinn's The Medical Assistant*, ed 13, St. Louis, 2017, Elsevier.)

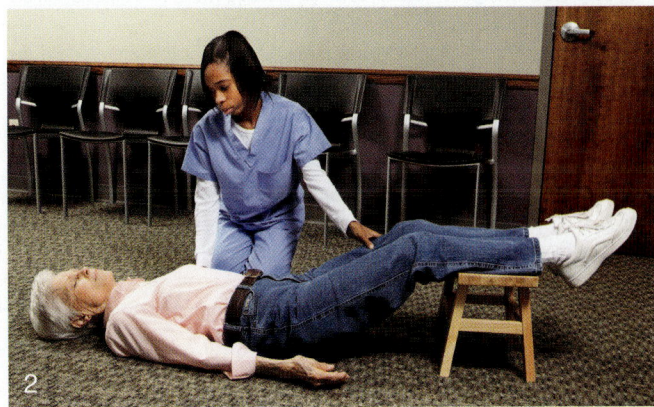

FIG. 40.22 Elevate the legs about 12 inches using pillows, blankets, or a small stool. (From Proctor D, et al: *Kinn's The Medical Assistant*, ed 13, St. Louis, 2017, Elsevier.)

BOX 40.24 Possible Causes of Syncope

- Too hot
- Dehydrated, alcohol use
- Standing up too quickly
- Drop in blood glucose
- Certain medications (diuretics, antihistamines, levodopa, calcium antagonists, angiotensin-converting enzyme [ACE] inhibitors, nitrates, antipsychotics, and narcotics)
- Neurologic condition (Parkinson's disease, postural orthostatic tachycardia syndrome [POTS], and diabetic neuropathy)
- Heart problem
- Vasovagal syncope: emotional stress, trauma, pain, reaction to the sight of blood, prolonged standing
- Carotid sinus syncope: constriction of the carotid artery in the neck (occurs with turning the head, shaving, or wearing tight clothing around the neck)
- Situational syncope: occurs during defecation, urination, and coughing

BOX 40.25 Symptoms of Shock

- Anxiety, agitation
- *Cyanosis* (sye uh NOH sis) (blue lips, fingernails)
- Chest pain
- Moist skin, *diaphoresis* (dye uh foh REE sis) (profuse sweating)
- Confusion
- Dizzy, faint, lightheaded
- Poor to no urine output
- Unconsciousness
- Shallow respirations; rapid, weak pulse

PROCEDURE 40.5 Provide First Aid for a Patient With a Bleeding Wound, Fracture, and Syncope

Tasks
Provide first aid to an individual with a suspected fracture, a bleeding wound, and syncope. Document the first aid you provide.

Scenario
You are returning from lunch and see a person fall at the entrance of the healthcare facility. He is an older man and is complaining of pain in his right lower arm. His arm looks deformed and is bleeding. You call for help. A provider comes, and coworkers bring supplies. The provider tells you to care for the wound and splint the arm before moving the individual. You have a coworker helping you.

Equipment and Supplies
- Gloves
- Sterile gauze
- Bandage
- Splinting material (e.g., SAM splint)
- Coban wrap or gauze roll

Procedural Steps

1. Wash hands or use hand sanitizer if possible. Identify yourself to the patient. Obtain the patient's name and date of birth as you put on gloves.
   Purpose: It is important to wear gloves when working with a wound. Obtaining the patient's name is important because the patient will be seen and you need to document the first aid provided.

2. Using sterile gauze, apply direct pressure over the wound to stop the bleeding. Make sure to immobilize the injured arm as you apply pressure. If possible, elevate the arm to help slow the bleeding. If the blood seeps through the gauze, apply another layer of gauze on the initial one. Continue with the direct pressure until the bleeding stops.
   Purpose: Applying pressure and elevating the arm will slow the bleeding.

3. Once the bleeding has stopped, cover the dressing with a bandage. Remember to immobilize the injured arm as you work.
   Purpose: It is important to cover the wound with a bandage in case the bleeding restarts. Immobilizing a suspected arm injury is important until the splint can be applied.

Scenario Update
As you apply the bandage to the injured arm, the patient states he does not feel good. He says he feels dizzy and thinks he is going to pass out. Your peer takes over by supporting his arm, and the man faints. He is still breathing and has a pulse.

4. Position the patient on his back. Continue to check his respirations and pulse rates.
   Purpose: If the patient is not breathing or does not have a pulse, administer rescue breathing and begin CPR.

5. Loosen any constrictive clothing around the neck and chest. Raise the legs above the heart level (about 12 inches).
   Purpose: Raising the legs allows the blood to return to the vital organs.

Scenario Update
After a few minutes, he starts to come around. He jokes that blood makes him faint. As he is lying on his back talking with you, you need to splint his injured arm.

6. Use the splint material and shape it to the injured arm. Do not straighten the arm. Apply the splint beyond the joint above and the joint below the injury.
   Purpose: It is important to keep the arm in the same position until the provider exams the arm and x-rays are taken.

7. Use Coban or a gauze role to secure the splint in place. Encourage the patient to hold the injured arm against his chest as he moves.
   Purpose: If the patient can hold the arm, it will decrease the pain.

8. Document the first aid measures you provided in the order that they occurred. Indicate the provider was at the scene.
   Purpose: Indicating the care provided along with details of the seizure activity will help the provider.

10/07/20XX 1215 Pt fell at the clinic entrance. He c/o pain in his lower right arm. Dr. Martin ordered for wound care and to splint the arm before moving the pt. Using sterile gauze, applied direct pressure over the wound until the bleeding stopped. Wound was covered with a bandage while arm was manually immobilized. Pt stated he felt dizzy and fainted. P: 68 regular, thready; R: 16 irregular, normal. Pt was positioned on his back with his feet elevated. Within a few minutes patient came to and started talking. SAM splint applied to right arm and coban applied to hold the splint. Pt held arm while transferring into wheelchair. Pt to see Dr. Martin immediately._____Gabe Garcia CMA (AAMA)

TABLE 40.12 Main Types of Shock

Types of Shock	Causes of Shock
Cardiogenic (KAR dee oh JEN ik)	Due to heart muscle damage caused by a *myocardial infarction* (mye oh KAR dee ul) (also known as MI, heart attack); the heart cannot pump enough blood to the other organs.
Hypovolemic (HYE poe voe LEE mik)	Due to heavy bleeding (i.e., accident or internal bleeding) or dehydration, blood volume is too low to provide nutrients and oxygen to the organs.
Anaphylactic	Caused by a severe allergic reaction (anaphylaxis); blood pressure drops and the airway narrows. Not enough blood gets to the vital organs, and the narrowed airway prevents adequate oxygenation.
Septic (SEP tik)	Caused by a severe infection (severe sepsis) that affects the functioning of vital organs (e.g., heart, brain, and kidneys). The blood pressure falls, and major organs can fail.
Neurogenic (NOO roe JEN ik)	Due to a central nervous system injury (e.g., spinal cord injury). Leads to vasodilation (not enough blood can return to the heart) and low blood pressure.

MEDICAL TERMINOLOGY
cyan/o: blue
myocardi/o: heart muscle
-osis: abnormal condition

the vital organs of the body. If the person has pain with raising the legs, keep the person flat. Make sure the person's head is flat. Loosen clothing and provide the appropriate first aid for the person's injuries (Procedure 40.6).

If a person goes into shock in the ambulatory healthcare facility, the provider will order that 911 be contacted. Oxygen and IV fluids are given. The vital signs are monitored, and the person's legs are elevated. Based on the medications available and the blood pressure, the provider may give IV medications that will increase the person's blood pressure. The goals are to keep the blood pressure high enough to sustain life and get the patient to the emergency department as quickly as possible.

Myocardial Infarction. Myocardial infarction (MI) is more commonly known as heart attack. Coronary arteries that bring blood to the heart muscle are blocked by a clot or narrowed from plaque. When the blood flow to an area of the heart is limited or stopped, the heart cells die and a MI occurs. The symptoms can vary. Pain, heartburn, and cold sweats are more common (Box 40.26).

First aid for a heart attack includes the following:
- Have the person sit down and rest; keeping the individual calm and loosening any tight clothing on the chest and neck area.
- Take nitroglycerin if prescribed (Box 40.27).
- Call 911 within 5 minutes of the onset of pain.
- Chew an aspirin (if not allergic).
- Monitor the person's respirations and pulse. Perform rescue breathing and CPR if needed (Fig. 40.23 and Procedure 40.7).

BOX 40.26 Symptoms of Myocardial Infarctions

- *Angina pectoris* (an JYE nuh PECK tore us) (chest pain)
- Upper body discomfort or pain in one or both arms, shoulders, neck, jaw, upper part of the abdomen, or back
- Pain qualities: mild or severe; sharp, burning, heaviness, squeezing, pressure; constant or *intermittent* (comes and goes)
- Shortness of breath with activity or rest
- Cold sweat
- Tiredness without a reason
- Heartburn, nausea, vomiting
- Dizziness, light-headedness
- Arrhythmia, palpitations

PROCEDURE 40.6 Provide First Aid for a Patient With Shock

Tasks
Provide first aid to an individual with who is in shock. Document the first aid you provide.

Scenario
You are working with Dr. Julie Walden. The administrative medical assistant at the reception desk notifies you that Robert Caudill (date of birth [DOB] 10/31/1940) is here and looks very ill. You bring the patient and his wife immediately back to the procedure room, as it is the only available room. He asks to move to the exam table, and you assist him as he transfers to the table. You obtain his vital signs, which are P: 92, R: 26, BP 72/48, and T: 103.2.

Equipment and Supplies
- Stethoscope
- Watch
- Pen
- Sphygmomanometer (blood pressure cuff)
- Pillows, blankets, or small stool to help elevate the feet
- Exam table

Procedural Steps
1. Call for help. Monitor the patient's breathing and pulse until the provider arrives.
   Purpose: It is important to have the provider see the patient immediately.

Situation Update
The provider examines the patient and suspects septic shock. You administer 2 L of oxygen per nasal cannula as the provider ordered. The triage RN inserts an IV and administers IV fluids. The provider directs another medical assistant to call 911.

2. Raise the patient's legs 12 inches.
   Purpose: Raising the person's legs helps the blood to return to the heart. Some tables will allow you to elevate the foot section. If this is not possible, use things such as pillows, blankets, or a small stool.

3. Make sure the patient's head is flat on the bed.
   Purpose: This helps the blood to flow to the head.
4. Loosen the person's clothing. Make sure the clothing does not restrict the neck and chest area.
   Purpose: Clothing that is tight can affect the breathing.
5. Obtain a pulse rate and respiration rate. Continue to monitor the patient's airway, pulse rate, and respiration rate.
   Purpose: Monitor vital signs. If the person is not breathing, provide rescue breathing. If the person has no pulse, start CPR.
6. While monitoring the patient, speak calmly with the patient. Use a gentle tone of voice. Demonstrate calming body language (e.g., do not appear scared, rushed, or out of control).
   Purpose: It is important to keep the patient calm during the crisis. Anxiety can be a symptom of shock.
7. Talk calmly with the patient's wife and explain what is occurring. Answer any questions the wife may have.
   Purpose: In an emergency, it is important to keep the family in the room updated on what is occurring. Depending on the emergency, sometimes a staff person will take the family members to another room.
8. Document the first aid measures you provided in the order that they occurred. Indicate which provider examined the patient. In addition, document the administration of oxygen and the vital signs obtained.
   Purpose: Indicating the care provided along with the vital signs will help the provider and the emergency responders.

10/07/20XX 1525 P: 92 irregular, thready; R: 26 regular, shallow; BP: 72/48 RA lying; T: 103.2 (TA). Notified Dr. Walden. Pt resting on table with his wife at his side. ———— Gabe Garcia CMA (AAMA)
10/07/20XX 1535 Administered 8 L of oxygen per mask per Dr. Walden's order. Raised legs about 12 inches, and head is flat.
P: 98 irregular, thready; R: 32 regular, shallow; BP: 70/42 RA lying.————
———————————————————— Gabe Garcia CMA (AAMA)

BOX 40.27 Nitroglycerin and Angina

Nitroglycerin is used for angina (chest pain). It dilates the coronary arteries, allowing more blood to move into the heart muscle. Nitroglycerin can be given as oral spray, sublingual (SL) powder, or sublingual tablets.

- Do not shake the spray. Prime (or release a test spray) 5 to 10 times for new bottles, up to 5 times for bottles not used within 3 months, and 1 to 2 times for bottles that have not been used in more than 6 weeks. Prime the bottles away from everyone. When administering the dose, spray onto or under the tongue. One to two sprays can be taken at the start of the pain. Then if the pain is not relieved in 5 minutes, give the third spray. Call 911 if the pain continues for an additional 5 minutes.
- Empty the pack of powder under the tongue. Allow the powder to dissolve without swallowing. Make sure the patient does not eat or rinse the mouth for 5 minutes.
- Tablets cannot be chewed or swallowed. Place the table under the tongue and let it dissolve. Usually they start providing relief within 1 to 5 minutes. If the pain is not relieved in 5 minutes, give another tablet. If the pain continues after 5 minutes, give a third tablet. Call 911 if the pain is not relieved 5 minutes after taking the third tablet. (Do not give more than three tablets within 15 minutes.)

Nitroglycerin works fast. The patient may feel dizzy, lightheaded, or faint after taking the medication.

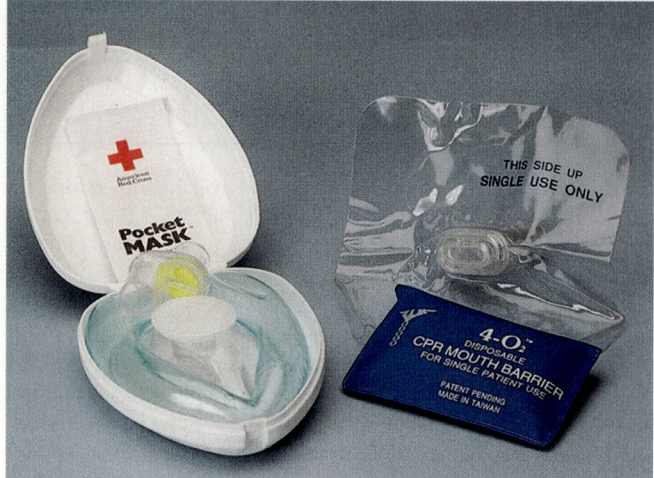

FIG. 40.23 Rescue breathing mouth barriers. (From Proctor D, et al: *Kinn's The Medical Assistant*, ed 13, St. Louis, 2017, Elsevier.)

PROCEDURE 40.7   Provide Rescue Breathing, Cardiopulmonary Resuscitation (CPR), and Automated External Defibrillator (AED)

Tasks
Perform rescue breathing and CPR. Use the AED machine.

Scenario
You are out jogging and find a person on the ground. No one is around.

Equipment and Supplies
- AED machine with adult pads
- Barrier ventilation device
- Mannequin
- Gloves (if available)

Procedural Steps

1. Check the scene for safety. Is it safe to approach and provide help to the victim?
   Purpose: It is important to look for toxic or electrical hazards. Also, look for other hazards that make the scene unsafe for you. If you find something, call 911 and wait for the emergency responders.
2. Check the person's response. Tap the individual on the shoulder and shout, "Are you all right?" Pause for a few moments for a response.
   Purpose: If the patient is responsive, the individual will talk, moan, move, or do something that indicates responsiveness.

Scenario Update
There is no response from the individual. A bystander comes up and you direct that person to find an AED machine.

3. Call 911 and answer the questions from the dispatcher.
   Purpose: The dispatcher needs to know what is occurring and where the emergency is located.
4. Put on gloves if available. Roll the person over if the person is face down. Roll the person as an entire unit, supporting the head, neck, and back. Open the airway and assess the respirations and the pulse for 5 to 10 seconds.

   Note: Occasional gasping is not considered breathing.
   - Person is breathing and has a pulse: If no head, neck, or spinal injury is suspected, then place the patient in the recovery position.
   - Person is not breathing and has a pulse: Give ventilations and monitor pulse.
   - Person is not breathing and has no pulse: Give CPR starting with compressions.

   Purpose: Before you initiate rescue breathing or CPR, you need to know if the person is breathing or has a pulse.

Scenario Update
The individual has a weak pulse and is not breathing. (Use a mannequin for the following steps.)

5. Use a barrier device if available. Pinch the person's nose and give each rescue breath over 1 second. Watch for the chest to rise. Give the appropriate amount of ventilations for the person's age (Table 40.13). Continue to monitor the pulse as you give rescue breaths.
   Note: For a situation in which a person had been choking, look in the mouth before giving a rescue breath. If you see the object, sweep it out with your finger. You can also provide nose ventilation, if the mouth is injured. Stoma ventilation must be done if the person has a stoma (in the throat area).
   Purpose: Adults get a rescue breath every 5 to 6 seconds. Children and infants get one every 3 seconds. If the chest does not rise, reposition and open the airway.

Scenario Update
When you check the pulse again, there is no pulse.

6. Place your hands at the correct location on the chest (Fig. 1). Bring your shoulders directly over the victim's sternum as you compress downward. Keep your elbows locked (Fig. 2).

PROCEDURE 40.7 Provide Rescue Breathing, Cardiopulmonary Resuscitation (CPR), and Automated External Defibrillator (AED)—cont'd

Purpose: The correct position will allow you to do the compressions at the depth they need to be.

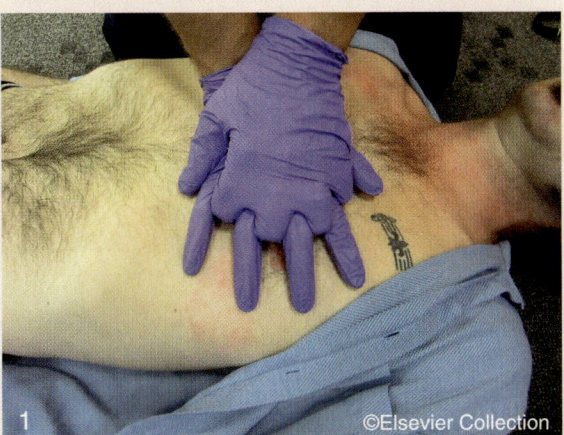

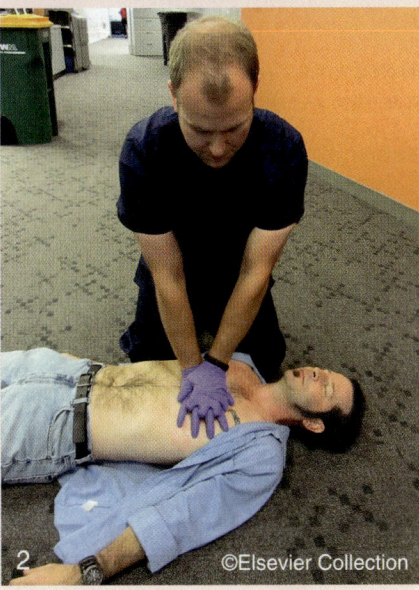

7. Give 30 compressions at the appropriate depth (see Table 40.13). Give 100 to 120 compressions per minute.
   Purpose: The appropriate depth is required to help compress the chambers of the heart.
8. Give two ventilations, and watch for the chest to rise. Continue with the cycle.
   Purpose: It is important to continue to provide ventilations and compressions until you are too exhausted, the person is breathing, an AED arrives, or emergency responders arrive.

Scenario Update
After two cycles, a bystander brings an AED but does not know how to use it. The bystander also does not know CPR. You need to stop the CPR and use the AED.

9. Turn on the AED and follow the directions. Attach the AED pads to the individual's bare dry chest (see Table 40.13) (Fig. 3). Attach the pads to the machine if required.
   Note: Make sure to remove any medication patches and medication residue from the chest before applying the pads.
   Purpose: The pads need to be placed on the bare, dry chest for the AED to work correctly.

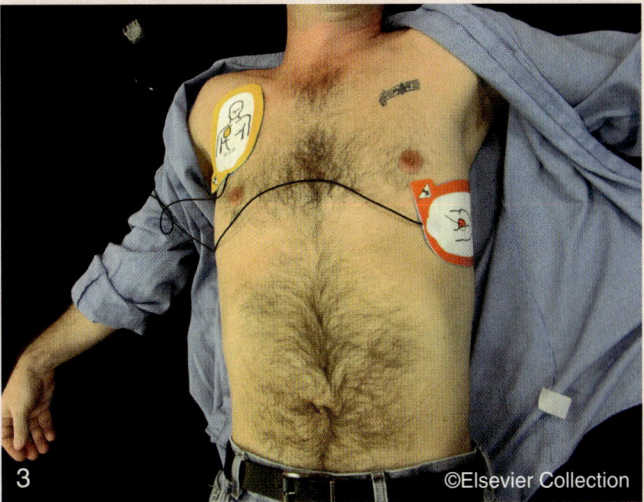

10. Have everyone stand back from the patient by announcing, "Stand clear." Push the analyze button and allow the machine to analyze the heartbeat.
    Purpose: "Stand clear" tells everyone to not touch the patient during this step.
11. Follow the prompts on the AED machine.
    - If a shock is advised, announce, "Stand clear" and make sure no one is touching the individual. Press the shock button. After the shock, do CPR for 2 minutes starting with compressions. Continue following the prompts until the emergency responders arrive.
    - If a shock is not advised, continue doing CPR for 2 minutes starting with compressions. Continue following the prompts until the emergency responders arrive.
    Purpose: The AED will prompt you as to what to do next.

If a patient arrives at the ambulatory care facility with chest pain or other MI type symptoms, bring the patient to a procedure or exam room immediately. Notify the provider at once. Usually the provider will order the following:
- One aspirin chewed and nitroglycerin administered sublingually
- Emergency 911 called
- Vital signs, pulse oximetry, ECG, oxygen to be administered while waiting for the ambulance to arrive.

The goals are to limit the damage to the heart muscle and transport the patient to the emergency department.

MEDICAL TERMINOLOGY
-is: structure
pector/o: chest

CRITICAL THINKING 40.7
Gabe is thinking of having a rescue breathing mouth barrier in each exam room and procedure room. He is also thinking of adding one to each of the first aid kits located in other parts of the clinic. Why is it important to make mouth barrier devices more available in the clinic?

TABLE 40.13 Summary of Rescue Breathing and Cardiopulmonary Resuscitation Differences

	Adult	Child	Infant
Check Responsiveness	Shout, "Are you all right?"		Tap the foot.
Open Airway	Head-tilt or if spinal injury is suspected, use the jaw thrust without head extension (Fig. 40.24).	Tilt head slightly past the neutral position.	Tilt head to the neutral position (Fig. 40.25A).
Assess Pulse	Feel for a carotid pulse near the middle of the throat (see Fig. 40.24).		Feel for a brachial pulse on the inside upper arm (Fig. 40.25B)
Give Rescue Breathing (Ventilation) Only	One rescue breath every 5–6 seconds, and deliver each breath for 1 second.	One breath every 3 seconds, and deliver each breath for 1 second.	
Chest Compression Hand Position	Heel of a hand is placed on the lower part of the chest (below the nipple line) and other hand is placed on top, so it overlaps the first hand.		Place two fingers just below the nipple line (see Fig. 40.25A)
Compressions	2–2.4 inches deep; 100–120 per minute.	2 inches deep; 100–120 per minute.	1.5 inches deep; 100–120 per minute.
Compression to Ventilation Ratio	One or two rescuers: 30 compressions and two ventilations.	One rescuer: 30 compressions and two ventilations; two rescuers: 15 compressions and two ventilations.	
Automated External Defibrillator (AED) Pads	Use only adult pads. Place one pad on the upper right chest and the second on the left side of the chest.	Use pediatric pads for children younger than 8 years; if not available use adult pads. If pads touch, place one on the back between the shoulder blades.	Use pediatric pads; if not available use adult pads. Place one pad on the chest and the other on the back.

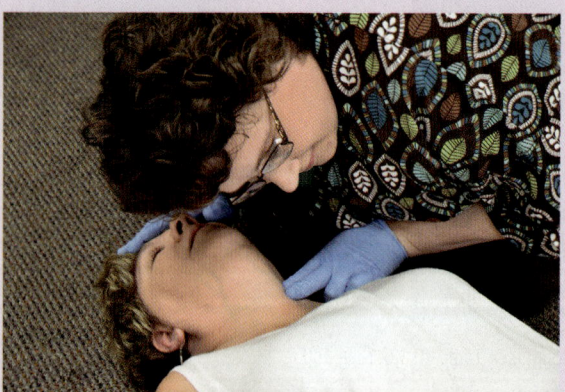

FIG. 40.24 Use the head-tilt position to open an adult's airway while checking the carotid pulse.

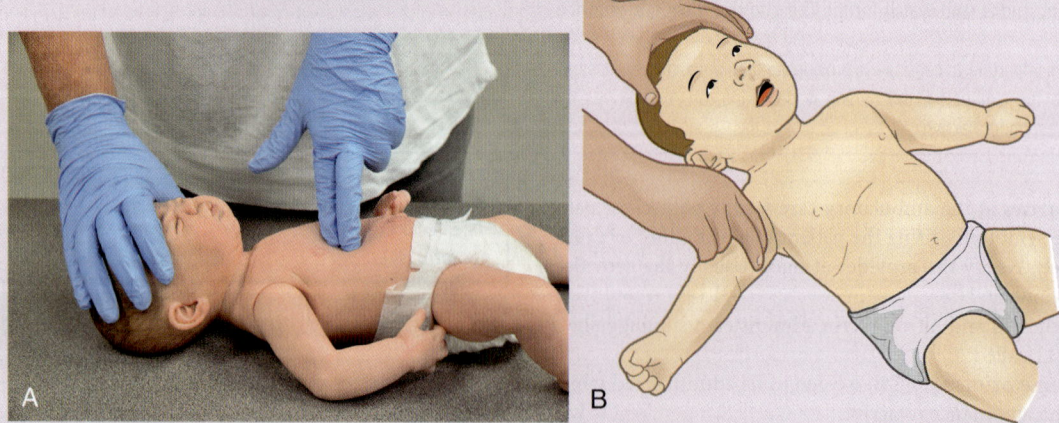

FIG. 40.25 (A) Open an infant's airway by tilting the head to a neutral position. For chest compressions, place two fingers below the nipple line. (B) In an infant, check for a brachial pulse. (B from Proctor D, et al: *Kinn's The Medical Assistant*, ed 13, St. Louis, 2017, Elsevier.)

CLOSING COMMENTS

A variety of emergencies can occur in the healthcare facility. It is important for the medical assistant to know which first aid actions to take. Knowing where the equipment and supplies are located is also vital in emergencies. Many agencies have mock codes to help prepare staff. These are training events that allow staff members to practice their skills. Often after mock events, the supervisors assess how the training went. They identify processes and procedures that need refinement and additional training.

Another method of improving processes comes after a real-life code situation. Usually a few days after a code, the staff involved will gather to debrief or discuss what occurred. They will usually talk about the following:
- How the code progressed, from the time the patient had symptoms to the time the patient was transported to the emergency department
- What went well and what was not so smooth
- Where more training is needed

These debriefings are extremely important after an emergency. Code situations can be anxiety inducing and stressful for staff members. It is important to talk through what occurred, while taking confidentiality into account. Besides talking, it is critical to manage one's stress by maintaining a healthy diet and getting adequate sleep and exercise.

An employee assistance program (EAP) is also helpful after stressful code situations. EAP is a work-based program designed to help employees resolve issues. These issues can be personal (e.g. financial, marital, or involving substance abuse) and professional (e.g., communication issues with coworkers and stress-related issues). The EAP services are confidential and designed to help the employee's work performance. EAP counselors help employees to deal with the aftereffects of an emergency.

EXCEPTIONAL CUSTOMER SERVICE

Medical emergencies are scary for patients and their families. We may be focused on providing emergency care, but we need to remember to communicate to the patient. Being sensitive to what patients are feeling is important. Remember to explain what you are doing. Ask the patient how he or she is doing.

Families of patients are often forgotten. In emergencies, often the family is moved to another room to allow more room for those helping with the code. It is helpful for the family to have a staff person wait with them. If this is not possible, then a staff person needs to report to the family and provide updates.

CHAPTER REVIEW

This chapter covers basic first aid in and out of the healthcare setting. In the healthcare setting, emergencies are communicated using special phrases (e.g., Code Blue). The healthcare team must respond immediately to the emergency and gather the crash cart and other required supplies. The first to respond to the emergency should initiate first aid. After the provider examines the patient, additional treatments may be done.

Many patients with environmental emergencies will contact or come to the ambulatory healthcare setting. In some cases, the most appropriate location for care is the emergency department. Hypothermia, heatstroke, full-thickness burns, and certain bites can be life threatening. These conditions are best treated in the emergency department. Heat cramps and heat exhaustion require electrolyte drinks and a cooler environment to bring down the body temperature. For minor burns, soaking the area in cool water immediately is important.

Diabetic emergencies occur when the blood glucose is too high or too low. Insulin will bring down elevated glucose levels, whereas carbohydrates (sugars and starches) will increase glucose levels.

Musculoskeletal emergencies are usually treated as fractures until the provider gives a diagnosis. First aid requires splinting the injured area. Applying pressure to stop bleeding and using ice packs to limit swelling are also steps to take.

Neurological emergencies range from minor to serious conditions. Frequently, patients can feel dizzy during or after procedures. Encouraging people to put their head between their legs will help relieve the dizzy or faint feeling. Having patients recline in a supine position and elevating their legs 12 inches will also help. With seizures, it is important to protect the patient from harm and get a provider immediately. Remember to time the length of a seizure. Strokes or CVAs can present with different symptoms. It is vital for the provider to see patients who have stroke-like symptoms immediately so treatment can begin.

Respiratory emergencies can also be life threatening. As with other life-threatening conditions, monitoring the airway, breathing, and pulse are important. Be ready to provide rescue breathing and CPR if it is required. With asthma attacks, help the person into a comfortable sitting position and give short-acting inhalers or nebulizer treatments.

Cardiovascular emergencies also range from minor to life threatening. With bleeding, apply direct pressure over the wound. Elevating the area and applying pressure over the artery between the wound and the heart can reduce the bleeding. Shock conditions require immediate medical attention. Managing the blood pressure and treating the condition that led to shock are important. The goal is to get the patient to the hospital for additional treatments. Myocardial infarction or heart attack requires early detection and treatment.

SCENARIO WRAP-UP

Gabe has been in his new position for only 2 weeks. Already he has a list of concerns and possible solutions he wants to address with his supervisor. Gabe also wants to discuss forming an emergency response team. This team would respond when a code is called throughout the building.

He hopes to have quarterly mock codes within the next 3 months. He wants to rotate the types of emergencies addressed by the mock codes. Gabe hopes that with additional training and more exposure to emergency supplies, the medical assistants will feel more comfortable with emergencies.

41

Assisting in the Clinical Laboratory

LEARNING OBJECTIVES

1. Discuss the role of the clinical laboratory personnel in patient care and the medical assistant's role in coordinating laboratory tests and results.
2. Describe the departments of the clinical laboratory.
3. Explain the three regulatory categories established by the Clinical Laboratory Improvement Amendments (CLIA), and identify CLIA-waived tests associated with common diseases.
4. Identify quality assurance practices in healthcare, document the results on a laboratory flow sheet, and discuss quality control guidelines.
5. List and discuss common safety signs and symbols seen in the laboratory, and compare the agencies that govern or influence practice in the clinical laboratory.
6. Summarize safety techniques to minimize physical, chemical, and biologic hazards in the clinical laboratory. Also, discuss the purpose of a Safety Data Sheet (SDS) and perform an emergency eyewash.
7. Describe the essential elements of a laboratory requisition.
8. Discuss specimen collection, including the importance of sensitivity to patients' rights and feelings when collecting a specimen. Also, discuss the steps for collecting specimens and informing patients of their results.
9. Discuss handling, processing, and storage of specimens. Also, explain chain of custody and why it is important.
10. Name common units used for measuring time, temperature, liquid volume, distance, and mass.
11. Complete the following related to the microscope:
    - Name the parts of a microscope, and describe their functions.
    - Summarize selected microscopy tests that may be performed in the ambulatory care setting.
    - Perform routine maintenance on a microscope.
12. Describe the safe use of a centrifuge.
13. Discuss the use of an incubator.

CHAPTER OUTLINE

1. Opening Scenario, 991
2. You Will Learn, 991
3. Introduction: The Clinical Laboratory and Patient Care, 991
    a. Personnel in the Clinical Laboratory, 991
    b. Clinical Laboratory Testing, 992
    c. Departments of the Clinical Laboratory, 993
        i. *Urinalysis, 993*
        ii. *Hematology, 993*
        iii. *Chemistry, 993*
        iv. *Microbiology, 993*
4. Government Legislation Affecting Clinical Laboratory Testing, 994
    a. Clinical Laboratory Improvement Amendments, 994
        i. *CLIA-Waived Tests and Laboratories, 994*
        ii. *Moderate- and High-Complexity Tests and Laboratories, 994*
5. Quality Assurance Guidelines, 996
    a. Three Stages of Quality Assurance in the Laboratory, 996
        i. *Preanalytic Stage, 996*
        ii. *Analytic Stage, 996*
        iii. *Postanalytic Stage, 996*
6. Quality Control Guidelines, 997
7. Laboratory Safety, 999
    a. Safety Standards and Governing Agencies, 1000
    b. Chemical Hazards, 1000
    c. Biohazards and Infection Control, 1001
        i. *Standard Precautions, 1001*
        ii. *Bloodborne Pathogens Standard, 1003*
        iii. *Safety Guidelines for Other Potentially Infectious Materials, 1003*
    d. Physical Hazards, 1004
8. Specimen Collection, Processing, and Storage, 1004
    a. Laboratory Requisitions and Reports, 1004
    b. Specimen Collection, 1005
        i. *Preventing Contamination, 1006*
    c. Handling, Processing, and Storing Specimens, 1007
        i. *Chain of Custody, 1007*
9. Laboratory Mathematics and Measurement, 1007
    a. Measuring Time, 1007
    b. Measuring Temperature, 1007
    c. Units of Measurement, 1008
    d. Measuring Liquid Volume, 1008
10. Laboratory Equipment, 1008
    a. Microscope, 1008
    b. Centrifuge, 1011
    c. Incubator, 1012
11. Closing Comments, 1013
12. Chapter Review, 1013
13. Scenario Wrap-Up, 1013

CHAPTER 41 Assisting in the Clinical Laboratory

OPENING SCENARIO

Greg Stuart, a certified medical assistant (CMA) through the American Association of Medical Assistants (AAMA), graduated from a medical assisting program 4 years ago and has been working at Walden-Martin Family Medical Clinic (WMFM) ever since. He enjoys working with patients and providers. Recently WMFM decided to expand its physician office laboratory (POL). Greg transferred into the phlebotomy laboratory area a few weeks ago and has really enjoyed it so far. He loves the patient contact during the phlebotomy procedures, and every day is just a little different. He really liked the laboratory portion of his medical assistant coursework in school and wanted a new challenge at work. It has been fun to brush up on his phlebotomy skills, and he has found that he has a real talent for putting people at ease.

He is working with another laboratory CMA, JulieAnn, as he trains in the laboratory. JulieAnn has worked in the POL for about 8 years and is happy to expand the services that are provided at WMFM. Today she is going to reintroduce Greg to the laboratory.

YOU WILL LEARN

1. To describe the role of the clinical laboratory in patient care and the medical assistant's role in coordinating laboratory tests and results.
2. To discuss the three regulatory categories established by the Clinical Laboratory Improvement Amendments (CLIA) and identify the CLIA-waived tests associated with common diseases.
3. To identify quality assurance practices in healthcare and document the results on a laboratory flow sheet.
4. To discuss the purpose of a Safety Data Sheet (SDS).
5. To summarize safety techniques to minimize physical, chemical, and biologic hazards in the clinical laboratory.
6. To discuss specimen collection, including the importance of sensitivity to patients' rights and feelings when collecting specimens.
7. To identify the metric units used for measuring liquid volume, distance, and mass.
8. To recognize parts of a microscope and describe their functions.

INTRODUCTION: THE CLINICAL LABORATORY AND PATIENT CARE

Laboratory medicine is the medical discipline that applies clinical laboratory science to the care and diagnosis of patients. Patient specimens can be collected at the laboratory or in an ambulatory care facility. Once in the laboratory, the specimen is processed and directed to the proper laboratory department. Each department of the lab will analyze and evaluate the specimen based on specific tests ordered by the provider. Tests can be performed manually (by hand) or with a variety of specialized automated (AW tuh meyt) instruments. Once test results are completed, they are reported to the provider.

> **VOCABULARY**
> **automated:** Measured by a machine or instrument. May involve human manipulation, coordination, or control.
> **specimen:** A sample of body fluid, waste product, or tissue collected for analysis.

Personnel in the Clinical Laboratory

Medical laboratories are in hospitals, ambulatory care facilities, public health departments, health maintenance organizations, and referral laboratories. The clinical laboratory could be staffed with the following:

- A director, who may be a pathologist (pah THOL uh jist) or a clinical laboratory scientist with a doctorate degree.
- Certified medical technologists (MTs) and certified medical laboratory technicians (MLTs)
- Medical laboratory assistants (MLAs), medical assistants (CMAs, RMAs), and *phlebotomists* (fluh BOT uh mists)

Phlebotomists and laboratory assistants have received specialized training in the collection of blood samples and the preparation of laboratory specimens. The agencies granting certifications and titles are listed in Table 41.1.

TABLE 41.1 Certifying Agencies for Laboratory Personnel

Certifying Agency	Title	Position
American Society for Clinical Pathologists (ASCP)	MT (ASCP)	Medical technologist
	MLT (ASCP)	Medical laboratory technician—certificate
	MLT-AD (ASCP)	Medical laboratory technician—associate's degree
American Medical Technologists (AMT)	MT (AMT)	Medical technologist
	MLT (AMT)	Medical laboratory technician
	MLA	Medical laboratory assistant
	RMA	Registered medical assistant
Department of Health and Human Services (DHHS)	CLT (HHS)	Clinical laboratory technologist
National Certification Agency for Medical Laboratory Personnel (NCA)	CLS (NCA)	Certified laboratory scientist
	CLT (NCA)	Certified laboratory technician
International Society for Clinical Laboratory Technology (ISCLT)	RMT (ISCLT)	Registered medical technologist
	RLT (ISCLT)	Registered laboratory technician
American Association of Medical Assistants (AAMA)	CMA (AAMA)	Certified medical assistant
National Healthcareer Association (NHA)	CCMA	Certified clinical medical assistant
	CPT	Certified phlebotomy technician
	CMLA	Certified medical laboratory assistant

From Proctor D, et al: *Kinn's The Medical Assistant*, ed 13, St. Louis, 2017, Elsevier.

TABLE 41.2 Comparison of Qualitative and Quantitative Testing

	Qualitative Test	Quantitative Test
Definition	A numeric value is not attached to the test results. May be used as a screening test.	Tests results represent the amount or quantity of an analyte in a certain volume of specimen.
Reported as	Positive or negative.	The test result is expressed as a number with units of measure attached.
Example	Negative fecal occult blood (FOB)—normal result; no blood found in the stool. Positive FOB—abnormal result; blood is found in the stool. Could indicate a cancerous colon lesion.	RBCs, 5 million per cubic millimeter ($5 \times 10^6/mm^3$) Hemoglobin 15 g per deciliter (15 g/dL) Hematocrit 45%

In ambulatory care facilities, the lab director may be the physician. These labs are referred to as *physician office laboratories* (POLs). Medical assistants are trained to properly collect patient specimens and perform specific testing procedures within the POL. They are also trained to properly collect specimens that are sent to outside reference laboratories for testing.

Laboratory tests may be used for four main purposes:
- To document good health of a patient
- To screen patients for diseases such as diabetes, high cholesterol, or urinary tract infection (UTI)
- To help the provider diagnose a medical disease, disorder, or condition
- To help the provider decide the most appropriate treatment and to monitor the effects of medications or a disease process

Only healthcare providers can request laboratory testing for a patient. The medical assistant is involved in the process of laboratory testing. To assume this responsibility, the medical assistant must know the following:
- Proper patient preparation
- Testing procedures common to the provider's practice
- Normal range of results for common testing

The medical assistant must carefully follow all laboratory instructions. This includes properly collecting and labeling patient specimens. Sending specimens to be tested at a laboratory will also require the medical assistant's attention to detail. Excellent communication between the team members and the patient is very important. The medical assistant should make the patient feel at ease with these procedures and hopefully gain the patient's cooperation and trust.

Clinical Laboratory Testing

Clinical laboratory testing is used in conjunction with a thorough health history and physical examination to obtain essential data for screening, diagnosis, or management of a patient's condition. The body is healthy when a state of equilibrium exists in the internal environment. This healthy state of equilibrium, called *homeostasis*, occurs when the physical and chemical characteristics of body substances are within a certain acceptable range, known as the *normal range*, or reference range. A change in the internal environment of the body often results in abnormal test values that are outside the population's reference range. When a provider uses a laboratory test for diagnosis, the patient's results are compared with the reference range of values. Reference values are also useful for assessing the progress of a patient's course of treatment.

Abnormal values for a particular test may be seen with more than one pathologic condition. For example, a decrease in the *hemoglobin* (HEE muh gloh bin) level in red blood cells (RBCs) is seen in iron-deficiency anemia, but also in *hyperthyroidism* (hahy per THAHY roi diz uhm) and *cirrhosis* (si ROH sis) of the liver. Therefore providers cannot rely solely on one laboratory test to make a diagnosis. They must use a combination of results obtained from the history, physical exam, and diagnostic and laboratory tests.

Tests performed in a clinical laboratory range from simple screening tests of one analyte (AN e lit) (e.g., measuring glucose to assess for diabetes) to complex profile testing, in which more than one analyte is related to an organ or disease (e.g., performing a lipid profile to determine the various fats in the blood). A *screening test* examines a specimen for the presence of an analyte that may indicate a disease state. Screening tests are not necessarily diagnostic for one particular disease but rather indicate that the disease state may exist. Screening tests are done routinely on patients based on their age, history, or gender. The results are often *qualitative* (KWOL I tey tiv), which means that a numeric value is not attached to the result. Qualitative tests are reported as positive or negative. A *fecal occult blood* (FOB) test is looking for blood in a stool specimen. A FOB test is an example of a screening test; if the test is positive, further testing is needed to diagnose the condition.

In a *quantitative* (KWON ti tey tiv) test, the test result is expressed as a number, usually with units of measure attached to numeric values. It is essential that the quantitative test results be reported with the units of measure. See Table 41.2 for a comparison of qualitative and quantitative testing.

CRITICAL THINKING 41.1

JulieAnn and Greg have been going over general information on laboratory testing this morning. It is important to know some terms used within the laboratory. JulieAnn asks Greg to define a qualitative test and a quantitative test in his own words. Take a few moments to write down these definitions in your own words. Be ready to share them in class.

VOCABULARY

analyte: The substance or chemical being analyzed or detected in a specimen.
pathologist: A physician specially trained in the nature and cause of disease.
profile testing: A series of laboratory tests associated with a particular organ or disease; also referred to as a "panel" of tests.
UTI: Urinary tract infection.
reference range: The numeric range of test values for which the general population consistently shows similar results 95% of the time.
referral laboratory: A laboratory that performs testing for another laboratory. Testing varies from high-volume routine testing to low-volume unique or unusual testing. Also called reference, diagnostic, or commercial testing laboratories. Often privately owned.

CHAPTER 41 Assisting in the Clinical Laboratory

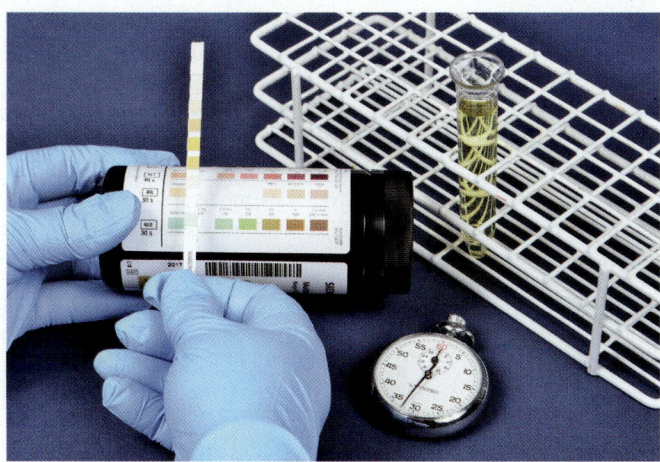

FIG. 41.1 Urinalysis.

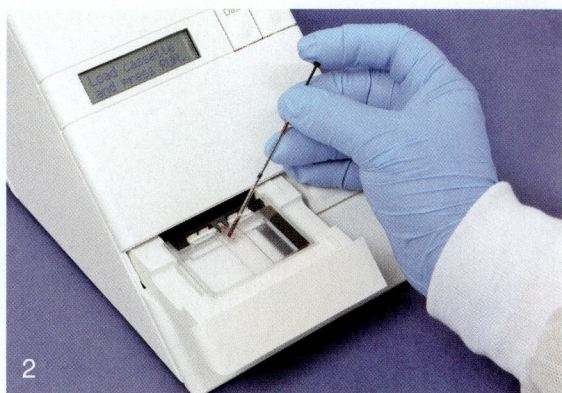

FIG. 41.2 Waived chemistry analyzer. (From Proctor D, et al: *Kinn's The Medical Assistant*, ed 13, St. Louis, 2017, Elsevier.)

Departments of the Clinical Laboratory

Large laboratories are divided into various departments, which may include urinalysis, hematology, chemistry, microbiology, specimen collection and processing, blood bank, coagulation, immunology/serology, **histology** (hi STOL oh jee), **cytology** (sahy TOL oh jee), **toxicology** (tok si KOL oh jee), and special chemistry. A POL generally performs test procedures in urinalysis, hematology, chemistry, and microbiology.

Urinalysis. *Urinalysis* (yoo r uh NAL uh sis) is the physical, chemical, and microscopic examination of urine (Fig. 41.1). As part of the physical examination, the color, clarity, and specific gravity are noted. The specimen's temperature may also be measured to verify that the sample is at body temperature and therefore recently collected. Urine is tested with a multiple test strip, also called a *dipstick*, which examines the following analytes in urine: glucose, protein, *ketones* (KEE tohns), blood, *bilirubin* (BIL ih roo bin), *urobilinogen* (YUR o bi lin e jen), *nitrites* (NAHY trahyts), and pH. We will go into the details of urinalysis in Chapter 42. Microscopically, the provider may examine urine for the presence of red blood cells (RBCs), white blood cells (WBCs), and epithelial cells, as well as mucus, casts, crystals, and microorganisms. Additional quantitative tests may be performed in the urinalysis department of a reference laboratory to confirm routine screening test results.

Hematology. *Hematology* (hee muh TOL uh jee) is the study of blood cells and *coagulation* (koh AG yuh ley shun). Laboratory testing in the hematology department may be qualitative or quantitative. In a POL, screening tests for hemoglobin, *hematocrit* (hi MAT uh krit), and the International Normalized Ratio (**INR**) (a coagulation test) are typically performed in the ambulatory setting. Reference laboratories perform blood cell counts that determine the number of RBCs, WBCs, and platelets in a blood sample. Microscopic tests determine the characteristics of cells, such as size, shape, and maturity. In addition, the hematology department performs tests to determine the coagulating ability of blood.

Chemistry. The clinical chemistry department analyzes the chemicals found in blood, cerebrospinal (suh ree broh SPAHYN l) fluid, urine, and joint fluid (synovial fluid). Specimen testing may be done manually or with complex chemistry instruments. In a POL, procedures may include single analyte tests (blood glucose) or multitest profiles. Chemistry profiles include tests for related analytes. Lipid profiles, for example, include assessments of total cholesterol, triglycerides, low-density lipoprotein (LDL), and high-density lipoprotein (HDL). POL chemistry analyzers are becoming more common in ambulatory care as technology becomes more compact and easier to use (Fig. 41.2).

Microbiology. Microbiology involves the study of very small, infectious organisms such as bacteria, fungi (FUHN jahy), yeasts, parasites, and viruses. Specimens used in microbiology include blood, urine, sputum, CSF, stool, wound, and other biologic sources. Specimens used for microbiology testing must be collected **aseptically** (ey SEP tick all ee) in **sterile** containers.

The goal of the microbiology department is to identify the microorganism that is causing the infection. The staff will also determine the most effective antimicrobial (an tee mahy KROH bee uh l) medications, which include antibiotics. This process is called identification and *sensitivity* (or susceptibility) testing.

Microbiology specimens may be grown on **culture media**. Once the organism is growing and in **pure culture**, it can be identified. Organism identification tests have changed with technology and will continue to change in the future. Various methods and technologies are used to identify microorganisms, including biochemical, molecular, and antigen-antibody complex testing.

Sensitivity testing is performed on organisms to establish an appropriate antibiotic therapy for that specific bacteria or fungus. Once again, a variety of techniques and technologies may be used to help determine which antibiotic would be most effective.

The following actions may be applied in a POL:
- Rapid strep testing may be performed to screen for strep throat.
- Microbiologic specimens may be aseptically collected and then sent to a reference laboratory.

VOCABULARY

aseptically: Free from living pathogenic organisms.
culture media: A solid, liquid, or semisolid medium designed to support the growth of microorganisms, especially bacteria and fungus.
cytology: The study of cells using microscopic testing methods.
histology: The study of tissues.
INR: International Normalized Ratio; is also called a prothrombin time (PT). Used to test the effectiveness of blood-thinning medication.
pure culture: The growth of only one microorganism in a culture or on a nutrient surface.
sterile: Free from all living organisms.
toxicology: The study and science dealing with the effects, antidotes, and detection of poisons or drugs.

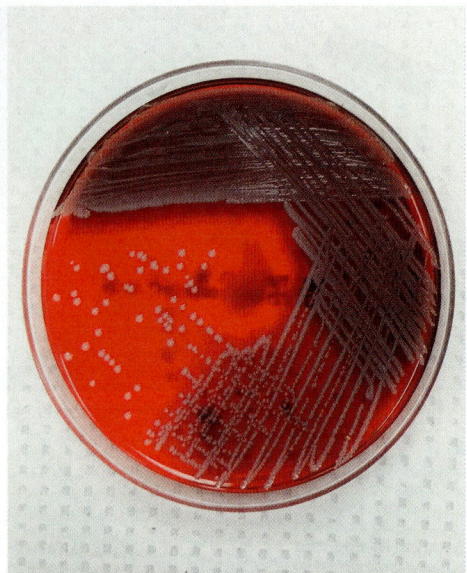

FIG. 41.3 Pure culture growing on culture media.

CRITICAL THINKING 41.2

Greg and JulieAnn have reviewed the different areas that are common in a POL. WMFM is now doing testing in microbiology, a new area that has been added to the POL in the past 6 months. As they talk about microbiology JulieAnn asks the question, "Why do microbiology samples need to be collected aseptically in a sterile container?" How would you answer this question in your own words?

- Microscope slides may be prepared for the provider to examine. Identification and sensitivity testing is usually performed in larger centralized ambulatory care, hospital, or reference laboratories (Fig. 41.3).

GOVERNMENT LEGISLATION AFFECTING CLINICAL LABORATORY TESTING

In 1988 Congress passed the Clinical Laboratory Improvement Amendments (CLIA). This law established quality standards for all clinical laboratory testing. CLIA is designed to ensure the accuracy, precision, reliability, and timeliness of patient test results, regardless of which laboratory performed the testing. A clinical laboratory is defined as any facility that performs laboratory testing on human specimens to provide information about the diagnosis, prevention, and treatment of disease or the impairment of health.

Clinical Laboratory Improvement Amendments

Under CLIA, all laboratories that perform even one type of test must meet certain federal requirements. They must register with the Centers for Medicare and Medicaid Services (CMS) as a laboratory. The registration application must be submitted to CMS with information about the laboratory's operations. The type of certificate that is issued is based on the information provided in the application. (Note: Most POLs are registered as CLIA-waived laboratories.)

The U.S. Food and Drug Administration (FDA) is responsible for categorizing commercially marketed tests performed in vitro (in VEE troh), based on the CLIA guidelines. The FDA has assumed primary responsibility for determining the CLIA complexity of all laboratory tests. Every laboratory test product is assigned to one of three CLIA categories based on the product's potential risk to public health. The CLIA categories are as follows: waived tests, moderate-complexity tests, and high-complexity tests. See Table 41.3 for common government acronyms in the clinical laboratory.

> **VOCABULARY**
> **in vitro:** Latin term meaning "in glass" and commonly known as "in the laboratory."

CLIA-Waived Tests and Laboratories. CLIA-*waived* (WEY ved) tests are defined as laboratory tests and procedures that have been approved by the FDA for home use or that are simple laboratory tests and procedures to perform. Waived tests are designed to have straightforward directions and procedures so that they have a minimal risk of incorrect results. Waived tests include tests that do the following:

- Use methodologies that are simple and accurate so that the likelihood of incorrect user results is negligible
- Pose no unreasonable risk of harm to the patient if it is performed incorrectly

Table 41.4 shows some common CLIA-waived tests performed in ambulatory care facilities registered as CLIA-waived laboratories.

The FDA's CLIA-waived database of tests is available to the public on the internet. This database contains the commercially marketed laboratory test systems categorized by the FDA since January 31, 2000, and tests categorized by the Centers for Disease Control and Prevention (CDC) before that date. The database can be searched by test system name, specialty or subspecialty, analyte, document number, qualifier, effective date, and complexity.

Moderate- and High-Complexity Tests and Laboratories. The CLIA program oversees the quality of nearly 200,000 different laboratory procedures. Most laboratory tests are categorized by the FDA as moderate-complexity tests. Some moderate-complexity tests that are performed in POLs include the following:

- Hematology and chemistry: testing done on an automated analyzer
- Microbiology: Gram stain procedures
- Urinalysis: microscopic analysis of urine sediment.

Moderate-complexity tests must be performed by qualified personnel as described by CLIA. High-complexity tests are generally not performed in a POL but rather in a hospital or reference laboratory.

Laboratories that perform moderate- to high-complexity testing must meet rigorous CLIA regulations and are subject to surprise inspections every 2 years. Each laboratory that performs these tests must do the following:

- Establish a system to maintain the identification of patients' specimens throughout the testing process and ensure accurate reporting of results.
- Establish and follow written quality control, quality assurance, and standard operating procedures (SOPs).
- Participate in *proficiency* (pruh FISH uh n see) *testing*, which is a form of external quality control. Three times a year, the laboratory must test samples provided by an approved proficiency-testing agency. The proficiency samples are tested in the same way as patient samples. Results are then reported to the proficiency-testing agency, and accuracy of testing is verified.

TABLE 41.3 Common Government Acronyms in the Clinical Laboratory

Acronym	Term	Application
BBPS	Bloodborne Pathogens Standard	OSHA standard that established precautions for dealing with all blood specimens
CDC	Centers for Disease Control and Prevention	Provides information for CLIA-waived laboratories in *Ready! Set! Test!* booklet
CLIA	Clinical Laboratory Improvement Amendments	Law that regulates all clinical laboratory testing products and sites
CMS	Centers for Medicare and Medicaid Services	Agency with which all labs must register and pay biannual fee based on complexity of tests performed in the lab
CoW	Certificate of waiver	The most common CLIA lab classification for physician office laboratories (POLs)
HHS	Department of Health and Human Services	Federal department that oversees the CMS, FDA, and CDC
FDA	Food and Drug Administration	Approves and categorizes CLIA-waived tests
HCS	Hazard Communication Standard	Standard regulated by OSHA that requires employers to communicate hazards to employees
HIPAA	Health Insurance Portability and Accountability Act	Law that enforces regulations for protected health information
HMIS	Hazardous Materials Information System	Identifies four color-coded chemical hazards (health, flammable, reactive, and other)
OPIM	Other Potentially Infectious Materials	Other materials related to bloodborne pathogens
OSHA	Occupational Safety and Health Administration	Regulates BBPS and HCS to ensure the safety of healthcare workers
PEP	Postexposure prophylaxis	Steps taken if a person is exposed to blood or OPIM
PHI	Protected health information	All test results are considered PHI and must be confidential
POL	Physician office laboratory	Located in ambulatory care facilities
PPE	Personal protective equipment	Gloves, gowns, and face protection worn when dealing with specimens
PPM	Provider-performed microscopy	CLIA moderate to complex microscopy tests available to POLs
QA	Quality assurance	
QC	Quality control	
SDS	Safety Data Sheet (formerly MSDS)	Must be in a uniform format with 16 section numbers, headings, and associated information to inform employees of chemical hazards in the laboratory

TABLE 41.4 CLIA-Waived Tests and Their Purposes

Specimen and Test	Purpose
Dipstick or tablet reagent urinalysis (manual or automated)	Urine screening to assess or diagnose diseases such as diabetes mellitus, kidney disease, and urinary tract infection
Urine pregnancy tests: visual color comparison tests	Diagnose pregnancy
Fecal occult blood	Colorectal screening to detect hidden blood in the stool
Erythrocyte sedimentation rate, nonautomated	Diagnose inflammatory process; increases in arthritis, infection, leukemia, and most cancers
Spun microhematocrit	Measures red blood cells; screening for certain types of anemia
STAT-CRIT hematocrit	Screening for certain types of anemia
Hemoglobin	Measure hemoglobin level in whole blood
Blood glucose by glucose-monitoring devices cleared by the FDA specifically for home use	Monitor blood glucose levels
Hemoglobin A_{1c} by single analyte instruments with self-contained or component features to perform specimen-reagent interaction	Measure A_{1c} levels to assess and manage long-term care of patients with diabetes
Cholestech LDX	Measures total blood cholesterol, triglycerides, HDL, and glucose levels
Whole-Blood i-STAT Chem8+ Cartridge	Measures ionized calcium, carbon dioxide, chloride, creatinine, glucose, potassium, sodium, urea nitrogen, and hematocrit in whole blood
Whole-blood thyroid-stimulating hormone (TSH) assay	Qualitative determination of TSH in whole blood
Blood mononucleosis antibodies	Rapid whole-blood test to detect heterophile antibodies to help diagnose infectious mononucleosis
Helicobacter pylori antibodies	Rapid whole-blood test to detect *H. pylori* antibodies to determine the cause of peptic ulcer
Borrelia burgdorferi antibodies	Rapid whole-blood test to detect *B. burgdorferi* antibodies to diagnose Lyme disease
Trinity Biotech Uni-Gold Recombigen HIV Test	Detects HIV-1 in a blood specimen
Nasal influenza A and B	Quick qualitative diagnosis of influenza antigens in nasal secretions or swab
Streptococcus A throat swab	Rapid strep test
Urine or blood drug tests	Multiple tests for the presence of a variety of substance abuse agents
Urine fertility and menopause tests	Detect follicle-stimulating hormone in urine
Ovulation tests; visual color comparison tests for luteinizing hormone	Detect ovulation

CLIA, Clinical Laboratory Improvement Amendments; *FDA*, U.S. Food and Drug Administration; *HDL*, high-density lipoprotein; *HIV-1*, human immunodeficiency virus type 1.
From the Centers for Medicare and Medicaid Services, *www.cms.gov/CLIA/downloads/waivetbl.pdf*.

- Employ personnel that meet CLIA regulations and specific qualifications for a moderate- to high-complexity laboratory. Requirements are most rigorous for high-complexity testing.

Medical assistants can perform all CLIA-waived tests and some specific moderate-complexity tests. Additional training will be required to perform moderate-complexity tests, depending on the certification of the POL where they work. Although medical assistants cannot perform high-complexity tests, they can be involved in preparing patients, sharing provider-directed patient education, collecting specimens, and documenting results in the patient's health record.

> ### CRITICAL THINKING 41.3
> The laboratory at WMFM is a registered waived facility. List five commonly performed waived tests. What is the difference between waived testing and moderate- or high-complexity testing? List three differences, and be ready to share them in the classroom.

QUALITY ASSURANCE GUIDELINES

Quality assurance (QA) is the promise of healthcare professionals to achieve the highest degree of excellence in the care given to every patient. QA includes a comprehensive set of policies developed to ensure excellent documentation and the reliability of laboratory testing. These policies benefit the provider by reducing the liability for inaccurate reporting of test results. QA also focuses on establishing a series of operating procedures for the benefit of the patient and the medical assistant who does the laboratory testing. The QA system enables the laboratory to assess, verify, and document the quality of the laboratory process. This documentation is a way of comparing what is happening with what should be happening.

As mandated by law, QA programs monitor all aspects of laboratory activity, from collecting specimens through processing, testing, and reporting steps. Programs check supplies, reagents, machinery, and actual test performance. The monitoring includes quality control, personnel orientation, laboratory documentation, knowledge of laboratory instrumentation, and enrollment in a proficiency testing program (if the lab performs moderate- or high-complexity tests).

Three Stages of Quality Assurance in the Laboratory

The overall process required to ensure QA in the laboratory is divided into three stages. These three stages must be applied to each test or procedure performed in the laboratory. If any of these steps are missed or performed incorrectly, QA has been broken.

Preanalytic Stage

1. The provider orders a test to screen, monitor, or diagnose a patient's condition.
2. A written or electronic requisition is filled out, showing the test requested, the specimen required, and where the specimen will be tested.
3. The specimen is collected, labeled, and processed.
4. The specimen is transported to the laboratory in the POL or properly prepared for offsite laboratory pickup.

Analytic Stage

1. Instruments are maintained and calibrated.
2. Controls are run and analyzed for each test method (part of ongoing quality control).
3. The specimen is tested, and the results are compared with reference ranges.
4. The test results are logged and documented in the patient's health record.

Postanalytic Stage

1. Specimens are properly discarded.
2. Analyses of control results are compared over time.
3. Patient reports from outside laboratories are logged or documented.
4. The provider interprets and signs all lab reports.
5. The patient is notified of the results in the office or is contacted by laboratory personnel.
6. The final report and all communication with the patient are documented in the patient's health record.

Accurate record keeping is one of the key responsibilities of a medical assistant. Various formats are available to record laboratory information. Most providers document patient information and testing results in the patient's electronic health record. Some POLs still use paper records, in which case the primary source of documentation is the *laboratory master logbook*. The logbook contains a written record for each procedure performed, the patient's identification number, results obtained, date performed, and personnel initials. The results are then sent to the provider for verification.

POLs are also required to have a procedure manual that describes how each test is performed and how the patient results are reported to the provider. Personnel are required to perform **calibration** (KAL uh brey shun) or **optics** (OP tiks) **checks** on laboratory instruments that use light detection or color change as part of the reaction process. In addition, they must run **quality control** or **control materials** each day before patient testing. Each manufacturer includes instructions for running control materials for its kit, procedure, or instrument. Quality control results must be documented and readily accessible. If errors or problems occur while completing quality control, the POL must perform and document remedial actions to correct errors or problems as they are identified.

Finally, **preventive maintenance** schedules must be followed and documented. Preventive maintenance prolongs the life of equipment

> ### VOCABULARY
> **calibration:** Occurs when the accuracy of an instrument is determined by comparing its output with that of a known standard or another instrument known to be accurate.
> **control materials:** Manufacturer-prepared samples that have a known quantity of a specific analyte. Used for quality control purposes. Testing results should fall within a manufacturer-defined range of results. Also called *controls* or *quality controls*.
> **optics checks:** A specific type of calibration that assesses the optics of an electronic testing instrument or system.
> **preventive maintenance:** Regularly scheduled care of equipment, which will decrease the likelihood of failure. Performed and documented at regular intervals while the equipment is in good working order.
> **quality assurance:** Written policies and procedures that ensure monitoring of all of the processes involved before, during, and after a laboratory test is performed to produce reliable patient test results.
> **quality control:** A process applied to ensure the reliability of test results, often using manufactured samples with known values.
> **standard operating procedures (SOP):** A set of step-by-step instructions to help employees carry out routine operations efficiently, with high quality, and uniformity of performance.

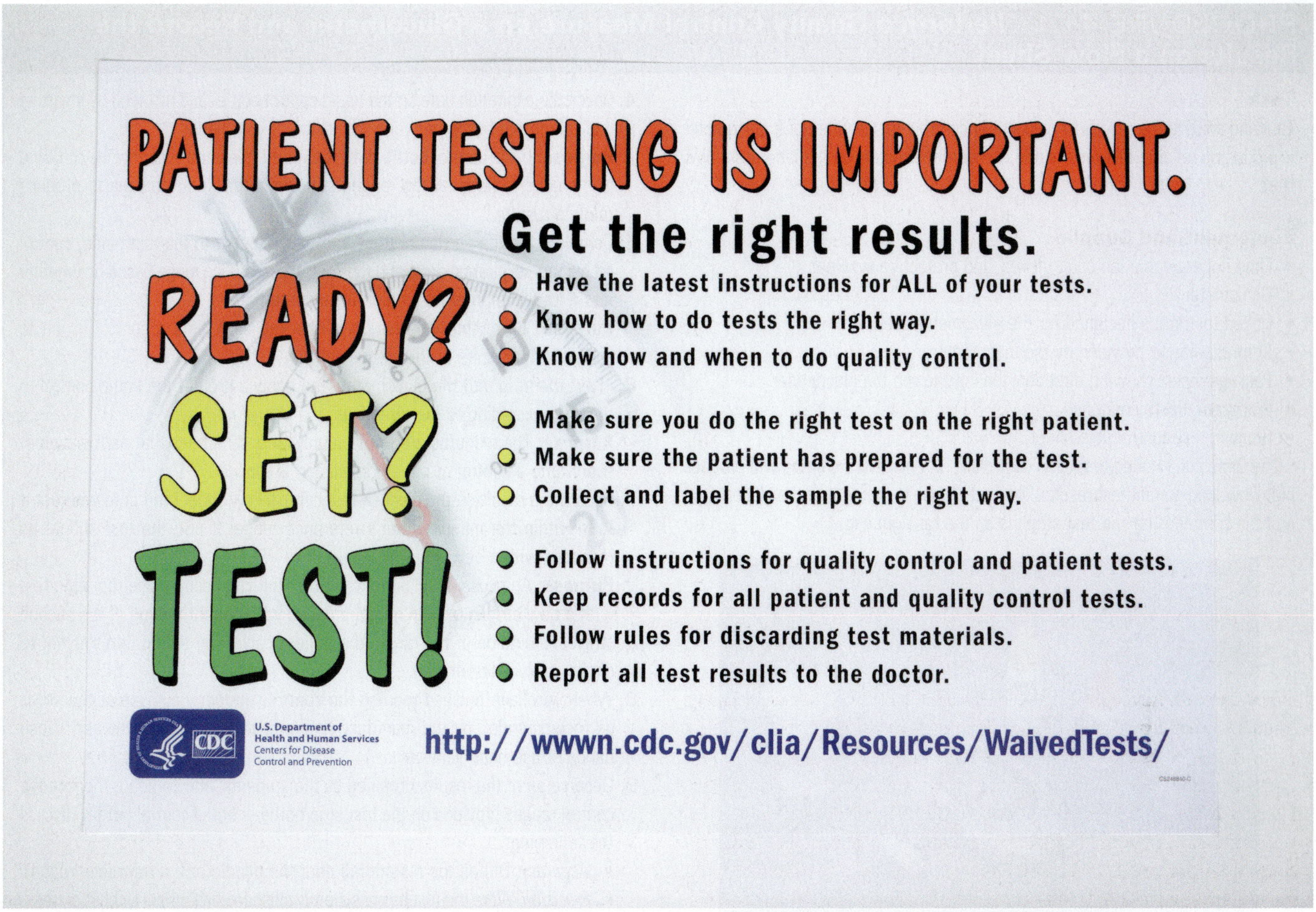

CHAPTER 41 Assisting in the Clinical Laboratory

PATIENT TESTING IS IMPORTANT.
Get the right results.

READY?
- Have the latest instructions for ALL of your tests.
- Know how to do tests the right way.
- Know how and when to do quality control.

SET?
- Make sure you do the right test on the right patient.
- Make sure the patient has prepared for the test.
- Collect and label the sample the right way.

TEST!
- Follow instructions for quality control and patient tests.
- Keep records for all patient and quality control tests.
- Follow rules for discarding test materials.
- Report all test results to the doctor.

CDC — U.S. Department of Health and Human Services, Centers for Disease Control and Prevention

http://wwwn.cdc.gov/clia/Resources/WaivedTests/

FIG. 41.4 Summary checklist from Ready? Set? Test? (From Proctor D, et al: *Kinn's The Medical Assistant*, ed 13, St. Louis, 2017, Elsevier.)

and reduces breakdown. Preventive maintenance includes daily cleaning and adjustment, as well as replacement of parts when necessary. Each instrument should have a paper or electronic log or worksheet for recording all changes, including daily maintenance details.

Ready? Set? Test! is an excellent online resource provided by the CDC for setting up and maintaining a CLIA-waived laboratory. Fig. 41.4 shows the checklist summary of the steps needed to assure proper CLIA-waived testing in a POL.

QUALITY CONTROL GUIDELINES

A crucial step in the QA process is running quality control (QC) specimens (Procedure 41.1). The purpose of QC in the laboratory is to ensure the reliability of test results while detecting and eliminating error. Here are a few important terms to remember:
- *Accuracy* is a measure of how close a test result is to the true value of the control material, as established by the manufacturer.
- *Precision* is the ability to consistently reproduce a test result.

When a series of control results show both accuracy and precision, the test is considered *reliable* and may be used for testing patients. QC monitoring is crucial because patient treatment is often based on or reinforced by the results of laboratory tests. Without QC monitoring, laboratory error is difficult to detect. Undetected laboratory errors may result in harm to the patient.

Prepared control samples are tested daily, along with patient samples. Control test results must fall within a preestablished range of results before patient results can be reported. QC samples are called *controls*. They are usually supplied with the manufacturer's prepackaged kits and are intended for use in a POL. Controls should be analyzed at specified intervals as recommended by the manufacturer. See Box 41.1 for some examples of routine QC testing.

BOX 41.1 Quality Control Examples

Examples of routine quality control testing in a POL include the following:
- Positive and negative controls supplied with pregnancy test kits are performed with each patient specimen.
- Urinalysis dipstick controls (used for chemical examination of urine) should be checked daily before patient testing and each time a new **reagent** (re AY jent) container is opened.
- Controls for automated chemistry analyses should be performed before patient testing and at specified intervals during the day, depending on the number of tests run per day and the manufacturer's recommendations. Consistent control results ensure constant conditions throughout the daily testing process.

VOCABULARY
reagent: A substance for use in a chemical reaction.

PROCEDURE 41.1 Perform a Quality Control Measure on a Glucometer and Record the Results on a Flow Sheet

Task
Test and analyze the results of glucometer controls to see whether a glucometer is producing reliable test results and to record the results on the laboratory flow sheet.

Equipment and Supplies
- Fluid impermeable lab coat, gloves, and protective eyewear
- Glucometer
- Coded test strips designed for the glucometer used
- Control solution provided by the manufacturer
- Package insert showing directions on how to run the glucometer
- Biohazard waste container
- Glucose test control flow sheet

The three color-coded bottles of controls (1, 2, and 3) in the figure will produce high, low, and normal test results. The test strip is to the right of the glucometer, and the container for the test strips is on the far right (Fig. 1).

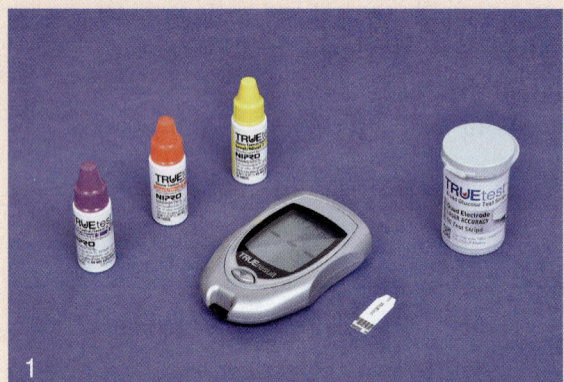

Procedural Steps
The following can be a class exercise in which all of the students participate.

1. Put on lab coat. Wash hands or use hand sanitizer. Put on gloves and eye protection.
   Purpose: Hand sanitization is an important step for infection control. PPE is necessary when working with any control or specimen material.
2. Take a coded strip out of the bottle and note the control level and range listed on the control bottle or the strip container.
3. Review the directions on the glucometer package insert, and calibrate the meter by inserting the precoded test strip into the monitor or by manually inserting the code number into the monitor (Fig. 2).
   Purpose: Manufacturers must provide directions on how to calibrate light-sensitive meters every time a new container of test strips is used. Note: The newer test strips will code themselves when inserted into the meter.

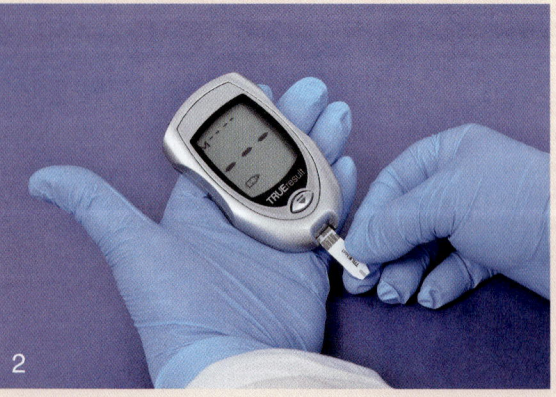

4. Check the expiration date on the liquid control bottle, and mix well by inverting and rolling the bottle between the palms of your hands.
   Purpose: If the control bottle date is expired, the control cannot be run. And it is crucial to have all the reagents in the bottle in suspension to produce reliable results.
5. Complete the top portion of the control log sheet with the test name, control lot number, expiration date, and the control's reference range based on whether it is a low-level, normal, or high-level control.
   Purpose: All of this information is checked each time a control is run to compare the results of the same control.
6. Insert the strip into the glucometer, and apply a drop of the liquid control to the strip according to the directions.
   Purpose: The manufacturer must supply clear directions that are consistent every time a control or patient specimen is run.
7. Record the result on the glucose test control flow sheet, and note whether it falls within the manufacturer's reference range. If not, the test should be repeated with a new strip.
   Purpose: An occasional "out of range" result can occur. If the repeated test with a new strip is back in range, proceed with patient testing. If the second strip falls outside of the range, the patient cannot be tested until the cause of the error is determined.
8. When you have finished running the controls, properly dispose of the strips as recommended by the manufacturer, remove gloves and eyewear. Wash hands or use hand sanitizer.
9. Observe all of the results obtained by the students, and compare them to the control ranges provided on the test strip bottle or liquid control bottle. Discuss the following:
   - *Accuracy:* Did all the results fall near the middle of the reference range?
   - *Precision:* Were the results consistently close to each other (without extreme highs and lows)?
   - *Reliability:* If both of the previous points are affirmed, the test is reliable and the glucometer may be used to test patient samples.

GLUCOSE TEST CONTROL FLOW SHEET						
Control Lot #: _____			Expiration Date: _____		
Control Range: _____			Level: Low/Normal/High		
Date	Student/ MA Initials	Result	Accept	Reject	Corrective Action	

BOX 41.2 Using a Graph for Quality Control Results

Many laboratories will use a graph to display daily quality control results. A paper graph or electronic graph file can be updated with daily QC values. Graphing advantages include the following:

- A graph is a physical representation of QC results that can display data irregularities in an easy-to-see format.
- It displays possible **trends** and **shifts** in data over time. See the labeled graph.

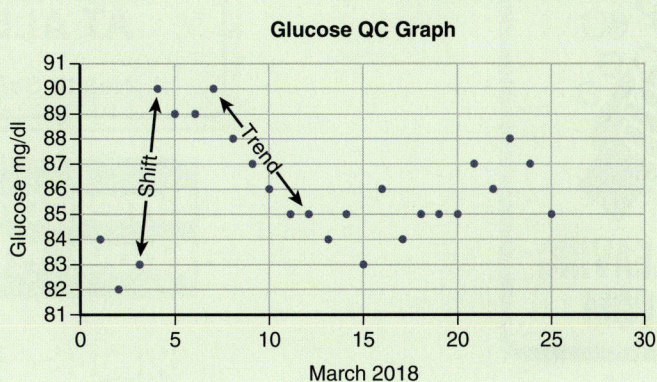

On every day that patient tests are performed, QC tests must also be performed and the results entered onto a paper or electronic graph or flow sheet. See Box 41.2 for more information on graphing QC results. When new control materials are opened and used, the results and dates must be entered on a new flow sheet, along with the expiration dates of the controls. These records must be retained for several years; the exact number of years is determined by state law and CLIA mandates.

Another part of quality control is routine preventive maintenance. All laboratory equipment should be on a routine preventive maintenance schedule so that equipment is serviced before a breakdown occurs. Any time equipment cannot be used is an inconvenience to the patient.

BOX 41.3 Preventive Maintenance Program for Laboratory Equipment

- Follow the manufacturer's instructions for calibrating instruments.
- Read and understand the instructions for routine instrument care.
- Perform all preventive maintenance specified by the manufacturer's instructions.
- Keep spare parts available for immediate use.
- Record the name, address, and phone number of a contact person for maintenance or repair.
- Create a maintenance form, or use the one provided by the manufacturer.

CRITICAL THINKING 41.4

As Greg and JulieAnn are reviewing quality assurance and quality control, Greg asks JulieAnn to clarify the difference between QA and QC. In your own words, define QA and QC. How are they different? Be ready to discuss your answer with the class.

See Box 41.3 for tips on preventive maintenance in the clinical laboratory.

LABORATORY SAFETY

The importance of safety in the laboratory cannot be overemphasized. Most laboratory accidents can be prevented by using proper techniques and common sense. Following safe practices in the laboratory requires a personal commitment and concern for others. An unsafe act may also harm an innocent bystander without harming the person who performs the act. See Box 41.4 for some common safety signs and symbols seen in the laboratory.

VOCABULARY

shift(s): Data results on a graph that make an abrupt change in value.
trend(s): Data results on a graph that are obtained over time, which continue to go upward or downward in value.

BOX 41.4 Common Safety Signs and Symbols Used in the Laboratory

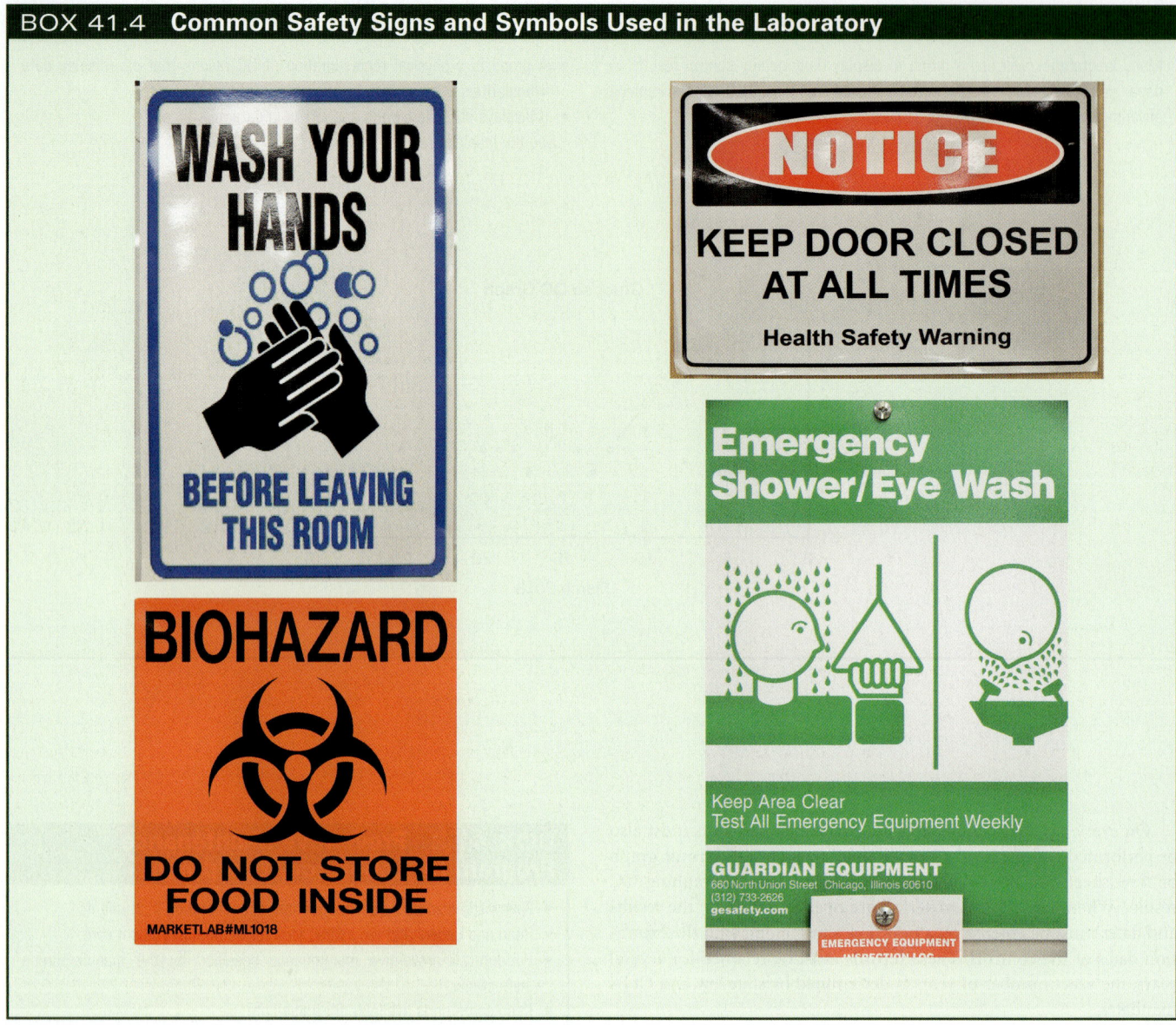

Safety Standards and Governing Agencies

The U.S. government created a system of safeguards and regulations under the Occupational Safety and Health Act of 1970. This system affects nearly every worker in the United States because the regulations apply to all businesses with one or more employees (the regulations are discussed in detail in Chapter 17). The Occupational Safety and Health Administration (OSHA) has mandated two programs intended to ensure the safety of personnel working in clinical laboratories. One covers occupational exposure to chemical hazards; the other covers exposure to bloodborne pathogens.

The CDC also established recommendations and resources in Standard Precautions and Transmission Precautions as they relate to specimen collection. (These recommendations were discussed in Chapter 28.)

Chemical Hazards

The clinical laboratory may have chemicals that are flammable, **caustic** (KAW stik), and/or potentially poisonous. Exposure to these dangerous chemicals can occur by breathing in fumes, direct absorption by contact with the skin, ingestion, direct contact with a mucous membrane, or entry through a cut, abrasion, or burn in the skin. OSHA is involved in regulating the standards directed at minimizing occupational exposure to hazardous chemicals in laboratories. OSHA's Hazard Communication Standard (HCS; known as the employee "right to know" rule) became law in 1991. It ensures that laboratory workers are made fully aware of the hazards associated with their workplace. The law requires the development of a comprehensive plan to put in place safe practices throughout the laboratory in regard to chemicals. All workers must be provided with information and training. A Safety Data Sheet (SDS) must also be on file for all chemicals used in the laboratory. SDS supply information about chemical safety and hazard information in case of an accident, spill, or fire, to the user or emergency personnel. OSHA requires the manufacturer of the chemical to make these sheets available, usually as a package insert or online

CHAPTER 41 Assisting in the Clinical Laboratory

> **BOX 41.5 Safety Data Sheet (SDS) Uniform Format**
>
> Since June 2015, OSHA has required all SDSs to use a uniform format that includes the following section numbers, headings, and information:
> Section 1. Identification
> Section 2. Hazard(s) identification
> Section 3. Composition/information on ingredients
> Section 4. First-aid measures
> Section 5. Fire-fighting measures
> Section 6. Accidental release measures
> Section 7. Handling and storage
> Section 8. Exposure controls/personal protection
> Section 9. Physical and chemical properties
> Section 10. Stability and reactivity
> Section 11. Toxicologic information
> Section 12. Ecologic information[a]
> Section 13. Disposal considerations[a]
> Section 14. Transport information[a]
> Section 15. Regulatory information[a]
> Section 16. Other information

[a]Sections 12 to 15 are regulated by agencies other than OSHA and are required of the manufacturers, not the employees.

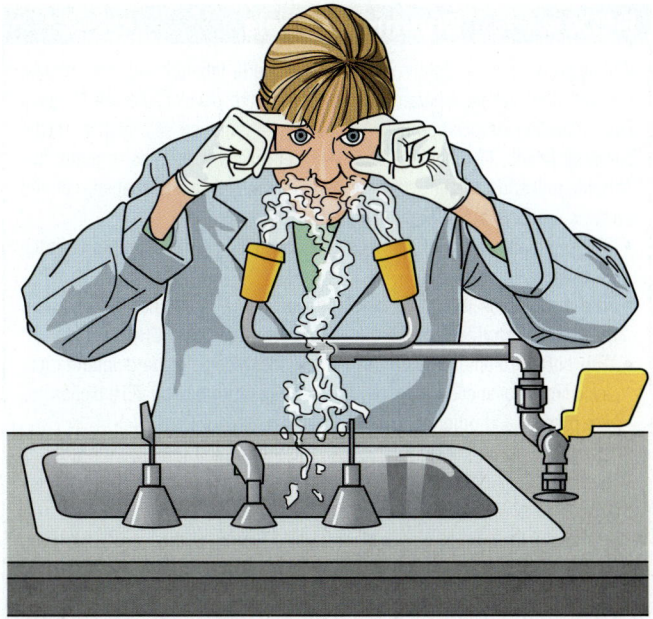

FIG. 41.5 Eyewash station. (From Proctor D, et al: *Kinn's The Medical Assistant*, ed 13, St. Louis, 2017, Elsevier.)

(Box 41.5). Employers must ensure that SDSs are readily accessible to employees.

In the POL, the most common hazardous chemicals are the following:
- Sodium *hypochlorite* (hahy puh KLAWR ahyt), commonly known as bleach, which is used for disinfecting laboratory work areas
- *Caviwipes* (KAH vee wahyps) and *glutaraldehyde* (gloo tuh RAL duh hahyd), which are disinfectants
- *Acetone* (AS i tohn) and dyes, which are used for staining slides

It should be noted that all of these disinfectants and dyes are available in premixed sprays or wipes to reduce chemical exposure during dilution.

Following principles of proper chemical handling reduces the risk of harmful effects. See Box 41.6 for additional information on chemical labels. The following are examples of proper chemical handling:
- If a chemical produces toxic or flammable vapors, work under a fume hood that exhausts air to the outside.
- In case of accidental exposure of the skin, rinse the affected area under running water for at least 5 minutes. Remove any contaminated clothing.
- If chemicals are splashed in the eyes, flush the eyes with water from an eyewash station (Fig. 41.5) for a minimum of 15 minutes. (See complete instructions on how to use an eyewash station in Procedure 41.2.)

Prompt medical attention must be given to victims of chemical exposure.

Biohazards and Infection Control

Biohazards, or biologic hazards, are materials or situations that present the possible risk of infection. Infection with biohazardous material can occur during specimen collection, handling, transportation, or testing. Specimens with the potential to be infectious include blood, body fluids, biologic specimens, **exudates** (EKS yoo deyts), bacterial cultures, and smears. Infection can be introduced into the body in many ways, including the following:
- Breathing in a pathogen
- Accidental inoculation by a needlestick or a **sharps** injury
- Aerosols created by uncapping specimen tubes
- Centrifuge accidents
- Entry of pathogens through a cut, abrasion, burn, or break in the skin

Standard Precautions. As described in Chapter 28, the CDC continuously monitors infection and disease in the United States. The CDC has also recommended preventive practices called **Standard Precautions**. These precautions apply to all patient care, regardless of the suspected or confirmed infection status of the patient. The precautions also apply to any setting where healthcare is delivered. The precautions are designed

> **VOCABULARY**
>
> **caustic:** Capable of burning, corroding, or damaging tissue by chemical action.
> **corrosive:** Causing or tending to cause the gradual destruction of a substance by chemical action.
> **exudates:** Fluids with high concentrations of protein and cellular debris that have escaped from the blood vessels and have been deposited in tissues or on tissue surfaces.
> **sharps:** Medical term for devices with sharp points or edges that can puncture or cut skin. Examples include needles, scalpels, or broken glass.
> **Standard Precautions:** A set of infection control practices used to prevent the transmission of diseases that can be acquired by contact with blood, body fluids, nonintact skin, and mucous membranes.

> **CRITICAL THINKING 41.5**
>
> Greg has a few hours to review WMFM's current laboratory safety policies and procedures on his own. There are policies that apply to the laboratory only, but there are also many policies that apply to the entire facility. Why is it so important for employees to be aware of safety policies and procedures? Write down five reasons for being safety aware in the laboratory, and be ready to discuss your thoughts with the class.

BOX 41.6 Chemical Labels

Chemicals should be tightly sealed and properly labeled with the original manufacturer's labels. A hazard identification system, developed by the National Fire Protection Association (NFPA), provides information at a glance on the potential health, flammability, and chemical reactivity hazards of materials. This identification system consists of four small, diamond-shaped, colored symbols grouped into a larger diamond shape.

- The top diamond is red and indicates flammability (the potential to catch on fire).
- The diamond on the left is blue and indicates a health hazard such as a dangerous **inhalant** (in HEY luh nt) or **corrosive** (kuh ROH siv) acid.
- The bottom diamond is white and provides special hazard information, including recommended **personal protective equipment** (PPE) if biohazards are present and other dangerous situations.
- The diamond on the right is yellow and indicates a reactivity or stability hazard. An example of reactivity is mixing an acid (e.g., bleach) with a base (e.g., ammonia), creating a dangerous gas.

The four-color system also indicates the severity of the hazard by using numbers imprinted in the diamonds from 0 to 4, with 0 representing no hazard and 4 representing an extremely hazardous substance (Fig. 41.6).

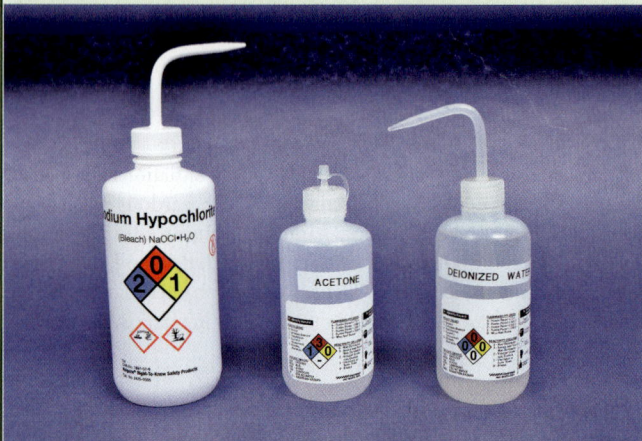

FIG. 41.6 Laboratory bottles with chemical labels. (From Proctor D, et al: *Kinn's The Medical Assistant*, ed 13, St. Louis, 2017, Elsevier.)

VOCABULARY
donning: Putting on.
inhalant: Any substance that can be breathed into the lungs.
personal protective equipment: Clothing, eye protection, gloves, or other garments or equipment designed to protect the wearer's body from injury or infection.

PROCEDURE 41.2 Use of the Eyewash Equipment: Perform an Emergency Eyewash

Task
Minimize the risk of occupational exposure to pathogens if body fluids contact the eyes.

Equipment and Supplies
- Plumbed or self-contained eyewash unit
- Gloves

Procedural Steps
1. Wash hands or use hand sanitizer. Remove contact lenses or glasses. Put on gloves.
   Purpose: To ensure flushing of all material in the eyes.
2. Following the manufacturer's directions, turn on the eyewash unit. If it is a plumbed unit, the control valve should remain on until the unit is manually shut off.
   Purpose: The unit must be plumbed so that it can remain on until manually turned off.
3. Hold the eyelids open with the thumb and index finger to ensure adequate rinsing of the entire eye and eyelid surface (Fig. 1).
   Purpose: The normal reflex is to close the eyes tightly, which prevents removal of all of the contaminated material.

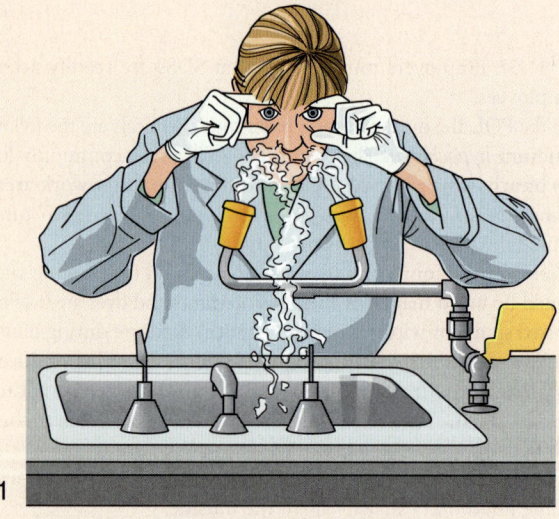

1

4. Avoid aiming the water stream directly onto the eyeball.
   Purpose: A direct water stream may cause discomfort or damage the eye.
5. Flush the eyes and eyelids for a minimum of 15 minutes, rolling the eyes periodically to ensure complete removal of the foreign material.
   Purpose: To completely remove the potentially dangerous substance from the eyes.
6. Properly remove gloves, dispose of them in a labeled biohazard waste container, and wash your hands or use hand sanitizer.
   Purpose: To prevent cross-contamination.
7. After completion of the eyewash, complete the postexposure follow-up procedures.
   Purpose: Depending on the type of exposure, the facility's policies may include provider completion of an exposure incident form and provider follow-up.

---

both to protect the healthcare provider and to prevent the healthcare provider from spreading infections among patients (Box 41.7).

According to the CDC, handwashing is the single most effective means of preventing infection. It is also the single most effective way to prevent the spread of infections. Proper hand sanitation protects you, your patient, and your coworkers because it removes or kills potentially pathogenic organisms from the skin surface. In the laboratory, it is essential to wash your hands with soap and water (Fig. 41.7) or use hand sanitizer in the following situations:

- When entering the laboratory or before leaving the laboratory
- Before **donning** gloves and after removing gloves

BOX 41.7 Standard Precautions

Standard Precautions include the following five elements:
- Hand hygiene
- Use of PPE (e.g., gloves, gowns, masks, eye protection)
- Safe needle practices
- Safe handling of potentially contaminated equipment or surfaces in the patient environment
- Respiratory hygiene/cough etiquette.

BOX 41.8 What Is Ebola?

In 2014 Ebola infections reappeared in Africa and were transmitted to several other continents. The Ebola virus is a bloodborne pathogen that causes bleeding throughout the body. In the United States, a key factor in stopping its spread was the rigorous training in donning and removing PPE that covered almost all parts of the healthcare worker's body. The CDC provided an Ebola bulletin for ambulatory healthcare practices on the evaluation of patients who may have been infected with the Ebola virus.

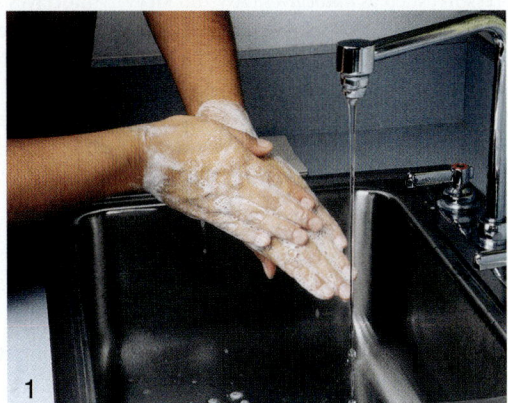

FIG. 41.7 Handwashing. (From Proctor D, et al: *Kinn's The Medical Assistant*, ed 13, St. Louis, 2017, Elsevier.)

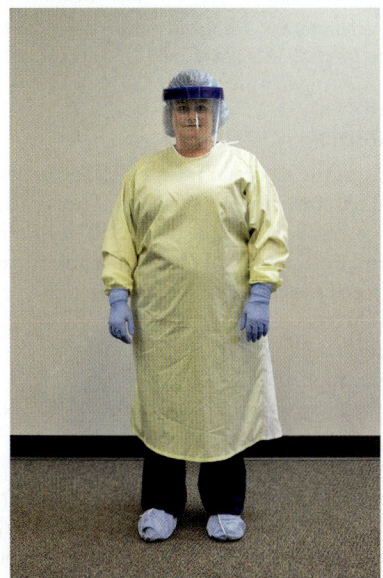

FIG. 41.8 Personal protective equipment (PPE). (From Proctor D, et al: *Kinn's The Medical Assistant*, ed 13, St. Louis, 2017, Elsevier.)

- After contact with body fluid
- Before and after eating
- Before and after using the restroom

After bloodborne pathogens were identified in the 1970s and 1980s, the CDC stepped up its infection control recommendations. The CDC acknowledged that all blood in all patients is potentially infectious. Therefore they required additional monitoring and regulation for the safety of both healthcare providers and patients. These guidelines became known as *Universal Precautions*. Regulation of the new law, referred to as the Bloodborne Pathogens Standard (BBPS), was delegated to OSHA (see Chapter 17 for additional information).

Bloodborne Pathogens Standard. OSHA's Bloodborne Pathogens Standard has been law since 1992. It regulates the handling of blood and blood products, but it also includes *other potentially infectious materials (OPIM)* that may contain bloodborne pathogens. Urine is the only fluid not specifically included in the standard. However, because blood and blood elements are frequently associated with urine, it must be included and considered a possible source of exposure.

The Bloodborne Pathogens Standard covers all employees who could "reasonably anticipate contact with blood and other potentially infectious materials as the result of performing their job duties." Hepatitis B virus (HBV), hepatitis C virus (HCV), and human immunodeficiency virus (HIV) are constant hazards to clinical laboratory personnel. *Ebola* (ee BOH luh) virus infections are very serious, although not common in the United States (Box 41.8). Bloodborne pathogens are transmitted through exposure to blood and body fluids, which are the primary substances handled in the laboratory. The Bloodborne Pathogens Standard requires that the laboratory employer have a written exposure control plan that proves the following steps have been taken to protect employees:

- Written job categories of employees at risk of exposure to blood (laboratory workers are considered "high risk")
- HBV vaccination guidelines and records for each employee at risk
- Record of initial and annual Universal Precautions training for bloodborne pathogens and safety training for each employee (including proper use of safety needles)
- Definition and listing of safe work practices: personal protective equipment (PPE) for all lab personnel (fluid-impermeable lab coats that do not leave the laboratory area, gloves, face protection [Fig. 41.8] and labeling of biohazardous sharps and waste containers and their proper disposal)
- Sharps injury log of all work-related needlesticks and exposures to blood, with medical intervention after exposure incidents
- Written plan to maintain the privacy of the individual exposed to blood
- Documentation of employee input on new safety devices

Safety Guidelines for Other Potentially Infectious Materials. The following guidelines are required for handling OPIM:

- Handle and process all specimens as if they contained infectious material.
- Wipe the outside of specimen containers with a germicide.
- Dispose of all infectious materials according to state and federal guidelines.
- Clean up spills using a disinfectant (see Chapter 28).
- Immediately dispose of any chipped or broken glassware into a sharps container using appropriate safety methods to prevent accidental punctures.

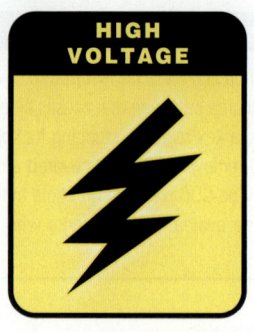 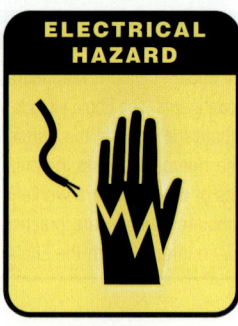

FIG. 41.9 High-voltage and electrical hazard labels. (From Proctor D, et al: *Kinn's The Medical Assistant*, ed 13, St. Louis, 2017, Elsevier.)

Physical Hazards

Physical hazards in the laboratory can be classified as electrical, fire, and mechanical hazards. Electric shock is a threat when any electrical equipment is in use. It is imperative to keep all electrical equipment in proper repair and to always to follow manufacturers' instructions.

Use these procedures for electrical hazards:
- Use surge protectors.
- Inspect all cords and plugs frequently.
- Never use extension cords.
- Do not overload circuits.

Unplug the electrical device before servicing, and never operate electrical instruments with wet hands. If a sink is nearby, make sure electrical cords do not come in contact with the water supply. Signs and labels should be placed on specific electrical hazards (Fig. 41.9).

Open flames are rarely used in a laboratory anymore, but the potential for fire still exists. Fires may be ignited by smoking, heating elements, and sparks from electrical connections. Flammable materials should not be stored near any source of ignition. All laboratory personnel should be familiar with the locations of fire extinguishers (ek STING gwi shers) and fire safety blankets. Fire extinguishers should be the carbon dioxide (CO_2), dry chemical, or *halon* (HAY lohn) type, known as the ABC type of extinguisher. ABC extinguishers can be used on all types of fires. Extinguishers should be inspected regularly by a licensed inspector and replaced or recharged if used. The medical assistant may be responsible for maintaining records on the care and maintenance of fire extinguishers (Procedure 41.3).

Fire safety blankets can be used to smother flames on burning clothing. However, a victim should not be wrapped in a fire blanket, because this may intensify burns. Instead, the flames should be patted out or the victim directed to stop, drop, and roll on the blanket.

Emergency phone numbers should be posted on the wall near the telephone, and all personnel should know the locations of fire alarms, the fire escape routes, and procedures to follow if exits are blocked. Periodic fire drills should be conducted, and hallways and exits should be kept free of clutter.

Mechanical hazards arise from the use of laboratory equipment. Care should be exercised when using equipment with moving parts, such as *centrifuges* (SEN truh fyooj es). Centrifuges, devices that separate liquids from solids, present a hazard not only from moving parts but also from glassware that might break during centrifugation and from aerosols that might be created if tubes are not capped tightly.

Care should also be exercised when using pieces of equipment that rely on pressure, such as *autoclaves* (AW tuh kleyv). Autoclaves are used to sterilize metal instruments, microbiologic media, and some microbiologic waste. Autoclaves present a danger if opened prematurely, before the pressure has come down to a safe level.

Although centrifuges and autoclaves often have built-in safeguards, such as locks that prevent entry until the environment is safe, improper care of the equipment can cause the safety measures to fail.

SPECIMEN COLLECTION, PROCESSING, AND STORAGE

Laboratory Requisitions and Reports

When the provider orders laboratory testing, an electronic or paper requisition must be generated. Patient information on the requisitions must be complete, accurate, and legible. The patient is then directed to the POL, or the specimen is collected, prepared, and sent to an outside laboratory.

Fig. 41.10 shows the electronic lab requisition form used in *SimChart for the Medical Office*. The following information typically is required on the requisition when specimens are sent to a reference laboratory:
- Provider's name, account number, address, and phone number
- Patient's full name, age, date of birth, sex, address, and insurance information
- Source of specimen
- Date and time of collection, and initials of the person collecting the specimen
- Specific test (or tests) requested
- Medications the patient is taking
- Whether the patient fasted or followed dietary restrictions if required; time of last intake
- Possible diagnosis
- Indication of whether the test is to be performed STAT (STAH t)

> **VOCABULARY**
> **STAT:** The medical abbreviation for the Latin term *statum*, meaning immediately; at this moment.

PROCEDURE 41.3 Evaluate the Laboratory Environment

Tasks
Evaluate the laboratory environment and identify unsafe working conditions. Identify compliance with safety signs, symbols, and labels.

Equipment and Supplies
Laboratory environment evaluation form
Pen

Procedural Steps
Observe use of safety signs, symbols, and labels in the laboratory setting. Document your findings on the work environment evaluation form.

Purpose: Safety signs, symbols, and labels must be used in the laboratory setting.
Explain if the laboratory personnel are complying with the safety signs, symbols, and labels.
Observe the environment for safety risks. Document your findings.
Purpose: Identifying and correcting safety risks is important in the workplace environment.
Based on your observations, summarize your findings. If risks are present, create a list of issues that need to be addressed. Describe what needs to be done for each risk.

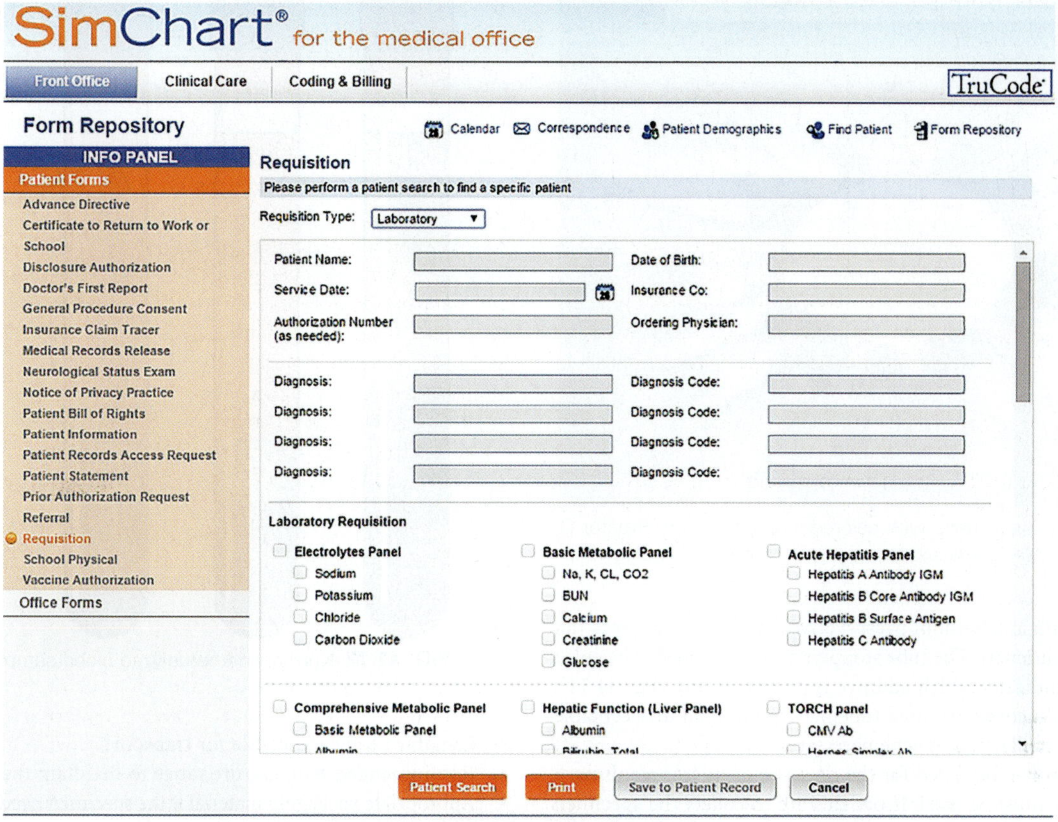

FIG. 41.10 Electronic laboratory requisition form.

When the results of the tests are obtained, a laboratory report is sent to the office. The laboratory reports can be distributed as follows:
- Sent directly from the referral laboratory to the patient's electronic health record (EHR)
- Sent electronically to the facility and then uploaded by staff to the EHR or printed out in order to be included in the paper medical record

A medical assistant is frequently responsible for making sure that all outside laboratory reports have been received and given to the provider for review. Testing results cannot be given to a patient until the provider has reviewed them. Any testing that is completed outside the POL at a reference lab must be tracked. This can be done by maintaining a master laboratory specimen log sheet or electronic file, which can be used to track patient specimens, tests ordered, designated lab, results, and provider response.

> **BOX 41.9 Tips for Labeling a Patient Specimen and Sample Container**
>
> When labeling a sample container, make sure you only use a black waterproof marker or pen, *never* pencil. All labels should include the following information, at a minimum:
> - Patient's name, surname, first, then middle initial
> - Identification number
> - Date (MM/DD/YYYY) and time of collection
> - Phlebotomist or collector's initials
>
> If affixing a computer-generated label, make sure to write the time and initial the specimen after the venipuncture has been completed.

Specimen Collection

The medical assistant is responsible for the collection of many different types of specimens. It is important to recognize that laboratory results are only as good as the specimen collected. The importance of proper specimen collection cannot be overemphasized. To ensure that test results are accurate indicators of the patient's state of health, it is critical that proper specimen collection is understood and followed exactly. The most common specimens are blood, urine, and swab samples collected from wounds or mucous membranes. Specimens that may be collected less frequently include feces, gastric contents, cerebrospinal fluid (CSF), tissue samples, semen, and *aspirates* (AS puh reyts).

Verifying the patient's identity before the specimen collection is a critical step in the collection process. Patient identification should follow the written procedure for your institution. Using a minimum of two patient *identifiers* (ahy DEN tuh fahy ehrs) before specimen collection is standard. If the patient is not identified properly, the laboratory results that are generated will be useless. See Box 41.9 for tips on labeling.

Another important step in specimen collection is the proper choice of a collection container. For example, blood may be collected using a vacuum tube system. Blood collection tubes are available in a variety of sizes, depending on the collection needs. Blood collection tubes are

> **VOCABULARY**
> **aspirate:** To withdraw fluid using suction, such as occurs, for example, when a specimen has been removed from the body using a needle and syringe.
> **identifiers:** Information unique to an individual. Common identifiers used for patient identification such as full name including middle initial, date of birth, medical identification number, or patient address.

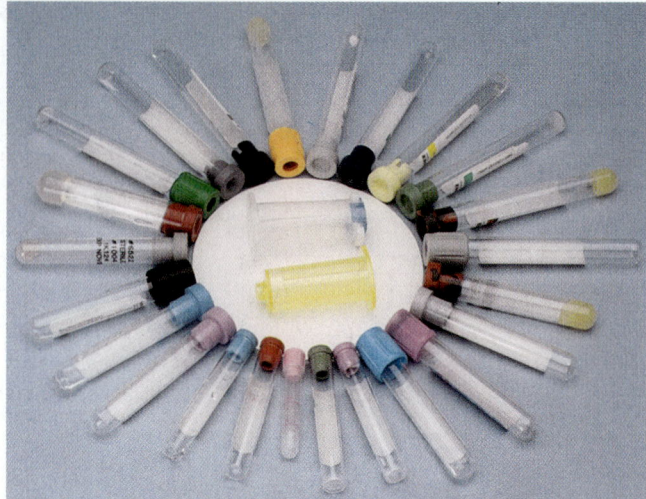

FIG. 41.11 Vacutainer tubes with colored stoppers. (From Proctor D, et al: *Kinn's The Medical Assistant*, ed 13, St. Louis, 2017, Elsevier.)

also available with and without **preservatives** and **anticoagulants** (an tee koh AG yuh luh nts). The tube stoppers are color coded. The color of the stopper indicates which additive is present, if any (Fig. 41.11). Collection in an incorrect colored tube may result in an unacceptable specimen, and recollection may be necessary.

If a specimen will be tested for the presence of microorganisms, a sterile container must be used. If patients are to collect the specimen at home, they should be provided with the appropriate container and complete instructions for collection. Patient education is an important role for the medical assistant. Each patient should receive clear instructions for proper home collection. Make sure your patients listen to the directions and ask them to repeat instructions back to you, so you know they understand the information. Remember to be sensitive to individual patient factors (e.g., hearing, sight, primary language, cognitive capacity). These can affect the patient's understanding of the instructions, as well as his or her ability to follow through. Giving patients written directions to take home can also be helpful and reassuring.

> **CRITICAL THINKING 41.6**
>
> As Greg has been working in phlebotomy, he has been reminded of the importance of patient identification. Write down three reasons why patient identification is critical to laboratory specimens. Be ready to share your reasons with the class.

The medical assistant should always check the laboratory's specimen requirements manual or reference laboratory website for any unfamiliar tests. A clear understanding of the specimen and collection requirements is very important. Any unanswered questions should be resolved by calling the reference laboratory before collecting the specimen. The container must be labeled properly at the time of collection. Unlabeled containers are not acceptable for laboratory testing and must be rejected. Labels should include the patient's full name, the date and time of collection, initials of the person collecting the specimen, and the specimen type.

Most offices have a laboratory courier service that picks up specimens periodically throughout the day. Specimens should be properly stored (some may require refrigeration) until the courier arrives. Instructions for properly obtaining, processing, and preparing a specimen for transport are usually supplied by the testing laboratory. If the instructions are not clear, or if you have a question about a particular test collection, the reference laboratory should answer the question over the phone. An understanding of the following criteria is necessary for the safe shipment of specimens:

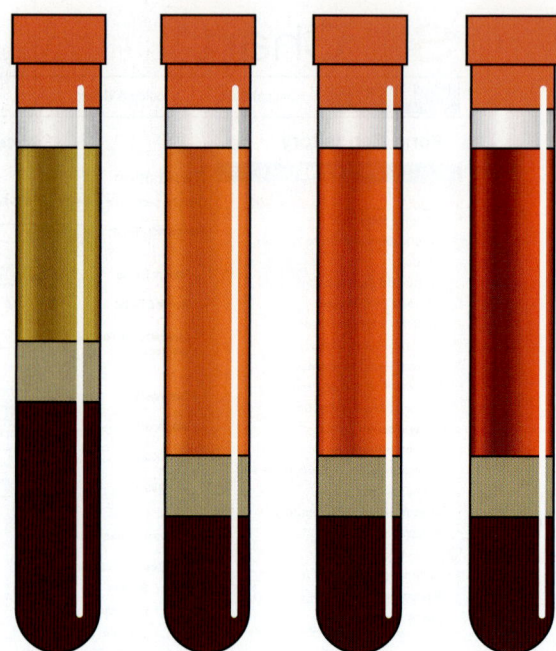

FIG. 41.12 Normal and hemolyzed blood sample graphic.

- Length of time acceptable for transport
- Recommended temperature range to maintain the specimen
- Appropriate packaging material if the specimen needs to be protected from light

If the specimen is to be mailed, it must be carefully packaged to prevent breakage, damage, or contamination (kuhn tam uh NEY shuh n) during handling. Follow the instructions for transport supplied by the reference laboratory. Do not ship specimens without proper packaging and labeling as specified by the test laboratory.

Preventing Contamination. Medical assistants must take care to prevent contamination of specimens and themselves. Expiration dates on swabs, tubes, transport media, and other collection containers should be checked before the items are used. Any expired materials should not be used and should be properly discarded. An improperly handled specimen may become contaminated or may contaminate the surrounding environment. Standard Precautions should be followed. All blood and body fluids from all patients should be considered infectious.

The specimen collected must be a true representative sample. A swab for a wound culture collected from the surface of the wound generally does not yield the same results as one taken from the depths of the wound. A **hemolyzed** (HEE muh lahyz d) blood specimen shows marked differences in many tests (Fig. 41.12). If a large volume of specimen is collected (e.g., a 24-hour urine specimen), the total volume or weight must be carefully measured and recorded. The specimen must be well mixed before an **aliquot** (AL i kwuh t) is removed and submitted for testing.

> **VOCABULARY**
> **aliquot:** A portion of a well-mixed sample removed for testing.
> **anticoagulants:** Substances (i.e., medications or chemicals) that prevent clotting of blood.
> **forensic:** Concerning the use of scientific tests or techniques regarding the detection of a crime.
> **hemolyzed:** Refers to a blood sample in which the red blood cells have ruptured.
> **preservatives:** Substances added to a specimen to prevent the deterioration of cells or chemicals.

Handling, Processing, and Storing Specimens

Specimens must be handled, processed, and stored according to the test manufacturer's guidelines to prevent any changes that would affect test results. In Chapters 42 through 45, specimen handling, processing, and storage will be discussed for each specific area of the laboratory. Each department in the lab has unique types of testing and specimen requirements. Some general guidelines to keep in mind include the following:

- The storage temperature of the specimen should follow the manufacturer's testing requirements.
- Serum must be separated from red blood cells as soon as possible after the specimen has clotted to prevent changes caused by the metabolism of the blood cells.
- Specimens for chemistry and liver panels may need to be protected from light.
- Specimens may need to be frozen to prevent chemical constituents (kuh n STICH oo oh nts) from changing. Follow manufacturer's guidelines for freezing specimens.
- The manufacturer's package inserts or reference laboratory specimen requirements should be consulted to ensure that each specimen is handled and processed properly.

Chain of Custody. When a specimen may be needed as evidence in a court case, certain procedures must be followed when collecting and handling the specimen. Forensic (fuh REN sik) or legal specimens should be collected, handled, and stored in a way that will allow them to be acknowledged in a court of law. Specimen processing must be documented precisely, ensuring that no tampering with evidence has occurred. *Chain of custody* refers to the stepwise method used to collect, process, and test a specimen. The documentation must be signed by every person who has any contact with the specimen, from collection to the final reporting of results. Blood alcohol level testing and drug screening often require chain of custody handling. Everything needed to collect the specimen is provided in a kit—the gloves, the vacuum tube, and the needle used to collect the blood specimen. Documentation is included and must be signed by all personnel. Medical assistants and phlebotomists can be subpoenaed (suh PEE nuhd) to testify in court about specimens they have collected. It is always in your best interest to follow chain of custody procedures exactly.

> ### CRITICAL THINKING 41.7
> What is the difference between a patient specimen and a forensic specimen? In your own words, describe *chain of custody*.

LABORATORY MATHEMATICS AND MEASUREMENT

All laboratory testing relies on the accurate use of values, units, and measurements. For example, values are used to report the time the sample was collected, the volume of the specimen, the amount of analyte found in a specimen, and dilutions used in sample preparation, and to record QC results.

Measuring Time

Time of day is a critical factor in patient care. Medications must be administered, diets must be followed, and specimens must be collected on a timed schedule. Many laboratories use the 24-hour clock when recording time; this method avoids the confusion that comes with the *Greenwich clock*, which uses a.m. (morning) and p.m. (afternoon) designations.

The 24-hour clock system, also known as *military time*, is expressed with four digits in terms of "hundred hours." Noon is referred to as 1200 (twelve hundred) hours; midnight is 0000 (zero hundred), or 2400 hours. The military clock is based on 24 60-minute hours, as is the Greenwich clock; therefore 5:35 p.m. is expressed as 1735 (seventeen thirty-five) hours (Table 41.5).

> ### CRITICAL THINKING 41.8
> If the time on the clock is 10:00 a.m., how would you write it in military time? If the time is 10:00 p.m., how would you write it in military time? If the time on a document were written as 1900 hours, how would you write it in Greenwich time? What if it were written as 0800 hours?

Measuring Temperature

Two scales are currently used for measuring temperature; each is divided into units called *degrees* (Table 41.6). The *Fahrenheit* (FAHR uhn hahyt) scale is considered part of the *English system* of measurement and is the scale most commonly used in the United States. The *Celsius* (SEL see uh s) *scale*, formerly called the centigrade scale, is used in countries that apply the *metric* (MEH trik) *system*. On the Celsius (C) scale, water freezes at 0°C and boils at 100°F. On the Fahrenheit (F) scale, water freezes at 32°F and boils at 212°F. Almost all laboratories in the United States use the Celsius scale for temperature. See Box 41.10 for examples of Fahrenheit and Celsius temperature conversions.

TABLE 41.5 Greenwich Time and Military Time

Greenwich Time	Military Time
1:00 a.m.	0100 hours
3:00 a.m.	0300 hours
5:00 a.m.	0500 hours
7:00 a.m.	0700 hours
9:00 a.m.	0900 hours
11:00 a.m.	1100 hours
1:00 p.m.	1300 hours
3:00 p.m.	1500 hours
5:00 p.m.	1700 hours
7:00 p.m.	1900 hours
9:00 p.m.	2100 hours
11:00 p.m.	2300 hours
12:00 a.m. (midnight)	2400 hours

> ### BOX 41.10 Converting Temperatures
>
> **To change from Fahrenheit to Celsius:**
>
> 98.6°F = _____ °C Solution
> Step 1: Subtract 32 from F temp   98.6 − 32 = 66.6
> Step 2: Divide number by 1.8   66.6/1.8 = 37°C
>
> **To change from Celsius to Fahrenheit:**
>
> 100°C = _____ °F Solution
> Step 1: Multiply C temp by 1.8   100 × 1.8 = 180
> Step 2: Add 32 to that number   180 + 32 = 212°F

TABLE 41.6 Common Laboratory Temperature Settings

	Fahrenheit	Celsius
Refrigerator	35°–46°	2°–8°
Freezer	32°	0°
Room	59°–86°	15°–30°
Incubator	98.6°	37°
Body temperature	98.6°	37°
Autoclave	254°	121°

Units of Measurement

The units of measurement that we commonly use in the United States differ from those used in the laboratory. In everyday life, we use the English system of measurement:
- Weight is measured in ounces and pounds
- Length is measured in inches and feet
- Volume is measured in cups and quarts

In the laboratory, the metric system and the Système International (SI) are used. It is important that medical assistants memorize and practice these systems so that they can communicate professionally (Table 41.7).

The metric system is based on a decimal system, which consists of basic units and prefixes that indicate a system of division in multiples of 10. Prefixes are added to each symbol to reduce or enlarge them by units of 10. See Tables 41.8 and 41.9 for an overview of the metric system measurements.

International organizations, such as the World Health Organization (WHO), officially recognize SI units. Many countries have adopted this system, but the United States has not completely converted to it. The SI is an adaptation of the metric system that uses several of the basic units, although some units are different for reporting results. For example, blood glucose is reported in *millimoles* (MIL uh mohls) per liter (mmol/L) using the SI system, but it is reported as mg/dL using the metric system. Therefore it is very important for the medical assistant to double-check the laboratory's standard and include the appropriate units of measurement when reporting test values.

> **CRITICAL THINKING 41.9**
>
> If you have 3.2 g of salt and you want to express it in milligrams, how will you write it? If the length of an item is 455 cm and you want to express it in meters, how will you write it?

Measuring Liquid Volume

Test tubes are used to test or hold liquid reagents, samples, or aliquots. Test tubes come in many sizes and are typically disposable. Test tubes may be sterile for use in microbiology. When liquids are measured into test tubes, the most common piece of glassware used is the **pipet** (pahy PET). A pipet is a hollow tube that can be made from glass or plastic. Pipets often have lines to indicate volume on the length of the tube. Some plastic pipets have a built-in bulb to help transfer fluids and are known as transfer pipets. This type of pipet usually does not have any measurement lines on the tube. Fig. 41.13 shows a variety of transfer pipets that are used in the laboratory. *Micropipets* (MAHY kroh pahy pets) are used to deliver very small volumes of liquid (Fig. 41.14). These pipetting devices must be fitted with an appropriate disposable tip. The device is equipped with a piston at the top, which must be depressed before the pipet is filled and when the pipet is drained. It is important to follow the manufacturer's instructions for use with all pipets and micropipets. Each type of pipet may be slightly different.

TABLE 41.7 Comparing the English System of Measurement With the Metric System

	English System of Measurement	Metric System
Weight	Ounces (oz) and pounds (lb)	Grams (g)
Length	Inches and feet	Meters (m)
Volume	Cups and quarts	Liters (L)

TABLE 41.8 Metric System: Prefixes of Measurements

Prefixes	Size	Or Another Way to Look At It	
Kilo (k)	1000 base units	1 kilo = 1000 base units	Larger than the base unit
Hecto	100 base units	1 hecto = 100 base units	
Deka	10 base units	1 deka = 10 base units	
Base Units (Meter, Liter, or Gram)			
Deci	0.1 unit	10 deci = 1 base unit	Smaller than the base unit
Centi (c)	0.01 unit	100 centi = 1 base unit	
Milli (m)	0.001	1000 milli = 1 base unit	
Micro (mc)	0.000001	1,000,000 micro = 1 base unit	

TABLE 41.9 Common Units of Measure Seen in Healthcare

Volume	Length	Weight
Liter (L)	Meter (m)	Gram (g)
Milliliter (mL or ml)	Centimeter (cm)	Kilogram (kg)
Cubic centimeter (cc)	Millimeter (mm)	Milligram (mg)
cc = mL		Microgram (mcg)

> **VOCABULARY**
>
> **pipet:** A slender tube attached to or including a bulb, for transferring or measuring small amounts of a liquid, often used in a laboratory.

LABORATORY EQUIPMENT

Microscope

Nearly every medical laboratory is equipped with a *microscope* (MAHY kruh skohp). This indispensable instrument is used to view objects too small to be seen with the naked eye (Fig. 41.15). The microscope is used to evaluate stained blood smears, urine sediment, vaginal secretions, and smears made from body fluids and microorganisms.

Microscopic procedures are not considered CLIA-waived because they require judgment and additional training. In addition, an error

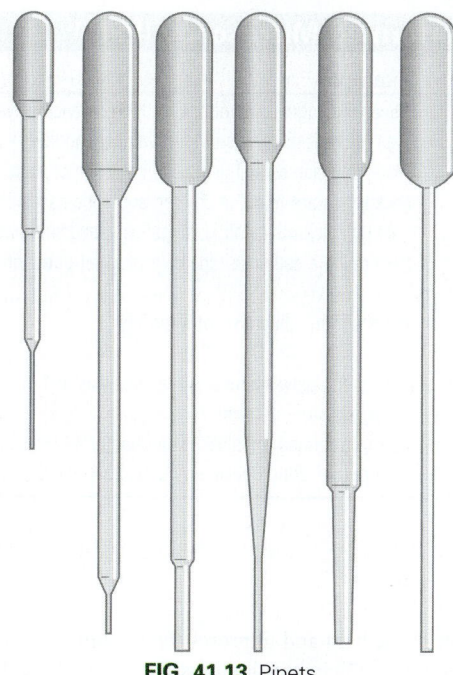

FIG. 41.13 Pipets.

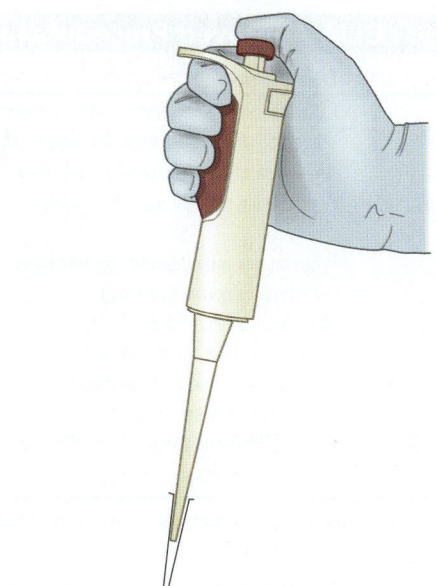

FIG. 41.14 Micropipet with disposable tips. (From Proctor D, et al: *Kinn's The Medical Assistant*, ed 13, St. Louis, 2017, Elsevier.)

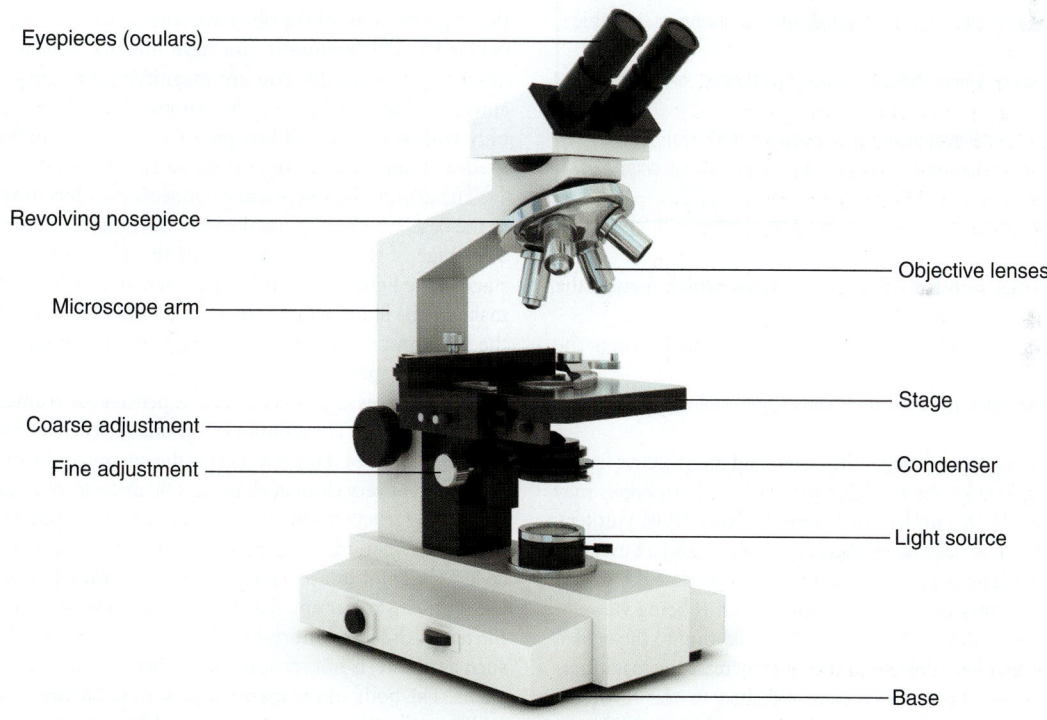

FIG. 41.15 The microscope. (Courtesy urfinguss/iStock/Thinkstock.)

in reading microscopic tests may have a detrimental effect on the patient's care. Providers petitioned the CMS to create a new laboratory category that would allow them to perform a set of simple microscopic tests in the ambulatory setting (Table 41.10). CMS approved the list and created an additional CLIA category called *provider-performed microscopy procedures (PPMP)*. Certified CLIA-PPMP laboratories must meet the same quality standards as laboratories that perform moderate-complexity tests, including passing three proficiency tests from an outside agency per year. The medical assistant is taught how to prepare the microscope slide and bring it into focus. See Box 41.11 for information on who can read a microscope slide.

Microscopes have three components:

TABLE 41.10 CLIA-Approved Procedures for Provider-Performed Microscopy (PPM)

Test Name	Description	Example
Direct wet mount	Examination of specimens for the presence or absence of bacteria, fungi, parasites, and human cellular elements	Observing vaginal secretions for the presence of yeast to assist with diagnosis of vulvovaginal candidiasis
KOH preparation	Any preparation using potassium hydroxide	Observing skin scrapings for the presence of fungi
Fecal leukocyte examination	Simple stain of fecal specimen; assists in diagnosis of diarrheal disease	Leukocytes are found in stool in antibiotic-associated colitis, ulcerative colitis, shigellosis, and salmonellosis
Pinworm examination	Preparations are observed for the presence or absence of *Enterobius vermicularis* eggs	Performing a cellulose tape collection for pinworms
Postcoital direct, qualitative examinations	Vaginal or cervical mucus is examined 4–10 hours after intercourse for the presence of live, motile sperm	Assists in the diagnosis of infertility
Qualitative semen analysis	Semen is examined for the presence or absence of spermatozoa; motility of the sperm is noted	Assists in postvasectomy semen analysis and in the diagnosis of infertility
Urine sediment examination	Urine sediment is examined for the presence or absence of formed elements	Part of a routine urinalysis (see Chapter 42, Procedure 42.6, Prepare a Urine Specimen for Microscopic Examination).

CLIA, Clinical Laboratory Improvement Amendments; *KOH*, potassium hydroxide.

BOX 41.11 Who Can Read a Microscope Slide?

The final analysis of a microscope slide must be made by one of the following personnel:
- Physician (medical doctor, doctor of osteopathy, or doctor of podiatric medicine)
- Midlevel practitioner (nurse midwife, nurse practitioner, or physician's assistant)
- Dentist (doctor of dental surgery or doctor of dental medicine)
- Trained laboratory professional with CLIA moderate- or high-complexity training

---

- *Magnification* (mag nuh fi KAY shuh n) system, which focuses the image
- *Illumination* (ih loo muh NEY shuh n) system, which brings the image from the slide to the viewer
- Framework, which includes all components responsible for positioning the slide

The magnification system includes the ocular and the objective lenses, plus the fine and coarse knobs to adjust the clarity. Microscopes may be *monocular* (muh NOK yuh ler) or *binocular* (bahy NOK yuh ler). A monocular microscope has one eyepiece for viewing, and a binocular microscope has two. The eyepiece, or ocular, is located at the top of the microscope and contains a lens to magnify what is being viewed.

The usual magnification is 10 times (10×). In addition to the ocular, compound microscopes have objective lenses that increase the magnification of the specimen. The objectives are attached to the revolving nosepiece. Most microscopes have four objectives, each with a different magnifying power:
- The shortest objective has the lowest power (4×) and is called the *scanning lens*. This lens is used to scan the field of interest and then focus on a particular object.
- Greater detail is observed with the next longest objective, which is low power (10×).
- The high or high dry objective usually has a magnification of 40× or 45×.
- The longest objective, oil immersion (100×), allows the finest focusing of the object and requires the use of a special oil that is placed directly on the slide. This special oil, called *immersion oil*, prevents refraction of the light and improves the resolution (clarity) of the magnified image. Oil immersion is used to view cells and extremely small materials (e.g., bacteria and platelets) and to examine stained specimens.

The total magnification of the specimen is determined by multiplying the magnification of the objective lens by 10 (the magnification of the ocular lens). Therefore if you have the 10× objective in place when observing blood cells, you are magnifying the image 100 times. Just above the base are the focusing knobs. The coarse adjustment is used only with scanning and low-power lenses, and the fine adjustment is used with high-power and oil immersion lenses.

The arm of the microscope connects the objectives and the oculars to the base, which supports the microscope and contains its light source. The stage of the microscope holds the slide to be viewed. Under the stage is the light source, the condenser, and the iris diaphragm, which make up the illumination system. The condenser directs light up through the slide, and the iris diaphragm regulates the amount of light passing through the specimen.

Microscopes are precise and expensive instruments that require careful handling. The amount of routine maintenance required depends on the amount of daily use. Dirt is the enemy of the microscope, which must be kept very clean at all times. Oil, makeup, dust, and eye secretions can all obstruct vision through the lens and may transmit infective organisms. The microscope should always be stored in a plastic dust cover when not in use. Lenses should be cleaned before and after each use with lens paper and lens cleaner. Any other type of tissue scratches the lenses or leaves lint residue behind. Routine use of solvent cleaners, such as xylene, is not recommended, because these cleaners may loosen a lens. The body of the microscope should be dusted with a soft cloth.

The microscope should be placed in a permanent location in the laboratory, on a sturdy table in an area where it cannot be bumped. If a microscope must be moved, it should be carried securely, with one hand supporting the base and the other holding the arm. When the microscope is stored, it should be left covered and with the low-power objective in the highest position. The stage should be centered.

Using a microscope involves focusing and illumination (Procedure 41.4). The image is focused by moving the objectives closer to the specimen using the fine and coarse knobs. Proper focusing begins with the objective at lowest power. The coarse adjustment moves the objective quickly. This knob is used first to bring the specimen into approximate focus. The fine adjustment focus knob then brings the specimen into

PROCEDURE 41.4 Perform Routine Maintenance on Clinical Equipment (Microscope)

Task
Focus the microscope properly by using a prepared slide under low power, high power, and oil immersion, then perform routine maintenance on the microscope before storing it.

Equipment and Supplies
- Microscope
- Lens cleaner
- Lens tissue
- Slide containing specimen
- Immersion oil

Procedural Steps
Note: Refer to the parts of a microscope shown in Fig. 41.15 if needed.
1. Wash your hands or use hand sanitizer.
2. Gather the needed materials.
3. Clean the lenses with lens tissue and lens cleaner.
   Purpose: Dust on lenses can obscure elements in the microscopic field.
4. Adjust the seating to a comfortable height.
5. Plug the microscope into an electrical outlet, and turn on the light switch.
6. Place the slide specimen on the stage, and secure it.
7. Turn the revolving nosepiece to engage the 4× or 10× lens.
   Purpose: Always begin microscopic observations at low power.
8. Carefully raise the stage while observing with the naked eye from the side.
   Purpose: Observing from the side prevents the slide from breaking if the coarse adjustment knob is advanced too far.
9. Focus the specimen using the coarse adjustment knob.
   Purpose: The coarse adjustment knob quickly brings the specimen into focus.
10. Adjust the amount of light by closing the iris diaphragm, by bringing the condenser up or down, or by adjusting the light from the source.
    Purpose: Too much light when the low-power objective is used can be irritating to the eyes.
11. Switch to the 40× lens. Use the fine adjustment knob to focus the specimen in detail.
12. Turn the revolving nosepiece to the area between the high-power objective and oil immersion.
13. Place a small drop of oil on the slide.
    Purpose: Immersion oil has nearly the same refractive index as glass and prevents refraction of the light, thus improving resolution.
14. Carefully rotate the oil immersion objective into place. The objective will be immersed in the oil.
15. Adjust the focus with the fine adjustment knob.
    Purpose: The fine adjustment knob moves the objective slowly, preventing damage to the microscope and the slide.
16. Increase the light by opening the iris diaphragm and raising the condenser.
    Purpose: Lighting is crucial to microscopy—the higher the magnification, the more light needed.
17. Identify the specimen.
18. Return to low power, but do not drag the 40× lens through the oil.
19. Remove the slide, and dispose of it in a biohazard sharps container.
20. Lower the stage.
21. Center the stage.
    Purpose: Returning the microscope to this position protects it during storage.
22. Switch off the light, and unplug the microscope.
23. Clean the lenses with lens tissue, and remove any oil with the lens cleaner.
    Purpose: Dust and oil must be removed from the lenses after a procedure.
24. Wipe the microscope with a cloth.
25. Cover the microscope.
26. Sanitize the work area.
27. Wash hands or use hand sanitizer.

---

precise focus. The fine focus moves the objective more slowly to allow the viewer to zero in on the specimen with greater accuracy. Illumination is accomplished by raising or lowering the condenser and by opening and closing the diaphragm on the condenser.

If the microscope is a binocular model, the eyepieces may need to be adjusted to accommodate the distance between the pupils and the individual's point of greatest visual acuity. A gentle push inward or pull outward adjusts the distance between the eyepieces.

Centrifuge

A centrifuge is an instrument that is used to separate solids from liquids. A centrifuge works by rapidly spinning the specimen, which increases the gravitational (grav i TEY shuhn uhl) force. The increased force pushes the heavier solids to the bottom of the specimen and lets lighter liquids remain at the top of the specimen. *Centrifugation* (SEN truh fyoo gahy shun) is used to separate blood cells from serum or plasma. It is also used to separate solid materials, such as cells and crystals, in urine specimens.

Centrifuges (Fig. 41.16) are designed for specific uses. They may be bench-top or floor models; some may be refrigerated. Some may have rotors or heads that are interchangeable to accommodate different sized sample tubes. Centrifuge configurations vary with the laboratory task that needs to be done. Three common configurations are used in the clinical laboratory:

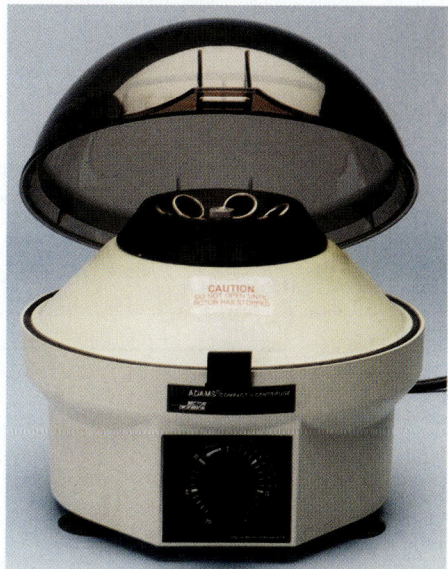

FIG. 41.16 A centrifuge. (From Proctor D, et al: *Kinn's The Medical Assistant*, ed 13, St. Louis, 2017, Elsevier.)

- A centrifuge that has a fixed-angle **rotor** (ROH ter), where specimen cups are held in a rigid position at a fixed angle
- A centrifuge that has horizontal head with buckets that swing out horizontally during centrifugation
- A centrifuge used for centrifuging capillary tubes for microhematocrit testing (see Chapter 44)

Directions for using a centrifuge usually are given in terms of revolutions per minute (rpm). Spinning generates centrifugal force, causing the heaviest particles in a liquid to migrate to the bottom of the tube. Centrifuges can be dangerous if not used correctly. The most important rule is to ensure that the centrifuge is balanced so that tubes of equal size and containing equal volume are directly across from one another in the rotor holders or buckets. Therefore there must always be an even number of tubes in the centrifuge. If a second specimen of the same volume in the same-sized tube is not available for balance, a tube of water may be used to balance the load. Tubes being centrifuged should be capped to prevent samples from creating aerosols during spinning. Rubber cups should be placed in the bottom of the carrier cups to keep the glass tubes from breaking.

Centrifuges should never be opened while they are in operation, nor should you attempt to slow a centrifuge with your hands. Most centrifuges are equipped with a brake, which should be used only in an emergency, the most common of which is a broken glass tube. In this case, wait until the centrifuge comes to a complete stop and follow the manufacturer's instructions for disinfecting the unit; also follow Standard Precautions to prevent injury and disease transmission.

Centrifuges should be checked, cleaned, and lubricated regularly to ensure proper operation. A certified technician must ensure the centrifuge's speed to comply with quality assurance guidelines set forth by the College of American Pathologists (CAP).

Incubator

Incubators (IN kyuh bey ters) are cabinets that maintain constant temperatures (Fig. 41.17) generally used in the microbiology laboratory. An incubator can be set to a specific temperature. Microbiology departments usually maintain a constant temperature of 35° to 37°C (95° to 98.6°F), although other temperatures may also be appropriate. Incubators usually have warning alarms that sound if the temperature exceeds or falls below a specified range. The temperature should be checked daily, and the cabinets should be cleaned regularly with a disinfectant approved by the manufacturer.

See Table 41.11 for an example of a laboratory maintenance log. All laboratory equipment that is temperature sensitive should have temperatures checked and recorded daily.

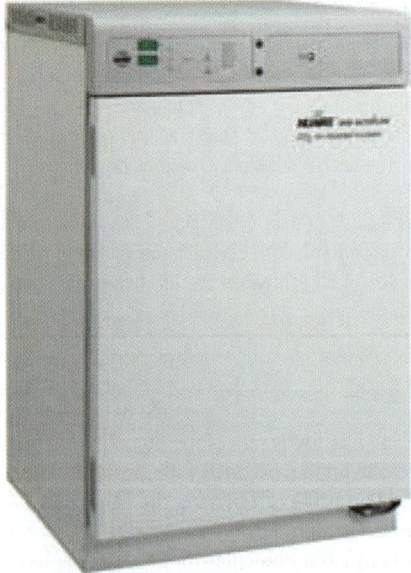

FIG. 41.17 An incubator. (Courtesy NuAire, Plymouth, Minnesota.)

VOCABULARY

rotor: The rotating member of a machine or device.

EXCEPTIONAL CUSTOMER SERVICE

For many testing procedures, patients must be given a specific set of instructions to follow. The provider often communicates the instructions to the patient, but he or she may also ask the medical assistant to reinforce the information. For example, patients may be required to fast 8 to 12 hours before blood samples are collected.

Often the medical assistant is responsible for communicating provider directions that need to be followed before laboratory testing. Make sure you have reviewed the provider's orders correctly before explaining the procedure to the patient. The patient should be given verbal and written instructions prior to testing. Also include a phone number on the instruction sheet so that the patient can call if he or she has questions after returning home. Maintaining a patient's privacy and confidentiality are crucial factors that must be considered when dealing with test results.

TABLE 41.11 Laboratory Maintenance Log

Medical Clinic

Daily Maintenance Control Chart

MONTH _____ **YEAR** _____

Day	Daily Refrig 2°–8° C	Freezer –0°–20° C	Room 15°–30°C	Incubator 34°–36° C	Bleach Counters	Monthly Eyewash Checked	Shower Checked	By
1								
2								
3								
4								
5								

CHAPTER 41 Assisting in the Clinical Laboratory

CLOSING COMMENTS

All health and safety risks to laboratory workers cannot be anticipated or eliminated, but the risks are greatly reduced when everyone who works in the laboratory is conscious of safety guidelines.

Use common sense and document everything. If it is not documented, in the eyes of the law it did not happen. If you have questions about a safety procedure, ask your supervisor. If you are aware of a potential safety problem, report it to the person in charge. Your welfare, the welfare of the patient, and the welfare of coworkers may depend on your commitment to safety.

If diseases did not exist, there would be little need for clinical laboratories. The fact that the human body is susceptible to disease creates a need for laboratory testing. The next four chapters discuss common CLIA-waived tests performed in the POL. They cover patient education, preparation, specimen collection, testing procedures, and proper documentation. All of these skills are aspects of a medical assistant's scope of practice within the laboratory.

CHAPTER REVIEW

In this chapter, you were introduced to the clinical laboratory and the role it plays in patient care. There are various categories of personnel that work in the laboratory. Categories are based on the education and certification of the individuals. Together, laboratory personnel work toward four purposes in patient care: to document good health, to screen patients for disease, to help the provider diagnose disease, and to help the provider decide on the most appropriate treatment and then monitor the effects of the treatment or disease.

Laboratory testing is one part of the information providers need in order to help patients maintain good health. We learned the definition for the term *homeostasis*, which is a state of internal balance the body needs to maintain proper function. This term is also applied to laboratory testing in defining a reference range. When testing for any particular analyte, a healthy person should test within the reference range of a test. Any test results that are out of the reference range should be investigated further in order to return the person to health, if possible. Laboratory tests can be quantitative, which means they have values associated with testing, or qualitative, which means they provide a positive or negative result.

There are different departments within the laboratory, but the areas most commonly seen in physician office laboratories (POLs) are urinalysis, hematology, chemistry, and microbiology. We also learned that government legislation affects the laboratory. Clinical Laboratory Improvement Amendments (CLIA) established quality standards for clinical laboratories, and the FDA categorizes all laboratory tests. There are three designations for testing: waived, moderate-complexity, and high-complexity testing. Each type of testing has designated personnel that can perform the tests. Medical assistants can perform waived testing of all types.

This chapter defined and discussed laboratory quality assurance (QA), comprehensive policies and procedures designed to ensure excellent documentation, and the reliability of laboratory testing. The three stages of QA are preanalytic, analytic, and postanalytic. Each stage is designed to ensure reliable patient testing results and documentation. Quality control (QC) was also defined and discussed in this chapter. QC includes the procedures that should be followed to prove and document test reliability, and therefore patient test result reliability. QA, QC, and preventive maintenance all work together to ensure that patient results are accurate and can be used by the provider with confidence.

This chapter also emphasized laboratory safety and safety standards regarding chemicals, biohazards, infection control, Standard Precautions, bloodborne pathogens, other potentially infectious materials (OPIM), and physical hazards.

As a continuation of safety and patient care, specimen collection, processing, and storage were discussed. Part of specimen handling is the process of documentation and maintaining accurate patient identification and tracking throughout specimen testing. The importance of patient identification cannot be stressed enough. Without proper identification, all testing results are questionable. Specimen storage is also important so that the integrity of the sample is maintained until testing can be completed.

In the laboratory documentation of test results, appropriate units of measurement must be included. In this chapter, we discussed mathematics as it relates to measuring and documenting time, temperature, volume, length, and weight.

Laboratory equipment is necessary to properly test and store samples or testing materials. The laboratory equipment discussed in this chapter included microscopes, centrifuges, and incubators. There is a good example of a daily maintenance control chart that can be used as part of an instrument quality assurance program.

This chapter wrapped up with a brief discussion about patient education and legal/ethical issues for the medical assistant related to the laboratory. Maintaining confidentiality and giving excellent patient care must be the focus of the medical assistant's work.

SCENARIO WRAP-UP

Greg has had a busy day in the laboratory. He has reviewed safety policies and procedures, reacquainted himself with waived laboratory testing, and had a refresher on units of measure. He is looking forward to another day training in the lab tomorrow—he will be running some urinalysis tests.

There is a lot to remember and learn, but with some extra effort, review with JulieAnn, and hands-on testing practice, Greg will become more comfortable in his new department. He thinks the change will be a good move for him.

42

Assisting in the Analysis of Urine

LEARNING OBJECTIVES

1. Describe the anatomy and physiology of the urinary tract, and discuss the formation and elimination of urine.
2. Show sensitivity to patients' rights and feelings when collecting specimens. Also, discuss collection containers, and instruct a patient on the collection of a 24-hour urine specimen.
3. Explain the various means and methods used to collect urine specimens. Also, instruct a patient on the collection of a clean-catch midstream urine specimen.
4. Discuss handling and transporting specimens.
5. Complete the following related to the physical examination of urine:
   - Examine and report the physical aspects of urine.
   - Assess urine for color and turbidity.
   - Perform quality control measures and differentiate between normal and abnormal results while determining the reliability of chemical reagent strips.
6. Examine and report on the chemical aspects of urine, and test urine with chemical reagent strips.
7. Discuss the limitations of reagent strip testing, and explain quality control and quality assurance related to urinalysis.
8. Prepare a urine specimen for microscopic evaluation, and understand the significance of casts, cells, crystals, and miscellaneous findings in the microscopic report.
9. Explain or perform the following CLIA-waived urine tests:
   - Glucose testing using the Clinitest method
   - Urine pregnancy test
   - Ovulation and menopause tests
   - Urine toxicology and drug tests
10. List the means by which urine could be adulterated before drug testing, and discuss chain of custody rules for drug testing.

CHAPTER OUTLINE

1. **Opening Scenario, 1015**
2. **You Will Learn, 1015**
3. **Introduction, 1015**
4. **Urine Formation, 1015**
   a. Elimination of Urine, 1015
5. **Collecting a Urine Specimen: Patient Sensitivity, 1017**
   a. Containers, 1017
   b. Methods of Specimen Collection, 1019
   c. Handling and Transporting a Specimen, 1019
6. **Routine Urinalysis, 1021**
   a. Physical Examination of Urine: Appearance, 1022
      i. *Color, 1022*
      ii. *Turbidity, 1022*
      iii. *Volume, 1022*
      iv. *Foam, 1023*
      v. *Odor, 1024*
      vi. *Specific Gravity, 1024*
   b. Chemical Examination of Urine, 1025
      i. *pH, 1025*
      ii. *Glucose, 1028*
      iii. *Ketones, 1028*
      iv. *Protein, 1028*
      v. *Blood, 1028*
      vi. *Bilirubin and Urobilinogen, 1029*
      vii. *Nitrite, 1029*
      viii. *Leukocyte Esterase, 1029*
   c. Limitations of Reagent Strip Testing, 1029
   d. Quality Assurance and Quality Control in Urinalysis, 1030
7. **Microscopic Preparation and Examination of Urine Sediment, 1030**
   a. Microscopic Preparation of Urine, 1030
   b. Microscopic Examination of Urine, 1032
      i. *Casts, 1032*
      ii. *Cells, 1032*
      iii. *Crystals, 1032*
      iv. *Miscellaneous Findings, 1034*
   c. Understanding the Results of Microscopic Examination, 1038
8. **Additional CLIA-waived Tests Performed on Urine, 1038**
   a. Clinitest
   b. Urine Pregnancy Testing, 1039
   c. Ovulation Testing, 1041
   d. Menopause Testing, 1041
   e. Urine Toxicology, 1041
      i. *Adulteration Testing and Chain of Custody, 1042*
9. **Closing Comments, 1045**
10. **Chapter Review, 1045**
11. **Scenario Wrap-Up, 1045**

CHAPTER 42 Assisting in the Analysis of Urine

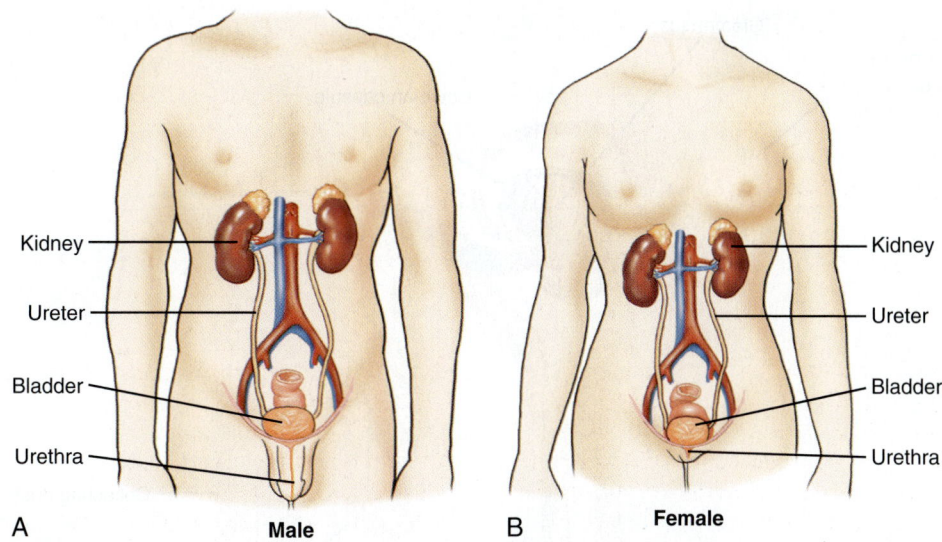

FIG. 42.1 The organs of the urinary system. (From Shiland B: *Mastering Healthcare Terminology*, ed 5, St. Louis, 2015, Elsevier.)

▶ OPENING SCENARIO

Becca Rundle is a medical assistant student who is observing at the Walden-Martin Family Medical (WMFM) Clinic physician office laboratory (POL) today. As part of an assignment, Becca needs to shadow an experienced medical assistant in an area that interests her. Becca is curious about the laboratory, so she will be spending a few hours with JulieAnn, a certified medical assistant (CMA) through the American Association of Medical Assistants (AAMA). JulieAnn is going to explain the tests that she will be performing in the urinalysis department. She has even saved a few interesting samples that came in earlier in the week.

YOU WILL LEARN

1. To describe urine collection procedures and discuss the choices of collection containers.
2. To instruct a patient in the proper collection of a 24-hour urine specimen and a clean-catch midstream urine specimen.
3. To examine and report on the physical and chemical aspects of urine.
4. To test and record quality control and chemical urinalysis using CLIA-waived methods.
5. To prepare a urine specimen for microscopic evaluation.
6. To explain the following CLIA-waived urine tests: Clinitest, urine pregnancy test, ovulation and menopause tests, and toxicology/drug tests.

INTRODUCTION

Urine is the second most common specimen analyzed in the laboratory. Only blood is tested more frequently. Urine is analyzed for several reasons:
- To detect diseases or disorders where the kidneys are working normally but are excreting abnormal substances that are the result of an imbalance of **homeostasis** (hoh mee oh STEY sis) in the body. An example would be an individual with diabetes mellitus who is excreting glucose.
- To detect diseases or disorders of the kidneys or urinary tract. Examples would be the presence of kidney stones or of a urinary tract infection (UTI).
- To detect medications or drugs that are excreted by the kidneys.

URINE FORMATION

Medical assistants must have a basic knowledge of kidney structure and urine formation to understand the results of a urinalysis (UA). For a helpful review of the urinary system, see Chapter 6.

The urinary tract consists of two kidneys, two ureters, one bladder, and one urethra (Fig. 42.1). Blood passes through microscopic structures in the kidneys called **nephrons** (NEF rons) (Fig. 42.2). In the nephrons blood is filtered to form a **filtrate** (FIL treyt). The composition of the filtrate is adjusted as it passes through the renal (REEN ahl) tubules of the nephron. Selective reabsorption (ree ab SAWRP shuh n) and secretion (se KREE shuh n) occurs in the renal tubules until the filtrate reaches its final composition. The final filtrate is known as *urine*. Table 42.1 is a quick structure and function review of the urinary system.

Elimination of Urine

Urine flows through a series of collection areas until it leaves the kidney through the ureter and is stored in the urinary bladder. Urine remains in the bladder until it is voided through the urethra. The average person voids about 1 to 2 liters of urine per day.

The largest component of urine is water. Normal waste products found in urine are as follows:
- Urea (yoo REE uh) and uric (yoo RIK) acid
- Creatinine (kree AT n een)

> **VOCABULARY**
> **filtrate:** Fluid and substances that are filtered out of the blood in the Bowman capsule. The fluid that remains after a liquid is passed through a filter.
> **homeostasis:** The internal environment of the body that is compatible with life. A steady state that is created by all the body systems working together to provide a consistent and unvarying internal environment.
> **nephron:** The functional unit of the kidney. Responsible for creating urine and adjusting it to maintain homeostasis.

> **MEDICAL TERMINOLOGY**
> **nephr/o:** kidney
> **ren/o:** kidney

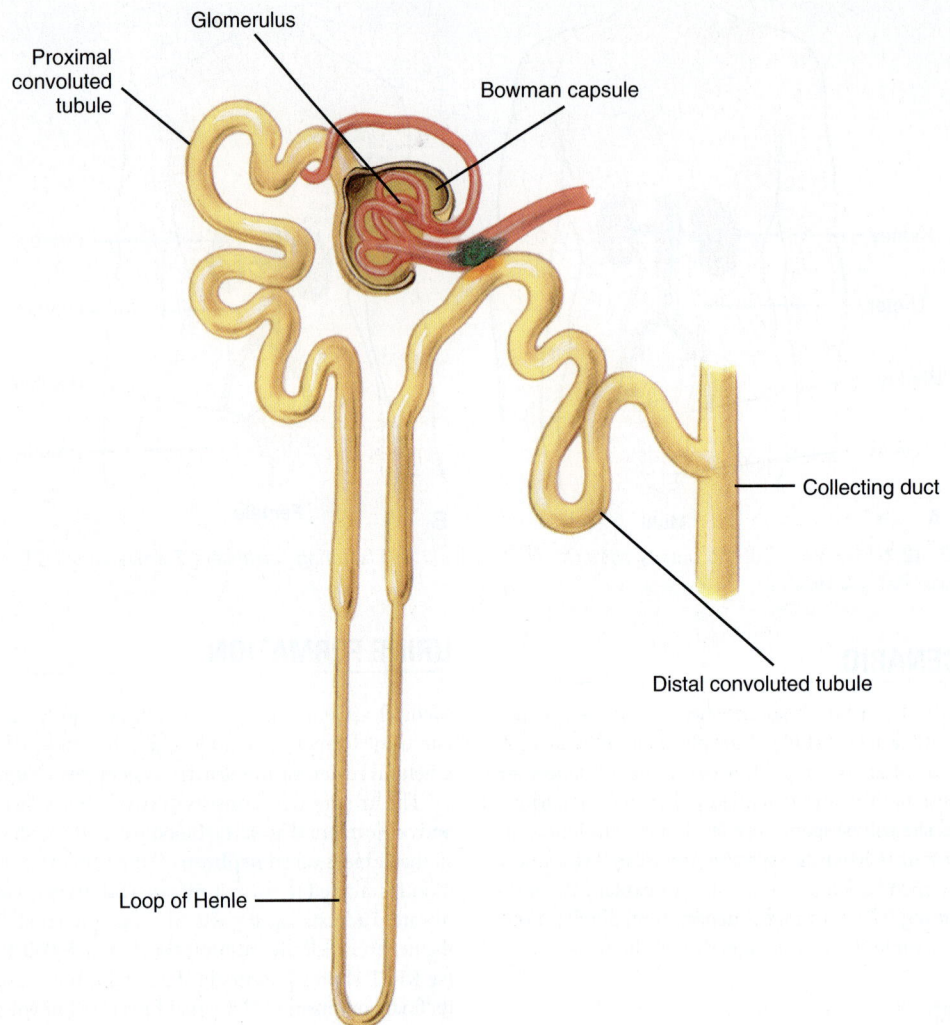

FIG. 42.2 The nephron. (From Applegate EJ: *The Anatomy and Physiology Learning System*, ed 4, Philadelphia, 2011, Saunders.)

TABLE 42.1	Review of Urinary Structures and Functions
Organs of the Urinary System	**Function**
Kidneys (2)	The primary organ of the urinary system, contains nephrons that produce urine.
Ureters (2) (yoo REE ters)	Tubes that lead from the kidney to the urinary bladder.
Urinary bladder	Hold urine until it is voided.
Urethra (yoo REE thruh)	The tube that is a passageway from the bladder to the outside environment.
Structures That Make Up a Nephron	**Function**
Glomerulus (gloh MER yuh luh s)	Filters the blood to create the *filtrate*, which normally contains water, urea, and electrolytes. See Box 42.1.
Bowman capsule	Filtrate collects in this structure. The glomerulus and Bowman capsule together are called the *renal corpuscle* (see Fig. 42.2).
Proximal convoluted tubules and loop of Henle (hehn LEE)	Reabsorb most of the water and glucose from the filtrate. See Box 42.1 for information on glucose reabsorption.
Distal convoluted tubules	Blood vessels selectively secrete additional products into the urine, such as potassium and hydrogen. See Box 42.2 for additional information on secretion.

> **BOX 42.1 Kidney Damage**
>
> Protein and blood cells are too large to be filtered by the glomerulus. So when these substances appear in the urine, it may indicate kidney damage.

> **BOX 42.2 Glucose Reabsorption**
>
> The reabsorption of glucose depends on its **renal threshold**. The renal threshold for blood glucose is below 160 mg/dL. This means that all the glucose will be reabsorbed into the blood if the blood glucose level is below 160 mg/dL. If the blood glucose level is higher than 160 mg/dL, the blood will not reabsorb the glucose. The filtered glucose then remains in the urine, which will show up as a positive test for glucose during urinalysis.

> **VOCABULARY**
>
> **renal threshold:** The blood level of a substance, above which the kidneys fail to reabsorb it, so the substance will appear in the urine. (See Box 42.2 for an example.)
>
> **polyethylene:** a plastic material used mostly for containers and packaging.

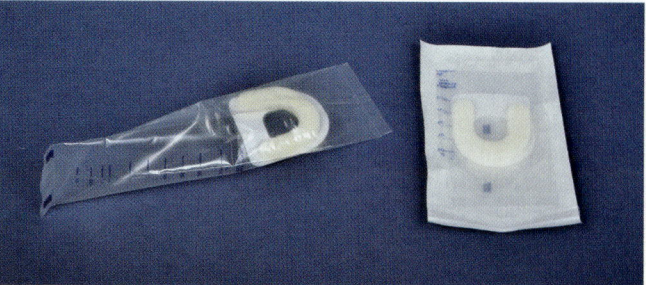

FIG. 42.3 Infant urine collection bag.

- Electrolytes such as chloride, sodium, and potassium

Abnormal waste products that can be found in urine include the following:
- Protein
- Glucose and ketones (KEE tohns)
- Red blood cells, white blood cells, bacteria, and nitrites (NAHY trahyts)
- Bilirubin (BIL uh roo bin) and urobilinogen (yoo roh by LIN uh jen)

COLLECTING A URINE SPECIMEN: PATIENT SENSITIVITY

The request for a urine specimen may create an uneasy moment for the patient. The request should be made in a private area, such as the exam room if possible. The patient should be given clear instructions so that he or she understands what is expected. The medical assistant should clearly communicate and explain the details of the procedure.

Be observant, and ask the patient to repeat the directions so you know he or she understands the procedure. Answer any questions with patience and clear directions to avoid confusion. If a language barrier exists, be creative but respectful of the patient's needs. Use an interpreter

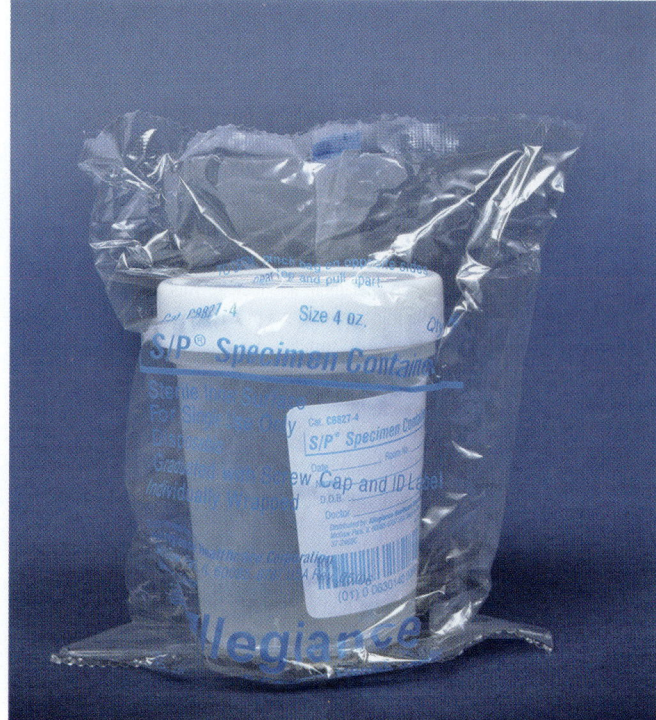

FIG. 42.4 Sterile urine container.

if one is available. Posting a picture with directions in a variety of languages in the patient restroom could also help.

Containers

The POL should provide the appropriate urine container for the patient. Patients should not use containers from home. Disposable, nonsterile, plastic, or coated paper containers are the most frequently used and are available in many sizes with tight-fitting lids. Most routine UA tests, pregnancy tests, and tests for abnormal analytes are performed on urine collected in nonsterile containers. Special flexible **polyethylene** (pol ee ETH uh leen) bags (Fig. 42.3) with adhesive are used to collect urine from infants and children who are not toilet trained (see Chapter 32). For specimens that must be collected over a stated time (24-hour urines), large, wide-mouth plastic containers with screw-cap tops are used (Procedure 42.1).

If the sample is being sent to the microbiology department of the laboratory for culture, it must be collected in a sterile container. Explain the collection procedure to the patient and make sure the patient understands how to collect the specimen and how to handle the sterile specimen cup. Sterile containers have a paper seal over the cap. If the seal is broken, the specimen cup may not be sterile and should be discarded. (Fig. 42.4).

> **CRITICAL THINKING 42.1**
>
> Becca and JulieAnn meet in the reception area and walk back to the POL. They talk about the need for proper PPE, and JulieAnn gives Becca a lab coat and protective eyewear. She also shows Becca where the gloves are near the UA counter. Becca will not be performing tests today, but anyone in the lab should wear proper PPE even if they are observing.
>
> There are a few specimens on the counter, and JulieAnn asks Becca if she has practiced giving instructions for UA collection procedures in any of her classes. Becca replies that she has, but thought it was a bit silly. JulieAnn talks about how patients can be embarrassed about collecting specimens and may not want to ask too many questions. JulieAnn asks Becca to write down three items that are important to include when explaining a UA collection procedure. Write down your own answer, and be ready to share with your class.

PROCEDURE 42.1 Instruct a Patient in the Collection of a 24-Hour Urine Specimen

Task
Collect a 24-hour urine sample to test for creatinine clearance.

Equipment and Supplies
- Patient's health record
- 3-L urine collection container
- Plastic cup or specimen collection pan for collecting urine (which is then poured into the collection container)
- Printed patient instructions
- Laboratory requisition

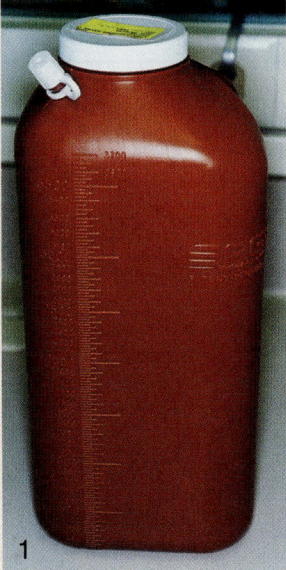

Procedural Steps

1. Greet the patient. Identify yourself. Verify the patient's identify with full name, ask the patient to spell the first and last name, and give their date of birth. Explain the procedure to be performed in a manner that the patient understands. Answer any questions about the procedure.
    Purpose: It is important to identify the patient in two different ways to ensure that you have the correct patient. Explaining the procedure can make the patient feel more comfortable and reduces anxiety.
2. Label the container with the patient's name and the current date, identify the specimen as a 24-hour urine specimen, and include your initials.
    Purpose: Labeling the container prevents a possible mix-up of specimens.
3. Explain the following instructions to adult patients or to the guardians of pediatric patients.

Patient Instructions: Obtaining a 24-Hour Urine Specimen

(1) Empty your bladder into the toilet in the morning without saving any of the specimen. Record the time you first emptied your bladder on the label.

(2) For the next 24 hours, each time you empty your bladder, all the urine should be collected into the plastic cup or collection pan that is placed on the toilet (also called a nun's cap or toilet hat). Then pour all the collected urine directly into the large specimen container (Fig. 1).
    Purpose: Do not urinate directly into the large specimen container. It may contain a preservative that could be caustic. You do not want to splash any of the preservative while urinating.

(3) Put the lid back on the container after each urination and rinse out the plastic cup or collection pan; store the container in the refrigerator or at room temperature, as directed, throughout the 24 hours of the study.
    Purpose: Refrigeration or the preservative inhibits microbial growth in the specimen.

(4) If at any time you forget to collect your specimen or if some urine is accidentally spilled, you must begin the test over again with a new container and a newly recorded start time.
    Purpose: The test will be inaccurate if you fail to collect all urine produced during the designated 24-hour period.

(5) Collect the final urine specimen at the same time you started the collection process on the previous day. This last collected specimen is placed in the large container. Collection ends with the voided morning specimen on the second day, which completes the 24-hour period.

(6) As soon as possible after completing collection, return the specimen container to the provider's office or the designated laboratory.

4. Give the patient the specimen container and supplies with written instructions to confirm understanding.
5. Document details of the patient education session in the patient's record.

Processing a 24-Hour Urine Specimen

1. Ask the patient whether he or she collected all voided urine throughout the 24-hour period or whether any problems occurred during the collection process.
    Purpose: To confirm the accuracy of the specimen.
2. Complete the laboratory request form. Make sure that all the information is filled out on the container label.
3. Wash hands or use hand sanitizer. Put on a fluid-impermeable lab coat, protective eyewear, and gloves before preparing the specimen for transport.
4. Store the specimen in the refrigerator until the laboratory picks it up.
5. Remove gloves, and discard them appropriately. Remove protective eyewear and lab coat. Wash hands or use hand sanitizer.
6. Document that the specimen was sent to the laboratory, including the type of test ordered, the date and time, the type of specimen, and your initials.

The label on all specimens must be printed in permanent marker or ink and must include the patient's name, the date and time of collection, and the type of specimen. If available, computer-generated labels should be placed on the container so that the information is easy to read. See Box 42.3 for additional information on specimen labeling. Always put on gloves before handling filled specimen containers.

> **BOX 42.3 Additional Labeling Information**
>
> A note about specimen labels: When a clinic sends specimens to multiple laboratories, it is important to have a system in place that meets the labeling and collection needs of all facilities. Each laboratory may require specific information and specific specimen containers. To avoid mistakes and possible specimen recollection issues, double-check the laboratory name and specimen requirements before patient collection. Patient insurance may direct laboratory usage or affiliation.

BOX 42.4 Additional Patient Instructions for At-Home 24-Hour Urine Collection

- Do not put anything but urine into the container.
- Do not pour out any liquid or powdered preservative from the container.
- If you accidentally spill some of the preservative on yourself, immediately wash with water and call the POL, provider's office, or testing laboratory.
- Always keep the collection container cool. Refrigerate the container, or keep it in an ice-filled cooler or pail.
- Keep the cap on the container.

Methods of Specimen Collection

Most tests are performed on freshly collected urine in clean containers; this is called a *random specimen*. If the specimen ordered should be collected when the patient first wakes up in the morning, it is called a *first morning specimen*. This type of specimen is more concentrated than a random sample and is best used when testing for nitrite, protein, pregnancy, and microscopic examination. First morning samples are also the preferred sample for possible UTI testing, but this is not a requirement. *Two-hour postprandial* (PPP) *urine specimens*, collected 2 hours after a meal, are used in diabetes screening and for home diabetes testing programs. A *24-hour urine specimen* is collected over 24 hours to provide a *quantitative* (KWON ti tey tiv) chemical analysis, such as hormone levels and *creatinine clearance rates*. The patient must understand the proper way to collect a 24-hour urine specimen (see Procedure 42.1 and Box 42.4).

A *second-voided specimen* usually is collected to determine glucose levels in urine. The first void of the morning is discarded, and the second void of the day is collected for testing. For a *catheterized* (KATH I tuh rahyz ed) *specimen*, the provider, nurse, or specially trained medical assistant inserts a sterile *catheter* (KATH i ter) into the bladder to collect the specimen (Fig. 42.5).

A *clean-catch midstream specimen* (CCMS) is ordered when the provider suspects a urinary tract infection. When a UTI is possible, the provider will order a urine *culture and sensitivity* (C&S). The clean-catch technique is used to eliminate microorganisms from the urinary *meatus* (mee EY tuh s). In the medical facility, CCMS samples start by instructing the patient to thoroughly cleanse around the meatus and then urinate a small amount into the toilet. This is done to flush out the distal portion of the urethra where *normal flora* (FLAWR uh) can accumulate. The patient then collects a CCMS specimen. Prior to collection, the medical assistant needs to give complete, understandable instructions to the patient on the method of collection (Procedure 42.2). Failure to do so may mean that the patient will have to return to the office to provide another specimen. For a urine culture and sensitivity, the urine is collected either by catheterization or by the clean-catch method into a sterile container.

Handling and Transporting a Specimen

Proper handling of specimens is essential. The chemical and cellular components of urine change if the urine warms to room temperature (Table 42.2). Urine specimens should therefore be kept refrigerated and should be processed within 1 hour of collection. If the specimen must be transported to a referral laboratory, evacuated transport tubes are available (Fig. 42.6). These tubes contain preservatives and look like blood collection tubes. The preservatives in the tube prevent the overgrowth of bacteria and will prevent chemical changes in the urine that may affect test results. Chemical reagent strip testing can be performed on preserved specimens within 72 hours. Tubes may be held at room temperature during this time.

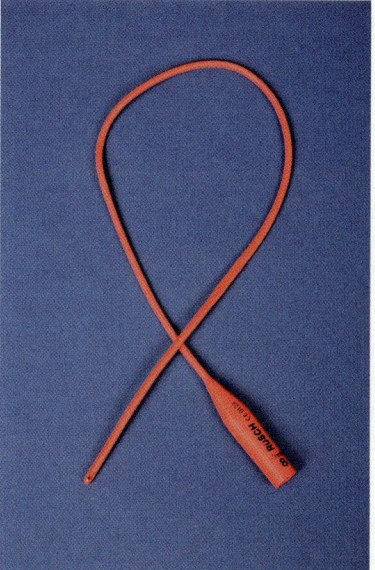

FIG. 42.5 Urinary catheter.

CRITICAL THINKING 42.2

As JulieAnn and Becca review the different types of UA specimens, JulieAnn asks, "Why is it so important that a CCMS be collected midstream? Why not start collecting the sample as soon as the void starts?" What would your answer be to that question? Write down your answer, and be ready to share in class.

A different preservative must be used for urine culture specimens. The preservative used for culture specimens helps maintain the number of bacteria present at the time of collection. This type of transport system should be used only for urine specimens that will be cultured.

VOCABULARY

catheter: A hollow, flexible tube that can be inserted into a vessel, organ, or cavity of the body to withdraw or instill fluid, monitor information, and visualize a vessel or cavity.

catheterized: Occurs when a catheter has been inserted into a vessel, organ, or cavity of the body (e.g., the urinary bladder).

creatinine clearance rates: Result from a procedure used to evaluate the glomerular filtration rate of the kidneys.

culture and sensitivity (C&S): A procedure in which a specimen is cultured on microbiologic media to detect bacterial or fungal growth. This is followed by screening for antibiotic sensitivity. C&S is performed in the microbiology department of a referral laboratory.

hemolyze: To cause the red blood cells in a blood sample to rupture.

meatus: A body opening or passage, especially the external opening of a structure.

normal flora: Microorganisms (mostly bacteria and yeast) that live on or in the body. Normal microscopic residents of the body.

quantitative: Describes a test result that is expressed as a number, usually with units of measure attached to numeric values.

random specimen: A urine specimen that can be collected at any time of the day into a nonsterile container.

PROCEDURE 42.2 Collect a Clean-Catch Midstream Urine Specimen

Task
Collect a contaminant-free urine sample for culture or analysis using the clean-catch midstream specimen (CCMS) technique.

Equipment and Supplies
- Patient's record
- Sterile container with a lid and label
- Antiseptic towelettes

Procedural Steps

1. Greet the patient. Identify yourself. Verify the patient's identify with full name, ask the patient to spell the last name, and give their date of birth. Explain the procedure to be performed in a manner that the patient understands. Answer any questions about the procedure.
   Purpose: It is important to identify the patient in two different ways to ensure that you have the correct patient. Explaining the procedure can make the patient feel more comfortable and reduce anxiety.

2. Label the sterile, sealed container, and give the patient the towelette supplies (Fig. 1).
   Purpose: Labeling the container prevents a possible mix-up of specimens.

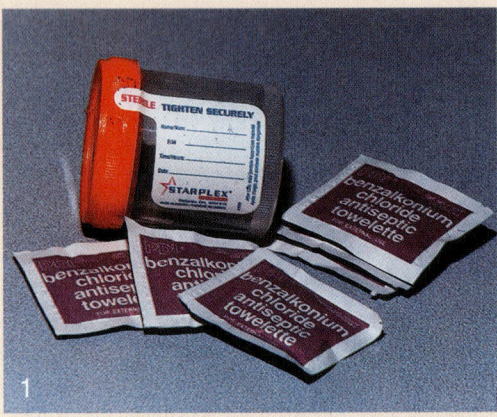

3. Explain the following instructions to adult patients or to the guardians of pediatric patients, making sure you show sensitivity to privacy issues.
   Purpose: Instructions must be understood if they are to be followed correctly. By talking to the patient, you can determine whether the patient understands or has any questions.

Patient Instructions: Obtaining a Clean-Catch Midstream Specimen (Female Patient)

(1) Wash your hands, and open the towelette packages for easy access.
(2) Remove the lid from the specimen container, being careful not to touch the inside of the lid or the inside of the container. Place the lid, facing up, on a paper towel.
   Purpose: The lid and the container must be handled carefully to maintain the internal sterility of the container and prevent contamination of the urine sample.
(3) Lower your underclothing, and sit on the toilet.
(4) Expose the urinary meatus by spreading apart the labia with one hand (Fig. 2A).
(5) Cleanse each side of the urinary meatus with a front-to-back motion, from the pubis toward the anus. Use a separate antiseptic wipe to cleanse each side of the meatus.

Purpose: Cleansing the area around the urinary meatus prevents contamination of the urine sample. Wiping in one stroke from front to back prevents the passage of microorganisms from the anal region to the area around the urinary meatus.

(6) Cleanse directly across the meatus, front to back, using a third antiseptic wipe (see Fig. 2A).
(7) Hold the labia apart throughout this procedure.
(8) Void a small amount of urine into the toilet (Fig. 2B).
   Purpose: Allowing the initial flow of urine to pass into the toilet flushes the opening of the urethra.

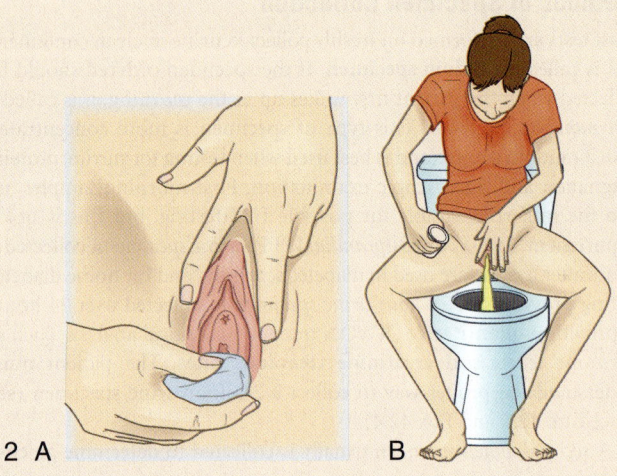

(9) Move the specimen container into position, and void the next portion of urine into it. Fill the container halfway. Remember, this is a sterile container. Do not put your fingers on the inside of the container.
(10) Remove the cup, and void the last amount of urine into the toilet. (This means that the first part and the last part of the urinary flow have been excluded from the specimen. Only the middle portion of the flow is included.)
(11) Place the lid on the container, taking care not to touch the interior surface of the lid. Wipe in your usual manner, redress, wash your hands, and return the sterile specimen to the place designated by the medical facility.

Patient Instructions: Obtaining a Clean-Catch Midstream Specimen (Male Patient)

(1) Wash your hands, and expose the penis.
(2) Retract the foreskin of the penis (if not circumcised).
(3) Cleanse the area around the glans penis (tip of the penis) and the urethral opening (meatus) by washing each side of the glans with a separate antiseptic wipe (Fig. 3A).
(4) Cleanse directly across the urethral opening using a third antiseptic wipe.
(5) Void a small amount of urine into the toilet or urinal (Fig. 3B).
(6) Collect the next portion of the urine in the sterile container, filling the container halfway without touching the inside of the container with the hands or the penis (Fig. 3C).
(7) Void the last amount of urine into the toilet or urinal.
(8) Place the lid on the container, taking care not to touch the interior surface of the lid. Wipe, wash your hands, and redress.
(9) Return the specimen to the designated area.

CHAPTER 42 Assisting in the Analysis of Urine

PROCEDURE 42.2 Collect a Clean-Catch Midstream Urine Specimen—cont'd

3 A B C

Processing a Clean-Catch Urine Specimen

1. Document the date, time, and collection type.
2. Wash hands or use hand sanitizer. Put on the fluid-impermeable lab coat, protective eyewear, and gloves.
   Purpose: Hand sanitization is an important step for infection control. PPE is part of Standard Precautions.
3. Process the specimen according to the provider's orders. Perform urinalysis in the office or prepare the specimen for transport to the laboratory. If it is to be sent to an outside laboratory, complete the following steps:
   - Make sure the label is properly completed with the patient's information and the date, time, test ordered, and your initials.
   - Place the specimen in a biohazard specimen bag.
   - Complete a laboratory requisition, and place it in the outside pocket of the specimen bag.
   - Keep the specimen refrigerated until pickup.
4. Remove gloves, protective eyewear, and lab coat. Dispose of gloves appropriately. Wash hands or use hand sanitizer.
   - Document that the specimen was sent.

TABLE 42.2 Changes in Urine After 1 Hour at Room Temperature

Constituent	Change
Clarity	Urine becomes cloudy as crystals precipitate and bacteria multiply
Color	May change if pH becomes alkaline
pH	Becomes alkaline as bacteria form ammonia from urea
Glucose	Decreases as it is metabolized by bacteria
Ketones	Decrease because of evaporation
Bilirubin and urobilinogen	Undergo degradation in light
Blood	May hemolyze; false-positive results are possible because of bacterial enzymes
Nitrite	Test result may change from negative to positive as bacteria multiply and reduce nitrates to nitrites
Casts	Lyse or dissolve in alkaline urine
Cells	Lyse or dissolve in alkaline urine
Bacteria	Multiply twofold approximately every 20 minutes
Yeasts	Multiply
Crystals	Precipitate as urine cools; may dissolve if pH changes

From Proctor D, et al: *Kinn's The Medical Assistant*, ed 13, St. Louis, 2017, Elsevier.

Results on the chemical reagent strip may be altered by the alternative preservatives. Culture and sensitivity testing should be performed within 72 hours. The C&S tubes can be held at room temperature.

A laboratory request form, paper or electronic, must be completed for all specimens that will be transported to another site for analysis. Typical forms include the following information:
- Patient's name and the date
- Type of urinalysis ordered
- Name of the provider requesting the examination
- Appropriate CPT (current procedural terminology) code for the diagnosis
- A line for the provider to sign after he or she has reviewed the results

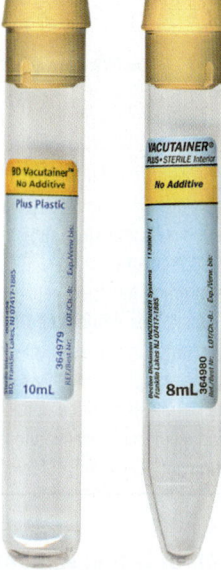

FIG. 42.6 Urine transport tubes. (Courtesy Becton, Dickinson & Co., Franklin Lakes, New Jersey.)

Specimens are sent to the laboratory in a plastic biohazard bag that zips closed and has an outside pocket, where a paper laboratory request is placed. After the test has been performed, the lab physically sends a paper report or electronically sends the results to the provider.

ROUTINE URINALYSIS

The minimum volume needed for a routine UA usually is about 10 to 12 mL, but more is preferred. A complete UA is an assessment of the following:
- Physical properties of the urine
- Selected chemical measurements that are important in the diagnosis of disease (Table 42.3).
- Microscopic contents of the urine and its sediment

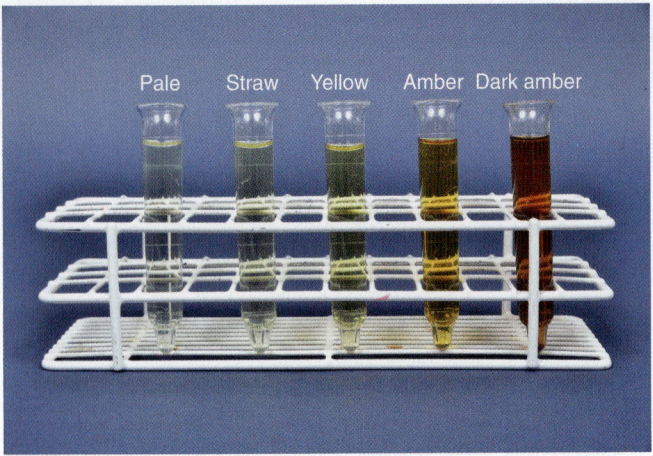

FIG. 42.7 Color of urine specimens.

TABLE 42.3	Components of Physical and Chemical Urinalysis
Physical Properties	**Chemical Properties**
Color	Protein
Clarity	Glucose
Specific gravity	Ketones
Volume[a]	Bilirubin
Odor[a]	Blood
Foam[a]	Nitrite
	pH
	Urobilinogen
	Leukocyte enzyme

[a]Not always assessed.
From Proctor D, et al: *Kinn's The Medical Assistant*, ed 13, St. Louis, 2017, Elsevier.

PROCEDURE 42.3 Assess Urine for Color and Turbidity: Physical Test

Task
Assess and record the color and clarity of a urine specimen.

Equipment and Supplies
- Patient's record
- Urine specimen
- Centrifuge tube
- Fluid-impermeable lab coat, protective eyewear, and gloves
- Biohazard waste container

Procedural Steps
1. Wash hands or use hand sanitizer. Put on the fluid-impermeable lab coat, protective eyewear, and gloves.
   Purpose: Hand sanitization is an important step for infection control. Wearing PPE is part of Standard Precautions.
2. Mix the urine by gently swirling the specimen.
   Purpose: Suspended substances settle when urine stands. If urine is not mixed before its appearance is assessed, the finding will be incorrect.
3. Label a centrifuge tube if a complete urinalysis is to be done.
   Purpose: If a complete urinalysis is to be done, a portion of the specimen will be centrifuged for microscopic examination. The centrifuged specimen must be labeled to prevent specimen confusion.
4. Pour the specimen into a standard-sized centrifuge tube.
   Purpose: Standard-sized containers are better for assessing color and clarity results.
5. Assess and record the color (refer to Fig. 42.7):
   - Pale straw or straw
   - Yellow
   - Amber or dark amber
6. Assess the clarity by placing a piece of white paper with fine, dark black print behind the specimen and see if you can see the print:
   Clear—Able to read through the specimen; no cloudiness
   Slightly turbid—Can barely see fine print on white paper through the tube
   Turbid—Cannot see fine print, dark print possibly seen through the tube, or see no print at all through the tube
7. Clean the work area, and dispose of procedure supplies in the biohazard waste container. Dispose of gloves. Remove lab coat and protective eyewear. Wash hands or use hand sanitizer.
   Purpose: To ensure infection control.
8. Record the results in the patient's record.
   Purpose: A procedure is not considered done until it is recorded.

Physical Examination of Urine: Appearance

The physical examination of urine involves observations regarding the appearance of the specimen (Procedure 42.3). This does not involve chemical analysis but rather observation of the following characteristics:
- Color
- Turbidity (TUR bid i tee)
- Volume
- The presence of foam, odor
- Specific gravity

Color. Normal urine is a shade of yellow that ranges from pale straw to yellow to amber (see Fig. 42.7). The color depends on the concentration of the pigment urochrome (YOO R uh krohm) and the amount of water in the specimen. A dilute specimen should be a pale straw color, and a more concentrated specimen should be a darker yellow or amber color. First morning specimens will likely be amber in color due to the concentration of the urochrome during the night. Variations in color may also be caused by diet, medication, and disease. Abnormal colors may be related to pathologic or nonpathologic factors (Table 42.4).

Turbidity. Both normal and abnormal urine specimens may range in appearance from clear to very cloudy (Fig. 42.8). Turbidity may be caused by cells, bacteria, yeast, vaginal contaminants, or crystals. It is possible for a urine specimen to be clear when voided, but then as crystals form and precipitate (pre SIP i teyt) out of the liquid, this causes the urine to become cloudy as it cools.

Volume. The amount of urine is rarely measured in a random specimen. With a timed specimen, volume is measured by pouring the complete collection into a large, graduated cylinder (Fig. 42.9). It is not accurate enough to use the markings on the side of the collection container. Once the volume has been measured and recorded, a portion of well-mixed specimen, called an *aliquot* (AL i kwuh t), is removed for testing. The remainder is discarded or stored, depending on the preference of the laboratory.

TABLE 42.4 Possible Causes of Urine Colors

Color	Pathologic Cause	Nonpathologic Cause
Straw	Diabetes	Diuretics; high fluid intake (coffee, beer)
Amber	Dehydration	Concentrated first morning specimen; Excessive sweating; low fluid intake
Bright yellow	—	Carotene, vitamins
Red	Blood, porphyrins	Menstruation, beets, drugs, dyes
Orange-yellow	Bile, hepatitis	Phenazopyridine (fen az oh PEER i deen) (Pyridium, Uristat), dyes, drugs
Greenish yellow	Bile, hepatitis	Senna (laxative), cascara (laxative), rhubarb
Reddish brown	Old blood, methemoglobin	—
Brownish black	Methemoglobin, melanin	Carbidopa-levodopa (kar buh DOH puh-lee vuh DOH puh) (Sinemet, Parcopa)
Salmon pink	—	Amorphous urates
White (milky)	Fats, pus	Amorphous phosphates
Blue-green	Biliverdin, infection with *Pseudomonas* organisms	Vitamin B, drugs, dyes

From Proctor D, et al: *Kinn's The Medical Assistant*, ed 13, St. Louis, 2017, Elsevier.

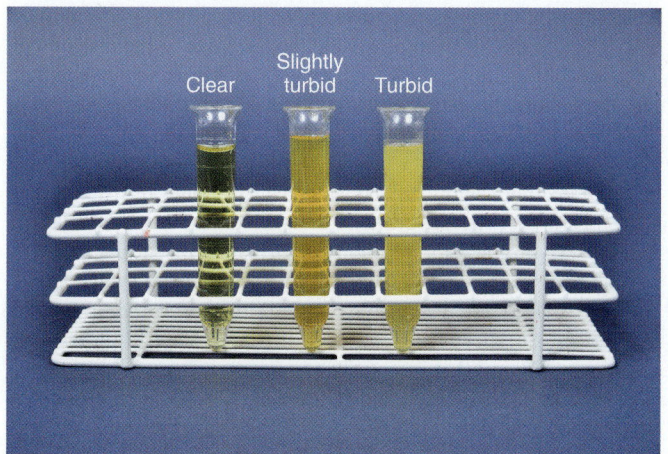

FIG. 42.8 Turbidity of urine specimens.

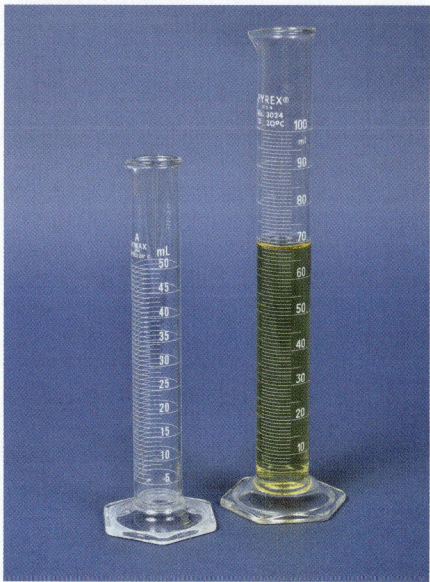

FIG. 42.9 Graduated cylinder.

The normal volume of urine produced every 24 hours varies according to the age of the individual. Infants and children produce smaller volumes than adults. The normal adult volume of urine produced is approximately 800 mL to 2000 mL in 24 hours. Excessive production of urine is called *polyuria* (pol ee YOO R ee uh). This is common in those who have diabetes mellitus, diabetes insipidus (in SIP i duhs), and certain kidney disorders. *Oliguria* (ol i GYOO R ee uh) is an insufficient production of urine, which can be caused by dehydration, decreased fluid intake, shock, renal disease, or urinary tract infections. The absence of urine production, *anuria* (an NOO R ee uh), occurs when there is renal obstruction and renal failure.

CRITICAL THINKING 42.3

Write down in your own words definitions for the following terms: anuria, oliguria, and polyuria. Be ready to share with your class.

VOCABULARY

crystals: Solid substances with a regular shape that is due to the structure of molecules.
bilirubinuria: The presence of bilirubin in the urine.
graduated cylinder: A narrow, tube-shaped container marked with horizontal lines to represent units of measurement used to precisely measure the volume of liquids.
precipitate: To separate a solid substance from a solution.
turbidity: A cloudy appearance; not clear.
urochrome: The yellow pigment normally found in urine; it is described as straw, yellow, or amber based on its concentration.

MEDICAL TERMINOLOGY

an: without
chrom/o: color or pigment
oligo-: a few, too little
poly-: many
ur/o-: urine

Foam. Normally the presence of foam is not recorded, but careful observation of this property can be a significant clue to an abnormality. Foam consists of small bubbles that persist for a long time after the specimen has been shaken. Foam must not be confused with any bubbles that rapidly disappear. White foam can indicate the presence of increased protein (Fig. 42.10). Greenish yellow foam can mean **bilirubinuria** (bih lee ROO bin yuhr e uh). Care should be taken in handling such urine specimens because the greenish yellow color may indicate that the patient has viral hepatitis, which is highly contagious. Always observe Standard Precautions, and wear appropriate personal protective equipment (PPE) when handling specimens. If foam is observed and seems significant, add a note in the comments field of a paper or electronic test report.

BOX 42.5 Ketones in Urine

A diabetic patient whose blood sugar is not well controlled or a person who is eating a low-carbohydrate diet may pass ketones in the urine. Ketones are the products of fat metabolism and give urine a slightly sweet or fruity smell. The following chemical compounds are examples of ketones produced in the body: *acetoacetate* (ah see toh AS I teyt), *acetone* (as i tohn), and beta *hydroxybutyric* (hayh DROK si byoo tir ik) acid; they are collectively called *ketone bodies*, or *ketones*.

BOX 42.6 Phenylketonuria

Phenylketonuria (PKU) is a rare hereditary condition in which the amino acid **phenylalanine** (fe nil AHL uh neen) is not properly metabolized, or broken down in the body. PKU that is undiagnosed or untreated can lead to severe cognitive disabilities. Accumulation of phenylalanine in the blood and urine gives body fluids the odor of wet fur. (Blood sampling for PKU is discussed in Chapter 43.)

BOX 42.7 Specific Gravity

A change in urine specific gravity may be an indication of underlying disease. For example, **glomerulonephritis**, the presence of glucose and protein in the urine, may increase the specific gravity. Chronic renal insufficiency or diabetes insipidus may lower the specific gravity in urine.

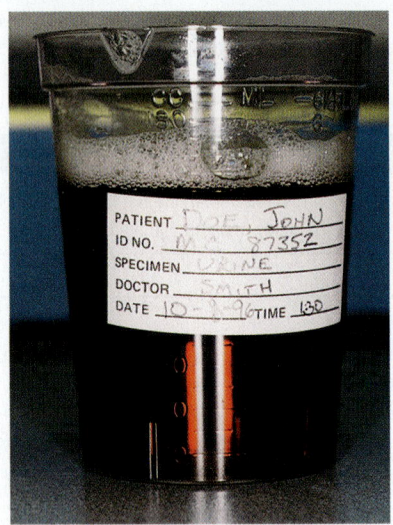

FIG. 42.10 Urine with foam. (From Proctor D, et al: *Kinn's The Medical Assistant*, ed 13, St. Louis, 2017, Elsevier.)

Odor. As with foam, odor is not normally recorded but can be an important clue to metabolic disorders. Normal urine is said to be **aromatic** (ar oh MAT ik). Changes in the odor of urine may be caused by disease, the presence of bacteria, or diet. A patient with diabetes may pass urine that has a fruity odor (Box 42.5). An ammonia or **putrid** (PYOO trid) smell in the urine can be caused by an infection. An ammonia smell may also be noticed in urine that has been at room temperature for too long before it is tested. Foods such as asparagus and garlic also can produce an abnormal odor in the urine. Urine from a child with *phenylketonuria* (fen l kee toh NOO r ee uh) *(PKU)* may smell "mousy" (Box 42.6). If odor seems significant, add a note in the comments field of a paper or electronic test report.

Specific Gravity. *Specific gravity* is defined as the weight of a substance compared with the weight of an equal volume of distilled water. In UA, specific gravity is the approximate measurement of the concentration of substances dissolved in the urine. The specific gravity of distilled water is 1.000. The normal specific gravity of urine ranges from 1.005 to 1.030, depending on the patient's fluid intake. Most samples fall between 1.010 and 1.025. The urine's specific gravity indicates whether the kidneys can concentrate the urine. A change in specific gravity is one of the first indications of kidney disease (Box 42.7). To measure the specific gravity, laboratories may use a refractometer or a chemical reagent strip that has been waived by the Clinical Laboratory Improvement Amendments (CLIA).

A *refractometer* (ree frak TOM I ter) measures the **refraction** (ri FRAK shuh n) of light through solids in a liquid. The result is called the *refractive index*, which, for our purposes, is the same as *specific gravity*. The refractometer requires only a drop of urine. One drop of well-mixed urine is placed under the hinged cover of the instrument. Then the value is read directly from a scale viewed through the eyepiece. Fig. 42.11 shows the refractometer on the left and the visual results of the urine in the circle on the right. The scale on the left side of the circle shows a urine specific gravity of 1.020. The refractometer must be calibrated daily with distilled water, which should read 1.000 (Fig. 42.12). Note that specific gravity carries no unit of measure after the number. See Box 42.7 for additional information on specific gravity.

The analysis that uses a **reagent strip**, also called a urine *dipstick*, is a CLIA-waived test. A reagent strip test is the most common method used for measuring specific gravity in the POL. The pad on the strip contains a chemical that is sensitive to positively charged **ions** (ahy uh n s), such as sodium (Na^+) and potassium (K^+). The pad detects the urine's specific gravity. Various color changes indicate values between 1.000 and 1.030 (see the *specific gravity* row of colors in the second figure in Procedure 42.4).

VOCABULARY

aromatic: Having a distinct, usually fragrant-smell.
glomerulonephritis: A kidney disease affecting the glomeruli of the nephron. Characterized by albumin in the urine, edema, and high blood pressure.
ion(s): An electrically charged atom or the smallest component of an element. (A cation has a positive charge, and an anion has a negative charge)
phenylalanine: An essential amino acid found in milk, eggs, and other foods.
phenylketonuria (PKU): A deficiency in the enzyme phenylalanine hydroxylase, which is responsible for converting phenylalanine into tyrosine.
putrid: Emitting a foul or decaying odor.
reagent strip: A plastic strip with paper pads that contain chemical reagents. Reagents react with analytes in the urine and are read by looking for a color change.
refraction: Bending of light waves when they pass through one substance into another substance of different density.

MEDICAL TERMINOLOGY

glomerul/o: glomerulus
-itis: inflammation
-meter: instrument used to measure
nephr/o: kidney
refract/o: bend, deflect

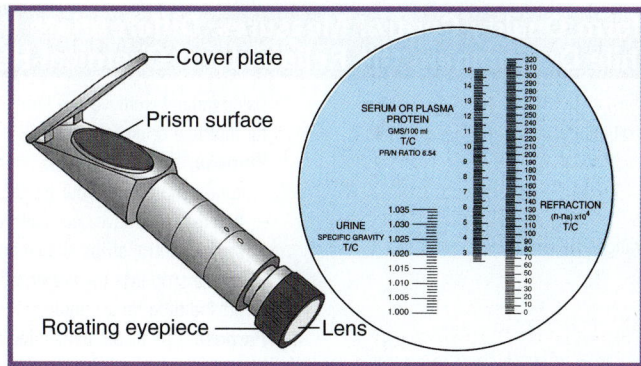

FIG. 42.11 Manual refractometer. (From Proctor D, et al: *Kinn's The Medical Assistant*, ed 13, St. Louis, 2017, Elsevier.)

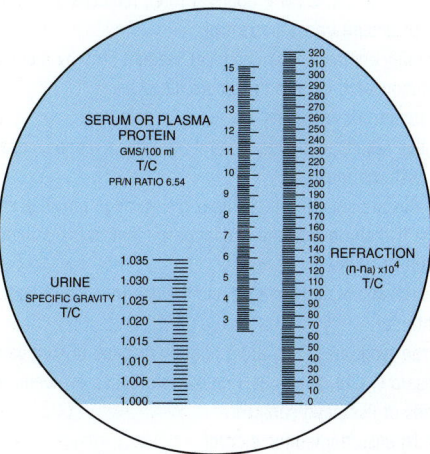

FIG. 42.12 Refractometer reading with distilled water. (From Proctor D, et al: *Kinn's The Medical Assistant*, ed 13, St. Louis, 2017, Elsevier.)

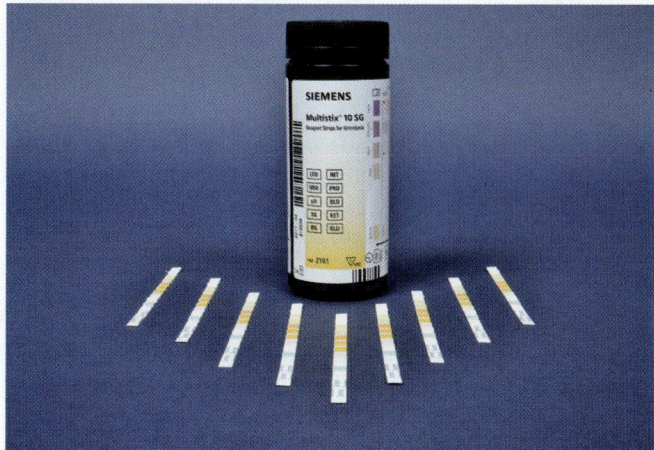

FIG. 42.13 Urine reagent strip test.

Chemical Examination of Urine

Tests can be performed on urine to detect the presence of certain chemicals, which can provide valuable information to the provider. In certain situations, these chemical test results can be critical to a diagnosis. Also, some urine dipstick results will turn positive before a patient has specific symptoms of a disease or disorder. That is one reason why a routine urinalysis can be a screening test for many conditions.

Reagent strip testing is the most widely used technique for detecting chemicals in the urine (Procedure 42.5). These strip tests are available in a variety of types (Fig. 42.13). Dipsticks are plastic strips with paper pads attached. The paper pads contain chemical reagents. The reagents react chemically with analytes in the urine. The chemical reaction is read by looking for a color change on each individual pad. See Table 42.3 for a listing of components on a routine UA reagent strip test. The presence or absence of these chemicals in the urine provides information on the status of carbohydrate metabolism, liver and kidney function, and the patient's acid-base balance.

Reagent strips are designed to be used once and then discarded in a biohazard waste container. The directions for each type of reagent strip test are included inside the package. Instructions must be followed exactly if accurate results are to be obtained. A color comparison chart is provided on the label of the container. In addition to reagent strips, a few tablet tests are available for chemically testing urine.

All strips and tablets must be kept in tightly closed containers in a cool, dry area and should be removed just before testing. To prevent contamination of the bottle, never touch a strip that has been exposed to urine against the color comparison chart on the bottle. If both a UA and a C&S have been ordered for a specimen, separate the sample. The original sample in the sterile container will go to microbiology and be used for the C&S. Pour off an aliquot into a nonsterile urine tube for the UA. If you were to introduce a reagent strip into the sterile urine sample, it would contaminate the specimen and make it unfit for C&S testing.

pH. The pH is a measurement of acidity or alkalinity of the urine. A urine specimen with a pH of 7 is neutral (Fig. 42.14). A value below 7 indicates acidity, and a value above 7 indicates alkalinity. Normal, freshly voided urine may have a pH range of 5.5 to 8. The urinary pH varies with an individual's metabolic status, diet, drug therapy, and disease. In the case of gross **bacteriuria** (bak teer ee YOO R ee uh), the urine pH is usually alkaline. Knowing the pH of the sample also helps when identifying crystals that may be found in the urine **sediment** (SED uh ment).

> **MEDICAL TERMINOLOGY**
> **bio:** life
> **micr/o:** small
> **-ology:** the study of

> **VOCABULARY**
> **bacteriuria:** The presence of bacteria in the urine (possible infection).
> **sediment:** An insoluble material that settles to the bottom of a urine specimen and to the bottom of centrifuged urine.

PROCEDURE 42.4 Perform Quality Control Measures: Differentiate Between Normal and Abnormal Test Results While Determining the Reliability of Chemical Reagent Strips

Task
Reconstitute a control sample, and test the reliability of the urinalysis chemical testing strip.

Equipment and Supplies
- Chek-Stix Control Strips with reference ranges for urinalysis
- Distilled water
- Capped tube with milliliter markings
- Test tube rack
- Forceps
- Timer
- Urine chemical strips for urine testing
- Color chart for interpreting the chemical strip results
- Fluid-impermeable lab coat, protective eyewear, and gloves
- Biohazard waste container
- Control reference sheet and control flow sheet

Procedural Steps
1. Assemble the equipment and supplies. Record the lot number and the expiration date of the Chek-Stix on the control log sheet.
   Purpose: Chek-Stix cannot be used if the expiration date has passed. Recording the lot number and expiration date is an important part of quality assurance.
2. Wash hands or use hand sanitizer. Put on the fluid-impermeable lab coat, protective eyewear, and gloves.
   Purpose: To ensure infection control. PPE is part of Standard Precautions.
3. Place a conical tube in a test tube rack, and remove the cap.
4. Pour 15 mL of distilled water into the tube.
5. Using forceps, remove one strip from the Chek-Stix bottle. Inspect the strips for mottling or discoloration.
   Purpose: The control strips have chemicals that you should not handle or contaminate with your hands. Any mottling or discoloration may mean that the strips have been exposed to moisture, light, or solvents. Improperly stored control strips should not be used.
6. Place the strip into the water, and tightly cap the tube.
7. Invert the tube for 2 minutes.
   Purpose: Chemicals embedded in the pads must be thoroughly dissolved in the water.
8. Allow the tube to sit in the rack for 30 minutes.
9. Invert the tube one more time, and remove the strip with forceps.
10. Discard the strip in the biohazard waste container. Once reconstituted, the control solution is stable for 8 hours at room temperature.
    Purpose: To ensure infection control.
11. Perform quality control of the chemical reagent strip by dipping it into the control solution according to Procedure 42.5.
12. Read and record the results.
13. Compare the results with the control reference ranges provided on the Chek-Stix package insert.
    Purpose: Results should fall within a given range provided by the manufacturer. If they do not, the chemical reagent strips cannot be used to test patients' urine.
14. Discard the chemical reagent strip and the control solution in the biohazard waste container.
15. Clean up the work area, and appropriately dispose of supplies and gloves in a biohazard waste container. Remove protective eyewear and lab coat. Wash hands or use hand sanitizer.
    Purpose: To ensure infection control.

PROCEDURE 42.5 Test Urine With Chemical Reagent Strips

Task
Perform chemical testing on a urine sample, and reassure the patient of its accuracy.

Equipment and Supplies
- Patient's record
- Urine specimen
- Reagent strips
- Timer
- Fluid-impermeable lab coat, protective eyewear, and gloves
- Biohazard waste container

Procedural Steps
1. Wash or sanitize your hands. Put on the fluid-impermeable lab coat, protective eyewear, and gloves.
   Purpose: To ensure infection control. PPE is part of Standard Precautions.
2. Check the time of collection, the container, and the mode of preservation.
   Purpose: Proper specimen identification and screening of specimens for appropriate collection containers and collection procedures prevent the testing of inappropriate specimens.
3. If the specimen has been refrigerated, allow it to warm to room temperature.
   Purpose: Certain tests are temperature dependent. Testing cold specimens may cause false-negative results.
4. Check the reagent strip container for the expiration date.
   Purpose: Do not use expired reagents.
5. Remove the reagent strip from the container. Hold it in your hand, or place it on a clean paper towel. Recap the container tightly.
   Purpose: Test strips are sensitive to moisture and light and must be stored in tightly sealed containers. Contamination from chemical residues on countertops can affect results.
6. Compare nonreactive test pads with the negative color blocks on the color chart on the container.
   Purpose: Discolored pads indicate that the product has not been properly stored and must not be used for testing.
7. Thoroughly mix the specimen by swirling.
   Purpose: If settling occurs, certain elements may not be detected.
8. Following the manufacturer's directions, note the time, dip the strip into the urine, and then remove it.
   Purpose: Tests are time dependent. Some pads darken over time.
9. Quickly remove the excess urine from the strip by pulling the back of the strip across the lip of the specimen container and then blotting the edge of the strip on a paper towel or the side of the specimen container.
   Purpose: Excess urine on the strip or prolonged dipping time affects test results.
10. Hold the strip horizontally (Fig. 1). At the required time, compare the strip with the appropriate color chart on the reagent container. *Do not touch the strip to the bottle.*

CHAPTER 42 Assisting in the Analysis of Urine

PROCEDURE 42.5 Test Urine With Chemical Reagent Strips—cont'd

11. Alternately, the strip can be placed on a paper towel.
    Purpose: Holding the strip horizontally prevents runover from one test pad to another and prevents interference from mixing chemicals in the test pads.

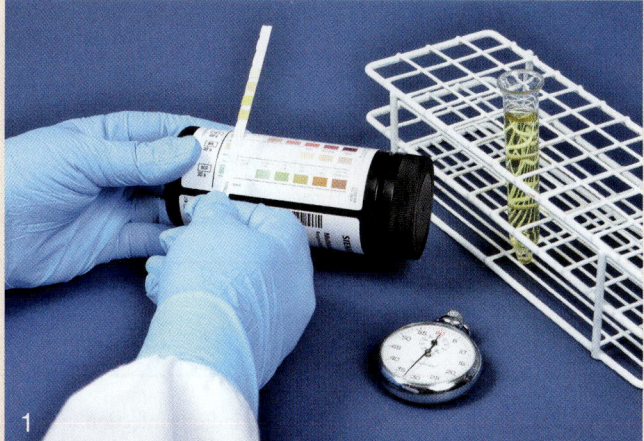

12. Read and record the first two results 30 seconds after dipping the strip (the indicated time to read the "Glucose" and "Bilirubin"). Compare the two reagent pads closest to your hand with the bottom two rows of the color chart (Fig. 2). Continue reading and recording each row of possible results with its appropriate reagent pad at its designated time.
    Purpose: Timing is critical. Allowing the strip to touch the bottle contaminates the bottle.
13. Clean the work area. If a paper towel was used, dispose of it and the reagent strip in an appropriate biohazard waste container. Remove gloves and dispose of them appropriately. Remove protective eyewear and lab coat. Wash hands or use hand sanitizer.
    Purpose: To ensure infection control.
14. Document the results in the patient's record, and reassure the patient of the accuracy of the test results.
    Purpose: A procedure is not complete until it has been documented.

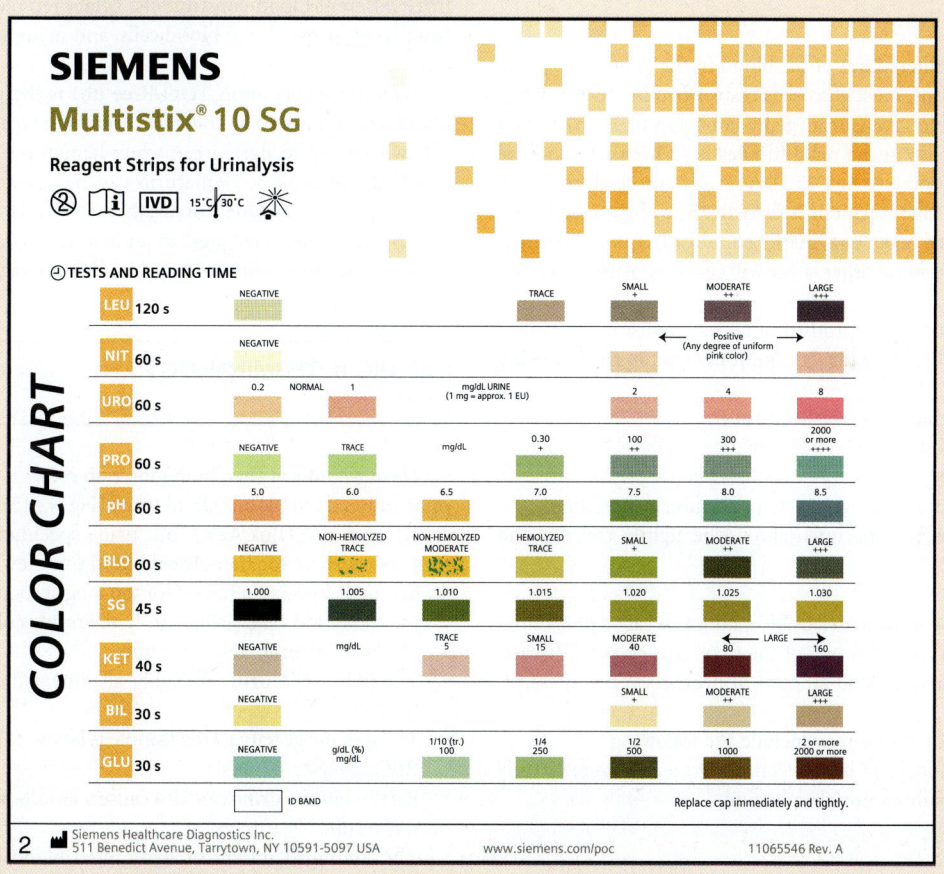

Fig. 2 ©Siemens Healthcare 2016. Used with permission.

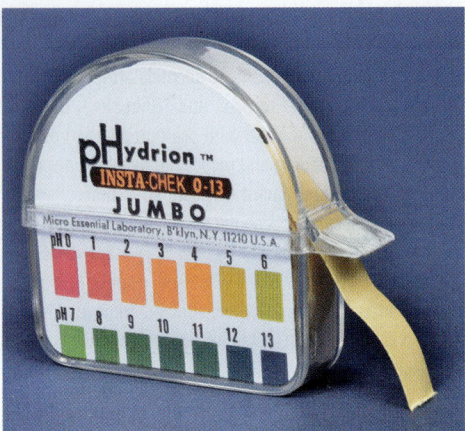

FIG. 42.14 The pH scale.

- Pregnancy: a common finding in pregnancy and must be monitored along with excessive weight gain and increased blood pressure (three possible symptoms of preeclampsia; see Chapter 31).
- After heavy exercise

The reagent strip is highly sensitive to urinary albumin and is less sensitive to the other proteins.

> **VOCABULARY**
> **bacteriuria:** The presence of bacteria in the urine (possible infection).
> **enzymatic reaction:** A specific chemical reaction controlled by an enzyme.
> **glycosuria:** An elevated urinary glucose level (possible diabetes mellitus).
> **ketonuria:** Results when there are ketones in the urine.
> **sediment:** An insoluble material that settles to the bottom of a urine specimen and to the bottom of centrifuged urine.

> **MEDICAL TERMINOLOGY**
> **orth/o:** straight, normal
> **-static:** inhibiting

Blood. The presence of blood in urine may indicate infection or trauma to the urinary tract. The blood test pad on the reagent strip reacts with three different blood constituents: intact red blood cells, hemoglobin from lysed (lahys d) red blood cells, and myoglobin (mahy uh GLOH bin).

Hematuria (hee muh TOO R ee uh) is the presence of intact red blood cells in urine. The color reaction on the reagent strip ranges from yellow to green to dark green when hematuria is present, revealing a speckled appearance. Hematuria can be caused by irritation of the kidneys, ureters, bladder, or urethra. It also is a common finding in cystitis (si STAHY tis) and in individuals passing kidney stones. A random specimen may contain blood from vaginal contamination if the woman is menstruating.

> **MEDICAL TERMINOLOGY**
> **cyst/o:** bladder

Hemoglobinuria (hee muh gloh buh NOO R ee uh) is the presence of hemolyzed red blood cells in urine (Fig. 42.15). True hemoglobinuria is not common (Box 42.8). But urine specimens that contain blood may test positive for hemolyzed blood for a few reasons:
- The urine specimen has sat for too long at room temperature, causing the red blood cells (RBCs) to lyse. Freshly collected specimens give the most accurate testing results.
- The pH of the urine is highly alkaline, which can cause RBCs to lyse.
- The specific gravity of the sample is below 1.010; this can also cause RBCs to lyse.
- Bacteria in the urine can also cause a false-positive hemolyzed blood test result.

The finding of blood or hemolyzed blood on the urine dipstick should be confirmed by microscopic examination of the urine. If intact RBCs are seen microscopically, it should be noted on the UA report to the provider.

Myoglobinuria occurs when muscle tissue is damaged or injured, as can occur with crushing injuries, myocardial infarctions, contact sports, or strenuous exercise. Patients with muscular dystrophy often have myoglobinuria. Hemoglobinuria cannot be distinguished from myoglobinuria by reagent strip testing. Both cause a uniform change in color from light green to dark green on the strip.

> **MEDICAL TERMINOLOGY**
> **glyco-:** sugar

Glucose. Glucose is filtered out of the blood in the glomerulus, and, under normal conditions, most glucose is reabsorbed in the tubules of the nephron. Detectable glycosuria (glahy kohs yoo REE uh) occurs when the filtered glucose in the renal tubules is so high it cannot be reabsorbed into the blood (see Box 42.2). A positive urine glucose may be the first indication that a patient is diabetic. The glucose pad on a reagent strip test is based on an enzymatic (en zahy MAT ik) reaction. It is specific for glucose, and no other sugar will cause a positive reaction.

Ketones. Ketones are the end product of fat metabolism in the body. Ketonuria (kee toh NOO R ee uh) is commonly seen in the following conditions:
- Diabetes mellitus that is not well controlled
- Very low-carbohydrate diets
- Excessive vomiting

Because ketones evaporate at room temperature, urine should be tested immediately, or the specimen should be tightly covered and refrigerated.

Protein. Protein in the urine in detectable amounts is called *proteinuria* (proh tee NOO R ee uh) and is one of the first signs of renal disease. We normally excrete a very small amount of protein every day that is undetectable.

Some causes of proteinuria may include the following:
- *Orthostatic* (awr thuh STAT ik) *proteinuria*: protein is excreted only when the patient is in an upright position.

> **CRITICAL THINKING 42.4**
> JulieAnn performs routine urinalysis as Becca observes. One sample has a high glucose level and a low ketone level. Becca knows that both analytes are associated with diabetes. How would you explain a high urine glucose and low urine ketone result? Write down your answer. Could there be more than one explanation? Discuss this question with your class.

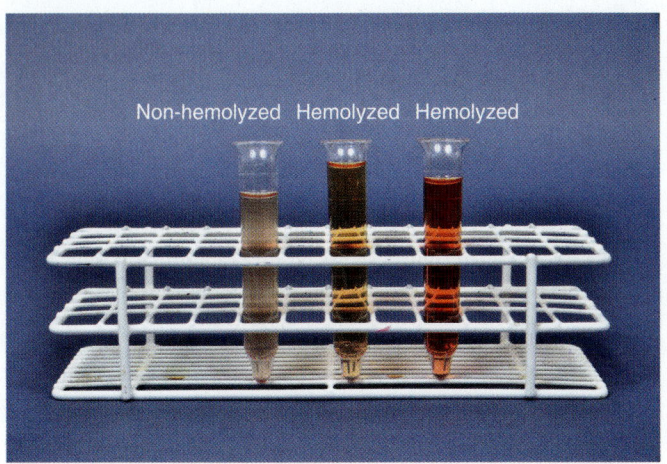

FIG. 42.15 Hemolyzed and nonhemolyzed blood in urine specimens.

BOX 42.8 True Hemoglobinuria

True hemoglobinuria is the result of intravascular red blood cell destruction and can be caused by blood transfusion reactions, malaria, drug reactions, snakebites, and severe burns.

Bilirubin and Urobilinogen. *Bilirubin* is a product of the breakdown of hemoglobin. Hemoglobin is released from old red blood cells and is gradually converted to bilirubin in the liver. The liver continues to convert bilirubin to *urobilinogen*, which is sent to the intestines for excretion. Bilirubin is a bile pigment not normally found in urine. Its

MEDICAL TERMINOLOGY
-globin: containing protein
myo-: muscle

presence in urine is one of the first signs of liver disease or other diseases in which the liver may be involved.

Bilirubinuria can occur even before jaundice (JAWN dis) or other symptoms of liver disease are evident. It is the result of liver cell damage or obstruction of the common bile duct by stones or tumors. Excessive bilirubin colors the urine yellow-brown to greenish orange. Because direct light causes bilirubin to break down, urine samples must be protected from light until testing is complete.

Urobilinogen normally is present in urine in small amounts. Elevated urobilinogen is seen with increased red blood cell destruction, liver disease, or total obstruction of the bile duct.

Nitrite. Nitrate is a common component of normal urine. *Nitrites* occur in urine when bacteria break down nitrate. A positive nitrite test result may indicate the presence of a urinary tract infection (UTI). However, not all bacteria are able to break down nitrate to nitrite. A negative nitrite test can occur when bacteria are in small numbers or when the urine has not been in the bladder long enough for the chemical breakdown to occur. *Escherichia coli* (ESCH ur reek ee ah co lye) (*E. coli*), the bacteria that is the most common cause of UTIs, does break down nitrate to nitrite. A positive reaction is any pink color on the nitrite dipstick pad.

Leukocyte Esterase. Leukocytes (white blood cells [WBCs]) are present in urine when a person has a UTI. The leukocyte esterase (ES tuh reys) test pad on the reagent strip takes 2 minutes to release esterase from white blood cells. Wait a full 2 minutes before reading the leukocyte esterase result. The test does not react with small numbers of white blood cells found in normal urine. A false-positive result could be caused by WBCs contaminants from the vagina, especially if the sample is allowed to sit at room temperature. It is very important to refrigerate urine specimens before testing or to test the samples as soon after collection as possible.

MEDICAL TERMINOLOGY
-cyte: cell
leuk/o: white

CRITICAL THINKING 42.5

One of yesterday's samples that JulieAnn saved in the laboratory refrigerator is ready to test. The sample gives a bright pink positive result for nitrites and a moderate positive result for leukocytes on the reagent strip test. What condition would give this result on a dipstick UA? Could there be more than one answer?

VOCABULARY
cystitis: Inflammation of the urinary bladder.
esterase: Any enzyme that breaks down esters (a type of organic molecule) into alcohols and acids.
intact: Complete or whole. Not broken or altered.
jaundice: Yellow discoloration of the skin, whites of the eyes, and mucous membranes due to an increase of bilirubin in the blood.
lysed: Broken apart or ruptured.
myoglobin: A type of hemoglobin found in the muscle.
myoglobinuria: The presence of myoglobin in the urine.

Limitations of Reagent Strip Testing

The reagent strip is a reliable method of testing urine if used properly. The normal urine reference ranges for a reagent strip are presented in Table 42.5. Errors can arise from several sources:
- The test strip is soaked in the specimen, and chemicals in the pads may be overly diluted.
- The test strip is not held horizontally while read, and colors from one pad may bleed onto another.
- The test pads on the strip are not read at the proper time, or the chemical reaction may be read incorrectly.
- Certain chemicals, such as vitamin C, also called *ascorbic acid* (uh SKAWR bik AC id), may affect the results of nitrite, glucose, bilirubin, and blood tests. Normal levels of vitamin C do not interfere with routine urinalysis (Box 42.9).

Urine reagent strip testing should also be performed as soon as possible after specimen collection, or samples should be refrigerated.

Visual interpretation of color on the reagent strip pads is likely to vary among individuals. Some laboratories use automated instruments to read the strips. Several companies manufacture instruments that detect the color change in the analysis of reagent strip. Once the strip has been placed in the instrument, a microprocessor controls the movement of the strip into the instrument. Light of a specific wavelength is beamed onto each of the test areas on the strip. The color change on each pad is analyzed by the microprocessor and converted into a digital reading, and the results are printed out (Fig. 42.16). The advantage of this method is that timing and color interpretation are consistent. The disadvantage is that the instrument is not able to identify and adjust for highly colored urine, leading to false results. The medical assistant should be aware of this and should manually test urine specimens that are darkly colored.

Quality Assurance and Quality Control in Urinalysis

The U.S. Food and Drug Administration (FDA) categorizes the chemical analysis of urine performed by an instrument or a reagent strip as a CLIA-waived test. The chemical analysis includes the reagent strip (dipstick) tests for bilirubin, glucose, hemoglobin or blood, ketones, leukocyte esterase, nitrite, pH, protein, specific gravity, and urobilinogen.

TABLE 42.5 Normal Urine Reference Ranges for Reagent Strips

Reference	Range
Color	Pale yellow to amber
Clarity	Clear to slightly turbid
Specific gravity	1.001–1.035
pH	4.6–8
Protein (mg/dL)	NEG
Glucose (mg/dL)	NEG
Ketone (mg/dL)	NEG
Bilirubin (mg/dL)	NEG
Blood (mg/dL)	NEG
Nitrite (mg/dL)	NEG
Urobilinogen (Ehrlich units)	0.1–1
White blood cells	NEG

From Proctor D, et al: *Kinn's The Medical Assistant*, ed 13, St. Louis, 2017, Elsevier.

BOX 42.9 Vitamin C

If a person consumes large amounts of vitamin C, a special strip can be used to detect interfering levels of vitamin C. If an elevated level is found, the patient should be instructed to discontinue vitamin C intake for 24 hours, and then another urine specimen should be collected for testing.

A commercially available control strip should be used to determine the reliability of the reagent strips used in chemical analysis. One such control strip is the Chek-Stix. The plastic control strip has seven pads, each of which contains synthetic ingredients that mimic human urine when reconstituted (ree KON sti too tid) in water. After reconstitution, a reagent test strip is immersed in the control solution, and the results are compared with a chart that accompanies the Chek-Stix. Both positive and negative Chek-Stix controls are available (see Procedure 42.4). The positive reconstituted control shows positive (abnormal) results when a test strip is inserted and read, whereas the negative reconstituted control shows normal urinalysis results along its test strip. It is important to observe and record the abnormal and normal results produced by the positive and negative controls. Also, make sure the test results are consistent with the Chek-Stix charts provided by the manufacturer before testing patient urine specimens.

The Chek-Stix is one type of commercial control, but others strips and prepared liquid controls are also available. Each POL should investigate the best commercial control for its needs and quality control program.

MICROSCOPIC PREPARATION AND EXAMINATION OF URINE SEDIMENT

Microscopic examination of urine consists of categorizing and counting cells, casts, crystals, and miscellaneous constituents in the sediment of a urine sample. The sediment is obtained after a measured portion of urine is centrifuged. The sediment will be pushed to the bottom of the tube containing urine. The sediment will be prepared for a microscopic exam, and the remaining liquid urine will be poured off and disposed of properly.

Many formed elements are found in the urine. Some are significant, and others are not. Most important, the microscopic examination should correlate with the physical and chemical analyses. For example, if the physical examination of the urine appeared reddish in color and the chemical reagent strip tested positive for blood, then seeing red blood cells during the microscopic examination would be consistent with physical and chemical results. Medical assistants should be familiar with the preparation of urine specimens for this test and with the possible test results (Procedure 42.6).

Microscopic Preparation of Urine

To perform the microscopic UA procedure, a laboratory must be certified to perform CLIA Provider Performed Microscopy Procedures (PPMPs),

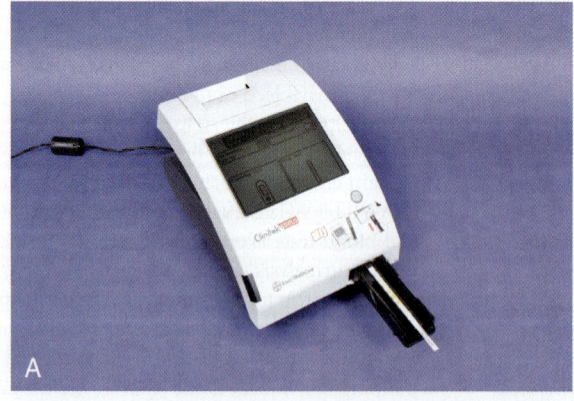
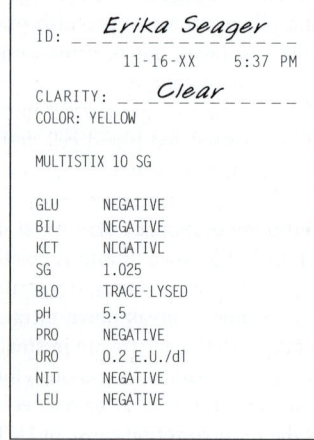

FIG. 42.16 Clinitek 50 urine chemistry analyzer and printout. (From Proctor D, et al: *Kinn's The Medical Assistant*, ed 13, St. Louis, 2017, Elsevier.)

PROCEDURE 42.6   Prepare a Urine Specimen for Microscopic Examination

Task
Prepare a urine specimen for the provider's microscopic examination to determine the presence of normal and abnormal elements.

Equipment and Supplies
- Patient's record
- Urine specimen
- Centrifuge tube
- Centrifuge
- Disposable pipet
- Sedi-Stain
- Microscope slide and coverslip
- Microscope
- Permanent marker
- Fluid-impermeable lab coat, protective eyewear, and gloves
- Biohazard waste container

Procedural Steps
1. Wash hands or use hand sanitizer. Put on the fluid-impermeable lab coat, protective eyewear, and gloves.
   Purpose: To ensure infection control. PPE is part of Standard Precautions.
2. Gently mix the urine specimen by swirling the covered specimen container.
   Purpose: If the urine is not well mixed, elements that have settled to the bottom of the specimen container will be missed.
3. Pour 12 mL of urine into a labeled centrifuge tube, and cap the tube.
4. Place the tube in the centrifuge (Fig. 1).

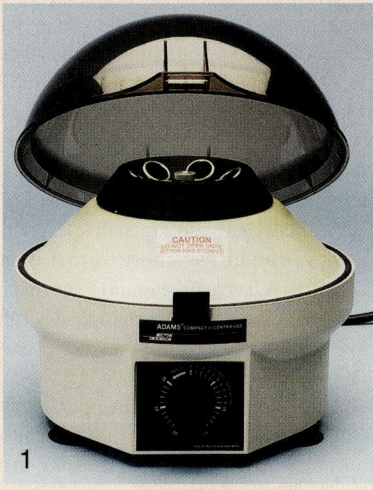

5. Place another tube containing 12 mL of urine or water in the opposite cup.
   Purpose: For proper operation, centrifuges must be carefully balanced. If not properly balanced, damage to the instrument can occur.
6. Secure the lid and centrifuge for 5 minutes or for the time specified for your instrument.
   Purpose: Timing varies according to the speed and the size of the centrifuge head.
7. Remove the tube from the centrifuge after the instrument has come to a full stop.
8. Pour off the clear supernatant from the top of the specimen by inverting the centrifuge tube over the sink drain while allowing the running water from the faucet to flush the urine down the drain. Turn the tube upright when the supernatant has been decanted, allowing a small amount to return to the sediment on the bottom of the tube without losing sediment down the drain (Figs. 2 and 3).
   Purpose: The sediment will be examined under the microscope.

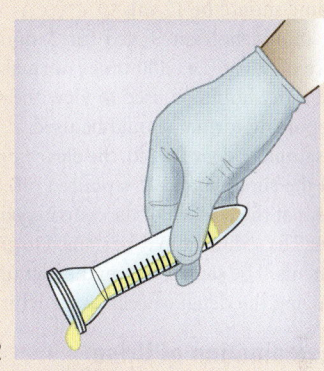

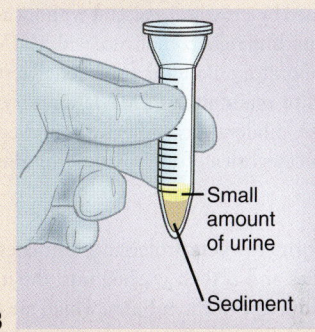

9. Thoroughly mix the sediment with a drop of Sedi-Stain by grasping the tube near the top and rapidly flicking it with the fingers of the other hand until all sediment is thoroughly resuspended.
   Purpose: Elements centrifuge at different rates. Failure to mix the entire sediment completely may result in evaluation errors. Sedi-Stain colors the sediment for easier viewing.
10. Transfer 1 drop of sediment to a clean, labeled slide using a clean, disposable transfer pipet.
11. Place a clean coverslip over the drop, and place the slide on the microscope stage. Remove eye protection.
12. Focus under low power and reduce the light.
    Note: Once the slide is focused under low power, the remaining steps of this procedure are performed by the trained healthcare provider or moderate/highly complex trained laboratory personnel.

Fig. 1 from Stepp CA, Woods MA: *Laboratory Procedures for Medical Office Personnel*, Philadelphia, 1998, Saunders.

a subcategory of CLIA moderate-complexity laboratories. Quality assurance is just as important in the microscopic examination as in the chemical analysis of urine. To ensure consistency and standardization, commercially available systems can be used, such as the KOVA System or the UriSystem. These systems may include specially designed, graduated centrifuge tubes with devices or pipets that allow easy **decanting** (dee KANT ihng) of **supernatant** (soo per NEYT nt) and retention of an exact amount of sediment. They also use specially designed plastic slides with wells or coverslips that accept only a given volume of sediment. Control solutions containing preserved cells are also available from KOVA. This type of solution provides quality control for cell identification too. Whatever system is used, the Clinical and Laboratory Standards Institute (CLSI) recommends the following:

- The urine volume should be 12 mL.
- The specimen should be centrifuged for 5 minutes at a relative centrifugal force of 400 *g* (i.e., 400 times normal gravity).
- A standardized slide should be used to view the sediment.
- A consistent reporting format should be used.

When a urine sample is centrifuged, the clear upper portion of the specimen is called the supernatant. It is poured off, and a drop of the well-mixed sediment at the bottom of the centrifuged tube is examined under a microscope. The sediment may be stained to give greater contrast to the formed elements. The stain assists in the identification of formed elements by improving the detail of cellular structures.

Microscopic Examination of Urine

The examination of urine is not categorized as CLIA waived; therefore it cannot be performed by a medical assistant without additional training, additional supervision, and rigid compliance with CLIA quality assurance protocols for the laboratory. Periodic proficiency testing must be successfully completed to maintain a PPMP laboratory certification. See Chapter 41 for CLIA moderate-complexity approved personnel.

The three main categories of microscopic findings are casts, cells, and crystals.

Casts. *Casts* are formed when protein accumulates and precipitates in the kidney tubules and is then washed into the urine. The protein takes on the size and shape of the tubules, which are called casts. Casts are cylindric (si LIN drik), with flat or rounded ends, and are classified according to the substances observed inside of them. Certain types of casts are connected to specific renal diseases and disorders. Other casts are physiologic (fi zee uh LOJ ik) and are generally caused by strenuous exercise (Table 42.6). Casts can dissolve in alkaline urine if the sample is not examined promptly. Microscopic exam should take place as soon as possible after specimen collection.

> **VOCABULARY**
> **crenate:** Having a cell surface that is bumpy, scalloped, or indented.
> **decanting:** Pouring a liquid gently so that it does not disturb the remaining sediment.
> **hyaline:** Glassy or transparent.
> **supernatant:** The clear liquid above the sediment in a centrifuged urine specimen.

> **MEDICAL TERMINOLOGY**
> **hyper-:** over, above, beyond
> **hypo-:** below, beneath, under
> **super-:** above or superior

Cells. Cells found in the urine include epithelial cells, which come from the lining of the genitourinary tract. Red blood cells and white blood cells come from the bloodstream. Cells are classified and counted under high-power magnification.

Red blood cells may enter the urinary tract at any point of inflammation or injury. They may be found in normal urine in small numbers. Persistent hematuria should be investigated. Red blood cells are smaller than white blood cells and have no nucleus (Fig. 42.17). If they are in *hypotonic* (dilute) urine, they swell and burst. In *hypertonic* (concentrated) urine, they may **crenate** (KREE neyt) and wrinkle.

> **CRITICAL THINKING 42.6**
> Becca is excited to look in the microscope and see a urine sediment that has been prepared for the nurse practitioner at WMFM, Jean Burke. As Becca looks in the microscope's eyepiece, she sees quite a few red blood cells. What could cause red blood cells to be present in the urine? Discuss your thoughts with the class.

Yeast cells in the urine may indicate vaginal contamination or a urinary yeast infection (Fig. 42.18). Yeast is common in the urine of patients with diabetes. Yeasts cells are oval shaped and may show budding.

White blood cells may occasionally be found in normal urine, but increased numbers are associated with a UTI or with vaginal contamination during specimen collection. White blood cells are larger than red blood cells and have a granular appearance. They may have a multilobed nucleus. Most white blood cells in the urine are neutrophils (Fig. 42.19).

Squamous epithelial cells line the lower portion of the genitourinary tract. When present in large numbers in female patients, they usually indicate vaginal contamination. Squamous epithelial cells are large, flat, and irregular. They have a single, small, round, centrally located nucleus and often occur in sheets or clumps (see Fig. 42.19).

Transitional epithelial cells line most of the urinary tract. They are round or oval and may have a tail. Occasionally, two nuclei are seen. They may be seen in diseases of the urinary system (Fig. 42.20).

Renal tubular epithelial cells are somewhat larger than white blood cells, are round or oval, and have a nucleus that is single, large, oval, and sometimes eccentric. A few may be found in normal urine specimens, but their presence in increased numbers indicates tubular damage of the nephrons (Fig. 42.21).

Crystals. Crystals are common in urine specimens, particularly if the specimen has been allowed to cool. Cooling causes solid crystals to precipitate out of the urine, which changes the urine's appearance from clear to cloudy. The presence of most crystals is not clinically

> **STUDY TIP**
> When looking at the different types of epithelial cell in urine, it is helpful to remember the appearance of eggs:
> - Squamous cells resemble fried eggs with a large nuclear "yolk" surrounded by the runny whites.
> - Transitional cells are much smaller and resemble poached eggs.
> - Renal tubular round epithelial cells resemble hard-boiled eggs that have been cut in half.

significant unless the crystals are found in large numbers. With only rare exceptions, abnormal crystals are seen in acidic urine. Abnormal crystals may be present because of certain disease states or an inherited metabolic condition. They may also be *iatrogenic* (ahy a truh JEN ik), which means they are present because of medication or treatment. Identification of crystals begins with noting the pH of the urine specimen. A history of medications and recent diagnostic testing may be helpful too.

Crystals are reported as occasional, few, moderate, or many per high-power field (Table 42.7). At times, crystals can be *amorphous* (uh MAWR fuh s) or lacking a defined shape. Frequently crystals are difficult to identify without additional chemical testing.

TABLE 42.6 Types of Urinary Casts

Name of Cast	Description	Associated With Disease or Disorder	Additional Notes	Photo Example
Hyaline casts (HAHY uh leen)	Pale, transparent, cylinder shaped, rounded ends and parallel sides	Found in individuals with kidney disease or in people who have exercised heavily	Easy to miss if lighting is too bright; adjust condenser to dim light	
White blood cell casts	Hyaline casts that contain WBCs	Occur in patients with pyelonephritis (pahy uh loh nuh FRAHY tis)	WBCs usually have a multilobed nucleus	
Red blood cell casts	Hyaline casts with embedded RBCs	Occur in patients with glomerulonephritis (gloh mer yuh loh nuh FRAHY tis)	They may appear brown	

Continued

TABLE 42.6 Types of Urinary Casts—cont'd

Name of Cast	Description	Associated With Disease or Disorder	Additional Notes	Photo Example
Renal tubular epithelial cell casts[a]	Hyaline casts with embedded renal tubular epithelial cells	Occur in patients with shock, renal ischemia (ih SKEE mee uh), heavy-metal poisoning, some allergic reactions, nephrotoxic (nef rot TOK sik) drugs, and excessive renal damage	Can be confused with WBC casts if cells have started to break down	
Finely and coarsely granular casts[b]	Hyaline casts with coarse or fine granular inclusions	May indicate renal disease	Granules are caused by protein clumping or a breakdown of cellular inclusions	
Waxy casts[b]	Glassy, brittle, smooth, uniform structures usually yellowish, have cracks and squared or broken ends	Occur in patients with severe renal disease	May be degenerated cellular casts, rarely seen	

[a]From Brunzel NA: *Fundamentals of Urine and Body Fluid Analysis,* ed 3, Philadelphia, 2013, Saunders.
[b]From Stepp CA, Woods MA: *Laboratory Procedures for Medical Office Personnel,* Philadelphia, 1998, Saunders.

VOCABULARY
nephrotoxic: Damaging or destructive to the kidneys.
renal ischemia: A blood flow deficiency to the kidney(s).

Miscellaneous Findings. *Oval fat bodies* are formed when renal tubular epithelial cells or macrophages absorb fats. The fat droplets in the cells vary in size. They are characteristic of kidney distress (Fig. 42.22).

MEDICAL TERMINOLOGY
a-: without, not
morph/o: form, shape, structure
nephr/o: kidney
-ous: possessing
tox/o: poison

TABLE 42.7 Normal and Abnormal Crystals Found in Urine

NORMAL CRYSTALS

Acid Urine	Alkaline Urine	Abnormal Crystals
Calcium oxalate[a] 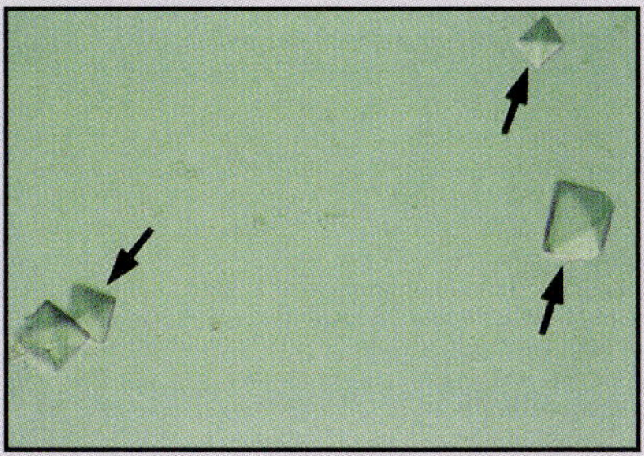	Ammonium biurate[b] 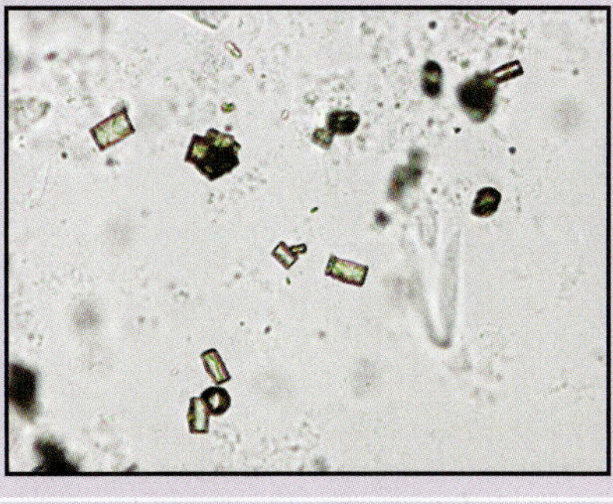	Sulfonamide 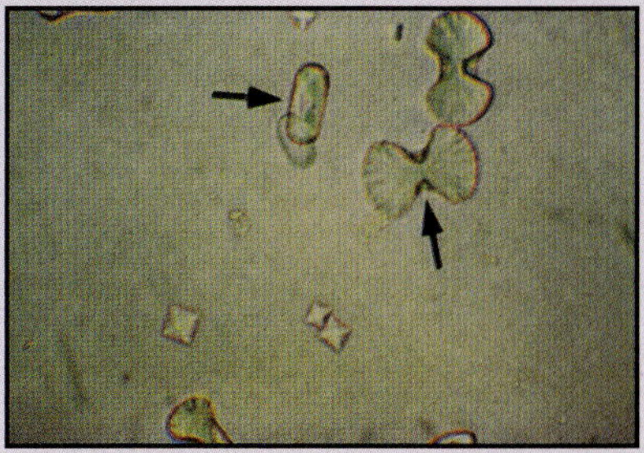
Uric acid[b] 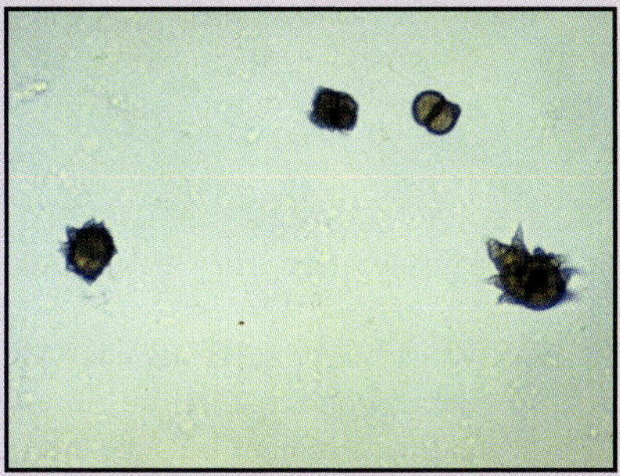	Triple phosphate[a] 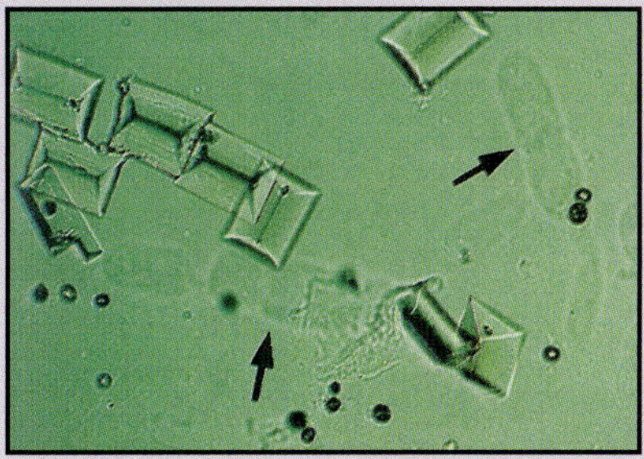	Cholesterol[a] 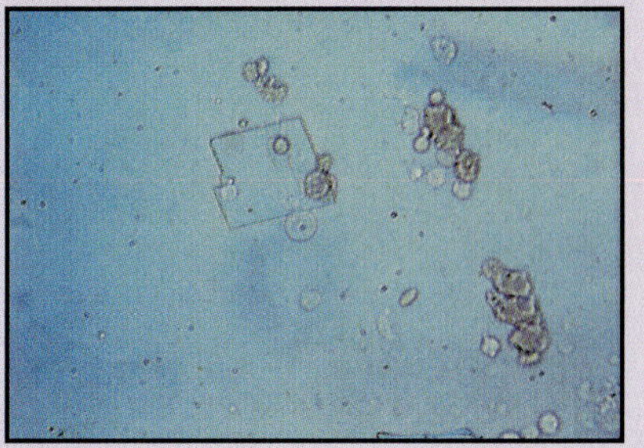

[a]From Stepp CA, Woods MA: *Laboratory Procedures for Medical Office Personnel,* Philadelphia, 1998, Saunders.
[b]From Brunzel NA: *Fundamentals of Urine and Body Fluid Analysis,* ed 3, Philadelphia, 2013, Saunders.

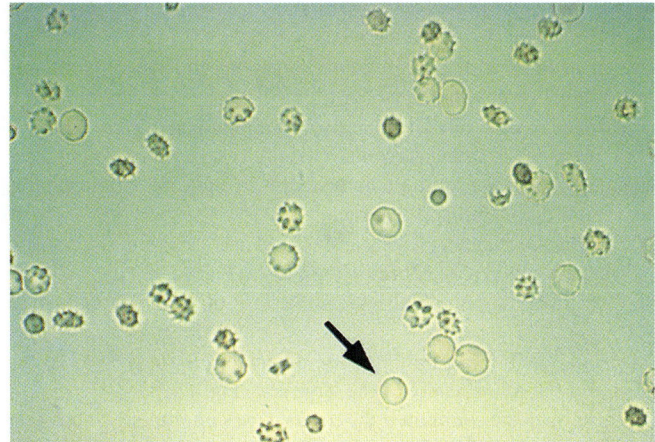

FIG. 42.17 RBCs in urine. (From Stepp CA, Woods MA: *Laboratory Procedures for Medical Office Personnel,* Philadelphia, 1998, Saunders.)

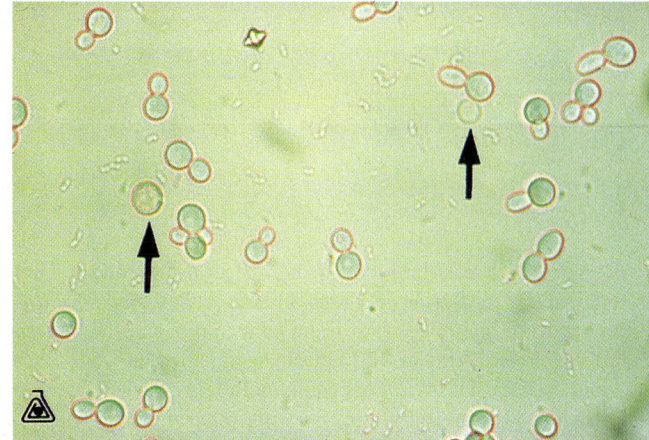

FIG. 42.18 Yeast cells in urine. (From Stepp CA, Woods MA: *Laboratory Procedures for Medical Office Personnel,* Philadelphia, 1998, Saunders.)

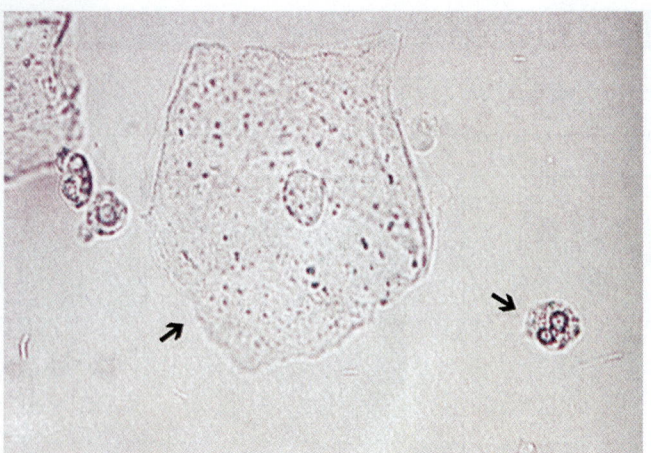

FIG. 42.19 WBCs and squamous epithelial cells in urine. (From Ringsrud KM, Linne JJ: *Urinalysis and Body Fluids: A Color Text and Atlas*, St. Louis, 1995, Mosby.)

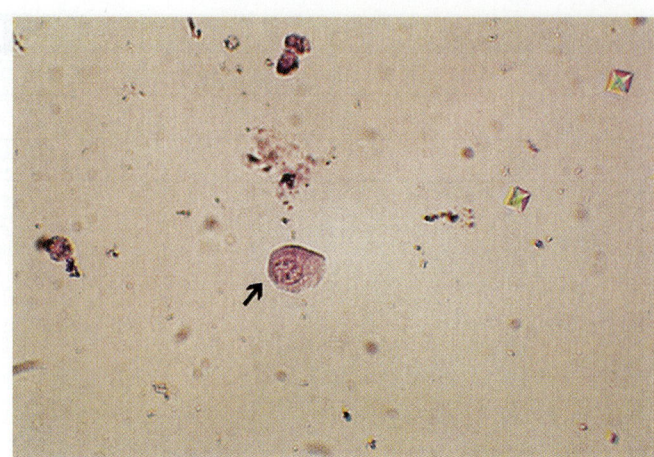

FIG. 42.21 Renal epithelial cells in urine. (From Ringsrud KM, Linne JJ: *Urinalysis and Body Fluids: A Color Text and Atlas*, St. Louis, 1995, Mosby.)

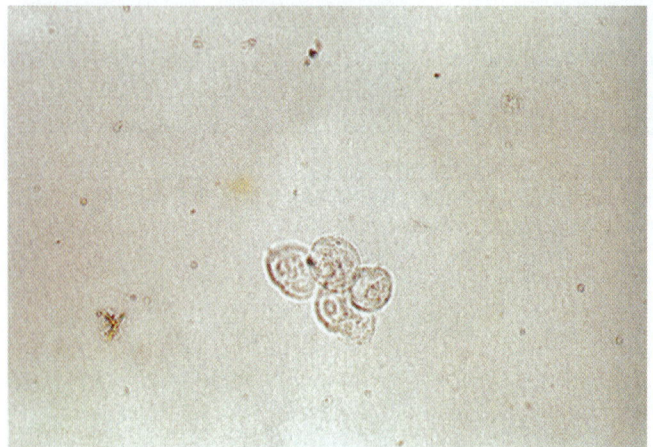

FIG. 42.20 Transitional epithelial cells in urine. (From Ringsrud KM, Linne JJ: *Urinalysis and Body Fluids: A Color Text and Atlas*, St. Louis, 1995, Mosby.)

have pointed, oval heads and long, whip-like tails. They may be motile in fresh urine.

Trichomonas vaginalis (trik uh MOH nuhs vaj IH nal uhs) is the most commonly encountered **protozoa** (proh tuh ZOH uh) in urine (Fig. 42.24). It is frequently a vaginal contaminant but may also be found in urine specimens from male patients. When urine is fresh and warm, trichomonas may be motile and move rapidly when viewed under the microscope. Trichomonas organisms are pear-shaped protozoa with four **flagella** (fluh JEL uh). They are larger than round epithelial cells but smaller than squamous cells. Trichomonas organisms die when the specimen cools.

Mucous threads can be found in most urine specimens. They appear as pale, irregular, threadlike structures with tapered ends. Beginners often confuse hyaline casts with mucous threads. They are frequently seen in patients with inflammation and in specimens contaminated with vaginal secretions (Fig. 42.25).

Artifacts (AHR tuh fakts) and contaminants are often found in urine sediment. Training is required to tell them apart from significant structures. Fibers are common in the sediment and come from clothing, diapers, or digested plant material:

- Clothing fibers often are long and twisted and sometimes are colored. Diaper fibers can be confused with casts (Fig. 42.26).
- Plant fibers appear in the urine because of fecal contamination (Fig. 42.27).
- Hair is distinct not only because of the visible rough look to the strand but also because of the large size (Fig. 42.28).
- Air bubbles are common if the coverslip was improperly placed over the sediment. Air bubbles are structureless and *refractile* (refracting light causing a glow) and have a dark outline (Fig. 42.29).

A few bacteria may be found in normal urine specimens. High bacterial counts in a urine specimen without white blood cells may indicate that the specimen sat at room temperature and the bacteria multiplied. Urine specimens with a putrid odor, numerous white blood cells, and bacteria (Fig. 42.23) are common in UTIs. Bacteria are seen under high-power magnification. They are often *motile* (MOH til) (moving).

Spermatozoa (spur mat uh ZOH uh) can be found in the urine specimens of both male and female patients. In a specimen from a female, their presence represents vaginal contamination. Sperm usually

---

MEDICAL TERMINOLOGY

proto-: first formed, primitive, original
-zoa: animal, organism

VOCABULARY

flagella: Thread-like or whip-like extensions of a cell that help the cell move.
protozoa: Single-celled organisms that are the most primitive form of animal life. Most are microscopic. Examples are amoebas, ciliates, flagellates, and sporozoans.

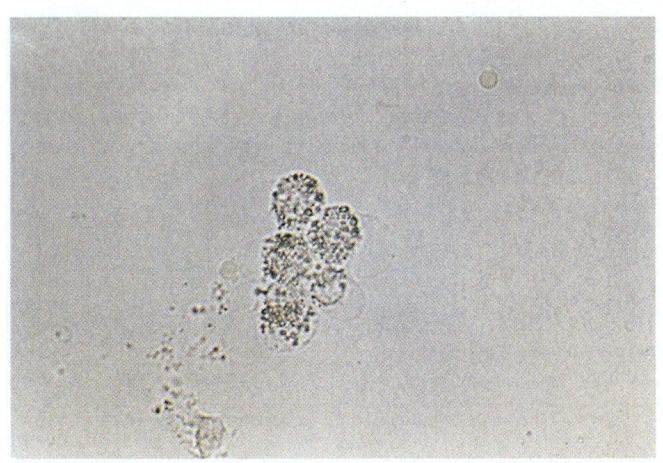
FIG. 42.22 Oval fat bodies in urine. (From Ringsrud KM, Linne JJ: *Urinalysis and Body Fluids: A Color Text and Atlas,* St. Louis, 1995, Mosby.)

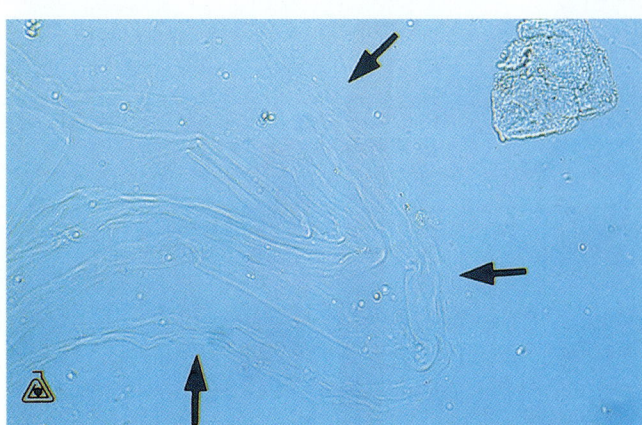
FIG. 42.25 Mucous threads in urine. (From Stepp CA, Woods MA: *Laboratory Procedures for Medical Office Personnel,* Philadelphia, 1998, Saunders.)

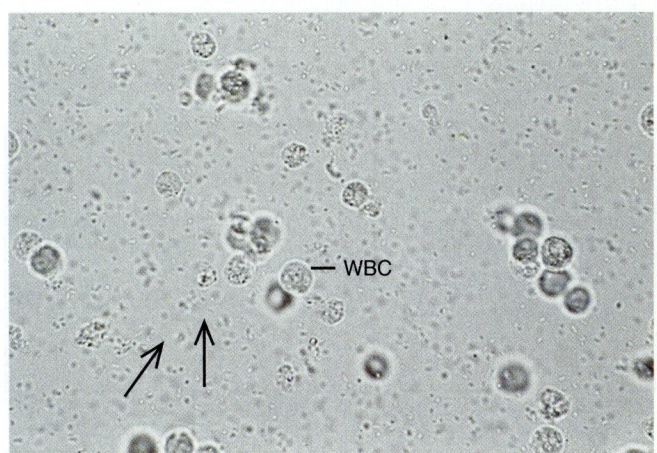
FIG. 42.23 Bacteria and WBCs in urine. (From Ringsrud KM, Linne JJ: *Urinalysis and Body Fluids: A Color Text and Atlas,* St. Louis, 1995, Mosby.)

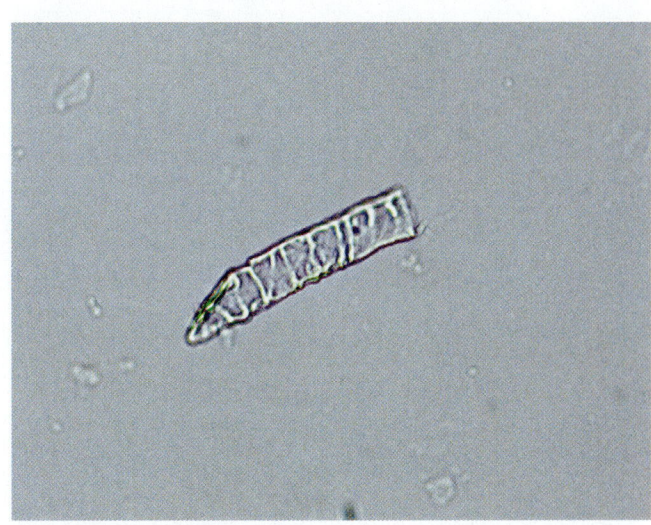
FIG. 42.26 Diaper fibers in urine. (From Brunzel NA: *Fundamentals of Urine and Body Fluid Analysis,* ed 3, Philadelphia, 2013, Saunders.)

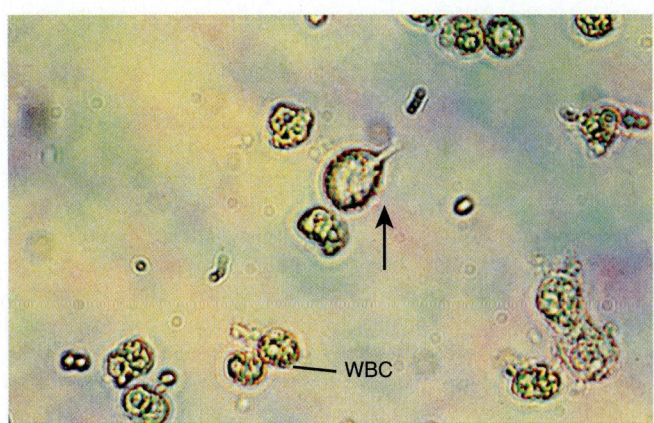
FIG. 42.24 *Trichomonas sp.* in urine. (From Stepp CA, Woods MA: *Laboratory Procedures for Medical Office Personnel,* Philadelphia, 1998, Saunders.)

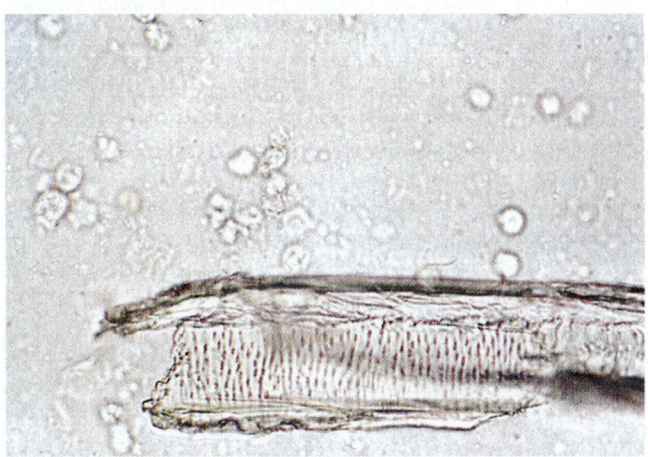
FIG. 42.27 Plant fiber from fecal contamination in urine. (From Ringsrud KM, Linne JJ: *Urinalysis and Body Fluids: A Color Text and Atlas,* St. Louis, 1995, Mosby.)

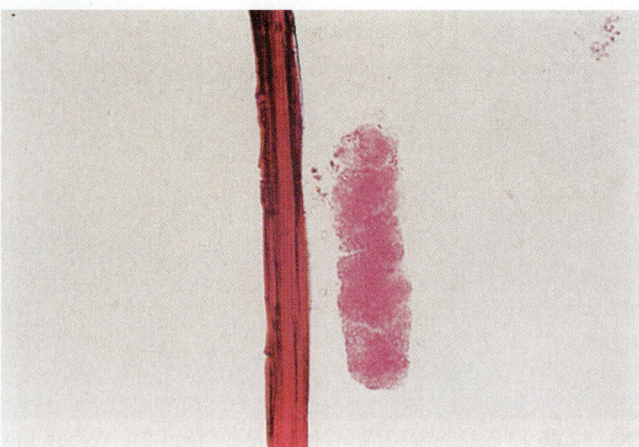

FIG. 42.28 Fiber, probably hair *(left)* and waxy cast *(right)* in urine. (From Ringsrud KM, Linne JJ: *Urinalysis and Body Fluids: A Color Text and Atlas,* St. Louis, 1995, Mosby.)

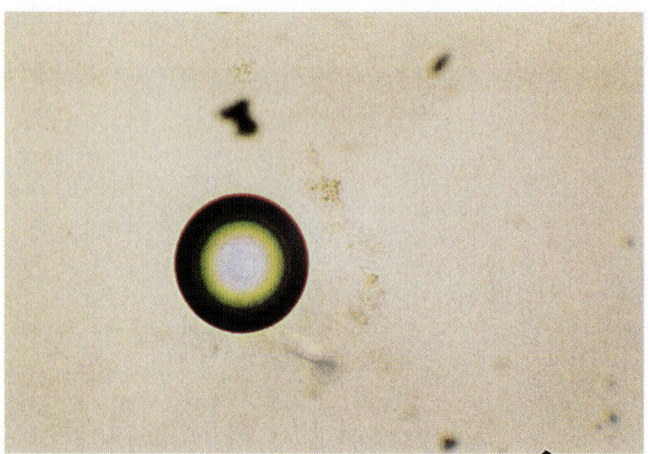

FIG. 42.29 Large air bubble in urine. (From Ringsrud KM, Linne JJ: *Urinalysis and Body Fluids: A Color Text and Atlas,* St. Louis, 1995, Mosby.)

BOX 42.10 Microscopic Examination: Casts, RBCs, and WBCs

Casts, white blood cells, and red blood cells are counted, totaled, and averaged. Casts, white blood cells, and red blood cells are reported using numeric ranges based on the average:
- 0
- 0–1
- 1–2
- 2–5
- 5–10
- 10–20 and so forth
- *TNTC:* too numerous to count

BOX 42.11 Microscopic Examination: Epithelial Cells

Epithelial cells are counted, totaled, and averaged, then they are reported as occasional, few, moderate, or many (per high-powered field), as follows:
- 1–3: occasional
- 4–6: few
- 7–12: moderate
- >12: many

BOX 42.12 Microscopic Examination: Miscellaneous

The miscellaneous elements are counted, then averaged, and estimated as occasional, few, moderate, or many, as follows:
- Occasional: not seen in every field
- Few: covers less than a quarter of the field
- Moderate: covers approximately half of the field
- Many: covers the entire field

BOX 42.13 Sugars in Urine

Certain metabolic disorders can result in the excretion of sugars such as *galactose* (guh LAK tohs), fructose, lactose, maltose, or pentose. *Galactosemia,* a rare pathologic condition, is a congenital deficiency in the body's ability to break down galactose to glucose. Galactosemia results in excretion of galactose in the urine. In an infant it results in failure to thrive, vomiting, and diarrhea. If detected early, galactose can be eliminated from the diet, and the child develops normally. Lactose may be found in the urine of pregnant women or premature infants, but it is not associated with disease. Maltose may be excreted in patients with diabetes.

Understanding the Results of Microscopic Examination

The medical assistant should understand how the microscopic findings of the sediment are reported. First, the sediment is examined under the low-power objective and low light to locate casts, which generally are found around the edges of the coverslip. From 10 to 15 low-power fields are scanned, and the number of casts is counted and reported.

Red and white blood cells, epithelial cells, yeasts, bacteria, and crystals are identified using the high-power objective and increased light. From 10 to 15 high-powered fields should be scanned and the number counted, averaged, and reported. The method of counting varies considerably among laboratories. It is important that all workers in the same laboratory use the same counting and reporting systems.

The results of the microscopic examination are reported as seen in Boxes 42.10 through 42.12.

ADDITIONAL CLIA-WAIVED TESTS PERFORMED ON URINE

Clinitest

The glucose test on the reagent strip detects only glucose, the most common sugar found in the urine. However, sugars other than glucose also can appear in the urine. See Box 42.13 for a brief overview of other sugars that can be found in the urine. Of the many sugars in the body, only the presence of glucose or galactose indicates possible pathologic conditions.

The *Clinitest* is based on the chemical reduction of copper. It is used to detect reducing substances (sugars) in the urine (Procedure 42.7). Copper reduction tests are based on the principle that reducing substances can chemically convert one form of copper into another form of copper. The chemical reaction produces a color change. The Clinitest uses a reagent tablet that is dropped directly into a test tube containing diluted urine. A heat-releasing reaction occurs and causes the Clinitest contents to boil. The reaction only takes a few seconds and then the boiling stops. After the reaction is complete, the color of the reaction is compared with the color chart supplied by the manufacturer. See Box 42.14 for additional information on reading Clinitest reactions.

Urine Pregnancy Testing

All pregnancy tests detect the presence of *human chorionic gonadotropin (hCG)*, a hormone produced by the placenta and present in urine during pregnancy (Procedure 42.8). After the fertilized egg has implanted in

> ### CRITICAL THINKING 42.7
> JulieAnn has three specimens that she needs to run a Clinitest, but first she needs to complete the quality control samples: one positive control and one negative control. She has Becca read the procedure and then put on gloves and protective eyewear. JulieAnn performs the quality control tests, and Becca watches as the tests bubble and boil. Why was it important for Becca to have on PPE during this test and during her whole time in the lab? Share your thoughts with your class.

PROCEDURE 42.7   Test Urine for Glucose Using the Clinitest Method

Task
Perform confirmatory testing for glucose and other simple sugars in the urine using the Clinitest procedure for reducing substances.

Equipment and Supplies
- Patient's record
- Urine specimen
- Clinitest tablet, test tube, and transfer pipet
- Distilled water
- Test tube rack
- Appropriate-sized plastic or metal forceps
- Color chart
- Timer
- Fluid-impermeable lab coat, protective eyewear, and gloves
- Biohazard waste container

Procedural Steps

1. Wash hands or use hand sanitizer. Put on fluid-impermeable lab coat, protective eyewear, and gloves.
2. Holding a transfer pipet vertically, add 10 drops of distilled water and then 5 drops of urine to a test tube.
   Purpose: Holding the transfer pipet vertically prevents alteration of the size of the drops.
3. Place the prepared tube in the test tube rack (Fig. 1).
   Purpose: The tube will become too hot to hold after the tablet is placed in the tube.

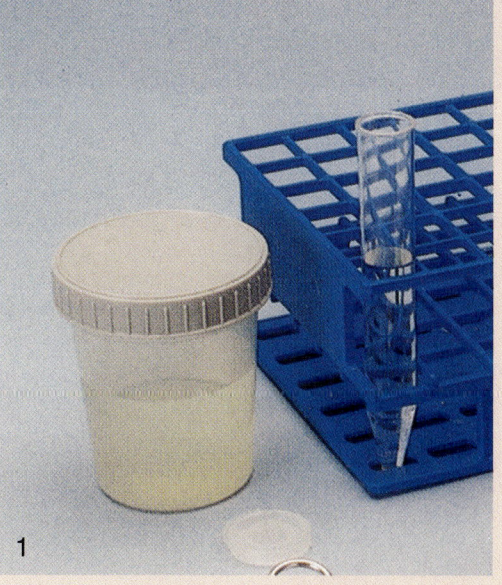

4. Remove a Clinitest tablet from the bottle by shaking a tablet into the bottle cap.
   Purpose: Clinitest tablets react with moisture and became caustic.
   Do not handle Clinitest tablets with your hands or gloved hands. Always use a forceps to transfer the tablet to the test tube.
5. Using a metal or plastic forceps, pick up the Clinitest tablet from the bottle cap, and drop the tablet into the prepared test tube. Recap the container.
6. With the test tube in the rack, observe the entire reaction to detect the rapid pass-through phenomenon, which indicates that the glucose level in the urine is very high (see the note in step 8).
   Purpose: If pass-through occurs but is not detected, the reading will be falsely low.
7. When boiling stops, time exactly 15 seconds and then gently shake the tube to mix all of the contents.
8. Immediately compare the color of the specimen with the five-drop color chart, and record your findings (Fig. 2).
   Note: If an orange color briefly develops during the reaction and then converts to a lower, darker color, rapid pass-through has occurred, meaning that the glucose was greater than the highest reading; this is recorded as "greater than 2%."
   Purpose: For accurate results, wait 15 seconds and then quickly read results. Color results will continue to darken over time.

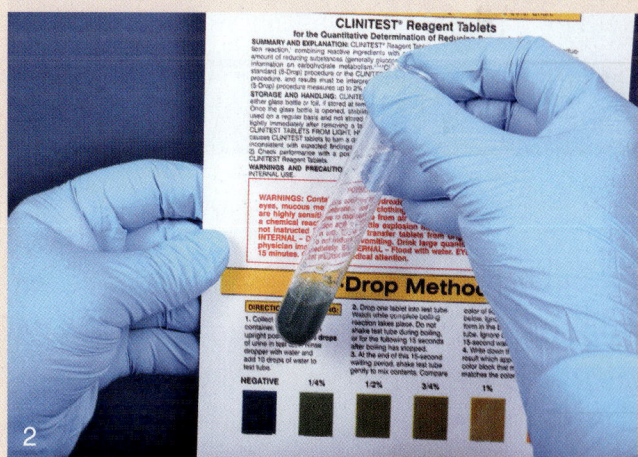

9. Record the results.
10. Clean up the work area, dispose of supplies in appropriate waste containers, then remove your gloves. Remove the fluid-impermeable lab coat and protective eyewear. Wash hands or use hand sanitizer.
    Purpose: To ensure infection control.
11. Record the results in the patient's record.
    Purpose: A procedure is not considered finished until it is recorded.

1040 UNIT 6 Medical Laboratory

> **BOX 42.14 Reading Clinitest Reactions**
>
> Clinitest Reaction Note: If the color change reaches the orange maximum color during the reaction and then ends in a lower color range, the test result is reported as "greater than" the highest positive result.

the uterus, the hCG levels in serum double every few days. This rapid rise occurs for approximately 7 weeks, and then the level begins to decline. Within 72 hours of delivery, the hormone disappears.

The most common type of test for pregnancy is the **lateral flow immunoassay** (im yuh noh uh SEY) test. Many brands are available

---

PROCEDURE 42.8   Perform a CLIA-Waived Urinalysis: Perform a Pregnancy Test

Task
Perform a pregnancy test on urine using the QuickVue pregnancy test method.

Equipment and Supplies
- Patient's record
- Urine specimen
- QuickVue test kit
- Fluid-impermeable lab coat, protective eyewear, and gloves
- Biohazard waste container

Procedural Steps
1. Wash hands or use hand sanitizer. Put on fluid-impermeable lab coat, protective eyewear, and gloves.
   Purpose: Hand sanitization is an important step for infection control. PPE is part of Standard Precautions.
2. Prepare the testing equipment (Fig. 1).

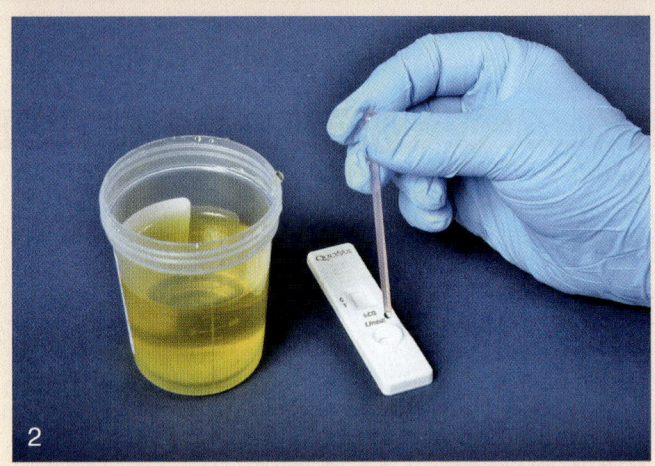

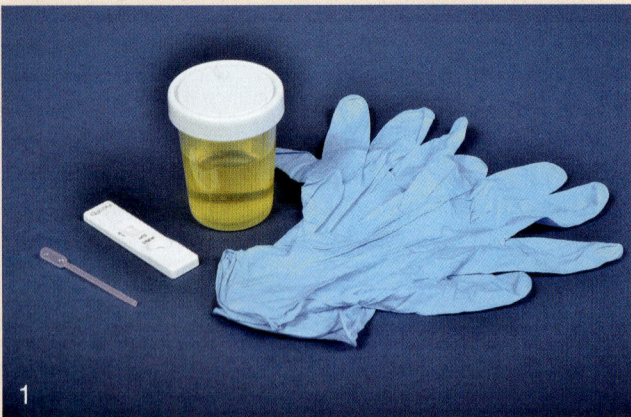

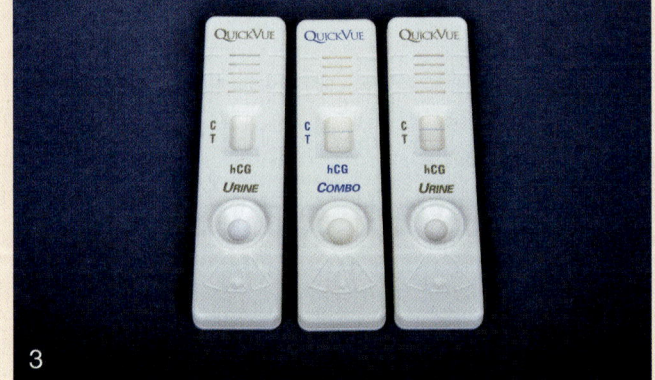

3. Collect the specimen (preferably a first morning specimen).
4. Remove the test cassette from the foil pouch.
5. Add 3 drops of urine using the transfer pipet (dropper) that accompanies the kit (Fig. 2).
   Purpose: To ensure accurate test results, the specimen amount must be added as indicated by the manufacturer's written procedure.
6. Dispose of the pipet in a biohazard sharps container.
7. Wait 3 minutes, and read the test results.
   Purpose: To ensure accurate test results, timing must be accurate.
8. Interpret the results as follows (Fig. 3):
   - *Negative:* A blue control line is next to the letter C; no line is seen next to the letter T. (See results in the middle.)
   - *Positive:* A blue control line is next to the letter C; a pink line is next to the letter T. (See results on the right)
   - *Invalid:* If a blue line does not appear in the C area, the test is invalid and the specimen must be retested using another kit. Check the expiration date of the kit before proceeding (See results on the left).
9. Discard the test cassette in the biohazard waste container, clean up testing area, then remove and discard gloves in a biohazard waste container. Remove lab coat and protective eyewear. Wash hands or use hand sanitizer.
   Purpose: To ensure infection control.
10. Record the results in the patient's record as either positive or negative for pregnancy.
    Purpose: A procedure is not considered finished until it is recorded.
    10/2/20—3:45 p.m.: Last menstrual period (LMP) 9/16/20—. QuickVue pregnancy test: Positive. JulieAnn Black, CMA (AAMA)

for laboratory use and are also available over the counter (OTC) for home use. These tests are sensitive enough to detect the presence of hCG in urine as early as 1 week after implantation, or 4 to 5 days before a missed menstrual period. The tests can be performed in as little as 5 minutes and are easy to interpret. Waived pregnancy tests or home pregnancy tests are read following the manufacturer's instructions. Tests are easy to read and often are as simple as reading a color change. For optimum results, the test should be performed on a first morning urine specimen because it is the most concentrated urine of the day.

The test is based on reactions that occur between **antibodies** (AN ti bod ee s) and **antigens** (AN ti jen s). Antibodies are proteins formed in response to antigens. Antibodies react against one specific antigen (e.g., like a lock and key). When antibodies and antigens come in contact, the antibody binds to the antigen. See Chapter 9 for more information on antibodies and antigens.

The pregnancy test cartridge contains a membrane with an absorbent pad. The urine sample is pipetted into the sample well of the test cartridge. The urine then moves along the absorbent pad, reaching the test area on the membrane. The following reactions can occur:

- All samples (positive or negative) cause the control zone (C) line to turn blue. The presence of this line indicates that the test has been carried out correctly. If the C control zone does not show a color reaction, the test is considered **invalid** (IN vahl id) and must be repeated using another test device.
- In a positive sample, the hCG antigen attaches to the antibodies in the test zone (T), forming a pink line.
- In a negative sample, there is no hCG antigen to attach to the antibodies in the test zone (T), and no line forms.

The QuickVue test (see Procedure 42.8) is a lateral flow pregnancy test that can be performed on urine. It is used routinely in many POLs.

Ovulation Testing

CLIA-waived lateral flow urine tests are available to predict ovulation for women attempting to conceive either naturally or using **artificial insemination** (in SEM uh ney shuhn). During the menstrual cycle, **luteinizing** (LOO tee uh nahyz ing) **hormone (LH)** remains at a relatively stable level. Approximately 14 days before menstruation, the body experiences the "LH surge," a brief, rapid increase in LH. This surge triggers the release of an ovum (egg) from the ovary. Two to 3 days after the surge, the LH level returns to the base level. Conception is most likely to occur within 36 hours after the LH surge. The principle behind this test is similar to that of the pregnancy test. The absorbent membrane contains anti-LH antibodies. A positive test result indicates a urine LH level of 20 mIU/mL or higher. Testing usually is performed for 5 consecutive days in the middle of a woman's cycle. Once the surge is detected, ovulation can be expected within 2 to 3 days.

Menopause Testing

A woman is said to have reached *menopause* when she has not had a menstrual period for at least 12 months. The time before menopause, called *perimenopause*, can last for years, bringing with it uncomfortable symptoms such as the following:

- Irregular periods
- Hot flashes
- Vaginal dryness
- Sleep problems

Some of this may be due to an increase in **follicle-stimulating hormone (FSH)**. Levels of FSH increase temporarily each month to stimulate the ovaries to produce an ovum (egg). When a woman enters menopause, the ovaries stop producing eggs, and the levels of FSH rise. CLIA-waived lateral flow tests detect FSH in the urine. A positive test result indicates that a woman may be in menopause; a negative test result, along with symptoms of menopause, may indicate that a woman is in perimenopause.

The qualitative lateral flow test should never be used to direct a woman to stop using birth control methods if she does not want to conceive. Pregnancy is still possible during perimenopause.

Urine Toxicology

Toxicology (tok si KOL uh jee) is the study of poisonous substances and drugs, and their effects on the body. The clinical laboratory performs testing on body fluids and tissues to monitor the use of therapeutic drugs such as the following:

- Antibiotics
- Anticonvulsants
- Antidepressants
- Barbiturates

They may also test for poisoning by using the following:

- Herbicides
- Metals
- Animal toxins
- Poisonous gases (e.g., carbon monoxide)

Laboratory testing for illegal drugs or alcohol is also done, most commonly due to an employment, insurance, or legal requirement (Table 42.8). A urine specimen is the most reliable choice for most routine

> ### CRITICAL THINKING 42.8
> Becca thinks the immunoassays are so fun, watching the quality control samples flow through the kit and then seeing the results develop right in front of you. Take a few moments and in your own words describe how a lateral flow immunoassay works. What substances interact to create the reaction in the test kit?

> ### VOCABULARY
> **antibodies:** Protein substances produced in the blood or tissues, in response to a specific antigen, that destroy or weaken the antigen. Part of the immune system.
> **antigens:** Substances that stimulate the production of an antibody when introduced into the body. Antigens include toxins, bacteria, viruses, and other foreign substances.
> **artificial insemination:** The injection of semen into the vagina or uterus using a catheter or syringe. Nonsexual.
> **follicle-stimulating hormone (FSH):** A glycoprotein hormone secreted by the anterior pituitary gland. It stimulates the growth of ovum (eggs) in the ovary and induces the formation of sperm in the testis.
> **invalid:** Not valid. A process or outcome that is not correct.
> **lateral flow immunoassay:** A laboratory or clinical technique that uses the specific binding between an antigen and an antibody to identify and quantify a substance in a sample. The sample in this technique moves in a sideways motion, usually on an absorbent paper.
> **luteinizing hormone (LH):** A hormone produced by the anterior pituitary gland. LH stimulates ovulation and the development of the corpus luteum in females and the production of testosterone in males.

TABLE 42.8 Commonly Abused Drugs and Body Retention Times

Drug	Retention Time
Alcohol	2–10 hours
Amphetamine	24–48 hours
Methamphetamine	3–5+ days
Barbiturates	
Phenobarbital	2–6 days
Secobarbital	24 hours
Cocaine, cocaine metabolites	12 hours–3 days
Opiates, heroin, morphine	3–4 days
Phencyclidine (PCP)	3–7+ days
Marijuana (tetrahydrocannabinol metabolites)	2 days–11 week
Oxycodone	3 days

From Proctor D, et al: *Kinn's The Medical Assistant*, ed 13, St. Louis, 2017, Elsevier.

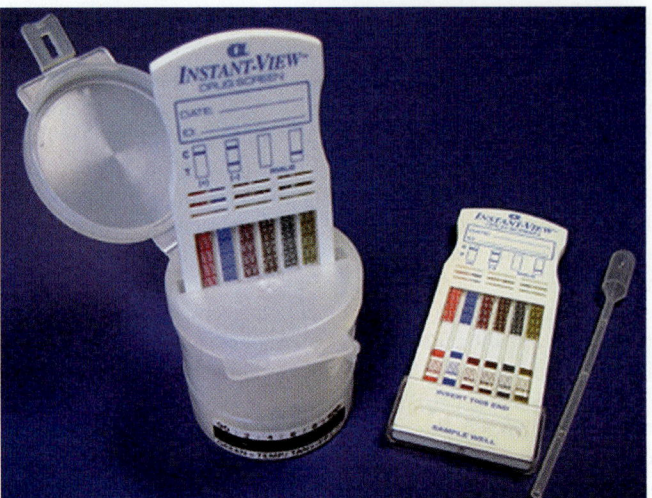

FIG. 42.30 Instant view drug screening test. (Courtesy Alfa Scientific, Poway, California.)

BOX 42.15 Detecting Drugs of Abuse

Urine multidrug screening tests may include the following drugs in a variety of combinations:

- Amphetamines
- Barbiturates
- Benzodiazepines (ben zoh dahy AZ uh peen)
- Cocaine
- Morphine
- Methadone (METH uh dohn)
- Phencyclidine (PCP)
- Tricyclic antidepressants
- Marijuana
- Ecstasy
- Methamphetamines
- Oxycodone
- Opiates

---

screening procedures. Urine drug tests detect drug **metabolites** and not the drug themselves. Urine samples will remain positive even after the effects of the drugs are gone. For routine screening, a random specimen is usually collected.

> **VOCABULARY**
> **metabolite:** A by-product of drug metabolism.

Often, the following safeguards are used to ensure that a specimen is fresh and is truly from the patient:
- Water may be temporarily unavailable in the restroom.
- Bluing agents may be added to the toilets.
- A sealed container with a temperature-sensitive strip may be provided for collection.
- Someone of the same gender may accompany the patient into the restroom during the collection.

Chain of custody protocol is required for any legal specimen. This means that everyone handling the specimen must document their interaction with the sample. The drugs and their metabolites often remain in urine much longer than the physical impairment lasts. This is one reason urine screening is favored over blood screening.

As a medical assistant, you may be responsible for collecting specimens for toxicology tests and for performing certain laboratory tests. Rapid drug screening devices are about the size and shape of a credit card (Fig. 42.30). The device is dipped into a urine sample, or urine is directly applied to the device. The results are read according to the manufacturer's instructions in just minutes. Negative results indicate that none of the targeted drugs were found in the urine sample at a detectable level. Inconclusive results indicate that the device reacted with something in the urine and confirmatory testing is needed.

Urine multidrug screening tests are a type of lateral flow immunoassay that tests for urine metabolites of a variety of drugs. See Box 42.15 for details. This type of testing is also an immunoassay where antibodies and antigens react to form a readable test result. By using antibodies specific to different drug classes, some test cartridges can simultaneously detect up to 10 different drugs from a single sample in 5 minutes.

Adulteration Testing and Chain of Custody. Drug testing has legal consequences; therefore additional testing may be necessary to ensure that samples have not been *adulterated* (uh DUHL tuh reyt ed). Adulteration is the intentional manipulation of a urine sample that allows someone to falsely pass a drug screening test. It may involve using urine from another person or an animal, diluting the sample with water, or adding other substances that would compromise the test procedure.

Sensitivity limits for drug screening are set by the U.S. Substance Abuse and Mental Health Services Administration (SAMHSA), the National Institute on Drug Abuse (NIDA), and the U.S. Department of Health and Human Services (DHHS). Positive results on urine drug samples should be confirmed with more specific confirmatory testing methods. See Box 42.16 for chain of custody rules for drug testing.

EXCEPTIONAL CUSTOMER SERVICE

Frequently, a medical assistant is called on to explain specimen collection techniques to the patient. Patients want to do the procedure correctly but often lack the knowledge of urinary terminology. They may be embarrassed or may not know how to ask questions about cleaning the genital area. When explaining a urinary collection procedure, use pictures and words that the patient will understand. If the procedure is explained in terms the patient is familiar with, he or she will feel comfortable asking you about important details that may have an impact on treatment. Providing the patient with a clearly written instruction sheet is also helpful. The instruction sheet should be personalized with the patient's name, the time to begin collection or testing (if applicable), what supplies should be used, and a phone number to call if questions arise.

BOX 42.16 Chain of Custody Rules

1. The individual being tested must provide a photo identification.
2. Indirect observation of specimen collection is important to make sure the patient being tested has provided the sample. Indirect methods of observation include the following:
   - Measuring the specimen's temperature
   - Securing water faucets in the restroom so that urine cannot be diluted
   - Having the patient remove outer clothing and leave personal belongings in the examination room
   - Not allowing water to be run or the toilet to be flushed in the restroom during the collection

   Note: If you suspect the sample has been adulterated, the patient may be asked to provide another specimen.
3. Within 4 minutes of receiving the specimen, check its temperature (range should be 32° to 38°C [90° to 100°F]). Sample volume should be a minimum of 30 to 45 mL. Inspect the sample for any indications of adulteration (e.g., an unusual color, the presence of foreign materials).
4. Pour the specimen into a specimen bottle and seal the lid with the tamper-evident label/seal provided at the bottom of the chain-of-custody form. The donor should be present when this is done and should see you write the date and your initials on the label (Fig. 42.31).
5. Ship the specimen to the testing laboratory as soon as possible. It must be sent the same day it was collected.
6. Individual testing method results may vary. Some tests have lower limits of detection, which can make some results positive at lower substance levels. Also, a person's diet, the volume of urine flow, and recent fluid intake can affect some results.
7. Because of the legal implications of drug testing, chain of custody must be strictly followed. Each step from collection of the specimen to reporting the test results must be strictly monitored and documented. Requirements include sealed specimen containers, supervised laboratory analysis throughout the process, and authorized signatures at each step.

Continued

UNIT 6 Medical Laboratory

BOX 42.16 Chain-of-Custody Rules—cont'd

FEDERAL DRUG TESTING CUSTODY AND CONTROL FORM

SPECIMEN ID NO. **1234567**   LAB ACCESSION NO. _____

OMB No. 0930-0158

STEP 1: COMPLETED BY COLLECTOR OR EMPLOYER REPRESENTATIVE

A. Employer Name, Address, I.D. No.

B. MRO Name, Address, Phone and Fax No.

C. Donor SSN or Employee I.D. No. _____

D. Reason for Test: ☐ Pre-employment   ☐ Random   ☐ Reasonable Suspicion/Cause   ☐ Post Accident
☐ Return to Duty   ☐ Follow-up   ☐ Other (specify)

E. Drug Tests to be Performed: ☐ THC, COC, PCP, OPI, AMP   ☐ THC & COC Only   ☐ Other (specify) _____

F. Collection Site Address:

Collector Phone No. _____

Collector Fax No. _____

STEP 2: COMPLETED BY COLLECTOR

Read specimen temperature within 4 minutes. Is temperature between 90° and 100° F? ☐ Yes ☐ No, Enter Remark

Specimen Collection: ☐ Split ☐ Single ☐ None Provided (Enter Remark)   ☐ Observed (Enter Remark)

REMARKS _____

STEP 3: Collector affixes bottle seal(s) to bottle(s). Collector dates seal(s). Donor initials seal(s). Donor completes STEP 5 on Copy 2 (MRO Copy)

STEP 4: CHAIN OF CUSTODY - INITIATED BY COLLECTOR AND COMPLETED BY LABORATORY

I certify that the specimen given to me by the donor identified in the certification section on Copy 2 of this form was collected, labeled, sealed and released to the Delivery Service noted in accordance with applicable Federal requirements.

X _____   AM/PM   Time of Collection
Signature of Collector

SPECIMEN BOTTLE(S) RELEASED TO:

(PRINT) Collector's Name (First, MI, Last)   Date (Mo./Day/Yr.)

Name of Delivery Service Transferring Specimen to Lab

RECEIVED AT LAB:

X _____
Signature of Accessioner

(PRINT) Accessioner's Name (First, MI, Last)   Date (Mo./Day/Yr.)

Primary Specimen Bottle Seal Intact ☐ Yes ☐ No, Enter Remark Below

SPECIMEN BOTTLE(S) RELEASED TO:

PRESS HARD - YOU ARE MAKING MULTIPLE COPIES

STEP 5a: PRIMARY SPECIMEN TEST RESULTS - COMPLETED BY PRIMARY LABORATORY

☐ NEGATIVE   ☐ POSITIVE for: ☐ MARIJUANA METABOLITE ☐ CODEINE ☐ AMPHETAMINE ☐ ADULTERATED
☐ DILUTE   ☐ COCAINE METABOLITE ☐ MORPHINE ☐ METHAMPHETAMINE ☐ SUBSTITUTED
☐ REJECTED FOR TESTING   ☐ PCP ☐ 6-ACETYLMORPHINE ☐ INVALID RESULT

REMARKS _____

TEST LAB (if different from above) _____

I certify that the specimen identified on this form was examined upon receipt, handled using chain of custody procedures, analyzed, and reported in accordance with applicable Federal requirements.

X _____
Signature of Certifying Scientist   (PRINT) Certifying Scientist's Name (First, MI, Last)   Date (Mo./Day/Yr.)

STEP 5b: SPLIT SPECIMEN TEST RESULTS - (IF TESTED) COMPLETED BY SECONDARY LABORATORY

Laboratory Name _____
Laboratory Address _____

☐ RECONFIRMED   ☐ FAILED TO RECONFIRM - REASON _____

I certify that the split specimen identified on this form was examined upon receipt, handled using chain of custody procedures, analyzed, and reported in accordance with applicable Federal requirements.

X _____
Signature of Certifying Scientist   (PRINT) Certifying Scientist's Name (First, MI, Last)   Date (Mo./Day/Yr.)

PEEL **1234567** A   SPECIMEN ID NO.
PLACE OVER CAP
1234567 SPECIMEN BOTTLE SEAL
Date (Mo. Day Yr.)   Donor's Initials

PEEL **1234567** B (SPLIT)   SPECIMEN ID NO.
PLACE OVER CAP
1234567 SPECIMEN BOTTLE SEAL
Date (Mo. Day Yr.)   Donor's Initials

COPY 1 - LABORATORY

Drug Form Part 1
Face Inks: 000 BLK / 000 RED
Date: 05/09/00
Not To Use For Colormatch
Follow PMS Guide For Colors

FIG. 42.31 First page of the five-page federal drug testing custody and control form.

CLOSING COMMENTS

There is a lot involved in urine testing, and the results can help the provider to diagnose diseases and disorders. The beneficial attributes of a laboratory professional performing urinalysis include the following:
- A discreet, respectful attitude when communicating with patients, coworkers, and supervisors
- Good eyesight and manual dexterity
- Accountability, honesty, and integrity when performing a urinalysis
- The ability to multitask, manage time, pay attention to details, and problem-solve if test results are suspicious

CHAPTER REVIEW

In this chapter, we covered urinalysis and the importance of this area of the laboratory. We started out with a brief review of the structure and function of the urinary system and how urine is formed and eliminated from the body.

Collecting a urine specimen is an important aspect of urinalysis. The testing is only as good as the specimen. A medical assistant often gives patients instructions on how to properly collect a urine sample. This can be a sensitive subject. Some patients may feel embarrassed talking about the topic, so we need to keep the feelings of our patients in mind. The medical assistant must be respectful, communicate clearly, and give patients a chance to ask questions and feel their concerns are important.

There are a variety of urine collection containers and methods. Being aware of which container is used for what method of collection is significant. Handling and transporting urine specimens are also areas that require the medical assistant to be detail oriented. Following proper labeling techniques is part of handling and transport. Also, sending samples in proper leak-proof containers is a necessary safety factor.

We looked at the procedures for performing a routine urinalysis. We first need to look at the physical characteristics and record our observations. Color, turbidity, volume, the presence of foam or odor, and specific gravity are all part of the physical analysis. Next, we looked at the chemical examination of urine. The most common urinalysis test is the reagent strip test, also called a urine dipstick. This test has 10 different analytes that can be analyzed simultaneously. The provider gains information about the patient's kidney and liver function, pH, sugar metabolism, and possible bacterial urinary tract infection—all from one small reagent strip test. We also discussed the limitations of routine UA and the need for quality assurance and quality control to ensure reliable patient test results.

Medical assistants must learn to process and prepare urine specimens for microscopic examination. In this chapter, we learned how to prepare the specimens, set up the specimen, and focus the microscope. We also discussed what may be seen microscopically in a urine sample and why some of the structures that we can see under the microscope may be present.

In addition to routine urinalysis, the chapter covered other CLIA-waived tests that can be performed on a urine specimen. The Clinitest, urine pregnancy tests, ovulation tests, menopause tests, and urine toxicology testing can all be done on urine samples. Each different type of testing is important and useful to the provider.

We closed the chapter by highlighting the importance of remembering our patients. Patient education is a key role for the medical assistant. We can inform patients about collection procedures and answer their questions. The hope is that the medical assistant will put the patient at ease and their conversations will be helpful and informative.

Urine is the second most tested sample in the laboratory. It is important to be confident in your knowledge of the sample and its testing process.

SCENARIO WRAP-UP

Becca has had a fun and busy time in the laboratory at WMFM. She has enjoyed learning about the laboratory. She has had a chance to see some of the testing, PPE, quality assurance, and quality control processes that are part of a day in the lab. It was also nice to see the general workflow of the lab and the need for organization, attention to detail, and manual dexterity in laboratory testing. With these observations fresh in her mind, Becca will finish her assignment later today. She is looking forward to graduating soon and working as a medical assistant. There are so many areas within ambulatory care to work as a medical assistant. Becca is excited for the future.

43

Assisting in Blood Collection

LEARNING OBJECTIVES

1. Discuss venipuncture equipment and personal protective equipment. Also, explain the purpose of a tourniquet, how to apply it, and the consequences of improper tourniquet application.
2. Discuss antiseptics, explain why the stopper colors on vacuum tubes differ, and state the correct order of the draw.
3. Discuss the needles and supplies used in phlebotomy.
4. Discuss needle safety and postexposure needlestick follow-up.
5. Complete the following related to routine venipuncture:
   - Discuss patient preparation for routine venipuncture.
   - List in order the steps of a routine venipuncture.
   - Detail patient preparation for venipuncture that shows sensitivity to the patient's rights and feelings.
- Perform a venipuncture using the vacuum tube method, syringe, and winged-infusion (butterfly) assembly.
6. Discuss possible solutions to venipuncture complications.
7. List situations in which capillary puncture would be preferred over venipuncture and discuss the equipment used.
8. Perform a capillary puncture.
9. Discuss pediatric phlebotomy, including typical childhood behavior and parental involvement during phlebotomy and general guidelines for pediatric venipuncture.
10. Describe handling and transport methods for blood after collection.

CHAPTER OUTLINE

1. **Opening Scenario, 1046**
2. **You Will Learn, 1047**
3. **Introduction, 1047**
4. **Venipuncture Equipment, 1047**
   a. Personal Protective Equipment, 1048
   b. Tourniquets, 1048
   c. Antiseptics, 1049
   d. Evacuated Collection Tubes, 1049
      i. *Tube Additives, 1050*
5. **Order of the Draw, 1052**
6. **Needles and Supplies Used in Phlebotomy, 1052**
   a. Multisample Needles, 1053
   b. Needle Holders, 1053
   c. Syringes, 1053
   d. Winged Infusion Sets (Butterfly Assembly), 1053
7. **Needle Safety, 1054**
   a. Postexposure Needlestick Follow-Up, 1056
8. **Routine Venipuncture, 1056**
   a. Patient Preparation, 1056
   b. Preparing for the Venipuncture, 1056
   c. Performing the Venipuncture, 1057
   d. Completing the Venipuncture, 1057
9. **Problems Associated With Venipuncture, 1066**
   a. Hematoma, 1066
   b. Nerve Damage and Other Complications, 1066
   c. Fainting, 1066
   d. Specimen Recollection, 1067
10. **Capillary Puncture, 1067**
    a. Equipment, 1068
       i. *Skin Puncture Devices, 1068*
       ii. *Collection Containers, 1069*
11. **Routine Capillary Puncture, 1069**
    a. Site Selection, 1069
    b. Patient Preparation, 1070
    c. Collecting the Specimen, 1070
    d. Specimen Handling, 1071
12. **Pediatric Phlebotomy, 1071**
13. **Handling the Specimen After Collection, 1074**
    a. Chain of Custody, 1074
14. **Closing Comments, 1074**
15. **Chapter Review, 1075**
16. **Scenario Wrap-Up, 1075**

OPENING SCENARIO

Maggie Brandt, CMA (AAMA), has been a medical assistant with the Walden-Martin Family Medicine Clinic (WMFM) for about 15 years. She has worked in many areas of the clinic, but for the past 8 years she has been the primary phlebotomist each morning from 8:00 a.m. until noon. Maggie has the right combination of skills to be a wonderful phlebotomist:
- She is warm, friendly, and can easily talk to patients.
- She is detail-oriented, a stickler for safety practices, and very organized.

- She has good small motor skills and that certain quality that seems to make her venipunctures so smooth that you hardly feel the needle go through the skin.
- She can explain procedures well in understandable terms and is willing to listen to her patients and put them at ease.

It is Monday morning, and the phlebotomy area is usually busy with patients who have scheduled venipunctures in advance. Let's see what is happening in the phlebotomy area today!

YOU WILL LEARN

- To assemble the equipment needed for a venipuncture and capillary puncture.
- To discuss the different colored stoppers on vacuum tubes and correctly state the order of the draw.
- To describe the types of safety needles and collection devices used in phlebotomy.
- To summarize postexposure management of accidental needlesticks.
- To perform a venipuncture using evacuated tubes, a syringe, and butterfly equipment, and also to perform a capillary puncture.
- To discuss problem-solving strategies related to blood collection.
- To discuss pediatric phlebotomy, including behavior, parental involvement during phlebotomy, and general guidelines for pediatric blood collection.

INTRODUCTION

Phlebotomy (fluh BOT uh mee) is performed primarily to:
- Aid in diagnosing disease
- Monitor a patient's condition, treatment, or medication levels
- Document the existing good health of a patient

According to the American Society of Clinical Pathologists (ASCP), nearly 80% of providers base at least part of their diagnostic decisions on the results of laboratory tests. The most common specimen used in the laboratory is blood. *Phlebotomy* is the process of acquiring blood from a patient. Phlebotomy involves highly developed skills, procedures, and equipment to ensure the patient's comfort and safety.

When it comes to phlebotomy, safety is an important concern. There are several bloodborne viral diseases that can be spread by exposure to infected blood and body fluids. The bloodborne viruses identified as possible bloodborne pathogen risks are:
- Hepatitis (hep uh TAHY tis) B virus (HBV)
- Hepatitis C virus (HCV)
- Human immunodeficiency (im yuh noh di FISH uh n see) virus (HIV)

These viruses are not the only diseases that can be spread by contaminated blood or body fluids, but they are considered a risk for healthcare workers and public safety personnel (such as firefighters, police, and first responders). The high standards necessary for the safe practice of phlebotomy led to the creation of the Bloodborne Pathogens Standard (overseen by the Occupational Safety and Health Administration [OSHA]) and by different organizations that develop additional standards for training (See Chapter 28, for more information on bloodborne pathogens).

Medical assistants are trained to perform phlebotomy. To be certified as a phlebotomist (fluh BOT uh mist), they must complete course work and training at an accredited institution, perform a specified number of witnessed venipunctures (VEN uh puhngk cher), and then pass a national medical assistant certification examination (Box 43.1).

The most common method of obtaining a blood specimen is by *venipuncture*, blood that is taken directly from a surface vein. The vein is punctured with a needle, and the blood is collected directly into a stoppered vacuum tube, or into a **syringe** and then transferred into the vacuum tube. The procedure is safe when performed by a trained professional, but it must be performed with care. Practice is required to become skilled and confident in the technique of venipuncture.

VENIPUNCTURE EQUIPMENT

Proper collection of blood requires specialized equipment. A complete list of materials used in routine venipuncture is shown in Box 43.2. Phlebotomists in hospitals generally carry the equipment in a portable

---

BOX 43.1 Phlebotomy Certifying Agencies

Phlebotomy certifying agencies include the American Society of Clinical Pathologists (ASCP), the International Academy of Phlebotomy Sciences (IAPS), the National Certification Agency (NCA), and the National Phlebotomy Association (NPA). Continuing education often is required to maintain certification. It is important that medical assistants become familiar with the guidelines of the states in which they work because not all states require a certificate to perform phlebotomy.

BOX 43.2 Equipment Used in Routine Venipuncture

- Personal protective equipment (PPE): gloves, fluid-impermeable (im PUR mee uh buh l) lab coat, and protective eyewear, or face shield (if necessary)
- Permanent marker
- Alcohol wipes
- Gauze
- Hypoallergenic (hahy poh al er JEN ik) self-stick wrap, tape, or bandages
- Nonlatex tourniquets (TUR ni kit)
- Double-pointed safety needles
- Winged infusion sets (butterfly needles)
- Disposable needle holders
- Evacuated (ih VAK yoo eyt ed), stoppered tubes
- Syringes (suh RINJ) and removable needles with safety devices
- Biohazard sharps container
- Biohazard waste container

MEDICAL TERMINOLOGY

hepat/o: liver
-itis: inflammation
-otomy: the process of cutting
phleb/o: vein
-puncture: to pierce the surface
syncop/o: faint, cut off, cut short **ven/i-:** vein

VOCABULARY

syringe: A device with a slender barrel and needle that is used to withdraw blood from a vein or an artery.

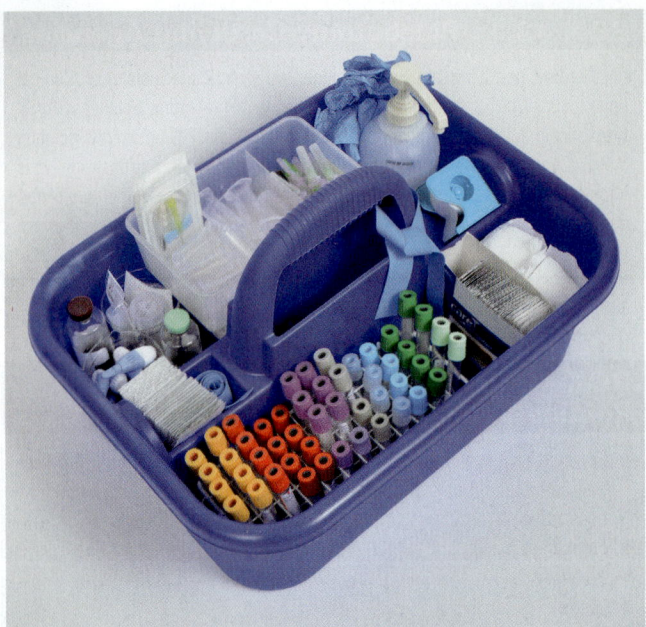

FIG. 43.1 A stocked venipuncture tray. (From Proctor D, et al: *Kinn's The Medical Assistant*, ed 13, St Louis, 2017, Elsevier.)

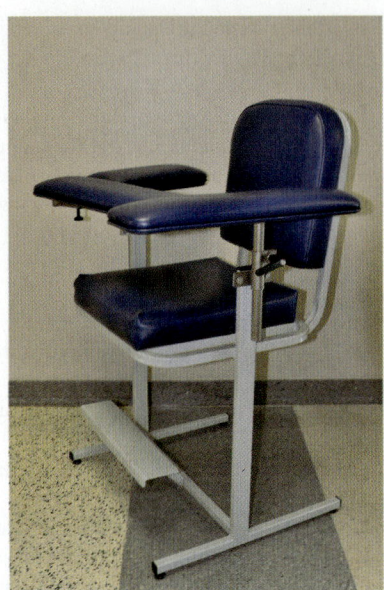

FIG. 43.2 A phlebotomy chair. (From Proctor D, et al: *Kinn's The Medical Assistant*, ed 13, St Louis, 2017, Elsevier.)

> **BOX 43.3 Latex-Free Supplies**
>
> All facilities must stock only latex-free supplies because of the potential for allergic responses in workers and patients. Some people with latex allergies can have life-threatening reactions with a latex exposure.

> **VOCABULARY**
>
> **syncope:** Fainting; a brief lapse of consciousness.

tray (Fig. 43.1). A physician office laboratory (POL) often has a permanent location where the same supplies are stored and venipuncture is performed. In such cases, you may use a phlebotomy chair, which has an adjustable locking armrest to protect the patient if he or she should faint (Fig. 43.2). However, if the patient has a history of syncope (SING kuh pee), it is best to perform phlebotomy while the patient is lying on an examination table or in a reclining phlebotomy chair.

Personal Protective Equipment

Employers must provide employees with personal protective equipment (PPE), such as gloves (Box 43.3), disposable fluid-impenetrable lab coats, protective eyewear, and face shields.

> **Critical Thinking Box 43.1**
>
> Maggie is in a little early on a Monday morning. She knows that Monday is usually busy, and she wants to make sure all her supplies are adequately stocked. Maggie cleans her protective eyewear and has it ready at the phlebotomy station. Why is it important to wear protective eyewear whenever drawing blood? Can you think of a few reasons and share them with your class?

OSHA requires healthcare workers to wear gloves during venipuncture. Because veins can be difficult to locate with gloved fingertips, the site may be palpated (PAL peyt ed) before gloves are put on, as long as the hands have been washed or sanitized. According to the standard procedure for venipuncture established by the Clinical and Laboratory Standards Institute (CLSI), gloves may be put on after vein palpation but before preparation of the site. Those who need the final assurance of one last palpation before the needle is inserted must remember that touching the prepared site, even with gloves, contaminates the area. To help yourself find the vein after the area has been cleansed, make note of any skin markers, such as creases, freckles, or scars. If the area is touched, *it must be cleansed again.* Keep in mind that the tourniquet should be tied for no longer than 1 minute at a time.

Tourniquets

Before blood can be drawn, a vein must be located. Most venipunctures are done in the *antecubital* (an TEE kyoo bih tul) *region,* or inner bend in front of the elbow. Application of a tourniquet is very helpful in locating veins in the antecubital region and any other area that may be drawn for venipuncture. Tourniquets prevent the venous blood flow out of the site, causing the veins to bulge or plump up. If the antecubital area is drawn, a tourniquet is tied around the upper arm so that it is tight but still comfortable and can be easily released with one hand. Single-use, nonlatex tourniquets are available (Fig. 43.3) and currently are recommended to:

- Reduce cross-contamination between patients and healthcare workers
- Help prevent nosocomial (nos uh KOH mee uh l) infections
- Prevent latex exposure

Other types of tourniquets with quick-release closures are available, but they must be disinfected after each use.

Tourniquets are applied 3 to 4 inches above the elbow immediately before the venipuncture procedure begins. Because a tourniquet slows blood flow, leaving it on for longer than 1 minute greatly increases the possibility of hemoconcentration (hee muh kon suh n TREY shuh n) and altered test results. The tourniquet should not be tied so tightly that it restricts arterial (ahr TEER ee uh l) blood flow. If arterial blood flow is restricted, then venous blood return is also restricted. This will result in veins that won't plump up. Checking the pulse at the wrist ensures that arterial flow is not restricted. Tourniquets also are used when blood is drawn from hand and foot veins and are tied on the wrist or ankle, respectively.

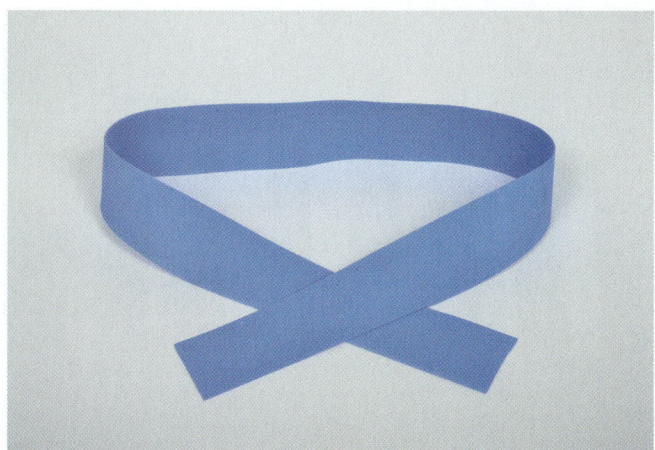

FIG. 43.3 A latex-free tourniquet. (From Proctor D, et al: *Kinn's The Medical Assistant*, ed 13, St Louis, 2017, Elsevier.)

Tourniquets can be uncomfortable for patients, especially those with heavy-set or hairy upper arms, if they are not applied correctly. Make sure the tourniquet is flat against the skin, and if necessary, tie it over the clothing if it is causing the patient discomfort. This may be especially important when blood is drawn on an elderly person because of the thinness or fragility of the skin.

Antiseptics

To prevent infection, a venipuncture site must be cleansed with an **antiseptic** (an tuh SEP tik). The most commonly used antiseptic is 70% isopropyl (ahy suh PROH pil) alcohol, also known as *rubbing alcohol*. Prepackaged alcohol wipes are the product used most often. An alcohol wipe is used to clean the puncture site, which is then allowed to air dry. Alcohol does not sterilize the skin; but it kills many of the existing bacteria that might contaminate the sample. To be most effective, the alcohol should remain on the skin for 30 to 60 seconds, and allowed to air dry. As the alcohol dries, it breaks open the bacterial cells and kills the bacteria. Alcohol wipes should not be used when collecting a blood alcohol sample (Box 43.4).

> **Critical Thinking Box 43.2**
>
> It is important to use a tourniquet to properly locate veins for phlebotomy. List three advantages of using a tourniquet to help locate veins. Be ready to share them with your class.

If a **blood culture** is ordered, additional preparation is needed at the venipuncture site to eliminate contaminating bacteria (Box 43.5).
- First 70% isopropyl alcohol wipes are used to clean the area, which is allowed to air dry.
- Then an iodine solution is used, such as chlorhexidine gluconate (klor hex IH dyn GLOO koh nayt). Benzalkonium (behn ZAHL koh nee uhm) chloride can be used for patients who are allergic to iodine.
- The iodine prep is also allowed to air dry.

Once the venipuncture site is properly prepared, the blood cultures must be drawn into a sterile tube or bottle specifically designed for the test (Fig. 43.4).

> **BOX 43.4 Collection for Blood Alcohol Test**
>
> Isopropyl alcohol wipes should not be used to clean the venipuncture site when a blood alcohol test is drawn. Sterile soap pads, benzalkonium chloride, or povidone-iodine (Betadine) can be used instead.

> **BOX 43.5 When Are Blood Cultures Ordered?**
>
> Blood cultures are ordered when a provider suspects that a bacterial infection is causing a fever of unknown origin (FUO).

Evacuated Collection Tubes

The most common collection system is the **evacuated** tube system (these tubes are also called *vacuum tubes*; a particular brand of vacuum tubes is the Vacutainer). It consists of evacuated tubes of various sizes that have color-coded stoppers. The colored stoppers indicate the tube's contents (Table 43.1). Venipuncture tubes must be either shatter-resistant glass or plastic. More traditional rubber tube stoppers have been replaced by safer plastic *Hemogard* (HEE moh gah rd) colored tops. Hemogard tops have the advantage of not splattering blood when removed from the tube (Fig. 43.5) Table 43.1 lists the colored stoppers and the chemical additives, **anticoagulants** (an tee koh AG yuh luh nt), **clot activators**, and/or **thixotropic** (THYH uh troh pik) **gel** that are contained in each type of tube. The different stopper colors indicate the unique contents

> **MEDICAL TERMINOLOGY**
>
> **-al:** pertaining to
> **ante-:** forward, before
> **anti-:** against
> **comi/o:** to care for
> **cubit/o:** elbow, forearm
> **nos/o:** disease
> **-sepsis:** infection

> **VOCABULARY**
>
> **anticoagulants:** Substances (i.e., medications or chemicals) that prevent the clotting of blood.
> **antiseptic:** A substance that inhibits the growth of microorganisms on living tissue (e.g., alcohol and povidone-iodine solution [Betadine]); it is used to cleanse the skin, wounds, and so on.
> **blood culture:** A microbiological procedure in which a blood sample is placed in a nutrient medium and held at body temperature. If bacteria are in the blood sample, the culture medium should encourage the growth of the infecting bacteria in the laboratory.
> **clot activators:** Substances added to a venipuncture tube to enhance and speed up blood clotting.
> **hemoconcentration:** A condition in which the concentration of blood cells is increased in proportion to the volume of plasma.
> **nosocomial:** An infection that is acquired in a healthcare setting. Also known as healthcare acquired infections (HAI).
> **thixotropic gel:** A chemically neutral gel added to evacuated blood tubes that creates a physical barrier between red blood cells and plasma or serum when the tube is centrifuged.
> **tourniquet:** A device for temporarily constricting blood flow.

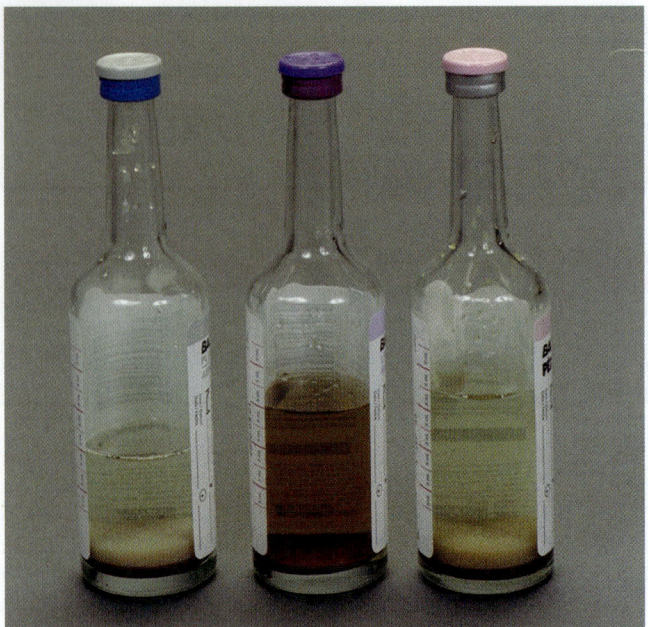

FIG. 43.4 An example of blood culture bottles. (From Proctor D, et al: *Kinn's The Medical Assistant*, ed 13, St. Louis, 2017, Elsevier.)

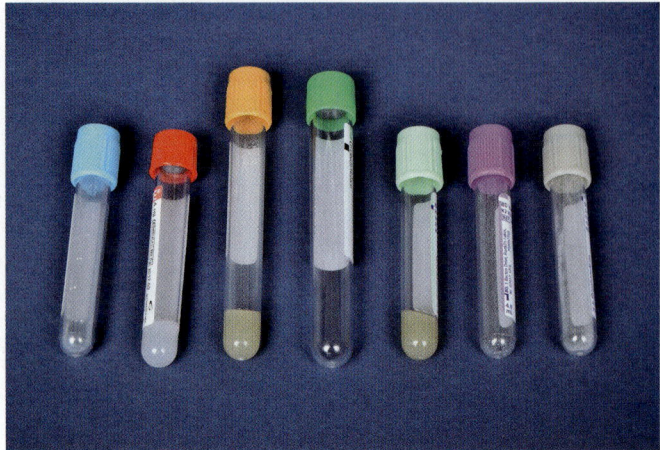

FIG. 43.5 Hemogard tube stoppers.

of that color-coded tube. The vacuum in each tube draws a measured amount of blood into the tube. Tube volumes range from 2 to 15 mL.

The size of the tube to be drawn depends on several factors. Each test performed in the laboratory requires a specific amount of blood. Blood volumes can often be combined, which reduces the number of tubes that must be drawn. For example, both a complete blood count and an erythrocyte sedimentation rate test (discussed in Chapter 44) are performed on a sample from a lavender-topped tube. The combined volume for both tests can be drawn with one lavender-topped tube, so you don't need to draw two tubes. When in doubt, call the laboratory. Keep in mind that blood is approximately half cells and half liquid. If a test requires 2 mL of serum, at least 4 mL of blood must be collected.

> **EXCEPTIONAL CUSTOMER SERVICE**
>
> Patients often express great concern when several tubes of blood must be drawn. It seems like they are losing a lot of blood. You can put their fears to rest by explaining that the average adult has a little less than 5 L of blood (10 pints). Most adults can relate to donating a unit of blood, which is about 500 mL (1 pint). Because the red-topped tube contains 10 mL, you would have to draw about 50 tubes to remove 500 mL of blood.

Tube Additives. Most vacuum tubes contain an additive. The plain red-topped tube contains nothing. It is a plain tube with no additives, and no anticoagulants or clot enhancers. A gold-topped tube contains silica to activate clotting and an inert gel to separate serum and cells after the sample is centrifuged. All the other color-topped plastic tubes contain some form of anticoagulant, which prevents blood from clotting. The additive may be a powder, a liquid visible in the tube, or a liquid sprayed inside the tube by the manufacturer and allowed to dry. The choice of anticoagulant depends on the test to be completed.

Anticoagulant additives prevent blood from clotting, which allows the contents of the tube to be used in two ways. First, the sample can be used as whole blood; second, the sample can be centrifuged, and the liquid portion, called *plasma,* can be used for testing. An example of a test that uses whole blood would be a complete blood count (CBC). An example of a test that uses plasma would be coagulation studies.

Ethylenediaminetetraacetic acid (EDTA) is the anticoagulant found in the lavender-topped tube. It prevents platelet clumping and preserves the appearance of blood cells for microscopic examination.

Clot activators promote blood clotting in the tubes with either a marbled red-gray or a gold top. For example, silica particles in the gold tubes enhance clotting by providing a surface for platelet activation. Thrombin from the platelets quickly promotes clotting and is used in tubes drawn for chemistry testing or in the event a sample is needed from a patient taking a prescribed anticoagulant, such as heparin.

If blood clots and then is centrifuged, the liquid portion is referred to as *serum.* Without a clot activator, blood clots in 15 to 60 minutes, after which it must be centrifuged. The serum must be quickly separated from the cells because cells may continue to metabolize glucose or may release substances that interfere with testing.

Thixotropic gel can be found in some tubes, including *serum separator tubes* (SST). SST tubes are identified by the marbled red-gray rubber stopper and the gold Hemogard top. The *plasma separator tube* (PST)

> **VOCABULARY**
>
> **evacuated:** A tube, flask, or reaction vessel in which a vacuum has been created.
> **glycolysis:** The chemical breakdown of carbohydrates (glucose) by enzymes, with the release of energy.
> **plasma:** The liquid portion of a whole blood sample that has not clotted due to an anticoagulant. The liquid portion of the blood that contains clotting factors. The liquid portion of the blood found in the body.
> **serum:** The liquid portion of a clotted blood specimen that no longer contains its active clotting agents.

> **MEDICAL TERMINOLOGY**
>
> **anti:** against
> **coagul/o:** coagulation or clotting
> **glyc/o:** glucose or sugar
> **iatr/o:** physician or treatment
> **-lysis:** breakdown, destruction, separation
> **ped/o:** child or foot

TABLE 43.1 Common Color-Coded Stoppers and Their Additives and Laboratory Uses

Vacuum Tube Color[a]	Color	Hemogard Color[b]	Additive and Its Function[c]	Laboratory Use
Blood culture bottles	No color for blood culture bottles (see Fig. 43.4)	Yellow Pale yellow	Sodium polyanethol sulfonate (pohl ee AHN eh thawl SUHL fuh neyt) (SPS); prevents blood from clotting and stabilizes bacterial growth. Yellow-topped tubes have specific uses. They cannot be used to collect all blood culture specimens.	Blood culture bottles – blood or body fluid cultures Yellow-topped tubes – mycobacteria (mahy koh bak TEER ee uh), fungus (FUHNG guh s), or acid-fast bacilli (buh SIL uh s) (AFB) blood cultures
Light blue		Light blue	Sodium citrate (SI treyt); removes calcium to prevent blood from clotting.	Coagulation (koh AG yuh ley shun) testing
Red		Red	None	Serum (SEER uh m) tests; chemistry studies, blood bank, immunology (im yuh NOL uh jee)
Red-gray (marbled)		Gold	No anticoagulant, but contains silica (SIL I kuh) particles to enhance clot formation, usually contain gel for serum separation.	Serum tests; chemistry studies, immunology
Green		Green	Heparin (HEP uh rin); inhibits thrombin (THROM bin) formation to prevent clotting.	Chemistry tests
Green-gray (marbled)		Light green	Lithium heparin and gel; for plasma separation.	Plasma (PLAZ muh) determinations in chemistry studies
Lavender		Lavender	Ethylenediaminetetraacetic (ETH uh leen DAHY uh meen TE truh uh SEE tik) acid (EDTA); removes calcium to prevent blood from clotting.	Hematology (hee muh TOL uh jee) tests
Gray		Gray	Potassium oxalate (OK suh leyt) and sodium fluoride; removes calcium to prevent blood from clotting; fluoride inhibits glycolysis (glahy KOL uh sis)	Chemistry testing, especially glucose and alcohol levels

[a]Stopper colors are based on BD Vacutainer tubes.
[b]Hemogard closures provide a protective plastic cover over the rubber stopper as an additional safety feature.
[c]Additives, additive functions, and laboratory uses are the same for both pediatric and adult tubes.
From Proctor D, et al: *Kinn's The Medical Assistant*, ed 13, St Louis, 2017, Elsevier.

also contains thixotropic gel. The glass tubes have a marbled green-gray top, and the Hemogard tubes have a light green top. Thixotropic gel, a synthetic gel, has a density between that of red cells and plasma or serum. The gel settles between the plasma/serum and cells during centrifugation. The gel forms a barrier that makes it easy to pour off the liquid portion of the sample without cells contaminating the specimen.

It is important to avoid a "short draw" (i.e., a tube that is not completely filled). Table 43.2 lists the consequences of underfilling tubes. Some tubes are designed to fill only partially, according to their preset vacuum. Having the proper ratio of blood to additive is crucial. Always check the tube for the expiration date. Outdated tubes may have a diminished vacuum, or the additive may have degraded and not be as effective.

Critical Thinking Box 43.3
In your own words, define plasma and serum.

TABLE 43.2 Effects of Underfilling Collection Tubes

Stopper Color	Effects of Underfilling
Yellow	Reduces possibility of bacterial recovery
Light blue	Coagulation test results falsely prolonged
Red	Insufficient sample
Marbled red-gray, and gold (SST tubes)	Poor barrier formation; insufficient sample
Green	False results because of excess heparin
Marbled green-gray, and light green (PST tubes)	False results because of excess heparin
Lavender	Falsely low blood cell counts and hematocrits; morphologic changes to red blood cells; staining changes
Gray	False results

Modified from Proctor D, et al: *Kinn's The Medical Assistant*, ed 13, St Louis, 2017, Elsevier.

> **BOX 43.6 Yellow-Topped Tubes**
>
> In addition to blood culture bottles, a yellow-topped tube can be drawn for blood cultures for mycobacteria, fungi, and acid-fast bacilli. These tubes are not drawn frequently in an ambulatory setting. If they are ordered, they would be drawn in the same place as blood culture bottles in the order of the draw.

ORDER OF THE DRAW

If more than one tube must be drawn during a venipuncture, a specified order must be followed. Carryover of additives from one tube to the next could cause sample alteration and incorrect results. CLSI has established a set of standards outlining the order of draw for a multitube draw. The same order applies to the filling of tubes when blood is collected in a syringe.

1. *Blood culture bottles* are filled first because they are sterile and should not be contaminated by the other tubes (Box 43.6).
2. *Light blue* top: These tubes, which contain sodium citrate, are next because other anticoagulants might contaminate the sample collected for coagulation studies. If no blood culture has been ordered, CLSI recommends that blood for the light blue–topped tube be drawn first if routine coagulation testing has been ordered (i.e., prothrombin time [PT] and activated partial thromboplastin time [APTT]). (See Chapter 44 for more details about coagulation testing). Some laboratories recommend that a red-topped "waste" tube with no additives be partially filled before the light blue–topped tube. This is done to remove any tissue thromboplastin that was released during the venipuncture. Thromboplastin interferes with coagulation testing. CLSI also recommends that, when a winged infusion (butterfly assembly) is used, blood be drawn into the red-topped tube even if the order does not call for it. This is done to fill the tubing's dead air space with blood before drawing the light blue–topped sodium citrate tube. A light blue tube must have an exact blood-to-citrate dilution. It is not necessary to completely fill the waste tube, because it will be discarded.
3. *Red* top or *Gold* top: Red serum tubes without clot activator, or gold serum tubes with clot activator, are filled next. These clotted specimens are drawn to test the serum after the specimens have clotted and been centrifuged. SSTs with thixotropic gel are also drawn at this time. SST tubes have a marbled red-gray stopper or a gold Hemogard stopper.
4. *Green* top: These tubes are drawn next because the plasma in their anticoagulated specimen is used for testing when STAT results are needed (usually in chemistry). The dark green tops contain no thixotropic gel. The tubes with marbled green-gray tops and light green Hemogard tops both contain the gel to help separate the plasma from the cells when centrifuged.

> **VOCABULARY**
>
> **STAT:** The medical abbreviation for the Latin term *statum*, meaning immediately; at this moment.

5. *Lavender* top: These tubes are drawn next. They contain an EDTA anticoagulant that preserves blood cell morphology. EDTA tubes are drawn near the end of the draw because the additive interferes with chemistry and coagulation specimens.
6. *Gray* top: This tube is drawn last, and the blood is used to test glucose or blood alcohol levels. Its additives may elevate electrolyte levels and damage cells if passed into the other tubes.

TABLE 43.3 Stopper Color and Inversion Mixing

Stopper Color	Mix by Gentle Inversion
Blood culture bottles or yellow-topped tubes	6–10 times
Light blue	6–10 times
Red, marbled red-gray, or gold	5–6 times
Green or marbled green-gray	6–10 times
Lavender	6–10 times
Gray	6–10 times

From Proctor D, et al: *Kinn's The Medical Assistant*, ed 13, St Louis, 2017, Elsevier.

To recap, Table 43.1 shows the order of draw of the colored tube tops, in addition to the additives, laboratory uses, and accepted volumes per tube. Table 43.2 lists the effects of underfilling the collection tubes. Table 43.3 shows how many times the various tubes need to be inverted after they have been filled with blood. It is important to gently mix the contents of the tubes well, after collection, by inverting them several times (do not shake the tubes).

> **STUDY TIP**
>
> Sometimes making up a saying or sentence can help you remember the order of a process. Here are a few sayings I have heard in the past to remember the order of the draw.
>
> The order of the draw is: **St**erile (blood culture bottles/tubes) – **l**ight blue-**r**ed/gold-**g**reen-**l**avender-**g**ray. Use the first letter for each tube color and make up a sentence that helps you remember the order of the draw.
>
> Examples: 1. Stop light red. Green light go. 2. Stan's light red glasses look gray. 3. Stella's lecture reading gives little giggles. 4. Street lights reveal green little gardens.

> **Critical Thinking Box 43.4**
>
> Can you make up your own saying or sentence to remember the order of the draw? Work with a group in your class and come up with a few different ways to remember the order of the draw.

NEEDLES AND SUPPLIES USED IN PHLEBOTOMY

A critical part of phlebotomy is knowing which needle and which tube or syringe should be used in each situation. All needles used in phlebotomy are sterile and have a safety device that is activated immediately after withdrawal from the vein. The needle is then discarded in a biohazard sharps container. Each needle is housed in a protected cover, which should be inspected before use to ensure that sterility has not been compromised (i.e., the seal should be intact) and that the needle has no manufacturing defects, such as burs, nicks, or bends.

Needles have two parts, the hub and the shaft. The hub of the needle is designed to attach the needle to the vacuum tube needle holder or a syringe. Shafts differ in length, ranging from $\frac{3}{4}$ inch to $1\frac{1}{2}$ inches (Fig. 43.6). The length of the shaft has no bearing on the venipuncture procedure. Some phlebotomists prefer a longer needle, and others prefer a shorter needle because it makes patients less uneasy. One end of the

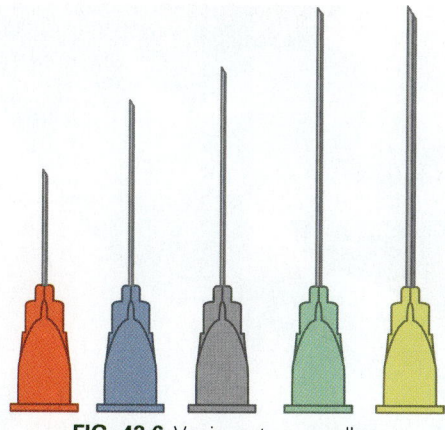

FIG. 43.6 Venipuncture needles.

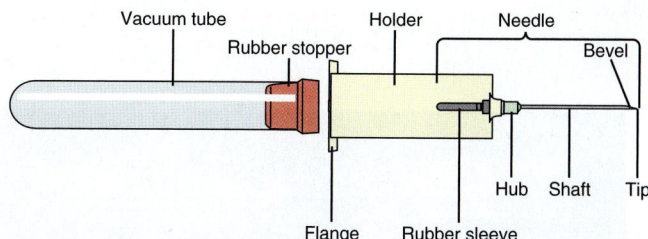

FIG. 43.8 Venipuncture assembly. (From Hunt SA: *Saunders Fundamentals Of Medical Assisting*, Revised Reprint, St. Louis, 2007, Saunders.)

Multisample Needles

Multisample (MUHL tee SAM puh l) needles are commonly used in routine adult venipuncture. They are used when several tubes need to be drawn during a single venipuncture. These needles are double pointed (Fig. 43.8). One point enters the patient's vein, and the other punctures the stopper of the collection tube. The point that enters the tube is sheathed with a retractable (ree TRAKT ah bul) rubber sleeve that allows tubes to be changed without blood leaking into the needle holder or tube holder.

> **Critical Thinking Box 43.5**
>
> Maggie has a few different gauge needles to use in phlebotomy. Why would she need different sized needles? The process is the same for each patient, why would the needle size be important? Share your ideas with the class.

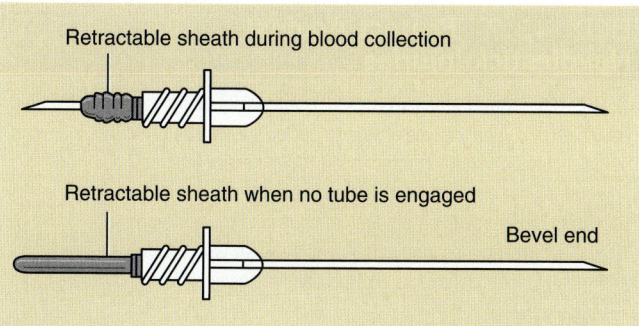

FIG. 43.7 Bevel of a venipuncture needle. (From Proctor D, et al: *Kinn's The Medical Assistant*, ed 13, St Louis, 2017, Elsevier.)

Needle Holders

Double-pointed needles must be firmly placed into a needle holder (see Fig. 43.8). Usually needle holders are translucent cylinders, and they come in different sizes to accommodate different-sized tubes. The holders often have a ring that indicates how far the tube can be pushed onto the needle without losing the vacuum. To prevent accidental needlesticks, OSHA requires that the needle holder, with its safety-activated needle still attached, must be discarded into a biohazard sharps container immediately after completing the venipuncture.

Syringes

Syringes are used when there is concern that the strong vacuum in a stoppered vacuum tube might collapse the vein. The syringe needle fits on the end of the syringe barrel. Syringe needles also come in different gauges. The amount of blood drawn into the syringe barrel depends on how much blood needs to be collected for testing. When blood is drawn into a syringe, it must be transferred immediately to the evacuated tube(s). Blood that sits in the syringe barrel could clot if not transferred quickly. The syringe needle safety device must be activated and discarded in the sharps container. A special transfer tube device is then used to transfer the blood to the vacuum tubes. This device connects to the top of the syringe; it contains an enclosed needle that punctures the vacuum tube's stopper and delivers the blood into the tube (Fig. 43.9).

Winged Infusion Sets (Butterfly Assembly)

Butterfly assemblies (Fig. 43.10) are designed for use on small veins. Butterfly needles are often used to draw veins in the back of the hand, or when drawing a pediatric patient. The most common butterfly needle size is a 22- or 23-gauge with a needle length of ½ to ¾ inch. A butterfly

shaft is cut at an angle and forms the *bevel* (BEV uh l), which creates a very sharp point. The bevel of the needle makes the entry into the skin much smoother (Fig. 43.7).

The bore, or hollow space, inside the needle is called the *lumen* (LOO muh n). Lumen size is important and is referred to as the *gauge* (geyj). A numeric value designates the gauge of the needle. The higher the gauge number, the smaller the lumen. Be sure to match the needle gauge to the size of the tube. A large vacuum tube is more likely to hemolyze the blood if a high-gauge needle (i.e., small lumen) is used. For example, blood banks use a large, 16-gauge needle to collect pints of blood for transfusions. The lumen is wide, which reduces the chance of hemolysis (hee MOL uh sis). A small, 23-gauge needle is used to collect blood from small or fragile veins, such as those in elderly and very young patients. Routine adult venipuncture requires a 20- to 21-gauge needle.

> **MEDICAL TERMINOLOGY**
>
> **hem/o:** blood
> **-lysis:** breakdown, separation, destruction

> **VOCABULARY**
>
> **hemolysis:** The breakdown of red blood cells with the release of hemoglobin.

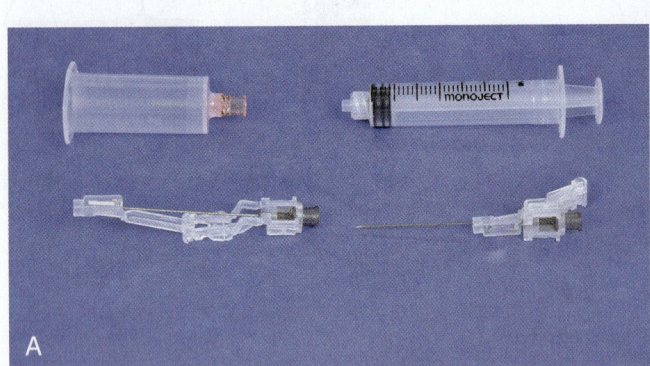
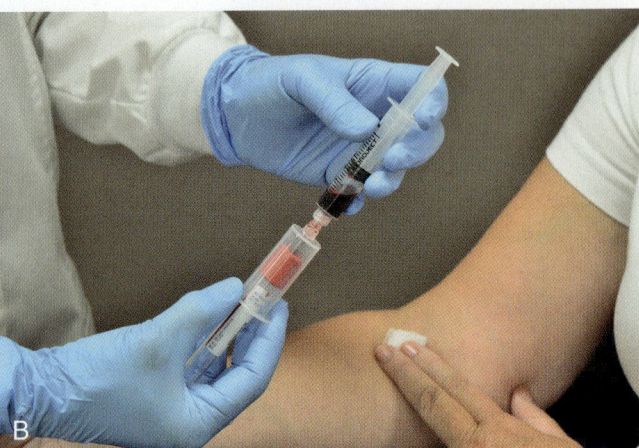

FIG. 43.9 Syringe assembly. (A from Proctor D, et al: *Kinn's The Medical Assistant*, ed 13, St Louis, 2017, Elsevier.)

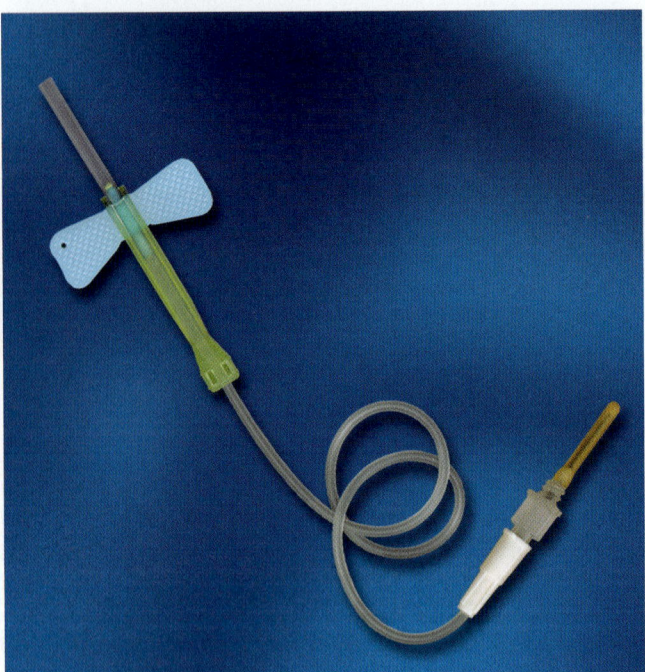

FIG. 43.10 Butterfly assembly. (Courtesy Becton, Dickinson, Franklin Lakes, NJ.)

> **BOX 43.7 Protect Against Needlestick Injuries**
>
> OSHA's Bloodborne Pathogens Standard emphasizes that phlebotomists should have direct input on the type of safety needles they will be using. The following steps should be taken to protect against needlestick injuries:
> - Help your employer evaluate and select devices with safety features.
> - Use devices with safety features provided by your employer.
> - Never recap a contaminated needle except with a safety device.
> - Plan for safe handling and disposal before beginning any procedure using needles.
> - Dispose of used needles and needle holders promptly in appropriate biohazard sharps containers.
> - Report all needlestick and other sharps-related injuries promptly to ensure that you receive appropriate follow-up care.
> - Tell your employer about hazards from needles that you observe in your work environment.
> - Participate in bloodborne pathogen training and follow recommended infection prevention practices, including vaccination against hepatitis B virus (HBV).

needle has a plastic, flexible, butterfly-shaped grip attached to a short length of tubing. The hub end is fitted into a syringe or a needle holder tube adapter. Syringes are frequently paired with butterfly needles because the syringe can create a gentle vacuum that can easily be controlled by the phlebotomist. The syringe blood sample must be transferred to the evacuated tubes using the transfer device described previously.

> **Critical Thinking Box 43.6**
>
> Describe the difference between a syringe and a winged infusion assembly. List two examples of when each type of equipment may be used.

NEEDLE SAFETY

Healthcare workers who use or may be exposed to needles are at increased risk of needlestick injury. Such injuries can lead to serious or fatal infections with blood-borne pathogens, such as HBV, HCV, and HIV. Needlestick injuries account for most accidental exposures to blood. As is discussed in Chapter 28 used needles should never be recapped. After use, needles should be covered with the appropriate engineered safety device that is part of the needle assembly.

According to OSHA, the best practice for preventing needlestick injuries after phlebotomy is to use safety needles that are activated with one hand immediately after use. The U.S. Food and Drug Administration (FDA), which is responsible for approving medical devices marketed and sold in the United States, recommends devices that provide a barrier between the hands and the needle, after use, in which the phlebotomist's hands remain behind the needle at all times. Safety shields that can be activated before or immediately after removal of the needle from the vein and that remain in effect after disposal should also be an integral part of the device. Finally, these devices should be as simple as possible, requiring little or no training to use (Box 43.7). Some examples of needle safety devices are:

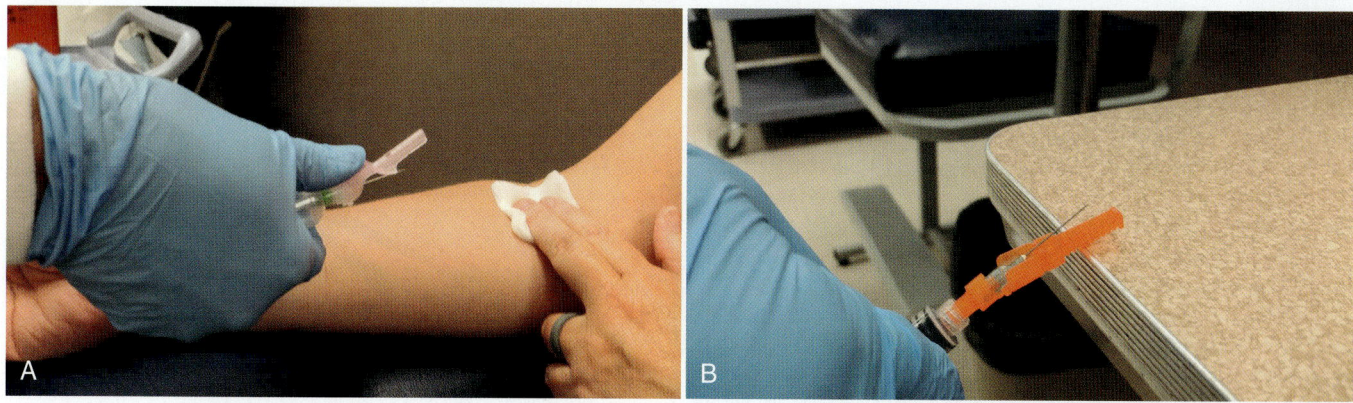

FIG. 43.11 One-handed safety needles. (A) Activated by sliding the thumb up at the base of the guard, causing it to cover the needle. (B) Activated by pressing the orange guard against a solid surface, causing it to cover the needle.

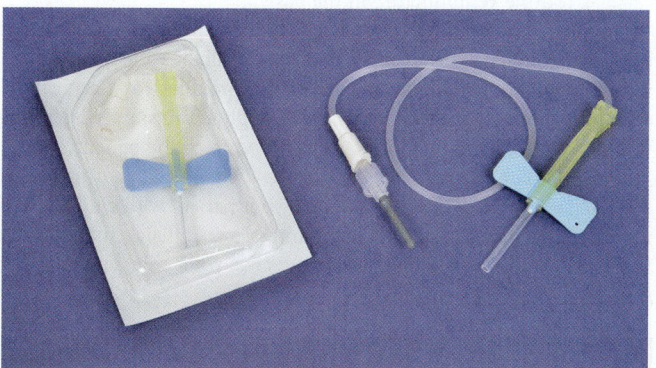

FIG. 43.12 Safety-Lok butterfly needle. (From Proctor D, et al: *Kinn's The Medical Assistant*, ed 13, St Louis, 2017, Elsevier.)

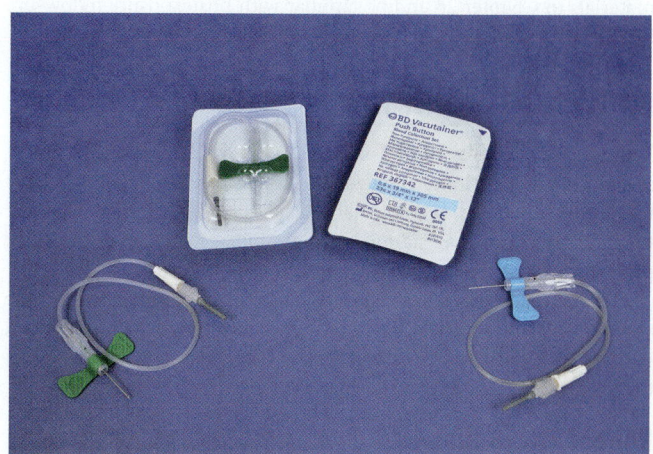

FIG. 43.13 Push-button butterfly needle. (From Proctor D, et al: *Kinn's The Medical Assistant*, ed 13, St Louis, 2017, Elsevier.)

- *One-handed vacuum tube needle:* After the needle has been used and removed from the vein, the thumb holding the vacuum tube holder slides under the base of the pink safety device, causing it to snap over the contaminated needle (Fig. 43.11A). Or, an orange needle shield on the holder is activated by pressing the device against a hard, flat surface (Fig. 43.11B).
- *Syringe needle safety devices* (see Fig. 43.9): These devices have a spring-activated shield attached to a disposable syringe needle. After the venipuncture, the phlebotomist activates the device with the thumb holding the syringe, and a spring locks a protective plastic tip into place, protecting the needle. The needle can then be removed and discarded. The syringe is attached to the safety transfer device to deliver the collected blood into the appropriate vacuum tubes (see Fig. 43.9).
- *Butterfly needle safety lock* (Fig. 43.12): After the venipuncture, the dominant hand holds the butterfly tail while the nondominant hand pulls back on the tubing, causing the needle to slide into the tubing and lock into place.
- *Push-button butterfly safety device* (Fig. 43.13): With the needle still in the arm, the medical assistant grasps the tail of the butterfly with the dominant hand while the nondominant hand presses the button just below the wings, causing the needle to retract into the butterfly body as it leaves the vein.

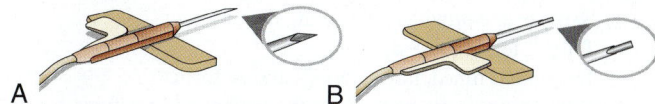

FIG. 43.14 Needle-blunting butterfly needle. (From Proctor D, et al: *Kinn's The Medical Assistant*, ed 13, St Louis, 2017, Elsevier.)

- *Needle-blunting butterfly set* (Fig. 43.14): A third "wing" is rotated after collection and before removal of the needle from the vein. As the third wing is rotated, it moves the blunt needle down the shaft before it is removed from the patient.

OSHA requires employers to establish and maintain a sharps injury log for recording injuries from contaminated sharps. This log should contain information about the device involved in the incident and the department or work area where the incident occurred, in addition to an explanation of the incident. Employee confidentiality must be maintained.

BOX 43.8 Postexposure Needlestick Management

- Immediately after injury, the wound is inspected and washed for 10 minutes with soap, 10% iodine solution, or chlorine-based antiseptic.
- The injury is reported to the supervisor, and an incident report is completed.
- The employee is referred to a physician for confidential assessment and follow-up. Baseline testing for hepatitis B virus (HBV), hepatitis C virus (HCV), and the human immunodeficiency virus (HIV) is recommended for both the employee and the source individual.
- Interim testing may be performed if the healthcare worker experiences symptoms of acute HIV exposure or hepatitis. Confidential follow-up care must include provisions for emotional support and counseling for the healthcare worker.

Postexposure Needlestick Follow-Up

An accidental needlestick is a medical emergency. OSHA-recommended management procedures are discussed in Chapter 28. Please review the materials in Chapter 28 and be familiar with postexposure follow-up. See Box 43.8 for a brief overview of postexposure management.

ROUTINE VENIPUNCTURE

Venipuncture involves a series of steps that are vital to collecting a good sample. In addition to learning good technique, we also want to be able to make our patients as comfortable as possible. As you read through the information you will start to become familiar with the venipuncture procedure and the details of the process.

The first step of the procedure is to select the proper method for venipuncture (evacuated tube, syringe, or butterfly assembly). Next, prepare your patient for the procedure. Then you are ready to collect the sample and the process the specimen appropriately.

Patient Preparation

All blood collections begin with a requisition, a form from the patient's provider requesting a test. Requisitions may be computer generated or handwritten, and at a minimum must include the following information:
- Patient's name
- Patient's date of birth
- Patient's identification number
- Name of the provider submitting the order
- Type of test requested
- Test status (timed, fasting, STAT, and so forth)

A venipuncture starts by greeting the patient and verifying his or her identity. According to CLSI, proper identification includes asking outpatients to (1) state and spell their first and last name, and (2) state their birth date. All the information must be compared and verified with the patient requisition. If communication with the patient is not effective due to any circumstances, a family member, guardian, or medical translator must provide the needed information. The name of the person assisting should be documented in the patient's medical record. Always follow your institution's procedures for assisted communication before completing the venipuncture procedure.

Briefly explain the venipuncture procedure to your patient, and make sure to ask him or her the following questions:
- Do you have any questions or concerns?
- Do you have an arm, vein, or site preference?
- Were you given any special instructions prior to the venipuncture (e.g., does the person need to be fasting?)

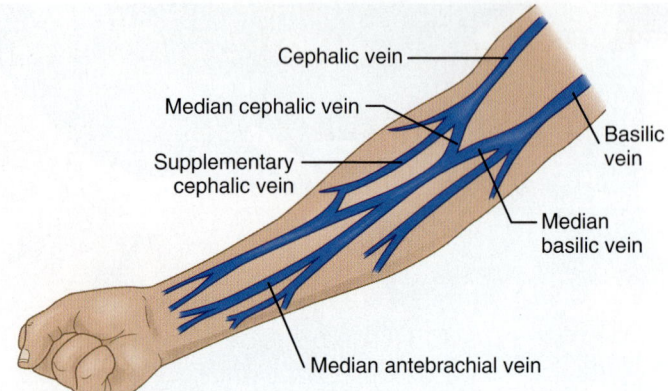

FIG. 43.15 The veins of the forearm. (From Stepp CA, Woods MA: *Laboratory Procedures For Medical Office Personnel*, Philadelphia, 1998, Saunders.)

- Have you ever experienced any problems or complications with a routine venipuncture in the past?

Answer questions and concerns, and take steps to prevent any past problems from recurring. If you cannot answer all the patient's questions, ask if he or she would like to talk to the provider for clarification. Obtain verbal consent to perform the venipuncture simply by asking whether you have permission to draw blood from the patient.

Your self-confidence in the procedure will help put your patient at ease. Act and speak professionally. Treat your patient with kindness and respect. Being pleasant and friendly is important. It makes your patients feel comfortable and shows that you take your role in their care seriously.

Critical Thinking Box 43.7

Why is patient identification so very important in phlebotomy? List four reasons and be ready to share them with the class.

EXCEPTIONAL CUSTOMER SERVICE

You may want to ask your patients how they would prefer to be addressed – by their first name? A nickname? Dr. Smith, Mr. Jones, Mrs. Blake, or Ms. Washington? – Don't assume that patients want to be called by their first name. Also, don't call patients "sweetie," "honey," or "dear." Be respectful.

Preparing for the Venipuncture

Seat the patient in a phlebotomy area. Ask the patient to extend an arm, and position his or her other hand under the elbow to help straighten the elbow, if necessary. Inspect both arms and ask whether the patient has an arm or site preference. Veins in the antecubital area are most commonly used for venipuncture (Fig. 43.15). According to CLSI standards, the veins in the center of the antecubital area should be located as a first choice before alternative veins within the antecubital area are considered. The puncture site should be carefully selected after both arms have been inspected. Alternative sites may be chosen if the area is scarred, bruised, burned, or swollen. You may use the veins on the back of the hand if the patient gives permission. For any other alternative site, consult the provider, and do not proceed without supervision.

When choosing the best available vein, palpate the area. Feel for a vein that has "bounce" when lightly palpated. The medial (MEE dee uh l) veins generally run at a slight angle to the fold in the antecubital

BOX 43.9 Two Most Common Phlebotomy Injuries

The most common injury patients suffer from phlebotomy is a **hematoma**; the second most common injury is nerve injury. If the patient complains of tingling, numbness, or a shooting pain, discontinue the procedure immediately! Attend to the patient and make sure he or she is okay. If you need to draw more blood, choose another site, and ask for the patient's permission before continuing. Do not blindly probe with the needle under any condition. Any attempt at relocating the needle puts the patient at risk of injury.

BOX 43.10 Palpating for Veins – With or Without Gloves?

According to the Clinical and Laboratory Standards Institute (CLSI), you can palpate veins without gloves on as long as the venipuncture site has not yet been cleaned. After locating the vein, clean the area with a 70% isopropyl alcohol wipe. While the site is drying, resanitize your hands, put on gloves, and continue with the rest of the procedure.

It is more efficient to put on gloves at the beginning of the procedure and continue. Also, if you learn to palpate veins with your gloves on, you will train your finger to recognize the veins with gloves on from the beginning.

BOX 43.11 Angle of Needle Entry

Why is the angle of the needle so important? If the needle is inserted at an angle greater than 15 degrees, it penetrates the vein quickly and may pass through the back side of the vein and enter other structures. Formation of a hematoma is more likely then.

If the angle is less than 15 degrees, the needle may skim on the top of the vein and not create a clean puncture. If the vein is just skimmed or scratched, there is a greater chance of creating a hematoma on the front of the vein.

The depth and position of the vein may require angle adjustment, but a 15-degree angle is a good place to start. The angle of entry is very important to a successful venipuncture.

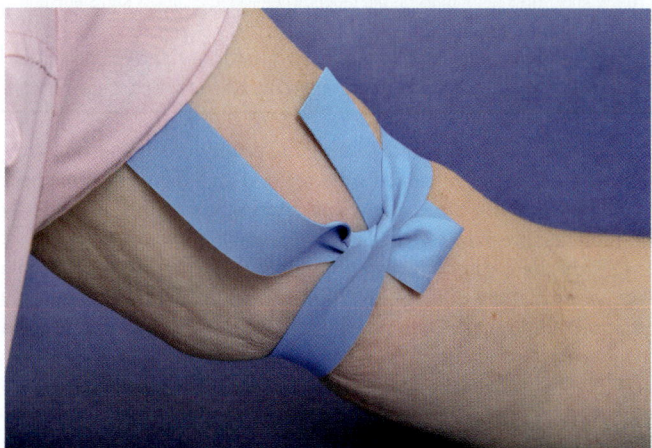

FIG. 43.16 Placement of the tourniquet on the arm. (From Proctor D, et al: *Kinn's The Medical Assistant*, ed 13, St Louis, 2017, Elsevier.)

area. The cephalic (suh FAL ik) veins are on the thumb side of the antecubital area. These veins are the veins of choice. The basilic (buh SIL ik) vein, which lies on the inside of the antecubital area (the little finger side), is very close to the brachial artery and median nerves and should *not* be used! If the medial or cephalic veins are not accessible, consult the provider. Only the most experienced phlebotomists should ever attempt a basilic venipuncture. The chance of injury to the patient is too great! See Box 43.9 for the most common phlebotomy injuries.

> **VOCABULARY**
> **hematoma:** An abnormal buildup of blood in an organ or a tissue of the body, caused by a leak or cut in a blood vessel.

The tourniquet should be placed about 3 to 4 inches above the patient's elbow. Make sure it is not twisted because that will cause discomfort to your patient (Fig. 43.16). Grasp the tourniquet ends, one in each hand, close to the patient's skin. Pull the ends apart to gently stretch the tourniquet, then cross one end over the other while maintaining the tension. Tuck the top portion of the tourniquet underneath the bottom portion, creating a loop with the upper flap free. The free end will be tugged on to release the tourniquet later in the draw. The tourniquet should be tight without being uncomfortable or pinching the patient's skin. Both ends of the tourniquet should be pointing upward on the arm. This way, the end of the tourniquet does not contaminate the venipuncture site.

When the tourniquet is in place, ask the patient to place his or her other hand or fist under the elbow of the arm that will be drawn if this aids in palpating the vein. Ask the person to just relax the arm. Palpate for an acceptable vein using your index finger. Palpate the vein through gloved fingers, and then continue with the phlebotomy process (Box 43.10).

Performing the Venipuncture

When you have located a vein, remove the tourniquet. A tourniquet can remain in place for 1 minute. After its removal, wait 2 minutes before reapplying it. During this time, sanitize your hands and put on gloves (if they are not already on). Then cleanse the antecubital area with a 70% alcohol wipe. Clean the area by using a back and forth motion. CLSI guidelines have been changed and now recommend cleansing the site with friction and not a circular motion. Do not touch this area after cleaning with alcohol. Assemble the equipment and place it within easy reach of the patient's arm.

Reapply the tourniquet. Do not have the patient clench or pump the fist. If the fist is relaxed, the venipuncture will feel less painful. Relocate the vein. Anchor the vein by gently stretching the skin downward below the collection site with the thumb of the nondominant hand. Smoothly and quickly insert the needle into the vein at about a 15-degree angle, depending on the depth and position of the vein (Box 43.11). The bevel should be facing up. Push the evacuated tube onto the double-pointed needle or pull back on the syringe plunger with your nondominant hand.

Critical Thinking Box 43.8

Maggie is drawing Ken Thomas this morning. The provider has ordered three different tests, so Maggie will need to draw three different-colored tubes. As Maggie puts on the tourniquet to locate a vein, Ken pumps his fist a few times to try to make the veins stand out. But Maggie asks him to just relax his hand. Why would relaxing his hand be better. List one or two reasons and be ready to share them with the class.

Completing the Venipuncture

Continue to draw the specimens, checking periodically on the patient's condition. As you remove each tube from the needle holder, gently invert it several times before placing it in a collection rack. Tubes with clot activator should be inverted 5 times. Tubes with anticoagulant should be inverted 6 to 10 times (see Table 43.3). If the tubes are not inverted immediately after collection, small clots can form in the specimen. When the last tube has started to fill, carefully release the tourniquet. Gently tug on the short portion of the tourniquet, and it should just fall open. Remove the final vacuum tube. Cover the venipuncture area with gauze, then smoothly and quickly remove the needle. Once the needle is out of the arm, apply pressure to the site. At the same time, activate the safety device to cover the needle. Dispose of the entire venipuncture assembly into a sharps container. Ask the patient to apply direct pressure to the gauze. **Do not** bend the arm.

While the patient applies pressure to the site, label the tubes with computer-generated labels or by writing the information in permanent marker. Make sure the label contains the following minimum information:
- Patient's last name, then first name
- Patient's date of birth
- Patient's ID number or medical insurance number
- Date and time of the draw, and the phlebotomist's initials
- Provider's name; also indicate if patient was fasting (optional)

Before putting on a bandage, perform a two-point check to make sure the site is not leaking. Observe the site for 5 to 10 seconds after releasing pressure and removing the gauze. If visible bleeding occurs or if the tissue around the puncture site rises, continue applying pressure until the bleeding has stopped. Special precautions must be taken for patients taking anticoagulants because the phlebotomy site will bleed longer than normal. Put on a pressure bandage by placing a folded gauze (not a cotton ball) over the site and then applying hypoallergenic self-stick wrap, stretchy gauze, or a bandage. Never leave the room or release an outpatient until all the tubes have been labeled. Make sure the patient is doing well, then escort him or her to the exit or to the reception area.

> ### Critical Thinking Box 43.9
> At the end of Ken's venipuncture, Maggie asks Ken to hold pressure on the draw site. She puts the computer-generated labels on the three tubes she drew and writes her initials on the labels. Then Maggie checks Ken's arm and wraps a gauze around the site.
>
> Why is it important to label the tubes immediately after finishing the venipuncture? List two reasons this is a good practice for a phlebotomist.

Procedures 43.1 and 43.2 outline the proper procedures for venipuncture using the evacuated tube method and the syringe method. Some patients may have small veins, and using a syringe or butterfly for venipuncture may work better than the standard evacuated assembly. Young children, chemotherapy patients, elderly patients, and people with veins that are difficult to draw may require syringe or butterfly equipment. Alternative equipment is always used to draw blood from hand veins (Procedure 43.3).

Text continued on p. 1066

PROCEDURE 43.1 Perform a Venipuncture: Collect a Venous Blood Sample Using the Vacuum Tube Method

Task
To collect a venous blood specimen by the vacuum tube technique.

Equipment and Supplies
- Patient's health record
- Provider's order and/or lab requisition
- Vacuum tube needle, needle holder, and proper tubes for requested tests
- 70% isopropyl alcohol wipes
- Gauze
- Tourniquet
- Hypoallergenic self-stick wrap, tape, or bandage
- Permanent marking pen and/or printed labels
- Fluid-impermeable lab coat, protective eyewear, and gloves
- Biohazard sharps container
- Biohazard waste container

Procedural Steps

1. Check the provider's order and/or requisition form to determine the tests ordered. Gather the appropriate tubes and supplies. Put on a fluid-impermeable lab coat.
   Purpose: Each test requires a specific tube color that is indicated on the requisition. Donning a lab coat is part of ongoing infection control.

2. Greet the patient. Identify yourself. Verify the patient's identity with full name; ask the patient to spell the first and last name and to give his or her date of birth. Explain the procedure to be performed in a manner that is understood by the patient. Answer any questions the patient may have on the procedure. Obtain permission for the venipuncture.
   Purpose: To make sure you have the right patient. Explanations help gain the patient's cooperation and show awareness of a patient's concerns related to the procedure being performed.

3. Wash hands or use hand sanitizer, then put on gloves and protective eyewear.
   Purpose: To ensure infection control.

4. Have the patient sit with the arm well supported in a slightly downward position. Ask the patient if he or she has a preference regarding which arm is used for the venipuncture.
   Purpose: The veins of the antecubital area are more easily located when the elbow is straight. Asking about a patient preference gives the patient a chance to participate in the procedure.

5. Apply the tourniquet around the patient's arm 3 to 4 inches above the elbow on the preferred arm. The tourniquet should never be tied so tightly that it restricts blood flow in the artery (Fig. 1). Tourniquets should remain in place no longer than 60 seconds.
   Purpose: The tourniquet is used to make the veins more prominent.

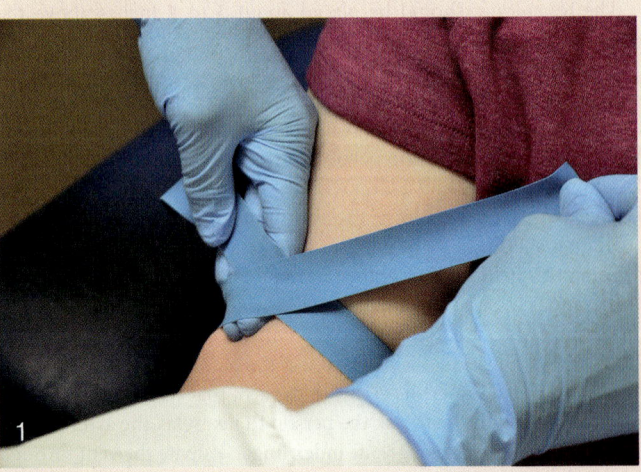

CHAPTER 43 Assisting in Blood Collection

PROCEDURE 43.1 Perform a Venipuncture: Collect a Venous Blood Sample Using the Vacuum Tube Method—cont'd

6. Select the venipuncture site by palpating the antecubital space. Use your index finger to trace the path of the vein and to judge its depth. The veins most often used are the medial or cephalic veins, which lie in the middle of the elbow (Fig. 2). Look at both arms and use your critical thinking skills to find the vein that will give you the greatest chance of success for the venipuncture.
   Purpose: The index finger is most sensitive for palpating the vein. Do not use the thumb because it has a pulse of its own. Spend time to properly locate the best vein available – your patient will thank you.

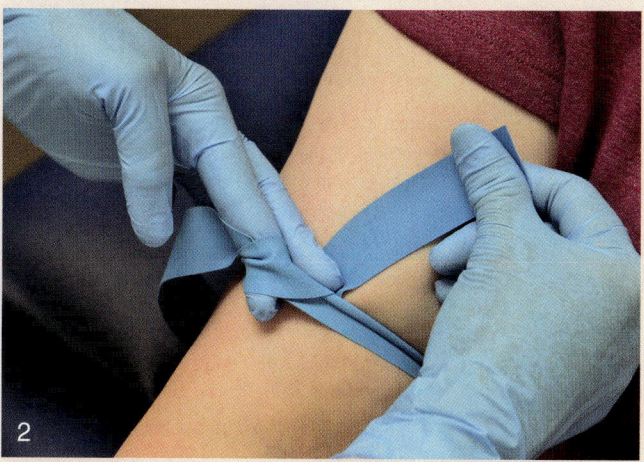

2

7. Remove the tourniquet and cleanse the site with a 70% alcohol wipe (Fig. 3).
   Purpose: The tourniquet should only be tied for 60 seconds.

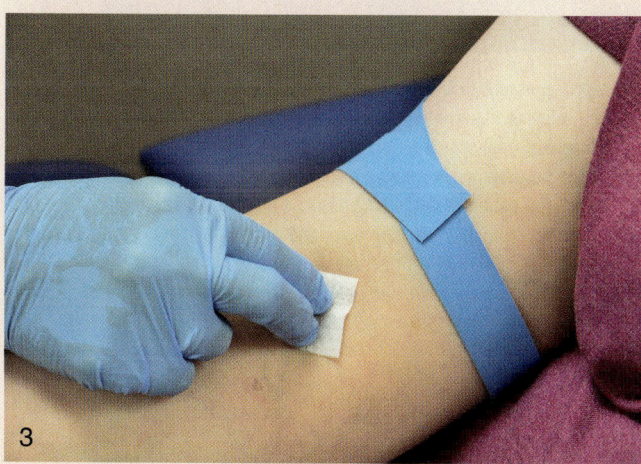

3

8. Assemble your equipment and supplies on the nondominant side of the patient's arm. The choice of needle size depends on your inspection of the patient's veins. Attach the needle firmly to the vacuum tube holder. Keep the cover on the needle.
   Purpose: If the needle is loose, it may turn during the procedure, causing the bevel of the needle to turn away from its upward position.
9. Reapply the tourniquet when the alcohol is dry.
   Purpose: Puncturing an area that is still wet with alcohol stings and can cause hemolysis of the sample.

10. Hold the vacuum tube assembly in your dominant hand. Your thumb should be on top and your fingers underneath (Fig. 4). You may want to lay the first tube to be drawn in the needle holder, but do not push it onto the double-pointed needle. Remove the needle sheath.
    Purpose: Positioning the hand in this manner provides the best visibility of the needle entering the vein and accessibility to insert and withdraw tubes with the nondominant hand. Pushing the tube into the double-pointed needle before it is in the arm causes air to rush into the tube, destroying the vacuum.

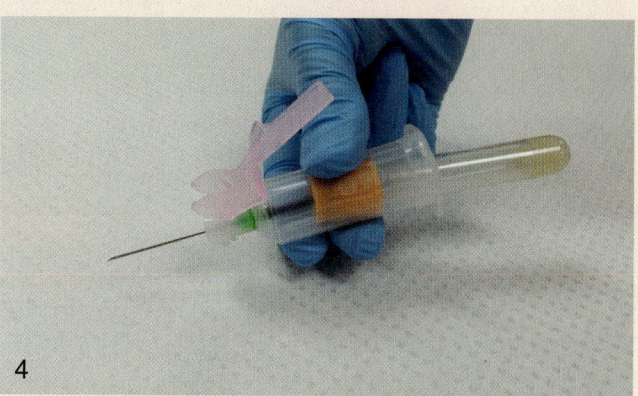

4

11. Grasp the patient's arm with the nondominant hand and anchor the vein by gently stretching the skin downward below the collection site with the thumb of the nondominant hand.
    Purpose: Failure to anchor the vein may cause the vein to move away from the needle as it enters the arm.
12. With the bevel up and the needle aligned parallel to the vein, insert the needle at a 15- to 20-degree angle through the skin and into the vein with a quick but smooth motion (Fig. 5).
    Purpose: The sharpest point of the needle is inserted first. Inserting the needle quickly minimizes pain.

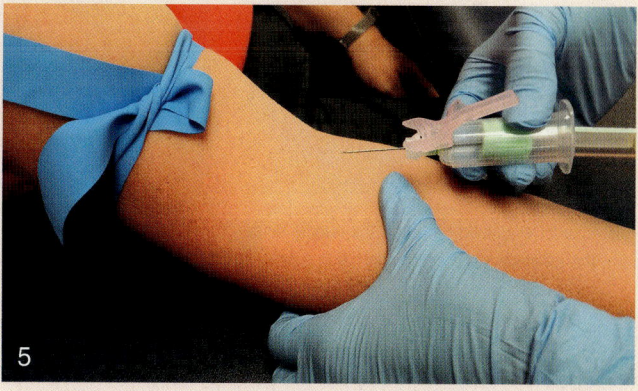

5

13. The dominant hand never lets go of the needle assembly once it is in the vein. Hold the assembly in place and steady through the venipuncture.
    Purpose: Holding the needle assembly steady will keep the needle from moving in the vein.
14. Place two fingers on the flanges of the needle holder and use the thumb to push the tube onto the double-pointed needle (Fig. 6). Make sure you do not change the needle's position in the vein.

Continued

PROCEDURE 43.1 Perform a Venipuncture: Collect a Venous Blood Sample Using the Vacuum Tube Method—cont'd

Purpose: The thumb has the strength to push the needle swiftly through the stopper. Be careful and keep the position of the needle steady so it is not pushed farther into the site when the tube is pushed.

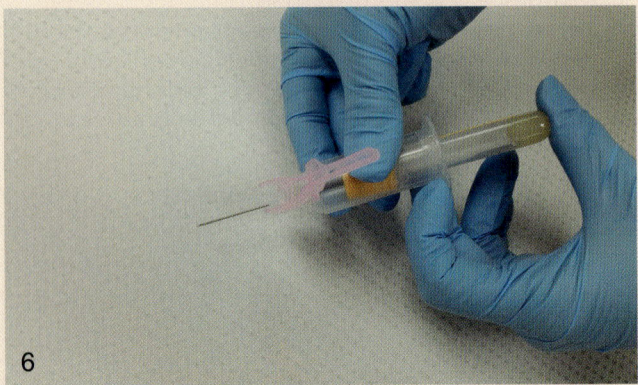
6

15. Allow the tube to fill to its maximum capacity. Remove the tube by placing the fingers at the end of the tube and pushing on the needle holder with the index finger (Fig. 7). Take care not to move the needle when removing the tube. Immediately after removing the tube from the needle holder, gently invert the tube to mix the additives and the blood.
Purpose: Tubes must be full to ensure the proper anticoagulant-to-blood ratio. Moving the needle may result in the needle advancing farther into the vein or slipping out of the vein. Gentle inversion prevents blood from clotting. Do not vigorously mix or shake the tubes, because this may cause hemolysis.

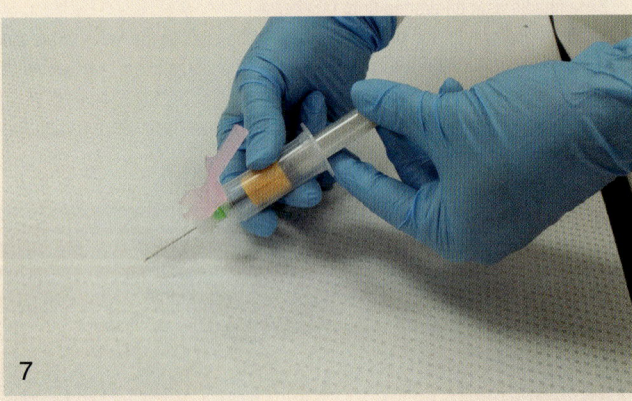
7

16. Insert the second tube into the needle holder, following the instructions in the previous steps. Continue filling tubes until the order on the requisition has been filled. Gently invert each tube after removing it from the needle holder. As the last tube begins filling, release the tourniquet. The tourniquet must be released before the needle is removed from the arm (Fig. 8).
Purpose: The tourniquet should remain in place for no longer than 1 minute to prevent hemoconcentration.

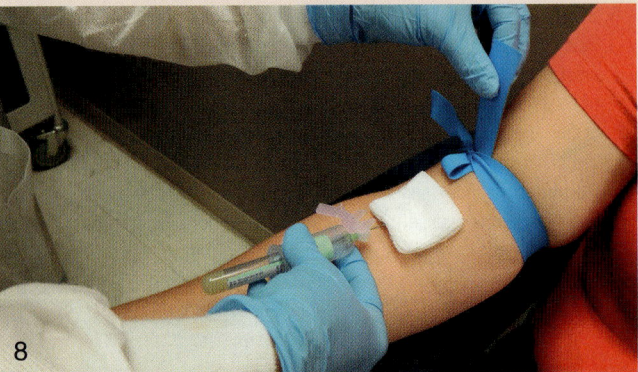
8

17. Remove the last tube from the holder. Place gauze over the puncture site and quickly remove the needle, engaging the safety device (Fig. 9). Dispose of the entire needle/holder assembly into the sharps container.
Purpose: The gauze over the puncture site and activation of the safety needle ensure infection control.

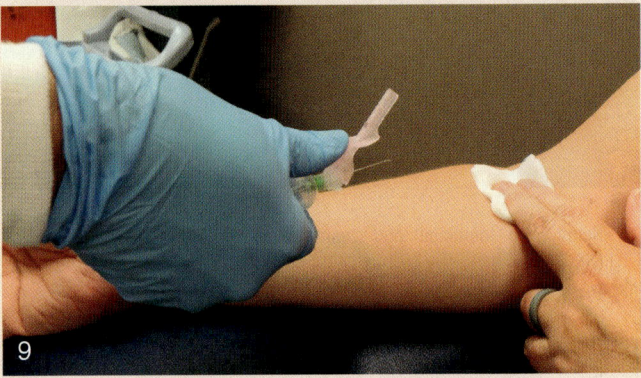
9

18. Apply pressure to the gauze or instruct the patient to do so. The patient may elevate the arm but should not bend the elbow.
Purpose: Applying direct pressure and elevating the arm above the heart is the best method to stop bleeding.
19. While the patient is applying pressure to the site, label the tubes with the patient's name and the date, time, and your initials, or affix the preprinted tube labels and print your initials on the label.
20. Check the venipuncture site. Make sure bleeding has stopped. Apply a hypoallergenic self-stick wrap, gauze and tape, or bandage (Fig. 10).

PROCEDURE 43.1   Perform a Venipuncture: Collect a Venous Blood Sample Using the Vacuum Tube Method—cont'd

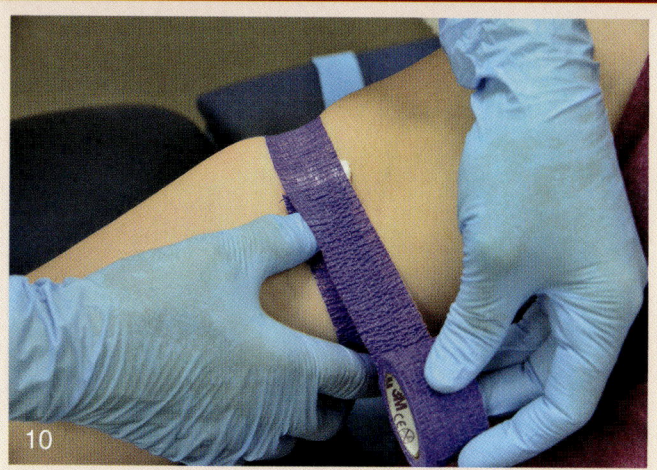

21. Disinfect the work area. Dispose of blood-contaminated materials (e.g., gauze and gloves) in the biohazard waste container. Remove your protective eyewear and gloves. Wash hands or use hand sanitizer.
    Purpose: To ensure infection control.
22. Complete the laboratory requisition form and route the specimen to the proper place. Record the procedure in the patient's record.
    Purpose: A procedure is not considered done until it is recorded in the patient record.

Documentation Example
10/05/20XX 1:45 p.m.: Venous blood drawn from antecubital space of ® arm. Lavender tube for CBC with differential, and red tube for Chemistry. Placed for pickup by Health Alliance Labs._____
_____Maggie Brandt, CMA (AAMA)

PROCEDURE 43.2   Perform a Venipuncture: Collect a Venous Blood Sample Using the Syringe Method

Task
To collect a venous blood specimen using the syringe technique.

Equipment and Supplies
- Patient's health record
- Provider's order and/or lab requisition
- Syringe with 21- or 22-gauge safety needle
- Vacuum tubes appropriate for tests ordered
- 70% isopropyl alcohol wipes
- Gauze
- Tourniquet
- Safety transfer device to transfer blood from syringe to vacuum tubes
- Hypoallergenic self-stick wrap, tape, or bandage
- Permanent marking pen or printed labels
- Fluid-impermeable lab coat, protective eyewear, and gloves
- Biohazard sharps container
- Biohazard waste container

Procedural Steps
1. Check the provider's order and/or requisition form to determine the tests ordered. Gather the appropriate tubes and supplies. Put on a fluid-impermeable lab coat.
   Purpose: To collect the specimen properly based on the tube requirements on the requisition. Donning a lab coat is part of ongoing infection control.
2. Greet the patient. Identify yourself. Verify the patient's identity with full name; ask the patient to spell the first and last name and to give his or her date of birth. Explain the procedure to be performed in a manner that is understood by the patient. Answer any questions the patient may have on the procedure. Obtain permission for the venipuncture.
   Purpose: It is important to identify the patient in two different ways to ensure that you have the correct patient. Explaining the procedure can make the patient feel more comfortable and helps to reduce anxiety.
3. Wash hands or use hand sanitizer. Put on gloves and protective eyewear.
   Purpose: To ensure infection control.
4. Have the patient sit with the arm well supported in a slightly downward position. Ask the patient if he or she has a preference regarding which arm is used for the venipuncture.
   Purpose: The veins of the antecubital area are more easily located when the elbow is straight. Asking about a patient preference gives the patient a chance to participate in the procedure.
5. Apply the tourniquet around the patient's arm 3 to 4 inches above the elbow on the preferred arm. The tourniquet should never be tied so tightly that it restricts blood flow in the artery (Fig. 1). Tourniquets should remain in place no longer than 60 seconds.
   Purpose: The tourniquet is used to make the veins more prominent.

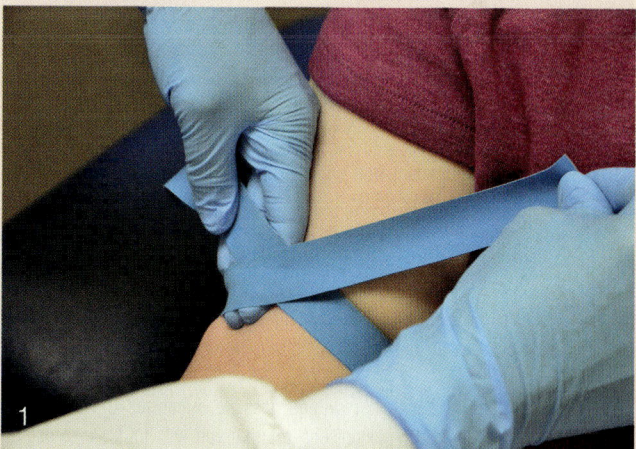

6. Select the venipuncture site by palpating the antecubital space. Use your index finger to trace the path of the vein and to judge its depth. The veins most often used are the medial or cephalic veins, which lie in the middle of the elbow (Fig. 2). Look at both arms and use your critical thinking skills to find the vein that will give you the greatest chance of success for the venipuncture.

Continued

PROCEDURE 43.2 Perform a Venipuncture: Collect a Venous Blood Sample Using the Syringe Method—cont'd

Purpose: The index finger is most sensitive for palpating the vein. Do not use the thumb because it has a pulse of its own. Spend time to properly locate the best vein available — your patient will thank you.

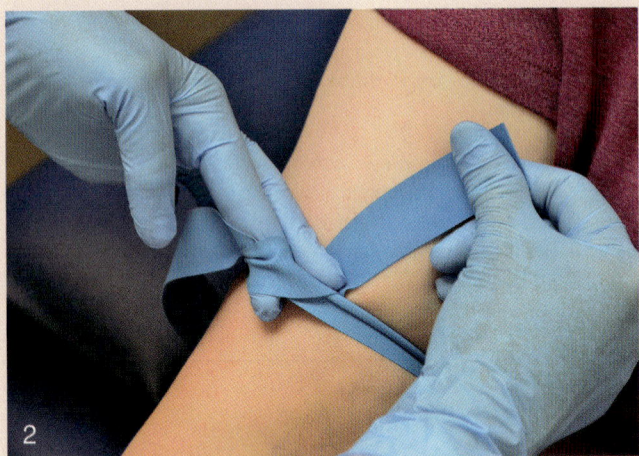

7. Remove the tourniquet and cleanse the site with a 70% alcohol wipe. (Fig. 3).
   Purpose: The tourniquet should only be tied for 60 seconds.

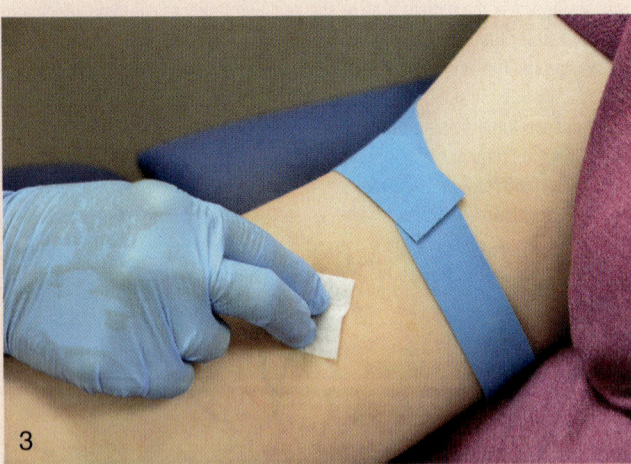

8. Assemble the equipment and supplies on the nondominant side of the patient's arm. Use your critical thinking skills to choose the proper syringe barrel size and needle size. This depends on the amount of blood required for the ordered tests and your inspection of the patient's veins. Attach the needle firmly to the syringe. Pull and depress the plunger several times to loosen it in the barrel while keeping the cover on the needle (Fig. 4). The plunger must be pushed in completely after you have loosened it in the barrel.
   Purpose: Using the smallest syringe possible minimizes the chance of hemolysis. Engaging the plunger ensures that you will not have to use as much force to pull the blood into the barrel, thereby minimizing the chance of hemolysis.

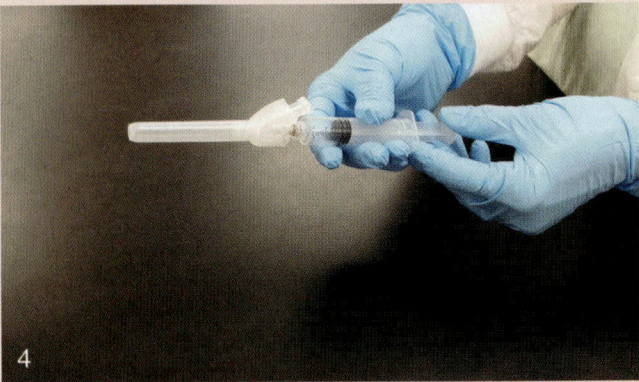

9. Reapply the tourniquet when the alcohol is dry.
   Purpose: Puncturing an area that is still wet with alcohol stings and can cause hemolysis of the sample.
10. Hold the syringe in your dominant hand. Your thumb should be on top and your fingers underneath, the same as in the vacuum tube method. Remove the needle sheath.
    Purpose: Positioning the hand in this manner provides the best visibility of the needle entering the vein and accessibility to the syringe plunger.
11. Grasp the patient's arm with the nondominant hand and anchor the vein by stretching the skin downward below the collection site with the thumb of the nondominant hand.
    Purpose: Failure to anchor the vein may cause the vein to move away from the needle when it is inserted, resulting in a missed vein.
12. With the bevel up and the needle aligned parallel to the vein, insert the needle at a 15- to 20-degree angle through the skin and into the vein with a quick but smooth motion (Fig. 5). Observe for a "flash" of blood in the hub of the syringe.
    Purpose: The sharpest point of the needle is inserted first. The angle ensures that the needle does not penetrate through the vein. The appearance (flash) of blood in the hub ensures that the needle is in the vein.

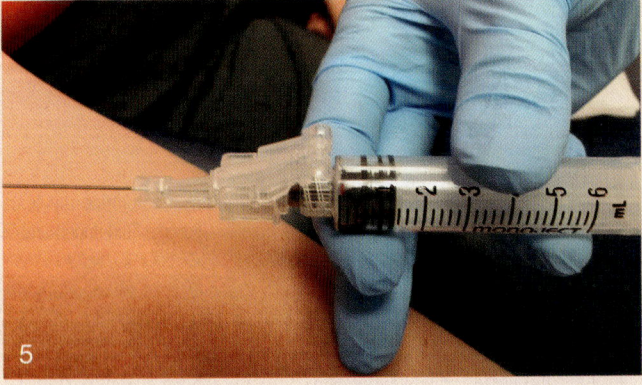

13. Slowly pull back the plunger of the syringe with the nondominant hand. Do not allow more than 1 mL of head space between the blood and the top of the plunger. Make sure you do not move the needle after entering the vein. Fill the barrel to the needed volume (Fig. 6).

PROCEDURE 43.2 Perform a Venipuncture: Collect a Venous Blood Sample Using the Syringe Method—cont'd

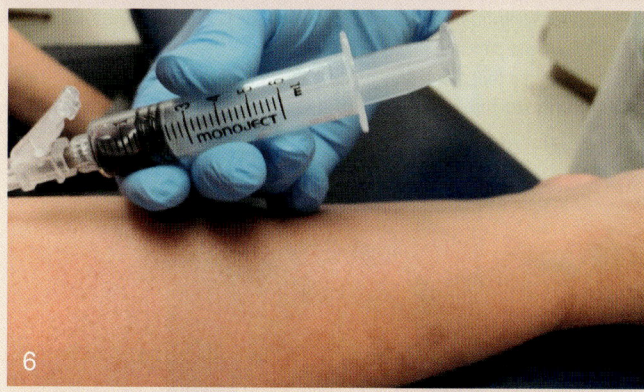
6

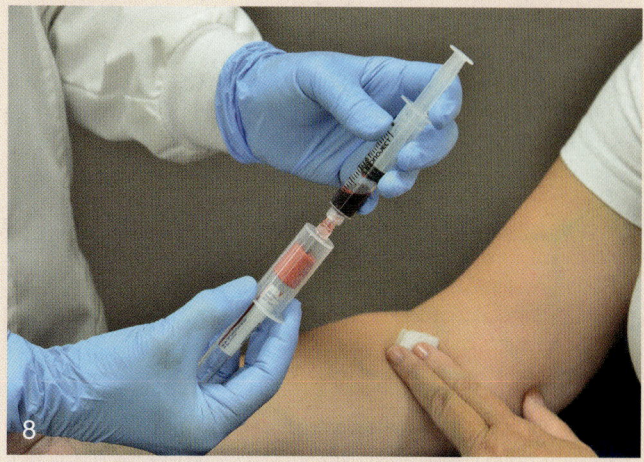
8

14. Release the tourniquet when the proper volume is reached. The tourniquet must be released before the needle is removed from the arm.
    Purpose: Removal of the tourniquet releases pressure on the vein and helps prevent blood from getting into adjacent tissues, causing a hematoma.
15. Place sterile gauze over the puncture site at the time of needle withdrawal (Fig. 7). Then, immediately activate the needle safety device using the syringe hand and apply pressure to the site with the nondominant hand.

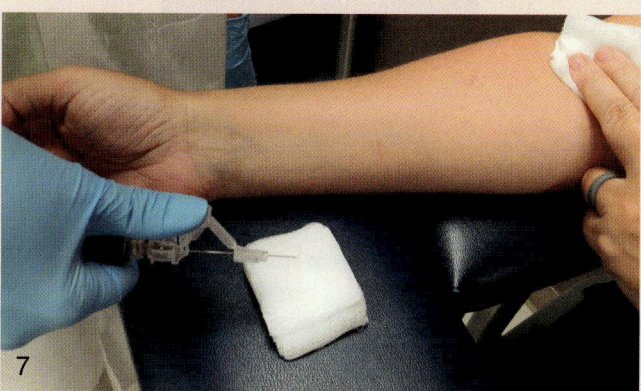
7

18. Check the venipuncture site. Make sure bleeding has stopped. Apply a hypoallergenic self-stick wrap, gauze and tape, or bandage (Fig. 9).

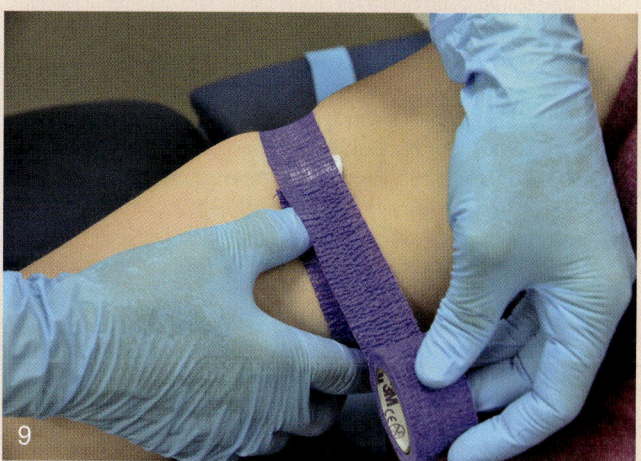
9

16. Instruct the patient to apply direct pressure on the puncture site with gauze. The patient may elevate the arm but should not bend the elbow.
    Purpose: Applying direct pressure and elevating the arm above the heart is the best method to stop bleeding.
17. Remove the syringe safety needle and transfer the blood immediately to the required tube or tubes using a safety transfer device. Do not push on the syringe plunger during transfer. Discard the entire unit in the sharps container when transfer is complete. Gently invert the tubes after the addition of blood. Label the tubes with the patient's name and the date, time, and your initials, or affix the preprinted tube labels and print your initials on the label. (Fig. 8).
    Purpose: The safety transfer device protects against accidental needlesticks and allows the correct amount of blood to be transferred into the tube by vacuum. Pushing the plunger hemolyzes the blood and may alter the amount of blood intended in each tube. Blood begins to clot shortly after collection, so it must be transferred into the vacuum tube and mixed with anticoagulant immediately after collection. Gently inverting the tubes ensures anticoagulation.

19. Disinfect the work area. Dispose of blood-contaminated materials (e.g., gauze and gloves) in the biohazard waste container. Remove your eyewear and gloves. Wash hands or use hand sanitizer.
    Purpose: To ensure infection control.
20. Complete the laboratory requisition form and route the specimen to the proper place. Record the procedure in the patient's record.
    Purpose: A procedure is not considered complete until it is recorded in the patient's record.

PROCEDURE 43.3   Perform Venipuncture: Obtain a Venous Sample With a Safety Winged Butterfly Needle Assembly

Task
To obtain a venous sample accurately from a hand or arm vein using a butterfly needle and syringe.

Equipment and Supplies
- Patient's health record
- Provider's order and/or lab requisition
- Safety winged (butterfly) needle set
- Syringe of appropriate volume for testing
- Vacuum tubes appropriate for tests ordered
- 70% isopropyl alcohol wipes
- Gauze
- Tourniquet
- Hypoallergenic self-stick wrap, tape, or bandage
- Permanent marking pen or printed labels
- Fluid-impermeable lab coat, protective eyewear, and gloves
- Biohazard waste container
- Biohazard sharps container

Procedural Steps

1. Check the provider's order and/or requisition form to determine the tests ordered. Gather the appropriate tubes and supplies. Put on a fluid-impermeable lab coat.
   Purpose: To collect the specimen properly based on the tube requirements on the requisition. Donning a lab coat is part of ongoing infection control.
2. Greet the patient. Identify yourself. Verify the patient's identity with full name; ask the patient to spell the first and last name and to give his or her date of birth. Explain the procedure to be performed in a manner that is understood by the patient. Answer any questions the patient may have on the procedure. Obtain permission for the venipuncture.
   Purpose: It is important to identify the patient in two different ways to ensure that you have the correct patient. Explaining the procedure can make the patient feel more comfortable and helps to reduce anxiety.
3. Wash hands or use hand sanitizer. Put on gloves and protective eyewear.
   Purpose: To ensure infection control.
4. *If drawing from the antecubital region:* Have the patient sit with the arm well supported in a slightly downward position. Ask the patient if he or she has a preference regarding which arm is used for the venipuncture.
   Purpose: The veins of the antecubital area are more easily located when the elbow is straight. Asking about a patient preference gives the patient a chance to participate in the procedure.
   a. *If drawing from the back of the hand:* Have the patient place the venipuncture hand over the other, fisted hand with the fingers lower than the wrist.
      Purpose: These positions help blood fill the veins in the hand; this makes it easier for you to identify the veins and choose the draw site.
5. *If drawing from the antecubital region:* Apply the tourniquet around the patient's arm 3 to 4 inches above the elbow on the preferred arm. The tourniquet should never be tied so tightly that it restricts blood flow in the artery. Tourniquets should remain in place no longer than 60 seconds.
   Purpose: The tourniquet is used to make the veins more prominent.
   a. *If drawing from the back of the hand:* Apply the tourniquet above the wrist just proximal to the wrist bone (Fig. 1). Do not apply the tourniquet so tightly that blood flow in the arteries is impeded.
      Purpose: The tourniquet is used to make the veins more prominent.

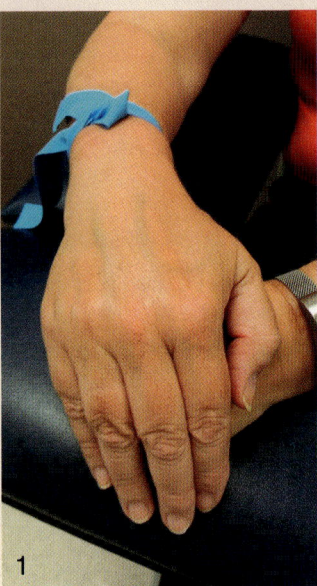

1

6. *If drawing from the antecubital region:* Select the venipuncture site by palpating the antecubital space. Use your index finger to trace the path of the vein and to judge its depth. The veins most often used are the medial or cephalic veins, which lie in the middle of the elbow. Look at both arms and use your critical thinking skills to find the vein that will give you the greatest chance of success for the venipuncture.
   Purpose: The index finger is most sensitive for palpating the vein. Do not use the thumb because it has a pulse of its own. Spend time to properly locate the best vein available — your patient will thank you.
   a. *If drawing from the back of the hand:* Select a vein on the back of the hand that is prominent, stable, and as straight as possible.
7. Remove the tourniquet and cleanse the site with a 70% alcohol wipe.
   Purpose: The tourniquet should only be tied for 60 seconds.
8. Assemble your equipment and supplies on the nondominant side of the patient's arm. Remove the butterfly device from the package and stretch the tubing slightly. Take care not to activate the needle-retracting safety device accidentally.
   Purpose: To keep the butterfly tubing from recoiling.
9. Attach the butterfly device firmly to the syringe (Fig. 2). If using a syringe, make sure to loosen the plunger a few times after the butterfly and syringe are attached.
   NOTE: The butterfly assembly can be attached to a needle holder OR a syringe (see Fig. 1). Make sure the connection is firmly in place. When a vein on the back of the hand is used for the draw, a butterfly-syringe combination is almost always used.

CHAPTER 43 Assisting in Blood Collection

PROCEDURE 43.3 Perform Venipuncture: Obtain a Venous Sample With a Safety Winged Butterfly Needle Assembly—cont'd

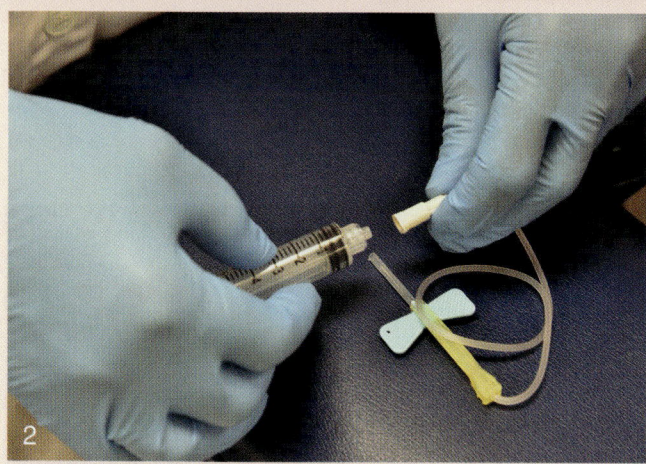

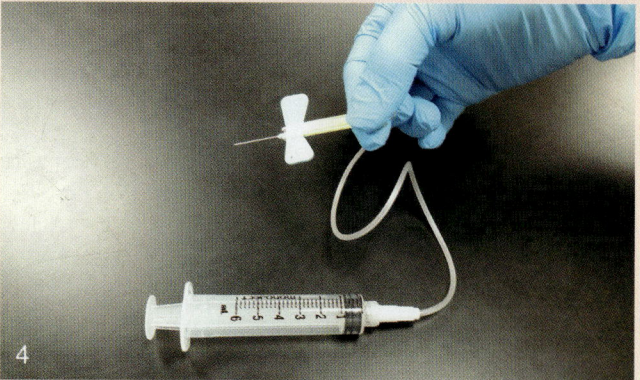

10. If using a needle assembly, lay the first tube in the vacuum tube holder and place the unit carefully where it will not roll away.
11. Reapply the tourniquet when the alcohol is dry.
    Purpose: Puncturing an area that is still wet with alcohol stings and can cause hemolysis of the sample.
12. Hold the butterfly wings pinched between your dominant hand thumb and index finger or hold the base of the needle (Figs. 3 and 4). Remove the needle sheath.
    Purpose: Positioning the hand in this manner provides the best visibility of the needle entering the vein and accessibility to insert and withdraw tubes with the nondominant hand.

13. *If drawing the antecubital region:* Grasp the patient's arm with the nondominant hand and anchor the vein by stretching the skin downward below the collection site with the thumb of the nondominant hand.
    Purpose: Failure to anchor the vein may cause the vein to move away from the needle when it is inserted, resulting in a missed vein.
    a. *If drawing from the back of the hand:* Using your thumb, pull the patient's skin taut over the knuckles.
       Purpose: Stretching the skin prevents the veins from rolling underneath.
14. With the bevel up and the needle aligned parallel to the vein, insert the needle at a 10- to 15-degree angle through the skin and into the vein with a quick but smooth motion (Fig. 5).
    NOTE: According to CLSI, after insertion of the needle, the wings should be held in place to keep the needle from moving until the butterfly needle is removed. Make sure the safety device is not activated.
    Purpose: The sharpest point of the needle is inserted first. The angle ensures that the needle does not penetrate through the vein.

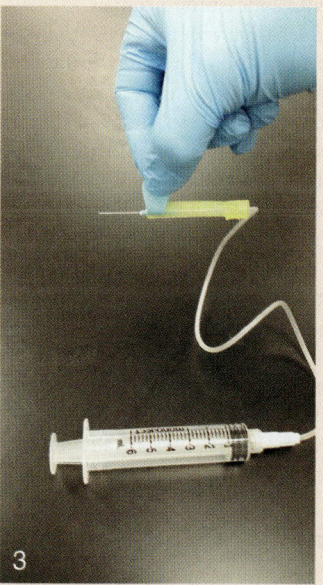

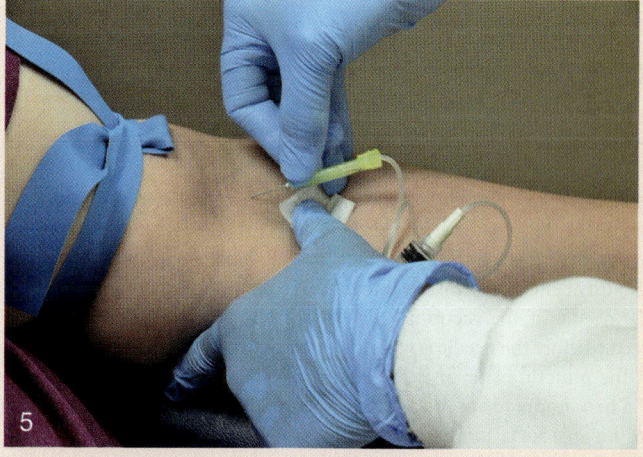

15. *If drawing with a needle holder assembly:* Push the blood collecting tube into the end of the holder. Note the position of the hands while drawing the blood.

Continued

PROCEDURE 43.3 Perform Venipuncture: Obtain a Venous Sample With a Safety Winged Butterfly Needle Assembly—cont'd

a. *If drawing with a syringe:* Make sure the vacuum you create is slow and steady and that no more than 1 mL of head space exists between the blood and the plunger. Slowly pull back the plunger of the syringe with the nondominant hand. Fill the barrel of the syringe to the needed volume (Fig. 6).

Purpose: Drawing blood too forcefully into the syringe may collapse the vein or hemolyze the blood.

Purpose: To prevent hemoconcentration, the tourniquet should remain in place no longer than 1 minute.

17. Always keep the tube and the holder in a downward position so that the tube fills from the bottom up.
18. Place a gauze over the puncture site and gently remove the needle, engaging the safety device. Dispose of the entire unit in the sharps container (Fig. 7).

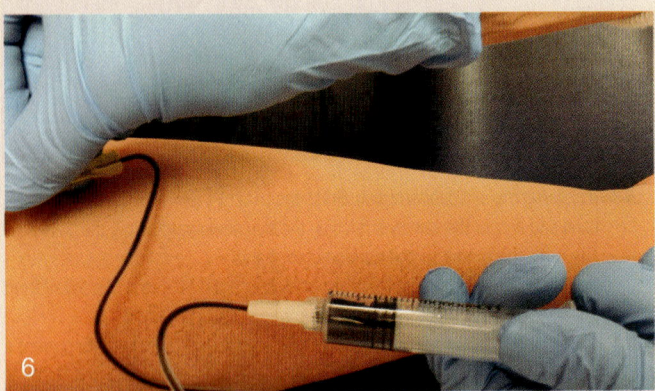

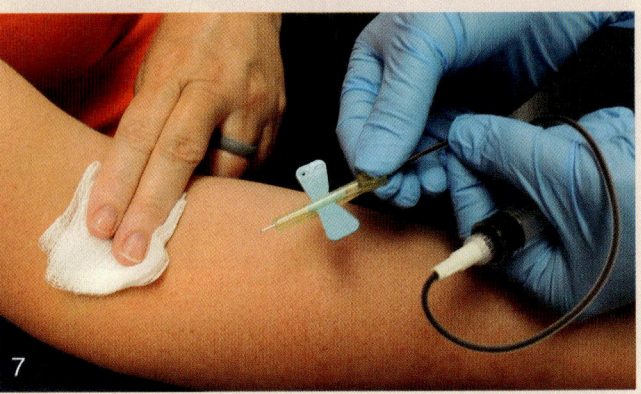

19. Complete the procedure as you would for an antecubital draw (see Procedure 43.1, Steps 18 through 22).

16. Release the tourniquet when the blood appears in the tubing or a "flash" of blood is seen in the hub of the syringe.

PROBLEMS ASSOCIATED WITH VENIPUNCTURE

Failure to obtain blood can occur due to several factors. Determining the cause of the problem may help you decide whether a second attempt would be successful. The first rule is to remain calm and professional. Remaining calm helps you think clearly about the situation and about the potential causes for not getting blood.

Hematoma

A hematoma (hee ma TOH muh) is a large, painful, bruised area at the puncture site caused by blood leaking into the tissue, which causes the tissue around the puncture site to swell. The most common causes of hematoma formation during the draw are excessive probing with the needle to locate a vein, failure to insert the needle far enough into the vein, and passing the needle through the vein. A hematoma can also form after a draw if the tourniquet is not removed before removing the needle; if the vacuum tube is not removed from the hub of the needle before the needle is withdrawn; if adequate pressure is not applied at the puncture site; or if the elbow is bent while pressure is applied. If a hematoma forms, discontinue the procedure STAT, apply pressure to the area for a minimum of 3 minutes, and then apply an ice pack to the area. Notify the provider and observe the site to determine whether the bleeding has stopped. Depending on the facility's policy, an incident report may have to be completed and documented in the patient's record. A hematoma may also occur if the puncture reopens and bleeds into the tissue due to heavy lifting with the venipuncture arm. Instruct the patient to be careful with the arm for several hours after the procedure.

MEDICAL TERMINOLOGY
hemat/o: blood
-oma: mass, fluid collection, tumor

Nerve Damage and Other Complications

Nerve damage can be a consequence of venipuncture, but the risk is very small. Preventive measures include:
- Avoiding the basilic vein for phlebotomy
- Refraining from "blind" probing if the vein is missed with the initial draw

Table 43.4 lists some workable solutions to complications. As a rule, it is wise to limit yourself to two venipuncture attempts for a patient. If a second attempt is unsuccessful, ask whether the patient would allow another phlebotomist to look at his or her arms. If another phlebotomist feels confident to attempt a venipuncture, that person will need to get permission from the patient first. If the patient doesn't give permission, it may be better to reschedule the venipuncture for another time. This strategy lets patients know that they have input into their care and some measure of control of the situation. At one time or another, everyone is unsuccessful in obtaining a blood sample, so do not feel badly. Make the best of the situation, learn from the experience, and treat the patient with kindness. We are all human, and our patients are usually quite understanding.

VOCABULARY
lymphostasis: Obstruction or interruption of normal lymph flow.
petechiae: Very small, round hemorrhage spots in the skin or mucous membrane.

Fainting

Fainting, or syncope, can have serious consequences, so the phlebotomist must always be prepared to take action quickly. Positioning the patient in a blood collection chair (by turning the armrest pad in front of the patient) prevents bodily injury if the person faints. Making eye contact and observing the patient before phlebotomy can help you estimate

TABLE 43.4 Managing Possible Blood Draw Complications

Complication	Management Strategies
Burned area	Choose another site because these areas are prone to infection.
Convulsions	Stay calm. Remove the needle and quickly dispose of it in a sharps container. Then help guide the patient to the floor, protecting him or her from injury. Call for help.
Damaged or scarred veins or infected areas	Look for an alternative site; do not draw blood from scarred or infected areas.
Edema	Avoid the area; look for an alternative site.
Hematoma	Adjust the depth of the needle or remove the needle and apply pressure.
Intravenous (IV) therapy or blood transfusion sites	Blood samples should not be drawn from an arm that is also the site for IV infusion or blood transfusion because of the dilution factor.
Mastectomy (ma STEK tuh mee)	Do not draw blood from the side of the mastectomy, because mastectomy surgery causes lymphostasis (lihm foh STEY sis), which may produce false results.
Nausea	Place a cold cloth on the patient's forehead, give the patient a basin in case of vomiting, and instruct him or her to take deep breaths. Alert the provider.
No blood	Manipulate the needle slightly or remove the vacuum tube and perform the blood draw again using a syringe or butterfly setup.
Petechiae (pih TEE kee uh)	Loosen the tourniquet because this complication usually results from the tourniquet being in place longer than 2 minutes.
Syncope	Position the patient's head between the knees (if in a sitting position). Check and record the patient's pulse, blood pressure, and respiration rate, and continue to observe the patient. Never leave the patient unattended.

From Proctor D, et al: *Kinn's The Medical Assistant*, ed 13, St Louis, 2017, Elsevier.

his or her level of comfort with the procedure. Constant light conversation with the patient during the venipuncture can help identify if the patient is distressed or anxious. As you finish the venipuncture, observe the patient's face, and assess the breathing rate if he or she seems anxious. Safety comes first. Make sure the patient is not in a position in which he or she can be hurt.

According to CLSI, the procedure for a fainting patient or one who is nonresponsive is as follows:
- If the patient begins to faint, quickly remove the tourniquet and needle from the arm, immediately activate the needle safety device, apply pressure to the site, and dispose of the unit in a sharps container to prevent an accidental exposure.
- Notify staff members for assistance.
- Lay the patient flat or lower the head if the patient is sitting.
- Loosen tight clothing.
- Do not use ammonia inhalants/capsules because these are associated with adverse effects and are no longer recommended.
- Apply a cold compress or washcloth to the patient's forehead and back of the neck.
- Stay with the patient until recovery is complete.
- Document the incident according to facility policies.
- When the patient regains consciousness, he or she must remain in the facility for at least 15 minutes and should not operate a vehicle for at least 30 minutes.

See Chapter 40 for information on what to do if a patient faints.

Specimen Recollection

Sometimes problems with a sample cannot be determined until the specimen is analyzed in the laboratory. Rejected specimens must be recollected. The laboratory may reject a specimen for reasons that include the following:
- Unlabeled or mislabeled specimen
- Insufficient specimen quantity
- Defective tube
- Incorrect tube used for the test ordered (incorrect stopper color)
- Hemolysis (Table 43.5)
- Clotted blood in an anticoagulated specimen
- Improper handling

Hemolysis is the major cause of specimen rejection. It cannot be detected until the blood cells are separated from the plasma or serum. It is crucial to take steps to prevent red blood cell damage during collection. Hemolyzed serum or plasma appears rosy to bright red because of the release of hemoglobin from the cells. Some routine tests that are adversely affected by hemolysis are chemistry tests for electrolytes (e.g., potassium, sodium), bilirubin (BIL uh roo bin), total protein, and liver enzymes.

> **MEDICAL TERMINOLOGY**
> **inter-:** between
> **-stitial:** pertaining to standing or positioned, to set

CAPILLARY PUNCTURE

Capillaries (KAP uh ler ee s) are small blood vessels that connect small arterioles (ahr TEER ee ohls) to small venules (VEN yool s). A capillary puncture is an efficient means of collecting a blood specimen when only a small amount of blood is needed. Capillary punctures are also used when a patient's condition makes venipuncture difficult, such as in a patient undergoing chemotherapy. Also, capillary punctures are performed on infants (as a heelstick) and some young children. The test requisition may not specify a capillary collection, so be familiar with the advantages, limitations, and appropriate uses of this technique. Capillary puncture is warranted in the following situations:
- Elderly patients
- Pediatric patients (especially younger than age 2)
- Patients who require frequent glucose monitoring
- Patients with burns or scars in venipuncture sites
- Obese patients
- Patients receiving intravenous (IV) therapy or chemotherapy
- Patients who have had a mastectomy
- Patients at risk for venous thrombosis (throm BOH sis)

TABLE 43.5 Major Causes of Hemolysis During Collection

Cause	Explanation	Prevention
Alcohol preparation	Transfer of alcohol into the specimen causes hemolysis.	Allow venipuncture site to dry completely.
Incorrect needle size	A high-gauge needle causes the blood to go through a small lumen with great force, causing hemolysis. A very-low-gauge needle causes a large amount of blood to suddenly enter the tube with great force, causing frothing.	Choose the correct needle for the job, aiming for a 19- to 23-gauge needle.
Loose connections on the vacuum tube assembly	If the connection between the needle holder and the double-pointed needle or the syringe and the needle is loose, air can enter the sample and cause frothing.	Make sure all connections are tight before beginning the venipuncture.
Removing the needle from the vein with the tube intact	The remaining vacuum in the tube can cause air to be drawn forcefully into the tube, causing frothing.	Remove the final tube from the needle holder before withdrawing the needle from the patient's vein.
Underfilled tubes	Underfilling tubes leads to an improper blood/additive ratio.	Permit blood to flow into the tubes until no more movement can be seen.
Syringe collections	Pulling back too rapidly on the plunger draws blood too quickly through the needle. This causes hemolysis.	Loosen the plunger before use. Use the smallest syringe possible. Gently draw the plunger so no more than 1 mL of air space is present. When transferring blood into the vacuum tube, use a transfer device. *Never* push on the plunger when transferring blood.
Mixing tubes too vigorously	All tubes should be gently inverted. (See Table 43.3.)	Gently invert tubes immediately after the draw. Vigorous mixing can hemolyze cells.
Temperature and transport problems	Trauma and temperature extremes can damage cells. Freezing will cause hemolysis.	Tubes should be transported in the upright position with as little trauma as possible. Control the temperature.
Separation of plasma or serum from red blood cells	Removing the serum/plasma from cells lowers the risk of contaminating the specimen with red blood cells (RBCs).	Blood samples that are centrifuged should have cells and plasma/serum separated as soon as possible.
Prolonged tourniquet time	Interstitial (in ter STISH uh l) fluid can leak into the veins and hemolyze RBCs.	Only leave the tourniquet on for up to 1 minute.
Poor collection; blood flowing too slowly into the tube	The needle lumen may be blocked because it is too close to the inner wall of the vein.	Withdraw the needle slightly to center it within the vein.

From Proctor D, et al: *Kinn's The Medical Assistant*, ed 13, St Louis, 2017, Elsevier.

- Patients who are severely dehydrated
- Tests that require a small volume of blood (i.e., some CLIA-waived tests)

> **MEDICAL TERMINOLOGY**
> **capillar/o:** capillary, tiniest blood vessels
> **thromb/o:** clot
> **-sis:** state of or condition

> **STUDY TIP**
> *Capillary puncture, dermal puncture,* and *fingerstick* are all terms for the same procedure.

Capillaries are connections between arteries and veins, so capillary blood is a mixture of the two. Small volumes of tissue fluid also are present in capillary blood, especially in the first drop. Analyte levels are usually the same in capillary and venous blood, with a few exceptions. Hemoglobin and glucose values are higher in capillary blood; potassium, calcium, and total protein are higher in venous blood.

Equipment

Capillary punctures are performed with specialized equipment. A look at the equipment is useful and can help you decide when a capillary puncture should be performed instead of a venipuncture.

Skin Puncture Devices. The device used to perform a dermal puncture is the *lancet* (LAHN sit), which delivers a quick puncture to a preset depth (Fig. 43.17). OSHA has directed that lancets must have retractable

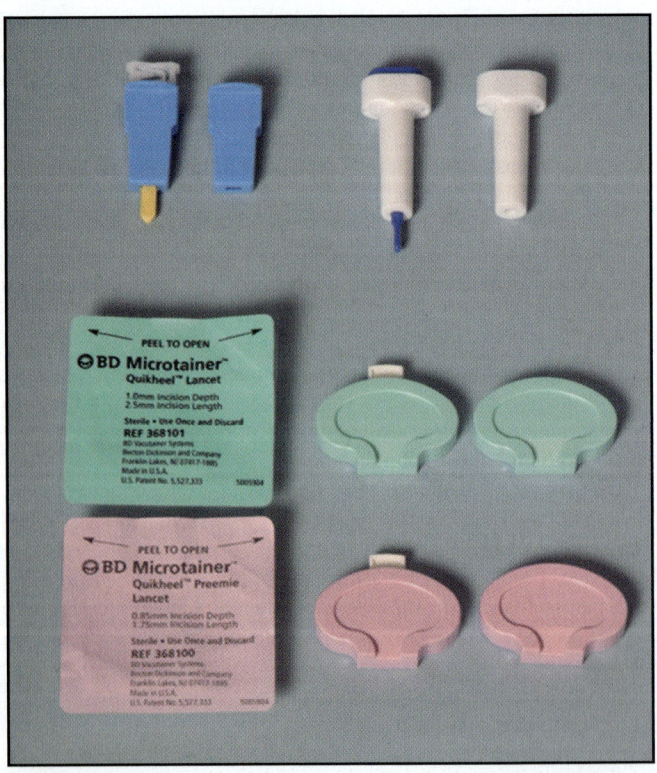

FIG. 43.17 Dermal puncture devices. (Courtesy Becton, Dickinson, Franklin Lakes, NJ.)

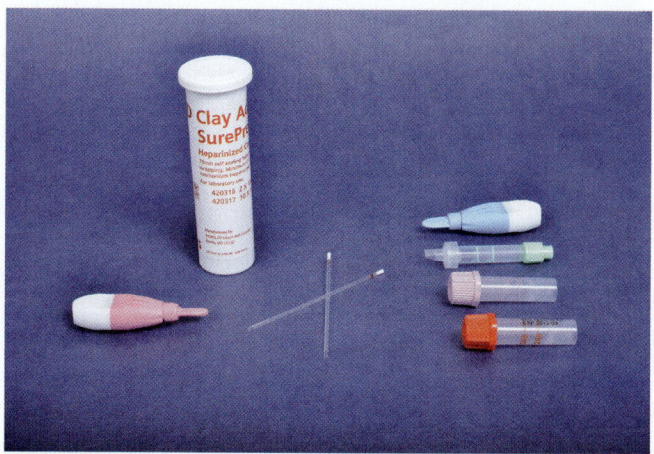

FIG. 43.18 Capillary collection containers, Microtainers, and self-sealing microhematocrit tubes. (From Proctor D, et al: *Kinn's The Medical Assistant*, ed 13, St Louis, 2017, Elsevier.)

blades. Safety lancets only puncture once and cannot be reused. Lancets are available as needle lancets and blade lancets. The choice of lancet should follow CLSI standards for puncture depth. Lancets should always be discarded in a sharps container immediately after use.

Collection Containers. Different types of containers and collection devices are available, and the ones used depend on the test to be performed. Microcollection tubes and Microtainers (MAHY kroh TEY ner) (Fig. 43.18) are available with a variety of anticoagulants and additives. Their color-coded tops indicate the same additives as evacuated tubes. Blood drops are collected into the Microtainers through a funnel-like device.

Capillary tubes are another type of blood collection tube used to get a capillary sample. A capillary tube is a glass tube surrounded by a protective plastic coating for safety. The blood is pulled into the tube by *capillary action*; this means that the blood fills these small, narrow tubes without the help of suction (SUHK shuh n). If the capillary tube is coated with the anticoagulant heparin, a red band will be seen at the top of the tube. A common, heparin-coated capillary tube is the microhematocrit (MAHY kroh hee MAT uh krit) tube. Microhematocrit tubes are used to determine the percentage of packed red blood cells in the blood. (discussed in Chapter 44). Fig. 43.19 shows a microhematocrit tube and centrifuge. Self-sealing capillary tubes are used in the microhematocrit test.

Manufacturers often provide collection devices for obtaining small amounts of blood for point-of-care testing (POCT), such as glucose, hemoglobin A_{1c}, and cholesterol (see Chapter 44). Blood is pulled into the collecting device by capillary action after the puncture, or it is applied to a reagent strip that has been inserted into the instrument to be analyzed.

Blood from a capillary puncture may also be deposited on paper cards. The Guthrie card (Fig. 43.20) is used to test babies for certain metabolic disorders, such as phenylketonuria (fen l kee toh NOO R ee uh) (PKU). Blood is deposited into circles on biologically inactive filter paper and is sent to a referral laboratory for analysis within 24 hours

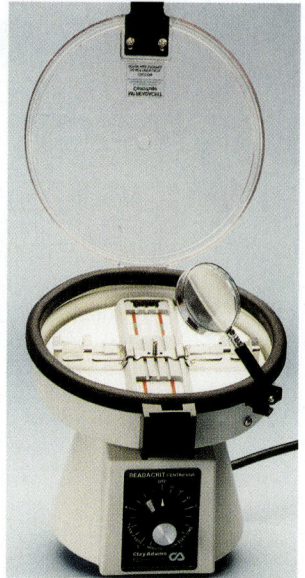

FIG. 43.19 Microhematocrit centrifuge with indicators for capillary tube placement. (From Proctor D, et al: *Kinn's The Medical Assistant*, ed 13, St Louis, 2017, Elsevier.)

BOX 43.12   Capillary Site Selection

Why do we just collect capillary samples from the middle and ring fingers? The thumb usually is too callused, and the index finger has sensitive nerve endings that make the puncture more painful. The fifth finger (pinky finger) has too little tissue for a successful puncture.

of sampling. Federal postal regulations for the mailing of biohazardous material must be followed.

ROUTINE CAPILLARY PUNCTURE

Site Selection

In adults and children (over 1 year old), capillary puncture sites include the ring or middle finger (Box 43.12). Dermal puncture of an infant should be done on the heel of the foot (Fig. 43.21). A capillary puncture is made on the palmar surface of the finger, near the tip and slightly to the side of the finger. Punctures should be made across the whorls of the finger. This helps to create a nice drop of blood to collect. Avoid areas that are callused, scarred, burned, infected, cyanotic, or edematous.

For children younger than 2 years of age, dermal puncture is performed on the medial or lateral areas of the *plantar* (PLAN ter) *surface* (bottom) of the heel or on the *palmar* (PAHL mer) *surface* of the ring or middle finger. Areas other than these are unsafe, and bone or nerve damage to an infant may occur. Blood flow from an infant's heel can be increased by applying a warm, moist towel (or other warming device) at a temperature no higher than 42° C (108° F) for 3 to 5 minutes. Never place bandages on the heel or anywhere on infants younger than age 2, because they may peel off and become a choking hazard.

VOCABULARY
interstitial: Between the cells.
suction: The production of a partial vacuum by the removal of air in order to force fluid into a vacant space.

MEDICAL TERMINOLOGY
derm/o: skin
plant/o: sole of the foot
palm/o: anterior surface of the hand

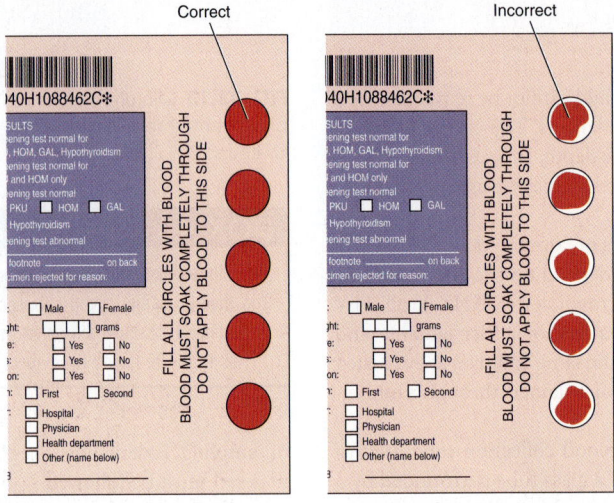

FIG. 43.20 (A) Guthrie card used in neonatal screening. (B) Correctly and incorrectly filled cards. (From Warekois RS, Robinson R: *Phlebotomy: Work Text And Procedures Manual*, ed 4, St Louis, 2016, Saunders.)

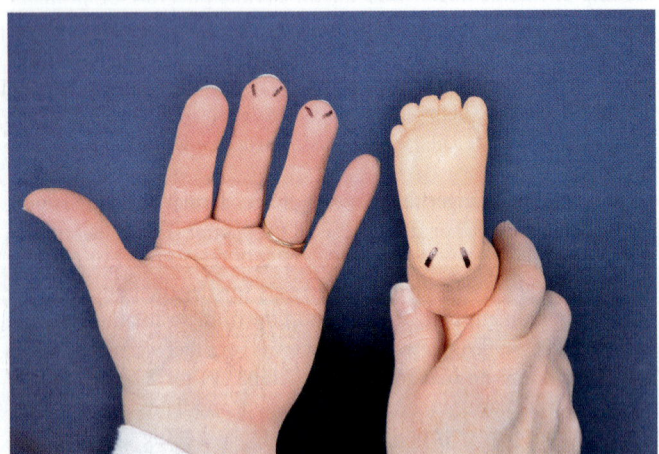

FIG. 43.21 Dermal puncture site selection and lancet placement.

Patient Preparation

Preparation for a capillary puncture is similar to that for a venipuncture. Put on a fluid-impermeable lab coat, wash your hands or use hand sanitizer, and put on gloves and protective eyewear. If the patient's hands are excessively soiled, ask the person to wash them before the procedure. If the patient's hands are cold, warm them in warm water and dry them thoroughly, or ask the person to rub or shake them vigorously. Cleanse the finger well with a 70% alcohol wipe.

You must work very efficiently when performing a capillary puncture because blood flow stops quickly. Be sure to have the supplies organized and within easy reach. Press the lancet firmly against the skin and quickly depress the plunger.

Collecting the Specimen

After the skin has been punctured, it is important to wipe away the first drop of blood with gauze. This drop contains tissue fluid that could interfere with test results. Fill the sampling containers according to the manufacturer's directions. Touch the container to the drop of blood as it is released from the puncture site, but do not touch the skin. If blood flow stops, wiping the site with gauze may restart the flow. Because you are working with blood that is free-flowing, make sure there are spare gloves, extra gauze, and disinfectant nearby. Be prepared if your gloves become contaminated with blood. After the containers have been filled, ask the patient to apply pressure to the gauze placed over the puncture site. Seal and mix the containers by gently inverting the tubes as recommended by the manufacturer.

> **Critical Thinking Box 43.10**
> Maggie is performing a capillary puncture on Johnny Parker, who is 7 years old. She is looking at his fingers to choose a site, and his hands are chilly. Which fingers would be the best choice for a child? If Johnny's hands are chilly, what can Maggie do to make sure they warm up?

Specimen Handling

Capillary collection containers are often too small for a label to be applied to the tube. The most efficient way to transport capillary tubes is to remove the stopper from a red-topped venipuncture tube, insert the capillary tubes, sealed-end down, replace the stopper, and label the red-topped tube. Microtainer tubes have plastic plugs that fit over the top. They may be placed in a labeled tube or in a labeled zipper-lock bag for transport. Always decontaminate collection containers before delivering them to the laboratory if blood was deposited on the surface during collection. The procedure for routine capillary collection is outlined in Procedure 43.4.

PEDIATRIC PHLEBOTOMY

Obtaining blood from children and infants may be difficult and potentially hazardous. The procedure should be performed by personnel trained in pediatric (pee dee A trik) phlebotomy. Successfully obtaining blood from children requires skill and an understanding of children and their development. Good communication skills are essential when dealing with children. The phlebotomist must gain the child's trust and often that of the parent or guardian. Parents frequently ask the phlebotomist to explain the tests being done and the reasons for testing. Be respectful when talking to parents. Defer to the provider if questions come up about specific information regarding possible diseases or conditions the child may have.

A parent or guardian may be helpful during phlebotomy. Ask the parent or guardian about the child's previous phlebotomy experiences and how cooperative the child has been in the past. Respectfully determine whether the parent or guardian seems comfortable assisting in restraint of an uncooperative child. Parental behavior greatly influences the child's behavior during the procedure. Children should never be restrained in a way that might cause physical injury or pain. If the parent or guardian is unable or unwilling to assist with the procedure, always refer to the office or laboratory policy on procedural holds for phlebotomy. Table 43.6 provides information on the typical fears and concerns of children during the procedure and suggested parental involvement.

Removing large amounts of blood, especially from premature infants, may result in anemia (Table 43.7). The amount of blood withdrawn must be recorded in the child's chart. Puncturing deep veins in children may result in:

- cardiac arrest
- hemorrhage (HEM er ij)
- venous thrombosis (throm BOH sis)
- damage to surrounding tissues
- infection

> **MEDICAL TERMINOLOGY**
> **hem/o:** blood
> **-rrhage:** bursting forth (of blood)

In addition, the child could be harmed during restraint. To prevent these problems, blood should be collected only by dermal puncture from children younger than age 2 unless the procedure warrants venous collection (lead levels or blood culture). Venipuncture on children younger than age 2 should be performed only on surface veins, including the dorsal hand vein, using a 23-gauge winged infusion set coupled to a syringe or a pediatric vacuum tube collection set.

When the medical assistant is required to perform pediatric phlebotomy, remember to:

- wear a colorful, fluid-impermeable jacket lab coat if possible
- be truthful about the discomfort the child will feel
- provide tokens and praise for bravery
- try to lessen the child's fears

Topical anesthetics (e.g., ethyl chloride [EC] spray or EMLA cream) may be used to reduce pain at the puncture site. In most cases a calm, professional phlebotomist who understands children and relates to them on their level can gain the trust needed. Work to perform a successful venipuncture or capillary puncture with a minimum of restraint and frustration.

PROCEDURE 43.4 Perform a Capillary Puncture: Obtain a Blood Sample by Capillary Puncture

Task
To collect a blood specimen suitable for testing using the capillary puncture technique.

Equipment and Supplies
- Patient's health record
- Provider's order and/or lab requisition
- Sterile, disposable safety lancet
- 70% alcohol wipes
- Gauze
- Hypoallergenic self-stick wrap, tape, or bandage
- Fluid-impermeable lab coat, protective eyewear, and gloves
- Appropriate collection containers (e.g., capillary tubes, Microtainer tubes)
- Permanent marking pen or printed labels
- Biohazard sharps container
- Biohazard waste container

Procedural Steps

1. Check the provider's order and/or requisition form to determine the tests ordered. Gather the appropriate tubes and supplies. Put on a fluid-impermeable lab coat.
   Purpose: To collect the specimen properly based on the tube requirements on the requisition. Donning a lab coat is part of ongoing infection control.

2. Greet the patient. Identify yourself. Verify the patient's identity with full name; ask the patient to spell the first and last name and to give his or her date of birth. Explain the procedure to be performed in a manner that is understood by the patient. Answer any questions the patient may have on the procedure. Obtain permission for the venipuncture.
   Purpose: It is important to identify the patient in two different ways to ensure that you have the correct patient. Explaining the procedure can make the patient feel more comfortable and helps to reduce anxiety.

3. Wash hands or use hand sanitizer. Put on gloves and protective eyewear.
   Purpose: To ensure infection control.

Continued

PROCEDURE 43.4 Perform a Capillary Puncture: Obtain a Blood Sample by Capillary Puncture—cont'd

4. Select a puncture site, depending on the patient's age and the sample to be obtained (e.g., palmar side of the middle or ring finger of the nondominant hand for an adult or child; medial or lateral curved surface of the plantar surface of heel for an infant).
   Purpose: The nondominant hand may have fewer calluses. The palmar side of the finger is less sensitive, and the skin usually is not as thick. Use great caution when performing capillary puncture on infants (see Fig. 43.21A and B).
5. Gently rub the finger or have your patient wiggle the fingers and open and close the hand.
   Purpose: To promote circulation. If the finger is very cold, you may immerse it in warm water or moisten it with warm towels.
6. Once the finger is warm, clean the site with a 70% alcohol pad and allow it to air dry (Fig. 1).
   Purpose: Puncturing skin that is wet with alcohol will sting and can hemolyze the specimen.

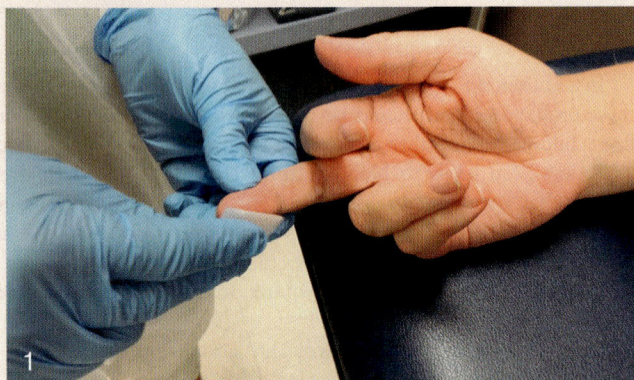

7. Hold onto the patient's finger above the puncture site with your nondominant hand.
   Purpose: Firmly holding the finger allows control of the puncture and will not let the patient pull the hand away.
8. Hold the safety lancet firmly against the patient's finger and press down on the safety trigger that activates the needle or blade to penetrate the skin. The sharp will then automatically retract into the plastic housing of the lancet. (Fig. 2).
   Purpose: Lancets are designed to puncture at specific depths that permit the free flow of blood.

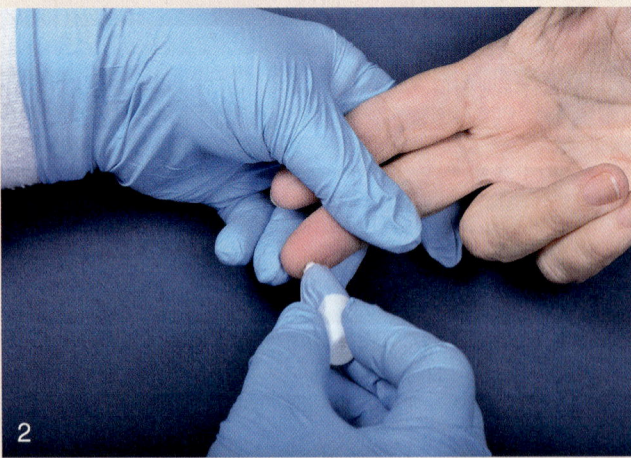

9. Dispose of the lancet in the sharps container. Wipe away the first drop of blood with gauze (Fig. 3).
   Purpose: The first drop of blood contains tissue fluid, which may alter test results. If there is any residual alcohol on the finger, it will hemolyze the blood.

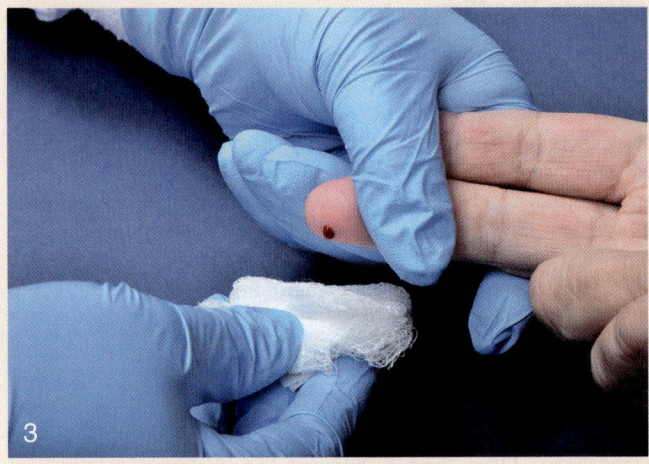

10. Apply gentle, intermittent pressure to cause the blood to flow freely (Fig. 4).
    Purpose: Forceful squeezing liberates fluid that dilutes the blood and causes inaccurate results. *Do not* milk the finger.

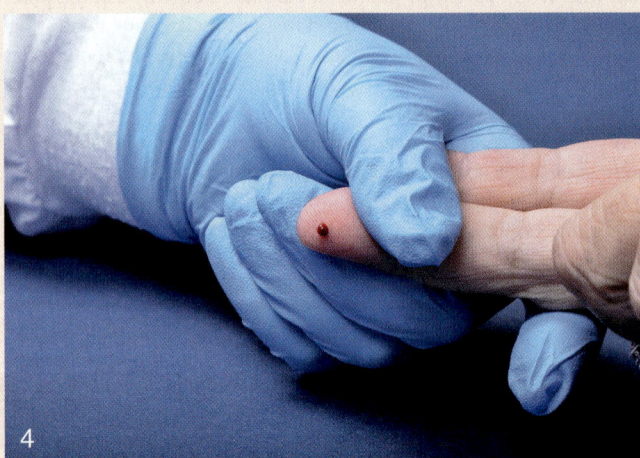

11. Collect the blood samples. Gently squeeze and release the finger two or three times to get a large drop of blood. Touch the capillary tube to the drop of blood. *Do not* scoop blood from the finger's surface. Fill the capillary to approximately three-fourths full or to the indicated line (Fig. 5). Then tip the tube with the presealed end down. When the blood flows down and touches the sealant, hold it for 30 seconds to allow it to seal automatically.
    Purpose: The specimen should be free of air bubbles and then sealed in preparation for centrifuging.

PROCEDURE 43.4 Perform a Capillary Puncture: Obtain a Blood Sample by Capillary Puncture—cont'd

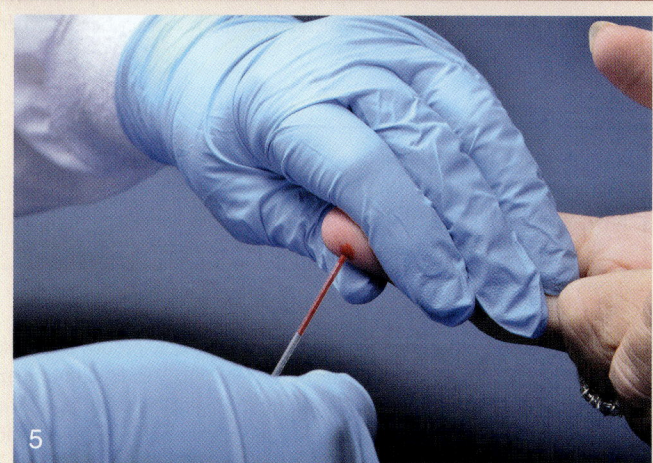

12. Wipe the patient's finger with gauze. Express another large drop of blood in the same way and fill a Microtainer (Fig. 6). Do not touch the container to the finger. If more blood is needed, gently squeeze and release the finger to get another drop. Cap the Microtainer tube when the collection is complete.
    Purpose: Touching the container to the finger irritates the puncture site and may cause infection. Touching the container also smears the blood in the fingerprint and doesn't allow the blood to form a good hanging drop.

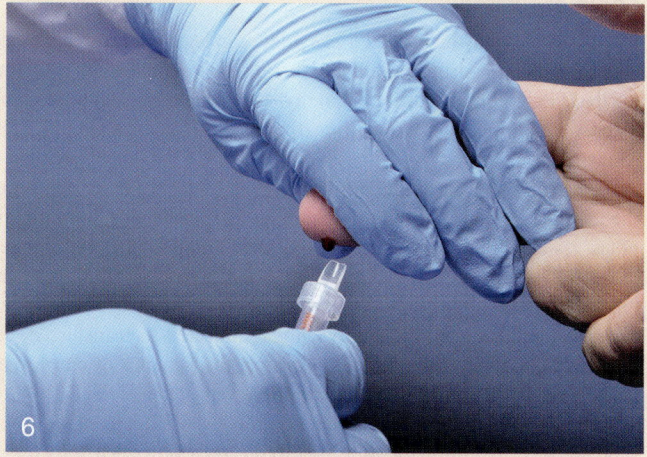

13. When collection is complete, apply pressure to the site with gauze (Fig. 7). The patient may be able to assist with this step.

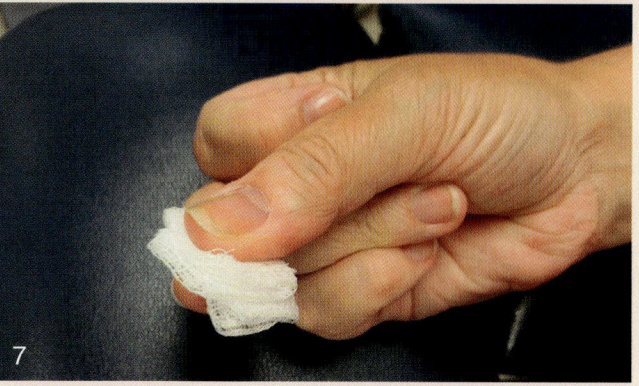

14. Select an appropriate means of labeling the containers. Sealed capillary tubes can be placed in a red-topped tube, which is then labeled. Microtainers can be placed in zipper-lock biohazard bags that are subsequently labeled. Follow your institution's procedures for labeling.
15. Check the patient for bleeding and clean the site if traces of blood are visible. Apply a folded gauze square to the puncture site and wrap with hypoallergenic self-stick wrap, tape, or bandage (Fig. 8).

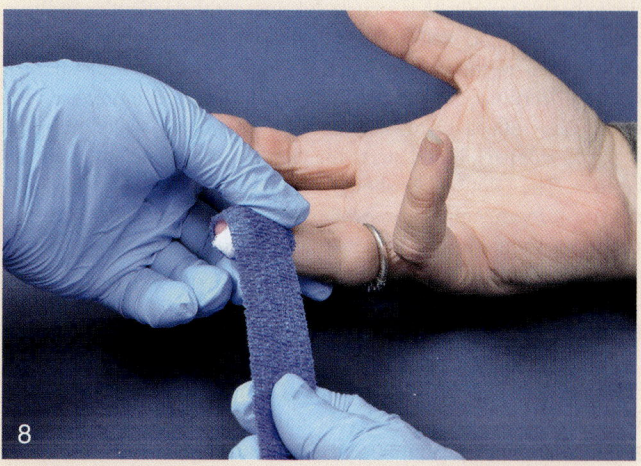

16. Disinfect the work area. Dispose of blood-contaminated materials (e.g., gauze and gloves) in the biohazard waste container. Remove your protective eyewear and wash hands or use hand sanitizer.
    Purpose: To ensure infection control.
17. Complete the laboratory requisition form and route the specimen to the proper location. Record the procedure in the patient's record.
    Purpose: A procedure is not considered done until it is recorded in the patient's record.

TABLE 43.6 Childhood Behavior and Parental Involvement During Phlebotomy

Age	Typical Mental State	Suggested Parental Involvement
Newborns (0–12 months)	Trust that adults will respond to their needs.	Parent should assist by cradling and comforting child.
Infants and toddlers (1–3 years)	Minimal fear of danger but fear of separation; limited language and understanding of procedure.	Parent should assist by holding the child and providing emotional support.
Preschoolers (3–6 years)	Fearful of injury to body; still dependent on parent.	Parent may be present to provide emotional support and to assist in obtaining child's cooperation.
School-aged children (7–12 years)	Less dependent on parent and more willing to cooperate; fear of loss of self-control (crying).	Child may not want parent present.
Teenagers (13–18 years)	Fully engaged in the process; embarrassed to show fear and may show hostility to cover emotions.	Teen may not want parent present.

From Proctor D, et al: *Kinn's The Medical Assistant*, ed 13, St Louis, 2017, Elsevier.

TABLE 43.7 General Guidelines for Pediatric Venipuncture

Weight (lb)	Single Draw Limit
8–10	3.5 mL
11–15	5 mL
16–40	10 mL
41–60	20 mL
61–65	25 mL
66–80	30 mL

From Proctor D, et al: *Kinn's The Medical Assistant*, ed 13, St Louis, 2017, Elsevier.

HANDLING THE SPECIMEN AFTER COLLECTION

The results of laboratory testing are only as good as the specimen sent for testing. Specimens handled improperly after collection may provide incorrect results. They may even compromise the patient's health. From the moment a specimen is collected, analytes in the blood begin to break down. By testing specimens as soon as possible, the laboratory tries to provide results that accurately represent the patient's condition at the time of blood collection. After collection, blood may need to be processed before the sample is tested. This may include separation of plasma or serum from the red blood cells. If the venipuncture tube contains no anticoagulant (i.e., tubes with a red, a marbled red-gray, or a gold stopper), blood starts the clotting process when it touches the tube. The "clot" tubes should sit upright in a rack for 30 to 60 minutes at room temperature while a solid clot forms. Tubes with clot accelerator should form a dense clot within 30 minutes. The presence of anticoagulants in the patient's blood, such as warfarin (Coumadin) or heparin, may delay clotting. Once the clot has formed, every effort should be made to remove the clot from the serum within 2 hours.

Removing the serum from a clot tube requires centrifugation. For thixotropic gel to form a barrier between the clot and the serum, certain requirements must be met. The tube must be centrifuged at a specified g-force, time, and temperature. A clinical centrifuge instruction manual should provide the appropriate settings for spinning blood specimens. The serum does not have to be removed from the tube after centrifugation because the gel has formed a barrier over the red blood cells. Once a tube with thixotropic gel has been centrifuged, it cannot be centrifuged again. The serum, however, can be decanted and centrifuged in another tube.

For tests that require plasma, the plasma should be removed from the cells as soon as possible. This can be done by centrifuging the tube and then aspirating (AS puh reyt ing) the plasma off the cells. The plasma is then transferred to another tube using a disposable transfer pipet. You can also use a PST tube with a marbled green-gray top, or a PST tube with a light green top. Both contain lithium heparin anticoagulant and a thixotropic gel, which forms the necessary barrier when centrifuged.

> **VOCABULARY**
> **aspirating:** To draw off or remove by suction.
> **g-force:** A force acting on an object because of gravity. Example: A centrifuge spins and exerts g-force.

Certain blood tests, such as a CBC, require whole blood. It is wise to check the specimen requirements of the laboratory that will perform the test and follow their instructions for transport and storage. The College of American Pathologists (CAP) recommends that whole blood for automated blood counts be refrigerated and tested within 72 hours.

Often specimens must be transported by courier to other facilities. The Hazardous Materials Shipping Regulations, established by the Department of Transportation, apply to the packaging and shipping of hazardous materials by ground transportation. POLs that ship human specimens must be trained to properly handle, pack, and ship biohazardous materials. Reference labs will frequently have couriers that pick up specimens. The specimens and their requisitions are typically placed in individual biohazard bags and sorted according to which reference lab is affiliated with the patient's insurance.

Chain of Custody

Blood samples may be collected as evidence in legal proceedings. Blood may be drawn for drug and alcohol testing, DNA analysis, or paternity testing. These samples must be handled according to special procedures to prevent tampering, misidentification, or interference with the test results.

Chain of custody is a legal term that refers to the ability to guarantee the identity and integrity of the specimen from collection to reporting of test results. It is a process used to maintain and document the history of a specimen. Documents should include the name or initials of the individual collecting the specimen, each person who tests or transports the specimen, the date the specimen was collected or transferred, the employer or agency, the specimen number, the patient's or employee's name, and a brief description of the specimen.

Collection kits are available that contain everything needed for the venipuncture, including the tube, the needle, the chain of custody forms and seals, the antiseptic, and even the tourniquet. Familiarize yourself with these kits before using them. Phlebotomists may be required to testify at legal proceeding if they are involved in the collection or testing of a legal sample.

CLOSING COMMENTS

Phlebotomy is an invasive procedure in which a sterile needle or lancet is inserted through the skin. Because the skin is penetrated, drawing blood becomes a surgical procedure and is subject to the laws and regulations of surgery. When a venipuncture is performed, the rules and regulations must be obeyed with no exceptions. Be sure to follow the written procedures in the laboratory. Become familiar with the regulations and standards established by CLSI and OSHA, and by state and local agencies. Deviations from the standards leave the medical assistant open to malpractice. Document any situations in which the standard of care comes into question.

CHAPTER REVIEW

In this chapter we covered phlebotomy and the importance of proper technique, safety measures, collection equipment, specimen labeling, and specimen handling.

We started out with a brief overview of a venipuncture. We then discussed personal protective equipment (PPE) and the role it plays in phlebotomy. When a healthcare worker is using a sharp and has the possibility of blood exposure, PPE is an important part of the procedure. Staying safe and protecting the patient are critical. Necessary PPE for venipunctures and capillary punctures include gloves, a fluid-impermeable lab coat, and protective eyewear.

We also covered information about tourniquets: proper placement on the arm and how to tie a one-handed release tourniquet. The use of antiseptics was also discussed as it refers to phlebotomy. Most procedures use 70% isopropyl alcohol wipes, but blood cultures require additional antiseptic procedures.

Evacuated collection tubes and the additives they contain were discussed in detail. Each evacuated collection tube has a colored stopper. The stopper color indicates which additive, if any, has been put into the tube. Table 43.1 lists the different stopper colors, anticoagulants and other additives in the tubes, and laboratory uses for each colored tube.

Once we had discussed the types of anticoagulants and additives in venipuncture collection tubes, we discussed the order of the draw. Collection tubes are not filled in a random order. Their collection order is important so that there is no cross-contamination between tubes. This ensures the best specimen possible, with no carryover from one tube to another.

We talked about the different types of needles used in phlebotomy, in addition to the length and lumen size (or gauge) and needle holders. We learned about the different equipment available for delicate or more difficult draws, such as a syringe and a winged infusion set (butterfly assembly).

Needlestick safety and postexposure follow-up are important when you work with sharps on a regular basis. Safety should always be in the forefront of the medical assistant's mind, but if a needlestick occurs, it is important to know what to do.

We went through the procedural steps for a routine venipuncture, syringe venipuncture, and butterfly assembly venipuncture. Using different equipment requires different skills. Patient preparation, work area preparation, and performing and completing a venipuncture have many steps in common. We covered common problems associated with venipunctures. Understanding what can go wrong and why hopefully will give you insight into how to prevent problems. Common patient problems include hematoma formation, nerve damage, and fainting. Common specimen problems include hemolyzed blood, short samples, and improperly labeled tubes. When specimens are not acceptable, recollection may be necessary.

Another phlebotomy procedure we talked about is the capillary puncture. The equipment used for capillary puncture is different. The puncture device used for dermal puncture is a lancet. Collection tubes are called *Microtainer tubes* and *microhematocrit tubes*. Capillary punctures should be performed on the ring or middle finger on the palmar surface of the distal end of the finger. Patient preparation, collecting the specimen, and specimen handling are all part of a complete capillary procedure.

The pediatric phlebotomy technique is just a bit different from an adult phlebotomy, but the communication skills component is important. Knowing how to interact with children and gain their trust is a significant aspect of pediatric phlebotomy.

Handling venipuncture specimens after collection and properly directing specimens to laboratory departments or to a referral laboratory complete the process of phlebotomy. For any legal specimens, chain of custody documentation needs to be strictly followed.

Phlebotomy is a vital part of the laboratory. Phlebotomy that is done correctly and with compassion for the patient is a great benefit to the laboratory. Proper specimen collection, labeling, processing, and handling all add up to an efficiently functioning laboratory. Patient satisfaction and trust increase with kind and respectful laboratory contact. Phlebotomy can be a very rewarding area of the clinical laboratory.

> **EXCEPTIONAL CUSTOMER SERVICE**
>
> Provide as much explanation as needed to ease the patient's anxiety. Often the patient can help by identifying the site of the last successful blood venipuncture. Follow the patient's suggestion in choosing the site for obtaining a blood specimen. When patients become active participants in the procedure, they remain more relaxed, talkative, and confident in your expertise as a phlebotomist.

SCENARIO WRAP-UP

Maggie has had a busy morning in the phlebotomy area! She likes it when it is busy, the morning seems to fly by. After the morning rush, Maggie restocks a few supplies and then is ready to sit down and take her lunch break. As she relaxes in the lunchroom for a few minutes, she thinks back on the morning with satisfaction. She helped a number of patients today. Norma Washington was in, and she is in her fourth week of chemotherapy. She was nervous about today's venipuncture. Maggie calmed her fears and was able to do a capillary puncture instead of a venipuncture. That made Norma's day!

Every patient who came into the phlebotomy area this morning left with a smile. That doesn't happen every day, but Maggie was so happy that this Monday morning went well.

44

Assisting in the Analysis of Blood

LEARNING OBJECTIVES

1. Name the main functions of blood.
2. Describe the appearance and function of erythrocytes, leukocytes, and platelets. Also, discuss plasma.
3. Explain the purpose of the microhematocrit test. Describe how to collect a microhematocrit specimen and perform a microhematocrit test.
4. Describe how to obtain a specimen for and perform a hemoglobin test.
5. Cite the reasons for performing an erythrocyte sedimentation rate (ESR) test, discuss the sources of error for ESR testing, and determine and record an erythrocyte sedimentation rate obtained by using a modified Westergren method.
6. Explain the purpose of a prothrombin time (PT) test, describe how to obtain a specimen for and perform a CLIA-waived prothrombin time/international normalized ratio (PT/INR) test, and explain how you could reassure a patient of the accuracy of PT/INR test results.
7. Identify the tests included in a complete blood count (CBC) and their reference ranges, and differentiate between normal and abnormal test results.
8. Explain the reasons for performing a white blood cell (WBC) count and differential.
9. Differentiate between the ABO blood groupings and the Rh blood groupings. Also, discuss legal and ethical issues related to blood transfusions.
10. Complete the following related to blood chemistry in the physician office laboratory:
    - Explain the reasons for testing blood glucose, hemoglobin A1c, cholesterol, liver enzymes, and thyroid hormones.
    - Assist a provider by performing a blood glucose test.
    - Determine a cholesterol level or lipid profile using a CLIA-waived chemistry analyzer.
    - Explain how to obtain a specimen and perform a blood glucose, hemoglobin A1c, and cholesterol test using CLIA-waived test methods.

CHAPTER OUTLINE

1. **Opening Scenario,** 1077
2. **You Will Learn,** 1077
3. **Introduction,** 1077
4. **Hematology,** 1077
    a. Plasma, 1078
5. **Hematology in the Physician Office Laboratory (POL),** 1078
    a. Hematocrit, 1078
    b. Hemoglobin, 1082
    c. Erythrocyte Sedimentation Rate, 1084
    d. Coagulation Testing, 1086
6. **Hematology in the Reference Laboratory,** 1086
    a. Complete Blood Count (CBC) Laboratory Reports, 1089
        i. *Red Blood Cell Count,* 1089
        ii. *Red Blood Cell Indices,* 1089
        iii. *White Blood Cell Count,* 1091
        iv. *Differential Cell Count,* 1091
    b. Identification of Normal Blood Cells, 1092
    c. Differential Examination, 1092
        i. *Red Blood Cell Morphology,* 1092
    d. Platelet Analysis, 1093
7. **Immunohematology,** 1093
    a. Blood Typing, 1093
    b. Other Blood Types, 1094
    c. Legal and Ethical Issues Related to Blood Transfusion, 1094
8. **Blood Chemistry in the Physician Office Laboratory,** 1094
    a. Blood Glucose Testing, 1095
    b. Hemoglobin A1c Testing, 1095
    c. Cholesterol Testing, 1096
    d. Alanine Aminotransferase (ALT) and Aspartate Aminotransferase (AST) Testing, 1097
    e. Thyroid Hormone Testing, 1097
9. **Reference Laboratory Chemistry Panels and Single Analyte Testing and Monitoring,** 1099
10. **Closing Comments,** 1102
11. **Chapter Review,** 1102
12. **Scenario Wrap-Up,** 1103

CHAPTER 44 Assisting in the Analysis of Blood

▶ OPENING SCENARIO

Anita James, CMA (AAMA), has been working at the Walden-Martin Family Medical (WMFM) Clinic for 16 years. She loves her position as a medical assistant in a family medicine clinic. Every day is different. Each patient is unique. She has seen a number of children grow up over the years. Children who were toddlers when she started are now driving and thinking about college. The time has flown by.

Anita is working with Dr. Perez today, and they have a very busy schedule. A number of patients are in for follow-up visits, and a few new patients have appointments today, too.

YOU WILL LEARN

- To identify the anticoagulant of choice for hematology testing and explain the purpose of the following tests: microhematocrit test, hemoglobin test, erythrocyte sedimentation rate (ESR).
- To explain the purpose of the prothrombin time (PT) in coagulation testing.
- To identify the tests included in a complete blood count (CBC) and their reference ranges, and to differentiate between normal and abnormal test results.
- To describe the red blood cell (RBC) indices.
- To explain the reasons for performing a white blood cell (WBC) count and differential.
- To describe the medical assistant's role in blood transfusions
- To explain the reasons for testing blood glucose, hemoglobin A1c, cholesterol, liver enzymes, and thyroid hormones.
- To summarize typical chemistry panels and the reason for performing each panel.

INTRODUCTION

The circulating blood supplies the body's cells with nutrients and oxygen. The blood also distributes **enzymes** (EN zahyms), **hormones** (HAWR mohns), and other chemicals needed for regulation of body activities.

> **VOCABULARY**
> **enzymes:** Special proteins that speed up the chemical reaction in the body.
> **hormones:** Chemical substances produced in an endocrine gland and transported in the blood to a specific tissue, where they have a specific effect.

In addition, the blood functions to maintain body temperature, keep body fluids in balance, and maintain pH. Maintaining a constant internal environment is called *homeostasis* (hoh mee uh STEY sis).

Blood tests are done routinely in the hematology (hee muh TOL uh jee), immunohematology (im YUH noh hee muh TOL uh jee) (used to be referred to as the blood bank), chemistry, and immunology (im yuh NOL uh jee) (also called *serology*) departments of the laboratory. The degree of blood testing performed by medical assistants depends on the level of service offered by the ambulatory care facility and the regulations established by the Clinical Laboratory Improvement Amendments (CLIA). As a medical assistant, you are qualified to perform the CLIA-waived procedures described in the physician office laboratory (POL) sections of this chapter. Moderate- and highly-complex CLIA blood tests are performed at reference and hospital laboratories and are not performed by medical assistants. This chapter explains more complex procedures to provide background information important to an understanding of the analysis of blood.

HEMATOLOGY

Whole blood is composed of visible formed elements suspended in *plasma* (a clear, yellow liquid). Plasma makes up approximately 55% of blood by volume. The remaining 45% consists of the following visible cellular elements:

- erythrocytes (RBCs)
- leukocytes (WBCs)
- thrombocytes (platelets)

The characteristics of blood and cellular components are described in Chapter 8. A brief review of the components is presented in Table 44.1.

All blood cells are made in the bone marrow. Most cells mature in the bone marrow and then are released into the blood (Box 44.1). Blood cells have a limited life span; they don't live forever. Once they become old and less efficient, they are broken down and the useful elements are recycled.

> **BOX 44.1 Thymus**
>
> T-cell lymphocytes are made in the bone marrow, but they mature in the *thymus* (THAHY muh s). The thymus is a small endocrine (EN duh krin) gland located behind the upper breastbone (*sternum*) in the chest. It produces a hormone called *thymosin* (THAHY moh sin), which helps T cells mature and understand their role in the immune system.

TABLE 44.1 Review of Blood Components

Blood Component	Function	Normal Values	Comments
Plasma	To transport nutrients to cells and waste products away from cells	Approximately 55% of blood total volume	Plasma is the liquid portion of the blood inside the body.
Red blood cells (RBCs)	To carry oxygen to the cells, helps carry some carbon dioxide away from cells	Approximately 4–6 million/mm^3; may be slightly higher for men and slightly lower for women	About 120-day life span
Platelets	Help with the process of blood clotting	150,000–450,000/mm^3	About 10-day life span
White Blood Cells (WBCs) – Granular			
Neutrophil (NOO truh fil)	Engulf and destroy foreign substances, particularly bacteria	Most abundant WBC in the blood, about 40%–60%	Also called *polymorphonuclear cells*, *PMNs*, *segs*, or *polys*
Eosinophil (ee uh SIN uh fil)	Helps in the destruction of parasites and fungi	About 1%–4% of WBCs in the blood	Also called *eos*

Continued

TABLE 44.1 Review of Blood Components—cont'd

Blood Component	Function	Normal Values	Comments
Basophil (BEY suh fil)	Helps in the destruction of allergens	About 0.5%–1% of WBCs in the blood	Also called *basos*
WBCs – Agranular			
Monocytes (MON uh sahyt)	Engulf and destroy foreign substances, particularly senescent (si NES uh nt) cells and malignant (muh LIG nuh nt) cells	About 2%–8% of WBCs in the blood	Monocytes are found in the blood, but once they migrate into tissue, they are called *macrophages*; (MAK ruh feyjs); also called *monos*
Lymphocyte (LIM fuh sahyt) B-cell	Destroy foreign substances by producing antibodies	B and T cells combined are the second most abundant WBC in the blood, about 20%–40%	Looking under the microscope, you cannot see the difference between B- and T-cell lymphocytes. They look the same, but they function differently. Also called *lymphs*
Lymphocyte T-cell	Destroy foreign substances – particularly intracellular pathogens		

Plasma

Plasma is the highly complex liquid that carries the formed elements plus other substances, such as:
- Plasma proteins, including albumin (al BYOO muh n), the clotting proteins *prothrombin* (proh THROM bin) and *fibrinogen* (fahy BRIN uh juh n), and immunoglobulins (im yuh noh GLOB yuh lins)
- Nutrients – carbohydrates, fats, and amino acids
- Hormones, enzymes, mineral salts, gases, and waste products

Plasma is composed of approximately 90% water, 9% protein, and 1% other chemical substances. The liquid portion of the blood in the body is plasma. Outside, the body plasma must have an added anticoagulant to remain part of whole blood. The liquid that remains after blood has clotted is called *serum*.

HEMATOLOGY IN THE PHYSICIAN OFFICE LABORATORY (POL)

For many POL hematology tests, an adequate blood sample can be obtained from capillary puncture of the finger. If a larger sample is required, blood can be obtained via venipuncture. For a complete blood count (CBC), venous blood is collected in a lavender-topped tube containing ethylenediaminetetraacetic (ETH uh leen DAHY uh meen TE truh uh SEE tik) acid (EDTA), an anticoagulant that prevents whole blood from clotting. EDTA is the anticoagulant of choice for hematology testing because it also acts as a preservative for the blood cells. It is very important to prevent blood from being hemolyzed (HEE muh lahyz d) during collection for hematology testing.

Hematocrit

The *hematocrit* (hee MAT uh krit) (abbreviated Hct) is a measurement of the percentage of packed RBCs in a volume of blood. The spun microhematocrit test is based on the principle of separating the cellular elements from plasma using a centrifuge (SEN truh fyooj) (Procedures 44.1 and 44.2). Two or three drops of blood are collected from a capillary puncture in two capillary tubes that are placed in a specially designed microhematocrit centrifuge (Fig. 44.1). Capillary tubes can also be filled with EDTA-anticoagulated blood from a lavender-topped vacuum tube. As required by the Occupational Safety and Health Administration (OSHA), capillary tubes must be safe. They are either made of plastic or plastic-coated glass to avoid sharps injuries. The most common type of microhematocrit tube is self-sealing at one end. A lesser used type is open on both ends. If the tube is self-sealing, it

MEDICAL TERMINOLOGY

bas/o: base, opposite of acid
-cyte: cell
eosin/o: red, rosy, dawn-colored
erythr/o: red
hemat/o: blood
immun/o: immune, protection, safe
intra-: within, into
leuk/o: white
-logy: study (process of)
neutr/o: neither, neutral, neutrophil
-phil: attraction for
thromb/o: clot

VOCABULARY

albumin: Most abundant plasma protein in human blood. It is important in regulating the water balance of blood.
centrifuge: A machine that rotates at high speed and separates substances of different densities by centrifugal force. Example: A tube of blood is separated into plasma/serum, white blood cells, platelets, and red blood cells.
immunoglobulins: A group of related proteins that function as antibodies. They are found in plasma and other body fluids.
intracellular pathogens: A disease-causing organism that is inside of a cell.
malignant: A cell with uncontrolled growth, rapidly spreading, and doing harm.
senescent cell: An old or aging cell that can no longer divide and reproduce.

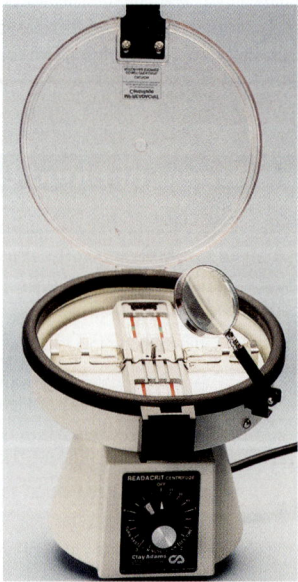

FIG. 44.1 Microhematocrit centrifuge. (From Proctor D, et al: *Kinn's The Medical Assistant*, ed 13, St Louis, 2017, Elsevier.)

PROCEDURE 44.1 Perform Preventive Maintenance for the Microhematocrit Centrifuge

Task:
To perform daily, monthly, semiannual, and annual maintenance on a microhematocrit centrifuge.

Equipment and Supplies
- Microhematocrit centrifuge
- Maintenance logbook
- Utility gloves
- Fluid-impermeable lab coat, eye protection, and gloves
- Disinfectant
- Biohazard waste container

Procedural Steps
- *Personal protective equipment (PPE):* Wash hands or use hand sanitizer. Put on fluid-impermeable lab coat, eye protection, and gloves. In all maintenance procedures, gloves are worn under the utility gloves.
- NOTE: These are generic recommendations. Always check the manufacturer's guidelines for specific instructions.
- Always unplug the power cord before cleaning or servicing the centrifuge.

Daily Maintenance
1. Clean the inside of the centrifuge and the gasket with a disinfectant recommended by the manufacturer. Plastic and nonmetal parts may be cleaned with a fresh solution of 5% sodium hypochlorite (bleach) mixed 1:10 with water (1 part bleach plus 9 parts water).
   Purpose: To remove any dried blood or shattered glass. Do not use bleach on the gasket because it may harden the rubber.

Monthly Maintenance
1. Check the reading device. Misuse and zeroing of the reading devices can result in considerable error. Always use a second, simple reading device as a cross-check. Use a ruler or a flat plastic card specially made for this purpose. To use these cards, lay the spun hematocrit tube on the card and align the red cells with a line on the card to obtain the reading.

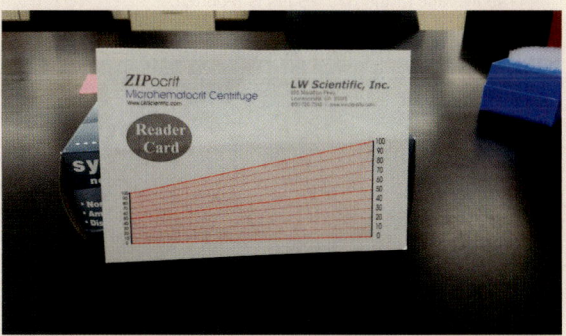

2. Check the rotor for cracks or corrosion and check the interior for signs of white powder.
   Purpose: Cracks, corrosion, or powder may indicate impending rotor failure; these findings require the immediate attention of a service technician.
3. Record all preventive maintenance in the laboratory logbook.
   Purpose: Recording maintenance is necessary to maintain warranties and to comply with regulations established by CLIA and other regulatory agencies.

Semiannual Maintenance
1. Check the gasket for cuts and breaks.
   Purpose: Cut gaskets allow tubes to leak and must be replaced.
2. Check the timer with a stopwatch to verify timer accuracy.
3. Perform a maximum cell pack to verify the time required for complete packing by reading a sample after centrifugation and then recentrifuging for 1 minute. The results should be the same. If they are not, perform preventive maintenance and/or call the service technician.
   Purpose: If the cells compact further during recentrifugation, the centrifuge is not rotating at the proper speed, and hematocrit results will be falsely elevated.
4. Record all preventive measures in the equipment maintenance log.
   Purpose: Recording maintenance is necessary to maintain warranties and to comply with regulations established by CLIA and other regulatory agencies.

Annual Maintenance (or Maintenance Performed as Needed)
1. The centrifuge functions and maintenance verification should be performed by qualified personnel. This includes checking the centrifuge mechanism, rotors, timer, speed, and electrical leads.
2. Record all professional service calls in the laboratory logbook.

MICROHEMATOCRIT CENTRIFUGE MAINTENANCE LOG		
DATE	SERVICE	INITIALS
10/7/20XX	Performed routine daily and monthly preventive maintenance	AJ

PROCEDURE 44.2 CLIA-Waived Hematology Testing: Perform a Microhematocrit Test

Task:
To perform a microhematocrit test accurately.

Equipment and Supplies
- Patient's health record
- Provider's order and/or lab requisition
- Microhematocrit lab log
- Fresh sample of blood collected in a tube containing ethylenediaminetetraacetic acid (EDTA) anticoagulant (or equipment for fingerstick specimen: lancet, alcohol wipe, gauze, bandage)
- Plastic-coated self-sealing capillary tubes, or plain capillary tubes (blue tipped)
- Sealing clay (if capillary tubes are not self-sealing)
- Gauze
- Microhematocrit centrifuge
- Fluid-impermeable lab coat, protective eyewear, and gloves
- Biohazard waste container
- Biohazard sharps containers

Procedural Steps

1. Wash hands or use hand sanitizer. Put on fluid-impermeable lab coat, protective eyewear, and gloves.
   Purpose: To ensure infection control.
2. Assemble the materials needed.
   a. *If the capillary tubes are self-sealing:* Fill two tubes by inserting the end opposite the sealed end into the well-mixed EDTA blood sample. **NOTE:** If the capillary tube and the EDTA tube are held almost parallel to the table, the capillary tubes fill easily by capillary action. When the self-sealing capillary tubes are two-thirds to three-fourths filled, tilt them upright, causing the blood sample to flow down the tube and meet the sealant. Continue to hold the tube vertical when the blood contacts the sealant for an additional 15 seconds.
   Purpose: Duplicates should always be done as a means of quality control.
   b. *Alternative:* Fill two plain (blue-tipped) capillary tubes two-thirds to three-fourths full of a well-mixed EDTA blood sample. Tip the blood tube slightly, touching the capillary tube into the blood using the side that is opposite the blue band. When enough blood has filled the capillary tube, tip the blue end of the tube down, causing the blood to flow towards the blue tip. Then readjust the tube horizontally while inserting the blue tip of the capillary tube into the clay sealant. Insert the tube as many times as needed to achieve a plug up to the blue band (Fig. 1).
   Purpose: Duplicates should always be done as a means of quality control. Tubes are not filled completely to provide space for the sealing clay.

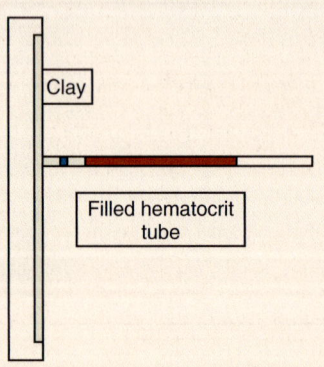

1

(From Keohane E et al: *Rodak's Hematology: Clinical Principles And Applications*, ed 5, St Louis, 2016, Saunders.)

3. Wipe the outside of the tubes with clean gauze without touching the wet open end of the tube.
   Purpose: Wiping the outside of the capillary tube removes any blood. Touching the blood inside the capillary tube with absorbent material removes more plasma than blood cells and can alter the hematocrit.
4. Place the tubes opposite each other in the centrifuge with the sealed ends securely against the gasket (see Fig. 44.1).
   Purpose: The centrifuge must always be balanced to prevent damage. If the clay ends of the capillary tubes are not outermost against the gasket, the sample will spin out of the tubes, contaminating the centrifuge.
5. Note the numbers on the centrifuge slots and record the numbers on the log sheet, along with the patient's name.
   Purpose: The sample must be identified throughout the entire procedure.
6. Secure the locking top, fasten the lid down, and lock it.
   Purpose: If the locking top is not firmly in place during the spinning cycle, the tubes will come out of their slots and break. The lid is always locked during centrifugation for safety purposes, to prevent the ejection of aerosols or broken glass.
7. Set the timer and adjust the speed as needed.
   Purpose: The prescribed time is 3 to 5 minutes at 11,000 to 12,000 rpm. Check the manufacturer's instructions for time and speed.
8. Allow the centrifuge to come to a complete stop. Unlock the outer locking top and then remove the inner lid.
   Purpose: Opening the centrifuge before it has stopped could result in harm to the user.
9. Remove the tubes immediately and read the results. If this is not possible, store the tubes in an upright position.
   Purpose: Tubes left in the centrifuge will show altered results because the red blood cell (RBC) layer will spread out horizontally.
10. Determine the microhematocrit values using one of the following methods:
    a. Centrifuge with built-in reader using calibrated capillary tubes.
       - Position the tubes as directed by the manufacturer's instructions.
       - Read both tubes.
       - The average of the two results is reported.
       - The two values should not vary by more than 2%.
    b. Centrifuge without a built-in reader.
       - Carefully remove the tubes from the centrifuge.
       - Place a tube on the microhematocrit reader.
       - Align the clay-RBC junction with the zero line on the reader. Align the plasma meniscus with the 100% line. The value is read at the junction of the red cell layer and the buffy coat. The buffy coat is not included in the reading (Fig. 2).
       - Read both tubes.
       - The average of the two results is reported.
       - The two values should not vary by more than 2%.

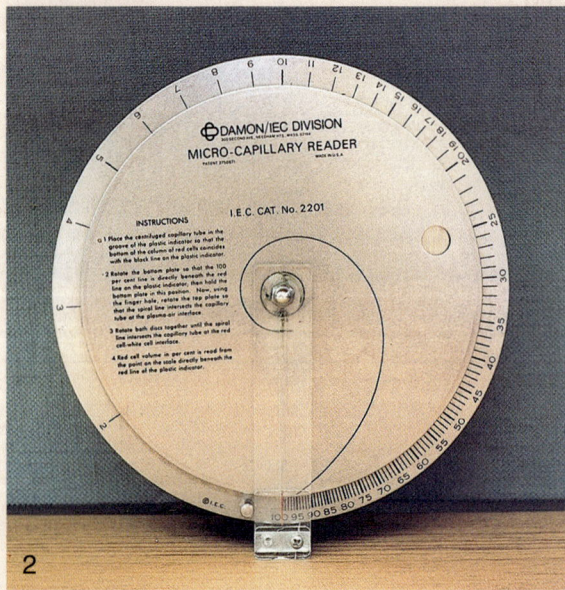

2

(From Keohane E et al: *Rodak's Hematology: Clinical Principles And Applications*, ed 5, St Louis, 2016, Saunders.)

11. Dispose of the capillary tubes in a biohazard sharps container.

PROCEDURE 44.2 CLIA-Waived Hematology Testing: Perform a Microhematocrit Test—cont'd

12. Disinfect the work area and properly dispose of all biohazardous materials. Remove your gloves, eyewear, and lab coat. Wash hands or use hand sanitizer.
   Purpose: To ensure infection control.

13. Record the results in the Hematocrit Patient Log and document the results in the patient's medical record, as shown below.
   Purpose: A procedure is not considered done until it is charted.

HEMATOCRIT—PATIENT LOG

Hematocrit expected values:
- Adult Males = 42–52%
- Adult Females = 36–48%
- Infants = 32–38%
- Children = increase to adult

DATE	TECH	PATIENT I.D.	SLOT #	RESULT	CHARTED
10/7/20–	dc	# 12345	1 & 4	44% & 44%	✓

Documentation Example
10/07/20XX 11:25 a.m.: Hct 44%. _____ Anita James, CMA (AAMA)

---

must be tilted upright, causing the blood sample to flow down the tube and come into contact with the seal, and then held in place for 15 to 30 seconds. The open-ended tubes must be sealed with special clay before centrifugation.

After centrifugation, the packed RBCs are at the bottom of the tube against the sealant, the WBCs and platelets are in the center **buffy coat**, and plasma is on top (Fig. 44.2). The microhematocrit is determined by comparing the volume of RBCs to the total volume of the whole blood sample. The percentage is read by placing the tubes on a special microhematocrit reader. Some microhematocrit centrifuges have a built-in reading scale that reads the calibrated capillary tubes. Microhematocrits should be performed in duplicate and the average of the two results reported.

Normal Hct values vary with gender and age (Table 44.2). They range from a low of 36% in women to a high of 52% in men. Low microhematocrit values can indicate **anemia** (uh NEE mee uh) or the presence of bleeding. High values may be caused by dehydration or **polycythemia vera** (pah lee sigh THEE mee uh VER uh). Values can be influenced by **physiologic** (fi zee uh LOJ ik), **pathologic** (path uh LOJ ik), and even geographic factors and by collection techniques (Box 44.2). The microhematocrit is a commonly performed test requested by providers either separately or as part of the CBC. Because it is a simple procedure that requires only a small amount of blood, it is an ideal screening test and often is part of a routine physical examination. Quality assurance includes care and maintenance of the microhematocrit instrument.

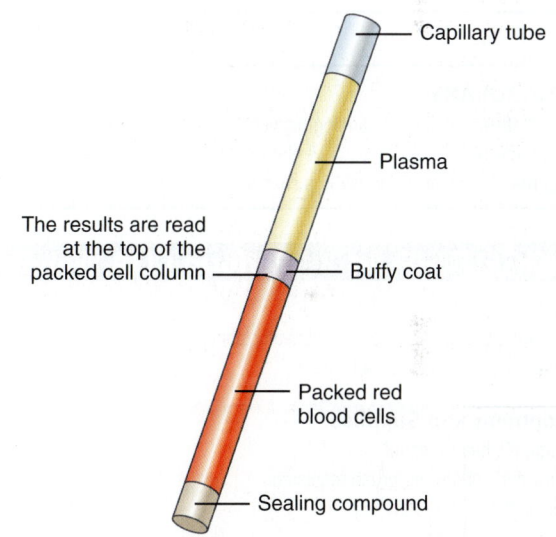

FIG. 44.2 Spun microhematocrit tube. (From Proctor D, et al: *Kinn's The Medical Assistant*, ed 13, St Louis, 2017, Elsevier.)

CRITICAL THINKING 44.1

One of Anita's patients today is Carl Bowden. Carl retired recently and has been enjoying his new, less hectic schedule. Carl is in good health, but he did mention at his physical today that he was feeling a little tired and lacked energy. Dr. Perez ordered a microhematocrit for Carl. The lab just sent the results to Carl's electronic health record.

Anita looks at the results and sees that his hematocrit is 38%. Is that value in the normal range for an adult male?

VOCABULARY

anemia: A deficiency of hemoglobin in the blood. It is accompanied by a reduced number of red blood cells, pale skin, weakness, and shortness of breath, among other symptoms.
buffy coat: The layer of white blood cells and platelets that separates red blood cells and plasma in a centrifuged sample of whole blood.
pathologic: Caused by or involving disease.
physiologic: Consistent with the normal function of the body.
polycythemia vera: A disorder characterized by an abnormal increase in the number of red blood cells in the blood.

TABLE 44.2 Hematocrit (Hct) Reference Values

Age/Gender	Hct Value (%)
Neonate (newborn–<1 mo)	44–64
Infant (1 mo–1 yr)	37–41
Child (1–10 yr)	35–41
Men (>10 yr)	42–52
Women (>10 yr)	36–45

From Proctor D, et al: *Kinn's The Medical Assistant,* ed 13, St Louis, 2017, Elsevier.

BOX 44.2 Hematocrit Geography

Normal hematocrit (Hct) ranges are affected by a person's geographic location. For example, people living at high altitudes have a higher percentage of RBCs, to compensate for the lower oxygen levels in the atmosphere.

MEDICAL TERMINOLOGY

an-: no, not, without
-emia: blood condition
poly-: many, much
cyt/o: cell
physi/o: nature, function
log/o: study
-ic: pertaining to
path/o: disease

VOCABULARY

hemoglobin: The oxygen-carrying pigment of red blood cells.
microcuvettes: A small tube or vessel used in laboratory experiments.
reagents: A substance for use in a chemical reaction.

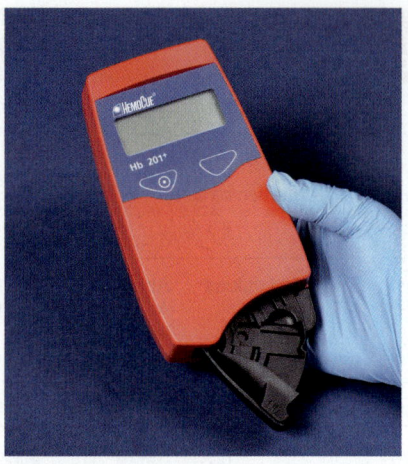

FIG. 44.3 Handheld hemoglobin monitor.

Hemoglobin

Hemoglobin (HEE muh gloh bin) (abbreviated Hgb) determination is another way to measure the oxygen-carrying capacity of blood. The hemoglobin concentration can be part of the CBC or an individual test.

CLIA-waived methods include the STAT-Site M Hgb, HemoPointH2, and HemoCue, all portable, battery-operated hemoglobin analyzers that fit in the palm of the hand (Fig. 44.3 and Procedure 44.3). The HemoCue uses plastic microcuvettes (MAHY kroh koo VETs) that contain reagents (ree EY juh nts) that *lyse* (break apart) the RBCs in the sample, releasing the hemoglobin. The hemoglobin reacts with the reagents and forms a colored compound. The color is detected and measured in the instrument, producing a digital readout. Capillary, venous, or arterial blood can be used in the disposable microcuvette. The cuvettes have a long shelf life.

PROCEDURE 44.3 Perform CLIA-Waived Hematology Testing: Perform a Hemoglobin Test

Task:
To accurately determine the level of hemoglobin present in a blood sample using the HemoCue B-Hemoglobin System.

Equipment and Supplies
- Patient's health record
- Provider's order and/or lab requisition
- Hemoglobin laboratory log
- HemoCue monitor
- HemoCue microcuvette
- Safety blood lancet
- Alcohol wipes
- Gauze
- Fluid-impermeable lab coat, protective eyewear, and gloves
- Biohazard waste container
- Biohazard sharps containers

Procedural Steps
1. Perform an instrument quality control check by inserting the control cuvette into the instrument. Make sure the reading is within acceptable limits before proceeding.
   Purpose: Only instruments that record values within acceptable control limits can be used for patient testing. If the value is outside the control limits, refer to the troubleshooting guide for the instrument or contact the manufacturer.
2. Wash hands or use hand sanitizer. Put on fluid-impermeable lab coat, protective eyewear, and gloves.
   Purpose: To ensure infection control.
3. Assemble all equipment and supplies needed.
4. Greet the patient. Identify yourself. Verify the patient's identity with the full name; ask the patient to spell the first and last name and to give his or her date of birth. Explain the procedure to be performed in a manner that is understood by the patient. Answer any questions the patient may have on the procedure. Obtain permission for the capillary puncture.
   Purpose: It is important to identify the patient in two different ways to ensure that you have the correct patient. Explaining the procedure can make the patient feel more comfortable and helps to reduce anxiety.
5. Examine the patient's fingers and choose the site to be used to obtain the blood sample.
   Purpose: The site must be free of trauma, calluses, and scarring.
6. Clean the site with an alcohol wipe or another recommended antiseptic preparation.
7. Perform a capillary puncture and wipe away the first drop of blood.
   Purpose: This drop may contain tissue fluid or antiseptic that may hemolyze the blood.
8. Obtain a large drop blood on the surface of the finger.
9. Touch the microcuvette to the drop of blood. Do not touch the finger. The correct volume is drawn into the cuvette by capillary action. Wipe off any excess blood from the sides of the cuvette (Figs.1 and 2).
   Purpose: Blood on the cuvette may alter the readings or contaminate the instrument.

PROCEDURE 44.3 Perform CLIA-Waived Hematology Testing: Perform a Hemoglobin Test—cont'd

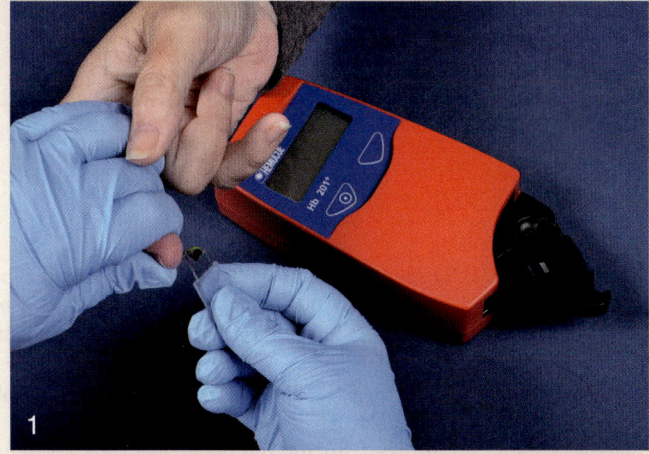

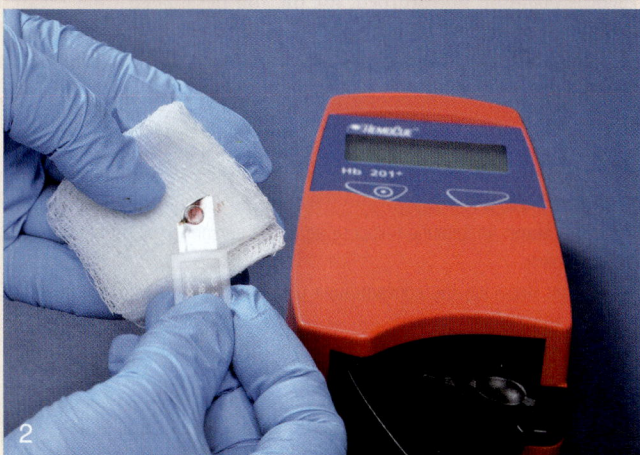

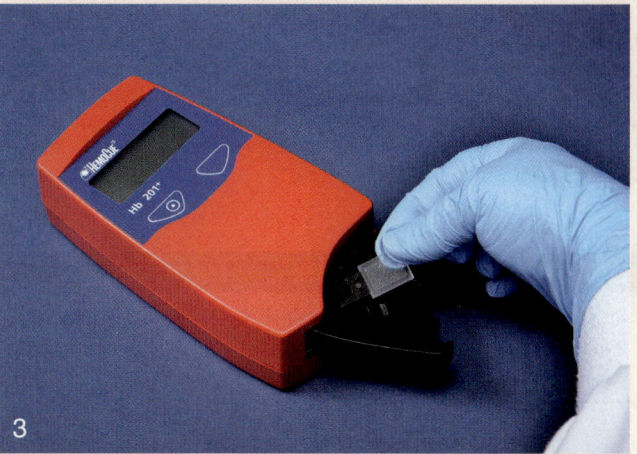

10. Place the cuvette in the cuvette holder of the HemoCue sample door and close the door of the instrument (Fig. 3).
11. Read the result and record it in the lab's hemoglobin log and the patient's health record.
    Purpose: A procedure is not completed until the results are recorded.
12. Dispose of biohazardous waste in biohazard waste containers. Turn off the instrument. Properly disinfect the work area.
13. Remove your gloves and dispose of them in the biohazard waste container. Remove the lab coat and protective eyewear. Wash hands or use hand sanitizer.
    Purpose: To ensure infection control.

HEMOCUE B HEMOGLOBIN SYSTEM PATIENT LOG

TEST: _____ KIT LOT # _____

Hemoglobin expected values=   Adult Males = 13.0–18.0 g/dL
                              Adult Females = 12.0–16.0 g/dL
                              Infants = 10.0–14.0 g/dL
                              Children = increase to adult

DATE	TECH	PATIENT I.D.	RESULT	CHARTED
10/09/20–	DC	# 12345	15.5 g/dL	✓

Documentation Example
10/09/20 9:30 a.m.: Hgb 15.5 g/dL._____Anita James, CMA (AAMA)

Normal hemoglobin values vary throughout a lifetime (Table 44.3). Factors that affect the hemoglobin level include age, gender, diet, altitude, and disease.

Hemoglobin and hematocrit tests are often performed together and are referred to as an "H&H." A quick mental calculation should always be done before H&H results are reported: the hemoglobin value × 3 (± 3) should equal the hematocrit value. For example, if the hemoglobin is 15 g/dL, calculate the hematocrit as:

$$15 \text{ g/dL} \times 3 = 45 \pm 3 = 42 \text{ to } 48$$

The hematocrit should be between 42% and 48%.

TABLE 44.3 Hemoglobin (Hgb) Reference Values

Age/Gender	Hgb Level (g/dL)
Neonate (newborn–<1 mo)	17–23
Infant (1 mo–1 yr)	9–14
Child (1–10 yr)	10–15
Female (>10 yr)	12–16
Male (>10 yr)	14–18

From Proctor D, et al: *Kinn's The Medical Assistant*, ed 13, St Louis, 2017, Elsevier.

TABLE 44.4 Erythrocyte Sedimentation Rate (ESR) Reference Values

	SEDIPLAST Test (mm/hr)
Men	≤50 yr: 0–15; >50 yr: 0–20
Women	≤50 yr: 0–20; >50 yr: 0–30

From Proctor D, et al: *Kinn's The Medical Assistant*, ed 13, St. Louis, 2017, Elsevier.

BOX 44.3 ESR Results

An increased erythrocyte sedimentation rate (ESR) is significant to the provider. It indicates the presence of inflammation in the body. A lower than normal ESR is not considered clinically significant.

Erythrocyte Sedimentation Rate

The *erythrocyte sedimentation rate* (ESR) is a laboratory test that measures the rate at which red blood cells gradually separate from plasma and settle to the bottom of a specially calibrated tube in 1 hour. The test is not specific for any disease in particular but is used as a general indicator of inflammation (Box 44.3). An increased ESR is seen in conditions such as:

- acute and chronic infections
- rheumatoid (ROO muh toid) arthritis, lupus erythematosus (LOO puhs er uh THEE muh toh sus), and other autoimmune (aw toh ih MYOON) conditions
- tuberculosis (too bur kyuh LOH sis), hepatitis, some cancers, multiple myeloma (mahy uh LOH muh), and rheumatic (roo MAT ik) fever

Normal values vary slightly with age and gender (Table 44.4). Several CLIA-waived methods of measuring the ESR are used, including the Sediplast procedure (Procedure 44.4). This closed system incorporates a pierceable (PEERS uh buhl) stopper that ensures a leakproof seal when punctured by a pipet (pahy PET). An automatic self-zeroing cap and reservoir accurately bring the blood level to the zero mark and prevent overfilling. A prefilled vial of sodium citrate reagent is provided for dilution (dih LOO shuh n) of blood before testing. A closed-tube Streck ESR method uses a Streck black-topped Vacutainer sample of blood that is directly placed in a Streck rack that provides results in 30 minutes (Fig. 44.4).

Many factors can affect the ESR. The tube must be filled with blood and must not have air bubbles. The tube must be allowed to sit in a vertical position, undisturbed, for the full designated time – careful timing is important. Tilting a tube a small amount may increase the sedimentation rate. Jarring or vibrations from nearby machinery will falsely increase the ESR.

VOCABULARY

autoimmune: An immune response against a person's own tissues, cells, or cell parts.
dilution: Reducing the concentration of a mixture or solution by adding a known volume of liquid.
pipet: A slender tube attached to or including a bulb, for transferring or measuring small amounts of a liquid, often used in a laboratory.

MEDICAL TERMINOLOGY

auto-: self, own
-globin: protein
hem/o: blood
immun/o: immune, protection, safe
micro-: small

PROCEDURE 44.4 Perform CLIA-Waived Hematology Testing: Determine the Erythrocyte Sedimentation Rate Using a Modified Westergren Method

Task:
Fill a Westergren tube properly, and observe and record an erythrocyte sedimentation rate (ESR) obtained by using a modified Westergren method.

Equipment and Supplies
- Patient's health record
- Provider's order and/or lab requisition
- Erythrocyte sedimentation rate (ESR) laboratory log
- Ethylenediaminetetraacetic acid (EDTA)–anticoagulated blood specimen
- Safety tube decapper (if tubes do not have Hemogard plastic tops)
- Disposable transfer pipet
- Sediplast ESR system (prefilled Sediplast vial)
- Sediplast rack
- Timer
- Fluid-impermeable lab coat, eye protection, and gloves
- Biohazard waste container
- Biohazard sharps container

Procedural Steps
1. Wash hands or use hand sanitizer. Put on a fluid-impermeable lab coat, eye protection, and gloves.
   Purpose: To ensure infection control.
2. Assemble the materials needed.
3. Check the leveling bubble of the Sediplast rack.
   Purpose: The rack must be horizontal on the table or bench to ensure that the tube is vertical.

PROCEDURE 44.4 Perform CLIA-Waived Hematology Testing: Determine the Erythrocyte Sedimentation Rate Using a Modified Westergren Method—cont'd

4. Bring the blood sample to room temperature if it has been refrigerated and mix the sample well by gently inverting the tube 6 to 8 times, making sure the tube has no bubbles.
   Purpose: Cells settle when a specimen stands, and blood must always be well mixed before sampling. Test results will be altered if refrigerated blood is not brought to room temperature.
5. Remove the plastic Hemogard stopper on the blood sample by twisting and slowly pushing up on the stopper with your thumbs (or by using a tube decapper on rubber-stoppered blood tubes). Also remove the stopper on the prefilled Sediplast vial.
   Purpose: Using the Hemogard cover or removing the rubber cap with a protective device blocks blood splashes and helps prevent aerosolization of the specimen.
6. Fill the Sediplast vial with blood to the indicated line using a disposable transfer pipet (Fig. 1). Replace the stopper on the prefilled vial and invert it several times to mix. Recap the blood collection tube with its stopper.
   Purpose: This dilutes the blood in accordance with the Westergren procedure.

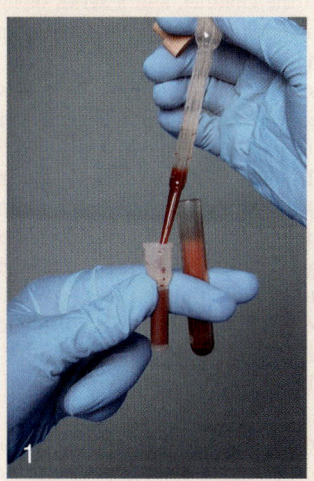

(Courtesy Polymedco, Cortland Manor, NY.)

7. Insert a Sediplast pipet through the pierceable stopper on the prefilled vial and push down until the pipet touches the bottom of the vial. The pipet automatically draws the blood up and over the zero mark (Fig. 2).

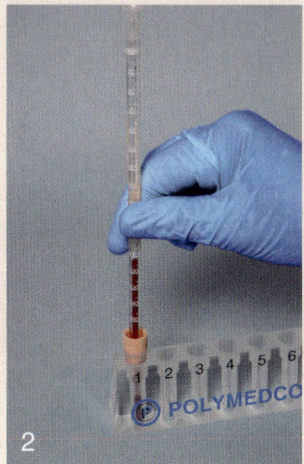

(Courtesy Polymedco, Cortland Manor, NY.)

8. Insert the filled Sediplast pipet and its vial into the Sediplast rack, making sure the vial is vertical.
   Purpose: A pipet that is not vertical produces incorrect results.
9. Note the start time on the ESR log sheet and allow the vial to stand undisturbed for 60 minutes.
   Purpose: Jarring or moving the vial increases the sedimentation rate.
10. After 60 minutes, measure the distance the erythrocytes have fallen at the top of the tube. The scale reads in millimeters – each line is 1 mm.
11. Properly dispose of all biohazardous materials. Disinfect the work area. Dispose of the plastic Sediplast pipet and its vial into a biohazard sharps container. Remove your gloves, protective eyewear, and lab coat. Wash hands or use hand sanitizer.
12. Record the findings in the lab's ESR log and the patient's health record. Remember: the Westergren ESR is reported in millimeters per hour (mm/hr).
    Purpose: A procedure is considered not done until it is recorded.

ESR—SEDIPLAST—PATIENT LOG

ESR expected values:
Adult Males < 50 years = 0–15 mm/hr
Adult Males > 50 years = 0–20 mm/hr
Adult Females < 50 years = 0–20 mm/hr
Adult Females > 50 years = 0–30 mm/hr

DATE	TECH	PATIENT I.D.	SLOT #	TIME	RESULT	CHARTED
10/09/20–	DC	# 12345	2	60 min	15 mm	✓

Documentation Example
10/09/20XX 9:30 a.m.: ESR 15 mm in 60 minutes. ———————————————————————————— Anita James, CMA (AAMA)

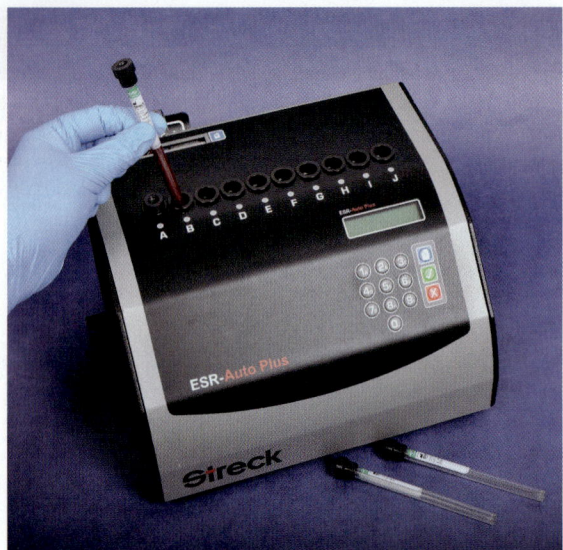

FIG. 44.4 30-minute Streck ESR CLIA-waived test (From Proctor D, et al: *Kinn's The Medical Assistant*, ed 13, St Louis, 2017, Elsevier.)

> **BOX 44.4 Prothrombin Time/International Normalized Ratio (PT/INR)**
>
> It is important to educate patients regarding their behaviors when a blood test such as the PT/INR is being monitored. Reassure these patients that follow-up testing is needed, accurate, and beneficial for their treatment. For example, if patients are taking the anticoagulant warfarin (Coumadin), they will need to follow up with the required lab work to monitor their PT/INR. Patients should understand how their vitamin K intake from food directly affects their lab results. Increased vitamin K can increase blood clotting time; this means that vitamin K is working against warfarin. Helping patients identify foods high in vitamin K is crucial to maintaining a proper PT/INR value. Many providers instruct patients to eat the same amounts of foods high in vitamin K consistently. Foods high in vitamin K include leafy greens (e.g., kale, collards, spinach, and turnip greens), Brussels sprouts, and broccoli.

capillary sample blood is dispensed into the channels of a testing strip. The blood is mixed with a thromboplastin reagent. The blood is pumped back and forth in the channel, and a series of light-emitting diodes (LEDs) detect formation of a clot when blood movement in the channels stop (Procedure 44.5).

PT test results are reported as the number of seconds blood takes to clot when mixed with the thromboplastin reagent. The international normalized ratio (INR) was created by the World Health Organization (WHO) because PT test results can vary, depending on the thromboplastin reagent used. The INR is a conversion unit that considers the different sensitivities of reagents. It is widely accepted as the standard unit for reporting PT results rather than actual clotting time. Normal PT values are 10 to 13 seconds, or an INR of 1 to 1.4. Patients who are taking warfarin to prevent the formation of blood clots or who have artificial heart valves should have an INR value of about 2 to 3. Their blood should take longer to clot than that of a normal healthy individual.

It is important that the medical assistant know how to accurately document INR follow-up and related warfarin dosages on a patient flow sheet. The provider will balance repeated INR levels with warfarin doses so the INR is maintained at about 2 throughout the anticoagulant treatment (Fig. 44.6).

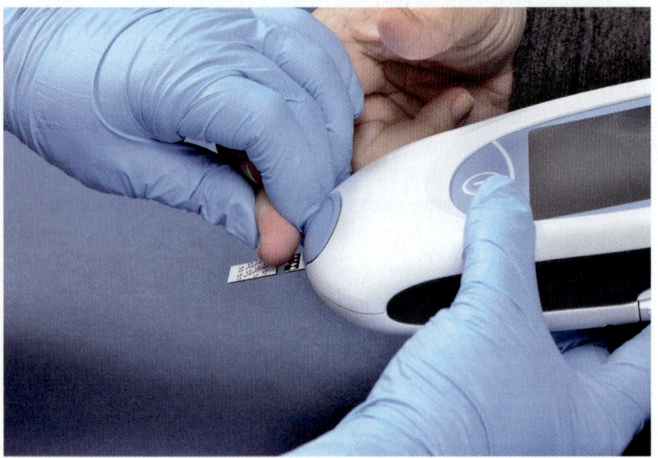

FIG. 44.5 Applying a blood sample to the CoagChek XS PT test monitor.

> **CRITICAL THINKING 44.2**
>
> Anita just roomed Janine Butler. She has an appointment today, and Dr. Perez would like to check her PT/INR results. Janine is on warfarin, but her INR is still a bit low. Anita checks her chart, and the INR completed in the lab is 1.7. Is this an acceptable result for someone who is on medication to prolong clotting time? Is it too high, too low, or normal?

HEMATOLOGY IN THE REFERENCE LABORATORY

The most frequently ordered reference laboratory procedure for hematology is the CBC. This test requires a lavender-topped EDTA blood specimen. It gives a comprehensive look at the cellular components of blood and can provide a wealth of information about a patient's condition. It routinely includes the following:
- RBC count, hematocrit, hemoglobin, and red cell indices (IN duh seez)
- WBC count and differential
- Platelet count

Coagulation Testing

The medical assistant may be asked to perform a CLIA-waived test called a *prothrombin time* (PT; also called a protime). This test can be performed using a handheld, CLIA-waived instrument that uses whole blood from a fingerstick (Fig. 44.5). A PT is a method of measuring how long it takes blood to clot. Prothrombin is a protein in the liquid part of blood *(plasma)* that is converted to thrombin as part of the clotting process. Thrombin then causes fibrinogen to be converted to fibrin (FAHY brin) during the clotting process.

The PT is often used in combination with the partial thromboplastin (throm buh PLAS tin) time (PTT) to screen for hemophilia (hee muh FIL ee uh) and other clotting disorders. The PT is also used to monitor patients taking the anticoagulant drug *warfarin* (Coumadin) and similar anticoagulants. Warfarin is given to prevent clots in deep veins of the legs and to treat a pulmonary embolism (Box 44.4).

The CLIA-waived CoaguChek XS PT (see Fig. 44.5) measures the time it takes a blood sample to form a fibrin clot. A precise amount of

PROCEDURE 44.5 Perform a CLIA-Waived PT/INR Test

Task:
Perform a coagulation test to determine PT/INR using the CoaguChek XS instrument with built-in quality control.

Directions:
Perform a protime/INR test on Connie Lange STAT.

Equipment and Supplies
- Patient's health record or flow chart (see Fig. 44.6)
- Provider's order and/or lab requisition
- PT/INR lab log
- Gauze, alcohol wipes, bandage
- CoaguChek XS PT Test monitor (see Fig. 44.5)
- CoaguChek lancet
- CoaguChek test strip container and code chip
- Package insert or flow chart with directions
- Fluid-impermeable lab coat, protective eyewear, and gloves
- Biohazard waste container
- Biohazard sharps containers

Procedural Steps
1. Wash hands or use hand sanitizer. Put on fluid-impermeable lab coat, protective eyewear, and gloves.
   Purpose: To ensure infection control.
2. Assemble the materials needed.
3. If you are using test strips from a new, unopened container, you must change the test strip code chip. The three-number code on the test strip container must match the three-number code on the code strip. To install the code strip, follow the instructions in the Code Chip section of the *User's Manual*.
   Purpose: To ensure that the instrument is calibrated correctly, to produce accurate, precise, and reliable results.
4. Place the meter on a flat surface so that it will not vibrate or move during testing.
   Purpose: The test results are based on the back-and-forth movement of the blood sample that stops when the clot has formed. Vibrations or other movements will result in an error message, and the test will have to be repeated.
5. Greet the patient. Identify yourself. Verify the patient's identity with full name; ask the patient to spell the first and last name and to give his or her date of birth. Explain the procedure to be performed in a manner that is understood by the patient. Answer any questions the patient may have on the procedure. Obtain permission for the capillary puncture.
   Purpose: It is important to identify the patient in two different ways to ensure that you have the correct patient. Explaining the procedure can make the patient feel more comfortable and helps to reduce anxiety.
6. Examine the patient's fingers and choose the site to be used to obtain the blood sample.
7. Prepare the site:
   - Warm the hand by placing it under the arm, using a hand warmer, and/or washing the hand in warm water.
   - Have the patient hold his or her arm down to the side so that the hand is below the waist.
   - Massage the palm of the hand toward the base of the finger and toward the tip until the fingertip has increased color.
   - If necessary, immediately after lancing, gently squeeze the finger from its base to encourage blood flow.

   Purpose: The hanging drop blood sample must be sufficient to travel down the three channels on the test strip. It must be free of contaminants, tissue fluids, and alcohol.
8. When you are ready to test, remove a test strip from the container and immediately close the container. Make sure it seals tightly. *Do not open the container or touch the test strips with wet hands or wet gloves.*
   Purpose: Exposure to moisture damages the test strips.
9. Insert the test strip as far as you can into the meter. This powers the meter ON (Fig. 1).

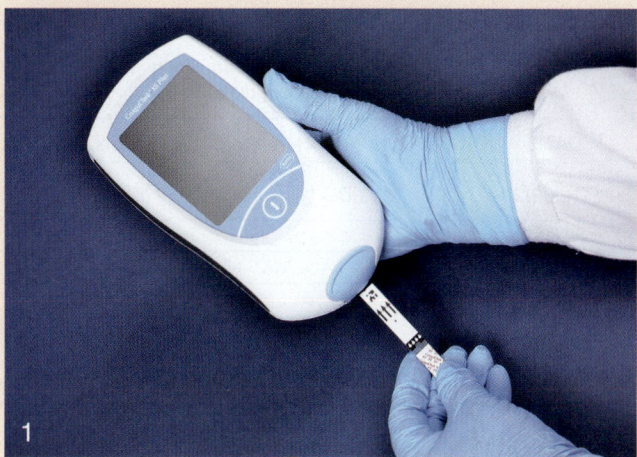

10. Disinfect the finger with an alcohol wipe and allow the finger to air dry. Perform the fingerstick.
11. Hold the finger with a blood drop very close to the target (the clear area of the test strip). Apply 1 drop of blood to the top or side of the target area and wait until you hear the beep. *You must apply a hanging drop of blood to the test strip within 15 seconds of the fingerstick. Do not add more blood. Do not touch or remove the test strip while the test is in progress.* The flashing blood drop symbol changes to an hourglass symbol when the meter detects a sufficient sample (see Fig. 44.5).
12. The result appears in approximately 1 minute. It may be displayed in three ways: as the international normalized ratio (INR); as the protime (PT) in seconds; or as %Quick (a unit used mainly in Europe). See the following chart.

Protime Expected Values for Normal and Therapeutic Whole Blood

	INR	PT (sec)
Normal	0.8–1.2	6.5–11.9[a]
Low anticoagulation therapy	1.5–2	Varies with method used
Moderate anticoagulation therapy	2–3	Varies with method used
High anticoagulation therapy	3–4	Varies with method used

[a]Laboratory reports and manufacturers must supply their own reference ranges for PT results along with each patient's results. This is because different methodologies may create different reference ranges and different units of measurement.

13. Record the result in the lab's PT/INR log and in the patient's warfarin therapy flow sheet and/or electronic health record. Circle any results that do not fall into the Desirable Ranges column of the preceding table based on a patient who is on "low anticoagulation therapy." You may add comments to the test result about the test conditions or the patient. Identify "critical values" and take appropriate steps to notify the provider.

Continued

PROCEDURE 44.5 Perform CLIA-Waived PT/INR Test—cont'd

Purpose: The provider needs to know the result while the patient is still in the office, for proper follow-up with the patient.

Purpose: To ensure infection control.

14. Dispose of all sharps into the biohazard sharps container. Dispose of regulated medical waste into the biohazard waste container. Disinfect the test area and remove your PPE. Wash hands or use hand sanitizer.

PROTIME—PATIENT LOG

Protime expected values for both normal and therapeutic whole blood:

	INR	PT seconds (ISI = 1.0)
Normal	0.8–1.2	10.4–15.7 sec
Low anticoagulation	1.5–2.0	19.6–26.1 sec
Moderate anticoagulation	2.0–3.0	26.1–39.2 sec
High anticoagulation	2.5–4.0	32.6–52.2 sec

DATE	TECH	PATIENT I.D.	INR	PT SECONDS	CHARTED
10/09/20–	DC	# 12345	1.0	19.7	✓

Documentation Example

10/09/20XX 9:30 a.m.: INR = 1.0 and PT = 19.7 seconds. Patient is on low anticoagulation therapy._____Anita James, CMA (AAMA)

Walden-Martin Family Medical Clinic
Warfarin Anticoagulant Record

Patient's Name: _____   DOB: _____
Address: _____   SSN: _____

Patient's Phone: _____
Dx for Anticoagulation: _____   ICDM Code: _____
Date Warfarin Started: _____   INR Goal: _____
Phone for Outside Lab: _____

Date	Warfarin Dose Pre-Test	PT	INR	Warfarin Dose Order	Next INR/PT	Signature

FIG. 44.6 Warfarin flow sheet. (From Proctor D, et al: *Kinn's The Medical Assistant*, ed 13, St Louis, 2017, Elsevier.)

TABLE 44.5 Reference Ranges for Complete Blood Count (CBC) Values[a]

Test	Neonates (Newborn–1 mo)	Infants (1 mo–1 yr)	Children (1–10 yr)	Men (>10 yr)	Women (>10 yr)
RBCs	4.8–7.1 million/mm^3	3.8–5.5 million/mm^3	4.5–4.8 million/mm^3	4.5–6 million/mm^3	4–5.5 million/mm^3
Hematocrit (Hct)	44%–64%	30%–40%	35%–41%	42%–52%	36%–45%
Hemoglobin (Hgb)	17–23 g/dL	9–14 g/dL	11–16 g/dL	15–17 g/dL	12–16 g/dL
WBCs	9000–30,000/mm^3	6000–16,000/mm^3	5000–13,000/mm^3	4000–11,000/mm^3	
RBC Indices					
MCV	96–108 fL			82–99 fL	
MCH	32–34 pg			26–34 pg	
MCHC	31–33 g/dL			31–37 g/dL	
WBC Differential					
Neutrophils	≥45% by age 1 wk	32%	60% for children ≥2 yr	50%–65%	
Bands	—	—	—	0%–7%	
Eosinophils	—	—	0%–3%	1%–3%	
Basophils	—	—	1%–3%	0%–1%	
Monocytes	—	—	4%–9%	3%–9%	
Lymphocytes	≥41% by age 1 wk	61%	59% for children ≥2 yr	25%–40%	
Platelets	140,000–300,000/mm^3	200,000–473,000/mm^3	150,000–450,000/mm^3	150,000–400,000/mm^3	

fL, Femtoliter; *MCH*, mean corpuscular hemoglobin; *MCHC*, mean corpuscular hemoglobin concentration; *MCV*, mean corpuscular volume; *pg*, picograms; *RBC*, red blood cell; *WBC*, white blood cell.
[a]Lab reports, both electronic and paper, must supply their own reference ranges, along with each patient's results. This is because different methodologies may create different reference ranges and different units of measurement.
From Proctor D, et al: *Kinn's The Medical Assistant,* ed 13, St Louis, 2017, Elsevier.

Complete Blood Count (CBC) Laboratory Reports

It is important that medical assistants understand the hematology laboratory reports that arrive from the reference laboratories. They should be able to distinguish between normal and abnormal results. Use the following references to complete the Critical Thinking Application exercise that follows:
- Hematology reference ranges (Table 44.5)
- The patient report form (Fig. 44.7), a sample lab report, also identifies the lab's reference ranges. Lab reports, both electronic and paper, must supply their own reference ranges, along with each patient's results.

CRITICAL THINKING 44.3

Using the reference ranges in Table 44.5 and the lab report form in Fig. 44.7, decide if the following results are normal or abnormal.
1. Grace Sifuentes, age 4, has a hematocrit of 38%. Is that normal, high, or low?
2. Christian Washington, age 45, has a WBC count of 14,200/mm^3. Is that normal, high, or low?
3. Brigitte Mulrooney, age 29, has a hematocrit of 32% and a hemoglobin of 10 g/dL. Are these results normal, high, or low?
4. Eleanor Jackson, age 81, has 23% bands in her white blood cell differential. Is that normal, high, or low?

Red Blood Cell Count.
The RBC count is part of the CBC (see Table 44.5). It approximates the number of circulating RBCs in a person's blood. The function of RBCs is to transport oxygen to tissues. The RBC count often is decreased in patients with anemia. Increased RBC counts are found in people with dehydration, polycythemia vera, or severe burns, and those living at high altitudes.

Normal RBC values range from approximately 4 million to 6 million cells/mm^3. RBC counts usually are higher in males than in females.

Red Blood Cell Indices.
A variety of calculations can be performed using the information obtained from the CBC. The red cell *indices* provide information about RBC disorders. The indices are used to classify anemias and to select additional tests that may help determine the cause of anemia. Red cell indices are also helpful to monitor the treatment of anemia. Because indices may change in response to treatment, they can be used as an indicator in the evaluation of treatment. The indices are mathematical calculations using the three red cell tests: Hct, Hgb, and the RBC count.
- *Mean cell volume (MCV)*: MCV = (Hct/RBC) × 10. The average size of the RBCs is the most important index for classifying anemias. Abnormally large RBCs are *macrocytic* (MAK ruh sih tik) and have a higher than normal MCV. Small RBCs are *microcytic* (MAHY kruh sih tik) and have a lower than normal MCV. The normal reference range is 82 to 108 femtoliters (fehm TOH lee turs) (fL).
- *Mean cell hemoglobin (MCH)*: MCH = (Hgb/RBC) × 10. The MCH is calculated to give the average weight of hemoglobin in the RBC. The reference range is 26 to 34 picograms (PEE kuh grams) (pg).
- *Mean cell ratio of Hgb and Hct (MCHC)*: MCHC = (Hgb × 100)/RBC. The MCHC indicates the average weight of hemoglobin compared with the cell size. The reference range is 32 to 37 g/dL. A decreased MCHC shows **hypochromic** (hahy puh KROH mik) RBCs in a stained blood smear. An increased MCHC is rare and should be flagged and brought to the attention of the provider.

VOCABULARY
hypochromic: Pale red blood cells. Lacking color.

MEDICAL TERMINOLOGY
hypo: deficient, below, under, less than normal
chrom/o: color

		DATE & TIME RECEIVED	ACCESSION NUMBER
		10/ 20/ 2013 20:45	
		LOCATION	DATE REPORTED
			10/ 21/2000

PHYSICIAN	PATIENT INFORMATION

TEST		RESULTS	REFERENCE RANGE	UNITS
HEMOGRAM	LO	2.9	4. 5-10. 5	CU.MM.
WHITE BLOOD COUNT	LO	2. 39	4.40-5.90	CU.MM.
RED BLOOD COUNT	LO	7.4	14.0-18.0	GM/100ML
HEMOGLOBIN	LO	22.3	40. 0-52.0 %	
MEAN CORPUSCULAR VOLUME		93	80-100	fL
MEAN CORPUSCULAR HGB		31.0	27. 0-32.0	PG
MEAN CORPUSCULAR HgB CONC		33.2	31.0-36.0	%
DIFFERENTIAL, WBC				
SEGMENTED NEUTROPHILS		57	38-80	%
LYMPHOCYTE		29	15-45	%
MONOCYTES		7	1-10	%
EOSINOPHILS		1	0-4	%
BAND NEUTROPHILS	HI	6	0-5	%
ANISOCYTOSIS	ABN	SLIGHT		
HYPOCHROMIA	ABN	SLIGHT		
PLATELET ESTIMATE	ABN	DECREASED		
PARTIAL THROMBOPLASTIN TIME				
PARTIAL THROMBOPLASTIN TIME		31.7	20.0-40.0	SECONDS
CONTROL PTT		30.4	20.0-40.0	SECONDS
PROTHROMBIN TIME				
PROTHROMBIN TIME		12.2	10.0-13.5	SECONDS
CONTROL PT		12.0	11.0-13.0	SECONDS
FINAL Report (Summary)				

FIG. 44.7 Sample lab report with normal and abnormal patient results. (From Proctor D, et al: *Kinn's The Medical Assistant*, ed 13, St Louis, 2017, Elsevier.)

White Blood Cell Count. The WBC count gives an estimate of the total number of leukocytes in circulating blood. The count is performed to help the provider determine whether an infection is present or to aid in the diagnosis of leukemia (loo KEE mee uh). It also may be used to follow the course of a disease and indicate if patient is responding to treatment.

The normal WBC count varies with age. It is higher in newborns and decreases throughout a lifetime. The average adult range is 4500 to 11,000 cells/mm^3. Many factors can affect the WBC count.

An increase in the number of normal WBCs is a condition called *leukocytosis* (loo koh sahy TOH sis). Increased WBC counts may normally be seen with pregnancy, stress, anesthesia, exercise, exposure to temperature extremes, and after treatment with corticosteroids (kawr tuh koh STER oids). Pathologic causes of leukocytosis include many bacterial infections, leukemia, appendicitis (uh pen duh SAHY tis), and pneumonia (noo MOHN yuh).

A decrease in the WBC count is called *leukopenia* (loo kuh PEE nee uh). This condition may be caused by viral infection or by exposure to radiation and certain chemicals and drugs.

Differential Cell Count. The purpose of the differential, or "diff," in the CBC is to analyze and count the types of WBCs found in a sample of blood. The differential can be manually performed using a stained blood smear and a microscope, or with an automated instrument. Automated cell counters have the ability to analyze the WBCs and gather information about cell size, internal structures, and density (DEN sih tee).

Preparation of blood smears for the differential. A *blood smear* enables the examiner to view the preserved cellular structures of blood. The morphology (mawr FOL uh jee) of WBCs, RBCs, and platelets can be studied. Their size, shape, and maturity can also be evaluated.

A blood smear is prepared by placing a drop of blood from a fingerstick or an EDTA tube (using a DIFF-SAFE blood dispenser) onto a clean glass slide (Fig. 44.8). The slide must be free of dust and grease. The best specimen for a blood smear is capillary blood that has no anticoagulant added. EDTA-anticoagulated blood can be used, provided the smear is made within 2 hours of specimen collection. Because timing is important, the medical assistant may be asked to prepare a smear during collection of the CBC specimen.

The wedge smear is used most frequently and would follow these steps:
- Place a small drop of blood ½ inch from the frosted end (placed to the right) of a glass slide.
- The end of a second glass spreader slide is placed in front (to the left) of the drop of blood at an angle of 30 to 35 degrees.
- The spreader slide is brought back into the drop with a quick but smooth gliding motion until the blood spreads along the edge of the spreader slide.
- The spreader slide is then pushed to the left with a quick, steady motion, spreading the blood across the slide (Fig. 44.9).

A good wedge smear should cover one half to three fourths of the slide. It should show a gradual transition from a thick to a thin end with a feathered edge (Fig. 44.10). It should have a smooth appearance with no ridges, holes, lines, streaks, or clumps. On microscopic examination, the cells should be evenly distributed.

After the smear has been made, it should be air dried (Box 44.5). Once dry, the patient's name is written on the frosted end of the slide with a pencil. After it has been labeled, the slide is *fixed*, which preserves and prevents changes in the cells. Many of the quick stains available on the market contain the fixative in the stain.

> **BOX 44.5 Blood Slide Artifacts**
>
> Do not blow on the blood slide to dry it. The moisture in your breath can cause artifacts (AHR tuh fakt) to form on the slide. Crystals in the stain can also be seen as artifacts on the slide!

> **VOCABULARY**
> **artifact:** A substance, structure, or event that does not naturally occur in a situation. Examples include interference, or electrical "garbage," on an ECG, or crystals, lint, or contamination of a staining technique.
> **density:** Describes how compact or concentrated something is.
> **morphology:** The study of the form, shape, and structure of an organism or a cell.

> **MEDICAL TERMINOLOGY**
> **morph/o:** shape, form
> **-logy:** study (process of)

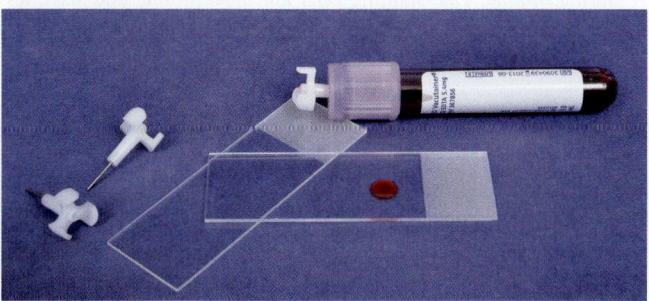

FIG. 44.8 DIFF-SAFE device used to make a blood smear.

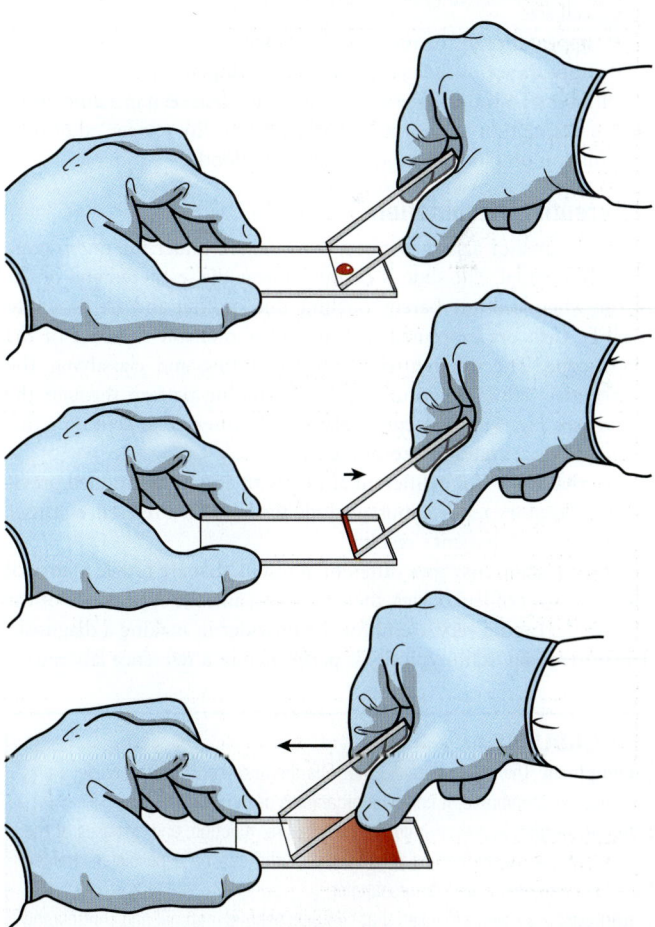

FIG. 44.9 Making a differential wedge smear.

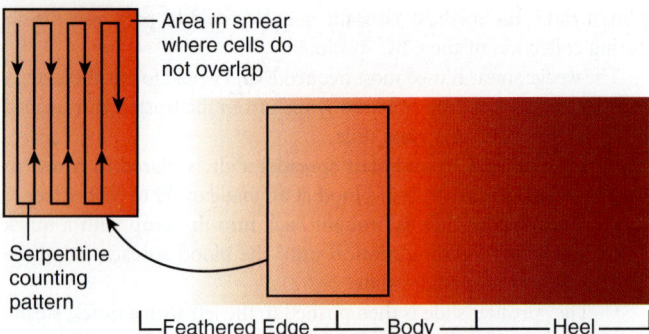

FIG. 44.10 *Right,* Appearance of a properly prepared wedge smear. *Left,* Serpentine pattern used to count the cells. (From Proctor D, et al: *Kinn's The Medical Assistant,* ed 13, St Louis, 2017, Elsevier.)

Staining blood smears. Stains commonly used to make blood smears are described as *polychromatic* (pol ee kroh MAR ik). They contain dyes that stain cell components different colors. These stains are attracted to different parts of the cell, which makes the cells and their structures easier to see and tell apart. The most commonly used differential blood stain is Wright's stain.

Identification of Normal Blood Cells

Useful information can be gathered from a microscopic evaluation of blood cells in a stained smear. The three features **hematologists** (hee muh TOL uh jists) look for in blood cells are:
- cell size
- appearance of the **nucleus** (NOO klee uh s)
- appearance of the **cytoplasm** (sahy tuh plaz uh m)

In Table 44.6 you will see a summary of the cells seen in a differential and a description of normal characteristics. To review additional information on blood cells, see Chapter 8, Blood.

Differential Examination

A specific area of a stained smear is examined under the microscope for a differential. The slide is examined near the feathered end of the smear, where cells are barely touching one another and are easiest to identify. Cells are examined with the oil immersion objective of the microscope. The differential involves counting and classifying 100 consecutive WBCs while moving in a winding pattern through the smear (see Fig. 44.10). A count of the cells observed is kept on a differential cell counter or a computer.

Normal values for a differential vary with age. As mentioned previously, laboratory reports must include the lab's own reference ranges, along with each patient's results.

Disease states may give differential results that are unlike a normal diff. The types of leukocytes, their maturity, and the appearance of the differential can be very useful for the provider in making a diagnosis. The differential exam typically is performed in a reference laboratory.

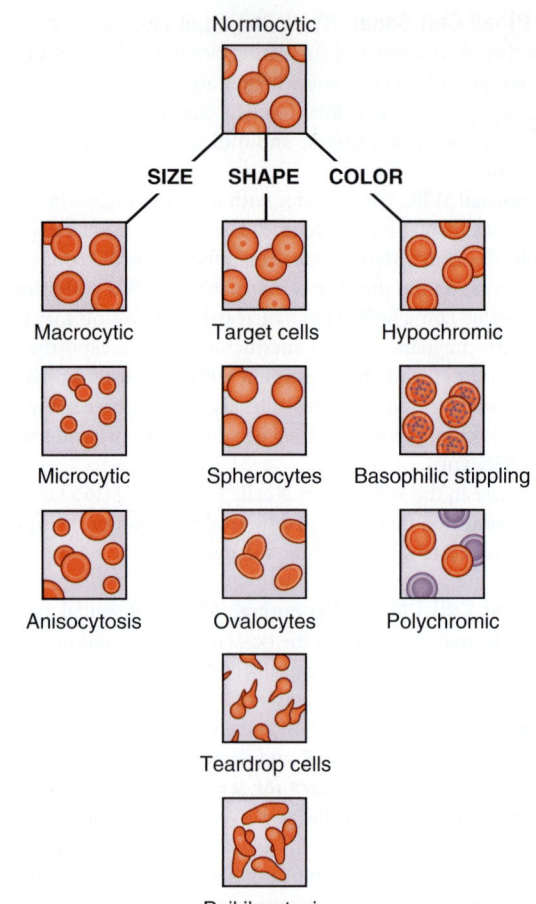

FIG. 44.11 Abnormal red blood cells. (From Proctor D, et al: *Kinn's The Medical Assistant,* ed 13, St Louis, 2017, Elsevier.)

Red Blood Cell Morphology. After the differential cell count has been determined, the RBCs are observed and evaluated. Normally, stained RBCs are the same size and shape and are well filled with hemoglobin. Any variations from the normal state are reported. (Fig. 44.11 shows examples of abnormal cells.) The appearance of the RBCs should correlate with the RBC indices.

Size. Normal-sized RBCs are said to be *normocytic*. If the cells are larger than normal, they are macrocytic; if the cells are smaller than normal, they are microcytic. The condition in which different sizes of RBCs are present is known as *anisocytosis* (ah nee soh sey TOH sis).

Shape. Normal RBCs are round or slightly oval. Cells may be shaped like sickles, targets, crescents, or burs. *Poikilocytosis* (poyh kee LOH sigh toh sis) is a significant variation in the shape of RBCs.

Content. An RBC with a normal amount of hemoglobin is said to be *normochromic*. Pale-staining cells are *hypochromic* and have less hemoglobin than normal. Any inclusions in red cells should be reported.

VOCABULARY

cytoplasm: The cell substance that fills the area between the nucleus and the cell membrane. It contains organelles of the cell.

hematologist: A person trained in the nature, function, and diseases of the blood and blood-forming organs. He or she can be a physician, trained laboratory personnel, or researcher.

nucleus: A structure in a cell that contains genetic material and controls the characteristics and growth of the cell.

CRITICAL THINKING 44.4

Anita checks Reuven Ahmad's CBC and differential results as she prepares information for Dr. Perez. Reuven's RBC count is 5.1 million/mm^3. Is that a normal value for an adult male? In the notes from the differential, the laboratory technologist comments that Reuven's RBCs are normocytic and slightly hypochromic. Define normocytic and hypochromic in your own words. Be ready to share your definitions with the class.

TABLE 44.6 Cells in a Differential

Cell Name	Normal Characteristics	Photograph of Normal Cell
Red blood cell	Most numerous cell on diff. A small, red, biconcave disk with no nuclei.	
Platelet	Smallest cell on diff. May be round or oval. Has no nucleus. A fragment of cytoplasm from a large bone marrow cell called a *megakaryocyte*. (From *Mosby's Dictionary of Medicine, Nursing, & Health Professions*, ed 8, St. Louis, 2009, Elsevier.)	
Neutrophil – mature	Most numerous white blood cell (WBC) on diff. Nucleus has many lobes. Increased numbers seen with bacterial infections.	
Neutrophil – immature	Called a *band* or *stab cell*. Horseshoe-shaped nucleus. Increased numbers seen with some types of leukemia, and infections.	
Eosinophil	Has large, red-orange granules. Increased numbers seen with allergies, asthma, and certain parasitic infections	
Basophil	Has large, dark blue/purple granules. Granules contain *histamine* (HIS tuh meen), which is involved in the inflammatory response. Natural anticoagulant.	
Lymphocyte	Smallest WBC, but most numerous in the blood. Large, dark blue/purple nucleus. Increased numbers seen with viral and some bacterial infections. Viral infections may show **atypical lymphs**.	
Monocyte	Largest WBC in the blood. Increased numbers seen with viral and some bacterial infections	

Platelet Analysis

On a stained smear, the platelets are observed for any abnormalities. Platelets are small and irregularly shaped and may vary considerably in size. The normal platelet count is 150,000 to 450,000/mm³. An increase in platelets is called *thrombocytosis*, and a decrease is called *thrombocytopenia*. Excessive clumping of platelets is also reported in a platelet analysis.

VOCABULARY
atypical lymphs: In many viral infections, stimulated or reactive lymphs are called *atypical lymphs*. They are commonly seen in infectious mononucleosis, commonly called *mono*.

MEDICAL TERMINOLOGY
norm/o: rule, order
macro-: large
micro-: small
anis/o: unequal
-osis: condition, usually abnormal
poikil/o: varied, irregular
thromb/o: clot
-penia: deficiency

IMMUNOHEMATOLOGY

Formerly called the *blood bank*, the immunohematology department of the laboratory is responsible for blood typing. The major reason for performing immunohematology tests is to prevent problems caused by blood types that are not compatible during blood transfusions. Compatibility testing (also called cross-matching) is performed to prevent transfusion reactions in patients receiving blood from a donor. Identifying potential Rh incompatibility problems in expectant mothers is another procedure done in immunohematology. Rh incompatibility between an expectant mother and the unborn child may result in hemolytic disease of the newborn (HDN). (See Chapter 8, for more details on HDN.)

Blood Typing

The two major blood antigen systems are the ABO system and the Rh system (See Chapter 8, for details). The ABO system has four major blood groups: A, B, O, and AB. Another major blood group is the Rh group. A person is either Rh-positive (Rh+) or Rh-negative (Rh−). Determinations of ABO and Rh blood groups are simple tests that can be performed easily. But because the consequences of performing the test incorrectly can be life-threatening, blood typing is not a CLIA-waived test. See Table 44.7 for blood transfusion compatibility types. See Box 44.6 for blood type frequency within ethnic populations in the United States.

TABLE 44.7 Blood Compatibility

Recipient Blood[a] RBC Antigen	Plasma Antibodies	Compatible With Donor Types[b]
Type O (no antigens)	Anti-A and anti-B	O
Type A (type A antigen)	Anti-B	O and A
Type B (type B antigen)	Anti-A	O and B
Type AB (type AB antigen)	None	O, A, B, and AB

RBC, Red blood cell.
[a]Patients with type AB blood are considered universal recipients.
[b]Patients with type O blood are considered universal donors.
From Proctor D, et al: *Kinn's The Medical Assistant,* ed 13, St Louis, 2017, Elsevier.

BOX 44.6 Blood Type Populations

This table gives you an idea of the blood type frequency in a few different populations in the United States.

Type	Caucasian	African-American	Hispanic	Asian
O+	37%	47%	53%	39%
O−	8%	4%	4%	1%
A+	33%	24%	29%	27%
A−	7%	2%	2%	0.5%
B+	9%	18%	9%	25%
B−	2%	1%	1%	0.4%
AB+	3%	4%	2%	7%
AB−	1%	0.3%	0.2%	0.1%

Data from the American Red Cross. www.redcrossblood.org/learn-about-blood/blood-types. Accessed July 5, 2017.

CRITICAL THINKING 44.5

Griffin Jones is in for a physical today, but she would also like to have her blood type tested. She and her husband are thinking of starting a family soon and would like to know her ABO/Rh type. She thinks she is A−. If Griffin is A−, what antigen or antigens are on her RBCs?

BOX 44.7 Beyond ABO and Rh Typing

There are many blood types beyond ABO and Rh. Here are a few blood antigens or antigen systems. Just so that you have seen the terms…

- Diego — Found only among East Asians and Native Americans
- MNS — Useful in maternity and paternity testing
- Duffy — The malarial parasite requires the Duffy antigen to enter the red blood cells. Lack of the antigen confers resistance to malaria. Duffy-negative blood is found only in descendants of African populations.
- Lewis — Antigens are soluble in blood rather than attached to the red blood cells. These are the only blood group antibodies that have never been implicated in hemolytic disease of the newborn.
- Other blood group systems — Colton, M, Kell, Kidd, Landsteiner-Wiener, P, Yt or Cartwright, XG, Scianna, Dombrock, Chido/Rodgers, Kx, Gerbich, Cromer, Knops, Indian, Ok, Raph, and JMH.

Other Blood Types

In addition to the A and B antigens that characterize the ABO blood grouping, more than 600 antigens and more than 20 other blood type systems are known. Many are named after the person or family in which the blood antigen system was discovered. Box 44.7 describes other blood systems.

Legal and Ethical Issues Related to Blood Transfusion

The Blood Safety Act was passed in 1991 to ensure that all donor blood is tested for the human immunodeficiency virus (HIV) and other bloodborne pathogens. The impact of this law can be seen in the ambulatory care environment. The law requires providers to explain to each elective surgery patient the chances that he or she may need a blood transfusion. The discussion must include positive and negative aspects of *autologous* (aw TOL uh guh s) *transfusion* (i.e., transfusion with a person's own blood). The pros and cons of transfusions from family, friends, or other donors should also be discussed. The conversation must be documented in the patient's health record. Before the surgery, the patient must sign a form giving consent to any needed blood transfusions. The medical assistant should be aware that certain populations (e.g., Jehovah's Witnesses) do not believe in blood transfusions.

If the patient decides to use autologous transfusions, this may require the patient to donate blood several weeks before the procedure. Usually autologous transfusions are performed for stable patients undergoing major orthopedic, vascular, cardiac, or thoracic surgery. The medical assistant might need to help make arrangements for the blood donation.

Another type of autologous transfusion can occur if the surgeon inserts an autologous drain in the surgical wound. The drain collects the blood from the surgical wound to prevent postoperative hematomas. The collected blood is then washed and reinfused into the patient.

BLOOD CHEMISTRY IN THE PHYSICIAN OFFICE LABORATORY

CLIA-waived chemistry tests using whole blood from capillary punctures have become popular in ambulatory practices. With the increase in diabetes and cardiovascular disease in the United States, both **metabolic** (met uh BOL ik) diseases benefit from early diagnosis. Treatment is based on continued monitoring of glucose and hemoglobin A1c for diabetes and of cholesterol, lipid panels, and liver enzymes for cardiovascular diseases related to fatty **plaque** in the arteries.

MEDICAL TERMINOLOGY

auto: self, own
log/o: study
-ous: pertaining to
orth/o: straight
ped/o: child, foot
vascul/o: vessel (blood)
thorac/o: chest
cardi/o: heart

VOCABULARY

metabolic: Relating to or resulting from metabolism (the chemical process in which cells produce the substances and energy needed to sustain life).
plaque: Any small abnormal patch on or within the body. A deposit of fatty material.

Blood Glucose Testing

Glucose is used as a fuel by all body cells. Under normal circumstances, it is the only substance used to nourish brain cells. Maintenance of blood glucose levels within a normal range is vital to homeostasis of the human body. Understanding the importance of glucose can help the medical assistant understand why glucose is the most frequently tested chemical analyte in the blood.

Elevated blood glucose levels are most often associated with diabetes mellitus. They also may indicate pancreatitis, endocrine disorders, or chronic renal failure. Diabetes mellitus is a disorder of carbohydrate metabolism that results in elevated blood and urine glucose levels. In diabetes mellitus, either the pancreas is unable to produce sufficient insulin to meet the body's needs, or insulin resistance develops at the cellular level (see Chapter 14).

For the initial screening of a patient for type 2 diabetes, a fasting blood sample is usually taken in the morning, after a fast of 10 to 12 hours. The patient's fasting blood glucose (FBG) level should be less than 100 mg/dL. If it is higher than 105 mg/dL, the provider may request a blood *glucose tolerance test* (GTT). For this test, the fasting patient receives a sugary liquid to drink that contains 100 g of glucose. (The amount may be adjusted according to the patient's weight.) A blood sugar level of less than 140 mg/dL after 2 hours is normal. A reading of more than 200 mg/dL after 2 hours may indicate diabetes. A reading between 140 and 199 mg/dL indicates impaired glucose tolerance, or prediabetes.

The medical assistant can screen a patient's blood glucose levels by using a glucometer cleared for home use by the FDA (Procedure 44.6). The blood glucose level is routinely monitored by patients with diabetes mellitus type 1 or type 2 (Box 44.8). Glucose levels may also be monitored by women with *gestational diabetes*, a condition seen during pregnancy in which the effect of insulin is partially blocked by hormones produced by the placenta (Fig. 44.12).

Hemoglobin A1c Testing

Hemoglobin A1c is also described as *glycosylated* (glahy KOH suh lay ted) *hemoglobin* (sugar-coated hemoglobin). Glycosylated hemoglobin is the result of glucose irreversibly binding to the hemoglobin molecules in the RBCs. It is also referred to as the A1c.

RBCs have a life span of approximately 120 days. Measuring the amount of glucose that has been irreversibly bound to hemoglobin provides an assessment of the average blood sugar during the 60 to 90 days before the test. The A1c test is performed every 3 months in patients with diabetes to monitor the person's average blood glucose level during those months. An A1c value higher than normal indicates that the average blood sugar has been elevated during the past 2 to 3 months. A normal A1c level for a person without diabetes ranges from 4% to 5.6%. For patients with diabetes, the goal is to maintain the glycosylated hemoglobin level below 7%. See Table 44.8, which associates glycosylated hemoglobin A1c levels with blood glucose levels. The goal for people with diabetes type 2 is to have A1c levels of 7% or lower. With higher levels, the risk of developing complications from diabetes increases.

Several methods can be used to measure the A1c level, and the medical assistant can perform A1c testing using several CLIA-waived

> **MEDICAL TERMINOLOGY**
> **glycos/o:** glucose, sugar

> **BOX 44.8   Blood Glucose Monitoring**
>
> Self-monitoring of blood glucose levels has become an important part of diabetes management. A very small amount of blood from a capillary puncture is drawn into a test strip in a glucose monitor. The test strip electronically calibrates the monitor and then tests the patient sample for blood glucose. These rapid-test glucose strips test the blood with the help of enzymes that convert glucose into a colored product that is measurable. The monitor detects and records the results and displays them on a small screen.

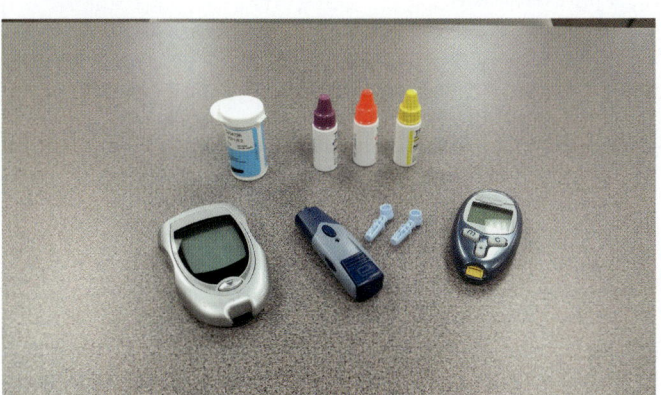

FIG. 44.12 Glucometer and supplies.

PROCEDURE 44.6   Assist the Provider with Patient Care: Perform a Blood Glucose TRUEresult Test

Task:
To perform a blood test for blood glucose accurately.

Equipment and Supplies
- Patient's record
- Provider's order and/or lab requisition.
- TRUEresult glucometer or similar glucose monitoring device
- TRUEtest strip
- Lancet and autoloading finger-puncturing device
- Alcohol wipes
- Gauze
- Fluid-impermeable lab coat, protective eyewear, and gloves.
- Biohazard waste container
- Biohazard sharps containers

Procedural Steps
1. Check the provider's order and collect the necessary equipment and supplies. Perform quality control measures according to the manufacturer's guidelines and office policy.
2. Wash hands or use hand sanitizer. Put on a fluid-impermeable lab coat, protective eyewear, and gloves.
   Purpose: To ensure infection control.
3. Greet the patient. Identify yourself. Verify the patient's identity with full name; ask the patient to spell first and the last name and to give his or her date of birth. Explain the procedure to be performed in a manner that is understood by the patient. Answer any questions the patient may have on the procedure. Obtain permission for the capillary puncture.

Continued

PROCEDURE 44.6 Assist the Provider with Patient Care: Perform a Blood Glucose TRUEresult Test—cont'd

Purpose: It is important to identify the patient in two different ways to ensure that you have the correct patient. Explaining the procedure can make the patient feel more comfortable and helps to reduce anxiety.

4. Ask the person to wash his or her hands in warm, soapy water, then rinse them in warm water, and finally dry them completely.
   Purpose: To clean the area that will be punctured; also, warming the fingers may increase peripheral blood flow.
5. Check the patient's middle and ring fingers and select the site for puncture (both forearm and fingertip testing can be done).
   Purpose: To make sure the site of puncture is free of trauma.
6. Turn on the TRUEresult glucometer by pressing the ON button (Fig. 1). No coding is necessary with this monitor; you do not have to match the code on the test strip vial with the code on the glucometer.

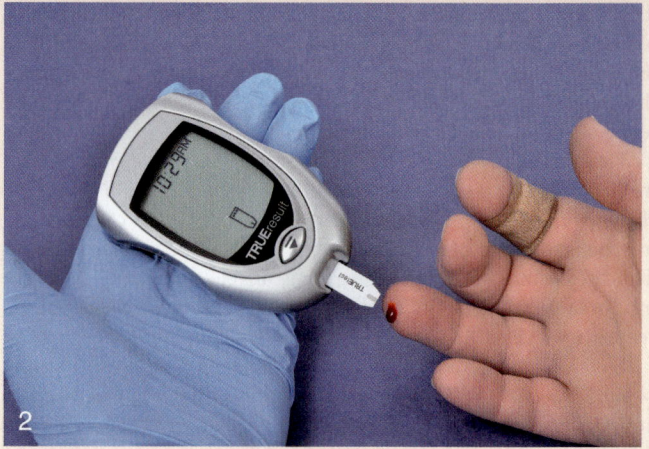

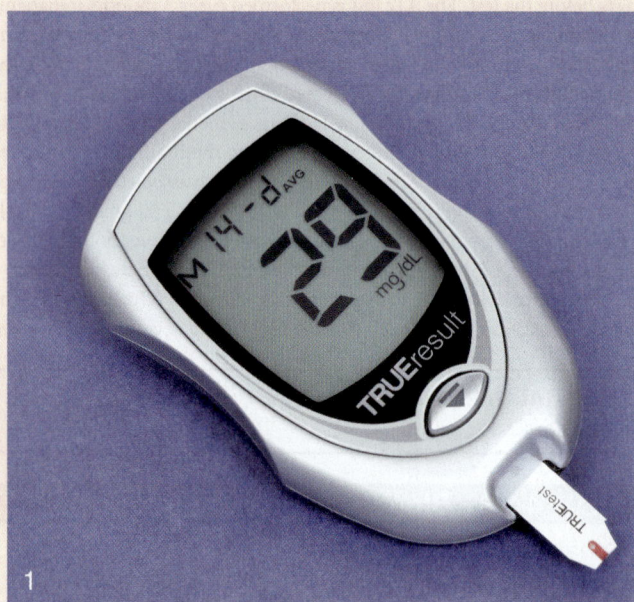

7. Check the expiration date on the test strip container. Take out a test strip and insert it into the glucometer.
8. Cleanse the selected site on the patient's fingertip with an alcohol wipe and allow the finger to air dry.
9. Perform the capillary puncture and wipe away the first drop of blood.
   Purpose: Tissue fluid may be present in the first drop of blood.
10. Apply a small blood sample (0.5 mL) to the end of the test strip (Fig. 2).
11. Give the patient gauze to hold securely over the puncture site; apply a hypoallergenic bandage or wrap if needed.
12. The glucometer automatically begins the measurement process, and results are obtained as soon as 4 seconds.
13. The test result is shown in the display window in milligrams per deciliter (mg/dL).
14. The patient can set up to four testing reminders on his or her personal glucometer; a ketone alarm signals when the blood glucose reading rises above a certain level.
15. The glucometer stores 30 daily average test results, up to 500 individual results, along with the date and time of each recording. Encourage patients to bring their personal glucometer to the clinic so the provider can review daily averages and previous test results.
16. The glucometer automatically turns off.
17. Discard all biohazardous waste in biohazard waste containers.
    Purpose: To ensure infection control.
18. Clean the glucometer according to the manufacturer's guidelines. Disinfect the work area. Remove your gloves and dispose of them properly. Remove protective eyewear and wash hands or use hand sanitizer
    Purpose: To ensure infection control.
19. Record the test results in the patient's health record.
    Purpose: A procedure is not done until the patient results are recorded.

Documentation Example
08/16/20XX 1:00 p.m.: Glucometer screening completed as ordered by Dr. Misha. NFBS 144. Pt took routine dose of 10 units Humalog insulin at noon. Pt had no questions._____Anita James, CMA (AAMA)

---

devices. The DCA A1cNOW+ for Professionals (Bayer Diagnostics) provides A1c values in 6 minutes from 1 drop of capillary blood obtained from a fingerstick. Patients also can perform A1c testing at home using FDA-approved instruments, such as the A1cNow SelfCheck (Bayer) and the in2it (II) Self-Test A1c System (Bio-Rad).

Cholesterol Testing

Cholesterol (kuh LES tuh rohl) is a fatlike substance (lipid) present in cell membranes. It is needed to form bile acids, steroid hormones, the coverings of our nerves, and some of our brain tissue. Cholesterol travels in the blood as distinct particles containing both lipid (LIP id) and proteins (PROH teen). These particles are called *lipoproteins* (lahy poh PROH teens). The cholesterol level in the blood is determined partly by inheritance and partly by acquired factors, such as diet, calorie and nutrient balance, and level of physical activity.

Patients often are confused by cholesterol testing. Cholesterol is often a catchall term for both the cholesterol a person eats and the cholesterol that is produced in the body. A high blood level of low-density lipoprotein, or LDL, cholesterol reflects an increased risk of heart disease. LDL cholesterol is often referred to as "bad" cholesterol. Lower levels of LDL cholesterol reflect a lower risk of heart disease. When too much LDL cholesterol circulates in the blood, it can slowly build up in the walls of arteries that feed the heart and brain. Together with other substances, it can form *plaque*, a thick and sticky deposit that can clog

TABLE 44.8 Relationship Between Glycosylated Hemoglobin Levels and Blood Glucose Levels

Glycosylated Hemoglobin A1c (%)	Blood Glucose (mg/dL)
14.0	380
13.0	350
12.0	315
11.0	280
10.0	250
9.0	215
8.0	180
7.0	150
6.0	115
5.0	80
4.0	50

From Proctor D, et al: *Kinn's The Medical Assistant,* ed 13, St Louis, 2017, Elsevier.

arteries. This condition is known as *atherosclerosis* (ath uh roh skluh ROH sis). If a clot (thrombus) forms at the site of plaque, blood flow can be blocked in the coronary arteries of the heart muscle, causing a heart attack. If a clot blocks blood flow to part of the brain, a stroke may result. LDL results are often interpreted as follows:

- LDL <100 mg/dL = Optimal
- LDL 100–129 = Near or above optimal
- LDL 130–159 = Borderline high
- LDL 160–189 = High
- LDL 190+ = Very high

About one-third to one-fourth of blood cholesterol is carried by high-density lipoprotein (HDL). HDL cholesterol is known as the "good" cholesterol. High levels of HDL cholesterol seem to protect against heart attack. HDL can carry cholesterol away from the arteries and back to the liver. It is believed that cholesterol is removed from the lining of the arteries when high levels of HDL exist. Low levels of HDL cholesterol (i.e., lower than 40 mg/dL) may result in a greater risk of heart disease.

CRITICAL THINKING 44.6

One of Anita's favorite patients is in today, Sophie McCoy. She is 86 years young, still lives in her own home, and works in her garden every chance she gets. Sophie had a cholesterol screen at a local senior citizens health fair recently, and her results were as follows:

Total cholesterol 202 mg/dL, LDL 104 mg/dL, HDL 42 mg/dL

Given Sophie's age and general good health, are the cholesterol results concerning? Are they normal, high, or low?

Adults older than 20 years of age should have a cholesterol test at least once every 5 years. Total cholesterol and the combination of LDL and HDL typically are screened and monitored (Procedure 44.7). All three tests are considered screening tests, and elevated results require additional testing. In general, total cholesterol levels under 200 mg/dL are considered normal. Results over 240 mg/dL are considered elevated and may place a person in the high-risk category for coronary heart disease. An HDL cholesterol level of 40 mg/dL or higher is considered acceptable for men, and values of 50 or higher are acceptable for women. HDL levels below 40 mg/dL for men and below 50 mg/dL for women place a person at risk of coronary heart disease.

Although total cholesterol and HDL cholesterol levels are not significantly affected by food consumption, most providers prefer that patients fast from food and liquids, with the exception of water, for 12 hours before cholesterol levels are checked. If the total cholesterol is elevated, the provider is likely to order a *lipid profile,* which is a series of tests that measures the total cholesterol, HDL and LDL cholesterol levels, and *triglyceride* (trahy GLIS uh rahyd) levels. Triglycerides are fat in the blood related to caloric intake. Therefore, the patient must be instructed to fast from all food and alcoholic beverages 12 hours before the triglyceride test and/or lipid profiles. Consistently high triglyceride levels may lead to heart disease, especially in people with low levels of "good" HDL cholesterol and high levels of "bad" LDL cholesterol, and in people with type 2 diabetes. Elevated levels of triglycerides are typically stored in the belly and are associated with central obesity.

CLIA-waived cholesterol monitors can measure total cholesterol from a fingerstick specimen. The Cholestech LDX analyzer performs a lipid panel and provides a risk assessment using a capillary blood sample (see Procedure 44.7). This system uses a cassette testing device capable of measuring glucose, total cholesterol (TC), HDL, LDL, very-low-density lipoprotein (VLDL), triglycerides, and the TC/HDL ratio. It uses a combination of testing methods to detect the color changes caused by each of the lipid panel analytes.

Alanine Aminotransferase (ALT) and Aspartate Aminotransferase (AST) Testing

Certain drugs can impair liver function and require the monitoring of two liver enzymes:

- alanine aminotransferase (AL uh neen uh mee noh TRANS fuh reys)
- aspartate aminotransferase (uh SPAHR teyt uh mee noh TRANS fuh reys)

These two liver enzymes will rise in the blood during liver damage. Drugs that cause liver damage include:

- statins (STAT n s), which are used to lower blood cholesterol
- fibrates (fahy BREYT s), a specific type of antidiabetic and antihypertensive drug

The provider will order liver function tests or panels to monitor the liver during therapy with drugs that have the potential to cause liver malfunction.

CLIA-waived liver enzyme testing for ALT and AST may be monitored on the same Cholestech LDX System using ALT/AST test cassettes.

Thyroid Hormone Testing

The thyroid gland is located anterior to the trachea in the throat. It produces the hormones triiodothyronine (trahy ahy oh doh THAHY ruh neen), or T_3, and thyroxine (thahy ROK seen), or T_4. These hormones are essential for life and regulate body metabolism, growth, and development. The thyroid gland is influenced by hormones produced by two other glands found in the brain, the pituitary (pi TOO I ter ee) gland and the hypothalamus (hahy puh THAL uh muh s). The pituitary gland produces thyroid-stimulating hormone (TSH), and the hypothalamus produces thyrotropin (thahy ruh TROH pin)-releasing hormone (TRH). (Regulation of thyroid hormone production and thyroid disorders are discussed in Chapter 14.)

CLIA-waived rapid diagnostic tests are available to qualitatively (KWOL I tey tiv lee) measure TSH. These tests are available for

PROCEDURE 44.7 Perform a CLIA-Waived Chemistry Test: Determine the Cholesterol Level or Lipid Profile Using a Cholestech Analyzer

Task:
To perform a Cholestech test for total cholesterol level and/or a lipid panel and accurately report the results.

Directions:
Perform a total blood cholesterol level or lipid panel on Connie Lange STAT.

Equipment and Supplies
- Patient's health record
- Provider's order and/or lab requisition
- Cholestech analyzer
- Package insert or flow chart with directions
- Optics check cassette
- Test cassettes (provided by Cholestech)
- Levels 1 and 2 liquid controls
- Capillary tubes and plungers for fingerstick sample (provided by Cholestech)
- Mini-Pet pipet and pipet tips for venipuncture sample (provided by Cholestech)
- Lancet, gauze, alcohol wipes, bandage for capillary blood, *or* lithium heparin (green-topped) tube for venous blood
- Safety tube decapper (if tubes do not have a Hemogard plastic top)
- Fluid-impermeable lab coat, protective eyewear, and gloves
- Biohazard waste container
- Biohazard sharps containers

Procedural Steps

1. Wash hands or use hand sanitizer. Put on a fluid-impermeable lab coat, protective eyewear, and gloves.
   Purpose: To ensure infection control.
2. Assemble the materials needed.
3. Perform quantitative quality control by performing a calibration check with the optics check cassette (Fig. 1). Then test level 1 and level 2 liquid controls if using a new set of cassettes.
   Purpose: To ensure instrument is reading results accurately, precisely, and reliably.

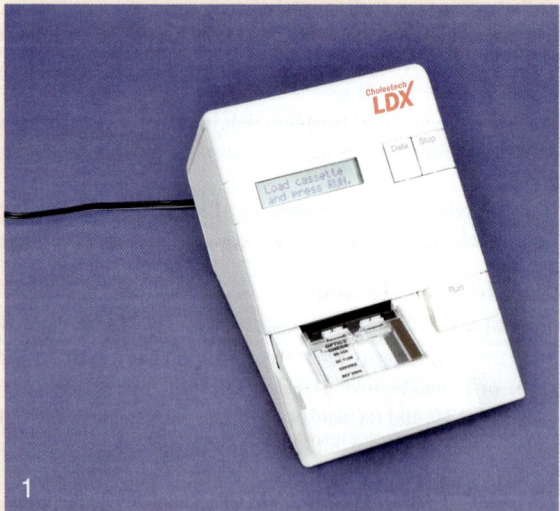

4. Allow refrigerated testing cassettes to come to room temperature (at least 10 minutes before opening).
   Purpose: Test is temperature and time sensitive when reading results.
5. Remove cassette from its pouch and place on flat surface without touching the black bar or magnetic strip.
   Purpose: The black bar is the testing area, and the magnetic strip must be read by the analyzer. Touching either may interfere with test results
6. Press RUN on the analyzer, allowing it to do a self-test; this will be followed by OK on the screen, and then the test drawer will open. The drawer will stay open for 4 minutes while the specimen is prepared.
7. Perform a fingerstick and collect the capillary blood to the black line of the Cholestech capillary tube with its plunger inserted into the red end of the tube. *Or* collect the fresh venous whole blood with the Cholestech Mini-Pet pipet.
   Purpose: Both collecting devices are provided by Cholestech to ensure that the exact volume of blood necessary is tested.
8. Place the whole blood sample into the well of the cassette. **NOTE:** The capillary specimen must be in the cassette within 5 minutes of collection (Fig. 2).
   Purpose: Fingerstick blood will clot if not tested within 5 minutes.

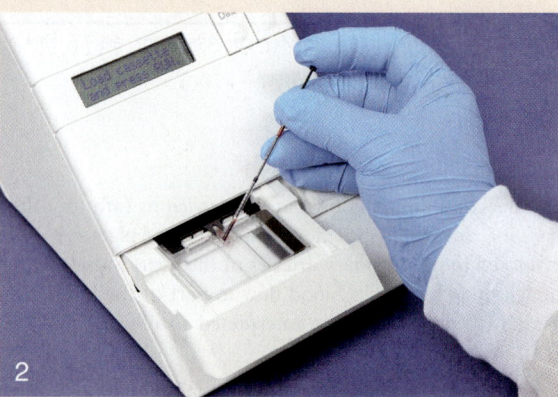

9. Immediately put the cassette into the drawer of the analyzer and press RUN. (**NOTE:** If the drawer has closed, press RUN again to open the drawer; load the specimen into the drawer and then press RUN to close the drawer.)
   Purpose: This is a test with a color reaction that continues to change over time.
10. When the test is complete, the analyzer beeps. The screen displays and then prints out the results (Fig. 3).

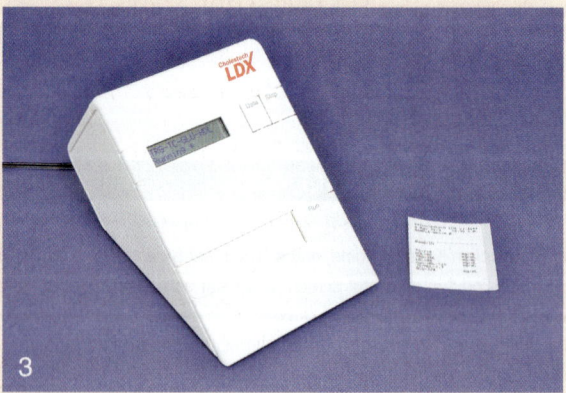

11. Record the findings in the laboratory log and in the patient's paper health record if they have not been transmitted electronically.
    Purpose: A procedure is considered not done until it is recorded.
12. Circle the results that do not fall within the Desirable Ranges column of the following table. Identify "critical values" and take appropriate steps to notify the provider.
    Purpose: The provider needs to know the results while the patient is still in the office, for proper follow-up with the patient.

CHAPTER 44 Assisting in the Analysis of Blood

PROCEDURE 44.7   Perform a CLIA-Waived Chemistry Test: Determine the Cholesterol Level or Lipid Profile Using a Cholestech Analyzer—cont'd

13. Dispose of all sharps in the biohazard sharps container (i.e., lancet and capillary pipet with plunger). Place all regulated medical waste into the biohazard waste container (i.e., gauze, alcohol wipes, and cassettes). Disinfect test area, remove PPE, and dispose of gloves in biohazard waste container. Wash hands or use hand sanitizer.
    Purpose: To ensure infection control.

CHOLESTECH LDX PATIENT/CONTROL LOG

Cassette Lot #: _____   Expiration Date: _____   LDX Serial #: _____

DATE	TECH	PT ID	TC	HDL	LDL	TRG	TC/HDL	GLU	CHARTED
10/09/20–	DC	#12345	190	50	120	135	4.3	80	✓

Documentation Example
Attach printed readout, or record results in the electronic chart:

Test	Results	Desirable
Total cholesterol (TC)	190	<200 mg/dL
HDL cholesterol	50	>40 mg/dL
LDL cholesterol	120	<130 mg/dL
Triglycerides	135	<150 mg/dL
TC/HDL ratio	4.3	≤4.5
Other		
Glucose	80	Fasting: 60–110 mg/dL
		Nonfasting: <160 mg/dL

NOTE: Laboratory reports and manufacturers must supply their own reference ranges, along with each patient's results. This is because different methodologies may create different reference ranges and different units of measurement.

---

point-of-care (POC) testing. Using whole blood from a fingerstick, CLIA-waived tests can screen patients for **hypothyroidism** (hahy puh THAHY roi diz uh m). Hypothyroidism is indicated with elevated TSH levels. The tests use **lateral flow immunoassay** technology housed in a plastic cassette. One such commercially available test is the ThyroTest Whole Blood TSH Test.

REFERENCE LABORATORY CHEMISTRY PANELS AND SINGLE ANALYTE TESTING AND MONITORING

Automated blood chemistry analyzers are often used to perform blood chemistry testing in a reference laboratory. It is common for several analytes to be detected at once. A provider may order a chemistry panel, such as a renal or liver panel, to determine the levels of several related analytes (Fig. 44.13). Analytes commonly detected in the chemistry department are listed in Table 44.9. In general, serum from a clotted specimen is needed to perform these tests. Typical panels are shown in Table 44.10. As noted previously, laboratory reports, both electronic and paper, must provide their own reference ranges, along with each patient's results. Different methodologies may generate different reference ranges and may use different units of measurement.

VOCABULARY

antibody: A protein produced in the blood or tissues in response to a specific antigen that destroys or weakens the antigen. Part of the immune system.
antigen: A substance that stimulates the production of an antibody when introduced into the body. Antigens include toxins, bacteria, viruses, and other foreign substances.
hypothyroidism: Deficient activity of the thyroid gland.
lateral flow immunoassay: A laboratory or clinical technique that uses the specific binding between an **antigen** and an **antibody** to identify and quantify a substance in a sample. The sample in this technique moves in a sideways motion, usually on an absorbent paper.

Physician's Medical Center
77332 E. Capital Drive
Anytown, USA 11123

Ronald J. Haldor, M.D.
Kaye M. Jones, M.D.
Nicholas P. Stepp, M.D.

PATIENT – PLEASE NOTE

☐

If this box is checked, don't eat or drink anything, except water, for 14 hours before going to the lab.

PATIENT NAME _____
                LAST   FIRST   M.I.
ADDRESS _____ DOB _____
CITY _____ STATE _____ ZIP _____ SEX: M F
TELEPHONE # _____ SOCIAL SECURITY # ___ – ___ – ___
ORDERING PHYSICIAN _____ DATE _____
BILLING: ☐ HMO ☐ MEDICARE ☐ MEDICAL ☐ OTHER # _____
    GUARANTOR (If other than patient) _____
  ☐ PHONE RESULTS TO _____
  ☐ SEND ADDITIONAL COPIES OF REPORT TO _____
        (Please attach copy of eligibilty card.)

Patient Diagnosis _____

☐ 906 ARTERIAL BLOOD GASES
       ROOM AIR _____
       RESP. ASSIST _____
☐ 105 BLOOD CELL PROFILE (Hgb + Hct)
☐ 862 BILIRUBIN (NEONATAL)
☐ 868 BILIRUBIN (TOTAL & DIRECT)
☐ 100 CBC (Complete Blood Count & Diff)
☐ 3000 ELECTROLYTES
☐   (NA, K, CO2, Cl)
☐   FANA
☐   GLUCOSE
☐ 915 GLUCOSE, PRE-NATAL DIABETIC SCR.
       (1 Hour Post-Glucola)
☐   GLUCOSE TOLERANCE TEST
       # OF HOURS _____ DOSE _____
☐ 3398 HEPATITIS PANEL
       (B-Surf Ag/Ab, B-Core Ab, A-Ab)
☐ 988 LIPID PROFILE
       (Chol, Trig, HDL, LDL, Cardiac Risk)
☐ 3380 LIVER PANEL
       (Alk Phos, Bili, TP, Alb, GGT, SGOT
       (AST) SGPT (ALT), & Consult)
☐ 3006 METABOLIC 7
       (Na, K, CO2, Cl, Glu, Mg)

☐ 3035 PANEL 17
       (Panel 13 + Na + K + Cl + CO2)
☐ 3020 METABOLIC 10
       (Na, K, CO2, Cl, Glu, BUN, Creat)
☐ 3015 METABOLIC 11
       (Met 10 & Phos)
☐ 3160 OBSTETRICAL PANEL 1
       (CBC, UA, ABO/Rh, Antibody
       Screen, Rubella, RPR)
☐ 3172 OBSTETRICAL PANEL 3
       (CBC, ABO/Rh, Antibody Screen,
       Rubella, RPR)
☐ 3445 OBSTETRICAL PANEL 7
       (ABO/Rh, Antibody Screen,
       Rubella, RPR)
☐ 3447 OBSTETRICAL PANEL 7A
       (ABO/Rh, Antibody Screen,
       Rubella, RPR, Hepatitis B Surt Ag)
☐ 3025 PANEL 13
       (Glu, BUN, Creat, Uric Acid, Ca,
       Tp, Alb, Bili, Chol, Alk, Phos,
       SGOT (AST), LDH, Phos)
☐ 3030 PANEL 15
       (Panel 13 + Na + K)

☐ 3010 METABOLIC 8
       (Na, K, CO2, Cl, Glu, BUN)
☐ 3040 PANEL 20 - SMAC
       (Panel 17 + SGPT (ALT) +
       GGT + Osmolality)
☐ 3043 S-1 Panel (Panel 20 + Triglyceride)
☐ 500 PROTHROMBIN TIME (PT)
☐ 505 Partial Thromboplastin Time (PPT)
☐ 7500 RPR
☐ 7515 RUBELLA
☐ 2030 THYROID SCREEN
       (T4, T3, Uptake, Adj T4)
☐ 704 URINALYSIS

BACTERIOLOGY

SPECIMEN SOURCE (REQUIRED) _____
COLLECTION DATE _____
☐ _____ ROUTINE CULTURE
☐ 8919 AFB CULTURE
☐ 8921 FUNGAL CULTURE

ADDITIONAL LABORATORY TESTS: _____
_____
_____
_____

2804 (4/93)

LABORATORY OUTPATIENT REQUEST

OFFICE USE ONLY

Telephone Order per _____
Order Received by _____

FIG. 44.13 Panel request form. (From Proctor D, et al: *Kinn's The Medical Assistant*, ed 13, St Louis, 2017, Elsevier.)

TABLE 44.9 Blood Chemistry Tests[a]

Test	Abbreviation	Normal Values	Description	Purpose
Alanine aminotransferase	ALT (SGPT)	<45 units/L	Enzyme found predominantly in the liver but also in the kidney	To detect liver disease
Albumin		3.5–5 g/dL	Protein	To assess kidney function
Alkaline phosphatase	ALP	20–70 units/L	Enzyme found in several tissues	To detect liver and bone disease
Aspartate aminotransferase	AST (SGOT)	<40 units/L	Enzyme found in several tissues	To detect tissue damage
Blood urea nitrogen	BUN	7–18 mg/dL or 2.5–6.4 mmol/L	Metabolic products of protein catabolism	To detect renal disease
Calcium	Ca	8.4–10.2 mg/dL or 2.1–2.6 mmol/L	Mineral	To assess parathyroid function and calcium metabolism
Chloride	Cl	98–106 mmol/L	Electrolyte	To determine acid-base and water balance
Cholesterol	CH, Chol	Total: <200 mg/dL or <5.18 mmol/L LDL: <130 mg/dL or <3.37 mmol/L HDL: >35 mg/dL or >0.91 mmol/L	Lipid	To screen for atherosclerosis related to heart disease
Creatine phosphokinase	CPK	Specific to testing method used	Enzyme found in several tissues	To assess source of muscle damage (myocardial infarct)
Creatinine	creat	0.2–0.8 mg/dL	Metabolic product of protein catabolism	To screen for renal function
Ferritin		20–50 ng/mL	Iron-carrying protein	To detect amount of iron stored in the body
Gamma glutamyl transferase	GGT	0–45 units/L	Enzyme found mainly in liver cells	To detect liver disease
Globulin	glob, Ig	Varies according to type	Protein	To detect abnormalities in protein synthesis and removal
Glucose fasting blood sugar	FBS	70–100 mg/dL or 3.9–6.1 mmol/L	Carbohydrate	To detect disorders of glucose metabolism (diabetes)
Glucose tolerance test	GTT	Varies with time	Carbohydrate	To detect disorders of glucose metabolism (diabetes)
Iron	Fe	35–140 mcg/dL	Mineral	To assist in diagnosis of anemia
Lactate dehydrogenase	LDH	<240 units/L	Enzyme found in several tissues	To assist in confirmation of myocardial or pulmonary infarct
pH	pH	7.35–7.45	Measurement of the acid-base (acidity and alkalinity)	To assess acidity or alkalinity of blood
Phosphorus	P	3–4.5 mg/dL or 0.97–1.45 mmol/L	Mineral	To assist in proper evaluation of calcium levels and to detect endocrine system disorders
Potassium	K	3.5–5.1 mmol/L	Mineral	To assist in diagnosis of acid-base and water balance
Sodium	Na	135–146 mmol/L	Mineral	To assist in diagnosis of acid-base and water balance
Total bilirubin	TB	0.2–1 mg/dL or 3.4–17.1 mmol/L	Metabolic product of hemoglobin catabolism	To evaluate liver function and to aid in diagnosis of anemia
Total iron-binding capacity	TIBC	245–400 mcg/dL		A measure of the potential to transport iron
Total protein	TP	6–8 g/dL; 60–80 g/L	Protein	To assess the state of hydration; to screen for diseases that alter protein balance
Troponin I and T		<0.4	Cardiac-specific protein found only with heart muscle damage	To aid in diagnosis of myocardial infarct
Thyroid-stimulating hormone (thyrotropin)	TSH	5–6 milliunits/L	Hormone produced by the pituitary	To assess thyroid and pituitary gland function
Thyroxine	T4	5–12 mcg/dL or 64–155 mmol/L	Hormone produced by the thyroid gland	To assess thyroid function
Triglycerides	Trig	30–190 mg/dL or 0.34–2.15 mmol/L		To screen for atherosclerosis related to heart disease
Triiodothyronine	T3	27%–47%	Hormone produced by the thyroid gland	To assess thyroid function
Uric acid	UA	Male: 3.4–7 mg/dL or 202–416 mcmol/L Female: 2.4–6 mg/dL or 143–357 mcmol/L	Metabolic product of protein catabolism	To evaluate renal failure, gout, and leukemia

[a]Lab reports, both electronic and paper, must supply their own reference ranges, along with each patient's results. This is because different methodologies may create different reference ranges and different units of measurement.

From Proctor D, et al: *Kinn's The Medical Assistant*, ed 13, St Louis, 2017, Elsevier.

TABLE 44.10 Typical Chemistry Panels

Panel	Component	Panel	Component
Liver	Alkaline phosphatase (ALP) Gamma glutamyl transferase (GGT) Aspartate aminotransferase (AST) Alanine aminotransferase (ALT) Lactate dehydrogenase (LDH)	Cardiac	Creatine phosphokinase (CPK) Troponin I Troponin T
Anemia	Iron Total iron-binding capacity Ferritin Transferrin	Electrolyte	Sodium Potassium Chloride
Thyroid	Thyroid-stimulating hormone (TSH) Thyroxine (T_4) Triiodothyronine (T_3)	Renal	Creatinine Blood urea nitrogen (BUN) Uric acid Glucose

From Proctor D, et al: *Kinn's The Medical Assistant,* ed 13, St Louis, 2017, Elsevier.

CLOSING COMMENTS

An ever-increasing number of CLIA-waived hematology and chemistry blood tests are relatively simple to perform and require minimal training. This has allowed the provider to share the results with the patient immediately. This results in greater patient compliance with the prescribed treatment plan. Proper patient care demands attention to detail in all three areas of the testing process:

- *Preanalytic:* Proper care of the testing supplies and equipment, and proper patient identification and specimen collection
- *Analytic:* Running the tests according to the specific manufacturer's instructions; recording and analyzing the controls and the test results
- *Postanalytic:* Proper disposal of biohazardous supplies; routing of test results to the provider and patient

The medical assistant is involved in all of these elements. He or she is responsible for the organization and documentation of each test performed on the appropriate lab flow sheet and in the patient's health record.

EXCEPTIONAL CUSTOMER SERVICE

As with all laboratory procedures, the test is only as good as the specimen! The medical assistant, as the provider's agent, is responsible for the authenticity of the sample when you instruct your patient regarding collection. You are also responsible for the patient results when you perform the test.

A medical assistant who is responsible for office laboratory testing must clearly understand the basic concepts of laboratory medicine. Therefore, you must stay current with the rapid technological advances in laboratory medicine and help establish testing protocols best suited to your provider-employer.

You are responsible for properly collecting specimens and testing them accurately. Patient confidentiality is paramount when testing is performed, as is following all the established quality control procedures.

Excellent customer service comes from dedicated, detail-oriented healthcare workers!

CHAPTER REVIEW

In this chapter, we covered areas in the laboratory where a medical assistant can perform waived testing. We also went over the medical assistant's role in reviewing patients' results and maintaining proper documentation for all laboratory results.

We started out looking at the hematology department and the testing done in that area of the laboratory. We had a short review of the components that make up the blood. Red blood cells, white blood cells, and platelets all have unique reference ranges that may change over a person's life span. We reviewed the composition of plasma and the importance of the liquid portion of blood to homeostasis. Waived hematology testing performed in a POL consists of four tests: hematocrit, hemoglobin, erythrocyte sedimentation rate, and the prothrombin time, which is a coagulation test.

Hematology in the reference laboratory consists of mostly moderate-complexity tests, which include a complete blood count. A CBC has a number of individual tests included in this automated analysis. A CBC can include the following tests: RBC count, WBC count, platelet count, hemoglobin, and hematocrit. Other important values are the RBC indices, which are calculations based on the RBC analytes. The RBC indices include the mean cell volume (MCV), the mean cell hemoglobin (MCH), and the mean cell ratio of hemoglobin and hematocrit (MCHC). These calculated indices help the provider to determine the possible type of anemia present and possible mode of treatment.

Hematology white blood cell counts can indicate a variety of disease states, such as infection, leukemia, lymphoma, or viral infections. Abnormal platelet counts that are too low may cause easy bruising and bleeding and can be life-threatening.

We also discussed the differential test. In this test, we take a drop of blood and spread it out thinly on a glass microscope slide, allow it to air dry, and then stain it with a specific stain. The stained slide is then examined under the microscope to look at the cells of the blood. Their shape, size, content, and overall appearance are noted. This useful information should agree with the automated analysis of the blood and will also give the provider additional clues to the person's health.

Discussing immunohematology is important. Blood typing and cross-matching blood for transfusion is precise work. Although type and cross-match testing is not waived testing, the medical assistant may be involved in collecting the specimen and documenting the test results in the patient's electronic medical record. ABO and Rh typing are the most common antigen systems in blood typing, but other blood systems do exist, and the terms should be easily recognized by a medical assistant.

The last department of the laboratory discussed was the chemistry department. There are many waived tests that can be performed in chemistry. They include blood glucose testing, hemoglobin A1c testing, cholesterol and lipid testing, alanine aminotransferase (ALT) and aspartate aminotransferase (AST) testing (i.e., liver enzyme testing), and thyroid hormone testing. Handheld chemistry monitors can do a variety of tests, and they have the added benefit of being quick and accurate. Patient samples can be tested in the provider's office, and results can be discussed in a timely manner. This may lead to better patient compliance.

We wrapped up the chemistry department by discussing some of the testing done in the reference laboratory. Chemistry profiles or panels are groups of analytes that are common to a particular organ or body system. Examples of chemistry profiles include a cardiac profile, liver profile, thyroid profile, and electrolyte panel. Most profile or panel testing makes use of complex automated equipment and is generally not CLIA-waived testing. However, individual analytes may be available in a waived kit or monitor.

We closed the chapter remembering our patients and our responsibility to work diligently in all areas as a medical assistant. Proper patient care requires attention to detail in all three areas of the testing process: preanalytic, analytic, and postanalytic. From greeting a new patient to recording results and documenting laboratory results, the medical assistant must always remain detail oriented and patient focused.

SCENARIO WRAP-UP

It has been another busy day for Anita at WMFM Clinic. She had a chance to see a variety of patients with a variety of concerns. It was a normal day at work! Anita enjoys the variety. She also enjoys the work she does with the laboratory. Anita prepares specimens for transport to the reference lab. She checks on results once they are posted in patients' electronic medical records. She knows that Dr. Perez and all the providers at WMFM Clinic rely on lab results as part of patient diagnosis and monitoring treatment.

Another good day at work. Now Anita is going to go home and try to get a little gardening done!

45

Assisting in Microbiology and Immunology

LEARNING OBJECTIVES

1. Discuss the classification of microorganisms, including how to name them.
2. Describe various characteristics of bacteria, including their staining properties, shapes, oxygen requirements, and physical structures. Also, explain the characteristics of common diseases caused by bacteria.
3. Describe the unusual characteristics of chlamydia, mycoplasma, and rickettsia organisms.
4. Identify the characteristics of common diseases caused by fungi, protozoa, parasites, and pathogenic helminths (worms). Also, instruct patients how to collect fecal specimens to be tested for ova and parasites.
5. Describe the characteristics of common viral diseases.
6. Discuss specimen collection and transport in the physician office laboratory. Also, explain how pinworm testing is done and when it is recommended.
7. Describe three microbiology CLIA-waived tests that use a rapid identification technique. Also, collect a specimen for a throat culture and perform a rapid strep test.
8. Complete the following related to CLIA-waived immunology testing:
   - Discuss the purpose of indirect immunology testing.
   - Describe four CLIA-waived immunology tests that can be done in the physician office laboratory.
   - Perform the QuickVue+ Infectious Mononucleosis Test.
9. Discuss the identification of pathogens in the microbiology reference laboratory, describe the staining process, and describe the reference laboratory assessment of a throat culture and a urine culture.

CHAPTER OUTLINE

1. Opening Scenario, 1105
2. You Will Learn, 1105
3. Introduction, 1105
4. Classification of Microorganisms, 1106
   a. Naming Microorganisms, 1106
5. Characteristics of Bacteria, 1107
   a. Bacterial Staining Properties, 1107
   b. Bacterial Shapes, 1107
   c. Bacterial Oxygen Requirements, 1108
   d. Bacterial Physical Structures, 1108
6. Unusual Pathogenic Bacteria: Chlamydia, Mycoplasma, and Rickettsia, 1108
7. Pathogenic Fungi, 1109
8. Pathogenic Protozoa, 1110
9. Pathogenic Parasites, 1110
10. Pathogenic Helminths (Worms), 1111
11. Pathogenic Viruses, 1111
12. Specimen Collection and Transport in the Physician Office Laboratory, 1111
    a. Collection of Pinworms, 1114
13. CLIA-Waived Microbiology Testing, 1116
    a. Rapid Strep Testing, 1116
    b. Influenza A and B Testing, 1116
    c. Respiratory Syncytial Virus Testing, 1116
14. CLIA-Waived Immunology Testing, 1119
    a. Infectious Mononucleosis Testing, 1119
    b. *Helicobacter pylori* Testing, 1121
    c. Lyme Disease Testing, 1121
    d. HIV Testing, 1121
15. Microbiology Reference Laboratory: Identification of Pathogens, 1122
    a. Staining, 1122
       i. *Gram Stain*, 1122
       ii. *Acid-Fast Stain*, 1122
    b. Inoculating Equipment, 1122
    c. Assessing a Culture, 1123
       i. *Throat Cultures*, 1123
       ii. *Urine Cultures*, 1124
    d. Microbiology Culture and Sensitivity Testing, 1124
16. Closing Comments, 1124
17. Chapter Review, 1125
18. Scenario Wrap-Up, 1125

CHAPTER 45 Assisting in Microbiology and Immunology

OPENING SCENARIO

Laura Piper, CMA (AAMA), has worked at Walden-Martin Family Medical (WMFM) Clinic for 6 years. She has seen many infectious diseases diagnosed over that time. Bacterial and viral infections are common, but Laura also knows that not all microorganisms are bad. Some diseases have been controlled using vaccines. Other infections can be treated with antibiotics. Not all infectious diseases can be treated with antibiotics, and improper use of antibiotics can lead to bacteria that are resistant to these very useful drugs. Laura knows that it is important to identify pathogens quickly so that proper treatment can begin. The identification of pathogens can involve various types of tests, many of which can be performed in the physician office laboratory (POL) where she works.

YOU WILL LEARN

1. To describe various bacterial shapes, oxygen requirements, and physical structures.
2. To describe the unusual characteristics of *Chlamydia*, *Mycoplasma*, and *Rickettsia* organisms.
3. To describe the characteristics of common viral diseases.
4. To describe the common methods for the collection, transport, and processing of microbiology and immunology specimens.
5. To describe three CLIA-waived microbiology tests that use a rapid identification technique.
6. To discuss the purpose of indirect immunology testing.
7. To describe three CLIA-waived immunology tests that could be done in the physician office laboratory.
8. To discuss the importance of the Gram stain and acid-fast stains in microbiology.
9. To describe the reference laboratory assessment of a throat culture and a urine culture.

INTRODUCTION

Infectious diseases caused by microorganisms (mahy kroh AWR guh niz uhms) and infectious agents have gotten a lot of publicity. We have heard news stories about Ebola (ee BOH luh), influenza, Zika (ZEE kuh), norovirus (NAWR oh vahy ruhs), antibiotic-resistant superbugs, and more. With news of food-borne illnesses, contaminated water supplies, tick-borne diseases, and communicable infections, it appears all microorganisms are harmful and can cause disease. Healthcare-associated infections (HAIs), such as methicillin (meth uh SIL in)-resistant Staphylococcus aureus (staf uh luh KOK uhs AWR ee uhs) (MRSA) and *Clostridium difficile* (klo STRID ee uhm dif i SEEL) (C. diff) infections, are becoming increasingly difficult to control. New strains of drug-resistant microorganisms are difficult to treat with existing antibiotics (an tee bahy ot iks). Bioterrorism has become a real concern worldwide. Antimicrobial (an tee mahy KROH bee uhl) products line the pharmacy and supermarket shelves and are going to keep us "germ free." It is no wonder many people have the impression that all microorganisms are harmful. In reality, less than 1% of known microorganisms are pathogens (PATH uh juhns).

Most microorganisms are good. Without microorganisms, we could not survive (Box 45.1). The normal flora (NAWR muhl FLAWR uh) in and on our bodies is needed for the following processes:
- Digesting food and making nutrients available to the body.
- Forming blood clots. Vitamin K is used in the clotting process and is made by bacteria (bak TEER ee uh) in our intestines.

BOX 45.1 Saprophytes

Beneficial microorganisms that are responsible for breaking down organic matter are called *saprophytes*. They help break down plants and organic waste in farming, water purification, composting, and gardening.

- Preventing pathogens from invading our skin, mucous membranes, and gastrointestinal and genitourinary tracts.

Normal flora take up space, require nutrients, and excrete waste. When pathogens try to populate the skin or areas of the body that have normal flora, they must compete with the existing organisms. This makes it harder for pathogens to cause disease. Normal flora discourages pathogen populations.

When the body's normal flora is weakened (e.g., by antibiotic overuse or hormonal changes), certain *opportunistic organisms* that are normally present in low numbers can overgrow. An example is *Candida albicans* (KAN di duh AHL bi kanz), which is a yeast (yeest) that is normally found in mucous membranes in the body. When a patient has been on broad-spectrum antibiotics for an infection, the antibiotics kill pathogens, along with some of the normal flora. If the patient is a woman and enough normal flora in the vagina is killed off, *Candida albicans* can increase in numbers, which causes a vaginal yeast infection. *Candida albicans* is not normally a problem, but given the opportunity, it can cause disease.

VOCABULARY

antibiotic: A substance or medication that can destroy or inhibit the growth of bacteria.

antimicrobial: A general term used to describe drugs, chemicals, or other substances that can destroy or inhibit the growth of microorganisms. Can be antibiotics or antiviral, antifungal, and antiparasitic drugs or agents (e.g., there are chemical antimicrobial additives in hand soap).

bacteria: Some of a large group of microorganisms that are single-celled, lack a nucleus, reproduce asexually, or can form spores. Some can cause disease. The most abundant life form on earth.

broad-spectrum antibiotics: Antibiotics that act against a wide range of disease-causing bacteria. Act against both Gram-positive and Gram-negative bacteria.

***Clostridium difficile* (C. diff):** A bacterium that can cause symptoms that range from diarrhea to severe inflammation of the colon (can be fatal). This condition is most commonly seen after antibiotic use.

healthcare-associated infections (HAIs): Infections that patients acquire while receiving treatment for other conditions within a healthcare setting (e.g., ambulatory care, long-term care, or rehabilitation facility).

infectious agents: Living and nonliving pathogens—such as bacteria, viruses, fungi, protozoa, parasite, helminths, and prions—that can cause disease. Also called infectious particles.

methicillin-resistant *Staphylococcus aureus*: (MRSA) A Gram-positive pathogen that is resistant to multiple antibiotics.

microorganism: Any living organism—such as bacterium, protozoan, fungus, parasite, or helminth—of microscopic size. Some definitions include viruses, which are not alive.

normal flora: Microorganisms (mostly bacteria and yeast) that live on or in the body. Normal microscopic residents of the body.

pathogens: Disease-causing organisms or agents.

yeast: Belongs to various single-celled fungi, which reproduce by budding and are able to ferment sugars.

As a medical assistant, you need to understand basic microbiology (mahy kroh bahy OL uh jee) and the role of microorganisms in both health and disease. The main objective in medical microbiology is to identify the organisms responsible for illness so that the provider can properly treat the patient. Your responsibilities will also include preventing HAIs by observing infection control. Microbiology testing procedures may be performed in the physician office laboratory (POL) or in the microbiology department of a medical referral laboratory.

Immunology (im yuh NOL uh jee) is the study of the immune system, which is closely tied to microbiology. Invasive microorganisms stimulate an immune response, leading to the production of **antibodies** (AN ti bod ees) that come to our defense. Often a bacterial or **viral** (VAHY ruh l) infection is diagnosed by testing for diagnosed by testing for a specific antibody that is produced to fight the infectious agent.

Chapter 28 discusses the chain of infection and how it can be broken by applying diligent infection control procedures, such as the following:
- Using proper hand hygiene
- Wearing appropriate personal protective equipment (PPE)
- Observing recommended precautions for infectious agent transmission
- Using appropriate **antiseptics** (an tuh SEP tiks) and **disinfectants** (dis in FEK tuh nts)
- Performing sterilization procedures

This chapter covers the following topics related to microbiology and immunology:
- Major categories of infectious agents
- Quality control issues regarding the collection and handling of microbiological specimens.
- Common CLIA-waived microbiology and immunology testing

The chapter concludes with an overview of the more complex microbiology procedures and tests performed in hospitals and reference laboratories.

Microorganisms are too small to be seen without magnification. Bacteria, **fungus** (FUHN gus), and **protozoa** (proh tuh zoh uh) are all microorganisms that can be seen with a **light microscope** (MAHY kruh skohp). **Parasitic** (par uh SIT ik) worm infections are also identified in the microbiology laboratory because their eggs are visible under the microscope. Viruses are the smallest microbe and are visible only with a highly magnified electron microscope.

Naming Microorganisms

Scientists use the **binomial** (bahy NOH mee uhl) system of **nomenclature** (NOH muh n-kley cher) (Box 45.2). This binomial system assigns two names; the first name is the *genus* (JEE nuh s) (plural, *genera*) and the second name is the *species* (SPEE sheez). Both names are either *italicized* or underlined when written. The genus begins with a capital letter, the species with a lowercase letter. When microbiology laboratory results are reported, it is essential that both the genus and species names be recorded. Different species may cause different symptoms or require different antibiotic treatment. For example, *Streptococcus pyogenes* (strep tuh KOK uhs PAHY uh jen eez) causes strep throat, whereas *Streptococcus viridans* (strep tuh KOK uhs VEER uh denz) is normal flora in the throat.

BOX 45.2   Nomenclature

Swedish botanist Carl Linnaeus developed the binomial system of nomenclature to name all living organisms: animals, plants, fungi, protozoa, and bacteria.

CLASSIFICATION OF MICROORGANISMS

Although the medical assistant is not responsible for identifying microorganisms, a working knowledge of the terminology used in naming microorganisms is essential.

MEDICAL TERMINOLOGY
anti-: against
bi/o: life
-coccus: berry-shaped bacterium
fung/i: fungus, mushroom
-gen: substance that produces
micro-: small
path/o: disease
parasit/o: parasite
prot/o: first
py/o: pus
-scope: instrument for visual examination
seps/o: infection
staphyl/o: clusters
strept/o: twisted chains
vir/o: virus
zo/o: animal life

VOCABULARY
antibodies: Protein substances produced in the blood or tissues in response to a specific antigen; they destroy or weaken the antigen. Part of the immune system.
antiseptics: Describes substances that inhibit the growth of microorganisms on living tissue (e.g., alcohol and povidone-iodine [Betadine]); they are used to cleanse the skin, wounds, and so on.
binomial: A name consisting of a generic and a specific term.
disinfectants: Chemical agents used on nonliving objects to destroy or inhibit the growth of harmful organisms.
fungus: Any of a diverse group of single-celled organisms, including mushrooms, molds, mildew, smuts, rusts, and yeasts and classified in the kingdom Fungi.
-gen: substance that produces
light microscope: An instrument that uses focused light and lenses to magnify a specimen, usually a cell.
nomenclature: A system of names or terms, used in science and art to categorize items.
parasitic: Pertaining to a parasite. (An organism that lives on or in another organism, known as the host. Benefits from the host; the host does not benefit from the parasite.)
protozoa: Single-celled organisms that are the most primitive form of animal life. Most are microscopic. Examples are amoebas, ciliates, flagellates and sporozoans.
viral: Relating to or caused by a virus.

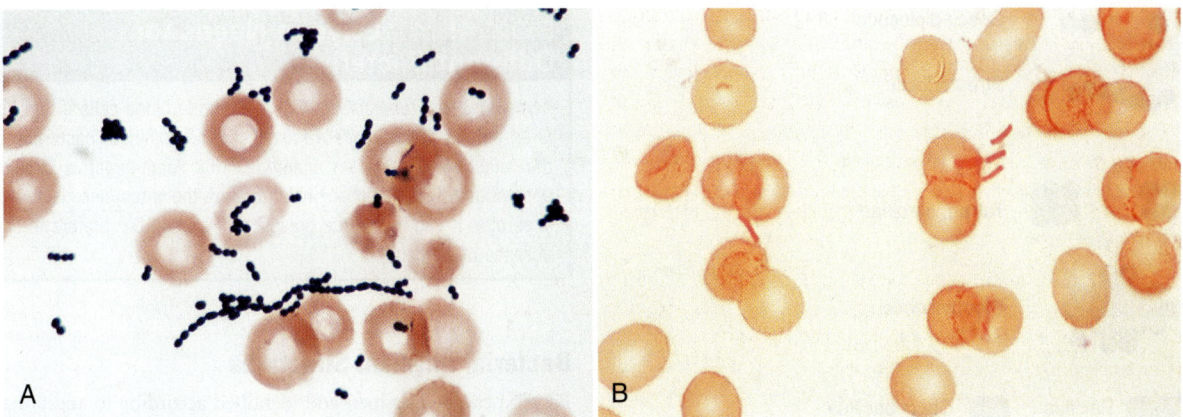

FIG. 45.1 (A) Gram stain A—red blood cells (RBCs) and Gram-positive cocci. (B) RBCs with Gram-negative bacilli. (From De la Maza LM, Pezzlo MT, Baron EJ: *Color Atlas of Diagnostic Microbiology*, St. Louis, 1997, Mosby.)

> **BOX 45.3 Bacteria Quickly Increase in Numbers**
>
> Because bacteria reproduce quickly, bacterial infections can swiftly overwhelm a person's immune system. Some bacteria reproduce in as little as 14 minutes, whereas other bacteria may take days. It is possible for a single *E. coli* cell, which reproduces about every 30 minutes, to produce about 3.5 trillion offspring in 24 hours.

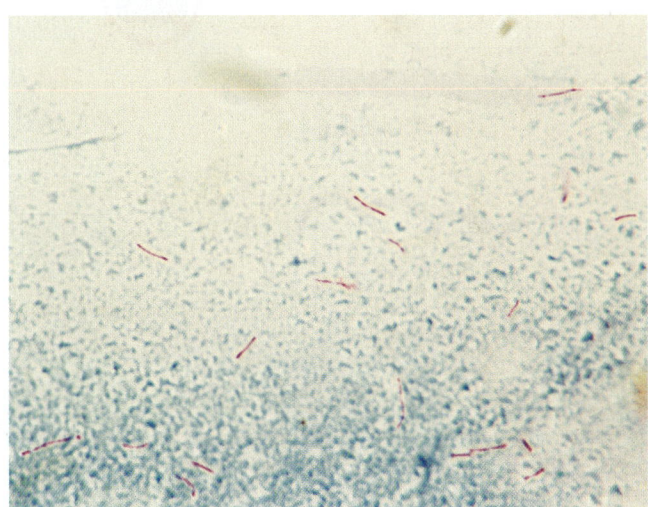

FIG. 45.2 Acid-fast stain. (From De la Maza LM, Pezzlo MT, Baron EJ: *Color Atlas of Diagnostic Microbiology*, St. Louis, 1997, Mosby.)

The genus name of the organism may be represented by a single letter, after the organism's full genus and species names have been written once in a report. For example, *Escherichia coli* (eh shu REEK e ah KOH lahy) is commonly referred to as *E. coli*.

CHARACTERISTICS OF BACTERIA

Bacteria are single-celled **prokaryote** (proh KAR ee oht) organisms that reproduce **asexually**, by **binary fission**. This process of reproduction results in large numbers of bacteria being formed from a single cell (Box 45.3).

Bacteria often are classified according to their staining characteristics, shape, and the environmental conditions in which they thrive. Both shape and staining characteristics are direct results of their cell wall composition.

Bacterial Staining Properties

Three types of cell wall structures are found among pathogenic bacteria: Gram-positive, Gram-negative, and acid-fast structures. These labels are based on reactions in specialized **stains** used to visualize the bacteria under the microscope. Bacterial cell walls are composed of *peptidoglycan* (pep tih DOH glahy kan) (PG), a **molecule** (MOL uh kyool) composed of carbohydrate and protein.

- *Gram-positive cells* contain a thick layer of PG, which produces a deep blue/violet when stained with Gram stain (Fig. 45.1A).
- *Gram-negative cells* contain a thin layer of PG, which produces a pinkish red color when stained with Gram stain (Fig. 45.1B).
- *Acid-fast cells* contain a thin layer of PG surrounded by a thick layer of waxlike lipids. Acid-fast bacteria do not stain well with a Gram stain, but they stain pink with the acid-fast stain (Fig. 45.2).

Bacterial Shapes

Bacteria assume three different shapes:
- Round bacteria are called *cocci* (KOK sahy).
- Rod-shaped bacteria are called *bacilli* (buh SIL ahy).
- Spiral-shaped bacteria are called *spirilla* (spahy RIL ah). Tightly coiled spirilla are called *spirochetes* (SPAHY ruh keets).

> **VOCABULARY**
>
> **asexually:** Describes reproduction that does not involve the fusion of male and female sex cells, such as in plant reproduction, fission, or budding.
> **binary fission:** Asexual reproduction in single-celled organisms during which one cell divides into two daughter cells.
> **molecule:** The simplest unit of a chemical compound that can exist, consisting of two or more atoms held together with chemical bonds.
> **prokaryote:** Any organism that is made up of at least one cell and has genetic material that is not enclosed in a nucleus. Bacteria are prokaryotes, primitive organisms.
> **stains:** Reagents or dyes used to treat specimens for microscopic examination.

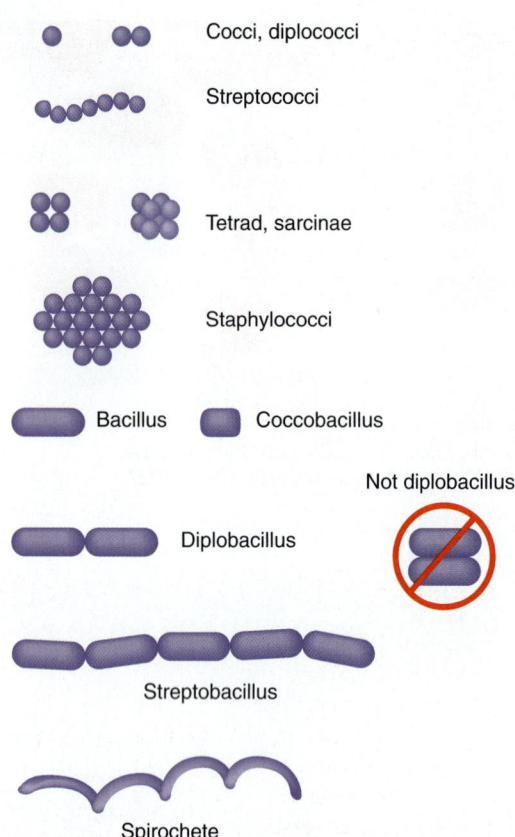

FIG. 45.3 Typical bacterial arrangement. (From Proctor D, et al: *Kinn's The Medical Assistant*, ed 13, St. Louis, 2017, Elsevier.)

> **BOX 45.4   Oxygen Needs for Different Bacteria**
>
> *Mycobacterium tuberculosis* thrives in white blood cells in the lungs and is an aerobe. *Bacteroides fragilis* is the predominant bacterium found in the intestines, and is an anaerobe. This Gram-negative bacillus is an anaerobe. *E. coli,* also an inhabitant of the intestines, is a facultative anaerobe. It can live in the presence of oxygen but prefers to live in the absence of oxygen.

Bacterial Physical Structures

Bacteria can be classified and identified according to additional physical structures. Some bacteria have long thin flagella (fluh jel uh) that help them move. Some bacteria have a thick, jelly-like substance that surrounds the cell wall called a *capsule*, which can make the bacteria more pathogenic. Other bacteria form intracellular structures called an endospore. An endospore allows the bacteria to remain viable (VAHY uh buhl) when environmental conditions are poor. *Clostridium tetani* (klo STRID ee uhm TET uh nee) produces spores, if spores enter a wound and grow, they cause the disease known as *tetanus* (TET nuhs).

See Tables 45.1 to 45.3 for a list of some important infectious diseases caused by pathogenic bacilli, cocci, and spirilla.

> **CRITICAL THINKING 45.1**
>
> In your own words, write a brief description of the term *capsule*. What advantage does a bacterium have if a capsule surrounds it? Share your thoughts with the class.

Certain arrangements are also seen with different bacteria. For example, when bacteria are in a chain formation, the prefix *strepto-* is used. When bacteria are found in pairs, the prefix *diplo-* is used, and when they are found in grapelike clusters, the prefix *staphylo-* is used. Cocci in packets of 4 are called *tetrads,* and in packets of 8 or 16 they are called *sarcinae* (SAHR suh nay) (Fig. 45.3).

Bacterial Oxygen Requirements

Bacteria are also classified according to oxygen requirements. Bacteria that require oxygen to live are called *aerobes* (AIR ohbs). Bacteria that die in the presence of oxygen are called *anaerobes* (an AIR ohbs). Some bacteria are flexible regarding their oxygen needs; they can survive in the presence of oxygen but prefer to live without oxygen. These bacteria are called *facultative anaerobes* (FAK uhl tey tiv an AIR ohbs). See Box 45.4 for some examples of oxygen needs for different bacteria.

UNUSUAL PATHOGENIC BACTERIA: CHLAMYDIA, MYCOPLASMA, AND RICKETTSIA

Typical pathogenic bacteria measure 1000 to 5000 nm in size. *Chlamydia* (kluh MID ee uh), *mycoplasma* (mahy koh PLAZ muh), and *rickettsia* (rih KET see uh) are tiny, unusual bacteria that fall between the size ranges of typical pathogenic bacteria and viruses (Table 45.4).

Chlamydia are tiny bacteria that require host cells for growth. They once were considered viruses. *Rickettsia* are tiny Gram-negative bacteria that are transmitted by blood-sucking insects. Rickettsia cannot multiply outside a living host cell. *Mycoplasmas* are unusual in that they have no PG in their cell wall.

> **MEDICAL TERMINOLOGY**
>
> **aer/o:** air
> **an-:** no, not, without
> **bacillus** (singular): bacilli (plural)
> **coccus** (singular): cocci (plural)
> **dipl/o:** double or two
> **spirillum** (singular): spirilla (plural)
> **tetra-:** four

> **VOCABULARY**
>
> **endospore:** An inactive form of certain bacteria that can withstand poor environmental conditions. When conditions improve, the bacteria become functional again.
> **flagella:** A long, whip-like outgrowth from a cell that helps the cell move.
> **viable:** Able to live and grow.

TABLE 45.1 Common Diseases Caused by Bacilli

Disease State	Causative Agent	Transmission
Botulism	Clostridium botulinum	Improperly cooked canned foods
Clostridium difficile (C. diff)	Clostridium difficile	May be healthcare-acquired infection (HAI), frequent antibiotic use increases likelihood. Idiopathic.
Diphtheria	Corynebacterium diphtheriae	Inhalation
Legionnaire's disease	Legionella pneumophilia	Grows readily in air conditioning systems (water)
Salmonella infection	Salmonella species	Food-borne illness
Tetanus (lockjaw)	Clostridium tetani	Open fractures, soil-contaminated wounds, open wounds, puncture wounds
Tuberculosis	Mycobacterium tuberculosis	Air-borne, inhalation
Urinary Tract Infection (UTI)	Various, most common include: Escherichia coli, Proteus species, Klebsiella species, Pseudomonas aeruginosa	Bacteria contaminate urethra, catheterization
Whooping cough	Bordetella pertussis	Respiratory secretions

TABLE 45.2 Common Diseases Caused by Cocci

Disease State	Causative Agent	Transmission
Gonorrhea	Neisseria gonorrhoeae	Sexually transmitted
Meningococcal meningitis	Neisseria meningitidis	Respiratory tract secretions
Methicillin-resistant Staphylococcus aureus (MRSA) infection	Methicillin-resistant Staphylococcus aureus	Healthcare-acquired infection (HIA), direct contact, fomites, carriers, poor hand washing technique
Pneumonia	Streptococcus pneumoniae	Direct contact, droplets
Staphylococcal food poisoning	Staphylococcus aureus	Poor hygiene, improper refrigeration of foods
Strep throat	Streptococcus pyogenes, also known as Group A Strep	Direct contact, droplets, fomites
Wound infections, abscesses, boils	Staphylococcus aureus	Direct contact, fomites, carriers, poor hand washing technique

TABLE 45.3 Common Diseases Caused by Spirilla

Disease State	Causative Agent	Transmission
Food-borne illness (most commonly seen in the United States)	Campylobacter jejuni	Contaminated and under cooked food, contaminated water and milk
Lyme disease	Borrelia burgdorferi	Tick bite
Pyloric ulcers	Helicobacter pylori	Unknown, possible food/water-borne
Syphilis	Treponema pallidum	Sexually or congenitally

TABLE 45.4 Common Diseases Caused by Rickettsia, Mycoplasma, and Chlamydia

Disease State	Causative Agent	Transmission
Atypical or walking pneumonia	Mycoplasma pneumoniae	Respiratory secretions
Inclusion conjunctivitis or pneumonia	Chlamydia trachomatis	During the birth process
Nongonococcal urethritis or vaginitis	Chlamydia trachomatis	Sexually
Rocky mountain spotted fever	Rickettsia rickettsii	Tick bite
Typhus (epidemic)	Rickettsia prowazekii	Body lice bite
Typhus (endemic)	Rickettsia typhi	Flea bite

> **STUDY TIP**
>
> *Mycoplasma pneumonia* is also referred to as "walking pneumonia."

PATHOGENIC FUNGI

Mycology (mahy KOL uh jee) is the study of fungi and the diseases they cause (Table 45.5). Fungi are **eukaryotes** (yoo KAR ee ohts) that are larger than bacteria and have a nucleus. Fungi include yeasts and **molds** (mohlds). Fungi are present in the soil, air, and water, but only a few species cause disease. They are transmitted by the following:
- Direct contact with infected persons
- Prolonged exposure to a moist environment
- Inhalation of contaminated dust or soil

Fungal infections may be superficial, affecting only the skin, hair, or nails. Some fungi can penetrate the tissues of the internal body structures and cause serious diseases of the mucous membranes, heart, and lungs. Fungal infections must be treated with specific antifungal medications.

> **VOCABULARY**
>
> **eukaryote:** Any single-celled or multicellular organism that has genetic material contained in a distinct membrane-bound nucleus.
>
> **mold:** A growth of tiny fungi forming on a substance. Often looks downy or furry and is associated with dampness or decay.

TABLE 45.5 Common Diseases Caused by Fungi

Disease State	Causative Agent	Transmission
Candidiasis, vulvovaginal, monilial, (vaginal yeast)	Candida species (yeast)	After antibiotic therapy, using hormonal birth control, diabetes-type I, II, gestational, AIDS
Cryptococcosis	Cryptococcus neoformans	Contact with poultry droppings
Fungal infections; Athlete foot, jock itch, ringworm	Tinea species and others	Direct contact with an infected person or animal, damp surfaces
Histoplasmosis	Histoplasma capsulatum	Inhaling dust contaminated with bird or bat droppings
Pneumocystis pneumonia	Pneumocystis jiroveci formerly known as Pneumocystis carinii	Contact with animals, most likely in immune-compromised patients, common in AIDS patients
Thrush (in the mouth)	Candida species (yeast)	Possibly during birth process, after antibiotic therapy, diabetes, or weakened immune system

TABLE 45.6 Common Diseases Caused by Protozoa and Parasites

Disease State	Causative Agent	Transmission
Amoebic dysentery	Entamoeba histolytica	Fecal contamination of food and/or water
Giardiasis	Giardia lamblia	Contaminated water, opportunist in intestinal tract
Lice	Pediculus humanus (head and body lice) Pthirus pubis (pubic lice)	Direct contact, contaminated clothing, bedding, furniture, personal items (combs, hats, etc.)
Malaria	Plasmodium species	Bite of the Anopheles mosquito
Pinworm	Enterobius vermicularis	Fecal-oral contamination
Scabies	Sarcoptes scabiei	Direct contact, contaminated clothing, bedding
Tapeworm – beef or pork	Taenia species	Eating undercooked beef or pork
Tapeworm - fish	Diphyllobothrium latum	Eating undercooked fish
Toxoplasmosis	Toxoplasma gondii	Fecal contamination of cat litter, congenitally
Trichinosis	Trichinella spiralis	Eating undercooked pork or bear

BOX 45.5 Ringworm

Tinea (TIN ee uh) means "ringworm" in Latin. Most tinea skin infections start out as a little dot on the skin that grows bigger in an ever-expanding circle. It looks like the pathogen is creating a large swirl on the skin. That is why it is called ringworm.

A superficial fungal infection often is referred to as *tinea* (TIN ee uh). See Chapter 4, which discusses the integumentary (in teg yuh MEN tuh ree) system, for a description of tinea infections (Box 45.5). A diagnosis of a fungal infection is usually based on culturing skin scrapings or microscopic observation of skin scrapings. Usually, before microscopic observation, the samples are treated with *potassium hydroxide* (puh TAS ee uhm hahy DROK sahyd) (KOH) to dissolve nonfungal material, making the fungal elements easier to observe.

CRITICAL THINKING 45.2

Fungi include two other types of organisms. Name these organisms. Share your answers with the class.

PATHOGENIC PROTOZOA

Protozoa are single-celled parasitic organisms that contain a nucleus. They range in size from microscopic to *macroscopic* (visible to the naked eye) (Table 45.6). They are present in moist environments and in bodies of water, such as lakes and ponds. Protozoa are transmitted through contaminated *feces* (FEE seez), food, and drink. Some pathogenic protozoa inhabit the bloodstream, others inhabit the intestines and genital tract. Diagnosis usually is based on the patient's signs and symptoms and on microscopic examination of stool or blood.

PATHOGENIC PARASITES

Parasitology includes the study of all parasitic organisms that live on or in the human body (see Table 45.6). In a parasitic relationship, the host is harmed and the parasite thrives. Parasites are transmitted by ingestion, direct penetration of the skin, and injection by an arthropod (AHR thruh pod). A parasite cannot be identified accurately based on a single test or specimen. Parasites are frequently identified in feces, blood, urine, sputum, tissue fluid, or tissue biopsy samples.

MEDICAL TERMINOLOGY
eu-: good, normal
fungi (singular), **fungus** (plural)
kary/o: nucleus
protozoan (singular), **protozoa** (plural)

VOCABULARY
arthropod: Any animal that lacks a spine, such as insects, crustaceans, arachnids, and others.

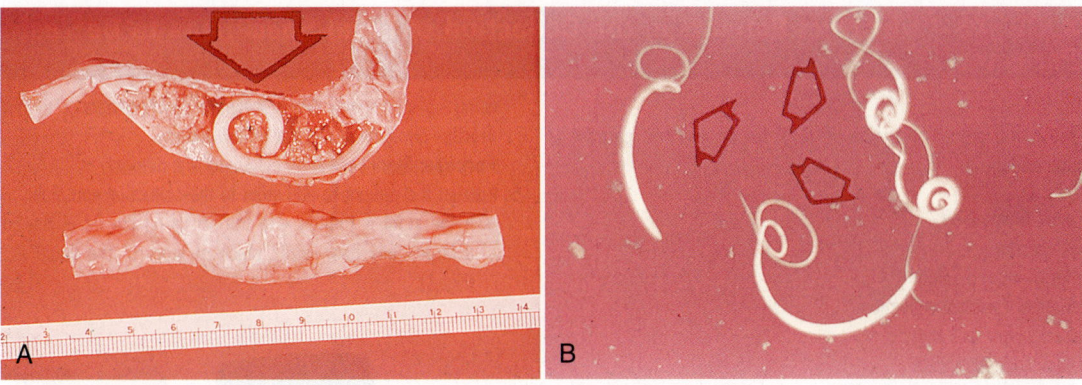

FIG. 45.4 (A) Roundworms. (B) Whipworms. (From Stepp CA, Woods MA: *Laboratory Procedures for Medical Office Personnel*, Philadelphia, 1998, Saunders.)

PATHOGENIC HELMINTHS (WORMS)

Helminths (HEL mihn th s) are parasites called worms. Helminths live on or in another living organism. They sustain themselves at the expense of the host organism. They can live in animals or humans. Worms are usually transmitted through the soil, by infected clothing or fingernails, contact with infected persons, or contaminated food/water. Helminths go through the same life cycle as other worms. The adult worm lays eggs (ova). The ova develop into **larvae** (LAHR vuh). Larvae grow into adult worms, and the cycle begins again. Diagnosis usually is based on microscopic examination of feces for ova (eggs) and parasites, and on patient signs and symptoms (Fig. 45.4).

Stool specimens are commonly examined for parasitic protozoa and helminths. The specimen is collected and placed into two vials, each with a preservative. From these preparations, a **wet mount** slide is made to observe moving organisms. A stained smear is made from a concentrated specimen. The smear is looked at under a microscope to observe **protozoal cysts** (sists) and helminth eggs. The medical assistant should always consult the procedure manual provided by the referral laboratory when an ova and parasites stool examination (O&P) is ordered to make sure that proper specimen collection and transport takes place (Procedure 45.1).

PATHOGENIC VIRUSES

Many scientists do not consider viruses to be microorganisms because they are not alive. Viruses consist of a genetic core covered by a protein coat called a *capsid* (KAP sid) (Box 45.6). Some viruses have an additional spiked layer of protection over the capsid called an envelope. Viruses are not able to metabolize or reproduce unless they are inside of a host cell. Viruses have their own enzymes but must use the host cell **organelles** (awr guh NELS) and **macromolecules** (mak ruh MOL uh kyools) to reproduce and metabolize. Because of the absolute need for a host cell, a virus can be considered an *obligate intracellular pathogen*. Viruses must be inside of a host cell to reproduce and cause disease (see Box 45.6).

A virus cannot be cultured on solid nutrient media, such as those used to culture bacteria and fungi. Viruses must be cultured in fertilized eggs or in a **tissue culture**, which is done by referral, research, or large hospital laboratories.

Usually, instead of culturing a specimen for a virus, the patient's blood sample is tested for a specific antibody related to the possible viral infection. For example, in the diagnosis of Lyme disease, patient serum is tested for the specific antibody produced in response to the Lyme **antigen** (AN ti juhn). This form of testing is referred to as *serology* or *immunology testing* (discussed later in the chapter). Table 45.7 lists common diseases caused by viruses.

> **BOX 45.6 Recipe for a Virus**
>
> A viral genetic core is made up of either *ribonucleic acid* (RAHY boh noo klee ik as id) (RNA) or *deoxyribonucleic acid* (dee auk see RAHY boh noo klee ik as id) (DNA). The RNA or DNA contains information about how and what the host cell needs to produce to form a new virus. The genetic material is like a recipe for a new viral particle.

SPECIMEN COLLECTION AND TRANSPORT IN THE PHYSICIAN OFFICE LABORATORY

Specimen collection and handling are very important considerations in patient care because the results are only as good as the quality of the

> **CRITICAL THINKING 45.3**
>
> Looking at Table 45.7, pick four viral diseases that you are familiar with. Write down the disease, the virus that causes it, and two ways to prevent the infection. Be ready to share your answers with the class.

> **MEDICAL TERMINOLOGY**
> **arthr/o:** joint
> **pod/o:** foot

> **VOCABULARY**
> **antigen:** A substance that stimulates the production of an antibody when introduced into the body. Antigens include toxins, bacteria, viruses, and other foreign substances.
> **larvae:** Immature free-living forms of many animals; develop into the adult form.
> **macromolecules:** The molecules needed for metabolism: carbohydrates, lipids, proteins, amino acids, and nucleic acids.
> **organelles:** Structures inside of the cell.
> **protozoal cyst:** A thick-walled protective membrane enclosing a cell, larva, or organism.
> **tissue culture:** The technique or process of keeping tissue alive and growing in a culture medium.
> **wet mount:** A glass slide that holds a specimen suspended in a drop of liquid for microscopic examination.

PROCEDURE 45.1 Instruct Patients in the Collection of Fecal Specimens to Be Tested for Ova and Parasites

Task

Instruct a patient in the proper collection of stool for an ova and parasite microscopic examination.

Equipment and Supplies
- Patient's health record
- Provider's order or lab requisition
- Clean, dry container for stool collection
- Plastic biohazard zipper-lock bag
- Two parasitology collection vials

Please note that several types of preservatives are available for the parasitology collection vials. Check with the referral laboratory to make sure the patient is given the proper vials for collection. Preservatives include low-viscosity polyvinyl alcohol (LV-PVA), zinc sulfite polyvinyl alcohol (ZN-PVA), sodium acetate acetic acid formalin (SAF), and 10% neutral buffered formalin.

Procedural Steps

1. Greet the patient. Identify yourself. Verify the patient's identity with full name, then ask the patient to spell first and the last name and to state his or her date of birth. Explain the procedure in a manner that the patient understands. Answer any general questions the patient may have about the collection procedures before you give detailed instructions.
2. Instruct the patient not to take any antacids, laxatives, or stool softeners before collecting the specimen.
   Purpose: Laxatives increase fecal transit time and may lead to a false-negative test result.
3. Instruct the patient to urinate before collecting the specimen.
   Purpose: This eliminates the possibility of the stool becoming contaminated by urine.
4. The patient then collects the specimen.
   Adults: Instruct the patient to defecate into the container provided. Stool cannot be retrieved from the toilet bowl. *Children:* Instruct parents/guardians to loosely drape the toilet rim with plastic wrap and lower the seat. The child should have a bowel movement into the toilet, onto the wrap. Remove the stool using a disposable plastic spoon.
   Purpose: The stool cannot be contaminated by or diluted with water. *Infants:* Fasten a "diaper" made of plastic wrap over the child using tape. Remove the plastic wrap immediately after a bowel movement and remove the stool using a plastic spoon. *Never leave the child unattended with the plastic wrap in place because of the risk of suffocation.*
   Purpose: Stool cannot be collected in a diaper.
5. Instruct the patient to add stool to the collection container.
   a. If the stool is formed, use the scoop on the lid of the container to add a large, jelly bean–sized piece of stool to the liquid in the containers (Fig. 1).

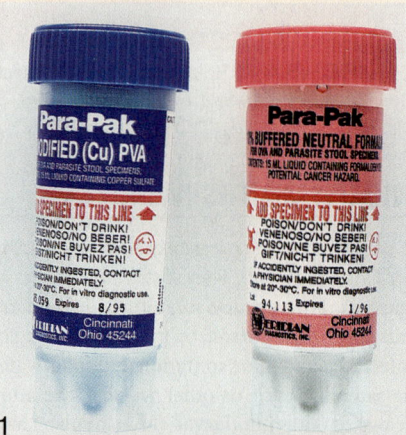

1 (Courtesy Meridian Bioscience, Cincinnati, Ohio.)

   b. If the stool is liquid, pour it into the container.
   c. In both of the previous cases, keep adding the specimen until the liquid preservative in the vial reaches the indicated level on the containers.
6. Instruct the patient to tighten the caps completely and wipe the outside of the vials with alcohol wipes or to wash carefully with soap and water.
   Purpose: To ensure infection control.
7. The vials should be labeled, placed in a biohazard bag with a zippered closure, and transported to the laboratory immediately, if possible. *The vials should not be refrigerated.*
8. Instruct the patient to wash his or her hands after the specimen collection process.
   Purpose: To ensure infection control.

TABLE 45.7 Common Diseases Caused by Viruses

Disease State	Causative Agent	Transmission
Acquired immunodeficiency syndrome (AIDS)	Human immunodeficiency virus (HIV)	Sexual intercourse/contact, sharing needles, at risk behavior
Common cold	Rhinovirus most common among many possible	Direct contact, inhaling droplets, fomites
Ebola	Ebola virus species (five identified)	Direct contact with infected blood and/or body fluids (bloodborne)
Infectious mononucleosis	Epstein-Barr virus	Direct contact and airborne
Influenza	Myxovirus, influenza A and B	Droplet and fomites
Measles	Paramyxovirus – measles virus	Direct contact, inhaling droplets
Molluscum contagiosum warts	Molluscipox virus	Direct contact with an infected person
Mumps	Paramyxovirus – mumps virus	Inhaling droplets, shared utensils with infected person
Polio	Poliovirus	Direct contact, via mouth
Rubella (German measles)	Rubella virus	Direct contact, inhaling droplets, congenitally
Warts (verruca)	Human papillomavirus (HPV)	Direct and indirect contact

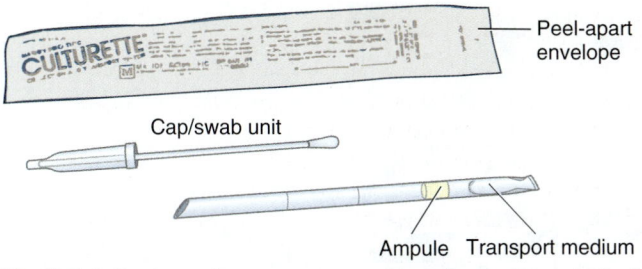

FIG. 45.5 Collection and transport system. (From Proctor D, et al: *Kinn's The Medical Assistant*, ed 13, St. Louis, 2017, Elsevier.)

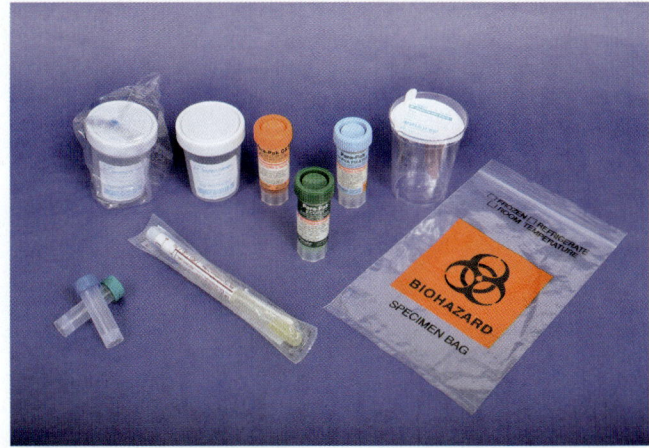

FIG. 45.6 Microbiology specimen containers. (From Proctor D, et al: *Kinn's The Medical Assistant*, ed 13, St. Louis, 2017, Elsevier.)

sample. Specimens for microbiology testing must be collected carefully so that contaminating microorganisms are not introduced into the specimen. This means not only using sterile collection and transport devices, but also taking steps to prevent contamination. Such steps include instructing a patient in the collection of a urine sample using the clean-catch midstream (CCMS) technique as described in Chapter 42. Also, the use of antiseptics on the skin to avoid contamination of the site as described in Chapter 43.

Before collecting specimens for microbiologic testing, you should ask yourself two questions:
1. How can I prevent contamination of this sample?
2. How can I protect myself from pathogen exposure while I collect this sample?

To prevent sample contamination, do the following:
- Wash hands properly, and wear gloves.
- Cleanse the area to be sampled with an antiseptic, if possible.
- Open sterile containers only when necessary.
- Never touch a sterile swab or collection device to a nonsterile surface.

To protect yourself from pathogen exposure, do the following:
- Use proper hand washing techniques.
- Wear gloves, a fluid-impermeable lab coat, a surgical mask (for droplet or airborne pathogens), protective eyewear, or a face shield.
- Always wear gloves when handling any patient specimen, even if you are not going to be testing the sample at that time.

Ideally, specimens should be collected during the acute phase of an illness and before antibiotics are prescribed. Many types of samples are collected. Some examples are as follows:
- Sterile swabs can be used to collect samples from wounds and the upper respiratory tract.
- Serum or whole blood can be used to test for infectious organisms.
- Urine samples are normally collected at the POL.
- Fecal samples can be collected by the patient at the POL or at home.

If patients are expected to collect a sample, it is crucial that they receive clear instructions on how to perform the procedure correctly and without contaminating the sample. The referral laboratory is responsible for providing a manual of written instructions to the POL, and the POL is responsible for providing clear oral and written instructions to the patient. If the patient will be collecting the sample in private or at home, written instructions that are simple and straightforward should be supplied.

The transport of specimens to referral laboratories is also crucial. Different types of transport devices are available. Close attention must be given to their proper use. Microorganisms are living organisms, so they must be given conditions that ensure their survival. Care must also be taken so that any normal flora in the sample will not multiply and overgrow possible pathogens. The type and number of microorganisms in the sample should reflect the type and number of microorganisms at the site of collection and at the time of collection.

Specialized transport media are often included with specimen collection swabs or devices (Fig. 45.5). Collection devices typically consist of a plastic tube that encases a sterile Dacron swab and a sealed vial of **transport medium**. After the specimen has been collected on the swab, it is placed in the plastic tube with the transport medium. It is essential to follow the manufacturer's directions to prevent the swab and specimen from drying out. Transport system swabs also have a label that must be filled out completely, indicating the patient's full name, the date and time of collection, the collector's initials, and the source of the specimen (e.g., deep wound sample from left leg abscess).

> **CRITICAL THINKING 45.4**
>
> Each time Laura collects a wound swab that needs to be sent to the reference laboratory, she needs to put the swab in a transport medium. List three reasons why we use transport media when wound specimens cannot be tested immediately. Be ready to share your ideas with the class.

If possible, a specimen should be placed on culture media immediately after collection. If this is not possible, then the transport device must be sent to a referral laboratory or held in the POL until it can be cultured. For specimens that will be transported by a courier, make sure the specimen is safely packaged in a leak-proof container marked with warning labels (Fig. 45.6). The proper time and temperature of storage are vital. Most pathogenic organisms prefer body temperatures, approximately 37°C (98.6°F). They will remain viable for up to 72 hours if held at room temperature or refrigerator temperature (4°C [39.2°F]). Some organisms die if exposed to cold temperatures. Always check the referral laboratory's procedure manual for directions regarding sample time and temperature of storage. See Fig. 45.7 for some commonly used microbiology collection devices.

Devices used for both aerobic and anaerobic blood collection are shown in Fig. 45.7A, and BACTEC blood culture bottles are pictured in Fig. 45.7B. Two other commonly used transportation devices are the JEMBEC plate for transporting *Neisseria gonorrhoeae* (see Fig. 45.7C) and a viral-chlamydial transport medium (see Fig. 45.7D).

See Table 45.8 for a description of the specimens, containers, patient preparation processes, and storage of specimens commonly collected or handled by medical assistants.

> **VOCABULARY**
>
> **transport medium:** A medium used to keep an organism alive during transport to the laboratory.

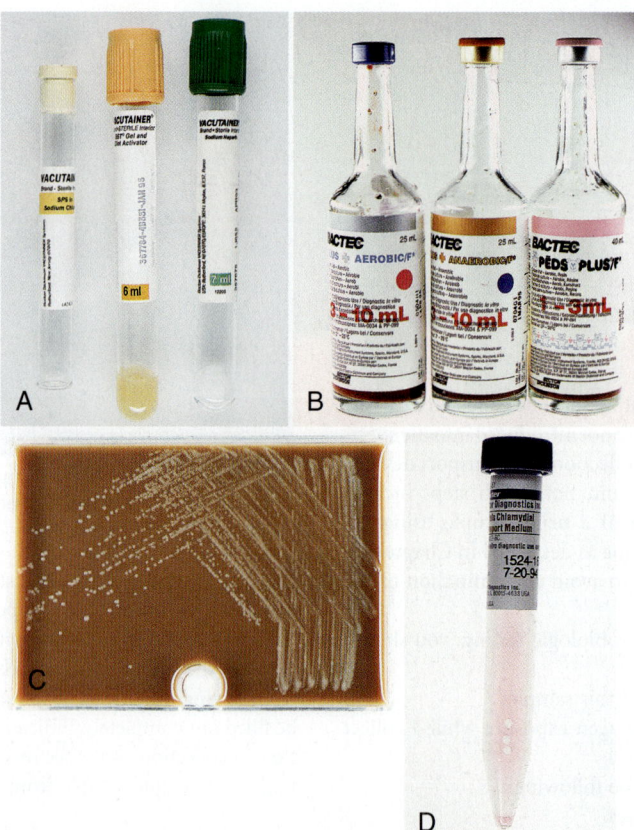

FIG. 45.7 (A) Blood collection Vacutainer tubes, one for aerobic and one for anaerobic. (B) BACTEC blood culture bottles. (C) JEMBEC plate. (D) Viral-chlamydial transport media. (From De la Maza LM, Pezzlo MT, Baron EJ: *Color Atlas of Diagnostic Microbiology*, St. Louis, 1997, Mosby.)

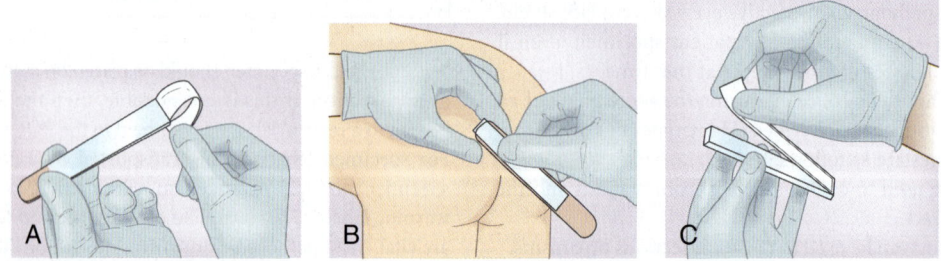

FIG. 45.8 The three steps for collecting a pinworm specimen from a child. (A) Place cellulose tape over a tongue depressor with the sticky side out. (B) Press the tape firmly against the right and left anal folds. (C) Place the tape with adhesive side down on to the microscope slide. (From Proctor D, et al: *Kinn's The Medical Assistant*, ed 13, St. Louis, 2017, Elsevier.)

Collection of Pinworms

Enterobius vermicularis (ehn tuh ROH bee uhs ver MIK yoo ler uhs) is commonly known as pinworm. This species of parasite primarily infects the colon of young children. Humans are infected by ingesting mature eggs through the following:
- Hand-to-mouth transfers
- Feces-contaminated fingers
- Feces-contaminated foods or liquids
- By inhaling eggs in air currents from infected areas

The eggs hatch in the small intestine, and the females migrate out of the anus, usually at night, to deposit the eggs. The eggs adhere to the skin and hair surrounding the anus, sleeping garments, and other clothing. Pinworms cause itching in the anal area, which may cause the eggs to come in contact with the hands and fingernails of the host.

In children, specimens are best collected late at night or early in the morning. Paraffin swabs impregnated with petroleum jelly or cellulose tape may be used to collect the eggs deposited by the adult worm during the night. The diagnosis is based on laboratory detection of the eggs in fecal smears. If the parent does not feel comfortable collecting the specimen, instruct the parent to bring the child to the office as soon as they wake up in the morning. Instruct the parent not to change the child's clothing or diaper before coming into the office. When the child arrives, have all the needed supplies ready to use, and perform the procedure immediately (Fig. 45.8).

TABLE 45.8 Collection, Transport, and Processing of Specimens Commonly Collected in the Physician Office Laboratory[a]

Specimen	Container	Patient Preparation	Special Instructions	Storage Before Processing
Throat	Transport swab (see Fig. 45.5)	Have patient sitting with head tilted back	Swab pharynx and tonsils, not mouth, tongue, or teeth	Transport and plate within 24 hr; room-temperature storage
Superficial wound	Aerobic transport swab (see Fig. 45.5)	Wipe area with sterile saline before collection	Rotate swab while gently swiping wound	Transport swab stored at room temperature
Eye	Aerobic transport swab (see Fig. 45.5)	Pull lower lid down while gently collecting exudate along rim	N/A	Transport swab may be stored up to 24 hr at room temperature
Ova and parasite (O&P)	O&P transport containers (with formalin and PVA) (see Fig. 45.6)	See Procedure 45.1 for collection of a stool specimen for ova and parasites	Wait 7–10 days if patient has been taking Pepto-Bismol, Kaopectate, or milk of magnesia	Store at room temperature and deliver to laboratory within 24 hr
Stool	Clean, leak-proof containers (see Fig. 45.6)	Outpatients: At minimum, three specimens are collected every other day	Transport to laboratory within 24 hr if storing at 4°C (39.2°F)	Laboratory must plate within 72 hr if storing at 4°C (39.2°F)
Sputum	Sterile, screw-cap container (see Fig. 45.6)	Patient should rinse or gargle with mouthwash before collection	Have patient collect from deep cough; do not collect saliva	Store at 4°C (39.2°F); laboratory must plate within 24 hr
Urine	Vacutainer collection system or sterile, screw-cap container (see Fig. 45.6)	Instruct patient in clean-catch midstream collection	Hold at 4°C (39.2°F) and deliver to laboratory within 24 hr	Hold at 4°C (39.2°F) and plate within 24 hr
Skin scraping (fungal culture)	Clean, screw-top tube (see Fig. 45.6)	Wipe skin with alcohol wipe	Scrape skin at leading edge of lesion	Can be held indefinitely at room temperature but best to process within 72 hr of collection
Blood	Blood culture tube with SPS medium (see Fig. 45.7A) or Vacutainer blood culture medium (see Fig. 45.7B)	Disinfect venipuncture site with alcohol wipe and Betadine	Draw blood during febrile episodes	Deliver to laboratory within 2 hr; incubate at 37°C (98.6°F) on receipt in the laboratory
Gonorrhea culture	JEMBEC transport system (see Fig. 45.7C)	Wipe away exudate before obtaining culture specimen, obtain culture specimen with swab	Do not refrigerate	Transport to laboratory within 2 hr
Chlamydia culture	Specialized antibiotic *Chlamydia* transport medium (see Fig. 45.7D)	Urogenital swabs preferred; necessary to obtain epithelial cells, not exudate	Transport immediately on ice to laboratory	Store up to 24 hr at 4°C (39.2°F); inoculate cultures within 15 min of collection if swab is not on ice
Body fluids (e.g., peritoneal, synovial, pleural)	Sterile, screw-cap container or anaerobic transporter	Disinfect aspiration site with alcohol wipe and Betadine	Needle aspirations are preferable to swab collections	Transport immediately to laboratory
Rectal swab	Swab placed directly into enteric transport medium	N/A	Insert swab approximately 1 inch past anal sphincter	Store at 4°C (39.2°F), transport within 24 hr to laboratory and plate within 72 hr
Deep wound or abscess	Anaerobic transport device	Wipe area with sterile saline or alcohol wipe before collection	Aspirate material, excise tissue, or insert swab deep into wound	Store at room temperature; transport to laboratory and plate within 4 hr

[a]Reference laboratories also have specific directions for collecting specimens based on their testing methods.
O&P, Ova and parasites; *PVA,* polyvinyl alcohol; *SPS,* Sodium polyanethole sulfonate.
Modified from Forbes BA, Sahm DF, Weissfeld AS: *Bailey and Scott's Diagnostic Microbiology,* ed 11, St. Louis, 2002, Mosby.

CLIA-WAIVED MICROBIOLOGY TESTING

Often, growing a pathogen on a nutrient media plate is difficult, and it takes time to grow and isolate the pathogen. A rapid direct immunology test demonstrates the presence of the antigen in a specimen that is placed in a test kit containing its specific antibody. If the pathogen is present, it produces a colored reaction, indicating a positive result.

POLs with appropriate CLIA-waived certification can perform many rapid identification tests for a variety of infectious diseases. Rapid tests are designed to give the provider positive test results quickly and efficiently, so that treatment can be started. If the test result is negative, the provider may need to order additional referral laboratory tests.

The first step in performing these tests is to review the package insert provided by the manufacturer. This gives the following valuable information about the test:
- Principle on which the test is based
- Reagents and equipment needed
- Proper specimen collection techniques
- Patient preparation requirements
- Test procedures
- Any precautions or warnings pertaining to the procedure

The insert also provides information about quality control, interpretation of results, limitations of the procedure, and references.

Rapid Strep Testing

Rapid strep testing is commonly performed in the POL and can be completed while the patient waits. The patient's throat is swabbed (Procedure 45.2). The test swab is placed in an extraction well, and the extract is tested for antigens found on the surface of *S. pyogenes* (also referred to as group A strep or GAS). The test kit uses a *lateral flow immunoassay*. This means that the specimen "flows" into the test area. If the strep A pathogen is present, there will be an antigen-antibody reaction with the group A strep antibodies in the testing area. The reaction of the strep A antigen and the strep A antibodies cause a color change that can be seen (Procedure 45.3).

Negative test results should be confirmed with a throat culture performed in the microbiology laboratory (explained later in the chapter). The rapid strep tests are highly specific, so if the test results are positive, there is confidence that *S. pyogenes* is present in the sample. If the test results are negative, the organism may not have been present in high enough numbers to be detected. Then a transport swab should be sent to the microbiology reference laboratory to be cultured.

> ### CRITICAL THINKING 45.5
> Frankie Burns, a 10-year-old, has a raw, sore throat, fever of 101°F and just feels awful. Laura is going to collect a throat swab for a rapid strep test from Frankie. What bacteria cause strep throat? What is the scientific name of the bacteria? Which of the two names is the genus, and which of the two names is the species? Write down your answers, and share them with your classmates.

Influenza A and B Testing

The *influenza* (in floo EN zuh) virus causes influenza, or "the flu." This is a highly contagious, acute viral infection of the respiratory tract. The infection is highly communicable through the respiratory route, and outbreaks are typically seen in the fall and winter. Type A viruses usually are more common than type B viruses. Type A viruses typically are associated with epidemics, and type B viruses cause a milder infection.

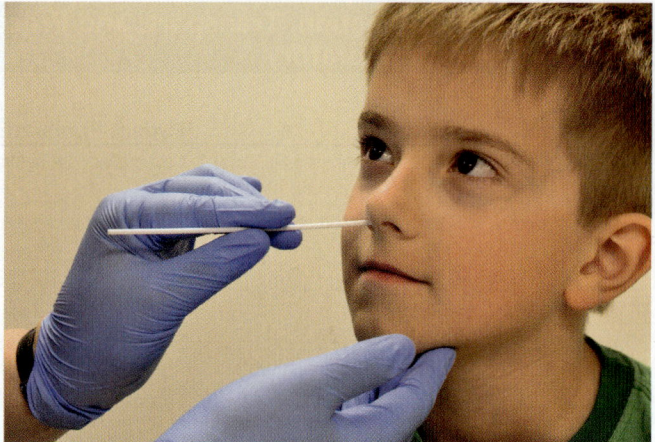

FIG. 45.9 Note the proper angle of insertion for the foam swab when collecting a nasal specimen. The swab is inserted at least 1 inch along the base of the nostril on the side that has the most discharge. Once inside, the swab is rotated and rocked back and forth gently for 5 to 10 seconds to obtain a sufficient specimen for influenza and respiratory syncytial virus (RSV) testing. (From Proctor D, et al: *Kinn's The Medical Assistant*, ed 13, St. Louis, 2017, Elsevier.)

A rapid diagnosis of influenza can help with the decision to give antiviral medications. They should be given early in the infection cycle to be the most effective. CLIA-waived rapid lateral flow immunoassays detect both influenza A and influenza B antigens from nasopharyngeal (ney zoh FAR in jee ahl) swabs or nasal washes.

Respiratory Syncytial Virus Testing

Respiratory *syncytial* (sin SISH ee ahl) virus (RSV) is a major cause of upper and lower respiratory tract infections. It is the major cause of bronchiolitis (bron kee o LIH tis) and pneumonia (noo MOHN nee uh) in children and infants. Outbreaks typically occur yearly in the fall, winter, and spring, and can be severe for very young children. The CLIA-waived rapid direct immunoassay for RSV uses a nasopharyngeal swab specimen or nasal washings to detect the virus. Because antiviral agents are available to treat RSV infection, rapid diagnosis can lead to the following:
- Shorter hospital stays
- Reduced need for antibiotic therapy to treat secondary bacterial infection
- Lower cost for hospital care

The tests are intended for children under age 5. Fig. 45.9 shows the proper placement of the swab when collecting a nasal specimen.

> ### VOCABULARY
> **bronchiolitis:** Occurs when the small airways of the lungs become inflamed because of a viral infection.
> **extract:** A certain substance that is taken out of a group or solution and is in a concentrated form.
> **extraction:** A process by which a specific substance is separated from a group or solution.
> **nasal wash:** Also called a nasal aspirate. A syringe is used to gently squirt a small amount of sterile saline into the nose, and the resulting fluid is collected into a cup (for a wash). Or after the saline is squirted into the nose, gentle suction is applied (for the aspirate).
> **nasopharyngeal:** Describes the part of the throat behind and above the soft palate and connected to the nasal passages.
> **pneumonia:** Inflammation of the lungs with congestion of the air sacs (alveoli). Can be caused by a bacterium or virus.

CHAPTER 45 Assisting in Microbiology and Immunology

PROCEDURE 45.2 Collect a Specimen for a Throat Culture

Task
Collect a throat culture, using sterile technique, for immediate testing or for transportation to the laboratory.

Equipment and Supplies
- Patient's health record
- Provider's order/or laboratory requisition
- Fluid-impermeable lab coat, face shield, and gloves
- Sterile swab if transporting to a reference laboratory, or sterile swab from the rapid strep test kit if testing patient in the POL
- Sterile tongue depressor
- Transport medium
- Biohazard waste container

Procedural Steps

1. Wash hands or use hand sanitizer. Put on a fluid-impermeable lab coat.
   Purpose: To ensure infection control.
2. Gather the materials needed.
3. Greet the patient. Identify yourself. Verify the patient's identity with full name, then ask the patient to spell the first and last name and to state his or her date of birth. Explain the procedure in a manner that the patient understands. Answer any questions the patient may have about the procedure.
   Purpose: It is important to identify the patient in two different ways to ensure that you have the correct patient. Explaining the procedure can make the patient feel more comfortable and reduces anxiety.
4. Put on face shield and gloves. Position the patient so that the light shines into the mouth.
   Purpose: To ensure infection control and to illuminate the area to be swabbed.
5. Remove the sterile swab from the sterile wrap with your dominant hand, and grasp the sterile tongue depressor with your nondominant hand.
   Purpose: To achieve better control of the swabbing process.
6. Instruct the patient to open the mouth and say, "Ah." Depress the tongue with the depressor.
   Purpose: Saying "Ah" helps elevate the uvula and reduces the tendency to gag. The tongue is depressed so that you can see the back of the throat and prevent contamination of the sterile swab.
7. Swab the back of the throat between the tonsillar pillars in a figure 8 pattern, especially any reddened, patchy areas of the throat, white pus pockets, purulent areas, and the tonsils; take care not to touch any other areas in the mouth (Fig. 1).
   Purpose: Pathogenic organisms are found in the back of the throat and on the tonsils.
8. Place the swab in the transport medium, label it, and send it to the laboratory (Fig. 2). If rapid strep testing is requested, return the labeled swab to the laboratory.
   Purpose: A transport medium prevents the swab from drying. Labeling immediately after collection prevents specimens from getting mixed up.
9. Dispose of contaminated supplies in the biohazard waste container.
   Purpose: To prevent the spread of infection.
10. Disinfect the work area.
11. Remove your gloves, and discard them in the biohazard waste container. Remove face shield.
12. Wash hands or use hand sanitizer.

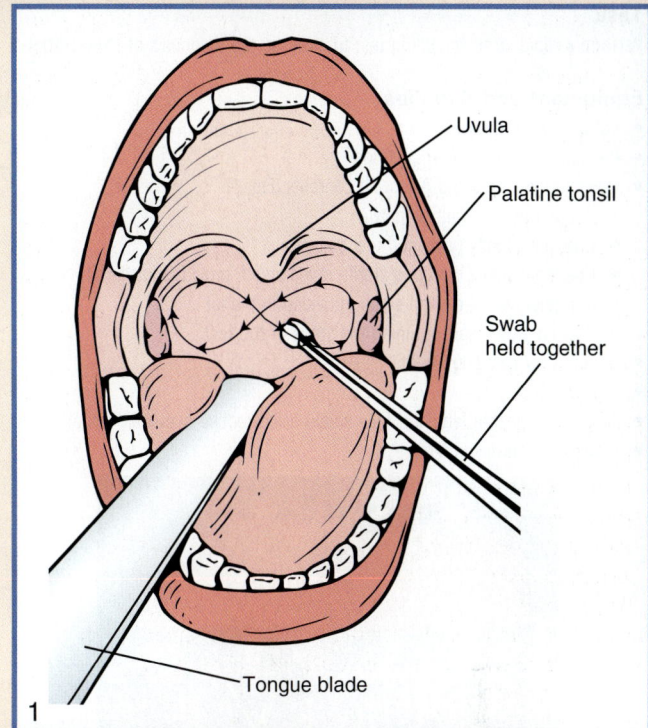

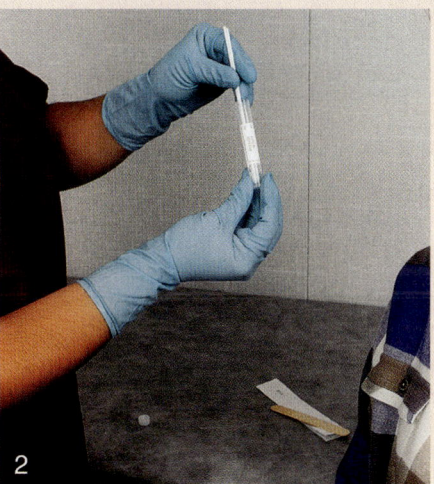

   Purpose: To ensure infection control.
13. Document the procedure in the patient's health record.
    Purpose: Procedures are not done until they are recorded.
    Documentation Example:
    8/14/20 8:35 a.m. Throat specimen collected via swab from tonsillar area. Sent to University Laboratories for strep testing. _____
    _____Laura Piper, CMA (AAMA)

PROCEDURE 45.3 Perform a CLIA-Waived Microbiology Test: Perform a Rapid Strep Test

Task
Perform a rapid strep screening test to assist in the diagnosis of strep throat.

Equipment and Supplies
- Patient's health record
- Provider's order or lab requisition
- QuickVue In-Line Strep A test kit contents (Fig. 1):
  - One extraction solution bottle
  - One individually packaged test cassette
  - One individually wrapped sterile rayon swab, provided in the kit
  - One positive (+) control swab, provided in the kit
  - A visual flow chart outlining the steps of the test
- Rapid Strep Test Log Sheet
- Stopwatch
- Fluid-impermeable lab coat, face shield or protective eyewear, gloves
- Biohazard waste container

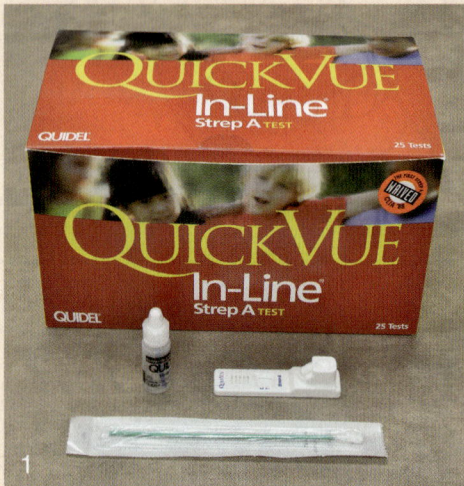

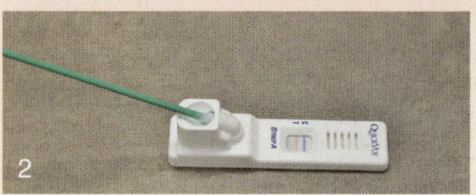

Procedural Steps

1. Collect all necessary supplies and equipment. Bring all reagents to room temperature. Check the expiration date on the test kit package.
2. Wash hands or use hand sanitizer.
   Purpose: To ensure infection control.
   Note: Before running the first patient test from a new test kit, positive and negative controls must be run using the control swabs provided in the kit. Confirm that both controls reacted correctly, and record the control results on the log sheet.
   Purpose: Both control swabs must be checked before patients are tested. If the controls show the appropriate results, the test kit is reliable.
3. Greet the patient. Identify yourself. Verify the patient's identity with full name, then ask the patient to spell the first and last name and to state his or her date of birth. Explain the procedure in a manner that the patient understands. Answer any questions the patient may have about the procedure. Obtain permission to collect a throat culture.
   Purpose: It is important to identify the patient in two different ways to ensure that you have the correct patient. Explaining the procedure can make the patient feel more comfortable and reduces anxiety.
4. Put on gloves and face shield or protective eyewear. Collect a throat specimen using the rayon swab provided in the test kit.
   Purpose: The test kit provides a rayon swab to avoid the use of cotton swabs, which can kill bacteria, possibly causing a false-negative result.
5. Remove the test cassette from the foil pouch and place it on a clean, dry, level surface. Using the notch at the back of the chamber as a guide, insert the patient's swab completely into the swab chamber (Fig. 2).
6. Place the extraction bottle between your thumb and forefinger, and squeeze once to break the glass ampule inside the extraction solution bottle. Vigorously shake the bottle 5 times to mix the solutions. The solution should turn green.
   Purpose: The color change is an indicator of extraction reagent integrity and that the extraction procedure was performed correctly.
7. Immediately remove the cap on the extraction solution bottle, hold the bottle vertically over the chamber, and quickly fill the chamber to the rim (approximately 8 drops).
   Purpose: The liquid extract reacts with the swab and then flows into the test cassette, passing through the test area (T) and then through the internal control area (C).
8. Remove your face shield. Wait 5 minutes to read the results, and record them in the lab log.
   Positive result: A pink line shows in the T area, indicating the presence of *Streptococcus pyogenes* antigen; a blue line appears in the C area, indicating that the fluid activated the internal control.
   Negative result: No pink line appears in the T test area; a blue line appears in the C control area, indicating that the internal control worked.
   Invalid result: The blue control line does not appear next to the letter C at 5 minutes. The test result cannot be reported.
9. Discard all the test materials in the appropriate biohazard waste container.
   Purpose: Items that come in contact with samples are considered potentially infectious.
10. Disinfect the work area. Remove your gloves. Wash hands or use hand sanitizer.
    Purpose: To ensure infection control.
11. Record the test results in the patient's health record.
    Purpose: A procedure is not done until the results are properly recorded.
12. If the test results are negative, a second throat swab should be obtained and sent to the reference laboratory for a throat culture. Often two swabs are used simultaneously when the sample is initially collected from the throat to prevent the need to re-collect a specimen.
    Purpose: Negative rapid strep test results should be confirmed with a throat culture.

Qualitative Control/Patient Log Sheet

TEST: ____STREP A TEST____
KIT NAME AND MANUFACTURER: __QuickVue In-Line Strep A Test – Quidel__
LOT # __12345__   EXPIRATION DATE: ____11/22/20XX____
STORAGE REQUIREMENTS: __Room Temp__   TEST FLOWCHART __yes__

Date	Specimen I.D. (Control/Patient)	Result (+ or –)	Internal Control Passed (Y or N)	Charted in Patient Record	Tech Initials
7/11/20XX	POSITIVE CONTROL	+	Y		LP
7/11/20XX	NEGATIVE CONTROL	–	Y		LP
7/11/20XX	PT ID: 5432	+	Y	✓	LP

Documentation Example:
10/9/20 9:30 a.m. Rapid Strep A Test performed with a positive result.
— Laura Piper, CMA (AAMA)

CLIA-WAIVED IMMUNOLOGY TESTING

Immunology testing provides information about past or present infections with bacteria or viruses. It also detects certain types of cancers. Testing done in the immunology department is designed to demonstrate the reaction between an antigen and its specific antibody. Antibodies are formed when the body encounters a foreign agent. In the **acute** (uh kyoot) **stage** of a disease, the antibody level is high. During the **convalescent** (kon vuh LES uh nt) **stage**, the antibody level declines. Once the immune system recognizes an antigen, then antibodies are made. The antibody will remain in the blood at a low but detectable level for a lifetime. The amount of antibody can be measured with **serologic** (si ROL uh jik) testing called a **titer** (TAHY ter).

Most serologic/immunologic testing performed in the ambulatory care center is done using individual test kits (e.g., strep, influenza, mononucleosis [mon uh nook lee OH sis], and HIV tests). The difference is the source of the specimen and what the test is looking for.

The direct immunologic tests in the previous section (strep test and influenza test) used a throat swab and nasal swab specimen. The test kits were detecting the antigen or pathogen causing the disease directly. In the indirect immunologic tests, the specimen is the patient's blood or serum. The blood or serum is tested to see whether the patient has produced the specific antibody to the pathogen in question. CLIA-waived immunology tests that can be performed by a medical assistant to detect antibodies to a pathogen include infectious mononucleosis, *Helicobacter pylori* (hee lih koh BAK tur pahy LAWR ee), Lyme disease, and human immunodeficiency virus (HIV) tests.

Infectious Mononucleosis Testing

Infectious mononucleosis, commonly called Mono, is an acute infectious disease caused by the *Epstein-Barr* (EP stahyn bahr) virus (EBV). EBV is one of the many herpes viruses. The virus is especially common in teenagers. It is found most frequently in people 10 to 25 years of age and is seen occasionally in adults over the age of 25. In the United States, about 95% of adults between 35 and 40 have already been infected.

In children, the infection may pass unrecognized or result in a mild illness lasting only a few days. It is marked by sore throat, fever, swollen tonsils, and enlarged lymph nodes in the neck. In young people, some of the most common complications include the abrupt onset of fatigue, headaches, very swollen tonsils, enlarged lymph glands, and loss of appetite often associated with nausea. There may be a short or prolonged period (days or weeks) after the initial illness when the fatigue continues. Occasionally, complications occur, including the development of a swollen spleen or liver, referred to as *hepatosplenomegaly*.

Testing for mononucleosis involves a complete blood count (CBC) and immunology tests. The CBC should reveal an increased number of lymphocytes that appear atypical on the blood smear. The infected lymphocytes undergo a cellular transformation, causing them to look like a monocyte (hence the name *mononucleosis*). Most patients exposed to EBV produce a nonspecific **heterophile** (HET er uh fihl) **antibody** response to the virus. These heterophile antibodies in the patient's blood react with the heterophile antigens supplied in the test kit, resulting in a positive color reaction in the testing area of the kit (Procedure 45.4).

MEDICAL TERMINOLOGY
ser/o: serum

VOCABULARY

acute stage: The phase during which rapid multiplication of the pathogen takes place. Symptoms are very distinct. A strong response of the immune system takes place during this stage.

convalescent stage: The phase during which the host recovers gradually and returns to baseline or normal health.

heterophile antibody: An antibody that has an affinity for an antigen other than the specific antigen that stimulated its production.

serologic: Pertaining to the science involving the immune properties and actions of serum.

titer: The lowest concentration of a serum solution containing a specific antibody where the antibody is still able to neutralize (or precipitate) an antigen.

PROCEDURE 45.4   Perform a CLIA-waived Immunology Test: Perform a QuickVue+ Infectious Mononucleosis Test

Task
Perform and interpret a rapid CLIA-waived test for infectious mononucleosis.

Equipment and Supplies
- Patient's health record
- Provider's order or lab requisition
- CLIA-waived QuickVue+ test kit for infectious mononucleosis and blood collecting supplies: (Fig. 1)
  - Package with supplies for 20 tests
  - Color-coded bottles of positive and negative controls and the developer
  - Test cassette in its foil-wrapped protective pouch
  - Alcohol wipes, gauze, and bandage
  - Pipets supplied in kit with black line indicating the amount of capillary blood to collect
  - Lancet
- Timer or wristwatch with sweep second hand
- Fluid-impermeable lab coat, protective eyewear, gloves
- Biohazard waste container

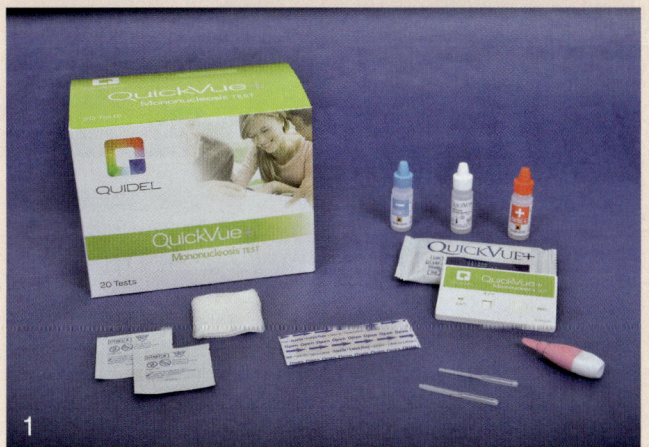

Continued

PROCEDURE 45.4 Perform a CLIA-Waived Immunology Test and Perform the QuickVue+ Infectious Mononucleosis Test—cont'd

Procedural Steps

1. Remove the test kit from the refrigerator, and allow the reagents to warm to room temperature. Check the expiration date of the kit.
   Purpose: Outdated or cold reagents do not react as expected.
2. Wash hands or use hand sanitizer. Put on the fluid-impermeable lab coat.
   Purpose: To ensure infection control.
3. Before running the first patient test from a new test kit, run the positive and negative liquid controls provided in the kit to see whether they react correctly. Record your control results on the log sheet.
   Purpose: Both control samples must be checked before patients are tested. If the controls show the appropriate results, the test kit is reliable.
4. Greet the patient. Identify yourself. Verify the patient's identity with full name, then ask the patient to spell the first and last name and to state his or her date of birth. Explain the procedure in a manner that the patient understands. Answer any questions the patient may have about the procedure. Obtain permission for the capillary puncture.
   Purpose: It is important to identify the patient in two different ways to ensure that you have the correct patient. Explaining the procedure can make the patient feel more comfortable and helps to reduce anxiety.
5. Put on gloves and protective eyewear. Remove the test device from its protective pouch, and label it with the patient's identification.
   Purpose: To ensure infection control. Label the test kit to ensure proper identity of the test being run.
6. Disinfect the patient's finger with an alcohol wipe. Allow it to dry, and then perform a capillary puncture.
7. Wipe away the first drop of blood, and then fill the disposable pipet provided in the kit to the calibration mark with capillary blood (see Chapter 43 for proper blood collection methods) (Fig. 2).
   Purpose: The plastic capillary tube measures the exact amount of sample, for accurate testing.

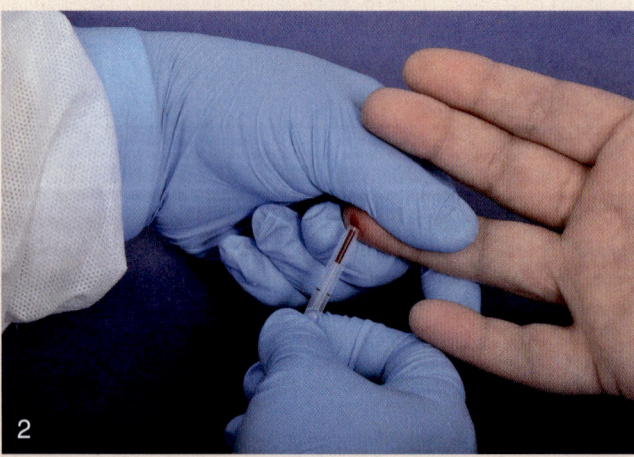

2

8. Dispense all the blood from the capillary tube into the "Add" well of the testing device. (Or, if you are using venous blood, transfer a large drop from the venous whole blood specimen using the longer capillary pipet provided in the kit.)
9. Hold the developer bottle vertically above the "Add" well, and allow 5 drops to fall freely.
   Purpose: Holding a dropper vertically ensures delivery of the same-size drop. If the dropper touches other materials, it becomes contaminated and the results will be inaccurate.

10. Read the results at 5 minutes. Note: The "Test Complete" box must be visibly colored by 10 minutes.
    Positive result: A vertical line in any shade of blue forms a plus sign in the "Read Result" window, along with a blue "Test Complete" line. Even a faint blue plus sign should be reported as a positive.
    Negative result: No vertical blue line appears, leaving a minus sign in the "Read Result" window, along with a blue "Test Complete" line.
    Invalid result: After 10 minutes, no line is visible in the "Test Complete" window, or a blue color fills the "Read Result" window. If either of these occurs, the test must be repeated with a new testing device. If the problem continues, request technical support.
11. Properly dispose of biohazardous waste material in the proper container, and disinfect the work area.
    Purpose: To ensure infection control.
12. Remove your gloves and protective eyewear. Wash hands or use hand sanitizer.
13. Document the patient's result and the control sample results in the lab logs and in the patient's health record.
    Purpose: A procedure is not done until the results are properly recorded.

Quality Control Procedures

External positive and negative liquid controls are provided with each new kit. Each new operator of the test should perform liquid positive and negative external controls once to confirm that his or her testing technique is correct. Also, external controls should be tested and charted when a new kit is used.

The *internal* control occurs in the "Test Complete" window built into each reaction unit. Chart the control results on the control log with the operator's initials.

Qualitative Control/Patient Log Sheet

TEST: ____MONONUCLEOSIS RAPID TEST_____
KIT NAME & MANUFACTURER: QUICK VUE+ Infectious Mononucleosis Test -QUIDEL
LOT # __12345_____   EXPIRATION DATE: ____11/22/20XX_____
STORAGE REQUIREMENTS: _REFRIGERATOR___ TEST FLOWCHART __yes_____

Date	Specimen I.D. (Control/Patient)	Result (+ or −)	Internal Control Passed (Y or N)	Charted in Patient Record	Tech Initials
7/11/20XX	POSITIVE CONTROL	+	Y		LP
7/11/20XX	NEGATIVE CONTROL	−	Y		LP
7/11/20XX	PT ID: 5432	−	Y	✓	LP

Documentation Example:
10/9/20 9:30 a.m. Mononucleosis rapid test performed with a negative result. Lavender-topped (EDTA) blood sample sent to lab for CBC and differential.
_____Laura Piper, CMA (AAMA)

> **CRITICAL THINKING 45.6**
>
> Allyson Anderson is 15 years old. She came into the clinic today with signs and symptoms of infectious mononucleosis. Laura is going to do a fingerstick on Allyson and do a Mono test. What are the typical signs and symptoms of Mono in a teenager? What is the Mono test checking for in Allyson's blood?

Helicobacter pylori Testing

H. pylori is a spiral-shaped bacterium that can infect the stomach's mucous layer or lining. *H. pylori* causes more than 90% of duodenal (doo uh DEEN l) ulcers and more than 80% of stomach ulcers (see Chapter 5). Several methods can be used to diagnose *H. pylori* infection. Serologic tests that measure specific *H. pylori* antibodies can determine whether a person has been infected. CLIA-waived rapid immunoassay tests use whole blood applied to a well in a test cartridge. The blood migrates from the well through the testing area of the cartridge. The presence of a line in the test area of the cartridge indicates the presence of antibodies to the pathogen *H. pylori*.

Lyme Disease Testing

Lyme disease is the most common insect-borne infectious disease in North America, and it is a significant public health concern. The spirochete bacterium *Borrelia burgdorferi* (buh REL ee uh buhrg DOR fuh rih) is the causative agent in Lyme disease.

The disease is contracted from an infected tick that bites a person. The bacteria are in the saliva of the tick. These ticks typically are found on deer, mice, dogs, horses, and birds. Infection occurs when the bacteria enter the tick bite. A characteristic bull's-eye rash, known as *erythema migrans* (er uh THEE muh MAHY grahns) (EM), develops at the bite site in 60% to 80% of patients. Lyme disease progresses in three stages. If the person is not treated, the disease progresses. The spirochete bacterium invades the skin, joints, central nervous system (CNS), heart, and other locations. Arthritic or CNS syndromes often accompany late-stage disease and may be the only clinical symptoms that indicate the infection.

Lyme disease can be detected early with a CLIA-waived test, such as the Wampole PreVue *B. burgdorferi* test. This immunoassay tests for antibodies in whole blood. A sample of blood is applied to a test cartridge, a diluent is added, and the results are read in 20 minutes. The microbiology reference laboratory should verify any positive results.

HIV Testing

HIV attacks and destroys the *T-helper (CD4) lymphocytes*. The T-helper lymphocytes play a critical role in protecting the body against infection. They work with the B lymphocytes to produce the specific antibodies that fight infections. As the HIV infection destroys more T-helper cells, the body becomes less able to fight off infections and more susceptible (suh SEP tuh buhl) to opportunistic infections. If HIV is not treated with antiretroviral (an tee reh TROH vahy ruhl) (ARV) medications, acquired immunodeficiency syndrome (AIDS) eventually develops. HIV infections become AIDS when life-threatening infections and cancers begin to appear (see Chapter 9 for more information on HIV and AIDS).

In 2013 the Centers for Disease Control and Prevention (CDC) and the World Health Organization (WHO) both advised preventive measures to control the disease. This requires early detection and early treatment of individuals infected with HIV. The sooner the virus is detected via immunology testing, the sooner treatment with ARV medications may begin.

Two CLIA-waived HIV tests are readily available to detect the presence of HIV antibodies in blood and in oral specimens.

Patients at risk of HIV infection are now strongly encouraged to take a blood test available in POLs or outpatient clinics. Note that HIV is a bloodborne pathogen. Therefore the medical assistant testing for HIV should strictly follow the Bloodborne Pathogens Standard established by the Occupational Safety and Health Administration (OSHA).

The patient may also choose to perform an oral self-test from a kit that is available at pharmacies (Fig. 45.10). The test kit includes a testing device that is rubbed once over the upper and lower gums. It then is inserted into the test vial, which is placed in a plastic stand. The test results are read in 20 minutes. The test includes an internal control band that verifies a specimen was added and that the test was run correctly (Box 45.7).

> **MEDICAL TERMINOLOGY**
>
> **hepat/o:** liver
> **hetero:** another, or different
> **-megaly:** enlargement
> **-phile:** to love or be attracted to
> **splen/o:** spleen

> **VOCABULARY**
>
> **diluent:** A liquid substance that dilutes or lessens the strength of a solution or mixture.
> **duodenal:** Describes the first section of the small intestines after the stomach.
> **opportunistic infections:** Microorganisms that normally do not cause disease but become pathogenic when the body's immune system is impaired and unable to fight off infection, as occurs with AIDS, malnutrition, and certain other diseases.

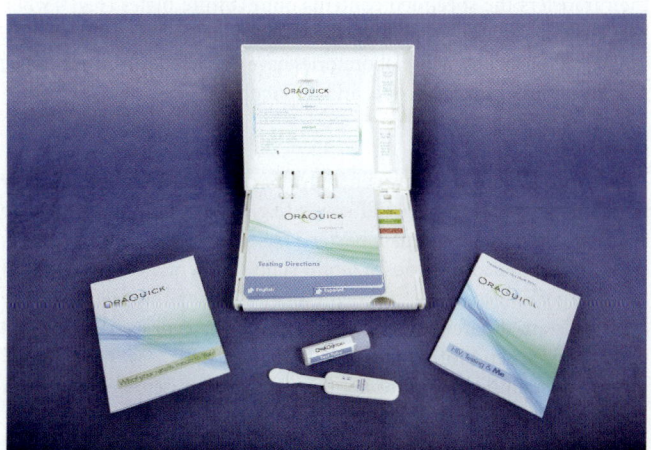

FIG. 45.10 HIV home testing kit. (From Proctor D, et al: *Kinn's The Medical Assistant*, ed 13, St. Louis, 2017, Elsevier.)

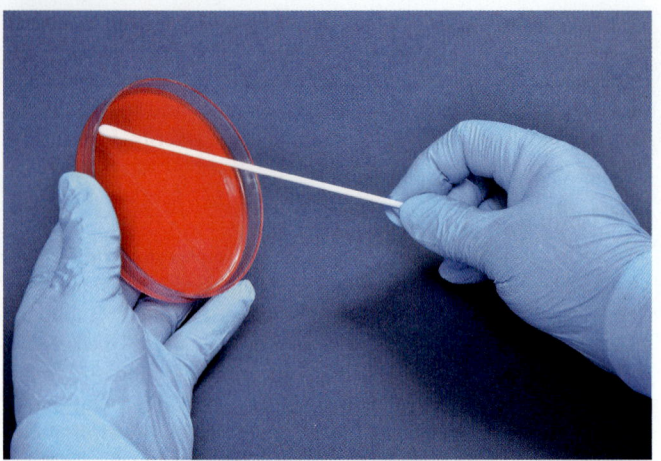

FIG. 45.11 Inoculating a blood culture plate with a swab.

BOX 45.7 HIV Testing

For both HIV testing methods, it is important to provide the patient with information or counseling regarding HIV infection and its relationship to AIDS. Be aware that patients being tested may be fearful; therefore proper knowledge presented in a therapeutic way can help them dispel the fear and take positive action toward preventive behavior and treatment. Positive HIV test results must be verified at a reference laboratory.

BOX 45.8 Fixing a Slide

Either heat or methanol can be used to *fix* the sample to the slide. Fixing results in the material (sample) adhering to the slide. Both heat (e.g., from a Bunsen burner or an incinerator) and methanol cause protein in the sample to break down and stick to the slide. It is similar to how an egg would stick to a hot frying pan.

MICROBIOLOGY REFERENCE LABORATORY: IDENTIFICATION OF PATHOGENS

After receiving the specimens collected in the POL described in the Specimen Collection and Transport in the Physician Office Laboratory section presented earlier in this chapter, the microbiology laboratory promptly prepares a smear of the specimen on a slide to be stained and then transfers the specimen contents onto culture plates (Fig. 45.11). The equipment and supplies in a microbiology laboratory vary with the size of the facility. Most laboratories have a refrigerator, an autoclave, a safety cabinet, a microscope, and an incubator.

Staining

Pathogenic microorganisms generally are colorless, and a microscope is needed to see them. Special stains (e.g., Gram stain and acid-fast stain) are used to differentiate bacteria based on cell membrane differences. As discussed previously, Gram stain differentiates bacteria into two categories according to chemical makeup of the cell wall. The acid-fast stain differentiates bacteria into two categories based on the presence or absence of a waxy lipid in the cell wall.

Before staining can be done, the specimen must be applied to a labeled slide. The slide is then air-dried and fixed (Box 45.8).

Gram Stain. The Gram stain, developed by Dr. Hans Christian Gram in the late 1800s, is still the most commonly used stain in microbiology.

This procedure involves applying a sequence of reagents: a primary stain, mordant (MAWR dnt), decolorizer, and counterstain to the slide. The dyes are taken up differently according to the chemical composition of the bacterial cell walls. Bacteria react best in the Gram stain when they are less than 24 hours old. Gram-positive bacteria stain purple, and Gram-negative bacteria stain pink or red (see Fig. 45.1). It is useful for the medical assistant to understand the procedures and the microscopic results obtained. For example, when a Gram stain report is called in, the terms *GPCs* and *GNBs* mean "Gram-positive cocci" (deeply blue-stained circular cells) and "Gram-negative bacilli," (pink/red stained rod-shaped cells).

CRITICAL THINKING 45.7

What are the four reagents used in the Gram stain? What color are Gram-positive organisms? What color are Gram-negative organisms? Share your answers with the class.

Acid-Fast Stain. The acid-fast stain is used in the identification protocol for *Mycobacterium* (mahy doh bak TEER ee uh) species. *M. tuberculosis* causes tuberculosis and can be isolated from sputum or tissue samples. *M. avium* complex (MAC) is a common soil organism that enters through the respiratory tract and spreads throughout the body. MAC is one of the causes of death among patients with AIDS. An overview of the acid-fast stain is listed here:

- A red primary dye, *carbolfuchsin* (kar BOL fyoo shin), is applied first
- Then the decolorizer, acid-alcohol, is applied
- Followed by a counterstain, *methylene* (meth uh leen) blue

Acid-fast positive microbes stain fuchsia-red. Acid-fast negative microbes stain baby blue. Bacilli that are acid-fast positive often are referred to as *acid-fast bacillus (AFB)* (see Fig. 45.2).

Inoculating Equipment

Next, the specimen must be spread on specific culture media based on the source of the specimen. The inoculated culture media are placed in a body temperature incubator to grow overnight. Inoculating needles and loops (Fig. 45.12) are used to transfer samples to culture media or microbes to slides for staining. Needles and loops may be disposable and presterilized. They may also be made of wire and can be heat sterilized before and after each transfer (Fig. 45.13). An inoculating loop is shaped like a bubble wand, and a thin film of liquid adheres to the loop. The amount of fluid held by the loop can be calibrated. For example, a urine culture uses a loop that delivers a 1-mcL sample. The urine in the loop is spread across the culture medium and allowed to grow overnight. The next day, each bacterium becomes a visible colony (KOL uh nee). Colonies can then be counted and analyzed to determine the cause of a urinary tract infection.

VOCABULARY

colony: A discrete group of organisms, such as a group of bacteria, growing on a solid nutrient surface.
decolorizer: A liquid that has the ability to wash out color.
mordant: Having the ability to fix, or set colors.

CHAPTER 45 Assisting in Microbiology and Immunology

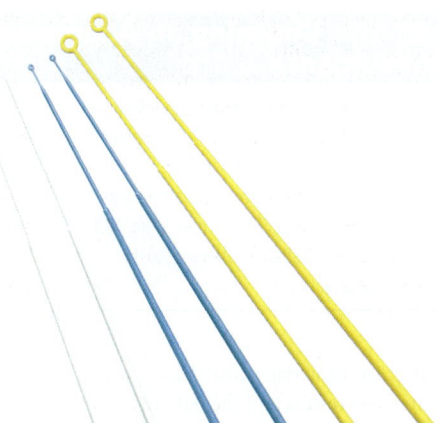

FIG. 45.12 *(Left)* Inoculating needles. *(Right)* Inoculating loops. (From Proctor D, et al: *Kinn's The Medical Assistant*, ed 13, St. Louis, 2017, Elsevier.)

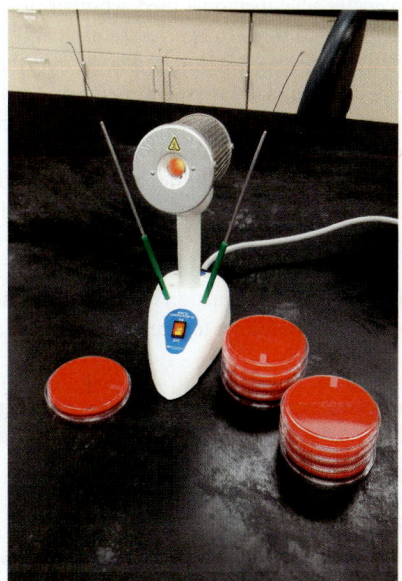

FIG. 45.13 Incinerator for sterilizing wire loops and needles.

Assessing a Culture

When the original (primary) culture has incubated at the appropriate temperature for 18 to 24 hours, it is examined for evidence of pathogens. Because normal flora is often present in samples in addition to pathogens, a trained eye is required to spot the organisms that might be causing an infection. Suspicious colonies are **subcultured** (suhb KUHL cher d) onto the appropriate medium to isolate them in **pure culture**. When the organism is in pure culture, staining and additional biochemical testing can be done to identify the organisms. Throat and urine cultures may be performed in POLs that have been CLIA certified to perform moderately-complex testing.

Throat Cultures. *Streptococcus pyogenes*, also known as *group A strep (GAS)* or *beta hemolytic streptococcus*, causes strep throat. If not diagnosed and treated promptly, this infection can cause severe complications, including scarlet fever, rheumatic (roo MAT ik) fever, and glomerulonephritis (gloh mer yuh loh nuh FRAHY tis). A throat swab is collected from the patient's throat. Then the swab is **streaked for isolation** on a **5% sheep's blood agar plate (BAP)** (Box 45.9). An antibiotic disk is placed on the first quadrant of the streaked plate (Fig. 45.14) and incubated overnight at 37°C (98.6°F). The antibiotic disk contains *bacitracin* (bas ih TREY sin), which prevents the growth of *S. pyogenes*. Complete clearing of the agar around the colonies indicates *beta hemolysis*, which is caused by a toxin produced by *S. pyogenes*. The toxin breaks down the red blood cells in the agar, causing the agar to be a clear

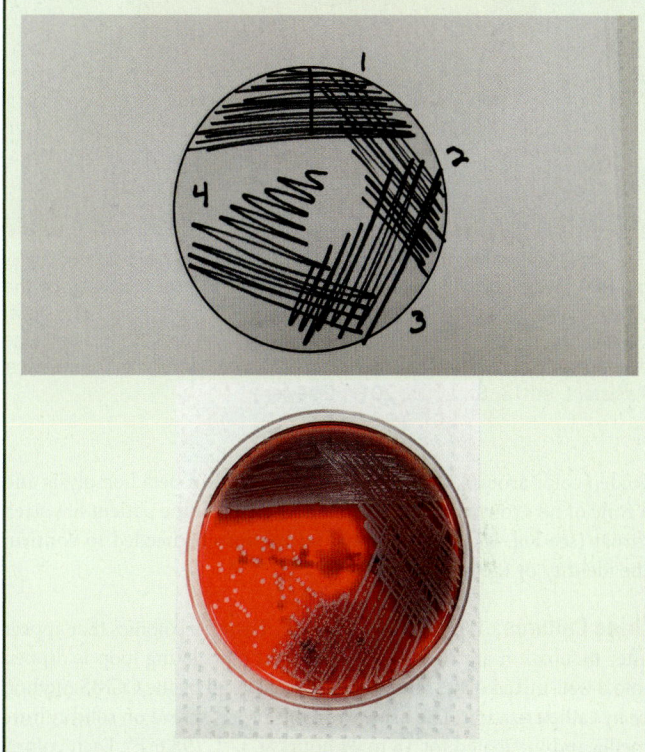

BOX 45.9 **Streaking for Isolation**

Streaking for isolation is also called a four-quadrant streak. It is a procedure that is performed with most microbiology specimens. By distributing bacteria across the agar plate and isolating bacterial colonies, laboratory personnel can see characteristics of the bacteria that are useful in the identification process.

VOCABULARY

5% sheep's blood agar plate (BAP): A solid agar medium that contains nutrients and 5% washed sheep's blood. The blood is added as an extra nutrient source for bacteria.

pure culture: The growth of only one microorganism in a culture or on a nutrient surface.

subcultured: Occurs when an organism (a bacterium) has been cultivated again on a new nutrient surface.

streaked for isolation: To have produced isolated colonies of an organism on an agar plate. Using an inoculating loop, pick one colony and methodically spread it out onto solid nutrient media. The goal is to have colonies that are separate from other colonies. See Box 45.9.

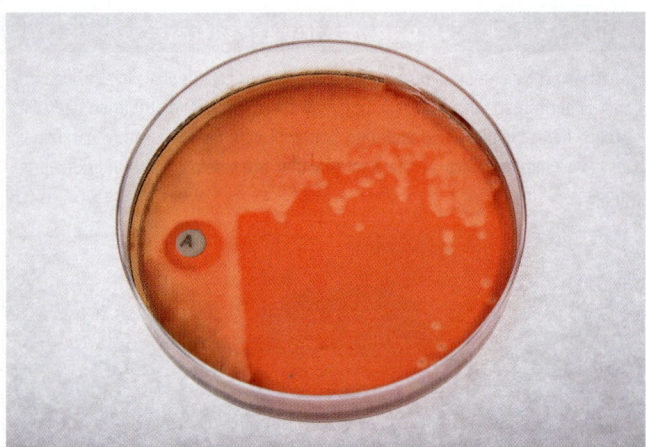

FIG. 45.14 Positive strep test result on blood agar (*left side of plate*) group A Streptococcus (GAS) shows beta hemolysis (clearing) of the blood agar below the growing colonies. Notice there is no hemolysis, or clearing of the blood around the white bacitracin disk. That is because bacitracin can destroy GAS. (From Proctor D, et al: *Kinn's The Medical Assistant*, ed 13, St. Louis, 2017, Elsevier.)

golden color around the colonies. The presence of beta hemolysis and a zone of no growth around the disk indicate that the patient has strep throat (see Fig. 45.14). Additional testing may be needed to confirm the identity of the organism.

Urine Cultures. With urine cultures, the bacterial colonies that appear after incubation are counted. A calibrated inoculating loop is dipped into a well-mixed urine sample that was collected by the CCMS method or by catheterization. The urine from the loop is spread on solid culture media and incubated for 18 to 24 hours at 37°C (98.6°F). Each colony that grows on the plate represents 1000 colony-forming units (cfu) per milliliter. The final cfu results are interpreted as follows:
- Normal: <10,000 cfu/mL of urine; no urinary tract infection (UTI) present.
- Borderline: 10,000 to 100,000 cfu/mL of urine; a chronic or relapsing infection may be present, and the test should be repeated.
- Positive: >100,000 cfu/mL of urine; a UTI is likely.

The medical assistant needs to be aware of the terminology and values reported for urine cultures.

Microbiology Culture and Sensitivity Testing

Once a bacterial infection has been identified additional steps are required for successful treatment. To determine the appropriate antibiotic to destroy the pathogen, the provider will order a culture and sensitivity (C&S) test. *Culture* refers to growing the organisms, and *sensitivity* refers to the organism's susceptibility to antibiotics.

> **BOX 45.10 Choosing an Appropriate Antibiotic Agent**
>
> The appropriate antibiotic agent meets the following criteria:
> - Destroys the infectious agent with a reasonable level of the drug
> - Is the least toxic to the patient
> - Has the least impact on normal flora of the body
> - Has the desired pharmacologic (fahr muh KOL loh jik) characteristics (preparation, route of delivery, effectiveness)
> - Is the most economical

The healthcare provider must decide which medication to order based on initial test results and the patient's physical examination. C&S test results provide vital information about which specific antibiotics work best against the particular infective pathogen.

There are many methods of performing sensitivity testing. Some methods involve culture media and antibiotic disks. Other methods are fully automated and require a very small amount of the pure culture to be tested. No matter what method is used, sensitivity testing is reported to the provider in one of three categories for each antibiotic tested:
- **S** means that the pathogen is *susceptible*, or that the antibiotic is effective in destroying that particular organism.
- **R** means that the pathogen is *resistant*, or that the antibiotic is not effective in destroying that particular organism.
- **I** means *intermediate*, or that additional testing must be performed to determine the dosage of antibiotic necessary for successful treatment.

Some testing methods may give additional information regarding the dosage tested *in vitro*. This information may be helpful as the providers choose the appropriate antibiotic for treatment (Box 45.10).

> **CRITICAL THINKING 45.8**
>
> Laura is looking over the reference laboratory results from the day. Mrs. Liz Darcy was in for an office visit yesterday and collected a urine specimen for C&S. Her preliminary culture report came back as 82,000 cfu/mL, pure culture. The identification and susceptibility report is due to follow tomorrow.
> - Does Mrs. Darcy have a urinary tract infection?
> - Does Mrs. Darcy need any additional testing for this condition?
> - In your own words, define pure culture.
> - Describe C&S in your own words.

> **VOCABULARY**
>
> **in vitro:** Latin term meaning "in glass" and commonly known as "in the laboratory."

CLOSING COMMENTS

Maintaining a laboratory in the office increases the physician's liability. By testing patients' specimens in the office, the physician assumes responsibility for the interpretation and accuracy of the results. As the person in the facility who runs the lab tests, you are responsible for maintaining accuracy in testing. A quality assurance (QA) program should include running, reading, and recording the controls supplied in each test kit. Both microbiology and immunology tests allow the patient to benefit from the convenience of POL testing. Strict confidentiality is essential. Never release information to anyone other than the patient or legal guardian.

Also note that certain infectious diseases must be reported to the CDC or to the local board of health. Each state legislature determines what diseases must be reported. Additional data for nationally notifiable diseases are published weekly in the CDC in the *Morbidity and Mortality Weekly Report* (MMWR). For additional information on infectious disease reporting, please review the reporting procedure presented in Chapter 17.

CHAPTER 45 Assisting in Microbiology and Immunology

EXCEPTIONAL CUSTOMER SERVICE

Microorganisms such as bacteria, viruses, fungi, and parasites are responsible for most human infectious diseases. Patient education plays an important role in helping the patient and family control the spread of infection. The teaching topics in the following list can help you educate a patient about infection control:

- An explanation of the patient's type of infection: bacterial, viral, fungal, or parasitic
- How infections spread
- Hand washing and sanitization, proper storage and cleaning of personal items, and disposal of contaminated supplies
- Risk factors for infection, such as poor nutritional habits or poor ventilation with airborne pathogens present
- The patient's role in specimen collection
- Patient preparation for laboratory tests, imaging tests, and other needed procedures

Explain to the patient that an infection can be transferred from person to person in many ways. Reinforce the importance of following directions for taking any medication. If patients do not follow the directions given to them by the provider and/or pharmacist, there is a real chance of the following:

- Developing complications
- Having a relapse of an infection
- Allowing an infection to spread to other areas or becoming systemic

Always listen to the patient. Be sure to answer all the patient's questions. Notify the provider of patient's concerns so that he or she can give further details or instructions before the patient leaves the facility.

CHAPTER REVIEW

In the chapter on assisting in microbiology and immunology, we learned a lot about microorganisms. Microorganisms are any microscopic organisms, such as bacteria, protozoa, fungi, parasites, and helminths (eggs). Because viruses are not alive, most scientists refer to them as infectious agents or infectious particles.

We discussed the classification of organisms and how microorganisms are named. There is a system of binomial nomenclature that gives names to all living organisms. The names consist of a genus, or more general name, and a species name, which is a specific name.

We also discussed a number of characteristics of bacteria, such as the following:

- Staining properties: including the Gram stain and acid-fast stain
- Bacterial shapes: cocci, bacilli, and spirilla
- Oxygen requirements: aerobic, anaerobic, and facultative anaerobic
- Physical structures: flagella and endospores

Some bacteria do not have all of the typical characteristics. This group includes chlamydia, mycoplasma, and rickettsia. These organisms have unique characteristics and therefore must be identified and treated differently. All three types of bacteria are pathogenic and must be considered when certain conditions and symptoms exist.

We discussed a variety of pathogenic (disease causing) fungi, protozoa, parasites, helminths, and viruses. These organisms or agents have unique characteristics and can cause disease. Microbiology includes all types of microorganisms, so we have to think beyond just bacteria when discussing possible pathogens.

Specimen collection is an important part of the medical assistant's job. If they are collecting a sample, medical assistants need to be aware of PPE and proper techniques to collect and not contaminate specimens. They also need to be aware of proper infection control. Proper collection, handling, and transport are critical to getting the correct specimen to its location safely and in a viable state.

We also went over CLIA-waived testing in microbiology and immunology. The microbiology testing methods discussed include rapid strep testing, influenza A and B testing, and respiratory syncytial virus (RSV) testing. The types of immunology testing discussed include infectious mononucleosis testing, *Helicobacter pylori* testing, Lyme disease testing, and HIV testing.

Testing that needs to be done in a reference laboratory related to microbiology and immunology includes the following:

- Gram and acid-fast stains
- Use and choices of inoculating equipment
- Assessing a culture: throat and urine
- Antibiotic sensitivity testing

We closed our discussion about microbiology and immunology testing with a look at infectious disease in general and the need for proper patient education regarding infection control and antibiotic use.

SCENARIO WRAP-UP

Laura has had another busy day at Walden-Martin Family Medical (WMFM) Clinic. Once again, she has seen infectious diseases in some of her patients today. Laura knows that most microorganisms are harmless, but knowing the signs and symptoms of common infectious diseases is important.

Laura knows how important it is to diagnose and treat infectious diseases. She knows that proper specimen collection is essential. She is also aware that rapid CLIA-waived tests can identify pathogens and help treat patients in a timely manner.

Microbiology and immunology tests have become useful in the physician office laboratory. Meeting the needs of patients and quickly addressing their concerns are benefits of CLIA-waived testing. Laura feels comfortable collecting specimens, testing patient samples, and reporting the results for the provider to review. As a certified medical assistant, she knows that the work she does throughout the day is helping every one of her patients.

46

Career Development

LEARNING OBJECTIVES

1. Describe personality traits important to employers.
2. Discuss personality traits, technical skills, and transferable job skills.
3. Describe how to develop a career objective and identify your personal needs.
4. Explain job search methods.
5. Create a resume and cover letter.
6. Complete an online profile and job application.
7. Describe how to create a career portfolio.
8. Describe how to prepare for a job interview.
9. Discuss the following related to the interview:
   - Describe tips when interviewing.
   - Practice interview skills during a mock interview.
   - List legal and illegal interview questions.
10. Explain how to follow up after an interview and create a thank-you note for an interview.
11. Describe ways to improve your job opportunities.
12. Explain common human resource hiring requirements, getting started on the job, maintaining your job, and leaving your job.

CHAPTER OUTLINE

1. Opening Scenario, 1127
2. You Will Learn, 1127
3. Introduction to Career Development, 1127
4. Understanding Personality Traits Important to Employers, 1127
    a. Collaboration and Interpersonal Skills, 1127
    b. Professionalism, 1128
    c. Compassion, 1128
    d. Genuine Interest, 1128
5. Assessing Your Strengths and Skills, 1128
    a. Personality Traits, 1128
    b. Technical Skills, 1129
    c. Transferable Job Skills, 1129
6. Developing Career Objectives, 1129
7. Identifying Personal Needs, 1130
8. Finding a Job, 1130
    a. Two Best Job Search Methods, 1130
        i. *Networking, 1130*
        ii. *Job Boards, 1130*
    b. Additional Job Search Methods, 1131
        i. *School Career Placement Offices, 1131*
        ii. *Newspaper Ads, 1131*
        iii. *Employment Agencies, 1131*
9. Developing a Resume, 1131
    a. Resume Formats, 1131
    b. Resume Content, 1132
        i. *Header, 1132*
        ii. *Education, 1133*
        iii. *Work Experience, 1134*
        iv. *Summary and Skills, 1135*
        v. *Certifications, 1135*
    c. Appearance of the Resume, 1135
10. Developing a Cover Letter, 1136
11. Completing Online Profiles and Job Applications, 1138
12. Creating a Career Portfolio, 1140
13. Job Interview, 1140
    a. Preparation for the Interview, 1140
        i. *Research the Healthcare Facility, 1140*
        ii. *Practice Answers to Questions, 1141*
        iii. *Decide on Your Interview Attire, 1141*
        iv. *Prepare for the Interview Day, 1141*
    b. During the Interview, 1142
        i. *Answering Interview Questions, 1142*
        ii. *Illegal Interview Questions, 1143*
        iii. *Phone Interview, 1144*
        iv. *Face-to-Face Interview, 1144*
        v. *Video Interview, 1144*
    c. Follow-up After the Interview, 1144
    d. Negotiation, 1145
14. Improving Your Opportunities, 1145
    a. Finding Job Postings, 1145
    b. Increasing Interview Opportunities, 1145
    c. Increasing Job Offers, 1145
15. You Got the Job!, 1146
    a. Human Resource Requirement, 1146
    b. Getting Started, 1146
    c. Maintaining Your Job, 1147
    d. Leaving a Job, 1147
16. Closing Comments, 1147
17. Chapter Review, 1147
18. Scenario Wrap-Up, 1148

CHAPTER 46 Career Development

OPENING SCENARIO

Michelle, Krysia, and Zacarias (or "Zac" to his friends) met during their first semester of college. They have developed a great friendship over the last few months. They will be graduating from the medical assistant program in less than 6 weeks. Michelle just graduated from high school a year ago. Krysia entered the military just after her high school graduation. She spent 10 years in the Marines. Zac has been out of high school for several years and worked in a factory. He started as a line worker and gradually advanced to supervisory positions. Due to downsizing, his position was eliminated. He went back to school. These friends are looking forward to graduation and getting jobs as medical assistants.

As these three friends discuss finding a job, Michelle is hesitant about the job search experience. Her only work experience is 2 years as a waitress at a local restaurant. She has never created a resume or a cover letter. She only had a very informal interview with the restaurant owner before she was given the job. Krysia is concerned about her military career. The positions she held were not related to health care. She managed inventory and supervised others. She was also deployed to many hot spots around the world. Zac has a lot of experience in the factory setting, but he feels that world is so different from health care. As they talk with each other, it is clear that each person has a unique situation, and they all must take a closer look at their past experiences as they prepare for their job search adventure.

YOU WILL LEARN

- The personality traits important to employers.
- The best job search methods.
- To develop a resume and cover letter.
- To complete a job application.
- How to prepare for an interview.

INTRODUCTION TO CAREER DEVELOPMENT

As you move toward graduation, you may be experiencing many emotions. You might be excited about finishing your medical assistant program. You might be scared of the future changes. The thought of finding a job might be overwhelming. These are common feelings of all graduates. The important step before graduation is to prepare for the next phase: getting a job.

Preparing for the job-seeking phase is very important. This chapter will help you:
- Understand the characteristics that employers want
- Identify your strengths, experiences, and skills
- Develop your career objectives

When you have done these things, you are ready to market yourself to potential employers. You will market yourself through your resume and interview experiences. Remember that an early job search, even before graduation, can be the key to landing a job soon after graduation.

UNDERSTANDING PERSONALITY TRAITS IMPORTANT TO EMPLOYERS

It is important to understand what employers are looking for in employees. Employers spend money and time training new employees. It is critical that they initially find the right employees. Many employers will agree that they can help refine technical skill proficiencies. It is more difficult to help grow or change personality traits. We will examine the four personality traits that are most important to employers.

Collaboration and Interpersonal Skills

Collaboration (kuh LAB uh rae shun) and interpersonal skills are crucial to the efficiency of the healthcare environment. Employers look for people who can blend well with the current staff. New employees need to be flexible, dependable, supportive of peers, and remain calm under pressure. Employers want employees who will provide excellent customer service by having outstanding interpersonal skills. These include verbal and nonverbal communication skills, listening skills, and good manners (Fig. 46.1). (Refer to Chapter 15, for more information on verbal and nonverbal communication skills.)

- Effective verbal communication involves using clear, thoughtful, and easily understood language.
- Nonverbal communication relays more information to patients and peers than any words you could use. Eye contact, posture, voice, and gestures provide insights into a person's attitude (Fig. 46.2). Being focused, calm, polite, and interested in the other person are traits of effective nonverbal communication.
- Listening is critical when working with peers and patients. For effective communication to occur, listening must occur. Appropriate questions can draw others into the conversation and show others you are listening and care. Communication techniques

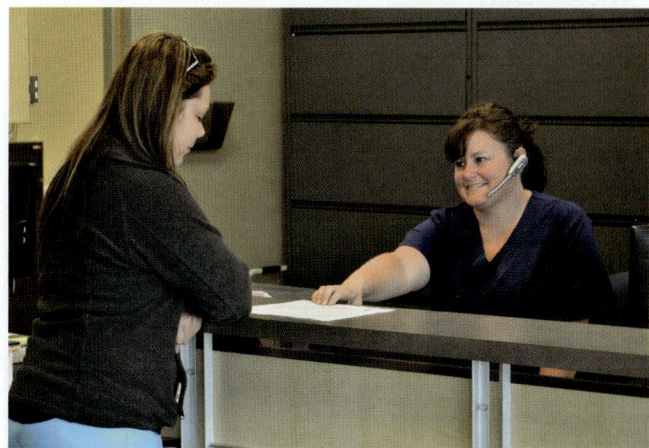

FIG. 46.1 Good communication skills and good manners are necessary to provide excellent customer service. (From Proctor D, et al: *Kinn's The Medical Assistant*, ed 13, St Louis, 2017, Elsevier.)

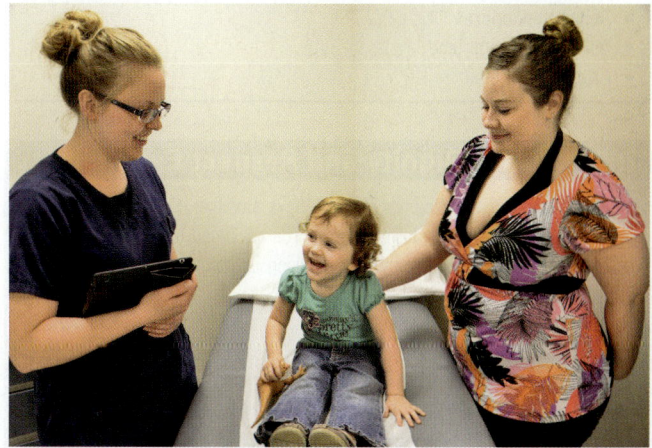

FIG. 46.2 It is important that medical assistants working in a family practice or pediatric setting have a positive attitude and enjoy working with children. (From Proctor D, et al: *Kinn's The Medical Assistant*, ed 13, St Louis, 2017, Elsevier.)

such as **reflecting**, **paraphrasing**, **summarizing**, and asking for **clarification** are also excellent ways of demonstrating active listening skills.
- Good manners and a basic understanding of the diversity of your patient population also help to facilitate communication.

Professionalism

A person's professionalism is being evaluated from the cover letter to the interview and beyond. Employers are looking for employees who project a professional image in all situations. Professionalism includes a person's appearance and behaviors (Box 46.1).

Compassion

Compassion is another trait employers look for. *Compassion* means to have a deep awareness of another's suffering and the desire to lessen it. **Dignity** and respect are part of providing compassionate care to others (Box 46.2). Many people go into health care to help others. They may like the technical skills involved with patient care. Providing dignity and respect during patient care is just as important. Compassion and respect help healthcare employees connect to patients and their families. Acts of kindness and thoughtfulness that lessen stress are welcomed by patients.

> **VOCABULARY**
> **clarification:** Allows the listener to get additional information.
> **collaboration:** The act of working with another or other individuals.
> **dignity:** Being worthy of honor and respect from others.
> **interpersonal skills:** The ability to communicate and interact with others; sometimes referred to as "soft skills."
> **reflecting:** Putting words to the patient's emotional reaction, which acknowledges the person's feelings.
> **paraphrasing:** Rewording a statement to check the meaning and interpretation; also shows you are listening and understanding the speaker.
> **summarizing:** Allowing the listener to recap and review what was said.

BOX 46.1 Professionalism Encompasses These Areas

- Dress and grooming habits
- Flexibility
- Punctuality
- Honesty
- Ability to follow directions
- Ability to prioritize
- Ability to manage time
- Attention to detail

BOX 46.2 Dignity and Respect Example

Imagine being a patient in your 70s. You have a walker. You spent 4 months in a wheelchair recovering from a stroke. You are proud to be walking today, even if you are slow. You know that walking is important so you don't get stiff and then can't walk.

The medical assistant calls you in for the visit. You slowly walk to her and then she takes you down the hall. She is far ahead of you as you slowly make your way. It appears the room is at the end of the long hall. You hear the medical assistant calling to a peer to get a wheelchair. She looks back at you and states, "We have a wheelchair for you to speed things up." How do you feel? Do you feel that she values you? Is she showing you respect?

If you reverse the roles, how could you, as a medical assistant, show her respect and that you value her?

Genuine Interest

Employers also look for people genuinely interested in the job. This trait can be seen during the interview. Does the person ask thoughtful questions regarding the position and the facility? Genuine interest in the job extends beyond the hiring phase into the day-to-day operations. Being interested in one's job is critical. Looking for ways to improve procedures and provide better patient care is an important behavior to demonstrate to the employer. This genuine interest is reflected in your attitude and performance in the workplace (Fig. 46.3). It helps ease your transition into a new job and promotes your success.

CRITICAL THINKING BOX 46.1

Think of the three friends. Michelle just graduated from high school and has 2 years of waitressing experience. Krysia has 10 years in the military, where she managed inventory, supervised others, and was deployed to many hot spots around the world. Zac has been working in a factory, advancing to supervisory positions. Now think about the personality traits that employers want. What personality traits might each friend possess? Explain your answer.
- Create your own list of the personality traits that employers want and you possess.

ASSESSING YOUR STRENGTHS AND SKILLS

As you prepare to market yourself to potential employers, you need to examine your strengths and skills in three different areas. What personality traits do you possess? What technical skills are your strengths? What are the transferable job skills that you possess?

Personality Traits

In addition to the typical personality traits required by employers, the job posting may list extra traits, including personality traits. Which of these skills and strengths do you possess? Many people will tell potential employers what they think employers want to hear. They claim to be "a team player," to "communicate well," to be "dependable," and so on. Listing these phrases on your resume or during the interview is not enough to convince the potential employer that you truly have those characteristics. They like "supporting evidence"!

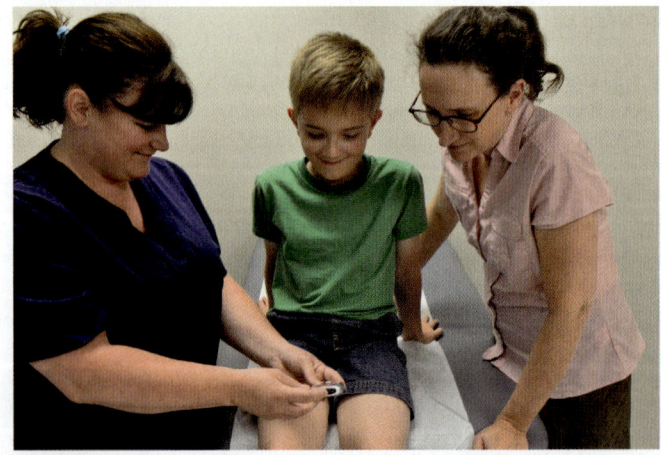

FIG. 46.3 Enjoyment of the job is paramount. Medical assistants should enjoy their work and give compassionate, friendly care to all patients. (From Proctor D, et al: *Kinn's The Medical Assistant*, ed 13, St Louis, 2017, Elsevier.)

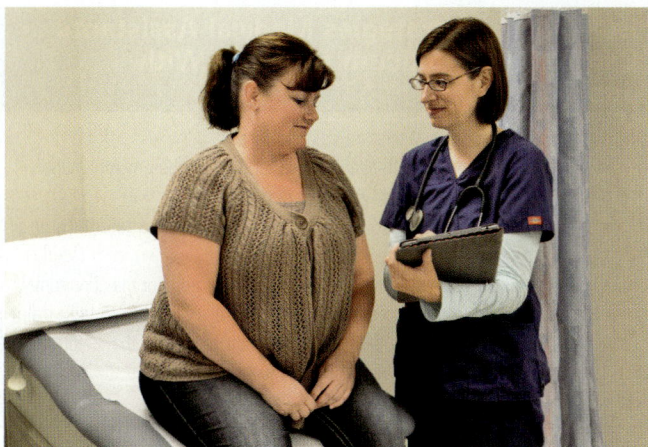

FIG. 46.4 The potential employer needs to know about the technical skills you have practiced in the classroom and the practicum setting. (From Proctor D, et al: *Kinn's The Medical Assistant*, ed 13, St Louis, 2017, Elsevier.)

Early on in the preparation phase, make a list of the qualities that you believe you possess. For each quality provide one or two pieces of "evidence" to support your claims. Your "evidence" may be a past job review or practicum evaluation in which the author indicates your strengths and characteristics. These are excellent documents to include in your portfolio, which will be discussed later in the chapter. Using stories of situations in which you portrayed those characteristics is another way to illustrate your qualities. It is important to share these during the interview, if pertinent to the questions asked.

Technical Skills

Employers are also interested in your technical skills. Technical skills for medical assistants can be related to clinical procedures, such as phlebotomy, injections, electrocardiograms (ECGs), and obtaining vital signs (Fig. 46.4). Technical skills can also be related to administrative procedures, including software proficiency, keyboard speed, reception duties, and coding procedures.

You may be able to provide supporting documentation of your technical skills through the use of practicum skill checklists or through a portfolio. Technical skills might also include skills that you developed outside of the medical assistant program but that still relate to your chosen career. For instance, if you worked as a pharmacy technician at a local hospital, several of the technical skills you acquired may relate to a clinic position.

Transferable Job Skills

Transferable job skills is the last area to examine. A person develops these skills in one job or experience. The skills can be "transferred" to another job. This means the person will use these skills in other jobs. Box 46.3 lists potential transferable skills. Many of these skills may sound familiar. They are also characteristics employers are looking for.

Identifying transferable job skills can be difficult for many people. Job descriptions for past experiences can be very useful. To start, make a list of your past jobs, military experience, and volunteer opportunities. Make a list of potential transferable skills you developed and used for each experience. Some examples of transferable skills for different jobs and situations include:
- Wait staff jobs: Strong communication and listening skills, prioritizing, and customer service skills
- Factory jobs: Communications skills, teamwork, and problem solving

> **BOX 46.3 Potential Transferable Skills**
> - Customer service
> - Compassion and empathy
> - Strong communication and listening skills
> - Computer skills
> - Leadership skills
> - Organizational skills
> - Teamwork
> - Time management and prioritizing skills
> - Creativity
> - Grace under pressure
> - Problem-solving skills

- Military experience: Strong communication skills, grace under pressure, and prioritizing
- Stay-at-home parent: Organization, prioritizing, and problem solving

This list of transferable job skills will be used as you create your resume and prepare for your interview.

> **CRITICAL THINKING BOX 46.2**
> What might be some transferable skills that the three friends, Michelle, Krysia, and Zac, possess? Explain your answer.
> - Using the list you have already started, add on the personality traits, technical skills, and transferable job skills that you possess. Also, indicate why you believe you have these skills (e.g., which job or experience helped you develop the skill).

DEVELOPING CAREER OBJECTIVES

Each medical assistant has a reason for entering the healthcare field. This basic desire should influence decisions concerning his or her career choices. Because medical assisting is such a versatile profession, a medical assistant has numerous options after graduation.

Medical assistant students should take some time to think about what they want from their careers. While the medical assistant is attending school and subsequently completing the practicum, ideas may surface about the area of health care or a specific facility in which she or he most wants to work.

When developing career objectives, the medical assistant should start by asking several questions:
- What areas and skills did I enjoy in practicum?
- Where do I want to be in 5 years?
- Where do I want to be in 10 years?
- What additional skills do I need to get where I want to go?

Write down the questions and answers and go into specific detail. Set realistic goals and develop a plan as to how and when they will be reached. Remember, career objectives are reached over time. It is important to know where you want to be, so you can start down the right path to reach your goals. Keep your list of goals available and visible so you can revisit it frequently.

> **CRITICAL THINKING BOX 46.3**
> For the following four questions, write down your answers and explain them. These answers will help you as you start the job search process.
> - What areas and skills did I enjoy in practicum?
> - Where do I want to be in 5 years?
> - Where do I want to be in 10 years?
> - What additional skills do I need to get where I want to go?

> **BOX 46.4   Certification Exams**
>
> - Certified Medical Assistant (CMA) through the American Association of Medical Assistants (AAMA)
> - Registered Medical Assistant (RMA) through the American Medical Technologists (AMT)
> - Medical Assistant Certification (CCMA) through the National Healthcareer Association
> - Medical Assistant (NCMA) through the National Center for Competency Testing (NCCT)

IDENTIFYING PERSONAL NEEDS

The next step in the process is to identify personal needs. What do you need in a job? Do you need a specific wage to meet your living expenses? What benefits do you need? What hours do you need to work? Some people need to consider day care and school hours for their children. How far are you willing to travel for a job? Do you have a reliable mode of transportation?

Evaluating your personal needs will help you find a job that matches your requirements.

> **CRITICAL THINKING BOX 46.4**
>
> What are your personal needs? Make a list identifying your needs that must be considered when seeking a new position.

FINDING A JOB

Finding employment and staying employed in health care are typically not difficult. Usually healthcare employment needs remain high, even in a poor economy. However, graduation from a medical assisting program does not guarantee employment. Completion of the program gives the medical assistant the job skills needed to work. A good attitude and positive outlook are essential for success in the job search. The medical assistant should always be open to new and better opportunities.

Some job seekers assume that potential employers will not interact with students until they have passed a credential examination (Box 46.4). However, searching for a job before graduation is a smart idea. Some employers do not require credentialing examinations. Others may hire a medical assistant before the exam is taken. They may have an agreement that the medical assistant obtain the credential within a specified period of time. Many employers are interested in hiring new graduates. They consider new graduates "teachable." This means they can train and "mold" them into the employee they require. Employers recognize that new graduates have more current knowledge and skills.

Two Best Job Search Methods

There are many ways to find employment. Networking and checking job boards are the best and most effective methods.

> **VOCABULARY**
>
> **job boards:** Websites where employers post jobs, that can be used by job seekers to identify open positions.

Networking. *Networking* is the exchange of information among others in your field. For medical assistant graduates or students searching for a job, networking involves meeting individuals in health care. It also involves sharing information on available opportunities. Through the medical assistant program, a student forms a network of friends and acquaintances (Fig. 46.5). Staying in contact with these people allows for networking opportunities. Email, LinkedIn, Facebook, Twitter, and other electronic advances make staying in touch very easy.

> **BOX 46.5   Strategies Medical Assistants Can Use in Practicum to Assist With Job Seeking**
>
> During practicum, medical assistant students can:
> - Inquire about potential job openings, either through their mentor, supervisor, or the facility's human resource department.
> - Ask their mentors if they would be willing to provide a reference or a letter of recommendation.
> - Show their gratitude by formally thanking their mentors for the opportunity. In most cases, the practicum agencies donate assistance to help train the medical assistant student. It is important to send a thank-you note to the mentor, the supervisor, and to the department.
> - Provide the supervisor with a resume and cover letter.

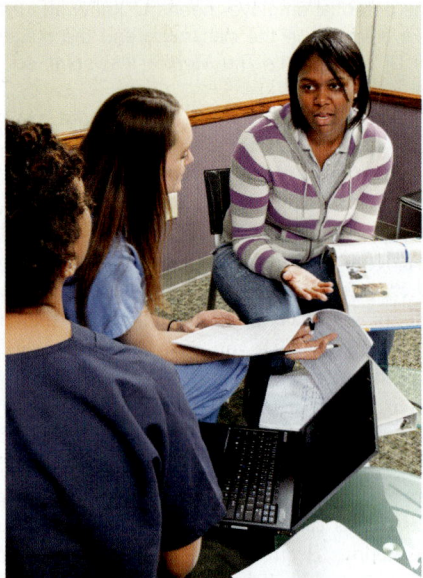

FIG. 46.5 Stay in touch with classmates. They are excellent networking contacts and may be able to provide job leads. (From Proctor D, et al: *Kinn's The Medical Assistant*, ed 13, St Louis, 2017, Elsevier.)

The practicum experience gives medical assistant students opportunities to network. During the practicum (externship), you will be working with many healthcare professionals. It is crucial that you look at the practicum as a continuous job interview (Box 46.5). It is important to be professional, follow the guidelines, and strive to do your very best. It is not uncommon that, when staff members find a student who portrays the characteristics of a professional medical assistant, they are willing to help the student find a job.

Another networking technique is to join a medical assistant organization. The members who attend regular meetings often know about job leads in the area. Creating connections with currently employed medical assistants can be helpful in the job search process.

> **CRITICAL THINKING BOX 46.5**
>
> Michelle, Krysia, and Zac know that networking is a great way to find employment. They make a list of people with whom they can share their resume or inform that they are now ready to seek employment as a medical assistant.
> - Who among your relatives would be good prospects for networking?
> - Who among your professional contacts would be good prospects for networking?

- *Facility job boards*: Larger healthcare facilities post job openings on their websites. The employment website can use different tools that make the process easier for the job seeker and the employer. Some sites allow the job seeker to register for a specific type of job. The software will generate emails to job seekers when new jobs are posted. Some websites allow job seekers to complete online profiles or applications and upload a resume and cover letter. These tools are useful to both the job seeker and the facility.
- *Public job boards*: These job boards include jobs from a variety of employers. The job boards can be local, state, or national. Local job boards may be found through your school or your community's media (i.e., newspaper, television, radio) agencies. These websites target the local audience. They are usually cheaper for employers. Smaller healthcare organizations tend to advertise using these boards. The Department of Workforce in each state addresses unemployment. They provide a job board for job seekers. National job boards, such as Monster and Indeed, provide job seekers the ability to search for openings across the country. Medical assistant jobs available in the federal government can be found at the website http://www.usajobs.gov.

Many positions for medical assistants use alternative job titles. Some agencies may use "technician" or "coordinator" for medical assistant jobs. It is important to research the local job titles that are used for medical assistants. If you do not know the local job title, try looking at the allied health positions. Look at a job posting and check the educational requirement. What are the educational requirements? Are the duties skills you have? Make a list of job titles related to medical assisting and search by those as you identify potential openings.

> **BOX 46.6 Being Organized in Your Job Search**
>
> As you submit your resume and cover letter for various positions, it is important that you keep organized. You should have a log to track the jobs you have applied for. You should also keep the original electronic files of your customized documents.
>
> Create a handwritten or electronic log of the jobs you apply for. Include the job title, number, and facility name. When you submit your resume and cover letter, update the log with the date of those activities. As you get notified about an interview, add the interview information (e.g., date, time, location, interview team members) to your log. Continually update the status of each job in the log.
>
> It is important for you to save the customized documents for each job position. If you are called for an interview, it is important to bring copies of your customized resume and cover letter. The easiest method is to create a job seeking folder on your computer. For each job you apply for, create a subfolder in the job seeking folder. Save your customized resume and cover letter in the subfolder. Save any other documents related to that job in that subfolder, including the job posting. If you get called for an interview, print the customized resume and cover letter for your interview portfolio and for the interviewer(s). You may also want to print the job posting as a reference during the interview.
>
> One of the most important things to remember with job searching is that it takes time, stamina, and persistence to find a job. Do not expect to get a job with the first resume and cover letter you send or with the first interview you have. By keeping good records, you will not apply for the same job twice or overlook job opportunities because you thought you had applied for them already.

> **CRITICAL THINKING BOX 46.6**
>
> Michelle, Krysia, and Zac make a list of possible job boards to review frequently for medical assistant postings. They know that sometimes the postings are only available for a short time, so they develop a schedule to review the sites.
> - Make a list of five job boards you would like to check for potential jobs.
> - What might be other titles that are used for medical assistants in your area?

Additional Job Search Methods

Besides using networking and checking job boards, the medical assistant can find job postings by other, more traditional methods. The school's placement office resources, newspaper ads (online and print), and employment agencies also can have medical assistant job postings.

School Career Placement Offices. Students usually have lifetime access to their school placement offices. Students and graduates should take advantage of the opportunities offered. Many schools offer resume building, job search classes, and interviewing assistance. School placement offices may also work with local employers to advertise their openings online to graduates. The school has a vested interest in helping you find employment. The placement office should be the first resource for the student's job search.

Newspaper Ads. Smaller healthcare facilities usually use newspaper ads to find potential employees. Many newspaper companies post their ads online. This allows more job seekers to view those positions.

Employment Agencies. Employment agencies hire staff to fill in at healthcare facilities. The employment agency is paid by the facility to staff different positions. Some employment agencies hire and pay the medical assistant. The medical assistants work in a healthcare facility as employment agency employees. After a period of time, if the medical assistant proves to be a good employee, the healthcare facility then hires that person. This allows the employment agency to do the hiring, firing, and managing of employees until the employees "prove themselves" to the healthcare facility (Box 46.6).

DEVELOPING A RESUME

The purpose of a resume is to "market" yourself. You want an employer interested in you. You want your resume to be included in those selected for an interview. A resume summarizes your qualifications, education, and experience. Medical assistants must determine what to include in the resume. The resume should be developed before the cover letter is written. Strengths for the posted job must be identified and highlighted on all documents. These documents include the resume, cover letter, and application.

Resume Formats

There are three commonly used resume formats: chronologic, combination, and targeted resumes. The resume format used will depend on the medical assistant's situation.

A *chronologic resume* is the most popular format used. It is useful when people are seeking employment in the same field as their education or prior experience. The chronologic resume focuses on the person's

Michelle Marison

1234 Cedar Way, Mytown, OH 45458
Home phone: 715.555.1899
Cell phone: 715.555.1355
mmarison@elsevier.net

Education

Community College, Mytown, OH
Medical Assistant Diploma, 20XX
- GPA 3.6

Health Care Experience

Family Practice Associates, Mytown, OH
Medical Assistant Practicum, April 20XX to May 20XX (220 hours)
- Performed injections, electrocardiogram, wound care, phlebotomy, throat swabs, and waived tests.
- Obtained vital signs and measurements on children and adults.
- Utilized an electronic health record to document patients' histories, test results and treatments.
- Answered calls, checked-in patients, and updated patients' demographic and insurance information.

Mytown Hospital, Mytown, OH
Volunteer, January 20XX to May 20XX
- Provided hospital information to visitors.
- Maintained confidentiality of patients.
- Assisted with deliveries of mail and flowers to patients.
- Assisted nursing staff as needed.

Work Experience

Mytown Family Diner, Mytown, OH
Waitress, June 20XX to present
- Provide efficient, accurate, and timely service to customers.
- Prioritize duties to meet customer needs.
- Provide exceptional customer service.

Special Skills

Fluent in Spanish.
Keyboarding speed: 73 wpm
Proficient in word processing and spreadsheet software

Credentials

Certified Medical Assistant, American Association of Medical Assistants (expires May 20XX)
BLS for Healthcare Providers, American Heart Association (expires March 20XX)

FIG. 46.6 Chronologic resume.

Zacarias Garcia

523 River Way, Mytown OH 45459
Cell phone: 715.555.5472
ZacGarcia@elsevier.net

Education

Community College, Mytown, OH
Medical Assistant Diploma, 20XX
- Medical Assistant Practicum at Mytown Orthopedic and Massage Center, Mytown, OH
  - o Obtained and charted history and vital signs in electronic health record.
  - o Assisted providers with tests and treatments.

Credentials

Certified Medical Assistant, American Association of Medical Assistants, expires May 20XX.
BLS for Healthcare Providers, American Heart Association, expires March 20XX.

Skills and Achievement

Strong communication skills
- Supervised 60 employees in a factory setting for over 3 years.
- Initiated procedures to improve communication between employees and management.
- Promoted in union to assist with negotiations with upper management.
- Fluent in Spanish.

Excellent problem-solving skills
- Problem-solved factory issues that delayed shipments to customers.
- Initiated solutions to expedite shipments and increased the profit margin of the company.

Excel in Teamwork
- Assisted team on assembly line, helping fill in when others were absent.
- Promoted to Team Lead within 6 months of hire.
- Received "Outstanding Employee" award in 20XX, 20XX, and 20XX.

Work Experience

Mytown Doors, Mytown, OH
Supervisor, (March 20XX – January 20XX)
Team Lead – Door Assembly, (January 20XX – March 20XX)
Door Assembler, (August 20XX – January 20XX)

FIG. 46.7 Combination resume.

employment history. Job duties for each position are bulleted out (Fig. 46.6). See Procedure 46.1 for the steps in creating a chronologic resume.

The *combination resume* is sometimes confused with a functional resume. A true functional resume showcases a person's skill sets. It does not include a work history. A combination resume is preferred over a functional resume. A combination resume:

- Lists a person's abilities and skill sets, as does the functional resume
- Includes the person's employment history, as does the chronologic resume (Fig. 46.7)

A combination resume may be used if a person is switching careers. Transferable skills related to the new position will be highlighted. It can also be used by applicants who have a gap in their work history. The focus is on the person's skills and ability, rather than the employment history.

The third type of resume is the *targeted resume.* This type of resume is customized to a unique job posting (Fig. 46.8). Targeted resumes:

- Detail key skills required for the position
- Indicate how the applicant has demonstrated those skills
- Take longer to create, but can be the most effective format

CRITICAL THINKING BOX 46.7

The three friends have very different backgrounds. Michelle has the waitressing experience, Krysia was in the military, and Zac worked in a factory. What type of resume might each use? Explain your answers.

- What type of resume would work best for you with your experience and background?

Resume Content

Between the resume formats, there are similarities and differences in the information presented. The following discussion will describe the content found in the different sections of a resume. See Procedure 46.1 for the steps in creating a chronologic resume.

Header. The person's contact information is found in the header of the document (Box 46.7). This information or a variation of the information should appear on each sheet if the resume is more than one page long.

Professional email addresses may include your first and last name or first initial and last name. Email addresses starting with expressions such as "one_hot_chick" or "party_dude" are not professional and are not used on resumes. If you do not have a professional email address, free email sites are available. Like professional emails, personal websites should be professional and contain a professional image of you (Boxes 46.8 and 46.9).

BOX 46.7 Information Found in the Header

The following applicant's information is found in the header:

- Name
- Mailing address
- Professional email address
- Phone number
- Personal websites (e.g., LinkedIn)

PROCEDURE 46.1   Prepare a Chronologic Resume

Task:
To write an effective resume for use as a tool in obtaining employment.

Equipment and Supplies
- Computer with word processing software and a printer
- Current job posting
- Resume paper
- Paper and pen

Procedural Steps

1. Apply critical thinking skills as you create a list of the personality traits (wanted by employers), technical skills, and transferable job skills you possess. Also write down your career goal(s).
   Purpose: To determine the strongest aspects of your abilities so that they can be highlighted on the resume.
2. Using the current job posting, identify the required and recommended qualifications and credentials needed for the position.
   Purpose: Identifying what the employer requires and would like will help you tailor your resume to address these qualifications and credentials.
3. Using the computer with word processing software, create a professional-looking header in the document's header. Include your name, address, telephone number(s), and email address. Select an appropriate font style for your name and a smaller font size for your contact information.
   Purpose: To make sure potential employers have a means of contacting you. Using a font style that is bold and a larger size for your name will help your name stand out. Make sure to have your contact information in a smaller, nonbold style so it will not detract from your name.
4. Create a section header for "Education." For the learning institution(s) you attended, list the school's name, city and state, degree obtained or coursework successfully completed, and the year. Include any additional educational information, such as grade point average (GPA), awards, and practicum information.
   Purpose: It is important to provide the school's name, city and state, along with the degree. Some employers may need to verify the information.
5. Create a section header for "Healthcare Experience" and/or "Work Experience." Provide details about your work experience, including the facility's name, city and state, title of your position, start and end date (month and year), and job duties. The job duties must start with an active verb using the appropriate tense (e.g., a past job would have past tense verbs and a current job would include present tense verbs).
   Purpose: The potential employer will need to know your employment history and all the details.
6. Create a section header for "Special Skills" and list your special language skills, computer proficiencies, and other unique skills you possess that relate to the position.
   Purpose: This section can be a "marketing" area where you highlight unique skills you possess.
7. Create a section header for "Certifications and Credentials" and list the active credentials and certifications you have. Include the title of the certification, awarding agency, and the expiration date.
   NOTE: You may want to consider adding in the date you are taking a credential examination. Employers like to know the status of your credential examination.
   Purpose: Employers need to know if you have your medical assistant credential (CMA or RMA). They also might like to know if you have an active cardiopulmonary resuscitation (CPR) card.
8. All information on the resume needs to appear in reverse chronologic order (i.e., newest information is on top). Work experiences should include both the start and end month and year.
   Purpose: Employers need to know how long you worked at a specific place. If the position was seasonal or temporary, it is important to note that.
9. The resume needs to look professional and interesting. Use font styles (e.g., bold, underline, italic) to highlight important words and phrases. Use professional-looking bullets to list out job duties and other information. Use the key words from the posting throughout the resume.
   Purpose: The more professional and interesting a resume appears, the better the chance that it will be reviewed by the potential employer.
10. Proofread the resume. Correct any spelling, grammar, punctuation, or sentence structure errors you find. If time allows, have another person review the resume and use the feedback to revise your resume.
    Purpose: Resumes submitted with errors often are discarded without consideration.
11. Print the resume on resume paper and proofread one final time. Any errors should be corrected, and the document should be reprinted or emailed to the instructor.

BOX 46.8   Are You Prepared to Be Contacted by a Potential Employer?

Before you give out your phone number to potential employers, make sure your voice mail message is appropriate and professional sounding. State your name clearly in the message so that the caller knows he or she has reached the right person.

BOX 46.9   Using an Objective on the Resume

Many experts consider the use of resume objective statements to be outdated. Typically, the objective statement is hard to write. They rarely provided valuable information to the employer. The space is better used to discuss your skills.

Education. The education section includes information on the schooling that the person has received after high school. The information should appear in *reverse chronologic order*. Information should include:

- *If a diploma was obtained:* List the school's name, city, and state, the degree, and the year it was obtained.
- *If no degree was obtained:* Summarize the coursework completed. List the school's name, city, and state, and the years of the coursework.
- *Practicum (externship) information:* Include the location, dates, and duties (optional; some will include this information in the Healthcare Experience section, discussed later in the chapter).
- *Academic recognition:* Include academic awards, scholarships, and overall GPA if greater than 3.0.

The location of the education section can differ based on the person's situation. For new graduates, the education section should appear toward the top of the resume. If the degree is not related to the position or the

> **VOCABULARY**
> **reverse chronologic order:** The most recent item is on top and the oldest item is last.

Krysia Debski
111 Mall Drive • Mytown, OH 45457
Cell phone: 715.555.6956 • Email: KDebski@elsevier.net

Education
Community College, Mytown, OH
A.S. in Medical Assisting, 20XX
- Medical Assistant Practicum at Mytown Associates, Mytown, OH
  o Obtained and charted patients' histories and vital signs in the electronic health record.
  o Assisted providers with tests and treatments in a busy internal medicine practice.
  o Performed injections, throat swabs, and phlebotomy.

Skills
ORGANIZATION SKILLS
- Organized supplies to expedited restocking procedures and decrease financial loss.
- Exceptional organizational and filing skills utilized to maintain purchase and delivery records from over 300 suppliers.
- Assisted with the install and training for inventory tracking software for warehouse.

TEAMWORK
- Refined teamwork skills with over ten years in the U.S. Marines.
- Taught teambuilding courses.
- Promoted teamwork among staff by incorporating incentives.

COMMUNICATION SKILLS
- Assertive when working with suppliers to meet deadlines.
- Utilized excellent listening skills to identify needs of various teams that impact the warehouse.
- Composed frequent emails and letters for supervisors.
- Fluent in Spanish and Polish

Credentials
Certified Medical Assistant, American Association of Medical Assistants, (expires May 20XX)

BLS for Healthcare Providers, American Heart Association (expires March 20XX)

Work Experience
United States Marines
  Supply Administration and Operations Specialist (May 20XX – September 20XX)
  Warehouse Clerk (August 20XX – May 20XX)

FIG. 46.8 Targeted resume customized for a medical assistant posting. The medical assistant should possess strong organizational skills, experience with teamwork, and exceptional communication skills. The posting indicated it required a person with a Certified Medical Assistant (CMA) credential and a current Basic Life Support (BLS) certification.

degree is older, the education section would come toward the end of the resume. Moving education to the end allows the person's achievements and work history to be emphasized.

Work Experience. This section can be titled several different ways. If a person is strictly including job information, then "Work Experience" or "Job Experience" can be used. Using the word "job" or "work," implies the person got paid for the position. If a person wants to include volunteer positions with job positions, then the section should be titled "Related Experience" or "Other Experience." Related means it relates to the position the person is applying for. If the section contains unrelated experience, then use "Other Experience." For healthcare experience, see Box 46.10. For those with military experience, it is recommended to add a special section to discuss the military experience.

BOX 46.10 What if You Have Prior Healthcare Experience?

If you have prior healthcare experience, you may want to separate your volunteer and job experiences into two sections. First, use "Healthcare Experiences". Include any healthcare jobs and volunteer positions you have had. Some students may opt to include their practicum in this section.

Second, use a topic header, such as "Other Experience" or "Additional Experience". Include all of your non-healthcare jobs and volunteer positions. Do not repeat information you included in prior sections.

The information in this section should be presented in reverse chronologic order. All three resumes discussed require the following elements for each position:
- Name of the facility
- City and state of the facility
- Title of position or positions held at that facility
- Dates in that position (include start date [month and year] and end date [month and year]; for a current position, include the start date and use "to present")

For those in the workforce for 10 years or longer, employers want to see 10 years of employment information. For those working at the same facility for over 10 years, it is important to list changes and advancements in the position over the duration of employment. Any gaps in the employment history should be explained to the potential employer during the interview or discussed in the cover letter.

For the chronologic resume, the most relevant job duties need to be listed. For instance, if you worked as a housekeeper in a motel, making beds is not related to medical assisting. Providing customer service would be relevant.

The statements regarding the duties should be bulleted and begin with an active verb. For present positions, use active verbs in the present tense (e.g., administer, provide). For past positions, use active verbs in the past tense (e.g., administered, provided) (Fig. 46.9).

The position of the work experience section is dependent on the resume format. Chronologic resumes typically have work experience near the top, whereas combination and targeted resumes list it toward the end of the resume.

Summary and Skills. A "Summary" section appears at the top in the targeted resume. This section summarizes why the applicant is the best candidate for the job. It is helpful to use key words from the job posting when describing skills one possesses. This helps to make the connection of why the person is the best candidate for the job.

A "Skills" or "Skills and Achievements" section is found in combination resumes. It showcases specific transferable skills that relate to the new position. These transferable skills may have been obtained in the military, by a stay-at-home parent, or by a person switching careers.

A "Special Skills" section is found in a chronologic resume. Information that may appear in this section includes:
- fluency in another language (e.g., fluent in Spanish)
- keyboarding speed (e.g., keyboarding speed: 85 wpm)
- computer skills and experiences (e.g., used electronic health records during practicum)

Certifications. Many employers may require specific certifications or credentials for a job position. It is important to include those that relate to the job position. When listing the information, include the:
- title of the certification or license
- awarding agency
- expiration date

An example for all resume formats would be: "BLS for Healthcare Providers, American Heart Association, expires 10/2022".

Appearance of the Resume

As you create your resume, keep in mind the eye appeal or interest the resume will create for the reader. It is recommended to bold-face only important information. A job title should be bold, whereas the facility should not be bold. Simple bullets help organize information and provide a neat appearance to the resume. Changing the font size in certain areas can emphasize more important elements and help keep content on one page.

Administered	Copied	Performed
Advocated	Developed	Posted
Aided	Distributed	Prepared
Answered	Documented	Processed
Arranged	Established	Provided
Assigned	Filed	Purchased
Assisted	Guided	Reconciled
Balanced	Helped	Restocked
Calculated	Instructed	Reviewed
Cared	Listened	Scanned
Coded	Logged	Scheduled
Collected	Mailed	Sorted
Compiled	Maintained	Supported
Composed	Monitored	Taught
Computed	Operated	Trained
Contacted	Ordered	Wrote
Coordinated	Organized	

FIG. 46.9 Action verbs in the past tense. (From Proctor D, et al: *Kinn's The Medical Assistant*, ed 13, St Louis, 2017, Elsevier.)

Spacing is crucial to the appearance of a resume. A lot of spacing creates too much "white space." This can give the reader a negative impression of the resume. Too little spacing creates a busy, text-heavy resume that is difficult to read. Make sure to use the same spacing between the sections. Use less spacing, but be consistent between subsections (e.g., different employment positions).

It is important to have resume paper available. Even if you submit your resume online, you should bring copies of your resume on resume paper to the interview. Use a light solid-colored resume paper (e.g., cream, light gray). The light colors will duplicate better than a pattern or dark-colored paper.

Before submitting your resume, have another person review it. Obtain the person's initial impression of the resume's appearance. Is there too much white space? Does the resume look too wordy? Does it look too plain? Does it look too busy? Then have the person read the content in the resume and provide you with feedback. Use the feedback to revise your resume. See Box 46.11 for additional tips on creating a resume.

> **CRITICAL THINKING BOX 46.8**
>
> Zac, Michelle, and Krysia drafted their resumes. They read each others' and provided feedback. Who else might they give their resumes to for proofreading and feedback?
> - Think of your circle of family and friends. List three people who might be great candidates to provide feedback on your resume.

BOX 46.11 Tips on Creating a Resume

- Don't add clipart or other pictures.
- Don't include personal information (e.g., married, children, and religious affiliation).
- Don't lie or exaggerate the truth.
- Don't add unrelated content, such as hobbies and interests.
- Don't include "References available upon request" or a similar statement, because it is understood references will be requested and required.
- Don't use personal pronouns, such as "I."
- Don't repeat content.
- Don't include any pay/salary information.
- Always keep the resume to one page, unless you have been in the workforce for multiple years. Then use an additional page, but your content must fill both pages.
- Be concise and clear.
- Use key terms found in the job posting or job description in your resume.
- Put important details first.
- Perform a grammar and spelling check on your resume.
- Limit abbreviations to only the abbreviations used in the job posting (i.e., BLS for basic life support, CPR for cardiopulmonary resuscitation).

DEVELOPING A COVER LETTER

A cover letter must always accompany the resume (Fig. 46.10). The cover letter is a critical tool that gains the reader's attention. The goal is to have the cover letter create enough interest that the reader wants to look at the resume. The cover letter gives the reader more information on the applicant's personality than the factual resume. Cover letters allow applicants to express themselves. Table 46.1 describes strategies and steps to follow when composing cover letters.

After writing the cover letter, review it for inaccuracies. Use the spell-check tool in your word processing software to help identify errors. Also **proofread** your letter. Make sure your spelling, punctuation, grammar, and sentence structure are correct. Common cover letter weaknesses include:

- Starting a majority of sentences with "I"
- Introducing yourself in the first sentence (for instance, "*Hi, I am Sally Green.*")

VOCABULARY
proofread: To read and mark corrections.

Michelle Marison

1234 Cedar Way, Mytown, OH 45458
Home phone: 715.555.1899
Cell phone: 715.555.1355
mmarison@elsevier.net

May 15, 20XX

Ms. Alex Brown
Medical Assistant Supervisor
Mytown Medical Clinic
555 Clover Drive
Mytown OH 45457

Dear Ms. Brown:

I was excited to see the posting on the Mytown Telegram job board for the medical assistant position (#1243) and would like to be considered for that position. I am graduating from Community College on May 30, 20XX and will be taking my AAMA CMA exam June 2, 20XX.

With two years of customer service experience and five months of being a hospital volunteer, I have learned the importance of prioritizing, teamwork, and communication. During my medical assistant practicum, I have utilized these skills along with my attention to detail and my medical assistant knowledge, as I assist providers with procedures and treatments. The knowledge and skills I am learning in practicum combined with the skills I have developed as a waitress and volunteer will help me provide the best care to my future patients.

I have heard excellent things about Mytown Medical Clinic and would love to be a part of the staff of such a caring agency. I am available for interviews whenever it is convenient for you. I am available either by phone or email.

Thank you so much for considering me for this position.

Sincerely,

Michelle Marison

Enclosure: 1

FIG. 46.10 Basic cover letter. (From Proctor D, et al: *Kinn's The Medical Assistant*, ed 13, St Louis, 2017, Elsevier.)

CHAPTER 46 Career Development

TABLE 46.1 Strategies When Writing a Cover Letter

Strategies	Steps
Match the appearance of the cover letter and resume	• Headers on both documents should be identical. • Font type and margins should be identical. • If using paper, use the same paper for both documents.
Address the inside address and the salutation (greeting) to a specific person	• Address the letter to the person who is hiring the new employee. This shows that you took time to find out the details. • Use the person's name and job title in the inside address. • Use a formal salutation (e.g., *Dear Mr. Jones:*). • Call the healthcare facility or use online resources, such as LinkedIn, to find out the information.
Start the body of your cover letter off with a bang!	• In the first paragraph: Show enthusiasm as you summarize why you believe you are the best candidate for the job. Also include the job title and the number for easy reference for the reader. • For example: *"Having a strong customer service background and a degree in medical assisting, I am confident that I can fulfill your expectations for the family practice medical assistant position (#123)."*
Sell yourself to the reader	• In the second paragraph: Provide a snapshot of your experiences. • Weave in the key "requirement" words from the job posting. Address the requirements first, followed by the lesser requirements or "would like" qualities. Some experts recommend using bold font for these key words. • You can bullet your qualifications and abilities, but limit the bullets to four or five points. • Be concise, yet clear. Do not repeat the resume. You want the reader to move onto the resume for the details.
Reaffirm that you are an excellent match for the job	• In the final paragraph: Use such phrases as "*I believe I have the qualities you require*" or "*I am confident I will meet your expectations.*" • If you include an action you will take (e.g., *I will call the week of…*), do not be overly aggressive in your tone. • Finish the paragraph by expressing your interest in and enthusiasm for an interview (e.g., "*I am very excited about this opportunity and would enjoy meeting with you to explore how my qualifications could meet your needs.*"). (See Fig. 46.10.)
Be professional	• Express your thanks to the reader for his or her consideration.

- Spelling, grammar, punctuation, and sentence structure errors
- Missing parts of the letter (e.g., date, inside address)
- Not including the position title and posting number
- Too busy (overuse of font styles), too wordy, or too much white space
- Inappropriate spacing that leads to the body of the letter being too high or too low on the page. Remember, the body should be centered vertically on the page.
- Creating a generic letter that does not contain the key requirement words from the job posting. (Many larger employers use software to screen letters and resumes for key words. Those with key words are reviewed more closely. Those that lack the key words are discarded.)

Create an error-free cover letter. It must have a professional tone and appearance. Also, have a few people proofread your letter. Use their advice as you make your changes. Refer to Chapter 21, if you need assistance with composing a business letter. Procedure 46.2 will help guide you in writing a professional cover letter.

PROCEDURE 46.2 Create a Cover Letter

Task:
To write an effective cover letter that will accompany the resume.

Equipment and Supplies
- Computer with word processing software and a printer
- Current job posting
- Resume paper
- Pen

Procedural Steps

1. Using the job posting, read through the job description. With a pen, circle the position requirements and the key phrases.
   Purpose: Your letter should contain the key phrases and position requirements that are found in the job posting.
2. Using the computer with word processing software, create a professional-looking header in the document's header that matches your resume header. Include your name, address, telephone number(s), and email address.
   Purpose: To ensure potential employers have a means of contacting you. You can increase the professional appearance of your documents by having the same header on each document.
3. Type the date in the correct location using the correct format. Have one blank line between the date line and the last line of the letterhead.
   Purpose: All letters require a date for legal purposes. The correct format would be month date, year (e.g., May 14, 2023).
4. Type the inside address using the correct spelling, punctuation, and location for the information. Leave 1 to 9 blank lines between the date and the inside address, depending on the location of the body of the letter.
   Purpose: The body of the letter needs to be centered vertically from top to bottom of the document. More blank lines can be added to move the body to the correct location.
5. Starting on the second line below the inside address, type the salutation using the correct format. Use a colon after the person's name.
   Purpose: A proper greeting helps set the tone of the letter.
6. Type the message in the body of the letter using the proper location and format. There should be a blank line after the salutation and between each paragraph. The message should be clear, concise, and professional. Use proper grammar, punctuation, capitalization, and sentence structure.
   Purpose: Proper grammar usage helps convey the message more accurately and professionally.

Continued

PROCEDURE 46.2 Create a Cover Letter—cont'd

7. The first paragraph should contain the title and number of the job posting. The middle paragraph(s) should summarize your strengths and include key phrases from the posting. The final paragraph should discuss your availability for an interview. The body should end with an expression of gratitude to the reader.
   Purpose: It is important to thank the reader for considering you for the position.
8. Type a proper closing, leaving one blank line between the last line of the body and the closing. Use the correct format and location.
   Purpose: The closing helps end the message with a proper tone.
9. Type the signature block using the correct format and location. There should be four blank lines between the closing and the signature block.
   Purpose: The four blank lines will provide you with space to sign your name.
10. Spell-check and proofread the document. Check for proper tone, grammar, punctuation, capitalization, and sentence structure. Check for proper spacing between the parts of the letter.
    Purpose: The spell-check tool will identify only certain errors; proofreading will help to identify incorrect word usage, improper tone, and errors in formatting. The tone of the letter should be professional, but not aggressive.
11. Make any final corrections. Print the document on resume paper and sign the letter, or email the document to your instructor or employer.
    Purpose: It is professional to use resume paper when submitting a resume and cover letter to an employer.

TABLE 46.2 Information Required for Online Profiles and Applications

Information	Details Needed
Education	Institution's name and address; dates and titles of coursework or diploma
Past and present jobs	Facility name and address; supervisors' names, titles, and contact information; job title, duties, start and end salary, start and end dates; and reason for leaving.
Certifications and credentials	Certifying agency's name and address; certification/credential; expiration date. (A copy of your certification and BLS card may be required by the employer.)
References	Name, title, facility, address, phone number, and email address (see Box 46.12)

BOX 46.12 References

An interested employer and many online profiles will require your references. This means you need to ask specific people if they would be a reference for you. If they agree, then obtain their contact information. It is not professional to use people's names without asking them.

Your reference list should include three or four names of people who know you as a person and as a professional. Select references based on someone who can speak to the following areas:
- Your skills and interactions with patients (e.g., practicum mentors)
- Your performance in the medical assistant program (e.g., instructors)
- Your work ethic, motivation, and professionalism (e.g., past and current co-workers or supervisors)

COMPLETING ONLINE PROFILES AND JOB APPLICATIONS

Many healthcare agencies use the internet during the employment process. The online human resource software may require applicants to create a profile before applying for open positions. The online profile collects the information that previously was collected by paper applications.

Online profiles have many advantages over paper applications for both the employer and the applicant. An applicant completes the profile once and updates the information as needed. Typically the agencies keep the profiles active for years. Employers can:
- Track the activities of applicants
- Easily read a person's information
- Advertise new postings to potential applicants whose profiles meet certain requirements

If a healthcare facility does not use online profiles, then the applicant will need to complete a job application (Fig. 46.11). Some organizations require the application to be submitted with the cover letter and resume. Others have applicants arriving for interviews complete the application. If you need to complete an application before an interview, come prepared with your information. Arrive at least 20 minutes before the interview so you can complete the application. See Procedure 46.3 for the steps in completing a job application.

Regardless of whether you need to complete a profile or an application, you will need to provide the same information. Even if you have the information on your resume, you still need to add it to the application or profile. Having the reference information in a word-processed document will save you time. If you are providing the information online, the copy and paste feature will speed up completion time. Table 46.2 contains the information you should include in the word-processed document (Box 46.12).

When filling out the application or profile, answer the questions carefully. When addressing your current and past employment, keep these points in mind:
- When giving your availability date, make sure you know how long you have to give notice at your current position. Most employers have a 2-week notice policy. If you are hired, your new employer will understand that you need to give a 2-week notice.
- When giving the reason you left prior positions, make sure to write the reason using a positive tone. For instance, *"Obtained a position that would advance my skill set"* or *"Resigned to focus on my education"* sounds more professional than *"I hated the job."*

If you have a unique situation (e.g., sick parent, new baby), ask the advice of your school's placement counselor if you are unsure what to say in these sections. Most employers require an explanation for time not employed.

As you complete the online profile or paper application, you will be required to read important legal statements and add your signature

APPLICATION FOR EMPLOYMENT

Date: _____
Name: (First, Middle Initial, Last) _____
Social Security No.: _____   Phone: _____
Address: _____

EDUCATION

	Name, City, State	Graduation Date	Degree Obtained
High School:			
College:			
Other:			

LICENSURE/CERTIFICATION/REGISTRATION

Type of Certification, License or Registration	Agency/State	Registration Name

List any special skills or qualifications which you possess and feel are relevant to health care and the position for which you are applying. _____

EMPLOYMENT HISTORY
May we contact and communicate with your present employer? ☐ Yes ☐ No

Employer:	Phone:
Address:	Supervisor:
Employed	Hourly Pay:
Position title and responsibilities:	
Reason for leaving:	

FIG. 46.11 Application for employment. (From Proctor D, et al: *Kinn's The Medical Assistant*, ed 13, St Louis, 2017, Elsevier.)

PROCEDURE 46.3   Complete a Job Application

Task:
To complete an accurate, detailed job application legibly so as to secure a job offer.

Equipment and Supplies
- Pen
- Application form
- Information regarding your past education, job experiences, and the skill sets you have developed (e.g., computer skills, keyboarding speed)
- Contact information for former supervisors and references
- Current resume

Procedural Steps
1. Read the entire job application before completing any part of the document.
   Purpose: Reading through the entire application helps prevent errors when filling out the document.
2. Refer to your information on past jobs, education experiences, and skill sets you have developed as you complete the application. Answers to the questions need to be accurate and honest.
   Purpose: The application is a legal document, and the answers must be correct and true.
3. Use proper grammar, sentence structure, punctuation, spelling, and capitalization. Handwriting should be legible to the reader.
   Purpose: Errors on the application or illegible sections may affect whether you are hired.
4. Do not leave any space blank. Answer each question on the document. If the question does not apply, write "not applicable."
   Purpose: Leaving a space blank on the application may suggest that the candidate did not want to answer a certain question or accidentally overlooked it. By writing "not applicable" on such questions, the candidate demonstrates competence and attention to detail.

Continued

PROCEDURE 46.3 Complete a Job Application—cont'd

5. Do not write "See resume" anywhere on the document.
   Purpose: Many supervisors view this practice as laziness. Always fill out the job application completely and do not leave blank spaces.
6. Include information on the application that exhibits dependability, punctuality, teamwork, attention to detail, a positive work ethic and initiative, the ability to adapt to change, a responsible attitude, and use of technology.
   Purpose: These phrases send an important message to employers. It is important to use words they are looking for.
7. Sign the document and date it.
   Purpose: Because this is a legal document, read the fine print before signing the document and dating it.
8. Proofread the document and make sure none of the information conflicts with the resume.
   Purpose: Proofreading helps the candidate to catch any errors before submitting the application.

BOX 46.13 Typical Items Found in Career Portfolios

Using a three-ring binder with plastic sheet protectors and divider tabs, include the following:
- Table of contents at the beginning with identified tabbed sections
- Cover letter and resume (a copy of what was sent to that facility)
- References
- Certifications (e.g., copy of BLS card, copy of credentials [e.g., CMA or RMA card])
- Education-related documents:
  - Copy of letters of recommendation
  - Copy of transcripts, awards, and honors
  - A list of the courses successfully completed with a short description of each course (optional, but consider if you are moving to another location where your institution may not be known)
  - Copy of practicum evaluation forms and skill document form
  - Scholarships awarded
  - Copy/details of school-related activities (e.g., officer in student medical assistant group, athlete, volunteer activities)
- Prior employment documents
  - Copy of past employment evaluations
  - Copy of letters of recommendations
- Documentation showing the student balancing work and education (This can help exhibit a strong work ethic, organizational skills, and prioritizing skills.)
- Examples of work or summary of projects that can provide evidence of abilities and skills
- Criminal background documentation, blood titers, vaccination history, and current tuberculosis (TB) skin or blood test (optional)

BOX 46.14 Topics to Research About the Healthcare Organization

- Mission and value statements
- Size of the organization
- Size of the department with the opened position
- Names and types of providers in the department

(or electronic signature). This is a legal document. It should be filled out accurately and completely.

CREATING A CAREER PORTFOLIO

Many job seekers claim to have the skill sets required by the potential employer. Very few actually show the employer evidence of those qualifications. A career portfolio is a fantastic tool to show that you have the skills required for the job.

The portfolio should be developed along with the cover letter and resume. Creating a different portfolio for each type of job applied for is a great strategy. A receptionist portfolio would look different from a phlebotomy portfolio. Box 46.13 identifies information that may be found in a portfolio. There will be similarities in the information for all portfolios, but different "evidence" of skills will be in each. The medical assistant should be prepared to leave the portfolio with the interviewer, so no originals should be included.

The documents placed in the career portfolio binder should be positive and helpful to you in your mission of getting a job. If you have not been very successful in school, you may not want to include your transcript. If you received negative performance evaluations, you should not include those in your portfolio. Be creative as you prepare your portfolio, keeping the appearance professional and neat.

Just before an interview, the medical assistant should customize the portfolio for that employer (Procedure 46.4). A copy of the cover letter and resume sent to the employer should be in the portfolio. A list of references should also be included. All three of these documents should be printed on the same type of resume paper. The medical assistant should do additional customization of the portfolio. The examples of work or the summary of projects should reflect the skills required and key words in the job posting.

JOB INTERVIEW

Interviewers can consist of one or two people or a panel of employees. The job seeker may interview with a human resource employee, the office manager, the provider, and/or potential peers. The job seeker may have a number of interviews before the actual decision is made.

For many people, the interview is a stressful part of the job search. Some individuals dread job interviews and become extremely nervous at the prospect of interviewing. Others are very comfortable and consider the interview to be as much for their own purposes as for the employer's. The more interviews people do, the more comfortable they become with each subsequent interview.

We will examine the four phases of an interview. These include preparation for the interview, the interview itself, the follow-up, and the negotiation.

Preparation for the Interview

When preparing for an interview, the job seeker needs to:
- Research the facility
- Practice answering potential questions
- Select interview attire
- Prepare for the day of the interview

We will discuss each of these in depth. The better prepared the job candidate is, the more comfortable he or she will be during the interview.

Research the Healthcare Facility. The job seeker should learn everything possible about the employer. The organization's website is an excellent source of information. Box 46.14 lists topics that the job

PROCEDURE 46.4 Create a Career Portfolio

Task:
To create a custom portfolio that provides potential employers evidence of your skills and knowledge as a medical assistant.

Equipment and Supplies
- Three-ring binder or folder
- Plastic sleeves for the three-ring binder
- Dividers with tabs for the three-ring binder
- Current resume and cover letter
- Documents providing evidence of your skills and knowledge (e.g., transcripts, job and practicum evaluation forms, practicum skill checklist, projects completed in school, letters of recommendation, copies of certifications [e.g., CPR card])

Procedural Steps
1. Group documents in a logical manner, putting similar documents together. Identify the arrangement for the portfolio. An arrangement could include cover letter and resume, education section (e.g., transcript, practicum evaluation form and skills checklist, awards), prior job-related documents (e.g., evaluations), reference letters, and work products (e.g., projects you created in your medical assistant program).
   Purpose: Organizing the documents in a logical manner will help the reader identify the important documents. The arrangement will also show the reader your ability to organize content.
2. Insert one document per plastic pocket. Place all documents in plastic pockets.
   Purpose: The plastic pockets will keep the documents clean and neat.
3. Neatly write the topic area on the tab of the dividers. Insert the tabbed dividers in the binder or folder.
   Purpose: This will help the reader find the content easier.
4. Place all documents in the binder or folder behind the correct divider. Place your cover letter and resume in the front of all the other documents.
   Purpose: The reader can review the letter and resume as needed before looking at the other documents in the portfolio.
5. Create a table of contents to identify the tabbed areas.
   Purpose: Organizing the documents in a logical manner will help the reader identify the important documents. The arrangement will also show the reader your ability to organize content.
6. After the portfolio is assembled, review the entire portfolio to ensure it looks professional and the documents provide positive support of your skill set and knowledge.
   Purpose: Minimize the negative documents in your portfolio. They will not help you obtain a job as much as the positive, supporting documents.

Practice Answers to Questions. Organizations need to follow federal and state hiring laws. The agencies cannot discriminate. During the interview phase, most organizations use a selected list of questions. All candidates are asked the same questions. You will not know the exact questions that will be asked. It is important to practice answering some standard interview questions (Fig. 46.12). This practice will help you prepare for the interview and also appear more confident during the actual interview.

When practicing your answers to standard interview questions, start by writing down your answer. Review your answer. Does it answer the question? What perception might you be giving to the interviewers by your answer? Is it the perception you want to be giving? How might you strengthen your answer? Is it really short or does it ramble on? Be clear and concise. Expand on the topic, but do not get too wordy. Provide examples to support what you say. When you have refined your answers, study your answers before the interview.

Decide on Your Interview Attire. Prior to the interview, it is important to select an interview outfit. Be conservative with wardrobe choices (Table 46.3). Be sure clothing is clean, wrinkle free, and well fitting, and that shoes are clean and shined. For a medical assistant, scrubs may be acceptable for an interview. (It is appropriate to ask the person arranging the interview if scrubs can be worn.) Take care in washing and pressing your scrubs, and use a lint roller on them, before wearing them on an interview.

Pay particular attention to other aspects of appearance. Make sure your hair is clean and styled attractively, your teeth are clean, and your breath is fresh. Nails should be clean and well-groomed. Nails should not be excessively long or painted in highly visible colors. Do not wear perfumes or colognes. Do not wear excessive jewelry or makeup. Do not chew gum during the interview. Do not smoke in your interview attire. Remember the appearance guidelines that applied to the practicum. Some employers will react negatively to tattoos, piercings, extravagant hairstyles, unnatural hair colors, or other excessive wardrobe choices. Always dress appropriately and conservatively for an interview. Once hired, the new employee may be allowed to wear more diverse styles that comply with the employee handbook or procedures manual.

Prepare for the Interview Day. Do a test run before the day of the interview to identify the travel time. Always arrive 15 minutes early for the interview. Never take anyone along on a job interview, especially children. Expect to be a little nervous. Any interview can be a stressful situation. If necessary, practice stress-relieving strategies that you can use before the interview. The better prepared a person is, the more successful the interview will be.

You should also prepare what you need to bring for the interview. These items include:
- An interview portfolio
- A copy of your cover letter and resume for each interviewer

seeker should research. It is important to ask questions at the interview. Possible questions can relate to your research on the facility:
- "I see that there are two providers in this department. Would I be working with both of them?"
- "There are three locations for your clinic on your website; how will I interact with the other locations?"
- "Given the size of your organization, is there an opportunity to interact with the other departments?"

Questions that relate to your research show the interviewer you are truly interested in the position (see Box 46.14). They also show that you prepared for the interview.

TABLE 46.3 Interview Attire

Females	Males
• Business suit; skirt or dress pants and blouse • Skirt or dress should be of modest length (i.e., at the knee or longer) • Blouse should not be sheer or show cleavage	• Business suit; dress pants and shirt • Conservative tie

1. Tell me about yourself.	16. What do you know about this facility and our competitors?
2. Why do you want to work for this company?	17. What has been your most rewarding experience at work?
3. Why should I hire you?	18. What was your single most important accomplishment for the company on your last job?
4. How do you work under pressure?	19. What was the toughest problem you have ever solved and how did you do it?
5. How do you handle criticism?	20. How do you see yourself fitting in with our company?
6. What do you think your co-workers think about you?	21. What skills did you learn on your last job that can be used here?
7. Describe your last supervisor.	22. What immediate contribution could you make if you came to work for us today?
8. What would you like to change about yourself?	23. Do you prefer working with others or by yourself?
9. What is your best asset?	24. Can you take instructions or criticism without being upset?
10. What adjectives would you use to describe yourself?	25. What job in this company would you choose if you could?
11. How would you describe the perfect job?	26. What have you done that shows initiative and willingness to work?
12. Why did you leave your last job?	27. What will previous supervisors say about you?
13. Why did you choose this type of profession?	28. Why would you be successful in this job?
14. What are your strongest and weakest personal qualities?	29. Can you explain the gap in your employment history?
15. What personal characteristics are necessary for success in your chosen field?	30. Are you a member of any professional organizations?

FIG. 46.12 Top 30 interview questions. (From Proctor D, et al: *Kinn's The Medical Assistant*, ed 13, St Louis, 2017, Elsevier.)

- A notepad and pen to take notes
- A list of references on resume paper
- A list of questions for the interviewer

If you will be completing an application, bring the information discussed in the prior section regarding completing online profiles and applications.

During the Interview

During the interview it is important to be professional. Your professionalism may be tested if the interviewer asks illegal questions. We will discuss how to answer interview questions. We will also discuss professionalism during the different types of interviews.

Answering Interview Questions. It is important to give the interviewers a good perception of you. As discussed in a prior section, it is important to practice answering questions before the interview. This will help you to prepare and to feel more confident during the interview. Box 46.15 provides a list of tips for successful interviews.

Many times the interview will start with a question such as, "Tell me about yourself." The temptation is to answer the question focusing on your personal life. For example, "I'm a recent graduate, and I am married and have two children." The answer to this question should not reflect information about personal issues. Answer instead with, "I am a recent graduate and completed a 6-week practicum in a family practice." Focus all answers on your career, your strengths and attributes, and what skills you have to bring to the healthcare setting. Be able to prove the skills you claim. You can provide examples either by relating professional situations you have handled well, or by using your interview portfolio. Before the interview ends, the medical assistant should ask when a decision will be made and if it would be acceptable to call to follow up (Procedure 46.5).

PROCEDURE 46.5 Practice Interview Skills During a Mock Interview

Task:
To project a professional appearance during a job interview and to be able to express the reasons the medical assistant is the best candidate for the position.

Equipment and Supplies
- Current job posting
- Resume
- Cover letter
- Interview portfolio (optional)
- Application (optional)
- Interviewer
- Mock interview questions

Procedural Steps

1. Wear interview-appropriate attire and be groomed professionally.
   Purpose: Your appearance will influence the first impression made on this potential employer. Most medical facilities prefer conservative dress.
2. Portray a professional image by shaking hands firmly prior to the start of the interview. Ensure that each interviewer has a copy of your resume and cover letter. Refrain from nervous behaviors (e.g., saying "um", tapping a pen or your foot) during the interview.
   Purpose: Many employers feel a firm handshake is important. Each interviewer may need a copy of your documents to reference during the interview.
3. Answer introductory questions by providing only professional information. This may include information about your education, experience, and career goals.
   Purpose: Many people are tempted to answer with personal information (e.g., if they are married, have children). Personal information should not be discussed during the interview.
4. Answer interview questions with open, honest, and positive responses. Completely answer questions, provide information or examples, and do not answer in single sentences or with limited responses.
   Purpose: The goal of the interview is for the employer to get to know you. Limited responses negatively impact this goal.
5. Use key words from the job posting when answering the interview questions.
   Purpose: This helps to prove the interviewee has exactly what the organization is looking for.
6. Ask the interviewer two to three appropriate questions about the facility or the position.
   Purpose: This demonstrates an interest in the organization and the position.
7. Express interest in the job and politely complete the interview by shaking hands and thanking the interviewer for the opportunity for the interview.
   Purpose: The employer wants to know that you are interested in the job. It is professional to thank the interviewer for the interview opportunity.

BOX 46.15 Tips for All Interviews

- For simple, straightforward questions, do not pause before you answer. Any pause would be hinting at insincerity.
- For complex questions, pause for a few seconds as you think about your answer. Write down some key words to help you focus and answer the question.
- Refrain from saying "um."
- Do not volunteer any negative information.
- Be honest and do not exaggerate experiences or lengths of employment.
- Never speak negatively about former employers.
- Write down the names of the interviewers to help you as you follow up after the interview.
- Avoid a "know-it-all" attitude, which indicates overconfidence and reluctance to take direction.
- Express a sincere interest in the employer and his or her projects, rather than in what the employer can do for the employee.
- Ask intelligent questions at the end of the interview if given the opportunity. Your first question should never be, "How much will I be paid?" Money, although important, cannot appear to be your primary concern.

Illegal Interview Questions. The interviewer should not ask any illegal questions. Table 46.4 lists such topics and potential illegal questions. Employers may either intentionally or accidentally ask illegal questions. The way that the medical assistant answers the questions can influence the employer's hiring decision. Here are some points to consider:
- If the medical assistant is openly offended: Employers may negatively conclude that the applicant will be offended by abrasive comments from patients.
- If the illegal question is answered: Discrimination may occur in the hiring process. The employer may use the information to weed out the medical assistant as a candidate.

The best approach is to politely address the question. Either answer the question or redirect the interviewer back to the job requirements. For example, an interviewer asks if the candidate plans to put his or her children in day care. This may be a way of determining the age of the dependent children. It could also provide information on the likelihood of absenteeism because of the children's illnesses. The medical assistant could answer, "I will be able to meet the work schedule and the responsibilities that this job requires."

TABLE 46.4 Illegal versus Legal Interview Questions

Topic	Examples of Illegal Questions	Examples of Legal Questions
Birthplace, ancestry, or national origin	When did you move to the United States?	Are you eligible to work in this state?
Marital status, children, or pregnancy	Who will look after your child when he is born?	Are you able to work an 8 a.m. to 5 p.m. schedule?
Physical disability, health or medical history	What medications are you on?	Can you perform the essential job functions of a medical assistant with or without reasonable accommodation?
Religion or religious days observed	Where do you attend church services?	Can you work on weekends?
Age, race, ethnicity, gender, or color	How old are you?	Are you 18 or older? (or whatever the minimum age is for the facility)
Criminal record	Have you ever been arrested?	Have you ever been convicted of a crime?

Some questions that might normally be considered illegal, such as, "What organizations are you a member of?" might be job related. The employer may be interested in knowing that the medical assistant is a member of various professional organizations, such as the AAMA or the AMT.

> **CRITICAL THINKING BOX 46.9**
>
> Krysia is enjoying a good interview when the interviewer, a male supervisor, asks her if she is married. When Krysia replies that she is not, he asks if she has a steady boyfriend.
> - What might the supervisor's motive be with this line of questioning?
> - How should Krysia respond?
> - Are these questions inappropriate or do they serve a purpose?

Phone Interview. Phone interviews are usually done by the supervisor or the human resource representative. A phone interview may be done to:
- Screen applicants and narrow the candidate pool
- Provide additional information (e.g., benefits, job description) and verify the applicant wants an interview
- Replace a face-to-face interview, especially if the candidate is from out of town

It is important to treat a phone interview as a regular interview. Box 46.16 provides a list of tips for phone interviews. Make sure to thank the interviewer at the end of the call.

Face-to-Face Interview. When you meet the interviewers, greet each person and shake hands. A firm handshake is recommended. Ensure each person has a copy of your resume and cover letter before the interview begins.

During the actual interview, maintain good eye contact. Many supervisors refuse to hire people who seem uncomfortable looking them directly in the eyes. Never take control of the interview. Allow the supervisor or panel members to ask questions at their own pace. Do not fidget in the chair or display any nervous habits (e.g., tapping your pen) (see Procedure 46.5).

Video Interview. A third interview possibility is a video interview using technology such as Skype. As with a phone interview, a video interview works well when the candidate is from out of town. There is a certain amount of technology needed for a video interview. Your school's placement office may be able to help you with that. The organization may have contacts for you to arrange your end of the interview. The benefit of a video interview over a phone interview is that the interviewers can actually see the interviewee. This allows the interviewers to assess the body language and the verbal message being presented.

> **BOX 46.16 Tips for Phone Interviews**
> - Prepare for the interview just as you would for a face-to-face interview.
> - Take the call in a quiet environment. Make sure no dogs or children are in the room. Be alone in the room.
> - Pay attention to the caller. Do not use other electronic devices or use the bathroom during the call.
> - Have a copy of your resume and cover letter.
> - Have your list of questions.
> - Have a glass of water available should you need it.

> **PROCEDURE 46.6 Create a Thank-You Note for an Interview**
>
> **Task:**
> To create a meaningful thank-you note to be sent after the interview process.
>
> **Equipment and Supplies**
> - Computer with word processing software and a printer
> - Job description
> - Contact name from interview
>
> **Procedural Steps**
> 1. Using word processing software, compose a professional letter using the business letter format. Include all of the required elements in the letter. Use correct spacing between the elements.
>   **Purpose:** Creating a letter that reflects a professional business letter shows the employer you pay attention to detail.
> 2. Highlight the particulars of the interview in the body of the letter.
>   **Purpose:** Providing highlights of the interview will assure the employer that you took the time to write an individual thank-you letter.
> 3. Include positive information you wish you had covered in the interview.
>   **Purpose:** This allows you to present any missed skills or details in a professional manner.
> 4. Create a message that is concise and to the point.
>   **Purpose:** Keep the letter short and concise. Employers look for employees who can summarize a message and communicate that message.
> 5. Proofread the letter and make any revisions as needed. Sign and send the thank-you note.
>   **Purpose:** It is important to make sure your note is written correctly. You want to leave a positive perception with the employer.

You should dress as you would for a face-to-face interview. You should have the same materials ready to access during the interview process. As with the face-to-face interview, you need to refrain from nervous habits.

Follow-Up After the Interview

Follow-up is critical after an interview. Always send a thank-you note, letter, or email to the person who conducted the interview (Procedure 46.6). It can be challenging to figure out what to send to the interviewer.
- *Send an email if:* the decision is going to be made quickly. Send an email later the day of the interview.
- *Send a written thank-you note or a letter if:* the facility is more conservative and formal. Also, it can be sent if the decision is going to be made in a week or two. Send the thank-you note within 24 hours of the interview.

Many employers see the thank-you as an expression of gratitude and professionalism. Even if you don't see yourself in that position, it is still important to send a thank you. This maybe their last perception of you, and it may help you in the future at that facility.

Typically, at the end of the interview, there will be a discussion of how quickly the decision will be made. Many agencies using online hiring software will indicate the status of the job on the posting. Candidates not selected for the position usually receive an email or letter.

After the initial interviews are completed with all the candidates, several things can occur. With some employers, the list of interviewed candidates will be narrowed. The top two or three may be asked to come back for a second interview with additional team members (e.g., providers, medical assistants). With other employers, the top candidate is selected and references are checked. These processes take time, and the deadline may be extended if vacations or out-of-office times occur.

If the interviewer indicates a decision would be made in 2 weeks, wait to hear from the facility. Give a few days after the deadline before you follow up. At that time you can call and ask the status of the job. Remember, following up prior to the deadline may not be in your best interest. The employer may perceive that you do not follow directions if you make extra phone calls. If you receive a job offer from another facility but are waiting for a decision on your favorite position, it is appropriate to contact the interviewer. Explain that you were offered another position and wondered about the status of this position. Many employers will let you know if you are in the running for the position.

Never place all your hope in one job. Make sure to continue to search and interview until an offer is made and accepted. In addition, always be on the lookout for the next job opportunity.

Negotiation

The negotiation stage of job acceptance can be as stressful as the actual interviews. The salary and benefits must be considered when determining whether to accept a position or not. When a job offer is made, there should also be a discussion of the other benefits. If the salary offered is a bit lower than expected, but the employee's share of the health insurance premium is less than expected, the salary offer becomes more attractive. Medical assistants should know the lowest salary/benefit combination they can afford. They should ask for a little more than that figure.

Bracket salary requests are often helpful in this. Instead of asking for $13 per hour, ask for a salary in the "mid to high twenties." Let the employer mention a figure or a range of salary first. Usually the person who mentions a salary range first has the disadvantage. For example, if the medical assistant requests $13 per hour, but the facility was willing to pay $16 per hour, the medical assistant probably will get $13.

Many organizations have a starting pay level for new medical assistants. If you hope to get a higher pay level, you may need to:
- Obtain a national medical assistant credential (e.g., CMA [AAMA] or RMA)
- Show an advanced skills level acquired from previous work experience in health care. Having a well-designed interview portfolio will allow you to show the interviewer all that you have accomplished.

Never say "no" to a job offer on the spot. Request at least 24 hours to consider the offer. Before accepting or rejecting a job offer, consider whether the position carries any authority, the benefits, the hours, the distance from home, and the potential for advancement. People accept jobs for reasons other than the salary; remember the value of experience.

> **CRITICAL THINKING BOX 46.10**
>
> Michelle has been on several interviews and likes the prospect of working for three different physicians. If an offer is made at each office, how can Michelle decide which to accept? What will help Michelle make this decision?

IMPROVING YOUR OPPORTUNITIES

Some people struggle finding jobs. We will examine ways to improve your opportunities for finding a job.

Finding Job Postings

Some students and graduates struggle to find jobs. They may not find job postings. This can be stressful, but it is important not to give up.

Those who are not having success with the job search may want to re-evaluate their search methods. Consider these questions:
- *Am I looking for a very selective opportunity?* For instance, are you looking for a dermatology medical assistant position in a specific facility? Those positions may be very limited. Try to broaden your search to other possible opportunities.
- *Am I looking for the correct job title?* Remember, employers may use a wide range of titles for a medical assistant.
- *Am I looking at all agencies that potentially could hire a person with my skill sets?* Depending on your area, medical assistants can be in many agencies besides a medical clinic, including a nursing home, hospital, school, or assisted-living facility.
- *Can I increase the geographical search area for employment opportunities?* Can I relocate to an area with greater employment opportunities?
- *Where can I network to increase my awareness of job openings?*
- *What job boards are being used by local employers?*

Increasing Interview Opportunities

For people who apply for jobs but never get calls for interviews, it is important to re-evaluate their information given to employers. Consider these questions:
- *Is your cover letter, resume, online profile, or application negatively impacting the job search?* It may be important to get another opinion on the content and presentation. Many times the school career placement officer will provide improvement tips.
- *Do you have spelling and grammar errors in your information?* Some employers may perceive that details are not important to you and overlook you. These mistakes are easy to fix.
- *Do your cover letter and resume need to be reformatted or revised?* Applicants need their letter and resume to stand out from the crowd. People get very creative in how they make this occur.
- *Are your cover letter and resume customized to the job posting?* Do your documents reflect the key words in the posting? Or do your documents look "generic"? With generic-looking documents, employers perceive that the person is not into details and wasn't interested enough to spend the time to customize the documents.
- *Are you following the directions in the job posting?* For instance, an employer may want a handwritten cover letter to be included. Sometimes the employer provides a mailing address and states that no calls or visits will be allowed. If applicants do not follow the directions, they may not be considered for the job.
- *Are you providing a professional image with your email address and on social media sites, such as Facebook?* Graduates struggling to find positions may want to review their social media sites. Consider tighter security settings to limit outside viewers. You may want to remove any questionable content and pictures.

Increasing Job Offers

If you are getting interviews but no job offers, re-evaluate your interview strategies. Again, the school's career placement office may have interview assistance. **Mock** interviews can help you refine your interview skills and behavior.

> **VOCABULARY**
>
> **mock**: Simulated; intended for imitation or practice.

The following is a ranked list of reasons interviewers do not hire job candidates, as expressed by surveyed career consultants and reported on the website http://www.workoplis.com:
- Not sufficiently differentiating themselves from others
- Failure to successfully transfer past experience to the current job opportunity
- Not showing enough interest and excitement
- Focusing too much on what they want and too little on what the interviewer is saying
- Feeling they can "wing" the interview without preparation
- Not being able to personally connect with the interviewer
- Appearing overqualified or underqualified for the job
- Not asking enough or the right questions
- Not researching a potential employer/interviewer
- Lacking humor, warmth, or personality during the interview process

It is always important to prepare for the interview, show enthusiasm for the position, and ask the right questions.

Other factors that may have negatively impacted the decision include:
- Inappropriate interview attire and grooming: The outfit was too tight, neckline was too low, pants dragged on the ground, or the shoes were too casual (e.g., flip-flops). The perfume or cologne was too strong. The hairstyle or color was too extreme.
- Didn't fit in the environment: Each facility has a corporate environment. The interviewer looks to see which candidate would fit best. If a person is too shy, too talkative, or too loud, he or she might not be the best fit. Or, a person may have worn too many piercings, or too many tattoos were visible.
- Used poor grammar: Some employers correlate good grammar with intelligence. Employers look for candidates who sound intelligent and who will positively represent their facility.

If you have heard or feel that your resume lacks skills needed for specific positions you want to obtain, you may want to increase your **skill sets**. This can occur through education and experience. Some people increase their job history and skill sets by obtaining temporary employment through temp agencies. Temporary jobs can provide experience and also help you refine your skills. Another way to increase your skill sets through experience is by volunteering at a healthcare facility or free clinic. Depending on the volunteer position, it may help increase your skill sets and also provide you with potential job leads. Volunteer activities should be added to the resume, because these valuable experiences often can be used in a healthcare setting. It does not matter that the position was not a paid job; experience counts, whether paid or not.

YOU GOT THE JOB!

Human Resource Requirements

When you obtain a job, you will be required to complete a number of documents (Table 46.5). You will be asked to bring in proof of identity and employment authorization (e.g., U.S. Passport, Social Security Account Number card, and driver's license). These documents are required for the employer's portion of the Form I-9. Form I-9 must be completed within a set time period to meet governmental regulations. Make sure to complete all the required forms in a timely manner. Meet the deadlines given to you by the human resource representative.

Getting Started

When you get your first job, it can be an exciting and scary time. You may feel excited for the new opportunities, yet scared of the new responsibilities. With any job, it takes time to learn the position. Most healthcare agencies have *probationary periods* for new employees. This time frame can vary. The purpose of the probationary period is to see if the new employee is the right fit for the job. If the employee is not able to do the job or is not the right person for the job, the employer can terminate the employee during the probationary period.

It is important for the medical assistant to do well during the probationary period. The first weeks to months of the job are usually devoted to orientation. The new employee learns the processes and becomes efficient and confident in the role. To be successful it is important for the medical assistant to:

> **VOCABULARY**
> **skill set**: A person's abilities or skills or expertise in an area.

TABLE 46.5 Forms to Complete When Hired

Form	Description
Form I-9: Employment Eligibility Verification Form	Form I-9 is used to verify a person's identity and employment authorization. All U.S. employers must ensure the form is completed by both the new hire and the employer. The form requires the new hire to provide the employer with documents that prove identity and employment authorization proof.
Form W-4: Employee's Withholding Allowance Certificate	New hires must provide their tax status (e.g., single) and how many allowances they are claiming. This information is used when the employer withholds money from their paycheck for income taxes.
Insurance benefit forms	Most agencies have health and life insurance benefits that the new hire can participate in. Completion of paperwork is required as part of the enrollment activities.
Background check forms	Many healthcare providers will pay for background checks on new hires. Some hiring may be contingent based on a clean background check. Some types of background checks include criminal, sexual offender registry, and caregiver.
Emergency contact form	The new employee gives the employer information on whom to contact in case of an emergency.
Handbook acknowledgement form	Some agencies have handbooks for each employee. They may require that the employee sign a form to acknowledge receiving the handbook.
Direct deposit form	Most healthcare agencies will pay the employees using the direct deposit method. Funds are transferred into the employee's bank account instead of the employee receiving a paper paycheck.
Agreement forms	The newly hired employee must sign agreement forms related to the Health Insurance Portability and Accountability Act (HIPAA) and computer security.

- Arrive 10 to 15 minutes prior to the start of the day. Limit absences, especially during the probationary period.
- Be groomed appropriately per the facility's dress code.
- Be honest, trustworthy, and respectful in all interactions with peers, patients, and providers.
- Be willing to try new things and ask questions.
- Take feedback professionally and with a positive attitude.
- Be motivated to do a good job and be willing to keep learning.
- Be a team player and be willing to help others.
- Provide safe care to patients, always working within the medical assistant scope of practice.
- Be open to new ideas, concepts, and procedures.
- Attempt to resolve simple differences with peers before involving the supervisor.
- Work with the supervisor to improve oneself and the department.
- Finish all assigned tasks in a timely manner, and look for additional duties if time is available.

Maintaining Your Job

For the medical assistant to continue with the facility, it is important to be a reliable employee. It is also important to improve one's weaknesses. The medical assistant will get regular feedback from supervisors through performance appraisals. The performance appraisals inform employees of their strengths and weaknesses on the job. These appraisals are done after the probationary period and annually thereafter. Types of performance appraisals include:

- *180-degree style*: Supervisors evaluate their employees based on their observations of the employees' performance over a given time period.
- *360-degree style*: Supervisors gather input from your co-workers and others whom you interact with on a regular basis.

Do not expect to receive a perfect appraisal. Employees are seldom perfect in all aspects of their jobs. If the supervisor gives perfect scores to an employee, there is no room for growth or improvement. The areas for growth are usually discussed during a meeting with the supervisor. You may be asked where you want to grow or improve and your goals for the coming year. It is important to consider these topics prior to the meeting with the supervisor.

Professional development is also important in maintaining one's job. Keeping updated and current is needed in the healthcare industry. It is important to meet the continuing education units (CEUs) needed to maintain your certification or registration. Information on the requirements can be found on the credentialing agency's website.

Leaving a Job

Always offer at least 2 weeks' notice when resigning from a job. Prepare a written notice of resignation and take it to the supervisor in person. Do not just leave it on a desk or place it in the interoffice mail.

Resigning from a job just as an attempt to get a salary increase is a dangerous practice. Once the employer doubts the employee's loyalty, the future is not usually bright for the employee at that facility. Resign only after a final decision has been made. If the medical assistant is resigning to take another position, the current employer may be expected to make a counteroffer. However, be wary about accepting counteroffers. What led you to look for a new job in the first place? Has the situation been resolved? Ask yourself these questions before agreeing to stay with the current employer. Often employees who accept a counteroffer and stay at their original job find that few changes are made, and the employee ends up leaving the position in the long run.

> **VOCABULARY**
> **counteroffer**: Return offer made by one who has rejected an offer or a job.

CLOSING COMMENTS

As you finish your medical assistant program, embrace the challenge of finding a job. Spend time preparing for the search. Design a professional resume and cover letter that positively set you apart from the other graduates. Network and check job boards for job openings. Apply for any jobs that interest you. Keep organized in your search so you don't overlook opportunities. Work with employment resources at your school to increase your confidence in interviewing. Your preparation and hard work will help you find your first medical assistant job!

> **EXCEPTIONAL CUSTOMER SERVICE**
>
> As you complete your practicum experience, make sure to focus on providing patients with excellent customer service. Observe how your mentors give that special service to the patients. How does your mentor help the patients feel respected and welcomed? As you observe others providing customer service, take those behaviors and incorporate them into your practice. Soon those behaviors will become part of your normal way of working with patients. Remember what you observed and practiced in practicum. Should a question about customer service come up in an interview, you will have a great conversation with the potential employer.

CHAPTER REVIEW

Employers spend a lot of time and money training their staff. It is important that they select the right employee initially. Employers look for specific personality traits when interacting with potential new employees. They seek people who already have collaboration and interpersonal skills, professionalism, compassion, and a sincere interest in the job.

Prior to job seeking, medical assistants need to prepare. They should identify the personality traits, technical skills, and transferable job skills that they possess. Medical assistants must consider what they want from their career and a job. What are the personal needs (e.g., wage, benefits, hours, locations)?

The two best methods to identify jobs are through networking and using job boards. Networking involves the medical assistant exchanging information with other professionals in hopes of obtaining possible job leads. Job boards are online sites that list positions posted by employers. Traditional job search methods include school career placement offices, newspaper ads, and employment agencies.

The three commonly used resume formats are chronologic, combination, and targeted resumes. As you create your resume, keep in mind the eye appeal or interest the resume will create in the reader. A cover letter should always accompany a resume, and much attention to detail is necessary.

The four phases of the interview process are the preparation, the actual interview, the follow-up, and the negotiation. It is important to write a thank-you note for an interview. It is a way to make you stand out from the other people who have interviewed for the same position. It shows that you are a courteous and conscientious person and also gives you another opportunity to show why you are the right person for the job.

SCENARIO WRAP-UP

Before graduation, Michelle was offered a job at Walden-Martin Family Medicine Center (WMFM). She took her instructor's advice and sent a thank-you note to those who interviewed her. When she was offered the job, the supervisor mentioned how thoughtful the note was. During the call, the supervisor summarized the benefits and the starting salary. She mentioned to Michelle that all medical assistants start at the same wage, but after they pass the CMA (AAMA) certification examination, they get a raise. Michelle took 2 days to consider the position and decided to accept the job offer. The wage was lower than what she was hoping for, but the benefits were much better.

Krysia interviewed for several medical assistant positions over the last few weeks. She found that employers respected her service to her country and valued the skills she learned in military service. She just received her third job offer within the last few days and has decided to accept the position at the local Veterans Affairs (VA) clinic. It is a full-time position with great benefits. The higher wage will help offset the extra mileage that she will be driving to work. She is very excited to be working with other veterans.

Zac has struggled identifying what type of clinic he wants to work for. With his strong leadership skills, he hopes to find a position where he can advance to a supervisory position. He has interviewed for job positions at small and large clinics. He is finding that he is more interested in working with surgeons than with family practitioners. He likes the complexity involved with surgical patients. He is hoping to receive a job offer shortly after graduation. He has decided that if his "dream job" is not offered to him, he will pursue a position in family medicine or internal medicine. This will give him a solid foundation for his new career and then someday he can move into orthopedics or surgery.

APPENDIX A

Word Parts and Definitions

Word Part	Meaning
-a	noun ending
a-	no, not, without
ab-	away from
abdomin/o	abdomen
-ablation	removal
-abrasion	scraping of
-ac	pertaining to
acid/o	acid
acous/o	hearing
acro-	heights, extremities
acromi/o	acromion
acu-	sharp
-acusis	hearing
-ad	toward
ad-	toward
aden/o	gland
adenoid/o	adenoid (pharyngeal tonsil)
adip/o	fat
adnex/o	accessory
adren/o	adrenal gland
aer/o	air
af-	toward
agglutin/o	clumping
agora-	marketplace
-al	pertaining to
albin/o	white
albumin/o	protein
-algia	pain
aliment/o	nutrition
allo-	other, different
alveol/o	alveolus
ambly/o	dull, dim
ambul/o	walking
amni/o	amnion
-amnios	amnion, inner fetal sac
amphi-	both
amyl/o	starch
-an	pertaining to
an-	no, not, without
an/o	anus
ana-	up, apart, away
andr/o	male
angi/o	vessel
ankyl/o	stiffening
ante-	forward, in front of, before
anter/o	front
anthrop/o	man

Word Part	Meaning
anti-	against
antr/o	antrum, cavity
aort/o	aorta (largest artery)
-apheresis	removal
aphth/o	ulceration
apic/o	pointed extremity, apex
apo-	separate, away from
append/o	vermiform appendix, that which is added
appendic/o	vermiform appendix, that which is added
-ar	pertaining to
-arche	beginning
arteri/o	artery
arteriol/o	arteriole (small artery)
arthr/o	articulation (joint)
articul/o	articulation (joint)
-ary	pertaining to
-ase	enzyme
astr/o	star
ather/o	fatty plaque
-atic	pertaining to
-ation	process of
atri/o	atrium
audi/o	hearing
aur/o	ear
auricul/o	ear
auto-	self
axill/o	axilla (armpit)
az/o	nitrogen
azot/o	nitrogen
bacteri/o	bacteria
balan/o	glans penis
bar/o	pressure, weight
bartholin/o	Bartholin gland
bas/o	base, bottom
bi-	two
bi/o	life, living
bil/i	bile
bin-	two
-blast	embryonic, immature
blast/o	embryonic, immature
blephar/o	eyelid
bol/o	to throw, throwing
brachi/o	arm
brachy-	short
brady-	slow

Continued

APPENDIX A Word Parts and Definitions

Word Part	Meaning	Word Part	Meaning
bronch/o	bronchus	cleid/o	clavicle (collarbone)
bronchi/o	bronchus	clitorid/o	clitoris
bronchiol/o	bronchiole	-coagulation	process of clotting
bucc/o	cheek	coccyg/o	coccyx (tailbone)
bunion/o	bunion	cochle/o	cochlea
burs/o	bursa	col/o	colon (large intestine)
calc/o, calc/i	calcium	coll/o	neck
calcane/o	calcaneus (heel bone)	colon/o	colon (large intestine)
calcul/o	stone, calculus	colp/o	vagina
cali/o	calyx, calix	commissur/o	connection
calic/o	calyx, calix	con-	together
calyc/o	calyx, calix	con/o	cone
cancer/o	cancer, malignancy	condyl/o	condyle, knob
canth/o	canthus (corner of eye)	coni/o	dust
capit/o	head	conjunctiv/o	conjunctiva
capn/o	carbon dioxide	contra-	opposite, against
carcin/o	cancer	cor/o	pupil
-carcinoma	cancer of epithelial origin	cord/o	cord, spinal cord
cardi/o	heart	cordi/o	heart
-cardia	condition of the heart	core/o	pupil
carp/o	carpus (wrist)	corne/o	cornea
cartilag/o	cartilage	coron/o	crown, heart
cata-	down	corpor/o	body
caud/o	tail	cortic/o	cortex (outer portion)
cauter/i	burning	cost/o	costa (rib)
cec/o	cecum (first part of large intestine)	cox/o	coxa (hip)
-cele	herniation, protrusion	crani/o	cranium (skull)
celi/o	abdomen	crin/o	to secrete, secreting
cellul/o	cell	-crine	to secrete, secreting
-centesis	surgical puncture	-crit	to separate, separating
cephal/o	head	crur/o	leg
cerebell/o	cerebellum	cry/o	extreme cold
cerebr/o	cerebrum	crypt-	hidden
cerumin/o	cerumen (earwax)	cubit/o	elbow, forearm
cervic/o	neck, cervix	culd/o	cul-de-sac (rectouterine pouch)
-chalasia	condition of relaxation, slackening	-cusis	hearing
-chalasis	relaxation, slackening	cut/o	skin
cheil/o	lips	cutane/o	skin
chem/o	drug, chemical	cyan/o	blue
-chezia	condition of stools	cycl/o	ciliary body, recurring, round
chol/e	bile, gall	-cyesis	pregnancy, gestation
cholangi/o	bile vessel	cyst/o	bladder, sac
cholecyst/o	gallbladder	cyt/o	cell
choledoch/o	common bile duct	-cyte	cell
cholesterol/o	cholesterol	-cytosis	abnormal increase in cells
chondr/o	cartilage	dacry/o	tear
chord/o	cord, spinal cord	dacryoaden/o	lacrimal gland
chori/o	chorion (outer fetal sac)	dacryocyst/o	lacrimal sac
chorion/o	chorion (outer fetal sac)	dactyl/o	digitus (finger or toe)
choroid/o	choroid, vascular membrane	de-	down, lack of
chrom/o	color	dendr/o	dendrite, tree
chromat/o	color	dent/i	teeth
chym/o	juice	derm/o	skin
circum-	around	dermat/o	skin
cirrh/o	orange-yellow	-desis	binding
-cision	process of cutting	dextr/o	right
-clasis	intentional breaking	di-	two, both
-clast	breaking down	dia-	through, complete
claustr/o	closing	diaphragm/o	diaphragm
clavicul/o	clavicle (collarbone)	diaphragmat/o	diaphragm

Word Part	Meaning
digit/o	finger or toe
dipl/o	double
dips/o	thirst
-dipsia	condition of thirst
dis-	bad, abnormal, apart
dist/o	far
diverticul/o	diverticulum, pouch
dors/o	back
-drome	to run, running
duct/o	to carry, carrying
duoden/o	duodenum
dur/o	dura mater, hard
-dynia	pain
dys-	bad, difficult, painful, abnormal
-e	noun ending
e-	outward, out
-eal	pertaining to
ec-	out, outward
echo-	sound, reverberation
-ectasia	condition of expansion, dilation
-ectasis	expansion, dilation
ecto-	outward, outer
-ectomy	removal, excision
-edema	swelling
ef-	away from
electr/o	electricity
-emesis	vomiting, vomit
-emia	blood condition
-emic	pertaining to blood condition
en-	in
encephal/o	brain
end-	within
endo-	within
endocardi/o	inner lining of the heart
endometri/o	endometrium
enter/o	small intestines, intestines
eosin/o	rosy-colored
epi-	above, upon
epicardi/o	epicardium
epicondyl/o	epicondyle
epididym/o	epididymis
epiglott/o	epiglottis
episi/o	vulva (external female genitalia)
epitheli/o	epithelium
erg/o	work
erythr/o	red
erythrocyt/o	red blood cell
eschar/o	scab
-esis	state of
eso-	inward
esophag/o	esophagus
esthesi/o	feeling, sensation
ethmoid/o	ethmoid bone
eu-	healthy, normal
ex-	out
exanthemat/o	rash
-exia	condition
exo-	outside
extra-	outside
faci/o	face
fallopi/o	fallopian tube
fasci/o	fascia
fec/a	feces, stool
femor/o	femur (thigh bone)
fer/o	to bear, carry
-ferous	pertaining to carrying
ferr/o	iron
fet/o	fetus
fibr/o	fiber
fibrin/o	fibrous substance
fibul/o	fibula (lower lateral leg bone)
-fida	to split, splitting
flex/o	to bend, bending
fluor/o	to flow, flowing
-flux	to flow, flowing
follicul/o	follicle, small sac
foramin/o	hole, foramen
fornic/o	arched structure, fornix
foss/o	hollow, depression
front/o	front, forehead
fund/o	fundus (base, bottom)
fung/i	fungus
-fusion	process of pouring
galact/o	milk
gastr/o	stomach
-gen	producing, produced by
gen/o	origin, originate
-genesis	production, origin
-genic	pertaining to, produced by
-genous	pertaining to, originating from
ger/o	old age
geus/o	taste
gingiv/o	gums
glauc/o	gray, bluish green
-glia	glia cell, glue
-globin	protein substance
-globulin	protein substance
glomerul/o	glomerulus
gloss/o	tongue
gluc/o	sugar, glucose
glute/o	gluteus (buttocks)
glyc/o	sugar, glucose
glycos/o	sugar, glucose
gnath/o	jaw, entire
gnos/o	knowledge
gon/o	seed
gonad/o	gonad, sex organ
goni/o	angle
-gram	record, recording
granul/o	little grain
-graph	instrument to record
graph/o	to write, writing
-graphy	process of recording
gravid/o	pregnancy, gestation
-gravida	pregnancy, gestation
gynec/o	female, woman
halit/o	breath
hal/o	to breathe, breathing
hedon/o	pleasure
hem/o	blood

Continued

Word Part	Meaning	Word Part	Meaning
hemangi/o	blood vessel	ischi/o	ischium (lower part of pelvic bone)
hemat/o	blood	-ism	condition, state of
hemi-	half	-ist	one who specializes
hemorrhoid/o	hemorrhoid	-itis	inflammation
hepat/o	liver	-itic	pertaining to
herni/o	hernia	-ium	structure, membrane
heter/o	different	-ive	pertaining to
hiat/o	an opening	-ization	process of
hidr/o	sweat	jejun/o	second part of small intestine, jejunum
hidraden/o	sudoriferous gland (sweat gland)	kal/i	potassium
hil/o	hilum	kary/o	nucleus
hist/o	tissue	kathis/o	sitting
home/o	same	kerat/o	hard, horny, cornea
homo-	same	ket/o	ketone
humer/o	humerus (upper arm bone)	keton/o	ketone
humor/o	liquid	-kine	movement
hydr/o	water, fluid	kinesi/o	movement
hymen/o	hymen	-kinin	movement substance
hyper-	excessive, above	klept/o	to steal, stealing
hypo-	deficient, below, under	kyph/o	round back
hypophys/o	hypophysis, pituitary	labi/o	lips, labia
hyster/o	uterus	labyrinth/o	labyrinth (inner ear)
-i	noun ending	lacrim/o	tear
-ia	condition, state of	lact/o	milk
-iac	pertaining to	-lalia	condition of babbling
-iasis	condition, presence of	lamin/o	lamina, thin plate
iatr/o	treatment	lapar/o	abdomen
-iatric	pertaining to treatment	-lapse	falling, dropping, prolapse
-iatrician	one who specializes in treatment	laryng/o	larynx (voice box)
-iatrist	one who specializes in treatment	later/o	side
-iatry	process of treatment	lei/o	smooth
-ic	pertaining to	leiomy/o	smooth muscle
ichthy/o	fishlike	-lepsy	seizure
-ician	one who studies	leuk/o	white
-icle	small, tiny	leukocyt/o	white blood cell
-id	pertaining to	levo-	left
idi/o	unique, unknown	lex/o	word, speech
-ile	pertaining to	ligament/o	ligament
ile/o	ileum (third part small intestines)	ligat/o	to tie, tying
ili/o	ilium (superior, widest pelvic bone)	lingu/o	tongue
immun/o	safety, protection	lip/o	fat
-in	substance	lipid/o	lipid, fat
in-	in, not	-listhesis	slipping
-ine	pertaining to	lith/o	stone, calculus
infer/o	downward	-lithotomy	removal of a stone
infra-	down	lob/o	lobe, section
inguin/o	groin	lobul/o	small lobe
insulin/o	insulin	log/o	study
inter-	between	-logist	one who specializes in the study of
interstit/o	space between	-logy	study of
intestin/o	intestine	long/o	long
intra-	within	lord/o	swayback
-ion	process of	lumb/o	lower back
-ior	pertaining to	lumin/o	lumen (space within vessel)
ipsi-	same	lymph/o	lymph
ir/o	iris	lymphaden/o	lymph gland (lymph node)
irid/o	iris	lymphangi/o	lymph vessel
-is	structure, thing, noun ending	lymphat/o	lymph
is/o	equal	lys/o	break down, dissolve
isch/o	hold back, suppress		

Word Part	Meaning
-lysis	breaking down, dissolving, loosening, freeing from adhesions
-lytic	pertaining to breaking down
macro-	large
macul/o	macula, macule, macula lutea, spot
mal-	bad, poor
-malacia	condition of softening
malle/o	malleus, hammer
malleol/o	distal process lower leg, little malleolus
mamm/o	breast
man/o	scanty pressure
mandibul/o	lower jaw
-mania	condition of madness
man/u	hand
mast/o	breast
mastoid/o	mastoid process
maxill/o	maxilla (upper jaw bone)
meat/o	meatus (opening)
medi/o	middle
mediastin/o	mediastinum (space between lungs)
medull/o	medulla, inner portion
-megaly	enlargement
melan/o	black, dark
men/o	menstruation, menses
mening/o	meninges
meningi/o	meninges
menisc/o	meniscus, crescent
menstru/o	menstruation
ment/o	mind, chin
meso-	middle
meta-	beyond, change
metacarp/o	metacarpal (hand bone)
metatars/o	metatarsal (foot bone)
-meter	instrument to measure
metr/o	uterus
metri/o	uterus
-metry	process of measurement
micro-	small
mid-	middle
-mission	to send, sending
mitochondri/o	mitochondria
mono-	one
morph/o	shape, form
muc/o	mucus
multi-	many
muscul/o	muscle
mut/a	change
my/o	muscle, to shut
myc/o	fungus
myel/o	bone marrow, spinal cord
myocardi/o	myocardium (heart muscle)
myos/o	muscle
myring/o	eardrum
myx/o	mucus
narc/o	sleep, stupor
nas/o	nose
nat/o	birth, born
natr/o	sodium
necr/o	death, dead
neo-	new
nephr/o	kidney
neur/o	nerve
neutr/o	neutral
nev/o	nevus, birthmark
nid/o	nest
noct/i	night
nod/o	node, knot
-noia	condition of mind
non-	not
nuch/o	neck
nucle/o	nucleus
nulli-	none
nyctal/o	night
nymph/o	woman, female
o/o	ovum, egg, female sex cell
occipit/o	occiput, back of head
occlus/o	to close, closing, a blockage
-occlusion	condition of closure
-occult	secret, hidden
ocul/o	eye
odont/o	teeth
-oid	resembling, like
olecran/o	elbow
olig/o	scanty, few
-oma	tumor, mass
omphal/o	umbilicus (navel)
onc/o	tumor
-on	structure
-one	hormone, substance that forms
onych/o	nail
oophor/o	ovary (female gonad)
ophthalm/o	eye
-opia	vision condition
-opsia	vision condition
-opsy	process of viewing
opt/o	vision
optic/o	vision
or/o	mouth, oral cavity
orbit/o	orbit
orch/o	testis, testicle (male gonad)
orchi/o	testis, testicle (male gonad)
orchid/o	testis, testicle (male gonad)
orex/o	appetite
organ/o	organ, viscus
orth/o	straight, upright
-ose	pertaining to, full of
-osis	abnormal condition
osm/o	sense of smell
oss/i	bone
osse/o	bone
ossicul/o	ossicle (tiny bone)
oste/o	bone
ot/o	ear
-ous	pertaining to
ov/o	ovum (egg)
ovari/o	ovary (female gonad)
ovul/o	ovum (female sex cell)
ox/i, ox/o	oxygen
oxy-	rapid

Continued

APPENDIX A Word Parts and Definitions

Word Part	Meaning
palat/o	palate, roof of mouth, palatine bone
palm/o	palm
palpebr/o	eyelid
pan-	all
pancreat/o	pancreas
papill/o	papilla, nipple, optic disk
papul/o	papule, pimple
par-	beside, near
-para	delivery, parturition
para-	near, beside, abnormal
parathyroid/o	parathyroid
parenchym/o	parenchyma
-paresis	slight paralysis
pariet/o	wall, partition
part/o	parturition (delivery)
-partum	parturition (delivery)
patell/o, patell/a	patella (kneecap)
path/o	disease
-pathy	disease process
-pause	stop, cease
pector/o	chest
ped/o	foot, child
pedicul/o	lice
pelv/i, pelv/o	pelvis
pen/i	penis
-penia	deficiency condition
-pepsia	digestion condition
per-	through
peri-	surrounding, around
pericardi/o	sac surrounding the heart
perine/o	perineum
peritone/o, periton/o	peritoneum
perone/o	lower, lateral leg bone, fibula
-pexy	fixation, suspension
phac/o	lens
phag/o	to eat, swallow
phak/o	lens
phalang/o	phalanx (finger/toe bones)
phall/o	penis
pharyng/o	pharynx (throat)
phas/o	speech
phe/o	dark
-pheresis	removal
-phil	attraction
phil/o	attraction
-philia	condition of attraction, increase
phleb/o	vein
-phobia	condition of fear, extreme sensitivity
phon/o	sound, voice
phor/o	to carry, to bear
phot/o	light
phren/o	diaphragm, mind
-phylaxis	protection
physi/o	growth, nature
-physis	growth, nature
phyt/o	growth, nature
pil/o	hair
pituitar/o	pituitary
placent/o	placenta
-plakia	condition of patches
plant/o	sole of foot
plas/o	formation
-plasia	condition of formation, development
-plasm	formation
plasm/o	plasma
plast/o	formation
-plastin	forming substance
-plasty	surgical repair
-plegia	paralysis
pleur/o	pleura, membrane surrounding lungs
plethysm/o	volume
plic/o	fold, plica
-pnea	breathing
pne/o	to breathe, breathing
pneum/o	lung, air
pneumon/o	lung
-poiesis	formation, production
-poietin	forming substance
pol/o	pole
poly-	many, much, excessive, frequent
polyp/o	polyp
poplite/o	back of knee
por/o	passage
post-	behind, after
poster/o	back
potass/o	potassium
prax/o	purposeful movement
pre-	before, in front of
preputi/o	prepuce (foreskin)
presby-	old age
press/o	pressure
primi-	first
pro-	forward, in front of, in favor of
proct/o	rectum and anus
prolactin/o	prolactin
prostat/o	prostate
prosth/o, prosthes/o	addition
proxim/o	near
psych/o	mind
-ptosis	drooping, prolapse, falling
-ptysis	spitting
pub/o	pubis, anterior pelvic bone
pulmon/o	lung
pupill/o	pupil
puerper/o	childbirth, puerperium
purpur/o	purple
pustul/o	pustule
py/o	pus
pyel/o	renal pelvis
pylor/o	pylorus
pyr/o	fever, fire
pyret/o	fever, fire
quadri-	four
rachi/o	spinal column, backbone
radi/o	radius (lower lateral arm bone)
radi/o	rays
radicul/o	nerve root, spinal nerve root
re-	back, backward, again
rect/o	rectum, straight

APPENDIX A Word Parts and Definitions

Word Part	Meaning
ren/o	kidney
reticul/o	network
retin/o	retina
retro-	backward
rhabd/o	striated
rhabdomy/o	striated (skeletal) muscle
rheumat/o	watery flow
rhin/o	nose
rhiz/o	spinal nerve root, nerve root
rhythm/o	rhythm
rhytid/o	wrinkle
rib/o	ribose
rot/o	wheel
-rrhagia, -rrhage	bursting forth
-rrhaphy	suture, repair
-rrhea	discharge, flow
-rrheic	pertaining to discharge
-rrhexis	rupture
rug/o	rugae, ridge
sacr/o	sacrum
sagitt/o	arrow, separating the sides
salping/o	tube, fallopian or eustachian
-salpinx	fallopian, tube
sarc/o	flesh
-sarcoma	connective tissue cancer
scapul/o	scapula (shoulder blade)
schiz/o	split
scler/o	sclera, hard
-sclerosis	abnormal condition of hardening
scoli/o	curvature
-scope	instrument to view
-scopic	pertaining to viewing
-scopy	process of viewing
scot/o	dark
scrot/o	scrotum (sac holding testes)
sebac/o	sebum, oil
seb/o	sebum, oil
semin/i	semen
seps/o	infection
-sepsis	infection
sept/o	septum, wall, partition
septic/o	infection
ser/o	serum
sial/o	saliva
sialaden/o	salivary gland
sider/o	iron
-siderin	iron substance
sigmoid/o	sigmoid colon
sin/o	sinus, cavity
sinistr/o	left
sinus/o	sinus, cavity
-sis	state of, condition
skelet/o	skeleton
somat/o	body
somn/o	sleep
son/o	sound
-spadias	a rent or tear
-spasm	spasm, sudden, involuntary contraction
sperm/o	spermatozoon (male sex cell)
spermat/o	spermatozoon (male sex cell)
sphenoid/o	sphenoid
spin/o	spine
spir/o	to breathe, breathing
splen/o	spleen
spondyl/o	vertebra, backbone, spine
squam/o	scaly
-stalsis	contraction
staped/o	stapes (third ossicle in ear)
-stasis	controlling, stopping
steat/o	fat
-stenosis	abnormal condition of narrowing
ster/o	steroid
stere/o	three-dimensional
stern/o	sternum (breastbone)
steth/o	chest
sthen/o	strength
-sthenia	condition of strength
stom/o	an opening, a mouth
stomat/o	mouth, oral cavity
-stomy	new opening
strom/o	stroma (supportive tissue)
sub-	under, below
sudor/i	sweat
sulc/o	sulcus, groove
super/o	upward
supra-	upward, above
sur/o	calf
sympath/o	to feel with
syn-	together, joined
syndesm/o	ligament (structure connecting bone)
synovi/o	synovium
tachy-	fast, rapid
tars/o	tarsal bone (ankle bone)
tax/o	order, coordination
tel/e	end, far, complete
tele/o	end, far, complete
tempor/o	temporal bone
ten/o	tendon (structure connecting muscles to bones)
tend/o	tendon (structure connecting muscles to bones)
tendin/o	tendon (structure connecting muscles to bones)
tens/o	stretching
-tension	process of stretching, pressure
terat/o	deformity
test/o	testis, testicle (male gonad)
testicul/o	testis, testicle (male gonad)
tetra-	four
thalam/o	thalamus
thalass/o	sea
thel/e	nipple
-therapy	treatment
therm/o	heat, temperature
thorac/o	thorax (chest)
-thorax	chest (pleural cavity)
thromb/o	clotting, clot
-thrombin	clotting substance

Continued

APPENDIX A Word Parts and Definitions

Word Part	Meaning
thrombocyt/o	clotting cell
thym/o	thymus gland, mind
-thymia	condition/state of mind
thyr/o	thyroid gland, shield
thyroid/o	thyroid gland
tibi/o	tibia (shinbone)
-tic	pertaining to
-tion	process of
toc/o	labor, delivery
-tocia	condition of labor, delivery
tom/o	section, cutting
-tome	instrument to cut
-tomy	incision, cutting
ton/o	tension, tone
tonsill/o	tonsil
top/o	place, location
tox/o	poison
toxic/o	poison
trabecul/o	little beam
trache/o	trachea (windpipe)
tract/o	to pull, pulling
trans-	through, across
-tresia	condition of an opening
tri-	three
trich/o	hair
trigon/o	trigone
-tripsy	process of crushing
-tripter	machine to crush
-trite	instrument to crush
trochanter/o	trochanter
trop/o	to turn, turning
troph/o	development, nourishment
-trophy	process of nourishment, development
tub/o	tube, pipe
tubercul/o	tubercle, a swelling
tympan/o	eardrum, drum
-ule	small
uln/o	ulna (lower medial arm bone)
ultra-	beyond
-um	structure, thing, membrane
umbilic/o	umbilicus (navel)
ungu/o	nail
uni-	one

Word Part	Meaning
ur/o	urine, urinary system
ureter/o	ureter
urethr/o	urethra
-uria	urinary condition
urin/o	urine, urinary system
-us	structure, thing, noun ending
uter/o	uterus
uve/o	uvea
uvul/o	uvula
vag/o	vagus nerve
vagin/o	vagina
valv/o	valve
valvul/o	valve
varic/o	varices
vas/o	vessel, ductus deferens, vas deferens
vascul/o	vessel
ven/o	vein
ventr/o	belly side
ventricul/o	ventricle
venul/o	venule, small vein
-verse	to turn
vers/o	to turn
-version	process of turning
vertebr/o	vertebra, spine
vesic/o	bladder
vesicul/o	small sac, seminal vesicle, blister
vestibul/o	vestibule (small space at entrance to canal)
vill/o	villus
vir/o	virus
viscer/o	viscera, organ
vitre/o	vitreous humor, glassy
vol/o	volume
vomer/o	vomer
vulgar/o	common
vulv/o	vulva (external female genitalia)
xen/o	foreign
xer/o	dry
xiph/i	xiphoid process, sword
-y	process of; condition
zo/o	animal
zygom/o	zygoma (cheekbone)
zygomat/o	zygoma (cheekbone)

APPENDIX B

Definitions and Word Parts

Meaning	Word Part
abdomen	abdomin/o, celi/o, lapar/o
abnormal	para-, dys-
abnormal condition	-osis
abnormal condition of hardening	-sclerosis
abnormal condition of narrowing	-stenosis
abnormal increase in cells	-cytosis
above, upon	epi-
accessory	adnex/o
acid	acid/o
acromion	-acromion
addition	prosth/o, prosthes/o
adenoid (pharyngeal tonsil)	adenoid/o
adrenal gland	adren/o
again	re-
against	anti-
air	aer/o, pneum/o
all	pan-
alveolus	alveol/o
amnion	amni/o
amnion (inner fetal sac)	-amnios
angle	goni/o
animal	zo/o
ankle bone (tarsal bone)	tars/o
antrum, cavity	antr/o
anus	an/o
aorta (largest artery)	aort/o
appendix, vermiform	append/o, appendic/o
appetite	orex/o
arm	brachi/o
armpit (axilla)	axill/o
around	circum-
arrow, separating the sides	sagitt/o
arteriole (small artery)	arteriol/o
artery	arteri/o
atrium	atri/o
attraction	phil/o, -phil
away from	ab-, ef-, apo-
back	dors/o, poster/o
backbone	rachi/o
back of knee	poplite/o
back, again	re-
backward	retro-, re-
bacteria	bacteri/o
bad, abnormal, apart	dis-
bad, difficult, painful, abnormal	dys-

Meaning	Word Part
bad, poor	mal-
Bartholin gland	bartholin/o
base, bottom	bas/o
bear, carry	fer/o, phor/o, duct/o
before, in front of	pre-
beginning	-arche
behind, after	post-
belly side	ventr/o
below	hypo-
bend, bending	flex/o
beside, near	par-
between	inter-
beyond	ultra-
beyond, change	meta-
bile, gall	bil/i, chol/e
bile vessel	cholangi/o
binding	-desis
birth, born	nat/o
black, dark	melan/o
bladder	vesic/o
bladder, sac	cyst/o
blister	vesicul/o
blood	hem/o, hemat/o
blood condition	-emia
blood vessel	hemangi/o
blue	cyan/o
bluish green	glauc/o
body	corpor/o, somat/o, som/o
bone	oss/i, osse/o, oste/o
bone marrow, spinal cord	myel/o
both	amphi-
brain	encephal/o
break down, dissolve	lys/o
break down, freeing from adhesions, dissolving, loosening	-lysis
breaking down	-clast
breast	mamm/o, mast/o
breastbone (sternum)	stern/o
breath	halit/o
breathe, breathing	pne/o
breathing, to breathe	-pnea, spir/o, hal/o
bronchiole	bronchiol/o
bronchus	bronch/o, bronchi/o
bunion	bunion/o
burning	cauter/i
bursa	burs/o

Continued

Meaning	Word Part	Meaning	Word Part
bursting forth	-rrhagia, -rrhage	condition of stools	-chezia
buttocks	glute/o	condition of strength	-sthenia
calcium	calc/o, calc/i	condition of the heart	-cardia
calf	sur/o	condition of thirst	-dipsia
calyx, calix	cali/o, calic/o, calyc/o	condition, presence of	-iasis
cancer	carcin/o	condition, state of	-exia, -ia, -ism, -y
cancer of epithelial origin	-carcinoma	condition/state of mind	-thymia, -noia
cancer, malignancy	cancer/o	condyle, knob	condyl/o
canthus (corner of eye)	canth/o	cone	con/o
carbon dioxide	capn/o	conjunctiva	conjunctiv/o
carry, carrying	duct/o	connection	commissur/o
carry, to bear	phor/o	connective tissue cancer	-sarcoma
cartilage	cartilag/o, chondr/o	contraction	-stalsis
cecum (first part of large intestine)	cec/o	controlling, stopping	-stasis
		cord, spinal cord	chord/o
cell	cellul/o, cyt/o, cyte	cornea	corne/o, kerat/o
cerebellum	cerebell/o	cortex (outer portion)	cortic/o
cerebrum	cerebr/o	crown	coron/o
cervix	cervic/o	curvature	scoli/o
change	mut/a	dark	phe/o, scot/o
cheek	bucc/o	death, dead	necr/o
cheekbone (zygoma)	zygom/o, zygomat/o	deficiency condition	-penia
chest (thorax)	pector/o, steth/o, thorac/o	deficient, below, under	hypo-
chest (pleural cavity)	-thorax	deformity	terat/o
child, foot	ped/o	delivery, parturition	-para
childbirth, puerperium	puerper/o	dendrite, tree	dendr/o
chin	ment/o	development	troph/o
cholesterol	cholesterol/o	diaphragm	diaphragm/o, diaphragmat/o
choroid	choroid/o	diaphragm, mind	phren/o
chorion (outer fetal sac)	chori/o, chorion/o	different	heter/o
ciliary body	cycl/o	digestion condition	-pepsia
clitoris	clitorid/o	discharge, flow	-rrhea
close, closing, a blockage	occlus/o	disease	path/o
closing	claustr/o	disease process	-pathy
clotting cell	thrombocyt/o	distal process lower leg, little malleolus	malleol/o
clotting substance	-thrombin		
clotting, clot	thromb/o	diverticulum, pouch	diverticul/o
clumping	agglutin/o	double	dipl/o
cochlea	cochle/o	down	cata-, infra-
collarbone (clavicle)	cleid/o, clavicul/o	down, lack of	de-
color	chrom/o, chromat/o	downward	infer/o
common	vulgar/o	drooping, prolapse	-ptosis
common bile duct	choledoch/o	drug, chemical	chem/o
condition of an opening	-tresia	dry	xer/o
condition of attraction; increase	-philia	dull, dim	ambly/o
		duodenum	duoden/o
condition of babbling	-lalia	dust	coni/o
condition of closure	-occlusion	ear	aur/o, auricul/o, ot/o
condition of expansion, dilation	-ectasia	earwax, cerumen	cerumin/o
		eardrum, drum	myring/o, tympan/o
condition of fear, extreme sensitivity	-phobia	eat, swallow	phag/o
		elbow	olecran/o
condition of formation, development	-plasia	elbow (forearm)	cubit/o
		electricity	electr/o
condition of labor, delivery	-tocia	embryonic, immature	-blast, blast/o
condition of madness	-mania	end, far, complete	tel/e, tele/o
condition of patches	-plakia	endocardium (inner lining of the heart)	endocardi/o
condition of relaxation, slackening	-chalasia		
		endometrium	endometri/o
condition of softening	-malacia	enlargement	-megaly

Meaning	Word Part
enzyme	-ase
epicardium	epicardi/o
epicondyle	epicondyl/o
epididymis	epididym/o
epiglottis	epiglott/o
epithelium	epitheli/o
equal	is/o
esophagus	esophag/o
ethmoid bone	ethmoid/o
excessive, above	hyper-
expansion, dilation	-ectasis
extreme cold	cry/o
eye	ocul/o, ophthalm/o
eyelid	blephar/o, palpebr/o
face	faci/o
falling, drooping, prolapse	-lapse, -ptosis
fallopian tube	fallopi/o, salping/o, -salpinx
far	tel/e, tele/o
fascia	fasci/o
fast, rapid	tachy-
fat	adip/o, lip/o, steat/o
fatty plaque	ather/o
feces, stool	fec/a
feel with	sympath/o
feeling, sensation	esthesi/o
female, woman	gynec/o, nymph/o
femur (thighbone)	femor/o
fetus	fet/o
fever, fire	pyr/o, pyret/o
fiber	fibr/o
fibrous substance	fibrin/o
fibula	fibul/o, perone/o
finger or toe (digitus)	dactyl/o, digit/o
finger/toe bones (phalanx)	phalang/o
first	primi-
fishlike	ichthy/o
fixation, suspension	-pexy
flesh	sarc/o
flow, flowing	fluor/o
fold, plica	plic/o
follicle, small sac	follicul/o
foot, child	ped/o
foreign	xen/o
foreskin (prepuce)	preputi/o
formation, production	plas/o, plast/o, -poiesis, -plasm
forming substance	-plastin, -poietin
fornix	fornic/o
forward, in front of	ante-, pro-
four	quadri-, tetra-
frequent	poly-
front, forehead	anter/o, front/o
fungus	myc/o, fung/i
fundus (base, bottom)	fund/o
gallbladder	cholecyst/o
gland	aden/o
glans penis	balan/o
glomerulus	glomerul/o
glue, glia cell	-glia
gonad, sex organ	gonad/o

Meaning	Word Part
groin	inguin/o
growth, nature	physi/o, -physis, phyt/o
gums	gingiv/o
hair	pil/o, trich/o
half	hemi-
hand	man/u
hard (dura mater)	dur/o
hard, horny, cornea	kerat/o
head	capit/o, cephal/o
healthy, normal	eu-
hearing	acous/o, audi/o, -acusis
heart	cardi/o, cordi/o, coron/o
heat, temperature	therm/o
heel bone (calcaneus)	calcane/o
heights, extremes, extremities	acro-
hemorrhoid	hemorrhoid/o
hernia	herni/o
herniation, protrusion	-cele
hidden	crypt-
hilum	hil/o
hip (coxa)	cox/o
hold back, suppress	isch/o
hole, foramen	foramin/o
hollow, depression	foss/o
hormone, substance that forms	-one
humerus (upper arm bone)	humer/o
hymen	hymen/o
ileum	ile/o
ilium (superior, widest pelvic bone)	ili/o
in	en-, in-
in favor of	pro-
incision, cutting	-tomy
infection	seps/o, -sepsis, septic/o
inflammation	-itis
inner ear (labyrinth)	labyrinth/o
instrument to crush	-trite
instrument to cut	-tome
instrument to measure	-meter
instrument to record	-graph
instrument to view	-scope
insulin	insulin/o
intentional breaking	-clasis
intestine	intestin/o, enter/o
inward	eso-
iris	ir/o, irid/o
iron	ferr/o, sider/o
iron substance	-siderin
ischium	ischi/o
jaw, entire	gnath/o
jejunum	jejun/o
joint (articulation)	arthr/o, articul/o
juice	chym/o
ketone	ket/o, keton/o
kidney	nephr/o, ren/o
kneecap (patella)	patell/o, patell/a
knowledge	gnos/o
labor, delivery	toc/o
lacrimal gland	dacryoaden/o

Continued

APPENDIX B   Definitions and Word Parts

Meaning	Word Part
lacrimal sac	dacrocyst/o
lamina, thin plate	lamin/o
large	macro-
large intestine (colon)	col/o, colon/o
left	levo-, sinistr/o
leg	crur/o
lens	phac/o, phak/o
lice	pedicul/i
life, living	bi/o
ligament	ligament/o, syndesm/o
light	phot/o
lipid, fat	lipid/o
lips	cheil/o
lips (labia)	labi/o
liquid	humor/o
little beam	trabecul/o
little grain	granul/o
liver	hepat/o
lobe, section	lob/o
long	long/o
lower back	lumb/o
lower jaw	mandibul/o
lumen (space within vessel)	lumin/o
lung	pneumon/o, pulmon/o, pneum/o
lymph	lymph/o, lymphat/o
lymph gland (lymph node)	lymphaden/o
lymph vessel	lymphangi/o
machine to crush	-tripter
male	andr/o
male sex cell, spermatozoon	spermat/o
malleus, hammer	malle/o
man	anthrop/o
many	multi-
many, much, excessive	poly-
marketplace	agora-
mass	-oma
mastoid process	mastoid/o
meatus (opening)	meat/o
mediastinum	mediastin/o
medulla	medull/o
meninges	mening/o, meningi/o
meniscus	menisc/o
menstruation, menses	menstru/o, men/o
metacarpal (hand bone)	metacarp/o
metatarsal (foot bone)	metatars/o
middle	medi/o, meso-, mid-
milk	galact/o, lact/o
mind	ment/o, phren/o, psych/o
mitochondria	mitochondri/o
mouth, oral cavity	or/o, stomat/o
movement	-kine, kinesi/o
movement substance	-kinin
mucus	muc/o, myx/o
muscle	muscul/o, my/o, myos/o
myocardium (heart muscle)	myocardi/o, cardiomy/o
nail	onych/o, ungu/o
near	proxim/o
near, beside, abnormal	para-, par-
neck	nuch/o, coll/o
neck, cervix	cervic/o
nerve	neur/o
nerve root	radicul/o, rhiz/o
nest	nid/o
network	reticul/o
neutral	neutr/o
nevus, birthmark	nev/o
new	neo-
new opening	-stomy
night	noct/i, nyctal/o
nipple	thel/e
nipple	papill/o
nitrogen	az/o, azot/o
no, not, without	a-, an-, in-, non-
node, knot	nod/o
none	nulli-
nose	nas/o, rhin/o
nourishment	troph/o
noun ending	-a, -e, -i, -is, -um, -on, -ium, -us
nucleus	kary/o, nucle/o
nutrition	aliment/o
occiput, back of head	occipit/o
old age	ger/o, presby-
one	mono-, uni-
one who specializes	-ist
one who specializes in the study of	-logist
one who specializes in treatment	-iatrician, -iatrist
optic disk	papill/o
one who studies	-ician
opening	hiat/o
opening, a mouth	stom/o
opposite, against	contra-
optic disk	papill/o
orange-yellow	cirrh/o
order, coordination	tax/o
organ, viscera	organ/o, viscer/o
origin, originate	gen/o
ossicle	ossicul/o
other, different	allo-
out, outward	ec-, ex-
outside	exo-, extra-
outward	e-, ecto-
ovary	oophor/o, ovari/o
ovum, egg	o/o, ovul/o, ov/o
oxygen	ox/i, ox/o
pain	-algia, -dynia
palate, roof of mouth, palatine bone	palat/o
palm	palm/o
pancreas	pancreat/o
papilla	papill/o
papule	papul/o
paralysis	-plegia
paralysis, slight	-paresis
parathyroid	parathyroid/o
parenchyma	parenchym/o
parturition, delivery	part/o, -partum

Meaning	Word Part
passage	por/o
pelvis	pelv/i, pelv/o
penis	pen/i, phall/o
perineum	perine/o
peritoneum	peritone/o, periton/o
peroneum	perone/o
pertaining to	-ac, -al, -an, -ar, -ary, -atic, -eal, -iac, -ac, -ic, -id, -ile, -ine, -ior, -itic, -ive, -ous, -tic
pertaining to blood condition	-emic
pertaining to breaking down	-lytic
pertaining to carrying	-ferous
pertaining to discharge	-rrheic
pertaining to originating from	-genous
pertaining to, produced by	-genic
pertaining to treatment	-iatric
pertaining to viewing	-scopic
pertaining to, full of	-ose
pimple	papul/o
pituitary, hypophysis	hypophys/o, pituitar/o
place, location	top/o
placenta	placent/o
plasma	plasm/a
pleasure	hedon/o
pleura (membrane surrounding lungs)	pleur/o
pointed extremity, apex	apic/o
poison	tox/o, toxic/o
pole	pol/o
polyp	polyp/o
potassium	kal/i, potass/o
pouch, diverticulum	diverticul/o
pregnancy, gestation	-cyesis, gravid/o, gravida
pressure	press/o
pressure, weight	bar/o
process of viewing	-opsy
process of	-ation, -ion, -ization, -tion, -y
process of clotting	-coagulation
process of crushing	-tripsy
process of cutting	-cision
process of measurement	-metry
process of nourishment, development	-trophy
process of pouring	-fusion
process of recording	-graphy
process of stretching, pressure	-tension
process of treatment	-iatry
process of turning	-version
process of viewing	-scopy
producing, produced by	-gen
production	-genesis
prolactin	prolact/o
prolapse	-ptosis
prostate	prostat/o
protection	-phylaxis
protein	albumin/o
protein substance	-globin, -globulin
pubis, anterior pelvic bone	pub/o

Meaning	Word Part
pull, pulling	tract/o
pupil	cor/o, core/o, pupill/o
purple	purpur/o
purposeful movement	prax/o
pus	py/o
pustule	pustul/o
pylorus	pylor/o
radius	radi/o
rapid, fast	oxy-, tachy-
rash	exanthemat/o
rays	radi/o
record, recording	-gram
rectouterine pouch (cul-de-sac)	culd/o
rectum and anus	proct/o
rectum, straight	rect/o
recurring, round	cycl/o
red	erythr/o
red blood cell	erythrocyt/o
relaxation, slackening	-chalasis
removal of a stone	-lithotomy
removal, excision	-ablation, -apheresis, -pheresis, -ectomy
renal pelvis	pyel/o
rent or tear	-spadias
repair	-rrhaphy
resembling, like	-oid
retina	retin/o
rhythm	rhythm/o
rib (costa)	cost/o
ribose	rib/o
right	dextr/o
rosy-colored	eosin/o
round back	kyph/o
rugae, ridge	rug/o
run, running	-drome
rupture	-rrhexis
sac surrounding the heart	pericardi/o
sacrum	sacr/o
safety, protection	immun/o
saliva	sial/o
salivary gland	sialaden/o
same	home/o, homo-, ipsi-
scab	eschar/o
scaly	squam/o
scanty, few	olig/o
scanty, pressure	man/o
sclera, hard	scler/o
scraping of	-abrasion
scrotum	scrot/o
sea	thalass/o
sebum, oil	seb/o, sebac/o
secret, hidden	-occult
secrete, secreting	crin/o, -crine
section, cutting	tom/o
seed	gon/o
seizure	-lepsy
self	auto-
semen	semin/i
send, sending	-mission
sense of smell	osm/o

Continued

APPENDIX B Definitions and Word Parts

Meaning	Word Part
separate, separating	-crit
separate, away	apo-
septum	sept/o
serum	ser/o
shape, form	morph/o
sharp	acu-
shinbone (tibia)	tibi/o
short	brachy-
shoulder blade (scapula)	scapul/o
side	later/o
sigmoid colon	sigmoid/o
sinus, cavity	sin/o, sinus/o
sitting	kathis/o
skeleton	skelet/o
skin	cut/o, cutane/o, derm/o, dermat/o
skull (cranium)	crani/o
sleep, stupor	narc/o, somn/o
slight paralysis	-paresis
slipping	-listhesis
slow	brady-
small	micro-, -ule
small intestines, intestines	enter/o
small lobe	lobul/o
small sac, seminal vesicle	vesicul/o
smooth	lei/o
smooth muscle	leiomy/o
sodium	natr/o
softening	-malacia
sole of foot	plant/o
sound	echo-, son/o
sound, voice	phon/o
space between	interstit/o
spasm	-spasm
speech	phas/o
spermatozoon	sperm/o
sphenoid	sphenoid/o
spinal column	rachi/o
spinal cord	cord/o, myel/o
spinal nerve root	rhiz/o, radicul/o
spine	spin/o, vertebr/o
spitting	-ptysis
spleen	splen/o
split	schiz/o, -fida
split, splitting	-fida
spot, macula lutea, macule	macul/o
stapes	staped/o
star	astr/o
starch	amyl/o
state of	-esis, -sis
state of relaxation	-chalasis
steal, stealing	klept/o
steroid	ster/o
stiffening	ankyl/o
stomach	gastr/o
stone (calculus)	calcul/o, lith/o
stop, cease	-pause
straight, upright	orth/o
strength	sthen/o
stretching	tens/o

Meaning	Word Part
striated	rhabd/o
striated (skeletal) muscle	rhabdomy/o
stroma (supportive tissue)	strom/o
structure, membrane, thing	-um, -ium
structure, thing, noun ending	-us, -on, -is
study	log/o
study of	-logy
substance	-in
sugar, glucose	glycos/o, gluc/o, glyc/o
sulcus, groove	sulc/o
surgical puncture	-centesis
surgical repair	-plasty
surrounding, around	peri-
suture	-rrhaphy
swallow, eat	phag/o
swayback	lord/o
sweat	hidr/o, sudor/i
sweat gland (sudoriferous gland)	hidraden/o
swelling	-edema, tubercul/o
synovium	synovi/o
tail	caud/o
tailbone (coccyx)	coccyg/o
taste	geus/o
tear	dacry/o, lacrim/o
teeth	dent/i, odont/o
temporal bone	tempor/o
tendon	ten/o, tend/o, tendin/o
tension, tone	ton/o
testis, testicle	orch/o, orchi/o, orchid/o, test/o, testicul/o
thalamus	thalam/o
thirst	dips/o
three	tri-
three-dimensional	stere/o
throat (pharynx)	pharyng/o
through	per-
through, across	trans-
through, complete	dia-
thymus gland, mind	thym/o
thyroid gland	thyroid/o
thyroid gland, shield	thyr/o
tissue	hist/o
throw, throwing	bol/o
tie, tying	ligat/o
to flow, flowing	fluor/o
together	con-
together, joined	syn-
tongue	gloss/o, lingu/o
tonsil	tonsill/o
to shut	my/o
toward	ad-, -ad, af-
treatment	iatr/o, -therapy
tree	dendr/o
trochanter	trochanter/o
trigone	trigon/o
tube, fallopian	-salpinx
tube, fallopian or eustachian	salping/o
tube, pipe	tub/o
tumor	onc/o

Meaning	Word Part	Meaning	Word Part
tumor, mass	-oma	vessel	angi/o, vascul/o, vas/o
tubercle	tubercul/o	vessel, ductus deferens, vas deferens	vas/o
turn, turning	trop/o, vers/o, -verse		
twisting	tors/o	villus	vill/o
two	bi-, bin-	vestibule	vestibul/o
two (both)	di-	virus	vir/o
ulceration	aphth/o	vision	opt/o, optic/o
ulna	uln/o	vision condition	-opia, -opsia
umbilicus (navel)	omphal/o, umbilic/o	vitreous humor, glassy	vitre/o
under, below	sub-, hypo-	voice box (larynx)	laryng/o
unique, unknown	idi/o	volume	plethysm/o, vol/o
up, apart, away	ana-	vomer	vomer/o
upper jaw bone (maxilla)	maxill/o	vomiting	-emesis
upward	super/o, supra-	vulva	episi/o, vulv/o
ureter	ureter/o	walking	ambul/o
urethra	urethr/o	wall, partition, septum	pariet/o, sept/o
urinary condition	-uria	water, fluid	hydr/o
urine, urinary system	ur/o, urin/o	watery flow	rheumat/o
uterus	hyster/o, metr/o, metri/o, uter/o	wheel	rot/o
		white	albin/o, leuk/o
uvea	uve/o	white blood cell	leukocyt/o
uvula	uvul/o	windpipe (trachea)	trache/o
vagina	colp/o, vagin/o	within	end, endo-, intra-
vagus nerve	vag/o	woman, female	nymph/o
valve	valv/o, valvul/o	word, speech	lex/o
varices	varic/o	work	erg/o
vas deferens	vas/o	wrinkle	rhytid/o
vein	phleb/o, ven/o	wrist (carpus)	carp/o
ventricle	ventricul/o	write, writing	graph/o
venule (small vein)	venul/o	xiphoid process	xiph/i
vertebra, spine	spondyl/o, vertebr/o		

Appendix C

Abbreviations

Abbreviation	Meaning
#	fracture
3DCRT	three-dimensional conformal radiation therapy
A	action
A&P	auscultation and percussion
A, B, AB, O	blood types
A1c	average glucose level
ABG	arterial blood gas
ABR	auditory brainstem response
Acc	accommodation
ACE	angiotensin-converting enzyme
ACS	anterior ciliary sclerotomy; American Cancer Society
ACTH	adrenocorticotropic hormone
AD	Alzheimer disease
ADH	antidiuretic hormone
ADHD	attention-deficit hyperactivity disorder
ADLs	activities of daily living
AEB	atrial ectopic beat
AF	atrial fibrillation
AFP	alpha fetoprotein
AHIMA	American Health Information Management Association
AI	artificial insemination
AICD	automatic implantable cardioverter-defibrillator
AIDS	acquired immunodeficiency syndrome
AK	astigmatic keratotomy
ALL	acute lymphocytic leukemia
ALS	amyotrophic lateral sclerosis
AMA	American Medical Association
AMI	acute myocardial infarction
AML	acute myelogenous leukemia
ANA	antinuclear antibody
ANS	autonomic nervous system
AP	anteroposterior
APA	American Psychiatric Association
ARF	acute renal failure; acute respiratory failure
ARMD, AMD	age-related macular degeneration
AS	aortic stenosis
ASD	atrial septal defect; autism spectrum disorder
ASHD	arteriosclerotic heart disease
ASL	American sign language
Astig, As, Ast	astigmatism
AV	atrioventricular
B2M	beta-2 microglobulin
BaS	barium swallow
basos	basophils
BBB	blood-brain barrier; bundle branch block
BCC	basal cell carcinoma
BCP	birth control pill
BD	bipolar disorder
BE	barium enema
BM	bowel movement
BMP	basic metabolic panel
BMT	bone marrow transplant
BP	blood pressure
BPH	benign prostatic hyperplasia, benign prostatic hypertrophy
bpm	beats per minute
BSE	breast self-examination
BTA	bladder tumor antigen
BUN	blood urea nitrogen
Bx	biopsy
C1-C7	first cervical through seventh cervical vertebrae
C1-C8	cervical nerves
Ca	calcium
CA	cancer
CA125	tumor marker primarily for ovarian cancer
CA15-3	tumor marker used to monitor breast cancer
CA19-9	tumor marker for pancreatic, stomach, and bile duct cancer
CA27-29	tumor marker used to check for recurrence of breast cancer
CABG	coronary artery bypass graft
CAD	coronary artery disease
CAM	complementary and alternative medicine
CAPD	continuous ambulatory peritoneal dialysis
CAT	computed axial tomography
Cath	(cardiac) catheterization
CBC	complete blood cell (count)
CCB	calcium channel blocker(s)
CCPD	continuous cycling peritoneal dialysis

Continued

APPENDIX C Abbreviations

Abbreviation	Meaning
CEA	carcinoembryonic antigen
CF	cystic fibrosis
CHF	congestive heart failure
CIN	cervical intraepithelial neoplasia
CIS	carcinoma in situ
CKD	chronic kidney disease
Cl	chloride
CLL	chronic lymphocytic leukemia
CML	chronic myelogenous leukemia
CMP	comprehensive metabolic panel
CNS	central nervous system
CO_2	carbon dioxide
COPD	chronic obstructive pulmonary disease
COX-2	cyclooxygenase-2
CP	cerebral palsy
CPAP	continuous positive airway pressure
CPK	creatine phosphokinase
CPR	cardiopulmonary resuscitation
CPT	Current Procedural Terminology
CR	closed reduction
CREF	closed reduction, external fixation
CRP	C-reactive protein
CS, C-section	cesarean section
CSF	cerebrospinal fluid; colony-stimulating factor
CST	contraction stress test
CT scan	computed tomography scan
CTA	clear to auscultation
CTR	certified tumor registrar
CTS	carpal tunnel syndrome
CV	cardiovascular
CVA	cerebrovascular accident
CVS	chorionic villus sampling
CWP	coal workers' pneumoconiosis
Cx	cervix
CXR	chest x-ray
D&C	dilation and curettage
D1-D12	first dorsal through twelfth dorsal vertebrae
DAP Test	Draw-a-Person Test
decub	decubitus ulcer
DEXA, DXA	dual-energy x-ray absorptiometry
DI	diabetes insipidus
diff	differential (WBC count)
DIP	distal interphalangeal joint
DJD	degenerative joint disease
DLE	disseminated lupus erythematosus
DM	diabetes mellitus
DMARD	disease-modifying antirheumatic drug
DNA	deoxyribonucleic acid
DOE	dyspnea on exertion
DRE	digital rectal exam
DSA	digital subtraction angiography
DSM	Diagnostic and Statistical Manual of Mental Disorders
DSM-5	Diagnostic and Statistical Manual of Mental Disorders, fifth edition
DT	delirium tremens
DTR	deep tendon reflex
DUB	dysfunctional uterine bleeding
DVT	deep vein thrombosis
EBV	Epstein-Barr virus
ECC	extracorporeal circulation
ECCE	extracapsular cataract extraction
ECG, EKG	electrocardiography, electrocardiogram
ECHO	echocardiography
ECP	emergency contraceptive pill
ECT	electroconvulsive therapy
ED	emergency department; erectile dysfunction
EDD	estimated delivery date
EEG	electroencephalography, electroencephalogram
EF	external fixation
EGD	esophagogastroduodenoscopy
ELISA	enzyme-linked immunosorbent assay
EM, Em	emmetropia
EMG	electromyography
ENT	ears, nose, and throat
EOC	epithelial ovarian cancer
EOM	extraocular movements
eosins	eosinophils
EP	evoked potential
ERCP	endoscopic retrograde cholangiopancreatography
ERT	estrogen replacement therapy
ESR	erythrocyte sedimentation rate
ESRD	end-stage renal disease
EST	exercise stress test
ESWL	extracorporeal shock wave lithotripsy
EVLT	endovenous laser ablation
FB	foreign body
FBS	fasting blood sugar
FEV	forced expiratory volume
FOBT	fecal occult blood test
FPG	fasting plasma glucose
FRC	forced residual capacity
FSH	follicle-stimulating hormone
FTA-ABS	fluorescent treponemal antibody absorption
FVC	forced vital capacity
Fx	fracture
G	grade, pregnancy
GAD	generalized anxiety disorder
GARS	gait assessment rating scale
GB	gallbladder
Gc	gonococcus
G-CSF	granulocyte colony-stimulating factor
GCT	germ cell tumor
GERD	gastroesophageal reflux disease
GFR	glomerular filtration rate
GGT	gamma-glutamyl transferase
GH	growth hormone
GHD	growth hormone deficiency
GI	gastrointestinal

Abbreviation	Meaning
GIFT	gamete intrafallopian transfer
GM-CSF	granulocyte-macrophage colony-stimulating factor
GN	glomerulonephritis
GPA	gravida, para, abortion
GRH	gonadotropin-releasing hormone
GU	genitourinary
H	hypodermic
H2RA	histamine-2 receptor antagonist
HAV	hepatitis A virus
Hb	hemoglobin
HBV	hepatitis B virus
hCG	human chorionic gonadotropin
Hct	hematocrit
HD	hemodialysis
HDL	high-density lipoprotein
HDN	hemolytic disease of the newborn
HF	heart failure
Hg	millimeters of mercury
Hgb	hemoglobin
hGH	human growth hormone
HHN	hand-held nebulizer
HIM	health information management
HIV	human immunodeficiency virus
HIVD	herniated intervertebral disk
hMG	human menopausal gonadotropin
HPV	human papillomavirus
HRT	hormone replacement therapy
HSG	hysterosalpingography
HSV	herpes simplex virus
HSV-1	herpes simplex virus-1
HSV-2	herpes simplex virus-2; herpes genitalis
HTN	hypertension
I&D	incision and drainage
IBD	inflammatory bowel disease
IBS	irritable bowel syndrome
IC	inspiratory capacity
ICCE	intracapsular cataract extraction
ICD	International Classification of Diseases
ICD-10	International Classification of Diseases, 10th revision
ICD-10-CM	International Classification of Diseases, 10th revision, Clinical Modification
ICL	implantable contact lens
ICP	intracranial pressure
ICSH	interstitial cell-stimulating hormone
ICSI	intracytoplasmic sperm injection
ID	intradermal
IDC	infiltrating ductal carcinoma
IDDM	insulin-dependent diabetes mellitus
IF	internal fixation
Ig	immunoglobulin
IMRT	intensity-modulated radiation therapy
IOL	intraocular lens
IOP	intraocular pressure
IQ	intelligence quotient

Abbreviation	Meaning
IUD	intrauterine device
IV	intravenous
IVF	in vitro fertilization
IVP	intravenous pyelography
IVU	intravenous urography; intravenous urogram
K	potassium
KS	Kaposi sarcoma
KUB	kidney, ureter, and bladder
L1-L5	lumbar vertebrae, first through fifth; lumbar nerves
LA	left atrium
Lap	laparoscopy
LASIK	laser-assisted in-situ keratomileusis
lat	lateral
LCA	left circumflex artery; left coronary artery
LDH	lactate dehydrogenase
LDL	low-density lipoprotein
LEEP	loop electrocautery excision procedure
LES	lower esophageal sphincter
LFT	liver function test
LGA	light for gestational age
LH	luteinizing hormone
LLL	left lower lobe
LLQ	lower left quadrant
LMP	last menstrual period
LP	lumbar puncture
LRQ	lower right quadrant
LUL	left upper lobe
LUQ	left upper quadrant
LV	left ventricle
LVAD	left ventricular assist device
lymphs	lymphocytes
MAOI	monoamine oxidase inhibitor
MCH	mean corpuscular hemoglobin
MCHC	mean corpuscular hemoglobin concentration
MD	muscular dystrophy; medical doctor
MDI	metered dose inhaler
MDRTB	multidrug-resistant tuberculosis
mets	metastases
MHA-TP	microhemagglutination assay-*Treponema pallidum*
MI	myocardial infarction
MIDCAB	minimally invasive direct coronary artery bypass
MMPI	Minnesota Multiphasic Personality Inventory
MR	mental retardation; mitral regurgitation
MRA	magnetic resonance angiography
MRI	magnetic resonance imaging
MS	multiple sclerosis; mitral stenosis; musculoskeletal
MSH	melanocyte-stimulating hormone
MSLT	multiple sleep latency test
MUGA	multigated (radionuclide) angiogram
MV	mitral valve

Abbreviation	Meaning
MVP	mitral valve prolapse
MY	myopia
N&V	nausea and vomiting
Na	sodium
neuts	neutrophils
NGU	nongonococcal urethritis
NIDDM	non–insulin-dependent diabetes mellitus (type 2 diabetes)
NIH	National Institutes of Health
NK	natural killer (cell)
NPDR	nonproliferative diabetic retinopathy
NSAID	nonsteroidal antiinflammatory drug
NSCLC	non–small cell lung cancer
NSE	neuron-specific enolase
NSR	normal sinus rhythm
NST	nonstress test
NTG	nitroglycerin
O	origin
O_2	oxygen
OA	osteoarthritis
OAE	otoacoustic emission
OCD	obsessive-compulsive disorder
OCP	oral contraceptive pill
ODD	oppositional defiant disorder
OGTT	oral glucose tolerance test
OM	otitis media
Ophth	ophthalmology
OR	open reduction
ORIF	open reduction, internal fixation
OSA	obstructive sleep apnea
OT	oxytocin
OTC	over the counter
Oto	otology
PA	physician's assistant; posteroanterior; pulmonary artery
PAC	premature atrial contraction
PACAB	port-access coronary artery bypass
Pap	Papanicolaou (test for cervical/vaginal cancer)
PCOS	polycystic ovary syndrome
PCV	packed-cell volume
PD	panic disorder; Parkinson disease
PDA	patent ductus arteriosus
PDD	pervasive developmental disorders
PDR	proliferative diabetic retinopathy
PEG	percutaneous endoscopic gastrostomy
PET scan	positron emission tomography scan
PFT	pulmonary function test
PGH	pituitary growth hormone
pH	acidity/alkalinity
PICC	peripherally inserted central catheter
PID	pelvic inflammatory disease
PIP	proximal interphalangeal joint
PK	penetrating keratoplasty (corneal transplant)
PKD	polycystic kidney disease
PKU	phenylketonuria
plats	platelets; thrombocytes
PMB	postmenopausal bleeding

Abbreviation	Meaning
PMDD	premenstrual dysphoric disorder
PMN	polymorphonucleocyte
PMNs, polys	polymorphonucleocytes
PMS	premenstrual syndrome
PNS	peripheral nervous system
pos	posterior
PPB	positive-pressure breathing
PPD	purified protein derivative
PRK	photorefractive keratectomy
PRL	prolactin
PSA	prostate-specific antigen
PSG	polysomnography
PT	prothrombin time
PTA	prothrombin activator
PTC/PTCA	percutaneous transhepatic cholangiography
PTCA	percutaneous transluminal coronary angioplasty
PTH	parathyroid hormone
PTSD	posttraumatic stress disorder
PTT	partial thromboplastin time
PTU	propylthiouracil
PUD	peptic ulcer disease
PUVA	psoralen plus ultraviolet A
PV	pulmonary vein
PVC	premature ventricular contraction
PVD	peripheral vascular disease
QFT	QuantiFERON-TB
RA	rheumatoid arthritis; right atrium
RAD	reactive airway disease
RAIU	radioactive iodine uptake
RBC	red blood cell (count)
RCA	right coronary artery
RF	rheumatoid factor
RFCA	radiofrequency catheter ablation
Rh	Rhesus (factor)
RIA	radioimmunoassay
RLL	right lower lobe (of the lung)
RLQ	right lower quadrant
RML	right middle lobe (of the lung)
RNA	ribonucleic acid
ROM	range of motion
RPR	rapid plasma reagin
RSV	respiratory syncytial virus
RUL	right upper lobe (of the lung)
RUQ	right upper quadrant
RV	right ventricle
Rx	prescribed
S1-S5	sacral vertebrae, first through fifth; sacral nerves
SA	sinoatrial
SAD	seasonal affective disorder
SARS	severe acute respiratory syndrome
SCC	squamous cell carcinoma
SCLC	small cell lung cancer
SG	skin graft; specific gravity
SIADH	syndrome of inappropriate antidiuretic hormone
SIRS	systemic inflammatory response syndrome

Continued

Abbreviation	Meaning
SLE	systemic lupus erythematosus
SNS	somatic nervous system
SOB	shortness of breath
SPECT	single-photon emission computed tomography
SPF	sun protection factor
SSRI	selective serotonin reuptake inhibitor
SSS	sick sinus syndrome
STD	sexually transmitted disease
STH	somatotropic hormone
STI	sexually transmitted infection
STSG	split-thickness skin graft
sup	superior
SVT	superficial vein thrombosis
sx	symptoms
T	tumor
T1-T12	thoracic vertebrae, first through twelfth; thoracic nerves
T_3	triiodothyronine
T_4	thyroxine
TA-90	tumor marker for spread of malignant melanoma
TAH-BSO	total abdominal hysterectomy with a bilateral salpingo-oophorectomy
TAT	Thematic Apperception Test
TB	tuberculosis
TCA	tricyclic antidepressant
TCC	transitional cell carcinoma
TEA	thromboendarterectomy
TEE	transesophageal echocardiography
TENS	transcutaneous electrical nerve stimulation
TFT	thyroid function test
THR	total hip replacement
TIA	transient ischemic attack
TKR	total knee replacement
TLC	total lung capacity
TM	tympanic membrane
TMJ	temporomandibular joint disorder
TMR	transmyocardial revascularization
TNM	tumor-node-metastases (staging)
tPA	tissue plasminogen activator
TS	tricuspid stenosis
TSE	testicular self-examination
TSH	thyroid-stimulating hormone
TTS	transdermal therapeutic system
TUIP	transurethral incision of the prostate
TUR	transurethral resection (of the prostate)
TURP	transurethral resection of the prostate
TV	tidal volume; tricuspid valve
UA	urinalysis
UAE	uterine artery embolization
UCL	ulnar collateral ligament
uE3	unconjugated estradiol
ULQ	upper left quadrant
UNHS	Universal Newborn Hearing Screening
URI	upper respiratory infection
URQ	upper right quadrant
UTI	urinary tract infection
UV	ultraviolet
VA	visual acuity
VBAC	vaginal birth after cesarean section
VCUG	voiding cystourethrography
VD	venereal disease
VDRL	Venereal Disease Research Laboratory
VEB	ventricular ectopic beat
VF	visual field
VHD	valvular heart disease
VMA	urine vanillylmandelic acid
VP	vasopressin
VSD	ventricular septal defect
WAIS	Wechsler Adult Intelligence Scale
WBC	white blood cell (count)
WHO	World Health Organization
ZIFT	zygote intrafallopian transfer

APPENDIX D

Medication Classifications

Classification	Information	Generic Name	Trade Names
Analgesics	**Indications for use:** Relieve pain. **Desired effects:** Reduce the sensory function of the brain; block pain receptors. **Side effects and adverse reactions:** *Nonnarcotic:* GI distress, liver and kidney disorders, and tinnitus. *Narcotic:* hypotension, decreased respirations, agitation, blurred vision, confusion, constipation, sedation, restlessness.	***Nonnarcotic over-the-counter (OTCs)***: **aspirin** (AS pir in) **acetaminophen** (a set a MEE noe fen) (APAP) **ibuprofen** (eye BYOO proe fen) ***Narcotic (opioids)***: **oxycodone** (ox i KOE done) **hydrocodone with acetaminophen** (hye droe KOE done, a set a MEE noe fen) **oxycodone with acetaminophen** (ox i KOE done, a set a MEE noe fen) **tramadol** (TRAH mah dole)	Ecotrin, Bayer Aspirin, Bufferin Tylenol, Tempra Advil, Motrin OxyContin Lortab, Norco, Vicodin Percocet, Oxycet, Roxicet Ultram, Conzip
Anesthetics	**Indications for use:** Produce local anesthesia (no loss of consciousness) or general anesthesia (loss of consciousness). **Desired effects:** Produce insensibility to pain or the sensation of pain; block nerve impulses to the brain, resulting in unconsciousness. **Side effects and adverse reactions:** Hypotension, cardiopulmonary depression, sedation, nausea, vomiting, headaches.	***Local:*** lidocaine (LYE doe kane) ***General:*** midazolam (MID ay zoe lam)	Xylocaine Versed
Antacids	**Indications for use:** Treat gastric hyperacidity. **Desired effect:** Neutralizes stomach acid. **Side effects and adverse reactions:** GI distress, increased urination, metallic taste.	**calcium carbonate** (KAL see um, KAR bon ate)	Os-Cal 500, Rolaids, Tums
Anti-Alzheimer	**Indications for use:** Alzheimer Disease **Desired effect:** Used to treat dementia be increasing naturally occurring substances in the brain. **Side effects and adverse reactions:** GI distress, frequent urination, muscle cramps, confusion, bradycardia, angina, bloody vomit or stools.	**donepezil** (doe NEP e zil) **memantine** (moh MAN teen)	Aricept Namenda

Continued

APPENDIX D Medication Classifications

Classification	Information	Generic Name	Trade Names
Antianxiety	**Indications for use:** Produce calmness and release muscle tension; sedation. **Desired effects:** Reduce anxiety and tension. **Types:** SSRI, SNRIs, tricyclic antidepressants (see antidepressants), and benzodiazepines. **Side effects and adverse reactions:** Drowsiness, weakness, blurred vision, GI distress, hypersensitivity, jaundice, arrhythmias.	**Benzodiazepines**: (used for short-term management of anxiety) lorazepam (lor AH zeh pam) alprazolam (al PRAY zoe lam) clonazepam (kloe NA ze pam)	Ativan Xanax Klonopin
Antiarrhythmic	**Indications for use:** Arrhythmias. **Desired effects:** helps the heart work better, controls heart rate. **Side effects and adverse reactions:** arrhythmias, weight gain, difficulty breathing, swelling of hands and feet.	amiodarone (a MEE oh da rone) procainamide (proe kane AE mide) flecainide (FLEK a nide) digoxin (di JOX in)	Cordarone, Pacerone Tambocor Lanoxin, Digitek, Cardoxin
Antibiotics	**Indications for use:** Treat bacterial infections. **Desired effects:** Kill or inhibit bacteria growth. **Side effects and adverse reactions:** Hypersensitivity reaction, GI distress	**Penicillins** (pen i SIL ins): amoxicillin (a mox i SIL in) amoxicillin and clavulanic acid (a mox i SIL in, KLAV yoo lan ic) **Cephalosporins** (sef a low spoe rins): (related to the penicillins) cephalexin (sef a LEX in) cefuroxime (se fyoor OX eem) **Macrolides** (MAK row lides): erythromycin (er ith roe MYE sin) clarithromycin (kla RITH roe mye sin) azithromycin (az ith roe MYE sin) **Fluoroquinolones** (FLOOR oh kwin oh lones): ciprofloxacin (sip roe FLOX a sin) levofloxacin (lee voe FLOX a sin) **Sulfonamide** (SUHL fon ah mides): co-trimoxazole (coe try MOX a zole) trimethoprim (trye METH oh prim) **Tetracyclines** (TET rah sye klenes): tetracycline (TET rah sye klene) doxycycline (dox i SYE kleen) **Aminoglycosides** (ah MEE noe glye kah sides): gentamicin (jen ta MYE sin) tobramycin (toe bra MYE sin)	Amoxil, Moxtag Augmentin Keflex Ceftin Ery-Tab Biaxin Zithromax, Zithromax Z-Paks, Zmak Cipro Levaquin Bactrim, Septra Primsol Sumycin Doryx, Oracea, Vibramycin Garamycin Tobrex

APPENDIX D Medication Classifications

Classification	Information	Generic Name	Trade Names
Anticholinergics	**Indications for use:** Dry secretions before surgery; prevent bronchospasm. **Desired effects:** Parasympathetic blocking agents; reduce spasms in smooth muscles. **Side effects and adverse reactions:** Blurred vision, confusion, reduced GI and genitourinary motility, dilation of pupils, fever, flushing, headache, increased heart rate.	**dicyclomine** (dye SYE kloe meen)	Bentyl
		propantheline (proe PAN the leen)	Pro-Banthine
		glycopyrrolate (glye koe PYE roe late)	Cuvposa, Robinul
Anticoagulants	**Indication for use:** Prevent blood clots from forming. **Desired effects:** Decrease blood clotting ability. **Side effects and adverse reactions:** Increased bleeding; blood irregularities; hypersensitivity	**heparin** (HEP ah rin)	
		enoxaparin (ee nox a PA rin)	Lovenox
		dabigatran (da bi GAT ran)	Pradaxa
		warfarin (WAR far in)	Coumadin
		rivaroxaban (riv a ROX a ban)	Xarelto
Anticonvulsants	**Indications for use:** Treat epilepsy and other neurologic disorders. **Desired effects:** Reduce the frequency and severity of seizures by reducing excessive stimulation of the brain. **Side effects and adverse reactions:** Sedation, vertigo, visual disturbances, GI disturbances, liver complications.	**lamotrigine** (la MOE tri jeen)	Lamictal
		topiramate (toe PYRE a mate)	Topamax
		valproic acid (val PROE ik)	Depakene, Depakote
		gabapentin (GAH bah pen tin)	Neurontin, Horizant
Antidepressants	**Indications for use:** Treat depression, anxiety, and other neurologic disorders. **Desired effect:** Treat depression. **Side effects and adverse reactions:** Anorexia, anxiety, sexual dysfunction, fatigue, drowsiness, vertigo, weight gain, confusion, blurred vision.	*Selective serotonin reuptake inhibitors (SSRIs)*: affects serotonin in the brain.	
		fluoxetine (floo OX e teen)	Prozac
		citalopram (sye TAL oh pram)	Celexa
		escitalopram (es sye TAL oh pram)	Lexapro
		sertraline (SER tra leen)	Zoloft
		Serotonin and norepinephrine reuptake inhibitors (SNRIs): affects serotonin and norepinephrine in the brain.	
		venlafaxine (VEN la fax een)	
		duloxetine (doo LOX e teen)	Cymbalta
		Atypical antidepressants: doesn't fit in other categories	
		bupropion (byoo PROE pee on)	Wellbutrin, Zyban
		Serotonin modulators: increases the amount of serotonin.	
		trazodone (TRAZ on done)	Oleptro
		Tricyclic antidepressants: affects serotonin, dopamine, and norepinephrine in the brain.	
		amitriptyline (a mee TRIP ti leen)	
		Monamine oxidase inhibitors (MAOIs): affects monamine, an enzyme in the brain. Interacts with foods and drugs.	
		phenelzine (FEN el zeen)	Nardil

Continued

APPENDIX D Medication Classifications

Classification	Information	Generic Name	Trade Names
Antiemetics	**Indications for use:** Prevent and relieve nausea and vomiting; manage motion sickness. **Desired effect:** Act on hypothalamic center in the brain to reduce or prevent nausea and vomiting. **Side effects and adverse reactions:** Dry mouth, sedation, drowsiness, diarrhea, blurred vision.	ondansetron (on DAN se tron)	Zofran, Zuplenz
Antifungals	**Indications for use:** Treat systemic or local fungal infections. **Desired effects:** Slow or retard multiplication of fungi. **Side effects and adverse reactions:** Anemia, chills, hypotension, vertigo, fever, kidney and liver damage, malaise, photophobia, muscle and joint pain.	fluconazole (floo KON na zole) Miconazole (mi KON a zole)	Diflucan Lotrimin, Monistat
Antigout	**Indications for use:** Gout **Desired effects:** Reduce the uric acid in the body. **Side effects and adverse reactions:** GI distress, eye irritation, itching, rash, blood in urine.	allopurinol (al oh PURE i nole) febuxostat (feb UX oh stat)	Zyloprim, Aloprim Uloric
Antihistamines	**Indications for use:** Relieve allergies. **Desired effects:** Blocks the action of histamine, which causes allergic symptoms. **Side effects and adverse reactions:** CNS depression, muscle weakness, GI distress, dry mouth.	loratadine (lor AT a deen) diphenhydramine (dye fen HYE dra meen) cetirizine (se TI ra zeen)	Claritin, Alavert Benadryl, Unisom Zyrtec, Alleroff
Antihyperglycemics (non-insulin)	**Indications for use:** Manage diabetes mellitus. **Desired effect:** Reduce blood glucose level. **Side effects and adverse reactions:** GI irritation, fatigue, hypoglycemia, vertigo; possible hypersensitivity reaction	*Oral (Type 2):* **rosiglitazone** (roe si GLI ta zone) **sitagliptin** (sit a GLIP tin) **glipizide** (GLIP i zide) **glyburide** (GLYE byoor ide) **metformin** (met FOR min) *Injectable (Type 2):* **exenatide** (ex EN a tide) **dulaglutide** (doo la GLOO tide) *Injectable (used with other Type 1 or 2 medications):* **pramlintide** (PRAM lin tide)	Avandia Januvia Glucotrol DiaBeta, Glynase Glucophage, Fortamet, Glumetza Byetta Trulicity SymlinPen 60

APPENDIX D Medication Classifications

Classification	Information	Generic Name	Trade Names
Antihypertensives	**Indications for use:** Reduce and control blood pressure. **Desired effects:** Lowers blood pressure **Side effects and adverse reactions:** Headache, vertigo, GI disturbances, rash, hypotension, nonproductive cough	***Beta-blockers:*** reduce the heart rate, the workload and the output of blood.	
		propranolol (proe PRAN oh lole)	Inderal
		atenolol (ah TEN oh lole)	Tenormin
		Angiotensin-converting enzyme (ACE) inhibitors: decrease angiotensin production which causes blood vessels to dilate.	
		quinapril (KWIN a pril)	Accupril
		benazepril (ben AY ze pril)	Lotensin
		lisinopril (lyse IN oh pril)	
		metoprolol (me TOE proe lole)	Lopressor
		carvedilol (KAR ve dil ol)	Coreg
		Angiotensin II receptor antagonists: block the effects of angiotensin and blood vessels dilate.	
		losartan (loe SAR tan)	Cozaar
		valsartan (val SAR tan)	Diovan
		Calcium channel blockers: prevent calcium from entering the heart and arteries' smooth muscles; decrease contraction force, dilates blood vessels, and reduces heart rate.	
		diltiazem (dil TYE a zem)	Cardizem, Cartia, Tiazac
		amlodipine (am LOE di peen)	Norvasc
		Alpha blockers: dilate arteries.	
		doxazosin (dox AY zoe sin)	Cardura
Anti-inflammatories	**Indications for use:** Treat arthritis and other inflammatory disorders (e.g., allergic rhinitis). **Desired effect:** Reduce inflammation. **Side effects and adverse reactions:** GI distress, GI bleeding, hepatitis, drowsiness, tinnitus, irregular heart rate, kidney disorders.	***Nonsteroidal anti-inflammatory drugs (NSAIDs):***	
		ibuprofen (eye BYOO proe fen)	Advil, Motrin, Midol
		naproxen (na PROX en)	Naprosyn
		meloxicam (mel OX i cam)	Mobic
		Steroidal:	
		prednisone (PRED ni sone)	Prednisone Intensol, Sterapred
		prednisolone (pred NIS oh lone)	Flo-Pred, Orapred, Pediapred
Antimigraines	**Indications for use:** Treatment or prevention of migraine headaches. **Desired effect:** Alter circulation to the brain. **Side effects and adverse reactions:** Confusion, psychomotor slowing, difficulty concentrating, memory problems, rare but serious cardiac events.	sumatriptan (soo ma TRIP tan)	Imitrex
		zolmitriptan (zohl mi TRIP tan)	Zomig

Continued

APPENDIX D Medication Classifications

Classification	Information	Generic Name	Trade Names
Antimuscarinics	**Indications for use:** Overactive bladder. **Desired effects:** Relaxes the bladder muscles. **Side effects and adverse reactions:** Blurred vision, dry mouth and eyes, GI disturbances, headache, confusion, arrhythmias.	**oxybutynin** (ox i BYOO ti nin) **solifenacin** (sol i FEN a cin) **fesoterodine** (fes oh TER oh deen) **tolterodine** (tole TER a deen)	Ditropan VESIcare Toviaz Detrol
Antineoplastics	**Indications for use:** Cancer chemotherapy and/or prevention. **Desired effects:** Slows or stops the growth of cancer cells. **Side effects and adverse reactions:** Nausea, vomiting, bone marrow depression, aplastic anemia, hair loss, GI ulcers.	**Cyclophosphamide** (sye kloe FOSS fa mide) **Methotrexate** (meth oh TREX ate) **Tamoxifen** (tah MOX I fen) **Imatinib** (i MAT in ib)	Amethopterin Nolvadex Gleevec
Antiplatelets	**Indications for use:** Post treatment of stroke, heart attack or angina. **Desired effect:** Inhibit the function of platelets (the formation of clots). **Side effects and adverse reactions:** GI distress, bleeding, weakness or numbness	**clopidogrel** (kloh PID oh grel)	Plavix
Antipsychotics	**Indications for use:** Treat the symptoms of schizophrenia and bipolar disorder. **Desired effect:** Alter chemical actions in the brain. **Side effects and adverse reactions:** GI distress, hypotension, electrocardiographic (ECG) changes, vertigo, sedation, headache, photosensitivity.	*Typical antipsychotics*: (older medications) **haloperidol** (ha loe PER i dole) **chlorpromazine** (klor PROE ma zeen) *Atypical antipsychotics*: (newer medications) **olanzapine** (oh LAN za peen) **lurasidone** (loo RAS i done) **aripiprazole** (ay ri PIP ray zole) **risperidone** (ris PER i done) **quetiapine** (kwe TYE a peen)	Zyprexa Latuda Abilify Risperdal Seroquel
Antitussives	**Indications for use:** Temporarily suppress a nonproductive cough; reduce the thickness of secretions. **Desired effect:** Inhibit the cough center. **Side effects and adverse reactions:** Codeine cough suppressants cause CNS depression and constipation.	**dextromethorphan** (dex troe meth OR fan)	Benylin
Antivirals	**Indications for use:** Treat viral infections, including oral and genital herpes, influenza, and HIV. **Desired effects:** Inhibit the growth or reduce the spread of viral cells. **Side effects and adverse reactions:** Confusion, diarrhea, headache, kidney disease, urticaria, vomiting.	**oseltamivir** (os el TAM i vir) **acyclovir** (ay SYE kloe veer)	Tamiflu Zovirax

APPENDIX D Medication Classifications

Classification	Information	Generic Name	Trade Names
Bronchodilators	**Indications for use:** Treat asthma, bronchospasm; promote bronchodilation. **Desired effect:** Relax the smooth muscle of the bronchi. **Side effects and adverse reactions:** CNS stimulation, tremors, tachycardia, increased blood glucose level, hypertension.	albuterol (al BYOO ter ole) tiotropium (tee oh TROH pee um)	Ventolin HFA, Proventil, ProAir HFA Spiriva Handihaler
Cholesterol-lowering agents	**Indications for use:** Reduce low-density lipoprotein (LDL) and triglycerides; increase high-density lipoprotein (HDL). **Desired effects:** Prevents absorption of cholesterol in the intestine. **Side effects and adverse reactions:** GI discomfort, muscle pain and weakness, liver complications, hypersensitivity, cataracts, myopathy.	ezetimibe (e ZET i mibe) atorvastatin (a TORE vas ta tin) rosuvastatin (roe soo vah STAT in) simvastatin (SIM va stat in)	Vytorin, Zetia Lipitor Crestor Zocor
Contraceptives	**Indications for use:** Prevent pregnancy. **Desired effect:** Inhibit conception. **Side effects and adverse reactions:** Breast enlargement and tenderness; cardiovascular risk; GI distress; headache; irregular menstrual bleeding; deep vein thrombosis; pulmonary embolus (PE).	**Progestin** (pro JES tin) **Ethinyl Estradiol, Norethindrone** (ETH in il es tra DYE ol, nor eth IN drone) **Ethinyl Estradiol, Levonorgestrel** (ETH in il es tra DYE ol, lee voe nor JES trel) **Ethinyl Estradiol, Norgestimate** (ETH in il es tra DYE ol, nor jes TI mate) **medroxyprogesterone acetate** (me DROX ee proe JES te rone)	Micronor, Jolivette, "minipill" Loestrin, Loestrin Fe, Ortho-Novum 1/35 Lessina, Triphasil Ortho Tri-Cyclen, Ortho Tri-Cyclen Lo, Ortho-Cyclen Depo-Provera
Corticosteroids (oral)	**Indications for use:** Used to treat chronic inflammatory diseases (e.g., arthritis) and acute conditions (e.g., poison ivy, asthma). **Desired effects:** Reduce inflammation. **Side effects and adverse reactions:** Headache, mood changes, difficulty falling asleep or staying asleep, increased sweating, vision problems, depression, and weight gain.	prednisone (PRED ni sone) prednisolone (pred NIS oh lone) methylprednisolone (meth ill pred NISS oh lone)	Prednisone Intensol, Sterapred Flo-Pred, Orapred, Pediapred Medrol
Corticosteroids (nasal and inhaled)	**Indications for use:** Long-term relief of asthma symptoms; decrease frequency of asthma attacks; manage chronic obstructive pulmonary disease (COPD) and seasonal allergies. **Desired effects:** Reduce airway inflammation and bronchial resistance. **Side effects and adverse reactions:** Headache, pharyngitis, myalgia, hypersensitivity, oral candidiasis. Diskus products are contraindicated in patients with a milk allergy.	fluticasone and salmeterol (floo TIK a sone, sal MEH te role) fluticasone (floo TIK a sone) budesonide (byoo DES oh nide) budesonide and formoterol (byoo DES oh nide, for MOH te rol) mometasone (moe MET a sone)	Advair Diskus Flovent Diskus, Flovent HFA, Flonase nasal spray Pulmicort Flexhaler, Pulmicort Respules, Rhinocort Symbicort Nasonex

Continued

APPENDIX D Medication Classifications

Classification	Information	Generic Name	Trade Names
Decongestants	**Indications for use:** Relieve nasal and sinus congestion caused by common cold, hay fever, or upper respiratory tract disorders. **Desired effect:** Relieve local congestion nasal and sinus tissues. **Side effects and adverse reactions:** Arrhythmias, hypertension, headache, nausea, dry mouth.	**pseudoephedrine** (soo doe e FED rin) **Phenylephrine** (fen il EF rin)	Sudafed Sudafed PE Congestion, PediaCare Children's Decongestant, Suphedrin PE
Diuretics	**Indications for use:** Increase urinary output; lower blood pressure. **Desired effects:** Inhibit reabsorption of sodium and chloride in the kidneys; promote excretion of excess fluid in the body. **Side effects and adverse reactions:** Dehydration, muscle weakness, fatigue, electrolyte imbalance.	**triamterene** (trye AM ter een) **furosemide** (fyoor OH se mide) **hydrochlorothiazide** (HCTZ) (hye droe klor oh THYE a zide)	Dyrenium Lasix Microzide, Oretic
Electrolytes	**Indications for use:** mineral supplement needed for certain diseases and medications. **Desired effect:** maintain normal electrolyte level; proper functioning of the body systems **Side effects and adverse reactions:** (depends on medication) confusion, listlessness, gray skin, black stools.	**potassium** (poe TASS i um) **ferrous sulfate** (FER us) (iron)	K-Tab, Klor-Con, K-Dur Feosol, Fer-in-Sol, Slow-Fe
Erectile Dysfunction agents	**Indications for use:** Facilitates an erection in patients with erectile dysfunction (impotence) and symptoms of benign prostatic hypertrophy (enlarged prostate). **Desired effect:** Facilitate an erection. **Side effects and adverse reactions:** Headache, flushing, nasal congestion, myalgia, prolonged erections, cerebrovascular accident (CVA), myocardial infarction (MI).	**Sildenafil** (sil DEN a fil) **Tadalafil** (tah DAY lay fil) **vardenafil** (var DEN a fil)	Viagra Cialis Levitra
Expectorants	**Indications for use:** Relieve upper respiratory tract congestion. **Desired effect:** Thin the secretions in the bronchial tubes to make it easier to cough up the mucus. **Side effects and adverse reactions:** GI distress.	**guaifenesin** (gwye FEN eh sin)	
Hematopoietics	**Indication for use:** Treat anemia in patients undergoing chemotherapy. **Desired effect:** Promote blood cell production. **Side effects and adverse reactions:** Headache, arthralgia, nausea, hypertension, diarrhea.	**pegfilgrastim** (peg fil GRA stim)	Neulasta
Hemostatics	**Indications for use:** Control acute or chronic blood-clotting disorder; promote formation of absorbable, artificial clot. **Desired effects:** Control bleeding; act as a blood coagulant (clots blood). **Side effects and adverse reactions:** Hypersensitivity reactions, transient flushing, dizziness; newborn hyperbilirubinemia.	**phytonadione** (fye toe na DYE one)	Vitamin K

APPENDIX D Medication Classifications

Classification	Information	Generic Name	Trade Names
Hormone Replacement (insulin)	**Indications for use:** Type 1 and Type 2 diabetes mellitus **Desired effects:** Lower the blood glucose level. **Side effects and adverse reactions:** Shortness of breath, blurred vision, tachycardia, sweating, weakness, muscle cramps, arrhythmias, and other hypoglycemic symptoms	*Short-acting Insulin:* regular insulin (IN su lin) *Rapid-acting Insulin:* insulin aspart (IN su lin AS part) insulin glulisine (IN su lin GLOO lis een) insulin lispro (IN su lin LYE sproe) *Intermediate-acting Insulin:* insulin isophane (IN su lin de GLOO dek) *Long-acting Insulins:* insulin degludec (IN su lin de GLOO dek) insulin detemir (IN su lin DE te mir) insulin glargine (IN su lin GLAR geen)	Humulin R, Novolin R Novolog, Novolog Mix 70/30 Apidra Humalog Humulin N, Novolin N Tresiba Levemir Lantus, Toujeo
Hormone Replacement	**Indications for use:** Maintain adequate hormone levels. **Desired effects:** Replace hormones or compensate for hormone deficiency. **Side effects and adverse reactions:** *Thyroid hormone replacement therapy:* Weight loss, tremor, headache, chest pain, arrhythmias *Estrogen replacement therapy:* Hot flashes, decreased sex drive, nausea, vomiting. *Estrogen and progestin replacement therapy:* Double vision, depression, unusual bleeding, acne, swelling of the hands and feet, nervousness, brown or black skin patches *Vasopressin replacement therapy:* Restlessness, seizures, hallucinations, slowed reflexes, tiredness	*Thyroid hormone:* (for hypothyroidism) levothyroxine (lee voe thye ROX een) *Estrogen:* (for menopause) Estrogen (ESS troe jen) *Estrogen and Progestin:* (for menopause) Estrogen and Progestin (ESS troe jen, pro JES tin) *Vasopressin:* (for diabetes insipidus) Desmopressin (des moe PRESS in)	Synthroid, Levothroid, Levoxyl Estrace, Ortho-est, Premarin Premphase, Prempro DDAVP
Laxatives	**Indications for use:** Increase and hasten bowel evacuation (defecation). **Desired effect:** Increase activity in the large intestine promoting stools. **Side effects and adverse reactions:** Nausea, bloating, flatulence, cramping.	bisacodyl (bis AK oh dil) psyllium (SIL i yum)	Dulcolax Fiberall, Genfiber, Konsyl, Metamucil, V-Lax
Leukotriene receptor antagonists	**Indications for use:** Asthma, exercise induced bronchospasms **Desired effect:** blocks the action of substances that cause asthma and allergic rhinitis **Side effects and adverse reactions:** headache, dizziness, heartburn, stomach pain, tiredness, hypersensitivity, numbness in arms and legs, swelling of the sinuses	montelukast (mon te LOO kast)	Singulair

Continued

APPENDIX D Medication Classifications

Classification	Information	Generic Name	Trade Names
Miotics	**Indications for use:** Glaucoma. **Desired effect:** Allows excess fluid to drain from the eye. **Side effects and adverse reactions:** Blurred vision, stinging and redness in the eye, headache, weakness, increase in saliva, muscle tremors.	pilocarpine (pye loe KAR peen)	Pilopine, Carpine
Muscle Relaxants	**Indications for use:** Painful musculoskeletal conditions (e.g., strains, sprains, muscle injuries). **Desired effect:** Decreases pain. **Side effects and adverse reactions:** drowsiness, clumsiness, tachycardia, GI intolerance, difficulty breathing, fever, weakness, burning in the eyes, seizures	carisoprodol (kar eye soe PROE dole) cyclobenzaprine (sye kloe BEN za preen)	Soma Flexeril
Mydriatics	**Indications for use:** Ophthalmic procedures. **Desired effect:** Dilate the pupil, some cause paralysis of the ciliary muscle. **Side effects and adverse reactions:** Stinging, burning, dry mouth, urine retention.	atropine (AH troe peen) cyclopentolate (sye kloe PEN toe late)	Isopto Atropine Cyclogyl, Pentolair
Osteoporosis agents	**Indications for use:** Promote bone mineral density and reverse progression of osteoporosis. **Desired effects:** Inhibit bone reabsorption and/or promote use of calcium. **Side effects and adverse reactions:** GI disorders, esophageal irritation.	alendronate (a LEN droe nate) risedronate (ris ED roe nate) ibandronate (i BAN droh nate) raloxifene (ral OX i feen)	Fosamax, Binosto Actonel, Atelvia Boniva Evista
Proton-Pump Inhibitors	**Indications for use:** Treat gastroesophageal reflux disease (GERD) and ulcers. **Desired effect:** Decrease the amount of acid produced in the stomach. **Side effects and adverse reactions:** Confusion, drowsiness, arrhythmias, sweating, flushing.	omeprazole (oh ME pray zol) pantoprazole (pan TOE pra zole) esomeprazole (es oh ME pray zol)	Prilosec Protonix Nexium
Sedative-Hypnotics	**Indications for use:** Treat insomnia; obtain sedation (lower doses). **Desired effects:** Slowing activity in the brain to allow sleep. **Side effects and adverse reactions:** Daytime sedation, confusion, dry mouth, hypersensitivity.	eszopiclone (es ZOE pi clone) temazepam (te MAZ e pam) zolpidem (ZOL pi dem)	Lunesta Restoril Ambien, Edluar, Zolpimist

Classification	Information	Generic Name	Trade Names
Stimulants	**Indications for use:** Treat attention deficit/hyperactivity disorder (ADHD) and narcolepsy. **Desired effects:** Stimulate the brain and body; making the messages move faster between the brain and the body. The person becomes more alert and physically active. **Side effects and adverse reactions:** arrhythmias, aggression, memory loss, flushing, hypertension, restlessness, fainting.	**atomoxetine** (AT oh mox e teen) **methylphenidate** (meth il FEN i date)	Strattera Concerta, Ritalin LA
Tumor-necrosis factor (TNF) inhibitors	**Indications for use:** Autoimmune disorders (e.g., rheumatoid arthritis) **Desired effect:** Blocks the action of TNF, preventing inflammation. **Side effects and adverse reactions:** GI distress, weakness, seizures, bleeding	**infliximab** (in FLIX i mab) **etanercept** (et a NER set)	Remicade Enbrel

GLOSSARY

5% sheep's blood agar plate: (BAP) A solid agar media that contains nutrients and 5% washed sheep blood. The blood is added as an extra nutrient source for bacteria.

A

abscesses: Localized collections of pus, which may be under the skin or deep in the body, that cause tissue destruction.

abstract: Collecting important information from the health record.

abuse: An action that purposely harms another person

accessory muscles: Muscles in the neck, abdomen, and back that assist in breathing in times of respiratory distress.

accounts payable: Money owed by a company to other companies for services and goods; pertains to paying the bills of the facility.

acetylcholine (ACh): A substance that is released at the junction between neurons and muscle fibers. A chemical messenger.

acuity: Test of the clearness or sharpness of vision.

acute stage: Phase of rapid multiplication of the pathogen, symptoms are very distinct. A strong response of the immune system is taking place during this stage.

Adam's apple: A projection of the thyroid cartilage at the front of the neck that is more noticeable in men than in women.

addiction: A disease that occurs when a person cannot stop or limit the use of a drug, even after negative consequences have been experienced.

adherence: The act of sticking to something.

adhesions: bands of scar tissue that can bind anatomical structures together

adjudicate: To settle or determine judicially.

adnexa: structures that are attached, adjacent, or adjoining to another structure

advance directives: Written instructions about healthcare decisions should a person be unable to make them.

afferent: Pertaining to carrying toward a structure.

age of majority: The age at which a person is recognized by law to be an adult; it varies by state.

albinism: A person with very pale skin, light or white hair, red of pinkish eyes. Caused by a genetic inability to produce the pigment melanin.

albumin: Most abundant plasma protein in human blood. It is important in regulating the water balance of blood.

aliquot: A portion of a well-mixed sample removed for testing.

alkaline: A substance that has a pH greater than 7.0 on the pH scale (0-14)

alphabetic filing: Any system that arranges names or topics according to the sequence of the letters in the alphabet.

alphanumeric: Systems made up of combinations of letters and numbers.

amenorrhea: Lack of menstrual flow

amino acids: Produced by the body and also obtained when protein foods are broken down; used to make proteins in the body.

analgesics: Category of medication used to relieve pain.

analyte: The substance or chemical being analyzed or detected in a specimen.

anaphylaxis: A rapidly progressing, life-threatening allergic reaction; characterized by hives, swelling of the mouth and airway, difficulty breathing, wheezing, and loss of consciousness.

anaplastic: A rapidly dividing cancer cell that has little to no similarity to normal cells.

anencephaly: Congenital absence of part or all of the brain.

anemia: A deficiency of hemoglobin in the blood. Accompanied by a reduced number of red blood cells, pale skin, weakness, and shortness of breath among other symptoms. Can be caused by a nutrient deficiency or inability to absorb vital nutrients.

anesthetic: Partial or complete loss of sensation.

anhedonia: The inability to feel or experience pleasure when doing a pleasurable activity.

aniridia: Condition where the iris in the eye is partially formed or fails to form.

anovulation: Failure of the ovaries to release an ovum at the time of ovulation.

answering service: A commercial service that answers telephone calls for its clients.

antibiotic: A substance or medication that can destroy or inhibit the growth of bacteria.

antibodies: Protein substances produced in the blood or tissues in response to a specific antigen, which destroys or weakens the antigen. Part of the immune system.

anticoagulants: Substances (i.e., medication of chemical) that prevents clotting of blood.

antigen: A substance that stimulates the production of an antibody when introduced into the body. Antigens include toxins, bacteria, viruses, and other foreign substances.

antihyperlipidemic: A substance (i.e., medication) that lowers the lipid levels in the blood.

antihypertensive: A substance (i.e., medication) that reduces high blood pressure.

antimicrobial: A general term for drugs, chemicals, or other substances that can destroy or inhibit the growth of microorganisms. Can be antibiotics, antiviral, antifungal, and antiparasitic drugs or agents.

antioxidant: Man-made or natural substances found in food and supplements; may prevent or delay some types of cell damage.

antipyretics: Category of medication used to reduce a fever.

antiseptics: Substances that inhibit the growth of microorganisms on living tissue (e.g., alcohol and povidone-iodine solution [Betadine]); they are used to cleanse the skin, wounds, and so on.

apnea: Abnormal, periodic cessation of breathing.

approximated: Near, close together.

arbitration: The process where conflicting parties of a dispute submit their differences to a court appointed person (arbitrator), who submits a legally binding decision.

aromatic: Having a distinct, usually fragrant smell.

arrhythmia: Abnormal heart rate or rhythm

arterioles: Small arteries

arteriosclerosis: Thickening, decreased elasticity, and calcification of arterial walls

auscultated: To listen with a stethoscope.

arteriovenous: Pertains to the arteries and veins

arteriovenous fistula: An abnormal joining of an artery and vein

arthropod: Any animal that lacks a spine, such as: insects, crustaceans, arachnids, and others.

artifact: A substance, structure, or event that does not naturally occur in a situation. Examples include interference, or electrical "garbage" on an EKG, or crystals, lint, or contamination of a staining technique.

artificial insemination: The injection of semen into the vagina or uterus using a catheter or syringe. Non-sexual.

aseptically: Free from living pathogenic organisms.

asexually: Reproduction not involving the fusion of male and female sex cells, as in plant reproduction, fission, or budding.

aspirate: To withdraw fluid using suction. Example: a specimen that has been removed from the body using a needle and syringe.

assets: All property available for the payment of debts.

ATP (adenosine triphosphate): A high-energy molecule found in every cell, that supplies large amounts of energy for various biochemical processes.

atrophy: Wasting away, degeneration from disuse. Attachment, and a hole where the spinal cord passes.

attenuated: Weakened or changed.

atypical lymphs: In many viral infections stimulated or reactive lymphs are called atypical lymphs. They are commonly seen in infectious mononucleosis.

audible: Capable of being heard.

audiologist: Allied healthcare professional who specializes in evaluation of hearing function, detection of hearing impairment, and determination of the anatomic site of impairment.

audit: A process done before claims submission to examine claims for accuracy and completeness.

auditory cortex: The region of the cerebral cortex that receives auditory data.

auscultate: To listen with a stethoscope.

authorized agent: A person who has written documentation that he or she can accept a shipment for another individual.

autoimmune: An immune response against a person's own tissues, cells, or cell parts, as in

GLOSSARY

autoimmune disease, leading to the deterioration of tissue.

automated: A process that is measured by a machine or instrument. May involve human manipulation, coordination, or control.

automatic call routing: A system that distributes incoming calls to a specific group or person based on customer need; for example, the customer presses 1 for appointments, 2 for billing questions, and so on.

autonomy: The ability to function independently.

avascular: Not supplied or associated with blood vessels.

B

backordered: An order placed for an item that is temporarily out of stock and will be sent at a later time.

bacteria: A large group of microorganisms that are single-celled, lack a nucleus, reproduce asexually, or can form spores. Some can cause disease. The most abundant life form on earth.

bacteriuria: The presence of bacteria in the urine (possible infection).

Bartholin cyst: A fluid-filled cyst in one of the vestibular glands located on either die of the vaginal orifice

basal: Bottom layer

belligerent: Hostile and aggressive.

beneficiary: A designated person who receives funds from an insurance policy.

benign: A non-cancerous condition, not malignant, harmless

biconvex: Having two outward curving surfaces, on a lens.

bilingual: ability to communicate effectively in two languages

bilirubin: A reddish pigment that results from the breakdown of red blood cells in the liver.

bilirubinuria: The presence of bilirubin in the urine.

billable service: Assistance (i.e., service) that is provided by a healthcare provider that can be billed to the insurance company and/or patient.

binary fission: Asexual reproduction in single-celled organisms where one cell divides into two daughter cells.

binocular: Involving, relating, or seeing with both eyes.

binomial: A name consisting of a generic and a specific term.

bioethicists: People who study the ethical effect of biomedical advances (e.g., drugs and genetic engineering).

biological product: Also known as biologics, they are made from a variety of natural resources that can be human, animal, or microorganism based.

biopsy: Process of viewing living tissue that has been removed for the purpose of diagnosis and/or treatment.

bipolar: Has two poles or electrical charges

blind spot: A small area on the retina that is insensitive to light. Where the optic nerve joins the retina.

blood culture: A microbiological procedure where a blood sample is placed in a nutrient media and held at body temperature. If bacteria are in the blood sample the culture media should encourage the growth of the infecting bacteria in the laboratory.

blood type: A person's blood is categorized based on the presence or absence of specific antigens on the red blood cell's surface. Also, known as blood groups. Blood type is inherited and is present before birth.

bonded: When an employer obtains a fidelity bond from an insurance company, which will cover losses from employee dishonest acts (e.g., embezzlement, theft).

bone marrow transplant: Is a procedure that replaces a person's bone marrow with bone marrow from a healthy donor (such as a sibling). Also called a stem cell transplant.

bookkeeping: The process of recording financial transactions.

bounding: A term used to describe a pulse that feels full because of increased power of cardiac contraction or as a result of increased blood volume.

bradycardia: A slow heartbeat; a pulse below 60 beats per minute.

bradypnea: Abnormally slow breathing.

brainstem: Part of the brain that is continuous with the top of the spinal cord, and is made up of the medulla oblongata, pons, and midbrain. Concerned with reflexes and vital functions of the body such as, respiration, heartbeat, swallowing.

breach: Disclosure of protected health information without a reason or permission and compromised the security or privacy of the information.

broad-spectrum antibiotics: An antibiotic that acts against a wide range of disease-causing bacteria. Acts against both Gram-positive and Gram-negative bacteria.

bronchiolitis: When the small airways of the lungs become inflamed because of a viral infection.

bronchodilators: Category of medication that relaxes smooth muscle contractions in the bronchioles to improve lung ventilation.

bruit: An abnormal sound or murmur heard on auscultation of an organ, vessel (e.g., carotid artery), or gland.

buffy coat: The layer of white blood cells and platelets that separates red blood cells and plasma is a centrifuged whole blood sample.

buying cycle: Refers to how often an item is purchased; depends on frequency of the use of the item and storage space available for the item.

C

calcium: A natural occurring element that is necessary for many body function, including strong bones and teeth, proper blood clotting, nerve conduction, and muscle contractions.

calculi: Stones formed in the kidneys, gallbladder, and other parts of the body.

calibrate: Determining the accuracy of an instrument by comparing its output with that of a known standard or another instrument known to be accurate.

caliper: A pocket-sized tool used for measuring the height and width of the ECG waves and intervals.

candidiasis: An infection caused by a yeast that typically affects the vaginal mucosa and skin.

cannula: A rigid tube that surrounds a blunt trocar or a sharp, pointed trocar, which is inserted into the body; when the trocar is withdrawn, fluid may escape from the body through the cannula, depending on the insertion site.

canthus: Angular junction of the eyelids at either corner.

capitation: A payment arrangement for health care providers. The provider is paid a set amount for each enrolled person assigned to them, per period of time, whether or not that person has received services.

caption: A heading, title, or subtitle under which records are filed.

carbon dioxide: A colorless, odorless gas, CO_2, that is present in the air we breathe. It is a waste product of cellular respiration and is removed from the body through exhaling via the lungs.

carbon: A naturally abundant, non-metallic element that occurs in all organic compounds and can be found in all known forms of life. A pure form of carbon is diamond.

cardiologist: A physician who has specialized in the study of the heart and its functions in health and disease.

cardiopulmonary resuscitation (CPR): Manual chest compressions and ventilations (also called rescue breathing) to patients who are not breathing nor have a pulse; also known as Basic Life Support (BLS).

cash on hand: The amount of money the healthcare facility has in the bank that can be withdrawn as cash.

cataract: Progressive loss of transparency of the lens of the eye.

catheter: Hollow, flexible tube that can be inserted into a vessel, organ, or cavity of the body to withdraw or instill fluid, monitor information, and visualize a vessel or cavity.

catheterized: To insert a catheter into a vessel, organ, or cavity of the body. (example: the urinary bladder)

caustic: Capable of burning, corroding, or damaging tissue by chemical action.

centrifuge: A machine that rotates at high speed and separates substances of different densities by centrifugal force. Example: a tube of blood is separated into plasma/serum, white blood cells, platelets, and red blood cells.

cerebrospinal fluid: A clear fluid that fills the ventricles of the brain, covers the surface of the brain and spinal cord, and subarachnoid space. It lubricates the tissues and cushions them from shock and injury.

cerumen: A waxy secretion in the ear canal; commonly called *ear wax*.

cessation: Bringing to an end.

Cheyne-Stokes respiration: Deep, rapid breathing followed by a period of apnea.

chief complaint: A statement in the patient's own words that describes the reason for the visit.

cholelithiasis: Presence of stones in the gall bladder.

chordae tendineae: Cord-like tendons that attach the papillary muscle to the heart valve.

chromosomes: Rod-shaped structures found in the cell's nucleus; contain genetic information.

chronic obstructive pulmonary disease (COPD): A progressive, irreversible lung condition that results in diminished lung capacity.

chronic: Developing slowly and lasting for a long time, generally 3 or more months.

chronological: Arranged in the order of time.

cicatrix: Early scar tissue that appears pale, contracted, and firm.

claim: A formal request for payment from an insurance company for services provided.

claims clearinghouse: An organization that accepts the claim data from the provider, reformats the data to meet the specifications outlined by the insurance plan, and submits the claim.

claim scrubbers: Software that finds common billing errors before the claim is sent to the insurance company.

clarification: Allows the listener to get additional information.

clone: A population of identical units, cells, or individuals that come from the same parent.

Clostridium difficile: (C. diff) A bacterium that can cause symptoms that range from diarrhea to severe inflammation of the colon (can be fatal). This condition is most commonly seen after antibiotic use.

clot: A mass of coagulated blood that is made up of red blood cells, white blood cells, and platelets in a protein (fibrin) mesh. It has a semi-solid consistency.

clot activators: Substances added to a venipuncture tube to enhance and speed up blood clotting.

clotting factors: Substances that are in the blood that interact in sequence to stop bleeding by for a clot. Examples include; prothrombin, fibrinogen, thromboplastin, and calcium.

clubbing: Abnormal enlargement of the distal phalanges (fingers and toes) associated with cyanotic heart disease or advanced chronic pulmonary disease.

CMS-1500 Health Insurance Claim Form (CMS-1500): The standard insurance claim form used for all government and most commercial insurance companies.

coaching: Provide information in a supportive environment that allows people to grow, change, or improve their situation.

coagulation: The process of changing a liquid into a solid.

code: Term used in healthcare settings to indicate an emergency situation and to summons the train team to the scene.

coding system: A system designed to use characters (i.e., numbers and letters) to represent something like a medical procedure or a disease.

coinsurance: After the deductible has been met the policyholder may need pay a certain percentage of the bill and the insurance company pays the rest. A typical split is 80/20 where the insurance company pays 80% and the policy holder pays 20%.

collaboration: The act of working with another or other individuals.

collagen: The most abundant structural protein found in skin and other connective tissues. It provides strength and cushioning to many parts of the body.

colonoscopy: A procedure in which a fiber optic scope is used to examine the large intestine.

colony: A discrete group of organisms, such as a group of bacteria, growing on a solid nutrient surface.

colostrum: The first milk secreted by mammals at birth. Different from the rest of the milk supply because it contains more protein and is rich in antibodies. Also called foremilk.

colposcopy: Using a microscope with a light source the vagina and cervix are visually examined to locate and evaluate abnormal cells. A biopsy of abnormal cells may be taken during this procedure.

combining forms: The "subjects" of most terms. That consists of the word root with its respective combining vowel.

common law: Unwritten laws that come from judicial decisions based on societal traditions and customs

communicable diseases: Diseases spread from person to person either by direct contact or nondirect contact (i.e., insects).

compact bone: Bone tissue that is the rigid, dense outer layer of bone that consists

compliance: Meeting the standards and regulations of the practice's established policies and procedures. Can also mean cooperation.

computer network: A system that links personal computers and peripheral devices to share information and resources.

computer on wheels (COW): Wireless mobile workstation; also called workstation on wheels (WOW).

computerized provider/provider order entry (CPOE): The process of entering medication orders or other provider instructions into the EHR.

concise: Using as few words as possible to express the message.

cone biopsy: an extensive cervical biopsy that removes a cone-shaped wedge of tissue from the cervix and examined under a microscopy. Abnormal tissue along with a small amount of normal tissue is removed.

congruence: Agreement; the state that occurs when the verbal expression of the message matches the sender's nonverbal body language.

conscientious: Meticulous, careful.

constrict: To contract or shrink

continuity of care: The smooth continuation of care from one provider to another. This allows the patient to receive the most benefit and no interruption or duplication of care.

contraindicate: Suggest that it should not be used.

control materials: Manufacturer prepared samples that have a known quantity of a specific analyte. Used for quality control purposes. Testing results should fall within a manufacturer defined range of results. Also called *controls* or *quality controls.*

convalescent stage: Phase when the host recovers gradually and returns to baseline or normal health.

copayment (copay): A set dollar amount that the patient must pay for each office visit. There can be one copayment amount for a primary care provider, a different copayment amount (usually higher) to see a specialist or be seen in the emergency department.

correlate: Establish an orderly relationship or connection.

corrosive: Causing or tending to cause the gradual destruction of a substance by chemical action.

corticosteroids: Group of steroid hormones produced in the body or given as a medication; some have metabolic functions and others decrease tissue inflammation. Glucocorticoids and mineralocorticoids are two types.

costochondral: The cartilage that joins the ribs and the sternum on the front of the rib cage.

counteroffer: Return offer made by one who has rejected an offer or a job.

crash cart: Emergency medications and equipment (e.g., oxygen, intravenous [IV], and airway supplies) stored in a cart, ready for an emergency.

creatinine clearance rates: A procedure for evaluating the glomerular filtration rate of the kidneys.

crenate: The cell surface is bumpy, scalloped, and/or indented.

crystals: A solid substance with a regular shape that is due to the structure of molecules.

culture and sensitivity (C&S): A procedure where a specimen is cultured on microbiological media to detect bacterial or fungal growth. This is followed by screening for antibiotic sensitivity. C&S is performed in the microbiology department of a referral laboratory.

culture media: A solid, liquid, or semi-solid medium designed to support the growth of microorganisms, especially bacteria and fungus.

cyanosis: Lack of O_2 in blood seen as bluish or grayish discoloration of the skin, nail beds, and/or lips

cyst: A small, capsule-like sac that is filled with a semisolid material, such as a keratinous or sebaceous cyst.

cystic fibrosis (CF): Affects all the exocrine cells, but it affects the respiratory system the most. Mucus is abnormally thick and it blocks the alveoli, causing dyspnea.

cystitis: Inflammation of the urinary bladder.

cytology: The study of cells using microscopic methods.

cytoplasm: The cell substance that fills the area between the nucleus and the cell membrane. Contains organelles of the cell.

D

damages: Monetary settlement the defendant pays the plaintiff in a civil case for loss or injury

data server: Computer hardware and software that perform data analysis, storage, and archiving; also called a *database server.*

debridement: The surgical removal of dead, damaged, or infected tissue to improve the function of healthy tissue.

debris: Remains of anything broken down or destroyed. Ruins, rubble.

decanting: To pour a liquid gently so that it does not disturb the remaining sediment.

declaratory judgement: A court judgement that defines the legal rights of the parties involved.

decolorizer: A liquid that has the ability to wash out color.

decongestants: Category of medication that is used for nasal congestion.

decryption: The computer process of changing encrypted text to readable or plain text after a user enters a secret key or password.

decubitus ulcers: Sores or ulcers that develop over a bony prominence as the result of ischemia from prolonged pressure; also called *bed sores* or *pressure sores*.

deductible: A set dollar amount that the policyholder must pay before the insurance company starts to pay for services.

de-escalating: To reduce the level or intensity; bring down a person's anger or elevated emotions.

defecation: To void waste from the bowels through the anus; have a bowel movement.

defendant: An individual or business against whom a lawsuit is filed.

defense: Strategy used by the defendant to avoid liability in a lawsuit.

dementia: Mental disorder in which the individual experiences a progressive loss of memory, personality alterations, confusion, loss of touch with reality, and stupor (seeming unawareness of, and disconnection with, one's surroundings).

demographics: Statistical data of a population. In healthcare this includes patient name, address, date of birth, employment, and other details.

density: Describes how compact or concentrated something is.

deoxygenated: Oxygen deficient; oxygen was removed

dependent adults: People between the ages of 18 and 64 who have a mental or physical impairment that prevents them from doing normal activities or cannot protect themselves.

deposition: A sworn testimony made before a court appointed officer; used in the discovery process and may be used in the trial.

depreciate: To diminish in value (of an item) over a period of time; concept used for tax purposes.

dermatome: Skin surface areas supplied by a single afferent spinal nerve.

desmopressin: A hormone that is injected into a vein (or given as a nasal spray) that may help stimulate a release of more clotting factor in the body to help stop bleeding.

detrimental: Harmful

diagnosis: Determining the cause of a condition, illness, disease, injury, or congenital defect

diagnostic procedures: Tests and procedures used to help diagnose or monitor a condition.

diagnostic statement: Information about a patient's diagnosis or diagnoses that has been taken from the medical documentation.

diaphragm: A broad dome-shaped muscle used for breathing that separates the thoracic and abdominopelvic cavities.

dictation: To say something aloud for another person to write down.

differentiate: To distinguish one thing from another, to make a distinction between items.

differentiated: Describes how malignant tissue looks like the normal tissue it came from; poorly differentiated means it doesn't look like the normal tissue and well differentiated means it looks like the normal tissue.

diffuse: To spread, scatter, disperse, or move.

dignity: Being worthy of honor and respect from others.

diluent: A liquid substance that dilutes or lessens the strength of a solution or mixture.

dilution: Reducing the concentration of a mixture or solution by adding a known volume of liquid.

diplopia: A pathological condition of vision where a single object is seen as two. Double vision.

direct filing system: A filing system in which materials can be located without consulting another source of reference.

discrepancies: A lack of similarity between what is stated and what is found; for instance, the computer inventory count is different than the physical count.

discretionary income: Money in a bank account that is not assigned to pay for any office expenses.

discrimination: Unfair treatment of another person based on the person's age, gender (sex), ethnicity, sexual orientation, disability, marital status, or other selective factors.

disinfectant: Any chemical agent used on nonliving objects to destroy or inhibit the growth of harmful organisms; not effective against bacterial spores.

disinfected: The state of having destroyed or rendered pathogenic organisms inactive; does not include spores, tuberculosis bacilli, and certain viruses.

disruption: An unexpected event that throws a plan into disorder; an interruption that prevents a system or process from continuing as usual or as expected.

dissect: To cut or separate tissue with a cutting instrument or scissors.

diuretic: A substance (i.e., medication) that increases the amount of urine produced.

diurnal variation: Fluctuations that occur during each day

donning: Putting on.

Down syndrome: Genetic disorder where abnormal cell division results in an extra chromosome 21.

dumb terminal: A personal computer that doesn't contain a hard drive and allows the user only limited functions, including access to software, the network, and/or the internet.

duodenal: The first section of the small intestines after the stomach.

dynamic equilibrium: Relating to balance when moving at an angle or rotating.

dyspnea: Difficult and/or painful breathing.

E

echocardiography: Use of ultrasonic waves directed through the heart to study the structure and motion of the heart. The visual record produced is called an echocardiogram.

ectopic: Occurring in an abnormal position or place; displaced. With ectopic pregnancy, the embryo implants outside of the uterus (e.g., in fallopian tube).

efferent: Pertaining to carrying away from a structure.

egress: Leaving a place; exit route.

elastin: A highly elastic protein in connective tissue and allows tissues to resume their shape after stretching or contracting. Found abundantly in the dermis of the skin.

electrocardiogram (ECG, EKG): A record or recording of electrical impulses of the heart as wave deflections of a needle on an electrocardiograph.

electrodes: Adhesive patches that conduct electricity from the body to the machine wires (e.g., ECG and TENS unit).

electrolyte: Inorganic compounds, mainly salts. A major factor in controlling fluid balance within the body.

electronic health record (EHR): An electronic record conforms to nationally recognized standards and contains health-related information about a specific patient. It can be created, managed, and consulted by authorized clinicians and staff from more than one healthcare organization.

electronic medical record (EMR): An electronic record of health-related information about an individual that can be created, gathered, managed, and accessed by authorized clinicians and staff members within a single healthcare organization. An EMR is an electronic version of a paper record.

electronic transaction: Electronic exchange of information between two agencies to accomplish financial or administrative healthcare activities.

eligibility: Meeting the stipulated requirements to participate in the health care plan.

emancipated minor: A minor who has been granted emancipation by the court; the minor can assume the rights and responsibilities of adulthood.

embezzlement: The misuse of a healthcare facility's funds for personal gain.

embolus: An air bubble, blood clot, or foreign body that travels through the bloodstream and blocks a blood vessel.

emergency: An unexpected, life-threatening situation that requires immediate action.

emphysema: thinning and eventual destruction of the alveoli; usually accompanies chronic bronchitis

emulsifies: When a substance suspends tiny droplets of one liquid in a second liquid. By creating an emulsion, you can mix two liquids that usually do not mix well, such as oil and water.

EMV chip technology: Global technology that includes imbedded microchips that store and protect cardholder data; also called *chip and PIN* and *chip and signature*.

encoder: Software that will apply diagnostic or procedure codes to medical conditions or procedures.

encounter form: A document used to capture the services/procedures and diagnoses for a patient visit. The fees for the services/procedures are usually included on the encounter form.

endemic: Part of the normal pathogen make-up of a specific geographical area

endocervical curettage: a small, spoon-shaped instrument (curette) or a thin brush is used to scrape a tissue sample from the cervix.

endocrine: A glandular secretion that is released into the blood or lymph directly, does not go through a duct.

endocrinologist: A physician who specializes in the treatment of the endocrine glands and their secretions, especially in relation to their processes or functions.

endoscope: A scope with a camera attached to a long, thin tube that can be inserted into the body.

endoscopy: Nonsurgical procedure that used an endoscope to view in the body

endospore: An inactive form of certain bacteria that can withstand poor environmental conditions. When conditions improve the bacteria becomes functional again.

endotracheal (ET) tube: Catheter that is inserted into the trachea through the mouth; provides a patent airway.

enunciation: The use of articulate, clear sounds when speaking.

enzymatic reaction: A specific chemical reaction controlled by an enzyme.

enzymes: Special proteins that speed up chemical reactions in the body.

epidemiological: The branch of medicine dealing with the incidence, distribution, and control of disease in a population and prevalence of disease in large populations and with detection of the source and cause of epidemics of infectious disease.

epiphyseal plate: A thin layer of cartilage located at the ends of a long bone where new bone forms.

epithelial cells: Form cellular sheets that cover surfaces, both inside and outside the body. Epithelial cells are closely packed, take on different shapes, and strongly stick to each other.

eponym: In medical terms, a medical diagnosis or procedure named for the person who discovered it.

e-prescribing: The use of electronic software to communicate with pharmacies and send prescribing information. It takes the place of writing a prescription by hand and giving it to a patient; most new or refill prescriptions can be submitted electronically, cutting down on fraud and errors.

equilibrium: A state of rest or balance due to the equal action of opposing forces.

ergonomics: An applied science concerned with designing and arranging things, needed to do your job, in an efficient and safe way.

erythropoietin: A hormone produced by the kidney cells and travels to the bone marrow to stimulate red blood cell formation.

essential hypertension: Elevated blood pressure of unknown cause that develops for no apparent reason; sometimes called *primary hypertension*.

established patient: A patient who has been treated previously by the healthcare provider within the past 3 years.

esterase: Any enzyme that breaks down esters (a type of organic molecule) into alcohols and acids.

ethernet: A communication system for connecting several computers so information can be shared.

ethics committees: A committee composed of members from a variety of disciplines that analyzes ethical issues

ethics: Rules of conduct

etiology: The study of the causes or origin of diseases.

eukaryote: Any single-celled or multicellular organism that has genetic material contained in a distinct membrane-bound nucleus.

evacuated: To create a vacuum in a tube, flask, or reaction vessel.

excoriation: Inflammation and irritation of the skin.

executor: An individual assigned to make financial decisions about the estate of a deceased patient.

exocrine: A glandular secretion released through a duct.

expediency: A means of achieving a particular end, as in a situation requiring urgency or caution.

expiration: Exhaling; movement of waste gases from the alveoli into the atmosphere

explanation of benefits (EOB): A document sent by the insurance company to the provider and the patient explaining the allowed charge amount, the amount reimbursed for services, and the patient's financial responsibilities.

explicit: Fully and clearly expressed or demonstrated; leaving nothing merely implied.

exploitation: The act of using another person for one's own advantage.

extension: Process of stretching out; increasing the angle of a joint.

extract: A certain substance that is taken out of a group or solution, and is in a concentrated form.

extraction: A process where a specific substance is separated from group or solution.

exudates: Fluids with high concentrations of protein and cellular debris that have escaped from the blood vessels and have been deposited in tissues or on tissue surfaces.

F

familial: Occurring in or affecting members of a family more than would be expected by chance.

fatigue: Extreme tiredness.

fatty acids: Results when fats are broken down; used by the body for energy and tissue development.

febrile: Pertaining to an elevated body temperature.

Federal Reserve Bank: The central bank of the United States. The Federal Reserve System consists of a seven-member Board of Governors with headquarters in Washington, D.C., and 12 Federal Reserve banks in major cities throughout the country.

fee schedule: A list of fixed fees for services.

fibrin sealants: Also known as fibrin glue. Is a topical medication that is applied directly to the skin. It is made up of substances that promote blood clotting and long-term healing. Can be used for a variety of wounds where stitches, bandages, or staples cannot be used.

filamentous: Composed of, or containing filaments or strands of a substance.

filtrate: The fluid that remains after a liquid is passed through a filter. Fluid and substances that are filtered out of the blood in the Bowman capsule.

fire doors: Doors made of fire-resistant materials; close manually or automatically during a fire to prevent the spread of the fire.

firewall: A program or hardware that acts as a barrier between the network and the internet.

fistula: An abnormal connection or passage, caused by disease or injury, between different body parts

flagella: A thread-like or whip-like extension of a cell that helps the cell move.

flexion: Process of decreasing the angle of a joint.

fluctuate: To shift back and forth.

follicle-stimulating hormone (FSH): A glycoprotein hormone secreted by the anterior pituitary gland. It stimulates the growth of ovum (eggs) in the ovary and induces the formation of sperm in the testis.

follow-up appointment: An appointment type used when a patient needs to see the provider after a condition should have been resolved or to monitor an ongoing condition, such as hypertension. Also known as a *recheck appointment*.

fontanelle: A space covered by thick membranes between the sutures of an infant's skull; called the baby's "soft spots"; there are both anterior and posterior fontanelles.

foramen magnum: A large opening in the base of the skull, forms the passage for the spinal cord.

forensic: Scientific tests or techniques used regarding the detection of crime.

form: How a medication comes (e.g., tablet and suspension).

fulminant: Rapid and aggressive disease state. Can cause complications, organ failure, rapid health decline, and death in a short period of time.

fungus: Any of a diverse group of single-celled organisms that include: mushrooms, molds, mildew, smuts, rusts, yeasts and classified in the kingdom Fungi.

G

gait: The manner or style of walking.

gamete: a mature sexual reproductive cell; spermatozoa or ovum

gatekeeper: The primary care provider, who is in charge of a patient's treatment. Additional treatment, such as referrals to a specialist, must be approved by the gatekeeper.

germicides: Agents that destroy pathogenic organisms.

g-force: A force acting on an object because of gravity. Example: A centrifuge spins and exerts g-force.

girth: The measurement around something; when referring to mail, it is the measurement around the middle of the package that is being shipped.

global services: For purposes of CPT coding, medical services and procedures performed for the patient before, during, and after a surgical procedure that is included with the assigned CPT code.

glomerulonephritis: A kidney disease affecting the glomeruli of the nephron. Characterized by albumin in the urine, edema, and high blood pressure.

glucagon: A hormone produced by the alpha cells in the pancreas; works on the liver to release glycogen to prevent dangerously low blood glucose levels.

glucose: Results when carbohydrates are broken down; main sugar found in the blood and used as the main source of energy. Also called blood sugar.

glycolysis: The chemical breakdown of carbohydrates (glucose) by enzymes, with the release of energy.

glycosuria: An elevated urinary glucose level (possible diabetes mellitus).

gonads: Organs that produce sex cells in both males and females.

graduated cylinder: A narrow, tube-shaped container marked with horizontal lines to represent units of measurement. Used to precisely measure the volume of liquids.

graft: Tissue taken from one area in the body and inserted into another area or person

gray matter: Brownish-gray nerve tissue, especially in the brain and spinal cord. Made up of nerve

cell bodies, their dendrites, and some supportive tissue.
gross: The amount earned before any tax deductions or adjustments.
guarantor: The person legally responsible for the entire bill. Usually the patient, but in the case of minor it would be a parent or legal guardian.

H

harassment: The continued, unwanted, and annoying actions done to another person.
hardware: Physical equipment of the computer system required for communication and data processing functions.
health insurance exchange: An online marketplace where you can compare and buy individual health insurance plans. State health insurance exchanges were established as part of the Affordable Care Act.
healthcare associated infections: (HAIs) Infections that patients acquire while receiving treatment for other conditions within a healthcare setting. Includes ambulatory care, long-term care, or rehabilitation facility.
hematologist: A person trained in the nature, function, and diseases of the blood and blood-forming organs. Can be a physician, trained laboratory personnel, or researcher.
hematoma: An abnormal buildup of blood in an organ or tissue of the body, caused by a leak or cut in a blood vessel.
hemoconcentration: A condition in which the concentration of blood cells is increased in proportion to the plasma.
hemoglobin: An oxygen-carrying pigment of red blood cells that contains iron. Gives red blood cells their color. Carries O_2 to the cells.
hemolysis: The breakdown of red blood cells with the release of hemoglobin.
hemolyzed: A blood sample in which the red blood cells have ruptured.
hemophilia: Group of inherited blooding disorders characterized by a deficiency of one of the factors necessary for the coagulation of blood.
hemostasis: The stoppage of bleeding.
hepatosplenomegaly: Inflammation of the liver and spleen. Can be severe.
hereditary: Passed from parents to offspring through the genes.
hernia: protrusion of a loop of intestine through a weakness in the abdominal wall.
hertz: The unit of measurement used in hearing examinations; a wave frequency equal to 1 cycle per second.
heterophile antibody: An antibody that has an affinity for an antigen other than the specific antigen that stimulated its production.
hierarchy: Things arranged in order or rank.
histology: The study of tissues.
history of present illness (HPI): Describes the signs and symptoms from the time of onset.
holistic: Considering the patient as a whole including the physical, emotional, social, economic, and spiritual needs of the person.
homeostasis: The internal environment of the body that is compatible with life. A steady state that is created by all the body systems working together to provide a consistent and unvarying internal environment.
hormone: A chemical substance produced in an endocrine gland and transported in the blood to a specific tissue, where it applies a specific effect.
hyaline: Glassy or transparent.
hydrocephaly: Enlargement of the cranium caused by abnormal accumulation of cerebrospinal fluid in the cerebral system.
hydronephrosis: A backup of urine that causes dilation of the ureters and calyces; can increase pressure on the nephron units.
hyperkalemia: High potassium levels in the blood
hyperlipidemia: An elevated level of lipids in the blood.
hyperpnea: Excessively deep breathing.
hyperventilation: Abnormally increased breathing
hypoalbuminemia: A decreased level of albumin (protein) in the blood.
hypochromic: Pale red blood cells. Lacking color.
hypospadias: Condition where the urethral opening is on the underside of the penis.
hypotension: Blood pressure that is below normal (systolic pressure below 90 mm Hg and diastolic pressure below 50 mm Hg).
hypothyroidism: Deficient activity of the thyroid gland.
hysterectomy: surgical removal of the uterus and cervix. The ovaries and fallopian tubes may also be removed.

I

identifiers: Information unique to an individual. Common identifiers used for patient identification include; full name including middle initial, date of birth, medical ID number, or patient address.
idiopathic: Of unknown cause.
immune: A person that has developed protective antibodies against a pathogen and is no longer at risk for acquiring the infection.
immunoglobulins: A group of related proteins that functions as antibodies. Are found in plasma and other body fluids.
impervious: Not permitting penetration.
in utero: The term means in the uterus. Referring to the fetus' time of development.
in vitro: Latin term meaning "in glass" and in commonly known as "in the laboratory"
inanimate: Not animate; lifeless.
incidence: How often something happens or occurs.
incompetence: The state of being incompetent or lacking the ability to manage personal affairs due to mental deficiency; an appointed guardian or conservator manages their affairs.
inconspicuous: not noticeable or prominent
incurred: To come into or acquire.
indigent: Poor, needy, impoverished.
infarction: Tissue death
infection: Invasion of body tissues by microorganisms, which then multiply and damage tissues.
infectious agents: Includes living and non-living pathogens such as bacteria, viruses, fungi, protozoa, parasite, helminths, and prions, that can cause disease. Also called infectious particles.
inflammation: Pathology with characteristic redness, swelling, pain, tenderness, heat and disturbed function of an area of the body. Especially a reaction of tissues to injury.
infusion: When a medication or treatment is given intravenously, but it needs to be given slowly. May be given through a port, catheter, or PICC line.
ingested: To take, as food, into the body.
inhalant: Any substance that can be breathed into the lungs.
inhalation: To breathe in.
initiative: The ability to start a task and energetically complete it.
injunction: A court order by which an individual or institution is required to perform or restrain from performing a certain act.
INR: INR stands for International Normalized Ratio, and is also called a prothrombin time (PT). It is used to test the effectiveness of blood thinning medication.
insidious: Stealthily treacherous.
inspiration: Inhaling; movement of oxygen from the atmosphere into the alveoli
insulin: A hormone produced by the beta cells in the pancreas; moves glucose into the cells so it can be used for energy.
intact: Complete or whole. Not broken or altered.
intangible: Something of value that cannot be touched physically.
integral: Essential; being an indispensable part of a whole.
integrity: Adhering to ethical standards or right conduct standards.
intercellular: Located between cells
intercostal muscles: Muscles located between the ribs that help with quiet respiration
interest: Money the bank pays the account holder on the amount in their account for using the money in the account.
interface: An interconnection between systems.
interferon: A protein formed when a cell is exposed to a virus; the protein blocks viral action on the cell and protects against viral invasion.
intermittent pulse: A pulse in which beats occasionally are skipped.
intermittent: Occurring in intervals
interoperability: The ability to work with other systems.
interpersonal skills: Ability to communicate and interact with others; sometimes referred to as "soft skills."
interrogatory: Written or oral questions that must be answered under oath.
interstitial cells: Testosterone-secreting cells of testes that are found in the spaces between the seminiferous tubules.
interstitial: Between the cells
interval: Space of time between events.
intracellular pathogens: A disease causing organism that is within or inside of a cell.
intravenously (IV): Through a vein; fluids and medications can be given through a vein.
invalid: Not valid. A process or outcome that is not correct.
inventory: Detailed list of equipment and supplies owned and stored; the process of counting the supplies in stock.
invoices: Billing statements that list the amount owed for goods or services purchased.
ion: An electrically charged atom or the smallest component of an element. (Cation has a positive charge, anion has a negative charge)

J

jargon: The vocabulary of a particular profession as opposed to common, everyday terms. Medical terminology and abbreviations can be considered jargon.
jaundice: Yellow discoloration of the skin, whites of the eyes, and mucous membranes, due to an increase of bilirubin in the blood.
job boards: Websites where employers post jobs and can be used by job seekers to identify open positions.
judicious: Using good judgement; being discreet, sensible.

K

ketones: A class of organic compounds that is a by-product of fatty acid metabolism. An example of a ketone is acetone.
ketonuria: Ketones in the urine.

L

lacrimation: The secretion or discharge of tears.
laparoscopy: a procedure to visually examine the abdomen
larvae: Immature free-living form of many animals that develops into an adult form.
larynx: voice box
lateral flow immunoassay: A laboratory or clinical technique that uses the specific binding between an antigen and antibody to identify and quantify a substance in a sample. The sample in this technique moves in a sideways motion, usually on an absorbent paper.
leads: Pictures created by electrical activity of the heart; leads can also refer to the lead wires attached to the electrodes.
lethargy: The state of being drowsy and dull, listless and unenergetic.
liability: State of being liable or responsible for something.
liable: Legally responsible or obligated.
libido: Sexual drive or instinct.
licensure: A mandatory process established by state law that ensures a person has met the legal standards for practicing an occupation in that state.
light microscope: An instrument that uses focused light and lenses to magnify a specimen, usually a cell.
litigious: prone to lawsuits
local: Affecting the area where it was applied.
locum tenens: A physician or advance practice professional temporarily contracted to provide healthcare services when a facility has a vacancy, vacation, or a leave of absence.
loop electrosurgical excision procedure (LEEP): after an injection of anesthetic to the cervix a high-frequency electrical current running through a wire is used to remove abnormal tissue from both the cervix and the endocervical canal.
lumen: the cavity, channel, or open space within a tube or tubular organ.
lumpectomy: removal of the breast tumor and a small amount of the surrounding tissue
luteinizing hormone (LH): A hormone produced by the anterior pituitary gland. LH stimulates ovulation and the development of the corpus luteum in females and the production of testosterone in males.
lymph: A clear, yellowish fluid containing white blood cells in a liquid similar to plasma. The fluid comes from the tissues of the body and is moved through the lymphatic vessels and the blood stream.
lymphoctyes: A type of white blood cell that has a large, round nucleus that is surrounded by a thin layer of agranular cytoplasm.
lymphostasis: Obstruction or interruption of normal lymph flow.
lysed: To break apart or rupture.
lysis: Destruction or break down of cells. Rupture or dissolution.

M

macromolecules: The molecules needed for metabolism: carbohydrates, lipids, proteins, amino acids, and nucleic acids.
macrophages: A large white blood cell that lives in the tissues and engulfs foreign particles, microorganisms, and cell debris.
maladaptive: Unacceptably adapted, or adapting poorly to a situation or purpose.
malaise: A condition of general bodily weakness or discomfort, often marking the onset of a disease.
malignant: A cell with uncontrolled growth, rapidly spreading, and doing harm.
malpractice: A type of negligence in which a licensed professional fails to provide the standard of care, causing harm to a person.
manipulation: Movement or exercise of a body part by means of an externally applied force.
mastectomy: removal of the entire breast
matrix: The environment where something is created or takes shape. A base on which to build.
mature minor: A person under the age of adulthood who demonstrates the maturity to make a personal healthcare decision and can give informed consent for treatment.
Meaningful Use requirements: Requirements established by the Centers for Medicare and Medicaid Services (CMS) as part of the Electronic Health Records (EHR) Incentives Program. The program provides financial incentives for healthcare organizations that "meaningfully used" their certified EHR technology. The requirements include implementing security measures to ensure the privacy of patients' EHRs.
meatus: A body opening or passage. Especially the external opening of a structure.
mechanism: A sequence of steps that allow something to be produced or a purpose to be accomplished.
media: A type of communication (e.g., social media sites); with computers, the term refers to data storage devices.
mediastinal: Location separating the right and left thoracic cavity.
mediastinum: the space in the thoracic cavity that lies between the lungs, containing the heart, trachea, and esophagus
mediation: The process of facilitating conflicting parties to make an agreement, settlement, or compromise.
medical necessity: CPT and HCPCS codes (services or supplies) used to treat the patient's diagnosis (indicated by the ICD code) meet the accepted standard of medical practice.
medulla oblongata: The lowest part of the brain, continuous with the top of the spinal cord.
melanocytes: Cells of the stratum germinativum that produce a brownish pigment called melanin. Melanin gives us our skin color.
menarche: first menstrual period
Ménière's disease: Chronic disease of the inner ear causing recurrent episodes of vertigo, progressive sensorineural hearing loss, and tinnitus.
meninges: The three membranes covering the brain and spinal cord.
meningiocele: The protrusion of the meninges through an opening in the spinal column or skull.
metabolic: relating to, or resulting from metabolism (the chemical process where cells produce the substances and energy needed to sustain life).
metabolism: The chemical processes that occur within a living organism in order to maintain life.
metabolites: Byproducts of drug metabolism
metastasizes: To spread from one part of the body (the primary tumor) to another part of the body forming a secondary tumor.
methicillin-resistant *Staphylococcus aureus*: (MRSA) A Gram-positive pathogen that is resistant to multiple antibiotics.
microbiome: The total collection of microorganisms and their genetic material present on/in the human body or a specific site in the human body.
microcephaly: Abnormally small head associated with incomplete brain development
microcuvettes: A small plastic or glass tube designed to hold samples for laboratory tests that detect light or color changes.
microorganisms: Any living organism, such as bacterium, protozoan, fungi, parasite, or helminth of microscopic size. Some definitions include viruses, which are not alive.
minor: One who has not reach adulthood; usually 18 or 21 depending on jurisdiction.
mitosis: A cell division process by which two daughter cells are formed from one parent cell; each daughter has a complete copy of parent's chromosomes.
mock: Simulated; intended for imitation or practice.
modem: Peripheral computer hardware that connects to the router to provide internet access to the network or computer.
mold: A growth of tiny fungi forming on a substance. Often looks downy or furry, and is associated with dampness or decay.
molecule: The simplest unit of a chemical compound that can exist, consisting of two or more atoms held together with chemical bonds.
monocytes: A large circulating white blood cell, formed in the bone marrow. Agranulocyte that engulfs foreign particles, microorganisms, and cell debris.
monotone: A succession of syllables, words, or sentences spoken in an unvaried key or pitch.
morals: Internal principles that distinguish between right and wrong.
mordant: Having the ability to fix, or set colors.
morphology: The study of the form, shape, and structure of an organism.
mortality: The relative frequency of deaths in a specific population

multiple-line telephone system: A business telephone system that allows for more than one telephone line.no-show: When a patient fails to keep an appointment without giving advance notice.

murmur: An abnormal sound heard during auscultation of the heart that may or may not have a pathologic origin; it is associated with valve disease or a congenital heart defect.

myalgia: Pain in a muscle or group of muscles.

mydriatic: A topical ophthalmic medication that dilates the pupil; it is used in diagnostic procedures of the eye and as treatment for glaucoma.

myelin sheath: Formed by Schwann cells, a protective insulation covering PNS nerve axons. Helps with the transmission of nerve impulses.

myocardium: Middle layer and the thickest layer of the heart; composed of cardiac muscles.

myofibrils: A contractile fiber of skeletal muscle, made up of mostly actin and myosin.

myoglobin: A type of hemoglobin found in the muscle.

myoglobinuria: The presence of myoglobin in the urine.

myositis: Inflammation of a muscle or group of muscles.

myxedema: Advanced hypothyroidism in adulthood

N

NAATs: Nucleic acid amplification tests (NAATs) are screening tests for chlamydia trachomatis, Neisseria gonorrhoeae infections and trichomoniasis. These tests can detect small amounts of DNA or RNA in test samples.

nasal wash: Also called a nasal aspirate. A syringe is used to gently squirt a small amount of sterile saline into the nose and the resulting fluid is collected into a cup (for a wash). Or after the saline is squirted into the nose, gentle suction is applied (for the aspirate).

nasopharyngeal: Part of the throat behind and above the soft palate, and connected to the nasal passages.

National Provider Identifier (NPI): An identifier assigned by the Centers for Medicare and Medicaid Services (CMS) that classifies the healthcare provider by license and medical specialties.

National Provider Identifier: An identifier assigned by the Centers for Medicare and Medicaid Services (CMS) that classifies the healthcare provider by license and medical specialties.

necrosis: Tissue death

negative feedback: An output or response affects the input of a system.

neglect: Failure to provide proper attention or care to another person.

negligence: Conduct expected of a reasonably prudent person acting under similar circumstances; it falls below the standards of behavior established by law for the protection of others against unreasonable risk of harm.

negotiable instrument: A document guaranteeing payment of a specific amount of money to the payer named on the document.

nephrectomy: Surgical removal of a kidney.

nephrologists: A physician who specializes in the treatment of the kidneys and their processes, function, and diseases.

nephron: Nephrons are the functional unit of the kidney. The job of the nephron is to create urine and adjust it to maintain homeostasis.

nephrotoxic: Damaging or destructive to the kidneys.

net: The amount someone is paid after taxes and other deductions have been subtracted.

neurons: Nerve cells

neuropathy: Nervous system disorder of the peripheral nerves causing discomfort, numbness, and weakness especially in the extremities.

neurotransmitter: A chemical that helps a nerve cell communicate with another nerve cell or muscle.

neutrophilia: An increase of neutrophilic white blood cells in blood or tissues.

nocturia: Frequent urination at night.

nodules: Small lumps, lesions, or swellings that are felt when the skin is palpated.

nomenclature: A system of names or terms, used in science and art to categorize items.

non-decodable terms: Words used in healthcare whose definitions must be memorized without the benefit of word parts.

noninvasive procedures: Those procedures that do not penetrate human tissue.

nonorganic: Refers to not having an organic or physiologic cause; a disorder that does not have a cause that can be found in the body.

serous: A thin, watery serum-like drainage.

normal flora: Microorganisms (mostly bacteria and yeast) that live on or in the body. Normal microscopic residents of the body.

nosocomial infections: Infections that are acquired in a healthcare setting.

Notice of Privacy Practices (NPP): A written document describing the healthcare facility's privacy practices. The patient must be provided with the NPP and sign an acknowledgment of receipt.

nucleus: A specialized portion of a cell that is encased in a membrane, and directs growth, metabolism, and reproduction of the cell.

numeric filing: The filing of records, correspondence, or cards by number.

O

objective information: Data obtained through physical examination, laboratory and diagnostic testing, and by measurable information.

obliteration: To remove or destroy all traces of; do away with; destroy completely.

obturator: A metal rod with a smooth, rounded tip that is placed in hollow instruments to reduce injury to body tissues during insertion.

occipital lobe: The lobe of the brain located at the back of the skull below the parietal lobe.

occlude: To close, shut, or stop up.

occult: Hidden or unseen.

oncologist: A specially trained doctor who diagnoses and treats cancer.

online provider insurance web portal: An online service provided by various insurance companies for providers to look up patient insurance benefits, eligibility, claims status, and explanation of benefits.

oophorectomy: Surgical removal of the ovaries.

opportunistic infections: A microorganism that normally does not cause disease but becomes pathogenic when the body's immune system is impaired and unable to fight off infection, as in AIDS, malnutrition, and certain other diseases.

optics checks: A specific type of calibration that assess the optics of an electronic testing instrument or system.

organelles: Structures within a cell that perform a specific function.

orthopnea: Condition of difficult breathing unless in an upright position.

orthostatic (postural) hypotension: A temporary fall in blood pressure when a person rapidly changes from a recumbent position to a standing position.

ossicles: The three small bones of the middle ear, that transmit sound vibrations from

ossification: The natural process of bone formation and hardening.

osteoporosis: Abnormal thinning of the bone structure causing bones to become brittle and weak

otitis externa: Inflammation or infection of the external auditory canal; commonly called *swimmer's ear.*

P

peripheral: A term that refers to an area outside of or away from an organ or structure.

otolaryngologist: A physician who has specialized in the study of anatomy, function, and diseases of the ear, nose, and throat.

otosclerosis: The formation of spongy bone in the labyrinth of the ear, which often causes the auditory ossicles to become fixed and unable to vibrate when sound enters the ears.

ototoxic: Medications that have a harmful effect on the eighth cranial nerve or the organs of hearing and balance.

outguides: A sturdy cardboard or plastic file-sized card used to replace a folder temporarily removed from the filing space.

output device: Computer hardware that displays the processed data from the computer (e.g., monitors and printers).

ovulation: The release of the ovum from the ovarian follicle.

oxygen: A colorless, odorless gas, O_2, that makes up about 25% of the air we breathe. It is essential for life and cellular respiration. Symbol on the periodic chart is O.

packing slip: A document that accompanies purchased merchandise and shows what is in the box or package.

palliative care: Care that is focused on providing relief from the symptoms and stress of a serious, possibly terminal illness. Improving the overall quality of life for the patient and their family.

palpation: The use of touch during the physical examination to assess the size, consistency, and location of certain body parts.

parameters: A rule that controls how something should be done, guidelines or boundaries.

GLOSSARY

paranasal sinuses: Hollow cavities filled with air located within the skull and facial bones and serve to lighten the weight of the skull and increase the tone or resonance of speech.

paraphrasing: Rewording a statement to check the meaning and interpretation; also shows you are listening and understanding the speaker.

parasitic: Pertaining to a parasite (An organism that live on in or another organism, known as the host. Benefits from the host, the host does not benefit from the parasite.)

parenteral: To take into the body by any route other than the digestive tract (e.g., subcutaneous, intravenous, or intramuscular administration).

participating provider: A physician or other healthcare provider who enters into a contract with a specific insurance company or program and by doing so agrees to abide by certain rules and regulations set forth by that particular insurance company.

patent: Open

pathogen: A disease-causing organism or agent.

pathologist: A physician specially trained in the nature and cause of disease.

pathology: Study of disease

patient abandonment: Form of medical malpractice and called negligent termination; provider ends the provider-patient relationship without reasonable or adequate notification.

patient account: A running balance of all financial transactions for a specific patient.

patient navigator: A person who identifies patients' needs and barriers; then assists by coordinating care and identifying community and healthcare resources to meet the needs. May also be called care coordinator.

patient portal: A secure online website that gives patients 24-hour access to personal health information using a username and password.

pegboard system: A manual bookkeeping system that uses a day sheet to record all financial transactions for the date of service and maintains patient account balances by using physical ledger cards.

pelvic girdle: A bowl-shaped complex of bones that connects the trunk and the legs. The pelvic girdle consists of the ilium, ischium, and pubis.

percutaneous: Puncture through the skin

perforated ulcer: A condition where an untreated ulcer can damage the wall of the stomach or small intestine creating a hole that allows digestive juices and food to leak into the abdominal cavity. Treatment generally requires immediate surgery.

performance measurement: The regular collection of data to assess whether the correct processes are being performed and desired results are being achieved.

perineal: Pertaining to the area between the vaginal opening and the rectum (perineum)

peripheral blood smear: A thin layer of blood is smeared on a glass microscope slide, then stained. This allows a trained laboratory technician or pathologist to examine various characteristics of the blood cells microscopically.

peripheral neuropathy: A problem with the function of the nerves outside the spinal cord; symptoms include weakness, burning pain, and loss of reflexes; a frequent complication of diabetes mellitus.

peristalsis: Rhythmic contraction of involuntary muscles lining the gastrointestinal tract.

peritoneum: Serous membrane lining of the abdominal cavity, folds inward to enclose the viscera (internal organs).

peritubular capillaries: Blood capillaries surrounding the proximal and distal convoluted tubules in the kidneys.

permeability: A quality or characteristic of a material that allows another substance to pass through it.

personal ethics: An individual's code of conduct.

personal protective equipment: Clothing, eye protection, gloves, or other garments or equipment designed to protect the wearer's body from injury or infection.

petechiae: Very small, round hemorrhage in the skin or mucous membrane.

Peyer patches: Small masses of lymphatic tissue found mostly in the ileum of the small intestine. They form an important part of the immune system by monitoring intestinal bacteria populations and preventing the growth of pathogenic bacteria in the intestines.

pharyngitis: Inflammation or infection of the pharynx, usually causing symptoms of a sore throat.

phenylalanine: An essential amino acid found in milk, eggs, and other foods.

phenylketonuria (PKU): A deficiency in the enzyme phenylalanine hydroxylase, which is responsible for converting phenylalanine into tyrosine.

physiologic: Consistent with the normal function of the body.

pipette: A slender tube attached to or including a bulb, for transferring or measuring small amounts of a liquid, often used in a laboratory.

pitch: The depth of a tone or sound; a distinctive quality of sound.

pituitary gland: Endocrine gland located in the skull responsible for producing luteinizing hormone (LH) and follicle-stimulating hormone (FSH).

plaintiff: An individual or party who brings the suit to court

plaque: Any small abnormal patch on or within the body. Deposit of fatty material.

plasma proteins: Proteins that circulate in the blood and are made in the liver

plasma: The liquid portion of a whole blood sample that has not clotted due to an anticoagulant. Liquid portion of blood that contains clotting factors. Liquid portion of the blood found in the body.

pleural effusion: Abnormal accumulation of fluid in the intrapleural space around the lungs.

plume: Vapor, smoke and particle debris produced from laser procedures.

pneumonia: Inflammation of the lungs with congestion of the air sacs (alveoli). Can be caused by a bacteria or virus.

point-of-care: Something designed to be used at or near where the patient is seen; point-of-care tools and apps are resources for the provider to use when working directly with the patient.

poised: Having a confident composure.

policy: A written agreement between two parties, where one party (the insurance company) agrees to pay another party (the patient) if certain specified circumstances occur.

polycythemia: A condition caused by an abnormally large number of red blood cells (RBCs) in the blood.

polyethylene: a plastic material used mostly for containers and packaging.

pores: A tiny opening in the surface of the skin that allows gases, liquids, or microscopic particles can pass.

portrait orientation: The most common layout for a printed page; the height of the paper is greater than its width.

postherpetic neuralgia: Nerve pain that occurs after a shingles outbreak and may become chronic.

practice management software: A type of software that allows the user to enter demographic information, schedule appointments, maintain lists of insurance payers, perform billing tasks, and generate reports.

preauthorization: A process required by some insurance carriers in which the provider obtains permission to perform certain procedures or services or refers a patient to a specialist.

precedence: Followed first.

precedent: A prior court decision that serves as a model for similar legal cases in the future.

precertification: The process of determining if a procedure or service is covered by the insurance plan and what the reimbursement is for that procedure or service.

precipitate: Solid particles that settle out of liquid.

preeclampsia: Abnormal condition of pregnancy with unknown cause, marked by hypertension edema, and proteinuria. May progress to eclampsia.

prefixes: Word parts that appear at the beginning of some terms.

pre-formed (antibodies): Antibodies are that formed before being introduced to an antigen. ABO antibodies are pre-formed.

premenstrual dysphoric disorder (PMDD): Mood disorder that includes depression, irritability, fatigue, changes in appetite or sleep, and difficulty in concentrating; occurs 1 to 2 weeks before the onset of the menstrual flow.

premenstrual syndrome (PMS): Poorly understood group of symptoms that occur in some women on a cyclical basis: breast pain, irritability, fluid retention, headache, and a lack of coordination are some of the symptoms.

preservatives: Substances added to a specimen to prevent deterioration of cells or chemicals.

preventive maintenance: Regularly scheduled care of equipment that will decrease the likelihood of failure. Performed and documented at regular intervals while the equipment is in good working order.

privacy filters: Devices attached to the monitor that allow visualization of the screen contents only if the user is directly in front of the screen; also called *monitor filters* or *privacy screens*.

privileged communication: Communication that cannot be disclosed without authorization of the person involved; includes provider-patient and lawyer-client communications.

productive cough: A cough that produces phlegm or mucus.

proficiency: Skilled as a result of training or practice.

profile testing: A series of laboratory tests associated with a particular organ or disease; also referred to as a "panel" of tests.

prognosis: The likely outcome of a disease including change of recovery.

progress notes: Documentation in the medical record to track the patient's condition and progress.

prokaryote: Any organism that is made up of at least one cell, has genetic material that is not enclosed in a nucleus. Bacteria are prokaryotes, primitive organisms.

proliferate: To increase in numbers or spread rapidly and often excessively.

proofread: To read and mark corrections.

protozoa: Single-celled organisms that are the most primitive form of animal life. Most are microscopic. Examples are amoebas, ciliates, flagellates and sporozoans.

protozoal cyst: A thick-walled protective membrane enclosing a cell, larva, or organism.

provider network: An approved list of physicians, hospitals, and other providers.

provisional diagnosis: A temporary diagnosis made before all test results have been received.

pruritus: Itching

pseudocyst: The formation of cyst-like pockets in the pancreas that are filled with fluid and debris. Acute pancreatitis can lead to the formation of pseudocysts that can rupture, causing complications such as internal bleeding and infection.

psoriasis: A usually chronic, recurrent skin disease marked by bright red patches covered with silvery scales.

psychiatrists: Medical doctors with special training to diagnose and treat patients with mental, emotional, and behavioral conditions.

puberty: The stage of life in which males and females become functionally capable of sexual reproduction.

pulmonary hypertension: High blood pressure that affects the pulmonary system (pulmonary arteries and the right side of the heart).

pulmonologists: A physician who specializes in the treatment of the lungs and their processes, function, and diseases.

pulse deficit: A condition in which the radial pulse is less than the apical pulse; it may indicate a peripheral vascular abnormality.

pulse oximetry: Noninvasive test used to measure the oxygen saturation in the blood.

pulse pressure: The difference between the systolic and diastolic blood pressures (30 to 50 mm Hg is considered normal).

purchase order number: Unique number assigned by the ordering facility that allows the facility to track or reference the order.

pure culture: The growth of only one microorganism in a culture, or on a nutrient surface.

purpura: A rash of purple spots on or under the skin often caused by internal bleeding from small blood vessels.

purulent: pus like

putrid: A foul or decaying odor

pyemia: The presence of pus-forming organisms in the blood.

pyrexia: A febrile condition or fever.

Q

qualified Medicare beneficiaries (QMBs): Low-income Medicare patients who qualify for Medicaid for their secondary insurance.

quality assurance: Written policies and procedures that ensure monitoring all the processes involved before, during, and after a laboratory test is performed in order to produce reliable patient test results.

quality control: A process to ensure the reliability of test results, often using manufactured samples with known values.

quantitative: The test result is expressed as a number, usually with units of measure attached to numeric values.

R

rales: An abnormal lung sound heard on auscultation, characterized by discontinuous bubbling noises.

random specimen: A urine specimen that can be collected at any time of the day, with special instructions, into a nonsterile container.

rapport: A relationship of harmony and accord between the patient and the healthcare professional.

reagent strips: Plastic strips with paper pads that contain chemical reagents. Reagents react with analytes in the urine. Read by looking for a color change.

refraction: Bending of light waves when they pass through on substance into another substance of different density.

reagent: A substance for use in a chemical reaction.

rebound pain: When a person feels abdominal pain as pressure is removed, rather than when pressure is applied to the abdomen. Also known as Blumberg's sign.

receptors: A structure or site on or in a cell that binds with substances such as hormones, antigens, or drugs.

recommended dietary allowance (RDA): Average daily level of intake needed to meet the nutrient requirements of most healthy people.

reconciliation: To bring into agreement.

reconciling: Comparing a document to ensure that it is consistent with another document.

reconstituted: Restored a dried substance (powder) to a fluid form so it can be injected.

recovery position: Position on the person's side that helps to keep the airway opened and clear.

red bone marrow: An active form of bone marrow that produces red and white blood

reference range: The numeric range of test values for which the general population consistently shows similar results 95% of the time.

referral laboratory: A laboratory that performs testing for another laboratory. Testing varies from high-volume routine testing to low-volume unique or unusual testing. Also called reference, diagnostic, or commercial testing laboratories. Often privately owned.

referral: An order from a primary care provider for the patient to see a specialist or get certain medical services.

reflecting: Putting words to the patient's emotional reaction, which acknowledges the person's feelings.

reflexes: Movement or process caused by a reflex response. An automatic response, doesn't require thought.

refracted: The bending of light rays

registered dietitian: A credentialed healthcare professional who is trained in nutrition and who has the ability to apply the information to the dietary needs of healthy and ill patients.

regular diet: What a person typically consumes with no dietary limitations.

regurgitation: Return of partly digested food or stomach contents, from the stomach to the mouth.

reimbursement: To make repayment to for expense or loss incurred

relapse: The recurrence of the symptoms of a disease after apparent recovery.

remission: The partial or complete disappearance of the clinical and subjective characteristics of a chronic or malignant disease.

release of information: A form completed by the patient that authorizes the medical office to release medical records to the insurance company for health insurance reimbursement.

reliable: Dependable, able to be trusted.

renal ischemia: A blood flow deficiency to the kidney(s).

renal thresholds: Blood level of a substance, above which the kidneys fail to reabsorb it, so the substance will appear in the urine.

replication: The production of exact copies of a complex molecule, such as DNA.

res ipsa loquitur: The thing speaks for itself

Res Judicata: "A thing decided"; once a case has been decided by the court, it cannot be litigated again.

residual urine: Urine that remains in the bladder after micturition or urination

resource-based relative value system (RBRVS): System used to determine how much providers should be paid for services rendered. Used by Medicare and many other health insurance companies.

respiratory arrest: Cessation of breathing

Respondeat Superior: Legal doctrine meaning "let the master answer"; the employer/provider is legally responsible for the wrongful actions or lack of actions of the employees if done within the scope of employment.

restock: Process of replacing the supplies that were used.

retaliation: Getting back at others for something they did to you.

retention schedule: A method or plan for retaining or keeping health records and for their movement from active to inactive to closed.

retribution: Punishment inflicted on someone as vengeance for a wrong or criminal act; the act of taking revenge.

reverse chronologic order: The most recent item is on top and oldest item is last.

review of systems: A list of questions related to each organ system, designed to uncover potential disease processes.

GLOSSARY

rheumatologist: A physician who specializes in the treatment of rheumatic diseases such as arthritis, systemic lupus erythematosus (SLE), scleroderma, and other joint and autoimmune diseases.
rhonchi: Abnormal rumbling sound heard on auscultation, caused by airways blocked by secretions or muscle contractions.
rotor: The rotating member of a machine or device.
route: The means by which a drug enters the body.
rugae: Folds in the wall of the organ; when organ (e.g., stomach, bladder, uterus) fills or needs to expand, the rugae unfold.

S

salaried: A fixed compensation periodically paid to a person for regular work.
salpingo-oophorectomy: surgical removal of the fallopian tube and ovary.
sanitize: The state of cleaning equipment and instruments with detergent and water, removing debris and reducing the number of microorganisms.
sclera: The white part of the eye that forms the orbit.
scope of practice: Range of responsibilities and practice guidelines that determine the boundaries within which a healthcare worker practices.
scored tablet: A tablet with a groove on the surface, used for splitting it into half.
screening: A system for examining and separating into different groups; in the healthcare facility, it means determining the severity of illness that patients experience and prioritizing appointments based on that severity.
seborrhea: An excessive discharge of sebum from the sebaceous glands, forming greasy scales or crusty areas on the body.
secondary storage devices: Media (e.g., jump drive, flash drive, hard drive) capable of permanently storing data until it is replaced or deleted by the user
security risk analysis: Identification of potential threats of computer network breaches, for which action plans for corrective actions.
sediment: Insoluble material that settles to the bottom of a urine specimen and to the bottom of centrifuged urine.
self-limiting viral infection: A viral infection that causes signs and symptoms, but after a period of time the person's immune system defeats the infection and is no longer ill. Example would be the common cold.
senescent cell: An old or aging cell that can no longer divide and reproduce.
sensitized: To make reactive to an antigen.
sensorineural: Involving the sensory nerves, especially as they affect hearing.
sentinel node biopsy: removal of a limited number of lymph nodes to determine if the cancer has spread to your lymph nodes
septicemia: Systemic infection with pathologic microbes in the blood as a result of an infection that has spread from elsewhere in the body
sequela (singular) sequelae (plural): An abnormal condition resulting from a previous disease.
sequestrum: A fragment of bone that has died as a result of disease or injury and has separated from the normal bone structure.
serologic: The science involving the immune properties and actions of serum.
serous: A thin, watery serum-like drainage.
serum: The liquid portion of a clotted blood specimen. It no longer contains active clotting agents.
sharps: Medical term for devices with sharp points or edges that can puncture or cut skin. Examples include needles, scalpels, or broken glass.
shift(s): Data results on a graph that make an abrupt change in value.
shoulder girdle: The shoulder girdle, or pectoral girdle, is the set of bones that connect the arm to the axial skeleton on each side. It consists of the clavicle and scapula.
sickle-cell anemia: Inherited anemia characterized by crescent shaped RBCs. The causes RBCS to block capillaries decreasing the oxygen supple to the cells.
side effects: Unpleasant effects of the drug in addition to the desired or therapeutic effect.
signs: Objective findings determined by a clinician, such as a fever, hypertension, or rash.
sinus: An air-filled cavity in a dense portion of a skull bone, lined with mucous-secreting cells.
sinus arrhythmia: An irregular heartbeat that originates in the sinoatrial node (pacemaker).
skill set: A person's abilities or skills or expertise in an area.
small claims court: A special court established to handle small claims or debts, without the services of lawyers.
small talk: Polite light conversation about uncontroversial matters.
software: A set of electronic instructions to operate and perform different computer tasks.
solvent: A liquid that is able to dissolve other substances. An example would be water.
special report: Additional medical documentation required to confirm the need for the use of unlisted, unusual, or newly adopted medical procedures code.
specificity: The quality or state of being specific.
specimen: A sample of body fluid, waste product, or tissue collected for analysis.
spermatozoa (sing. spermatozoon): mature male reproductive cell
spina bifida: Condition in which the spinal column has an abnormal opening that allows protrusion of the meninges and/or the spinal column.
spirometer: An instrument that measures the volume of air inhaled and exhaled.
spongy bone: Light and porous bone tissue that contains bone marrow. Also called
spore: A thick-walled, dormant form of bacteria that is very resistant to disinfection measures.
staged or staging: The process of determining how much cancer is in the body and where it is located. Staging describes the severity of an individual's cancer.
stains: A reagent or dye used to treat specimens for microscopic examination.
standard operating procedures: Or SOP, is a set of step-by-step instructions to help employees carry out routine operations efficiently, with high quality, and uniformity of performance.
Standard Precautions: A set of infection control practices used to prevent transmission of diseases that can be acquired by contact with blood, body fluids, non-intact skin, and mucous membranes.
STAT: The medical abbreviation for the Latin term *statum*, meaning immediately; at this moment.
static equilibrium: Relating to balance when moving in a straight line.
stem cells: Undifferentiated cells that can become specialized cells in the body.
sterile: Free of all microorganisms, pathogenic and nonpathogenic.
sterilize: The state of removing all microorganisms.
stertorous: Heavy snoring.
stoma: A temporary or permanent surgically created opening used for drainage (i.e., urine, stool)
strata: Naturally or artificially formed layers of material, usually multiple layers
streaked for isolation: To produce isolated colonies of an organism on an agar plate. Using an inoculating loop, you pick one colony and methodically spread it out onto solid nutrient media. The goal is to have colonies that are separate from other colonies.
stretch receptor: Sensory nerve ending that responds to a stretch stimuli
striated: Striped in appearance
stridor: High-pitched inspiratory sounds from the larynx; a sign of upper airway obstruction.
stylus: A pen-shaped device with a variety of tips that is used on touchscreens to write, draw, or input commands. A metal probe that is inserted into or passed through a catheter, needle, or tube used for clearing purposes or to facilitate passage into a body orifice.
subcultured: To cultivate an organism (a bacteria) again on a new nutrient surface.
subjective information: Data or information obtained from the patient, including the patient's feelings, perceptions, and concerns; obtained through interview or questions.
subpoena duces tecum: A legal document commanding a person to bring a piece of evidence (like the plaintiff's health record) to court
subpoena: A court order requiring a person to appear in court at a specific time to testify in a legal case.
subsequent: Occurring later or after.
suction: The production of a partial vacuum by the removal of air in order to force fluid into a vacant space.
suffixes: Word parts that appear at the end of some terms.
summarizing: Allowing the listener to recap and review what was said.
supernatant: The clear liquid above the sediment in a centrifuged urine specimen.
suppurative: Characterized by the formation and/or discharge of pus
surface area: Total area of the surface of a three-dimensional object. Measured in square units. Example; the surface area of ball was 14 cubic millimeters.
surfactant: A mixture of protein and fats that lines the alveoli and prevents the tissues from sticking together and collapsing during exhalation.
suture lines: Where the bones of the skull meet.
symmetry: similarity in size, form and arrangement of parts on opposite sides of the body

symptoms: Subjective complaints reported by the patient, such as pain or nausea.
syncope: Fainting; a brief lapse in consciousness.
synthesis: Formation of a chemical compound from simpler compounds or elements.
synthesize: To make whole by combining parts or constituents.
syringes: A device with a slender barrel and needle used to withdraw blood from a vein or artery.
systemic: Affecting the entire body.

T

T cells: T cells are formed from stem cells in bone marrow and then migrate to the thymus where they mature and learn their role in the immune system. They are effective against intracellular pathogens.
tachycardia: A rapid but regular heart rate; one that exceeds 100 beats per minute.
tachypnea: Rapid, shallow breathing
tactful: The quality of having a sense of what to do or say to maintain good relations with others or to prevent offense.
triage: To sort out and classify the injured; used in the military and emergency settings to determine the priority of a patient to be treated.
target tissue: The destination, or intended tissue in the nervous impulse, e.g., a muscle.
telemedicine: The use of telecommunication technology to provide healthcare services to patients at a distance; usually used in rural communities.
termination letters: Documents sent to patients explaining that the provider is ending the physician-patient relationship and the patients need to see other providers.
testes (sing. Testis) or testicles (TESS tick kuls): male gonads
testosterone: Male sex hormone produced by the interstitial cells in the testes.
thalamus: The middle part of the brain through which sensory impulses pass to reach the cerebral cortex.
therapeutic range: Blood concentrations of the medication are high enough for the therapeutic effect to occur.
third-party administrator (TPA): An organization that processes claims and provides administrative services for another organization. Often used by self-funded plans.
thixotropic gel: A chemically neutral gel added to evacuated blood tubes, that creates a physical barrier between red blood cells and plasma or serum, when centrifuged.
thoracentesis: Aspiration of a fluid from the pleural cavity.
thready: A term describing a pulse that is thins and feeble.
thrombus: A blood clot that blocks the flow of blood.
tickler file: A chronologic file used as a reminder that something must be dealt with on a certain date.
tinea: Any fungal skin disease that results in scaling, itching, and inflammation. Examples; ringworm, athlete's foot.
tissue culture: The technique or process of keeping tissue alive and growing in a culture medium.
titer: The lowest concentration of a serum solution containing a specific antibody where the antibody is still able to neutralize (or precipitate) an antigen.
tort: A civil wrongdoing that causes harm to a person or property, excludes breach of contract.
tortfeasor: An individual who committed the tort.
tourniquet: A device for temporarily constricting blood flow.
toxicity: Harmful and deadly effects of the medication that can develop due to the buildup of medication or byproducts in the body.
toxicology: The study and science dealing with the effects, antidotes, and detection of poisons or drugs.
toxins: Substances created by microorganisms, plants, or animals and are poisonous to humans
transcription: To make a written copy of dictated material.
transient: not lasting, enduring or permanent; transitory
transillumination: Inspection of a cavity or organ by passing light through its walls.
transitional epithelium: Type of cells found in the lining of hollow organs; have the ability to stretch with the contraction and distention of organ
transmission: To pass or spread disease.
transport medium: A medium used to keep an organism alive during transport to the laboratory.
trauma: A physical injury or wound caused by an external force or violence.
trend(s): Data results on a graph that are obtained over time, which continue to go upward or downward in value.
triage: To sort out and classify the injured; used in the military and emergency settings to determine the priority of a patient to be treated.
triaging flow map: A written flow map to make triage decision; based on answers to questions the person moves through the map until a triage decision is made.
tripod position: The standing position when using crutches; crutch tips are 4 to 6 inches to the side and front of each foot.
trustee: The coordinator of financial resources assigned by the court during a bankruptcy case.
tunics: A coat or layer covering an organ or part of an organ
turbidity: A cloudy appearance. Not clear.
turgor: A term referring to normal skin tension; the resistance of the skin to being grasped between the fingers and released. Turgor is decreased with dehydration and increased with edema.

U

undescended testicles: Condition where one or both testicles do not descend into the scrotum.
unipolar: Has one pole or electrical charge
unsecured debt: Debt that is not guaranteed by something of value; credit card debt is the most common type of unsecured debt.
urgent: An acute situation that requires immediate attention but is not life-threatening.
urochrome: The yellow pigment normally found in urine; it is described as straw, yellow, or amber based on its concentration
urostomy: A surgically created opening on the abdominal wall used to drain urine
urticaria: Hives.
utilization management: A decision making process used by managed care organizations. Used to manage healthcare costs through a case-by-case assessments of the appropriateness of care.

V

valvulitis: Inflammatory condition of a valve, caused most commonly by rheumatic fever, bacterial endocarditis or syphilis; results in valve stenosis and obstructed blood flow.
vascular access: Surgical procedure that creates vein to remove and return blood during the hemodialysis procedure.
vascular: Having (blood) vessels that conduct or circulate liquids (blood).
vasoconstriction: Contraction of the muscles causing the narrowing of the inside tube of the vessel.
vectors: Animals or insects (e.g., ticks) that transmit a pathogen.
vendors: Companies that sells supplies, equipment, or services to another companies or individuals.
ventricles: A series of connecting cavities in the brain.
venule: A very small vein
verification of eligibility: The process of confirming health insurance coverage for the patient.
vertebrae: a series or small irregular shaped bones that form the backbone or spine.
vertigo: Dizziness; abnormal sensation of movement when there none.
vested: Granted or endowed with a particular authority, right or property; to have a special interest in.
viable: Able to live and grow.
vigilance: Keenly watchful to detect danger.
viral: Relating to or caused by a virus.
viscosity: Resistance to flow; the thicker the liquid, the higher the viscosity.
visual cortex: The portion of the cerebral cortex of the brain that receives and processes impulses from the optic nerve.

W

waiting period: The amount of time a patient waits for disability insurance to pay after the date of injury.
wet mount: A glass slide holding a specimen suspended in a drop of liquid for microscopic examination.
wheezing: Whistling sound made during breathing
whistleblower: A person (usually an employee) who reports a violation of the law within the organization. The person reports the information to the public or a person in authority.
white noise: The sounds from a television or stereo that muffle or mute the conversation of others, thus helping to protect the confidentiality of patients.
whole blood: Plasma and the formed elements of blood in a free-flowing liquid form.
workplace emergencies: Unforeseen situations that threaten the employees and visitors; can disrupt services provided.

Y

yeast: Belong to various single-celled fungi, which reproduce by budding and are able to ferment sugars.
yellow bone marrow: An inactive, fatty form of bone marrow, it does not produce blood cells.

Z

zone: A region or geographic area used for shipping.

INDEX

A
A1c, 330*t*, 337*t*
AAAs. *See* Abdominal aortic aneurysms
AAMA. *See* American Association of Medical Assistants
AAT deficiency. *See* Alpha-1 antitrypsin deficiency
Abbreviations, 3
　for blood, 185*t*
　for cardiovascular system, 236*t*
　for digestive system, 120*t*
　for ear, 322*t*
　for endocrine system, 340*t*
　for eye, 321*t*
　for integumentary system, 93*t*
　for lymphatic and immune systems, 205*t*
　medical, for physical examination, 676*t*
　for mental and behavioral health, 293*t*
　for musculoskeletal system, 68*t*
　for nervous system, 292*t*
　for prescriptions
　　measurements, 870*t*
　　medications, 871*t*
　　miscellaneous, 871*t*
　　route and form, 869*t*
　　timing, 870*t*
　for reproductive system, 163*t*–164*t*
　for respiratory system, 259*t*
　for urinary system, 143*t*
ABCDE Rule, for malignant melanoma, 812*t*
Abdomen, physical examination of, 690
Abdominal aortic aneurysms (AAAs), 814
Abdominal examination, in gynecology, 706
Abdominopelvic quadrants and regions, 22–23, 23*f*, 23*t*–24*t*, 33*t*
Abduction, 52*t*–53*t*
ABHES. *See* Accrediting Bureau of Health Education Schools
Abilify (aripiprazole), 863*t*–867*t*
ABN. *See* Advanced Beneficiary Notice
ABO blood typing, 1093, 1094*b*, 1094*t*
Abortions, 372*b*, 406, 407*b*
Abruptio placentae, 162*t*
Abscesses, 759, 759*b*
Absorbable sutures, 767
Absorption, drug, 855, 855*t*
Absorption, of digestive system, 101
Abstract, 538
Abuse
　accurate diagnostic coding preventing, 577–578
　adult, 392–393
　child, 389*t*, 391–392, 391*b*–392*b*, 740, 740*b*
　domestic, signs of, 719–720
AC interference artifacts, 947–948, 947*f*
ACA. *See* Affordable Care Act
Acai, 872*t*–873*t*
Acalculia, 281*t*
Access restrictions, 477*t*
Account maintenance fees, 604*t*
Account numbers, in checks, 606
Accounting management software, for banking in ambulatory care setting, 611*b*
Accounts payable (A/P), 510, 510*b*, 604–614
　banking and, 604–605
　　account types in, 605
　　in ambulatory care setting, 609–611
　　bank statements and, 611–613, 612*f*–613*f*
　　checks in, 605–606, 608–611, 608*b*, 611*t*
　　debit cards in, 608, 608*b*
　　Federal Reserve Bank and, 604–605, 604*f*, 605*b*
　　fees common to, 604*t*
　　online, 605
　　signature cards and, 605
　checks in, 605–606, 608–611, 608*b*, 611*t*
　direct deposit for, 614
　invoices and statements for, 614

Accounts payable (A/P) *(Continued)*
　online bill pay for, 614
　patient payment management in, 606–609
　　cash payments in, 606
　　checks and, 608, 608*b*
　　contactless payment systems for, 608–609
　　credit cards in, 608–609, 609*f*
　　debit cards in, 608, 608*b*
　　online payment options for, 609
　paying bills to maximize cash flow in, 613–614
Accounts receivable (A/R), 589–604
　collection procedures for, 598–604
　　bankruptcy and, 601
　　claims against estates and, 601
　　collection agencies and, 601–602, 602*f*, 603*b*
　　letters and, 600
　　personal finance interviews and, 600, 600*f*
　　preparing patient accounts for, 598, 599*f*
　　small claims court and, 603–604, 603*b*
　　special, 601
　　starting, 598
　　telephone techniques and, 598–600, 598*b*
　　tracing skips and, 601, 601*b*
　monthly patient account statements and, 597–598, 597*b*
　　billing minors and, 597
　　fees in hardship cases and, 598, 598*b*
　　medical care for those who cannot pay and, 597
　patient ledger and, 589–597, 591*f*
　　credit balances in, 595–596, 596*b*
　　entering and posting transactions in, 589
　　NSF checks and, 595*b*, 595*f*
　　payment agreements in, 596–597
　　payment at time of service in, 596, 596*b*, 596*f*
　　pegboard system for, 589, 589*b*, 591*b*, 592*f*
　　posting adjustments in, 593–596, 595*b*, 595*f*
　　posting charges in, 591, 592*b*–593*b*
　　posting payments in, 592–593, 592*b*–593*b*, 594*f*
　　TILA and, 596–597, 597*f*
Accreditation, in practice requirements, 378
Accrediting Bureau of Health Education Schools (ABHES), 378
ACE inhibitors. *See* Angiotensin converting enzyme inhibitors
Acetaminophen (Tylenol), 872*t*
Acetylcholine (ACh), 51, 51*b*
Achalasia, 117*t*
Achilles tendon, definition of, 3
Achondroplasia, 65*t*
Achromatopsia, 318*t*
Acid-base balance, 24–25, 242
Acid-fast stain, 1122
Acne vulgaris, 77–78, 78*f*
Acoustic neuroma, 320*t*
Acquired immunity, 194–195, 195*f*
Acquired immunodeficiency syndrome (AIDS), 152, 154*t*, 198–201. *See also* Human immunodeficiency virus
　diagnostic coding of, 543–544
　nutrition needs for, 847
Acromegaly, 332*f*, 332*t*–333*t*
Acronyms, 3, 888*b*
Acrophobia, 291*t*
ACS. *See* Anterior ciliary sclerotomy
ActHIB, 730*t*
Action potentials, 263, 264*b*, 264*f*
Action verbs, in resumes, 1135, 1135*f*
Active immunity, 194, 195*f*, 620*b*
Active listening, 354, 355*b*, 355*f*, 442, 442*b*, 668–669
Activities of daily living (ADLs), 277*t*
Activity codes, 546
Acuity, 691
Acupressure/acupuncture, 823
Acute, definition of, 3, 25
Acute bronchitis, 246–247
Acute cystitis, 130–131, 131*b*
Acute infections, 621, 621*b*
Acute intoxication, 271*t*
Acute lymphocytic leukemia, 180–181, 180*f*, 204*t*

Acute myelogenous leukemia, 180–181, 180*f*, 204*t*
Acute psychotic disorders, 290*t*
Acute respiratory failure, 256*t*–257*t*
Acute stage, of infections, 621*b*, 1119, 1119*b*
Acute tubular necrosis, 141*t*–142*t*
Adam's apple, 326, 326*b*
Adaptive coping mechanisms, 358–359, 359*t*
Addendum, 429
Addiction, 857*t*
Addison disease, 335, 335*f*, 335*t*
Adduction, 52*t*–53*t*
Adenocarcinoma, 31*t*, 119*t*
Adenoidectomy, 198*t*
Adenosine triphosphate (ATP), 51, 51*b*
ADHD. *See* Attention deficit/ hyperactivity disorder
Adherence, definition of, 252, 800, 800*b*
Adhesions, 160, 160*b*
Adipose tissue, 70, 71*f*
Adjective forms
　for blood, 184*t*
　for cardiovascular system, 235*t*
　definition of, 480, 480*t*
　for digestive system, 119*t*
　for ear, 322*t*
　for endocrine system, 340*t*
　for eye, 321*t*
　for lymphatic and immune systems, 204*t*
　for mental and behavioral health, 292*t*
　for nervous system, 292*t*
　for reproductive system, 163*t*
　for respiratory system, 258*t*
　for urinary system, 143*t*
Adjective suffixes, 5, 6*t*
Adjudicate, 572–573, 573*b*
Adjustment disorder, 291*t*
ADLs. *See* Activities of daily living
Administrative law, 362
Administrative simplification, 381–382
Adnexa, 99, 99*b*, 100*f*
Adolescents, 723
　examination challenges with, 739
　therapeutic approaches to, 725*b*
Adoption, 407, 407*b*, 408*t*
Adrenal gland diseases, 333–336, 335*t*
Adrenal glands, 325, 325*f*, 327, 328*t*
Adrenalectomy, 331*t*
Adrenaline, 328*t*, 968*t*
Adrenocorticotropic hormone, 327*t*
Adult abuse, neglect, and exploitation, 392–393
Adult respiratory distress syndrome, 256*t*–257*t*
Adult signature restricted delivery, USPS, 489*t*
Advance care planning, 408–409, 409*b*
Advance directives, 390, 390*b*, 409, 409*b*, 409*t*
Advanced Beneficiary Notice (ABN), 584*b*
Advanced practice professionals, practice requirements for, 376*t*
Advanced Practice Registered Nurse (APRN), 376*t*
Adverbs, 480, 480*t*
Advice, in patient interviews, 672
Advil (ibuprofen), 863*t*–867*t*, 872*t*
AED. *See* Automated external defibrillator
Aerobes, 1108
Aerobic conditioning, 51*t*
Aesthetic needs, 358, 358*f*
Affect, 271*t*, 276*b*
Affective domain, of learning, 802, 803*f*, 803*t*
Afferent, definition of, 123, 124*b*
Affirmative defense, 366, 367*b*
Affordable Care Act (ACA), 372, 373*b*–376*b*, 373*f*, 388, 522, 530–531
Afluria, 730*t*
African American patients, cultural differences with, 805*b*
Age
　blood pressure and, 651*t*
　diversity in, 345*t*
　nutrition needs by, 847*t*
　pulse rates related to, 647*t*

Page numbers followed by "*f*" indicate figures, "*t*" indicate tables, and "*b*" indicate boxes.

Age Discrimination in Employment Act of 1967, 395t–396t
Age of majority, 424–425
Agent Orange exposure, 137b
Ageusia, 281t
Aggressive communicators, 354, 354t
Aging. See Geriatrics
Agnosia, 281t
Agoraphobia, 291t
Agranulocytes, 169–170, 171f, 190, 190b
Agraphia, 281t
AHA. See American Heart Association
AICD. See Automatic implantable cardioverter-defibrillator
AIDS. See Acquired immunodeficiency syndrome
AIDS tests, 197t
Air bubbles, in urine examination, 1038f
Air lock technique, in intramuscular injections for medication administration, 927
Akathisia, 289t
Alanine aminotransferase (ALT) testing, 1097
Albinism, 90t–91t, 297t
Albumin, 167, 167t, 1078, 1078b
Albuterol (Ventolin HFA, Proventil HFA, ProAir), 863t–867t
Alcohol, in medications, 888b
Alcohol misuse screening, 815
Aleve (naproxen), 872t
Aliquot, 1006
Alkaline, 101, 101b
Allergens, 842, 846–847, 846b, 973t
Allergic rhinitis, 256t–257t
Allergies, 29, 195b
Allergists, 348t
Allergy testing, 197f, 197t, 921, 921b, 922f
Allis tissue forceps, 762t–764t, 764f
Allograft, 81t
Aloe vera, 872t–873t
Alopecia areata, 199t–200t, 200f
Alpha-1 antitrypsin (AAT) deficiency, 248b
Alphabetic color coding, 435, 435f
Alphabetic filing, 432–433, 432b, 434b
Alphabetic Index
 of CPT, 550, 551f, 552–554, 554b
 of ICD-10-CM, 534–536, 535f, 539–542, 543f
Alpha-blockers, 136t, 231t
Alphanumeric, definition of, 434–435, 434b
Alprazolam (Xanax), 863t–867t
ALS. See Amyotrophic lateral sclerosis
ALT testing. See Alanine aminotransferase testing
Alveoli, 240–241, 240f
Alzheimer's disease, 3, 285–287
 geriatrics and, 749–750, 750t
Ambien (zolpidem), 863t–867t
Amblyopia, 317t
Ambulatory allied health occupations, 347t
Ambulatory care center
 drug laws and, 857–859, 858t
 technology in
  advances in, 478–479, 478f–479f, 479b
  introduction to, 469
Amenorrhea, 162t, 707, 707b
American Association of Medical Assistants (AAMA), 350t, 402, 402b–403b, 991t
American Heart Association (AHA), 845, 845t
American Medical Technologists (AMT), 350t, 991t
American Society for Clinical Pathologists (ASCP), 991t
Americans with Disabilities Act Amendments Act of 2008, 355, 397b
Americans with Disabilities Act and the Rehabilitation Act of 1973, 397b
Americans with Disabilities Act of 1990, 355, 395t–396t
Amino acids, 834, 834b, 836
Amiodarone (Cordarone, Pacerone), 968t
Amlodipine (Norvasc), 863t–867t
Amnesia, 280t–281t, 289t
Amniocentesis, 718–719, 719f
Amnion, 150, 151f
Amniotic fluid, 150, 151f
Amoxicillin (Amoxil, Moxatag), 863t–867t
Amphiarthrotic joints, 44
Ampules, for parenteral medication administration, 904, 904f, 905b–906b
Amsler grid, 304f, 304t–305t
AMT. See American Medical Technologists

Amylase, 101
Amyotrophic lateral sclerosis (ALS), 283b, 283t
Anabolism, 834
Anacusis, 320t
Anaerobes, 1108
Anal fissure, 117t
Analgesics, 251, 872t
Analyte, definition of, 992, 992b
Analyte testing, reference laboratory blood chemistry panels and, 1099, 1100f, 1101t–1102t
Anaphylactic shock, 984t
Anaphylaxis, 846, 846b
 environmental emergencies and, 972–973, 973b, 973f, 973t
Anaplastic, definition of, 30b, 30t
Anastomosis, 104f, 104t–105t
Anatomy
 abdominopelvic quadrants and regions in, 22–23, 23f, 23t–24t, 33t
 of blood, 167–170, 167f
 body cavities in, 22–23, 23f, 23t–24t, 33t
 body planes in, 23–24, 24f, 33t
 of cardiovascular system, 208–215, 934
 definition of, 13
 of digestive system, 96–98
 of ear, 299–300, 300f
 of endocrine system, 325–329, 325f
 of eye, 296–299
 geriatrics changes in, 744–755, 744t
 of integumentary system, 70–73
 of lymphatic and immune systems, 188–190
 of musculoskeletal system, 36–46
 of nervous system, 261–263
 positional and directional terminology in, 18, 20t
 of reproductive system, 146–148
 of respiratory system, 238–241
 structural organization of body and, 14–18
  body systems in, 16, 17t
  cells in, 14–15, 14t, 15f
  medical terminology related to, 32t–33t
  organism, 16–18
  organs in, 16, 16t–17t
  tissues in, 15, 15t–16t
 surface terminology in, 18, 18f, 19t–20t
 of urinary system, 123–125
Andrology, 146b
Anemias, 1081, 1081b
 aplastic and hemolytic, 183t
 deficiencies, 183t
 definition of, 173, 173b
 iron deficiency, 173–175, 175f
 sickle-cell disease, 175–176, 176f, 715, 715b
Anencephaly, 715, 715b
Anesthesiologists, 348t
Anesthetics, 759
Aneurysms, 234f, 234t
Angina pectoris, 218t–219t, 231, 232f, 986b
Angiocardiography, 219t–221t
Angioma, 92t
Angioplasty, 221t–223t, 222f
Angiosarcomas, 234t
Angiotensin converting enzyme (ACE) inhibitors, 185t
Angiotensin II receptor blockers, 185t
Anhedonia, 815, 815b
Animal bites, 974, 974b, 974t
Aniridia, 134t
Anisocoria, 317f, 317t
Ankylosing spondylitis, 65t
Anorchism, 155t–156t, 158t
Anorectal abscess, 117t
Anorexia nervosa, 291f, 291t, 848–849, 848b, 848f
Anosmia, 256t–257t, 281t
Anovulation, 709
Answering services, 452, 496, 496b
Antagonistic muscles, 45
Anterior ciliary sclerotomy (ACS), 306t
Anterior pituitary hormones, 326f, 327t
Anterior prolapse, 141t–142t, 142f
Anthracosis, 256t–257t
Anthropometric measurements, 658–661. See also Vital signs
 in health records, 418, 637
 height, 658–661, 659b
 weight, 658–661, 659b–660b, 660f, 660t
Anthropophobia, 291t

Antibiotic resistance, 618b
Antibiotics, 1105, 1105b
Antibodies, 29, 29b, 170, 191, 192b, 619, 619b–620b, 1041, 1099b, 1106
 blood, 170–172, 171b
 preformed, 170–171, 172b
Anti-CCP. See Cyclic citrullinated peptide antibody
Anticholinergics, 136t
Anticoagulants, 135, 135b, 168, 854, 863t–867t, 1005–1006, 1005b, 1049–1050
Anticonvulsants, 863t–867t
Antidepressants, 863t–867t
Antidiuretic hormone, 327t
Antigens, 29, 29b, 170, 191, 192b, 619, 1041, 1099b, 1111, 1111b
 blood, 170–172, 171b
Antihistamines, 863t–867t, 872t
Antihyperglycemics, 863t–867t
Antihyperlipidemics, 135, 135b
Antihypertensives, 133, 133b, 863t–867t
Antiinflammatory drugs, 863t–867t
Antimicrobials, 1105, 1105b
Antimuscarinics, 136t
Antinuclear antibody testing, 197t
Antioxidants, 837b–838b, 838t
Antiplatelets, 863t–867t
Antipsychotics, 863t–867t
Antipyretics, 251, 872t
Antiseptics, 617, 617b, 1106
 venipuncture and, 1049, 1049b, 1050f
Antitussives, 872t
Anus, 98, 99f
Anxiety, 271t
Anxiety disorders, 291t
Aorta, coarctation of, 227f, 227t
Aortic regurgitation, 230t
Aortic valve, 209, 211f, 934, 935f
A/P. See Accounts payable
Apgar score, 729, 733t
Aphasia, 280t–281t
Apheresis, 175t
Aphonia, 243t
Apical pulse, 646, 647b, 648–649
Aplastic anemia, 183t
Apnea, 243t, 649–650
Apocrine glands, 72
Appeals phase, in civil lawsuit, 368b
Appearance, diversity in, 345t
Appendicitis, 102–106, 102f
Appendicular skeleton, 37, 38f, 39–40, 40t, 42f, 42t, 43f
Appendix, 189, 189f
Application software, 476t
Appointment book scheduling, 455, 456f
Appointment cards, 464, 465f
Appointment matrix, 453–454, 454b, 455f
Appointment scheduling, 452–466
 appointment matrix in, 453–454, 454b, 455f
 cancellations and, 465–466
 customer service and, 466b
 delays and, 465–466
 emergency situations, 464
 for established patients, 459, 460b–461b, 460f
 facility availability in, 454
 failed appointments and, 464
 increasing appointment show rates and, 464–465, 465f
 for inpatient surgeries, 461
 late patients and, 463
 law and, 456
 methods of, 454–455
  appointment book scheduling, 455, 456f
  computerized, 454–455
  self-scheduling, 455
 for new patients, 457–459, 458b–459b, 458f
 no-show policies and, 464, 464b
 for outside visits, 461
 patient needs in, 453
 for patient procedures, 461, 462b–463b
 for pharmaceutical representatives, 461–463
 provider preferences and habits for, 453
 rescheduling and, 463
 for salespeople, 463
 telephone techniques for, 457
 types of, 456–457
Appointment show rates, increasing, 464–465, 465f
Approximated, definition of, 790, 790b

INDEX

Apraxia, 281t
APRN. *See* Advanced Practice Registered Nurse
Aqueous humor, 297, 298f, 299
A/R. *See* Accounts receivable
Arbitration, 366
Aricept (donepezil), 750t
Aripiprazole (Abilify), 863t–867t
Arms, ventral surface anatomy terms for, 18f, 19t
Aromatic, definition of, 1024, 1024b
Arrhythmias, 224, 224t
    definition of, 948, 948b
    ECG identification of, 948–950
        atrial arrhythmias, 948–949, 949b
        heart block, 949
        implantable device rhythms, 950, 950f–951f
        sinus arrhythmias, 948
        ventricular arrhythmias, 949–950, 949f
    sinus, 646, 646b, 948
ART. *See* Assisted reproductive technology
Arterial blood gas, 244t–245t
Arteries, 208, 208f, 209t, 210f
Arterioles, 123, 124b, 208
Arteriosclerosis, 234t, 651, 745
Arteriovenous, 132–133, 133b
Arteriovenous fistula, 132–133, 133b
Arthritis, 4, 59, 59t–60t
Arthrography, 54t
Arthropathies, 65t
Arthroplasty, 4–5
Arthropod, 1109b, 1110
Arthroscopy, 26t–27t, 54t
Artifacts, 937, 937b, 1091b
    ECG troubleshooting of, 947–948
        AC interference, 947–948, 947f
        interrupted baseline, 948, 948f
        somatic tremor, 947, 947f
        wandering baseline, 947, 947f
Artificial insemination, 1041
Asbestosis, 256t–257t
Ascending colon, 98, 99f
ASCP. *See* American Society for Clinical Pathologists
ASD. *See* Autism spectrum disorder
Asepsis, 630–631
Aseptic techniques
    for infection control, 630–634
        customer service and, 634b
        disinfection and, 634, 634b
        hand hygiene, 632, 632b
        MA role in, 634
        sanitization and, 632–634, 633b
        sterilization and, 634
    for minor surgery, 769
Aseptically, definition of, 993
Asexual reproduction, 1107, 1107b
Asian ginseng, 872t–873t
Aspartate aminotransferase (AST) testing, 1097
Aspirates, definition of, 1005, 1005b
Aspiration
    definition of, 904, 904b
    in intramuscular injections for medication administration, 926
    in subcutaneous injections for medication administration, 922, 923b
Aspirin, 872t
Assault, 365t
Assertive communicators, 354, 354t
Assessment. *See* Patient assessment, in physical examination
Assets, 601
Assignment of benefits, 526, 573t
Assisted reproductive technology (ART), 406, 406b, 406t
Assistive devices, coaching on, 823–828, 824b
    canes, 828, 828f, 829b–830b
    crutches, 824–825, 824f–825f, 826b
    walkers, 825–828, 827b–829b, 827f
    wheelchairs, 828
Assumption of risk, 367b, 367t
AST testing. *See* Aspartate aminotransferase testing
Asthma, 2, 245–246, 246f, 246t
Asthmatic attacks, 981, 981b
Astigmatic keratotomy, 306t
Astigmatism, 302b, 691–693
Astrocytes, 263
Astrocytomas, 286t
Asystole, 949f, 950

Atelectasis, 256t–257t
Atenolol (Tenormin), 863t–867t
Atherectomy, 221t–223t
Atheromas, 225, 226f
Atherosclerosis-related diseases, 225, 225t, 226f
Athetosis, 280t–281t
Atopic dermatitis (eczema), 85–86
Atorvastatin (Lipitor), 863t–867t
ATP. *See* Adenosine triphosphate
Atrial arrhythmias, 948–949, 949b
Atrial myxomas, 234t
Atrial septal defect, 227t
Atrioventricular block, 224t
Atrioventricular node, 215f, 216, 936f
Atrioventricular septal defect, 227t
Atrophy, 74f, 283b, 747
Atropine, 968t
Attention deficit/hyperactivity disorder (ADHD), 289t
Attenuated organisms, 727, 727b
Attorneys, 364
Atypical lymphs, 1093t
Audible, definition of, 301, 301b
Audiology/audiologists, 296b, 347t, 700–702, 700b
Audiometric testing, 303b, 303f, 699–702, 700b, 701f
Audit trails, 477t
Auditory canal, 299, 300f
Auditory cortex, 301, 301b
Audits, 571, 571b
Augmented leads, 939, 940t
Aura, 280t–281t
Auricle, 299, 300f
Auscultated, definition of, 649, 649b, 678b, 678t
Auscultation, in physical examination, 687, 688f
Authorized agents, 488b, 489t
Autism spectrum disorder (ASD), 289t, 728b
Autoantibody testing, 197t
Autoclave, 770–775, 771f
    biologic sterilization indicators in, 774
    chemical sterilization indicators in, 774, 774f
    effectiveness of, factors influencing, 771, 771t
    loading, 774, 775b
    quality-assurance records for office sterilization in, 774
    steam temperature for, 771, 771b
    tips for improving techniques with, 772t
    unloading, 774–775, 775b
    wrapping instruments for, 774
    wrapping materials for, 771, 772b–773b, 773f
Autograft, 81f, 81t
Autoimmune, definition of, 1084, 1084b
Autoimmune acquired hemolytic anemia, 183t
Autoimmune diseases, 195–198, 617
    common types of, 199t–200t
    definition of, 36b
    diagnostic procedures for, 196
    etiology of, 195–196
    prevention of, 198
    prognosis of, 198
    signs and symptoms of, 196
    treatment for, 198
Autoimmunity, 29
Autoinflammatory diseases, 29
Autologous bone marrow transplant, 198t
Autologous transfusion, 175t, 1094
Automated call reminders, 464
Automated external defibrillator (AED), 967, 967f, 986b–987b
Automated files, 431
Automated instruments, definition of, 991, 991b
Automatic call routing, 452, 452b
Automatic implantable cardioverter-defibrillator (AICD), 221t–223t
Automatic log-off, 477t
Autonomic nervous system, 262, 262f, 269–270, 270f
Autonomy
    definition of, 724, 724b
    ethics and, 404, 404b
Autotransfusion, 175t
Avascular, definition of, 299
Avian flu, 256t–257t
Avulsion fracture, 56t–57t
Axial skeleton, 37–39, 38f–39f, 38t, 40t, 41f
Axillary crutches, 824–825, 824b, 824f, 826b
Axillary temperature, digital thermometer for, 642b
Azithromycin (Zithromax, Zmax), 863t–867t

B

B_{12} deficiency, 183t
Babinski's reflex, 277t
Bacille Calmette-Guérin (BCG) vaccine, 252, 918
Bacilli, diseases caused by, 1109t
Backorders, 510
Bacteria, 618, 618b, 1105
    characteristics of, 1107–1108, 1107b
        oxygen requirements, 1108, 1108b
        physical structures, 1108
        shapes, 1107–1108, 1108f
        staining properties, 1107, 1107f
    diseases caused by, 1108, 1109t
    "good", 25
    in urine examination, 1036, 1037f
Bacteriuria, 1025
Baker cyst, 65t
Balance of power, 362, 363t
Ball-and-socket joint, 44t, 45f
Bandages, for wound care, 796–797, 796f–797f, 797b
Bank statements, 611–613, 612f–613f
Banking, 604–605
    account types in, 605
    in ambulatory care setting, 609–611
        accounting management software for, 611b
        check endorsements for, 609–611, 611t
        deposits for, 609, 610b, 610f–611f
        overdrafts and, 611
        stop-payments and, 611
    bank statements and, 611–613, 612f–613f
    checks in, 605–606, 608–611, 608b, 611t
    debit cards in, 608, 608b
    Federal Reserve Bank and, 604–605, 604f, 605b
    fees common to, 604t
    online, 605
    signature cards and, 605
Bankruptcy, collection procedures and, 601
Bariatric surgery, 104t–105t
Barium enema, 103t
Barium swallow, 103t, 111f
Barrier methods, of contraception, 708, 709f
Barrier protection, Standard Precautions and, 625, 625b–626b, 625f, 627f
Bartholin cysts, 706
Basal cell carcinoma, 80–83, 82f
Basal cells, 81
Basal layer, 71, 71b
Basal metabolic rate (BMR), 834, 834b
Basophils, 169
Battery, 365t
BCG vaccine. *See* Bacille Calmette-Guérin vaccine
Bead packs, 821t–822t, 822b
Bedsores, 83
Behavior, understanding, 357–359
Behavioral health, 271
Behavioral therapy, 286t
Belligerent, definition of, 599, 599b
Bell's palsy, 284b, 284f, 284t
Benadryl (diphenhydramine), 872t, 968t
Benazepril (Lotensin), 863t–867t
Bender Gestalt Test, 283
Beneficence, ethics and, 404
Beneficiaries, 529–530
Benign, definition of, 90t–91t
Benign prostatic hyperplasia (BPH), 141t–142t, 153–155, 157f
Benylin (dextromethorphan), 872t
Beta-3 adrenergic agonists, 136t
Bexsero, 730t
Biconvex, 299, 299b
Bicuspid valve, 209, 211f, 934, 935f
Bile, 100, 100b
Bilingual, definition of, 450, 450b
Bilirubin, 169, 169b
    in urine specimens, 1029
Bilirubinuria, 1023, 1024b
Bill inquiries, phone calls regarding, 448–449
Billable service, 505, 505b
Billing. *See* Medical billing
Billing minors, 597
Binary fission, 1107, 1107b
Binge eating disorder, 849
Binocular vision, 296, 296b
Binomial, definition of, 1106
Bioethicists, 404

INDEX

Biohazard safety, in clinical laboratory, 1001–1003, 1003b, 1003f
Biohazard waste collection, 628, 629f
Biologic product, blood as, 176b–177b
Biologic sterilization, 774
Biological chemical disposal, 629b
Biopsy
  cervical, 710–711, 711b
  cone, 158b, 159t–160t
  definition of, 30, 103t–104t
  of lymphatic structures, 198t
  needle biopsy setup, 789t
  sentinel node, 158b, 159t–160t
  types of, 83t
Biopsy forceps, 766f, 766t
Biotin, 839t
Bipolar disorder, 289t
Bipolar (standard) leads, 939, 940f
Birth control implants, 708t, 710
Bites
  animal, 974, 974b, 974t
  insect, 973, 973b–974b
Black cohosh, 872t–873t
Bladder
  anatomy of, 125
  cancer of, 128–130, 130f
  neurogenic, 135–136, 136b, 136t
Bladder outlet obstruction (BOO), 141t–142t
Bland diet, 843
Blank endorsements, 611t
Bleeding, 983, 984b
Blepharedema, 315t
Blepharitis, 315t
Blepharochalasis, 315t
Blepharoplasty, 92t, 305t
Blepharoptosis, 315t
Blepharorrhaphy, 305t
Blind spot, 298
Blood. *See also* Capillary puncture; Hematology; Phlebotomy; Venipuncture
  abbreviations for, 185t
  adjective forms for, 184t
  anatomy of, 167–170, 167f
    plasma, 167–168, 167t
    RBCs, 168–169
    thrombocytes, 170, 170f
    WBCs, 169–170, 171f
  antibodies, 170–172, 171b
  antigens, 170–172, 171b
  as biologic product, 176b–177b
  chemistry of, in POL, 1094–1099
    ALT and AST testing and, 1097
    blood glucose testing and, 1095, 1095b–1096b, 1095f
    cholesterol testing and, 1096–1097, 1098b–1099b
    hemoglobin A_{1c} testing and, 1095–1096, 1097t
    thyroid hormone testing and, 1097–1099
  chemistry panels of, in reference laboratory, 1099, 1100f, 1101t–1102t
  CO_2 in, 24
  combining forms for, 184t
  components of, 1077t–1078t
  cultures, 174t, 1049, 1049b
  deoxygenated, 211–212, 212f–213f, 213b
  diseases and disorders of, 173–183
    anemia, aplastic and hemolytic, 183t
    anemia, deficiencies, 183t
    anemia, iron deficiency, 173–175, 175f
    anemia, sickle-cell disease, 175–176, 176f
    hemophilia, 177–178
    idiopathic thrombocytopenic purpura, 178, 178f
    infectious mononucleosis, 179–180
    interventions for, 175t
    laboratory tests for, 174t
    leukemia, acute lymphocytic/acute myelogenous, 180–181, 180f, 204t
    leukemia, chronic lymphocytic/chronic myelogenous, 181–182, 204t
    leukocytic disorders, 184t
    systemic infections, 184t
    thrombophlebitis, 182–183, 182f
  flow, 211–215, 935, 936f
    blood pressure and resistance to, 225
    conduction system and, 216–217, 216t
    coronary circulation and, 213, 213f
    fetal circulation and, 214–215, 214f

Blood (*Continued*)
    hepatic portal circulation and, 213
    pulmonary circulation and, 211–213, 212b, 212f
    systemic circulation and, 211–213, 212f
  introduction to, 166–167
  life span changes to, 184
  oxygenated, 211–212, 212f–213f
  physiology of, 170–172
    coagulation and hemostasis, 172, 172b, 173f
    RBC blood types, 170–172, 171f, 172b
    WBC phagocytosis, 172, 172f
  prefixes for, 184t
  Rh-factor in donation of, 171, 171b
  specimens
    capillary puncture for collection of, 1070–1071, 1071b–1073b
    chain of custody for, 1074
    customer service and, 1102b
    handling after collection of, 1074
    hemolysis and rejection of, 1067, 1068t
    venipuncture and recollection of, 1067, 1068t
  structure and function of, 17t
  suffixes for, 185t
  transfusion, 175t, 1094
  types, 170–172, 171f, 172b, 1093–1094, 1094b, 1094t
  in urine specimens, 1028, 1029b, 1029f
Blood alcohol testing, 275t
Blood bank. *See* Immunohematology
Blood glucose testing, 26t–27t, 1095, 1095b–1096b, 1095f
Blood pressure, 217
  blood flow resistance and, 225
  blood volume and, 217
  diastolic, 651
  measuring, 219t–221t
  regular screenings for, 812, 814t
  stages of, 185t
  systolic, 651
  urinary system and, 128
  ventricular contractions and, 217
  vital sign readings for, 651–657
    age and, 651t
    body position for measurement of, 654–656, 657f
    errors in measurement of, 657b
    evaluation in, 651–653, 652b, 652t
    factors affecting, 651
    Korotkoff sounds and, 656–657
    measurement in, 653–656, 653f–654f, 654t, 655b–656b
    palpatory method in, 657
    personal systems for, 656f
Blood Safety Act, 1094
Blood slide artifacts, 1091b
Blood smears, in differential cell count for CBC reports, 1091–1092, 1091b, 1091f–1092f
Blood tuberculin testing, 921
Blood urea nitrogen (BUN) test, 130t
Blood vessels, 208–209, 208f, 209f, 210f
Blood volume, blood pressure and, 217
Bloodborne Pathogens Standard. *See* Standard Precautions, OSHA
Bluetooth headsets, 478, 478f
Blunted affect, 276b
BMI. *See* Body mass index
BMR. *See* Basal metabolic rate
Body cavities, 22–23, 23f, 23t–24t, 33t
Body mass index (BMI), 660, 660b, 660t
Body mechanics
  for patient transfer, 679–680, 680f, 681b
  principles of, 679–680, 679f–680f, 680b
  safety and, 512–513, 512f, 513b
Body planes, 23–24, 24f, 33t
Body systems, structure of, 16, 17t
Body temperature
  average adult, 639t
  converting, 639
  digital thermometers for, 639–640, 640f, 641b–642b
  factors influencing, 637–638
  febrile illnesses and, 638, 638b
  fever and, 191, 638, 638f
  integumentary system regulation of, 73
  sites for, 638–640
  temporal artery thermometers for, 640, 640f, 644b
  tympanic thermometers for, 640, 640f, 643b
Bonded deliveries, 511, 511b

Bone
  density, regular screenings for, 812, 814t
  diseases and disorders of, 65t
  scans, 54t
  types and shapes of, 37, 38f, 38t
Bone marrow transplant, 175t, 176, 177b, 198t
BOO. *See* Bladder outlet obstruction
Bookkeeping, in healthcare facilities, 588–589, 589b. *See also* Accounts payable; Accounts receivable
Borderline personality disorder, 290t
Bounding pulse, 646–647, 647b
Bowman capsule, 124, 127t
Bozeman sponge forceps, 762t–764t, 764f
BPH. *See* Benign prostatic hyperplasia
Brachial pulse, 644–645, 645f
Bradycardia, 218t–219t, 646
Bradypnea, 243t, 649–650
Brain, 265–266, 265f
  cerebellum of, 266
  cerebrum of, 265–266, 266f
  diencephalon of, 266
  injuries to, 266b
  interventions for, 278t
Brain scan, 273t
Brainstem, 265–266, 265b, 265f
Brand name medications, generic medications compared to, 859–860, 860b
Breach notification, 386–387, 386b
Breach of contract, 370–371
Breasts, female, 147–148
  cancer of, 159t–160t, 809b
  gynecology and examination of, 705–706
  physical examination of, 690–691
  self-exams of, 809, 809b–810b, 810f
Broad-spectrum antibiotics, 1105
Bronchi, 240, 240f
Bronchiectasis, 256t–257t
Bronchioles, 240–241, 240f
Bronchiolitis, 256t–257t, 1116
Bronchitis, 246–247, 256t–257t
Bronchodilators, 248, 248b, 863t–867t
Bronchoscopy, 26t–27t, 244t–245t, 250f, 777
Broselow, James, 967
Bruit, 218t–219t, 687, 687b
Buccal medication administration, 890
Buerger disease, 234t
Buffered medications, 889t
Buffers, 24
Buffy coat, 1081, 1081b, 1081f
Buildings evacuations, 516
Bulimia nervosa, 291t, 849, 849b
Bulla, 74f
BUN test. *See* Blood urea nitrogen test
Bundle branch block, 224t
Bundle of His, 215f, 216, 936f
Bunion, 65t
Burns, 78–80
  diagnostic coding for, 545–546
  environmental emergencies and, 970–971, 971f, 972t
  rule of nines for, 78, 79b, 971f, 972t
  treatment of, 80t
Bursae, 44
Bursitis, 59–61
Business associates, 382b
Business checks, 606
Business letter formats, 484–485, 484t, 485b, 486f
Butterfly assemblies (winged infusion sets), 1053–1054, 1054f
Butterfly assembly method, for venipuncture, 1064b–1066b
Buying cycle, 506, 506b
Buzzy, 917f

C

C & S. *See* Culture and sensitivity
CAAHEP. *See* Commission on Accreditation of Allied Health Education Programs
CABG. *See* Coronary artery bypass graft
Calcitonin, 327t
Calcium, 326, 326b, 838t
Calcium channel blockers, 231t
Calcium chloride, 968t
Calculi, renal, 139–140, 139b, 139f–140f, 141t–142t
Calibration, definition of, 653, 654b, 996, 996b
Calipers, 940, 940b, 941f

INDEX

Call forwarding, 441t
Callus, 90t–91t
Calyces, 124, 124f
Cambodian patients, cultural differences with, 805b
Canadian crutches, 824
Canals of Schlemm, 299
Cancellations, appointment scheduling and, 465–466
Cancellous bone, 36–37, 37b
Cancer
  of bladder, 128–130, 130f
  breast, female, 159t–160t, 809b
  cervical, 159t–160t
  classifications of, 30, 30f, 31t
  colorectal, regular screenings for, 812, 814t
  of digestive system, 107–108, 107t
  of female reproductive system, 158–161, 159t–160t
  grade of, 32
  of kidneys, 133–135, 133f–134f, 134t
  laryngeal, 256t–257t
  of lungs, 249–250, 250f, 250t, 813, 814t
  neoplasms and, 30–32, 30t
  nutrition needs for, 847–848
  oral, 107t, 812, 812b
  ovarian, 159t–160t
  of prostate, 137–138, 138f, 141t–142t, 155–158, 814t
  of skin, 80–83
    diagnostic procedures for, 82, 83t
    etiology of, 81
    prevention of, 83
    prognosis of, 83
    risk factors of, 812b
    signs and symptoms of, 81–82, 82b, 82f
    treatment of, 76t, 82–83
  stages of, 32, 32t
  testicular, 158, 812b
Candidiasis, 90t–91t, 161t, 618, 707
Canes, coaching on, 828, 828f, 829b–830b
Cannula, 765b, 765t–766t
Canthus, 893b–895b
CAP. See College of American Pathologists
Capillaries, 208, 208f
Capillary puncture, 1067–1069
  equipment for, 1068–1069
    collection containers, 1069, 1069f
    Guthrie cards, 1069, 1070f
    lancets, 1068–1069, 1068f
    microhematocrit tubes and centrifuge, 1069, 1069f, 1080
  routine, 1069–1071
    patient preparation, 1070
    site selection for, 1069, 1069b, 1070f
    specimen collection and handling, 1070–1071, 1071b–1073b
Capitalization, 480–481
Capitation, 527t, 571
Caplet medications, 889f, 889t
Capsule, 124, 124f
Capsule endoscopy, 26t–27t
Capsule medications, 889f, 889t
Captions, 424b, 431
Carbohydrates, 835–836, 835b–836b, 835t
Carbon, 168b
Carbon dioxide (CO_2), 166, 167b
  in blood, 24
Carcinomas, 31t
Carcinomas, of skin, 80–83. See also Skin, cancer of
Card files, 431
CARD (Check, Assign, Reverse, and Define) method, 3–4, 3f
Cardiac ablation, 221t–223t
Cardiac arrhythmias. See Arrhythmias
Cardiac catheterization, 219t–221t, 220f
Cardiac cell states, 216
Cardiac defibrillator, 221t–223t
Cardiac enzymes test, 219t–221t
Cardiac event recorders, 952–953
Cardiac muscles, 45, 46f, 215
Cardiac myxosarcoma, 234t
Cardiac pacemaker, 221t–223t, 222f
Cardiac tamponade, 234t
Cardinal signs, 637
Cardiodynia, 218t–219t
Cardiogenic shock, 233t, 984t
Cardiology/cardiologists, 188b, 208b
Cardiomegaly, 218t–219t

Cardiomyopathy, 225–226
Cardiopulmonary resuscitation (CPR), 221t–223t, 964b, 964t, 986b–987b, 986f, 988t
Cardiovascular system
  abbreviations for, 236t
  adjective forms for, 235t
  anatomy of, 208–215, 934
    blood flow, 211–215, 935, 936f
    blood vessels, 208–209, 208f, 209f, 210f
    heart, 209–211, 934, 935f
  combining forms for, 235t
  diseases and disorders of, 217–235
    additional, 234t, 235
    arrhythmias, 224, 224t
    atherosclerosis-related diseases, 225, 225t, 226f
    cardiomyopathy, 225–226
    CHF, 228
    congenital heart defects, 226–228, 227f, 227t
    diagnostic procedures for, 219t–221t
    DVT, 182–183, 182f, 228–229, 229f
    heart valve diseases, 182–183, 184t
    hypertension, 182, 185t, 231t, 652, 652b, 652t
    myocardial infarction, 231–232, 231f–232f, 232t
    POTS, 232–233
    shock, 233, 233t
    signs and symptoms of, 218t–219t
    treatment for, 221t–223t
  emergencies of, 982–987
    bleeding, 983, 984b
    myocardial infarction, 985–987, 985b–987b, 986f
    shock, 983–985, 983b–985b, 984t
    syncope, 982–983, 983b–984b, 983f
  geriatrics changes in, 744–745, 745t
  life span changes to, 235, 235t
  physiology of, 215–217
    blood pressure, 217
    conduction system, 215–217, 936–937, 936f
  prefixes for, 235t
  structure and function of, 17t
  suffixes for, 235t
Cardioversion, 221t–223t
Cardoxin (digoxin), 863t–867t
Care coordination, 828–830, 829b–831b
Career development
  career portfolios and, 1140, 1140b–1141b
  introduction to, 1127
  job interviews and, 1140–1145
    answering questions in, 1142, 1143b
    attire for, 1141, 1141f
    face-to-face, 1144, 1144b
    follow-up after, 1144–1145, 1144b
    healthcare facility research for, 1140–1141, 1140b
    illegal interview questions in, 1143, 1143t
    negotiation after, 1145
    opportunities increased for, 1145
    on phone, 1144, 1144b
    practice answers to questions for, 1141, 1142f
    preparation for, 1140–1142
    professionalism during, 1142–1144
    on video, 1144
  job search and, 1130–1131
    certification exams and, 1130, 1130b
    employment agencies for, 1131, 1131b
    finding job postings in, 1145
    improving opportunities for, 1145–1146
    job interview opportunities increased in, 1145
    networking for, 1130, 1130b, 1130f
    newspaper ads for, 1131
    offers increased for, 1145–1146
    school career placement officers for, 1131
  jobs in, 1146–1147
    human resource requirements for, 1146, 1146t
    leaving, 1147
    maintaining, 1147
    starting, 1146–1147
  objectives for, 1129
  online profiles and job applications and, 1138–1140, 1138b–1140b, 1138f, 1139f
  personal needs in, 1130
  personality traits for, 1127–1128
    collaboration and interpersonal skills, 1127–1128, 1127f, 1128b
    compassion, 1128, 1128b
    genuine interest, 1128, 1128f

Career development (Continued)
  professionalism, 1128, 1128b
  strengths and skills in, 1128–1129
  resumes and, 1131–1135
    action verbs in, 1135, 1135f
    appearance of, 1135, 1136b
    certifications in, 1135
    content in, 1132–1135, 1133b
    cover letters for, 1129f, 1136–1137, 1137b–1138b, 1137t
    education in, 1133–1134
    formats for, 1131–1132, 1132f, 1133b
    header in, 1132, 1132b–1133b
    summary and skills in, 1135
    work experience in, 1134–1135, 1134b
  strength and skill assessment for, 1128–1129
    personality traits, 1128–1129
    technical skills, 1129, 1129f
    transferrable job skills, 1129, 1129b
Career portfolios, 1140, 1140b–1141b
Carisoprodol (Soma), 863t–867t
Carotid artery, 209, 211f
Carotid artery disease, 225t
Carotid endarterectomy, 221t–223t, 222f
Carotid pulse, 643–644, 645f
Carpal tunnel syndrome, 61, 61f
Carpals, 42t
Carvedilol (Coreg), 863t–867t
Case law, 362
Cash flow, paying bills to maximize, 613–614
Cash on hand, 589, 589b
Cash payments, 606
Cashier's checks, 606
Casts, coaching on, 818–820, 820t
Casts, in urine, 1032, 1033t–1034t, 1038b
Catabolism, 834
Cataract extraction, 307f, 307t
Cataracts, 2, 309–310, 310f, 543, 543b, 751
Catatonia, 289t
Catheterized, definition of, 1019
Catheters, 131b, 1019
Caustic, definition of, 775, 775b, 1000–1001
Cauterization, 76t
CBC. See Complete blood count
CC. See Chief complaint
CCK. See Cholecystokinin
CCMA. See Certified Clinical Medical Assistant
CDC. See Centers for Disease Control and Prevention
Cecum, 98
CEJA. See Council of Ethical and Judicial Affairs
Celexa (citalopram), 863t–867t
Celiac disease, 199t–200t
Cell phones, 442
Cell-mediated immunity, 190f, 193, 619
Cells
  in microscopic examination of urine, 1032, 1035f–1036f
  structure of, 14–15, 14t, 15f
Cellulitis, 90t–91t
Center for Medicare and Medicaid Services (CMS), 389t, 523
Centers for Disease Control and Prevention (CDC), 389b, 389t
  disinfectant levels of, 634b
  growth charts of, 735f–736f
  hand hygiene and, 622–624, 622f, 623b
  infection prevention checklist for, 630, 631t
  Needlestick Safety and Prevention Act and, 622
  Universal Precautions of, 622
  weight status categories of, 723, 723b
Central nervous system (CNS), 261, 262f, 265–267
  brain in, 265–266, 265f
    cerebellum of, 266
    cerebrum of, 265–266, 266f
    diencephalon of, 266
    injuries to, 266b
    interventions for, 278t
  brainstem in, 265–266, 265b, 265f
  meninges in, 266–267, 267f
  spinal cord in, 266–267, 267f
Central processing unit (CPU), 473t
Centrifuges, 173, 174b, 175f, 1011–1012, 1011f, 1078–1081, 1081b. See also Hematocrit centrifuge
Centrioles, 14t
Cephalexin (Keflex), 863t–867t

Cerebellum, 266
Cerebral angiography, 273f, 273t
Cerebral palsy, 281t–282t
Cerebrospinal fluid (CSF), 266–267, 267b, 277t
Cerebrovascular accident (CVA), 272–274, 272b, 980, 980b
Cerebrum, 265–266, 266f
Certificate of mailing, USPS, 489t
Certification
    exams, job search and, 1130, 1130b
    in practice requirements, 378
    in resumes, 1135
Certified Clinical Medical Assistant (CCMA), 350t
Certified mail, 489f, 489t
Certified Medical Administrative Assistant (CMAA), 350t
Certified Medical Assistant (CMA), 350t
Certified Nurse Midwife (CNM), 376t
Certified nurse midwives, 347t
Certified ophthalmic assistants, 347t
Certified ophthalmic technicians, 347t
Certified Registered Nurse Anesthetist (CRNA), 376t
Certifying agencies, for clinical laboratory personnel, 991t
Cerumen, 299, 640, 640b
    impacted, 698–699
Ceruminoma, 320t
Cervarix, 730t
Cervical biopsy, 710–711, 711b
Cervical caps, 708, 708t, 709f
Cervical sponges, 708, 708t
Cervicitis, 161t
Cervix, 147, 149f
    cancer of, 159t–160t
Cessation, definition of, 409, 409b, 800, 800b
CF. See Cystic fibrosis
Chain of command, 349
Chain of custody, for specimen handling, processing and storing, 1007, 1042, 1043b, 1074
Chain of infection, 617–620, 617f
Chalazion, 316f, 316t
CHAMPVA. See Civilian Health and Medical Program of the Veterans Administration
Chaperones, during physical examination, 689b
Check, Assign, Reverse, and Define (CARD) method, 3–4, 3f
Check fraud, 613b
Check scanner, mobile, 611f
Check-in procedures, for all patients, 500
Checking accounts, 605
Checkout, patient, 502
Checks, 605–606, 608–611, 608b, 611t
Checks, in clinical laboratory, 996, 996b
Cheeks, 96, 96f
Chek-Stix, 1031
Chemical cold packs, 821t, 822b
Chemical digestion, 99–101, 99b–101b, 100f
Chemical hazards, clinical laboratory safety and, 1000–1001, 1001b–1002b, 1001f
Chemical hot pack, 822t
Chemical labels, 1002b
Chemical peel, 92t
Chemical sterilization, 774–775, 774f
Chemistry, 993, 993f
Chest, physical examination of, 690
Chest (precordial) leads, 939, 941f
Chest x-rays, 244t–245t
Chewable tablet medications, 889f, 889t
Cheyne-Stokes respiration, 243t, 650
CHF. See Congestive heart failure
Chief complaint (CC), 538, 560, 560b, 663–664, 663b
Child abuse, neglect, and exploitation, 389t, 391–392, 391b–392b, 740, 740b
Child Abuse Prevention and Treatment Act, 740
Childbirth complications, diagnostic coding of, 545, 545b
Childhood issues, ethics and, 407–408, 407b
Children. See Minors; Pediatrics
Children's Health Insurance Program (CHIP), 524
Chinese patients, cultural differences with, 805b
CHIP. See Children's Health Insurance Program
Chiropractic care, 59b, 823
Chlamydia, 152, 153t, 707, 1108, 1109t
Chloride, 838t
Choking, 981, 981b–982b

Cholangitis, 118t
Cholecystectomy, 104t–105t
Cholecystitis, 118t
Cholecystography, 103t
Cholecystokinin (CCK), 100
Cholelithiasis (gallstones), 107–108, 108f, 554, 554b
Cholesteatoma, 320t
Cholesterol, regular screenings for, 812, 814t
Cholesterol testing, for blood chemistry in POL, 1096–1097, 1098b–1099b
Cholesterol-lowering agents, 863t–867t
Chondromas, 66t
Chondrosarcomas, 66t
Chordae tendineae, 209, 209b
Chordee, 155f, 155t–156t
Chorionic villus sampling (CVS), 719, 719f
Choroid, 297, 299, 301t
Choroidal hemangioma, 318t
Chromium, 838t
Chromosomes, 14–15, 404, 404b
Chronic, definition of, 3, 25, 535, 535b
Chronic infections, 621
Chronic kidney disease, 225t
Chronic lymphocytic leukemia, 181–182, 204t
Chronic myelogenous leukemia, 181–182, 204t
Chronic obstructive pulmonary disease (COPD), 247–248, 248f, 649–650
Chronologic order, 664, 665b
Chronologic resumes, 1131–1132, 1132f, 1133b
Chyme, 98
Cicatrix, 793, 793b
Cigarettes, 247b, 808b
Cilia, 14t, 25
Ciliary body, 297, 297b, 298f, 301t
Circulatory system. See Cardiovascular system
Circumcision, 149
Circumduction, 52t–53t
Cirrhosis, 118f, 118t
Citalopram (Celexa), 863t–867t
Citrucel, 836b
Civil law, 363, 364t
Civil lawsuit, stages of, 368b
Civil Rights Act of 1964, 355, 395t–396t
Civil Rights Act of 1991, 395t–396t
Civilian Health and Medical Program of the Veterans Administration (CHAMPVA), 525
Claim scrubbers, 580, 580b
Claims, 522, 522b
    accurate diagnostic coding preventing fraud and abuse in, 577–578
    clearinghouses, 381–382, 382b, 566, 566b, 571–572
    CMS-1500 and, 566, 566b, 572–577, 576t–577t
        guidelines for reviewing, 580b
        Section 1: Carrier - Block 1, 572, 572f
        Section 2: Patient and Insured Information - Blocks 1a through 13, 572–573, 573b, 573f
        Section 3a: Physician or Supplier Information - Blocks 14 Through 23, 573–574, 574b, 574f
        Section 3b: Physician or Supplier Information - Blocks 24 Through 33, 575–577, 575f, 575t, 578b, 579f
    customer service and, 584b
    denied, 581–582, 582b–583b
    against estates, 601
    medical necessity and, 581, 581b–583b
    rejection of, preventing, 580
    status of, checking, 581
    third-party requirements for, 580
Claims-made policy, 369
Clamping and grasping instruments, 761, 762t–764t
Clarification, 355t, 668, 668b, 1127–1128, 1128f
Claudication, 218t–219t
Claustrophobia, 291t
Clavicle, 42t
Clean claims, 580
Clean-catch midstream urine specimens, 1019, 1020b–1021b
Clear liquid diet, 842, 842t
Clearinghouses, claims, 381–382, 382b, 566, 566b, 571–572
Cleft palate, 116f, 116t
CLIA. See Clinical Laboratory Improvement Amendments

Clinical diagnosis, 663–664
Clinical laboratory
    CLIA and, 994–996, 995t
    customer service and, 1012b
    departments of, 993–994
    equipment in, 1008–1012
        centrifuges, 1011–1012, 1011f
        incubators, 1012, 1012f
        maintenance log for, 1012, 1012t
        microscopes, 1008–1011, 1009f, 1010b–1011b, 1010t
    introduction to, 991–994
    mathematics and measurement for, 1007–1008
        liquid volume measurement, 1008, 1009f
        temperature measurement, 1007, 1007b, 1008t
        time measurement, 1007, 1007t
        units in, 1008, 1008t
    personnel in, 991–992, 991t
    QA stages in, 996–997, 997f
    QC guidelines for, 997–999, 997b–999b
    requisitions and reports of, 1004–1005, 1005f
    safety in, 999–1004
        biohazards and infection control for, 1001–1003, 1003b, 1003f
        chemical hazards and, 1000–1001, 1001b–1002b, 1001f
        OSHA's Standard Precautions for, 1001–1003, 1003b, 1003f
        physical hazards and, 1004, 1004f
        signs and symbols for, 1000b
        standards and governing agencies for, 1000
    specimen collection in, 1005–1006, 1005b, 1006f
        contamination prevention for, 1006, 1006f
    specimen handling, processing and storing in, 1007
        chain of custody and, 1007, 1042, 1043b, 1074
    testing
        introduction to, 992
        qualitative compared to quantitative, 992t
Clinical Laboratory Improvement Amendments (CLIA), 219t–221t, 244t–245t, 388–389, 389t, 1077
    clinical laboratory and, 994–996, 995t
    immunology testing and, 1119–1121
        Helicobacter pylori testing, 1121
        HIV testing, 1121, 1121f, 1122b
        infectious mononucleosis testing, 1119, 1119b–1120b
        Lyme disease testing, 1121
    microbiology testing and, 1116
        influenza A and B testing, 1116
        rapid strep testing, 1116, 1117b–1118b
        RSV testing, 1116, 1116f
Clinical Nurse Specialist (CNS), 376t
Clinitest, 1038–1039, 1038b–1040b
Clitoris, 147, 149f
Clonazepam (Klonopin), 863t–867t
Clones, 192–193
Cloning, 405
Clopidogrel (Plavix), 863t–867t
Closed fracture, 56t–57t
Closed questions, 670
Clostridium difficile, 1105, 1105b
Clot activators, 1049–1050
Clots, 168
Clotting factors, 167, 167t, 168b
Clubbing, 243t, 249, 249b, 250f, 689
CMA. See Certified Medical Assistant
CMAA. See Certified Medical Administrative Assistant
CMP. See Comprehensive metabolic panel
CMS. See Center for Medicare and Medicaid Services
CMS-1500 Health Insurance Claim Form (CMS-1500), 566, 566b, 572–577, 576t–577t. See also Claims
    guidelines for reviewing, 580b
    Section 1: Carrier - Block 1, 572, 572f
    Section 2: Patient and Insured Information - Blocks 1a through 13, 572–573, 573b, 573f
    Section 3a: Physician or Supplier Information - Blocks 14 Through 23, 573–574, 574b, 574f
    Section 3b: Physician or Supplier Information - Blocks 24 Through 33, 575–577, 575f, 575t, 578b, 579f
CNM. See Certified Nurse Midwife
CNS. See Central nervous system; Clinical Nurse Specialist
CO_2. See Carbon dioxide

INDEX

Coaching, 842b
  areas in, 800
  on assistive devices, 823–828, 824b
    canes, 828, 828f, 829b–830b
    crutches, 824–825, 824f–825f, 826b
    walkers, 825–828, 827b–829b, 827f
    wheelchairs, 828
  care coordination and, 828–830, 829b–831b
  for community resources, 800, 831b
  on diagnostic tests, 800, 817, 818t–819t
  on disease prevention, 800, 806–807, 807b–808b
  health belief model and, 801, 801b
  on health maintenance and wellness, 800, 809–815
    additional screenings for, 815, 815b–817b, 816f
    breast self-exams and, 809, 809b–810b, 810f
    one-time screenings for, 814–815
    oral cancer self-exams and, 812, 812b
    regular screenings for, 812–813, 814t
    self-exams and, 809–812
    skin self-exams and, 810–812, 812b, 813f
    testicular self-exams and, 810, 811b–812b
  learning domains and, 802
    affective, 802, 803f, 803t
    cognitive, 802, 802f, 803t
    psychomotor, 802, 803t
  patient adaptations for, 802–806
    communication barriers and, 806, 806b
    cultural diversity and, 803–805, 804b–805b, 805f
    developmental levels and, 802–803, 804f, 804t
  for specific needs, 800
  stages of grief and dying and, 801, 801t
  teaching-learning process and, 806, 806b, 807t
  on treatment plans, 800, 817–828
    assistive devices and, 823–828, 824b
    casts and splints and, 818–820, 820t
    cold therapy and, 820–821, 820b, 821t, 822b
    complementary therapies and, 823
    exercise therapy and, 823, 823f
    hot therapy and, 820–821, 820b, 821f, 822t
    medication administration at home and, 818, 819b, 819f
    RICE therapy and, 822–823
    ultrasound therapy and, 821–822
CoaguChek XS PT test monitor, 1086, 1086f
Coagulation, 167, 167f
  platelets and, 172, 172b, 173f
Coagulation testing, 1086, 1086b–1088b, 1086f, 1088f
Coarctation of the aorta, 227f, 227t
Cobalamin, 839t
Cocci, diseases caused by, 1109t
Cochlea, 300, 300f
Cochlear implants, 302b, 309f, 309t
COD. *See* Collect on delivery
Code, definition of, 964, 964b
Code modifiers, in CPT, 551–552, 552t
Code of ethics
  for medical assistants, 402, 402b
  for physicians, 401–402, 402f
Coding systems, 381, 382b
Cognitive ability, 749
Cognitive domain, of learning, 802, 802f, 803t
Cognitive needs, 358f
Cognitive therapy, 286t
Co-insurance, 522, 566, 583t
  calculation of, 582, 583f
Cold compress, 821t
Cold therapy, coaching on, 820–821, 820b, 821t, 822b
Cold-related emergencies, 970, 970t
Colic, 725
Colitis, 117t
Collaboration, 1127–1128, 1127f, 1128b
Collagen, 72, 72b, 746–747, 747b
Collect on delivery (COD), 489t
Collecting duct, 124, 127t
Collection agencies, 601–602, 602f, 603f
Collection letters, 600
Collection procedures, 598–604
  bankruptcy and, 601
  claims against estates and, 601
  collection agencies and, 601–602, 602f, 603f
  letters and, 600
  personal finance interviews and, 600, 600f
  preparing patient accounts for, 598, 599f
  small claims court and, 603–604, 603f
  special, 601

Collection procedures *(Continued)*
  starting, 598
  telephone techniques and, 598–600, 598b
  tracing skips and, 601, 601b
College of American Pathologists (CAP), 378
Cologuard stool DNA test, 819t
Colon cancer, 107t
Colonoscopy, 26t–27t, 668, 668b, 777
Colony, definition of, 1122, 1123b
Color, sensation, motion, and temperature (CSMT), 820, 820t
Color, urine, 1022, 1022b, 1022f, 1023t
Color blindness testing, 318b
Color coding, 435, 435b, 435f
Colorectal cancer, regular screenings for, 812, 814t
Colorectal surgeons, 348t
Colostomy, 104f, 104t–105t
Colostrum, 192b
Colposcopy, 26t–27t, 158b, 159t–160t, 710–711, 712f
Comas, 282t
Combination resumes, 1132f, 1133
Combining forms
  for blood, 184t
  for cardiovascular system, 235t
  common types of, 12t
  definition of, 1b, 2
  for digestive system, 119t
  for ear, 322t
  for endocrine system, 340t
  for eye, 321t
  for integumentary system, 93t
  for lymphatic and immune systems, 204t
  for mental and behavioral health, 292t
  for musculoskeletal system, 67t
  for nervous system, 292t
  for reproductive system, 163t
  for respiratory system, 258t
  suffixes added to, 3–4, 3t–4t
  for urinary system, 143t
Commas, 481, 482t
Commercial liability insurance, 369
Comminuted fracture, 56t–57t
Commission on Accreditation of Allied Health Education Programs (CAAHEP), 378
Commissurotomy, 221–223t
Common law, 362, 362b
Communicable diseases, 390b, 391
Communication. *See also* Patient interviews; Written communication
  coaching patients with barriers in, 806, 806b
  for geriatrics, 755b
  nonverbal, 350–353, 442b
    cultural differences in, 352–353, 353t
    delivery factors in, 352, 352t
    for patient communication, 669, 669b–671b, 669t, 670f
    physical boundaries to, 351–352, 352t
    positive and negative behaviors in, 351t
  with patients, 665–670
    active listening for, 668–669
    closed questions for, 670
    nonverbal communication for, 669, 669b–671b, 669t, 670f
    obtain and document information from, 667b
    open-ended questions/statements for, 669–670
    self-boundaries with, 345, 666b, 701b
    sensitivity to diversity in, 666–667, 668b, 668f
    therapeutic techniques for, 668–671, 672f
  self-boundaries with, 345, 666b, 701b
  verbal, 353–357
    barriers to, 355–357, 356t–357t
    communication cycle, 353, 353f
    oral communication, 353–354, 354t
    therapeutic communication, 354–355, 355t
Communication cycle, 353, 353f
Community resources, coaching for, 800, 831b
Compact bone, 36–37, 37b
Compactible files, 431
Comparative negligence, 367t
Compartment syndrome, 820
Compassion, 344, 1128, 1128b
Compensatory damages, 368
Complement, 167, 167f, 191, 191b
Complementary therapies, 823

Complete blood count (CBC), 26t–27t, 103t–104t, 174t, 197t, 275t
  reference laboratory reports of, 1086–1093, 1089t, 1090f
  differential cell count in, 1091–1092, 1091b, 1091f–1092f
  RBC counts in, 1089
  RBC indices in, 1089
  WBC counts in, 1091
Compliance, definition of, 420, 420b, 800, 800b
Compliance reporting, 391–396. *See also* Law
  employment concerns with, 394–396, 394b–397b, 395t–396t
  environmental safety concerns with, 396, 397b
  financial concerns with, 393–394, 394b–395b, 394t
  patient safety concerns with, 396, 398b–399b
  programs for, 393–396
  with public health statutes, 391–393, 391b
    adult abuse, neglect, and exploitation, 392–393
    child abuse, neglect, and exploitation, 389t, 391–392, 391b–392b
    reportable diseases, 391, 391t, 392b
    wounds of violence, 391
  for vaccination issues, 393
Comprehensive chemistry panel, 103t–104t
Comprehensive metabolic panel (CMP), 26t–27t, 174t, 197t, 275t
Compression fracture, 56t–57t
Computed tomography (CT), 26t–27t, 54, 103t, 130t, 196t, 244t–245t, 273t, 331t, 818t
Computer networks, 474, 474b
  privacy and security for, 476–478, 477b, 477t
Computer on wheels (COWs), 478, 478b
Computerized physician/provider order entry (CPOE), 420, 420b
Computerized scheduling, 454–455
Computers. *See* Personal computers
COMVAX, 730t
Concerta (methylphenidate), 863t–867t
Concise, definition of, 416–418, 416b
Concussions, 282t, 978, 978b–979b
Condoms, 708, 708t
Conduct disorder, 289t
Conduction system, 215–217
  blood flow and, 216–217, 216t
  cardiac cell states and, 216
  cardiac muscle and, 215
  nervous system and, 217
  structures of, 215–216, 215f, 936–937, 936f
Conductive hearing loss, 302b, 320t, 698
Condyloid joint, 44t, 45f
Cone biopsy, 158b, 159t–160t
Cones, 298, 301t
Confabulation, 289t
Conference calls, 441t
Confidential healthcare for minors, 407–408, 408b
Confidentiality, phone call management and, 444
Confirmation calls, 464–465
Conflict of interest, 394, 394t, 395b
Congenital disorders
  of male reproductive system, 152–158, 155t–156t
  of nervous system, 281t–282t
Congenital heart defects, 226–228, 227f, 227t
Congenital hip dysplasia, 65t
Congestive heart failure (CHF), 228
Congruence, definition of, 669, 669b
Conjunctiva, 296
Conjunctiva disorders, 316t
Conjunctivitis, 316f, 316t, 727b
Connective membranes, 70t
Conscientious, definition of, 343, 758, 758b
Consent, 371–372, 371b–372b, 778
Consequences, legal, 364t
Constipation, 102t
Constitutional law, 362
Constrict, definition of, 172
Consumer Credit Protection Act, 596
Contact dermatitis, 90t–91t
Contactless payment systems, 608–609
Continuing education, 349–350, 350t
Continuity of care, 414
Continuous fevers, 638, 638f

INDEX

Contraception, 707–710
  barrier methods of, 708, 709f
  hormonal, 708–710
  IUDs and, 708t, 710, 711f
  permanent methods of, 710
  types of, 708t
Contract law, 364t, 369–371
  breach of contract in, 370–371
  contract elements, 369
  provider-patient relationship in, 370, 370t
Contractures, 66t
Contraindication, definition of, 539–542
Contrast media, 26t–27t
Contributory negligence, 367t
Control materials, 996, 996b
Controlled substance prescriptions, 871, 871t
Controlled Substances Act (CSA), 388, 388t, 858–859, 859b–860b, 859t
Contusions, cerebral, 282t
Convalescent stage, of infections, 621b, 1119, 1119b
ConZip (tramadol), 863t–867t
Coombs antiglobulin test, 174t
Cooperation, for helping others, 347–348
Copayment (co-pay), 449, 522, 566, 583t
COPD. See Chronic obstructive pulmonary disease
Coping mechanisms, 358–359, 359t
Copper, 838t
Cordarone (amiodarone), 968t
Cordotomy, 280t
Coreg (carvedilol), 863t–867t
Coreoplasty, 308t
Cornea, 296–297, 298f, 301t, 306t
Corneal incision procedure, 306t
Corneal transplants, 297b, 306t
Corneal ulcer, 317t
Coronary artery bypass graft (CABG), 221t–223t, 222f
Coronary circulation, 213, 213f
Coronary heart disease, 225t
Coronary microvascular disease, 225t
Corpora cavernosa, 149
Corpora spongiosum, 149
Corrosions, diagnostic coding of, 545–546
Corrosive, definition of, 1001b–1002b
Cortex, of kidney, 124, 124f
Corticosteroids, 135, 135b, 246b, 246t, 863t–867t
Costal cartilage, 750
Costochondral cartilage, 37, 41f
Cough etiquette, 807b
Coumadin (warfarin), 863t–867t, 1088f
Council of Ethical and Judicial Affairs (CEJA)
  on abortion, 406b
  on adoption, 407b
  on advance care planning, 409b
  on advance directives, 409b
  on confidential healthcare for minors, 408b
  duties of, 402
  on euthanasia, 410b
  on genetic testing, 405b
  on organ transplantation from deceased donors, 411b
  on withholding or withdrawing life-sustaining treatment, 410b
Counterfeit, definition of, 606, 606b
Counteroffers, 1147, 1147b
Courtesy, 344
Courts, 364t
Cover letters, for resumes, 1129f, 1136–1137, 1137b–1138b, 1137t
Covered entities, 382b
Cowper glands, 146, 148f
COWs. See Computer on wheels
Coxsackievirus, 727b
CPOE. See Computerized physician/provider order entry
CPR. See Cardiopulmonary resuscitation
CPT. See Current Procedural Terminology
CPT Assistant, 550
CPU (central processing unit), 473t
Cranial nerves, 267, 268t
Craniectomy, 278t
Craniotomy, 278t
Cranium, bones of, 37–39, 40t
Crash carts, 964–965, 965f
Crash cast, 503
C-reactive protein (CRP), 26t–27t, 55t, 87t, 103t–104t, 197t
Cream medications, 889t

Create Your Plate method, 844–845, 844f
Creatinine clearance rates, 1019
Creatinine tests, 130t, 819t
Credentials, for medical assistants, 349–350, 350t
Credit, 589, 589b
Credit balances, 595–596, 596b
Credit cards, 608–609, 609f
Crenate, definition of, 1032
Crestor (rosuvastatin), 863t–867t
Cretinism, 334t
Criminal law, 362–363, 364t
Criticism, responding to, 349
CRNA. See Certified Registered Nurse Anesthetist
Crohn disease, 108–109, 109f
Croup, 253t–254t
CRP. See C-reactive protein
Crushing medications, 888b
Crust, 74f
Crutches, 824–825, 824f–825f, 826b
Cryosurgery, 76t, 777
Cryotherapy, 710
Cryptorchidism, 155f, 155t–156t
Crystals, 1022, 1023b, 1032–1033, 1035t
CSA. See Controlled Substances Act
CSF. See Cerebrospinal fluid
CSMT (color, sensation, motion, and temperature), 820, 820t
CT. See Computed tomography
Cued-speech interpreters, 356t
Cultural diets, 850b
Cultural differences, in nonverbal communication, 352–353, 353t
Cultural diversity, 344t, 803–805, 804b–805b, 805f
Culture and sensitivity (C & S), 26t–27t, 1019, 1019b, 1124, 1124b
Culture media, 993
Curettage, 76f, 76t
Current Procedural Terminology (CPT), 549, 549t
  Alphabetic Index of, 550, 551f, 552–554, 554b
  category I codes of, 549–550, 549b
  category II codes of, 550, 550b
  category III codes of, 550
  code modifiers in, 551–552, 552f
  coding guidelines for, 551–552
  conventions of, 552, 552f
  customer service and, 563b
  documentation for, 552, 553f
  Evaluation and Management codes of, 555–561
    complexity in, 560–561
    patient status identification in, 555
    POS in, 558, 559t, 575, 575t
    service level provided in, 555–560, 559f, 560t
  for integumentary system lesion excision, 561
  introduction to, 549
  for maternity care and delivery, 561–562
  for musculoskeletal system, 561–562
  for office visits, 558b
  organization of, 550
  Pathology and Laboratory section of, 562, 562b
  Surgery section of, 556b–557b, 561–562
  for surgical package, 561
  Tabular List of, 550, 551f, 554–555, 555b
  Unlisted Procedures and Services in, 550–551
Cushing disease, 335–336, 335t, 336f
Customer service
  appointment scheduling and, 466b
  aseptic techniques for infection control and, 634b
  blood specimens and, 1102b
  care coordination and, 830b
  clinical laboratory and, 1012b
  CPT and, 563b
  definition of, 343
  diabetes mellitus and, 339b
  diagnostic coding and, 546b
  ECG and, 962b
  emergencies and, 989b
  exceptional, 360b
  financial management in healthcare facilities and, 614b
  geriatrics and, 756b
  gynecology and, 720b
  health insurance and, 531b
  health records and, 436b
  healthcare facilities and, 519b
  medical billing and claims and, 584b
  medication administration and, 932b

Customer service (Continued)
  microbiology and, 1125b
  minor surgery and, 797b
  obstetrics and, 720b
  PCs and, 491b
  pediatrics and, 740b
  physical examination and, 701b
  prescriptions and, 883b
  urine specimen collection and, 1042b
  venipuncture and, 1050b
  vital sign measurement and, 661b
Customers, definition of, 343
Cutting and dissecting instruments, 761, 761f–762f, 761t–762t
CVA. See Cerebrovascular accident
CVS. See Chorionic villus sampling
Cyanosis, 218t–219t, 243t, 248f
Cyclic citrullinated peptide antibody (anti-CCP), 55t
Cyclobenzaprine (Flexeril), 863t–867t
Cyclothymia, 289t
Cymbalta (duloxetine), 863t–867t
Cyst removal setup, 789t
Cystadenomas, 118t
Cystic fibrosis (CF), 248–249, 249b, 715, 715b
Cystitis, 130–131, 131b, 1028, 1029b
Cystoscopy, 26t–27t, 130f, 130t
Cysts, 75t, 542, 542b
  Bartholin, 706
  ovarian, 162t
  protozoal, 1111
  pseudocysts, 114, 115b
Cytology, 993, 993b
Cytoplasm, 14t, 189, 190b, 1092, 1092b

D

Dacryoadenitis, 316t
Dacryocystitis, 316f, 316t
Dacryocystorhinostomy, 305t
Damages, 363b, 364t, 367–368
Daptacel, 730t
DASH. See Dietary Approaches to Stop Hypertension
Data servers, 473, 473b
Data shifts and trends, 999b
Database, 664
DEA. See Drug Enforcement Agency
Debit, 589, 589b
Debit cards, 608, 608b
Debridement, 55–58, 76t
Debris, 188
Debt, unsecured, 601b
Decanting, definition of, 1030–1032
Declaratory judgment, 363b, 364t
Declining stage, of infections, 621b
Decodable terms
  samples of, 4t
  types of, 2, 2f
Decongestants, 255t, 872t
Decryption, 477b, 477t
Decubitus ulcers, 83–84, 84f, 748, 749b
Deductibles, 522, 566, 583t
  calculation of, 582, 583f
Deep massage, 823
Deep tendon reflex, 277t
Deep vein thrombosis (DVT), 182–183, 182f, 228–229, 229f
De-escalation, definition of, 514b
Defamation, 365b, 365t
Defecation, 619, 619b
Defendants, 362, 364t, 604
Defense mechanisms, 289t, 358, 359t, 672, 673b
Defenses, 366, 366t
Defibrillators, 965–967, 967f, 986b–987b
Degenerative joint disorder (DJD), 62
Deglutition, 96
De-identify, 382b, 382t
Delirium, 272t
Delirium tremens, 271t
Delivery zone, 487
Deltoid site, for intramuscular injections for medication administration, 927–928, 927f
Delusion, 272t
Dementia, 285–287, 289t, 537, 749
Demographic information, in prenatal record for obstetrics, 713
Demographics, definition of, 453, 453b, 664, 665b

INDEX

Denial, 359t, 673b
Denial defense, 366
Denied claims, 581–582, 582b–583b
Density, definition of, 54b, 1091
Dental caries, 117t
Dental exam, 813, 814t
Deoxygenated blood, 211–212, 212f–213f, 213b
Department of Agriculture (USDA), 840
Department of Health and Human Services (DHHS), 991t
Dependability, 344–345
Dependence syndrome, 271t
Dependent adults, 392–393, 395b
Dependent clauses, 480, 480t
Depo-Provera (DMPA), 708t, 710
Deposition, 367b–368b
Deposits, for banking in ambulatory care setting, 609, 610b, 610f–611f
Depreciate, definition of, 503, 503b
Depression, geriatrics and, 752, 753f
Depression fracture, 56t–57t
Depression screening, 815, 816f
Depressive disorders, 287–288
Dereliction, 367
Dermabrasion, 92t
Dermal papillae, 71
Dermal-epidermal junction, 71
Dermatofibroma, 92t
Dermatology/dermatologists, 70b, 348t
Dermatomes, 81f, 81t, 268, 270f, 748f
Dermatophytosis (ringworm infections), 84–85, 85b, 1110b
Dermatoplasty, 92t
Dermis, 71f, 72
Descending colon, 98, 99f
Desktop computers, 470f, 470t
Desmopressin, 177, 177b
Detoxification, 286t
Detrimental behavior, 343, 343b
Development patterns, normal, 723–725, 724b–725b
Developmental levels, coaching adaptation for, 802–803, 804f, 804t
Developmental theories, 725
Deviated septum, 256t–257t
DEXA scan. See Dual energy x-ray absorptiometry scan
Dextromethorphan (Benylin, Robitussin), 872t
Dextro-transposition of the great arteries, 227t
DHHS. See Department of Health and Human Services
Diabetes insipidus, 141t–142t, 332t–333t
Diabetes mellitus
  complications of, 338b
  customer service and patient education for, 339b
  diagnostic coding of, 545
  geriatrics management of, 746b
  type 1, 199t–200t, 337, 337t
  type 2, 337, 337t, 814t
Diabetic eating plans, 843–845, 844f, 844t
Diabetic emergencies, 974–976, 975b–976b, 975f–976f, 975t
Diabetic ketoacidosis (DKA), 974–976, 975t
Diabetic retinopathy, 318f, 318t
Diagnosis
  clinical, 663–664
  definition of, 2, 533, 533b
  differential, 663–664
  in health records, 418
  provisional, 418, 418b
Diagnostic cardiac sonographers, 347t
Diagnostic coding. See also ICD-10-CM
  activity codes and, 546
  of AIDS/HIV, 543–544
  of burns and corrosions, 545–546
  customer service and, 546b
  definition of, 533
  of diabetes mellitus, 545
  etiology and manifestation in, 543
  fraud and abuse prevention with accurate, 577–578
  guidelines for, 543–546
  for health status and contact with health services, 546
  for morbidity, external causes, 546
  of neoplasms, 544–545, 544b, 544f
  of organism-caused diseases, 543, 543f
  place of occurrence code and, 546
  of pregnancy, childbirth, and puerperium complications, 545, 545b

Diagnostic coding *(Continued)*
  preparing for, 538–539
    discharge summary and, 538–539
    encounter forms and, 538, 538b
    medical history and physical examination and, 538
    operative report and, 539
    progress notes and, 538
    radiology, laboratory, and pathology reports and, 539
  providers and accurate, 546
  signs and symbols in, 543
  steps in, 539–542, 539t, 540b–541b
Diagnostic medical sonographers, 347t
Diagnostic procedures
  for autoimmune diseases, 196
  for cardiovascular system diseases, 219t–221t
  definition of, 14, 25
  for ear disorders, 699–702, 699f
  for eye diseases and disorders, 304t–305t, 693–697
  for fractures, 54t, 55
  for HIV, 200–201
  for MBHDs, 279–283
  for nervous system diseases and disorders, 277t
  for respiratory system diseases, 244t–245t
  for skin cancer, 82, 83t
  suffixes for, 8, 8t
  types of, 26t–27t
  for urinary system diseases, 130t
Diagnostic statement, 533
Diagnostic tests, coaching on, 800, 817, 818t–819t
Diapedesis, 170b
Diaper fibers, in urine examination, 1036, 1037f
Diaphoresis, 218t–219t
Diaphragm
  definition of, 22b, 241b
  respiration and, 241, 241f
Diaphragms, contraception, 708, 708t
Diarrhea, 102t, 725–726
Diarthrotic joints, 44, 44t, 45f
Diastole, 217
Diastolic blood pressure, 651
Diazepam (Valium), 863t–867t, 968t
Dictation, of health records, 429–430, 429b
Diego blood antigens, 1094b
Diencephalon, 266
Dietary Approaches to Stop Hypertension (DASH), 845, 845t
Dietary changes, patient instruction on, 849–851, 849b–850b
Dietary Guidelines, USDA, 840
Dietary nutrients, 834–840
  carbohydrates and, 835–836, 835b–836b, 835t
  fats and, 837, 837b, 837t
  GI and, 836, 836f
  minerals and electrolytes and, 837, 838t
  protein and, 836, 836b
  vitamins and, 838, 838b, 839t, 840b
  water and, 838–840, 840b
Dietary supplements, 840b
Diets, medically ordered. See Medically ordered diets
Differential cell count, 174t, 197t, 275t
  in CBC reports, 1091–1092, 1091b, 1091f–1092f
  examination, in reference laboratory, 1092
  RBC morphology in, 1092, 1093f
  summary of cells in, 1093t
Differential diagnosis, 663–664
Differentiated, definition of, 30b, 30t, 190
Diffuse, definition of, 329, 330b
Digestive system
  abbreviations for, 120t
  adjective forms for, 119t
  anatomy of, 96–98
    esophagus, 97, 98f, 117t
    large intestine, 98, 99f, 117t
    oral cavity, 96–97, 96b, 96f–97f, 117t
    small intestine, 98, 117t
    stomach, 97–98, 98f, 117t
    throat, 97, 97b, 97f
  combining forms for, 119t
  diseases and disorders of, 102–116
    appendicitis, 102–106, 102f
    cancer, 107–108, 107t
    congenital disorders, 116t
    Crohn disease, 108–109, 109f
    diverticulitis, 109–110, 109f

Digestive system *(Continued)*
    gallstones, 107–108, 108f
    GERD, 110–111, 110f–111f
    hemorrhoids, 111–112
    hepatitis, viral, 112, 112t–113t
    hernias, 118t
    hiatal hernia, 113–114, 114f
    imaging of, 103t
    laboratory tests for, 103t–104t
    neoplasms, 118t–119t
    oral cavity disorders, 117t
    pancreatitis, 114
    peptic ulcers, 115–116, 115f
    signs and symptoms of, 102t
    therapeutic interventions for, 104t–105t
  geriatrics changes in, 746
  introduction to, 95–96, 95f
  lifespan changes in, 119
  physiology of, 99–101
    absorption and excretion, 101
    chemical digestion, 99–101, 99b–101b, 100
  prefixes for, 120t
  structure and function of, 17t
  suffixes for, 120t
Digital communication devices, 350, 351t
Digital rectal examination (DRE), 130t, 138, 138f, 154, 157f
Digital subtraction angiography (DSA), 219t–221t
Digital thermometers, 639–640, 640f, 641b–642b
Digitalis, 854
Digitek (digoxin), 863t–867t
Dignity, 344, 1128
Digoxin (Lanoxin, Digitek, Cardoxin), 863t–867t
Dilated eye exam, 813, 814t
Dilators and probes, 765, 765f–766f, 765t–766t
Diluent, definition of, 758, 909–911, 911b
Dilution, definition of, 1084, 1084b
Diopters, 304t–305t
Diovan (valsartan), 863t–867t
Diphenhydramine (Benadryl), 872t, 968t
Diphtheria, 256t–257t, 730t
Diplegia, 285t
Diplomacy, 344
Diplopia, 309, 309b, 317t
Direct cause, 367
Direct deposit, 614
Direct filing system, 432–433, 432b
Direct medical billing, 571
Direction request phone calls, 447
Directional anatomy terminology, 18, 20t
Directory assistance, for outgoing calls, 452
Dirty claims, 580
Disability insurance, 529–530
Discharge summary, 538–539
Disciplinary action, 377–378, 378b
Disclosure authorization process, 383–384, 384f, 385b
Discoid lupus erythematosus, 90t–91t
Discovery phase, in civil lawsuit, 368b
Discrepancies, 507, 507b
Discretionary income, 605
Discrimination, 394, 394b
Diseases
  bacterial, 1108, 1109t
  of blood, 173–183
  of cardiovascular system, 217–235
  causes of, 28–32
  coaching for prevention of, 800, 806–807, 807b–808b
  definition of, 25, 617
  of digestive system, 102–116
  of ear, 301, 313–315
  of endocrine system, 330–338
  environmental agents of, 30
  of eye, 301, 309–313, 691–693
  fungi causing, 1109–1110, 1110b, 1110t
  genetic, 28, 28t
  of integumentary system, 73–89
  of lymphatic and immune systems, 195–203
  of musculoskeletal system, 52–63, 54b
  of nervous system, 271–279
  parasitic, 1110, 1110t
  in pediatrics, 725–727
  protozoa causing, 1110, 1110t
  of reproductive system, 151–161
  of respiratory system, 242–253

Diseases (Continued)
　types of, 617
　of urinary system, 128–141
　viruses causing, 1111, 1111b, 1112t
Disinfectants, 628, 629b, 1106
　CDC levels of, 634b
Disinfection, 634, 634b, 770
Dislocation, joint, 58, 58f, 58t
Disorders
　of blood, 173–183
　of cardiovascular system, 217–235
　definition of, 25
　of digestive system, 102–116
　of ear, 301, 313–315
　of endocrine system, 330–338
　of eye, 301, 309–313, 691–693
　of lymphatic and immune systems, 195–203
　mental and behavioral health, 270–271
　of musculoskeletal system, 52–63, 54b
　of nervous system, 271–279
　in pediatrics, 725–727
　of reproductive system, 151–161
　of urinary system, 128–141
Displaced fracture, 56t–57t
Displacement, 359t
Disposable scalpels, 761, 762f
Disruption, 456
Dissecting and cutting instruments, 761, 761f–762f, 761t–762t
Dissocial personality disorder, 290t
Dissociative identity disorder, 291t
Distal convoluted tubule, 124, 127t
Distance visual acuity (DVA), 694–696, 694b–695b, 695f
Distribution, of drugs, 855–856, 855b
Diuretics, 135, 135b, 185t, 863t–867t
Diurnal variation, 637
Diversity, 344, 344t–345t
　cultural, coaching adaptations for, 803–805, 804b–805b, 805f
　patient communication and sensitivity to, 666–667, 668b, 668f
Diverticulitis, 109–110, 109f
Divider guides, 431
Dizziness, 977–978
DJD. See Degenerative joint disorder
DKA. See Diabetic ketoacidosis
DMPA. See Depo-Provera
DNR. See Do not resuscitate
DO. See Doctor of Osteopathy
Do not resuscitate (DNR), 409t
Doctor of Medicine (MD), 376t
Doctor of Osteopathy (DO), 376t
Domestic abuse signs, 719–720
Domestic shipping sizes, 487t
Donepezil (Aricept), 750t
Dopamine (Intropin), 968t
Doppler, for checking pulse, 218f, 218t–219t, 649, 649f
Dorsal body cavity, 22–23, 23t
Dorsal recumbent position, 683, 683b
Dorsal surface anatomy, 18, 18f, 20t
Dorsalis pedis pulse, 646, 649, 649f
Dorsiflexion, 52t–53t
Dorsogluteal site, for intramuscular injections for medication administration, 930b
Dorsopathies, 65t
Double-booking, 457
Doulas, 146b
Down syndrome, 715, 715b
Drapes, in minor surgery, 767–769, 767f
Draw-a-Person Test, 283
Drawer files, 430
DRE. See Digital rectal examination
Dress code, 345–346, 345f, 346t
Dressings, 791b–792b, 796–797
Drug abuse screening, 815, 815b
Drug Enforcement Agency (DEA), 388, 388t, 858
Drugs, 854. See also Medication administration; Medication math; Medication orders; Pharmacology basics; Prescriptions
　absorption of, 855, 855b
　action of, 856–857
　　adverse reactions of, 857, 857t
　　factors influencing, 856, 856b, 856t
　　therapeutic effects of, 857
　distribution of, 855–856, 855b

Drugs (Continued)
　excretion of, 856
　herbal, 871, 872t–873t
　laws on, 388, 388b, 388t
　　in ambulatory care setting, 857–859, 858t
　　CSA, 388, 388t, 858–859, 859b–860b, 859t
　　Food, Drug, and Cosmetic Act, 388, 858, 858t
　metabolism and, 856, 856b
　names of, 859–860, 860b
　OTC, 871, 872t
　pregnancy and lactation labeling rule for, 838b
　reference information of, 860–862
　　classification, 860–861, 861t
　　terminology, 861–862, 862t–867t
　sources of, 854
　urine toxicology and, 1041–1042, 1042b–1043b, 1042f, 1042t
　uses of, 854, 855t
DSA. See Digital subtraction angiography
Dual energy x-ray absorptiometry (DEXA) scan, 54t
Ductus arteriosus, 214–215, 214f
Ductus deferens, 146, 148f
Ductus venosus, 214, 214f
Duffy blood antigens, 1094b
Duloxetine (Cymbalta), 863t–867t
Dumb terminal, 473
Duodenal, definition of, 1121
Duty of care, 367
DVA. See Distance visual acuity
DVT. See Deep vein thrombosis
Dwarfism, 332t–333t, 333f
Dying, stages of, 357t, 801, 801t
Dynamic equilibrium, 300, 300b
Dysfunctional uterine bleeding, 162t
Dyslexia, 281t
Dyspepsia, 102t
Dysphagia, 280t–281t
Dysphonia, 243t
Dysphoria, 271t
Dyspnea, 218t–219t, 243t, 649–650
Dyssomnias, 280t–281t, 754
Dysthymias, 289t

E
Ear
　abbreviations for, 322t
　adjective forms for, 322t
　anatomy of, 299–300, 300f
　　inner, 300
　　middle, 299–300
　　outer, 299
　bones of, 37, 40t
　combining forms for, 322t
　diseases and disorders of, 301, 313–315
　　hearing loss disorders, 320t
　　hearing tests for, 308t
　　inner ear disorders, 320t
　　Ménière's disease, 313–314, 751, 752b
　　middle ear disorders, 320t
　　neoplasms, 320t
　　otosclerosis, 314
　　outer ear disorders, 319t
　　presbycusis, 314–315
　　symptomatic disorders, 319t
　　therapeutic interventions for, 309t
　geriatrics and, 751–752, 752b, 753b
　irrigation of, 898b–899b
　life span changes to, 315
　medication administration into, 894, 895b–896b
　physical examination of, 689–690
　physiology of, 301
　prefixes for, 322t
　vision and hearing screenings for disorders of, 698–699
　　audiometric testing for, 699–702, 700b, 701f
　　diagnostic procedures in, 699–702
　　hearing loss and, 698–699, 698f–699f, 699b
　　tuning fork testing for, 699
Ear curettes, 766f, 766t
Eating disorders, 848–849
　anorexia nervosa, 291f, 291t, 848–849, 848b, 848f
　binge, 849
　bulimia nervosa, 291t, 849, 849b
EBV. See Epstein-Barr virus
Ecchymosis, 75t

Eccrine glands, 72
ECG. See Electrocardiography
Echinacea, 872t–873t
Echocardiography, 219t–221t, 220f, 934, 934b
Echoencephalography, 273t
Echolalia, 289t
E-Cigarettes, 248t, 808b
Eclampsia, 162t
Economic status, diversity in, 345t
ECT. See Electroconvulsive therapy
Ectopic, definition of, 335
Ectopic beats, 224t
Ectopic pregnancy, 106, 106b, 715
Ectropion, 315f, 315t
Eczema (atopic dermatitis), 85–86
Edema, 203t, 218t–219t
Edluar (zolpidem), 863t–867t
Education, in resumes, 1133–1134
EEG. See Electroencephalography
Efferent, definition of, 123, 124b
Effervescent tablets, 889t
EGD. See Esophagogastroduodenoscopy
EHR. See Electronic health record
Ejaculatory duct, 146, 148f, 149
Elastin, 72, 72b, 750, 750b
Elation, 271t
Elbow crutches, 824, 824f
Elderly. See Geriatrics
Elderly safety screening, 809, 815b
Elective procedures, 522
Electrical issues, for safety, 514, 515b
Electrical muscle stimulation, 823, 823f
Electrocardiography (ECG), 219t–221t, 677, 677b
　arrhythmia identification in, 948–950
　　atrial arrhythmias, 948–949, 949b
　　heart block, 949
　　implantable device rhythms, 950, 950f–951f
　　sinus arrhythmias, 948
　　ventricular arrhythmias, 949–950, 949f
　artifact troubleshooting in, 947–948
　　AC interference, 947–948, 947f
　　interrupted baseline, 948, 948f
　　somatic tremor, 947, 947f
　　wandering baseline, 947, 947f
　cardiac event recorders and, 952–953
　customer service and, 962b
　definition of, 934
　in exercise stress tests, 951–952, 951f
　Holter monitor and, 952, 952b–953b
　implantable loop recorders and, 953–954
　introduction to, 934
　in nuclear stress tests, 952
　portable handheld monitors for, 954
　procedure of, 942–950, 944b–945b
　　electrode and lead wire application in, 945, 946f, 946t
　　finishing, 950
　　patient preparation for, 942–945, 943b, 945f
　　tracing evaluation, 948, 948t–949t
　　tracing in, 946–947, 947b
　supplies and equipment for, 939–942
　　calipers, 940, 940b, 941f
　　ECG machine, 941–942, 942t, 943b, 943f
　　electrodes, 934, 941, 942f
　　thermal ECG paper, 940, 940b, 941f
　tracing, 937–938
　　evaluating, 948, 948t–949t
　　intervals in, 938
　　running, 946–947, 947b
　　terminology in, 937, 937f
　　waves and segments in, 937–938, 938t
　TTM and, 954
　12-lead, 939, 939f
　　augmented leads, 939, 940t
　　bipolar (standard) leads, 939, 940f
　　chest (precordial) leads, 939, 941f
Electroconvulsive therapy (ECT), 286t
Electrodes, in ECG, 934, 941, 942f
　application and placement of, 945, 946f, 946t
Electroencephalography (EEG), 276f, 276b
Electrolyte panel, 26t–27t
Electrolytes, 837, 838t, 863t–867t
Electromyography (EMG), 54t
Electroneurodiagnostic technologists, 347t
Electronic checks, 606

INDEX

Electronic claims submissions, 571–572
Electronic health record (EHR), 381, 381b, 413, 413b, 469, 469b, 475–476. *See also* Health records
  backup systems for, 424
  capabilities of, 420–422, 421f–422f
  documentation in, 428, 429f
  EMR compared to, 419–420, 419t
  integrity of, protecting, 423b
  for medical history, 665f
  patient connection maintained when using, 422–423, 423f
  phone message documentation for, 446, 446b, 448f
  upload documents to, 423b
Electronic medical record (EMR), 419–420, 419t, 475–476, 479b
Electronic transaction, 381–382, 382b
Electrosurgery, 776, 776b, 776f
Electrosurgical unit (ESU), 776, 776f
Eligibility, 566, 566b
Elimination diet and food allergies, 846–847, 846b
ELISA. *See* Enzyme-linked immunosorbent assay
Elmasonic E ultrasonic cleaner unit, 770f
E-mails, 350, 351t
  professional, 488–490, 491b
  reminder, 465
Emancipated minors, 369b, 369t, 597, 597b
Embezzlement, 608, 608b
Embolus, 172b, 177
Embryo, 151f, 152
Emergencies
  appointment scheduling and, 464
  cardiovascular, 982–987
    bleeding, 983, 984b
    myocardial infarction, 985–987, 985b–987b, 986f
    shock, 983–985, 983b–985b, 984t
    syncope, 982–983, 983b–984b, 983f
  CPR and rescue breathing for, 986b–987b, 986f, 988t
  customer service and, 989b
  definition of, 444, 445b
  diabetic, 974–976, 975b–976b, 975f–976b, 975t
  documentation for, 964b
  environmental, 970–974
    anaphylaxis, 972–973, 973b, 973f, 973t
    animal bites, 974, 974b, 974t
    burns, 970–971, 971f, 972t
    foreign body in eye, 974
    insect bites and stings, 973, 973b–974b
    poisonings, 969b, 971–972, 972b
    temperature-related, 970, 970t–971t
  equipment and supplies for, 964–968
    crash carts, 964–965, 965f
    defibrillators, 965–967, 967f, 986b–987b
    medications, 967, 967f, 968t
    oxygen and airway supplies, 965, 965f, 966b
    pediatric supplies, 967–968, 968f–969f
  handling, 968–987, 969b
  introduction to, 964
  musculoskeletal, 976–977, 977b, 977t
  neurological, 977–980
    concussions, 978, 978b–979b
    CVA, 980, 980b
    seizures, 978–980, 979b–980b
    vertigo and dizziness, 977–978
  respiratory, 980–981, 980t
    asthmatic attacks, 981, 981b
    choking, 981, 981b–982b
    hyperventilation, 980–981, 980t
  staff roles in, 964, 964t
  triaging flow map for, 969, 969b, 969f
Emergency physicians, 348t
Emergency response plans, 514–518, 515t–516t
Emesis, 218t–219t
EMG. *See* Electromyography
Emotional barriers to communication, 356f, 356t
Empathy, 344
Emphysema, 673, 690b
Employee payroll, 614
Employee Retirement Income Security Act of 1974, 395t–396t
Employer group insurance plans, 525–526, 526b
Employment agencies, for job search, 1131, 1131b
Employment concerns, with compliance reporting, 394–396, 394b–397b, 395t–396t
EMR. *See* Electronic medical record
Emulsifies, definition of, 100

EMV chip technology, 608
Encephalitis, 284t
Encoder software, 533, 542
Encounter forms, 538, 538b, 589, 590f
Encryption software, 477t
Endocarditis, 5
Endocardium, 209, 211f, 934, 935f
Endocervical curettage, 158b, 159t–160t
Endocrine gland, 101b
Endocrine system
  abbreviations for, 340t
  adjective forms for, 340t
  anatomy of, 325–329, 325f
    adrenal glands, 325, 325f, 327, 328t
    pancreas, 98, 101, 101b, 325, 325f, 328
    parathyroid glands, 325, 325f, 327, 327f
    pineal gland, 325, 325f, 329
    pituitary gland, 148, 150b, 325–326, 325f–326f, 326b, 327t
    reproductive glands, 325, 325f, 329
    thymus gland, 188, 189f, 325, 325f, 328
    thyroid gland, 325–326, 325f, 327t
  combining forms for, 340t
  diseases and disorders of, 330–338
    adrenal gland diseases, 333–336, 335t
    excisions for, 331t
    imaging for, 331t
    laboratory tests for, 330t
    pancreatic diseases, 336–338, 337t
    pituitary gland diseases, 330–331, 332t–333t
    signs and symptoms of, 330b, 331t
    thyroid gland diseases, 332–333, 334t
  geriatrics changes in, 745–746, 746b
  introduction to, 325
  life span changes to, 339
  nervous system connection to, 325b
  physiology of, 329
  prefixes for, 340t
  structure and function of, 17t
  suffixes for, 340t
Endocrinology/endocrinologists, 188b, 325b
End-of-life issues
  ethics and, 408–410
  laws for, 390, 390t
Endometriosis, 160–161
Endorsement, 377t
Endoscope, definition of, 26t–27t
Endoscopic retrograde cholangiopancreatography (ERCP), 26t–27t, 103t, 108f
Endoscopy
  definition of, 103t, 570b
  for minor surgery, 777, 777f
  types of, 26t–27t
Endospore, 1108, 1108b
Endotracheal (ET) tube, 965, 965b–966b
Endovenous laser ablation (EVLT), 221t–223t
End-stage renal disease (ESRD), 131–133, 132t
Enema, 104t–105t
Engerix-B, 730t
English language origins, 1–2, 2t
Enoxaparin (Lovenox), 923t
Enteric coated tablets or capsules, 889t
Enterobius vermicularis (pinworms), 1114, 1114f
Entropion, 315f, 315t
Enucleation of the eye, 305t
Enunciation, 442, 442b
Environmental agents of disease, 30
Environmental distractions, to communication, 356t
Environmental emergencies, 970–974
  anaphylaxis, 972–973, 973b, 973f, 973t
  animal bites, 974, 974b, 974t
  burns, 970–971, 971f, 972t
  foreign body in eye, 974
  insect bites and stings, 973, 973b–974b
  poisonings, 969b, 971–972, 972b
  temperature-related, 970, 970t–971t
Environmental protection, OSHA Standard Precautions and, 625–627
Environmental safety concerns, with compliance reporting, 396, 397b
Enzymatic reactions, 1028
Enzyme-linked immunosorbent assay (ELISA), 197t
Enzymes, 834, 834b, 1077
EOB. *See* Explanation of benefits
Eosinophils, 169

Epicardium, 209, 211f, 934, 935f
Epidemiological, definition of, 533, 533b
Epididymis, 146, 148f
Epigastric region, 23f, 24t
Epiglottitis, 255f, 255t
Epilepsy, 274–275, 847
Epinephrine, 328t, 968t
EpiPen, 906, 908f, 973f
Epiphora, 316t
Epiphyseal plates, 723, 723b
Epistaxis, 243t, 256t–257t
Epithelial cells, 70, 1038b
Epithelial tissue, 15, 15t
Epithelial-cutaneous membranes, 70t
Epithelial-mucous membranes, 70t
Epithelial-serous membranes, 70t
EPO. *See* Exclusive provider organization
Eponyms, definition of, 3
E-prescribing, 420, 420b, 479, 479f, 494b–495b, 495f
Epstein-Barr virus (EBV), 1119
Equal Pay Act of 1963, 395t–396t
Equilibrium, definition of, 300
Equipment, of healthcare facilities, 503–511
  inventory of, 503, 504b, 504f
  maintenance logs for, 503–504, 505f, 506b
  purchasing, 505–506, 506b
  warranties and service calls for, 504
ERCP. *See* Endoscopic retrograde cholangiopancreatography
Erectile dysfunction, 158t
Ergonomics, 440, 440b
  PC workstations and, 475, 476f
Erikson, Erik, 355, 357t, 725, 803, 804t
Erythema infectiosum, 727b
Erythrocyte sedimentation rate (ESR), 26t–27t, 55t, 87t, 174t, 197t, 275t
  for hematology POL testing, 1084, 1084b–1085b, 1084t, 1086f
Erythrocytes, 168–169
Erythropoietin, 128, 169
Eschar, 75t
Escharotomy, 76t
Escitalopram (Lexapro), 863t–867t
Esomeprazole (Nexium), 863t–867t
Esophageal atresia, 116f, 116t
Esophageal varices, 234t
Esophagogastroduodenoscopy (EGD), 5, 5f, 26t–27t
Esophagus, 97, 98f, 117t, 239–240, 239f
Esotropia, 317f, 317t
ESR. *See* Erythrocyte sedimentation rate
ESRD. *See* End-stage renal disease
Essential hypertension, 652, 652b, 652t
Established patients, appointment scheduling for, 459, 460b–461b, 460f
Estates, claims against, 601
Esteem needs, 358, 358f
Esterase, 1029, 1029b
ESU. *See* Electrosurgical unit
ET tube. *See* Endotracheal tube
Ethernet, 474
Ethics
  autonomy and, 404, 404b
  beneficence and, 404
  childhood issues with, 407–408, 407b
  definition of, 381b, 401
  end-of-life issues with, 408–410
  genetics issues with, 404–406
    cloning, 405
    genetic engineering, 405–406, 405b, 405t–406t
  introduction to, 401
  justice and, 404
  nonmaleficence and, 404
  personal, 401, 401t
  principles of, 403–404
  professional, 401–402, 401t, 402f
  reproductive issues with, 406
  separation plan for, 402–403, 403b
Ethics committees, 407b
Ethnic diversity, 344t
Etiology
  definition of, 25, 533–534
  in diagnostic coding, 543
Eukaryotes, 1109, 1110b
Euphoria, 271t
Eupnea, 243t

INDEX

Eustachian tube, 299–300, 300f
Euthanasia, 410, 410b, 410t
Euthymia, 271t
Evacuated collection tubes, venipuncture and, 1049–1052, 1050f, 1051f
Evacuation chairs, 515
Evacuation procedures, 514–516, 516b–517b, 516f, 517t
Evaluation and Management codes, of CPT, 555–561
Eversion, 52t–53t
Evisceration of the eye, 305t
EVLT. *See* Endovenous laser ablation
Evoked potential, 276t
Evzio (naloxone), 968t
Examination room
    escorting patients to, 500–501, 501b
    preparation of, for physical examination, 675–676
Excisional biopsies, 83f, 83t
Exclusive provider organization (EPO), 527, 528t
Excoriation, 725
Excretion
    of digestive system, 101
    of drugs, 856
    of integumentary system, 73
Executive branch, of government, 363t
Executors, 601
Exelon (rivastigmine), 750t
Exenteration of the eye, 305t
Exercise
    benefits of regular, 51, 51b, 51t
    stress test, 219t–221t
        ECG in, 951–952, 951f
    therapy, 823, 823f
Exfoliation, 83t
Exhalation, 649
Exocrine function, 328, 328b
Exocrine glands, 72, 101b
Exophthalmia, 317t, 331t
Exotropia, 317f, 317t
Expediency, definition of, 466, 466b
Expert witnesses, 367b–368b
Expiration, 241, 241b, 241f
Explanation of benefits (EOB), 524, 566, 592–593, 593b, 594f
Expletives, 599, 599b
Explicit, definition of, 745
Exploitation
    adult, 392–393
    child, 389t, 391–392, 391b–392b
Expressed contracts, 369
Extended cycle pills, 709
Extended release tablets or capsules, 888b, 889f
Extension, 52t–53t, 688, 688b
Extension crutches, 824
Extensor muscles, 45
External customers, 343
External hard drives, 424
External ocular muscles, 301t
External respiration, 649
Extracorporeal circulation, 221t–223t
Extract, definition of, 1116, 1116b
Extraction, definition of, 1116, 1116b
Extraocular muscles, 297
Exudates, definition of, 1001, 1001b
Eye
    abbreviations for, 321t
    adjective forms for, 321t
    anatomy of, 296–299
        eyeball, 297–299, 298f, 305t
        ocular adnexa, 296–297, 297f, 305t
    combining forms for, 321t
    dilated eye exam, 813, 814f
    diseases and disorders of, 301, 309–313, 691–693
        cataracts, 2, 309–310, 310f, 751
        conjunctiva disorders, 316t
        diagnostic procedures for, 304t–305t, 693–697
        eye muscle and orbital disorders, 317t
        eyelash disorders, 316t
        eyelid disorders, 315t
        glaucoma, 310–311, 311f, 751
        interventions for, 305t–308t
        lens and retina disorders, 318t
        macular degeneration, 311–313, 312f, 751
        neoplasms, 318t–319t
        optic nerve disorders, 318t
        refractive errors, 302b, 302f, 691–693, 693b, 693t

Eye *(Continued)*
        sclera disorders, 317t
        tear gland disorders, 316t
        uvea disorders, 317t
    foreign body in, 974
    geriatrics and, 750–751, 751b, 751t
    irrigation of, 897b–898b
    life span changes to, 315
    medication administration into, 893, 894b–895b
    physical examination of, 689
    physiology of, 301, 301f
    prefixes for, 321t
    vision and hearing screenings for disorders of, 691–693
        diagnostic procedures for, 693–697
        DVA tests for, 694–696, 694b–695b, 695f
        Ishihara color vision test for, 696–697, 697b
        NVA tests for, 696, 696f
Eye muscle disorders, 317t
Eyeball, 297–299, 298f, 305t
Eyelash disorders, 316t
Eyelid, 301t
Eyelid disorders, 315t
Eyewash stations, 1001f, 1002b

F

Face-to-face job interviews, 1144, 1144b
Facets, 39, 41f
Facial bones, 37–39, 39f, 40t
Facilities. *See* Healthcare facilities
Fact witnesses, 367b–368b
Facultative anaerobes, 1108
FAERS. *See* FDA Adverse Event Reporting System
Failed appointments, 464
Failure to thrive, 726
Fainting, venipuncture and, 1066–1067
Fair Debt Collection Practices Act, 598, 598b
Fair Labor Standards Act of 1938, 395t–396t
Fallopian tubes, 147, 149f
Falls
    geriatrics and, 748–749
    preventing, 514
False Claims Act, 394t
False imprisonment, 365t
False ribs, 37, 41f
Familial, definition of, 664, 665b
Familial dilated cardiomyopathy, 234t
Family history, 664, 715–716
Family law, 364t
Family Medical Leave Act of 1991, 395t–396t
Family practice physicians, 348t
Farsightedness. *See* Hyperopia
Fasciculation, 280t–281t
FAST, for stroke, 980b
Fast dissolving tablets or film strips, 889f
Fasting blood glucose, 330t
Fatigue, 621b
Fats, 837, 837b, 837t
Fatty acids, 328, 328b, 834, 834b, 836b
Faxed communication, 490–491
FDA. *See* Food and Drug Administration
FDA Adverse Event Reporting System (FAERS), 858
Febrile illnesses, 638, 638b
Fecal immunochemical test (FIT), 26t–27t, 819t
Fecal occult blood test, 103t–104t, 109, 109f
Feces, 98
Federal Anti-Kickback Law, 394t
Federal Insurance Contributions Act of 1935, 395t–396t
Federal Reserve Bank, 604–605, 604f, 605b
Fee adjustments, 598, 598b
Fee inquiries, phone calls regarding, 449
Fee schedules, 524, 524b, 528, 591, 592b
Fee-for-service plans, 526
Fees in hardship cases, 598, 598b
Felonies, 364t
Female pelvis, male pelvis compared to, 43b, 43f
Female reproductive system
    abbreviations for, 164t
    additional diseases of, 162t
    adjectives for, 163t
    anatomy of, 147–148, 149f
    cancers of, 158–161, 159f–160f
    combining forms for, 163t
    infections of, 161, 161t

Female reproductive system *(Continued)*
    life span changes to, 162
    physiology of, 149–151, 151f
    prefixes for, 164t
    suffixes for, 164t
Femoral hernia, 118t
Femoral pulse, 645, 649
Femur, 42t
Fetal circulation, 214–215, 214f
Fetal heart tones, 717
Fetus, 152
Fever, 191, 638, 638f
Fiber, 835, 835t, 836b
    diet high/low in, 846, 846t
FiberCon, 836b
Fibers, in urine examination, 1036, 1037f–1038f
Fibrillation, 224t
Fibrin sealants, 177, 177b
Fibroids, 162t
Fibromyalgia, 66t
Fibula, 42t
Fifths disease, 727b
Filamentous, definition of, 172
File folders, 431
File organization, for health records, 435–436
Filing equipment, 430–431, 431f
Filing methods, for health records, 432–435
    alphabetic filing, 432–433, 432b, 434b
    color coding, 435, 435b, 435f
    numeric filing, 433–434, 433b
    subject filing, 434–435
Filing supplies, 431
Filtrate, definition of, 124, 1015, 1015b
Filtration, in urinary system, 126
Financial concerns, with compliance reporting, 393–394, 394b–395b, 394t
Financial management, in healthcare facilities, 588–589, 614b. *See also* Accounts payable; Accounts receivable
Financial responsibilities, of patient, 582–584
    allowed amount in, 583, 583f
    co-insurance and deductible calculation for, 582, 583f
    comparison of, 583t
    discussion of, 583–584, 584b, 585f
    sensitivity when discussing, 584, 585f
Finely and coarsely granular casts, 1033t–1034t, 1034f
Fire doors, 514
Fire extinguishers, 518b
Fire prevention, for safety, 514, 515b
Fire response actions, 516–518, 517b–519b, 519t
Firewalls, 477b, 477t
First morning urine specimens, 1019
First-class mail, 487t
First-degree burns, 78, 80t
Fissure, 74f, 75t
Fistula, 108, 109b
FIT. *See* Fecal immunochemical test
Fixation, for fractures, 57, 57f
Flagella, 14t, 1108, 1108b
Flail chest, 256t, 256t–257t
Flap, 81t
Flap procedure, 306t
Flash memory devices, 474f, 474t
Flat affect, 276b
Flatus, 102t
Flaxseed, 872t–873t
Flexeril (cyclobenzaprine), 863t–867t
Flexion, 52t–53t, 688, 688b
Flexor muscles, 45
Flonase nasal spray (fluticasone), 863t–867t
Flora, 631–632, 1019, 1019b, 1105
Flovent Diskus (fluticasone), 863t–867t
Flovent HFA (fluticasone), 863t–867t
Flu vaccine, intradermal, 916b
Fluad, 730t
Fluarix, 730t
Flublok, 730t
Flucelvax, 730t
Fluctuation, definition of, 638
FluLaval, 730t
FluMist, 730t
Fluorescein angiography, 304t–305t
Fluorescein staining, 304t–305t
Fluoride, 838t
Fluoroscopy, 26t–27t

INDEX

Fluticasone (Flonase nasal spray, Flovent HFA, Flovent Diskus), 863t–867t
Flutter, 224t
Fluvirin, 730t
Fluzone, 730t
Foam, in urine, 1023, 1024f
Foerster sponge forceps, 762t–764t, 764f
Folate, 839t
Folate deficiency, 183t
Follicle-stimulating hormone, 148, 327t, 1041, 1041b
Follicle-stimulating hormone (FSH), 26t–27t
Follicular phase, of menstrual cycle, 150
Folliculitis, 90t–91t
Follow-up appointment, 453
Follow-up files, 436
Fontanelles, 738, 739b
Food, Drug, and Cosmetic Act, 388, 858, 858t
Food allergies, elimination diet and, 846–847, 846b
Food and Drug Administration (FDA), 388, 388b, 389t, 858, 858t
Food labels, 840–842, 841f
Foot care, peripheral neuropathy screening for, 815, 815b–817b
Foramen magnum, 265, 265b
Foramen ovale, 214, 214f
Forearm crutches, 824, 824f
Foreign body in eye, 974
Forensic, definition of, 1007
Foreskin, 149
Form, definition of, 862, 862b, 885, 885b
Fortamet (metformin), 863t–867t
Four-point crutch gait, 824, 825f
Fourth-degree burns, 78, 80t
Four-wheel walkers, 827
Fovea centralis, 298, 298f, 301t
Fowler position, 682, 682b
Fractures, 54–58
　diagnostic procedures for, 54t, 55
　etiology of, 54
　fixation for, 57, 57f
　prevention of, 58
　signs and symptoms of, 54–55
　treatments for, 55–58, 57f
　types of, 56t–57t
Fragments, 480t
Fraternal twins, 151
Fraud, 365t, 394, 394b–395b, 394t, 613b
　accurate diagnostic coding preventing, 577–578
Freud, Sigmund, 725
Friction sounds, 244t
Frostbite, 970, 970t
FSH. *See* Follicle-stimulating hormone
Full block letter format, 484–485, 484t, 486f
Full liquid diet, 842, 842t
Full server backup, 424
Full-thickness graft, 81t
Full/wide range of affect, 276b
Fulminant, definition of, 112t–113t, 113b
Functional status screening, 815
Fundal height measurement, 717, 717f
Fungal tests, 75t
Fungi, 618, 1106, 1106b
　pathogenic, 1109–1110, 1110b, 1110t
Furosemide (Lasix), 863t–867t
Furuncle, 90t–91t

G

Gabapentin (Neurontin, Horizant), 863t–867t
GAD. *See* Generalized anxiety disorder
Gait
　abnormal, 280t–281t
　assessment rating scale for, 277t
　definition of, 686, 686b
Galantamine (Razadyne), 750t
Gallbladder, 98, 100, 118t
Gallstones. *See* Cholelithiasis
Gametes, 146
Gardasil, 730t
Garlic, 872t–873t
GAS. *See* General adaptation syndrome
Gastrectomy, 104t–105t
Gastric gavage, 104t–105t
Gastric juice, 99
Gastritis, 117t
Gastroenteritis, 5
Gastroenterology/gastroenterologists, 96b
Gastroesophageal reflux disease (GERD), 110–111, 110f–111f
Gastrointestinal system. *See* Digestive system
Gastroscopy, 777
Gatekeepers, 526
Gel packs, 821t–822t, 822b
Gender, diversity in, 345t
Gene therapy, 405–406
General adaptation syndrome (GAS), 518
General appearance, physical examination for, 689
General correspondence, 435
General damages, 368
General liability insurance, 369
Generalized anxiety disorder (GAD), 291t
Generic medications, brand name medications compared to, 859–860, 860t
Genetic diseases, 28, 28t
Genetic engineering, 405–406, 405b, 405t–406t
Genetic Information Nondiscrimination Act (GINA), 387, 395b–396b
Genetic testing, 405, 405b, 405t
Genetics, ethical issues with, 404–406
　cloning, 405
　genetic engineering, 405–406, 405b, 405t–406t
Genital herpes, 152, 154f, 154t
Genital warts, 152, 154t
Genitourinary surgery, 777
Genuine interest, 1128, 1128f
GERD. *See* Gastroesophageal reflux disease
Geriatrics
　Alzheimer's disease and, 749–750, 750t
　anatomy and physiology changes in, 744–755, 744f
　　cardiovascular system, 744–745, 745t
　　digestive system, 746
　　ear, 751–752, 752b, 753f
　　endocrine system, 745–746, 746b
　　eye, 750–751, 751b, 751t
　　integumentary system, 746–747, 747f, 748b
　　musculoskeletal system, 747–749, 748b
　　nervous system, 749–750, 750t
　　reproductive system, 754
　　respiratory system, 750
　　sensory system, 750–752, 751b–752b, 751t
　　urinary system, 753–754
　communication for, 755b
　customer service and, 756b
　depression and, 752, 753f
　diabetes mellitus management and, 746b
　elderly safety screening and, 815, 815b
　falls and, 748–749
　introduction to, 742–743
　living arrangements and, 754–755
　MAs and, 755, 755b
　nutritional status and, 752
　osteoporosis and, 748
　physical and sensory changes in, 743, 743b
　sleep disorders and, 754
　stereotypes and myths about, 743b
　taste and smell and, 752
Germicides, 619
Germline cells, 406, 406b
Gestational diabetes, 337–338, 337t
Gestational wheel, 716, 716f
gFOBT. *See* Guaiac fecal occult blood test
GI. *See* Glycemic index
Gigantism, 332t–333t, 333f
GINA. *See* Genetic Information Nondiscrimination Act
Ginger, 872t–873t
Gingivae, 96
Gingivitis, 117t
Ginkgo biloba, 872t–873t
Girth, in mail, 487t
Glands, 71f, 72
Glans penis, 149
Glaucoma, 310–311, 311f, 751
Glia, 263
Gliding joint, 44t, 45f
Global services, 561
Globulins, 167, 167t
Glomerulonephritis, 133, 141t–142t, 1024b
Glomerulus, 124, 127t
Gloves, 678t
　minor surgery and sterile procedure for, 785b–786b
　Standard Precautions and, 625, 626b
　for venipuncture, 1057, 1057b
Glucagon, 835, 835b, 968t, 975t, 976f
Glucocorticoids, 328t
Glucometer, 330t
Glucophage (metformin), 863t–867t
Glucose, 834–835, 834b
　blood glucose testing, 26t–27t, 1095, 1095b–1096b, 1095f
　reabsorption of, 1017b
　in urine specimens, 1028, 1039b
Glucose tests, 819t
Glucosuria, 331t
Glumetza (metformin), 863t–867t
Gluten-free diet, 847, 847b
Glycated hemoglobin test, 26t–27t
Glycemic index (GI), 836, 836t
Glycolysis, 1050b, 1051t
Glycosuria, 1028
Goiter, 331t, 334f, 334t
Golgi apparatus, 14t
Gonads, 146, 329, 329b
Goniometry, 55t
Gonioscopy, 304t–305t
Goniotomy, 308t
Gonorrhea, 152, 152f, 153t
"Good" bacteria, 25
Good Samaritan law, 366t, 390
Gossip, 350, 350f
Gout, 59t–60t
Government branches, 363t
Government managed care plans, 524
Graduated cylinder, 1022, 1023b, 1023f
Grafts
　definition of, 132–133, 133b
　skin, 81t
Grains, 835b
Gram stain, 1122
Grammatical errors, 480t
Granulocytes, 169, 169b, 171f, 189, 189b
Grasping and clamping instruments, 761, 762t–764t
Graves' disease, 199t–200t, 334t
Gray matter, 265, 266b
Green tea, 872t–873t
Greenstick fracture, 56t–57t
Greenwich time, 1007, 1007t
Greetings, patient interviews and, 671, 671f
Grief
　responses of, 409b
　stages of, 357t, 801, 801t
Gross, definition of, 588, 614b
Grouping procedures, 457
Growth hormone, 327t
Growth patterns, normal, 723–725, 723b, 723t
Guaiac fecal occult blood test (gFOBT), 26t–27t, 819t
Guarantor, 583, 597, 597b
Guillain-Barré syndrome, 179b, 283t
Gums, 96, 96f
Gustatory sense, 296b
Guthrie cards, 1069, 1070f
Gynecologic surgery, 777
Gynecologists, 146b, 348t
Gynecology, 146b, 348t, 704–712
　abdominal examination and, 706
　breast examination and, 705–706
　contraception and, 707–710
　　barrier methods of, 708, 709f
　　hormonal, 708–710
　　IUDs and, 708t, 710, 711f
　　permanent methods of, 710
　　types of, 708t
　customer service and, 720b
　examination in
　　duties following, 710
　　MAs assisting with, 704–705, 705b
　　preparation for, 704, 705b
　　setting up for, 704
　menopause and, 711–712
　patient education for, 707b
　pelvic examination in, 706, 706f
　special procedures in, 710–711
　　cervical biopsy and, 710–711, 711b
　　colposcopy and, 710–711, 712f

Gynecology *(Continued)*
   cryotherapy and, 710
   LEEP and, 711, 713*f*
   specimen collection in
      maturation index for, 707
      Pap tests for, 705*b*, 706–707, 707*b*
      vaginal infections and, 707, 707*b*
Gynecomastia, 158*t*

H

H1N1 (influenza A) infection, 256*t*–257*t*
Habit and impulse disorders, 292*t*
Hair, 71*f*, 72
Hair fibers, in urine examination, 1036, 1038*f*
Halitosis, 102*t*
Hallucination, 272*t*
Hand hygiene, 622–624, 622*f*, 623*b*, 632, 632*b*
Hand-foot-and-mouth disease, 727*b*, 727*f*
Hands-free crutch, 824, 824*f*
Harassment, 394, 394*b*
Hard copy statement fees, 604*t*
Hard drives, 473*t*
Hard palate, 96, 96*f*
Hardship cases, fees in, 598, 598*b*
Hardware, PC, 469–474. *See also* Personal computers
Harmful use, 271*t*
Hashimoto thyroiditis, 199*t*–200*t*, 334*t*
HAV. *See* Hepatitis A virus
Havrix, 730*t*
HBV. *See* Hepatitis B virus
hCG. *See* Human chorionic gonadotropin
HCPCS. *See* Healthcare Common Procedure Coding System
HCV. *See* Hepatitis C virus
HDLs. *See* High-density lipoproteins
HDN. *See* Hemolytic disease of the newborn
Head
   physical examination of, 689
   skeletal muscles of, 47*t*, 50*f*
   ventral surface anatomy terms for, 18*f*, 19*t*
Header, in resumes, 1132, 1132*b*–1133*b*
Headsets, telephone, 440, 441*f*
Health belief model, 801, 801*b*
Health care professionalism. *See* Professionalism, in health care
Health information management professionals, 347*t*
Health Information Technology for Economic and Clinic Health (HITECH) Act, 386–387, 387*b*, 420, 477
Health insurance. *See also* Claims; Medical billing
   ACA and, 372, 373*b*–376*b*, 373*f*, 388, 522, 530–531
   benefits in, 522
   CMS-1500 and, 566, 566*b*, 572–577, 576*t*–577*t*
      Section 1: Carrier - Block 1, 572, 572*f*
      Section 2: Patient and Insured Information - Blocks 1a through 13, 572–573, 573*b*, 573*f*
      Section 3a: Physician or Supplier Information - Blocks 14 Through 23, 573–574, 574*b*, 574*f*
      Section 3b: Physician or Supplier Information - Blocks 24 Through 33, 575–577, 575*f*, 575*t*, 578*b*, 579*f*
   customer service and, 531*b*
   exchanges, 526
   fee schedules and, 524, 524*b*, 528
   government plans for, 523–525
      CHAMPVA, 525
      CHIP, 524
      government managed care plans, 524
      Medicaid, 524, 524*b*
      Medicare, 523–524, 523*b*, 523*t*
      TRICARE, 524–525, 525*t*
      workers' compensation, 525
   identification card for, 528, 529*f*
   introduction to, 522
   MAs and, 528–529
   MCOs and, 526–527
      EPO, 527, 528*t*
      HMOs, 526–527, 527*t*–528*t*
      medical billing and policies and procedures of, 569–571, 569*b*
      PPO, 527, 528*t*
      utilization management and, 527, 527*b*
   PARs and, 527–528
   primary and secondary determination with, 573*b*

Health insurance *(Continued)*
   private plans for, 525–526
      employer group plans, 525–526, 526*b*
      individual, 526
   traditional, 526
   verification of eligibility and, 500, 500*b*, 528–529, 530*f*
Health Insurance Portability and Accountability Act of 1996 (HIPAA), 381–386
   appropriate communication according to, 498*t*
   disclosure authorization process and, 383–384, 384*f*, 385*b*
   Privacy Rule of, 382–385, 383*t*
   records release process and, 383, 385, 385*b*, 386*f*, 387*b*
   Security Rule of, 386
   sign-in register and, 499*t*
   standards of, 382
   terminology of, 382*b*
Health maintenance and wellness, coaching on, 800, 809–815
   additional screenings for, 815, 815*b*–817*b*, 816*f*
   one-time screenings for, 814–815
   regular screenings for, 812–813, 814*t*
   self-exams and, 809–812
      breast, 809, 809*b*–810*b*, 810*f*
      oral cancer, 812, 812*b*
      skin, 810–812, 812*b*, 813*f*
      testicular, 810, 811*b*–812*b*
Health maintenance organizations (HMOs), 526–527, 527*t*–528*t*
Health records
   accuracy of, importance of, 414
   contents of, 414–419
   corrections and alterations to, 428–429, 430*f*
   customer service and, 436*b*
   dictation and transcription of, 429–430, 429*b*
   electronic, 381, 381*b*, 413, 413*b*, 469, 469*b*, 475–476
      backup systems for, 424
      capabilities of, 420–422, 421*f*–422*f*
      documentation in, 428, 429*f*
      EMR compared to, 419–420, 419*t*
      integrity of, protecting, 423*b*
      for medical history, 665*b*
      patient connection maintained when using, 422–423, 423*f*
      phone message documentation for, 446, 446*b*, 448*f*
      upload documents to, 423*b*
   file organization for, 435–436
   filing methods for, 432–435
      alphabetic filing, 432–433, 432*b*, 434*b*
      color coding, 435, 435*b*, 435*f*
      numeric filing, 433–434, 433*b*
      subject filing, 434–435
   HITECH Act and, 420
   indexing rules for, 432, 434*t*
   MA's role with, 418–419, 419*b*
   objective information in, 414, 414*b*, 418
      diagnosis in, 418
      laboratory and radiology reports in, 418
      treatment prescribed and progress notes in, 418, 418*b*
      vital signs and anthropometric measurements in, 418, 637
   organization of, 425–428
      POR, 425–428, 427*f*
      SOR, 425
   ownership of, 419
   paper, 413
      documentation in, 428
      management system for, 430–431, 433*b*
      phone message documentation for, 446, 446*b*, 447*f*
   personal, 420
   releasing, 425, 426*f*
   retention and destruction of, 424–425
   subjective information in, 414–418, 414*b*
      past health, family, and social history in, 414–418, 416*f*–417*f*
      personal demographics in, 414, 414*b*, 415*f*, 417*b*
   technological terms in, 419–420, 419*t*
   types of, 413
Health status and contact with health services coding, 546
Healthcare Common Procedure Coding System (HCPCS), 549, 549*t*
   code set and manual of, 562, 562*b*–563*b*, 563*f*
   guidelines for, 563

Healthcare ethics. *See* Ethics
Healthcare facilities. *See also* Patient processing tasks
   availability of, appointment scheduling and, 454
   bookkeeping in, 588–589, 589*b*
   closing, 502–503, 503*f*
   customer service and, 519*b*
   equipment of, 503–511
      inventory of, 503, 504*b*, 504*f*
      maintenance logs for, 503–504, 505*f*, 506*b*
      purchasing, 505–506, 506*b*
      warranties and service calls for, 504
   financial management in, 588–589
   job interview preparation with research on, 1140–1141, 1140*b*
   mail to, 511
      incoming, 511, 511*f*
      private delivery services for, 511
   opening, 494–497, 495*f*
      MA tasks in, 494–497, 495*b*
      reception area in, 497, 497*b*, 497*f*
   safety and security in, 512–518
      body mechanics and, 512–513, 512*f*, 513*b*
      electrical issues and fire prevention for, 514, 515*b*
      emergency response plans for, 514–518, 515*t*–516*t*
      evacuation procedures for, 514–516, 516*b*–517*b*, 516*f*, 517*t*
      evaluation for, 513–514, 515*b*
      fire response actions for, 516–518, 517*b*–519*b*, 519*t*
      preventing falls and injuries for, 514
      safe environment and, 513, 513*b*
      stress and, 518, 519*b*
      workplace violence and, 513, 513*b*–514*b*
   supplies of, 503–511
      inventory control systems for, 507, 507*f*
      inventory management for, 506, 506*f*, 507*b*
      ordering, 509, 509*b*
      receiving order for, 509–511, 510*b*, 510*f*–511*f*
      taking inventory for, 507, 508*b*–509*b*, 508*f*
   telephone identification of, 444
Healthcare Fraud Statute, 394*t*
Healthcare proxy, 409*t*
Healthcare-associated infections, 1105, 1105*b*
Health-related correspondence, 435
Health-related websites, 479*b*
Hearing aids, 309*t*
Hearing impaired, communication and, 356*t*
Hearing loss, 302*b*–303*b*, 303*f*, 698–699, 698*f*–699*f*, 699*b*
Hearing loss disorders, 320*t*
Hearing tests, 308*t*
Heart
   anatomy of, 209–211, 934, 935*f*
   chambers of, 209, 211*f*
   heartbeat of, 209–211
   valves of, 209, 211*f*
Heart block, 949
Heart sounds, listening for, 219*t*–221*t*
Heart transplantation, 221*t*–223*t*
Heart valve diseases, 182–183, 184*t*
Heartbeat, 209–211
Heart-healthy diet, AHA's, 845, 845*t*
Heat cramps, 970, 971*t*
Heat exhaustion, 970, 971*t*
Heat lamp therapy, 821
Heat stroke, 970, 971*t*
Heating pad, 822*t*
Heat-related emergencies, 970, 970*t*
Height, anthropometric measurement of, 658–661, 659*b*
Helicobacter pylori testing, 103*t*–104*t*, 1121
Helminths, 619, 1111, 1111*f*, 1112*b*
Hematemesis, 102*t*
Hematochezia, 102*t*
Hematocrit, microhematocrit test and, 1078–1081, 1080*b*–1082*b*, 1081*f*, 1082*t*
Hematocrit centrifuge, 173, 174*f*, 175*f*
   microhematocrit centrifuge, 1069, 1069*f*, 1078–1081, 1078*f*, 1079*b*
Hematocrit/packed-cell volume, 174*t*
Hematologists, 1092*b*, 1102
Hematology, 993, 1077–1078
   blood components and, 1077*t*–1078*t*
   immunohematology, 1093–1094
      blood typing and, 1093–1094, 1094*b*, 1094*t*
      legal and ethical issues with, 1094
   microhematocrit centrifuge maintenance and, 1078–1081, 1078*f*, 1079*b*

Hematology (Continued)
  plasma and, 1078
  in POL, 1078–1086
    coagulation testing, 1086, 1086b–1088b, 1086f, 1088f
    ESR, 1084, 1084b–1085b, 1084t, 1086f
    hematocrit and microhematocrit test, 1078–1081, 1080b–1082b, 1081f, 1082t
    hemoglobin test, 1082–1083, 1082b–1083b, 1082f, 1084t
  in reference laboratory
    blood chemistry panels and analyte testing, 1099, 1100f, 1101t–1102t
    CBC reports, 1086–1093, 1089t, 1090f
    differential cell count examination, 1092, 1093f
    differential cell count in, 1091–1092, 1091b, 1091f–1092f
    normal blood cell identification in, 1092, 1093t
    platelet analysis, 1093
    RBC counts in, 1089
    RBC indices in, 1089
    WBC counts in, 1091
Hematoma, 75t, 282f, 282t, 1057b
  venipuncture and, 1066–1067
Hematuria, 1028
Hemi walkers, 827, 827f
Hemianopsia, 318t
Hemiparesis, 285t
Hemiplegia, 285f, 285t
Hemoccult test, 103t–104t
Hemoconcentration, 1048
Hemogard tube stoppers, 1049–1051, 1050f, 1051t
Hemoglobin, 168, 169b, 174t, 1082
Hemoglobin A_{1c} testing, 1095–1096, 1097t
Hemoglobin electrophoresis, 174t
Hemoglobin fractionation by high-pressure liquid chromatography, 174t
Hemoglobin isoelectric focusing iron studies, 174t
Hemoglobin test, 1082–1083, 1082b–1083b, 1082f, 1084t
Hemoglobinuria, 1028, 1029b
Hemolysis, 1053, 1053b
  specimen rejection and, 1067, 1068t
Hemolytic anemia, 183t
Hemolytic disease of the newborn (HDN), 162t, 171–172, 716b, 717f
Hemolyzed, definition of, 1006
Hemophilia, 177–178, 715, 715b
Hemoptysis, 243t
Hemorrhoidectomy, 104t–105t, 221t–223t
Hemorrhoids, 111–112
Hemostasis, 172, 172b, 173f, 793
Hemostatic forceps, 762t–764t, 763f
Hemothorax, 256t–257t, 257f
Henle loop, 124, 127t
Heparin, 169, 854
Hepatic function panel, 103t–104t
Hepatic portal circulation, 213
Hepatitis, viral, 112, 112t–113t
Hepatitis A virus (HAV), 730t
Hepatitis B virus (HBV)
  childhood immunization guidelines for, 730t
  postexposure follow-up for, 629, 630b
  vaccination for, 629, 630f
Hepatitis C virus (HCV), 630b, 815
Hepatobiliary scan, 103t
Hepatocellular carcinoma, 119t
Hepatosplenomegaly, 179, 179b
Herbal medications, 871, 872t–873t
Hereditary patterns, 415, 415b, 617
Hernias, 118t, 539b
Herniated intervertebral disk, 65t, 282t
Herniorrhaphy, 104t–105t
Herpes simplex virus (HSV), 90t–91t
Herpes zoster (shingles), 87–88, 88b, 88f, 268b, 748b
Herpetic stomatitis, 117t
Hertz, 699, 699b
Heterophile antibody, 1119
Hiatal hernia, 113–114, 114f
Hiberix, 730t
Hiccups, 244t
Hidradenitis, 90t–91t
Hierarchy, definition of, 357, 357b
Hierarchy of needs, Maslow's, 357–358, 358f
High-density lipoproteins (HDLs), 837
Hinge joint, 44t, 45f

HIPAA. See Health Insurance Portability and Accountability Act of 1996
Hirschsprung disease, 116t
Hirsutism, 336, 336f
Hispanic patients, cultural differences with, 805b
Histamine, 169
Histology, definition of, 15, 993, 993b
Histoplasmosis, 256t–257t
History of present illness (HPI), 664, 665b
HITECH Act. See Health Information Technology for Economic and Clinic Health Act
HIV records, confidentiality of, 385, 385b
HIV testing, 275t, 814, 1121, 1121f, 1122b
Hmong patients, cultural differences with, 805b
HMOs. See Health maintenance organizations
Hodgkin's lymphoma, 31t, 201–202
Hold for pickup, USPS, 489t
Holistic, definition of, 663, 663b
Holter monitor, 219f, 219t–221t, 952, 952b–953b
Homeostasis, 15, 15b, 166–167, 188, 329, 330b, 637, 637b, 1015, 1015b
Homologous bone marrow transplant, 175t, 198t
Homonyms, 480, 481t
Honesty, 344–345
Hordeolum, 316t, 316t
Horizant (gabapentin), 863t–867t
Horizontal evacuations, 516
Horizontal recumbent (supine) position, 683, 683b
Horizontal shelf files, 430, 431f
Hormonal contraception, 708–710
Hormonal patch, 708t, 709
Hormone replacement medications, 863t–867t
Hormone tests, 330t
Hormones, 1077
  nonsteroid, 329
  regulation of, 329
  steroid, 329
Hospice care, 408b
Hot compress, 822t
Hot soak, 822t
Hot therapy, 820–821, 820b, 821f, 822t
Household system, for medication math measurement, 874, 874b, 874t, 875t
Housekeeping controls, OSHA Standard Precautions and, 627–628, 628f–629f, 629b
HPI. See History of present illness
HPV. See Human papillomavirus
HSV. See Herpes simplex virus
Huddles, for team members, 349b
Human chorionic gonadotropin (hCG), 103t–104t, 275t, 1039–1040
Human immunodeficiency virus (HIV), 152, 154t, 198–201, 814
  diagnostic coding of, 543–544
  diagnostic procedures for, 200–201
  etiology of, 198–200
  nutrition needs for, 847
  postexposure management of, 630b
  prevention of, 201
  prognosis of, 201
  records of, confidentiality of, 385, 385b
  risk after exposure to, 630b
  signs and symptoms of, 200
  testing for, 275t, 814, 1121, 1121f, 1122b
  treatment for, 201
Human papillomavirus (HPV), 730t
Humerus, 42t
Humoral immunity, 190f, 192–193, 619, 620b
Huntington's chorea, 281t–282t
Hyaline casts, 1033f, 1033t–1034t
Hydrocele, 158t
Hydrocephalus, 281f, 281t–282t
Hydrocephaly, 734, 734b
Hydrochloric acid, 99
Hydrochlorothiazide (Microzide, Oretic), 863t–867t
Hydrocodone (Vicodin, Norco, Lortab), 863t–867t
Hydronephrosis, 139b, 141t–142t
Hydroxyurea, 176b–177b
Hymen, 147
Hyperalimentation, 104t–105t
Hypercapnia, 243t
Hyperemesis gravidarum, 162t
Hyperglycemia, 338t
Hyperhidrosis, 90t–91t
Hyperinsulinism, 337t

Hyperkalemia, 133
Hyperlipidemia, 135
Hyperopia, 302b, 691, 693f
Hyperpnea, 243t, 649–650
Hypersensitivity reactions, 194, 194b
Hypersplenism, 203t
Hypertension, 182, 185t, 231t
  DASH and, 845, 845t
  essential, 652, 652b
  race and risk of, 652b
  signs and symptoms of, 652b
  stages and treatment of, 652t
Hyperthyroidism, 199t–200t, 332–333, 334t
Hypertrichosis, 90t–91t
Hypertrophy, 744
Hyperventilation, 24, 243t, 649–650, 980–981, 980t
Hyphema, 317t
Hypnosis, 286t
Hypoalbuminemia, 135
Hypocalcemia, 331t
Hypochromic RBCs, 1089, 1089b
Hypodermic needles, 899–900, 899f–900f
Hypodermic syringes, 900, 900f–901f, 901b–902b
Hypogastric region, 23f, 24t
Hypoglycemia, 331t, 338t
Hypokalemia, 331t
Hypokinesia, 280t–281t
Hyponatremia, 331t
Hypophysectomy, 331t
Hypoplastic left heart syndrome, 227t
Hypopnea, 243t
Hypospadias, 134t, 155t–156t, 156f
Hypotension, 653, 653b
Hypothalamus, 325, 325f
Hypothermia, 970, 970t
Hypothyroidism, 199t–200t, 333, 334t, 1097–1099, 1099b
Hypovolemia, 183t
Hypovolemic shock, 233t, 984t
Hypoxemia, 243t
Hypoxia, 243t
Hysterectomy, 158b, 159t–160t
Hysteroscopy, 777

I
IBD. See Inflammatory bowel disease
IBS. See Irritable bowel syndrome
Ibuprofen (Advil, Motrin, Midol), 863t–867t, 872t
ICD-10-CM
  activity codes and, 546
  AIDS/HIV coding in, 543–544
  Alphabetic Index of, 534–536, 535f, 539–542, 543f
  burns and corrosions coding in, 545–546
  coding steps in, 539–542, 539t, 540b–541b
  diabetes mellitus coding in, 545
  encoder software and, 533, 542
  etiology and manifestation in, 543
  guidelines for, 543–546
  health status and contact with health services coding in, 546
  morbidity coding in, external causes, 546
  neoplasms coding in, 544–545, 544b, 544f
  organism-caused diseases coding in, 543, 543f
  place of occurrence code and, 546
  pregnancy, childbirth, and puerperium complications coding in, 545, 545b
  signs and symbols in, 543
  structure and format of, 533–534, 533b, 534f, 534t
  Tabular List of, 536–538, 536f, 537b, 542, 542f
  third-party reimbursement and, 546
ICD-10-PCS. See International Classification of Diseases, Tenth Revision, Procedural Coding System
Ice bags, 821f
Identical twins, 151
Identification card, for health insurance, 528, 529f
Identifiers, definition of, 1005, 1005b
Idiopathic, definition of, 178b, 652, 652b
Idiopathic thrombocytopenic purpura, 178, 178f
Ileus, 117t
Ilium, 42t
Illegal interview questions, in job interviews, 1143, 1143b
Illiteracy, communication and, 356t
Illusion, 272t
Immune, definition of, 179, 179b
Immune system. See Lymphatic and immune systems

INDEX

Immunizations, 620
  pediatrics and, 727–729
    documentation for, 729, 731b
    guidelines for, 729, 730t
    schedules for, 727, 728f
    storage for, 729, 731b
Immunodeficiency, 29
Immunoglobulins, 192, 192b, 1078, 1078b
Immunohematology, 1093–1094
  blood typing and, 1093–1094, 1094b, 1094t
  legal and ethical issues with, 1094
Immunologists, 188b
Immunology, 188b
  CLIA-waived testing, 1119–1121
    Helicobacter pylori testing, 1121
    HIV testing, 1121, 1121f, 1122b
    infectious mononucleosis testing, 1119, 1119b–1120b
    Lyme disease testing, 1121
  introduction to, 1105–1106
Impacted cerumen, 319t
Impacted fracture, 56t–57t
Impervious, definition of, 628, 629b, 771, 773b
Impetigo, 90f, 90t–91t
Implantable device rhythms, 950, 950f–951f
Implantable loop recorders, 953–954
Implied contracts, 369, 370f
In utero, definition of, 177, 177b
In vitro
  definition of, 168b, 994, 994b, 1124, 1124b
  fertilization, 406t
In vivo, definition of, 168b
Inactive poliovirus (IPV), 730t
Inanimate objects, 619
Incarcerated hernia, 118t
Incidence, definition of, 25, 414
Incision and drainage, 76t
Incisional biopsies, 83f, 83t
Incompetence, 369t
Incomplete sentences, 480t
Inconspicuous, 688–689
Incontinence, urinary, 140–141, 140t
Incubation stage, of infections, 621b
Incubators, 1012, 1012f
Incurred, definition of, 589, 589b
Incus, 299–300, 300f
Indexing rules, 432, 434t
Indigent, 523, 597
Infanrix, 730t
Infants, therapeutic approaches to, 724b
Infarction, 172b, 177
Infection control
  aseptic techniques for, 630–634
    customer service and, 634b
    disinfection and, 634, 634b
    hand hygiene, 632, 632b
    MA role in, 634
    sanitization and, 632–634, 633b
    sterilization and, 634
  CDC checklist for prevention and, 630, 631t
  in clinical laboratory, 1001–1003, 1003b, 1003f
  introduction to, 617
  OSHA Standard Precautions for
    compliance guidelines of, 625–630
    definition of, 622
    environmental protection and, 625–627
    hand hygiene and, 622–624, 622f, 623b
    HBV vaccination and, 629, 630f
    housekeeping controls and, 627–628, 628f–629f, 629b
    OPIM and, 622, 622b
    postexposure follow-up and, 629–630, 630b
    PPE, barrier protection and, 625, 625b–626b, 625f, 627f
    summary of, 624, 624f
  in reception area, 499
Infections, 59t–60t, 769, 769b
  chain of, 617–620, 617f
  of female reproductive system, 161, 161t
  healthcare-associated, 1105, 1105b
  inflammatory response process and, 620–621, 620f
  of nervous system, 284t
  nosocomial, 632, 632b, 1048
  opportunistic, 622, 1121
  stages of, 621b

Infections *(Continued)*
  of upper respiratory tract, 256t–257t
  vaginal, specimen collection and, 707, 707b
  viral, 1106
Infectious agents, 617f, 1105, 1105b
  bacteria, 618, 618b
  fungi, 618
  helminths, 619
  protozoa, 619
  viruses, 617
Infectious mononucleosis, 179–180, 203t, 249
Infectious mononucleosis testing, 1119, 1119b–1120b
Infectious myringitis, 320t
Inflammation, 54b, 189, 190b, 191
  of nervous system, 284t
Inflammatory bowel disease (IBD), 108, 117t
Inflammatory response, 28–29, 29b
  process of, 620–621, 620f
Influenza, 253t–254t
  childhood immunization guidelines for, 730t
Influenza A and B testing, 1116
Influenza A (H1N1) infection, 256t–257t
Informed consent, 371–372, 371b–372b, 778
Infusion, definition of, 177, 177b
Ingested, definition of, 617
Inguinal hernia, 118t
Inhalants, definition of, 1001b–1002b
Inhalation, 619, 649
Inhaled medication administration, 892
Initial pleading phase, in civil lawsuit, 368b
Initiative, 347, 347b, 503
Injunction, 363b, 364t
Injuries
  to brain, 266b
  pediatrics and prevention of, 739–740
  personal injury insurance and, 369
  phlebotomy and, 1056–1057, 1057f
  preventing workplace, 514
Inkjet printers, 472, 472t
Inner ear, 300
Inner ear disorders, 320t
Inorganic substances, 168b
Inpatient procedures, appointment scheduling for, 461, 462b–463b
Inpatient surgeries, appointment scheduling for, 461
Input devices, 469–472, 471f–472f
INR. *See* International Normalized Ratio
Insect bites and stings, 973, 973b–974b
Insidious, definition of, 745, 745b
Insoluble fiber, 835, 835b
Inspection, in physical examination, 686
Inspiration, 241, 241b, 241f
Instrument suffixes, 8–9, 8t
Insulin, 835, 835b, 854
  mixing two, for parenteral medication administration, 913, 913b–914b, 913f
Insulin shock, 974–976, 975t
Insurance. *See also* Health insurance
  assistance requests, phone calls regarding, 449
  cards, interpretation of information on, 567b
  law, 388
  professional, 368–369
Insurer, 368–369
Intact, definition of, 1028, 1029b
Intangible services, 600
Integral, definition of, 453
Integrity, 343
Integumentary system
  abbreviations for, 93t
  anatomy of, 70–73
    accessory structures, 72–73
    glands, 71f, 72
    hair, 71f, 72
    membranes of the body, 70, 70t
    nails, 72–73, 73f
    skin, 73
  body temperature regulation of, 73
  combining forms for, 93t
  CPT for lesion excision in, 561
  diseases and disorders of, 73–89
    acne vulgaris, 77–78, 78f
    additional, 89, 90t–92t
    burns, 78–80, 79b, 80t, 545–546
    decubitus ulcers, 83–84, 84f
    dermatophytosis, 84–85, 85b

Integumentary system *(Continued)*
    eczema, 85–86
    psoriasis, 86–87, 86b, 86f–87f, 87t
    shingles, 87–88, 88b, 88f, 268b, 748b
    signs and symptoms of, 73b
    skin cancer, 80–83
    skin infestations, 88–89, 88f–89f
    skin lesions, 74f, 75, 75t–76t
  excretion of, 73
  geriatrics changes in, 746–747, 747f, 748b
  life span changes to, 92
  physiology of, 73
  prefixes for, 93t
  protection of, 73
  sensory receptors of, 73
  skin, 73
    cancer of, 80–83, 812b
    dermal-epidermal junction of, 71
    dermis of, 71f, 72
    epidermis of, 71f, 73
    grafts, 81f
    infestations, 88–89, 88f–89f
    lesions, 74f, 75, 75t–76t
    physical examination of, 689
    self-exams of, 810–812, 812b, 813f
    subcutaneous tissue of, 70, 71f, 72
  structure and function of, 17t
  suffixes for, 93t
  vitamin D synthesis of, 73
Intellectual and developmental disabilities, 289t
Intellectual disability, communication and, 356t
Intentional torts, 363–364, 365t
Interatrial septum, 209
Intercalated discs, 934
Intercellular material, 15, 15b
Intercom, 441t
Intercostal muscles, 241, 241b, 649
Interest, 604, 604f
Interface, definition of, 421
Interferons, 617, 617b
Intermittent, definition of, 134t
Intermittent fevers, 638, 638f
Intermittent pulse, 646, 646b
Internal distractions, to communication, 356t
Internal respiration, 649
International Classification of Diseases, Tenth Revision, Procedural Coding System (ICD-10-PCS), 549, 549t
International Normalized Ratio (INR), 26t–27t, 993, 1086, 1086b–1088b, 1086f
International Society for Clinical Laboratory Technology (ISCLT), 991t
Internet access devices, 473–474
Internists, 348t
Interoperability, 419t, 421b
Interpersonal skills, 1127–1128, 1127f, 1128b
Interpreters, 356t
Interrogatory, definition of, 367b–368b
Interrupted baseline artifacts, 948, 948f
Interstitial cells, 148, 150b
Interstitial cystitis, 141t–142t
Interstitial fluid, 126, 1068t
Intervals, 453
  in ECG tracing, 938
Intervening cause, 367t
Interventricular septum, 209
Interview questions, illegal, 396b
Interviews. *See* Job interviews; Patient interviews
Intimate partner violence screening, 815
Intracellular pathogens, 1077t–1078t
Intradermal injections, for medication administration, 896–899, 915–921
  allergy testing and, 921, 921b, 922f
  of flu vaccine, 916b
  sites for, 917f
  summary of, 915f
  tuberculin testing and, 917–921, 917b–920b, 918t, 921f
Intramuscular injections, for medication administration, 896–899, 926–928, 926f
  giving, 929b–930b
  sites for
    deltoid site, 927–928, 927f
    dorsogluteal site, 930b
    vastus lateralis site, 928, 928f
    ventrogluteal site, 928, 930f
  for small children, 928b

INDEX

Intramuscular injections, for medication administration (Continued)
  summary of, 926t
  techniques in, 926–927
    air lock technique in, 927
    aspiration in, 926
    Z-track technique in, 927, 927f, 931b–932b
Intraocular lenses, 307t
Intraocular melanoma, 319f, 319t
Intraocular pressure, 299
Intrauterine devices (IUDs), 708t, 710, 711f
Intrauterine insemination (IUI), 406t
Intravenous (IV), 128b, 130t
  for medication administration, 931
Intravenous pyelogram, 130t
Intrinsic factor, 99, 99b
Intropin (dopamine), 968t
Intussusception, 117t
Invalid, definition of, 1041
Invasion of privacy, 365t, 394b
Inventory
  of equipment, 503, 504b, 504f
  of supplies
    control systems for, 507, 507f
    management for, 506, 506f, 507b
    taking, 507, 508b–509b, 508f
Inversion, 52t–53t
Invoices, 509, 509b, 614
Iodine, 838t
Iodoform gauze strips, 760b, 760f
Ions, 936b, 1024, 1024b
Ipol, 730t
IPV. See Inactive poliovirus
Iris, 297, 298f, 301t, 308t
Iron, 838t
Iron deficiency, anemia, 173–175, 175f
Irrigation routes, in medication administration, 893–896, 896f, 897b–899b
Irritable bowel syndrome (IBS), 117t
Ischemia, 218t–219t
Ischium, 42t
ISCLT. See International Society for Clinical Laboratory Technology
Ishihara color vision test, 318b, 696–697, 697b
Islet cell carcinoma, 337t
Isometric muscle contractions, 51
Isotonic muscle contractions, 51
IUDs. See Intrauterine devices
IUI. See Intrauterine insemination
IV. See Intravenous

J

Jargon, 443, 443b
Jaundice, 118t, 1029, 1029b
Jobs, 1146–1147
  human resource requirements for, 1146, 1146t
  leaving, 1147
  maintaining, 1147
  starting, 1146–1147
Job applications, online profiles and, 1138–1140, 1138b–1140b, 1138t, 1139f
Job boards, 1130–1131, 1130b
Job interviews, 1140–1145
  answering questions in, 1142, 1143b
  face-to-face, 1144, 1144b
  follow-up after, 1144–1145, 1144b
  illegal interview questions in, 1143, 1143t
  mock, 1143b, 1145, 1145b
  negotiation after, 1145
  opportunities increased for, 1145
  on phone, 1144, 1144b
  preparation for, 1140–1142
    attire decisions in, 1141, 1141t
    healthcare facility research in, 1140–1141, 1140b
    practice answers to questions in, 1141, 1142f
  professionalism during, 1142–1144
  on video, 1144
Job postings, 1145
Job search, 1130–1131
  certification exams and, 1130, 1130b
  employment agencies for, 1131, 1131b
  improving opportunities for, 1145–1146
    finding job postings, 1145
    job interviews increased, 1145
    offers increased, 1145–1146

Job search (Continued)
  networking for, 1130, 1130b, 1130f
  newspaper ads for, 1131
  school career placement officers for, 1131
Joint Commission, 378
Joints, 40–44, 44f–45f, 44t
  dislocation of, 58, 58f, 58t
Judicial branch, of government, 363
Judicious, definition of, 671b
Justice, ethics and, 404
Juxtaglomerular cells, 128

K

Kaposi sarcoma, 90t–91t
K-Dur (potassium), 863t–867t
Keflex (cephalexin), 863t–867t
Kegel exercises, 136b
Keloid scar, 75t
Keratin, 71
Keratinous cyst, 90t–91t
Keratitis, 317t
Ketoacidosis, 331t
Ketones, 328, 328b
  in urine specimens, 330t, 1024b, 1028
Ketonuria, 331t, 1028
Keyboards, 469–471, 471f
Kidneys
  anatomy of, 123–124, 124f
  cancer of, 133–135, 133f–134f, 134t
  damage to, 1017b
  PKD and, 136–137, 137f, 141t–142t
  renal calculi and, 139–140, 139f, 139f–140f, 141t–142t
Kissing disease, 179–180
Kleptomania, 292t
Klonopin (clonazepam), 863t–867t
Klor-Con (potassium), 863t–867t
Knee joint, 44, 44f
Knee walkers, 827, 827f
Knee-chest position, 685, 687b
Korotkoff sounds, 656–657
K-Tab (potassium), 863t–867t
Kübler-Ross, Elizabeth, 356–357, 801
Kyphosis, 63, 64f, 64t

L

L&A test. See Light and accommodation test
Labels, 431, 885, 886f, 1002b
Labia majora, 147, 149f
Labia minora, 147, 149f
Labile affect, 276b
Laboratory. See Clinical laboratory
Labyrinthitis, 320t
Lacrimal glands, 296, 297f, 301t
Lacrimation, 751, 751b
Lactation
  labeling rule of drugs for, 838b
  nutrition needs for, 847
Lacteals, 101
Lactose-intolerance diet, 847
Laminae, 39, 41f
LAN (local area network), 473–474
Lancets, for capillary puncture, 1068–1069, 1068f
Language, diversity in, 345
Lanoxin (digoxin), 863t–867t
Laparoscopic surgery, 104t–105t, 160, 777
Laparotomy, 104t–105t
Laptop computers, 470f, 470t
Large intestine, 98, 99f, 117t
Larvae, 1111
Laryngeal cancer, 256t–257t
Laryngitis, 255t
Laryngologic surgery, 777
Laryngopharynx, 97, 97f, 239–240, 239f
Larynx, 239–240, 239f–240f, 643–644, 644b
Laser peripheral iridotomy, 308t
Laser printers, 472, 472f
Laser surgery, 776
Laser therapy, 76t
Laser-assisted in-situ keratomileusis (LASIK), 306f, 306t
LASIK (Laser-assisted in-situ keratomileusis), 306f, 306t
Lasix (furosemide), 863t–867t
Late patients, appointment scheduling and, 463
Latent infections, 621
Lateral flow immunoassay test, 1040–1041, 1097–1099, 1099b

Latino patients, cultural differences with, 805b
Law. See also Compliance reporting
  appointment scheduling and, 456
  balance of power and, 362, 363t
  civil, 363, 364t
  consent and, 371–372, 371b–372b, 778
  contract, 364t, 369–371
    breach of contract in, 370–371
    contract elements, 369
    provider-patient relationship in, 370, 370t
  criminal, 362–363, 364t
  drug, 388, 388b, 388t
    in ambulatory care setting, 857–859, 858t
    CSA, 388, 388t, 858–859, 859b–860b, 859t
    Food, Drug, and Cosmetic Act, 388, 858, 858t
  end-of-life issues and, 390, 390t
  family, 364t
  Good Samaritan, 366t, 390
  insurance, 388
  introduction to, 362, 381
  medical laboratory regulations and, 388–389, 389t
  Patient's Bill of Rights and, 372, 373b–376b, 373f
  practice requirements and, 372–378, 376t
    accreditation in, 378
    certification and registration in, 378
    disciplinary action and, 377–378, 378b
    licensure and, 377, 377b, 377t
    Medical Practice Act and, 377–378
    scope of practice and, 366, 366b, 377, 377b–378b
  privacy and confidentiality in, 381–387
    amendments related to, 381b
    GINA and, 387, 395t–396t
    HIPAA and, 381–386
    HITECH Act and, 386–387, 387b, 420, 477
  procedural, 362
  property, 364t
  safe haven infant protection, 407
  sources of, 362
  substantive, 362
  tort, 363–369, 364t
    damages in, 363b, 364t, 367–368
    defenses in, 366, 366t–367t
    intentional, 363–364, 365t
    negligent, 364–369, 365t
    professional insurance and, 368–369
    proving malpractice in, 366–368, 368b
  types of, 362
  workplace safety, 389–390
LDLs. See Low-density lipoproteins
Lead paint exposure, 733b
Lead wire, ECG application of, 945, 946f, 946t
Leading questions, in patient interviews, 672
Learning
  domains, 802
    affective, 802, 803f, 803t
    cognitive, 802, 802f, 803t
    psychomotor, 802, 803t
  perceptual difficulties and, 281t
  teaching-learning process and, 806, 806b, 807t
LEEP. See Loop electrosurgical excision procedure
Left bundle branch, 215f, 216, 936f
Left hypochondriac region, 23f, 24t
Left iliac region, 23f, 24t
Left lower quadrant (LLQ), 23
Left lumbar region, 23f, 24t
Left upper quadrant (LUQ), 23, 23f
Left ventricular assist device (LVAD), 221t–223t
Legionnaires' disease, 256t–257t
Legislative branch, of government, 363
Legs, ventral surface anatomy terms for, 18f, 19f
Leiomyomas, 66t, 118t
Leiomyosarcomas, 66t
Lens, 298f, 299, 301t, 307t
Lens disorders, 318t
Lesion excision, in integumentary system, 561
Lethargy, 725, 725b
Letter delivery, 486–487, 487t, 488f, 489t
Letter templates, 485–486
Letters, collection procedures and, 600
Leukemia, 31t
  acute lymphocytic/acute myelogenous, 180–181, 180f, 204t
  chronic lymphocytic/chronic myelogenous, 181–182, 204t
Leukocyte esterase, in urine specimens, 1029

INDEX

Leukocytes, 169–170, 171f
Leukocytic disorders, 184t
Leukocytosis, 184t
Leukopenia, 184t
Leukoplakia, 117f, 117t
Leukotriene receptor antagonists, 863t–867t
Levels of defense, immune system, 190–193, 190f
Levothyroxine (Synthroid, Levothroid, Levoxyl), 863t–867t
Lewis blood antigens, 1094b
Lexapro (escitalopram), 863t–867t
Liability, 363, 363b, 370, 370b
Liability insurance, 369, 530
Libido, 289t, 336, 336b
Lice, 88–89, 89f
Licensed healthcare professions, 347t
Licensed Practical Nurse (LPN), 347t, 376t
Licensing exam, 377t
Licensure, 377, 377b, 377t
Lidocaine, 968t
Life insurance, 530
Life-sustaining treatment, withholding or withdrawing, 410, 410b
Ligation, 104t–105t
Light and accommodation (L&A) test, 693b
Light microscope, 1106, 1106b
Light therapy, 286f, 286t
Limited data set, 382b, 382t
Limited or no harm, 367t
Lipase, 101
Lipectomy, 92t
Lipid profile, 26t–27t, 219t–221t, 819t
Lipids, 101
Lipitor (atorvastatin), 863t–867t
Lipoma, 92t
Liposuction, 92t
Lips, 96, 96f
Liquid medication doses, in medication math, 879, 879b, 880f
 pediatric doses, 879, 881b, 882f
 solutions, 879
 when units do not match, 879, 881b
Liquid volume measurement, clinical laboratory, 1008, 1009f
Lisinopril, 863t–867t
Listening, active, 354, 355b, 355f, 442, 442b, 668–669
Lister bandage scissors, 761f, 761t–762t
Lithotomy position, 684, 684b
Litigious, definition of, 362
Liver, 98, 100, 101b, 118t
 cancer of, 107t
 coagulation and, 172, 172b
 function panel, 26t–27t, 103t–104t
Living arrangements, geriatrics and, 754–755
Living will, 409t
LLQ. See Left lower quadrant
Lobectomy, 250f, 250t
Local, definition of, 890, 890b
Local anesthetics, 759, 759b
Local area network (LAN), 473–474
Local evacuations, 515
Lockdown procedures, 514b
Locum tenens, 377, 377b
Lofstrand crutches, 824, 824f
Log-in activity, monitoring of, 477t
Long bone, 36–37, 36f
Long-distance calling, 451–452
Longitudinal fracture, 56t–57t
Long-term care insurance, 530
Loop electrosurgical excision procedure (LEEP), 158b, 159t–160t, 711, 713f, 776
Lopressor (metoprolol), 863t–867t
Lordosis, 63, 64f, 64t
Lortab (hydrocodone), 863t–867t
Love and belongingness needs, 358, 358f
Lovenox (enoxaparin), 923t
Low-density lipoproteins (LDLs), 837
Lower extremities, skeletal muscles of, 47t, 48f–49f
Lower respiratory tract, 240–241, 240f–241f
 diseases of, 253, 253t–254t
Low-protein diet, 846, 846t
Low-sodium diet, 845, 845b
Lozenges, 889t
LPN. See Licensed Practical Nurse
Lumbar puncture, 277f, 277t

Lumen, 98, 98b
Lumpectomy, 158b, 159t–160t
Lung ventilation/perfusion scan, 244t–245t
Lungs, 240f, 241
 abnormal sounds of, 244t
 cancer of, 249–250, 250f, 250t, 813, 814t
LUQ. See Left upper quadrant
Luteal phase, of menstrual cycle, 150
Luteinizing hormone, 148, 327t, 1041
LVAD. See Left ventricular assist device
Lyme disease, 59t–60t
 blood antibodies, 55t
 testing, 1121
Lymph, 188, 188b, 1093t
Lymphadenectomy, 198t
Lymphadenitis, 203t
Lymphadenography, 196t
Lymphadenopathy, 203t
Lymphangiography, 196f, 196t
Lymphangitis, 203t
Lymphatic and immune systems
 abbreviations for, 205t
 acquired immunity and, 194–195, 195f
 adjective forms for, 204t
 anatomy of, 188–190
  immune system cells, 189–190
  lymphatic fluid flow, 188
  organs of, 188–189, 189f
 combining forms for, 204t
 diseases and disorders of, 195–203
  additional, 203, 203t
  allergies, 195b
  autoimmune diseases, 195–198
  HIV/AIDS, 198–201
  imaging for, 196f, 196t
  interventions for, 198t
  laboratory tests for, 197f, 197t
  lymphomas, 31t, 201–202
  multiple myeloma, 202–203
  neoplasms, 204t
  signs and symptoms of, 194b
 introduction to, 188
 life span changes to, 204
 malfunctions of, 29
 physiology of, 190–194
  cell-mediated immunity, 190f, 193, 619
  humoral immunity, 190f, 192–193, 619, 620b
  hypersensitivity reactions, 194, 194t
  levels of defense, 190–193, 190f
  nonspecific immunity, 190–191, 190f, 192f
  specific immunity, 190f, 191–193, 193f
 prefixes for, 205t
 structure and function of, 17t
 suffixes for, 205t
Lymphatic fluid flow, 188
Lymphedema, 203f, 203t
Lymphocytes, 170, 188, 188b
Lymphocytopenia, 203t
Lymphocytosis, 203t
Lymphomas, 31t, 201–202
Lymphostasis, 1066b, 1067t
Lysed, definition of, 1028, 1029b
Lysis, 104t–105t, 171, 172b

M
Macromolecules, 1111, 1111b
Macrophages, 188, 188b
Macrotia, 319t
Macula lutea, 298, 298f, 301t
Macular degeneration, 311–313, 312f, 751
Macule, 74f
Magnesium, 838t, 968t
Magnetic resonance imaging (MRI), 26t–27t, 54t, 103t, 196t, 219t–221t, 244t–245t, 273t, 331t, 818t
Magnetic storage devices, 474t
Mail, to healthcare facilities, 511
 incoming, 511, 511f
 private delivery services for, 511
Mailed reminders, 465
Maintenance logs
 for clinical laboratory equipment, 1012, 1012t
 for healthcare facilities equipment, 503–504, 505f, 506b
Maladaptive coping mechanisms, 358–359, 359t
Maladaptive response, 271, 271b

Malaise, 54b, 621b, 638, 638b
Male pelvis, female pelvis compared to, 43b, 43f
Male reproductive system
 abbreviations for, 163t
 adjectives for, 163t
 anatomy of, 146, 148f
 combining forms for, 163t
 congenital disorders of, 152–158, 155t–156t
 life span changes to, 162
 physiology of, 148–149
 prefixes for, 163t
 suffixes for, 163t
Malfeasance, 365t
Malignant, definition of, 80, 80b, 1077t–1078t
Malignant melanoma, 80–83, 82b, 82f, 812t
Malleolus, 42t
Malleus, 299–300, 300f
Malpractice, 365, 365b
 proving, 366–368, 368b
Mammary glands, 147–148
Mammograms, 813, 814t, 818t
Managed care organizations (MCOs), 526–527
 EPO, 527, 528t
 HMOs, 526–527, 527t–528t
 medical billing policies and procedures of, 569–571, 569b
 precertification/preauthorization processes, 569–570, 570b
 referrals and, 571
 training in, 569b
 PPO, 527, 528t
 utilization management and, 527, 527b
Manifestation, in diagnostic coding, 543
Manipulation, in physical examination, 688, 688b
Manipulative communicators, 354, 354t
Mantoux tuberculin skin test, 917–921, 917b–918b, 918t
Manubrium, 39, 41f
Marfan syndrome, 234t
MAs. See Medical Assistants
Masks, for oxygen therapy, 958, 960t, 961b, 961f
Maslow, Abraham, 357–358, 358f
MAST. See Multiple-antigen simultaneous testing
Mastectomy, 158b, 159t–160t
Mastication, 96
Mastoidectomy, 309t
Mastoiditis, 320f, 320t
Maternity care and delivery, CPT for, 561–562
Math. See Clinical laboratory, mathematics and measurement for; Medication math
Matrix, appointment, 453–454, 454b, 455f
Maturation index, 707
Mature minors, 371, 371b
MBHDs. See Mental and behavioral health disorders
MCOs. See Managed care organizations
MD. See Doctor of Medicine
MDIs. See Metered-dose inhalers
Mean corpuscular hemoglobin concentration, 174t
Meaningful use requirements, 477
Means of exit and entry, 619, 619b
Meatus, 1019, 1019b
Mechanical digestion, 96
Mechanical soft diet, 842–843, 843t
Mechanical washing of instruments, 769, 770f
Mechanisms, definition of, 329, 330b
Media, 469
Media mail, 487t
Median cubital vein, 209
Mediastinal, definition of, 188
Mediastinum, 96, 96b, 240, 328
Mediation, 366
Medicaid, 524, 524b
Medical asepsis, 630
Medical Assistant (NCMA) certification, 350t
Medical Assistants (MAs), 376t, 378b
 aseptic techniques and role of, 634
 code of ethics for, 402, 402b
 credentials for, 349–350, 350t
 geriatrics and, 755, 755b
 gynecology examination assistance of, 704–705, 705b
 health insurance role of, 528–529
 health records and, 418–419, 419b
 healthcare facility opening tasks of, 494–497, 495b
 job description of, 347t

INDEX

Medical Assistants (MAs) (Continued)
  minor surgery assistance of, 777–793
    completing surgical procedure in, 790, 791f
    follow-up and, 793, 794b
    informed consent in, 778
    passing instruments in, 787–790, 790f
    patient positioning in, 778
    patient preparation in, 777–778, 778b
    postoperative instructions and care in, 792–793, 793f
    postoperative responsibilities in, 790–792, 792b
    procedure room preparation in, 778
    setups for, 789t
    skin prep for, 778, 779b
    specimen collection in, 790
    sterile dressing application in, 791b–792b
    sterile field preparation in, 782b–784b, 786, 786f, 787b
    sterile gloves procedure for, 785b–786b
    sterile technique in, 778–786
    during surgery, 786–793, 787b–789b
    surgical hand scrub in, 780b–782b
    two-person sterile tray setup in, 784b
    warning signs and, 793
  pediatrics role of, 733–739, 734f
    examination and, 734–739, 738t, 739f
    measurements and, 734, 735f–736f, 737b–738b
    urine sample collection and, 739, 739f
  physical examination responsibilities of, 680–691, 692b
  prescription role of, 867–871, 868f, 869b
  professional characteristics of, 343–345
Medical billing. See also Claims
  customer service and, 584b
  cycle, 597b
  direct, 571
  electronic claims submissions and, 571–572
  EOB and, 524, 566, 592–593, 593b, 594f
  MCO policies and procedures with, 569–571, 569b
    precertification/preauthorization processes, 569–570, 570b
    referrals and, 571
    training in, 569b
  patient financial responsibilities and, 582–584
    allowed amount in, 583, 583f
    co-insurance and deductible calculation for, 582, 583f
    comparison of, 583t
    discussion of, 583–584, 584b, 585f
    sensitivity when discussing, 584, 585f
  patient information form and, 567, 567f
  process of, 566, 567b
  third-party claims and, 571
Medical care for those who cannot pay, 597
Medical durable power of attorney, 409t
Medical emergencies. See Emergencies
Medical geneticists, 348t
Medical history, 664–665
  collecting, 664
  components of, 664–665
  diagnostic coding preparation with, 538
  EHR for, 665f
  in prenatal record for obstetrics, 714–715
  ROS and, 665, 666f
Medical laboratory. See also Clinical laboratory
  assistants, 991
  blood tests, 26t–27t
  regulations, 388–389, 389t
  technicians, 991
Medical malpractice insurance, 369
Medical necessity, 581, 581b–583b
Medical Practice Act, 377–378
Medical scribes, 419b
Medical specialists, 348t
Medical technologists, 347t, 991
Medical terminology
  abbreviations and symbols in, 3
  for body cavities, planes and abdominopelvic quadrants and regions, 33t
  combining forms in
    common types of, 12t
    definition of, 1b, 2
    suffixes added to, 3–4, 3t–4t

Medical terminology (Continued)
  decodable terms in
    CARD method for, 3–4, 3f
    samples of, 4t
    types of, 2, 2f
  nondecodable terms in, 2–3, 2b
  in patient interviews, 672
  prefixes in
    definition of, 1b, 2
    types of, 9, 10t–11t
  pronunciation of unusual letter combinations in, 11t
  roots of, 1–2, 2t
  singular/plural ending rules in, 9, 11t
  spelling rules for, 4–5, 5f
  for structural organization of body, 32t–33t
  suffixes in
    adjective, 5, 6t
    combining forms added to, 3–4, 3t–4t
    definition of, 1b, 2
    diagnostic procedure, 8, 8t
    instrument, 8–9, 8t
    noun-ending, 5, 6t
    pathology, 6t–7t, 7f, 8
    specialty and specialist, 9, 9t
    therapeutic intervention, 8, 8t
  types of, 2–3
Medical Waste Tracking Act, 629b
Medically necessary services, 522, 533
Medically ordered diets, 842–847
  AHA's heart-healthy diet, 845, 845t
  bland diet, 843
  clear liquid diet, 842, 842t
  diabetic eating plans, 843–845, 844f, 844t
  elimination diet and food allergies, 846–847, 846b
  full liquid diet, 842, 842t
  gluten-free diet, 847, 847b
  high/low-fiber diets, 846, 846t
  lactose-intolerance diet, 847
  low-protein diet, 846, 846t
  low-sodium diet, 845, 845b
  soft and mechanical soft diet, 842–843, 843t
  weight control diet, 843, 843b, 843t
Medicare, 523–524, 523b, 523t
Medication administration
  customer service and, 932b
  for emergencies, 967, 967f, 968t
  at home, coaching on, 818, 819b, 819f
  intradermal injections for, 896–899, 915–921
    allergy testing and, 921, 921b, 922f
    of flu vaccine, 916b
    sites for, 917f
    summary of, 915t
    tuberculin testing and, 917–921, 917b–920b, 918t, 921f
  intramuscular injections for, 896–899, 926–928, 926f
    air lock technique in, 927
    aspiration in, 926
    deltoid site for, 927–928, 927f
    dorsogluteal site for, 930b
    giving, 929b–930b
    for small children, 928b
    summary of, 926t
    techniques in, 926–927
    vastus lateralis site for, 928, 928f
    ventrogluteal site for, 928, 930f
    Z-track technique in, 927, 927f, 931b–932b
  introduction to, 885
  IV for, 931
  medication forms and, 887–889, 888b, 889t–890t
  needles and syringes in, 899–903
    hypodermic needles, 899–900, 899f–900f
    hypodermic syringes, 900, 900f–901f, 901b–902b
    plunger handling with, 903, 903f
    reading syringes, 901b–902b
    switching needles, 903, 904f
    uncapping and recapping needles, 903, 904f
    unpackaging and removing, 903, 903f
    working with, 900–903
  Nine Rules of, 885–887, 885f
    right documentation, 887, 888b
    right dose, 885
    right education, 887, 887b
    right medication, 885, 886f
    right patient, 886–887
    right route, 886, 886f

Medication administration (Continued)
    right technique, 887, 888f
    right time, 886, 886b
    right to refuse, 887
  parenteral, giving, 914–915
    guidelines for, 915, 916b, 916f–917f
    route of, 896–899
    special situations in, 915, 916b
  parenteral, preparation of
    ampules for, 904, 904f, 905b–906b
    mixing insulins for, 913, 913b–914b, 913f
    prefilled sterile cartridge for, 906, 906f, 907b–908b
    preparation of, 904–913
    reconstituting powdered medication for, 909–911, 911b–912b, 912f
    specialty syringe units for, 906, 908f
    vials for, 908–909, 908f, 909b–910b
  routes of, 889–899
    inhaled, 892
    irrigation, 893–896, 896f, 897b–899b
    nasal, 893
    ocular, 893, 894b–895b
    oral, 890, 891b–892b
    otic, 894, 895b–896b
    parenteral, 896–899
    rectal, 893, 893b
    sublingual and buccal, 890
    topical, 892–893, 892b
    transdermal, 890, 890b, 892f
    vaginal, 893, 893b
  subcutaneous injections for, 896–899, 922–924, 922b, 922f
    aspiration for, 922, 923b
    giving, 924b–925b
    sites for, 924
    summary of, 923t
    techniques in, 922
Medication math, 871–879
  guidelines for, 872–874, 873t
    Roman numerals in, 874, 874b
    rounding numbers in, 872, 873f, 874b
  liquid medication doses in, 879, 879b, 880f
    pediatric doses, 879, 881b, 882f
    solutions, 879
    when units do not match, 879, 881b
  measurement systems for, 874–876
    household system, 874, 874b, 874t, 875f
    metric system, 874–876, 874b, 875f–876f, 875t, 876b
  tablets per dose in, 877–878, 878f, 879b
  temperature conversion in, 876, 876b, 877f
  total tablets needed in, 876–877, 877b, 877f
Medication orders, 862–871
  herbal, 871, 872t–873t
  OTC, 871, 872t
  prescriptions and, 867–871, 868f
    controlled substance, 871, 871t
    customer service and, 883b
    MA's role with, 867–871, 868f, 869b
    measurement abbreviations for, 870t
    medication abbreviations for, 871t
    miscellaneous abbreviations for, 871t
    route and form abbreviations for, 869t
    timing abbreviations for, 870t
  types of, 868t
Medrol (methylprednisolone), 863t–867t
Medulla, of kidney, 124, 124f
Medulla oblongata, 301, 301b, 649
Medullary pyramid, 124, 124f
Medulloblastomas, 286t
Megakaryocytes, 170
Melanocytes, 71, 71b, 81
Melanoma, malignant, 80–83, 82b, 82f, 812t
Melena, 102t
Memantine (Namenda), 750t, 863t–867t
Membranes of the body, 70, 70t
Membranous glomerulonephritis, 141t–142t
Memorandums, 488, 490f
Menactra, 730t
Menarche, 149–150, 704, 704b
MenHibrix, 730t
Ménière's disease, 313–314, 751, 752b
Meninges, 266–267, 267b, 267f
Meningiomas, 285t
Meningitis, 284t
  meningococcal vaccine for, 730t

INDEX

Meningocele, 715, 715b
Meningococcal vaccine for meningitis, 730t
Meningomyelocele, 281t–282t, 282f
Meniscus, 44
Menomune, 730t
Menopause, 147, 162t, 711–712
Menopause testing, 1041
Menstrual cycle
  follicular phase of, 150
  luteal phase of, 150
  menstrual phase of, 150
  pregnancy and delivery and, 150–151, 151f
Menstrual history, in prenatal record for obstetrics, 713
Menstrual phase, of menstrual cycle, 150
Mensuration, in physical examination, 687–688, 688f
Mental and behavioral health disorders (MBHDs), 270–271, 279–288
  abbreviations for, 293t
  adjective forms for, 292t
  adjustment disorder and, 291t
  Alzheimer's disease and, 3, 285–287, 749–750, 750t
  anxiety disorders and, 291t
  combining forms for, 292t
  depressive disorders and, 287–288
  diagnostic procedures for, 279–283
  disorders first diagnosed in childhood, 289t
  eating disorders and, 291f, 291t
  habit and impulse disorders and, 292t
  life span changes to, 288
  mood disorders and, 271, 271t, 289t
  personality disorders and, 271, 272t, 290t
  physiology of, 270–271
  psychotherapy for, 286t
  substance-related disorders of, 271, 271t
  suffixes for, 293t
  symptoms of, 289t
  terminology for, 271
  therapeutic methods for, 286t
Mental illness, 271
Mental status examination, 279
Message therapy, 823
Metabolic, definition of, 1094–1095, 1094b
Metabolic syndrome, 234t, 652, 652b
Metabolism, 834, 834b
  drugs and, 856, 856b
Metabolites, 126, 856, 856b, 1041–1042, 1042b
Metacarpals, 42t
Metamucil, 836b
Metastasizes, definition of, 30b, 30t
Metatarsals, 42t
Metered-dose inhalers (MDIs), 892, 956–958, 958b–959b, 958f
Metformin (Glucophage, Fortamet, Glumetza, Riomet), 863t–867t
Methicillin-resistant *Staphylococcus aureus* (MRSA), 1105, 1105b
Methylphenidate (Concerta, Ritalin LA), 863t–867t
Methylprednisolone (Medrol), 863t–867t
Metoprolol (Lopressor), 863t–867t
Metric system
  for clinical laboratory measurement, 1008, 1008t
  for medication math measurement, 874–876, 874b, 875f–876f, 875t, 876b
Microbiology, 993–994, 994f
  classification of, 1106–1107
  CLIA-waived testing of, 1116
    influenza A and B testing, 1116
    rapid strep testing, 1116, 1117b–1118b
    RSV testing, 1116, 1116f
  customer service and, 1125b
  introduction to, 1105–1106
  in reference laboratory, 1122–1124, 1122f
    C&S testing, 1124, 1124b
    culture assessment for, 1123–1124, 1123b, 1124f
    inoculating equipment for, 1122, 1123f
    staining for, 1122, 1122b
Microbiome, 195, 195b
Microcephaly, 162t, 707–708, 734, 734b
Microcuvettes, 1082
Microglia, 263
Microhematocrit centrifuge, 1069, 1069f, 1080
Microhematocrit test, 1078–1081, 1080b–1082b, 1081f, 1082t
Micro-K (potassium), 863t–867t

Microorganisms, 188, 1105, 1105b. *See also* Bacteria
  classification of, 1106–1107
  naming, 1106–1107, 1106b
Micropipets, 1008, 1009f
Microscopes
  in clinical laboratory, 1008–1011, 1009f, 1010b–1011b, 1010t
  light, 1106, 1106b
  urine examination by, 1030–1038
    air bubbles in, 1038f
    bacteria, 1036, 1037f
    casts in, 1032, 1033t–1034t, 1038b
    cells in, 1032, 1035f–1036f
    crystals in, 1032–1033, 1035t
    fibers in, 1036, 1037f–1038f
    miscellaneous findings in, 1034–1036
    mucous threads in, 1036, 1037f
    oval fat bodies in, 1034, 1037f
    preparation for, 1030–1032, 1031b
    spermatozoa in, 1036
    Trichomonas vaginalis in, 1036, 1037f
    understanding results of, 1038, 1038b
Microsurgery, 279t, 777
Microtia, 319t
Microvilli, 14t
Microzide (hydrochlorothiazide), 863t–867t
MIDCAB. *See* Minimally invasive direct coronary artery bypass
Middle ear, 299–300
Middle ear disorders, 320t
Midol (ibuprofen), 863t–867t, 872t
Midwives, 146b, 347t
Migraine headache, 285b, 285t
Military time, 1007, 1007f
Mineralocorticoids, 328t
Minerals, 837, 838t
Minimal change disease, 141t–142t
Minimally invasive direct coronary artery bypass (MIDCAB), 221t–223t
Ministrokes, 272b
Minnesota Multiphasic Personality Inventory, 283
Minor surgery
  aseptic techniques for, 769
  customer service and, 797b
  drapes in, 767–769, 767f
  instruments for, 759–761
    care and handling of, 769–797
    classification of, 761–765
    cutting and dissecting, 761, 761f–762f, 761t–762t
    grasping and clamping, 761, 762t–764t
    mechanical washing of, 769, 770f
    miscellaneous, 766, 766t
    names of, 761
    passing, 787–790, 790f
    probes and dilators, 765, 765f–766f, 765t–766t
    retractors, 761–765, 765f
    ring-handle, spring-handle, thumb-handle/grasp, 759, 760f
    with serrations, 760, 760f
    surgical staples, 768, 768f
    toothed, 760–761, 760f
  introduction to, 758
  MAs assisting with, 777–793
    completing surgical procedure in, 790, 791f
    follow-up and, 793, 794b
    informed consent in, 778
    passing instruments in, 787–790, 790f
    patient positioning in, 778
    patient preparation in, 777–778, 778b
    postoperative instructions and care in, 792–793, 793f
    postoperative responsibilities in, 790–792, 792b
    procedure room preparation in, 778
    setups for, 789t
    skin prep for, 778, 779b
    specimen collection in, 790
    sterile dressing application in, 791b–792b
    sterile field preparation in, 782b–784b, 786, 786f, 787b
    sterile gloves procedure for, 785b–786b
    sterile technique in, 778–786
    during surgery, 786–793, 787b–789b
    surgical hand scrub in, 780b–782b
    two-person sterile tray setup in, 784b
    warning signs and, 793

Minor surgery *(Continued)*
  needles in, 768, 768f
  procedure room for, 758, 758f, 778
  solutions and medications in, 758–759, 759b–760b
  sterilization of instruments for, 770–775, 778–786
    autoclave, 770–775, 771f
    utility room and, 770b
  Steri-Strips in, 768, 768f
  surgical procedures in, 775–777
    cryosurgery, 777
    electrosurgery, 776, 776b, 776f
    endoscopy, 777, 777f
    laser surgery, 776
    microsurgery, 777
  surgical staples in, 768, 768f, 794b
  sutures in, 767–768, 767b, 767f, 794b
  tissue adhesives in, 768–769, 769b
  wound care and, 793–797
    bandages for, 796–797, 796f–797f, 797b
    dressings for, 796–797
    wound healing, 793–796
    wound types and, 793, 795f
Minors. *See also* Pediatrics
  age of majority and, 424–425
  billing, 597
  confidential healthcare for, 407–408, 408b
  definition of, 369t
  emancipated, 369b, 369t, 597, 597b
  mature, 371, 371b
Miscellaneous files, 435–436
Misdemeanors, 364t
Misfeasance, 365t
Mitochondria, 14t
Mitosis, 14–15
Mitral valve prolapse, 230f, 230t
Mixed connective tissue disorder, 199t–200t
Mixed hearing loss, 698
Mixed tumors, 31t
M-M-R II, 730t
MNS blood antigens, 1094b
Mobile check scanners, 611f
Mock interviews, 1143b, 1145, 1145b
Mode of transmission, 617f, 619
Modems, 474, 474b
Modified block letter format, 484t, 485, 486f
Modified wave scheduling, 456–457
Modifiers, CPT code, 551–552, 552t
Mohs surgery, 76t, 77f
Molds, 1109, 1110b
Molecules, definition of, 1107
Mon pubis, 147, 149f
Money market savings accounts, 605
Money orders, 606
Monitoring of log-in activity, 477t
Monitors, 472
Mono, 179–180
Monocytes, 170, 188, 188b
Monofilament foot test, 815, 816b–817b
Monoparesis, 285t
Monoplegia, 285t
Monospot, 174t
Monotone, voice, 442, 442b
Montelukast (Singulair), 863t–867t
Monthly patient account statements, 597–598, 597b
  billing minors and, 597
  fees in hardship cases and, 598, 598b
  medical care for those who cannot pay and, 597
Mood disorders, 271, 271t, 289t
Morals, 401
Morbidity
  definition of, 25
  diagnostic coding for external causes of, 546
Morphology, definition of, 1091, 1091b
Mortality, definition of, 25, 533, 533b, 744, 744b
Morula, 152
Motherboards, 473t
Motion sensitivity/sickness, 300
Motor neurons, 46
Motrin (ibuprofen), 863t–867t, 872t
Mouse, 471, 471f
Mouth. *See* Oral cavity
Moxatag (amoxicillin), 863t–867t
MRI. *See* Magnetic resonance imaging
MRSA. *See* Methicillin-resistant *Staphylococcus aureus*
Mucositis, 117t

INDEX

Mucous threads, in urine, 1036, 1037f
Mucus, 25
MUGA scan, 219t–221t
Multiple myeloma, 202–203
Multiple sclerosis, 199t–200t, 283t
Multiple sleep latency test, 276t
Multiple-antigen simultaneous testing (MAST), 197t
Multiple-line telephone system, 440, 440f
Multisample needles, for venipuncture, 1053, 1053f
Murmurs, 218t–219t, 687, 687b
Muscle relaxants, 863t–867t
Muscle tissue, 15, 16t
Muscles, 45–46
  actions of, 51, 52t–53t
  aging impact on, 52b
  cardiac, 45, 46f
  contraction of, types of, 51
  naming conventions of, 46, 47t
  skeletal
    attachments of, 45, 46f
    exercise benefits on, 51, 51b, 51t
    of human body, 46, 47t, 48f–50f
    structure of, 45–46, 46f
  smooth, 45, 46f
Muscular dystrophy, 62–63
Musculoskeletal emergencies, 976–977, 977b, 977f
Musculoskeletal system
  abbreviations for, 68t
  anatomy of, 36–46
    joints, 40–44, 44f–45f, 44t
    muscles, 45–46
    skeleton, 36–40
  combining forms for, 67t
  connections in, 37b
  CPT for, 561–562
  diagnostic testing for, 55t
  diseases and disorders of, 52–63, 54b
    arthritis, 4, 59, 59t–60t
    arthropathies, 65t
    bone diseases and disorders, 65t
    bursitis, 59–61
    carpal tunnel syndrome, 61, 61f
    congenital, 65t
    DJD, 62
    dorsopathies and spondylopathies, 65t
    joint dislocation of, 58, 58f, 58t
    kyphosis, 63, 64f, 64t
    lordosis, 63, 64f, 64t
    muscle disorders, 66t
    muscular dystrophy, 62–63
    neoplasms, 66t
    osteoporosis, 63
    scoliosis, 63, 64f, 64t
    sprains and strains, 58, 58f, 58t
    subluxation, 58, 58t
  fractures of, 54–58
    diagnostic procedures for, 54t, 55
    etiology of, 54
    fixation for, 57, 57f
    prevention of, 58
    signs and symptoms of, 54–55
    treatments for, 55–58, 57f
    types of, 56t–57t
  geriatrics changes in, 747–749, 748b
  imaging of, 54t
  life span changes in, 63–66
  physiology of, 46–51
    cells in, 46–51
    exercise benefits on, 51, 51b, 51t
    muscle action types in, 51, 52t–53t
    muscle contractions in, 51
  prefixes for, 67t
  structure and function of, 17t
  suffixes for, 68t
Myalgia, 54b
Myasthenia gravis, 66t, 199t–200t
Mycoplasma, 1108, 1109t
Mydriatic eyedrops, 694, 694b
Myelin sheath, 263
Myelograms, 54t
Myelography, 273t
Myeloma, 31f, 31t
Myocardial infarction, 231–232, 231f–232f, 232t, 985–987, 985b–987b, 986f
Myocardial perfusion imaging, 219t–221t

Myocardium, 209, 211f, 651, 651b, 934, 935f
Myofibrils, 46, 46b
Myoglobin, definition of, 1028, 1029b
Myoglobinuria, 1028, 1029b
Myomas, 162t
Myopia, 302b, 691, 693f
Myositis, 54b
MyPlate, 840, 840f, 841t
Myxedema, 334t, 543, 543b

N

NAATs. *See* Nucleic acid amplification tests
Nails, 72–73, 73f
Naloxone (Evzio, Narcan), 968t
Namenda (memantine), 750t, 863t–867t
Naproxen (Aleve, Naprosyn), 872t
Narcan (naloxone), 968t
Narcosynthesis, 286t
Nasal cannula, 958, 959f, 960t, 961b, 961f
Nasal polyps, 256t–257t
Nasal route, in medication administration, 893
Nasal washes, 1116
Nasogastric intubation, 104t–105t
Nasolacrimal duct, 296, 297f
Nasopharyngeal carcinoma, 256t–257t
Nasopharyngeal swabs, 1116
Nasopharynx, 97, 97f, 239, 239f
National Center for Competency Testing (NCCT), 350t
National Certification Agency for Medical Laboratory Personnel (NCA), 991t
National Committee for Quality Assurance (NCQA), 378
National Healthcareer Association (NHA), 350t, 991t
National Labor Relations Act, 395t–396t
National Organ Transplant Act (NOTA), 390t, 410–411
National Provider Identifier (NPI), 574, 574b, 869, 869b
National Uniform Claim Committee (NUCC), 574
Nationality, 344t
Native American patients, cultural differences with, 805b
Natural killer (NK) cells, 191, 191b
Nausea, 102t, 218t–219t
NCA. *See* National Certification Agency for Medical Laboratory Personnel
NCCT. *See* National Center for Competency Testing
NCMA (Medical Assistant) certification, 350t
NCQA. *See* National Committee for Quality Assurance
Near visual acuity (NVA), 696, 696f
Nearsightedness. *See* Myopia
Nebulizer treatment, 958, 959b–960b
Neck
  physical examination of, 690
  skeletal muscles of, 47t, 50f
Necrosis, 973, 973b
Needle aspiration, 83t
Needle biopsy setup, 789t
Needle holders, 762t–764t, 763f
Needles, in minor surgery, 768, 768f
Needles and syringes
  in medication administration, 899–903
    hypodermic needles, 899–900, 899f–900f
    hypodermic syringes, 900, 900f–901f, 901b–902b
    plunger handling with, 903, 903f
    reading syringes, 901b–902b
    switching needles, 903, 904f
    uncapping and recapping needles, 903, 904f
    unpackaging and removing, 903, 903f
    working with, 900–903
  in phlebotomy, 1052–1054
    butterfly assemblies, 1053–1054, 1054f
    multisample needles, 1053, 1053f
    needle angle of entry, 1057
    needle holders, 1053, 1053f
    needle structure, 1052–1053, 1053f
    safety, 1054–1056, 1054b, 1055f, 1056b
  syringes, 1053, 1054f
Needlestick Safety and Prevention Act, 389–390, 390f, 622
Negative feedback, 329, 330b
Neglect
  adult, 392–393
  child, 389t, 391–392, 391b–392b
Negligence, 365, 365b
Negligent torts, 364–369, 365t
Negotiable instruments, 606

Neoplasms
  benign compared to malignant, 30–32, 30t
  diagnostic coding of, 544–545, 544b, 544f
  of digestive system, 118t–119t
  of ear, 320t
  of eye, 318t–319t
  of lymphatic and immune systems, 204t
  of musculoskeletal system, 66t
  of nervous system, 285t–286t
Nephrectomy, 134t
Nephrologists, 188b
Nephrons, 124, 127t, 1015, 1015b, 1016f
Nephrotic syndrome, 135
Nephrotoxic, definition of, 1033t–1034t
Nephroureterectomy, 134t
Nerve block, 280t
Nerve conduction test, 276t
Nerve damage, venipuncture and, 1066, 1067t
Nervous system. *See also* Mental and behavioral health disorders
  abbreviations for, 292t
  adjective forms for, 292t
  anatomy of, 261–263
    cells of, 262–263
    organization of, 261–262, 262f
  autonomic, 262, 262f, 269–270, 270f
  central, 261, 262f, 265–267
    brain in, 265–266, 265f, 278t
    brainstem in, 265–266, 265b, 265f
    meninges in, 266–267, 267b, 267f
    spinal cord in, 266–267, 267f
  combining forms for, 292t
  conduction system and, 217
  diseases and disorders of, 271–279
    brain and skull interventions for, 278t
    congenital disorders, 281t–282t
    CVA, 272–274, 272b
    degenerative disorders, 283f, 283t
    diagnostic procedures for, 277t
    electrodiagnostic procedures for, 276t
    epilepsy, 274–275
    general interventions for, 279t
    imaging techniques for, 273t
    infectious diseases and inflammations, 284t
    laboratory tests for, 275t
    learning and perceptual difficulties, 281t
    life span changes to, 288
    neoplasms, 285t–286t
    nondegenerative disorders, 284t
    pain management for, 280t
    paralytic conditions, 285f, 285t
    Parkinson's disease, 275–278
    signs and symptoms of, 272b, 280t–281t
    traumatic conditions, 282t
    vascular disorders, 285b, 285t
  endocrine system connection to, 325b
  geriatrics changes to, 749–750, 750t
  introduction to, 261
  life span changes to, 288
  parasympathetic, 270, 270f
  peripheral, 261, 262f, 267–268, 268t
  somatic, 262, 262f
  structure and function of, 17t
  suffixes for, 292t
  sympathetic, 269, 270f
Net, definition of, 588, 614b
Network access devices, 473–474
Network privacy and security, PCs and, 476–478, 477b, 477t
Networking, for job search, 1130, 1130b, 1130f
Neuralgia, 280t–281t
Neurectomy, 279t
Neuritis, 284t
Neuroblastomas, 286t
Neuroendoscopy, 277t
Neurofibromas, 285t
Neurogenic bladder, 135–136, 136b, 136t
Neurogenic shock, 233t, 984t
Neuroglia, 263
Neurological emergencies, 977–980
  concussions, 978, 978b–979b
  CVA, 980, 980b
  seizures, 978–980, 979b–980b
  vertigo and dizziness, 977–978
Neurology/neurologists, 261b

Neurolysis, 279t
Neuromas, 285t
Neuromuscular junction (NMJ), 46
Neurons, 15, 15b, 262–263, 262f–263f
Neurontin (gabapentin), 863t–867t
Neuropathy, 136
  peripheral, 678b, 678t
Neuroplasty, 279t
Neurorrhaphy, 279t
Neurosurgeons, 348t
Neurotomy, 279t
Neurotransmitters, 46, 263, 263b, 265b
Neutral communication, 355t
Neutropenia, 184t
Neutrophilia, 106, 106b
Neutrophils, 169
New patients
  appointment scheduling for, 457–459, 458b–459b, 458f
  registration of, 499, 499b–501b, 499f
Newspaper ads, for job search, 1131
Nexium (esomeprazole), 863t–867t
NHA. See National Healthcareer Association
Niacin, 839t
Nicotine, 854
Nicotine screening, 815
Nine Rules of Medication Administration, 885–887, 885f
  right documentation, 887, 888b
  right dose, 885
  right education, 887, 887b
  right medication, 885, 886f
  right patient, 886–887
  right route, 886, 886f
  right technique, 887, 888f
  right time, 886, 886b
  right to refuse, 887
Nitrite, in urine specimens, 1029
Nitroglycerin, 968t, 986b
NK cells. See Natural killer cells
NMJ. See Neuromuscular junction
Nocturia, 754, 754b
Nocturnal enuresis, 141t–142t
Nodules, 74f, 75t, 689
Nomenclature, definition of, 1106, 1106b
Nominal damages, 368
Nonabsorbable sutures, 767
Nondecodable terms, 2–3, 2b
Nondisplaced fracture, 56t–57t
Non-English speaking, 356t
Nonfeasance, 365t
Non-Hodgkin's lymphoma, 31t, 201–202
Noninvasive procedures, 632
Nonmaleficence, ethics and, 404
Nonorganic, definition of, 726
Non-rebreather masks, 958, 960t, 961b, 961f
Nonspecific immunity, 190–191, 190f, 192f
Nonsteroid hormones, 329
Nonsufficient funds (NSF) checks, 595b, 595f
Nonsufficient funds (NSF) fees, 604t
Nonverbal communication, 350–353, 442b
  cultural differences in, 352–353, 353t
  delivery factors in, 352, 352t
  for patient communication, 669, 669b–671b, 669t, 670f
  physical boundaries to, 351–352, 352t
  positive and negative behaviors in, 351t
Noradrenaline, 328t
Norco (hydrocodone), 863t–867t
Norepinephrine, 328t
Normal flora, 1019, 1019b, 1105
Norvasc (amlodipine), 863t–867t
Nose, physical examination of, 690
Nose coverage, 369
No-show policies, 464, 464b
Nosocomial infections, 632, 632b, 1048
NOTA. See National Organ Transplant Act
Notice of Privacy Practices (NPP), 449b, 459
Noun-ending suffixes, 5, 6t
Nouns, 480, 480t
NovoPen, 908f
NP. See Nurse Practitioner
NPI. See National Provider Identifier
NPP. See Notice of Privacy Practices
NSF checks. See Nonsufficient funds checks
NSF fees. See Nonsufficient funds fees
NUCC. See National Uniform Claim Committee
Nuclear medicine technologists, 347t

Nuclear scans, 26t–27t
Nuclear stress tests, ECG in, 952
Nuclei, 14t
Nucleic acid amplification tests (NAATs), 153b, 153t
Nucleolus, 14t
Nucleus, 329, 330b, 1092, 1092b
Numbers, rules for, 480–481
Numeric color coding, 435, 435b
Numeric filing, 433–434, 433t
Nurse anesthetist, 347t
Nurse Practitioner (NP), 347t, 376t
Nutrition
  dietary changes and, patient instruction on, 849–851, 849b–850b
  dietary nutrients and, 834–840
    carbohydrates and, 835–836, 835b–836b, 835t
    fats and, 837, 837b, 837t
    GI and, 836, 836t
    minerals and electrolytes and, 837, 838t
    protein and, 836, 836b
    vitamins and, 838, 838b, 839t, 840b
    water and, 838–840, 840b
  eating disorders and, 848–849
    anorexia nervosa, 291f, 291t, 848–849, 848b, 848f
    binge, 849
    bulimia nervosa, 291t, 849, 849b
  food labels and, 840–842, 841f
  geriatrics and, 752
  imbalances, 29
  introduction to, 834
  medically ordered diets and, 842–847
    AHA's heart-healthy diet, 845, 845t
    bland diet, 843
    clear liquid diet, 842, 842t
    diabetic eating plans, 843–845, 844f, 844t
    elimination diet and food allergies, 846–847, 846b
    full liquid diet, 842, 842t
    gluten-free diet, 847, 847b
    high/low-fiber diets, 846, 846t
    lactose-intolerance diet, 847
    low-protein diet, 846, 846t
    low-sodium diet, 845, 845t
    soft and mechanical soft diet, 842–843, 843t
    weight control diet, 843, 843b, 843t
  metabolism and, 834, 834b
  MyPlate and, 840, 840f, 841t
  needs with, for various populations, 847–848
    by age, 847t
    for cancer, 847–848
    for epilepsy, 847
    for HIV and AIDS, 847
    for pregnancy and lactation, 847
  USDA Dietary Guidelines and, 840
NVA. See Near visual acuity
Nystagmus, 318t

O

O & P. See Stool parasitic examination
Obesity, 726
Objective data, 674–675
Objective information, in health records, 414, 414b, 418
  diagnosis in, 418
  laboratory and radiology reports in, 418
  treatment prescribed and progress notes in, 418, 418b
  vital signs and anthropometric measurements in, 418, 637
Oblique fracture, 56t–57t
Obliteration, definition of, 428, 428b
Obsessive-compulsive disorder (OCD), 291t
Obstetricians, 146b, 348t
Obstetrics, 146b, 348t, 713–719
  customer service and, 720b
  domestic abuse signs and, 719–720
  first prenatal examination in, 716, 716b, 716f–717f
  patient education for, 719b
  postpartum visit and, 717
  prenatal record and, 713–716
    demographic information for, 713
    family history for, 715–716
    medical and surgical history in, 714–715
    menstrual history in, 713
    obstetric history in, 713–714, 714f, 715t
    return prenatal visits and, 716–717
      fetal heart tones in, 717
      fundal height measurement in, 717, 717f

Obstetrics (Continued)
  special tests and procedures in, 717–719
    amniocentesis for, 718–719, 719f
    CVS for, 719, 719f
    laboratory testing for, 718
    ultrasound for, 718, 718f
Obstructive sleep apnea, 256t–257t
Obturators, 765b, 765f, 765t–766t
Occipital lobe, 301, 302b
Occludes, definition of, 648–649, 649b
Occlusive therapy, 76t
Occult, definition of, 108, 109b
Occupational Safety and Health Act of 1970 (OSH Act), 389, 512
Occupational Safety and Health Administration (OSHA), 389, 389t, 397b
  Standard Precautions of
    for clinical laboratory safety, 1001–1003, 1003b, 1003f
    compliance guidelines of, 625–630
    definition of, 622
    environmental protection and, 625–627
    hand hygiene and, 622–624, 622f, 623b
    HBV vaccination and, 629, 630f
    housekeeping controls and, 627–628, 628f–629f, 629b
    for needlestick injuries, 1054–1055, 1054b
    OPIM and, 622, 622b
    postexposure follow-up and, 629–630, 630b
    PPE, barrier protection and, 625, 625b–626b, 625f, 627f
    summary of, 624, 624f
Occupational therapists, 347t
Occurrence policy, 369
OCD. See Obsessive-compulsive disorder
Ocular adnexa, 296–297, 297f, 305t
Ocular route, in medication administration, 893, 894b–895b
Odontectomy, 104t–105t
Odontogenic tumor, 118t
Odor, of urine, 1024, 1024b
Offense/wrong called, 364t
Office sterilization, quality-assurance records for, 774
Oil glands, 70, 71f, 72
Ointment medications, 889t
Oleptro (trazodone), 863t–867t
Olfactory sense, 296b
Oligodendrocytes, 263
Oligospermia, 158t
Omega-3 fatty acids, 836b
Omeprazole (Prilosec), 863t–867t
Omnibus Budget Reconciliation Act of 1989, 523b
Oncologists, definition of, 30
Online
  backup system, 424
  banking, 605
  bill pay, 614
  insurance web portal, 528, 528b
  payment options, 609
  profiles, job applications and, 1138–1140, 1138b–1140b, 1138t, 1139f
Onychectomy, 76t
Oophorectomy, 748, 748b
Open fracture, 56t–57t
Open office hours, 457
Open-ended questions/statements, 669–670
Operating scissors, 761f, 761t–762t
Operative report, 539
Ophthalmia neonatorum, 316t
Ophthalmic sonography, 304t–305t
Ophthalmologic surgery, 777
Ophthalmology/ophthalmologists, 296b, 348t
Ophthalmoscopy, 304t–305t, 678t
OPIM. See Other potentially infectious materials
Opportunistic infections, 622, 1121
Optic disk, 298, 298f
Optic nerve, 301t
Optic nerve disorders, 318t
Optic neuritis, 318t
Optical drives, 473t
Optical storage devices, 474t
Optics, 996, 996b
Oral cancer, 107t, 812, 812b
Oral cavity, 96–97, 96b, 96f–97f, 117t, 239, 239f, 690
Oral communication, 353–354, 354t

INDEX

Oral contraceptives, 708t, 709
Oral glucose tolerance tests, 330t
Oral interpreters, 356t
Oral medication administration, 890, 891b–892b
Oral temperature, digital thermometer for, 641b
Orbital disorders, 317t
Order of draw, in venipuncture, 1051t–1052t, 1052
Ordinances, 362
Oretic (hydrochlorothiazide), 863t–867t
Organ donation, 409t, 410–411, 410b–411b
Organ of Corti, 300
Organelles, 14, 14b, 329, 330b, 1111, 1111b
Organic substances, 168t
Organism, structure of, 16–18
Organism-caused diseases, diagnostic coding of, 543, 543f
Organs, structure of, 16, 16t–17t
Orifice, 147
Oropharynx, 97, 97f, 239, 239f
Orthopedics/orthopedists, 36b
Orthopnea, 218t–219t, 243t, 649–650
Orthostatic (postural) hypotension, 653, 653b, 745
Orthostatic vital signs, 233
OSH Act. See Occupational Safety and Health Act of 1970
OSHA. See Occupational Safety and Health Administration
Ossicles, 37, 299–300, 300f
Ossification, definition of, 36
Osteitis deformans, 65t
Osteoarthritis, 62, 747
Osteogenesis imperfecta, 65t
Osteomalacia, 65t
Osteomas, 66t
Osteomyelitis, 65t
Osteoporosis, 63, 712, 712b, 748b
    geriatrics and, 748
Osteosarcomas, 66t
Otalgia, 319t, 698
OTC medications. See Over-the-counter medications
Other potentially infectious materials (OPIM), 622, 622b
Otic route, in medication administration, 894, 895b–896b
Otitis externa, 319t, 640, 640b
Otitis media, 320f, 320t, 698, 698f–699f, 726–727, 726f–727f
Otolaryngologists, 188b, 348t
Otologic surgery, 777
Otoplasty, 309t
Otorhinolaryngology/otorhinolaryngologists, 296b
Otorrhea, 319t
Otosclerosis, 314, 698, 751
Otoscopy, 308t, 678t
Ototoxic medications, 698, 751, 752b
Out guides, 431, 431b, 432f
Outer ear, 299
Outer ear disorders, 319t
Outpatient procedures, appointment scheduling for, 461, 462b–463b
Output devices, 469, 472, 472f
Outside visits, appointment scheduling for, 461
Ova, 147
Ova and parasite examination, 103t–104t
Oval fat bodies, in urine, 1034, 1037f
Oval window, 299–300, 300f
Ovarian cysts, 162t
Ovaries, 147, 149f, 329
    cancer of, 159t–160t
Overdraft fees, 604t
Overdrafts, 611
Over-the-counter (OTC) medications, 871, 872t
Ovulation, 150
Ovulation testing, 1041
Oxycet (oxycodone), 863t–867t
Oxycodone (Percocet, Oxycet, Roxicet), 863t–867t
Oxygen, 166, 167b
    bacteria requirements with, 1108, 1108b
    supplies of, for emergencies, 965, 965f, 966b
    therapy, 958, 959f, 960t, 961b, 961f
Oxygenated blood, 211–212, 212f–213f
Oxytocin, 327t

P

PA. See Physician Assistant
PACAB. See Port-access coronary artery bypass
Pacemakers, 950, 950f–951f
Pacerone (amiodarone), 968t
Packing slips, 509
Pain Ease, 916f
Palatine tonsils, 239, 239f
Palliative care, 182, 182b, 283b, 408b
Pallor, 218t–219t
Palpation, in physical examination, 686, 686b, 688f
Palpatory method, for blood pressure measurement, 657
Palpitations, 218t–219t
Pancreas, 98, 101, 101b, 325, 325f, 328
Pancreatectomy, 331t
Pancreatic cancer, 107t
Pancreatic diseases, 336–338, 337t
Pancreatitis, 114
Pancreatoduodenectomy, 331t
Pancytopenia, 183t
Panhypopituitarism, 332t–333t
Panic disorder, 291t
Pantothenic acid, 839t
Pap tests, 705b, 706–707, 707b, 814t, 819t
Paper health records, 413
    documentation in, 428
    management system for, 430–431, 433b
        filing equipment, 430–431, 431f
        filing supplies, 431
    phone message documentation for, 446, 446b, 447f
Papule, 74f, 75t
Paracentesis, 104t–105t
Paracusis, 320t
Paraffin bath therapy, 821, 821f
Paralytic conditions, 285f, 285t
Parameters, definition of, 420, 452
Paranasal sinuses, 239, 239b, 239f
Paranoid personality disorder, 290t
Paraparesis, 285t
Paraphrasing, 355t, 1127–1128, 1128b
Paraplegia, 285f, 285t
Parasites
    definition of, 1106, 1106b
    pathogenic, 1110, 1110t
Parasympathetic nervous system, 270, 270f
Parathyroid glands, 325, 325f, 327, 327f
Parathyroidectomy, 331t
Parenteral, definition of, 622, 622b
Parenteral medication administration. See also Intradermal injections, for medication administration; Intramuscular injections, for medication administration; Subcutaneous injections, for medication administration
    giving, 914–915
        guidelines for, 915, 916b, 916f–917f
        route of, 896–899
        special situations in, 915, 916b
    preparation of, 904–913
        ampules for, 904, 904f, 905b–906b
        mixing insulins for, 913, 913b–914b, 913f
        prefilled sterile cartridge for, 906, 906f, 907b–908b
        reconstituting powdered medication for, 909–911, 911b–912b, 912f
        specialty syringe units for, 906, 908f
        vials for, 908–909, 908f, 909b–910b
Paresthesia, 280t–281t, 331t
Parietal pleura, 241
Parkinson's disease, 275–278
Parotid salivary glands, 97, 97f
PARs. See Participating providers
Partial thromboplastin time (PTT), 26t–27t, 174t
Participating providers (PARs), 449, 449b, 527–528, 583, 583f
Parts of speech, 480, 480t
PASS, for fire extinguishers, 518b
Passive communicators, 354, 354t
Passive immunity, 194–195, 195f, 620b
Passive-aggressive communicators, 354, 354t
Passwords, 477b
Past health, family, and social history, in health records, 414–418, 416f–417f
Past medical history, 664
Paste medications, 889t
Patch, 75t
Patella, 42t
Patent airway, 965, 965b
Patent ductus arteriosus, 227t
Patent foramen ovale, 227t
Pathogens, 25, 166, 167b, 188, 1105, 1105b
    common infectious, 28, 28t
    definition of, 25b, 70, 70b, 759
    transmission of, 29t
Pathologic fracture, 56t–57t
Pathologists, definition of, 30, 348t, 991
Pathology
    definition of, 14, 25, 1081, 1081b
    disease causes in, 28–32
    predisposing factors in, 25–28
    protection mechanisms in, 25
    reports, diagnostic coding preparation and, 539
    suffixes for, 6t–7t, 7f, 8
    terminology in, 25
Pathology and Laboratory section, of CPT, 562, 562b
Patient abandonment, 370, 370b
Patient accounts, 589
Patient assessment, in physical examination, 674–675, 674b
Patient assistance, for physical examination, 676–677, 679–680, 680f, 681b
Patient checkout, 502
Patient communication, 665–670. See also Patient interviews
    active listening for, 668–669
    closed questions for, 670
    nonverbal communication for, 669, 669b–671b, 669t, 670f
    obtain and document information from, 667b
    open-ended questions/statements for, 669–670
    self-boundaries with, 345, 666b, 701b
    sensitivity to diversity in, 666–667, 668b, 668f
    therapeutic techniques for, 668–670
Patient financial responsibilities and. See Financial responsibilities, of patient
Patient Health Questionnaire (PHQ), 815
Patient information form, medical billing and, 567, 567f
Patient interviews, 670–674
    advice in, 672
    barriers in, 671–672
    defense mechanisms and, 672, 673b
    environment preparation for, 671b
    greetings and, 671, 671f
    leading questions in, 672
    across life span, 672–674, 673f
    medical terminology in, 672
    privacy and, 673–674
    therapeutic communication techniques for, 671, 672t
    unwarranted assurance and, 671
    verbal overload in, 672
Patient ledger, 589–597, 591f
    credit balances in, 595–596, 596b
    entering and posting transactions in, 589
    NSF checks and, 595b, 595f
    payment agreements in, 596–597
    payment at time of service in, 596, 596b, 596f
    pegboard system for, 589, 589b, 591b, 592f
    posting adjustments in, 593–596, 595b, 595f
    posting charges in, 591, 592b–593b
    posting payments in, 592–593, 592b–593b, 594f
    TILA and, 596–597, 597f
Patient navigators, 829, 829b
Patient payment management, 606–609
    cash payments in, 606
    checks and, 608, 608b
    contactless payment systems for, 608–609
    credit cards in, 608–609, 609f
    debit cards in, 608, 608b
    online payment options for, 609
Patient portal, 418, 499, 499b, 664
Patient positioning and draping, for physical examination, 680–685
    dorsal recumbent position, 683, 683b
    Fowler position, 682, 682b
    knee-chest position, 685, 687b
    lithotomy position, 684, 684b
    prone position, 684, 686b
    semi-Fowler position, 682, 682b
    Sims position, 684, 685b
    supine (horizontal recumbent) position, 683, 683b
    Trendelenburg position, 685, 687f
Patient procedures, appointment scheduling for, 461, 462b–463b

INDEX

Patient processing tasks, 497–502
  challenging situations in, 501–502, 502b
  escorting patients to exam room in, 500–501, 501b
  patient checkout in, 502
  patient's arrival in, 497–500, 498f
    check-in procedures for all patients, 500
    HIPAA appropriate communication for, 498t
    infection control in reception area, 499
    names and greetings, 498b
    new patient registration, 499, 499b–501b, 499f
    sign-in register, 498, 498f, 499t
    special needs patients, 500
    patient's time considerations in, 500, 501f
Patient Protection and Affordable Care Act. *See* Affordable Care Act
Patient safety concerns, with compliance reporting, 396, 398b–399b
Patient Self-Determination Act (PSDA), 390t, 408–409, 409b
Patient tracking systems, 478
Patient transfer, body mechanics for, 679–680, 680f, 681b
Patient-centered medical home (PCMH), 349b, 578b
Patient's Bill of Rights, 372, 373b–376b, 373f
Paying bills, to maximize cash flow, 613–614
Payment agreements, 596–597
Payment at time of service, 596, 596b, 596f
PBS. *See* Prune belly syndrome
PCMH. *See* Patient-centered medical home
PCPs. *See* Primary care providers
PDR. *See* Physician Desk Reference
PE. *See* Pulmonary embolism
Peak flow monitor, 244f, 244t–245t
Peak flow rate measurement, 955, 955b–956b, 955f
Pediatricians, 348t
Pediatrics. *See also* Minors
  Apgar score and, 729, 733t
  child abuse signs and, 740, 740b
  customer service and, 740b
  development patterns in, normal, 723–725, 724b–725b
  developmental theories and, 725
  diseases and disorders in, 725–727
    ASD, 728b
    colic, 725
    conjunctivitis, 727b
    diarrhea, 725–726
    failure to thrive, 726
    fifths disease, 727b
    hand-foot-and-mouth disease, 727b, 727f
    obesity, 726
    otitis media, 726–727, 726f–727f
    Reye's syndrome, 727b
  doses for, medication math for liquid medication, 879, 881b, 882f
  emergency supplies for, 967–968, 968f–969f
  growth patterns in, normal, 723–725, 723b, 723t
  immunizations and, 727–729
    documentation for, 729, 731b
    guidelines for, 729, 730t
    schedules for, 727, 728f
    storage for, 729, 731b
  injury prevention and, 739–740
  introduction to, 722–723
  MA's role in, 733–739, 734f
    examination and, 734–739, 738f, 739f
    measurements and, 734, 735f–736f, 737f–738b
    urine specimen collection and, 739, 739f
  phlebotomy and, 1071, 1073t–1074t
  sick-child visits in, 733, 733t
  vital signs in, 738t
  well-child visits in, 729, 733b
Pediculosis, 88–89, 89f
PedvaxHIB, 730t
Pegboard system, 589, 589b, 591b, 592f
Pelvic examination, in gynecology, 706, 706f
Pelvic girdle, 52f
Pelvic inflammatory disease, 161t
Pelvis, male and female compared, 43b, 43f
Penicillin, 854
Penis, 146, 148f, 149
Pepsin, 99
Peptic ulcers, 115–116, 115f
Percocet (oxycodone), 863t–867t
Percussion, in physical examination, 686–687, 688f
Percutaneous, definition of, 112t–113t, 113b
Percutaneous endoscopic gastrostomy, 104t–105t

Percutaneous transhepatic cholangiography (PTC), 103t
Percutaneous transluminal coronary angioplasty (PTCA), 221t–223t
Perforated ulcers, 116, 116b
Performance measurement, 550
Pericardiocentesis, 221t–223t, 223f
Pericarditis, 234t
Pericardium, 209, 211f
Perimenopause, 712
Perineal areas, 683, 684b, 706, 706b
Perineum, female, 147, 149f
Periodontal disease, 117t
Peripheral artery disease, 225t
Peripheral blood smear, 174t, 176, 177b
Peripheral nervous system (PNS), 261, 262f, 267–268, 268t
Peripheral neuropathy, 678b, 678t
Peripheral neuropathy screening, 815, 815b–817b
Peripheral pulse, 641, 643b
Peripheral vascular disease, 234t
Peristalsis, 15b, 16t, 45, 746, 746b
Peritoneum, 123, 123b
Peritonitis, 117t
Peritubular capillaries, 123, 124b
Permeability, definition of, 51, 51b, 126, 189, 190b, 771, 773b
Permission, 382b
PERRLA chart, 693b
Persistent delusional disorders, 290t
Persistent mood disorders, 289t
Personal checks, 606
Personal communication, 350, 351t
Personal computers (PCs)
  customer service and, 491b
  hardware for, 469–474
    input devices, 469–472, 471f–472f
    internal components, 472, 473t
    maintaining, 474, 474b–475b
    network and Internet access devices, 473–474
    output devices, 469, 472, 472f
    secondary storage devices for, 473, 474t
  network privacy and security for, 476–478, 477b, 477t
  software for, 469, 469b, 475–476, 476b
  types of, 470f, 470t
  workstation ergonomics, 475, 476f
Personal demographics, in health records, 414, 414b, 415f, 417b
Personal ethics, 401, 401t
Personal finance interviews, 600, 600f
Personal health record (PHR), 420
Personal identification number (PIN), 608
Personal injury insurance, 369
Personal problems/baggage, 350
Personal protective equipment (PPE), 1001b–1002b, 1003f
  OSHA Standard Precautions and, 625, 625b–626b, 625f, 627f
  for venipuncture, 1048, 1048b
Personality disorders, 271, 272t, 290t
Personality traits, for career development, 1127–1128
  collaboration and interpersonal skills, 1127–1128, 1127f, 1128b
  compassion, 1128, 1128b
  genuine interest, 1128, 1128f
  professionalism, 1128, 1128b
  strengths and skills in, 1128–1129
Pertussis, 253t–254t, 730t
Pessary medications, 889t
PET. *See* Positron emission tomography scan
Petechiae, 75t, 1066b, 1067t
Petty cash, 614b
Peyer patches, 188–189, 188b, 189f
Peyronie disease, 141t–142t
PFTs. *See* Pulmonary function tests
pH, 24–25
  of urine specimens, 1025, 1028f
Phacoemulsification and aspiration of cataract, 307t
Phagocytic cells, 169
Phagocytosis, 172, 172f, 191
Phalanges, 42
Phalen test, 55t
Pharmaceutical representatives, appointment scheduling for, 461–463
Pharmacogenetics, 405
Pharmacogenomics, 856b

Pharmacokinetics, 854–856
  absorption, 855, 855t
  distribution, 855–856, 855b
  excretion, 856
  metabolism, 856, 856b
Pharmacology basics, 854–857. *See also* Drugs; Medication administration; Medication math; Medication orders
  drug action in, 856–857
    adverse reactions of, 857, 857t
    factors influencing, 856, 856b, 856t
    therapeutic effects of, 857
  drug sources in, 854
  drug uses in, 854, 855t
  pharmacokinetics in, 854–856
    absorption, 855, 855t
    distribution, 855–856, 855b
    excretion, 856
    metabolism, 856, 856b
Pharmacotherapy, 286t
Pharmacy technicians, 347t
Pharyngeal tonsils, 239, 239f
Pharyngitis, 255t–257t, 543
Pharynx, 97, 97b, 97f
Phenylalanine, 1024b
Phenylketonuria, 715, 715b, 1024b
Pheochromocytoma, 335t
PHI. *See* Protected health information
Phlebectomy, 221t–223t
Phlebography, 219t–221t
Phlebotomists, 991
Phlebotomy. *See also* Capillary puncture; Venipuncture
  certification agencies for, 1047b
  common injuries associated with, 1056–1057, 1057f
  needles and syringes in, 1052–1054
    butterfly assemblies, 1053–1054, 1054f
    multisample needles, 1053, 1053f
    needle angle of entry, 1057b
    needle holders, 1053, 1053f
    needle structure, 1052–1053, 1053f
    safety, 1054–1056, 1054b, 1055f, 1056b
    syringes, 1053, 1054f
  pediatric, 1071, 1073t–1074t
  purpose of, 1047
Phone calls, 350, 351t
Phone interviews, for job interviews, 1144, 1144b
Phonetic alphabet, 442b
Phosphorus, 838t
Photodynamic therapy, 76t
Photophobia, 317t
Photorefractive keratectomy, 306t
Phototherapy, 76t
PHQ. *See* Patient Health Questionnaire
PHR. *See* Personal health record
Phrases, 480, 480t
Physiatrists, 348t
Physical examination, 675–678. *See also* Medical history; Patient interviews; Vision and hearing screenings
  body mechanics principles and, 679–680, 679f–680f, 680b
  chaperones during, 689b
  customer service and, 701b
  diagnostic coding preparation and, 538
  documentation guidelines for, 675, 676t
  examination room preparation for, 675–676
  MA responsibilities with, 680–691, 692b
  medical abbreviations for, 676t
  methods of, 685–688
    auscultation, 687, 688f
    inspection, 686
    manipulation, 688, 688b
    mensuration, 687–688, 688f
    palpation, 686, 686b, 688f
    percussion, 686–687, 688f
  patient assessment in, 674–675, 674b
  patient assistance for, 676–677, 679–680, 680f, 681b
  patient positioning and draping for, 680–685
    dorsal recumbent position, 683, 683b
    Fowler position, 682, 682b
    knee-chest position, 685, 687b
    lithotomy position, 684, 684b
    prone position, 684, 686b
    semi-Fowler position, 682, 682b

INDEX

Physical examination (Continued)
    Sims position, 684, 685b
    supine (horizontal recumbent) position, 683, 683b
    Trendelenburg position, 685, 687f
  patient transfer for, 679–680, 680f, 681b
  provider assistance for, 677
  sequence of, 688–691
    abdomen, 690
    breast and testicles, 690–691
    chest, 690
    ear, 689–690
    eye, 689
    general appearance, 689
    head, 689
    neck, 690
    nose and sinuses, 690
    oral cavity and throat, 690
    rectum, 691
    reflexes, 690
    skin, 689
    speech, 689
  supplies and instruments needed for, 677–678, 677f, 678t
  vision and hearing screenings for, 691–702
Physical hazards, in clinical laboratory safety, 1004, 1004f
Physical therapists, 347t
Physician Assistant (PA), 347t, 376t
Physician Desk Reference (PDR), 860
Physician office laboratory (POL)
  blood chemistry in, 1094–1099
    ALT and AST testing and, 1097
    blood glucose testing and, 1095, 1095b–1096b, 1095f
    cholesterol testing and, 1096–1097, 1098b–1099b
    hemoglobin A_{1c} testing and, 1095–1096, 1097t
    thyroid hormone testing and, 1097–1099
  hematology in, 1078–1086
    coagulation testing, 1086, 1086b–1088b, 1086f, 1088f
    ESR, 1084, 1084b–1085b, 1084t, 1086f
    hematocrit and microhematocrit test, 1078–1081, 1080b–1082b, 1081f, 1082t
    hemoglobin test, 1082–1083, 1082b–1083b, 1082f, 1084t
  specimen collection in, 1111–1114, 1113f–1114f, 1115t
Physician Orders for Life-Sustaining Treatment (POLST), 409b
Physician-assisted suicide, 410, 410t
Physicians
  code of ethics for, 401–402, 402f
  practice requirements for, 376t
Physiological needs, 357, 358f
Physiology
  of blood, 170–172
  of cardiovascular system, 215–217
  definition of, 13, 1081, 1081b
  of digestive system, 99–101
  of ear, 301
  of endocrine system, 329
  of eye, 301, 301t
  geriatrics changes in, 744–755, 744t
  of integumentary system, 73
  of lymphatic and immune systems, 190–194
  of mental health, 270–271
  of musculoskeletal system, 46–51
  of reproductive system, 148–151
  of respiratory system, 242
  of urinary system, 126–128
Pilonidal cyst, 90t–91t
PIN. See Personal identification number
Pineal gland, 325, 325f, 329
Pinkeye, 727b
Pinna, 299, 300f
Pinworms (Enterobius vermicularis), 1114, 1114f
Pipets, 1008, 1008b, 1009f, 1084, 1084b
Pitch, voice, 442, 442b
Pituitary gland, 148, 150b, 325–326, 325f–326f, 326b, 327f
Pituitary gland diseases, 330–331, 332t–333t
Pivot joint, 44t, 45f
PKD. See Polycystic kidney disease
Place of occurrence code, 546
Place of service (POS), 558, 559b, 575, 575t
Placenta, 150, 151f
Placenta previa, 162t
Plain-thumb forceps, 762t–764t, 763f
Plaintiffs, 362, 364t, 604

Plant fibers, in urine examination, 1036, 1037f
Plantar fasciitis, 66t
Plantar flexion, 52t–53t
Plaque, 74f, 75t, 1094–1095, 1094b
Plasma, 167–168, 167t, 1050b, 1051t, 1078
Plasma glucose levels, 337t
Plasma membrane, 14t
Plasma protein, 167, 167t, 168b
Plasma separator tubes (PSTs), 1050–1051, 1051t
Plastic surgeons, 348t
Platelets
  analysis of, in reference laboratory, 1093
  anatomy of, 170, 170f
  in coagulation and hemostasis, 172, 172b, 173f
Platform crutches, 824
Platform walker attachments, 827b, 827f
Plavix (clopidogrel), 863t–867t
Pleura, 240f–241f, 241
Pleural effusion, 253b, 253t–254t
Pleurisy, 253t–254t
Pleurodynia, 243t
Plicae, 101
Plume, definition of, 776, 776b
Plural/singular ending rules, 9, 11t
PMDD. See Premenstrual dysphoric disorder
PMS. See Premenstrual syndrome
Pneumococcal pneumonia, 730t
Pneumonectomy, 250f, 250t
Pneumonia, 251, 251b, 1116
Pneumothorax, 253t–254t, 254f
Pneumovax 23, 730t
PNS. See Peripheral nervous system
PO numbers. See Purchase order numbers
Point-of-care, 478, 478b
Point-of-sale (POS) purchases, 608
Poise, 351b, 351t
Poisonings, environmental emergencies and, 969b, 971–972, 972b
POL. See Physician office laboratory
Policies, 381, 522, 522b
Poliomyelitis, 284t
POLST. See Physician Orders for Life-Sustaining Treatment
Polycystic kidney disease (PKD), 136–137, 137f, 141t–142t
Polycystic ovary syndrome, 162t
Polycythemia, 217, 217b
Polycythemia vera, 183t, 1081, 1081b
Polydactyly, 65t
Polydipsia, 331t
Polyethylene, 1017
Polymyalgia rheumatica, 66t
Polymyositis, 66t, 199t–200t
Polyneuritis, 284t
Polypectomy, 104t–105t
Polyphagia, 331t
Polyps, 118t
Polysomnography, 276t
Polyuria, 331t
Popliteal pulse, 645–646, 649
POR. See Problem-oriented medical record
Pores, 71f, 72
Portable handheld ECG monitors, 954
Port-access coronary artery bypass (PACAB), 221b–223b
Portal of exit and entry, 619, 619b
Portion size, 843, 843b, 843t
Portrait orientation, 487b, 488
POS. See Place of service
POS purchases. See Point-of-sale purchases
Positional anatomy terminology, 18, 20t
Positron emission tomography (PET) scan, 26t–27t, 196t, 219t–221t, 273f, 273t, 818t
Post discovery phase, in civil lawsuit, 368b
Postage options, 487, 487t, 489f
Postal Service. See US Postal Service
Posterior pituitary hormones, 326f, 327t
Postexposure follow-up, Standard Precautions and, 629–630, 630b
Postherpetic neuralgia, 748t
Postpartum depression (PPD), 718b
Postpartum visit, obstetrics and, 717
Posttraumatic stress disorder (PTSD), 291t
Postural (orthostatic) hypotension, 653, 653b, 745

Postural orthostatic tachycardia syndrome (POTS), 232–233
Postvoid residual (PVR) urine test, 130t
Potassium, 838t
Potassium (K-Tab, Klor-Con, K-Dur, Micro-K), 863t–867t
POTS. See Postural orthostatic tachycardia syndrome
Powder medications, 889t
PPD. See Postpartum depression
PPE. See Personal protective equipment
PPMP. See Provider-performed microscopy procedures
PPO. See Preferred provider organization
Practice management files, 435
Practice management software, 454, 454b, 476t
Practice requirements, 372–378, 376t
  accreditation in, 378
  certification and registration in, 378
  disciplinary action and, 377–378, 378b
  licensure and, 377, 377b, 377t
  Medical Practice Act and, 377–378
  scope of practice and, 366, 366b, 377, 377b–378b
Preauthorization process, 459, 459b, 526, 526b
Precedents, 362, 362b, 381
Precertification/preauthorization processes, 459, 459b, 566, 566b, 569–570, 570b
Precipitate, definition of, 1022, 1023b
Precordial (chest) leads, 939, 941f
Prediabetes, 337t
Predisposing factors, 25–28
Preeclampsia, 162t, 338, 338b, 715, 715b
Preferred provider organization (PPO), 527, 528t
Pre-filing phase, in civil lawsuit, 368b
Prefilled sterile cartridge, for parenteral medication administration, 906, 906f, 907b–908b
Prefixes
  for blood, 184t
  for cardiovascular system, 235t
  definition of, 1b, 2
  for digestive system, 120t
  for ear, 322t
  for endocrine system, 340t
  for eye, 321t
  for integumentary system, 93t
  for lymphatic and immune systems, 205t
  of metric measurement, 874–876, 875f
  for musculoskeletal system, 67t
  for reproductive system, 163t–164t
  for respiratory system, 258t
  types of, 9, 10t–11t
  for urinary system, 143t
Preformed antibodies, 170–171, 172b
Pregnancy and delivery, 150–151, 151f
  conditions related to, 162t
  labeling rule of drugs for, 838b
  nutrition needs for, 847
Pregnancy complications, diagnostic coding of, 545, 545b
Pregnancy Discrimination Act of 1978, 395t–396t
Pregnancy tests, 150b
  urine and, 1039–1041, 1040b
Premature atrial contractions, 224t
Premature ventricular contractions (PVCs), 224t, 949, 949f
Premenstrual dysphoric disorder (PMDD), 162t, 709, 709b
Premenstrual syndrome (PMS), 162t, 709, 709b
Premium, 368–369
Prenatal record, obstetrics and, 713–716
  demographic information for, 713
  family history for, 715–716
  medical and surgical history in, 714–715
  menstrual history in, 713
  obstetric history in, 713–714, 714f, 715f
Prepositions, 480, 480t
Prepuce, 149
Presbycusis, 302b, 314–315, 698
Presbyopia, 302b, 691
Prescription pads, 494, 495b
Prescriptions, 867–871, 868f
  abbreviations for
    measurements, 870t
    medications, 871t
    miscellaneous, 871t
    route and form, 869t
    timing, 870t

INDEX

Prescriptions *(Continued)*
   controlled substance, 871, 871*t*
   customer service and, 883*b*
   MA's role with, 867–871, 868*f*, 869*b*
   refill request phone calls for, 447
Preservatives, definition of, 1005–1006, 1005*b*
Prevalence, definition of, 25
Preventative maintenance, 996–997, 996*b*
Prevention, definition of, 25
Preventive care, 522, 522*b*
Prevnar 13, 730*t*
Priapism, 158*t*
Prilosec (omeprazole), 863*t*–867*t*
Primary care providers (PCPs), 526
Primary memory, 473*t*
Primary skin lesions, 74*f*, 75*t*
Printers, 472, 472*t*
Prioritizing, time management skills and, 348–349
Priority mail, 487*t*
Priority mail express, 487*t*
Privacy
   computer networks and, 476–478, 477*b*, 477*t*
   confidentiality and, 381–387
      amendments related to, 381*b*
      GINA and, 387, 395*t*–396*t*
      HIPAA and, 381–386
      HITECH Act and, 386–387, 387*b*, 420, 477
   filters, 477, 497
   patient interviews and, 673–674
Privacy Rule, HIPAA, 382–385, 383*t*
Private delivery services, 511
Privileged communication, 391–392, 391*b*
ProAir (albuterol), 863*t*–867*t*
Probes and dilators, 765, 765*f*–766*f*, 765*t*–766*t*
Problem solving, 349
Problem-oriented medical record (POR), 425–428, 427*f*
Procedural coding, 549, 549*t*. *See also* Healthcare Common Procedure Coding System; International Classification of Diseases, Tenth Revision, Procedural Coding System
Procedural law, 362
Procedure room, for minor surgery, 758, 758*f*, 778
Procedures, 381
Proctitis, 117*t*
Proctologists, 96*b*
Prodromal stage, of infections, 621*b*
Prodrugs, 856*b*
Productive cough, 247, 247*b*
Professional e-mails, 488–490, 491*f*
Professional ethics, 401–402, 401*t*, 402*f*
Professional insurance, 368–369
Professional letters, 482–484, 483*f*, 483*t*, 484*b*
Professional liability insurance, 369
Professionalism, in health care, 343–350. *See also* Appointment scheduling; Career development; Telephone techniques
   appearance, 345–346, 345*f*, 346*t*
   barriers to, 350, 350*f*
   continuing education and, 349–350, 350*t*
   in job interviews, 1142–1144
   medical assistants and professional characteristics, 343–345
   nonverbal communication and, 350–353, 442*b*
      cultural differences in, 352–353, 353*t*
      delivery factors in, 352, 352*t*
      physical boundaries to, 351–352, 352*t*
      positive and negative behaviors in, 351*t*
   as personality trait for career development, 1128, 1128*b*
   team members and, 346–349, 346*f*, 349*b*
   understanding behavior and, 357–359
   verbal communication and, 353–357
      barriers to, 355–357, 356*t*–357*t*
      communication cycle, 353, 353*f*
      oral communication, 353–354, 354*t*
      therapeutic communication, 354–355, 355*t*
      written communication, 353, 354*t*
Proficiency, definition of, 454
Profile testing, 992, 992*b*
Prognosis, definition of, 3, 25, 414
Progress notes, 496, 496*b*, 538
   in health records, 418, 418*b*
   incoming calls on, 448
Projection, 359*t*, 673*b*
Prokaryote, 1107, 1107*b*

Prolactin, 327*t*
Prolactinoma, 332*t*–333*t*
Proliferate, definition of, 192–193
Promethazine (Promethegan), 863*t*–867*t*
Pronation, 52*t*–53*t*
Prone position, 684, 686*b*
Pronunciation of unusual letter combinations, 11*t*
Property law, 364*t*
ProQuad, 730*t*
Prostaglandins, 329
Prostate gland, 125, 146, 148*f*
   cancer of, 137–138, 138*f*, 141*t*–142*t*, 155–158, 814*t*
Prostatitis, 141*t*–142*t*
Proteases, 101
Protected health information (PHI), 382*b*–383*b*, 382*t*, 386*b*, 420
Protein, 836, 836*b*
   diet low in, 846, 846*t*
   in urine specimens, 1028
Prothrombin time (PT), 26*t*–27*t*, 174*t*, 1086, 1086*b*–1088*b*, 1086*f*
Proton-pump inhibitors, 863*t*–867*t*
Protozoa, 619, 1106, 1106*b*
   pathogenic, 1110, 1110*t*
Protozoal cysts, 1111
Protraction, 52*t*–53*t*
Proventil HFA (albuterol), 863*t*–867*t*
Provider assistance, for physical examination, 677
Provider networks, 526
Provider-patient relationship, 370, 370*t*
Provider-performed microscopy procedures (PPMP), 1008–1009, 1010*t*
Provisional diagnosis, 418, 418*b*
Proximal convoluted tubule, 124, 127*t*
Prune belly syndrome (PBS), 141*t*–142*t*
Pruritus, 90*t*–91*t*, 132, 132*b*
PSDA. *See* Patient Self-Determination Act
Pseudocysts, 114, 115*b*
Pseudoephedrine (Sudafed), 872*t*
Psoralen plus ultraviolet A (PUVA) therapy, 76*t*
Psoriasis, 86–87, 86*b*, 86*f*–87*f*, 87*t*, 199*t*–200*t*
PSTs. *See* Plasma separator tubes
Psychiatry/psychiatrists, 261*b*, 348*t*
Psychoanalysis, 286*t*
Psychological testing, 283
Psychology/psychologists, 261*b*
Psychomotor domain, of learning, 802, 803*t*
Psychosis, 272*t*
Psychosocial development stages, Erikson's, 357*t*, 804*t*
Psychotherapy, 286*t*
Psychotherapy notes, confidentiality of, 385*b*
PT. *See* Prothrombin time
PTC. *See* Percutaneous transhepatic cholangiography
PTCA. *See* Percutaneous transluminal coronary angioplasty
PTSD. *See* Posttraumatic stress disorder
PTT. *See* Partial thromboplastin time
Puberty, 148, 150*b*
Pubis, 42*t*
Public health statutes, compliance reporting with, 391–393, 391*b*
Puerperium complications, diagnostic coding of, 545, 545*b*
Pulmonary abscess, 256*t*–257*t*
Pulmonary angiography, 244*t*–245*t*
Pulmonary atresia, 227*t*
Pulmonary circulation, 211–213, 212*b*, 212*f*
Pulmonary congestion, 218*t*–219*t*
Pulmonary edema, 256*t*–257*t*
Pulmonary embolism (PE), 182, 251–252
Pulmonary function tests (PFTs), 954–956, 954*t*
   peak flow rate, 955, 955*b*–956*b*, 955*f*
   spirometry tests, 955–956, 956*t*, 957*b*–958*b*, 957*t*
Pulmonary hypertension, 251, 251*b*
Pulmonary resections, 250*f*, 250*t*
Pulmonary system. *See* Respiratory system
Pulmonary treatments, 956–958
   MDIs, 956–958, 958*b*–959*b*, 958*f*
   nebulizer treatment, 958, 959*b*–960*b*
   oxygen therapy, 958, 959*f*, 960*t*, 961*b*, 961*f*
Pulmonary valve, 209, 211*f*, 934, 935*f*
Pulmonology/pulmonologists, 188*b*, 239*b*

Pulse, 641–649
   apical, 646, 647*b*, 648–649
   bounding, 646–647, 647*b*
   brachial, 644–645, 645*f*
   carotid, 643–644, 645*f*
   characteristics of, 646–647
   deficit, 646
   Doppler for checking, 218*f*, 218*t*–219*t*, 649, 649*f*
   dorsalis pedis, 646, 649, 649*f*
   femoral, 645, 649
   intermittent, 646, 646*b*
   peripheral, 641, 643*b*
   popliteal, 645–646, 649
   radial, 645, 646*f*, 648–649, 648*b*
   rate of, 646, 647*t*, 648–649, 648*b*, 649*f*
   rhythm of, 646
   sites of, 643–646, 645*f*
   temporal, 643, 645*f*
   thready, 646–647, 647*b*
   volume of, 646–647, 648*b*
Pulse oximetry, 244*t*–245*t*, 245*f*, 246, 658, 658*b*, 658*f*
Pulse pressure, 651
Punch biopsies, 83*f*, 83*t*
Punctuality, 347
Punctuation, 480–481
Punitive damages, 368
Pupil, 297, 298*f*, 299
Purchase order (PO) numbers, 509, 509*b*
Pure culture, 993, 1123
Pure tone audiometry, 308*t*
Purging, 424
Purkinje fibers, 215*f*, 216, 936*f*
Purpura, 75*t*
   definition of, 178*b*
   idiopathic thrombocytopenic, 178, 178*f*
Pustule, 74*f*, 75*t*
Putrid, definition of, 1024, 1024*b*
PUVA (Psoralen plus ultraviolet A) therapy, 76*t*
PVCs. *See* Premature ventricular contractions
PVR urine test. *See* Postvoid residual urine test
Pyelonephritis, 138–139
Pyemia, 621
Pyloric stenosis, 116*t*
Pyloromyotomy, 104*t*–105*t*
Pyorrhea, 117*t*
Pyothorax, 256*t*–257*t*
Pyrexia, 191, 243*t*, 638
Pyridoxine, 839*t*
Pyromania, 292*t*
Pyrosis, 102*t*

Q

QA. *See* Quality assurance
QC. *See* Quality control
QFT-GIT. *See* QuantiFERON-TB Gold In-Tube test
QMBs. *See* Qualified Medicare Beneficiaries
Quadriparesis, 285*t*
Quadriplegia, 285*f*, 285*t*
Qualified endorsements, 611*t*
Qualified medical interpreters, 356*t*
Qualified Medicare Beneficiaries (QMBs), 524, 524*b*
Qualitative testing, quantitative testing compared to, 992*t*
Quality assurance (QA)
   in clinical laboratory, 996–997, 997*f*
   records, for office sterilization, 774
   in urinalysis, 1026*b*, 1030
Quality control (QC), 413, 494, 494*b*, 996, 996*b*
   clinical laboratory guidelines for, 997–999, 997*b*–999*b*
   in urinalysis, 1026*b*, 1030
QuantiFERON-TB Gold In-Tube test (QFT-GIT), 921
Quantitative chemical analysis, 1019
Quantitative testing, qualitative testing compared to, 992*t*
Quetiapine (Seroquel), 863*t*–867*t*
QuickVue pregnancy test, 1040*b*
Quinidine, 854

R

RAAS. *See* Renin-angiotensin aldosterone system
Rabies, 974, 974*b*, 974*t*
Rabies immune globulin (RIG), 974*t*
Rabies vaccine, 974*t*
RACE, for fires, 517*b*
Race, hypertension risk and, 652*b*
Racial diversity, 344*t*
Radial artery, 209, 211*f*

INDEX

Radial pulse, 645, 646f, 648–649, 648b
Radiculitis, 284t
Radioactive iodine uptake scans, 331t
Radiography, 331t
Radioimmunoassay studies, 330t
Radiologists, 348t
Radiology reports
 diagnostic coding preparation and, 539
 in health records, 418
 incoming calls regarding, 448
Radiology technicians, 347t
Radius, 42t
Rales, 244t, 650
Random access memory (RAM), 473b, 473t
Random specimens, 1019
Range of motion (ROM), 40, 55t
Rapid strep testing, 1116, 1117b–1118b
Rapport, 354, 354b, 670
Rationalization, 359t, 673b
Raynaud phenomenon, 234t
Razadyne (galantamine), 750t
RBCs. *See* Red blood cells
RBRVS. *See* Resource-based relative value scale
RDA. *See* Recommended dietary allowance
Reabsorption, in urinary system, 126–128, 127f, 127t
Reaction formation, 359t, 673b
Read-only memory (ROM), 473t
Reagent strip testing, 1024–1025, 1024b, 1025f, 1026b–1027b
 limitations of, 1029–1030, 1030b, 1030f, 1030t
Reagents, 997b, 1082
Reasonable person standard, 365
Rebound pain, 106, 106b
Reception area. *See also* Healthcare facilities; Patient processing tasks
 escorting patients to exam room from, 500–501, 501b
 infection control in, 499
 opening facility and, 497, 497b, 497f
 patient's time considerations in, 500, 501f
Receptors, definition of, 329, 330b
Recheck appointment, 453
Reciprocity, 377t
Recombivax HB, 730t
Recommended dietary allowance (RDA), 838, 838b
Reconciliation, 611–613, 611b, 859, 859b
Reconstituted, definition of, 909–911, 911b
Reconstituting powdered medication, for parenteral medication administration, 909–911, 911b–912b, 912f
Records release process, 383, 385, 385f, 386f, 387b
Recovery position, 975b, 975f, 975t
Rectal route, in medication administration, 893, 893b
Rectal temperature, digital thermometer for, 642b
Rectum, 98, 99f
 physical examination of, 691
Red blood cell casts, 1033f, 1033t–1034t, 1038b
Red blood cells (RBCs)
 anatomy of, 168–169
 blood types and, 170–172, 171f, 172b
 counts of, in CBC reports, 1089
 deficiencies related to, 183t
 hypochromic, 1089, 1089b
 indices of, in CBC reports, 1089
 morphology of, in differential cell count, 1092, 1093f
Red bone marrow, 36–37, 37b
Reference laboratory, hematology in, 1086–1093
 blood chemistry panels and analyte testing, 1099, 1100f, 1101f–1102f
 CBC reports, 1086–1093, 1089t, 1090f
  differential cell count in, 1091–1092, 1091b, 1091f–1092f
  RBC counts in, 1089
  RBC indices in, 1089
  WBC counts in, 1091
 differential cell count examination, 1092
  RBC morphology in, 1092, 1093f
  normal blood cell identification in, 1092, 1093f
  platelet analysis, 1093
Reference laboratory, microbiology in, 1122–1124, 1122f
 C&S testing, 1124, 1124b
 culture assessment for, 1123–1124, 1123b, 1124f
 inoculating equipment for, 1122, 1123f
 staining for, 1122, 1122b
Reference range, 992, 992b
References, in online profiles, 1138b

Referral laboratories, 991
Referrals, 449, 526, 526b, 571
Refined grains, 835b
Reflection, 355f, 1127–1128, 1128f
Reflex hammers, 678t
Reflexes, physical examination of, 690
Reflux nephropathy, 141t–142t
Refracted, definition of, 691, 691b, 1024, 1024b
Refractive errors, 302b, 302f, 691–693, 693b, 693f
Registered dietitians, 347t, 842, 842b
Registered mail, 489t
Registered Medical Assistant (RMA), 350t
Registered Nurse (RN), 347t, 376t
Registration, in practice requirements, 378
Regression, 359t, 673b
Regular diet, 842
Regular referrals, 571
Regulatory law, 362
Regurgitation, 110, 111b
Rehabilitation Act of 1973, 395t–396t
Reimbursements, 533, 533b
Relapse, definition of, 621, 621b
Release of information form, 567, 567b
Release of tortfeasor, 366t
Reliability, 347, 347b
Religion, diversity in, 345t
Remission, definition of, 621, 621b
Remittent fevers, 638, 638f
Renal calculi, 139–140, 139f–140f, 141t–142t
Renal cell carcinoma, 133, 134t
Renal column, 124, 124f
Renal corpuscle, 124, 127t
Renal ischemia, 1033t–1034t
Renal threshold, 1017b
Renal tubular epithelial cell casts, 1033t–1034t, 1034f
Renal tubular epithelial cells, in urine, 1032, 1036f
Renal tubule, 124
Renin, 128, 128b
Renin-angiotensin aldosterone system (RAAS), 128, 128b
Replication, definition of, 191, 191b
Reportable diseases, 391, 391t, 392b
Reports, of clinical laboratory, 1004–1005, 1005f
Repression, 359t
Reproductive glands, 325, 325f, 329
Reproductive issues, ethics and, 406
Reproductive system
 abbreviations for, 163t–164t
 adjectives for, 163t
 anatomy of, 146–148
  female, 147–148, 149f
  male, 146, 148f
 combining forms for, 163t
 diseases and disorders of, 151–161
  BPH, 141t–142t, 153–155, 157f
  congenital disorders of male reproductive system, 152–158, 155t–156t
  endometriosis, 160–161
  female reproductive system additional diseases, 162t
  female reproductive system cancers, 158–161, 159t–160t
  female reproductive system infections, 161, 161t
  pregnancy-related conditions, 162t
  prostate cancer, 137–138, 138f, 141t–142t, 155–158
  STIs, 151–152, 152b, 153t, 807b
  testicular cancer, 158
 geriatrics changes to, 754
 life span changes to, 162
 physiology of, 148–151
  female, 149–151, 151f
  male, 148–149
 prefixes for, 163t–164t
 structure and function of, 17t
 suffixes for, 163t–164t
Requisitions, of clinical laboratory, 1004–1005, 1005f
Res ipsa loquitur, 368, 368b
Res judicata, 366t
Rescheduling appointments, 463
Rescue breathing, 986b–987b, 986f, 988t
Reservoir host, 617f, 619, 619b
Resident flora, 631–632
Residual urine, 125, 125b
Resistance training, 51t
Resource-based relative value scale (RBRVS), 523, 523b
Respect, 344

Respiration, 649–651
 characteristics of, 649–650
 Cheyne-Stokes, 243t, 650
 counting, 648b, 650–651, 651f
 depth of, 650
 external and internal, 649
 rate of, 648b, 650, 650f, 650t
 rhythm of, 650
Respiratory arrest, 242, 242b
Respiratory distress syndrome, 256t–257t
Respiratory syncytial virus pneumonia, 252–253
Respiratory syncytial virus (RSV) testing, 1116, 1116f
Respiratory system, 954–958
 abbreviations for, 259t
 adjective forms for, 258t
 anatomy of, 238–241
  lower respiratory tract, 240–241, 240f–241f
  upper respiratory tract, 239–240, 239f–241f
 combining forms for, 258t
 diseases of, 242–253
  abnormal lung sounds, 244t
  acute bronchitis, 246–247
  additional, 253, 256t–257t
  asthma, 2, 245–246, 246f, 246t
  CF, 248–249, 249b
  COPD, 247–248, 248f, 649–650
  diagnostic procedures for, 244t–245t
  infectious mononucleosis, 179–180, 203t, 249
  lower respiratory tract diseases, 253, 253t–254t
  lung cancer, 249–250, 250f, 250t, 813, 814t
  PE, 182, 251–252
  pneumonia, 251, 251b
  respiratory syncytial virus pneumonia, 252–253
  symptoms of, 243t
  TB, 252, 252t
  upper respiratory tract diseases, 253, 255t
 emergencies of, 980–981, 980t
  asthmatic attacks, 981, 981b
  choking, 981, 981b–982b
  hyperventilation, 980–981, 980t
 geriatrics changes to, 750
 life span changes to, 258
 PFTs for, 954–956, 954t
  peak flow rate, 955, 955b–956b, 955f
  spirometry tests, 955–956, 956f, 957b–958b, 957t
 physiology of, 242
  acid-base balance, 242
  ventilation, 242
 prefixes for, 258t
 pulmonary treatments for, 956–958
  MDIs, 956–958, 958b–959b, 958f
  nebulizer treatment, 958, 959b–960b
  oxygen therapy, 958, 959f, 960t, 961b, 961f
 structure and function of, 17t
 suffixes for, 258t
Respiratory therapists, 347t
Respondent superior, 370, 370b
Responsibility, 344–345
Restatement, 355t
Restock, definition of, 502, 502b
Restricted delivery, USPS, 489t
Restrictive endorsements, 611f, 611t
Resumes, 1131–1135
 action verbs in, 1135, 1135f
 appearance of, 1135, 1136b
 certifications in, 1135
 content in, 1132–1135, 1133b
 cover letters for, 1129f, 1136–1137, 1137b–1138b, 1137f
 education in, 1133–1134
 formats for, 1131–1132, 1132f, 1133b
 header in, 1132, 1132b–1133b
 summary and skills in, 1135
 work experience in, 1134–1135, 1134b
Retail ground shipping, 487t
Retaliation, 393, 393b
Retention schedule, 424, 424b
Retina, 297–298, 298f, 301t, 308t
Retina disorders, 318t
Retinal photocoagulation, 308t
Retinal tear/detachment, 318t
Retinitis pigmentosa, 318t
Retinoblastoma, 319f, 319t
Retraction, 52t–53t
Retractors, 761–765, 765f

INDEX

Retribution, 393, 393b
Return receipt, USPS, 489t
Returned deposit fees, 604t
Reverse chronologic order, 425, 425b
Review of systems (ROS), 559, 559b, 665, 666f
Reye's syndrome, 727b
RF test. *See* Rheumatoid factor test
Rh blood typing, 1093, 1094b, 1094t
Rh immunoglobulin (RhIg), 172b
Rhabdomyomas, 66t
Rhabdomyosarcomas, 66t
Rheumatic fever, 230t
Rheumatoid arthritis, 59t–60t, 199t–200t
Rheumatoid factor (RF) test, 55t, 87t
Rheumatologists, 188b
Rheumatology/rheumatologists, 36b
Rh-factor, in blood donation, 171, 171b
Rhinologic surgery, 777
Rhinomycosis, 256t–257t
Rhinorrhea, 243t
Rhizotomy, 280t
Rhonchi, 244t, 650
Riboflavin, 839t
Ribosome, 14t
Ribs, 37, 41f
RICE therapy, 822–823
Rickettsia, 1108, 1109t
RIG. *See* Rabies immune globulin
Right bundle branch, 215f, 216, 936f
Right hypochondriac region, 23f, 24t
Right iliac region, 23f, 24t
Right lower quadrant (RLQ), 23
Right lumbar region, 23f, 24t
Right upper quadrant (RUQ), 23, 23f
Ring-handle instruments, 759, 760f
Ringworm infections (dermatophytosis), 84–85, 85b, 1110b
Rinne tuning fork test, 308t
Riomet (metformin), 863t–867t
Ritalin LA (methylphenidate), 863t–867t
Rivastigmine (Exelon), 750t
RLQ. *See* Right lower quadrant
RMA. *See* Registered Medical Assistant
RN. *See* Registered Nurse
Robitussin (dextromethorphan), 872t
Rods, 298, 298b, 301t
Rollators, 827
ROM. *See* Range of motion; Read-only memory
Roman numerals, 874, 874b
Rorschach inkblot test, 283, 290f
ROS. *See* Review of systems
Rosacea, 90t–91t
Rosuvastatin (Crestor), 863t–867t
Rotarix, 730t
Rotary circular files, 430
Rotation, 52t–53t
Rotavirus, 730t
Rotors, 1012, 1012b
Rough endoplasmic reticulum, 14t
Rounding numbers, 872, 873f, 874b
Routers, 474
Routing numbers, 606
Roxicet (oxycodone), 863t–867t
RSV testing. *See* Respiratory syncytial virus testing
Rugae, 125
Rule of nines, burns and, 78, 79b, 971f, 972t
Rumors, 350, 350f
Ruptured tympanic membrane, 320f, 320t
RUQ. *See* Right upper quadrant
Russian patients, cultural differences with, 805b

S

Saddle joint, 44t, 45f
Safe haven infant protection laws, 407
Safety
    clinical laboratory, OSHA's Standard Precautions for, 1001–1003, 1003b, 1003f
    in clinical laboratory, 999–1004
        biohazards and infection control for, 1001–1003, 1003b, 1003f
        chemical hazards and, 1000–1001, 1001b–1002b, 1001f
        physical hazards and, 1004, 1004f
        signs and symbols for, 1000b
        standards and governing agencies for, 1000

Safety *(Continued)*
    in healthcare facilities, 512–518 (*See also* Healthcare facilities, safety and security in)
    needs, 358, 358f
    for phlebotomy needles and syringes, 1054–1056, 1054b, 1055f, 1056b
Safety Data Sheet (SDS), 1000–1001, 1001b
Salaries, 588, 614b
Salespeople, appointment scheduling for, 463
Saliva, 25
Salivary glands, 97, 97f
Salpingo-oophorectomy, 158b, 159t–160t
Sanitization, 632–634, 633b, 770
Sanitize, definition of, 502, 502b
Saprophytes, 1105b
Sarcoidosis, 256t–257t
Sarcomas, 31t
SARS. *See* Severe acute respiratory syndrome
Saturated fats, 837t
Savings accounts, 605
Scabies, 88–89, 88f
Scales, 74f
Scalpels, disposable, 761, 762f
Scanners, 472
Scapula, 42t
Scars, 74f, 75t
Scheduling appointments. *See* Appointment scheduling
Schilling test, 174t
Schirmer tear test, 304t–305t
Schizoid personality disorder, 290t
Schizophrenia, 290t
School career placement officers, for job search, 1131
School-aged children, therapeutic approaches to, 724b
Schwann cells, 263
Sciatica, 284f, 284t
Scissors, 761, 761f, 761t–762t
Sclera, 297, 298f, 301t, 306t, 689, 689b
Sclera disorders, 317t
Scleral buckling, 308f, 308t
Scleroderma, 65t, 90t–91t, 199t–200t
Sclerotherapy, 221t–223t
Scoliosis, 63, 64f, 64t
Scope of practice, 366, 366f, 377, 377b–378b
Scored tablet medications, 889f, 889t
Scotoma, 318t
Screening, definition of, 464
SDS. *See* Safety Data Sheet
Seasonal affective disorder, 289t
Sebaceous glands, 70, 71f, 72
Seborrheic dermatitis, 90t–91t
Seborrheic keratosis, 92t, 747, 747f
Sebum, 72
Secondary skin lesions, 74f, 75t
Secondary storage devices, 469, 473, 474t
Second-degree burns, 78, 80t
Second-voided urine specimens, 1019, 1019f
Secretion, in urinary system, 128
Security. *See also* Healthcare facilities, safety and security in
    computer networks and, 476–478, 477b, 477t
    in healthcare facilities, 512–518
Security risk analysis, 477, 477t
Security Rule, HIPAA, 386
Sedative-hypnotics, 863t–867t
Sediment, 1025
Segmental resection, 250f, 250t
Segments, in ECG tracing, 937–938, 938t
Seizures, 274–275, 280t–281t, 978–980, 979b–980b
Selenium, 838t
Self-actualization needs, 358, 358f
Self-boundaries, with patient communication, 345, 666b, 701b
Self-exams, 809–812
    of breasts, 809, 809b–810b, 810f
    for oral cancer, 812, 812b
    of skin, 810–812, 812b, 813t
    of testicles, 810, 811b–812b
Self-limiting viral infection, 179, 179b
Self-scheduling, 455
Selye, Hans, 518
Semen, 146
Semi-block letter format, 484t, 485, 486f
Semicircular canals, 300, 300f
Semi-Fowler position, 682, 682b
Seminal vesicles, 146, 148f

Seminiferous tubules, 146, 148f
Semisolid medications, 889t
Senescent cells, 1077t–1078t
Senn retractors, 765, 765f
Sensitized, definition of, 192–193
Sensorineural hearing loss, 302b, 698
Sensory system
    ear
        abbreviations for, 322t
        adjective forms for, 322t
        anatomy of, 299–300, 300f
        bones of, 37, 40t
        combining forms for, 322t
        diseases and disorders of, 301, 313–315
        geriatrics and, 751–752, 752b, 753f
        irrigation of, 898b–899b
        life span changes to, 315
        medication administration into, 894, 895b–896b
        physical examination of, 689–690
        physiology of, 301
        prefixes for, 322t
        vision and hearing screenings for disorders of, 698–699
    eye
        abbreviations for, 321t
        adjective forms for, 321t
        anatomy of, 296–299
        combining forms for, 321t
        diagnostic procedures for, 693–697
        dilated eye exam, 813, 814f
        diseases and disorders of, 301, 309–313, 691–693
        foreign body in, 974
        geriatrics and, 750–751, 751b, 751t
        irrigation of, 897b–898b
        life span changes to, 315
        medication administration into, 893, 894b–895b
        physical examination of, 689
        physiology of, 301, 301f
        prefixes for, 321t
        vision and hearing screenings for disorders of, 691–693
    geriatrics changes to, 750–752, 751b–752b, 751t
    introduction to, 296–297
    structure and function of, 17t
Sentinel node biopsy, 158b, 159t–160t
Separation plan, ethics, 402–403, 403b
Septic shock, 184t, 984t
Septicemia, 138, 138b, 184t
Septum, 209, 934, 935f
Sequela, definition of, 3
Sequestrum, 55–58, 58b
Serologic testing, 1119, 1119b
Seroquel (quetiapine), 863t–867t
Serous otitis media, 726, 726b, 726f
Serrations, instruments with, 760, 760f
Sertraline (Zoloft), 863t–867t
Serum, 1050b, 1051f
Serum calcium, 55t
Serum separator tubes (SSTs), 1050–1051, 1051t
Service calls, for equipment, 504
Severe acute respiratory syndrome (SARS), 256t–257t
Sex hormones, 328t
Sexually transmitted infections (STIs), 151–152, 152b, 153t, 807b
Sharps, definition of, 1001, 1001b
Shaving/paring, 76t
5% sheep's blood agar plate, 1123–1124, 1123b
Shelter-in-place evacuations, 515
Shifts, in data, 999b
Shingles (herpes zoster), 87–88, 88b, 88f, 268b, 748b
Shock, 233, 233t, 983–985, 983b–985b, 984t
Shortness of breath, 218t–219t, 243t
Shoulder girdle, 41b, 52f
SI. *See* Système International
SIADH. *See* Syndrome of inappropriate antidiuretic hormone
Sick sinus syndrome, 224t
Sick-child visits, in pediatrics, 733, 733t
Sickle-cell disease, anemia, 175–176, 176f, 715, 715b
Side effects, 854, 854b
Sideropenia, 183t
Sigmoid colon, 98, 99b, 99f
Sigmoidoscopy, 26t–27t
Sign language interpreters, 356t
Signature cards, 605

INDEX

Signature confirmation, USPS, 489t
Signature pads, 472, 472f
Sign-in kiosks, 478
Sign-in register, 498, 498f, 499t
Signs, definition of, 3, 674–675, 675b
Silence, 355t
Silicosis, 256t–257t
Simple sugars, 835, 835t
Sims position, 684, 685b
Simvastatin (Zocor), 863t–867t
Single-photon emission computed tomography (SPECT), 273t
Singulair (montelukast), 863t–867t
Singular/plural ending rules, 9, 11t
Sinoatrial node, 215–216, 215f, 936f
Sinus arrhythmias, 646, 646b, 948
Sinuses, 37, 39b, 39f, 40t
   physical examination of, 690
Sinusitis, 255t
SIRS. See Systemic inflammatory response syndrome
Sjögren syndrome, 199t–200t
Skeletal muscles
   attachments of, 45, 46f
   exercise benefits on, 51, 51b, 51t
   of human body, 46, 47f, 48f–50f
   structure of, 45–46, 46f
Skeleton, 36–40
   appendicular, 37, 38f, 39–40, 40t, 42f, 42t, 43b
   axial, 37–39, 38f–39f, 38t, 40t, 41f
   bone types and shapes in, 37, 38f, 38t
   divisions of, 38t
   formation and structure of, 36–37, 36f
Skill sets, 1146, 1146b
Skin, 25, 73. See also Integumentary system
   cancer of, 80–83
      diagnostic procedures for, 82, 83t
      etiology of, 81
      prevention of, 83
      prognosis of, 83
      risk factors of, 812b
      signs and symptoms of, 81–82, 82b, 82f
      treatment of, 76t, 82–83
   dermal-epidermal junction of, 71
   dermis of, 71f, 72
   epidermis of, 71f, 73
   grafts, 81t
   infestations, 88–89, 88f–89f
   lesions, 74f, 75, 75t–76t
   physical examination of, 689
   self-exams of, 810–812, 812b, 813f
   subcutaneous tissue of, 70, 71f, 72
Skin prep, for minor surgery, 778, 779b
Skin tags, 92t
Skips, collection and tracing, 601, 601b
Skull
   bones of, 37–39, 39f, 40t
   interventions for, 278t
Slapped cheek disease, 727b
SLE. See Systemic lupus erythematosus
Sleep disorders, geriatrics and, 754
Slit lamp examination, 304f, 304t–305t, 694, 694f
Slow-release tablets, 888b
Small claims court, 603–604, 603b
Small intestine, 98, 117t
Small talk, 519b
Smell, 296b
   geriatrics and, 752
Smoking/smokeless tobacco, 247b, 808b
Smooth endoplasmic reticulum, 14t
Smooth muscles, 45, 46f
Snellen charts, 304t–305t, 305f, 695–696, 696b
SOAP progress notes, 425–428, 428f
Social diversity, 344t
Social history, 664
Social media, 350, 351t
Sodium, 838t, 845, 845b
Sodium bicarbonate, 968t
Soft diet, 842–843, 843t
Soft palate, 96, 96f
Software, 469, 469b, 475–476, 476t
Solid medications, 889t
Soluble fiber, 835, 835t
Solvent, 167–168, 168b
Soma (carisoprodol), 863t–867t
Somali patients, cultural differences with, 805b

Somatic cells, 406, 406b
Somatic nervous system, 262, 262f
Somatic tremor artifacts, 947, 947f
Somatoform disorder, 291t
Somnambulism, 289t
SOPs. See Standard operating procedures
SOR. See Source-oriented record
Sound cards, 473t
Source-oriented record (SOR), 425
Space, types of, 351–352, 352t
Spasms, 280t–281t
Speakerphone, 441t
Special damages, 368
Special endorsements, 611t
Special handling, USPS, 489t
Special needs patients, processing, 500
Special report, 550–551, 551b
Specialty and specialist suffixes, 9, 9t
Specialty syringe units, for parenteral medication administration, 906, 908f
Specific gravity, urine, 1024, 1024b, 1025f
Specific immunity, 190f, 191–193, 193f
Specific needs, coaching for, 800
Specificity, definition of, 536b–537b, 550
Specimens
   blood
      capillary puncture for collection of, 1070–1071, 1071b–1073b
      chain of custody for, 1074
      customer service and, 1102b
      handling after collection of, 1074
      hemolysis and rejection of, 1067, 1068t
      venipuncture and recollection of, 1067, 1068t
   clinical laboratory collection of, 1005–1006, 1005b, 1006f
      contamination prevention for, 1006, 1006f
   clinical laboratory handling, processing and storing of, 1007
   chain of custody and, 1007, 1042, 1043b, 1074
   definition of, 991, 991b
   gynecology collection of
      maturation index for, 707
      Pap tests for, 705b, 706–707, 707b
      vaginal infections and, 707, 707b
   minor surgery collection of, MAs assisting with, 790
   pinworm collection, 1114, 1114f
   POL collection of, 1111–1114, 1113f–1114f, 1115t
   from throat, 1116, 1117b–1118b, 1123–1124, 1123b, 1124f
   urine, 1124
      appearance of, 1022–1024, 1022b
      bilirubin and urobilinogen in, 1029
      blood in, 1028, 1029b, 1029f
      clean-catch midstream, 1019, 1020b–1021b
      color of, 1022, 1022b, 1022f, 1023t
      containers for, 1017–1018, 1017f–1018f, 1018b
      first morning, 1019
      foam and, 1023, 1024f
      glucose in, 1028, 1039b
      handling and transporting, 1019–1021, 1021f–1022f, 1021f
      ketones in, 330t, 1024b, 1028
      leukocyte esterase in, 1029
      methods of, 1019, 1019b, 1019f
      nitrite in, 1029
      odor of, 1024, 1024b
      patient sensitivity and, 1017–1021
      in pediatrics, 739, 739f
      pH of, 1025, 1028f
      protein in, 1028
      second-voided, 1019, 1019f
      specific gravity of, 1024, 1024b, 1025f
      sugars in, 1038b
      turbidity of, 1022, 1022b, 1023f
      24-hour, 1018b, 1019
      two-hour postprandial, 1019
      volume of, 1022–1023, 1023f
SPECT. See Single-photon emission computed tomography
Specula, 765t–766t, 766f
Speech, physical examination for, 689
Speech audiometry, 308t
Spelling rules, for medical terminology, 4–5, 5f
Sperm, 146, 147f, 148
Spermatogenesis, 146, 148

Spermatozoa, 146, 146b
   in urine examination, 1036
Sphincter, 125, 125t
Sphygmomanometers, 653, 653f–654f, 654f, 655b–656b
Spina bifida, 281t–282t, 715, 715b
Spina bifida occulta, 65t
Spinal column, 39, 41f
Spinal cord, 266–267, 267f
Spinal nerves, 268, 269f
Spinal stenosis, 65t
Spine
   abnormal curvatures of, 63, 64f, 64t
   bones of, 39, 40t, 41f
Spinous processes, 39, 41f
Spiral fracture, 56t–57t
Spirilla, diseases caused by, 1109t
Spiriva (tiotropium), 863t–867t
Spirometer, 650, 650f, 956f
Spirometry tests, 244t–245t, 245f, 955–956, 956f, 957b–958b, 957t
Spleen, 188, 189f
Splenectomy, 198t
Splenic arteriography, 196t
Splenomegaly, 203f, 203t
Splinter forceps, 762t–764t, 763f
Splints
   application of, 977b
   coaching on, 818–820, 820t
Split-thickness skin graft, 81t
Splitting, 359t
Spondylolisthesis, 65t
Spondylopathies, 65t
Spongy bone, 36–37, 37b
Spores, 618, 618b, 770, 770b
Sports massage, 823
Sprains, 58, 58f, 58t
Spring-handle instruments, 759, 760f
Sputum, 243t
Sputum culture, 244t–245t
Sputum cytology, 244t–245t
Squamous cell carcinoma, 31f, 31t, 80–83, 82f
Squamous cells, 81
SSTs. See Serum separator tubes
St. John's wort, 872t–873t
Staged/staging, definition of, 181, 181b
Stains, definition of, 1107
Standard insurance, USPS, 489t
Standard (bipolar) leads, 939, 940f
Standard of care, 365, 964b
Standard of proof, 364t
Standard operating procedures (SOPs), 994
Standard Precautions, OSHA
   for clinical laboratory safety, 1001–1003, 1003b, 1003f
   compliance guidelines of, 625–630
   definition of, 622
   environmental protection and, 625–627
   hand hygiene and, 622–624, 622f, 623b
   HBV vaccination and, 629, 630f
   housekeeping controls and, 627–628, 628f–629f, 629b
   for needlestick injuries, 1054–1055, 1054b
   OPIM and, 622, 622b
   postexposure follow-up and, 629–630, 630b
   PPE, barrier protection and, 625, 625b–626b, 625f, 627f
   summary of, 624, 624f
Standard walkers, 827, 827b, 827f
Stapedectomy, 309t
Stapes, 299–300, 300f
Staples, surgical, 768, 768f
Starches, 835, 835t
Stark Law, 394t
STAT, 448, 448b, 1004, 1004b, 1052, 1052b
STAT referrals, 571
Statements, invoices and, 614
Static equilibrium, 300, 300b
Statute of limitations, 366t
Statutes, 362, 391–393, 391b
Statutory law, 362
Stem cells, 169, 169b, 192–193, 328, 405, 406t
Stereotaxic radiosurgery, 278t
Sterile, definition of, 993
Sterile dressing, application of, 791b–792b
Sterile field preparation, 782b–784b, 786, 786f, 787b
Sterile tray setup, two-person, 784b

Sterilization
  aseptic techniques for infection control and, 634
  autoclave, 770–775, 771f
    biologic sterilization indicators in, 774
    chemical sterilization indicators in, 774, 774f
    effectiveness of, factors influencing, 771, 771t
    loading, 774, 775b
    quality-assurance records for office sterilization in, 774
    steam temperature for, 771, 771b
    tips for improving techniques with, 772t
    unloading, 774–775, 775b
    wrapping instruments for, 774
    wrapping materials for, 771, 772b–773b, 773f
  biologic, 774
  chemical, 774–775, 774f
  of instruments for minor surgery, 770–775, 778–786
    autoclave, 770–775, 771f
    utility room and, 770b
  sterile field preparation and, 782b–784b, 786, 786f, 787b
  sterile gloves procedure and, 785b–786b
  surgical hand scrub for, 780b–782b
  two-person sterile tray setup for, 784b
Sterilize, definition of, 502, 502b, 617
Steri-Strips, 768, 768f
Sternum, 39, 41f
Steroid hormones, 329
Stertorous, definition of, 650
Stethoscopes, 654, 678f, 678t
Stimulants, 863t–867t
STIs. See Sexually transmitted infections
Stoma, 136, 136b, 820b
Stomach, 97–98, 98f, 117t
Stomach acid, 25
Stomach cancer, 107t
Stomatoplasty, 104t–105t
Stool culture, 103t–104t
Stool guaiac, 103t–104t
Stool parasitic examination (O & P), 26t–27t
Stool specimens, 1111, 1112b
Stop-payments, 611
Strabismus, 317t
Strains, 58, 58f, 58t
Strangulation, 118t
Strata/stratum, 70–71, 71f
Stratum corneum, 71, 71f
Streaked for isolation, 1123–1124, 1123b
Stream scheduling, 456
Strength and skill assessment, for career development, 1128–1129
  personality traits, 1128–1129
  technical skills, 1129, 1129f
  transferrable job skills, 1129, 1129b
Strep throat, 255t
Stress, 518, 519b
Stretch receptors, 125, 125b
Stretching, 51t
Striated, definition of, 15b, 16t
Stridor, 244t
Stroke, 272, 980, 980b
Stylus, 471–472, 471b, 765b, 765t–766t
Subcultured, definition of, 1123
Subcutaneous injections, for medication administration, 896–899, 922–924, 922b, 922f
  aspiration for, 922, 923b
  giving, 924b–925b
  sites for, 924
  summary of, 923t
  techniques in, 922
Subcutaneous tissue, 70, 71f, 72
Subject filing, 434–435
Subjective data, definition of, 25, 674
Subjective information, in health records, 414–418, 414b
  past health, family, and social history in, 414–418, 416f–417f
  personal demographics in, 414, 414b, 415f, 417f
Subjects, 480, 480t
Sublimation, 673b
Sublingual medication administration, 890
Sublingual salivary glands, 97, 97f
Subluxation, 58, 58t
Submandibular salivary glands, 97, 97f
Subpoena, 367b–368b
Subpoena duces tecum, 367b–368b

Subsequent, definition of, 418
Substance abuse records, confidentiality of, 385b
Substance-related disorders, 271, 271t
Substantive law, 362
Suction, definition of, 1069, 1069b
Sudafed (pseudoephedrine), 872t
Sudoriferous glands, 70, 71f, 72
Suffixes
  adjective, 5, 6t
  for blood, 185t
  for cardiovascular system, 235t
  combining forms added to, 3–4, 3t–4t
  definition of, 1b, 2
  diagnostic procedure, 8, 8t
  for digestive system, 120t
  for endocrine system, 340t
  instrument, 8–9, 8t
  for integumentary system, 93t
  for lymphatic and immune systems, 205t
  for mental and behavioral health, 293t
  for musculoskeletal system, 68
  for nervous system, 292t
  noun-ending, 5, 6t
  pathology, 6t–7t, 7f, 8
  for reproductive system, 163t–164t
  for respiratory system, 258t
  specialty and specialist, 9, 9t
  therapeutic intervention, 8, 8t
  for urinary system, 143t
Sugars, in urine, 1038b
Sulfur, 838
Summarizing, 355t, 1127–1128, 1128b
Summary and skills, in resumes, 1135
Summary judgment, 367
Supernatant, definition of, 1030–1032
Supination, 52t–53t
Supine (horizontal recumbent) position, 683, 683b
Supplies, of healthcare facilities, 503–511
  inventory control systems for, 507, 507f
  inventory management for, 506, 506f, 507b
  ordering, 509, 509b
  receiving order for, 509–511, 510b, 510f–511f
  taking inventory for, 507, 508b–509b, 508f
Suppository medications, 889t
Suppression, 359t, 673b
Suppurative, definition of, 90t–91t, 92b, 698
Suppurative otitis media, 726, 726b, 727f
Supreme Court, U.S., 362f
Surface anatomy, 18, 18f, 19t–20t
Surface area, definition of, 169, 169b
Surfactant, 240–241
Surgeons, 348t
Surgery section, of CPT, 556b–557b, 561–562
Surgical asepsis, 630–631
Surgical hand scrub, 780b–782b
Surgical history, in prenatal record for obstetrics, 714–715
Surgical package, 561
Surgical staples, in minor surgery, 768, 768f, 794b
Surgical technologists, 347t
Surrogacy, 406t
Susceptible host, 620
Suture lines, 40, 44b
Suture repair setup, 789t
Suture scissors, 761f, 761t–762t
Sutures, in minor surgery, 767–768, 767b, 767f, 794b
Swan-Ganz catheter, 219t–221t
Sweat glands, 70, 71f, 72
Swedish massage, 823
Swing through crutch gait, 825, 825f
Swing to crutch gait, 825, 825f
Symbols, 3
Symmetry, definition of, 673, 690b, 706
Sympathectomy, 280t
Sympathetic nervous system, 269, 270f
Symptoms, definition of, 3, 674, 674b
Synapses, 46, 263, 263f
Synaptic cleft, 46
Synarthrotic joints, 40
Syncope, 218t–219t, 280t–281t, 653, 653b, 982–983, 983b–984b, 983f, 1047–1048, 1048b
Syndactyly, 65t
Syndrome of inappropriate antidiuretic hormone (SIADH), 332t–333t
Syndromes, definition of, 25

Synergistic muscles, 45
Synthesis, 70, 70b
Synthesize, definition of, 101
Synthroid (levothyroxine), 863t–867t
Syphilis, 152, 153t
Syphilis testing, 275t
Syringe method, for venipuncture, 1061b–1063b
Syringes, 1047, 1053, 1054f. See also Needles and syringes
System software, 476t
Système International (SI), 1008
Systemic, definition of, 890, 890b
Systemic circulation, 211–213, 212f
Systemic inflammatory response syndrome (SIRS), 184t
Systemic lupus erythematosus (SLE), 65t, 90t–91t, 199f, 199t–200t
Systems review, 665, 666f
Systole, 217
Systolic blood pressure, 651

T
Tablet computers, 470f, 470t, 478f
Tablet medications, 889f, 889t
Tablets needed, medication math and total, 876–877, 877b, 877f
Tablets per dose, in medication math, 877–878, 878f, 879b
Tabular List
  of CPT, 550, 551f, 554–555, 555b
  of ICD-10-CM, 536–538, 536f, 537b, 542, 542f
Tachycardia, 218t–219t, 646
Tachypnea, 243t, 649–650
Tact, 344
Tactful, definition of, 443, 443b
Tail coverage, 369
Talipes, 65t
Tape measures, 678t
Target cells, 329
Target resumes, 1133, 1134f
Target tissue, 263, 263b
Tarsals, 42t
Taste, 296b
  geriatrics and, 752
TB. See Tuberculosis
T-cells, 193b, 328, 1077, 1077b
Teaching-learning process, 806, 806b, 807t
Team members, professionalism for, 346–349, 346f, 349f
Tear gland disorders, 316t
Tears, 25
Technical defense, 366
Technology, in ambulatory care center. See also Personal computers
  advances in, 478–479, 478f–479f, 479b
  introduction to, 469
Teeth, 96, 96b, 96f
Telangiectasia, 75t
Telemedicine, 377, 377b
Telephone techniques, 440–452, 440f
  for appointment scheduling, 457
  call management for, 443–446
    caller identification, 444
    confidentiality, 444
    facility identification, 444
    placing callers on hold, 445
    prompt answering, 444
    provider information, 445
    screening incoming calls, 444–445
    thinking ahead, 443
    transferring calls, 445
  collection procedures and, 598–600, 598b
  effective use of, 442–443
    active listening, 442, 442b
    pleasing personality, 442–443, 442b–443b
  equipment for, 440–442
    cell phones, 442
    features, 440, 441t
    headsets, 440, 441f
    multiple-line telephone system, 440, 440f
  for incoming calls
    angry callers, 450
    bill inquiries, 448–449
    complaints about care or fees, 450
    difficult, 450–451
    direction requests, 447
    fee inquiries, 449
    friends or family of staff members, 450

INDEX

Telephone techniques (Continued)
    insurance assistance requests, 449
    language challenges, 450–451
    non-patient-related calls, 449
    patients who refuse to discuss symptoms, 449
    prescription refill requests, 447
    progress notes, 448
    radiology and laboratory reports, 448
    screening of, 444–445
    special, 449–450
    test results requests, 449–450
    third party callers, 450
    typical, 447–449
    unauthorized inquiry calls, 450
  messages in, 445–446
    electronic record of, 446, 446b, 448f
    paper record of, 446, 446b, 447f
    retaining record of, 446
    taking action on, 446
  for outgoing calls, 451–452
    answering services, 452, 496, 496b
    automatic call routing, 452, 452b
    directory assistance, 452
    long-distance calling, 451–452
    time zones, 451, 451f
Temperature
  body
    average adult, 639t
    converting, 639b
    digital thermometers for, 639–640, 640f, 641b–642b
    factors influencing, 637–638
    febrile illnesses and, 638, 638b
    fever and, 191, 638, 638f
    integumentary system regulation of, 73
    sites for, 638–640
    temporal artery thermometers for, 640, 640f, 644b
    tympanic thermometers for, 640, 640f, 643b
  conversion, in medication math, 876, 876b, 877f
  emergencies related to, 970, 970t–971t
  measurement, clinical laboratory, 1007, 1007t, 1008t
Temporal artery thermometers, 640, 640f, 644b
Temporal pulse, 643, 645f
Temporary files, 436
Temporomandibular joint disorder (TMJ), 65t
Tenaculum forceps, 762t–764t, 764f
Tendinitis, 65t
Tendons, 45
Tenia fungal infections, 84–85, 85b
Tenormin (atenolol), 863t–867t
TENS. See Transcutaneous electrical nerve stimulation
Termination letters, 487, 488b
Terminology. See Medical terminology
Testes, 146, 146b, 148f, 329
Testicles, 148f
  cancer of, 158, 812b
  definition, 146, 146b
  physical examination of, 690–691
  self-exam of, 810, 811b–812b
  undescended, 134t
Testicular torsion, 158t
Testosterone, 148, 150b, 329
Tetanus, childhood immunization guidelines for, 730t
Tetany, 331t
Tetralogy of Fallot, 227f, 227t
Text messaging, 350, 351t
Thalamus, 301, 301b
Thalassemia, 183t
Thematic Apperception Test, 283
Therapeutic communication, 354–355, 355t, 668–671, 672t
Therapeutic intervention suffixes, 8, 8t
Therapeutic range, 857, 857b
Thermal ECG paper, 940, 940b, 941f
Thermometers
  digital, 639–640, 640f, 641b
  temporal artery, 640, 640f, 644b
  tympanic, 640, 640f, 643b
Thiamine, 839t
Third party callers, 450
Third-degree burns, 78, 80t
Third-party administrator (TPA), 526b
Thixotropic gel, 1049–1051
Thoracentesis, 253b, 253t–254t
Thoracic surgeons, 348t
Thoracic vertebrae, 37, 41f

Thoracodynia, 243t
Thready pulse, 646–647, 647b
Three-dimensional (3D) printing, 479
Three-point crutch gait, 825, 825f
Three-wheel walkers, 827
Thrill, 218t–219t
Throat, 97, 97b, 97f, 690
  specimen collection from, 1116, 1117b–1118b, 1123–1124, 1123b, 1124f
Thrombocytes, 170, 170f
Thromboendarterectomy, 221t–223t
Thrombophlebitis, 182–183, 182f
Thrombus, 172b, 177
Thumb-handle/grasp instruments, 759, 760f
Thymomas, 204t
Thymus gland, 188, 189f, 325, 325f, 328, 1077, 1077b
Thyroid carcinoma, 334t
Thyroid function tests, 330t
Thyroid gland, 325–326, 325f, 327t
Thyroid gland diseases, 332–333, 334t
Thyroid hormone testing, 1097–1099
Thyroid nodule, 334t
Thyroidectomy, 331t
Thyroiditis, 334t
Thyroid-stimulating hormone, 327t
Thyroxine, 327t
TIAs. See Transient ischemic attacks
Tibia, 42t
Tickler files, 436, 436b, 600, 600b
TILA. See Truth in Lending Act
Tilt table test, 233
Time management skills, 348–349
Time measurement, clinical laboratory and, 1007, 1007t
Time zones, 451, 451f
Time-specified scheduling, 456
Timing, of vaccinations, 886, 886b
Tinea, 618
Tinnitus, 319t
Tiotropium (Spiriva), 863t–867t
Tissue adhesives, in minor surgery, 768–769, 769b
Tissue culture, 1111, 1111b
Tissues, structure of, 15, 15t–16t
Titers, 620, 1119, 1119b
TMJ. See Temporomandibular joint disorder
Tobacco, smoking/smokeless, 247t, 808b
Tobacco screening, 815
Toddlers, therapeutic approaches to, 724b
Tolerance, 271t
Tongue, 96, 96f
Tongue depressors, 678t
Tonometry, 304t–305t
Tonsillitis, 256t–257t
Tonsils, 189, 189f
Toothed instruments, 760–761, 760f
Toothed tissue forceps, 762t–764t, 764f
Topical medication administration, 892–893, 892b
Tort, 363, 363b
Tort law, 363–369, 364t
  damages in, 363b, 364t, 367–368
  defenses in, 366, 366t–367t
  intentional, 363–364, 365t
  negligent, 364–369, 365t
  professional insurance and, 368–369
  proving malpractice in, 366–368, 368b
Tortfeasor, 363b, 364t
Torticollis, 65t
Total bilirubin, 103t–104t
Total calcium, 330t
Touch pads, 471, 471f
Touch screens, 471–472
Tourette's syndrome, 284t
Tourniquets, 1048–1049, 1049b, 1057, 1057f
Towel clamps, 762t–764t, 764f
Toxicity, definition of, 854, 855b
Toxicology, 993, 993b
  urine, 1041–1042, 1042b–1043b, 1042f, 1042t
Toxins, 28b
TPA. See Third-party administrator
Trabeculotomy, 308t
Trachea, 239–240, 239f–240f
Tracing skips, collection and, 601, 601b
Tracking, USPS, 489t
Traditional health insurance, 526
Tramadol (Ultram, ConZip), 863t–867t
Trans fatty acids, 837t

Transaction fees, 604t
Transcendence needs, 358, 358f
Transcription, of health records, 429–430, 429b
Transcutaneous electrical nerve stimulation (TENS), 280f, 280t, 823, 823f
Transdermal medication administration, 890, 890b, 892f
Transferrable job skills, 1129, 1129b
Transient flora, 631–632
Transient ischemic attacks (TIAs), 272b
Transient microorganisms, 759
Transient psychotic disorders, 290t
Transillumination, 690
Transitional cell carcinoma, 133, 134f, 134t
Transitional epithelial cells, in urine, 1032, 1036f
Transitional epithelium, 125
Transitory files, 436
Transmission, mode of, 617f, 619
Transmyocardial revascularization, 221t–223t
Transtelephonic monitoring (TTM), 954
Transurethral resection of the prostate (TURP), 155, 157f
Transverse colon, 98, 99f
Transverse fracture, 56t–57t
Transverse processes, 39, 41f
Trauma, 30, 54, 682–683, 683b. See also specific traumas
Trazodone (Oleptro), 863t–867t
Treatment
  for autoimmune diseases, 198
  of burns, 80t
  for cardiovascular system diseases, 221t–223t
  definition of, 25
  for fractures, 55–58, 57f
  health records of prescribed, 418, 418b
  for HIV, 201
Treatment plans, coaching on, 800, 817–828
  assistive devices and, 823–828, 824b
    canes, 828, 828f, 829b–830b
    crutches, 824–825, 824f–825f, 826b
    walkers, 825–828, 827b–829b, 827f
    wheelchairs, 828
  casts and splints and, 818–820, 820t
  cold therapy and, 820–821, 820b, 821t, 822b
  complementary therapies and, 823
  exercise therapy and, 823, 823f
  hot therapy and, 820–821, 820b, 821f, 822t
  medication administration at home and, 818, 819b, 819f
  RICE therapy and, 822–823
  ultrasound therapy and, 821–822
Tremors, 280t–281t
Trendelenburg position, 685, 687f
Trends, in data, 999b
Triage, 444, 444b, 497, 969, 969b
Triaging flow map, 969, 969b, 969f
Trial phase, in civil lawsuit, 368b
TRICARE, 524–525, 525t
Triceps crutches, 824
Trichomonas vaginalis, in urine, 1036, 1037f
Trichomoniasis, 152, 153t, 707
Trichotillomania, 292t
Tricuspid valve, 209, 211f, 934, 935f
Trigeminal neuralgia, 283f, 283t
Trigger point massage, 823
Triglycerides, 837, 837b
Triiodothyronine, 327t
Tripod position, 824, 825b
Trocar, 104t–105t, 105f
Trocars, 765f, 765t–766t
True ribs, 37, 41f
Trumenba, 730t
Trunk
  skeletal muscles of, 47t, 50f
  ventral surface anatomy terms for, 18f, 19t
Trustees, 601b
Truth in Lending Act (TILA), 596–597, 597f
T-SPOT TB test (T-Spot), 921
TTM. See Transtelephonic monitoring
Tubal ligations, 710
Tuberculin testing
  blood, 921
  Mantoux tuberculin skin test, 917–921, 917b–920b, 918t
  two-step, 921, 921f
Tuberculosis (TB), 252, 252t
Tubular necrosis, acute, 141t–142t

INDEX

Tumors, 74f, 75t
  benign compared to malignant, 30, 30t
Tunica vaginalis testis, 146, 148f
Tunics, 96, 96b
Tuning fork testing, 699
Tuning forks, 678f, 678t
Turbidity, urine, 1022, 1022b, 1023f
Turgor, 689
TURP. *See* Transurethral resection of the prostate
12-lead ECG, 939, 939f
  augmented leads, 939, 940t
  bipolar (standard) leads, 939, 940f
  chest (precordial) leads, 939, 941f
24-hour urine specimens, 1018b, 1019
Twins, 151
Two-hour postprandial urine specimens, 1019
Two-person sterile tray setup, 784b
Two-point crutch gait, 824, 825f
Two-wheel walkers, 827, 827f
Tylenol (acetaminophen), 872t
Tympanic membrane, 299, 300f
Tympanic thermometers, 640, 640f, 643b
Tympanogram, 698, 699f
Tympanometry, 308t
Tympanoplasty, 309t
Tympanostomy, 309f, 309t
Tympanotomy, 309t
Tympany, chest, 244t

U

UAGA. *See* Uniform Anatomical Gift Act
UCR. *See* Usual, customary, and reasonable
UDDA. *See* Uniform Determination of Death Act
Ulcerative colitis, 117t
Ulcers
  decubitus, 83–84, 84f
  definition of, 74f, 75t
  peptic, 115–116, 115f
  perforated, 116, 116b
Ulna, 42t
Ultram (tramadol), 863t–867t
Ultrasonic sanitization, 632–634
Ultrasound, 26t–27t, 27f, 103t, 130t, 331t, 718, 718f, 818t
Ultrasound therapy, 821–822
Ultraviolet (UV) light, 71
Umbilical cord, 150–151, 151f
Umbilical hernia, 118t
Umbilical region, 23f, 24t
Undescended testicles, 134t
Undoing, 673b
UNHS. *See* Universal Newborn Hearing Screening test
Uniform Anatomical Gift Act (UAGA), 390t, 410, 411b
Uniform Determination of Death Act (UDDA), 390t, 409–410
Unipolar, definition of, 939, 939b
Universal Newborn Hearing Screening (UNHS) test, 308t
Universal Precautions, CDC, 622. *See also* Standard Precautions, OSHA
Universal serial bus (USB) port, 473t
Unlisted Procedures and Services, in CPT, 550–551
Unsaturated fats, 837t
Unsecured debt, 601b
Unusual letter combinations, pronunciation of, 11t
Unwarranted assurance, patient interviews and, 671
UPJ obstruction. *See* Ureteropelvic junction obstruction
Upper extremities, skeletal muscles of, 47t, 48f–49f
Upper respiratory tract, 239–240, 239f–241f
  diseases of, 253, 255t
  infections of, 256t–257t
Ureter, segmental resection of, 134t
Ureterocele, 141t–142t
Ureteropelvic junction (UPJ) obstruction, 141t–142t
Ureteroscopy, 26t–27t, 130t
Ureters, 125
Urethra, 125, 125t, 146, 148f, 149
Urethritis, 141t–142t
Urgent, definition of, 445, 445b
Urgent referrals, 571
Urinalysis, 26t–27t, 103t–104t, 130t, 197t, 275t, 330t, 993, 993f. *See also* Urine
  chemical examination in, 1025–1029, 1025f, 1026b–1027b
  components of, 1022t
  physical examination in, 1022–1024, 1022f
  purpose of, 1015

Urinalysis *(Continued)*
  QA and QC for, 1026b, 1030
  reagent strip testing limitations in, 1029–1030, 1030b, 1030f, 1030t
  routine, 1021–1030
Urinary incontinence, 140–141, 140t, 753–754
Urinary system
  abbreviations for, 143t
  adjective forms for, 143t
  anatomy of, 123–125
    bladder, 125
    female, 123f
    kidneys, 123–124, 124f
    male, 123f
    ureters, 125
    urethra, 125, 125t
  combining forms for, 143t
  diseases and disorders of, 128–141
    additional, 141, 141t–142t
    bladder cancer, 128–130, 130f
    cystitis, acute, 130–131, 131f
    diagnostic procedures for, 130t
    ESRD, 131–133, 132f
    glomerulonephritis, 133
    incontinence, 140–141, 140t, 753–754
    kidney cancer, 133–135, 133f–134f, 134t
    nephrotic syndrome, 135
    neurogenic bladder, 135–136, 136b, 136t
    PKD, 136–137, 137f, 141t–142t
    prostate cancer, 137–138, 138f, 141t–142t, 155–158, 814t
    pyelonephritis, 138–139
    renal calculi, 139–140, 139b, 139f–140f, 141t–142t
    signs and symptoms of, 129t
  geriatrics changes to, 753–754
  life span changes to, 141–142
  physiology of, 126–128
    blood pressure, 128
    erythropoietin, 128
    filtration, 126
    reabsorption, 126–128, 127f, 127t
    renin, 128, 128b
    secretion, 128
    vitamin D, 128
  prefixes for, 143t
  structure and function of, 17t
  suffixes for, 143t
Urine, 25. *See also* Urinalysis
  Clinitest for, 1038–1039, 1038b–1040b
  elimination of, 1015–1017
  formation of, 126, 127f, 1015–1017, 1015f–1016f
  introduction to, 1015
  menopause testing and, 1041
  microscopic examination of, 1030–1038
    air bubbles in, 1038f
    bacteria, 1036, 1037f
    casts in, 1032, 1033t–1034t, 1038b
    cells in, 1032, 1035f–1036f
    crystals in, 1032–1033, 1035t
    fibers in, 1036, 1037f–1038f
    miscellaneous findings in, 1034–1036
    mucous threads in, 1036, 1037f
    oval fat bodies in, 1034, 1037f
    preparation for, 1030–1032, 1031b
    spermatozoa in, 1036
    Trichomonas vaginalis in, 1036, 1037f
    understanding results of, 1038, 1038b
  ovulation testing and, 1041
  pregnancy tests and, 1039–1041, 1040b
  reagent strip testing of, 1024–1025, 1024f, 1025f, 1026b–1027b
  specimen collection of, 1124
    appearance of, 1022–1024, 1022f
    bilirubin and urobilinogen in, 1029
    blood in, 1028, 1029b, 1029f
    clean-catch midstream, 1019, 1020b–1021b
    containers for, 1017–1018, 1017f–1018f, 1018b
    customer service and, 1042b
    first morning, 1019
    foam and, 1023, 1024f
    glucose in, 1028, 1039b
    handling and transporting, 1019–1021, 1021f–1022f, 1021t
    ketones in, 330t, 1024b, 1028
    leukocyte esterase in, 1029

Urine *(Continued)*
  methods of, 1019, 1019b, 1019f
  nitrite in, 1029
  odor of, 1024, 1024b
  patient sensitivity and, 1017–1021
  in pediatrics, 739, 739f
  pH of, 1025, 1028f
  protein in, 1028
  second-voided, 1019, 1019f
  specific gravity of, 1024, 1024b, 1025f
  specimen collection of, color of, 1022, 1022b, 1022f, 1023f
  sugars in, 1038b
  turbidity of, 1022, 1022b, 1023f
  24-hour, 1018b, 1019
  two-hour postprandial, 1019
  volume of, 1022–1023, 1023f
  structures and functions of, 1016t
  toxicology, 1041–1042, 1042b–1043b, 1042f, 1042t
Urine culture, 130t
Urine drugs of abuse screening test, 275t
Urine glucose, 330t
Urobilinogen, in urine specimens, 1029
Urochrome, 1022, 1023b
Urology/urologists, 123b, 146b, 348t
Urostomy, 136, 136b
Urticaria, 90t–91t, 729, 729b
US Postal Service (USPS)
  domestic services of, 487t
  domestic shipping sizes of, 487t
  optional services of, 489f, 489t
  postage options of, 487, 487t, 489f
  street abbreviations of, 483t
USB (universal serial bus) port, 473t
USDA. *See* Department of Agriculture
Usual, customary, and reasonable (UCR), 526
Uterine curette, 762f, 762t–764t
Uterus, 147, 149f
Utility room, sterilization and, 770b
Utilization management, MCOs and, 527, 527b
UV light. *See* Ultraviolet light
Uvea, 297, 297b
Uvea disorders, 317t
Uveitis, 317t
Uvula, 96, 96f

V

Vaccinations, 620
  compliance reporting for, 393
  flu, intradermal, 916b
  HBV, 629, 630f
  rabies, 974t
  timing of, 886, 886b
Vaccine Adverse Event Reporting System (VAERS), 393
Vaccine Information Statement (VIS), 393, 887, 887b
Vaccine Injury Compensation Program (VICP), 393
Vaccine storage guidelines, 509–510, 510b, 510f
Vacuum tube method, for venipuncture, 1058b–1061b
Vacuum tubes. *See* Evacuated collection tubes, venipuncture and
VAERS. *See* Vaccine Adverse Event Reporting System
Vagina, 147, 149f
Vaginal infections, specimen collection and, 707, 707b
Vaginal ring, 708t, 709–710
Vaginal route, in medication administration, 893, 893b
Vagotomy, 279f, 279t
Valium (diazepam), 863t–867t, 968t
Valsartan (Diovan), 863t–867t
Valvular diseases, 182–183, 184t
Valvuloplasty, 221t–223t
Vaping, 248b
Vaqta, 730t
Varicella, 730t
Varicocele, 158t
Varicose veins, 234t
Varivax, 730t
Vas deferens, 146, 148f
Vascular, definition of, 297, 298b
Vascular access, 132–133, 133b
Vascular disorders, 285b, 285t
Vascular technologists, 347t
Vasculitis, 234t
Vasectomies, 710
Vasoconstriction, definition of, 15b, 16t, 191, 759, 820, 820b, 973, 973b

Vastus lateralis site, for intramuscular injections for medication administration, 928, 928f
VCUG. See Voiding cystourethrogram
Vectors, 619
Veins, 208, 208f, 209t, 210f
Vendors, 508–509, 508b
Venipuncture
　customer service and, 1050b
　equipment for, 1047–1052, 1047b, 1048f
　　antiseptics, 1049, 1049b, 1050f
　　evacuated collection tubes, 1049–1052, 1050f, 1051t
　　PPE, 1048, 1048b
　　tourniquets, 1048–1049, 1049f
　needles in
　　angle of entry, 1057b
　　holders, 1053, 1053f
　　multisample, 1053, 1053f
　　safety, 1054–1056, 1054b, 1055f, 1056b
　　structure of, 1052–1053, 1053f
　order of draw in, 1051t–1052t, 1052
　pediatric, 1074t
　problems associated with
　　fainting, 1066–1067
　　hematoma, 1066–1067
　　nerve damage and complications, 1066, 1067t
　　specimen recollection, 1067, 1068t
　routine, 1056–1058
　　butterfly assembly method, 1064b–1066b
　　completion, 1057–1058
　　gloves for, 1057, 1057b
　　needle angle of entry, 1057b
　　patient preparation, 1056
　　performing procedure, 1057
　　procedure preparation, 1056–1057, 1056f–1057f, 1057b
　　syringe method, 1061b–1063b
　　tourniquet placement, 1057, 1057f
　　vacuum tube method, 1058b–1061b
Venous distention, 218t–219t
Ventilation, of respiratory system, 242
Ventolin HFA (albuterol), 863t–867t
Ventral body cavity, 22–23, 23t
Ventral surface anatomy, 18, 18f, 19t
Ventricles, 266–267, 267b
Ventricular arrhythmias, 949–950, 949f
Ventricular contractions, blood pressure and, 217
Ventricular fibrillation, 949f, 950
Ventricular septal defect, 227t
Ventricular tachycardia, 224t, 949–950, 949f
Ventriculoperitoneal shunt, 278f, 278t
Ventriculostomy, endoscopic, 278t
Ventrogluteal site, for intramuscular injections for medication administration, 928, 930f
Venules, 123, 124b, 208
Verbal communication, 353–357. See also Written communication
　barriers to, 355–357, 356t–357t
　communication cycle, 353, 353f
　oral communication, 353–354, 354t
　therapeutic communication, 354–355, 355t
Verbal overload, in patient interviews, 672
Verbs, 480, 480t
Verification of eligibility, 500, 500b, 528–529, 530f
Vermiform appendix, 98
Vertebrae, 39, 40b, 41f
Vertical evacuations, 516
Vertigo, 280t–281t, 319t, 650, 650b, 977–978
Vesicle, 74f, 75t
Vesicoureteral reflux, 141t–142t
Vested, definition of, 419, 419b
Vestibule, 300, 300f
Viability, definition of, 191, 714f, 715t, 1108, 1108t
Vials, for parenteral medication administration, 908–909, 908f, 909b–910b
Vicodin (hydrocodone), 863t–867t
VICP. See Vaccine Injury Compensation Program
Video cards, 473t
Video job interviews, 1144
Vietnamese patients, cultural differences with, 805b
Vigilance, 778–780, 780b
Villi, 101
Violence, workplace, 513, 513b–514b
Viral hepatitis, 112, 112t–113t
Viral hepatitis-serum antibody and antigen testing, 103t–104t

Viral infections, 1106
Virus protection software, 477t
Viruses, 617
　pathogenic, 1111, 1111b, 1112t
VIS. See Vaccine Information Statement
Visceral pleura, 241
Viscosity, 899, 899b
Vision and hearing screenings, 691–702
　ear disorders and, 698–699
　　audiometric testing for, 699–702, 700b, 701f
　　diagnostic procedures in, 699–702, 699f
　　hearing loss and, 698–699, 698f–699f, 699b
　　tuning fork testing for, 699
　eye disorders and, 691–693
　　diagnostic procedures for, 693–697
　　DVA tests for, 694–696, 694b–695b, 695f
　　Ishihara color vision test for, 696–697, 697f
　　NVA tests for, 696, 696f
Visual acuity assessment, 304t–305t, 305f, 694–696, 694b–695b, 695f
Visual cortex, 301, 302b
Visual field test, 304t–305t
Visually impaired, communication and, 356t
Vital signs. See also Anthropometric measurements
　blood pressure readings for, 651–657
　　age and, 651f
　　body position for measurement of, 654–656, 657f
　　errors in measurement of, 657b
　　evaluation in, 651–653, 652b, 652t
　　factors affecting, 651
　　Korotkoff sounds and, 656–657
　　measurement in, 653–656, 653f–654f, 654t, 655b–656b
　　palpatory method in, 657
　　personal systems for, 656f
　body temperature
　　average adult, 639t
　　converting, 639b
　　digital thermometers for, 639–640, 640f, 641b–642b
　　factors influencing, 637–638
　　febrile illnesses and, 638, 638b
　　fever and, 191, 638, 638f
　　integumentary system regulation of, 73
　　sites for, 638–640
　　temporal artery thermometers for, 640, 640f, 644b
　　tympanic thermometers for, 640, 640f, 643b
　customer service and measurement of, 661b
　factors influencing, 637
　in health records, 418, 637
　introduction to, 637
　in pediatrics, 738t
　pulse, 641–649
　　apical, 646, 647b, 648–649
　　bounding, 646–647, 647b
　　brachial, 644–645, 645f
　　carotid, 643–644, 645f
　　characteristics of, 646–647
　　deficit, 646
　　Doppler for checking, 218f, 218t–219t, 649, 649f
　　dorsalis pedis, 646, 649, 649f
　　femoral, 645, 649
　　intermittent, 646, 646b
　　peripheral, 641, 643b
　　popliteal, 645–646, 649
　　radial, 645, 646f, 648–649, 648f
　　rate of, 646, 647b, 648–649, 648b, 649f
　　rhythm of, 646
　　sites of, 643–646, 645f
　　temporal, 643, 645f
　　thready, 646–647, 647b
　　volume of, 646–647, 648f
　pulse oximetry, 244t–245t, 245f, 246, 658, 658b, 658f
　respiration, 649–651
　　characteristics of, 649–650
　　Cheyne-Stokes, 243t, 650
　　counting, 648b, 650–651, 651f
　　depth of, 650
　　external and internal, 649
　　rate of, 648b, 650, 650f, 650t
　　rhythm of, 650
Vitamin deficiency anemia, 183t

Vitamins, 838, 838b, 840b
　A, 839t
　B, 839t
　C, 839t
　D, 839t
　　integumentary system and synthesis of, 73
　　urinary system and, 128
　E, 839t
　K, 839t
Vitiligo, 90t–91t, 91f, 199f, 199t–200t
Vitrectomy, 308t
Vitreous humor, 298f, 299
Voice mail, 441t
Voice recognition software, 429–430
Voiding cystourethrogram (VCUG), 130t, 131f
Volume, urine, 1022–1023, 1023f
Volvulus, 117t
Vomiting, 102t
Voucher checks, 606, 607f
Vulva, 147, 149f

W

Waiting period, 529–530
Walkers, coaching on, 825–828, 827b–829b, 827f
WAN (wide area network), 473–474
Wandering baseline artifacts, 947, 947f
Warfarin (Coumadin), 863t–867t, 1088f
Warranties, 504
Warts, 90t–91t
Water, 838–840, 840b
Wave scheduling, 456
Waves, in ECG tracing, 937–938, 938t
Waxy casts, 1033t–1034t, 1034f
WBCs. See White blood cells
Weber tuning fork test, 308t
Websites, health-related, 479b
Wechsler Adult Intelligence Scale, 283
Wedge resection, 250f, 250t
Weight
　anthropometric measurement of, 658–661, 659b–660b, 660f, 660t
　CDC status categories for, 723, 723b
　obesity and, 726
Weight control diet, 843, 843b, 843t
Well-child visits, in pediatrics, 729, 733b
Wellness. See Health maintenance and wellness, coaching on
Western blot test, 197t
Wet mount, 1111
Wheal, 74f, 75t
Wheelchairs, coaching on, 828
Wheezing, 244t, 649–650
Whirlpool bath, 822t
Whistleblowers, 394–395, 394b–395b
White blood cell casts, 1033t, 1033t–1034t, 1038b
White blood cells (WBCs)
　agranular, 190, 190b
　anatomy of, 169–170, 171f
　count of, 174t, 197t, 275t
　　in CBC reports, 1091
　granular, 189, 189b
　phagocytosis and, 172, 172f
　in urine, 1032, 1036b
White noise, 497
Whole blood, 167, 168b
Whole grains, 835b
Wide area network (WAN), 473–474
Wide ear forceps, 766f, 766t
Willingness to help others, 347–348
Wilms tumor, 133, 133f, 134t
Winged infusion sets. See Butterfly assemblies
Withdrawal state, 271t
Withholding or withdrawing life-sustaining treatment, 410, 410b
Wong-Baker FACES Pain Scale, 739, 739f, 887, 888f
Wood light examination, 75f, 75t
Word origins, 1–2, 2t
Work ethic, 347
Work experience, in resumes, 1134–1135, 1134b
Workers' compensation, 525
Workplace emergencies, 514, 514b
Workplace injuries, preventing, 514
Workplace safety law, 389–390
Workplace violence, 513, 513b–514b
Workstation ergonomics, PCs and, 475, 476f

Workstations on wheels (WOWs), 478, 478b
Wound and abscess cultures, 75t
Wound care, minor surgery and, 793–797
    bandages for, 796–797, 796f–797f, 797b
    dressings for, 796–797
    wound healing, 793–796
    wound types and, 793, 795f
Wounds of violence, 391
WOWs. *See* Workstations on wheels
Wristbands, with bar code technology, 478
Written communication, 353, 354t
    business letter formats in, 484–485, 484t, 485b, 486f
    faxes and, 490–491
    fundamentals of, 480–481
        capitalization, numbers, and punctuation, 480–481
        parts of speech, 480, 480t
        word use, appropriate, 480, 481b, 481t

Written communication *(Continued)*
    letter delivery in, 486–487, 487t, 488f, 489t
    letter templates in, 485–486
    memorandums in, 488, 490f
    professional e-mails in, 488–490, 491b
    professional letters in, 482–484, 483f, 483t, 484b
Wrong act against, 364t
Wrongful termination, 394b

X

Xanax (alprazolam), 863t–867t
Xenograft, 81t
Xenotransplantation, 411
Xerophthalmia, 316t
Xiphoid process, 39, 41f
X-rays, 26t–27t, 54t, 111f, 196t, 818t

Y

Yeast cells, 1032, 1035f, 1105
Yeast infection, 707
Yellow bone marrow, 36–37, 37b

Z

Zika virus, 162t
Zinc, 838t
Zithromax (azithromycin), 863t–867t
Zmax (azithromycin), 863t–867t
Zocor (simvastatin), 863t–867t
Zoloft (sertraline), 863t–867t
Zolpidem (Ambien, Edluar, Zolpimist), 863t–867t
Zone, delivery, 487
Z-track technique, in intramuscular injections for medication administration, 927, 927f, 931b–932b
Zygote, 152